Hysterectomy

Ibrahim Alkatout • Liselotte Mettler
Editors

With the Assistance of Dawn Rüther

Hysterectomy

A Comprehensive Surgical Approach

Volume 1

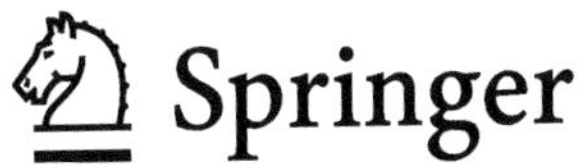

Springer

Editors
Ibrahim Alkatout
Gynecology and Obstetrics
University Hospitals Schleswig-Holstein
Campus Kiel
Kiel
Germany

Liselotte Mettler
Gynecology and Obstetrics
University Hospitals Schleswig-Holstein
Campus Kiel
Kiel
Germany

ISBN 978-3-319-22496-1 ISBN 978-3-319-22497-8 (eBook)
DOI 10.1007/978-3-319-22497-8

Library of Congress Control Number: 2017949291

Printed on acid-free paper

This Springer imprint is published by Springer Nature
The registered company is Springer International Publishing AG
The registered company address is: Gewerbestrasse 11, 6330 Cham, Switzerland

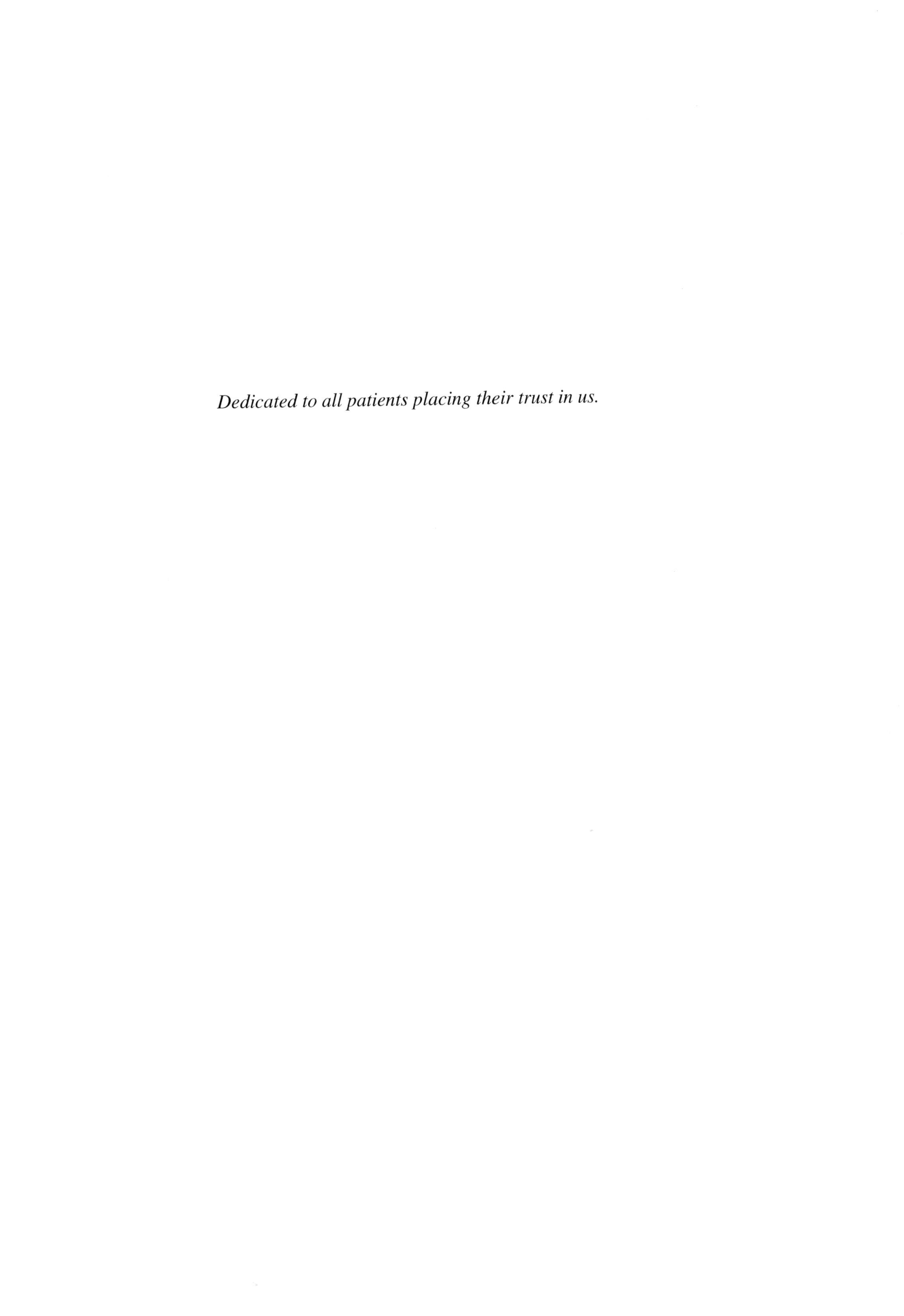

Dedicated to all patients placing their trust in us.

Foreword 1

The most common gynecological surgeries performed in the world are hysterectomies which date back to ancient time and were mainly associated with noncancerous conditions. The Italian anatomist Berengario da Carpi of Bologna carried out the first authenticated vaginal hysterectomy in 1507. In Manchester, England, Charles Clay performed the first recorded abdominal hysterectomy in 1843, and in 1853, by accident Walter Burnham performed the first successful abdominal hysterectomy in Lowell, Manchester. The early hysterectomies, either vaginal or abdominal, were performed without anesthesia, and with a fatality rate ranging from 70 to 90 %. In the absence of an alternative management of cervical cancer, the radical hysterectomy was introduced. The first radical hysterectomy was performed by John Clark at Johns Hopkins in 1985, and in 1898, Ernst Wertheim of Vienna performed the first extended radical hysterectomy. The more radical extension of vaginal hysterectomy was developed by Karl Schuchardt of Gottingen, and in 1901, Friedrich Schauta described radical vaginal hysterectomy in detail. With the advent of antiseptics, anesthesia, antibiotics, blood transfusion, new technologies, and advances in surgical techniques, by the 1940s, total abdominal hysterectomy had become the norm, and hysterectomy had become a safer surgical procedure for women worldwide. The fatality rate dropped significantly.

As science and technology advanced, Kurt Semm, in Kiel, Germany, in 1984, was the first to describe a technique for laparoscopic assistance in vaginal hysterectomy, thereby laying the foundation for all endoscopic procedures. Laparoscopic hysterectomy is increasingly performed in many countries in the world; however, conservative and less invasive operative managements, such as hysteroscopic surgery and the application of ulipristal acetate, may reduce the traditional indications for hysterectomy. The limitations of conventional laparoscopy and advances in robotic surgery have led to the increased use of robotic techniques in hysterectomy. Diaz-Arrastia reported the first series of successful robotic laparoscopic hysterectomies in 2002, and surgeries using robotic techniques for hysterectomy are now rapidly expanding.

The indication and performance of hysterectomies in general have changed with the change in techniques and procedures and have been adapted to the request of women to retain their uterus; therefore, the need for a comprehensive textbook on hysterectomy to improve the knowledge, skills, and competencies of surgeons has become very evident.

Ibrahim Alkatout and Liselotte Mettler have compiled the very first comprehensive medical textbook of its kind, *Hysterectomy*: *A Comprehensive Surgical Approach*, dealing with all surgical techniques of hysterectomy (vaginal, abdominal, laparoscopic, and robotic-assisted) and their extended operations, such as lymphadenectomy and omentectomy, with excellent illustrations. This textbook contains 132 chapters contributed by over 100 renowned international authors. This book is an important addition to the literature on hysterectomy techniques, accessible to gynecologists worldwide, and thereby contributing towards the global improvement of healthcare for women.

I believe this textbook will be very valuable and find extensive use in developed and developing countries. I am honored and privileged to write this foreword.

Windhoek, Namibia

Prof. Quazi Monirul Islam, MBBS, MPH, FRCOG
WHO Representative to Namibia

Foreword 2

Hysterectomy ranks among the most frequently performed procedures in gynecology. Since modern surgical techniques have allowed the reduction of intra- and postoperative complications to a considerable degree, it has become a well-established option in the treatment of a wide variety of conditions, including cancers of the reproductive system, certain types of endometriosis and adenomyosis, uterus myomatosus, chronic pelvic pain, or uncontrollable bleeding.

The range of procedures used is broad, not only in regard to surgical techniques – laparoscopic, robotic-assisted, vaginal, abdominal – but also in regard to the extent of the surgery, depending on which organs are included, in addition to the uterus itself, e.g., the cervix, the vagina or parts of it, the parametrium, the lymph nodes, the fallopian tubes, the ovaries, or the omentum.

With its comprehensive overview of all surgical techniques and its illustrated step-by-step descriptions, this book will provide not only a valuable decision aid for surgeons in their choice of method but also a training guide for surgeons at every level of education and experience. It can be considered an additional advantage that this book also covers anatomical and diagnostic aspects of hysterectomy, including questions of when hysterectomy is indicated.

This book is the successor to Liselotte Mettler's *Manual of New Hysterectomy Techniques* (2007), an indispensable handbook on vaginal and laparoscopic hysterectomy. This new volume, edited by a team, Ibrahim Alkatout and Liselotte Mettler, benefits in a similar way from the high standards of the Kiel School of Gynaecological Surgery, of which Liselotte Mettler is one of the distinguished protagonists. Along with Kurt Semm, she initiated the "minimally invasive revolution" of laparoscopic hysterectomy, thus establishing the foundation of today's procedures in the field.

This book's widened scope, now including all available techniques, diagnostic guidance, and in-depth background information, puts itself forward as a standard reference in the field of gynecological medicine.

Prof. Dr. Diethelm Wallwiener
Executive Director of the Department of Women's Health, Tübingen, Germany

Medical Director of the Tübingen University Women's Hospital, Tübingen, Germany

President of the German Society of Gynaecology and Obstetrics
(Deutsche Gesellschaft für Gynäkologie und Geburtshilfe, DGGG), Tübingen, Germany

Prof. Dr. Sara Brucker
Deputy Executive Director of the Department of Women's Health, Tübingen, Germany

Medical Director of the Tübingen Research Centre for Women's Health, Tübingen, Germany

Foreword 3

It is with great pleasure that I write a forward for this book edited by Ibrahim Alkatout and Liselotte Mettler. Liselotte Mettler has lived on the cutting edge of advanced laparoscopic surgery from its beginning, and by beginning, I mean 1985 when we presented together at AAGL, known previously as a tubal ligation society. The next year, we were both teaching the advanced course at the AAGL. She has continuously worked as a leader to advance the surgical care of women and still does. She is active as a teacher worldwide, especially concerning hysterectomy, and was a founder of the Kiel School of Gynaecological Endoscopy, one of the first training centers in this specialty.

I have known and worked with Liselotte Mettler for over 30 years. Her work with Kurt Semm progressed along parallel paths with mine until we met in 1985–1986. Kurt and Lilo called me Mr. Electrosurgery at that time as Kurt used sutures for oophorectomy, while I pioneered the use of bipolar desiccation for large vessel hemostasis. It was then that Kurt told me, "If I learned to suture, I would be king." So I learned how to suture!

Somewhat lost in these discussions is that I started as a vaginal surgeon. Vaginal surgery was my passion! Abdominal mutilation was our common enemy. After 10 years of doing vaginal hysterectomy surgery with the occasional use of the laparoscope for salpingo-oophorectomy, I began to do the whole operation using laparoscopic visualization with desiccation of both the uterine arteries and the ovarian arteries in 1988. Laparoscopic supracervical hysterectomy came soon thereafter by Kurt and Lilo.

Now, Lilo and her associates from the Kiel School of Gynaecological Endoscopy have put everything about hysterectomy together with this textbook describing different techniques in a relatively comprehensive manner. I must admit that my favorites are both the vaginal and the laparoscopic approaches. So, I look forward to reading those sections to determine if the difference between a colpotomy and a culdotomy has been finally resolved.

I believe that this is a much-needed textbook, and I am sure that most gynecologists will benefit from reading it.

Harry Reich, MD, FACOG, FRCOG
Pioneer in the Development of Laparoscopic Hysterectomy, Shavertown, PA, USA

Honorary Member of AAGL, Pennsylvania, USA

Foreword 4

Hysterectomy is the most common major surgical procedure in modern gynecology. In the USA alone, approximately 600,000 hysterectomies are performed each year. All gynecologists will, at some stage of their training, learn how to perform the hysterectomy procedure independently. What is so special about a hysterectomy, compared to most other surgical procedures, is that there is such a variation of methods and surgical routes for this surgery. More than 90 % of all hysterectomy procedures are performed for benign indications. Thus, there are special needs concerning safety, efficiency, and cost-effectiveness in relation to this nonvital, quality of life-enhancing surgery.

A hysterectomy procedure can take anytime from 15 min to several hours. However, a hysterectomy that spans several hours may be as rewarding for the patient and the surgeon as a quick hysterectomy. I personally have probably performed the longest hysterectomy procedure. In a series of nine abdominal total hysterectomies that took place in 2013, the surgical duration was between 10.5 and 13 h. What is also so special is that these nine abdominal hysterectomies were performed to increase the quality of life of another woman and not the operated woman herself.

My co-surgeon, Pernilla Dahm-Kähler, and I performed the surgery through a midline incision and apart from the uterus also long extensive vascular pedicles, including the uterine and internal iliac arteries and veins, were harvested. The hysterectomy specimen was flushed and cooled ex vivo, before transplantation into the pelvis of the recipient (in most cases the daughter). Up until today, five healthy babies have been born from these transplanted uteri, and three out of these five recent mothers also grew themselves inside the same uterus as their babies.

Dr. Dahm-Kähler and I would never have been able to conduct these successful hysterectomies and uterus transplantations without a structured training in several different hysterectomy procedures during our early years of surgical training and more importantly, without the parallel acquisition of a great understanding of the anatomy of the pelvis. All these important aspects are covered in this comprehensive book. Another important point is that a prolonged duration of surgery does not necessarily equate with inadequate surgical skills. During my early training, I would closely record the time and would not be satisfied by a long duration of a seemingly easy hysterectomy. Today, I try to teach the residents in training that they should strive for minimal bleeding and follow the natural anatomic layers to minimize the tissue damage and thereby shorten the recovery time of the patient.

The editors, Ibrahim Alkatout and Liselotte Mettler, have been able to recruit a large number of absolute top clinicians/scientists in the field of gynecology and surgical hysterectomy to contribute chapters to this book. The impressive list of authors guarantees the readers not only up-to-date information on each aspect of hysterectomy but also that the opinions and surgical tips have passed the critical eyes of world-renowned doctors in academic medicine. Notably, this book covers not only the surgical techniques of all various hysterectomy procedures but also the important aspects of indications and presurgical diagnostics.

I am convinced that *Hysterectomy: A Comprehensive Surgical Approach* will become one of the classic books in the field of gynecology.

Mats Brännström
Professor and Chairman of Obstetrics and Gynecology,
University of Gothenburg, Gothenburg, Sweden

Visiting Professor of Obstetrics and Gynecology,
Mayo Clinic, USA and Karolinska Institute, Gothenburg, Sweden

Visiting Professor of Transplantation Surgery,
Harvard Medical School, Boston, MA, USA

Director, Stockholm IVF, Gothenburg, Sweden

Preface

This comprehensive surgical approach to hysterectomy rests on the pillars erected by the great masters in our specialty. The first hysterectomy was performed as a vaginal hysterectomy and dates back to ancient times. The procedure was performed in the time of Soranus of Ephesus, 120 years after the birth of Christ. There were many reports of its use in the Middle Ages, nearly always for the extirpation of an inverted uterus, and the patients rarely survived. Hysterectomy became safer with the introduction of anesthesia, antibiotics and antisepsis, blood transfusions, and intravenous therapy. During the 1930s, Richardson introduced the total abdominal hysterectomy to avoid serosanguinous discharge from the cervical remnant and the risk of cervical carcinoma developing in the stump.

Apart from this innovation, and the transverse abdominal incision introduced by Johannes Pfannenstiel of Kiel in the 1900s, there was little advance in hysterectomy techniques until the advent of endoscopic surgery and the performance of the first laparoscopic hysterectomy by Kurt Semm in Kiel in 1984 and Harry Reich in Kingston, Pennsylvania, in 1988. With his never-ending dedication to the teaching of laparoscopy, Kurt Semm stimulated his coworkers in Kiel and courageous followers around the world to move forward with laparoscopic total and radical hysterectomy.

Thoralf Schollmeyer was a pupil of Semm and head of the Kiel School of Gynaecological Endoscopy from 2007 until his early death at the age of 52 in 2014. He continues to inspire us and was the driving force behind the decision of the Kiel School to go ahead with the second edition of the *Manual of New Hysterectomy Techniques* (2007).

In this age of global communication, it is a great privilege to publish a specialist surgical book on hysterectomy which features the leading surgeons, researchers, and teachers as contributing authors. With the assistance of over 200 multidisciplinary authors, we have been able to compile a book that hopefully meets the requirements of a broad base of readers.

This book brings into balance theoretical background, clinical experience, and scientific findings in a readily comprehensible form with numerous illustrations and tables. For the beginner, this book could become a reliable companion, providing background information and assistance for all procedures associated with hysterectomy. This includes abdominal, vaginal, conventional laparoscopic, and robotic-assisted surgical procedures. But also the experienced surgeon will be able to broaden his spectrum and learn experimental and innovative surgical approaches as this is the first textbook on hysterectomy including traditional, up-to-date, and innovative surgical methods.

Additionally, the book contains a large proportion of interdisciplinary aspects, and we believe it will make a substantial contribution to meeting the growing requirements of interdisciplinary medical treatment. It offers related disciplines (especially general surgery and urology) the opportunity to describe the areas of common overlap and how these can be treated. This multidisciplinary approach is of advantage not only for gynecologists but also for general surgeons and urologists.

The wide range of the contents developed in the course of the conception of the book. Extended hysterectomy procedures cannot be separated from procedures on the internal genital organs or those involving the anatomical and functionally relevant surrounding area.

Finally, we would like to thank Joni Fraser for her continuous support and valuable assistance in preparing the book for production. Special thanks also go to Lizzy Raj, Julia Megginson, and Melissa Morton at Springer International Publishing for allowing us the freedom to design a book according to our ideas and supporting us in the realization of what turned out to be a mammoth project. Tribute is also due to the illustrators for their creative visual implementation of complex issues.

The editors are conscious of the privilege of having access to the most advanced treatment concepts of our time. In an unstable world, our foremost intention is to share the greatest good, the ability to cure one's fellow human beings.

Kiel, Germany, 2017 Ibrahim Alkatout and Liselotte Mettler

Contents

Contributors

Karolina Afors Obstetrics and Gynaecology, King's College Hospital NHS Trust, London, UK

Wael Agur University of Glasgow, Glasgow, UK
Obstetrics and Gynecology, University Hospital Crosshouse, Kilmarnock, UK

Bahriye Aktas Department of Gynecology and Obstetrics, University Hospital Essen, Essen, Germany

Ibrahim Alkatout Gynecology and Obstetrics, Kiel School of Gynaecological Endoscopy, University Hospitals Schleswig-Holstein, Kiel, Germany

Céline D. Alt-Radke Department of Diagnostic and Interventional Radiology, Medical Faculty, University Duesseldorf, Duesseldorf, Germany

Zouhair Amarin Faculty of Medicine, Mutah University, Karak, Jordan

Michael Anapolski Obstetrics and Gynaecology, Community Hospital Dormagen, Dormagen, Germany

Massaki Andou Obstetrics and Gynecology, Kurashiki Medical Center, Kurashiki, Okayama, Japan

Katrin S. Arnolds Department of Gynecology, Cleveland Clinic Florida, Weston, FL, USA

Masout Azodi Department of Obstetrics and Gynecology, Yale University, Yale New Haven Hospital, New Haven, CT, USA

Erika Balassiano Department of Gynecology, Center for Special Minimally Invasive and Robotic Surgery, Palo Alto, CA, USA

Marc Banerjee Praxis für Orthopädie und Unfallchirurgie, Media Park Klinik, Cologne, Germany

Emma L. Barber Obstetrics and Gynecology, Division of Gynecologic Oncology, University of North Carolina, Chapel Hill, North Carolina, USA

Sven Becker Department of Gynecology and Obstetrics, University Hospital Frankfurt, Kiel, Germany

Dragan Belci Department of Gynecology and Obstetrics, General Hospital Pula, Pula, Croatia

Giorgio Bogani Gynecologic Oncology, National Cancer Institute, Milan, Italy

John F. Boggess Obstetrics and Gynecology, Division of Gynecologic Oncology, University of North Carolina, Chapel Hill, NC, USA

Bernd Bojahr Klinik für MIC Minimal Invasive Chirurgie, Berlin, Germany

António Braga Department of Obstetrics and Gynaecology, Centro Materno-Infantil do Norte/Centro Hospitalar do Porto, Largo da Maternidade Júlio Dinis, Porto, Portugal

Jvan Casarin Obstetrics & Gynecology Department, University of Insubria, Varese, Italy

Vito Cela Obstetrics and Gynecology Unit, Department of Maternal Fetal, University of Pisa, Pisa, Italy

Gabriele Centini Molecular and Developmental Medicine, Obstetrics and Gynaecology, University of Siena, Ospedale santa Maria alle scotte, Siena, Italy

Karen K.L. Chan Department of Obstetrics and Gynaecology, The University of Hong Kong, Queen Mary Hospital, Hong Kong, Hong Kong SAR

Vito Chiantera Department of Oncologic Surgery, Gynecologic Oncologic Unit, Campobasso, Italy

Gun Oh Chong Gynecologic Cancer Center, Kyungpook National University Medical Center, Daegu, South Korea

Ettore Cicinelli Department of OB/GYN, University Medical School of Bari, Bari, Italy

Siamak Daneshmand Urologic Oncology, Institute of Urology, University of Southern California/Norris Comprehensive Cancer Center, Los Angeles, CA, USA

Alexander A. Danilov Institute of Numerical Mathematics, Russian Academy of Sciences, Moscow, Russia

Moscow Institute of Physics and Technology (MIPT), Moscow, Russia

Alexander Di Liberto Department of Gynecology and Obstetrics, Leverkusen Municipal Hospital, Teaching Hospital of the University of Cologne, Leverkusen, Germany

Silvia Di Tommaso Division of Medical Genetics, Department of Biomedical Sciences and Human Oncology, Università "AldoMoro", Bari, Italy

Berta Diaz-Feijoo Department of Obstetrics and Gynecology, Hospital Universitari Vall d'Hebron Universitat Autònoma de Barcelona, Passeig Vall d'Hebron, Barcelona, Spain

Marie-Madeleine Dolmans Department of Gynecology, IREC, UCL, Cliniques Universitaires St. Luc, Brussels, Belgium

Lindsay Clark Donat Department of Obstetrics and Gynecology, Rhode Island Hospital, Warwick, RI, USA

Jacques Donnez SRI (Société de Recherche sur l'Infertilité), Brussels, Belgium

Olivier Donnez Gynecology, Polyclinique Urbain V, Avignon, France

Nadja Dornhöfer Department of Obstetrics and Gynecology, Leipzig University Clinic, Leipzig, Saxony, Germany

Andreas du Bois Gynecology & Gynecological Oncology, Kliniken Essen Mitte (KEM), Essen, NRW, Germany

Werner Dürr, DEGUM II – Kursleiter Department of Gynecology, Nürtingen, Baden-Württemberg, Germany

Jan-Hendrik Egberts Department of Visceral-, Thoracic, Transplantation-, and Pediatric Surgery, University Hospitals Schleswig-Holstein, Campus Kiel, Kiel, Germany

Mohamed Elessawy OB/GYN, University Hospitals Schleswig-Holstein, Campus Kiel, Kiel, Germany

Marina Eliseeva Peoples' Friendship University of Russia, Department of Obstetrics and Gynecology, Moscow, Russia

Mohamed I. Ellaithy Obstetrics and Gynecology, Ain Shams University Faculty of Medicine, Cairo, Egypt

Jörg Engel Department of OB/Gyn, Klinikum Aschaffenburg, Aschaffenburg, Germany

Kubilay Ertan Department of Gynaecology and Obstetrics, Leverkusen Municipal Hospital, Leverkusen, Germany

Amanda Nickles Fader Kelly Gynecologic Oncology Service, Department of Gynecology and Obstetrics, Johns Hopkins Medicine, Baltimore, Maryland, USA

Anna Fagotti Division of Minimally Invasive Gynecological Surgery, Santa Maria Hospital, University of Perugia, Terni, Italy

Tommaso Falcone Department of Obstetrics, Gynecology, and Women's Health Institute, Cleveland Clinic, Cleveland, OH, USA

Francesco Fanfani Division of Gynecologic Oncology, Policlinico Gemelli, Catholic University of Sacred Heart of Rome, Rome, Italy

Giovanni Favero Department of Advanced Surgical and Oncologic Gynecology, Asklepios Hospital Hamburg, Hamburg, Germany

Alessandro Favilli Department of Obstetrics and Gynecology, University of Perugia, Perugia, Italy

Rodrigo P. Fernandes Department of Gynecology Oncology, Instituto do Câncer do Estado de São Paulo – ICESP FM USP, São Paulo, Brazil

Helder Ferreira Gynaecological Endoscopy Unit, Department of Gynecology, Centro Materno-Infantil do Norte/Centro Hospitalar do Porto, Largo da Maternidade Júlio Dinis, Porto, Portugal

Gwenael Ferron Surgical Oncology, Institut Claudius Regaud – Institut Universitaire du Cancer, Toulouse, France

Gerald Feuer Department of Gynaecologic Oncology, Northside Hospital, Atlanta, GA, USA

Daniel Fink Department of Gynecolocy, University of Zurich, Switzerland, Zurich, Switzerland

Markus C. Fleisch Department of Obstetrics & Gynaecology, Heinrich-Heine-University, Duesseldorf, Northrhine-Westfalia, Germany

Christina Fotopoulou Surgery and Cancer, Imperial College London, London, UK

Rene Pareja Franco Department of Gynecologic Oncology and Reproductive Medicine, University of Texas MD Anderson Cancer Center, Houston, TX, USA

Letizia Freschi Obstetrics and Gynecology Unit, Department of Maternal Fetal, University of Pisa, Pisa, Italy

Robert S. Furr Minimally Invasive Gynecology, Obstetrics and Gynecology, University of Tennessee College of Medicine at Chattanooga, Chattanooga, TN, USA

Yamini M. Gadkari Minimal Invasive Surgery, Galaxy Care Laparoscopy Institute Pune, Pune, India

Garri Tchartchian Klinik für MIC Minimal Invasive Chirurgie, Berlin, Germany

Sandro Gerli Department of Obstetrics and Gynecology, University of Perugia, Perugia, Italy

Fabio Ghezzi Obstetrics & Gynecology Department, University of Insubria, Varese, Italy

Blanca Gil-Ibañez Department of Obstetrics and Gynecology, Hospital Universitari Vall d'Hebron Universitat Autònoma de Barcelona, Passeig Vall d'Hebron, Barcelona, Spain

Antonio Gil-Moreno Department of Obstetrics and Gynecology, Hospital Universitari Vall d'Hebron Universitat Autònoma de Barcelona, Passeig Vall d'Hebron, Barcelona, Spain

Ali S. Gözen Urology, SLK Kliniken Heilbronn, Heilbronn, Germany

Bindiya Gupta Department of Obstetrics and Gynecology, UCMS and GTB Hospital, Delhi, India

Andreas Hackethal Gynecology and Obstetrics, University Clinic Wuerzburg, Wuerzburg, Germany

Sergio Haimovich Head of the Hysteroscopy Unit, Del Mar University Hospital, Barcelona, Spain

Engelberg Hanzal Gynecology and Gynecologic Oncology, Medical University of Vienna, Vienna, Austria

Oz Harmanli Division of Urogynecology and Pelvic Surgery, Tufts University School of Medicine Baystate Medical Center, Springfield, MA, USA

Philipp Harter Gynecology and Gynecologic Oncology, Kliniken Essen-Mitte, Essen, NRW, Germany

Saad Hatahet Department of Urology, The Ohio State University, Wexner Medical Center, Columbus, OH, USA

Sebastian F.M. Häusler Universitätsfrauenklinik Würzburg, Universitätsklinikum Würzburg, Würzburg, Germany

Florian Heitz Gynecology and Gynecologic Oncology, Kliniken Essen-Mitte, Essen, NRW, Germany

Philip M. Hepp Department of Obstetrics & Gynaecology, Heinrich-Heine-University, Duesseldorf, Germany

Martin Heubner Genecology and Obstetrics, University Hospital Essen, Essen, Germany

Amanda M. Hill Department of Obstetrics and Gynecology, Yale University, Bridgeport Hospital, Bridgeport, CT, USA

Anne K. Höhn Division of Breast, Perinatal & Gynecologic Pathology, Institute of Pathology, University Hospital of Leipzig, Leipzig, Germany

Bernd Holthaus Department of OB/GYN, Krankenhaus St. Elisabeth, Damme, Germany

Lars-Christian Horn Institute of Pathology, Division of Breast, Perinatal and Gynecologic Pathology, University Hospital of Leipzig, Leipzig, Germany

Marcel Hruza Urology, SLK Kliniken Heilbronn, Heilbronn, Germany

Lu Huang Department of Gynecology, Zhejiang Provincial People's Hospital, Hangzhou, Zhejiang, China

Wolfram Jaeger Urogynecology, University of Cologne, Köln, Germany

Stephen T. Jeffery Obstetrics and Gynaecology, University of Cape Town, Cape Town, Western Cape, South Africa

Ingolf Juhasz-Böss Gynecology and Obstretrics, Homburg University Hospital, Homburg, Saarland, Germany

Hiroyuki Kanao Gynecologic Oncology, Cancer Institute Hospital, Tokyo, Japan

Seok-Ho Kang Department of Urology, Korea University College of Medicine, Seongbuk-gu, Seoul, South Korea

Tomoyasu Kato Gynecology Department, National Cancer Center Hospital, Chuo-ku, Tokyo, Japan

Kimberly Kenton Department of Obstetrics and Gynecology and Urology, Female Pelvic Medicine and Reconstructive Surgery, Northwestern University Feinberg School of Medicine, Prentice Women's Hospital, Chicago, IL, USA

Jieun Kim Samsung Medical Center, Sungkyunkwan University Medical School, Seoul, South Korea

Seon-Hahn Kim Department of Colorectal Surgery, Korea University College of Medicine, Seongbuk-gu, Seoul, South Korea

Rainer Kimmig Gynecology and Obstetrics, West German Cancer Center, University Hospital Essen, University Duisburg-Essen, Essen, NRW, Germany

Jan T. Klein Urology, SLK Kliniken Heilbronn, Heilbronn, Germany

Günter Köhler Department of Obstetrics and Gynaecology, University Greifswald, Greifswald, Germany

Christhardt Köhler Department of Advanced Surgical and Oncologic Gynecology, Asklepios Hospital Hamburg, Hamburg, Germany

Stephen R. Kovac Department of Gynecology/Obstetrics, Emory University School of Medicine, Atlanta, GA, USA

Hsin-Hong Kuo Obstetrics and Gynecology, Chang Gung Memorial Hospital, Linko, Taiwan, Taoyuan City, Taiwan

Satoru Kyo Department of Obstetrics and Gynecology, Shimane University Faculty of Medicine, Izumo, Shimane, Japan

Hung-Cheng Lai Obstetrics and Gynecology, Shuang Ho Hospital, Taipei Medical University, New Taipei City, Taiwan

Nisha Lakhi Department of Obstetrics and Gynaecology, Richmond University Medical Center, Island, NY, USA

Florian Langer II. Medizinische Klinik und Poliklinik, Universitätskliniken Eppendorf, Hamburg, Germany

Roy Lauterback Obstetrics and Gynecology, Rambam Medical Center, Haifa, Israel

Yoon S. Lee Gynecologic Cancer Center, Kyungpook National University Medical Center, Daegu, South Korea

Sanghoon Lee Department of Obstetrics and Gynecology, Korea University College of Medicine, Seongbuk-gu, Seoul, South Korea

Chyi-Long Lee Chang Gung Memorial Hospital, Keelung Branch, Keelung City, Taiwan

Jun Ho Lee Samsung Medical Center, Sungkyunkwan University Medical School, Seoul, South Korea

Verena Limperger Fachärztin für Laboratoriumsmedizin, Institute of Clinical Chemistry, University Hospital Schleswig Holstein, Kiel, Germany

Melissa H. Lippitt Kelly Gynecologic Oncology Service, Department of Gynecology and Obstetrics, Johns Hopkins Medicine, Baltimore, Maryland, USA

C.Y. Liu Minimally Invasive Gynecology, Obstetrics and Gynecology, University of Tennessee College of Medicine at Chattanooga, Chattanooga, TN, USA

Farah Lone Obstetrics and Gynaecology, Royal Cornwall Hospital, Truro, Cornwall, UK

Celine Lõnnerfors Department of Obstetrics and Genecology, Skåne University Hospital, Lund, Sweden

Lior Lowenstein Obstetrics and Gynecology, Rambam Medical Center, Haifa, Israel

Alessandro Lucidi Department of Oncologic Surgery, Gynecologic Oncologic Unit, Campobasso, Italy

Javier F. Magrina Mayo Clinic, Phoenix, AZ, USA

Bernard Malavaud Surgical Oncology, Institut Claudius Regaud – Institut Universitaire du Cancer, Toulouse, France

Narendra Malhotra Department of Obstetrics and Gynecology, Rainbow Hospitals, Agra, Uttar Pradesh, India

Antonio Malvasi Department of Gynecology and Obstetrics, Santa Maria Hospital, Bari, Italy

Abhishek P. Mangeshikar Mangeshikar Minimal Access Gynecology Infertility Clinic for Women, 8 Laburnum Road, Gamdevi, Mumbai 400007, India

Prashant Mangeshikar Mangeshikar Minimal Access Gynecology Infertility Clinic for Women, 8 Laburnum Road, Gamdevi, Mumbai 400007, India

Andrea Mariani Gynecologic Surgery, Mayo Clinic, Rochester, MN, USA

Alejandra Martinez Surgical Oncology, Institut Claudius Regaud – Institut Universitaire du Cancer, Toulouse, France

Emad Matanes Obstetrics and Gynecology, Rambam Medical Center, Haifa, Israel

Russalina Mavrova Gynecology and Obstretrics, Homburg University Hospital, Homburg, Saarland, Germany

Ivan Mazzon Unit of Gynecology and Obstetrics, "Arbor Vitae" Centre, Clinica Nuova Villa Claudia, Rome, Italy

Sumita Mehta Obstetrics & Gynaecology, Babu Jagjivan Ram Memorial Hospital, Jahangir Puri, Delhi, India

Rauf Melekoglu Department of Obstetrics and Gynecology, Inönü University, School of Medicine, Turgut Ozal Medical Center, Malatya, Turkey

Rolf Mesters Medizinische Klinik und Poliklinik A, University Hospital Münster, Münster, Germany

Liselotte Mettler Department of Obstetrics and Gynecology, University Hospitals Schleswig-Holstein, Kiel, Germany

Emad Mikhail Obstetrics and Gynecology, University of South Florida, Tampa, FL, USA

Charles E. Miller Department of Obstetrics & Gynecology, University of Illinois at Chicago, Chicago, IL, USA

Minimally Invasive Gynecologic Surgery, Advocate Lutheran General Hospital, Park Ridge, IL, USA

The Advanced Gynecologic Surgery Institute, Naperville, IL, USA

Shanti I. Mohling Minimally Invasive Gynecology, Obstetrics and Gynecology, University of Tennessee College of Medicine at Chattanooga, Chattanooga, TN, USA

John E. Morrison Department of Surgery, Louisiana State University Health Sciences Center, New Orleans, LA, USA

Dimitrios Moschonas Department of Urology, Royal Surrey County Hospital, Guildford, UK

Margaret G. Mueller Department of Obstetrics & Gynecology, Division of Female Pelvic Medicine & Reconstructive Surgery, Northwestern University Feinberg School of Medicine, Prentice Women's Hospital, Chicago, IL, USA

Atul P. Munshi Department of Obstetrics and Gynecology, Munshi Hospital, GCS Medical College, Ahmedabad, Gujarat, India

Sujal A. Munshi Department of Obstetrics and Gynecology, Munshi Hospital, PS Medical College, Karamsad, Gujarat, India

Rouba Murtada Department of Gynecology and Obstetrics, Hôpital Jean Verdier, AP-HP, Bondy, France

Ospan A. Mynbaev The Department of Obstetrics, Gynecology and Reproductive Medicine, Peoples' Friendship University of Russia, Moscow, Russia

Arun Nagrath Department of Obstetrics and Gynecology, U. P. Rims & R. Saifai, Etawah, India

Laila Najjari Department of Obstetrics and Gynecology, University Hospital Aachen, Aachen, Germany

Suyash S. Naval Minimal Invasive Surgery, Galaxy Care Laparoscopy Institute Pune, Pune, India

Klaus Neis Klinik für Frauenheilkunde, Geburtshilfe und Reproduktionsmedizin der Universität des Saarlandes, Homburg, Saar, Germany

European Training Center for Gynecologic Endoscopy, Saarbrücken, Germany

Felix Neis Universitätsfrauenklinik Tübingen, Tübingen, Germany

Azadeh Nezhat Nezhat Medical Center, Center for Special Minimally Invasive and Robotic Surgery, Palo Alto, CA, USA

Camran Nezhat Center for Special Minimally Invasive and Robotic Surgery, Palo Alto, CA, USA

Ceana H. Nezhat Nezhat Medical Center, Atlanta, GA, USA

Siew Fei Ngu Department of Obstetrics and Gynaecology, The University of Hong Kong, Queen Mary Hospital, Hong Kong, Hong Kong SAR

Katherine A. Nixon Obstetrics and Gynaecology, Queen Charlotte's and Chelsea Hospital, London, UK

Karl-Günter Noé Department of OB/GYN, University of Witten/Herdecke, Hospital Dormagen, Dormagen, Germany

Ulrike Nowak-Göttl University Hospital Schleswig-Holstein, Intitute of Clinical Chemistry, Thrombosis and Haemostatsis treatment Unit, Kiel, Germany

John A. Occhino Division of Urogynecology, Department of Obstetrics and Gynecology, Mayo Clinic, Rochester, MN, USA

Funlayo Odejinmi Department of Obstetrics and Gynaecology, Whipps Cross University Hospital, Barts Health NHS Trust, London, UK

Agnieszka Oleszczuk-Cosse Department of Gynecology, Charité University Hospital Charitéplatz 1, Berlin, Germany

Reeba Oliver Whipps Cross University Hospital, Barts Health NHS Trust, London, UK

Peter Oppelt Gynecology & Obstetrics, Women's and Children's Hospital Linz, Linz, Austria

Mona E. Orady Robotic Surgery Education, Women's Health Institute, Cleveland, OH, USA

Kurush P. Paghdiwalla Breach Candy, Saifee, Masina, and B.D. Petit Parsee General Hospitals, Mumbai, Maharashtra, India

Andrea Papadia Gynecologic Oncology, National Cancer Institute, Milan, Italy

René Pareja Clinica de Oncología ASTORGA, Medellin, Antioquia, Colombia

William H. Parker Obstetrics and Gynecology, UCLA School of Medicine, Santa Monica, CA, USA

Resad Pasic Minimally Invasive Gynecologic Surgery OB/GYN, University of Louisville, Louisville, KY, USA

Jan Persson Department of Genecology and Obstetrics, Skåne University Hospital, Lund, Sweden

Marco Petrillo Department of Oncologic Surgery, Gynecologic Oncology Unit, Campobasso, Italy

Nicola Pluchino Obstetrics and Gynecology, University Hospital of Geneva, Geneva, Switzerland

Christophe Pomel Surgical Oncology, Jean Perrin Cancer Centre, Clermont-Ferrand, France

Marco Fabián Puga Departamento de Ginecología, Unidad de Oncología Ginecológica, Instituto Nacional del Cancer- Clínica Alemana de Santiago-Universidad del Desarrollo, Vitacura, Santiago, Chile

Shailesh P. Puntambekar Minimal Invasive Surgery, Galaxy Care Laparoscopy Institute Pune, Pune, India

Seema S. Puntambekar Minimal Invasive Surgery, Galaxy Care Laparoscopy Institute Pune, Pune, India

D. Querleu Surgery, Institut Bergonié, Bordeaux, France

Julia C. Radcsa Gynecology and Obstretrics, Homburg University Hospital, Homburg, Saarland, Germany

Shalini Rajaram Department of Obstetrics and Gynecology, University College of Medical Sciences & Guru Teg Bahadur Hospital, Shahdara, Delhi, India

Pedro T. Ramirez Department of Gynecologic Oncology and Reproductive Medicine, University of Texas MD Anderson Cancer Center, Houston, TX, USA

Francesco Raspagliesi Gynecologic Oncology, National Cancer Institute, Milan, Italy

Jens J. Rassweiler Urology, SLK Kliniken Heilbronn, Heilbronn, Germany

Stephan Rimbach Department of Obstetrics and Gynecology, Krankenhaus Agatharied, Hausham, Germany

Marcella L. Roenneburg Eastern Shore Ob/Gyn, Salisbury, MD, USA

Cristiano Rossitto Division of Gynecologic Oncology, Policlinico Gemelli, Catholic University of Sacred Heart of Rome, Rome, Italy

Ralf Rothmund Universitäts-Frauenklinik, Tübingen, Germany

Sabina Salicru Department of Obstetrics and Gynecology, Hospital Universitari Vall d'Hebron Universitat Autònoma de Barcelona, Passeig Vall d'Hebron, Barcelona, Spain

Giovanni Scambia Division of Gynecologic Oncology, Policlinico Gemelli, Catholic University of Sacred Heart of Rome, Rome, Italy

Ana-Maria Schmidt Department of Gynecolocy, University of Zurich, Zurich, Switzerland

Achim Schneider Institute for Cytology and Dyplasia, MVZ im Fürstenberg-Karree Berlin, Berlin, Germany

Carol E.H. Scott-Conner Department of Surgery, University of Iowa Carver College of Medicine, Iowa City, IA, USA

Julia Serno Obstetrics and Gynecology, University Hospital RWTH Aachen, Aachen, Germany

Shikha Seth Department of Obstetrics and Gynecology, U. P. Rims & R. Saifai, Etawah, Uttar Pradesh, India

Ahmad Shabsigh Department of Urology, The Ohio State University Wexner Medical Center, Columbus, OH, USA

Vikrant C. Sharma Minimal Invasive Surgery, Galaxy Care Laparoscopy Institute Pune, Pune, India

Shirish S. Sheth Department of Gynecology, Sheth Nursing Home, Mumbai, Maharashtra, India

Linda-Dalal J. Shiber Minimally Invasive Gynecologic Surgery OB/GYN, University of Louisville, Louisville, KY, USA

Dan-Arin Silasi Obstetrics, Gynecology and Reproductive Sciences, Gynecologic Oncology, Yale Universty School of Medicine, New Haven, CT, USA

Sergei S. Simakov Department of Applied Mathematics, International Translational Medicine and Biomodelling Research Group, Moscow Institute of Physics and Technology (MIPT), Moscow, Russia

Natasha U. Singbal Minimal Invasive Surgery, Galaxy Care Laparoscopy Institute Pune, Pune, India

Anshuja Singla Obstetrics & Gynaecology, University College of Medical Sciences and Guru Teg Bahadur Hospital, Delhi, India

Noam Smorgick Obstetrics and Gynecology, Assaf Harofe Medical Center, Tzrifin, Israel

Manol B. Sokolov Medical University, University Hospital Alexandrovska, Sofia, Bulgaria

Erich Franz Solomayer Gynecology and Obstretrics, Saarland University Hospital, Homburg, Saarland, Germany

Jae Yun Song Department of Obstetrics and Gynecology, Korea University College of Medicine, Seongbuk-gu, Seoul, South Korea

Michael Sonntagbauer Department of Anaesthesia, Intensive Care Medicine and Pain Therapy, Frankfurt University Hospital, Frankfurt, Germany

Petros Sountoulides Department of Urology, Royal Surrey County Hospital, Guildford, UK

Michael L. Sprague Department of Gynecology, Cleveland Clinic Florida, Weston, FL, USA

Elmar Spüntrup Department of Radiology, Klinikum Saarbrücken, Saarbrücken, Saarland, Germany

Carolin Spüntrup Endoscopic Gynecology, Pelvic School Saarbrücken, Saarbrücken, Saarland, Germany

Michael Stark The New European Surgical Academy (NESA), Berlin, Germany

Courtney J. Steller Minimally Invasive Gynecologic Surgery, Obstetrics and Gynecology, Advocate Lutheran General Hospital, Park Ridge, IL, USA

Alexander Strauss Department of Obstetrics and Gynecology, Kiel University Hospital, Kiel, Germany

Christopher J.G. Sutton Professor of Gynaecological Surgery, Faculty of Health and Social Sciences, Guilford, Surrey, UK

Tsutomu Tabata Obstetrics and Gynecology, Mie University School of Medicine, Tsu-City, Mie, Japan

Nobuhiro Takeshima Cancer Institute Hospital, Department of Gynecologic Oncology, Tokyo, Japan

Karl Tamussino Division of Gynecology, Department of Obstetrics & Gynecology, Medical University of Graz, Graz, Austria

Edward J. Tanner III Kelly Gynecologic Oncology Service, Department of Gynecology and Obstetrics, Johns Hopkins Medicine, Baltimore, Maryland, USA

Artin M. Ternamian Gynecologic Endoscopy Division, Obstetrics and Gynecology, Saint Joseph's Health Centre – University of Toronto, Toronto, Ontario, Canada

Raffaele Tinelli Department of OB/GYN, Perrino Hospital, Brindisi, Italy

Andrea Tinelli Obstetrics and Gynecology, Division of Experimental Endoscopic Surgery, Imaging, Technology and Minimally Invasive Therapy, Vito Fazzi Hospital, Lecce, Italy

Hans-Rudolf Tinneberg University Clinic Giessen, Department of Gynecology and Obstetrics, Giessen, Germany

Juan J. Torrent Gynecology, Hospital Universitari Germans Trias y Pujol, Badalona, Spain

Ralf Ulrich Hematology and Oncology, Ev. Diakonie-Krankenhaus gemeinnützige GmbH, Bremen, Germany

Ilgin Türkgüoglu Department of Obstetrics and Gynecology, Inönü University, School of Medicine, Turgut Ozal Medical Center, Malatya, Turkey

Stephano Uccella Obstetrics & Gynecology Department, University of Insubria, Varese, Italy

Roberta Venturella Gynecologyst, Department of Obstetrics and Gynecology, Magna Graecia University of Catanzaro, Catanzaro, Italy

Daniele Vergara Department of Biological and Environmental Sciences and Technologies, University of Salento, Via Monteroni, Lecce, Italy

Giuseppe Vizzielli Department of Oncologic Surgery, Gynecologic Oncologic Unit, Campobasso, Italy

Yu-Chi Wang Obstetrics and Gynecology, Tri-Service General Hospital, Taipei, Taiwan

Megan N. Wasson Mayo Clinic, Phoenix, AZ, USA

Arnaud Wattiez OB GYN, University of Strasbourg, Strasbourg, France
GYN Department, Latifa Hospital, Dubai, United Arab Emirates

Thilo Wedel Institute of Anatomy, Center of Clinical Anatomy, Christian-Albrechts-University of Kiel, Kiel, Germany

Benjamin E. Wolf Department of Obstetrics and Gynecology, Leipzig University Clinic, Leipzig, Saxony, Germany

Monika Martina Wölfler Obstetrics and Gynecology, Medical University of Graz, Graz, Austria

Sheng Xu Department of Gynecology, Zhejiang Provincial People's Hospital, Hangzhou, Zhejiang, China

Magdalena Zalewski Klinik für Gynäkologie und Geburtsmedizin, Uniklinik RWTH Aachen, Aachen, Germany

Xiaofeng Zhao Department of Gynecology, Zhejiang Provincial People's Hospital, Hangzhou, Zhejiang, China

Stephen E. Zimberg Department of Gynecology, Cleveland Clinic Florida, Weston, FL, USA

Carl W. Zimmerman Department of Obstetrics and Gynecology, Vanderbilt University Medical Center, Nashville, TN, USA

Marek T. Zygmunt Department of Obstetrics and Gynaecology, University Greilswald, Greifswald, Germany

Part I

Historical Background

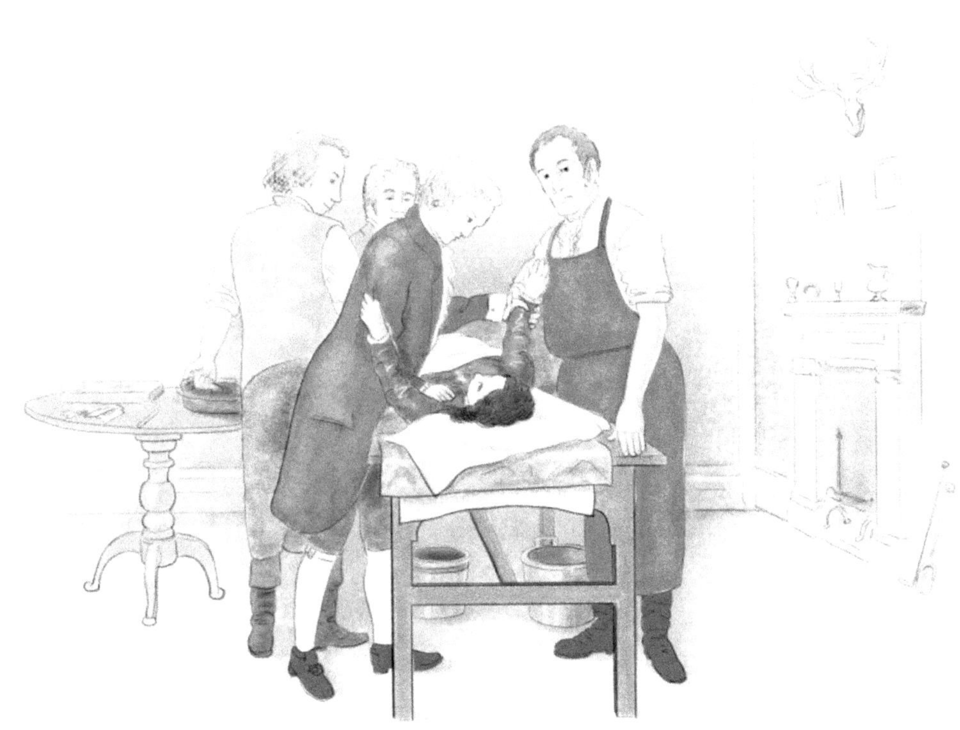

1 The History of Hysterectomy

Christopher J.G. Sutton

Introduction: The Ancient Greek Understanding of Female Pelvic Anatomy

There was a certain mystique about female anatomy in ancient times so the Greeks believed that the uterus (hysteros) was the seat of the soul. The Pythagoreans believed that the uterus was bifid which almost implies a knowledge of embryology but probably arose from the fact that they were permitted to dissect animals but human dissection was forbidden. They hypothesised that the left uterine horn represented the west, or darkness, from which females were derived whereas the right side represented the east, or light, in which males developed. They believed that the uterus wandered around the abdominal cavity and that when the organ was displaced the poor woman developed signs of hysteria [1]. Such male orientated thinking persisted until the late nineteenth Century allowing gynaecologists to remove normal ovaries, popularised by the American Surgeon Robert Battey – for a range of dubious indications ranging from hysteria, menstrual madness, insanity and even nymphomania and masturbation [2]. Such a practice performed at a time when operative mortality was around 75 % represented the zenith of morality in the specialties of gynaecological surgery and psychiatry and was probably the greatest scandal in medical history [3].

The First Vaginal Hysterectomies

Although the history of vaginal hysterectomy is shrouded in the mists of antiquity there are reports of it having been performed 50 years before the birth of Christ by Themison of Athens [4, 5]. Most of our knowledge of surgery in Greek and Roman times is derived from *Gynaecology*, the oldest published work on obstetrics and gynaecology written by Soranus [6]. Soranus (Fig. 1.1) was born in Ephesus in Asia Minor, and being situated between India and Greece absorbed the early medical ideas of these two great cultures [7]. Ephesus, which has a well preserved stone amphitheatre, was originally a Greek city but is now situated in Turkey on the Aegean Sea north of Izmir.

Soranus received his medical training in Alexandria in Egypt and later worked in Rome during the reigns of Emperor Trajan (AD 98–117) and Emperor Hadrian (AD 117–138).

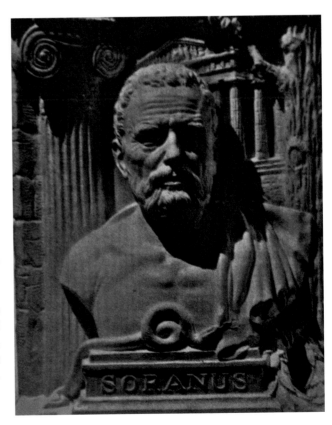

Fig. 1.1 Soranus of Ephesus (AD 98–138) who wrote the first textbook of Gynaecology and described a vaginal hysterectomy he performed (Photo: Dr. Chris Sutton taken at the Amphitheatre in Ephesus,Turkey)

C.J.G. Sutton, MA (Cantab), MB BChir, FRCOG
Professor of Gynaecological Surgery, Faculty of Health and Social Science, Gunners Farm, Stringers Common, Guilford, Surrey GU4 7PR, UK
e-mail: chrislasersutton1@btinternet.com

I. Alkatout, L. Mettler (eds.), *Hysterectomy*, DOI 10.1007/978-3-319-22497-8_1

In his book *Gynaecology* there is a well documented case of a vaginal hysterectomy which explained in detail an operation performed by the author which involved the removal of an inverted uterus that had become gangrenous and had turned black in colour [8]. The ureters, and often the bladder, were part of these early surgical excisions and the patients invariably died [1, 9].

Nevertheless in the writing of the eleventh century Arabian physician, Alsaharavius he clearly states that if the uterus had prolapsed externally and could not be reinserted, then he advised his pupils that it should be surgically excised and it is unlikely that he would have advocated this practice if death was the inevitable result of such intervention.

There is another report from a Latin translation of a Hebrew text in 1287 that Abumeron Avenzoar (?1092–1162), generally regarded as the greatest Moslem physician of the Western Caliphate was the first to attempt total extirpation of the uterus [10].

The Middle Ages

In fact there are several reports of patients surviving vaginal hysterectomy in the Middle Ages, and these are referred to in medical writings in the sixteenth and seventeenth centuries. The first authenticated case was reported by Giacomo Berengario da Carpi who lived in Bologna, the site of one of the oldest medical schools in Europe. In 1507 he was reputed to have performed a partial vaginal hysterectomy and added that his father had also performed one in the same year [11].

Schenck of Grabenberg reported 26 cases during the early part of the seventeenth century and the operation was also performed by Andreas da Crusce in Italy in 1560 and by Valkaner of Nuremberg in Germany in 1675, when the patients appear to have survived [12]. Modern medical historians are somewhat sceptical about some of these early reports and, as usual, have largely ignored the contribution of the midwives of Europe who, from time to time, amputated prolapsed or inverted puerperal uteri. They have also overlooked an early example of self-help: Faith Howard, a 46 year old peasant woman who performed the operation on herself. This case was well documented and reported in 1670 by Percival Willoughby, an early male midwife and lifelong friend of William Harvey, who famously discovered the circulation of blood. Apparently, while she was carrying a heavy bucket of coal one day, Faith's uterus prolapsed completely and, frustrated by this frequent occurrence, she grabbed the offending organ, pulled as hard as possible and "cut the whole lot off with a short knife". In his report, Willoughby states that "there was a mighty bleeding which eventually stopped" and Faith lived on for many years after this "with water passing from her insensible day and night", obviously from a vesico-vaginal fistula [13, 14].

The famous French *accoucheur,* Jean- Louis Baudeloque , the inventor of the pelvimeter, introduced the technique of artificially prolapsing the uterus and then, in favourable cases cutting it off together with the adnexal organs and he performed 23 of these procedures over 10 years from 1800. He was a fervent supporter of Caesarean Section, as opposed to symphysiotomy, and his external pelvimeter was used to measure the diameter of the external conjugate to predict those women who were likely to have an obstructed labour. He attended the first confinement of Napoleon's wife, Empress Marie-Louise, and his reputation in Paris was such that he was called '*le grand Baudeloque*' [15].

It seems that the first vaginal hysterectomy on a non-puerperal uterus was an unfortunate accident. Dr. G.B.Paletta of Milan carried out the operation on 13 April 1812 assisted by an eminent Milanese surgeon Dr. D.B. Monteggia. He intended to amputate what he thought was a cervical cancer, but to his great surprise found that he had removed the entire uterus vaginally. Unfortunately the patient died 3 days later from peritonitis [7].

The First Elective Vaginal Hysterectomies

Most of these procedures were performed on puerperal uteri and were undertaken on an emergency basis, but the first planned elective hysterectomy was by Friedrich Osiander (1759–1822) of Gottingen in Lower Saxony in Germany just over two hundred years ago in 1801 who employed the vaginal approach. He did not report the case until he had operated on his ninth patient [16].

It is interesting to reflect that almost all women subjected to caesarean section at this time died from shock, haemorrhage or sepsis. In the early 1800's Ossiander wrote: "Before undertaking this procedure, one should allow the patient to draw up her will and grant her time to prepare herself for death" [15]. A rather extreme example of informed consent long before the modern epidemic of litigation might make this seem reasonable in certain circumstances.

The first deliberate planned vaginal hysterectomy for endometrial carcinoma was by Conrad Langenbeck (Fig. 1.2) who, interestingly, also came from Gottingen and was possibly the most distinguished surgeon of his time and the Surgeon-General of the Hanoverian army. He performed this operation in 1813 but did not report it until 4 years later [17].

Langenbeck, the inventor of the retractor that is familiar to all surgeons, was himself a surgeon of such supreme swiftness that he once amputated the shoulder of a wounded infantry officer whilst a colleague who had come to watch the procedure had turned around to take a pinch of snuff thereby totally missing the operation he had travelled far to observe [18, 19].

Having little precedent to follow, Langenbeck had to devise his own plan for the removal of the entire uterus. He

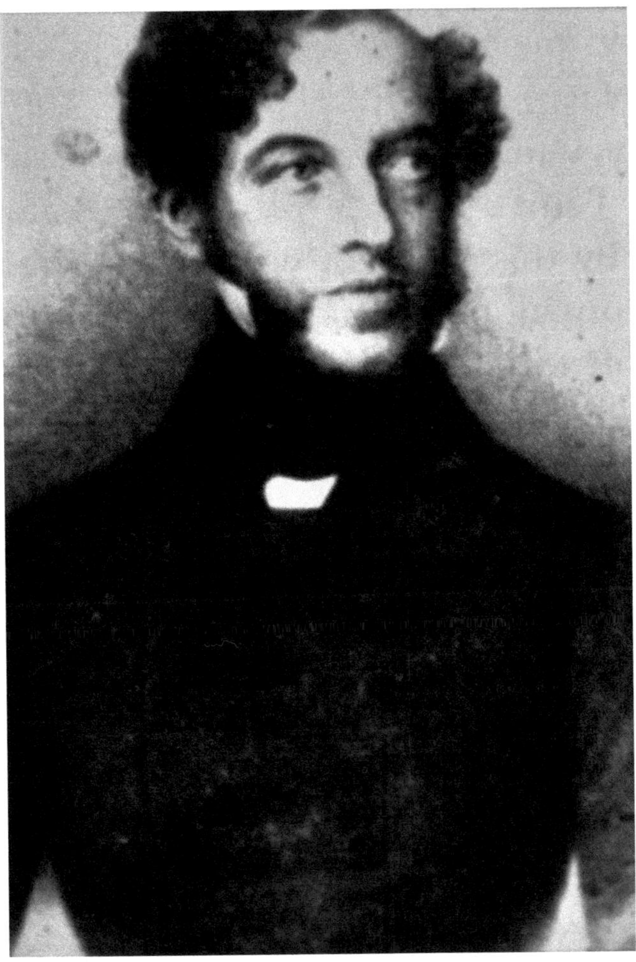

Fig. 1.2 Conrad Langenbeck from Gottingen, Lower Saxony, Germany: Surgeon General to the Hanoverian Army, who performed the first elective vaginal hysterectomy for endometrial cancer in 1813 (Reproduced with permission of Jaypee Brothers Medical Publishers, India)

performed a retroperitoneal dissection taking great care not to enter the peritoneal cavity. Towards the end of the procedure he encountered uncontrollable bleeding from the uterine artery and called upon his assistant, a Surgeon Commander afflicted with gout, to come and help but the gentleman was enormously overweight and could not rise from his chair. Langenbeck had no alternative but to compress the bleeding artery with his left thumb and forefinger and with his right hand he placed a ligature- carrying needle through the tissues behind the bleeding point and tied the ligature by grasping one end between his teeth and secured the pedicle with a one handed slip knot tied with his right hand. Following the procedure he could detect no opening into the peritoneal cavity and the patient made a surprising and uneventful recovery but after this extraordinary display of technical virtuosity, none of his colleagues believed that the operation had taken place since there was no visible scar. As is so often the case the operative specimen had been lost on the way to the pathology laboratory, the Surgeon Commander with gout died the following week and the patient herself was demented so was unable to provide reliable testimony. For the next 26 years Langenbeck was subjected to ridicule and the jibes of his colleagues and accused of being a liar and a charlatan and was only finally able to substantiate his claim when the patient died of senility and an autopsy showed that she had indeed had her uterus removed in its entirety [9].

The First Laparotomy: Christmas Day 1809

In order to put these events into historical perspective the vaginal hysterectomy for endometrial cancer performed by Conrad Langenbeck described above took place in 1813 at the time when Napoleon's *Grande Armée* was retreating from Moscow after the failure of his Russian Campaign. It was only 4 years before, on Christmas day 1809, that the human abdomen was deliberately opened for the first time in order to remove a diseased organ, in this case a massive ovarian cyst.

Until the beginning of the nineteenth Century there was no possible way of removing a large tumour because it was considered that surgical opening of the peritoneal cavity resulted in certain death. A little over 200 years ago an event took place which has had a momentous impact on our survival as individuals and as a species and yet it has been remembered by relatively few. That day saw the birth of operative abdominal surgery which has saved countless lives, yet it did not take place in one of the great University Teaching Hospitals but in the front parlour of the house of an American country doctor in the small frontier town of Danville in Kentucky [20, 21].

On the morning of Christmas Day 1809 the brave surgeon Ephraim McDowell (Fig. 1.3) performed the world's first elective laparotomy to remove a massive tumour from the equally brave patient, Jane Todd Crawford (Fig. 1.4) who had to withstand the horrific pain of a large abdominal incision without the benefit of an anaesthetic. The doctor was brave because the abdominal cavity had never been deliberately opened with a surgical knife before and it was widely accepted that such an intervention would inevitably result in death.

Legend has it that the townsfolk of Danville had gathered in the square outside his house on the morning of the operation and were erecting a gallows so that if Jane Todd Crawford died at the hands of the "dreadful doctor" he would be hanged in public [22].

The Father of Abdominal Surgery: Ephraim McDowell

McDowell's family were of mixed Irish and Scottish extraction and he was born in Rockbridge County, Virginia in 1771, the ninth of twelve children. When he was 13 years old the

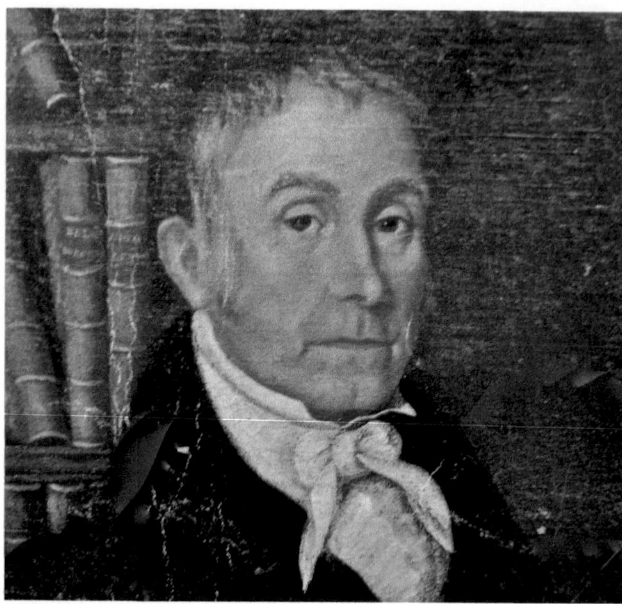

Fig. 1.3 Ephraim McDowell (1771–1830): The Father of Abdominal Surgery. Performed the First Laparotomy on Christmas day 1809. Painting by P.W. Davenport in McDowell House. Note the three volumes on Surgery by John Bell, one of McDowell's teachers in Edinburgh (Photo: Chris Sutton with permission McDowell House and Museum, Danville, Kentucky)

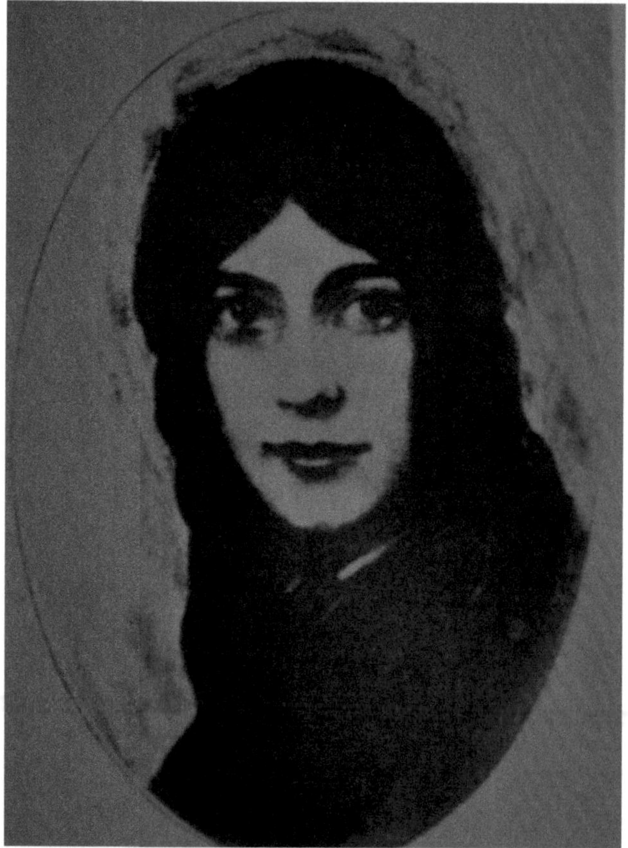

Fig. 1.4 Jane Todd Crawford (1763–1842) From a painting of young Jane of unknown origin. McDowell House, Danville, Kentucky (Reproduced courtesy of McDowell House and Museum, Danville, Kentucky)

family moved to Danville, a frontier town that was the first capital of the State of Kentucky, where his father was appointed Judge of the small community of some "150 homes and some tolerably good buildings" [23]. The young Ephraim decided on a career in medicine early in his life and served as an apprentice to a family physician, Dr. Alexander Humphreys in Staunton, Virginia. When he was 22 he spent 2 years studying anatomy in Edinburgh under Alexander Munro and surgery under the tutelage of John Bell. For financial reasons he had to return home to Danville without earning a medical degree but even without the letters after his name the prestige of being educated at one of the most famous Medical Schools in the world ensured that he rapidly built up an extensive surgical practice and he came to be regarded as "the best doctor west of Philadelphia" [24] He was renowned for his swift amputations, hernia repairs and lithotomies and would typically operate in the homes of patients with family members gathered round to hold the unfortunate sufferer down. One of his patients was James Polk who, as a 14 year old boy had several bladder stones removed, and later became the eleventh president of the United States [25].

McDowell's fame spread locally among the frontier people because this was an area that was expanding rapidly after Dr. Thomas Walker had opened up the Wilderness Trail through the Cumberland Gap from Virginia into Kentucky accompanied by frontiersmen and Indian fighters such as Daniel Boone and Davy Crockett [21].

The Patient: Jane Todd-Crawford

Jane Todd-Crawford lived with her family of five children in a small log cabin in Motley's Glenn near Greensburg, Kentucky, some 60 miles from Danville and at the age of 44 she was thought to be carrying another child and was causing concern with the local doctors and midwives because she was 2 months beyond her due date and " she was afflicted with excrutiating pains similar to those of labour, which were incessant" [26]. The two attending physicians were in despair and had tried various potions and enemas used to induce labour and in desperation had even employed two midwives to jump up and down on her extremely distended abdomen. All this was to no avail and the poor woman had such a swollen abdomen that she could barely breathe and in desperation they decided to summon the "surgeon from Danville to assist with the delivery".

Although the journey from Danville to Greensburg can nowadays be easily accomplished in an hour or so using modern highways, in 1809 it required a lengthy and difficult journey on horseback, crossing many mountain ridges and fording deep rivers and when McDowell set out on this arduous journey the snow had already fallen deeply and there were added hazards from bands of skirmishing Indians, to say nothing of predatory wolf packs and bears. When he

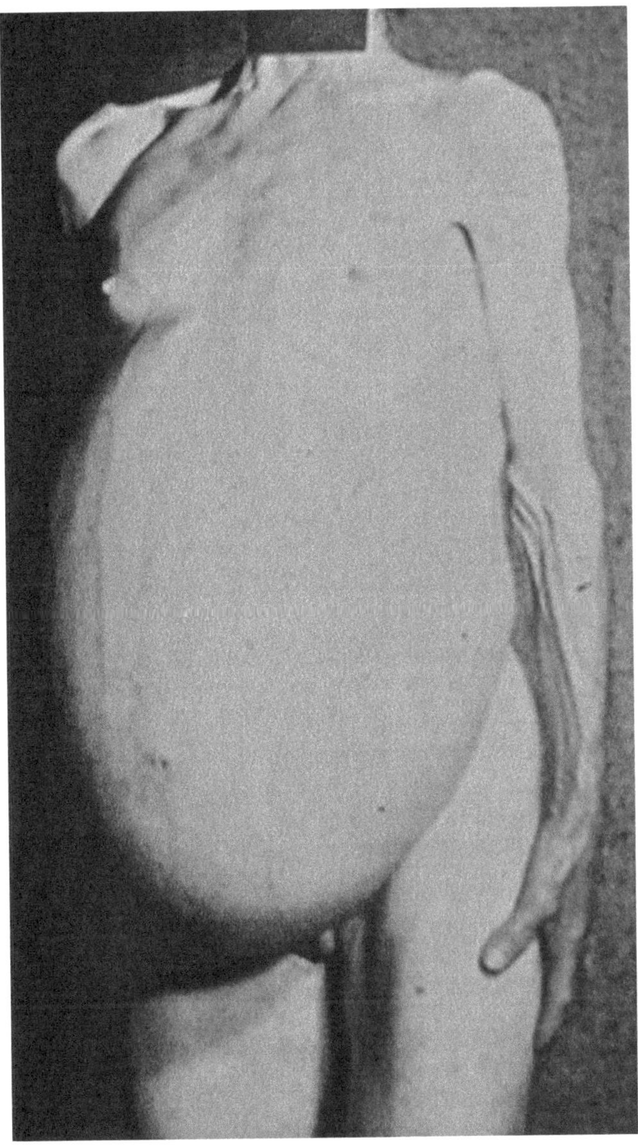

Fig. 1.5 Massive ovarian cyst. When removed it weighed half of the weight of the patient (Photo: Chris Sutton. St. Luke's Hospital, Guildford)

arrived he quickly appraised the situation and saw that the swollen abdomen did, indeed, have the appearance of a pregnancy, possibly a multiple one, with a size that was indeed making it difficult for the patient to breathe.

Without recourse to sophisticated imaging techniques it is often difficult clinically to distinguish a massive fibroid from a large ovarian tumour (Fig. 1.5) or, indeed, from a term pregnancy [27]. Possibly because of his education in Edinburgh under the tutelage of the anatomist Alexander Monroe (Secundus), he performed a more thorough examination than had been performed by the local physicians and this included a vaginal examination where he found that the mass was inclined to one side and was mobile and his examining fingers felt a normal sized uterus and cervix which were pushed to the other side, all of which indicated that the mass was an "enlarged ovarium".

Clearly, he was very depressed by his findings and in an account written many years later to a medical student, Robert Thompson, he wrote "I told the lady that I could do her no good and candidly stated to her, her deplorable situation; informed her that John Bell, Hunter, Hay and A Wood, four of the first and most eminent surgeons in England and Scotland, had uniformly declared in their lectures that such was the danger of peritoneal inflammation that opening the abdomen to extract the tumour led to inevitable death."

She was clearly devastated by this pronouncement but told him that it was impossible to continue to live in her present situation since she was almost unable to breathe and felt that she would die anyway. He therefore continued "but, notwithstanding this, if she thought herself prepared to die, I would take the lump from her if she would come to Danville." He ended this account by stating simply "she appeared willing to undergo an experiment" [28]. This must surely be the first documented case in the world of informed consent.

The Operation on McDowell's Kitchen Table

Dr. McDowell returned to Danville expecting to hear no more from her because the journey with the increasing snowfall that winter was long and difficult and dangerous by horseback, but she was a tough frontier woman and a few days later appeared on his doorstep. Unfortunately the arduous journey had caused considerable bruising over the lower abdomen, where she had rested the enormous tumour on the pommel of her saddle. He therefore determined to wait for a few days before deciding to perform the operation and, being a deeply religious man, he timed the procedure to occur on the morning of Christmas Day when many of the townsfolk were in church so that they could bring the efforts of their combined prayers onto his endeavour. He was joined by his nephew, Dr. James McDowell, who had graduated a few months previously from the first Medical School in America, in Philadelphia, to join the practice as a partner and he did his best to dissuade his uncle from "the experiment". The kitchen table was dragged into the front room and Jane Todd Crawford was placed on her back on the table and tilted slightly to the right side (Fig. 1.6) and then "he removed all her dressing which might in any way impede the operation". He then offered up a prayer saying " Direct me, O God, in performing this operation, for I am but an instrument in thy hands, and am but thy servant, and if it is thy will, oh! spare this poor afflicted woman."

Many years later when he wrote about the procedure he described it as follows: "I made an incision about 3 inches from the rectus abdominus muscle on the left side, continuing the same 9" in length, parallel with the fibres of the above-named muscle, extending into the cavity of the abdomen. The tumour then appeared full in view but was so large that we could not take it away entire. We put a strong ligature around the fallopian tube near the uterus and then cut open

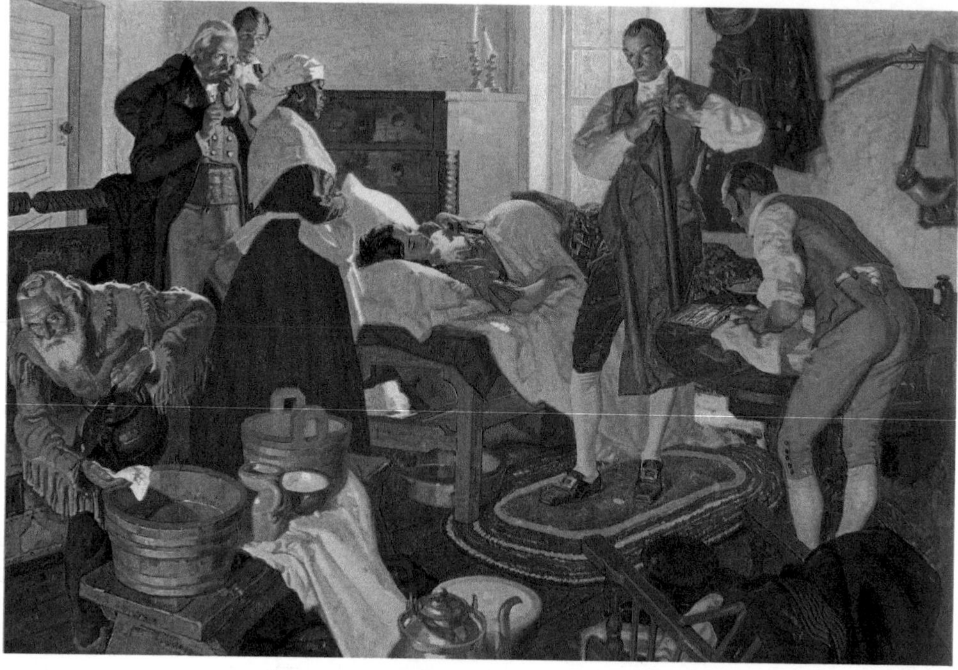

Fig. 1.6 The first laparotomy in the world on Christmas Day 1806 performed on the kitchen table in Ephraim McDowell's House in Danville, Kentucky. Painting by Dean Cornwell *" the Dawn of Abdominal Surgery"* (Reproduced courtesy of McDowell House and Museum, Danville, Kentucky)

the tumour, which was the ovarium and fimbrious part of the fallopian tube, very much enlarged. We took out 15 lbs of a dirty gelatinous-looking substance, after which we cut through the fallopian tube and extracted the sac, which weighed 7 lb and one-half. As soon as the external opening was made the intestines rushed out upon the table and so completely was the abdomen filled by the tumour that they could not be replaced during the operation which was terminated in about 25 minutes. We then turned her upon her left side so as to permit the blood to escape, after which we closed the external opening with the interrupted suture, leaving out at the lower end of the excision the ligature which surrounded the fallopian tube."

During the whole of this ghastly painful procedure Jane Todd-Crawford remained motionless and merely recited the Psalms in order to calm herself during her ordeal.

She stayed in McDowell's house and the bed in which she lay can still be seen because the entire house and gardens have been turned into a museum to commemorate this amazing feat of pioneering surgery. Several years ago the American College of Obstetricians and Gynaecologists donated the wooden door knocker from the front door of McDowell House to the Royal College of Obstetricians and Gynaecologists in London and it is still used to this day as a gavel on ceremonial occasions.

Ephraim McDowell visited Mrs. Crawford on a daily basis and on the 5th day he found her making her own bed and reprimanded her severely. She continued to make an excellent recovery and 25 days later she returned home in good health by the same route that she had come, which is now a long distance footpath named "The Jane Todd Crawford Trail".

The two of them never met again during their lives. Ephraim McDowell died at the age of 59 years of "an acute attack of inflammation of the stomach" which was probably appendicitis and long before the time when a laparotomy could be performed to remove the infected organ. Jane Todd Crawford outlived him and died at the age of 78 years and a picture of her in her old age (Fig. 1.7) shows her displaying a locket with the picture of Abraham Lincoln, who was born in a log cabin at Sinking Spring Farm very close to where she grew up in Greensburg County and to whom she was related as a cousin when he married one of her sisters who thus became America's First Lady as Mary Todd Lincoln.

The often repeated story that the townsfolk had gathered in the square outside his house and had erected a gallows to hang him in the event of Jane Todd Crawford dying during the operation is almost certainly anecdotal and untrue for several reasons. Firstly he was considered the most famous, knowledgeable, and skilful surgeon in that frontier area which probably had few doctors and he would have been treated with the greatest respect and unlikely to have been publicly hanged. Furthermore his father was the County Judge and his elder brother was the Sheriff of Danville who was sadly killed a few weeks later when he was involved, along with Davy Crockett and Daniel Boone, in a skirmish with a local Indian tribe at Blue Lick in Kentucky [21].

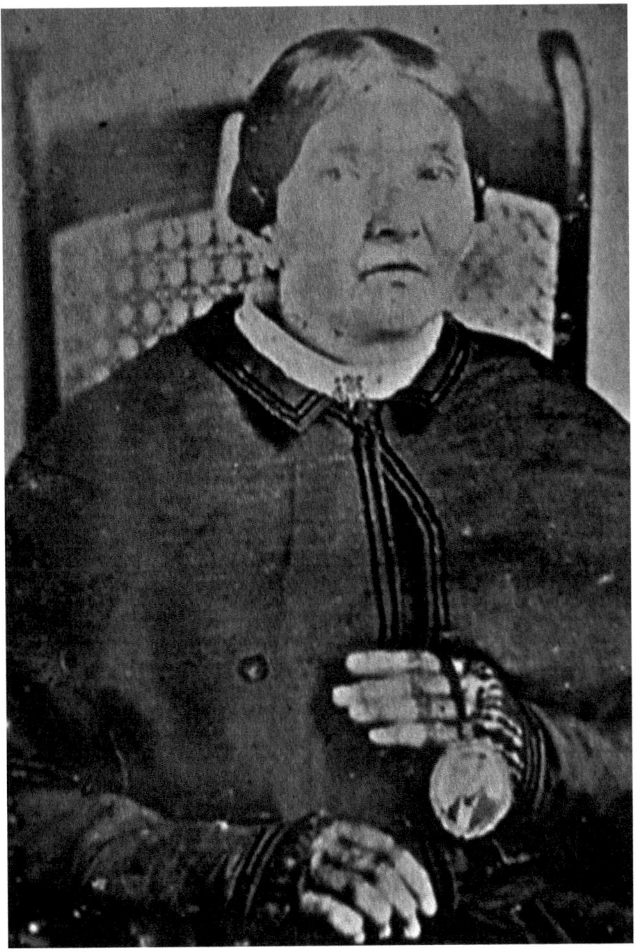

Fig. 1.7 Jane Todd Crawford. A daguerreotype of her as an old lady a few months before her death in 1842.She is holding a locket with a portrait of Abraham Lincoln, a distant relative by marriage to one of her cousins, who became America's First Lady as Mary Todd Lincoln (Photo: Chris Sutton with permission McDowell House and Museum, Danville, Kentucky)

The Ovariotomists: Pioneers of Ovarian Surgery

Unlike his modern counterparts, Ephraim McDowell did not immediately rush off to get this operation published and waited until he had performed two more successful operations on ovarian tumours in 1813 and 1816 before reporting it in a journal with a limited readership, "The Eclectic Repertory and Analytical Review of Philadelphia" [29]. Two years later he published two further cases in the same journal, one of whom survived, but the other died of peritonitis on the third post-operative day. During his lifetime he performed three further ovarian operations between 1822 and 1826. One involved merely drainage but the patient lived for a long time afterwards, the second underwent complete excision, but the third had to be abandoned because of extensive adhesions.

There were a further three that are mentioned in letters and on reading his descriptions it does seem that, although he styled himself as an ovarian surgeon, at least two of his cases were large pedunculated myomas [30, 31]. News of great surgical advances took a long time to percolate across the Atlantic and, even in America, McDowell's achievement was greeted with a certain amount of scepticism and even outright disbelief [32]. It was 14 years later that the first ovariotomy was carried out in Europe by John Lizars, a fellow student from Edinburgh, but the patient died and he then made three more successful attempts [33]. It appears that the Edinburgh Surgeon, J.Y.Simpson, the inventor of the anaesthetic agent chloroform was the first to introduce the word 'ovariotomy', a strange choice for the name of this operation in an age when most surgeons were reared in the classics and therefore etymologically correct [32]. The initial years of abdominal surgery were associated with an enormous mortality rate, mainly due to uncontrolled haemorrhage or peritonitis and sepsis but the few women that survived spawned a new generation of pioneering surgeons who finally realised that opening the human abdomen with a surgical incision did not result in certain death.

The World's First Abdominal Hysterectomy November 17th 1843

The greatest of the ovariotomists in Europe was Charles Clay of Manchester, in the North of England [34]. He studied at the Manchester Royal Infirmary and, like Ephraim McDowell received part of his medical education in Edinburgh. Like McDowell he also started in surgical practice in a small rural community, Ashton-under-Lyne under the shadow of the Pennine Hills in Cheshire. After 16 years he moved to the industrial city of Manchester where he established his surgical reputation. He was a member of the Reform Club and was a friend of my great grandfather, William Sutton, who was a successful businessman in this thriving Victorian metropolis. Charles Clay is shown in Fig. 1.8 at the peak of his surgical career, profoundly confident and appearing dapper with his top hat.

The first four of his ovariotomies survived but with the fifth he was not so lucky and this turned out to be the first abdominal hysterectomy recorded and it was a complete disaster. The operation was performed on 17 November 1843 in the first floor room above his Consulting Rooms in Piccadilly, the large square in the centre of Manchester. As was usual in those days he was accompanied by several

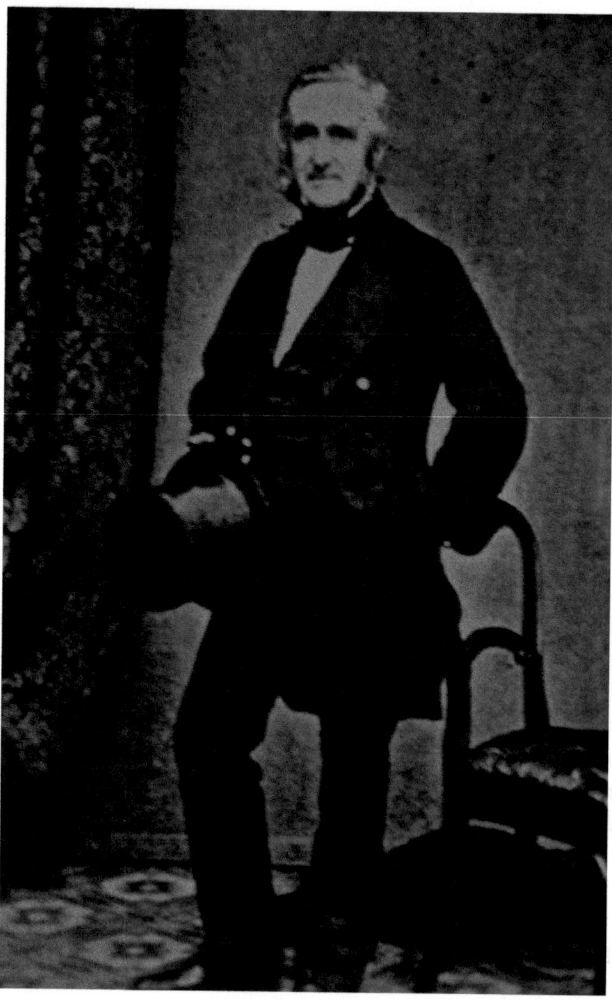

Fig. 1.8 Charles Clay (1801–1893) who performed the first successful abdominal hysterectomy in Europe on 2nd January 1863 (Copyright of the Rylands Library, University of Manchester, England)

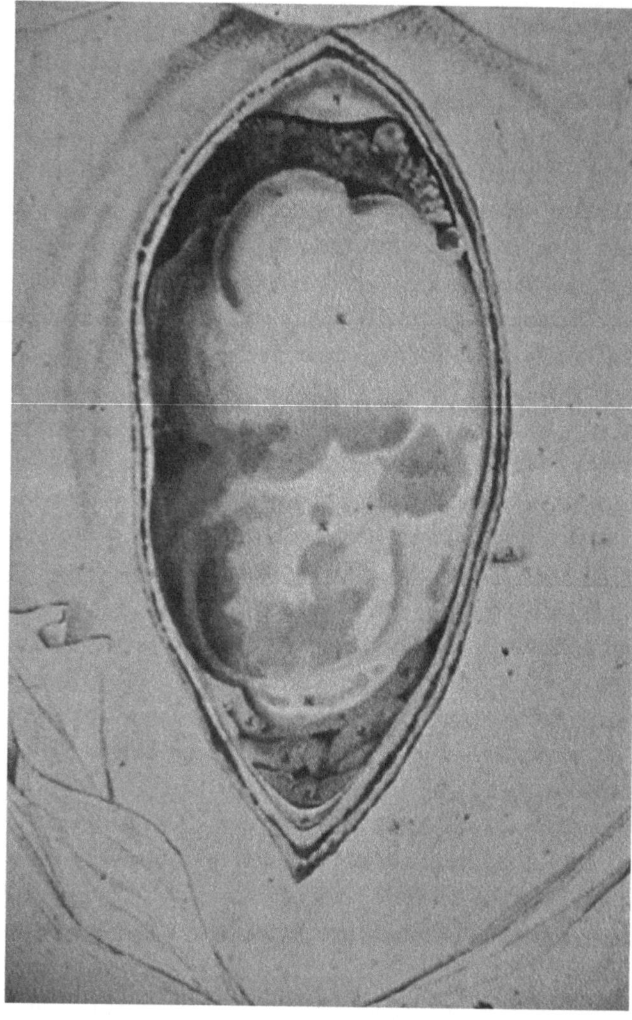

Fig. 1.9 Massive fibroid exposed at laparotomy (Photo: Chris Sutton)

friends and medical students as spectators and since it was before the time of Pasteur or Lister no one wore masks or surgical gloves and the patient was given brandy and milk to alleviate the pain of the operation since this was a long time before anaesthesia was introduced by WRT Morton at the Massachusetts General Hospital in Boston in 1846 [35]. He was certain that he was dealing with a massive ovarian cyst so he made a long 60 cm surgical incision from the xiphisternum to the pubis. Unfortunately once the peritoneum was entered the patient coughed and the massive tumour was extruded (Fig. 1.9) and he realised to his horror that it was a huge fibroid and since the patient was now struggling and had to be forcibly restrained by the medical students and it was impossible to replace the hugely enlarged uterus back in the abdominal cavity he had no option but to proceed and performed a subtotal hysterectomy. By an extraordinary coincidence a few days later on the 21st of November, A M Heath who was also an ovarian surgeon in Manchester, found himself in a similar situation operating on a huge fibroid instead of an ovarian cyst. Unfortunately both patients died of a massive haemorrhage a few hours later [19].

The next year, Clay was more successful with a similar case but on this occasion he placed a ligature of Indian hemp around the supra-vaginal cervix to prevent haemorrhage from the uterine arteries. The patient lived for 15 days when she fell out of bed in a coma and never regained consciousness. Although this was tragic for the patient it was also sad for Clay since she had survived the critical post-operative period and not succumbed to sepsis which was the usual cause of death following a laparotomy.

From reading contemporary accounts of this woman's post-operative course it is difficult to determine the exact mode of death. She could have had a pulmonary embolus or she could have fallen out of bed in uraemic coma due to occlusion of both ureters by the ligature but popular Mancunian folklore suggests that she was dropped on the floor by a couple of incompetent porters whilst the nurses changed her bed linen. If this is true then her death was entirely unrelated to the operation and Charles Clay could have claimed to have performed the first successful hysterectomy in the world [22, 36].

In fact it was not for a further 20 years that he attempted another hysterectomy and this time the patient survived. Interestingly he mentioned this almost as an aside during his important presentation to the Obstetrical Society of London in 1863 when he presented his experience of 395 ovariotomies with only 25 deaths [37].

The First Successful Abdominal Hysterectomy in the World

The first successful removal of a fibroid uterus was by Walter Burnham in Lowell, Massachusetts in 1853 [18, 38, 39]. The patient, a 42 year old woman, was referred to him by another physician who had observed a slowly growing abdominal mass over the previous 6 years that was without any other symptoms but had recently become persistently painful. Burnham diagnosed an ovarian cyst but told her there was no treatment available other than surgical removal and even '… this course of action could not be adopted without placing her life in imminent danger'. He advised her to seek a second opinion and ' also to consult her friends as to the propriety of running so great a risk' [15].

Nevertheless she elected to have the operation which took place on 25 June 1853 with two surgical assistants and in the presence of a large number of medical gentlemen as was often the case with these early surgical interventions. This operation took place in the early days of anaesthesia and the chloroform caused the patient to vomit so when he made a long midline incision from the sternum to the pubis, a large pedunculated fibroid attached to an enlarged fibroid uterus was extruded through the incision when in fact Burnham was anticipating a massive ovarian cyst. It proved impossible to replace the large fibroid and he had little choice but to proceed with a subtotal hysterectomy tying off both ovarian and uterine arteries. The patient recovered, apparently with the aid of brandy and opium, and the fact that the original diagnosis was incorrect should not detract from his achievement.

Early records of the first abdominal hysterectomies read like a disaster saga until Burnham produced the first survivor, but even in that instance the diagnosis was wrong (Table 1.1).

However, later the same year Gilman Kimball (Fig. 1.10) who, also resided in Lowell, carried out the first deliberate hysterectomy to remove a fibroid, and the patient survived the operation [40]. In this particular case the surgeon correctly diagnosed a large fibroid of about the size of a 6 month pregnancy but it was not the size that was the problem but the severe menorrhagia that was causing the loss of a large quantity of blood each month which had become life-threatening.

Table 1.1 A summary of the abdominal hysterectomies performed in the early years (1843–1863)

Date	Operator	Diagnosis	Outcome
1843	Clay	Ovarian tumour	Massive haemorrhage a few hours after the operation and died
1843	Heath	Ovarian tumour	Massive haemorrhage a few hours after the operation and died
1844	Clay	Ovarian tumour	Dropped on the floor on day 15 and died
1846	Bellinger	Fibroids	Haemorrhaged on day 5 and died
1853	Burnham	Ovarian tumour	Survived but diagnosis wrong
1853	Kimball	Fibroids	Survived and diagnosis correct
1863	Clay	Fibroids	Survived. First successful operation in Europe
1863	Koeberle	Fibroids	Survived

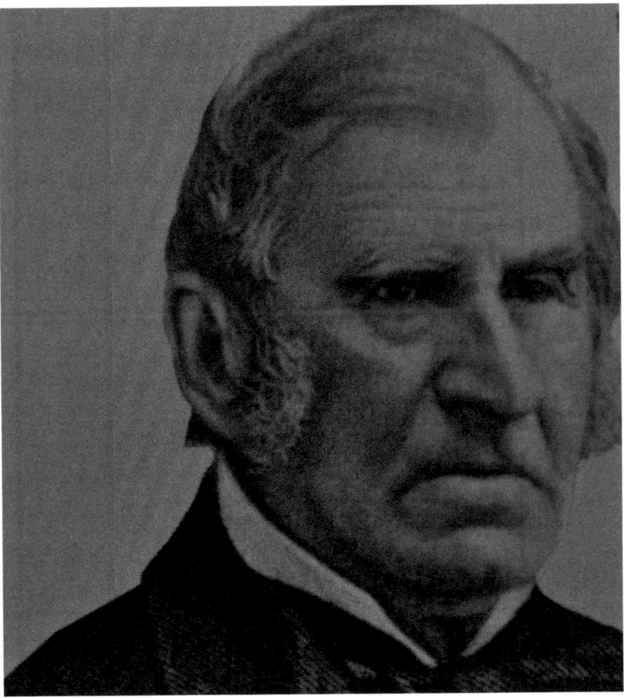

Fig. 1.10 Gilman Kimball (1804–1892) from Lowell, Massachusetts who performed the first successful hysterectomy in the world with the correct pre-operative diagnosis on 1 September 1853 (Reproduced with permission from RCOG Press, London)

During the consultation with her other physicians Kimball felt that ' Rather than give up the case as utterly hopeless, I would propose, as a last resort, the removal of the uterus itself …. Extraordinary and hazardous as this suggestion seemed, the feeling was unanimously and unhesitatingly expressed by everyone present at the consultation, that this procedure offered the only possible chance of saving the patient from impending death. This conclusion was no sooner made known to the patient, than it was readily consented to – both she and her husband claiming that a chance of life by an operation however small that chance might be, was better than the certainty of a speedy death" [40].

They wasted no time and the same afternoon the patient was anaesthetized with chloroform and a relatively small incision was made through the linea alba directly over the most prominent part of the tumour. Kimball's plan was to perform a myomectomy and having reduced the size of the uterus to then proceed to sub-total hysterectomy. This is essentially what he achieved and the patient made a full and complete recovery, although the protruding ligatures were still causing inconvenience 8 months later.

It is interesting that these two surgeons came from a small town in rural Massachusetts and considering that hysterectomy is the second most common operation performed on women, second only to Caesarean Section, that enquiries I made at the tourist office last year as to where these operations actually took place lead nowhere and it seems that the burghers of that small town of Lowell are quite unaware of the fame that should be the just due of these two pioneering surgeons.

Walter Burnham was the son of a doctor and studied medicine under the tutelage of his father and graduated from the University of Vermont in 1829. He moved to Lowell in 1846 and carried out general and gynaecological surgery and was one of the early advocates of ovariotomy having performed 300 procedures in 30 years with a survival rate of 75 % which were excellent results for those times. His hysterectomy results were not so good and after the first survivor he performed a further 15 hysterectomies during the following 13 years but only two survived – the rest succumbing to sepsis, peritonitis, haemorrhage and exhaustion.

Walter Burnham was a member of the Massachusetts House of Representatives and was instrumental in securing the passage of the Anatomy Act in 1855,which authorised the medical profession to obtain bodies of dead paupers for dissection and anatomical research. During the American Civil War (1862–1870) he was surgeon to the Sixth Massachusetts Regiment of Volunteers. He died at his home in Lowell on 16 January 1883 at the age of 75 [41].

Gilman Kimball also served as a Brigade Surgeon in the American Civil War and was Medical Director to General Butler. Following his first successful operation at the Lowell Hospital he became Professor of Surgery at the Berkshire Medical Institute and the Vermont Medical College and was awarded an honorary MD at Yale College in Connecticut in 1856. In 1877 he was elected to Fellowship of the American Gynaecological Society and became President of that Society in1883. He died in his 88th year in 1892 [41].

The First Successful Abdominal Hysterectomy in Europe

Eugene Koeberle from Strasbourg was one of the greatest surgeons in Europe in the latter half of the nineteenth Century and the French usually claim that he performed the first successful hysterectomy in Europe. The operation was for fibroids and the diagnosis was correct and in order to obtain haemostasis he used a device of his own invention called a serre-noeud which was a wire loop tightened by a screw device (Fig. 1.11) that held the cervix like a clamp and allowed it to be exteriorised through the wound (Fig. 1.12). Eventually the avascular cervical stump necrosed and fell back into the pelvis [22]. This operation took place on 2 April 1863 and was certainly the first in Continental Europe but in his lecture to the Obstetrical Society of London Charles Clay had briefly mentioned a successful case of "the entire removal of the uterus and its appendages" which he had performed in Manchester a couple of months earlier on 3 January 1863 [37]. It would appear there-

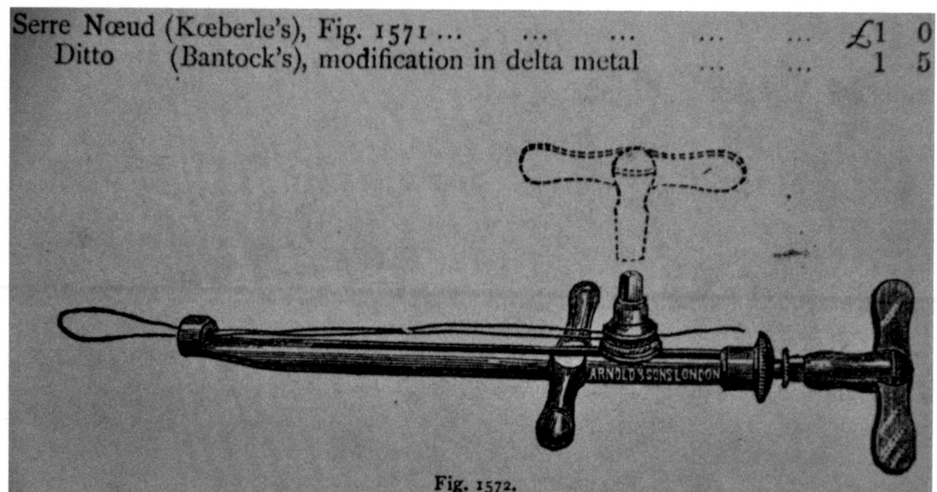

Fig. 1.11 The serre-noeud from a commercial catalogue of Arnold and Sons, Instrument Makers, London priced at £1 (1.38 Euros) (Photo by Chris Sutton. Company no longer in existence)

fore that the first successful hysterectomy in Europe was performed by an English surgeon albeit by only 3 months.

Anaesthesia was employed regularly and Lister had promulgated the theory of antisepsis and had devised a carbolic spray to prevent infection and peritonitis [42], although there is no actual reference in Clay's writings that he used these methods. In this particular case, which was deliberately undertaken to remove a uterine fibroid, he determined to cut through the cervix and not to open the vagina. The case is well authenticated by three doctors from Preston, Sheffield and Manchester, and immediately after the operation, Professor J Y Simpson, (Fig. 1.13) the inventor of chloroform, arrived unexpectedly from Edinburgh. He was greatly interested in the case and took the specimen back to Edinburgh from whence, some time later, he returned a description and a sketch, ending his letter with 'your case may turn out as a precedent for operative interference in some exceptional cases of large fibroids of the uterus and I congratulate you most sincerely on the happy recovery of your patient' [22].

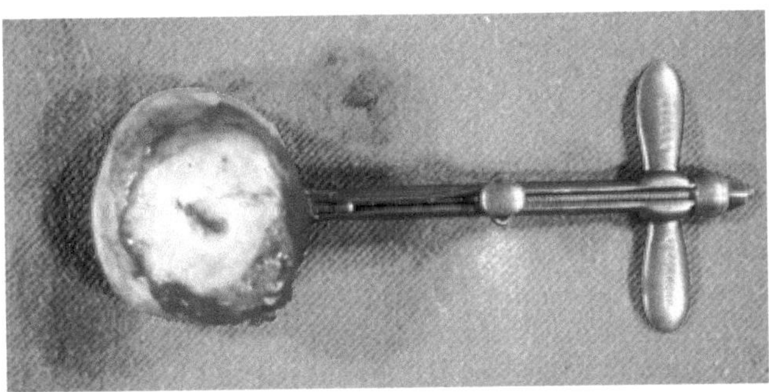

Fig. 1.12 The serre-noeud introduced by Koeberle of Strasbourg, who performed the first successful hysterectomy in continental Europe on 2nd April 1863 (Photo: Chris Sutton taken at St. Luke's Hospital, Guildford)

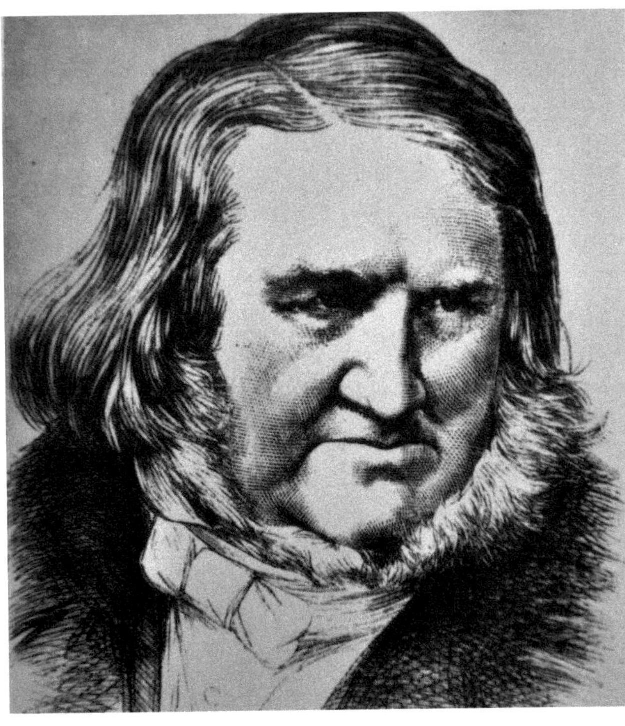

Fig. 1.13 James Young Simpson, Professor of Midwifery at the University of Edinburgh and inventor of chloroform and Simpson's Forceps (Photo: Chris Sutton from a contemporary portrait)

James Young Simpson was the Professor of Midwifery in Edinburgh where he had enrolled in the University at the tender age of 14 initially to study the arts. He had difficulties with administering ether to patients in prolonged labour and sought an alternative solution by inventing chloroform [43] which could more easily be given as a small droplet inhaled on a handkerchief. He famously experimented on himself and his guests after a dinner party in his house, among them Matthew Duncan (of placenta fame) and George Keith, the brother of Thomas Keith (*vide infra*) and all the guests slid off their chairs and were found next morning soundly asleep on the floor.

He used it on many patients having prolonged painful labours and on children undergoing surgery but had to face criticism from religious objectors who quoted the Bible citing Genesis 3:16 '.... *in sorrow and suffering thou shalt bring forth children....*' With his wide knowledge of literature and the scriptures Simpson was able to quote back to them Genesis 2:21: ' *And the lord God caused a deep sleep to fall upon Adam, and as he slept he took one of his ribs and closed up the flesh instead thereof* ' [44].

The criticism continued until Dr. John Snow successfully administered chloroform to Queen Victoria during the birth of Princess Charlotte and after this widely publicised regal event, ' *Chloroform à la Reine* ', the technique became widely accepted and for that and other contributions to Midwifery such as the design of Simpson's Forceps he was eventually made a Knight of the Realm [41].

Gynaecological Surgery in the Late Nineteenth Century

The initial mortality in these operations was extremely high since many of the early abdominal surgeons employed the long ligature hanging out of the lower part of the incision in order to allow the drainage of '*laudable pus*' from the peritoneal cavity, in much the same way as when they were amputating limbs in battlefield surgery. Charles Clay used the long ligature procedure throughout his career but Lawson Tait, (Fig. 1.14) of Birmingham, the first surgeon to successfully operate on an ectopic pregnancy, believed that if the ligature was short and the wound completely closed, the mortality rate would probably fall to 6 or 8 %. Such results were achieved by Isaac Baker Brown who cauterized the ligated ovarian pedicle before closure of the abdominal wound on 40 patients with only four deaths. He was a Consultant Gynaecological Surgeon at London's greatest teaching hospital, St. Mary's Hospital in Paddington (Fig. 1.15) and sadly went the way of so many in the medical profession in the past. He somehow went off at a tangent and in 1865 published a paper on 'The cureability of some forms of insanity, epilepsy and hysteria by clitoridectomy' [45]. Unfortunately, he also advertised the success of this procedure and as a result he fell from grace and was expelled from the Obstetrical Society of London and died in obscurity [46]. Because of this, his technique of ovariotomy failed to be adopted and it fell to Thomas Keith, an apprentice of James Young Simpson, to rediscover this manoeuvre.

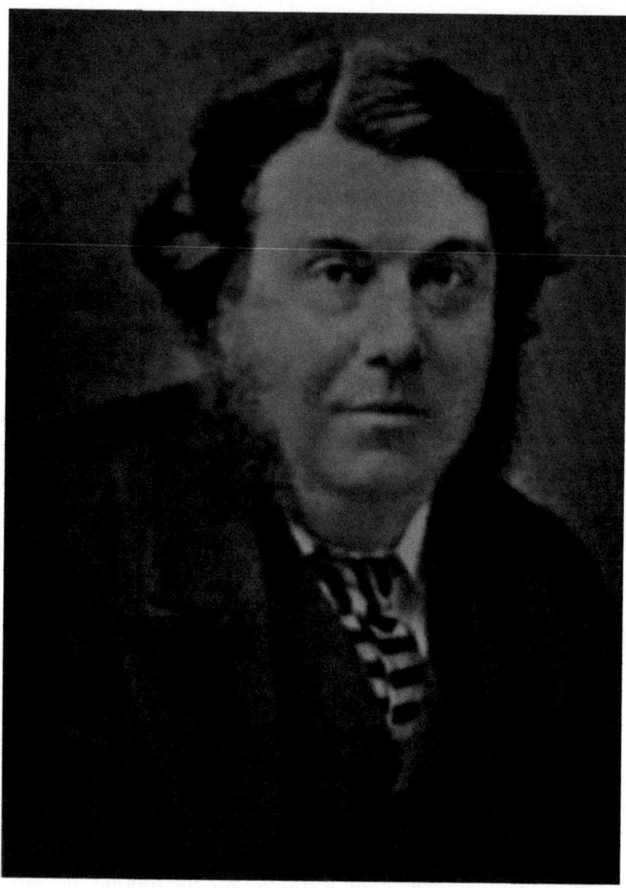

Fig. 1.14 Lawson Tait from Birmingham , an industrial city in the Midlands of England was one of the greatest surgeons of his generation and had a low mortality due to rigorous attention to cleanliness and aseptic principles (Figure reproduced courtesy of Jaypee Brothers Medical Publishers, India)

Dr. Keith Ends the Dark Period of Appallingly High Mortality

Thomas Keith was probably the greatest analytical surgeon in our speciality during the late nineteenth-century. He was a wild looking man, born in the Manse of St. Cyrus, near Montrose in the Scottish Borders and was a lifelong sufferer from cysteine stones for which he required many operations which probably accounts for his rather startling appearance (Fig. 1.16). Thomas Keith performed his first ovariotomy in September 1862, but his initial mortality was high. This was around the time that Lister was advocating antiseptic surgery, although Keith found that the carbolic spray did not help to reduce his operative mortality. He therefore turned his attention to the method of wound closure, abandoning the long ligature and exteriorized clamp that Koeberle and, later, Spencer Wells (Fig. 1.17) had popularized and instead cauterized the pedicle and dropped it into the peritoneal cavity, which he then drained.

He was also a vigorous opponent of the technique of blood-letting, and out of 156 cases reported only six deaths (3.8 % mortality). His hysterectomy results were no less impressive and by the time he left Edinburgh for London he had recorded 33 cases with only three deaths [22].

Appalling results were achieved by Spencer Wells, a society dilettante who considered himself the greatest

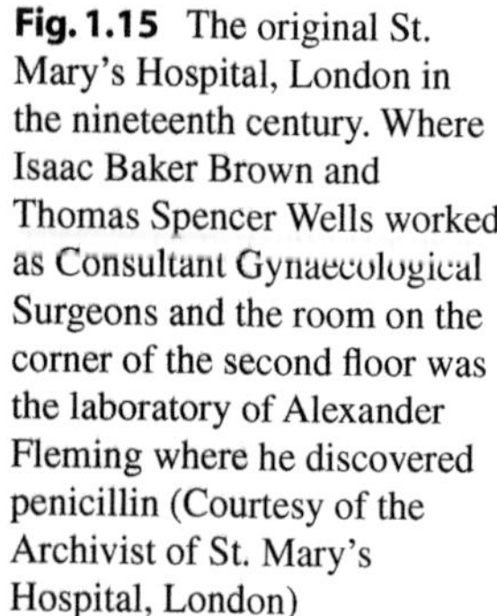

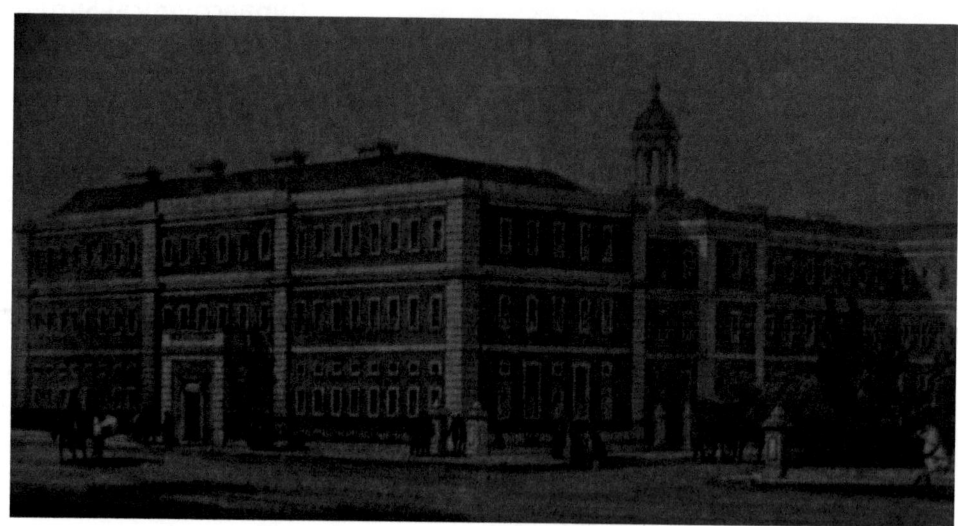

Fig. 1.15 The original St. Mary's Hospital, London in the nineteenth century. Where Isaac Baker Brown and Thomas Spencer Wells worked as Consultant Gynaecological Surgeons and the room on the corner of the second floor was the laboratory of Alexander Fleming where he discovered penicillin (Courtesy of the Archivist of St. Mary's Hospital, London)

gynaecological surgeon in Europe at that time and drove from hospital to hospital in London in his 'brougham and four silver grey horses' and produced results that were appalling and out of 40 hysterectomies performed for fibroids, there were 29 deaths–a mortality rate of 73 % [47].

His poor results were vigorously criticized in public by Charles Clay and he was joined in his disapproval by Lawson Tait, a rather aggressive Surgeon from Birmingham in the Midlands. Tait loathed Spencer Wells, and found that despite using the carbolic spray he still had a 38 % mortality with his first 50 ovariotomies. He then realized that it was not the spray that had given Keith his excellent results (indeed there is no evidence that Keith ever used it) but the intra-peritoneal method of dealing with the pedicle. He immediately adopted this technique, abandoned the carbolic spray and of his next 73 patients only two died – a remarkable achievement at that time. Lawson Tait also learned the value of cleanliness from both Lister and Keith that was unusual in those days, as no surgeons wore gloves and very few washed their hands before operating. He also preferred to operate in the home of the patient because hospitals at that time, and sadly now, are riddled with infection and before closing rinsed the abdominal and pelvic cavity with sterile water.

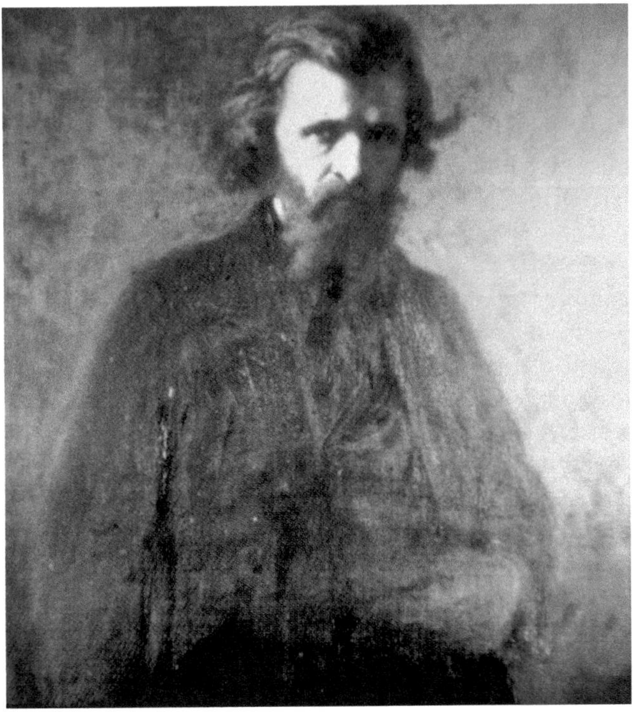

Fig. 1.16 Thomas Keith from Melrose, Scotland, who drastically reduced the mortality and morbidity of hysterectomy by his treatment of the cervical stump (Figure reproduced courtesy of Jaypee Brothers Medical Publishers, India)

Lawson Tait was a formidable character in the history of gynaecological surgery and was without doubt one of the most audacious and talented surgeons of his generation. He was aggressive and opinionated and successful and, as is often the case with large men of short stature, he was arrogant but often right. As can be seen from Fig. 1.14 his physical appearance was remarkably similar to that of Sir James Young Simpson (Fig. 1.13) with whom he lived after entering Edinburgh University at the tender age of 15 and also assisted him with his operations when still a teenager. Since Lawson Tait was born in Edinburgh in 1845 at the time of antidisestablishmentarianism when many clergymen were on strike against the idea of disestablishment of the church so no birth certificates were issued at this time thus fuelling speculation that Lawson Tait was the illegitimate son of JY Simpson [22].

Tait was prominent in the movement to start the Birmingham and Midland Hospital for Women and established many 'firsts' in gynaecological surgery including the first successful treatment of ectopic pregnancy in 1881, the first oophorectomy for sepsis, first bilateral oophorectomy for intractable menorrhagia as well as the removal of hepatic hydatid cysts and an appendicectomy in 1880.

Not only was he a gifted surgeon but he wrote more than 200 scientific papers and several books and also produced leading articles in the *Birmingham Morning News* and was

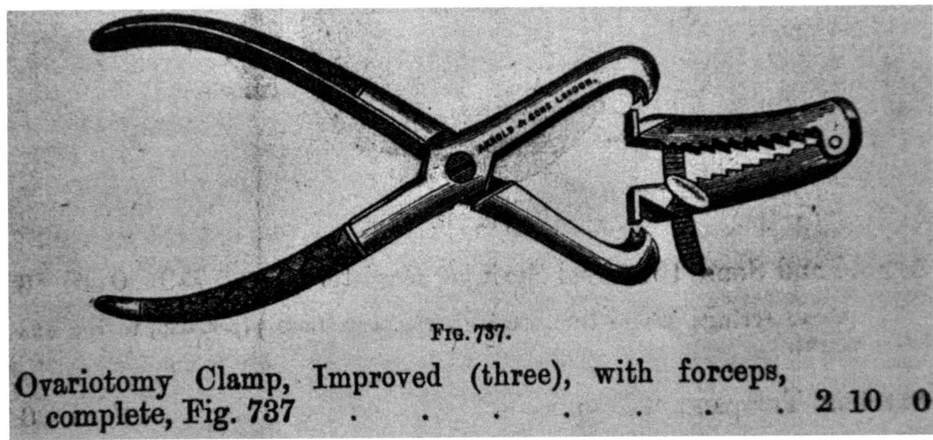

Fig. 1.17 The Spencer Wells Ovariotomy Clamp from a commercial catalogue of Arnold and Sons, Instrument Makers, London priced at £2.10 (2.80 Euros) (Photo by Chris Sutton. Company no longer in existence)

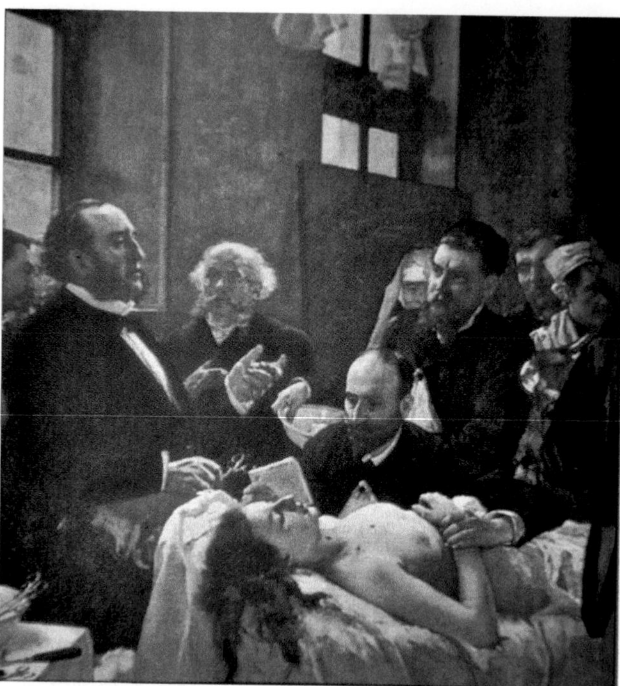

Fig. 1.18 Jules Pean, a renowned French gynaecological surgeon performing an early hysterectomy before a crowd of spectators in Paris. Note the absence of gloves and masks (Figure reproduced courtesy of Jaypee Brothers Medical Publishers, India)

elected to the Birmingham Town Council but was unsuccessful in his bid to be elected as a Member of Parliament. He founded and became the first President of the Medical Defence Union to counter the growing number of litigation cases against doctors. He was appointed Professor of Gynaecology at Queen's College in Birmingham and founded the British Gynaecological Society and was the first President in 1886.

He lived well and ate, drank and smoked excessively and was enormously successful and very wealthy owning two mansions and two luxury yachts and his own nursing home for his private patients. In the end this proved to be his undoing since he personally employed several nurses who were sexually attractive and it is alleged that three of them became pregnant by him and one of them cited him in a paternity case and at the same time he lost a libel case. Such behavior was not tolerated in times of strict Victorian prudery and his fall from grace was swift and coincided with declining health due to chronic pyelonephritis. He became anuric and died in Llandudno in North Wales after smoking his last cigar '… a very good Laranga - and the last I shall ever smoke'. Lawson Tait was cremated and his ashes laid in Warriston Cemetery, Edinburgh close to the grave of James Young Simpson [41].

The early hysterectomies were sociable affairs and it was considered good form to bring along friends, both medical and non-medical, to witness these momentous surgical events. Figure 1.18 shows the legendary French surgeon

Table 1.2 A summary of the hysterectomies performed for fibroids (1880–1884)

Operator	Date	Cases	Deaths	Mortality (%)
Lawson Tait	1882	30	10	33
Spencer Wells	1882	40	29	73
Koeberle	1882	19	10	52
Schroder	1884	100	32	32
Pean	1881	51	18	35
Keith	1883	25	2	8

Jules Pean operating. There are a large number of onlookers, many wearing beards and Pean himself wears neither a mask nor surgical gloves. Since this operation occurs in a Paris Hospital the painter has been given a certain amount of artistic liberty in allowing the lovely French patient to display her *très jolie poitrines* whilst the anaesthetist, in keeping with modern practice, appears to be busy with the crossword puzzle.

Lawson Tait summed up the end of this rather dark era in gynaecological surgery as "the ovarian tumour was the battlefield whereupon the first abdominal engagements were fought. Whereas ovariotomy undoubtedly opened the gateway to abdominal surgery, Spencer Wells by his outmoded technique and resultant mortality of 73% for abdominal hysterectomies undoubtedly held back progress, because no one would submit women to such fearful risk unless life were already threatened. Dr Thomas Keith ended this dark period by showing us how to operate on the abdomen without fear and with little risk" [27]. (Table 1.2).

Refinements of Technique at the End of the Nineteenth Century

The latter years of the nineteenth century witnessed further development and technique for abdominal hysterectomy which was refined and standardised by Freund who performed the first successful abdominal hysterectomy for cervical cancer and was the first German surgeon to use Lister's Carbolic Spray [48]. Czerny following Langenbeck's original description, did the same for vaginal hysterectomy [49].

The first planned hysterectomy performed on a gravid uterus took place in 1876 and was performed by Porro from Milan in Italy [50].

In spite of advances in anaesthesia and antisepsis in the latter part of the nineteenth century the incidence of fatal haemorrhage and peritonitis remained high. Eduardo Porro (1842–1902) was an analytical surgeon who reviewed his own cases of contracted pelvis, mainly from rickets, and after experimental operations on pregnant rabbits and cadavers offered an alternative solution by removing the uterus after delivering the baby by caesarean section. He sutured the cervical stump to the abdominal incision thus diverting the potentially septic contents of the cervix and vagina away from the peritoneal cavity. He performed this operation at his clinic for the first time on 21 May 1876 when he was presented with a rachitic primigravida in obstructed labour with a true conjugate of 4 cm and the woman survived and left hospital with her baby 6 weeks later [51].

For a time after his publication this approach found favour but later Ferdinand Kehrer and Max Sänger found that careful suture allowed the uterus to be reconstituted and allow for its conservation [52]. With the introduction of specially modified instrumentation, anaesthesia and antisepsis, the mortality rate for vaginal hysterectomy dropped precipitously and by 1886 was approximately 15 %; by 1890 it had reached 10 % and by 1910 it was as low as 2.5 %.

Unfortunately, abdominal hysterectomy lagged far behind and even as late as 1872 the mortality was so high that the procedure was formally condemned by the Academy of Medicine in Paris. In spite of this it was still performed though more often for fairly tenuous indications such as the relief of menstrual hysteria and 8 years after this pronouncement from Paris, TG Thomas reported on 365 consecutive cases with a mortality of 70 % [53].

In spite of these disastrous results, progress in abdominal hysterectomy was being made. Mikulicz abandoned the *serre-noeud* after using it for 13 years and instead placed triple ligatures on the broad ligaments and tied them off separately [53].

In 1878, Freund introduced techniques for packing off the intestines, ligating the major blood vessels and covering the cervical stump with peritoneum, which, in the same year, had been practised independently by both Schroeder and Spencer Wells.

In 1889 Lewis Stimpson had advocated the systematic ligation of the main ovarian and uterine vessels separately rather than tying off the entire broad ligament in one large ensnaring suture, and 3 years later Bare, of Philadelphia, the father of the modern subtotal hysterectomy, tied the uterine vessels 'outside of, but close to, the cervix'. He was also the first to advise gynaecological surgeons to 'take care' to avoid the ureter [54] then described an immaculate technique for subtotal hysterectomy little different from that employed today. Thus in the space of one decade, exterior fixation of the cervix by the *serre-noeud*, the Spencer Wells clamp or long ligature had been replaced by the intraperitoneal treatment of the cervical stump, which itself was modified and became extraperitoneal again, by covering the stump with pelvic peritoneum. These new techniques are reflected in the dramatic fall in mortality shown in the figures from the London teaching hospitals in 1896 and 1906 showing an impressive drop in mortality from 22 to 3.5 % [54] (Table 1.3).

Table 1.3 A summary of the abdominal hysterectomies performed for fibroids in London Teaching Hospitals (1896 and 1906)

	1896		1906	
Hospital	Cases	Deaths	Cases	Deaths
St Bartholomew's	7	3	26	4
St George's	1	0	8	0
St Thomas'	5	2	40	2
Middlesex	6	1	50	0
University College	3	0	21	1
Soho Hospital	1	0	60	1
St Mary's (Samaritan)	17	4	37	2
Chelsea	9	1	80	1
Total	49	11 (22 %)	322	11 (3.4 %)

Radical Hysterectomy for Cervical Cancer

Radical hysterectomy for cervical cancer was first performed by Dr. John G Clark of the Johns Hopkins Medical School in Baltimore in the United States of America who published details of two cases in which all of the parametra were removed [55]. The operation was refined by the addition of lymphadenectomy in certain cases and popularised by Ernst Wertheim (Fig. 1.19) the famous Austrian gynaecological cancer surgeon from Vienna, after whom the operation is now somewhat unfairly named [56]. Clark at the time was a 28 year old second year resident in gynaecology and had made a careful pathological study of cervical cancer and found that in most specimens that he examined the broad ligaments were cut too close to the uterus and too small a portion of the vagina had been removed [57].

Ernst Wertheim (1864–1920) was born in Graz in Austria and worked as assistant to Friedrich Schauta at the German University in Prague and later they moved to Professorial Chairs at the First and Second University Departments of Obstetrics and Gynaecology in Vienna, initially on an amicable basis but later disagreed due to the inability of Schauta's Radical Vaginal Hysterectomy to adequately remove the lymph nodes even though the vaginal approach was undoubtedly safer [58]. Even with the enlarged perineal relaxing incision introduced by Karl Schuchardt (1856–1901) who, like Ossiander and Langenbeck came from Gottingen, there was sufficient view to remove the parametrium but it was still not possible to remove all the involved lymph nodes [59]. Karl Schuchardt became a Professor at Stettin State Hospital but sadly died at the young age of 45 from sepsis following a surgical needle stick injury in the same way as Semmelweiss a few years later.

Ernst Wertheim performed his first radical abdominal hysterectomy and pelvic lymphadenectomy on Madame Rudd on 16th November 1898. He had carefully studied the

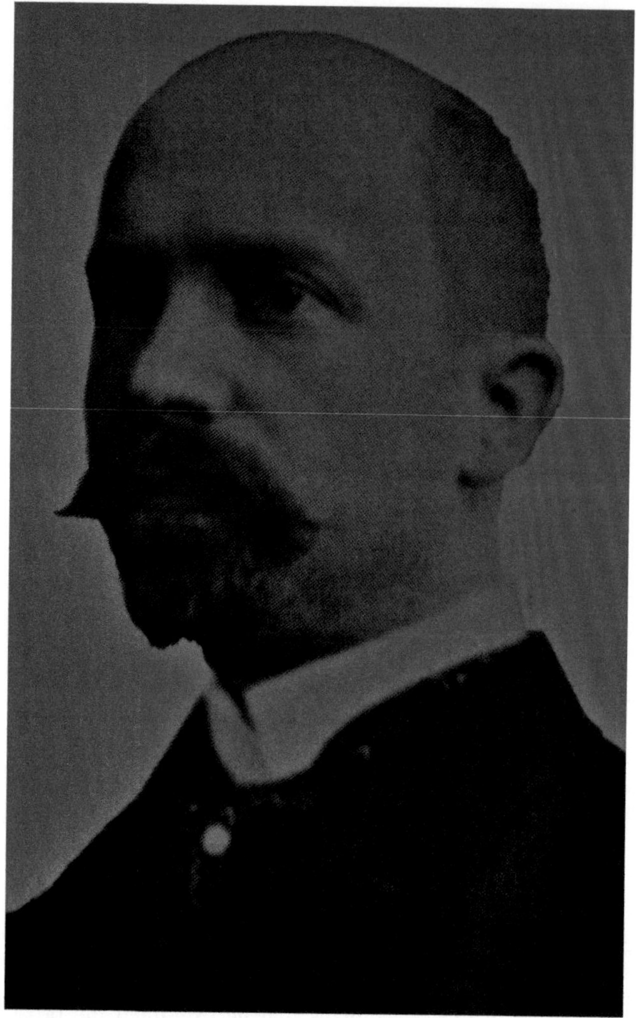

Fig. 1.19 Ernst Wertheim, Professor of the First Gynaecology Clinic of the University of Vienna, who ultimately performed 1300 radical hysterectomies with complete follow up (Photo courtesy of RCOG Press, London)

pathology and usual mode of lymphatic spread of cervical cancer and the procedure was based on an operation designed in 1878 by William Alexander Freund of Breslau who had carried out 66 radical operations with appalling results that included 55 deaths which occurred during the operation. These were mainly due to haemorrhage since this was before the introduction of blood transfusion since Landsteiner, from Vienna, only discovered the first four blood groups in 1900 [7].

The mortality rate in Wertheim's first 100 patients was high at 30 % [60] but as time went on his technique improved and when he had performed 500 radical hysterectomies the mortality rate had dropped to 19 % [61]. In those days there were no trained anaesthetists and patients died of shock due to the length of the procedures as well as blood loss and some were so feeble they were unable to bear the strain of the operation. In addition there were ureteric injuries, vesico-vaginal fistulas, pyelonephritis and recurrences. In those pre-antibiotic days there was still a high mortality from peritonitis and sepsis from the abdominal wound. It has to be said however that the infection rate could have been lowered had Wertheim adhered to some of the aseptic principles used by Keith and Lawson Tait because although surgical rubber gloves were available since 1900 Wertheim refused to wear them since he claimed they interfered with his sense of touch.

During his visit to London to deliver a lecture at the Royal College of Obstetricians and Gynaecologists a Consultant Gynaecologist from one of the poorer communities in the East End of London asked him to operate on a suitable patient with cervical cancer. Wertheim agreed and they set off for the hospital in their horse-drawn carriages and Wertheim examined the patient and later demonstrated his technique of radical hysterectomy. At one stage he needed an extra assistant and one of the junior doctors who was performing a post-mortem in the mortuary was summoned to come up to the operating theatre to help. As was the custom in England at the time the young doctor started to wash his hands prior to putting on a gown and surgical gloves but Wertheim admonished him and told him that was not necessary since he was needed immediately to assist in the surgery. The patient survived the operation but died 5 days later from peritoneal sepsis.

Ernst Wertheim was an expert skier and skater and once crossed the Alps in a hot-air balloon. He was prone to bouts of depression and was a difficult man to deal with and had an abrupt and defensive demeanour. He died at the age of 56, a victim of the pandemic of Spanish Influenza, and was buried in the Vienna City Cemetery next to the grave of Friedrich Schauta [41].

The Development of Hysterectomy in the Twentieth Century

As late as the mid-1940s the universal approach to hysterectomy was the subtotal procedure which involved retaining the cervix with the reduced chance of pelvic infection and ureteric injury but mainly, in the pre-antibiotic era, to reduce the chance of ascending infection and peritonitis, which was almost invariably fatal. Once the problem of ascending infection and peritonitis had been eradicated by the development of antibiotics, hysterectomy almost invariably included removal of the cervix.

The first total hysterectomy was performed by E.H. Richardson of the USA in 1929 [62]. His main concern in moving away from the traditional subtotal procedure, was to prevent the occurrence of cervical stump carcinoma, yet even in the days before cervical screening with Papanicolaou smears was available, the actual incidence of neoplastic change in retained cervical stumps was only 0.4 % in 6600 cases in the USA [63] and only 0.1 % in Finland [64]. As Thomas Lyons from Atlanta, Georgia, USA , a keen advocate of laparoscopic subtotal hysterectomy has pointed out, this is similar to the rate of vaginal cancer following total abdominal hysterectomy and yet no one has seriously recommended the removal of the vagina at hysterectomy as prophylaxis against this [65].

During the past 100 years the introduction of antibiotics, intravenous therapy, anticoagulation, safe anaesthesia and blood transfusion has reduced the mortality for both vaginal and abdominal hysterectomy to around 0.1 %. There has also been a concomitant reduction in morbidity, reflected by a shorter hospital stay and the use of the transverse incision introduced by Johannes Pfannenstiel from Breslau in 1900 which gives a stronger and better cosmetic result [66]. Nevertheless, it took many years for this incision with its higher tensile strength making it less prone to wound dehiscence and incisional hernia, to gain universal acceptance.

Hermann Johann Pfannenstiel (1862–1909) received his medical degree from the University of Berlin and later moved to the Breslau Frauernklinic then to the University of Giessen and in 1907 became Chairman of the University Department of Obstetrics and Gynaecology at Kiel University where he remained until his premature death. Sadly Pfannenstiel died at the age of 47 following a needle-stick injury to the middle finger of his left hand sustained during the removal of a tubo-ovarian abscess [41].

Other famous surgeons including Karl Schuchardt, who was also from Breslau, had died at a relatively early age from similar injuries and it is salutatory to note that these injuries are not uncommon during various surgeries, and many doctors would have suffered a similar fate were it not for the revolutionary, but accidental, discovery of penicillin by Alexander Fleming at my own teaching hospital, St Marys Hospital in London.

Increased surgical skill and prowess from an apprenticeship type of training has ensured that the operation now is extremely safe with an incidence of ureteric injury of 0.2–0.5 % and a mortality of 0.12 % [67, 68].

The advent of prophylactic anticoagulants and antibiotics has further increased the safety of this procedure. Dicker et al. showed the superiority of vaginal hysterectomy (morbidity, 24.5 %) compared with abdominal hysterectomy (morbidity, 42.8 %). Although these statistics appear favourable to the vaginal approach they are, in fact, an eloquent testimony to the efficacy of prophylactic antibiotics, since those who had a vaginal hysterectomy had the benefit of these drugs, whereas those who had an abdominal hysterectomy did not [69].

Inevitably the increased safety of the operation with a mortality rate of approximately 12 per 10,000 led to an explosive increase in the number of hysterectomies performed so that it is now the second most common operation undertaken in the USA with over 650,000 being performed annually at a cost of approximately three billion dollars. With this increased safety the indications for the procedure had become wider, to the extent that up to 50 % of American women at the end of the past decade underwent hysterectomy [70]. Not only had the procedure become open to a certain amount of abuse, but technological advances, apart from endometrial ablation and embolization of fibroids, had largely by-passed hysterectomy and up until the mid part of twenty-ninth century, gynaecological surgery was in the doldrums.

The Modern Era: The Introduction of Laparoscopic Surgery

During the middle part of the twentieth century apart from a more conservative approach to the treatment of ovarian cysts and fibroids and the surgical refinements in instrumentation and technique introduced by tubal microsurgeons, few technical advances were made in gynaecological surgery.

A revolution in surgical technique could not occur until a different way of accessing the peritoneal cavity was invented and essentially this involved a method whereby the contents of the abdominal cavity could be visualised.

In 1901 Dr. Georg Kelling (Fig. 1.21) who was a Professor in Dresden in an address he gave to the German Biological

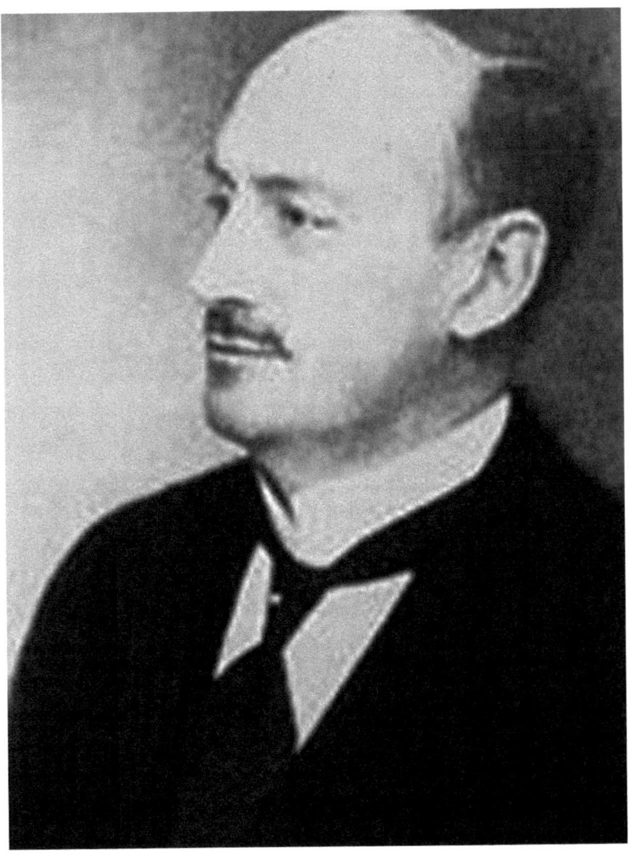

Fig. 1.20 Hans Christian Jacobaeus of Stockholm.The first person to perform laparoscopy on humans (Photo from the Archives of the Minimal Access Therapy Training Unit, Guildford, UK)

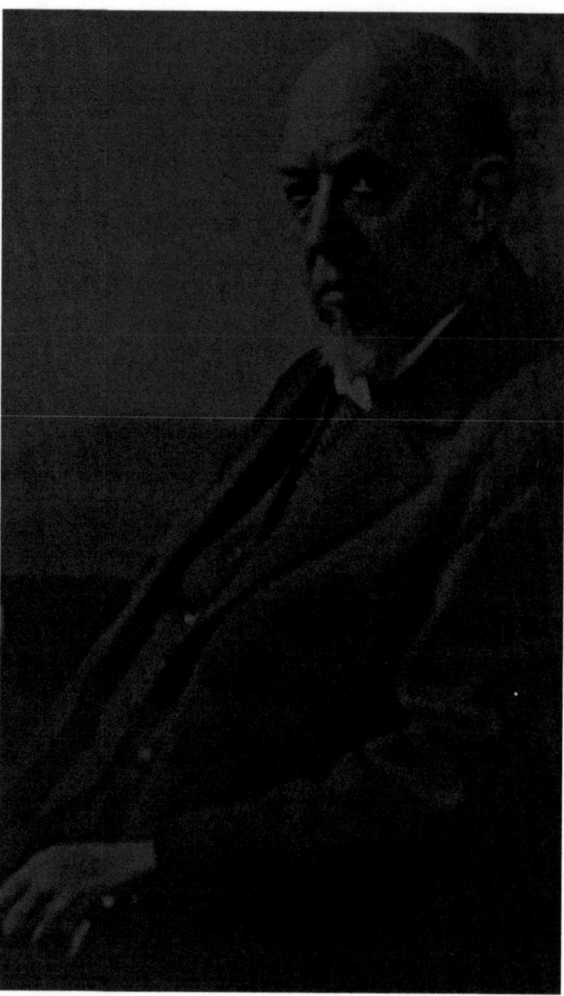

Fig. 1.21 Professor Dr. Georg Kelling (1866–1945) of Dresden, one of the "fathers of laparoscopy" (Photo by Chris Sutton from an original supplied by Prof. Dr. Liselotte Mettler)

and Medical Society in Hamburg described the visual examination of the stomach and oesophagus in the human and additionally the use of a cystoscope to visualise the viscera of a dog using air filtered through cotton wool to produce a pneumoperitoneum [71].

In that same year of 1901 von Ott from Saint Petersburg in Russia published a different technique of viewing the pelvis of a pregnant woman by way of culdoscopy through an incision in the posterior vaginal fornix and using as his light source reflected light from a head mirror. He called this technique Ventroscopy [72].

However the credit for the first true laparoscopy on a human goes to Hans Christian Jacobaeus (Fig. 1.20) from Stockholm who coined the term 'laparoscopy' and in 1910 described his technique for the inspection of the human peritoneal, thoracic and pericardial cavities [73]. Only 1 month later Kelling reported a series 45 laparoscopies and described the appearance of the liver, tumours and tuberculosis.

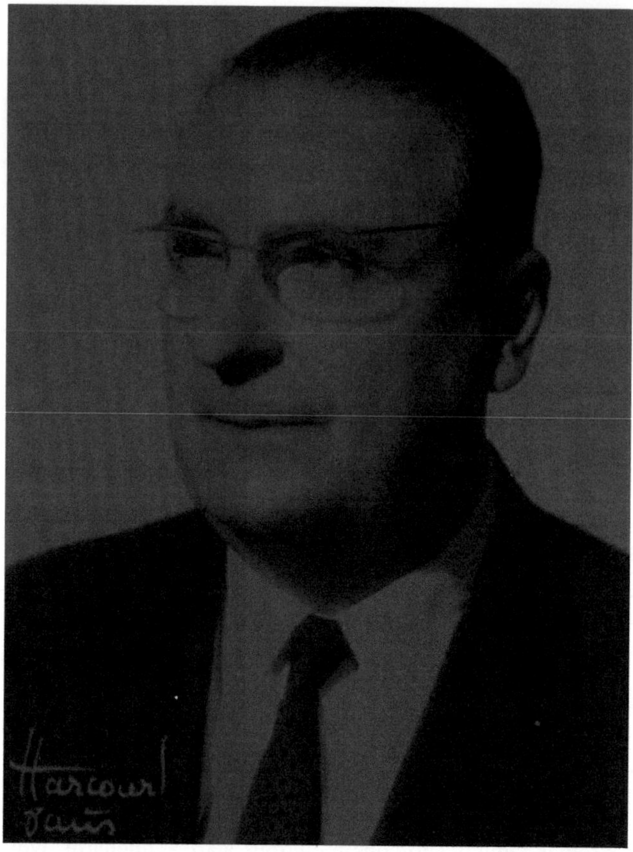

Fig. 1.22 Dr. Raoul Palmer from Paris. Generally considered the " Father of Operative Laparoscopy" (Photo by kind permission of the late Mme Elizabeth Palmer)

Laparoscopy became popular mainly with general physicians or internists for the diagnosis and treatment of tuberculosis and liver disease and to them must go the credit for the development of laparoscopy over the next 40 years [74].

This changed radically with the introduction of laparoscopic surgery by pioneers in Europe such as Raoul Palmer (Fig. 1.22) in Paris [75] and Hans Frangenheim in Konstanz [76] in the 1940s but such advances were hampered by the lack of communication across the Atlantic during the Second World War and the Americans, although using laparoscopy in the 1930's, had mysteriously reverted to culdoscopy for visualization of the pelvis. It required the publication of the first text book on this new technique in the English language in 1967 by Patrick Steptoe (Fig. 1.23) one of the pioneers of In-Vitro Fertilisation, working in a small district hospital in Oldham, near Manchester in Lancashire, to allow the widespread dissemination of this new technique to the English speaking world after he had learned the technique from Frangenheim and Palmer in Continental Europe [77].

Initially laparoscopy was used for diagnosis and relatively simple therapeutic procedures such as female sterilisation and puncture or fenestration of benign ovarian cysts but gradually became more sophisticated owing much to the

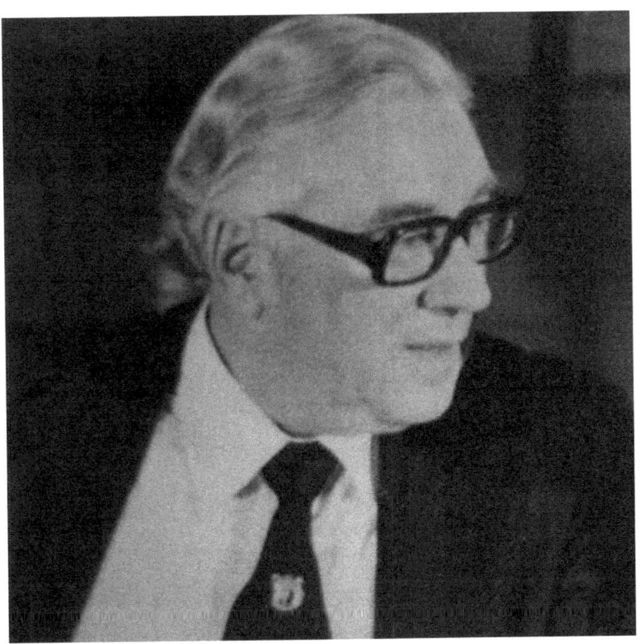

Fig. 1.23 Patrick Steptoe from Oldham, near Manchester, England, One of the pioneers of In-Vitro Fertilisation who wrote the first book in English on Laparoscopy (Photo supplied by the late Patrick Steptoe)

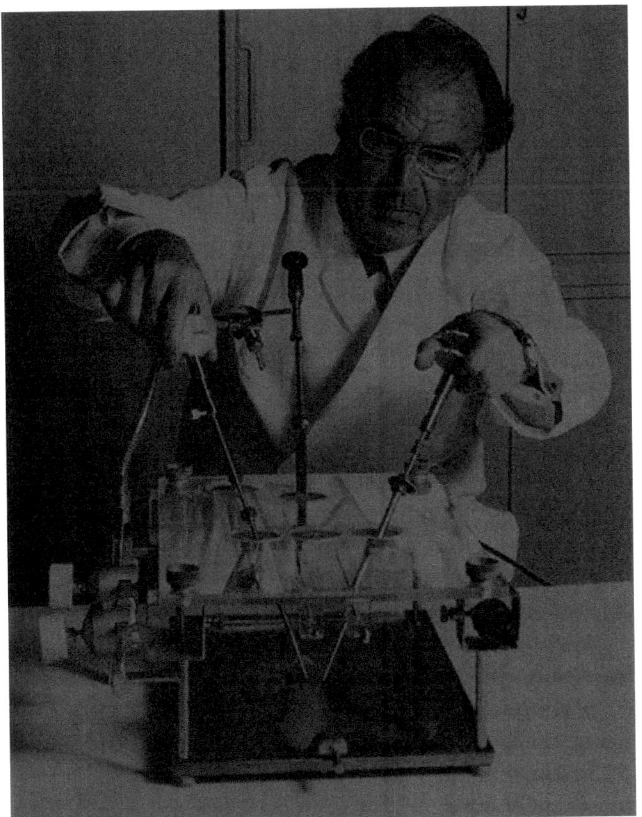

Fig. 1.24 Professor Kurt Semm from Kiel one of the great advocates and teachers of laparoscopic surgery and an inventor of much of the original equipment (Photo taken by Chris Sutton on a visit to the Minimal Access Therapy Training Unit in Guildford, UK)

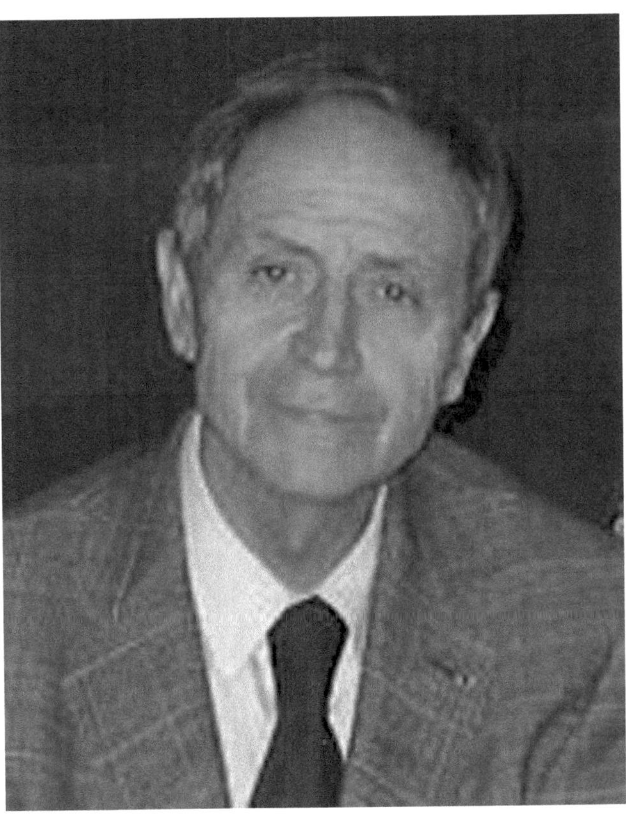

Fig. 1.25 Professor Maurice Bruhat from the University of the Auvergne in Clermont Ferrand in France who performed the first laparoscopic removal of an ectopic pregnancy with Dr. Hubert Manhes (Photo given to Chris Sutton by the late Maurice Bruhat)

pioneering work of Professor Kurt Semm (Fig. 1.24) of Kiel University in Northern Germany who could claim to have performed the first Laparoscopic Hysterectomy using the CISH (Classic Intrafascial Supracervical Hysterectomy technique using the SEMM (Serrated Edged Macro Morcellator) [78, 79] although this would not be strictly classified as a total laparoscopic hysterectomy[80].

Professor Maurice Bruhat (Fig. 1.25) and Hubert Manhes and their gifted team from the University of Clermont Ferrand in the Auvergne in the Massif Central in France were a major influence on the development of laparoscopic surgery and were the first to treat ectopic pregnancy laparoscopically[81].

By the 1980s, minimally invasive surgery had become a reality but for a long time gynaecologists struggled with primitive equipment relying on advances in laser technology and electrosurgical devices to achieve cutting and coagulation. This was before the time of disposable instruments and self-sharpening scissors and it was necessary to return laparoscopic scissors to the factory and wait several weeks whilst they were sharpened.

The advent of laparoscopic cholecystectomy and its rapid uptake by our general surgical colleagues enabled industry to see the full potential of this new type of surgery and there were rapid developments in the quality of instrumentation and sophistication in optics with the introduction of the rod lens system and external cold light source by Professor Harold Hopkins [82] of Reading University in the UK and later with the development of silicone chip cameras and high resolution television monitors to enable surgeons to operate comfortably and to usefully employ assistants to help with the operation.

In a remarkably short time these techniques were adopted universally to the extent that at least 80 % of gynaecological operations can now be performed using endoscopic techniques with several small incisions for the access of surgical instruments resulting in less pain, shorter hospital stays and rapid recovery compared with conventional laparotomy [83]. Nevertheless these techniques required special visual skills and hand-eye coordination which can not be achieved by all surgeons and the universal uptake of minimal access surgery, which was so confidently predicted in the 1990s, has not become a reality and conventional techniques are still employed by the majority of practicing gynaecological surgeons in the UK and USA although the adoption of this surgical revolution has been more successful in France and Germany.

Dr. Reich Performs the First Total Laparoscopic Hysterectomy

With the increasing skill of laparoscopic surgeons and the sophistication of the equipment laparoscopic operations became increasingly complex and it was only a matter of time before the first total laparoscopic hysterectomy was performed and this was in the Autumn of 1988 at the William Nesbit Memorial Hospital in Kingston, Pennsylvania by Dr.Harry Reich (Fig. 1.26). He published a description of this technique the following year [84].

The original operation proposed by Reich was an impressive display of technical virtuosity since the whole procedure was performed laparoscopically, including dissecting out part of the ureter and individually ligating and tying off the uterine artery and veins with extracorporeal sutures. He also performed the colpotomy incision laparoscopically in order to remove the uterus and repaired it with laparoscopic sutures. As a routine at the end of all advanced laparoscopic procedures he performs a cystoscopy, after injection of Methylene blue dye, to check that there had been no damage to the ureters.

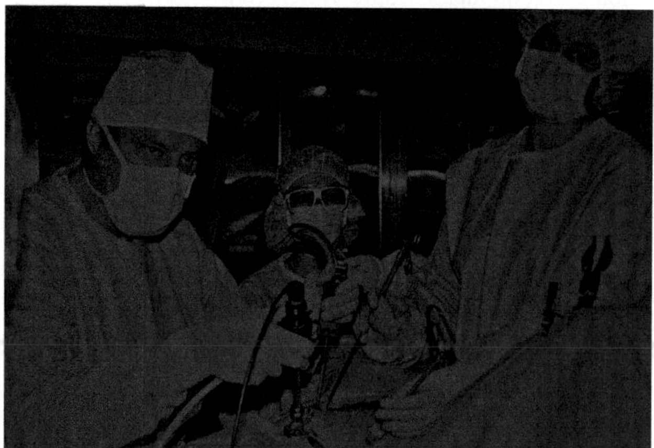

Fig. 1.26 Dr. Harry Reich who performed the world's first Total Abdominal Hysterectomy at the William Nesbit Memorial Hospital, Kingston, Philadelphia in October, 1988 (Photo by Chris Sutton)

After the success of his first total laparoscopic hysterectomies he toured the United States demonstrating this new operation and then travelled the world, demonstrating it in the different countries that practiced laparoscopic surgery at that level. He performed the first demonstration in the UK in my own Department at the Royal Surrey Hospital in Guildford and I had the honour of being able to act as first assistant. The patient did extremely well and went home the following day with little pain and required only mild analgesics such a paracetamol and ibuprofen and was able to return to work 2 weeks after the operation. Nevertheless the procedure took five and a half hours occupying an entire morning operating session in which we would normally be expected to perform five or six laparoscopic operations of various types and difficulties.

At around this time I was performing about 35 laparoscopic operations per week whereas various American surgeons I had spoken to performed only 2–3 so clearly this procedure was more suited to a private based medical system than the socialised healthcare system operating in most European countries [85].

Laparoscopic hysterectomy was designed to replace abdominal hysterectomy and if a vaginal hysterectomy could be performed then that was clearly the minimal access procedure of choice. Nevertheless the original total laparoscopic hysterectomy (TLH) was too complicated and time consuming and required a very high level of laparoscopic skills so was soon replaced by many surgeons with the laparoscopic assisted vaginal hysterectomy (LAVH) whereby the upper pedicles were ligated, electrocoagulated or stapled while the remaining part of the operation was performed as a routine vaginal hysterectomy. It soon became evident that none of the laparoscopic part of the operation did anything to make the vaginal approach easier and because there is no descent until the utero-sacral and cardinal ligaments are transected. Most surgeons found that, with the limited access involved, the procedure became a very difficult vaginal hysterectomy. Cynics pointed out that this was in fact a complicated way of performing a vaginal hysterectomy, but it certainly had the advantage of honing vaginal surgical skills and allowed dissection of bowel adhesions laparoscopically, as well as the treatment of any existing endometriosis, particularly deep infiltrating endometriosis in the recto-vaginal septum, and the easier removal of ovaries where this was indicated.

It also had the advantage that the internal incision could be inspected at the completion of the procedure and any residual bleeding vessels could be sealed by bipolar diathermy ensuring at the end of the procedure the field was absolutely dry. Theoretically this had the advantage of preventing secondary haemorrhages occurring a few days later and preventing subsequent haematoma formation but in reality this was not always achieved.

Advances in instrumentation such as the ultrasonic scalpel, more effective techniques to coagulate large vessels using plasma kinetic energy and ingenious uterine manipulators and vaginal tubes to delineate the vaginal fornices have led some surgeons to persevere with the total laparoscopic approach and in recent years the time taken to perform these procedures has been considerably decreased but it remains a difficult procedure and one that can only really be performed by highly trained laparoscopic surgeons with a high level of skill.

These various criticisms led some laparoscopic surgeons to search for a simpler approach that could be universally employed by laparoscopic surgeons who had slightly lower skill levels or who were required by hospital administrators to perform the operation in a much shorter time and also discharge patients earlier, preferably on a day case basis. The simplest way to do this was to devise a simpler procedure that avoided any possibility of a secondary haemorrhage from the vaginal vault after the patient had left hospital and this meant performing a laparoscopic version of the outmoded subtotal hysterectomy.

Development of Laparoscopic Subtotal Hysterectomy and Introduction of New Laparoscopic Instrumentation for Hysterectomy

In 1993 Semm developed the intra-fascial laparoscopic supra-cervical hysterectomy with a technique of coring out the whole of the transformation zone and the central core of the uterus using a macro-morcellator with a serrated edge reamer turned manually in a clockwise direction to achieve cutting. The idea of this was to remove the entire transformation zone to avoid the subsequent development of cancer and also to decrease the chance of post-operative bleeding and monthly sero-sanguinous discharge [86, 87].

In 1991, we published our initial experience of supracervical laparoscopic hysterectomy and removal of the transformation zone using a modification of Semm's technique using the artificial sapphire tip of an ND-YAG laser (Laserscope, Cwmbran, UK) and endocoagulating the vaginal aspect of the cervical stump at the end of the procedure. Our technique also differed from the one described by Semm because he used sutures to secure the vascular pedicles whereas we used the Endo GIA 30 stapler (Autosuture Ltd., Ascot, UK) which was quick and effective and in those patients where it was not technically possible to secure the uterine vessels with the device, we used bipolar diathermy [88]. The mean operating time in our small series of eleven procedures was 111 min, with a mean blood loss of 185 ml. The mean duration of hospital stay was 3 days and the mean time to full recovery was 20 days and there were no complications. The reason for the long operating time was due to the fact that the SEMM (Serrated Edged Macro-Morcellator) was a manual device requiring long and arduous rotation and several of my Residents developed an occupational disease unique to laparoscopic surgical assistants – morcellator's thumb. This condition, which fortunately was only temporary, was due to injury to the peroneal nerve to the thumb causing numbness and hyperaesthesia in the skin distribution of that nerve.

Lyons [89] described a slightly different technique of laparoscopic supracervical hysterectomy also using the artificial sapphire tip of the ND-YAG laser but he did not merely coagulate the ascending branches of the uterine arteries, but actually included the main branch of the uterine artery and divided the utero-sacral ligaments making an inverted cone through the cervix, also removing the transformation zone but effectively leaving only the rim of the cervix. This was a slightly more radical procedure but almost certainly resulted in less long-term problems involving bleeding or serosanguinous discharge from the cervical stump [90, 91]. The team from UCH-Louvain in Brussels published a large series of 500 cases which also used the Nd:YAG laser to cut across the cervical stump but removed the transformation zone by a large loop electrosurgical excision in much the same way as that used for the removal of the transformation zone when treating cervical intra-epithelial neoplasia [92].

Further refinements have been made in recent years with the introduction of the Lap-Loop™ (Medsys, Gembloux, Belgium) invented by Jacques Dequesne in Lausanne [93]. whereby an electric wire loop is threaded around the cervix once the ascending branches of the uterine artery have been coagulated and cut and the bladder pushed down slightly. After making sure that there is no bowel close to the wire posteriorly, a 100–120 W cutting current is applied and the "noose" formed by the wire is slowly tightened as the heated wire slices through the tissue coagulating many small vessels and providing a very effective method of rapidly severing the cervix from the uterine fundus. In a study comparing the loop device with conventional methods (laparoscopic monopolar scissors or ultrasonic scalpel) the mean time for detaching the cervix from the fundus with the loop electrode was 6.6 min compared with 14.4 min in the control group [94].

Further advances have been made with more effective laparoscopic ligation instruments to effectively seal even large arteries and veins (Ligasure, Covidien Commercial Ltd., Gosport, UK; Enseal· Ethicon Endo-Surgery, Edinburgh, UK; Plasma Kinetic energy system, Olympus, KeyMed Ltd.,

Southend, UK; Gyrus International, Berkshire,UK) thus reducing the risk of secondary haemorrhage from major vessels and with the decreased operating time makes laparoscopic sub-total hysterectomy eminently suitable for day case surgery.

Some of these recently introduced electrosurgical devices that operate in a liquid field use the word plasma when describing their *modus operandi* but in reality use radiofrequency electrosurgery via specially designed bipolar electrode systems to seal vessels. Examples of this is the so-called PlasmaKinetic technology used in the Olympus (Gyrus ACMI) Plasma-Knife and the ArthroCareCoblation device, which only generates non-thermal plasma within the tiny bubbles formed in the fluid on the surface of their electrodes but in reality relies on basic electrosurgery for its tissue effect. Another new device, the Peak PlasmaBlade may generate a non-thermal plasma at the interface of the handpiece blade with the tissue or fluid medium in which it is used but, notwithstanding this, it is the rapid pulses of high-voltage energy that create the surgical effect [95]. All of these devices allow rapid sealing of large vessels and allow a new generation of gynaecological surgeons to dispense with the need for traditional sutures. It remains to be seen whether these new vessel sealing devices will have a wider application and increase the uptake of vaginal hysterectomy or if they are only used by laparoscopic surgeons because traditional abdominal and vaginal surgeons seem to have more faith in traditional sutures to seal vessels. Virtually all of these vessel sealing devices are single use only and add considerably to the cost of the procedure although they contribute to a shorter operating time.

The remaining problem is the removal of the detached fundus which can be via a colpotomy incision but this adds to the complexity and difficulty of the operation. High speed electromechanical morcellators such as the Gynecare X-Tract Ethicon Inc., Somerville, New Jersey) are not only very expensive but require considerable care and skill to operate and have been associated with serious accidents many of which have been fatal and will be described later.

Nevertheless in spite of these caveats laparoscopic subtotal hysterectomy (LSH) underwent a massive upsurge in popularity particularly in California where the rate increased from 6.9 to 20.8 % between 1997 and 2003 [96] and also in Scandinavia, particularly in relatively conservative countries such as Denmark when in a similar time frame it increased by 375 % so that 22 % of all hysterectomies were subtotal [97].

It is generally assumed that retaining the cervix enables a quicker procedure than TAH, and several laparoscopic series have confirmed this. If the cervix is retained, the surgeon needs only to secure the ascending branches of the uterine artery and vein, thus averting the need for dissection in the highly vascular tissue in the paravaginal area close to the ureter. It is claimed that STH is associated with fewer perioperative complications, in particular, hemorrhage because the main uterine artery is not ligated and the vaginal angles are left untouched.

In the 1980s a plethora of extravagant claims about other advantages of retaining the cervix had arisen, mainly from Finland, backed up by some poorly designed comparative clinical trials [98]. Among the claims of the advantages of STH over TAH are the reduced intra-operative complications, particularly ureteric injury, and no possibility of vault dehiscence but it was also claimed that there are fewer difficulties with post-operative bladder function, less subsequent pelvic floor complications and, particularly, less dyspareunia. It was also suggested that there was a considerable increase in sexual satisfaction, increased libido and better quality of orgasm and even an increased number of multiple orgasms. It was this latter suggestion that was seized on by the popular press and encouraged many women to come forward to seek this particular variety of hysterectomy if given the choice.

Although these claims seem compelling on superficial reading, we live in an age of evidence-based medicine largely due to the example shown by Dr. Archie Cochrane of Wales, and until recently these advantages have not been supported by adequate randomized controlled trials (RCTs) that have fulfilled the conditions required by the Cochrane Collaboration. However one study by St. George's Hospital in London [99] assessed urinary, bowel, and sexual function in great detail before surgery and at 6 and 12 month intervals afterwards with a series of carefully validated questionnaires. In addition, urinary function was determined with the use of twin-channel subtracted cystometrography and uroflowmetry, and definitions of urinary incontinence conformed to those of the International Continence Society.

There was no significant difference in any of the urinary symptoms between women who underwent TAH or STH. Urodynamic studies demonstrated a reduction in stress incontinence after surgery in both groups. Insofar as bowel symptoms were concerned the rates of constipation, hard stools, urgency, straining, use of laxatives, and incontinence of flatus were similar in the two groups after surgery.

Sexual function , which in the studies by Kilkku and colleagues [100] was greatly improved after STH, was remarkably similar in both groups in this study, which reasonably included only women who were sexually active at all three points in time: preoperatively and 6 and 12 months postoperatively. The frequency of intercourse, desire for intercourse, and initiation of intercourse did not differ significantly between the two groups; however, there was a significant increase in the frequency of intercourse in both groups (p 5.01). The type of surgery had a similar outcome insofar as frequency of orgasm, frequency of multiple orgasms, extent of vaginal lubrication, and rating of the sexual relationship with a partner. Deep dyspareunia was reduced significantly in both groups at 6 and 12 months, whereas superficial dyspareunia decreased at 6 months but increased in both groups at 12 months, the reasons for which were not clear.

From the results of this carefully planned double-blind, randomized, prospective, controlled trial with adequate patient numbers and duration of follow-up, there was little to chose between the two types of abdominal hysterectomy other than the shorter operating time and decreased perioperative complications associated with subtotal abdominal hysterectomy. This brilliant study, published in arguably the most prestigious medical journal in the world, The New England Journal of Medicine, sadly did not include laparoscopic subtotal hysterectomy (LSH). We are therefore left to wonder whether its inclusion would have resulted in different conclusions, although it is clear from this study that abdominal hysterectomy, whether performed as a total or subtotal procedure, with the large painful scar associated with it and the prolonged recovery period, resulted in considerable patient satisfaction at 12 months of follow-up. It is a great shame that this otherwise excellent study which was conducted by urogynaecologists did not include an arm with laparoscopic subtotal hysterectomy because St. George's Hospital has some highly skilled laparoscopic surgeons who, I am sure, would have been happy to have taken part in this trial.

This was a great shame because the last time I did a thorough search of the literature I was only able to find one prospective randomized study comparing surgical complications and clinical outcomes after supracervical vs total laparoscopic hysterectomy in 141 patients followed up for 2 years, and that article was published only in Italian [101]. There were no statistically significant differences in the rates of complications, degree of symptom improvement, or activity limitation, although patients assigned to STH tended to have more hospital readmissions. Patients weighing more than 100 kg at study entry were more than twice as likely to be readmitted to the hospital during the 2 years of follow-up.

The Introduction of Robotic Laparoscopic Surgery

The most recent development in endoscopic hysterectomy is the development of hysterectomy techniques using robotic arms with wristed instruments rather than "straight sticks" with limited movements and a high fulcrum. This both exaggerates movement and requires the movement outside the body to be in the opposite direction as that inside the abdominal cavity, which is a primary reason for the learning curve in laparoscopic surgery. The wristed instruments powered by the robotic arms enable both a full range of movement and this movement can be slowed for fine manipulation. The only commercially available robotic systems the da Vinci S and the da Vinci SI (Intuitive Surgical, Inc., Sunnyvale, California) are equipped with a double optic, which gives the operator who works from a distant console, but not any of the observers, 3-dimensional vision, enabling much improved visualisation of the pelvis, which compensates for the loss of haptic feedback using the robotic arms. This is probably the main advantage of robotic surgery since it enables the operator to work with virtually no fatigue enabling several cases to be performed in one operating session. The wristed instruments, however, mean that the more recently available "safe" power sources such as the ultrasonic devices and bladed instruments are not available, and the only power sources are monopolar or bipolar diathermy, the latter now available with impedance feedback control. There have been several important publications that relate to the use of robotic techniques but they are primarily in surgery to treat malignant disease although recently increasingly they include benign disease particularly advanced stage endometriosis [102] and the thorny issue of cost effectiveness [103]. In this study from Lund in Sweden a randomized controlled trial (Canadian Task Force classification 1) of 122 women with a uterine size of less than 6 weeks who were scheduled to undergo minimally invasive hysterectomy for benign disease, who were not considered candidates for vaginal surgery, were assessed for hospital costs and short term clinical outcomes to compare laparoscopic hysterectomy with robot-assisted hysterectomy. All women underwent surgery as randomized and vaginal hysterectomy was possible in 41 % at a mean hospital cost of $4579 compared to $7509 for traditional laparoscopic hysterectomy and, surprisingly given that the robot is a pre-existing investment, the use of the robot only added $993 per case. If the calculation included the share of the purchase of the robot and maintenance this increased to $1607 extra per case but the robotic group had less blood loss and postoperative complications. The Robotic arms facilitate suturing in difficult situations such as the prostatic capsule in radical prostatectomy, and has been adopted in institutions that perform many of these procedures, predominantly by urologic oncologists. Case series have demonstrated that in appropriately skilled hands, radical hysterectomy performed using robotic techniques was comparable with laparotomy, and required significantly shorter time than laparoscopy, with equal lymph node harvest and significantly reduced blood loss and length of stay (2 days) [104].

Robotic hysterectomy to treat benign disease has now also become popular after the initial reports by Reynolds and Advincula of 16 consecutive patients with no conversions to laparotomy, a short hospital stay, and a complication rate comparable with routine laparoscopic (straight stick) surgery [103]. Their experience now includes patients with obliterated pelvic cul-de-sacs, six of whom have undergone hysterectomy with resection of the underlying disease safely and with no conversions to laparotomy, which demonstrates that with the appropriate experience and training, robotic surgery is a useful tool for dealing with this associated disease [104].

An early limitation of robotic surgery was the need to dock the robot between the patient's legs, which meant that access to the vagina for uterine manipulation was difficult; however, this has been overcome by repositioning the robotic arms and docking the robot to the side of the patient where the surgeon would stand. The ports are relatively big, 8 mm for the robotic arm ports and 12 cm for the optical and accessory ports, and they need to be placed high in the abdomen, resulting in more obvious scarring.

Although robotic surgery is an exciting advance with great possibilities, it comes at considerable financial cost. The robot and optic cost $2 million, and limited-life reusable instruments cost $2000 each plus associated support costs. Despite the costs, there are now hundreds of units in place in the United States, and in the hands of enthusiasts, the techniques are gaining popularity in Europe and the United Kingdom.

The Choice of the Best Route for Hysterectomy

The last 80 years has witnessed a revolution in surgery from operations performed through a large painful abdominal incision with long hospital stays to minimal access procedures which are essentially the same operations but owing to the small incisions allow surgery often to be undertaken on a day care basis with much less pain and discomfort, rapid recovery and early return to work or domestic activity.

In this chapter I have described the amazingly brave interventions of pioneering surgeons when an abdominal incision was almost tantamount to a sentence of death and slowly seeing an improvement throughout the ages with the gradual reduction of associated morbidity and mortality until we final arrive in the modern era, when laparoscopic hysterectomy is performed to improve quality of life rather than to remove a threat to life as in former times. The sophistication of new instrumentation and optics together with the long training of the surgeon has ensured that the complication rate is low and technological progress is still continuing so that surgery can now be performed with the assistance of robots.

There has also been a steady progression from early reports from pioneers of each type of surgery and then a collected series by individual experts or teams from centres of excellence which have invariably given a favourable outcome for the procedure they are describing and finally a more evidence based approach with well constructed prospective comparative studies which, I feel sure, will be dealt with in detail in other chapters in this book. Some of these studies such as the excellent eVALuate Study have shown that when some of these procedures are put into general use the complication rate is inevitably higher than when a series is reported from an individual expert or centre of excellence [105]. Although this can result in unfair criticism from some quarters it is nevertheless essential that we face the obvious truth that the complication rate is likely to increase when the procedure is universally adopted but this is important when confronting the patient with the likelihood of complications associated with each type of procedure.

Much of this can be addressed by adequate training and experience but it must be realized that laparoscopic surgery requires special skills and excellent hand – eye coordination and this appears not to be available to all surgeons and it is essential that all surgical practitioners are aware of their own limitations. The ultimate choice of the type of hysterectomy to be chosen depends on a frank discussion between the patient and the doctor keeping the above factors in mind.

It is difficult to predict the future for however much increasing popularity seems to support a particular operation such was the case with laparoscopic subtotal hysterectomy in the past decade there was a severe setback when morcellation, which is a convenient way to rapidly remove the uterus after is has been severed from the cervix, has been associated with reports of dissemination of malignant material and, suddenly, the leader of the pack suffers a reversal of fortune until adequate ways are found to prevent this problem [106].

The ingenuity of doctors and scientists never ceases to amaze me and I remember some times ago being fascinated when seeing a video of an appendicectomy performed endoscopically by the passage of a multi channeled endoscope via the nose and entering the peritoneal cavity through a small incision in the stomach and finally removing the appendix without any abdominal incision and retrieving the specimen through the nose after repairing the small hole in the stomach. Thus a new chapter was born in this ongoing saga under the general title of Natural Orifice Endoscopic Surgery but gynaecologists should always remember that the vagina provides the natural orifice of our specialty and allows us to access the pelvis without painful abdominal incisions and in spite of all the advances that I have described it would appear that vaginal hysterectomy throughout the ages has remained the best, quickest and safest way of performing minimal access hysterectomy.

References

1. Lameras K. Galen and hippocrates. Athens: Papyrus; 1975.
2. Studd J. Ovariotomy for menstrual madness and premenstrual syndrome – 19th century history and lessons for current practice. Gynaecol Endocrinol. 2006;22(8):411–5.
3. Barker-Benfield GI. The horrors of the half-known life. London: Routledge; 2000.
4. Adler RE. Medical firsts: from Hippocrates to the human genome. Hobokin: Wiley; 2004.

5. Leonardo RA. History of gynecology. New York: Foben Press; 1944.
6. Temkin O (1956). Soranus' Gynaecology. (Translated). Baltimore: The Johns Hopkins University Press; 1991. Softshell Books edition.
7. O'Dowd MJ, Philipp EE. The history of obstetrics and gynaecology. Carnforth: Parthenon Press; 1994.
8. Soranus (of Ephesus). De arte obstetrician morbisque mulierum quae superaunt. Ex apogropho F.R. Dietze. Regimontii Pr: Graef et Unzer; 1838.
9. Senn N. The early history of vaginal hysterectomy. JAMA. 1895; 25:476–82.
10. Avenzoar A. L iber Teiser, sive rectification medication et reg*iminus*. J & G de Gregoriis, Venice.
11. Berengario da Carpi G. Commentaria cum amplissimis additionibus super anatomia Mundini., per H de Benedictus, Bononiae; 1521.
12. Benrubi GI. History of hysterectomy. J Fla Med Assoc. 1988; 75:533–42.
13. Sutton CJG. The history of vaginal hysterectomy. In: Sheth SS, editor. Vaginal hysterectomy, vol. 1. 2nd ed. New Delhi: Jaypee Publishers; 2014. p. 1–8.
14. Thornton JL, Want PC. William Harvey (1578 – 1657), 'Father of British Obstetrics', and his friend Percival Willughby (1596 – 1685). Br J Obst Gynaecol. 1978;85(4):241–5.
15. Baskett T. On the shoulders of giants. Eponyms in obstetrics and gynaecology. 1st ed. London: Butterworths; 1998.
16. Ricci JV. One hundred years of gynaecology 1800–1900. Philadelphia: Bakiston Company; 1945.
17. Langenbeck CJM. Geschichte einer von mir glucklich verichteten extirpation der ganger gebarrmutter. Bibliotyh Chir Opth Hannover. 1817;1:557–62.
18. Matthieu A. History of hysterectomy. West J Surg Obstet Gynecol. 1934;1(8):333–49.
19. Sutton CJG. Hysterectomy: a historical perspective. In: Wood C, Maher P, editors. Baillières clinical obstetrics and gynaecology, Hysterectomy, vol. 1. London: Bailliere Tindal; 1997. p. 1–23.
20. Ricci JV. Genealogy of gynaecology. Philadelphia: Blakiston; 1950. p. 350–2.
21. Gray L. The life and times of Ephraim McDowell. Louisville: VG Reid Printers; 1987.
22. Sutton CJG. The Royal College of Obstetricians and Gynaecologists historical lecture 1993. 150 years of hysterectomy: from Charles Clay to laparoscopic hysterectomy. Year Book of the Royal College of Obstetricians and Gynaecologists. London: RCOG Press; 1994.
23. Ellis H. Ephraim McDowell and the first elective successful laparotomy. Br J Hosp Med(Lond). 2009;70(2):107.
24. Tan SY, Wong C. Ephraim McDowell (1771 – 1830): pioneer of ovariotomy. Singapore Med J. 2005;46(1):4–5.
25. Graham S Jr D. Ephraim McDowell (1771 – 1830). The President's lithotomist. Invest Urol. 1981;19(3):216–7.
26. Bernhard CM. Presidential address: Dr. Ephraim McDowell: father of abdominal surgery. Am Surg. 1980;46(1):1–5.
27. Tait L. Diseases of the ovaries. New York: William Wood; 1883.
28. Othersen Jr HB. Ephraim McDowell: the qualities of a good surgeon. Ann Surg. 2004;239:648–50.
29. McDowell E. Initial observations on abdominal extirpation of tumours of the ovaria: a report of three cases. The Eclectic Repertory and Analytical Review of Philadelphia; 1819.
30. Sutton CJG: (2014). In: Reidy J, Hacking N, McLucas B, editors. Radiological interventions in obstetrics and gynaecology. Ch. 1; 3–16. Berlin: Springer.
31. Speert H. Obstetrics and gynaecology in America: a history. Baltimore: Waverly Press; 1980.
32. Morton LT. (1965). Garrison and Morton's medical Bibliography. Andre Deutsch London , 527–537.
33. Lizars J. Observations on extirpation of the ovaria with cases. Edinburgh Med Surg J. 1824. 22 October.
34. Bosdin Leech E. Some Manchester Medical Authors and their works. The Manchester University Medical School Gazette; 1956a, p. 102–6.
35. Fenster JM. Ether day: the strange tale of America's greatest medical discovery and the haunted men who made it. New York: Harper Collins; 2001.
36. Bosdin Leech E. Some Manchester Medical Authors and their Works. III – Charles Clay. The Manchester University Medical School Gazette; 1956b, p. 152–6.
37. Clay C. Observations on ovariotomy statistical and practical: also a successful case of entire removal of the uterus. Trans Obstet Soc London. 1863;5:58–74.
38. Burnham W. Extirpation of the uterus and ovaries for sarcomatous disease. Am Lancet. 1845:147–51.
39. Graham H. Eternal Eve. London: W Heinemann; 1950. p. 153–4.
40. Kimball G. Successful case of extirpation of the uterus. Boston Med Surg J. 1855;52:249–55.
41. Baskett TF. On the shoulders of giants. eponyms and names in obstetrics and gynaecology. 2nd ed. London: RCOG Press; 2008.
42. Lister J. On a new method of treating compound fractures, abscess, etc. with observations on the condition of suppuration. Lancet 1867;1867:326–9.
43. Simpson JY. Discovery of a new anaesthetic agent, more effective than sulphuric ether. Lancet. 1847;2:549–51.
44. Simpson JY. Answer to the religious objections advanced against the employment of anaesthetic agents in midwifery and surgery. Sutherland and Knox: Edinburgh; 1857. p. 23–5.
45. Baker BI. On the curability of certain forms of insanity, epilepsy, catalepsy, and hysteria in females. J Obstet Soc. London 1866:107–11.
46. Fennel P. Treatment without consent. Law, Psychiatry and treatment of mentally disordered people since 1845. London: Taylor and Francis; 2002.
47. Shepherd JA. Spencer Wells. The life and work of a Victorian Surgeon. Edinburgh: E & S Livingstone; 1965.
48. Freund WA. Eine neue Methode der Exstirpation des ganzen uterus. Berlin Med Surg J. 1878;15:417–8.
49. Czerny V. Ueber die Ausrottung des Gebarmutterkrebses. WienMedWahrc. 1879;29:1171–4.
50. Porro E. Della amputazione utero-ovarica come complement di taglio cesareo. Ann Univ Med Chir (Milan). 1876;237:289–350.
51. Caffarato TM. Ricordo di Eduardo Porro nell'centenario del'suo operazione. Minerva Ginecol. 1976;28:1033–40.
52. Baskett TF. Hysterectomy: evolution and trends. Best Pract Res Clin Obstet Gynaecol. 2005;10:295–305.
53. Ricci JV. The development of gynaecological surgery and instruments. Philadelphia: Blackiston; 1949. p. 297–301.
54. Sutton CJG. The past present and future of hysterectomy. J Minim Inv Gynecol Surgery. 2010;17(4):421–35.
55. Clark JG. A more radical method of performing hysterectomy for cancer of the uterus. Johns Hopkins Hospital Bulletin. 1895;6: 120–4.
56. Wertheim E. Zur Frage der Radicaloperation beim Uteruskrebs. Arch Gynakol. 1900;61:627–68.
57. Webb MJ. Radical Hysterectomy. Baillieres Clin Obstet Gynaecol. 1997;11(1):149–66.
58. Schauta F. Die erweiterte vaginale totalexstirpation des Uterus bei Kollumkarzinom. Leipzig: J Safar; 1908.
59. Schuchardt K. Eine neue Methode der Gerbärmutterextirpation. Zentralbl Chir. 1893;20:1121–6.
60. Mikuta JJ. A history of the centennial of the first radical hysterectomy and its developer – Dr. John Goodrich Clark. J Pelvic Surg. 1995;1:3–7.
61. Wertheim E. The extended abdominal operation for carcinoma uteri. Am J Obstet. 1912;66:169–232.

62. Richardson EH. A simplified technique for abdominal panhysterectomy. Surg Gynaecol Obstet. 1929;48:248–51.
63. Cutler EC, Zolenger RM, editors. Atlas of surgical operations. 1949. New York: McMillan & Co.; 1949.
64. Kilkku P, Gronroos M, Rauramo L. Supravaginal uterine amputation with pre-operative electro coagulation of endocervical mucosa. Acta Obstetrica et Gynaecologica Scandinavica. 1985;64: 175–7.
65. Lyons TL. Laparoscopic supracervical hysterectomy using the contact Nd:YAG laser. Gynecol Endosc. 1993;2:79–81.
66. Pfannenstiel HJ. Uber die vortheile des suprasymphsaren Fascienquerschnitts fur die gynakogischen Koliotomein zugleich ein Beitrag zu der Indikationstellung der Operationswerge. Samml Klin Vortr Leipzig. 1900;268:1735–56.
67. Amirikiah M, Evans TN. Ten year review of hysterectomies: trends indications and risks. Am J Obstet Gynecol. 1979;124:431–7.
68. Daly JW, Higgins KA. Injury to the ureter during gynaecological procedures. Surgical Gynaecology and Obstetrics. 1988;167: 19–21.
69. Dicker RC, Greenspan JR, Strauss LT, et al. Complications of abdominal and vaginal hysterectomy among women of reproductive age in the United States. The collaborative review of sterilisation. Am J Obstet Gynecol. 1982;144:841–8.
70. Bachmann G. Hysterectomy: a critical review. J Reprod Med. 1990;35(9):839–62.
71. Kelling G. Uber oesophagoskopie, gastroskopie und koelioskopie. Munch Med Wochenschr. 1902;49:21–4.
72. Von Ott D. Die direkte Beleuchtung der Bauchhohle, der Harnblase, des Dickdarms und des Uterus zu diagnostischen Zwecken. Rev Med Tcheque (Prague). 1901;2:27.
73. Jacobaeus HC. Uber due Moglichkeit die Zystosco;ie bei Untersuchlung seroser Hohlungen anzerwerden. Munchen Medizinische Wochenschrift. 1910;57:2090–2.
74. Gordon AG, Taylor P. History and development of endoscopic surgery. In: Sutton C, Diamond M, editors. Endoscopic surgery for gynaecologists. 2nd ed Ch 1. London: W B Saunders; 1998. p. 1–8.
75. Palmer R. La coelioscopie gynécologique. Acad Chir. 1946;72: 363–8.
76. Frangenheim H. Die tuben sterilization unter sicht mit dem laparoscope. Gerbutsh Frauenheilk. 1964;24:470–3.
77. Steptoe PC. Laparoscopy in gynaecology. Edinburgh/London: Livingstone; 1967.
78. Semm K. Hysterectomy by pelviscopy: an alternative approach without colpotomy (CASH). In: Garry R, Reich H, editors. Laparoscopic hysterectomy. Oxford: Blackwell; 1993. p. 118–32.
79. Semm K O'Neill-Freys L. Conventional operative laparoscopy (pelviscopy). In: Sutton CJG, editors. Laparoscopic surgery; Baillière's Clinical Obstetrics and Gynaecology; Baillière Tindall, London. vol. 3: 3; 1989, p. 451–85.
80. Garry R, Reich H. Laparoscopic hysterectomy – definitions and indications. Gynaecol Endosc. 1994;4(2):77–9.
81. Bruhat MA, Manhes H, Mage G, Pouly JL. Treatment of ectopic pregnancy by means of laparoscopy. Fertil Steril. 1980;33:411–4.
82. Hopkins HH. Optical principles of the endoscope. In: Berci G, editor. Endoscopy. New York: Appleton-Century-Crofts; 1976. p. 3–27.
83. De Cherney AH. The leader of the band is tired. Fertil Steril. 1985;44:299–302.
84. Reich H, De Caprio J, McGlynn F. Laparoscopic hysterectomy. J Gynecol Surg. 1989;5(2):213–5.
85. Sutton CJG. Wither Hysterectomy? Curr opin gynaecol. 1994;6: 203–5.
86. Semm K. Hysterectomy via laparotomy or pelviscopy. a new CISH method without colpotomy. Geburtshilfe Frauenheilkd. 1991;51:996–1003.
87. Mettler L, Ahmed-Ebbiary N, Scollmeyer T. Laparoscopic hysterectomy: challenges and limitations. Min Invas Ther & Allied Technol. 2005;14:145–59.
88. Ewen SP, Sutton CJG. Initial experience with supra-cervical laparoscopic hysterectomy and removal of the transformation zone. Br J Obstet Gynaecol. 1994;101:225–8.
89. Lyons TL. Laparoscopic supra-cervical hysterectomy. A comparison of morbidity and mortality results with laparoscopic assisted vaginal hysterectomy. J Reprod Med. 1993;38:738–63.
90. Okara EO, Jones KD, Sutton CJG. Long term outcome following laparoscopic supracervical hysterectomy. Br J Obstet Gynaecol. 2001;108:1017–20.
91. Lieng M, Qvigstat E, Istre O, Langebrekke A, Ballard K. Long term outcomes following laparoscopic supracervical hysterectomy. Br J Obstet Gyanaecol. 2008;115:1605–10.
92. Donnez J, Nisolle N, Smets M, et al. Laparoscopic supracervical (subtotal) hysterectomy: a first series of 500 cases. Gynaecol Endosc. 1997;6:73–6.
93. Dequesne J, Schmidt N, Fryman R. A new electrosurgical loop technique for laparoscopic supra-cervical hysterectomy. Gynaecol Endosc. 1998;7:29–32.
94. Pasic R, Abdelmomen A, Levine R. Comparison of cervical detachment using monopolar lap loop ligature and conventional methods in laparoscopic supracervical hysterectomy. JSLS. 2006;10:226–30.
95. Sutton C, Abbott J. History of power sources in endoscopic surgery. J Minimally Invasive Gynecol. 1995;20(3):271–8.
96. Merrill RM. Hysterectomy surveillance in the United States: 1997 through 2005. Med Sci Monit. 2008;14:24–31.
97. Gimbel H, Settiness A, Tabor A. Hysterectomy for benign conditions in Denmark 1988 – 1998. Acta Obstet Gynecol Scand. 2001;80:267–72.
98. Kilkku P, Gonroos M, Hirvonen T, Rauramo L. Supravaginal uterine amputation vs hysterectomy: effect on libido and orgasm. Acta Obstet Gynaecol Scand. 1983;62:147–52.
99. Thakar R, Ayers S, Clarkson P, Stanton S, Manyonda I. Outcomes after total versus subtotal hysterectomy. N Engl J Med. 2002;347: 11318–24.
100. Morelli M, Noia R, Mocciaro R, et al. Laparoscopic supracervical hysterectomy versus laparoscopic total hysterectomy: a prospective randomized study. Minerva Gynecol. 2007;59:1–10.
101. Nezhat CR, Stevens A, Balassiano E, Soliemannjad BS. Robotic-assisted laparoscopy vs conventional laparoscopy for the treatment of advanced stage endometriosis. J Minim Invasive Gynecol. 2015;22:40–4.
102. Magrina JF, Kho R, Weaver L, Montero P, Magtibay P. Robotic radical hysterectomy: comparison with laparoscopy and laparotomy. Gynaecol Oncol. 2008;109:86–91.
103. Reynolds R, Advincula A. Robot-assisted laparoscopic hysterectomy technique and initial experience. Am J Surg. 2006;191:555–60.
104. Advincula A, Reynolds R. The use of robot-assisted laparoscopic hysterectomy in the patient with a scarred or obliterated anterior cul-de-sac. JSLS. 2005;9:287–91.
105. Garry R, Fountain J, Mason S, et al. The eVALuate study: two parallel randomised trials, one comparing laparoscopic with abdominal hysterectomy, the other comparing laparoscopic with vaginal hysterectomy. BMJ. 2004;328:129–33.
106. Brown J, Taylor K, Ramirez PT, et al. Laparoscopic supracervical hysterectomy with morcellation: should it stay or should it go? J Minim Invas Gynaecol. 2015;22:185–92.

2 History of Radical Hysterectomy

Karl Tamussino

At the end of the nineteenth century, cervical cancer was a scourge for which there was no early detection and no cure. In an era where the average life expectancy was about 50 years, cervical cancer was the most common cause of cancer death in women, as it still is today in parts of the world. "It is enough to make a physician's heart sink within him to make the diagnosis of cancer uteri," wrote Charles Meigs in [12], "for such a diagnostic is ipso facto a prognostic of death."

This dire state of affairs led to heroic efforts to remove uteri to cure cancer. The first abdominal removal of a cancerous uterus was apparently performed in 1878 by W. A. Freund in Breslau (Wroclaw, then Germany, now Poland). Three mass ligatures were placed on each side of the uterus. The ligatures contained the ovarian ligaments, the round ligaments, and the paracervical tissue. The last ligature was placed by "leading a suture from in front of the base of the ligamentum latum through the anterior lateral part of the vaginal fornix behind the base of the ligamentum latum into the pouch of Douglas" [7]. The patient went home 19 days after surgery. Sixty-six Freund operations performed by 1880 entailed 49 perioperative deaths (72 %) [3].

Surgeons worked to improve the Freund operation. In 1881 Linkenheld, an assistant of Freund's, noted that all the patients who survived the Freund operation developed a recurrence within two and a half years at the latest. He ascribed this to the fact that "in all these cases, the neoplasia exceeded the limits of the uterus and spread to the adjacent parametria, and that the operation had not removed all diseased tissue." Like surgeons who removed the tissue in the axilla of patients undergoing surgery for cancer of the breast, Linkenheld suggested "removing the parametria, of course avoiding injury to the ureters, under all circumstances." This entailed omitting the mass ligatures, since "they present a barrier to outward dissection. Instead, after circumcision of the portio, the uterus must be removed like a tumor, and the various vessels ligated individually. The parametria should then be removed bluntly, as is done in the removal of the axillary tissue" [10].

Consistent with the philosophy of extended mastectomy envisioned and advocated by William Halsted for women with breast cancer, surgeons continued to push the limits of parametrial excision. Brunet [1], in studies of Mackenrodt's surgical specimens, found that 60 % of those that were considered negative at palpation contained disease. Also, 42 % of the specimens showed spread to the upper third of the vagina. Increasing resection of the parametrial tissue soon led to the issue of the ureter [4, 20, 21]. The work of these surgeons built the foundation for what is today known and thought of as radical hysterectomy.

In the late 1890s, Ernst Wertheim (1864–1920) in Vienna began to standardize the operation that later came to bear his name. Wertheim was born and studied medicine in Graz, then moved to Vienna and Prague to train with Friedrich Schauta. He performed his first radical operation in 1898 and reported on the first 29 patients in 1900 [30]. His rationale was that simple removal of the uterus was providing poor results for patients with uterine cancer and that "to obtain better results – as for the surgical approach to cancers in other organs – in addition to the primary focus one should remove as much as possible of the surrounding tissue". This was the Halstedian vision applied to uterine cancer.

Wertheim's famous monograph describing 500 radical abdominal operations appeared in 1911 [31] and was soon translated into English [32]. The monograph is a monumental effort. It assiduously tabulates his first 500 patients, including their postoperative courses and outcomes. It provides detailed descriptions of the clinical findings. Descriptions such as "cauliflower like", "infiltration to the pelvic wall", "cervix replaced by neoplasia", "portio replaced by necrotic mass" are the rule. Obviously none of these were screening-detected lesions and many we today would not

K. Tamussino, MD, FACS
Division of Gynecology, Department of Obstetrics and Gynecology, Medical University of Graz, Graz, Austria
e-mail: karl.tamussino@medunigraz.at

I. Alkatout, L. Mettler (eds.), *Hysterectomy*, DOI 10.1007/978-3-319-22497-8_2

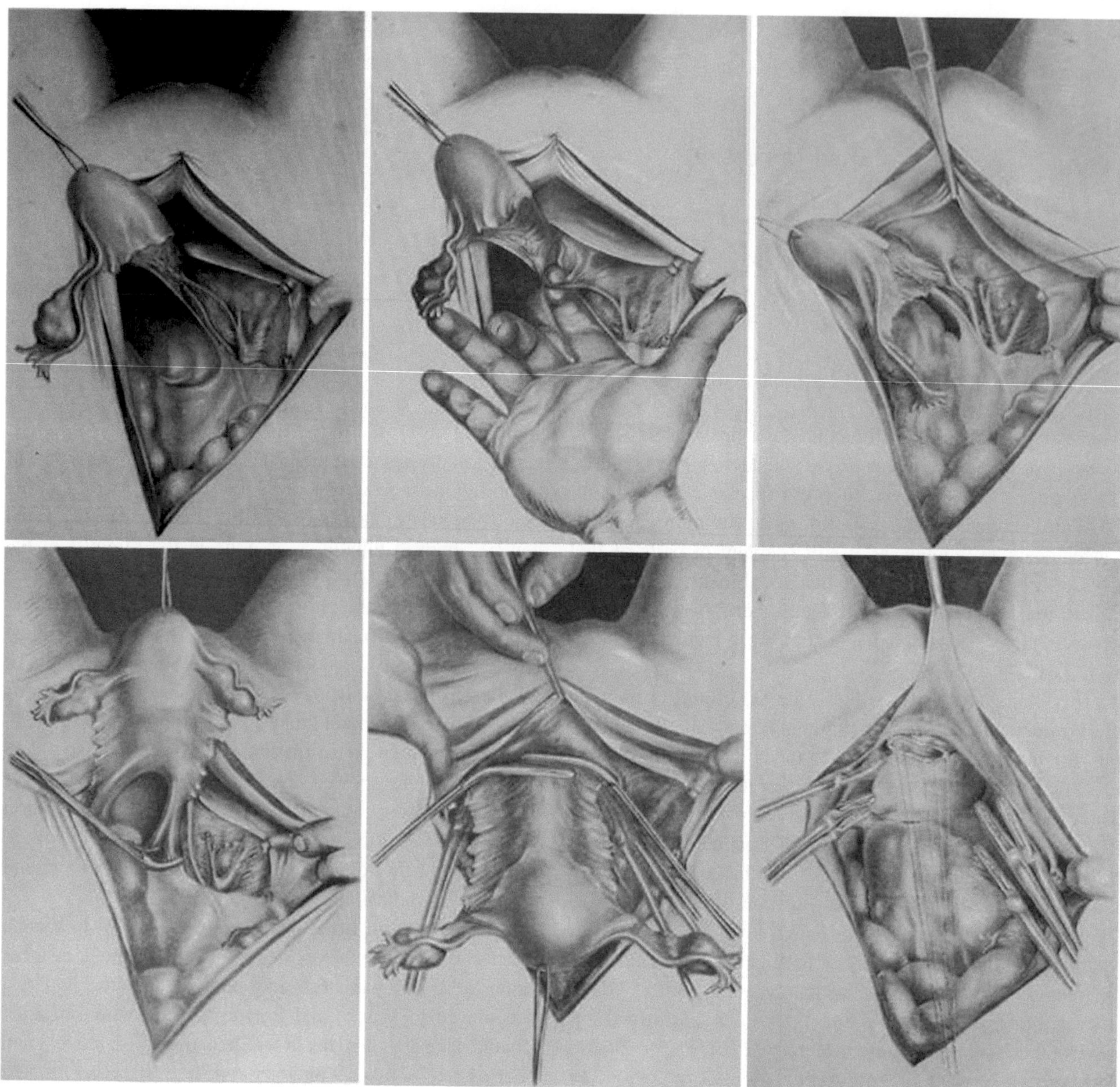

Fig. 2.1 Plates from Wertheim's original description of his extended hysterectomy (Wertheim [31])

consider for surgical treatment at all. The monograph lists the operating times (consistently under 2 h), the postoperative course (including 38 % mortality amongst the first 50 patients), and follow-up with information on time and site of recurrence.

Key steps of Wertheim's technique were digital separation of the leaves of the broad ligament, isolation of the ureter down to its entrance into the parametrium, a maneuver of poking the index finger through the parametrium along the ureter to isolate and ligate the uterine vessels, dissection of the bladder, dissection of the rectum, division of the parametria "from" the pelvic wall with specially designed clamps. Finally, the vagina was clamped and divided below the clamps to excise the specimen without contaminating the surgical field with malignant cells (Fig. 2.1).

Notably, Wertheim performed the hysterectomy first and then did a "search for and extirpation of enlarged lymph glands". Spaces were not systematically developed, and lymph nodes not removed systematically. Thus, a key feature of Wertheim's technique was that he did the hysterectomy first and then turned his attention to the lymph nodes, and then removed only enlarged nodes. Of course, issues regarding the indications for lymphadenectomy and which nodes to remove are still avidly debated for many cancers more than 100 years later.

Latzko and Schiffmann [9] in Vienna, like Peiser [17] before them but in contrast to Wertheim, began the operation

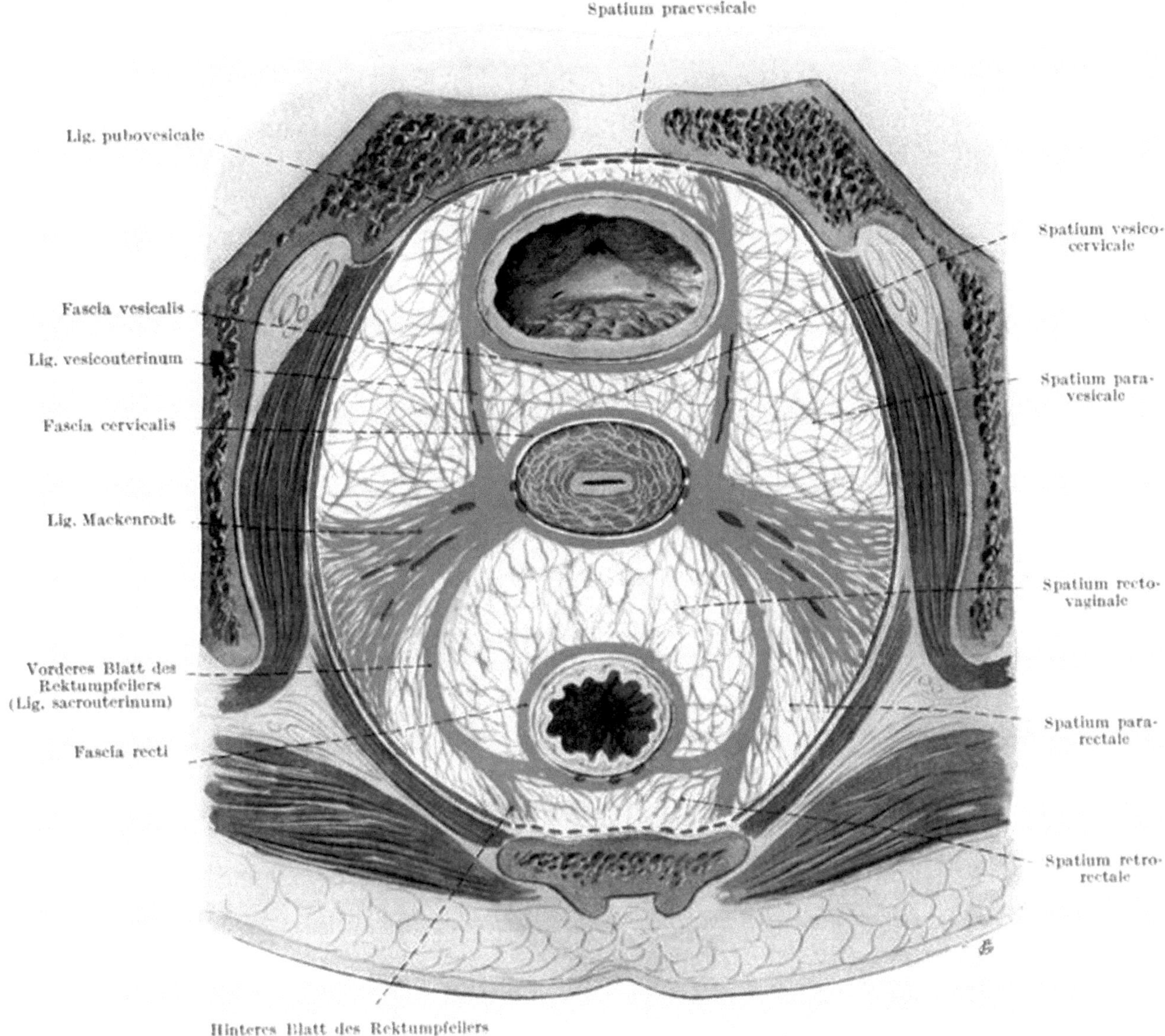

Fig. 2.2 Original schema of the potential spaces in the pelvis (Reprinted from Peham and Amreich [16], with permission from Elsevier)

with systematic lymphadenectomy. Thus, "the object of the operation was isolated according to the anatomic conditions." This was done by opening the paravesical and pararectal spaces (although these were not named) and freeing the ureter from its attendant tissue. The sacrouterine ligament was completely demonstrated and divided close to the sacrum. Isolating the specimen in this way made it possible to resect the parametrial tissue directly at the pelvic wall. By systematically removing lymph nodes before removing the uterus, and thereby "setting up" the operation, Latzko and Schiffmann [9] describe the radical hysterectomy much as we think of it today, but did not name the potential spaces they developed to set up the operation.

The schema with the names of the potential spaces in the pelvis that is the basis of today's surgical anatomy of the pelvis was first described by Peham and Amreich of Vienna in a classic textbook published in [15] (Fig. 2.2).

Lymphadenectomy was associated with radical hysterectomy from early on. The impulse came from anatomic studies by Wagner [29] and Cruveilhier [5] that had found involved nodes in more than 50 % of women who died of cervical cancer. Veit [28] and Mackenrodt [11] repeatedly found tumor deposits in the lymphatics of the parametrial tissue, even before the cervix was "completely infiltrated by tumor to its outer layers." Macroscopically normal parametrial tissue was therefore capable of containing tumor.

General surgeons were already working on removing all accessible regional lymph nodes (not just palpable nodes) in patients undergoing surgery for cancer. Schuchardt [25] stipulated this requirement for cancers of the uterus. In 1898,

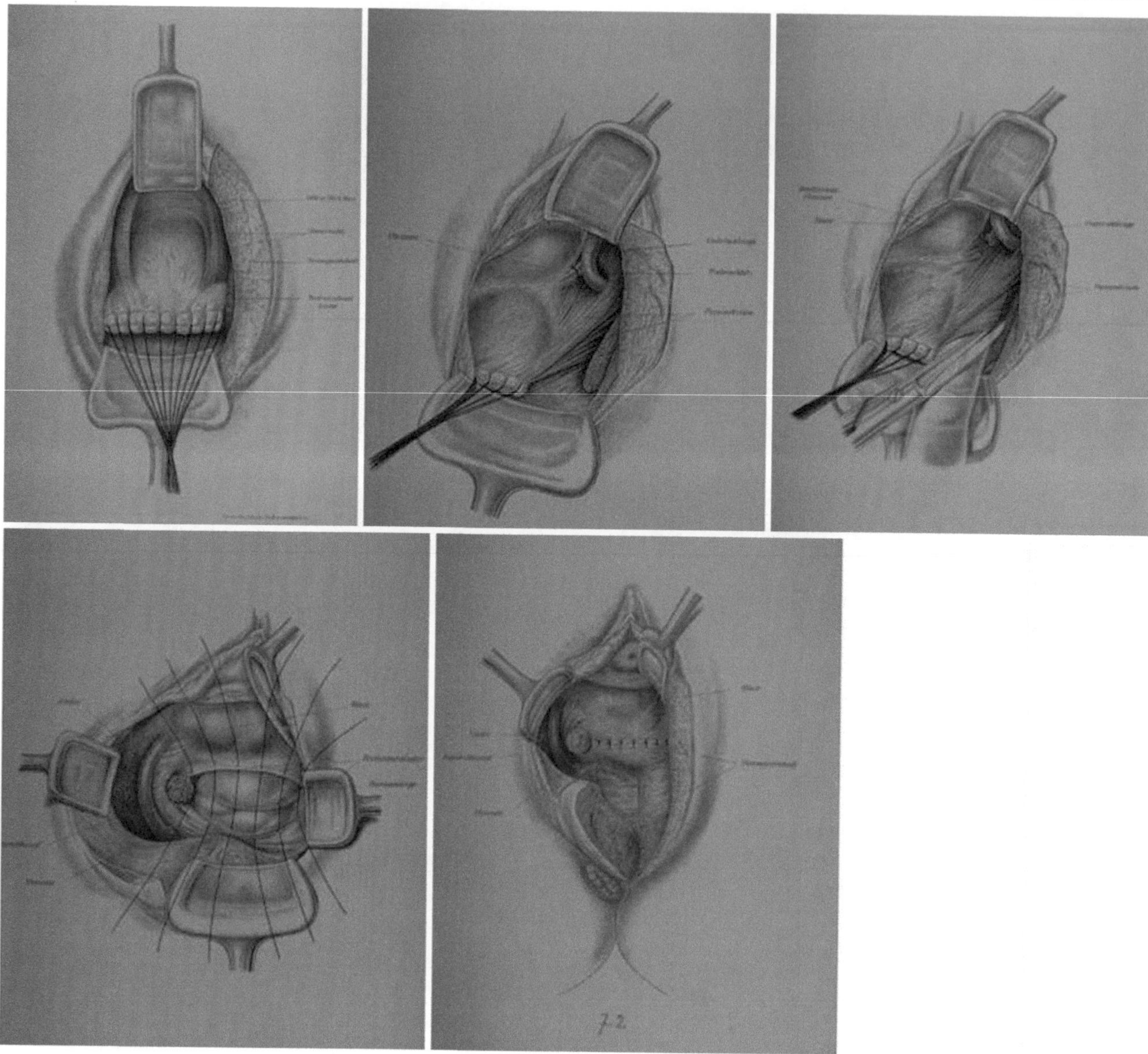

Fig. 2.3 Plates from Schauta's original description of extended vaginal hysterectomy (Schauta [22, 24])

Peiser published anatomical and clinical studies of the lymphatic system of the uterus. He saw a need for systematic lymphadenectomy by also removing the lymphatic channels between the cervix and the pelvic wall. This amounted to total excision of the parametrial tissue. Peiser's publication prompted Wertheim to make "a search for lymph nodes" part of his operation. Schauta [22–24], a proponent of radical vaginal hysterectomy, came out against the "needless search for glands," and stated that, at autopsy, nonenlarged and impalpable nodes could contain cancer. Thus, he unintentionally provided the rationale for systematic removal of the nodes. Latzko and Schiffmann [9] stated that searching for enlarged nodes was fundamentally different from their systematically rempoving node bearing tissue. This still holds true. In contrast to Wertheim, Latzko and Schiffmann performed lymphadenectomy at the beginning of the operation, thereby setting up the subsequent radical hysterectomy.

While Wertheim and others were pursuing an abdominal approach, Friedrich Schauta, Wertheim's erstwhile teacher, was working on the radical vaginal procedure first described by Schuchardt [25]. Schauta, also of Vienna, did for radical vaginal hysterectomy what Wertheim did for radical abdominal hysterectomy. In 1908 he published an assiduous and beautifully illustrated monograph with a list of 258 consecutive operations (Fig. 2.3). Like Wertheim, Schauta provides clinical descriptions, perioperative results and complications, and follow-up (25 % considered cured at 5 years).

Interestingly, Schauta and Wertheim were first teacher (Schauta) and student (Wertheim), later bitter rivals. Their dispute concerned the approach to radical hysterectomy (vaginal vs. abdominal) and the issue of lymphadenectomy. Wertheim considered the removal of involved glands therapeutic, Schauta was not convinced. Of course, these arguments continue to the present day, and not just for cervical cancer. Both Schauta and Wertheim devote passages in their monographs to disparaging the other's approach. The tone is not friendly. It is ironic that the two rivals received honorary graves in the Vienna Zentralfriedhof, almost next to each other.

The exacting and self-critical work done by Schauta and Wertheim – with clinical descriptions, perioperative morbidity and mortality, and long-term outcome – also remind us that evidence-based surgery is not new.

Late in his life, in the late 1910s, Wertheim was despondent at the thought that his life's work on the treatment of cervical cancer was being made obsolete by the advent of radium treatment for this disease. Wertheim's last publication, which appeared in 1919, the year before he died, was a monograph on a vaginal, uterine-sparing operation for uterovaginal prolapse.

In the United States, Taussing [26] and Meigs [13] were influential in making lymphadenectomy a part of radical surgery for cervical cancer. An influential book edited by Joe V. Meigs of Boston, *Surgical Treatment of Cancer of the Cervix* [14], pulled together authors and the arguments for surgical treatment of cervical cancer and led to a renaissance of surgical treatment for this disease.

Improvements in surgical technique, anesthesiology, blood replacement, perioperative care and technology made possible longer and more complex operations. Pelvic exenterations were a further push to extend the reach of surgical treatment of cervical cancer. These were pioneered by Alexander Brunschwig (1901–1969) of New York [2]. These are complex operations with considerable complication rates and sequelae but continue to have a place in the surgical treatment of recurrent cervical cancer.

Differences in surgical approaches, anatomical concepts and terminologies have led to some confusion and attempts to classify what is understood under the term "radical" or "extended" hysterectomy. The classification put forth by Piver et al. in [18], which distinguished five classes of extended hysterectomy, has probably gained the most traction. Class I (which they called the the TeLinde modification) amounts to a standard total hysterectomy and was used for in situ and microinvasive carcinomas. Class II is a "moderately extended radical hysterectomy", with removal of the medial half of the cardinal ligament. A Class III procedure is the classic Latzko-Meigs concept with pelvic lymphadenectomy and excision of the cardinal ligaments at the pelvic wall, of the uterosacral ligaments at the sacrum, and of the upper half of the vagina. Class IV radical hysterectomy entails excision of three-fourths of the vagina and class V hysterectomy includes resection of involved areas of the ureter and bladder (but is short of exenteration). In Querleu and Morrow [19] developed a more detailed (and thus more complex) classification.

With the advent of cytologic screening after the Second World War, based on the work of George Papanicolaou, the spectrum of cervical cancers seen in developed shifted toward early, screening-detected lesions. Simultaneously, advances in radiation and chemoradiation therapy were made for the treatment of bulky or locally advanced disease. Accordingly, instead of continuously extending radicality, surgeons began to explore whether certain patients with smaller lesions could undergo less aggressive surgery and thus be spared morbidity. This was the basis for nerve-sparing radical hysterectomies [27], radical trachelectomies (with preservation of the uterus and thus of fertility) [6], and sentinel lymph node biopsy. Also, Japanese surgeons developed an anatomical approach to nerve-sparing radical hysterectomy that dates back to Okabayashi in the 1930s [8]. Evidence that small cervical cancers infrequently involve the parametrial tissue is the basis for an ongoing multinational randomized trial of simple vs. radical hysterectomy for early cervical cancer.

The story of radical history contains much of the history of gynecologic surgery and gynecologic oncology and reflects the enormous progress that has been made in combating what was once the leading cause of cancer death in women. The operation is fundamental to our understanding of the surgical anatomy of the pelvis. Wertheim need not have worried, the operation continues to evolve to serve the needs of women with cervical cancer.

References

1. Brunet G. Ergebnisse der abdominalen Radikaloperation des Gebärmutterscheidenkrebses mittels Laparotomia hypogastrica. Z Geburtshilfe Gynäkol. 1905;56:1–87.
2. Brunschwig A. Total and anterior pelvic exenterations: report of results based on 315 operations. Surg Gynecol Obstet. 1954;99:324–30.
3. Burghardt E. Radical abdominal hysterectomy: historical background. In: Burghardt E, Webb MJ, Monaghan JM, Kindermann G, editors. Surgical gynecologic oncology. Stuttgart: Thieme; 1993. p. 275–6.
4. Clark JG. A more radical method of performing hysterectomy for cancer of the uterus. Bull Johns Hopkins Hosp. 1895;6:120.
5. Cruveilhier J. Traité d'anatomie descriptive. Paris: Bechet Jeune; 1834. p. 3.
6. Dargent D, Querleu D, Plante M, Reynolds K. Vaginal and laparoscopic vaginal surgery. Boca Raton: CRC Press; 2004.
7. Freund WA. Zu meiner Methode der totalen Uterus-Exstirpation. Z Gynäkol. 1878;2:265.
8. Fuji S, Takakura K, Matsumura N, Higuchi T, Yura S, Mandai M, Baba T, Yoshioka S. Anatomic identification and functional outcomes of the nerve sparing Okabayashi radical hysterectomy. Gynecol Oncol. 2007;107:4–13.
9. Latzko W, Schiffmann J. Klinisches und Anatomisches zur Radikaloperation des Gebärmutterkrebses. Zbl Gynäkol. 1919;34: 689–705.

10. Linkenheld J. Zur Totalexstirpation des Uterus. Z Gynäkol. 1881; 5:169.
11. Mackenrodt A. Beitrag zur Verbesserung der Dauerresultate der Totalexstirpation bei Carcinoma uteri. Z Geburtshilfe Gynäkol. 1894;29:157.
12. Meigs CC. Woman, her diseases and remedies. Philadelphia: Lea and Blanchard; 1850.
13. Meigs JV. Wertheim operation for carcinoma of cervix. Am J Obstet Gynecol. 1945;49:542.
14. Meigs JV, editor. Surgical treatment of cancer of the cervix. New York: Grune & Stratton; 1954.
15. Peham H, Amreich J. Gynäkologische Operationslehre. Berlin: S. Karger; 1930 .766 pp
16. Peham H, Amreich J. Operative gynecology. Philadelphia: J.B. Lippincott; 1934 .779 pp.
17. Peiser E. Anatomische und klinische Untersuchungen über den Lymphapparat des Uterus mit besonderer Berücksichtigung der Totalexstirpation bei Carcinoma uteri. Z Geburtshilfe Gynäkol. 1898;39:259–78.
18. Piver MS, Rutledge F, Smith JP. Five classes of extended hysterectomy for women with cervical cancer. Obstet Gynecol. 1974;44:265–72.
19. Querleu D, Morrow CP. Classification of radical hysterectomy. Lancet Oncol. 2008;9:297–303.
20. Ries E. Eine neue Operationsmethode des Uteruscarcinoms. 1. Beitrag. Z Geburtshilfe Gynäkol. 1895;32:266.
21. Ries E. Modern treatment of cancer of the uterus. Chicago Med Rec. 1895;9:284.
22. Schauta F. Die Operation des Gebärmutterkrebses mittels des Schuchardt'schen Pravaginalschnittes. Monatschr f Geburtsh u Gynakol. 1902;15:133.
23. Schauta R. Die Operation des Gebärmutterkrebses mittels des Schuchardtschen Paravaginalschnittes. Monatsschr Geburtshilfe Gynäkol. 1902;15:133–52.
24. Schauta F. Die erweiterte vaginale Totalexstirpation des Uterus beim Kollumkarzinom. Vienna: Safar; 1908.
25. Schuchardt K. Eine neue Methode der Gebärmutterexstirpation. Zbl Chir. 1893;20:1121.
26. Taussig FJ. Iliac lymphadenectomy for group II cancer of the cervix. Am J Obstet Gynecol. 1943;45:733.
27. Trimbos JB, Maas CP, Deruiter MC, Peters AAW, Kenter GG. A nerve-sparing radical hysterectomy: guidelines and feasibility in Western patients. Int J Gynecol Cancer. 2001; 11:180.
28. Veit P. Operation bei fortgeschrittenem Gebärmutterkrebs. Dtsch Med Wochenschr. 1891;40.
29. Wagner N.. Gebärmutterkrebs. Eine pathologisch-anatomische Monographie. Leipzig. 1858.
30. Wertheim E. Zur Frage der Radikaloperation beim Uteruskrebs. Arch Gynäkol. 1900;61:627–68.
31. Wertheim E. Die erweiterte abdominale Operation bei Carcinoma colli uteri. Berlin: Urban and Schwarzenberg; 1911 .223 pp
32. Wertheim E. The extended abdominal operation for carcinoma uteri (based on 500 operative cases). Am J Obstet Dis Women Children. 1912;66:169–32.

Part II

Topographical Anatomy

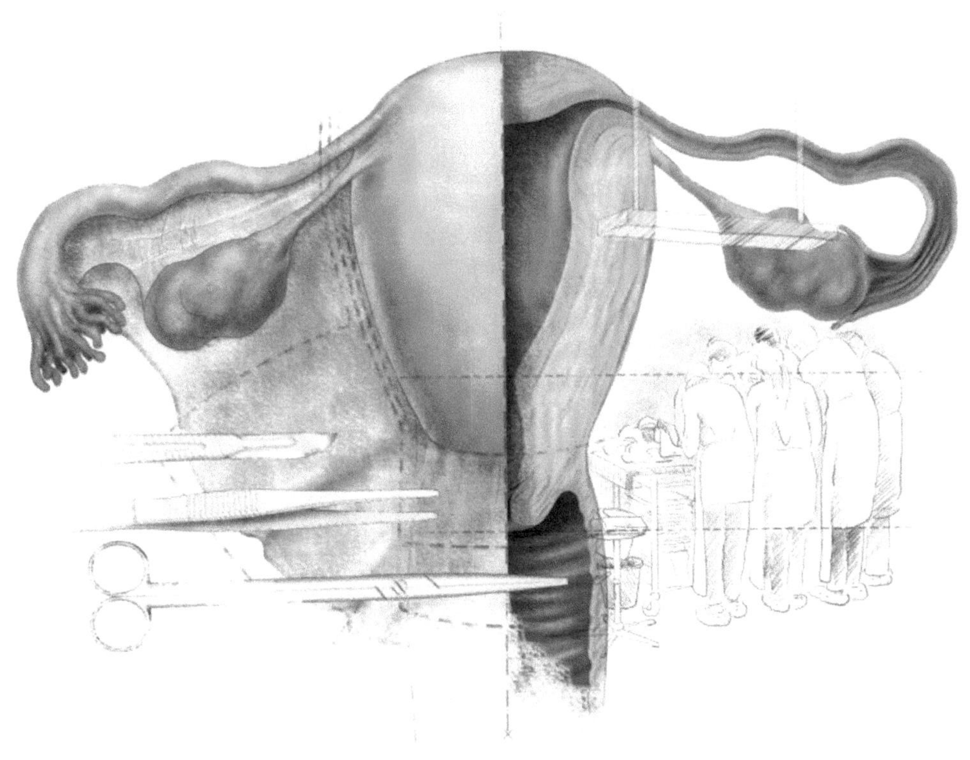

3 Topographical Anatomy for Hysterectomy Procedures

Thilo Wedel

Compartments of the Female Pelvic Cavity

The female pelvic cavity is divided into an anterior, middle and posterior compartment (Fig. 3.1). In contrast to the male pelvic cavity which is confined to two compartments and contains parenchymatous organs (e.g. prostate and seminal glands), all three female compartments consist of hollow visceral organs resting upon the pelvic floor:

- Anterior compartment: urinary bladder and urethra
- Middle compartment: uterus with uterine adnexa and vagina
- Posterior compartment: rectum and anal canal

The peritoneum covers the organs contained in these pelvic compartments from above. While the urinary bladder and rectum are only partially lined by peritoneal serosa, almost the entire uterus and the complete adnexa including the ovaries and uterine tubes are wrapped by peritoneum and, thus, readily accessible by transperitoneal approach. The peritoneum reflects from the uterine body anteriorly on to the fundus of the urinary bladder forming the vesicouterine pouch delimited laterally by the vesicouterine folds and posteriorly on to the rectal wall forming the rectouterine pouch delimited laterally by the rectouterine folds. Except for the posterior vaginal fornix directly facing the rectouterine pouch, the vagina is located extraperitoneally. Both peritoneal pouches are often filled with small intestinal loops, sigmoid colon or greater omentum, thus requiring proper exposure by moving the content upwards.

The pelvic compartments are separated by septa mainly composed of connective tissue and intermingled smooth muscle tissue. Between the anterior vaginal wall and both the urinary bladder and urethra extends the vesico–/urethrovaginal septum, between the posterior vaginal wall and the anterior rectal wall extends the rectovaginal septum. The connective tissue septa are devoid of major blood vessels and serve as separating gliding layers between the three pelvic compartments reflecting the different ontogenetic origins of the urinary, genital and digestive tract. Thus, if surgical dissection follows these self-opening planes between the pelvic compartments, the uterovaginal complex can be readily delineated from the urinary bladder and urethra anteriorly and the anorectum posteriorly without relevant bleeding risk [1–3].

Female Pelvic Floor

The female pelvic floor (Fig. 3.2) is of larger dimension than in males displaying a wider urogenital opening, although its muscle strength is generally lower and its nerve supply less developed. These peculiar features allow vaginal delivery, but also predispose to an higher susceptibility for structural and functional insufficiency and pelvic organ prolapse.

The pelvic floor is composed of a pelvic diaphragm consisting of the levator ani muscle and a urogenital diaphragm comprising the transverse perineal muscles. The levator ani muscle corresponds to a flattened and funnel-shaped muscle closing most of the lower pelvic aperture. However, along the ventral midline openings are left for the urethra and vagina (urogenital hiatus) and the anal canal (anal hiatus).

The largest portion of the levator ani muscle are the ileococcygeal muscles extending from the pelvic side walls to a midline raphe. The rather thin muscle layer originates at the tendinous arc of the levator ani muscle formed by condensed

Note In regards to the nomenclature of anatomical structures, eponymes although commonly used in medical literature (e.g. Lee/Frankenhäuser ganglion, Poupart ligament, Mackenrodt ligament, Cooper ligament, Denonvillier fascia, Waldeyer fascia, Sampson artery, Richard fimbria, Latzko and Okabayashi spaces, etc.) are avoided to prevent confusions frequently resulting from misinterpretation of the historical descriptions.

T. Wedel
Institute of Anatomy, Center of Clinical Anatomy,
Christian-Albrechts-University of Kiel, Kiel, Germany
e-mail: t.wedel@anat.uni-kiel.de

I. Alkatout, L. Mettler (eds.), *Hysterectomy*, DOI 10.1007/978-3-319-22497-8_3

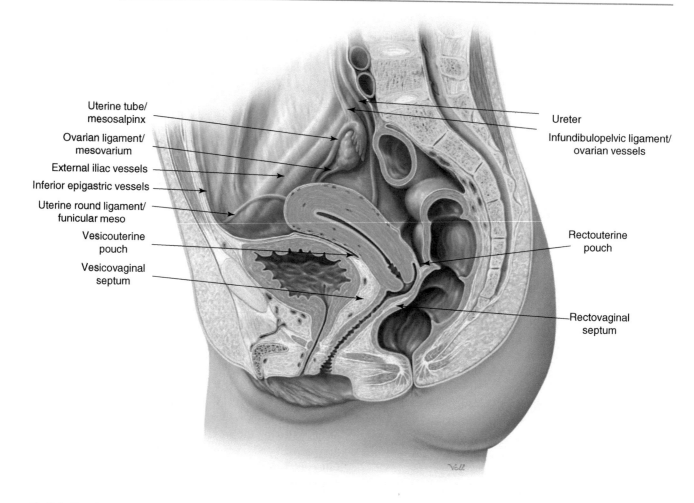

Fig. 3.1 Female pelvic cavity. Midsagittal section, view from left side (Reproduced from Schünke et al. [24])

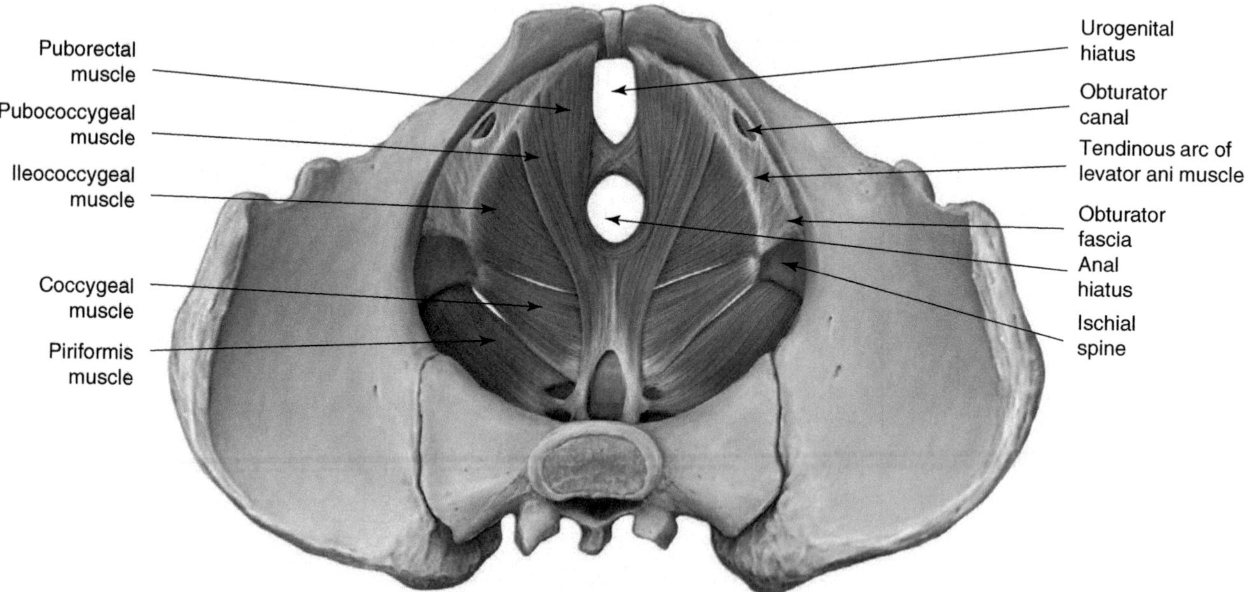

Fig. 3.2 Female pelvic floor. Cranial view. Content of pelvic cavity removed (Reproduced from Schünke et al. [24])

connective tissue of the obturator fascia ("white line"). The hammock-shaped pubococcygeal muscle originates from the pubic bone and extends towards the coccygeal bone, whereas the sling-shaped puborectal muscle bends arround the anal canal to produce the anorectal angle.

Innervation of the pelvic floor muscles is mainly provided by infralevatory branches of the pudendal nerve. In addition, also direct nerve branches the from sacral spinal nerves S3–S4 contribute and extend from the sacral concavity to reach the levator ani muscle from above. Thus, when exposing the pelvic floor muscle during extended deep lymphadenectomy, care must be taken to preserve these direct supralevatory nerve branches [1–3].

Uterus

The uterus (Fig. 3.3) is a pear-shaped hollow muscular organ of 7–9 cm length with its long axis nearly at right angle to that of the vagina (anteversion of uterine cervix plus anteflexion of uterine corpus) depending on the filling state of the urinary bladder. The anteroposteriorly flattened uterine corpus narrows caudally and continues into the cylindrical uterine cervix. The convex upper part of the uterine corpus is defined as the uterine fundus. On either side, a uterine cornu is formed to receive the uterine tube. Anterior to the uterine cornu inserts the uterine round ligament, posteroinferior to it attaches the ovarian ligament. The uterine cervix is 2–3 cm long, far less mobile than the uterine corpus due to its fixating ligaments and divided into a supravaginal and vaginal portion. Posteriorly the uterine cervix is covered by peritoneum, laterally it is in close relationship to the uterine arteries and the ureters flanking the uterine cervix at a distance of ca. 1–2 cm. The uterine cervical canal connects the uterine cavity with the vaginal lumen [3].

Uterine Adnexa

The uterine adnexa comprise the ovaries, ovarian tubes and ligaments adjacent to the uterus on both sides (Figs. 3.1 and 3.3). The ovaries lie in the ovarian fossae posterolateral to the uterus and medial to the external iliac vessels. They are attached to the uterus by the ovarian ligaments extending from the uterine pole of the ovary to the uterine cornu. The peritoneal fold raised by the ovarian ligament corresponds to the mesovarium containing the ovarian branch of the uterine artery (Figs. 3.5 and 3.8).

The tubal pole of the ovary is connected to the fimbriated end of the uterine tube. Between the tubal pole and the dorsolateral pelvic wall extends the infundibulopelvic ligament corresponding to a peritoneal fold raised by the ovar-

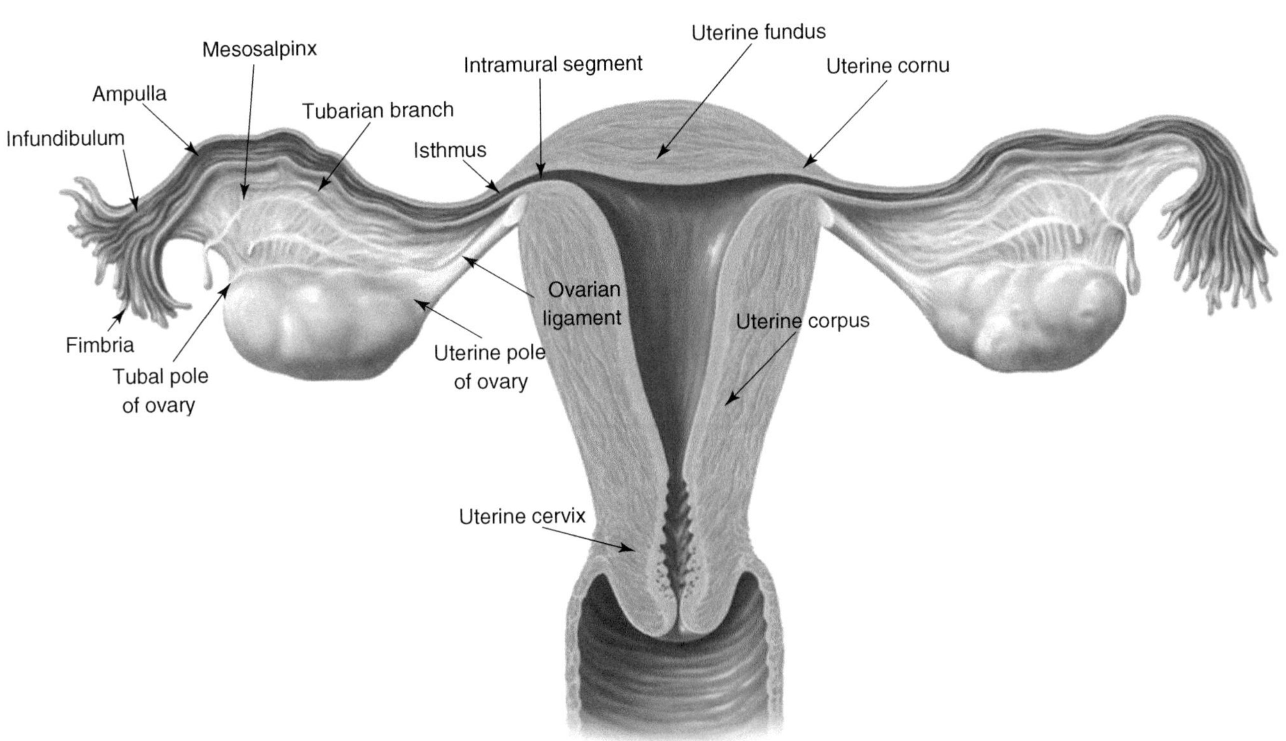

Fig. 3.3 Internal female genital organs. Frontal section, dorsal view. Broad ligament, parametrium and paracolpium removed (Reproduced from Schünke et al. [24])

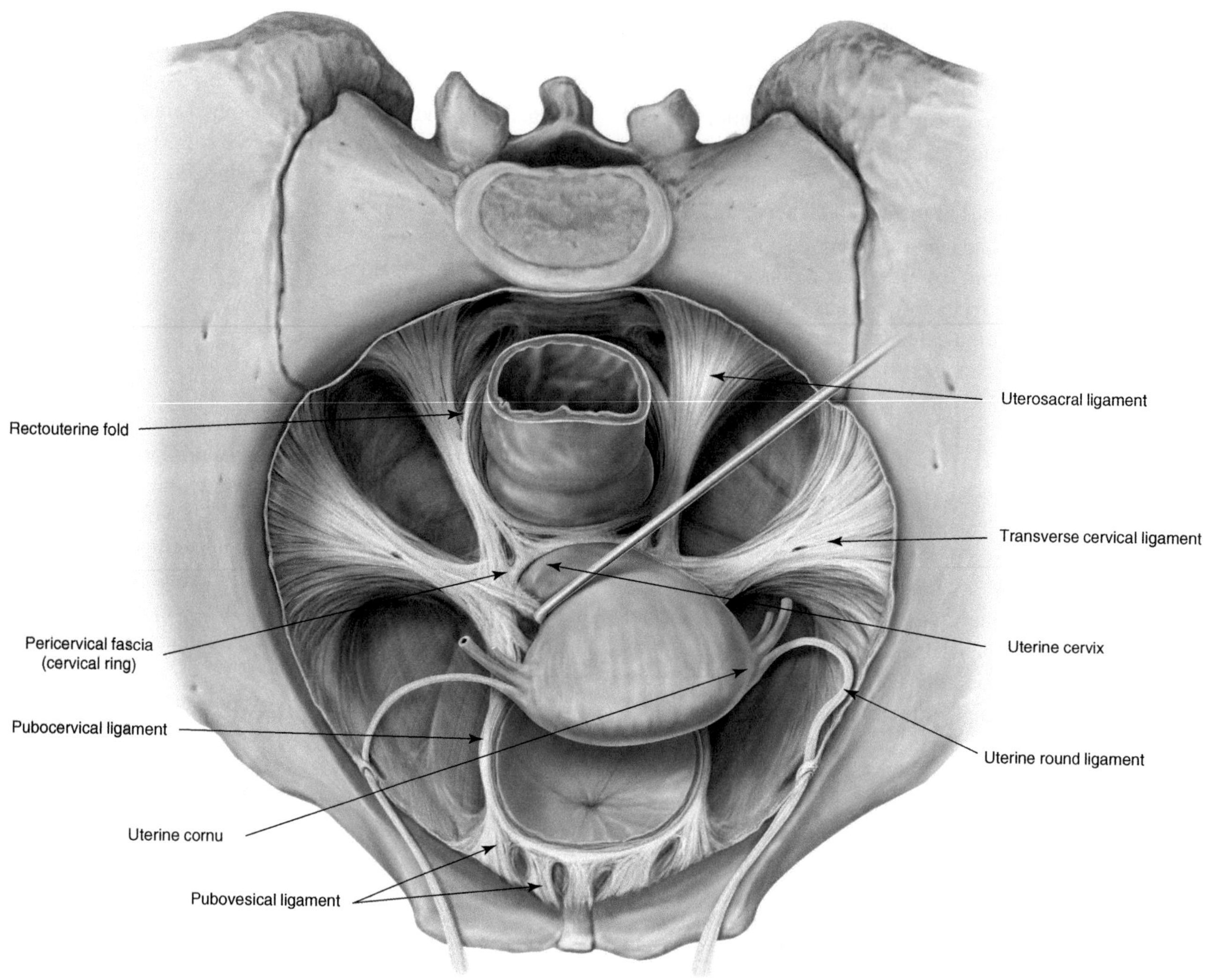

Fig. 3.4 Uterine ligaments. Cranial view. Rectum and urinary bladder are cut transversely, the uterus is shifted to the left side (Reproduced from Schünke et al. [24])

ian blood vessels. The synonym "suspensory ligament of the ovary" is inadequate, as the ovary is not substantially suspended by this peritoneal duplicature. When mobilizing the uterine adnexa, attention should be paid to the fact that the infundibulopelvic ligament together with the ovarian blood vessels cross the external iliac blood vessels ca. 1–2 cm anterolateral to the ureter. Moreover, due to its considerable intraperitoneal mobility the ovary may come into close proximity to both the external and internal iliac vessels and the ureter at the pelvic brim (Figs. 3.1, 3.5, 3.6, 3.9, and 3.7).

The uterine tube is ca. 9–11 cm long and connects the tubal pole of the ovary with the uterus. The infundibulum of the uterine tube is funnel-shaped and displays several fimbriae of which the ovarian fimbria is attached to the tubal pole of the ovary. The widened ampulla shows a luminal diameter of up to 10 mm and narrows at the isthmus to 0.1–0.5 mm. The uterine or intramural portion of the uterine tube is ca. 10 mm long and opens into the uterine cavity via the uterine os located at the uterine cornu. The peritoneal fold raised by the uterine tube corresponds to the mesosalpinx and contains the tubal branch of the uterine artery (Figs. 3.3, 3.5, and 3.8) [3].

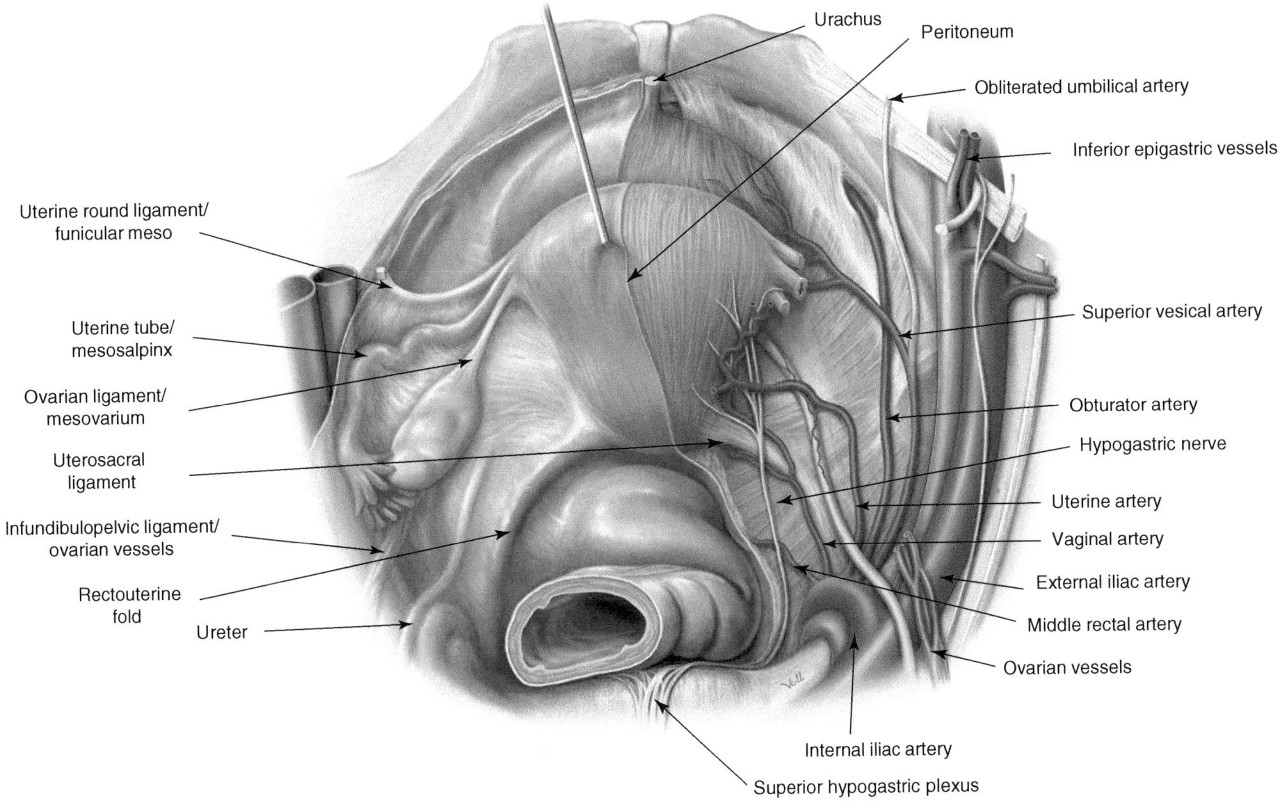

Fig. 3.5 Female pelvic cavity. Cranial view. The peritoneum, uterine adnexa and parametrial tissue are removed on the right side to expose the pelvic arteries and the ureter (Reproduced from Schünke et al. [24])

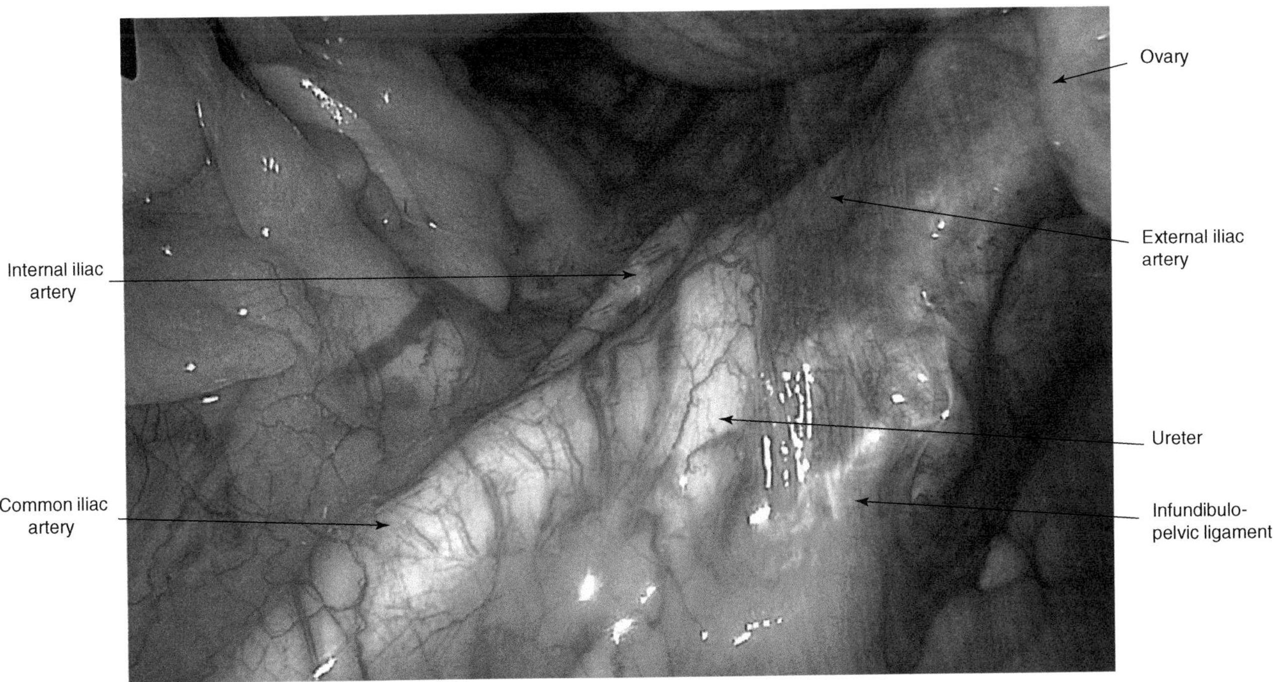

Fig. 3.6 Iliac vessels at the entrance into the right-sided female pelvis. Laparoscopic cranial view. The ureter crosses the pelvic brim running over the external iliac artery and medially to the infundibulopelvic ligament and the ovary

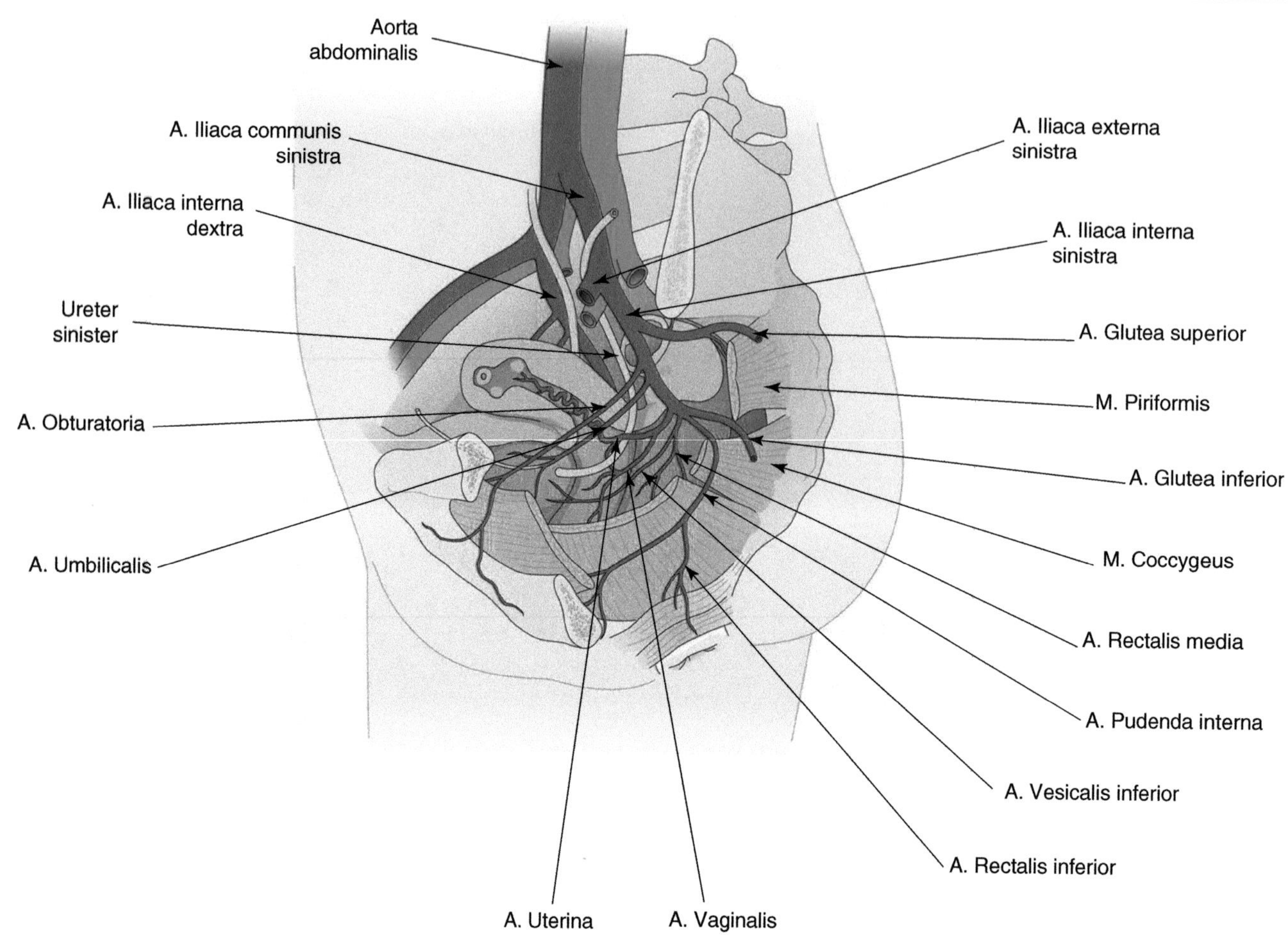

Fig. 3.7 Branches of the internal iliac artery in a female pelvis. Parasagittal section, view form left side. The left broad ligament is sectioned (Reproduced from Schünke et al. [24])

Uterine Ligaments, Parametrium and Mesometrium

Fixation of the uterovaginal complex is achieved on the one hand by the support of the pelvic floor (Fig. 3.2), on the other hand by uterine ligaments providing connections either to other pelvic organs or to the pelvic wall (Fig. 3.4). There is still an ongoing discussion about the exact tissue composition, topographic anatomy, functional relevance and terminology of these ligamentous, parauterine structures [1, 2, 4–7].

Broad Ligaments

The broad ligaments are named according to the fact that they provide a wide-stretched and ample connection between the middle pelvic compartment and the pelvic side walls. The peritoneal covering is lifted up by the broad ligaments and descends anteriorly to cover the paravesical space (anterior leaf) and posteriorly to cover the pararectal space (posterior leaf) on both sides. When viewed from above, the broad ligaments display three peritoneal folds on each side converging from different origins of the inner abdominal and pelvic walls towards the uterine cornu (Fig. 3.5):

- Funicular meso (anterior fold)
- Mesosalpinx (middle fold)
- Mesovarium (posterior fold)

The funicular meso corresponds to the peritoneal fold raised by the uterine round ligament extending from the uterine fundus below and lateral to the uterine cornu to the deep inguinal ring. The fibromuscular bands pass along the paravesical fossa and are accompanied by a branch from the uter-

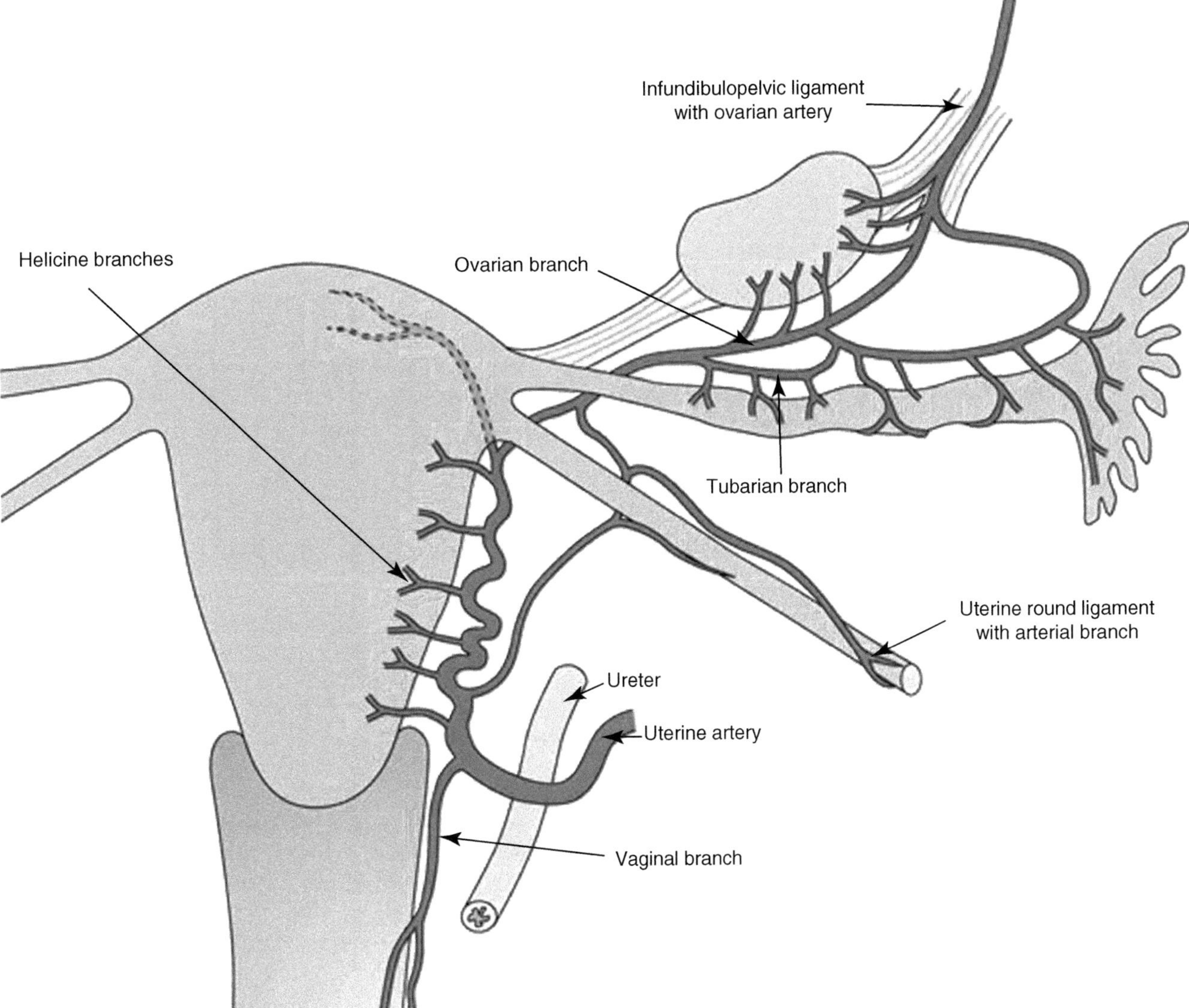

Fig. 3.8 Arterial supply of internal female organs. Ventral view. Branches of the left ovarian and uterine artery (Reproduced from Schünke et al. [24])

ine artery and lymphatic vessels draining to superficial inguinal lymph nodes. The mesovarium and mesosalpinx have been described previously (see section "Uterine Adnexa").

Parametrium and Transverse Cervical Ligaments

Beneath the peritoneal covering the broad ligaments consist of condensed connective tissue connecting the pelvic side walls with the uterus (parametrium) and the vagina (paracolpium) – comparable to those densifications of connective tissue extending lateral to the urinary bladder (paracystium) and rectum (paraproctium). The fibrous tissue contained within the parametrium/paracolpium corresponds to the transverse cervical ligaments (cardinal ligaments) which predominantly attach to the uterine cervix and vaginal fornix. Although composed of connective tissue providing a certain degree of mechanical suspension, the transverse cervical ligaments primarily resemble a mesentery-like structure serving as main routes of vascular, lymphatic and nervous supply of the uterus. The transverse cervical ligaments and parametrial tissue compartment are ca. 10 cm long and traversed by the ureter at its intermediate segment (Figs. 3.3, 3.4, 3.5, 3.10, 3.11, and 3.12) [4–6].

Uterosacral Ligaments

The uterosacral ligaments (Figs. 3.3, 3.4, and 3.5) attach to the uterine cervix and upper vagina and are often confluent with the uterine insertion site of the transverse cervical ligaments.

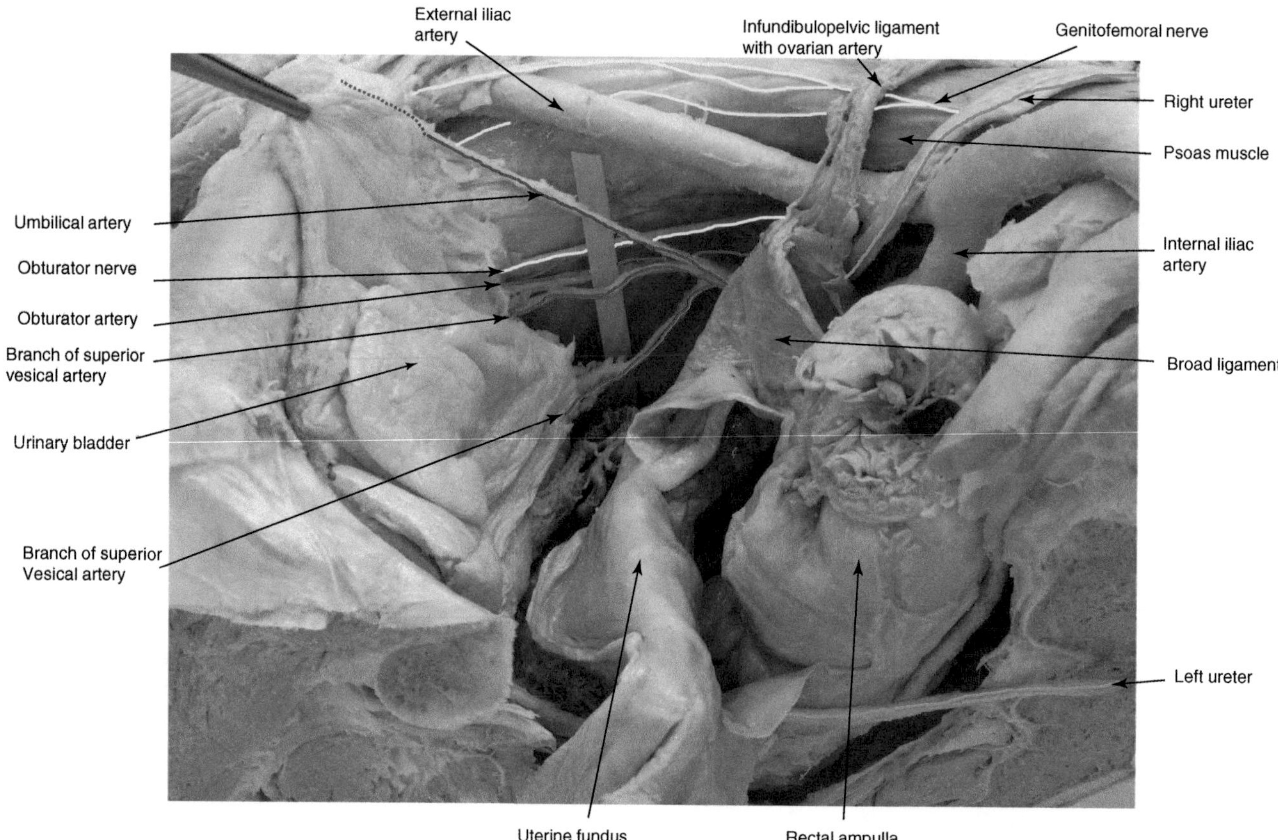

Fig. 3.9 Female right-sided hemipelvis. Parasagittal section, view from left side. The peritoneum is partially removed and incised, the anterior leaf of the right broad ligament is reflected dorsally, the urachus and the bladder roof are pulled upwards by a forceps, the obturator artery and nerve are marked by a yellow plastic strip. Arteries are highlighted by *red lines*, nerves by *yellow lines*, the ureter by *green line*. Formaldehyde-fixed specimen (same specimen also displayed in Fig. 3.10)

The fibrous bands extend dorsally along the rectal sidewalls to reach the sacrum. On their way to the sacrum they create the rectouterine folds and fan out before inserting at the sacral vertebrae S2–S4. The uterosacral ligaments serve as suspension of the uterine cervix and the vaginal tube ensuring the craniodorsal orientation of its long axis. In close proximity extend autonomic nerve fibers of the inferior hypogastric plexus passing immediately lateral to the uterosacral ligaments [4, 7–9].

Pubocervical Ligaments

The pubocervical ligaments (Fig. 3.4) connect the back side of the pubic bone with the uterine cervix. On their way to the uterus the pubocervical ligaments diverge around the urethra and bladder neck. In fact, all uterine ligaments – transverse cervical ligaments from both sides, uterosacral ligaments from behind, and pubocervical ligaments from front – insert at the uterine cervix. The insertion site is reinforced by a connective tissue condensation radially running around the uterine cervix termed cervical ring or pericervical fascia.

Mesometrium

The term mesometrium refers to the embryologically defined tissue compartment of the middle pelvic compartment that contains the neurovascular supply and major lymphatic drainage routes of the uterus – comparable to the mesorectum wrappend around the rectum in the posterior pelvic compartment. The mesometrium actually corresponds to the parametrial tissue, however further emphasizing its mesentery-like function provided by the lymphofatty tissue and accompanying uterine blood vessels and its clear delineation by fascial envelopes preventing early tumor transgression [6, 10].

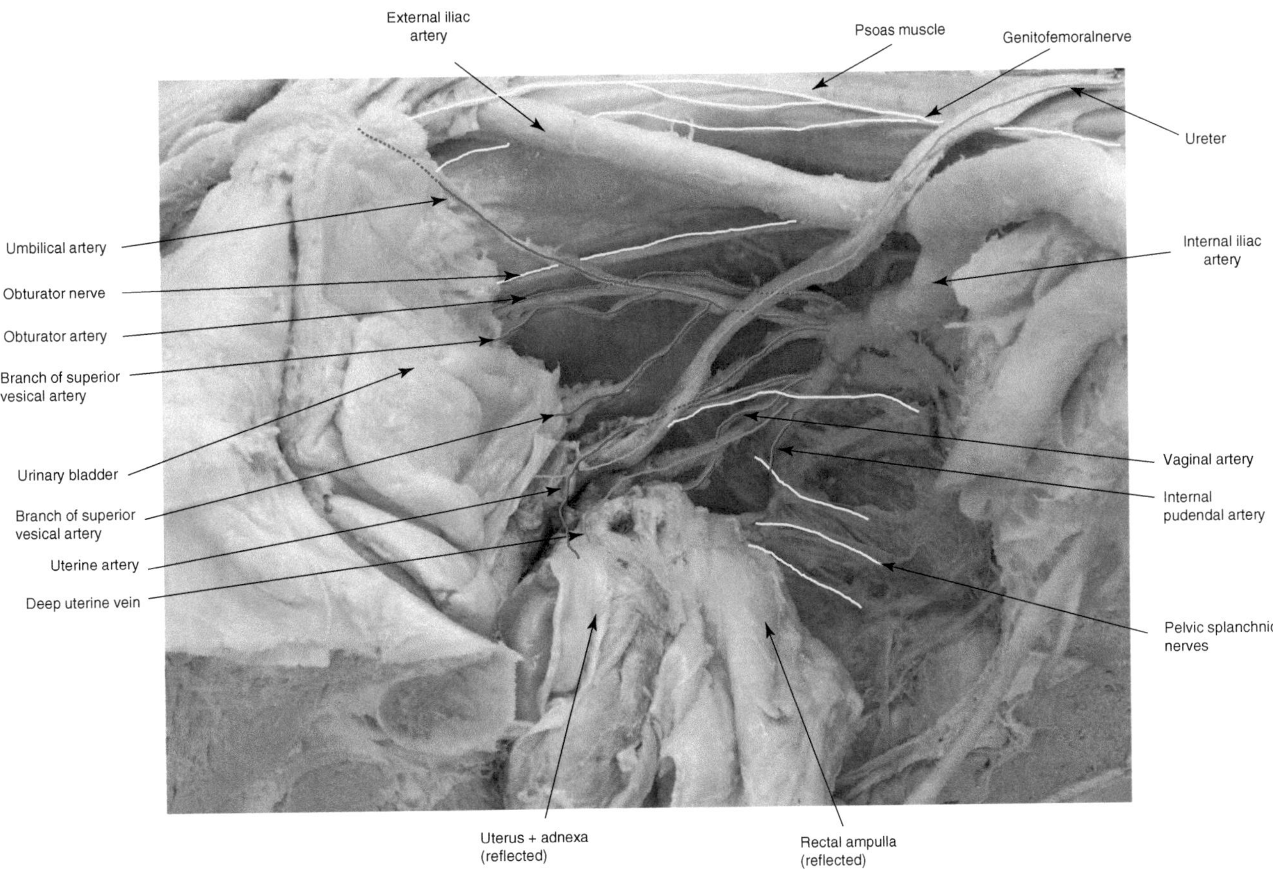

Fig. 3.10 Female right-sided hemipelvis. Parasagittal section, view from left side. The peritoneum is partially removed and incised, uterus and rectum are shifted to the left side to expose the blood vessels, nerves and ureter at the right pelvic sidewall. Arteries are highlighted by *red lines*, veins by *blue lines*, nerves by *yellow lines*, the ureter by *green line*. Formaldehyde-fixed specimen (same specimen also displayed in Fig. 3.9)

The clinical significance of the mesometrium has received special attention after the introduction of total mesometrial resection (TMME) for uterine cancer – in turn comparable to total mesorectal excision (TME) [11] carried for rectal cancer or complete mesocolic excision (CME) [12] recently introduced for colon cancer. All these surgical approaches are commonly based on the concept that tumor spread is initially confined to permissive ontogenetic compartments and its corresponding lymh node basins, so that complete removal of these embryologically defined packages will result in both optimal tumor control and low morbidity, if the resection margins are properly respected [10, 13, 14].

The uterine tubes, uterus and upper vagina are derivates of the paramesonephric ducts (Müllerian ducts). The distal fusion of the Müllerian ducts induces the development of the uterovaginal canal and the formation of the broad ligaments and the mesometrial tissue. According to Höckel the mesometrium can be subdivided into a vascular mesometrium containing the uterine vessels and surrounding lymphofatty tissue with mesometrial lymph nodes and a ligamentous mesometrium corresponding to the uterosacral ligaments and rectovaginal septum [10].

Blood Vessel Supply of Female Pelvic Viscera

The female pelvic viscera are mainly supplied by the internal iliac arteries (Figs. 3.5, 3.6, and 3.7) [3] The common iliac arteries originate at the aortic bifurcation in front of the left side of the fourth lumbar vertebra. They pass along the medial borders of the psoas major muscle without giving off branches and diverge into external and internal iliac arteries. Whereas the external iliac arteries follow the psoas major muscle until traversing the lacuna vasorum through the femoral ring to reach the lower limb, the internal iliac arteries descend into the pelvic cavity in posterocaudal direction over ca. 4 cm and then divide into an anterior and posterior trunk. To expose the inter-

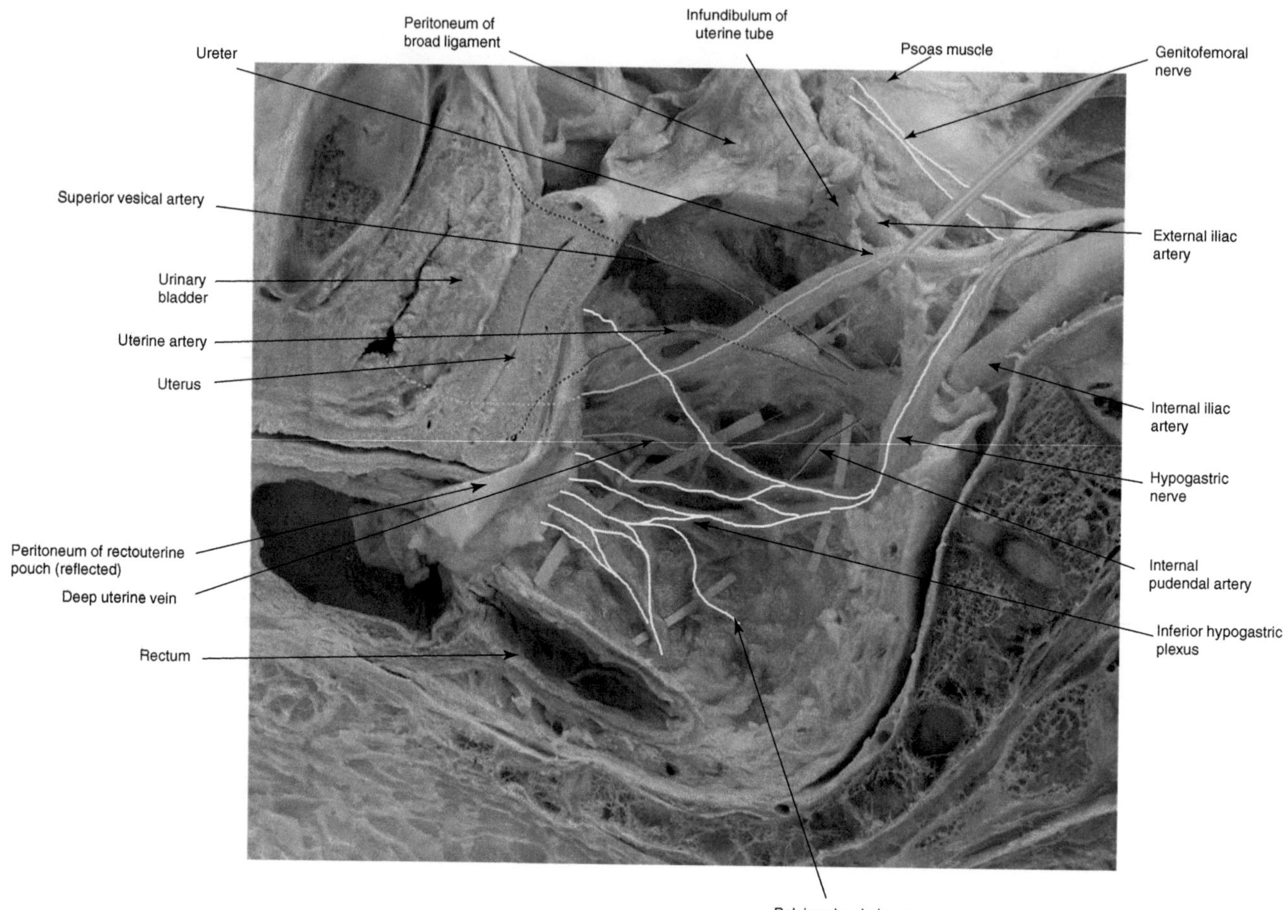

Fig. 3.11 Female right-sided hemipelvis. Midsagittal section, view from left side. The peritoneum is partially removed and shifted to the left side to expose the blood vessels, nerves and ureter at the right pelvic sidewall. The ureter is marked by a green vessel loop, the pelvic autonomic nerve plexus by yellow plastic strips, the uterine artery by a red plastic strip, the uterine vein by a blue plastic strip. In addition, arteries are highlighted by *red lines*, veins by *blue lines*, nerves by *yellow lines*, the ureter by *green line*. Formaldehyde-fixed specimen

nal iliac artery the adjacent and sometimes overlying infundibulopelvic ligament and ovary have to be shifted upwards. The common, external and internal iliac veins are located medially or dorsomedially to their arterial counterparts.

The anterior trunk or division of the internal iliac artery comprises the following branches:

Superior Vesical Artery

The superior vesical artery (Figs. 3.5, 3.7, 3.8, 3.9, 3.10, 3.11, and 3.12) is the first visceral branch and corresponds to the proximal, patent segment of the fetal umbilical artery. The artery follows the pelvic sidewall medially to the obturator vessels and nerve and craniolaterally to the urinary bladder. Before reaching the urinary bladder the superior vesical artery splits into various branches mostly for the vesical fundus and corpus but also for the distal ureter. The obliterated segment corresponds to the medial umbilical ligament ascending from the vesical fundus along the anterior abdominal wall to the umbilicus thereby forming the medial umbilical fold underneath the parietal peritoneum (Figs. 3.20 and 3.21). Gentle traction applied to the medial umbilical ligament allows easy identification of the superior vesical artery and usually thereby also of the uterine artery, as both arteries originate either from a common trunk or close to each other.

Uterine Artery

The uterine arteries supply (Figs. 3.5, 3.7, 3.8, 3.10, 3.11, 3.12, and 3.13) the entire uterus including the uterine tubes and uterine round ligaments and also the upper third of the vagina. The uterine artery originates from the internal iliac artery either as a separate branch or as a common trunk together with the superior vesical artery. Although the superior vesical and uterine arteries supply different pelvic compartments, vesicovaginal anastomoses are often observed, in particular regarding the corresponding veins.

The uterine artery runs through the parametrial tissue covered by the broad ligament towards the uterine cervix. The ureter crosses underneath the uterine artery ca. 1–2 cm lateral to the uterine cervix and lateral vaginal fornix and receives a supplying branch. Whereas in most of the cases one single uterine artery is present on each side, multiple uterine veins of different sizes can be observed which drain the uterine venous plexus. The uterine veins often do not directly follow the course of the uterine artery, but often pass underneath the ureter. The most caudally located vein is also termed deep uterine vein.

The main branch of the uterine artery ascends lateral to the uterus in meander-like course towards the uterine cornu where it gives off an ovarian branch running within the mesovar and a tubal branch running within the mesosalpinx. These branches establish anastomoses with the ovarian artery. An additional branch originates at the uterine cornu to follow and supply the uterine round ligament.

From the tortuous segment of the uterine artery multiple helicine branches enter in the uterine wall, divide into arcuate arteries and supply the myometrial and endometrial layers by giving off radial and spiral branches. The right and left uterine arteries establish extensive intramural anastomotic connections across the midline, so that the uterine blood supply is not seriously compromised after unilateral ligation. At the level of the uterine cervix branches descend to the vagina and anastomose with branches of the vaginal artery to form two longitudinal vessels. These vaginal azygos arteries run along the anterior and posterior vaginal wall.

Vaginal Artery

In addition to vaginal branches of the uterine artery one or more arteries originating from the internal iliac artery directly run to the vagina. These vaginal arteries (Figs. 3.5, 3.7, and 3.10) correspond to the inferior vesical artery in males and supply thc vagina, vaginal vestibule as well as the vesical trigone and urethra.

Middle Rectal Artery

The last visceral branch of the internal iliac artery is the middle rectal artery (Figs. 3.5 and 3.7) running above the levator ani muscle within the lateral rectal pedicles together with autonomic nerve fibers of the rectal plexus to reach the rectal wall. However, in contrast to both the superior vesical and uterine arteries the middle rectal arteries are much smaller in size and inconstantly present, as the rectal blood supply is mainly provided by the more promiment superior rectal artery running within the mesorectum (Figs. 3.17 and 3.18).

Obturator Artery

The obturator artery (Figs. 3.5, 3.7, 3.9, 3.10, and 3.13) is one of the first branches of the internal iliac artery. However, it does not primarily supply the pelvic viscera, but leaves the pelvic cavity via the obturator canal to approach the adductor muscles of the medial thigh. In the pelvis the artery passes medially to the internal obturator muscle and caudally to the obturator nerve which converges with the obturator vascular pedicle at the entrance foramen of the obturator canal. At its proximal segment the obturator artery is located in close proximity both to the ureter and the ovary and it gives off iliac branches supplying the iliopsoas muscle. From the distal segment vesical branches may ramify and pass medially to the urinary bladder.

Frequently, an anastomotic connection between the obturator and inferior epigastric artery is provided by a pubic branch running across the pubic bone over the pectineal ligament (Figs. 3.13, 3.14, and 3.20). A prominent pubic branch is also termed corona mortis ("crown of death"), because in earlier times an inadvertent injury of this vessel during inguinal or femoral hernia repair has led to serious bleedings. In up to one third of cases the obturator artery does not originate from the internal iliac artery but from the inferior epigastric artery or even the external iliac artery sending an enlarged pubic branch directly towards the obturator canal. In any case, special attention should be payed to these vascular variations, when operating in the obturator fossa and paravesical space, e.g. for extended pelvic lymphadenectomy.

Internal Pudendal Artery

The internal pudendal artery (Figs. 3.7, 3.10, and 3.11) is one of the terminal branches of the anterior division of the internal iliac artery and supplies the perineal region, anal canal, external genital organs, and pelvic floor muscles. The artery descends laterally in front of the piriformis muscle and sacral nerve plexus roots, leaves the pelvis through the infrapiriform hiatus of the greater sciatic foramen and bends around the ischial spine to enter into the ischioanal fossa via the lesser sciatic foramen. The artery is accompanied medially by the internal pudendal vein and pudendal nerve. Branches of the internal pudendal artery include muscular branches for the pelvic and gluteal region, inferior rectal artery, perineal arteries, posterior labial branches, branches to the vestibular bulb and vaginal introitus, deep and dorsal artery of the clitoris.

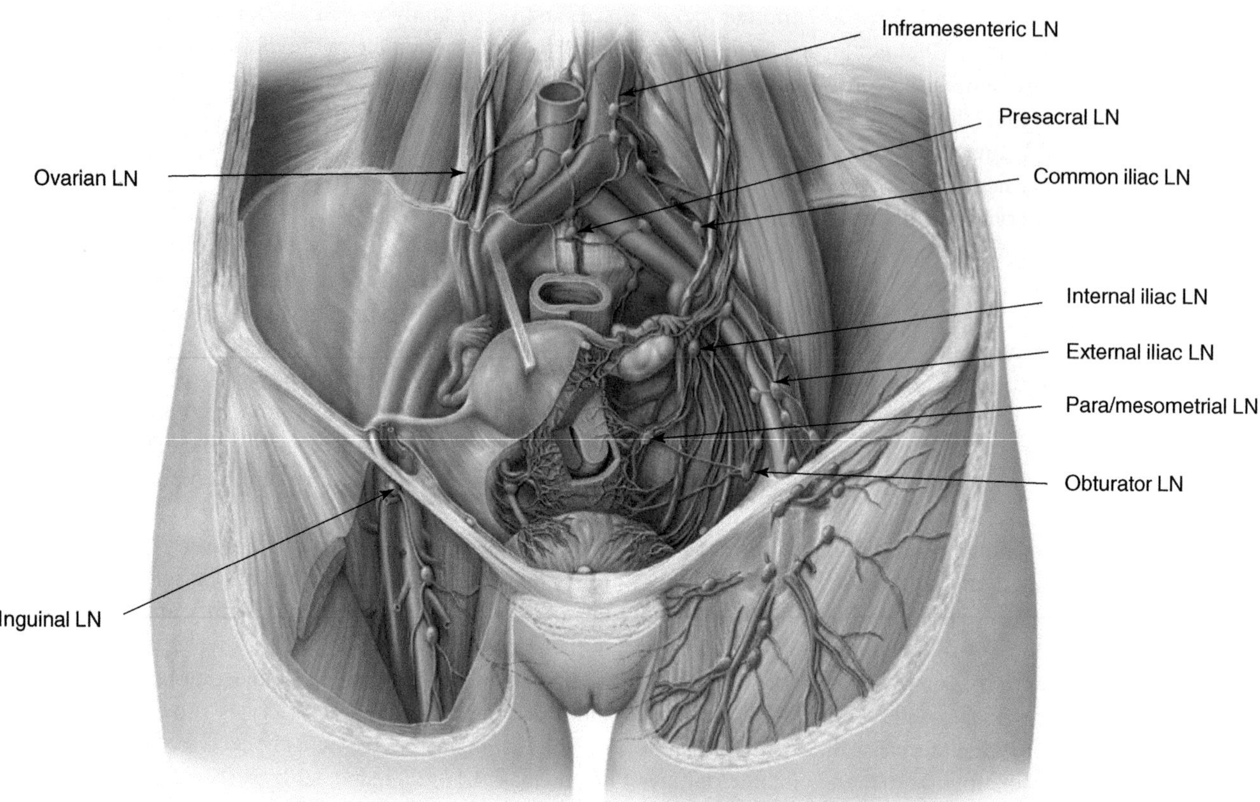

Fig. 3.12 Lymph nodes (LN) and lymphatic drainage of female genital organs. Ventral view. The uterus is shifted to the right side, the peritoneum is removed on the left side and above the aortic bifurcation (Reproduced from Schünke et al. [24])

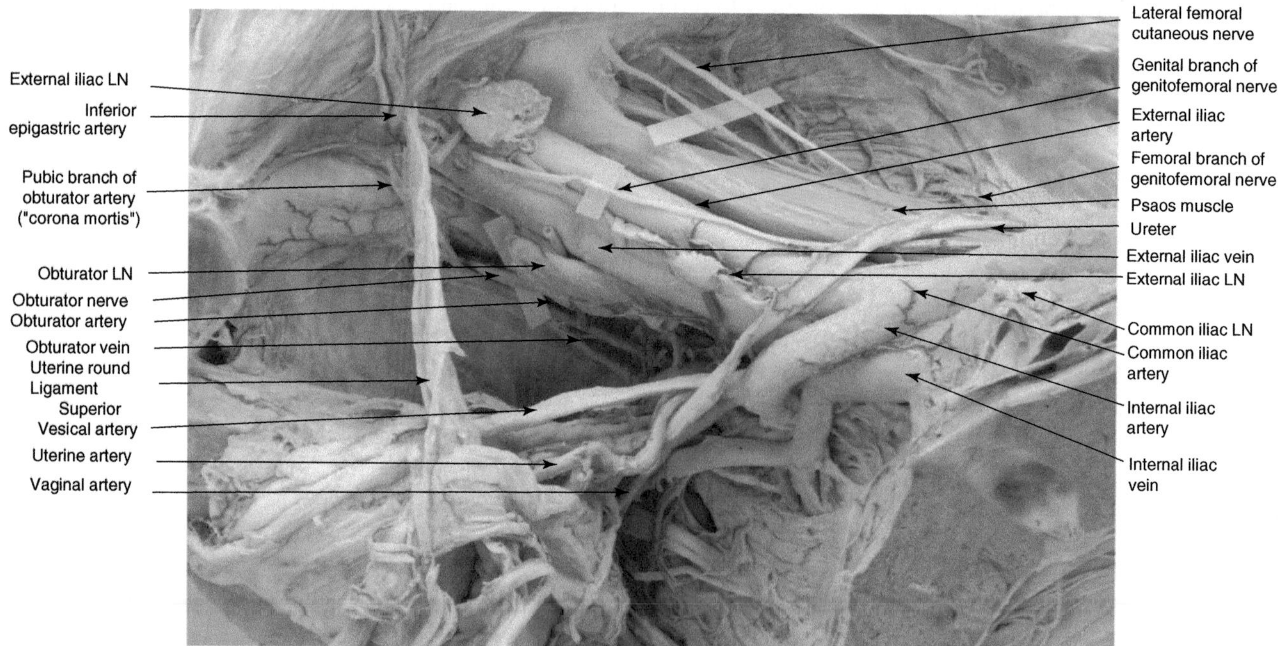

Fig. 3.13 Female right-sided hemipelvis, view from left side. The peritoneum is completely removed and the pelvic viscera are shifted to the left side to expose the blood vessels, nerves and ureter at the right pelvic sidewall. Lymph nodes (LN) are marked by green plastic tubes, nerves by yellow plastic strips. Formaldehyde-fixed specimen

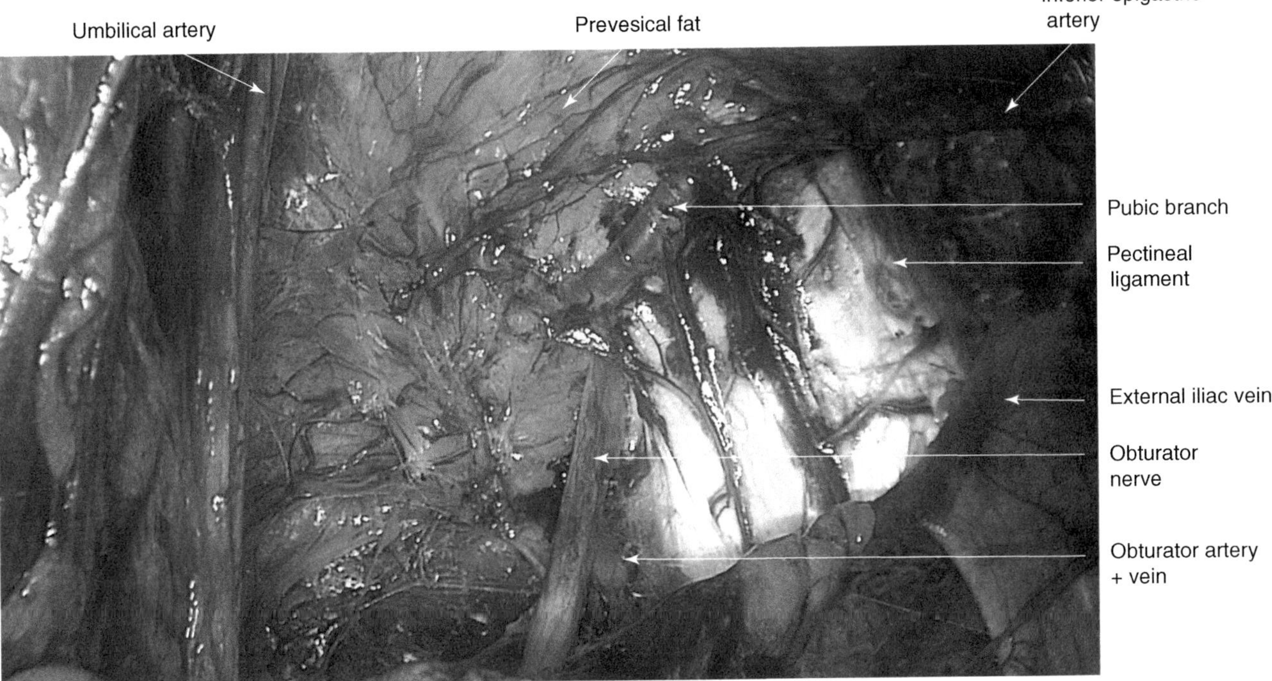

Fig. 3.14 Exposure of right-sided prevesical space and obturator fossa. Laparoscopic cranial view. A prominent pubic branch is visible crossing the pectineal ligament and the superior pubic ramus

Inferior Gluteal Artery

The inferior gluteal artery (Fig. 3.7) is the other terminal branch of the anterior division of the internal iliac artery, however often originating from a common stem together with the internal pudendal artery. It also decends anterior to the piriformis muscle and sacral nerve plexus, but then passes posteriorly between the ventral rami of the sacral spinal nerves and traverse the infrapiriform hiatus of the greater sciatic foramen to reach the gluteal and posterior femoral region.

The posterior trunk or division of the internal iliac artery comprises the following branches:

Iliolumbar Artery

The iliolumbar artery is the only ascending branch of the internal iliac artery passing posterior to the external iliac vessels and obturator nerve in front of the sacroiliac joint to reach the psoas muscle. The iliac and lumbar branches supply the muscles of the corresponding regions and establish anastomoses with the gluteal and deep circumflex iliac arteries.

Lateral Sacral Arteries

Usually a superior and inferior branch originate from the internal iliac artery, descend and approach the anterior sacral foramina to supply the sacral canal and dorsal sacral region. The lateral sacral arteries anastomose from both sides with the median sacral artery.

Superior Gluteal Artery

The superior gluteal artery (Fig. 3.7) corresponds to the terminal branch of the posterior division of the internal iliac artery. Immediately after its origin the large vessel traverses between the first ventral rami of the sacral spinal nerves to leave the pelvis via the suprapiriform hiatus of the greater sciatic foramen. Deep and superficial branches of the superior gluteal artery supply the gluteal and sacral region and anastomose with the inferior gluteal, deep circumflex iliac and circumflex femoral arteries.

Pelvic Veins

As a general rule, larger veins such as the common, external and internal iliac veins follow the course of their arterial counterparts. In most cases, the veins run medially or dorsomedially to the arteries. The same observation holds true for most of the parietal branches (e.g. obturator, pudendal, gluteal veins) of the internal iliac artery, whereas the visceral branches display different features: the urinary bladder, uterus and vagina are drained by venous plexus which are interconnected with each other and release the blood into multiple vesical, vaginal and uterine veins. These veins do

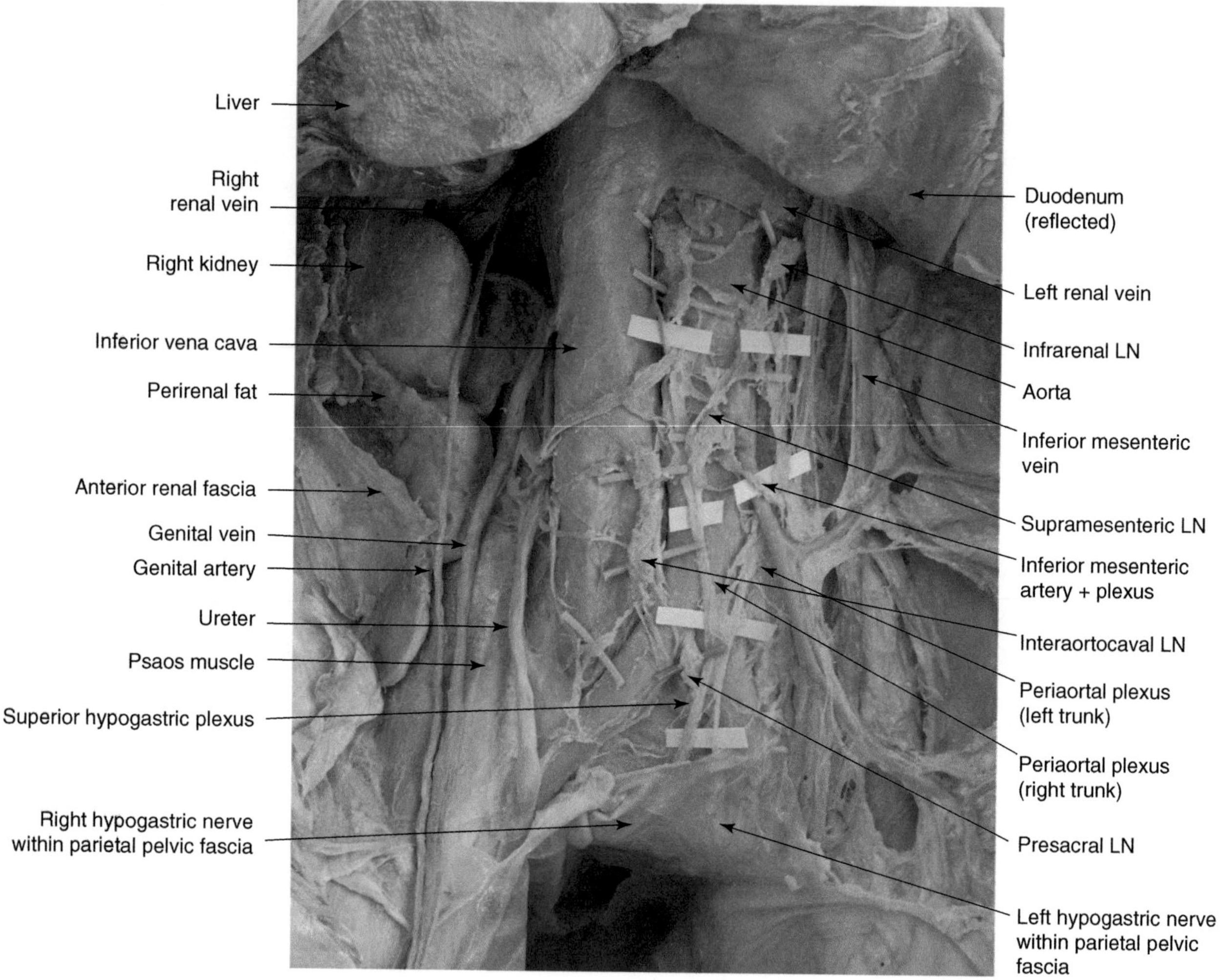

Fig. 3.15 Prevertebral and retroperitoneal region. Ventral view. The parietal peritoneum is removed down to the entrance into the pelvic cavity on both sides, the anterior renal fascia is removed on the left side. Lymph nodes (LN) are marked by green plastic tubes, nerves by yellow plastic strips. Formaldehyde-fixed specimen

not strictly accompany and parallel the arteries until they have entered into the internal iliac vein.

It has to be emphasized that during laparoscopic or roboter assisted surgery, pelvic veins often collapse due to the intraperitoneal pressure exerted by gas insufflation onto the thin venous walls. Thus, special care must be taken to clearly identify and respect the pelvic veins, because injury may occur inadvertently and lead to troublesome bleeding sometimes only evident after diminishing the intraperitoneal pressure.

Lymph Nodes and Lymphatic Drainage of the Uterus and Uterine Adnexa

In general, lymphatic drainage follows the blood supply of the corresponding organs and is realized by a network of rather thin-walled lymphatic vessels and lymph nodes grouped along the nutrient vascular branches and enveloped by fatty and loosely arranged connective tissue. As the arterial supply of the uterus and uterine adnexa originates from two sources (uterine and ovarian arteries), the main lymphatic drainage involves both pelvic and paraaortic routes and is therefore complex and multidirectional due to the peculiar ontogenetic anatomy of the female genital tract [3]. However, direct lymphatic drainage pathways into the anterior pelvic compartment via the vesicouterine ligaments or into the posterior compartment via the uterosacral ligaments could not be demonstrated [15, 16].

Lymphadenectomy is considered to be an integral component of the surgical treatment for uterine carcinoma. Due to the topographic complexity of lymphatic drainage and close proximity between lymph nodes and both blood vessels and nerves, pelvic and paraaortic lymph node dissection are challenging and often time consuming procedures. Therefore, profound anatomical knowledge of the different lymph node

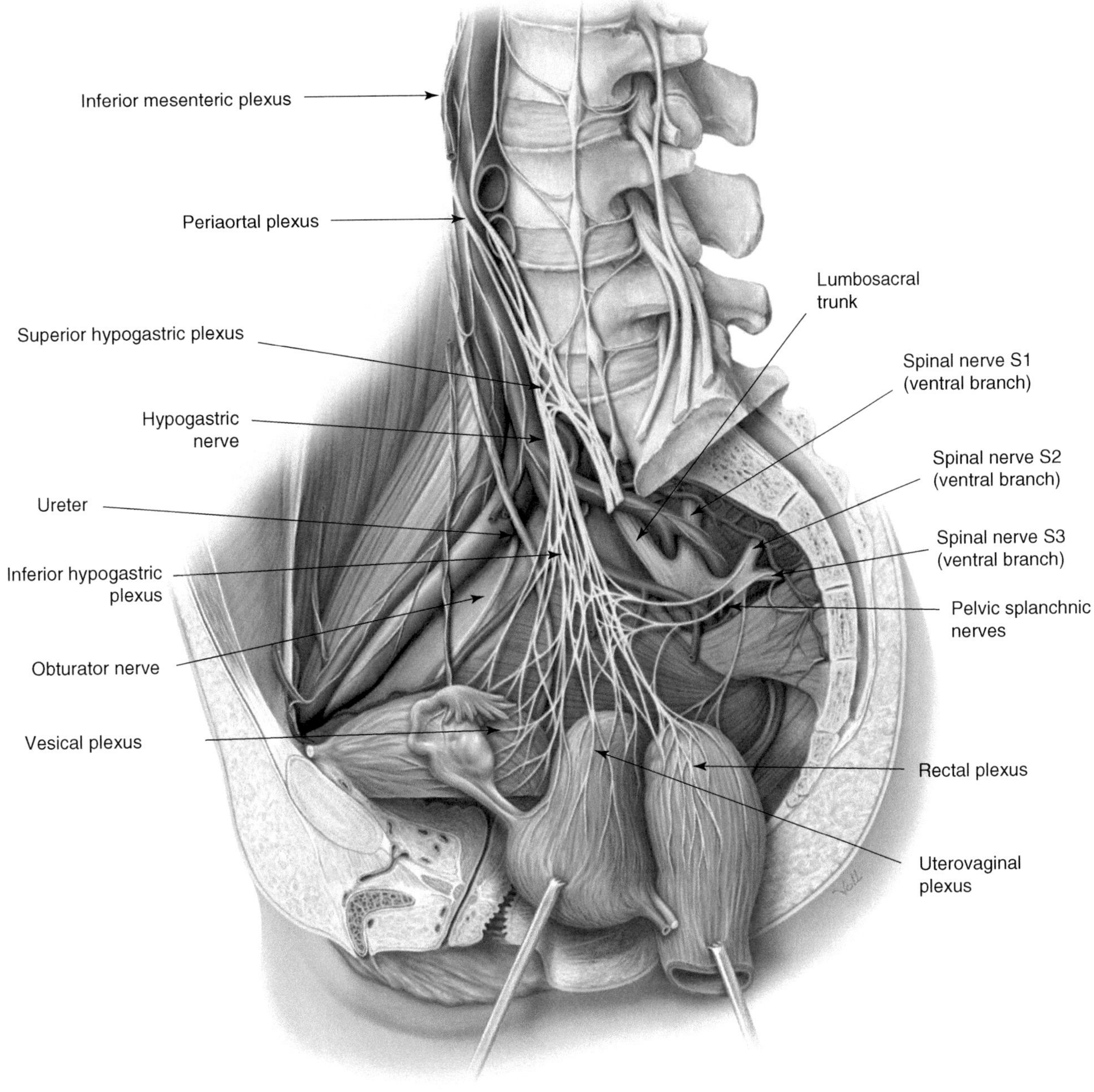

Fig. 3.16 Nerve supply of female pelvic viscera. Midsagittal section, view from left side. Uterus and rectum are shifted to the left side to expose the pelvic autonomic nerve plexus, (Reproduced from Schünke et al. [24])

regions is required to be familiar with the anatomical landmarks which help to identify and preserve structures at risk when removing the areolar fibrofatty tissue pads harbouring the relevant lymph nodes.

The pelvic lymphatic system is composed of parietal lymph nodes and trunks following the major pelvic blood vessels and of organ-related lymph nodes intercalated into the different mesenteries supplying the pelvic viscera. The following pelvic lymph node compartments or basins can be described: [13, 17, 18].

External Iliac Lymph Nodes

The external iliac lymph basin (Figs. 3.9, 3.10, 3.12, and 3.13) extends from the common iliac bifurcation down to the femoral ring along the psoas muscle. The medial border of the compartment is defined by the paravesical and obturator fossa. Lymph nodes may be further subdivided into a lateral group located between the external iliac vessels and the psoas muscle, an intermediate group between the artery and vein, and a medial group between the vein and the pelvic

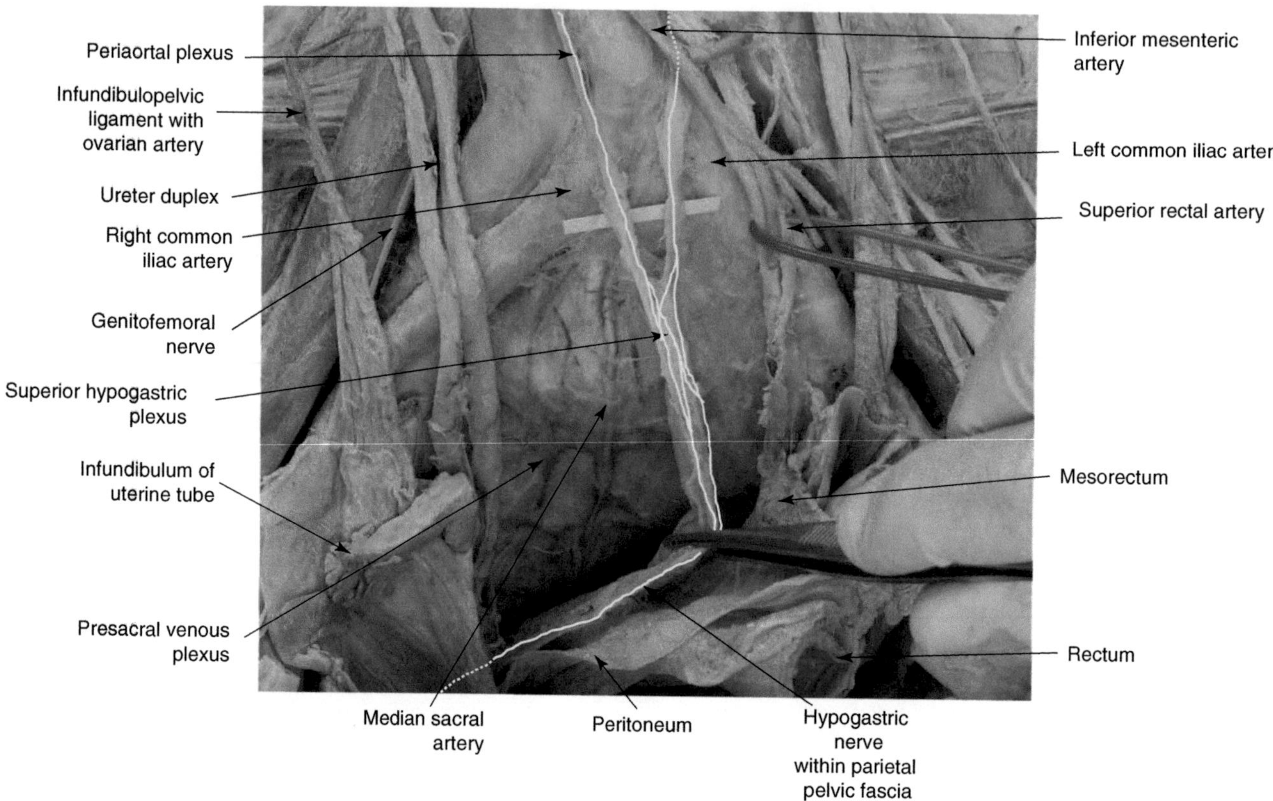

Fig. 3.17 Presacral region of a female pelvis. Ventral view. The peritoneum is removed, the rectum and mesorectum are shifted ventrally towards the left side, the pelvic parietal fascia is grasp by a forceps and also pushed ventrally to left side. The superior rectal artery is marked by a red vessel loop, the autonomic nerves are highlighted by *yellow lines* and plastric strip. Formaldehyde-fixed specimen

sidewall. Structures at risk during lymph node dissection are the external iliac vessels, in particular the vein when lifted up for harvesting medial lymph nodes, and the genitofemoral nerve when harvesting lymph nodes lateral to external iliac vessels. In some instances, minor branches originating from external iliac vessels to supply the psoas muscle may be torn and bleed during lymph node removal in this compartment.

Internal Iliac Lymph Nodes

Internal iliac lymph nodes (Figs. 3.10, 3.11, 3.12, and 3.13) follow the anterior and posterior trunk of the internal iliac artery and its corresponding branches, thus collecting lymphatic fluid from parietal/somatic structures, e.g. gluteal, perineal, sacral regions, as well as visceral organs, e.g. bladder, uterus, rectum. The compartment originates at the common iliac bifurcation and extends dorsally onto the piriformis muscle, caudally down to the levator ani muscle and ventrally to the origin of the visceral arterial branches for the urinary bladder and uterus. Most important for lymph node dissection is the direct vicinity of both the ureter and the delicate branches of the inferior hypogastric plexus approaching the internal iliac branches and lymph nodes from the medial side.

Common Iliac Lymph Nodes

The common iliac lymph nodes (Figs. 3.9, 3.10, 3.12, and 3.13) drain the external and internal iliac lymph nodes and follow the common iliac vessels towards the aortic bifurcation. Like the external iliac lymph nodes, they can be further subdivided into a lateral group facing the iliolumbar fossa, an intermediate group intercalated between the common iliac vessels adjacent to the lumbosacral trunk, and a medial group located along the pelvic brim underneath the common iliac vein. Structures at risk during lymph node dissection are the genitofemoral nerve on the lateral side, the lumbosacral trunk and obturator nerve at the dorsocaudal aspect and the ureter crossing the common iliac bifurcation.

Presacral Lymph Nodes

In front of the promontorium and underneath the aortic bifurcation the bilateral common iliac lymph routes drain into presacral lymph nodes (Figs. 3.12, 3.15, 3.16, 3.17, and 3.18), also termed promontory, midsacral or subaortic lymph nodes. The presacral compartment extends from the aortic bifurcation down to the end of the second sacral vertebra.

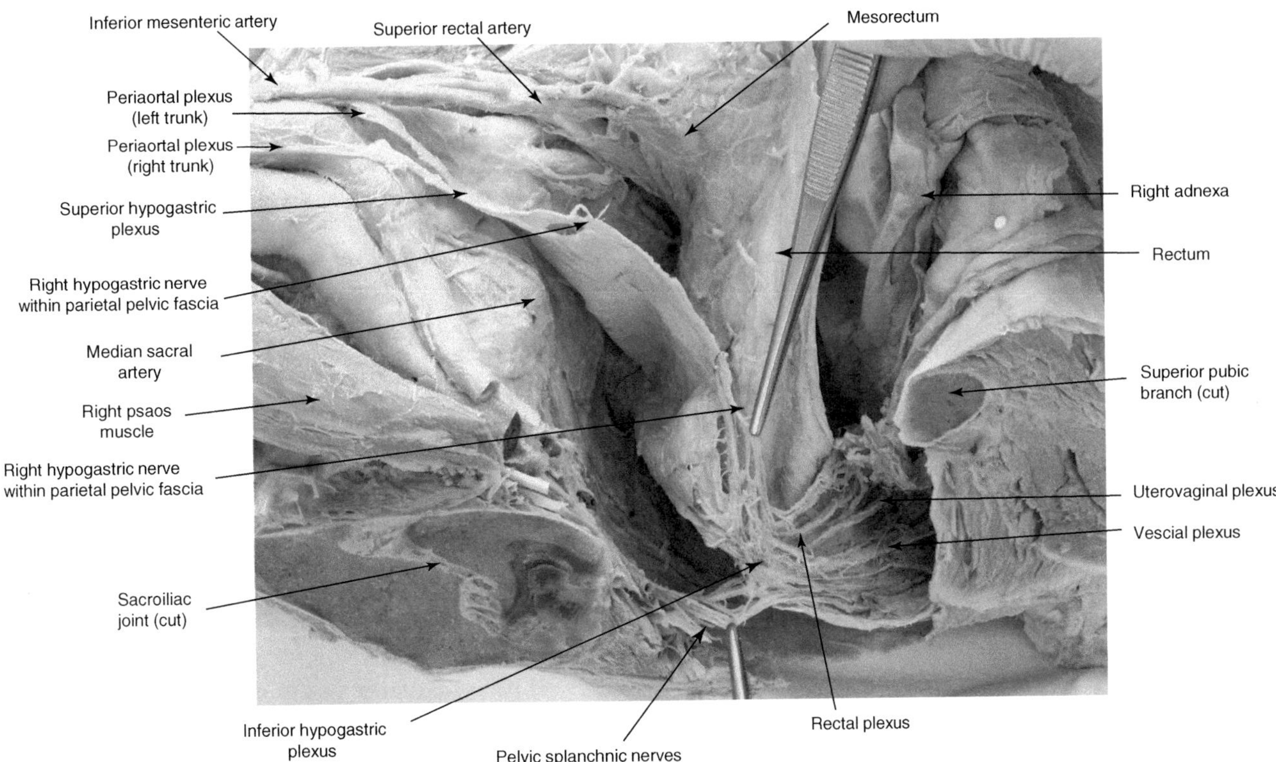

Fig. 3.18 Female left-sided hemipelvis. Parasagittal section, view from right side. The peritoneum is removed, the rectum and uterine adnexa are shifted ventrally, the forceps grasps the right hypogastric nerve embedded within the parietal pelvic fascia. Formaldehyde-fixed specimen with previous hysterectomy

Structures at risk during lymph node dissection are the median sacral artery and the presacral venous plexus as well as the thin-walled common iliac veins, in particular the left one due its exposed course running above the promontorium. Moreover, the promontorium region is crossed slightly left by the superior hypogastric plexus giving off the hypogastric nerves on both sides.

Obturator Lymph Nodes

The obturator lymph nodes (Figs. 3.9, 3.10, 3.12, 3.13, and 3.14) are distributed within the areolar fibrofatty tissue pad extending along the pelvic sidewall formed by the internal obturator muscle, the tendinous arcs of levator ani muscle and parietal pelvic fascia, and the levator ani muscle itself. The upper border is defined by the pelvic brim and the external iliac vessels, the dorsal border by the common iliac bifurcation, and the medial border by the visceral branches of the internal iliac artery. The obturator fossa is traversed by the neurovascular obturator pedicle composed of the obturator nerve recognizable by its pearl-white colour and the obturator artery and vein which join the nerve coming from below. The neurovascular obturator pedicle enters into the obturator canal beneath the superior pubic branch and frequently displays a pubic branch anastomosing with the inferior epigastric artery.

Lymph nodes in this compartment may be further subdivided into supraobturator (superficial) and infraobturator (deep) lymph nodes according to its position related to the obturator pedicle. Complete lymphadenectomy of the obturator fossa requires also subtle clearance of infraobturator nodes located below the obturator pedicle and along the upper surface of levator ani muscle. However, care must be taken not to injure the obturator pedicle itself as well as the neurovascular pedicles of the urinary bladder, in particular the vesical venous plexus.

Obturator and internal iliac lymph nodes may also be subsumed as paravisceral lymph nodes, as they are located adjacent to pelvic visceral organs which they drain – that is the urinary bladder and the uterus.

Parametrial/Mesometrial Lymph Nodes

Those lymph nodes located in close topographical vicinity to the uterus underneath the broad ligament (parametrium) and intercalated into the uterine mesentery (mesometrium)

correspond to the parametrial/mesometrial lymph nodes (Figs. 3.10, 3.11, and 3.12). They are embedded in areolar fibrofatty tissue and follow the branches of the uterine artery (vascular mesometrium). On the one hand, the aim of oncologic surgery is to completely remove these organ-related lymph nodes. On the other hand, the vesical neurovascular pedicles supplying the urinary bladder and the ureters crossing the parametrial compartment have to be preserved during lymphadenectomy of the parametrial/mesometrial tissue.

The paraaortic lymphatic system composed of the lumboaortic lymphatic chains extends beyond the pelvic lymph nodes and may be affected by lymphatic spread of tumors involving the uterine body and/or fundus and uterine adnexa. In these cases, lymphadenectomy should include removal of the lymph routes following the infundibulopelvic ligament and the ovarian vessels up to the paraaortic lymph basins. The following paraaortic lymh node compartments can be described:

Inframesenteric Lymph Nodes

Inframesenteric lymph nodes (Figs. 3.12 and 3.15) extend from the origin of the inferior mesenteric artery along the aorta and inferior vena cava down to the aortic and caval bifurcation. The lateral borders of this compartment are defined by the ureters running in front of the psoas muscles and undercrossing the ovarian vessels. On the left side, the ureter also undercrosses the root of the sigmoid mesocolon and the inferior mesenteric pedicle which has to be lifted up to achieve full exposure and protection of the ureter. The paraaortic lymph nodes are grouped into a readily discernible ventral chains including interaortocaval lymph nodes and less obvious dorsolateral chains. Thus, complete inframesenteric lymph node removal requires full exposure of both pericaval and periaortal tissue compartments.

However, dissection should be carried out carefully avoiding a too rigorous "cleaning" of the large prevertebral vessels to preserve or at least minimize the damage of the perivascular autonomic nervous network. Nerve fibers emerge from paravertebral sympathetic ganglia and form an aortic plexus composed of a left and right periaortal trunk with multiple interconnecting fibers crossing in front of the aortal wall. While the inferior mesenteric plexus follows the corresponding artery into the inferior mesenteric pedicle for the left and rectosigmoid colon, the superior hypogastric plexus descends in front of the aorta to divide in front of the promontorium into the left and right hypogastric nerves. Preservation of these autonomic nerve plexus is best achieved, when both the inferior mesenteric pedicle and superior hypogastric plexus are gently lifted up to gain access to the paraaortic lymph nodes. Care should also be taken to preserve the segmental lumbar arteries and veins and the small blood vessels approaching the ureter from the medial side.

Supramesenteric/Infrarenal Lymph Nodes

Supramesenteric lymph nodes (Fig. 3.15) include those lymph nodes of the paraaortic compartment located superior to the inferior mesenteric root and inferior to the left renal vein. Like in the inframesenteric compartment, supramesenteric lymph nodes are grouped around and in between the large vessels. Additionally, lymph nodes from the renal hilus drain into this compartment and autonomic nerve fibers derived from the aortic nerve plexus diverge to both sides to form the renal nerve plexus following the corresponding vessels (Fig. 3.12).

Autonomic Nerves of the Female Pelvis

As pointed out in the introduction, the challenge of oncologic surgery is twofold: aiming at the highest radicalness to ensure curative therapy and lowest loss of function to maintain quality of life after surgery. The latter one depends essentially on the preservation of those autonomic sympathetic and parasympathetic nerves mediating urogenital and anorectal functions [8, 9, 19–21].

Sympathetic nerves support the filling phase of the urinary bladder under resting conditions by relaxing the detrusor vesicae muscle and closing the internal urethral sphincter and bladder neck, thereby contributing to urinary continence. For controlled micturition, parasympathetic nerves suppress the sympathetic input and initiate contraction of the detrusor vesicae muscle and opening of the urethra and bladder neck. Thus, injury of the vesical nerve plexus may lead to both urinary incontinence and urinary bladder dysfunction.

Similar actions of autonomic nerves are also exerted for the control of anorectal function: While sympathetic nerves contribute to fecal continence by mediating internal anal sphincter contraction and rectal filling, parasympathetic nerves initiate defecation by relaxing the internal anal sphincter and enhancing rectal motility.

Moreover, both sympathetic and parasympathetic nerves are involved in regulating sexual functions. Sympathetic nerves mediate contraction of the musculature of the clitoris, vagina and uterus. Parasympathetic nerves are responsible for the lubrification of external genital organs and the filling of cavernous bodies thereby inducing swelling of the clitoris. Sexual dysfunctions due to surgically induced pelvic autonomic nerve injury are generally more evident in male patients, e.g. leading to erectile dysfunction and impaired ejaculation. However, the impact of autonomic nerve damage in female patients, such as inability to experience orgasm and insufficient lubrification, should not be underestimated.

The extent of autonomic nerve injury that will result in definite postoperative impairment of urinary and fecal continence as well as sexual functions remains unclear. The autonomic innervation of pelvic organs is characterized by its functional redundancy, anatomically reflected by a bilateral organization of intrapelvic nerve plexus abundantly ramifying and connecting both sides with each other. Thus, partial or unilateral damage may be compensated by the remaining intact contralateral nervous input.

Sympathetic Nerves

The preganglionic sympathetic nerve fibers emerge from lower lumbar and upper sacral spinal cord segments and pass along the descending aorta on both sides as periaortal trunks. The periaortal nervous network fuses ventrolaterally to form the inferior mesenteric and superior hypogastric plexus. In front of the promontorium and slightly left to the midline the superior hypogastric plexus divides into the left and right hypogastric nerves. The hypogastric nerves often consist of various nerve bundles and are embedded within the parietal pelvic fascia extending in front of the sacral concavity. Gentle traction of the hypogastric nerve will lift up this fascial sheath in a tent-like fashion thereby illustrating its course along the pelvic side wall down to the inferior hypogastric plexus (Figs. 3.11, 3.15, 3.16, 3.17, and 3.18) [22].

Parasympathetic Nerves

Parasympathetic nerves derive from the sacral part of the parasympathetic nervous system residing in the sacral spinal cord. Together with ventral branches of the sacral spinal nerves S2–S4, these pelvic splanchnic nerves leave the ventral sacral foramina and pierce the parietal pelvic fascia on both sides to join the hypogastric nerves. The pelvic splanchnic nerves coming from dorsocaudally and the hypogastric nerves coming from dorsocranially converge to form the inferior hypogastric plexus (Figs. 3.10, 3.11, 3.16, and 3.18).

Inferior Hypogastric Plexus

The inferior hypogastric plexus is a mixed autonomic nerve plexus composed of both sympathetic and parasympathetic nerves. As this abundant nerve network provides the autonomic nerve supply to all pelvic viscera, the inferior hypogastric plexus is also termed pelvic plexus. In fact, several subgroups of delicate nerve fiber bundles diverge from the main plexus towards the different pelvic compartments to supply the corresponding organs: rectal plexus, uterovaginal plexus, vesical plexus.

Like the hypogastric and pelvic splanchnic nerves, the inferior hypogastric plexus is embedded within the parietal pelvic fascia covering the pelvic sidewalls. The nervous meshwork extends medially to the internal iliac artery and follows its branches to the pelvic organs. Posteriorly, the rectal plexus diverges at the level of the rectal ligaments/pedicles and enters into the rectal wall accompanied by the middle rectal artery. Anteriorly, the inferior hypogastric plexus widens in a fan-like manner and releases a lateral and medial trunk. The lateral trunk corresponds to the vesical plexus running to the bladder lateral and underneath the ureter. The nerve bundles follow the branches of the vesical artery and further ramify to innervate the distal ureter, urinary fundus and neck, and internal urethral sphincter. The medial trunk corresponds to the uterovaginal plexus passing to the uterine cervix and vagina medial and underneath the ureter. The nerve bundles follow the uterine artery after its intersection with the ureter and innervate the uterus and urinary bladder from both sides (Figs. 3.11, 3.16, and 3.18).

Ureter

Special attention should be paid to the topographic anatomy of the ureter [3, 23] due to its high vulnerability to intraoperative injury for the following reasons:

- considerably long course (25–30 cm) along the interface between the retro- und intraperitoneal space exhibiting segments susceptible to damage at virtually all levels.
- hampered identification caused by obesity, previous surgery or radiation, inflammatory or neoplastic events, scarce peristaltic movements.
- morphological appearance and size similar to vascular structures.
- relatively common congenital anomalies (e.g. ureter duplex, ureter fissus, crossed ureter, retrocaval ureter).

Abdominal Segment

The abdominal segment (Figs. 3.12, 3.15, and 3.16) extends from the renal pelvis to the pelvic brim in front of the psoas muscle. The course of the ureter may vary from a paravertebral position close to either the vena cava or aorta to a lateral position along the outer border of the psoas muscle. The ureter is crossed anteriorly by the ovarian vessels and posteriorly by the genitofemoral nerves. On the left side, the ureter additionally undercrosses the root of the sigmoid mesocolon and the inferior mesenteric pedicle. Inspite of the close proximity between the ureter and the digestive tract, both are clearly separated by the anterior renal fascia delimiting the intraperitoneal from the retroperitoneal organs to which the ureter belongs.

While the ovarian vessels extend further laterally to form the infundibulopelvic ligaments, the ureters run medially creating ureteric peritoneal folds. Thus, at the pelvic brim the

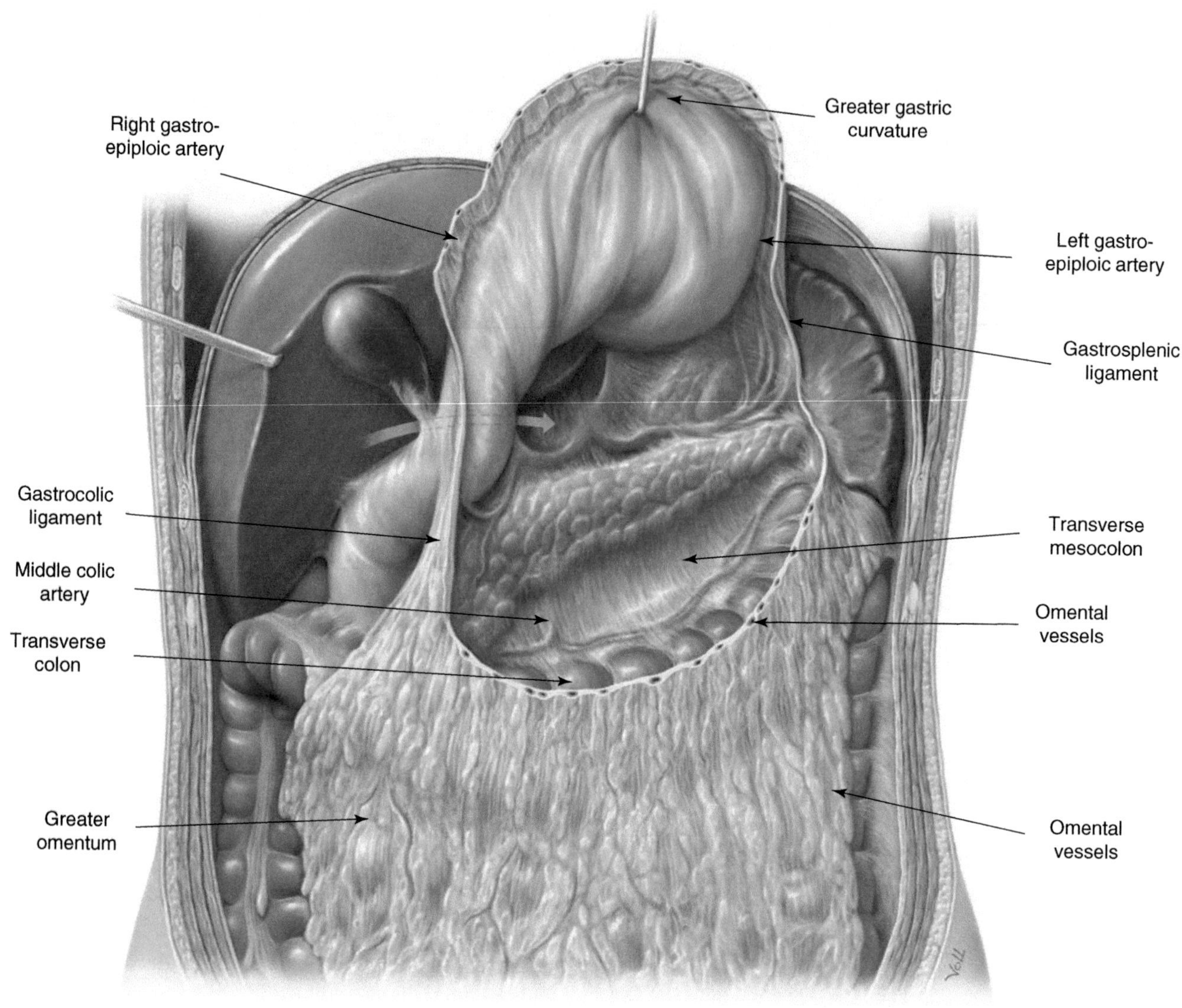

Fig. 3.19 Greater omentum. Ventral view. The gastrocolic ligament is partially cut, the stomach is flipped upwards to expose the lesser sac (Reproduced from Schünke et al. [24])

ureteric fold is closely related to and located medially to both the infundibulopelvic ligament and the ovary, so that care should be taken to protect the ureter underneath its peritoneal fold when mobilizing the uterine adnexa (Figs. 3.6, 3.9, 3.11, 3.12, and 3.17).

Pelvic Segment

In most cases the ureter enters the pelvic cavity anterior to the common iliac artery on the left side and anterior to the external iliac artery on the right side. The ureter further descends underneath the peritoneum and is related laterally to the branches of the internal iliac artery (obturator, superior vesical and uterine artery) and the obturator nerve and medially to the uterosacral ligament and its corresponding rectouterine fold as well as to the inferior hypogastric plexus.

Before the ureter reaches the urinary bladder via the vesicouterine ligament, the parametrium has to be traversed at the level of the uterine cervix (paracervix). The distance of the ureter from the uterine cervix and lateral vaginal fornix is ca. 1–2 cm. While the uterine artery bends medially to reach the uterine cervix, the ureter undercrosses the vessel in anterior oblique direction. As this area is a common site of ureter injury, the distance between the ureter and both the uterine cervix and artery can be enlarged by shifting the uterus to the contralateral side, e.g. by means of a uterus manipulator (Figs. 3.5, 3.8, 3.10, 3.11, 3.12, 3.13, and 3.17).

Blood Vessel and Nerve Supply

Due to its considerable length the ureter is supplied by various sources of blood vessels including branches from the aorta, renal, ovarian and internal iliac arteries. Of note is the observation that the nutrient arteries approach the abdominal segment from the medial side and the pelvic segment from the lateral side. Consequently, when mobilizing or dissecting the ureter, special care has to be taken to preserve the blood vessels at the medial side of the ureter above the pelvic brim and at its lateral side below the pelvic brim. Moreover, excessive denudation of the ureter over a long distance should be avoided to preserve the adventitial layer together with the mesoureter which contain an elaborated vascular plexus. Due to this intramural anastomotic system interruption of one blood supply can be compensated by the remaining vascular sources given that the periureteric tissue is left intact.

The autonomic innervation of the ureter mediates its peristaltic movements and pain perception. The nerve fibers derive from the aortic, superior and inferior hypogastric plexus. The distal ureter is innervated by nerve fibers originating from the lateral trunk of the inferior hypogastric plexus and running within the superior portion vesical plexus. To prevent bladder and sexual dysfunctions due to injury of the vesical plexus, manipulation of the distal ureter at the region of the vesicoureteric junction and vesical trigone should be avoided.

Greater Omentum

Both infragastric and infracolic omentectomy require knowledge of the topographic anatomy of the greater omentum (Fig. 3.19). Embryologically, the greater omentum is part of the dorsal mesogastrium which descends from the greater gastric curvature to cover the small intestinal loops and ascends back to reach the transverse colon and become adherent with the transverse mesocolon. The portion extending between the greater gastric curvature and the transverse colon is also termed the gastrocolic ligament. The gastrosplenic ligament corresponds to the continuation of the greater omentum at its left border connecting the stomach with the spleen. Although the greater omentum is fused to the transverse colon, both structures can be separated from each other by gently detaching the adherent peritoneal surfaces. Once the greater omentum has been released from the transverse colon or the gastrocolic ligament has been split, the omental bursa is opened.

At a distance of approximately 1–2 cm and parallel to the greater gastric curvature, the right and left gastroepiploic arteries run within the gastrocolic ligament and give off nutrient branches to the gastric wall. Descending branches of the gastroepiploic arc traverse the greater omentum to supply both the infragastric and infracolic parts.

The space between the peritoneal layers is usually filled with adipose tissue which may be massive in obese patients. On the other hand, the greater omentum may be thin, translucent or even congenitally absent. Beside fat storage the greater omentum functions as immuncompetent organ by means of its high content of macrophages and the ability to cover and thereby limit intraperitoneal inflammations [3].

Anterior Abdominal Wall

The topographic anatomy of the anterior abdominal wall (Figs. 3.20 and 3.21) [3] is particularly relevant, when multiple trocar incisions are applied in minimal invasive techniques bearing the risk of vascular, nerve or organ injuries. The abdominal wall is composed of the following layers:

- Skin
- Subcutaneous tissue
- Musculofascial layer
- Transversalis fascia
- Preperitoneal space
- Parietal peritoneum

Below the umbilicus the peritoneal layer displays five folds:

- 1 median umbilical fold (obliterated urachus)
- 2 medial umbilical folds (obliterated umbilical arteries)
- 2 lateral umbilical folds (inferior epigastric vessels)

The median umbilical fold is continuous with the urinary bladder fundus and sometimes stretches the urinary bladder cavity cranially which may lead to inadvertent injury of the urinary bladder wall during suprapubic trocar placement. The medial umbilical folds separate the supravesical from the medial inguinal fossae. Although the umbilical arteries are mostly obliterated, in some cases these vessels are still patent and may cause bleeding when the medial umbilical folds are perforated inadvertently by trocars.

While both the median and medial umbilical folds converge upwards to reach the umbilicus, the lateral umbilical folds pass laterally to the umbilicus behind the rectus abdominis muscle. The lateral umbilical folds extend between the medial and lateral inguinal fossae – the latter ones corresponding to the deep inguinal rings into which the uterine round ligaments enter. The inferior epigastric vessels originate medially to the deep inguinal ring and ascend under-

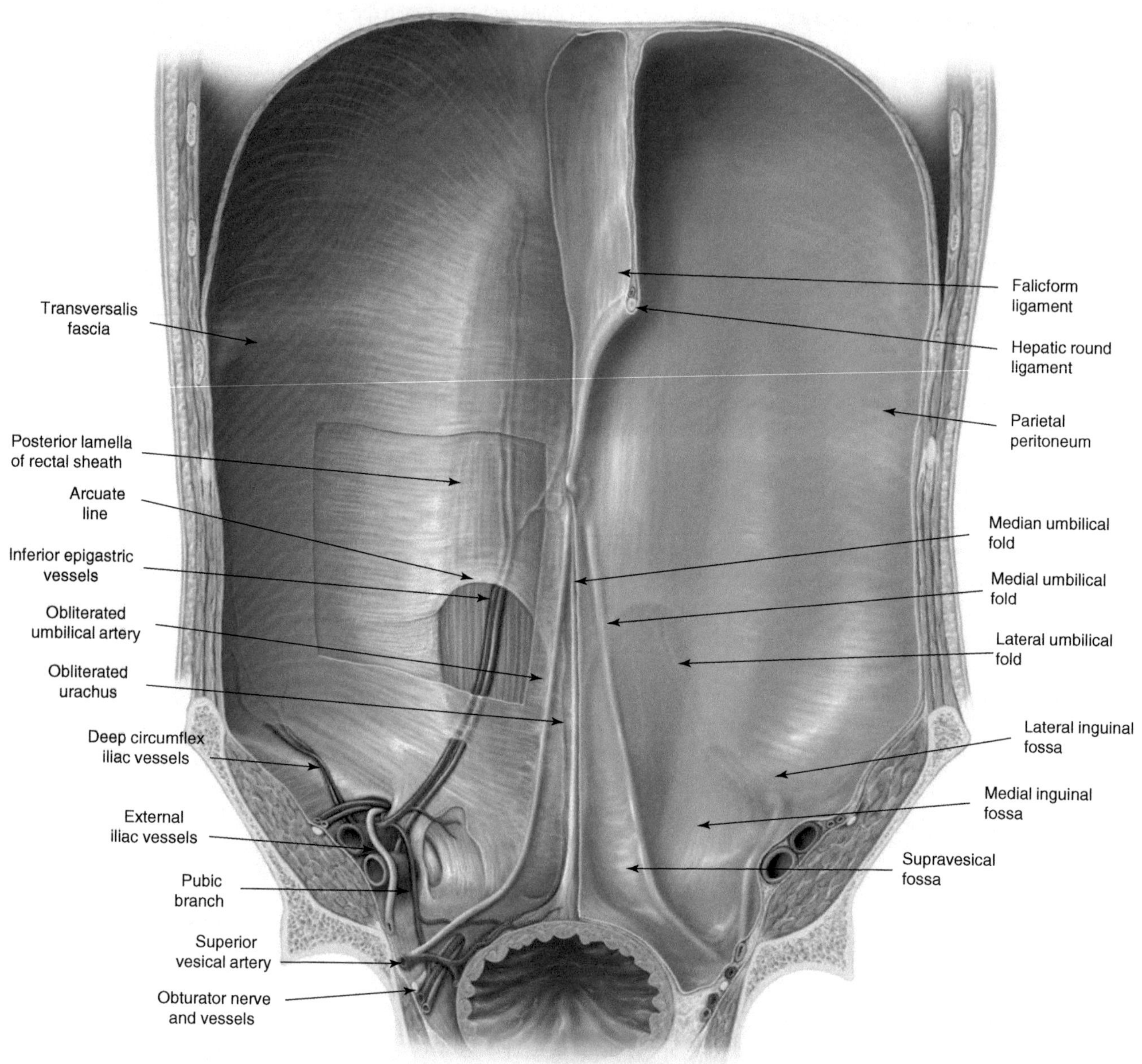

Fig. 3.20 Backside of the anterior abdominal wall. Frontal section, dorsal view. On the left side the peritoneum and part of the transversalis fascia are removed

neath the peritoneum and transversalis fascia to reach and enter into the rectus abdominis muscle. Frequently, the inferior epigastric vessels give off a pubic branch which passes along the femoral fossa and over the pectineal ligament to anastomose with the obturator vessels.

Whereas the transversalis fascia is ubiquitously present and most developed in the lower abdominen, the posterior lamella of the rectus sheath is only present in the upper addomen and fades out at the level of the arcuate line below the umbilicus. The preperitoneal space extends between the transversalis fascia and the parietal peritoneum and is filled by fat. In obese patients an increased content of adipose tissue may considerably thicken the preperitoneal space – which has to be considered during trocar placement to avoid unwanted insufflation of this tissue compartment.

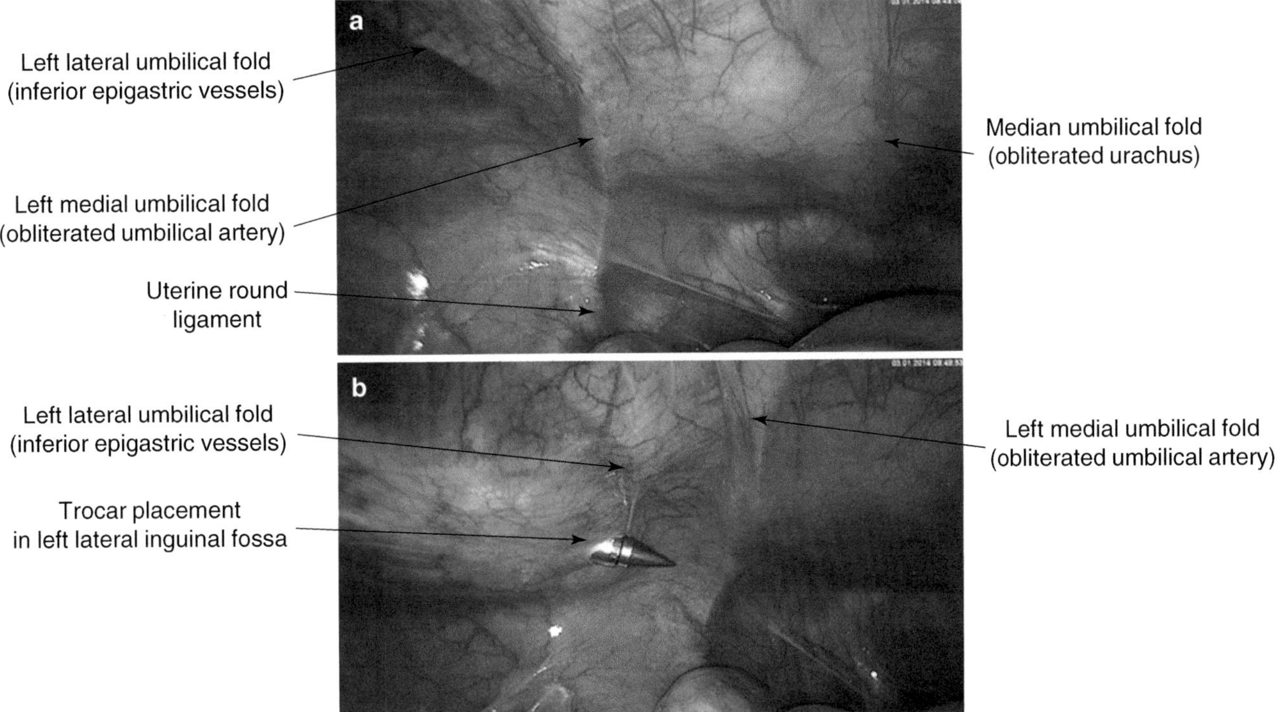

Fig. 3.21 Backside of the left anterior abdominal wall. Laparoscopic view. The three umbilical folds are discernible (**a**), the entry site of the trocar (**b**) is lateral to the lateral umbilical fold

References

1. Ashton-Miller JA, DeLancey JO. Functional anatomy of the female pelvic floor. Ann N Y Acad Sci. 2007;1101:266–96.
2. Fritsch H, Lienemann A, Brenner E, Ludwikowski B. Clinical anatomy of the pelvic floor. Adv Anat Embryol Cell Biol. 2004;175:III–X. 1–64.
3. SGH S, editor. Gray's anatomy: the anatomical basis of clinical practice. 40th ed. New York: Churchill Livingstone/Elsevier; 2008.
4. Ramanah R, Berger MB, Parratte BM, DeLancey JO. Anatomy and histology of apical support: a literature review concerning cardinal and uterosacral ligaments. Int Urogynecol J. 2012;23:1483–94.
5. Samaan A, Vu D, Haylen BT, Tse K. Cardinal ligament surgical anatomy: cardinal points at hysterectomy. Int Urogynecol J. 2014; 25:189–95.
6. Touboul C, Fauconnier A, Zareski E, Bouhanna P, Darai E. The lateral infraureteral parametrium: myth or reality? Am J Obstet Gynecol. 2008;199:242.e241–6.
7. Yabuki Y, Sasaki H, Hatakeyama N, Murakami G. Discrepancies between classic anatomy and modern gynecologic surgery on pelvic connective tissue structure: harmonization of those concepts by collaborative cadaver dissection. Am J Obstet Gynecol. 2005;193: 7–15.
8. Mauroy B, Demondion X, Bizet B, Claret A, Mestdagh P, Hurt C. The female inferior hypogastric (= pelvic) plexus: anatomical and radiological description of the plexus and its afferences–applications to pelvic surgery. Surg Radiol Anat. 2007;29:55–66.
9. Raspagliesi F, Ditto A, Fontanelli R, Solima E, Hanozet F, Zanaboni F, Kusamura S. Nerve-sparing radical hysterectomy: a surgical technique for preserving the autonomic hypogastric nerve. Gynecol Oncol. 2004;93:307–14.
10. Hockel M, Horn LC, Manthey N, Braumann UD, Wolf U, Teichmann G, Frauenschlager K, Dornhofer N, Einenkel J. Resection of the embryologically defined uterovaginal (mullerian) compartment and pelvic control in patients with cervical cancer: a prospective analysis. Lancet Oncol. 2009;10:683–92.
11. Heald RJ, Ryall RD. Recurrence and survival after total mesorectal excision for rectal cancer. Lancet. 1986;1:1479–82.
12. Hohenberger W, Weber K, Matzel K, Papadopoulos T, Merkel S. Standardized surgery for colonic cancer: complete mesocolic excision and central ligation–technical notes and outcome. Colorectal Dis. 2009;11:354–64. ; discussion 364–5.
13. Hockel M, Horn LC, Tetsch E, Einenkel J. Pattern analysis of regional spread and therapeutic lymph node dissection in cervical cancer based on ontogenetic anatomy. Gynecol Oncol. 2012;125:168–74.
14. Kimmig R, Wimberger P, Buderath P, Aktas B, Iannaccone A, Heubner M. Definition of compartment-based radical surgery in uterine cancer: radical hysterectomy in cervical cancer as 'total mesometrial resection (tmmr)' by m hockel translated to robotic surgery (rtmmr). World J Surg Oncol. 2013;11:211.
15. Ercoli A, Delmas V, Iannone V, Fagotti A, Fanfani F, Corrado G, Ferrandina G, Scambia G. The lymphatic drainage of the uterine cervix in adult fresh cadavers: anatomy and surgical implications. Eur J Surg Oncol. 2010;36:298–303.
16. Kraima AC, Derks M, Smit NN, Van Munsteren JC, Van der Velden J, Kenter GG, DeRuiter MC. Lymphatic drainage pathways from the cervix uteri: implications for radical hysterectomy? Gynecol Oncol. 2014;132:107–13.
17. Cibula D, Abu-Rustum NR. Pelvic lymphadenectomy in cervical cancer–surgical anatomy and proposal for a new classification system. Gynecol Oncol. 2010;116:33–7.

18. Kimmig R, Iannaccone A, Buderath P, Aktas B, Wimberger P, Heubner M. Definition of compartment based radical surgery in uterine cancer-part i: therapeutic pelvic and periaortic lymphadenectomy by michael hockel translated to robotic surgery. ISRN Obstet Gynecol. 2013;2013:297921.
19. Baader B, Herrmann M. Topography of the pelvic autonomic nervous system and its potential impact on surgical intervention in the pelvis. Clin Anat. 2003;16:119–30.
20. Park NY, Cho YL, Park IS, Lee YS. Laparoscopic pelvic anatomy of nerve-sparing radical hysterectomy. Clin Anat. 2010;23: 186–91.
21. Stelzner S, Holm T, Moran BJ, Heald RJ, Witzigmann H, Zorenkov D, Wedel T. Deep pelvic anatomy revisited for a description of crucial steps in extralevator abdominoperineal excision for rectal cancer. Dis Colon rectum. 2011;54:947–57.
22. Runkel N, Reiser H. Nerve-oriented mesorectal excision (nome): autonomic nerves as landmarks for laparoscopic rectal resection. Int J Colorectal Dis. 2013;28:1367–75.
23. Frober R. Surgical anatomy of the ureter. BJU Int. 2007;100: 949–65.
24. Schünke M, Schulte E, Schumacher U. Prometheus atlas of anatomy, vol. 2. Stuttgart: Thieme Publisher; 2015.

Part III

Imaging and Diagnostics

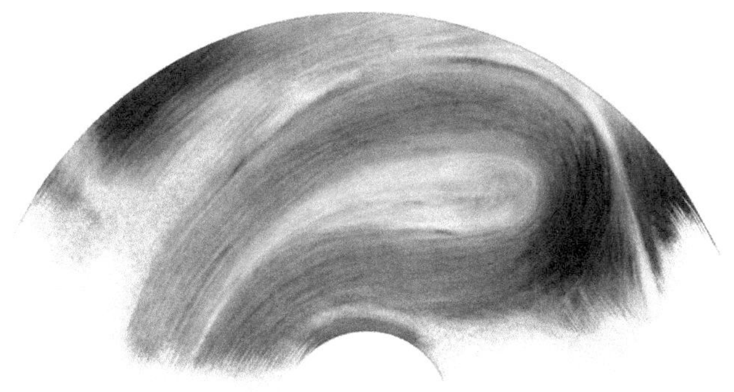

Clinical Diagnostics Before Hysterectomy

4

Stefan Rimbach

Introduction

Diagnostic measures before hysterectomy aim to ensure patients general perioperative safety with regard to risk management as well as to prepare accuracy, safety and success of the planned surgical procedure.

In order to be efficient, tools and extent of diagnostics should allow to

- prove the indication for hysterectomy
- assess general pre-operative risk (including co-morbidity and anaesthesiological factors)
- reveal individual (risk-) factors referring to
  - surgical procedure planning
  - individualized surgical strategy (e.g. interdisciplinary procedure)
  - ressource management (e.g. operating room time)
  - individualized perioperative management
- reveal/exclude unsuspected additional findings (e.g. adnexal masses)
- reveal/exclude unsuspected malignancy
- exclude contraindications
- save as a basis for patient information to achieve informed consent

Diagnostic Tools Overview

Basic (mandatory):

- anamnesis/patient history
- physical examination
- gynecological examination: inspection, palpation
- cervical cytology

S. Rimbach
Department of Obstetrics and Gynecology, Krankenhaus Agatharied, Norbert-Kerkel-Platz, D-83734, Hausham, Germany
e-mail: stefan.rimbach@khagatharied.de

Additional (optional):

- colposcopy
- vaginal ultrasonography (endometrium, intracavitary pathology, myometrium, myometrial pathology, adnexa, pouch of douglas
- renal sonography
- MRI
- (MR) urography

Laboratory investigations:

- according to institutional standard
- and to individual risk profile
- pregnancy test in premenopausal women

Patient History

Patient history comprises personal as well as family history. Familial disorders may influence surgical and perioperative planning. E.g. hereditary diseases of the blood coagulation system may be of utmost importance for perioperative thrombosis prevention, choice of anaesthesia and pain therapy as far as catheter methods are concerned, and for coagulation management during surgery; rare conditions such as HLRCC-syndrom (hereditary leiomyomatosis and renal cell carcinoma) predispose to malignancy such as sarcoma in case of presumed benign myoma. Personal patient history informs the surgeon about individual risks such as co-morbidity, previous surgery (e.g. leading to adhesions), medication influencing procedural planning (e.g. anti-coagulation), but also feasibility aspects for the planned hysterectomy (e.g. history of vaginal births vs cesarean sections influencing the route of hysterectomy in terms of vaginal vs abdominal approach). Menstrual history may not only lead to the hysterectomy indication itself in case of bleeding disorders, but also add information on the risk of malignancy in case of irregular bleeding. A typical history of dysmenorrhea may lead to the suspicion

I. Alkatout, L. Mettler (eds.), *Hysterectomy*, DOI 10.1007/978-3-319-22497-8_4

of endometriosis. Inquiring about bladder and intestinal function may reveal (pre-)existing incontinence problems and play a role for procedure planning as well as for the evaluation of potential post-surgical conditions or presumed complications. The same applies for anamnestic pain or neurological symptoms. Psycho-social aspects should not lack in a complete patient history.

Physical and Gynecological Examination

Gynecological examination including inspection and bimanual palpation allow to evaluate size, position and mobility of the uterus, as well as the adnexa, parametria and pouch of douglas.

Inspection of the vaginal fornix may e.g. reveal vaginal endometriosis (Fig. 4.1), malformations like a vaginal septum (Fig. 4.2) or raise suspicion of vaginal infection, usually rendering hysterectomy contraindicated until successfully treated.

In some instances, such as suspected endometriosis, rectovaginal palpation may additionally give informations on the rectovaginal septum . Palpation may be focally painful, reveal induration or resistance, caused at level of the sacro-uterine ligaments (Fig. 4.3) or the rectovaginal space (Fig. 4.4).

Size and mobility of the uterus as determined by palpation may decide about the surgical approach to hysterectomy or indicate further imaging such as MRI. In case of prolapse, inspection and palpation may allow differentiation between levels and compartments affected and different forms of cele formation. Depending on the clinical impression further functional testing such as urodynamics and ultrasound may be indicated.

Physical examination does also comprise inspection and palpation/percussion of the abdomen, the inguinal regions, back with renal beds and case depending the breast/thoracic area, extremities and head/neck area.

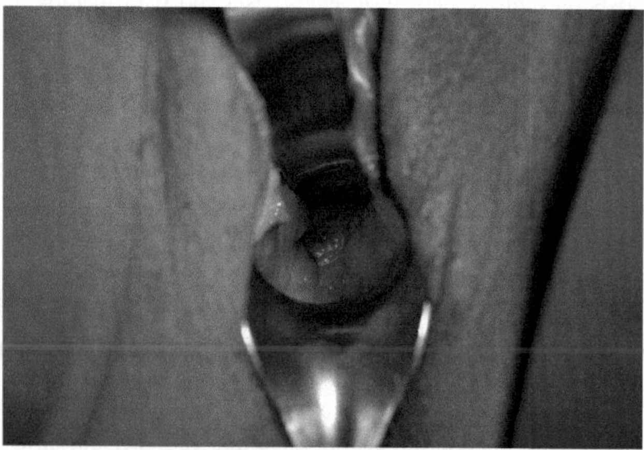

Fig. 4.1 Inspection of the vaginal fornix: blue spots as a sign of vaginal endometriosis

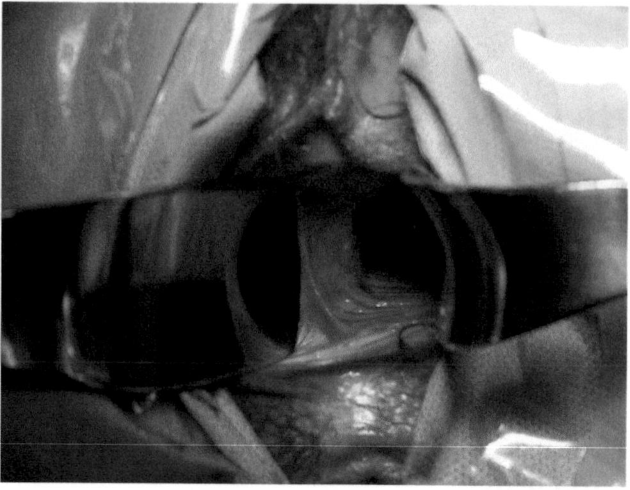

Fig. 4.2 Inspection of the vagina (foto taken during surgery): vaginal septum

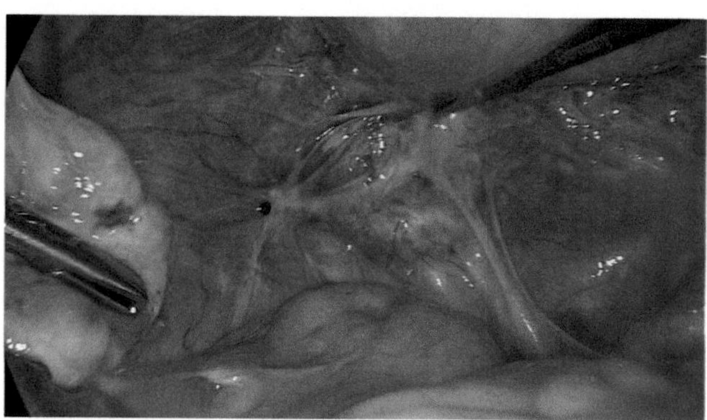

Fig. 4.3 Laparoscopic aspect of the palpatory painful and indurated sacro-uterine ligament on the left side affected by deep infiltrating endometriosis

Cervical Cytology and Colposcopy

Cervical cytology is important to exclude cervical pathology before hysterectomy, and colposcopy may add detailed information relevant to surgical strategies, e.g. when discussing total versus supracervical procedure. HPV-testing may also add helpful information.

Imaging Techniques: Ultrasonography and MRI

Vaginal sonography as an adjunct to clinical examination allows to double check clinical information on size and position of the uterus, but especially gives further insight to the structure of the endometrium and myometrium [1, 2]. Thus, intracavitary pathology such as polyps, submucous fibroids or irregular formations suspect for malignancy can be detected and hysterectomy indication adapted, or further

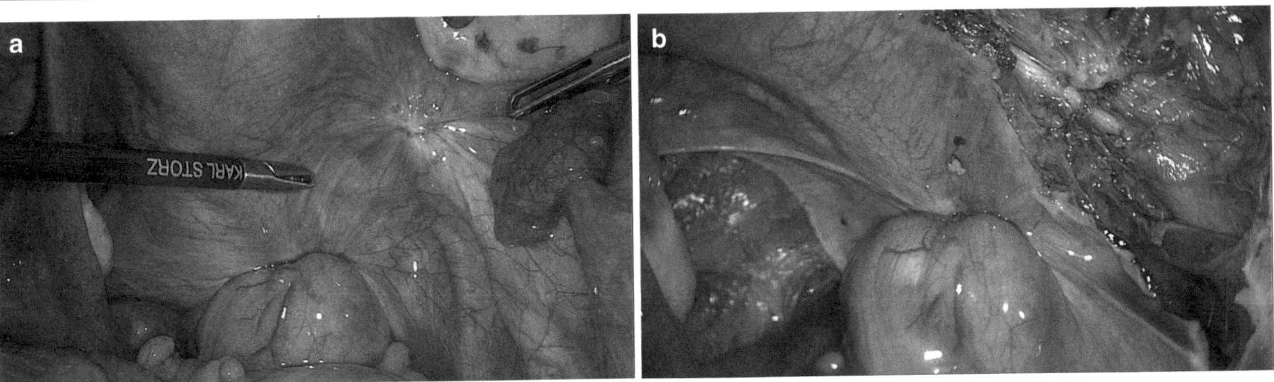

Fig. 4.4 Laparoscopic aspects (**a** = overview, **b** = close-up during preparation) of the palpatory painful and indurated recto-vaginal septum affected by a nodule of deep infiltrating endometriosis

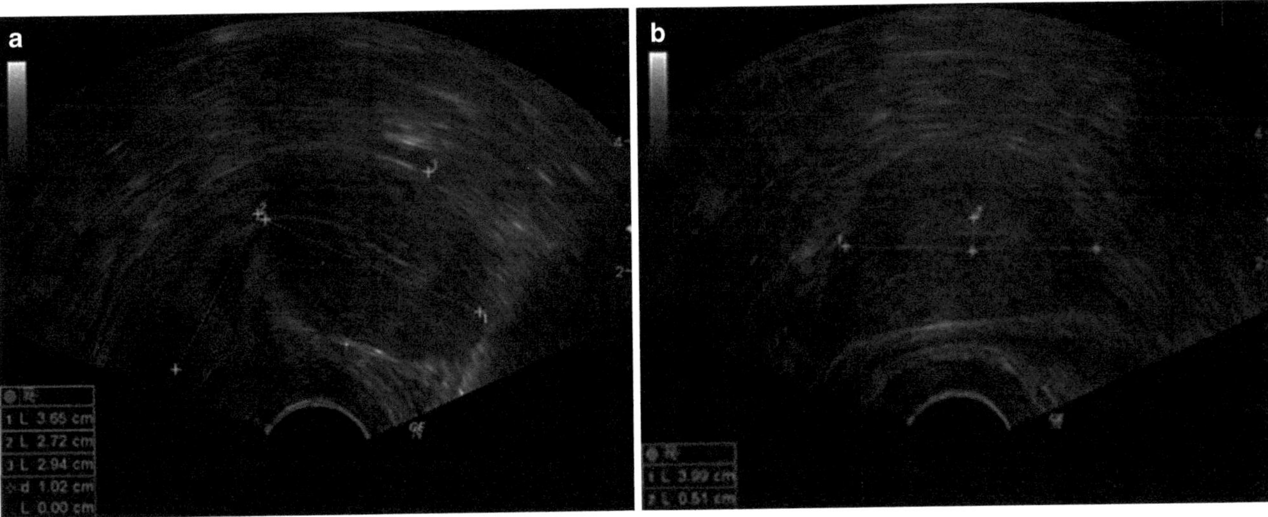

Fig. 4.5 (**a**, **b**) Preoperative vaginal sonography of a regular uterus

investigations such as hysteroscopy or endometrial biopsy scheduled prior to hysterectomy [3].

Figure 4.5 shows the vaginal-sonographic appearance of a uterus before hysterectomy (in this case for dysfunctional uterine bleeding). Detectable pathologies are absent. Size and position of the organ, endometrium and myometrium can be described.

Figures 4.6, 4.7, and 4.8 show examples of endometrial, myometrial and intracavitary pathology as can be detected and described by vaginal sonography.

With regard to additional findings such as endometriosis, ovarian tumors, ascites, sonographic investigation of the adnexa, pouch of douglas, and kidneys may be helpful. Examples are given in Figs. 4.9, 4.10, and 4.11, showing cystic adnexal tumors of tube and ovary.

MRI may play a role in diagnosing and staging endometrial tumors, e.g. in case of an endometrial carcinoma as shown in Fig. 4.12.

Large fibroids may be better visualized by MRI than sonography, if relevant to the projected surgery (Fig. 4.13). MRI may also add valuable informations to vaginal sonography and Doppler results when findings are suspicious for sarcoma [4–7], a question which is most relevant before hysterectomy when morcellation is discussed.

Ureteral compression with subsequent renal dilation may be detected by urography, which is advisable especially if obstruction is presumed or ureters shall be visualized by intraoperative preparation (Figs. 4.14 and 4.15). Postoperative control may be advisable when there was a risk of ureteral impairment during hysterectomy.

Laboratory Investigations

Laboratory investigations are done above all to exclude individual risks with regard to anaesthesia. Usually there exist institutional standards or individual risk profile requires serum specimens [8]. In order to exclude pregnancy, a serum or urinary test is performed in premenopausal women.

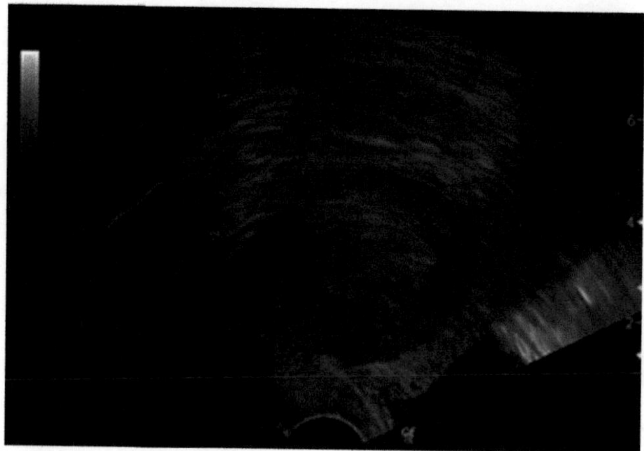

Fig. 4.6 Vaginal sonograpy: suspect endometrium, postmenopausal patient; histology: endometrioid adenocarcinoma

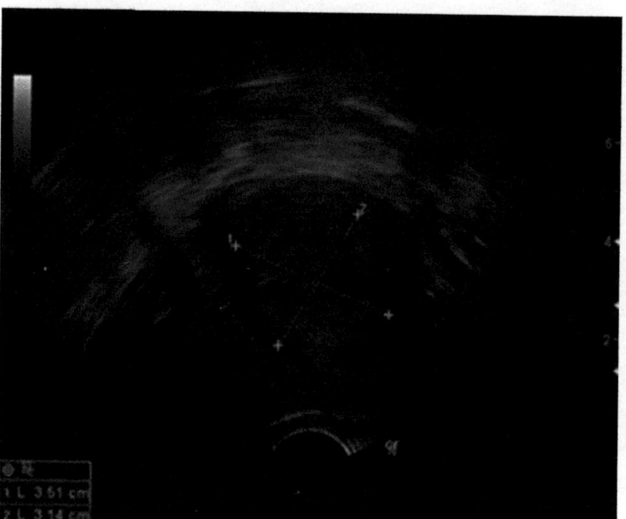

Fig. 4.7 Vaginal sonography: fundal fibroid 3.5 × 3.2 cm

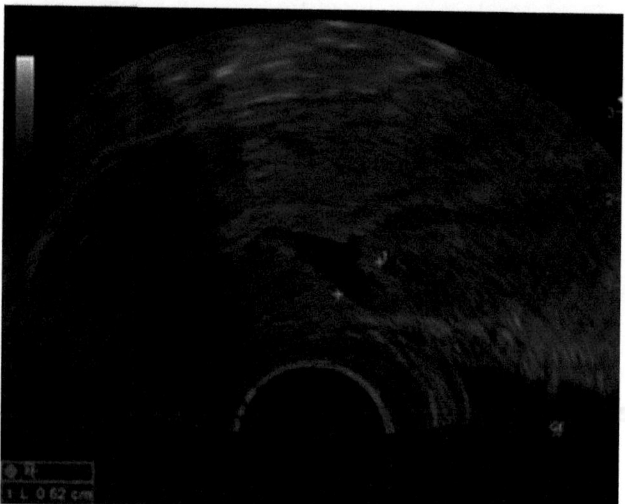

Fig. 4.8 Menorrhagia because of dehiscent cesarean scar

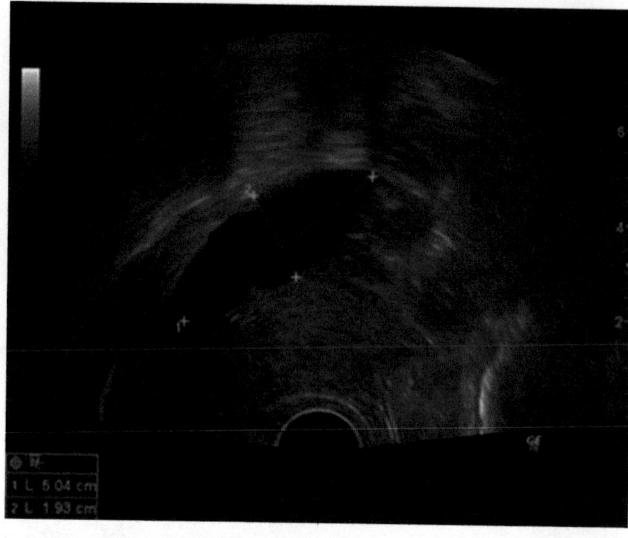

Fig. 4.9 Hydrosalpinx (right adnexa)

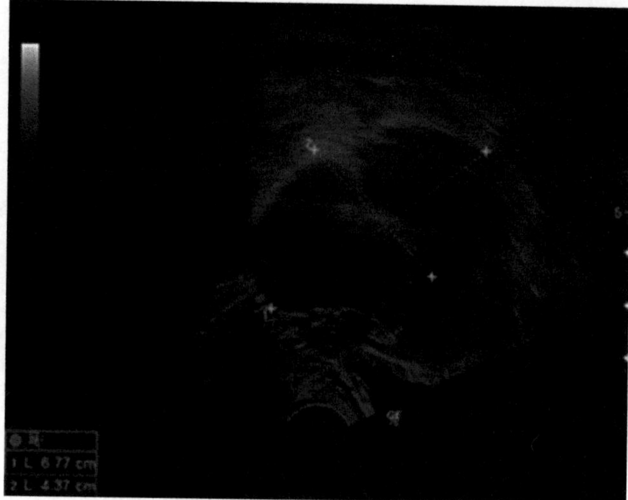

Fig. 4.10 Cystic adnexal mass of unclear dignity

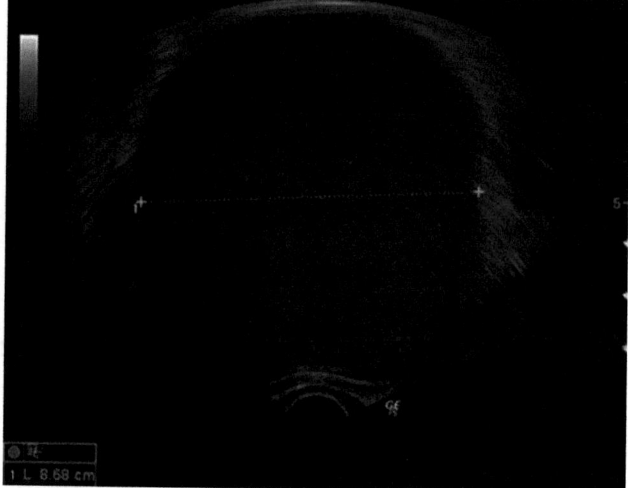

Fig. 4.11 Ovarian endometriosis

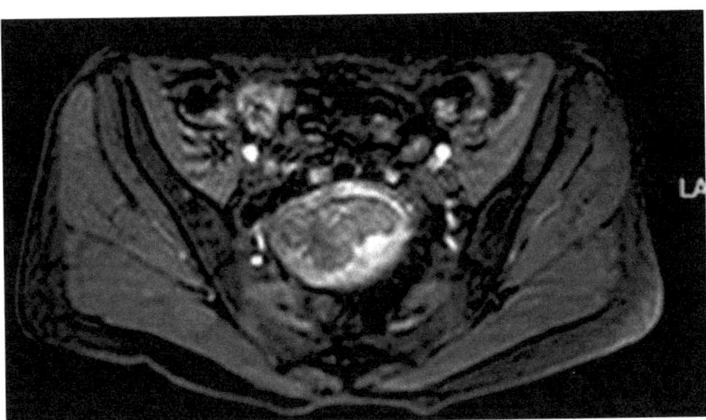

Fig. 4.12 Pelvic MRI: endometrial carcinoma

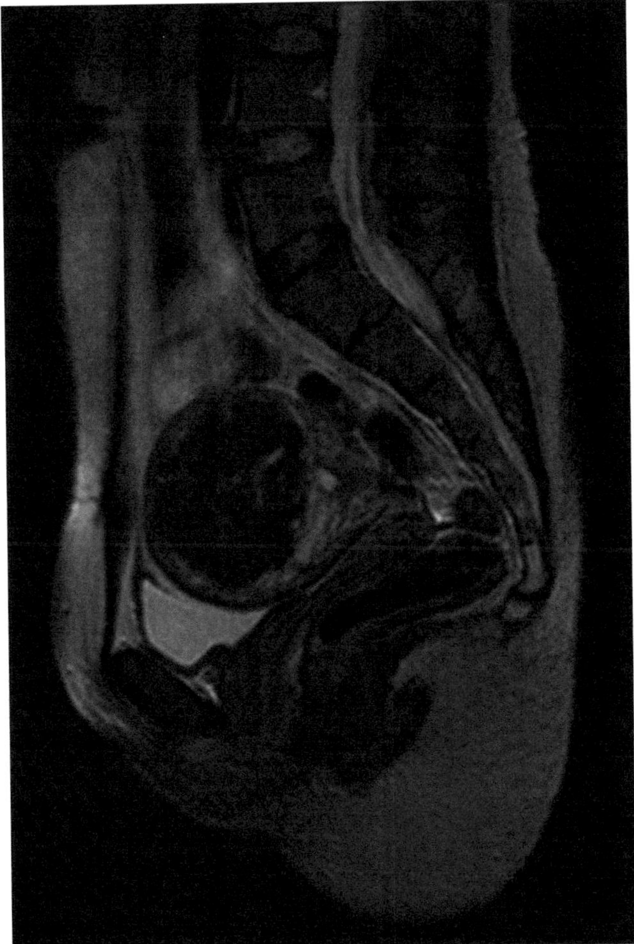

Fig. 4.13 MRI showing an uterus with a large intramural myoma

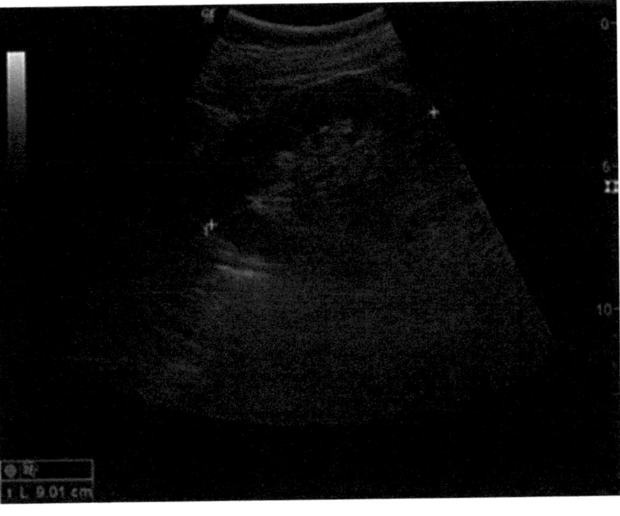

Fig. 4.14 Renal sonography

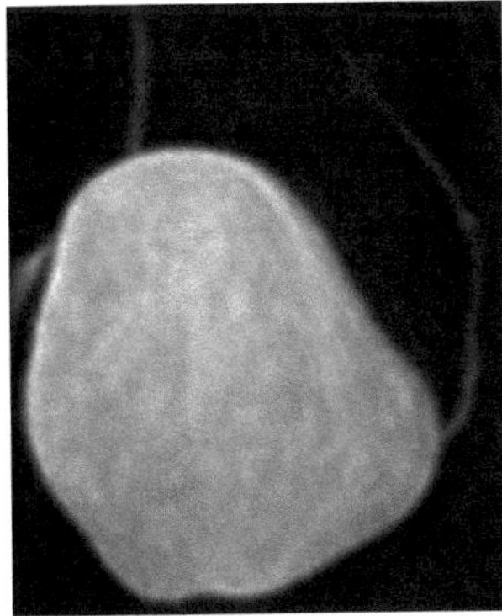

Fig. 4.15 MR-Urography

Conclusion

As a basis for clinical indication, counselling and decision making, patient history and physical examination are required when hysterectomy is considered. Cervical cytology seems mandatory in order to exclude or diagnose cervical dysplasia. Imaging serves as an adjunct to clinical examination. Vaginal sonography will be helpful and applied in most cases before hysterectomy. In selected circumstances, MRI may add valuable information. The necessity of laboratory investigations beyond a pregnancy test in fertile patients varies depending on the indication and co-morbidity of the individual patient. The results of clinical examinations before hysterectomy serve to verify the indication and exclude contraindications, minimize risks, and allow individualized procedure planning as well as adequate patient information in order to achieve informed consent.

References

1. Munro MG, Dickersin K, Clark MA, Langenberg P, Scherer RW, Frick KD. The Surgical Treatments Outcomes Project for Dysfunctional Uterine Bleeding: summary of an Agency for Health Research and Quality-sponsored randomized trial of endometrial ablation versus hysterectomy for women with heavy menstrual bleeding. Menopause. 2011;18(4):445–52.
2. Guideline NG. Diagnosis and treatment of endometrial carcinoma. (S2 k). 2010;Registry No. AWMF 032/034 (Band I):185–92.

3. Dijkhuizen FP, Mol BW, Brölmann HA, Heintz AP. The accuracy of endometrial sampling in the diagnosis of patients with endometrial carcinoma and hyperplasia: a meta-analysis. Cancer. 2000;89(8):1765–72.
4. Sato K, Yuasa N, Fujita M, Fukushima Y. Clinical application of diffusion-weighted imaging for preoperative differentiation between uterine leiomyoma and leiomyosarcoma. Am J Obstet Gynecol. 2014;210(4):368.e1–8. doi:10.1016/j.ajog.2013.12.028. Epub 2013 Dec 22.
5. Amant F, Coosemans A, Debiec-Rychter M, Timmerman D, Vergote I. Clinical management of uterine sarcomas. Lancet Oncol. 2009;10(12):1188–98. doi:10.1016/S1470-2045(09)70226-8. Review.
6. Beckmann MW, Juhasz-Böss I, Denschlag D, Gaß P, Dimpfl T, Harter P, Mallmann P, Renner SP, Rimbach S, Runnebaum I, Untch M, Brucker SY, Wallwiener D. Surgical Methods for the Treatment of Uterine Fibroids – Risk of Uterine Sarcoma and Problems of Morcellation: Position Paper of the DGGG. Geburtshilfe Frauenheilkd. 2015;75(2):148–64.
7. Brölmann H, Tanos V, Grimbizis G, Ind T, Philips K, van den Bosch T, Sawalhe S, van den Haak L, Jansen FW, Pijnenborg J, Taran FA, Brucker S, Wattiez A, Campo R, O'Donovan P, de Wilde RL. European Society of Gynaecological Endoscopy (ESGE) steering committee on fibroid morcellation. Options on fibroid morcellation: a literature review. Gynecol Surg. 2015;12(1):3–15. Epub 2015 Feb 7.
8. Geldner G ME, Wappler F et al. Präoperative Evaluation erwachsener Patienten vor elektiven, nicht kardiochirurgischen Eingriffen. http://www.dgaide/eev/EEV_2011_S_129-142pdf.

5 Ultrasound Imaging

Werner Dürr

Abbreviations

EMJ	Endometrial-myometrial junction [1]. Anatomically, an inner layer of myometrium surrounding the endometrium differentiated sonographically and by MRI from the other myometrium by lower echogenity (Figs. 5.2 and 5.3). This layer is also part of the endometrial-subendometrial unit "archimetra" [2], which evolutionary is an old part of the uterus. According to the theory of Leyendecker, the EMJ is of importance for uterine peristalsis by performing contractions and is believed to play a role in fertility and the development of adenomyosis and endometriosis [3].
Glass body	3D glass-body rendering. Grey values in a transparent mode and color presentation together give a glass-like image of vascularization (Fig. 5.5). Color Doppler alone without grey values shows the vascularization without any surrounding tissue (Fig. 5.6).
Inversion mode	Image presentation of surfaces in a technically inverted way. Findings of low or no echogenity present echogenic (Fig. 5.7) whereas echogenic structures present low echogenic.
OmniView	Image presentation on the basis of a stored volume and a chosen plane of section.Used to render structures in planes not ordinarily visible in real time e.g. the uterus can be shown in a frontal scan in its whole length without its usual flexure, so to say "stretched" (Fig. 5.1).
TAS	Transabdominal sonography
TUI	Tomographic ultrasound imaging. Imaging of a sonographic finding in diverse, simultaneously presented parallel planes of section on the basis of a stored volume (Fig. 5.4)
TVS	Transvaginal sonography
US	Ultrasound
VCI	Volume contrast imaging. Image presentation in a certain selectable slice thickness for better contrast and suppression of artifacts on the basis of a special technique with assemblage of diverse, parallel scans of close vicinity and their following superposition with the effect of better discrimination between structures of different echogenity (Fig. 5.1).

W. Dürr
Gynecologist, Sonographically Specialized,
Nürtingen, Baden-Württemberg, Germany
e-mail: duerrwe@aol.com

I. Alkatout, L. Mettler (eds.), *Hysterectomy*, DOI 10.1007/978-3-319-22497-8_5

Introduction

Independent of the indication for hysterectomy, each operating surgeon will be highly interested in the detailed information on the uterus given by preoperative imaging methods, such as sonographic imaging.

To know what to expect enables the surgeon to define an adequate surgical management and prevents unexpected intraoperative findings. This is one of the most important reasons for preoperative sonographic imaging.

Especially transvaginal sonography (TVS), more so than transabdominal sonography (TAS), gives us the opportunity to closely approach the regions of interest within the minor pelvis. Because of the short distances within the minor pelvis, probes of high frequency with corresponding high resolution can be used to discover even very small uterine alterations.

Developments such as color Doppler and volume scan give additional diagnostic extensions and refinements.

As sonography is an imaging method, this chapter will be primarily image-based appropriate to the saying, "A good image tells more than a thousand words".

Normal Findings

It is important to know the normal sonographic appearance of the uterus (Figs. 5.8 and 5.9) to be able to identify uterine alterations as findings deviating from the norm. In addition to the classic B-mode sonography, other techniques, such as OmniView and VCI, are demonstrated in this section (see Fig. 5.1). Normal findings of the so-called EMJ are also demonstrated by images (Figs. 5.2 and 5.3).

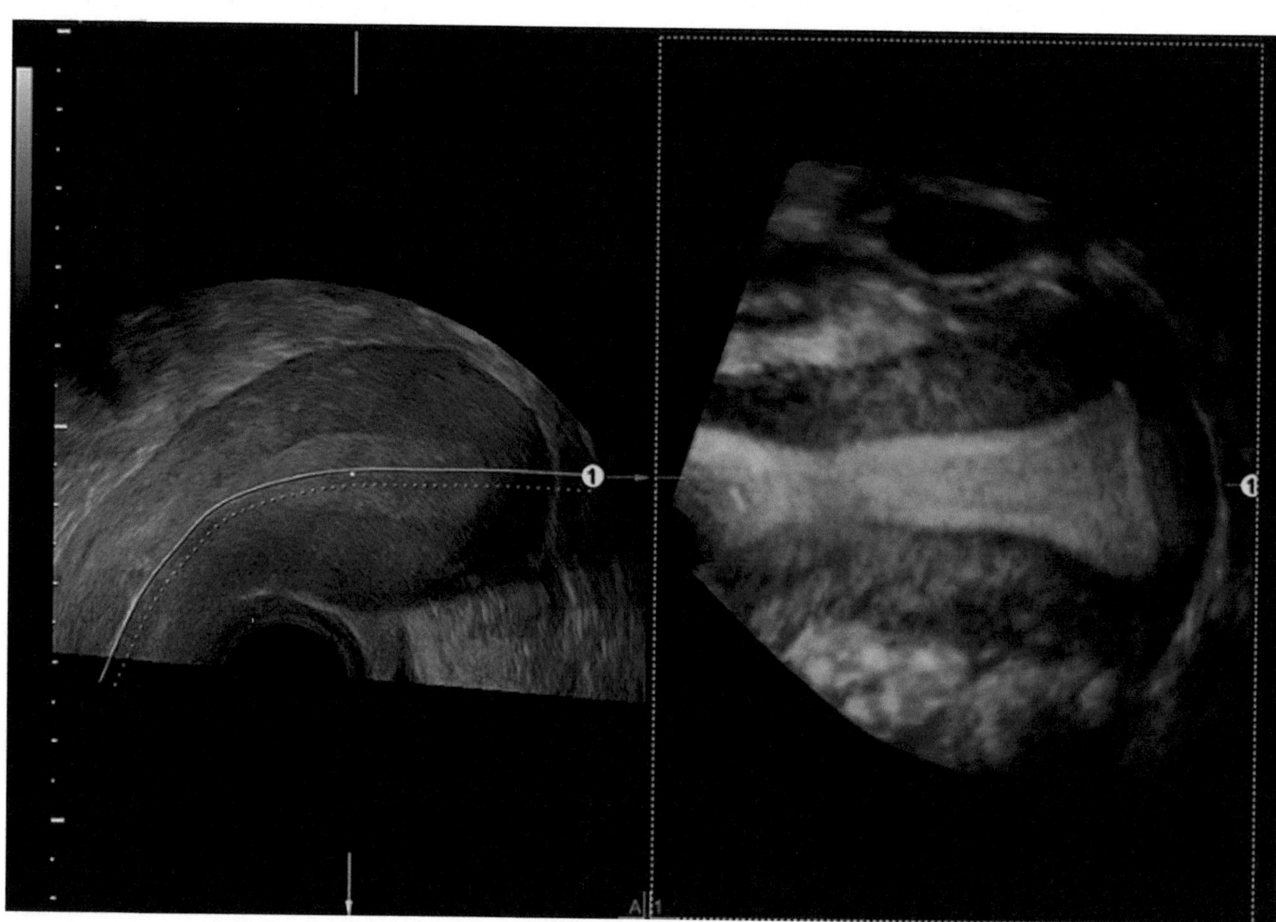

Fig. 5.1 To demonstrate OmniView and VCI technique, a frontal scan to present the uterus in its total length, so to speak "stretched" (*right image*). VCI technique is used to give a more plastic impression of the endometrium (*right image*) (Image from Dürr, Transvaginale Sonographie in der Gynäkologie, De Gruyter, 2nd Edition, 2015)

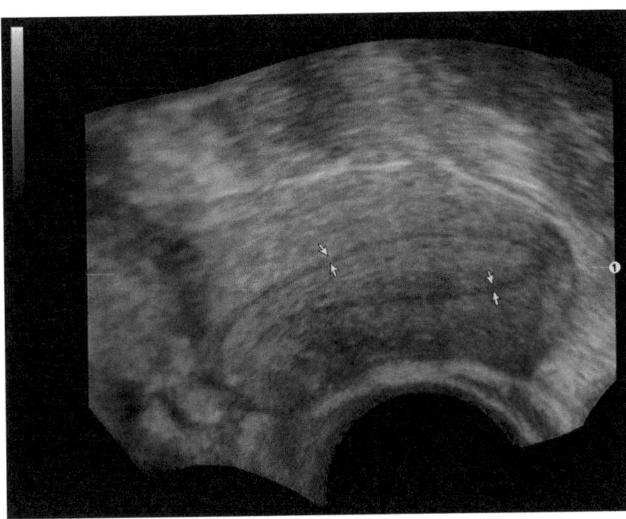

Fig. 5.2 This longitudinal scan in 3D technique shows an anteverted, anteflected, normal sized uterus with a remarkably clear and sharp demarcation, in comparison to endometrium and myometrium hypoechoic line (*arrows*) which represents the inner layer of myometrium, surrounding the endometrium. This endometrial-myometrial junction (EMJ) is of importance for uterine peristalsis by performing contractions and is believed to play a role in fertility and the development of adenomyosis and endometriosis [2–4]. It is unusual to see the EMJ as clear and demarcated as in this image (Image from Dürr, Transvaginale Sonographie in der Gynäkologie, De Gruyter, 2nd Edition, 2015)

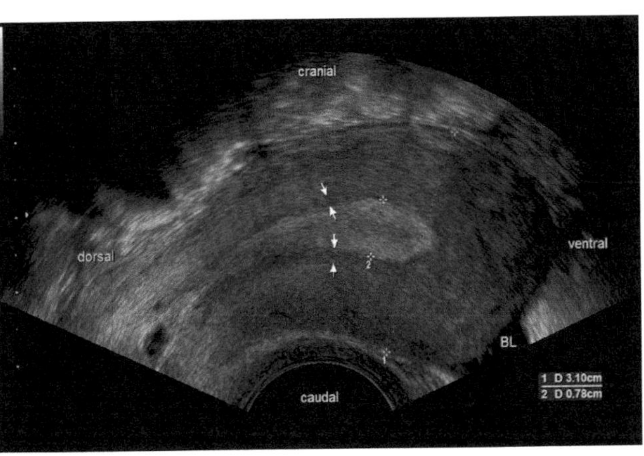

Fig. 5.3 This longitudinal scan shows an anteverted, anteflected, normal sized uterus with a fundal uterine wall thicker than expected, in comparison to the anterior and the posterior uterine wall. As an additional finding, a normal EMJ (*arrows*) (Image from Dürr, Transvaginale Sonographie in der Gynäkologie, De Gruyter, 2nd Edition, 2015)

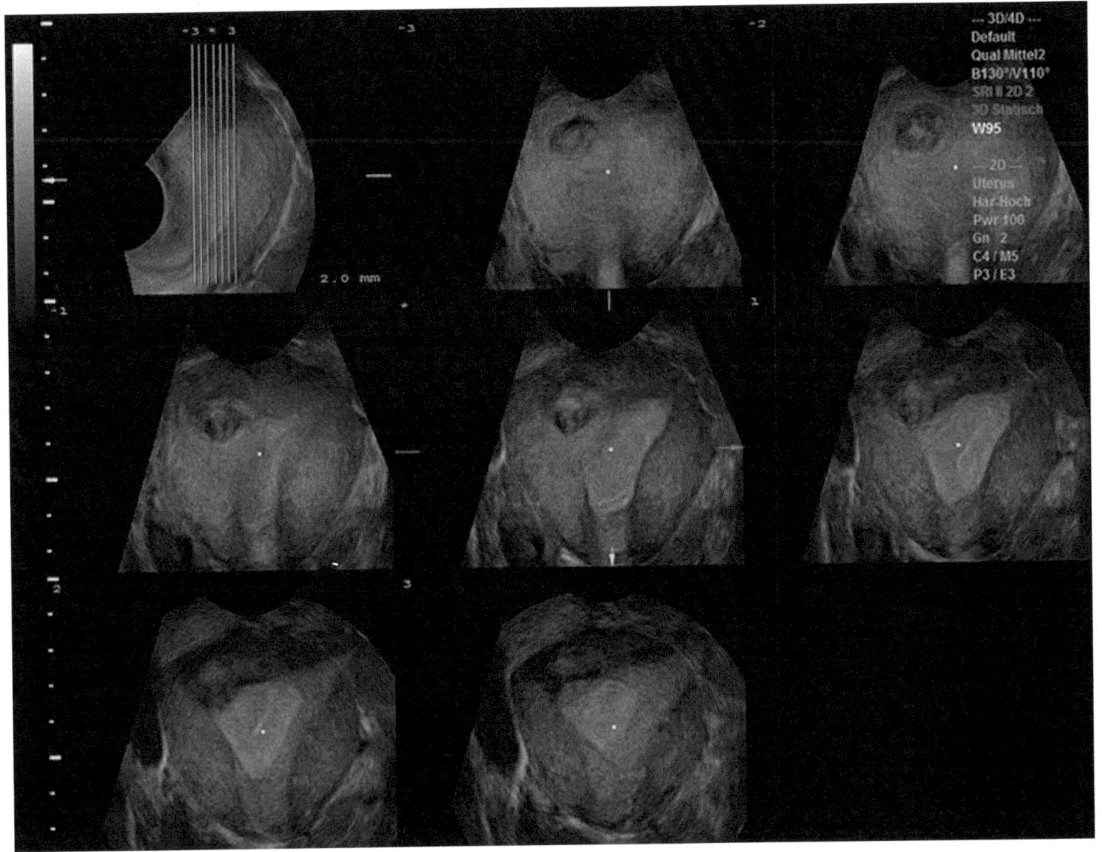

Fig. 5.4 A myoma, for example, as shown by Figs. 5.19, 5.20, and 5.21, can also be presented by a tomographic technique, such as TUI, as shown in this image (Image from Dürr, Transvaginale Sonographie in der Gynäkologie, De Gruyter, 2nd Edition, 2015)

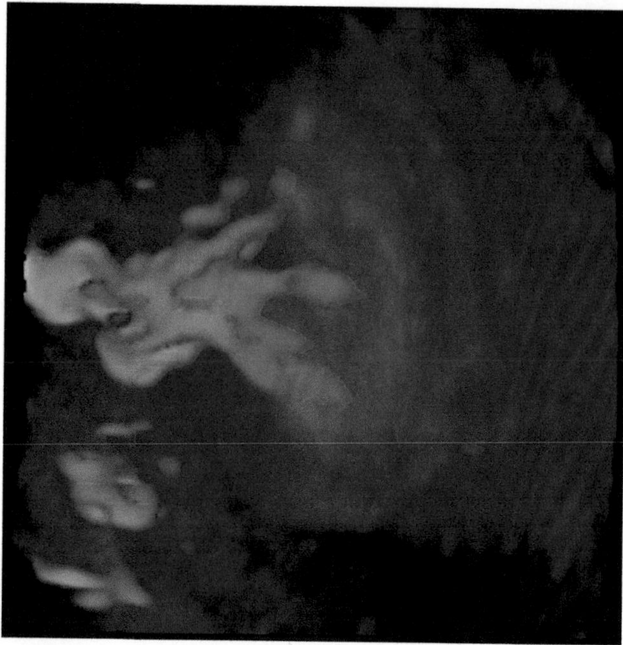

Fig. 5.5 3D color Doppler glass body modus shows impressively pedicle vessels and their branching as well as the diminuating echogenity of endometrial polyp, endometrium and myometrium

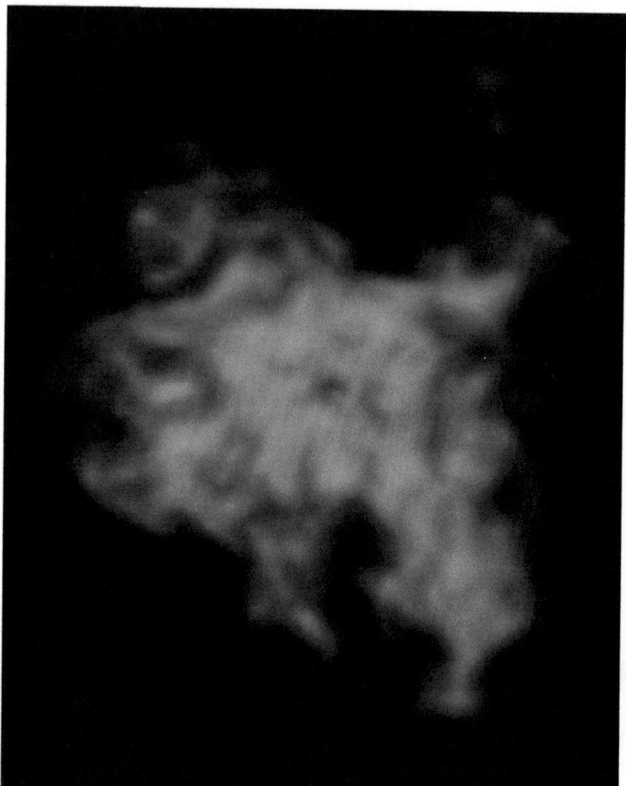

Fig. 5.7 3D presentation of a deep infiltrating endometriosis, inversion modus. The very irregular surface and the pedicle-like extensions give an impression of the highly aggressive potential of this kind of endometriosis and its suspected tendency to progress (Image from Dürr, Transvaginale Sonographie in der Gynäkologie, De Gruyter, 2nd Edition, 2015)

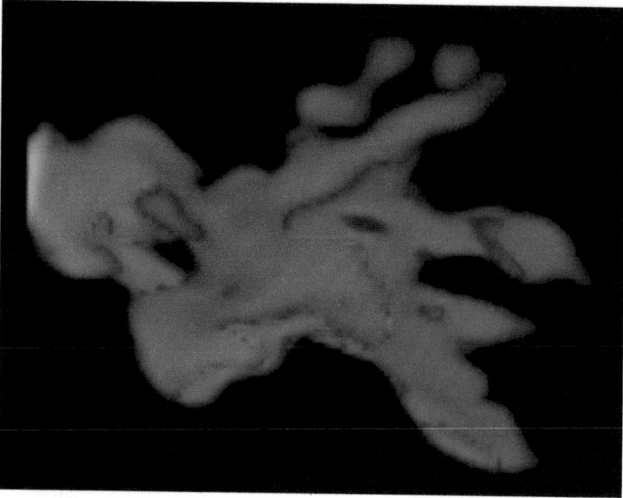

Fig. 5.6 Pure color Doppler without any surrounding tissue shows precisely the branching pedicle vessels (Images from Dürr, Transvaginale Sonographie in der Gynäkologie, De Gruyter, 2nd Edition, 2015)

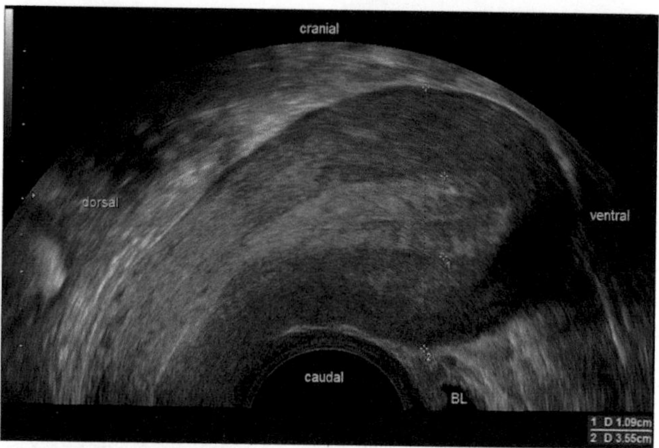

Fig. 5.8 Longitudinal scan of anteverted, anteflected, normal sized uterus with nearly homogeneous echodense endometrium typical for the progestogenic second phase of the cycle

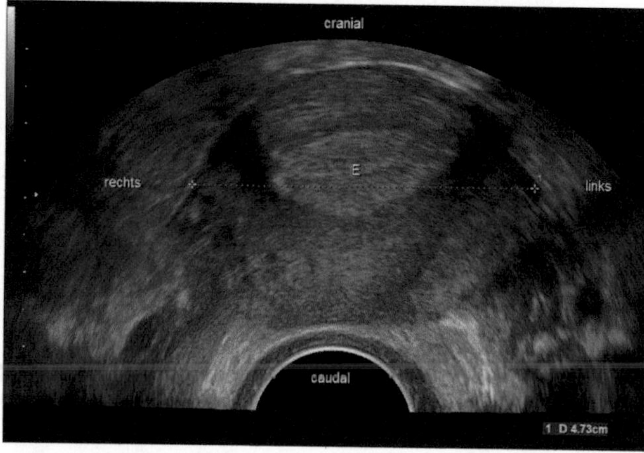

Fig. 5.9 The same uterus, transverse scan through the corpus uteri at its widest lateral extension. See above additionally Fig. 5.1 which demonstrates OmniView and VCI techniques (Images from Dürr, Transvaginale Sonographie in der Gynäkologie, De Gruyter, 2nd Edition, 2015)

Congenital Uterine Anomalies

Some of these anomalies can easily be missed by US if only a longitudinal scan, showing a normal uterus, is performed. Once the investigator has documented a normal uterus he does not always think of a second one, such as a uterus duplex or bicornis or a septate uterus. By performing a transverse scan, it is hard to miss such uterine malformations. Within a few seconds the transverse scan reveals these anomalies, here for example an arcuate uterus (Figs. 5.10, 5.11, and 5.12), see also Fig. 5.3, and a septate uterus (Figs. 5.13 and 5.14). Additionally, an overview of uterine malformations is given by schematic drawings (Fig. 5.15).

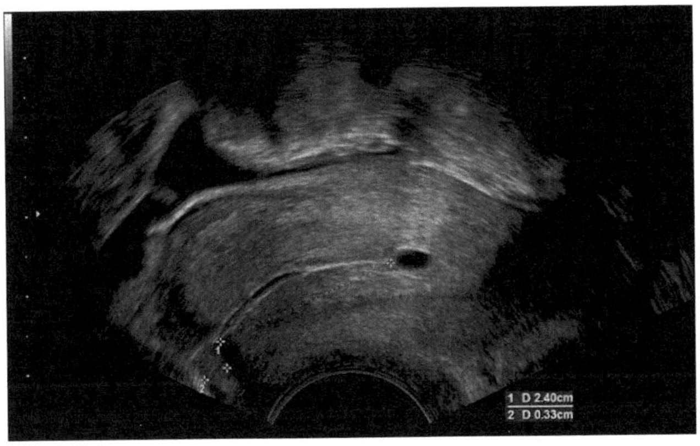

Fig. 5.10 Additionally to Fig. 5.3 a longitudinal scan of the same uterus presenting the cervical part, showing the cervical channel with a small amount of (anechoic) mucus and, at the level of the internal os, a small retention cyst. The distance from internal to external os, here measured at 2.4 cm, corresponds to the cervical length. Close to, but distinct from the external uterine orifice, the dorsal vaginal wall can be seen, here indicated by the two measuring points which demonstrate the wall- thickness of 3.3 mm

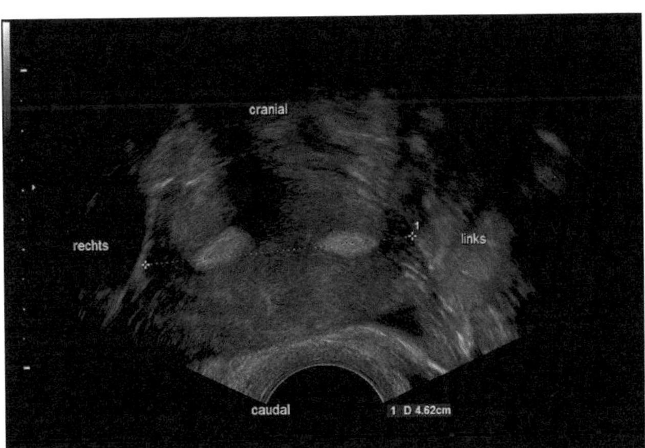

Fig. 5.11 Also additionally to Fig. 5.3 a transverse scan at the fundal region of the corpus uteri clearly showing two endometrial parts separated from each other

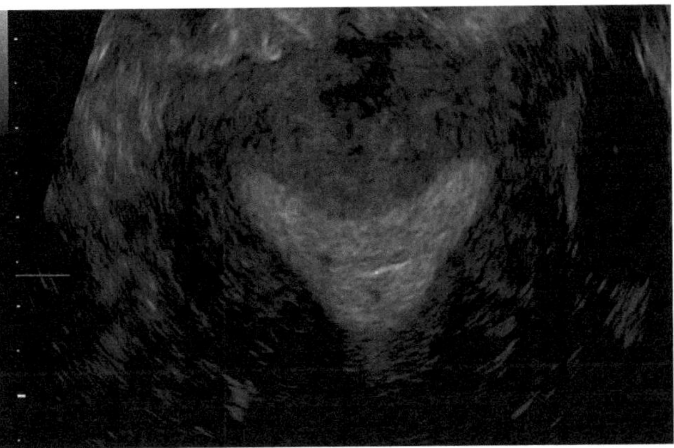

Fig. 5.12 Representation of the endometrium in the fundal region by 3D sonography indicates an arcuate uterus which explains the thicker than expected fundal uterine wall, see above Fig. 5.3 (Images from Dürr, Transvaginale Sonographie in der Gynäkologie, De Gruyter, 2nd Edition, 2015)

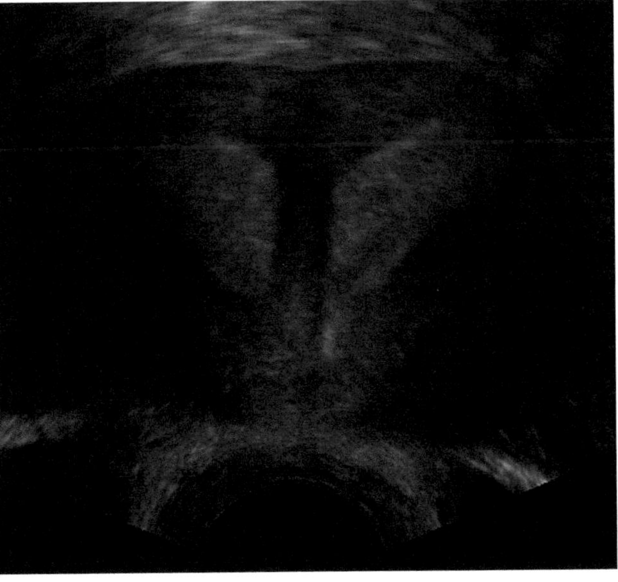

Fig. 5.13 Corpus uteri, transverse scan, showing two parts of endometrium separated from each other. Suspicion of a septate uterus becomes firmer by performing continuous transverse scans from the fundal to the cervical uterine region and reverse

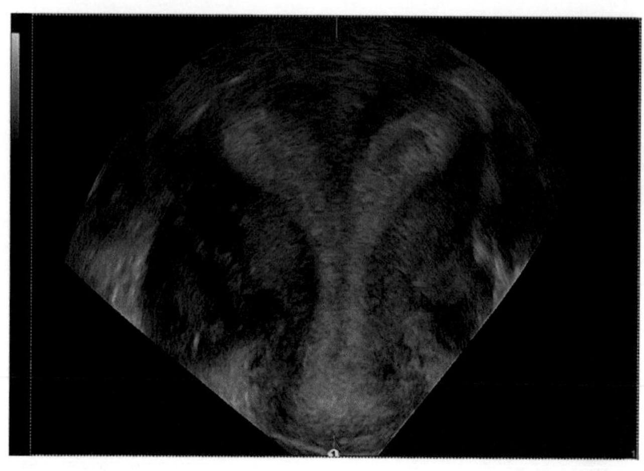

Fig. 5.14 Presentation of the whole uterus in its length by a frontal scan, using the 3D OmniView technique, impressively demonstrates the septate uterus (Images from Dürr, Transvaginale Sonographie in der Gynäkologie, De Gruyter, 2nd Edition, 2015)

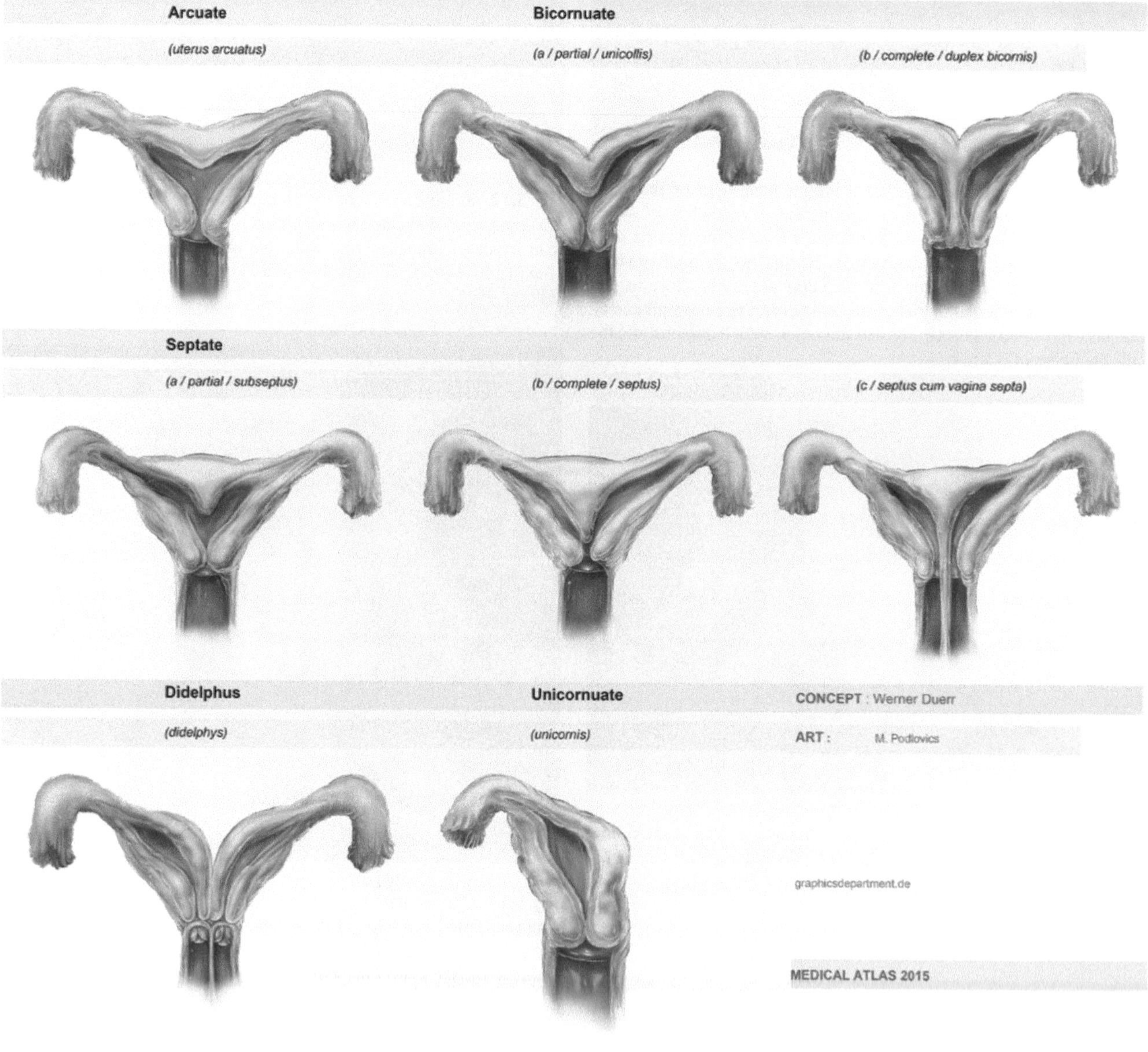

Fig. 5.15 An overview of uterine malformations by schematic drawings

Uterine Myomata

Uterine myomata are the most common benign uterine alterations.

Their location can be intramural, subserosal, submucosal, subserosal-intramural, submucosal-intramural (Fig. 5.16) and subserosal-intramural-submucosal (Figs. 5.17 and 5.18), however, all begin to develop within the uterine wall. Similar to congenital uterine malformations, small myomata, located laterally from the uterine midline, can be missed by TVS in a longitudinal scan whereas a transverse scan reveals the myoma within a few seconds. To prevent overlooking uterine myometrial or intracavitary alterations not located in the midline, it is necessary, or at least helpful, to perform not only a longitudinal but also a transverse scan. This is illustrated by images and additional information gained by 3D (Figs. 5.19, 5.20, 5.21, and 5.22) and TUI techniques, see Fig. 5.4.

To differentiate between myomata and other myometrial or intracavitary alterations, e.g. adenomyosis or endometrial polyps, the use of color Doppler is helpful because myomata usually present typical surrounding blood vessels feeding the myoma (Fig. 5.23). This is in contrast to the more diffuse vascularization of adenomyosis (Figs. 5.24 and 5.25) and the very characteristic vascular pedicle of mostly pedunculated endometrial polyps (Fig. 5.26).

Some examples of myomata and their vascularization are given by the images Figs. 5.16, 5.17, 5.18, 5.23, 5.27, and 5.28.

In some cases the differentiation between subserosal myoma and adnexal tumor can be very difficult by US (Fig. 5.29); however, this is very important with regard to the further diagnostic and therapeutic proceeding. If, using color Doppler, a vascular connection between the suspected adnexal tumor and the uterus is found, the diagnosis would be subserosal myoma (Fig. 5.30). If no vascular connection exists or can be found by color Doppler, further diagnostic and therapeutic steps have to be performed.

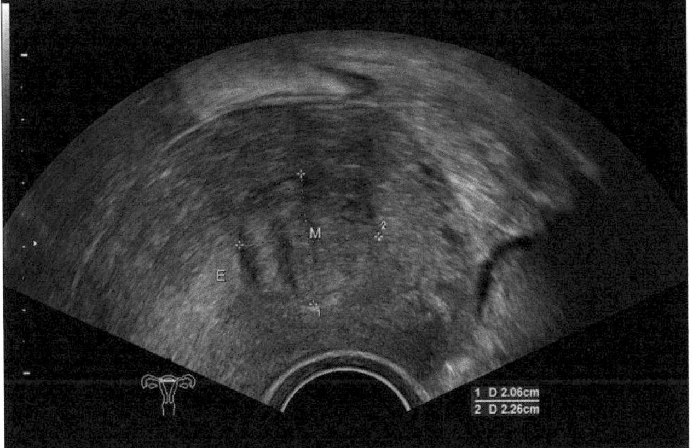

Fig. 5.16 Corpus uteri with a partial submucosal myoma left of the more echodense endometrium, transverse scan

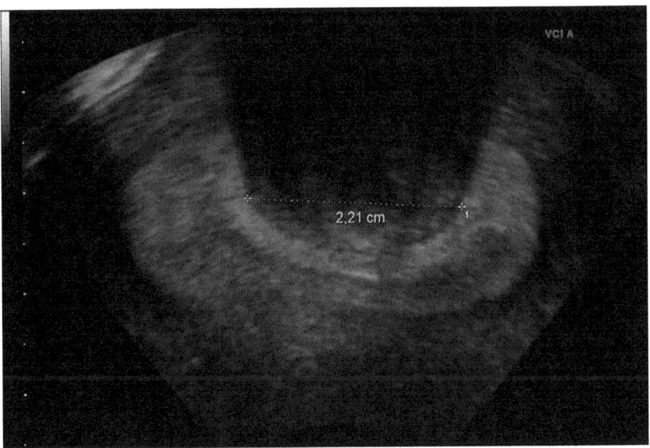

Fig. 5.18 Corpus uteri, transverse scan using 3D and VCI technique to show more impressively the relationship between endometrium and the submucosal part of the myoma

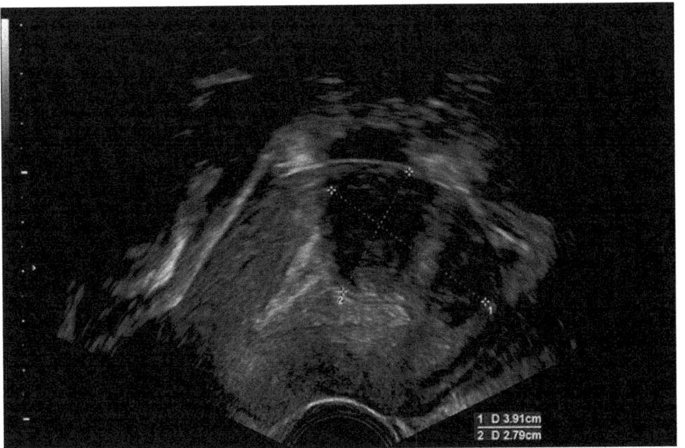

Fig. 5.17 Corpus uteri with a subserosal-intramural-submucosal myoma impressing the endometrium. This image shows the typical differences of echogenity between myometrium which is of middle echodensity, endometrium with its mostly higher echodensity and myoma which is usually hypoechoic in comparison to both

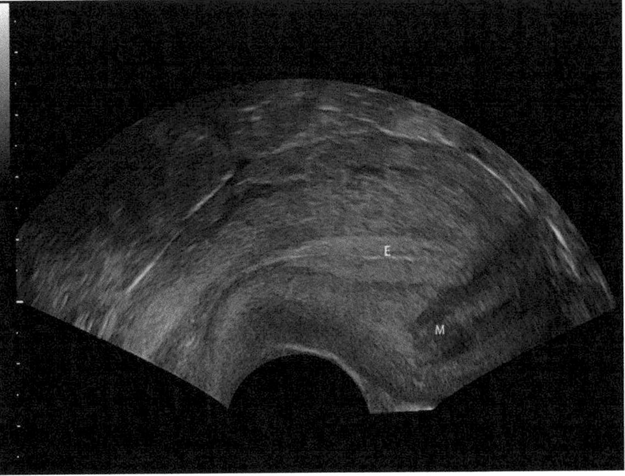

Fig. 5.19 Normal-sized, anteverted, anteflected uterus in a slightly oblique longitudinal scan, including the right paramedian anterior uterine wall, showing a small intramural myoma in the anterior uterine wall, right of the midlinc

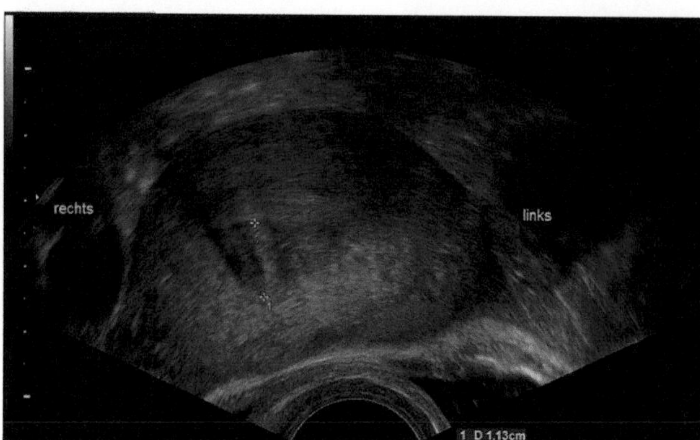

Fig. 5.20 The transverse scan reveals not only the intramural but also the submucosal location of the myoma on the right side

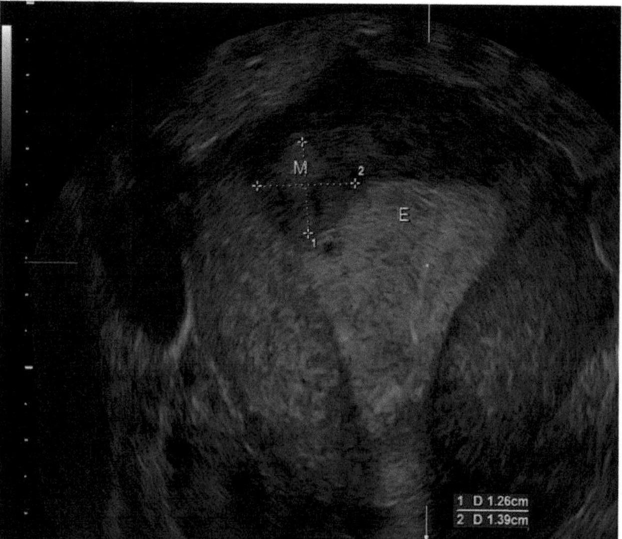

Fig. 5.21 The additional 3D image confirms the intramural and submucosal location of the myoma, at the right tubal angle with possible negative effects on the patency of the interstitial tubal part. Such detailed information is important, especially in cases of fertility disorder. See above also Fig. 5.4, showing the myoma presented by a tomographic technique, such as TUI

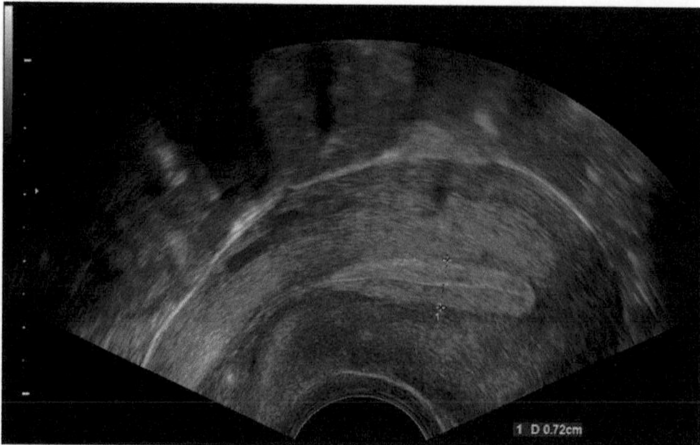

Fig. 5.22 Here, to demonstrate how easily this myoma could have been missed by TVS, a longitudinal scan exactly in the midline where the myoma cannot be seen. This emphasizes the necessity of a transverse scan in addition to the obligatory longitudinal scan when investigating the uterus by US (Images from Dürr, Transvaginale Sonographie in der Gynäkologie, De Gruyter, 2nd Edition, 2015)

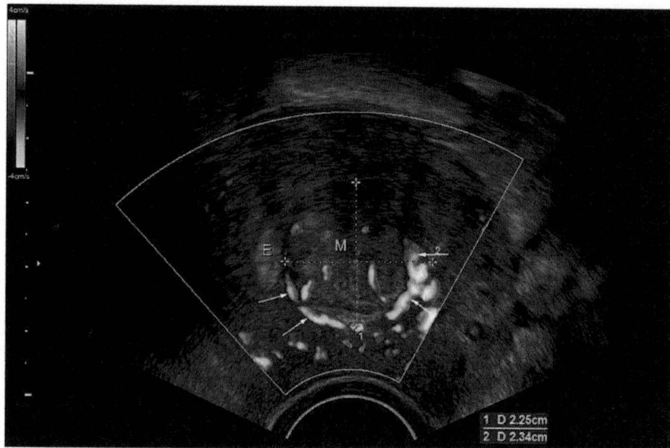

Fig. 5.23 Colour Doppler impressively shows the typical feeding vessels surrounding the myoma and some vessels entering the myoma. See above Fig. 5.16, which presents this myoma without colour Doppler (Images from Dürr, Transvaginale Sonographie in der Gynäkologie, De Gruyter, 2nd Edition, 2015)

Endometrial Polyps

Endometrial polyps are to be found in the uterine cavity, seldom sessile, mostly pedunculated, possibly reaching into the cervical channel and presenting there. The echogenity of these polyps is usually higher than in the endometrium (Fig. 5.31). The differentiation from submucosal myoma is easy by color Doppler when the typical vessel in the vascular pedicle can be seen. This feeding vessel begins in the myometrium, crosses the EMJ and ends within the polyp, see Fig. 5.26. The branching of this feeding vessel within the polyp is shown by Fig. 5.32, see also Figs. 5.5 and 5.6.

Endometrial Hyperplasia

Endometrial hyperplasia is predominantly found in the adolescent and climacteric transitional phase when, because of anovulatoric cycles with corresponding progestagenic deficiency, usually as a result of follicular persistence, the endometrial proliferation, induced by ovarian estrogen, is not opposed sufficiently by progesterone and, therefore, no endometrial transformation with following regular menstrual discharge is

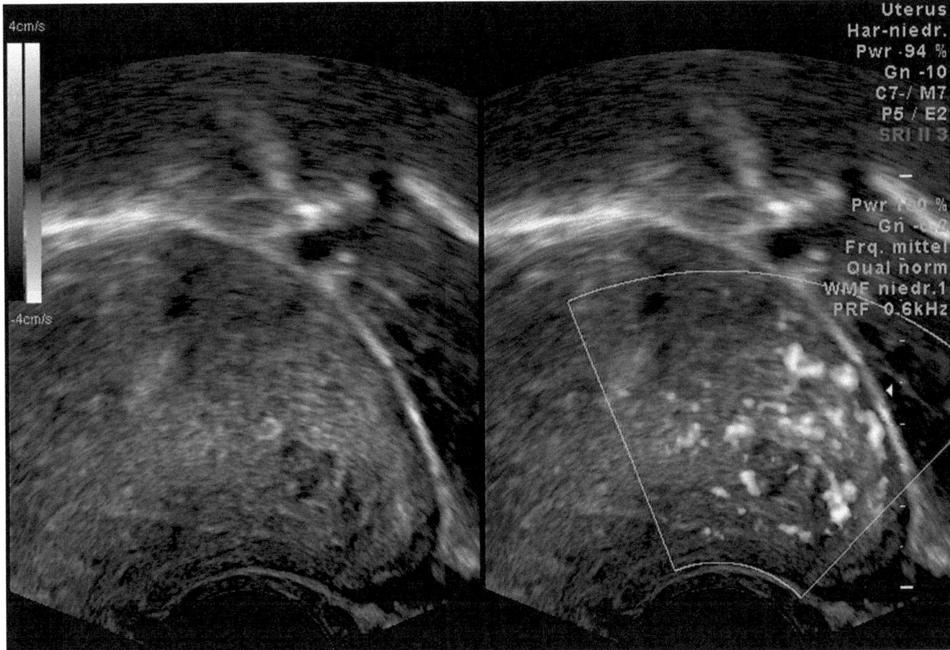

Fig. 5.24 Color Doppler shows a markedly higher and more irregular vascularization of the area affected by adenomyosis in comparison to the regular vascularization by preexisting vessels (Images from Dürr, Transvaginale Sonographie in der Gynäkologie, De Gruyter, 2nd Edition, 2015)

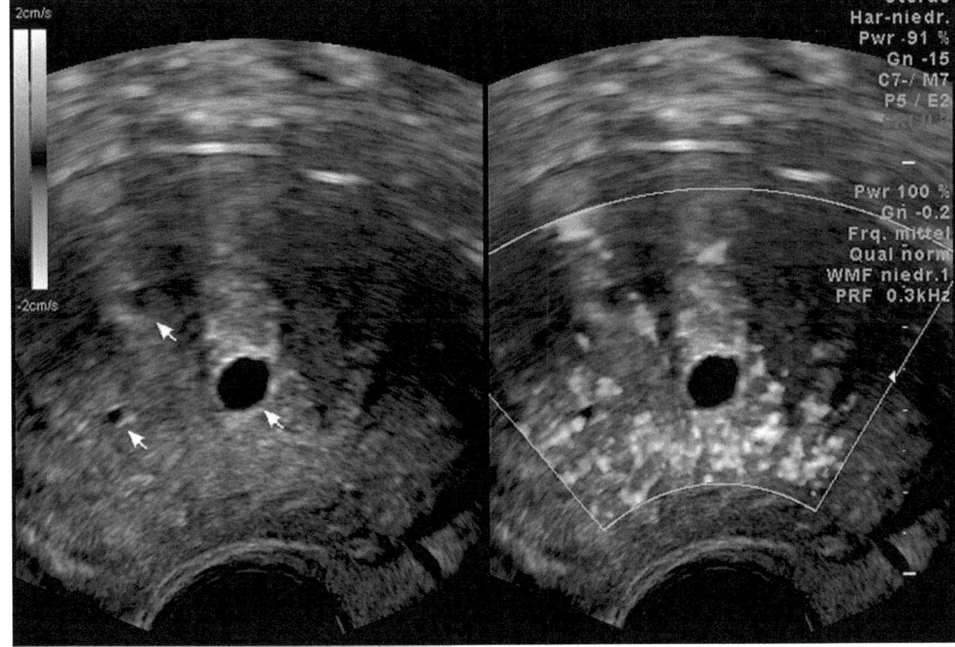

Fig. 5.25 In another area of the same uterus as shown by Fig. 5.72, cystic structures, surrounded by an echogenic endometrium-like margin, are to be found. Color Doppler shows a very marked and diffuse neovascularization in the cystic area as a sign of adenomyosis with a tendency to progress. It seems to be that streaky shadows indicate older processes and cystic findings more recent afflictions of adenomyosis (Images from Dürr, Transvaginale Sonographie in der Gynäkologie, De Gruyter, 2nd Edition, 2015)

possible. Instead of this continuous bleedings occur as a result of highly proliferated endometrium which is no longer fed in its upper layers whereas proliferation continues.

High resolution TVS can show the typical microcysts within an endometrial hyperplasia, well known from the histological term "cystic glandular hyperplasia" (Fig. 5.33).

Endometrial hyperplasia can be treated with progestin to induce an endometrial transformation and withdrawal bleeding. This is an alternative to possible sequential curettages (Figs. 5.33, 5.34, and 5.35).

Endometrial Carcinoma

Endometrial carcinoma, the most common malignant gynecological tumor, can be detected and described in its extension by sonography, especially TVS, with the help of color Doppler. The sonographic finding is mostly an inhomogeneous intracavitary echo which shows an irregular vascularization, such as neovascularization typical for malignant tumors. The EMJ is penetrated by tumor vessels in areas where myometrial invasion has taken place (Figs. 5.36, 5.37, 5.38, 5.39, and 5.40).

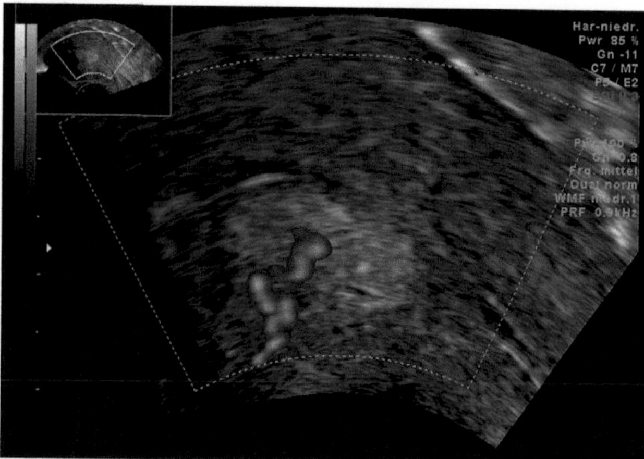

Fig. 5.26 Color Doppler demonstrates a well-defined feeding vessel crossing the EMJ, ending in an intracavitary echodense clearly demarcated mass. This pedicle vessel indicates an endometrial polyp and makes sure that indeed the finding is doubtless nothing else, no submucous myoma, no endometrial hyperplasia, for example

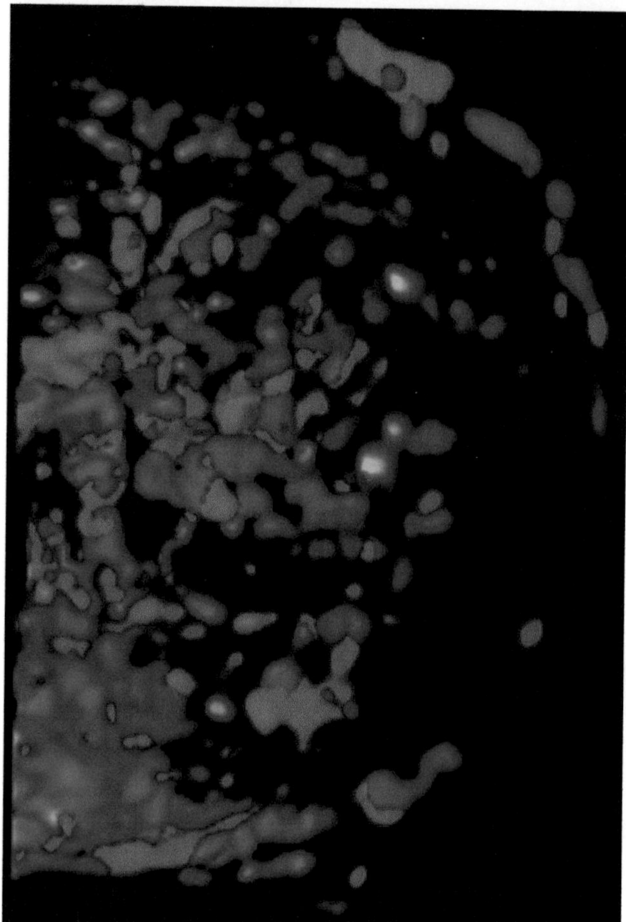

Fig. 5.28 3D color flow shows a very intense vascularization and perfusion of the myoma (see Figs. 5.17 and 5.18) as a possible sign of its tendency to grow. In this case the tendency was confirmed by comparison of the actual findings with the preceding findings (Images from Dürr, Transvaginale Sonographie in der Gynäkologie, De Gruyter, 2nd Edition, 2015)

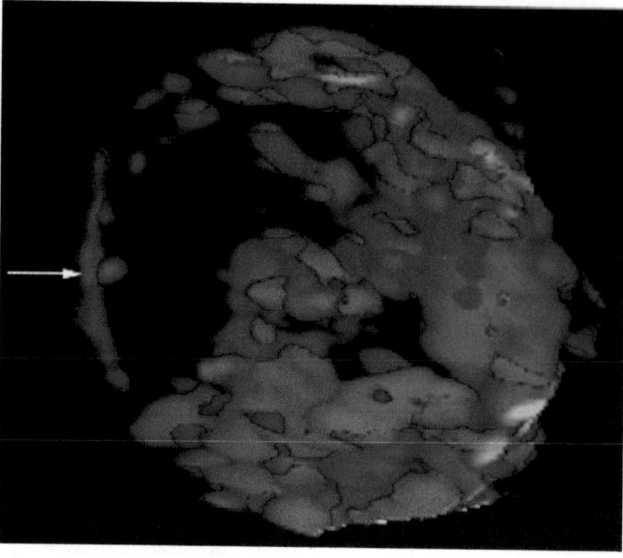

Fig. 5.27 3D color flow demonstrates, like an angiogram, the relatively intense vascularization of this myoma (see Figs. 5.16 and 5.23) as a possible expression of its tendency to grow (Images from Dürr, Transvaginale Sonographie in der Gynäkologie, De Gruyter, 2nd Edition, 2015)

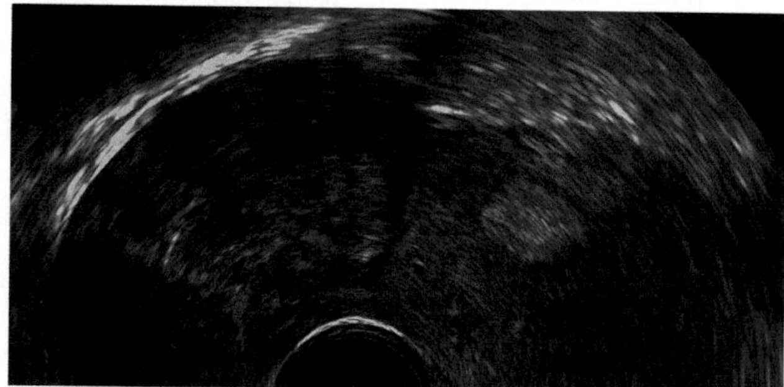

Fig. 5.29 A tumor-like mass in the right adnexal region, as large as the corpus uteri, seems to displace the corpus uteri (identifiable by the echogenic endometrium) from the midline to the left side. Echogenity and clear demarcation of this mass as well as its close vicinity to the corpus uteri give suspicion of a subserosal myoma

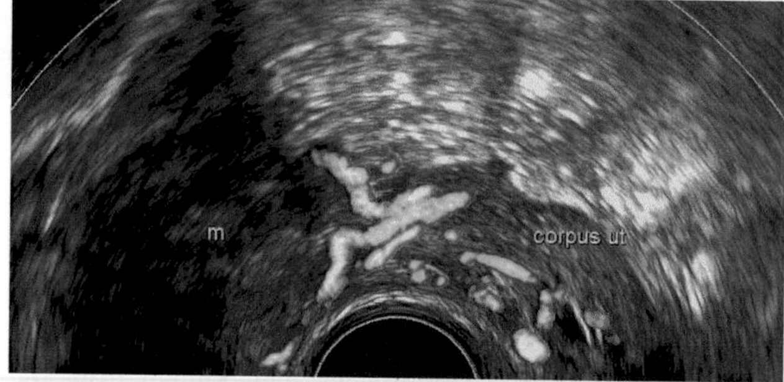

Fig. 5.30 Intensive search by color Doppler succeeded in showing not only a vascular connection between corpus uteri and tumor-like mass but also the typical feeding vessels surrounding the myoma, originating from the corpus uteri. Thus, the diagnosis subserosal myoma could be confirmed and a tumor, originating from the right adnexal region, was excluded (Images from Dürr, Transvaginale Sonographie in der Gynäkologie, De Gruyter, 2nd Edition, 2015)

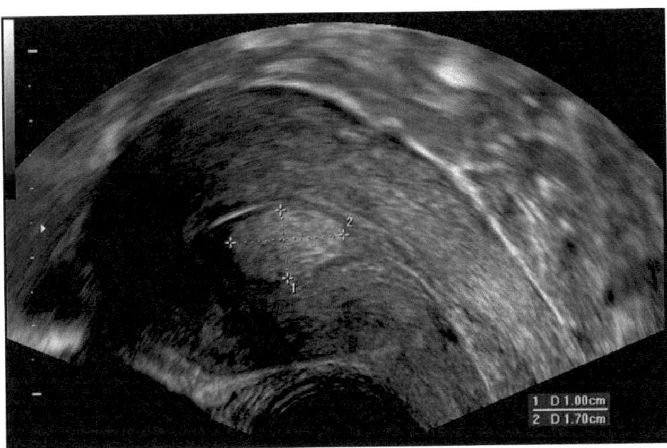

Fig. 5.31 Uterus in a longitudinal scan showing an intracavitary, echodense, clearly demarcated mass, at first sight resembling an endometrial polyp. Additional Color Doppler – see Fig. 5.26 – demonstrates a well-defined feeding vessel crossing the EMJ. This pedicle vessel indicates an endometrial polyp

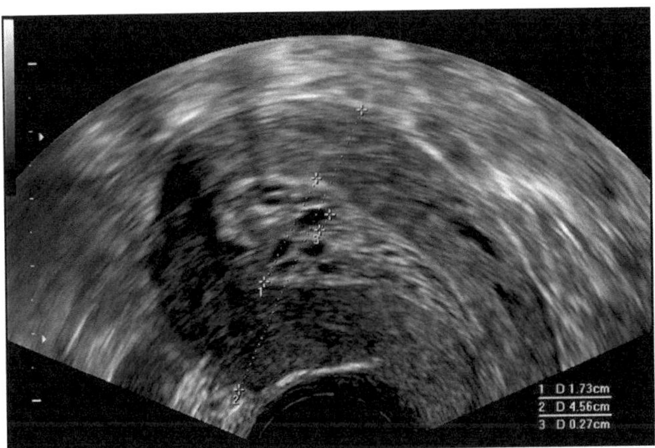

Fig. 5.33 Uterine longitudinal scan shows a microcystic intracavitary echo, thickness a.-p. 17.3 mm. In connection with an existing follicular persistence in a 47-year-old woman with continuous bleeding, this finding should be an endometrial hyperplasia

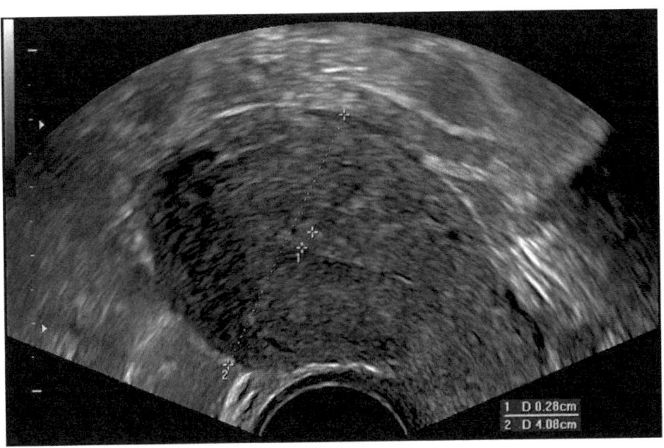

Fig. 5.35 Thus, as endometrial hyperplasia was expected on the basis of sonographic diagnostics in connection with anamnestic data, administration of an exogenous progesterone agent should therapeutically be at least as helpful as a curettage. The image demonstrates the uterine cavity as nearly empty after gestagen-induced transformation and following withdrawal bleeding (Images from Dürr, Transvaginale Sonographie in der Gynäkologie, De Gruyter, 2nd Edition, 2015)

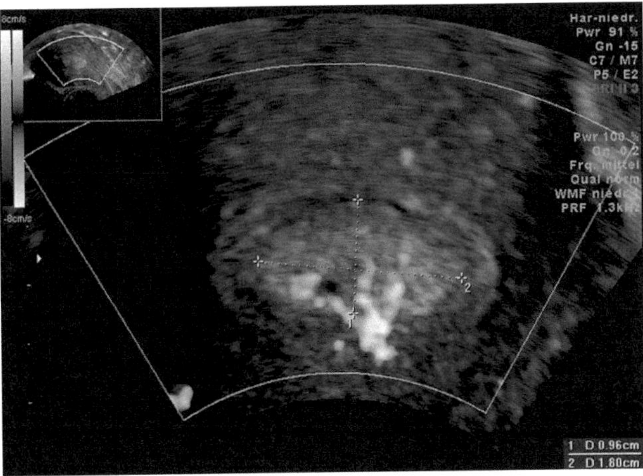

Fig. 5.32 The transverse scan shows a branching of the pedicle vessel within the endometrial polyp. See above additionally Figs. 5.5 and 5.6 which demonstrate sonographic-technical possibilities and are less part of the daily routine proceedings (Images from Dürr, Transvaginale Sonographie in der Gynäkologie, De Gruyter, 2nd Edition, 2015)

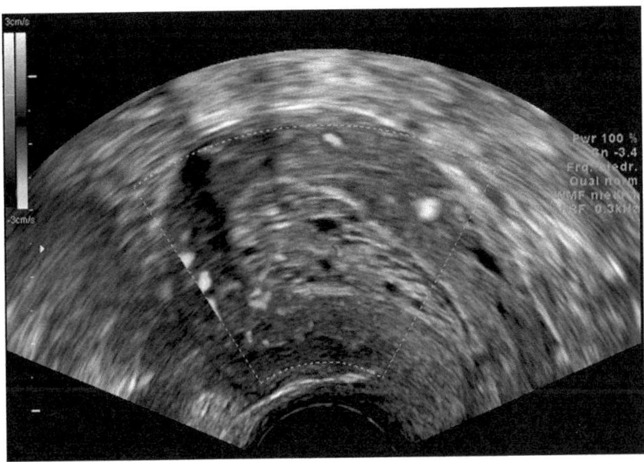

Fig. 5.34 To exclude an endometrial polyp, which looks very similar when of cystic-fibrous texture, color Doppler is used. Only a spiral artery-like vessel, no pedicular vessel typical for an endometrial polyp, can be found

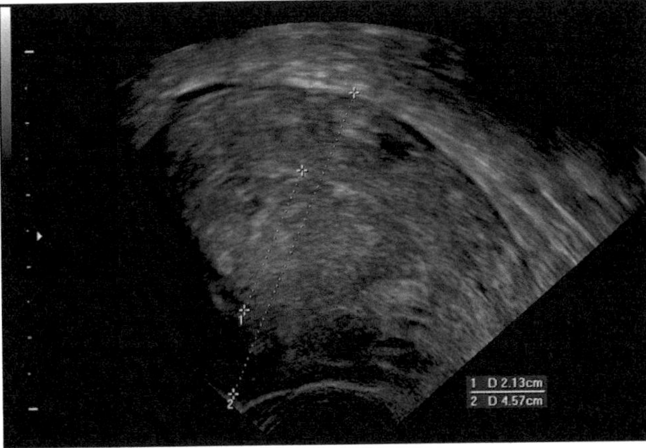

Fig. 5.36 Uterus of a 55-year-old woman with postmenopausal bleeding. The longitudinal scan shows a markedly thickened inhomogeneous endometrium of 21.3 mm which seems distinctly demarcated from the myometrium

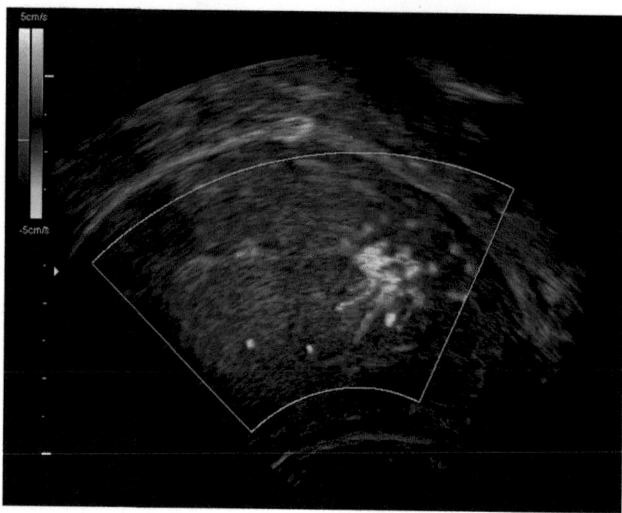

Fig. 5.37 Transverse scan in the fundal region of the corpus uteri. The color Doppler reveals on the left side a chaotic neovascularization typical for malignant growth, with vessels penetrating the EMJ in this zone of myometrial invasion

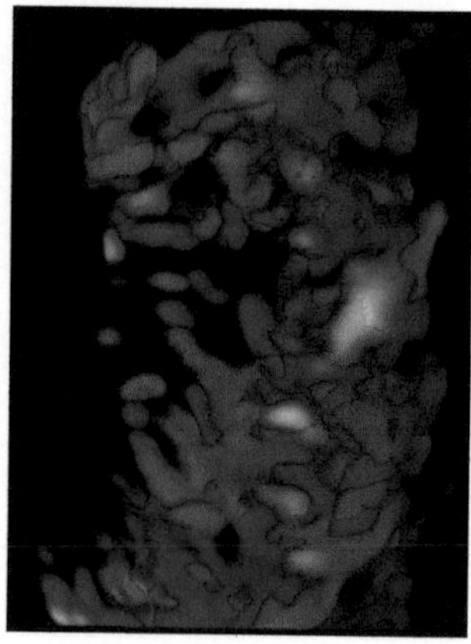

Fig. 5.38 3D color presentation of this zone confirms the tumor-suspicious neovascularization. Postoperative histological diagnosis: endometrial carcinoma pT1a (Images from Dürr, Transvaginale Sonographie in der Gynäkologie, De Gruyter, 2nd Edition, 2015)

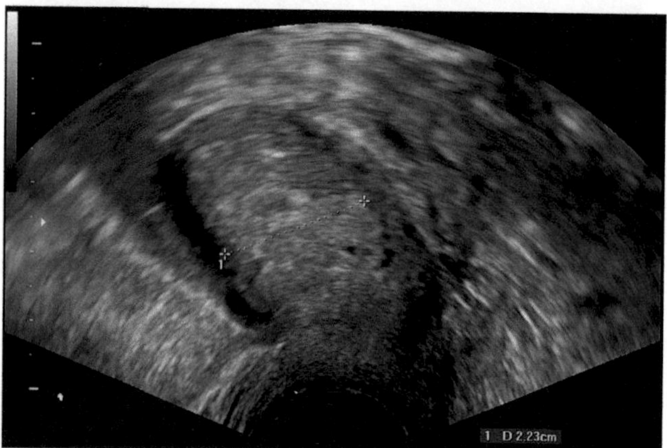

Fig. 5.39 Corpus uteri with endometrial cancer, longitudinal scan. The extension and respective myometrial invasion of the tumor can easily be estimated and measured when, as in this case, there is a clear demarcation by markedly different echogenities between tumor (higher echogenity) and the non-invaded myometrium (lower echogenity)

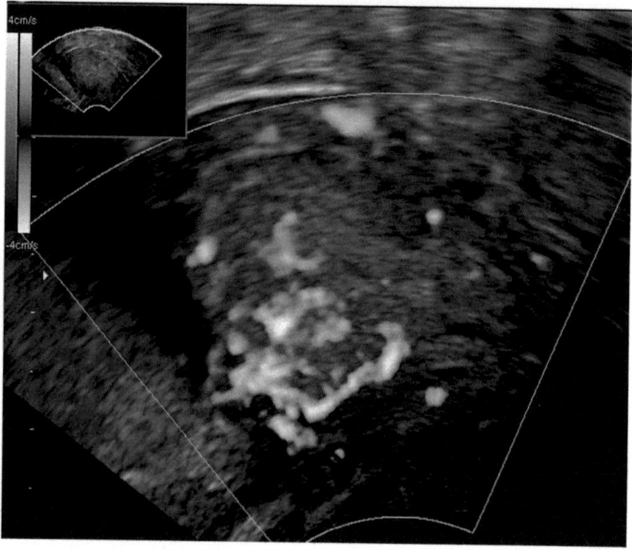

Fig. 5.40 Color Doppler shows the irregular vessels of a typical tumor neovascularization which involves the endometrium and the myometrium (Images by courtesy of Dr. Isabel Wallrafen)

Uterine Sarcoma

Uterine sarcoma, a very rare tumor, is often mistaken for a fast growing myoma. Color Doppler can be helpful to confirm the suspicion of malignancy when an extraordinarily high vascularization of tumor-like pattern is detected. Every fast-growing uterine tumor, even in the case of well-known myomata, warrants further evaluation for uterine sarcoma. Myomata do not exclude sarcoma; however, not all sarcomas grow markedly fast and not all sarcomas present the typical tumor neovascularization.

Other sonographic signs of malignancy could be central anechoic or low echogenic areas, caused by tumor-necrosis or hemorrhage; however, these findings are sonographically indistinguishable from very similar looking areas of central liquefaction in myomas without any additional malignancy.

In summary, we have no really reliable sonographic signs to diagnose or exclude uterine sarcomas preoperatively. Nevertheless, sonography with the help of color Doppler is and will most likely remain an important diagnostic tool in the preoperative differentiation of benign from malignant uterine mass. If sonographically there is any suspicion of malignancy, morcellation should not be performed and no other uterine incision except for total hysterectomy to prevent, as far as possible, tumor tissue or cell dissemination.

In future, a risk score for uterine sarcomas, based not only on imaging parameters, but including all other known

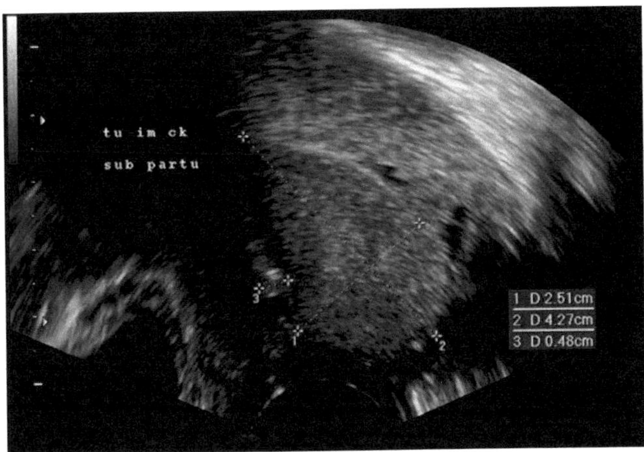

Fig. 5.41 Longitudinal scan of the uterine cervix showing a tumor in the cervical channel, seeming to be "sub partu"

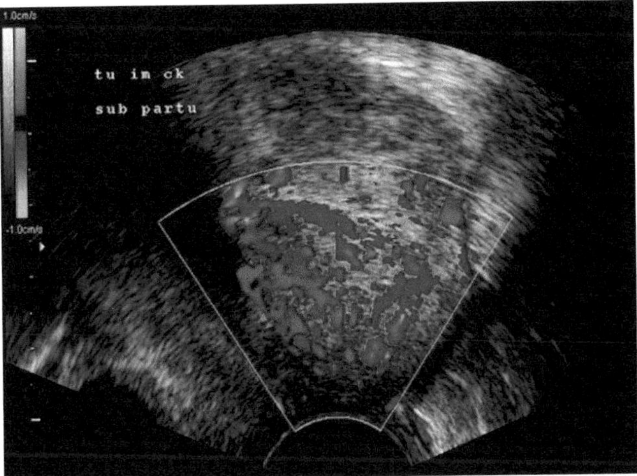

Fig. 5.42 Color Doppler shows a remarkably high but totally irregular perfusion of this polyp-like tumor. Postoperative histological diagnosis: "leiomyosarcoma of low malignancy" (Images from Dürr, Transvaginale Sonographie in der Gynäkologie, De Gruyter, 2nd Edition, 2015)

relevant risk factors, could be helpful in decreasing the number of coincidentally, intraoperatively or postoperatively, histologically found sarcomas, by increasing the number of preoperatively suspected and thus adequately operated tumors.

Examples of uterine sarcomas and their vascularization are given by the images Figs. 5.41, 5.42, 5.43, and 5.44.

Cervical Carcinoma

The diagnosis of cervical carcinoma is not the domain of sonography although more progredient tumors can be estimated sonographically (Figs. 5.45, 5.46, and 5.47). It has been successfully proven that early diagnosis of cervical cancer is still the domain of cytology and histology after biopsy.

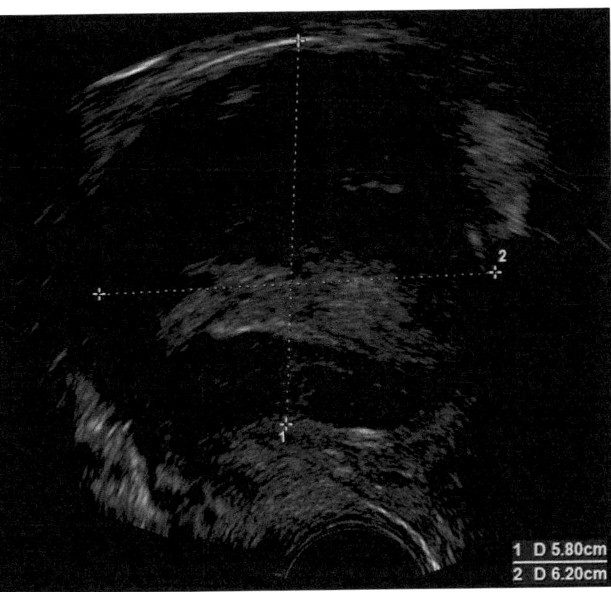

Fig. 5.43 Cross section of a previously known myoma which seems to have grown markedly since the last control some months ago

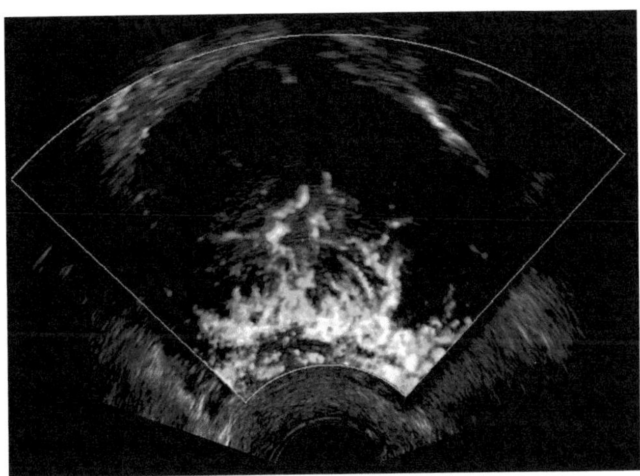

Fig. 5.44 Color Doppler reveals an extremely high vascularization with the pattern of typically chaotic tumor neovascularization. The postoperative histological diagnosis was uterine sarcoma.(Images by courtesy of Dr. Isabel Wallrafen)

Tamoxifen-Induced Intrauterine Alterations

Sonographically, uterine alterations under Tamoxifen treatment usually look like cystic intracavitary proliferations, but in reality are subendometrial extended cysts with atrophy of the endometrium. The uterine cavity is often totally smooth except when additional intracavitary proliferations, such as endometrial polyps, are present. The subendometrial cysts can differ in size from very small, similar to the microcysts in cystic glandular hyperplasia or cystic fibrous endometrial polyps, to relatively large, as shown in the image (Fig. 5.48).

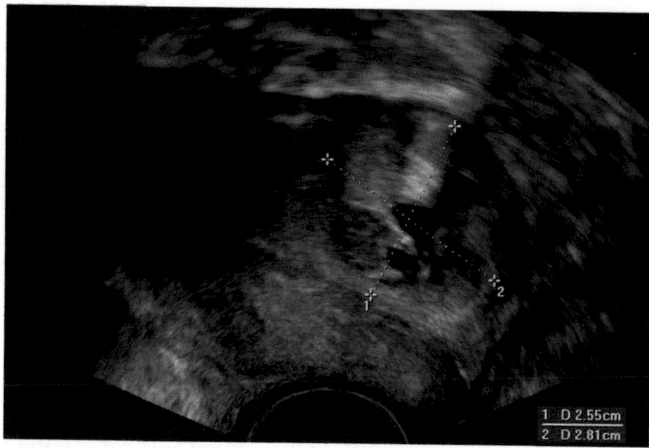

Fig. 5.45 In this image, left is anterior and right is posterior. The longitudinal scan of a cervix shows a clear, demarcated area in the posterior wall with different echogenities from echodense to anechoic. The described finding is also palpable as a strong knot similar to a cervical myoma. Diverse, previously known myomata are palpable as subserosal myomata originating from the uterine corpus

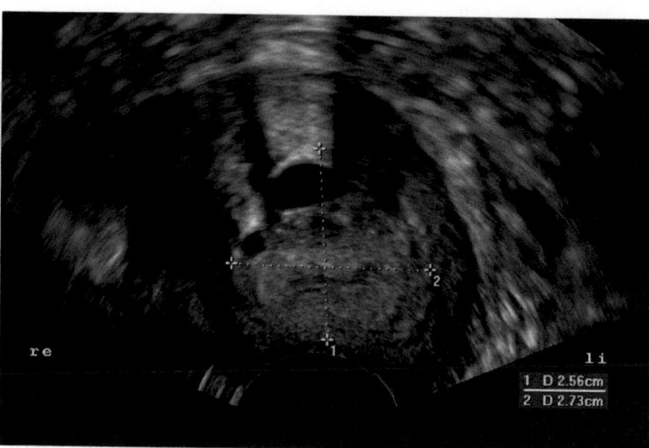

Fig. 5.46 Transverse scan demonstrates that the alteration also includes, but to a lower degree, the anterior cervical wall without direct connection to the cervical channel. The intact-looking circular layer of cervical endometrium around the cervical channel may correspond to an inconspicuous pap smear taken some months previously. Therefore, the differential diagnosis could tend more to a cervical myoma with zones of liquefaction rather than cervical carcinoma

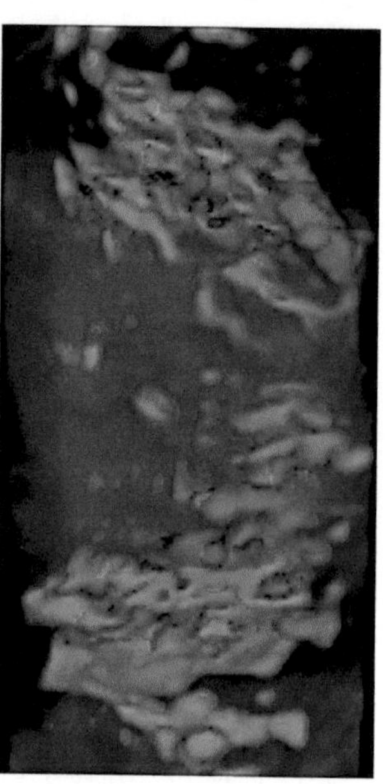

Fig. 5.47 3D color Doppler in glass body modus reveals a very remarkable vascularization over the whole cervix with the pattern of typical tumor neovascularization, corresponding to a cervical carcinoma, as was histologically confirmed

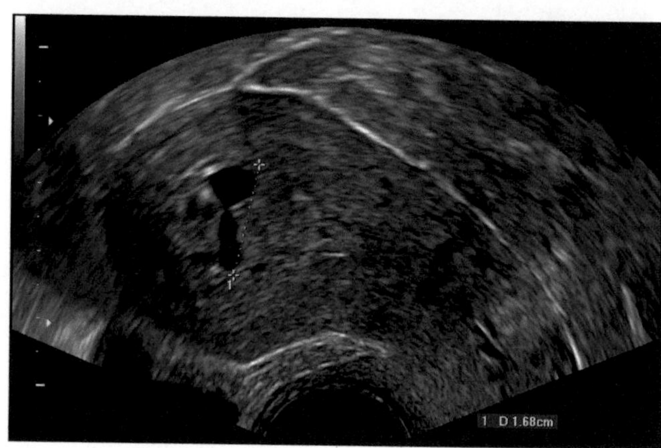

Fig. 5.48 Uterus in a longitudinal scan with intracavitary-looking cystic proliferations which in reality are typical subendometrial cysts under Tamoxifen treatment, whereas the endometrium is atrophic (Image by courtesy of Dr. Annette Philippi)

Intrauterine Fluid Collection (Serometra)

Intrauterine fluid collection presents sonographically as anechoic. Sonographically confirmed intrauterine fluid collection is often seen by chance in postmenopausal women with cervical stenosis (Fig. 5.49). In these cases no further treatment is necessary, provided there are no other intracavitary findings.

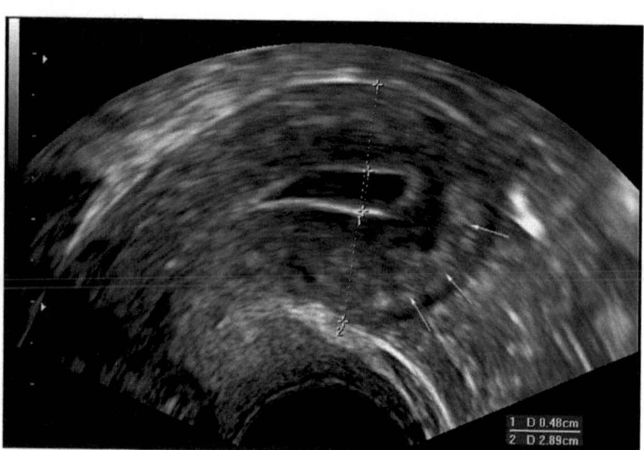

Fig. 5.49 Intrauterine fluid collection (Serometra) in a 75-year-old woman. Noticeable is not only the small amount of intracavitary serous liquidity but also the hyperechoic zones in the outer myometrial region (*arrows*) as a sign of atheromatous alterations in the arcade arteries (Image from Dürr, Transvaginale Sonographie in der Gynäkologie, De Gruyter, 2nd Edition, 2015)

Hematometra

Hematometra refers to a uterus with an intracavitary accumulation of blood. The causes for this condition vary and must be clarified. The intracavitary echo is homogenous because of the corpuscular contents of blood and, as to be expected, intracavitary vascularization will not be found (Figs. 5.50 and 5.51).

Pyometra presents sonographically very similar to hematometra.

Adherent Placental Remnants

Remnants of pregnancy can remain intrauterine after delivery and after abortion. Sonographic controls can be helpful to detect and remove them, if necessary. Remaining placental tissue has the potential for malignant degeneration and must be removed (Fig. 5.52).

The leading sign of a vital and therefore potentially dangerous placental remnant is vascularization within the sonographic finding. Vessels can be seen crossing the EMJ, usually reaching deep into the myometrium (Figs. 5.52 and 5.53). This is not found in blood clots. Another sign of a remaining "vital" placental remnant is possible hormonal activity. Both signs, vascularization and hormonal activity, can easily be assessed, the one by color Doppler, the other by serodiagnosis of HCG.

If, to prevent possible uterine damage, expectant management with regard to a possible spontaneous resolving of the suspected placental remnant is chosen, sonographic and serodiagnostic short time controls are strongly indicated. If there is no rapid decrease in vascularization and especially in HCG-values, operative removal has to be performed sooner rather than later.

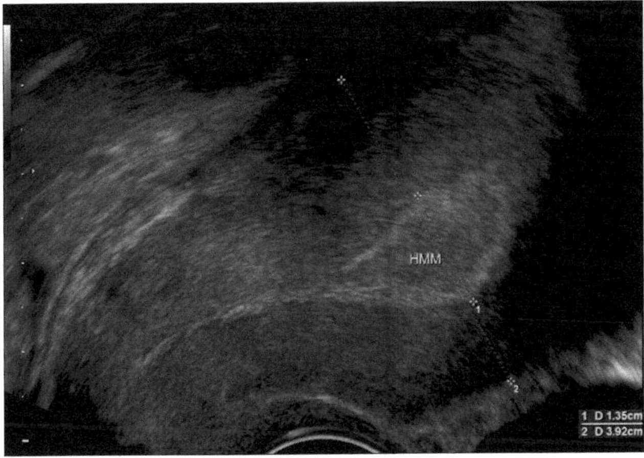

Fig. 5.50 Hematometra after spontaneous abortion. Homogenous intracavitary echo as a sign of liquid, not yet clotted blood

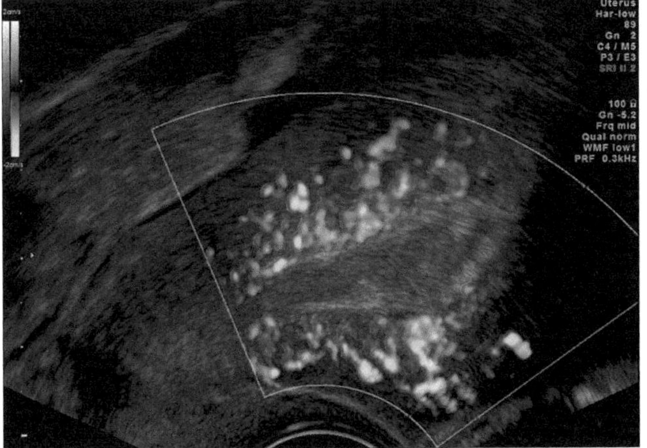

Fig. 5.51 Color Doppler shows, as expected, no intracavitary vascularization. The increased myometrial and subendometrial vascularization ends exactly at the wall of the uterine cavity (Images from of Dürr, Transvaginale Sonographie in der Gynäkologie, De Gruyter, 2nd Edition, 2015)

Intrauterine Adhesions

Intrauterine adhesions can develop after intrauterine surgery, e.g. curettage, and can be a cause of infertility. They disrupt the EMJ and present sonographically as endometrial defects (Figs. 5.54, 5.55, 5.56, 5.57, 5.58, and 5.59).

Subendometrial Fibrosis

Subendometrial fibrosis can occur after intrauterine surgery, such as a curettage, and seems to be without significant effect on endometrial function. Sonographically subendometrial fibrosis presents as echogenic foci in the basal endometrium [1] (Fig. 5.60).

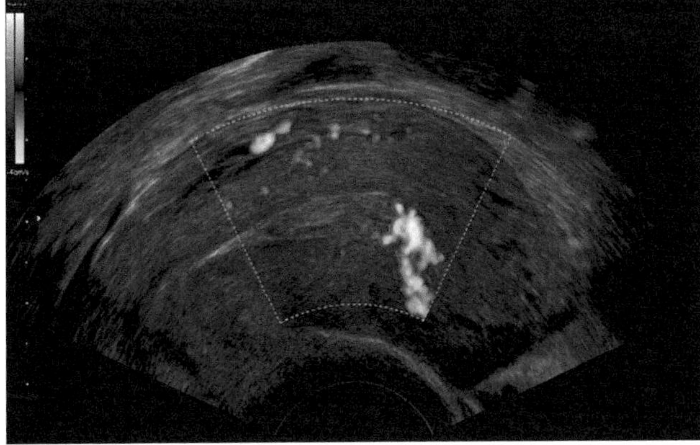

Fig. 5.52 Uterus was scanned because of continuous bleeding 3 months after spontaneous abortion. An intracavitary, spindle-like mass with a very marked vascularization in the fundal part crosses the EMJ and reaches deep into the myometrium

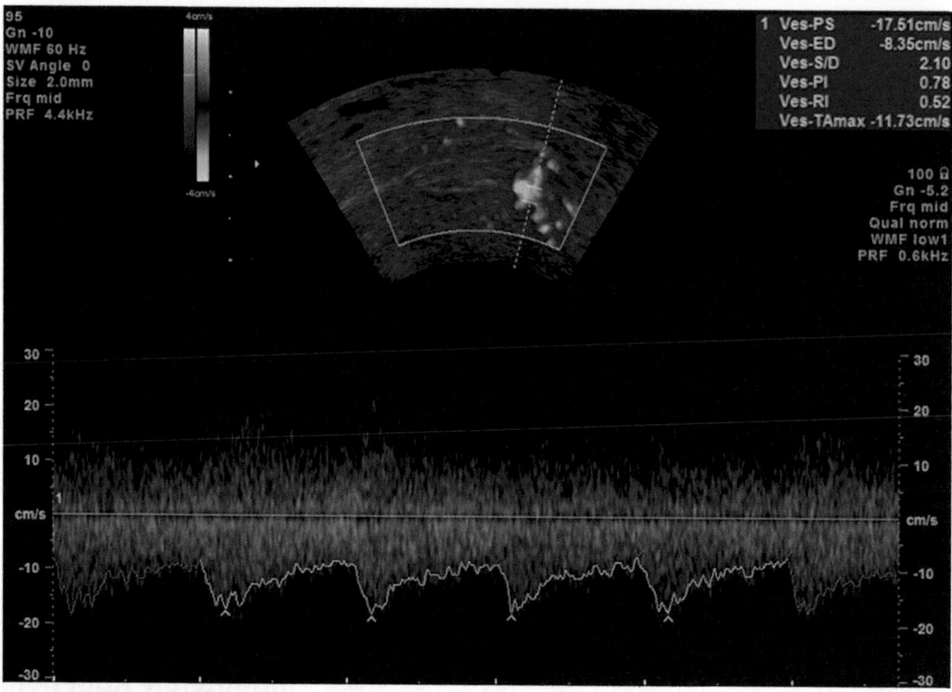

Fig. 5.53 Spectral Doppler shows the typical low impedance of neovascularization. This, in connection with the color flow image and the anamnestic information, leads to the suspicion of hormonal active "vital" placental remnants. Corresponding to this suspicion, beta-HCG was 720 mIE/ml and the histologically confirmed diagnosis after curettage: "regressive altered abortion material with partial mole-like degeneration of the villi. In the presented material no signs of malignant growth." (Images from Dürr, Transvaginale Sonographie in der Gynäkologie, De Gruyter, 2nd Edition, 2015)

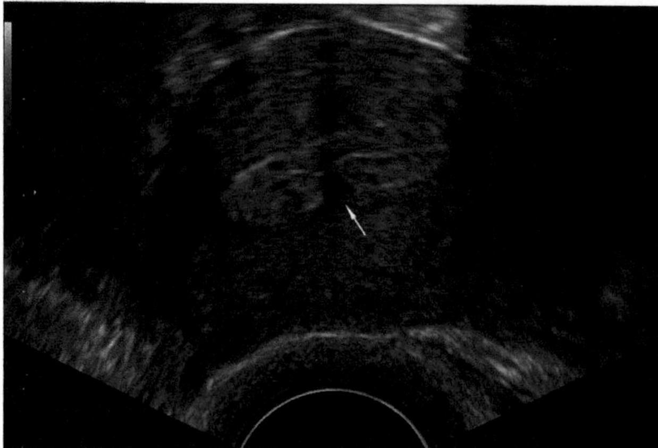

Fig. 5.54 The image shows an endometrial defect (*arrow*) with focal interruption of the EMJ, typical for intrauterine adhesion

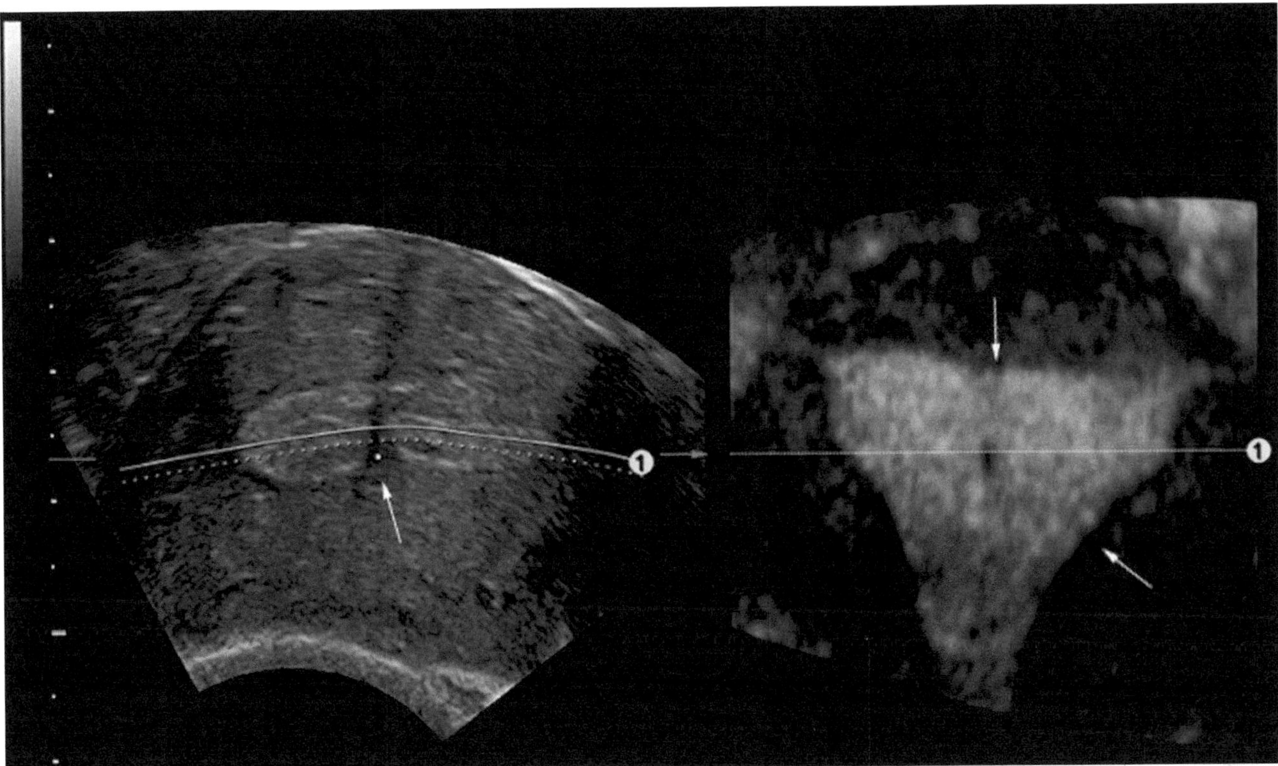

Fig. 5.55 Frontal scan by 3D OmniView technique for better localization and presentation of the very thinly marked adhesion

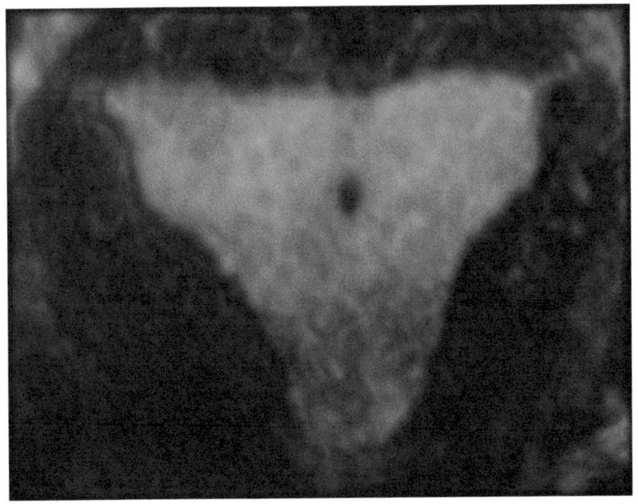

Fig. 5.56 The same frontal scan augmented and colored for better optical perception. Supplementary case history: state after curettage because of abortion (Images from Dürr, Transvaginale Sonographie in der Gynäkologie, De Gruyter, 2nd Edition, 2015)

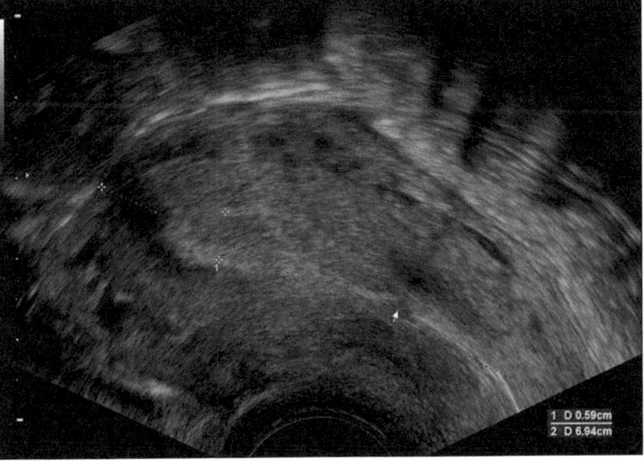

Fig. 5.57 A second example of an endometrial defect with focal interruption of the EMJ, located in the lower part of the uterine cavity (*arrow*), suspicious for intrauterine adhesion

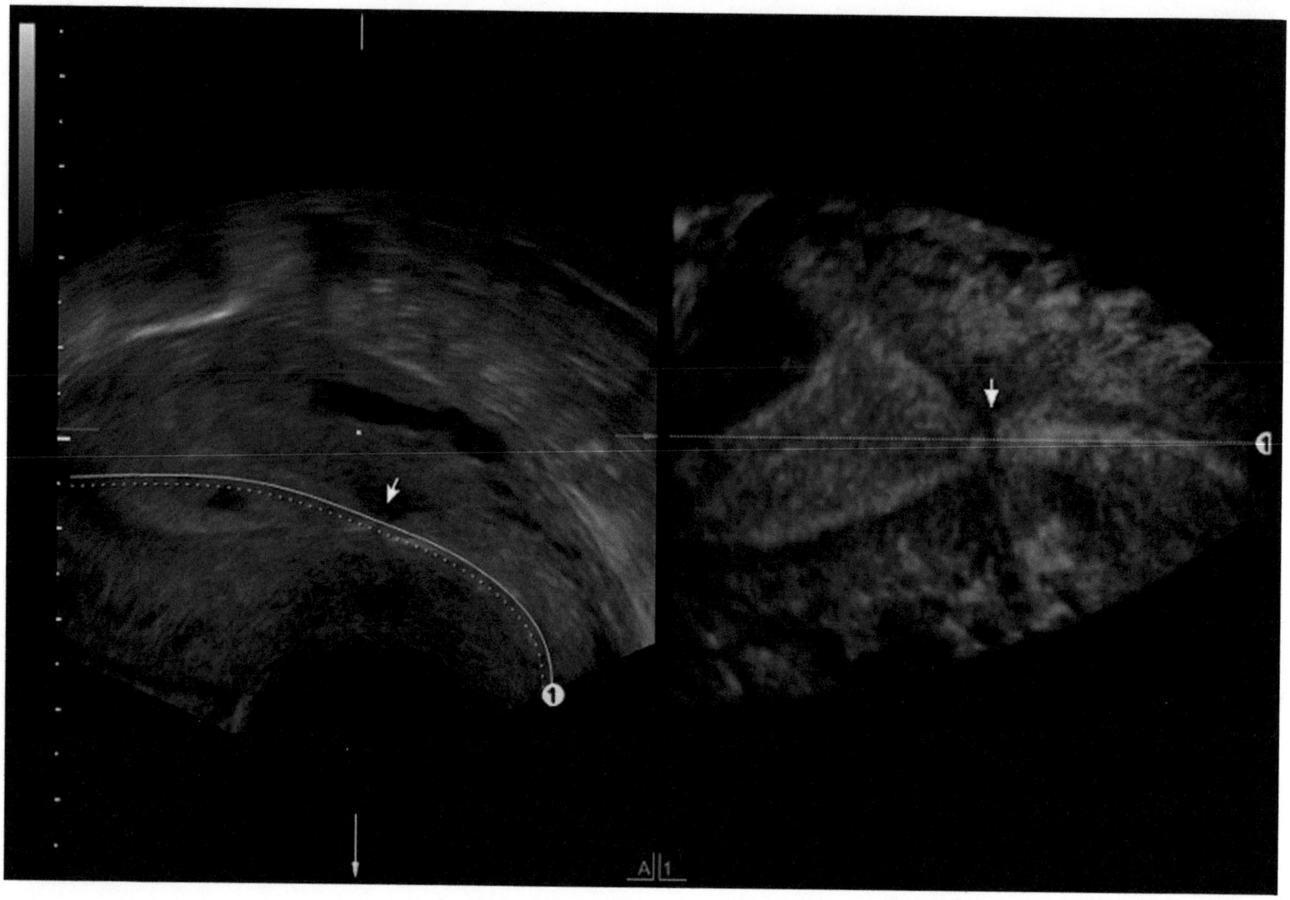

Fig. 5.58 Frontal scan by 3D OmniView technique shows the suspected adhesion (*arrow*) better than a 2D scan

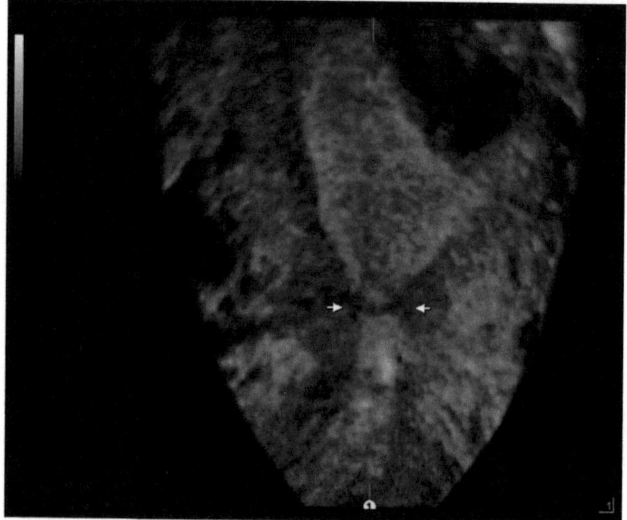

Fig. 5.59 The same frontal scan augmented and turned in the usual position for frontal scans impressively shows the endometrial interruption at the expected level (*arrows*). Supplementary case history: At this level (*arrows*) a strong, impenetrable obstacle was found when a sounding test was made before insertion of an intrauterine contraceptive device. These findings are to be seen in connection with a state after curettage due to retained pregnancy remnants (Images by courtesy of Dr. Isabel Wallrafen)

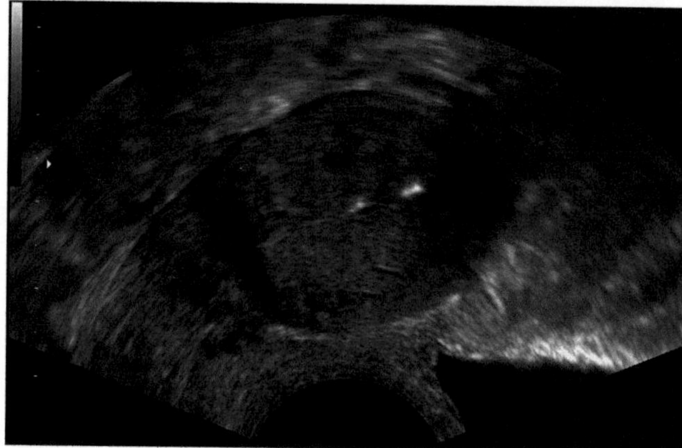

Fig. 5.60 Uterus with two echogenic foci as signs of subendometrial fibrosis (Image from Dürr, Transvaginale Sonographie in der Gynäkologie, De Gruyter, 2nd Edition, 2015)

Cesarean Section Scar

Cesarean scars are usually found in the lower uterine segment of the anterior uterine wall and present sonographically as a structure of low echo density reaching from the uterine serosa to the endometrium, interrupting the endometrial-myometrial continuity (Fig. 5.61).

Scar defects (dehiscences, niches) of smaller and larger size (Figs. 5.62, 5.63, and 5.64) are common sonographic findings after cesarean section. Different authors have published different findings on the prevalence of scar defects, but agree that the defects occur not seldom but more or less frequently. For example, O. Vikhareva Osser et al. found scar defects "in 61 % (66/108), 81 % (35/43) and 100 % (11/11) of the women who had undergone one, two and at least three cesarean sections" [4].

The larger the defect the greater is the loss of myometrial thickness at the level of the scar defect, with possible negative effects on the stability of the anterior uterine wall during pregnancy. But, quite astonishingly, even in more advanced pregnancies, where sonographically the remaining myometrium at the defect is found to be very thin (Fig. 5.64), its stability is usually better than expected. Nevertheless, uterine rupture is possible and sequential sonographic surveillance is obligatory.

Another consequence of scar defects, depending on their extension and shape, can be the retaining of menstrual blood and therefore irregular bleedings.

But the most severe aspect of cesarean scar defects are cesarean scar pregnancies (CSP) with the high risk of developing placental attachment disorders, such as placenta accreta, increta, and especially percreta.

These developments could be due to the loss of normal endometrium at the level of the scar with its interrupted EMJ. "The loss of functional endometrium results in inadequate decidualization at the scar site; the absence of decidua is considered to be the main factor explaining the propensity of trophoblast to penetrate deep into myometrium, beyond the EMJ, when future pregnancies are implanted into a deficient cesarean scar" [5].

As cases of CSP are described with placental implantation "on" the scar as well as cases with placental implantation "in" the niche of a defect scar [6], it seems that not only scar defects but also scars without (sonographically visible) defects are a risk for CSP.

Because of the high risk of CSP developing the above-mentioned severe placental disorders with all their severe consequences of blood loss, loss of uterus and fertility, all pregnant patients with previous cesarean section should have an early first trimester TVS, preferably between 6 and 8 weeks (p.m.), to localize the gestational sac and placental insertion. If a CSP is found, the patient should be counseled in detail "to enable

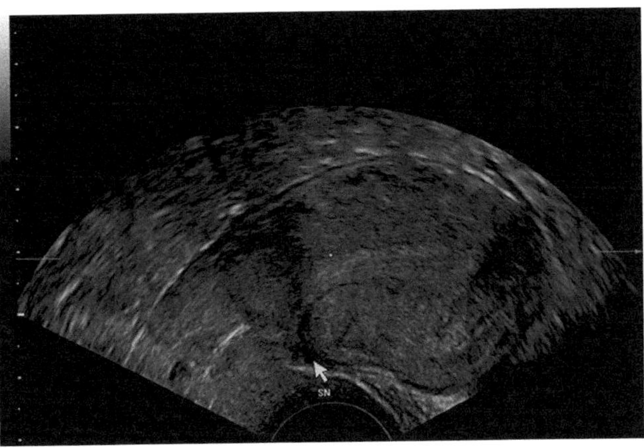

Fig. 5.61 Typical cesarean scar in the anterior wall of the lower uterine segment (Image from Dürr, Transvaginale Sonographie in der Gynäkologie, De Gruyter, 2nd Edition, 2015)

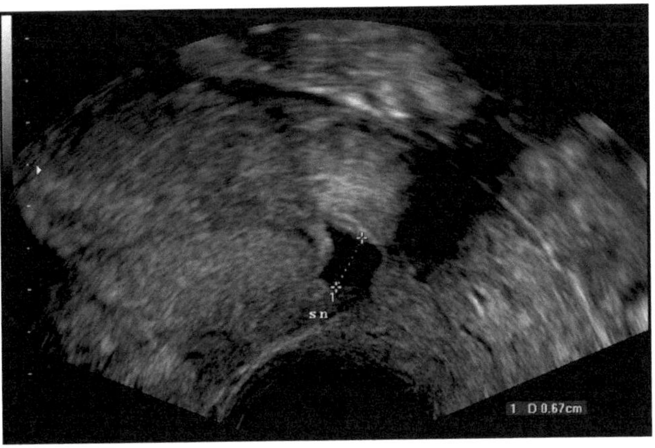

Fig. 5.62 Longitudinal scan of the lower part of the uterus (in this image, left is anterior and right is posterior). Cesarean scar defect filled with anechoic fluid, no pregnancy (Image from Dürr, Transvaginale Sonographie in der Gynäkologie, De Gruyter, 2nd Edition, 2015)

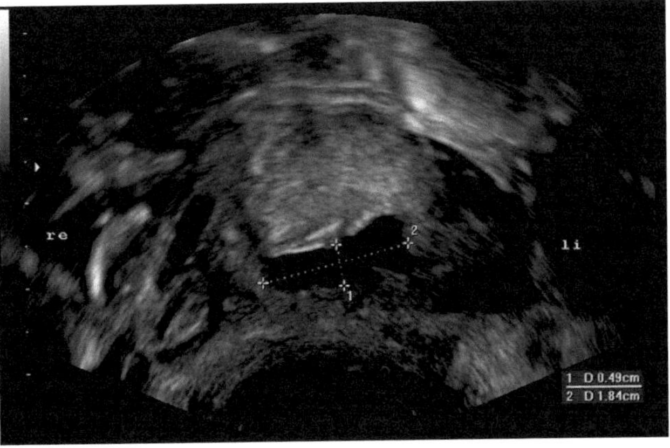

Fig. 5.63 The same case: transversal scan at the level of the scar defect (Image from Dürr, Transvaginale Sonographie in der Gynäkologie, De Gruyter, 2nd Edition, 2015)

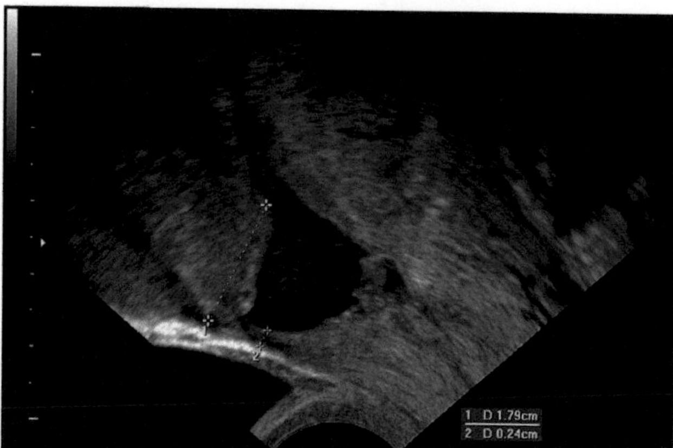

Fig. 5.64 A different case. Longitudinal scan of the lower part of the uterus (in this image, left is anterior and right is posterior). Cesarean scar defect during pregnancy at 26 weeks. The defect is much extended and sharply delineated by amniotic fluid. The remaining myometrial thickness at the scar level is very thin, only 2.4 mm compared to the normal thickness of 17.9 mm at this level (measurements within the image). The course of this pregnancy with sequential sonographic controls was finally terminated by cesarean re-re-section at 36 weeks. The intraoperatively found anterior uterine wall at the level of the cesarean scar was paper-thin but not ruptured. The newborn baby was in good condition (Image from Dürr, Transvaginale Sonographie in der Gynäkologie, De Gruyter, 2nd Edition, 2015)

her to make an informed choice between first trimester termination and continuation of the pregnancy, with its risk of premature delivery and loss of uterus and fertility " [6]. In this connection, it is well worth reading the article of Timor-Tritsch et al. with its very instructive images of cesarean scar pregnancies and their development in the course of pregnancy [6].

Intrauterine Ectopic Pregnancy

Ectopic pregnancies can be implanted not only extrauterine but also ectopic within the uterus, which is a life-threatening condition and a challenge for therapeutic treatment (Figs. 5.65 and 5.66).

Intrauterine Contraceptive Devices

The position of these devices within the uterus can easily be documented by 2D-sonography and more accurately by 3D sonography (Figs. 5.67,5.68, 5.69, and 5.70).

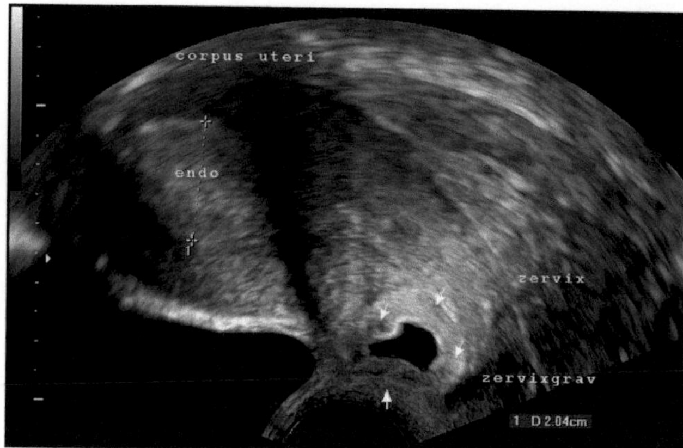

Fig. 5.65 In this longitudinal scan the anterior uterine wall is on the left side of the image. Within the anterior cervical wall a round, in comparison to the surrounding myometrium, more echodense area with a central liquid zone can be seen

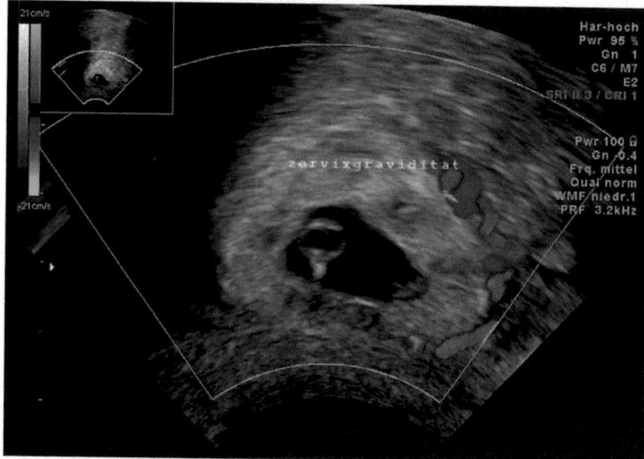

Fig. 5.66 Color Doppler and augmentation show the finding of a vital early pregnancy with the typical neovascularization around the trophoblast (Images by courtesy of Drs. Sibylle Haase and Isabel Wallrafen)

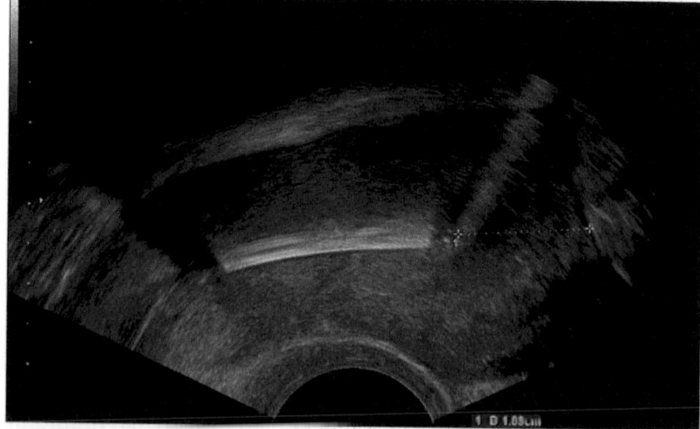

Fig. 5.67 As far as can be estimated by 2D sonography, the image shows a correctly positioned intracavitary IUD. The marked echo indicates a copper-armed IUD

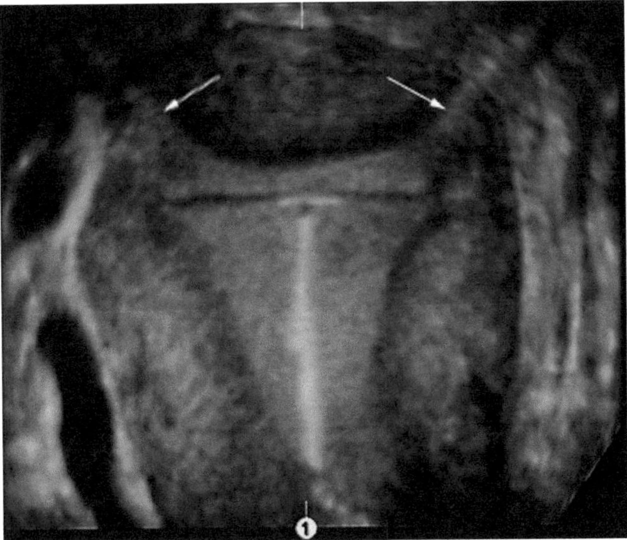

Fig. 5.68 The frontal scan by the 3D OmniView technique demonstrates the correctly extended side arms of this "Copper-T" IUD (Images from Dürr, Transvaginale Sonographie in der Gynäkologie, De Gruyter, 2nd Edition, 2015)

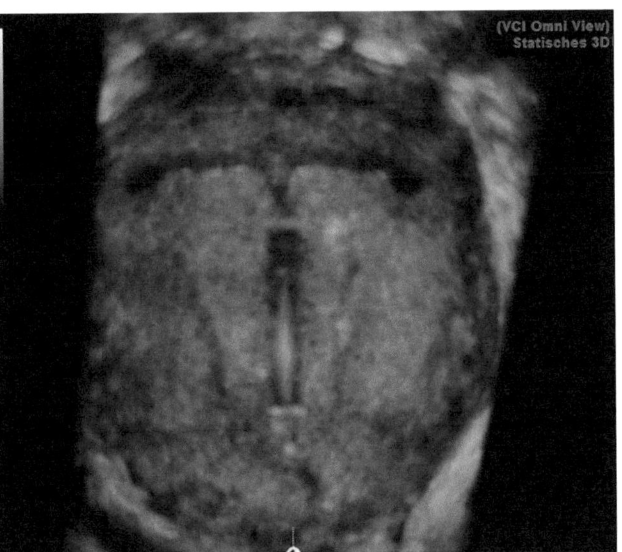

Fig. 5.70 The frontal scan by the 3D OmniView technique demonstrates the correctly extended side arms of the levonorgestrel-bearing IUD Mirena (Images from Dürr, Transvaginale Sonographie in der Gynäkologie, De Gruyter, 2nd Edition, 2015)

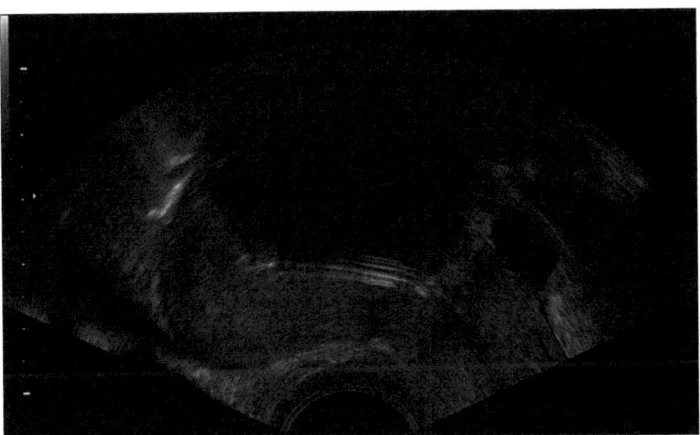

Fig. 5.69 As far as can be estimated by 2D sonography, the image shows a correctly positioned intracavitary IUD. The very marked shadowing behind the IUD indicates a gestagen-delivering IUD

Adenomyosis Uteri Interna or Endometriosis Interna

Adenomyosis is a uterine disease, caused by protrusion of vital endometrium from the basal layer into the myometrium, forming focal or widespread alterations within the myometrium on the other side of the EMJ. This disease is characterized by endometrial glands and stroma, surrounded by hypertrophic myometrium. Each focus can be seen as a "mini-uterus" within the uterus.

According to the theory of Leyendecker, autotraumatization of the uterus, caused by hyperperistalsis and dysperistalsis of the EMJ (archimetra) with consecutive increase of intrauterine pressure, leads to the dislocation of basal endometrium [3]. If basal endometrium fragments settle within the myometrium, the term adenomyosis uteri interna or endometriosis uteri interna is used. If the fragments enter the cavum uteri and from there by retrograde menstruation the peritoneal cavity and settle there, the term endometriosis externa is used.

A common trait of adenomyosis (interna) and endometriosis (externa) is an "infiltrative expansion of the archimetra" into the surrounding uterine wall. Consequently, a disease of the archimetra, that is a disease of the uterus, is the primary phenomenon and "endometriosis of the peritoneal cavity is not an obligatory secondary phenomenon" (Leyendecker).

So much for the shortened theory of Leyendecker.

The spreading of adenomyosis can be focal or multifocal diffuse, with a more infiltrative expansion which, contrary to myomata, shows no clear demarcation from the surrounding tissue. In contrast to myomata the vascularization (angiogenesis) is increased more within the affected area and less around this area. Calcifications are not found within adenomyosis.

A very easy and immediately recognizable sonographic sign of adenomyosis, even with older or low grade ultrasound equipment, is a marked asymmetry between the non or less affected and the more affected uterine wall (Fig. 5.71), provided that the asymmetry is not caused by myomata.

Streaky shadowing within the affected areas, caused by marked differences in sonographic impedances, indicates the older, advanced processes (Fig. 5.72) whereas cystic, clear demarcated adenomyotic islands indicate the more recent processes, see above Fig. 5.25.

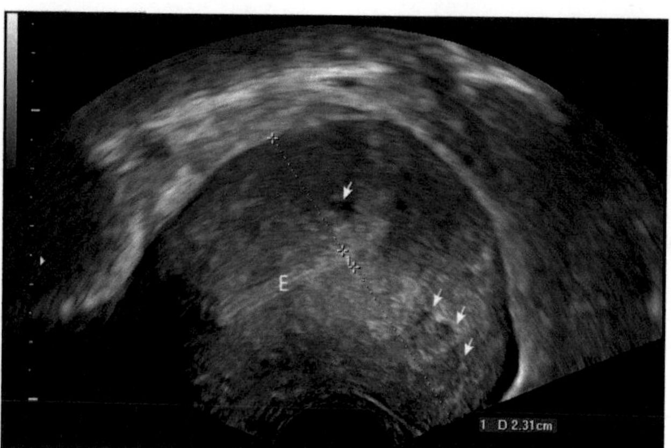

Fig. 5.71 This longitudinal scan demonstrates the common finding of a uterine asymmetry in a case of adenomyosis. "*E*" in the image indicates the mid uterus. One uterine wall contains more adenomyotic foci (*arrows*) than the other, with only one focus (*arrow*), and therefore is markedly thicker. This sign of asymmetric uterine walls can easily be assessed even by low grade US equipment. See above also Fig. 5.24 Color Doppler shows a markedly higher and more irregular vascularization of the affected area in comparison to the regular vascularization by preexisting vessels (Images from Dürr, Transvaginale Sonographie in der Gynäkologie, De Gruyter, 2nd Edition, 2015)

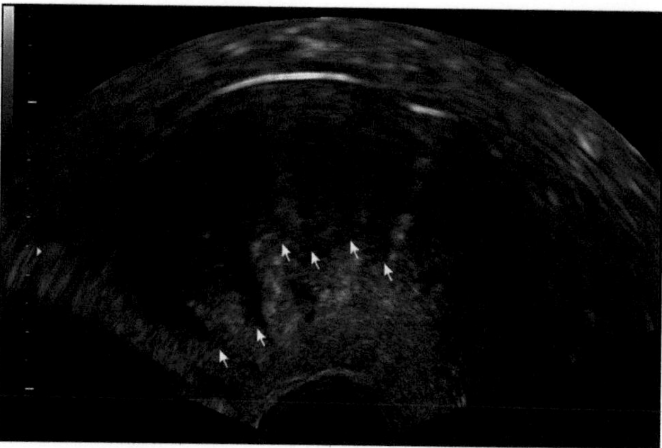

Fig. 5.72 In this longitudinal scan streaky shadowing indicates a widespread adenomyosis. See above also Fig. 5.25: In another area of the same uterus cystic structures, surrounded by an echogenic endometrium-like margin, are to be found. Color Doppler shows a very marked and diffuse neovascularization in the cystic area as a sign of adenomyosis with a tendency to progress. It seems to be that streaky shadows indicate older processes and cystic findings more recent afflictions of adenomyosis (Images from Dürr, Transvaginale Sonographie in der Gynäkologie, De Gruyter, 2nd Edition, 2015)

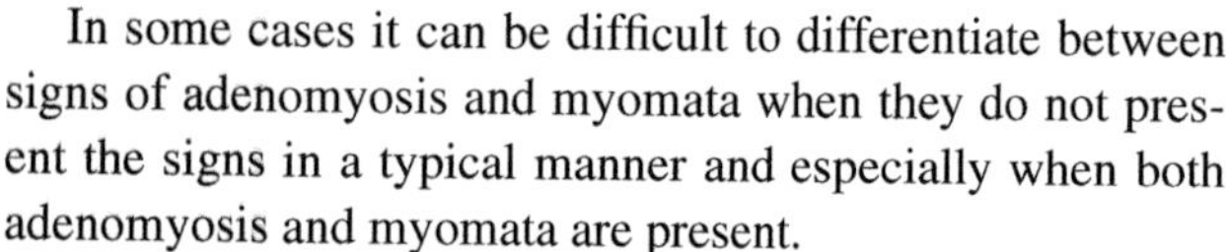

In some cases it can be difficult to differentiate between signs of adenomyosis and myomata when they do not present the signs in a typical manner and especially when both adenomyosis and myomata are present.

The symptoms and consequences of adenomyosis vary, depending on the progression of the disease, from very heavy dysmenorrhea, algopareunia, continuous pain, sterility, to a more or less symptomless course of the disease with normal or only slightly reduced fertility.

Therapeutically medical treatment can be attempted in the form of drugs often given in cases of endometriosis (externa), but it is not really effective. More promising seems to be the intrauterine application of levonorgestrel by means of the intrauterine device Mirena (Schering).

Hysterectomy is the surgical choice for reliably removing all foci. However, if fertility should be conserved as far as possible, organ-preserving methods with excision or electric coagulation of the foci could be considered, depending on the extent of the disease.

Adenomyosis is a very common disease and is detected increasingly more by high resolution TVS in the hands of well-trained investigators whereas in earlier times diagnosis was usually made by chance, histologically.

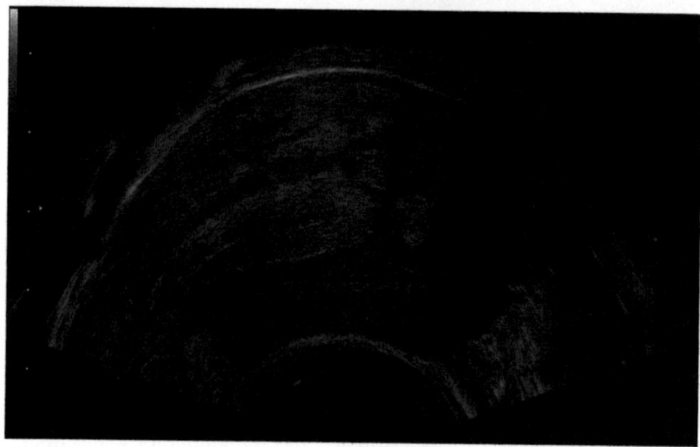

Fig. 5.73 The longitudinal scan shows two adenomyotic foci close to the endometrium

The examples of adenomyosis presented here (Figs. 5.71, 5.72, 5.73, 5.74, 5.75, 5.76, and 5.77), and see above Figs. 5.24 and 5.25, demonstrate the high value of TVS and color Doppler in the diagnosis and assessment of this disease. In addition to this today's primary tools, MRI can be necessary for special demands, such as "mapping" before surgical treatment.

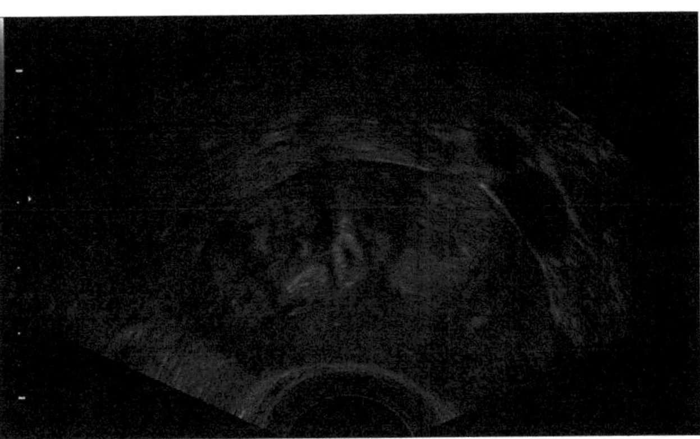

Fig. 5.74 The transverse scan in the fundal region shows some larger and many smaller adenomyotic foci which are more distant from the endometrial part where protrusion into the myometrium has begun

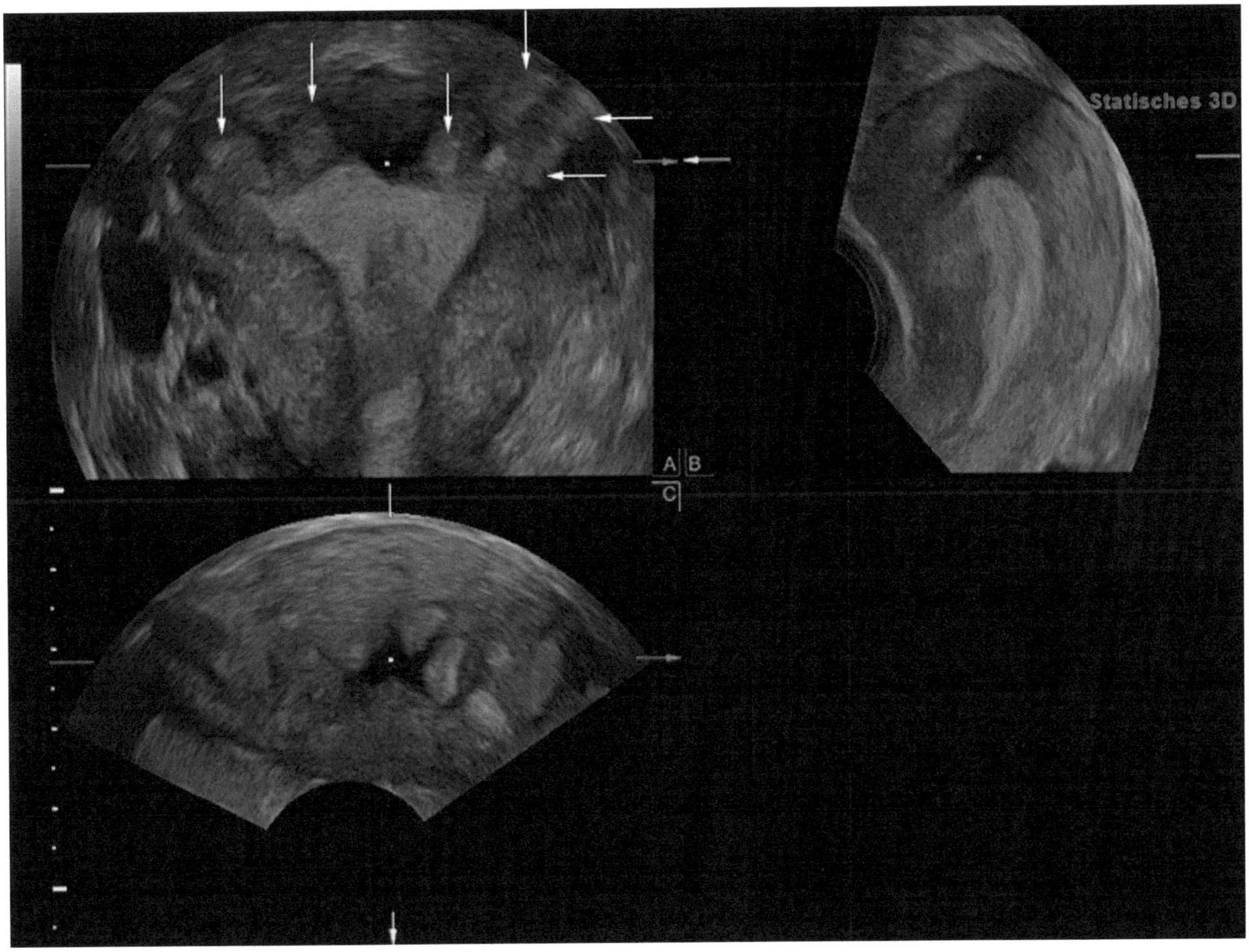

Fig. 5.75 The 3D frontal scan shows multiple adenomyotic foci (*arrows*) which obviously started from the fundal endometrium, as is often found in cases of adenomyosis

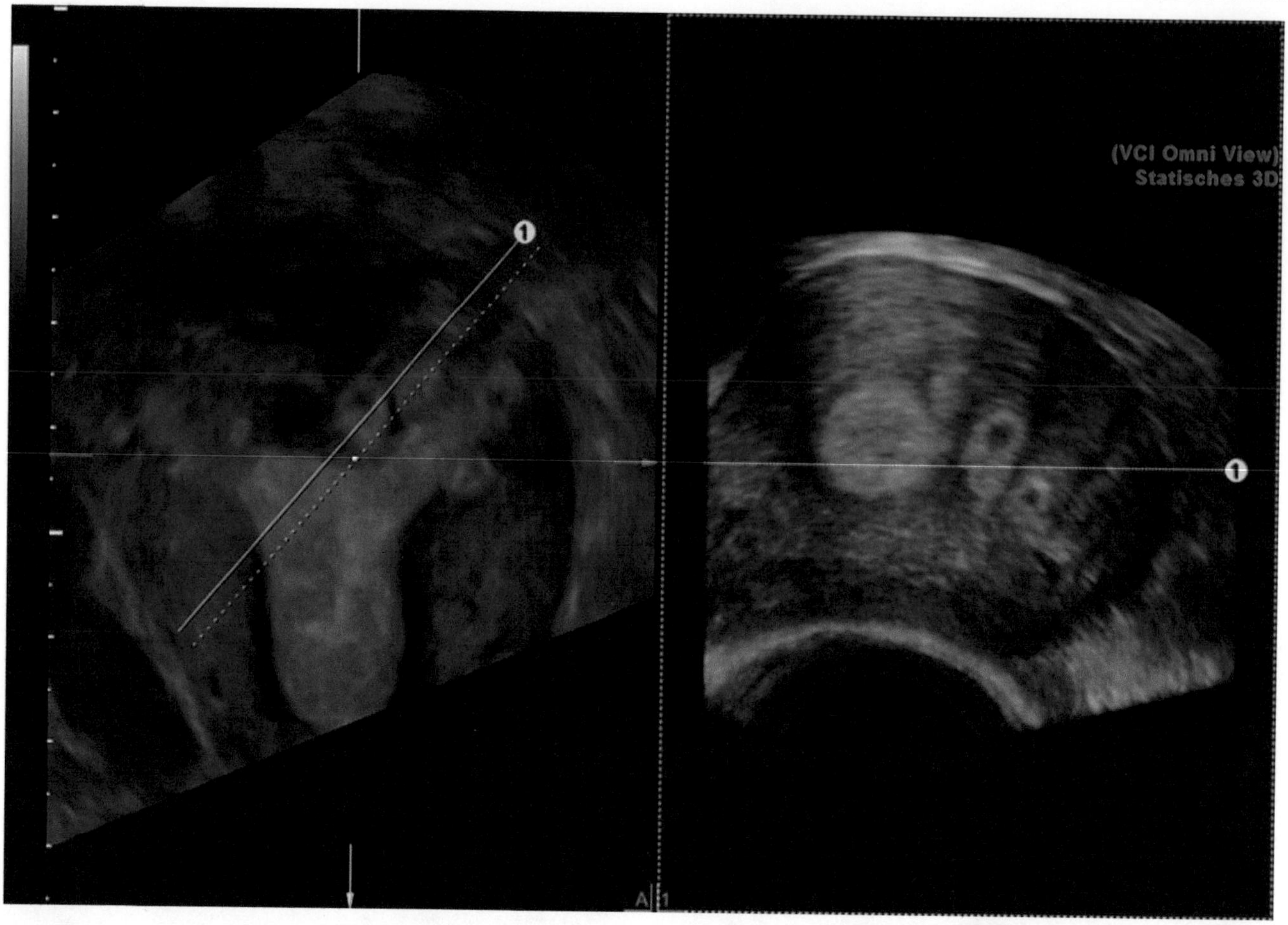

Fig. 5.76 The frontal scan on the left side of the image shows the EMJ as a low echogenous seam surrounding the middle and lower part of the endometrium. In the fundal region the EMJ is no longer visible because of multiple adenomyotic activities with their partially destroying effect on the EMJ. On the right part of the image endometrium and adenomyotic islands are presented more vividly by using OmniView and VCI techniques. The chosen plane of section is indicated by the line 1

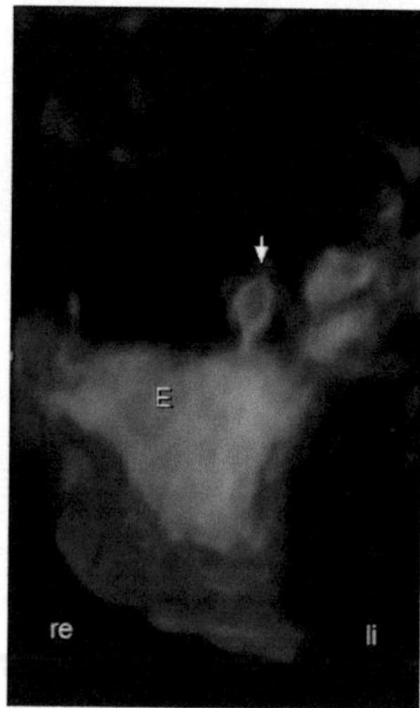

Fig. 5.77 This frontal scan in the fundal region demonstrates an adenomyotic focus in the early phase of development, still connected to the endometrium (Images from Dürr, Transvaginale Sonographie in der Gynäkologie, De Gruyter, 2nd Edition, 2015)

Deep Infiltrating Endometriosis or Adenomyosis Externa

Deep infiltrating endometriosis, described by Donnez et al. [7] as a form of "adenomyosis" invading deep into the rectovaginal space, affects the bowel wall in the rectosigmoid area, the uterus with its ligaments and the paraprocticum. Sonographically, the nodular alteration can be shown as a low echogenic, relatively clear demarcated structure between the cervical part of the uterus and the anterior rectal wall that is invaded in its muscular part (Fig. 5.78), see also Figs. 5.79, 5.80, 5.81, 5.82, and 5.83. To improve the surgical management, the extension of deep infiltrating endometriosis should be assessed by TVS before surgical treatment.

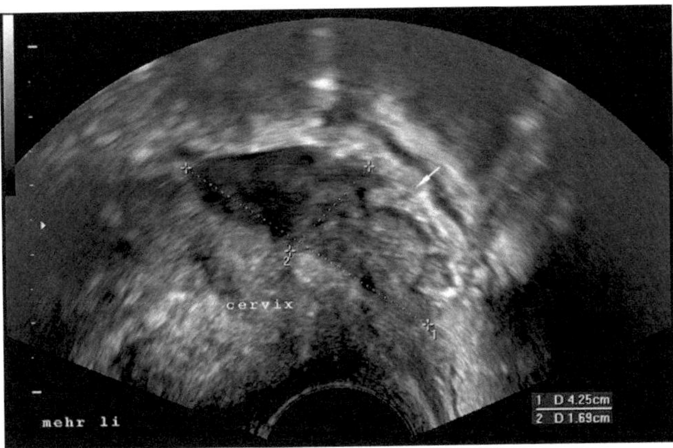

Fig. 5.78 Longitudinal cervical scan, left paramedian. In this and the following images, left is anterior and right is posterior. A retrocervical, rectovaginal deep endometriosis is shown sonographically as a relatively clear, demarcated structure of low echogenity, extended between the posterior cervical wall and the vicinal bowel (rectum) which is infiltrated in its frontal muscular wall. The non-affected mucosal part of the bowel is indicated by high echogenity (*arrow*). Measurements within the image

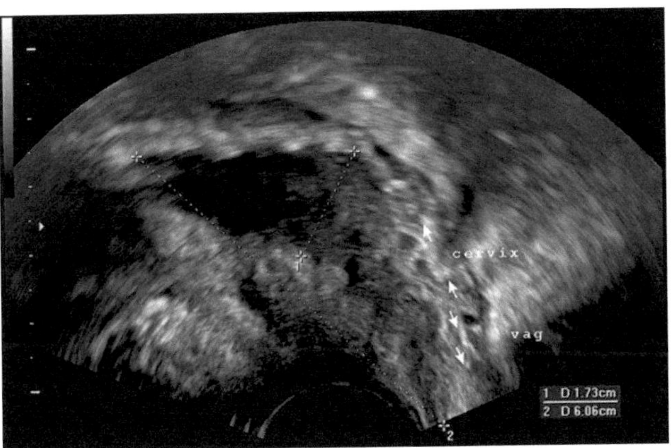

Fig. 5.79 The wide spread of the endometriosis towards the vagina is indicated by two *arrows* and towards the *cervix* by one *arrow*. Measurements within the image

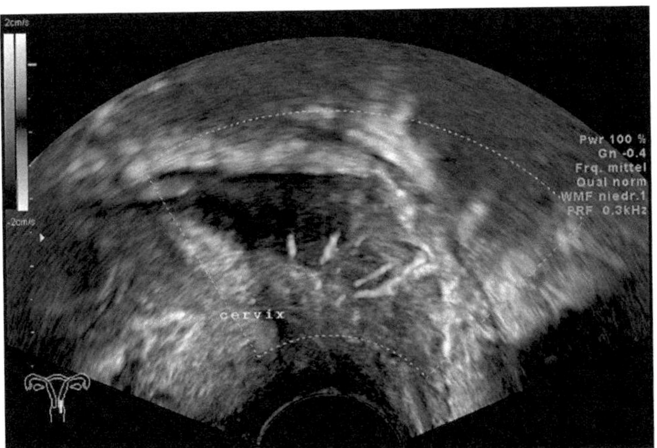

Fig. 5.80 Color Doppler shows vascularization as a possible sign of "vitality" and a tendency to progress

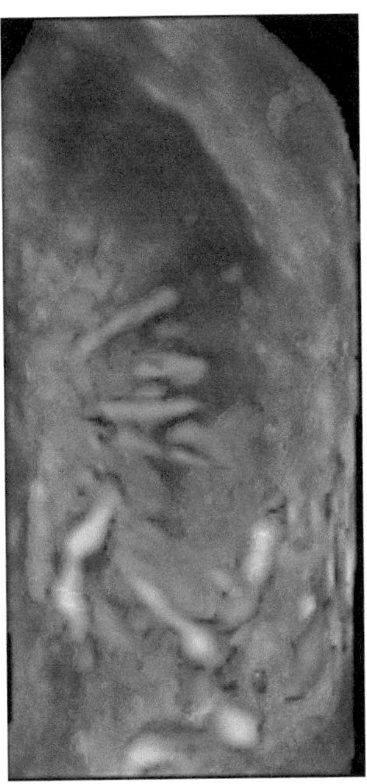

Fig. 5.81 Vascularization demonstrated by color Doppler glass body mode

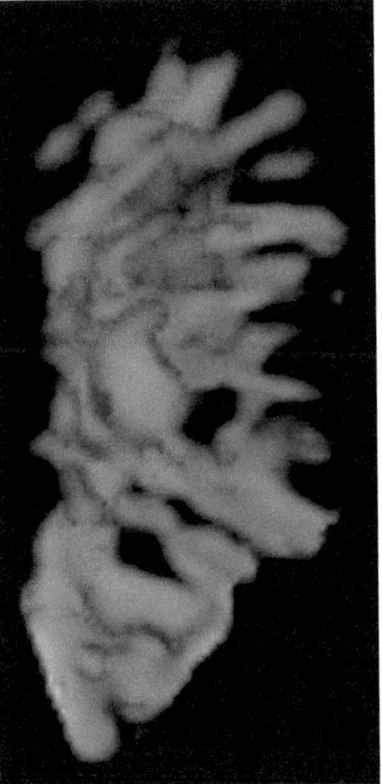

Fig. 5.82 Vascularization demonstrated by solely color, without any surrounding tissue. See above also Fig. 5.7 3D presentation of the endometriosis, inversion modus: The very irregular surface and the pedicle-like extensions give an impression of the highly aggressive potential of this kind of endometriosis and its suspected tendency to progress (Images from Dürr, Transvaginale Sonographie in der Gynäkologie, De Gruyter, 2nd Edition, 2015)

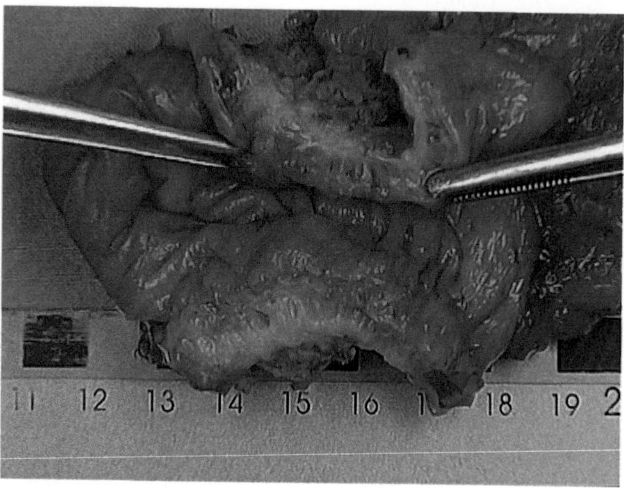

Fig. 5.83 The postoperative image shows the opened endometriotic node, extended in the anterior muscular part of the rectum (Courtesy of Prof. Dr. J. Keckstein)

References

Book

Dürr, W: Transvaginale Sonographie in der Gynäkologie. De Gruyter, 2. Auflage 2015.

Journal Articles

1. Naftalin J, Jurkovic D. Editorial.The endometrial- myometrial junction: a fresh look at a busy crossing. Ultrasound Obstet Gynecol. 2009;34:1–11.
2. Leyendecker G, Kunz G, Noe M, Herbertz M, Mall G. Endometriosis: a dysfunction and desease of the archimetra. Hum Reprod Update. 1998;4:752–62.
3. Leyendecker, G, Herbertz M, Kunz, G. Neue Aspecte zur Pathogenese von Endometriose und Adenomyose. Frauenarzt 43. 2002 Nr.3 297–307.
4. Vikhareva Osser O, Jokubkiene O, Valentin L. High prevalence of defects in Cesarean section scars at transvaginal ultrasound examination. Ultrasound Obstet Gynecol. 2009;34:90–7.
5. Ben-Nagi J, Helmy D, Ofili-Yebovi J, Jazbek J, Sawyer E, Yurkovic D. Reproductive outcomes of women with a previous history of Caesarean scar ectopic pregnancies. Hum Reprod. 2007;22:2012–5. Cited out of (1).
6. Timor-Tritsch IE, Monteagudo A, Cali G, Vintzileos A, Viscarello R, Al-Khan A, Zamudio S, Mayberry P, Cordoba MM, Dar P. Caesarean scar pregnancy is a precursor of morbidly adherent placenta. Ultrasound Obstet Gynecol. 2014;44:346–53. doi:10.1002/uog. 13426.
7. Donnez J, Nissole M, Smets M, et al. Rectovaginal septum adenomyotic nodule: a distinct entity: a series of 460 cases. In: Sutton C, Diamond M, editors. Endoscopic surgery for gynecologists. 2nd ed. London: WB Saunders; 1998. p. 357–62.

Radio-Imaging for Benign Uterine Disease

6

Céline D. Alt-Radke

Introduction

Magnetic Resonance Imaging (MRI)

Native high-resolution T2-weighted images (T2WI) are essential for morphological differentiation of pelvic organ tissue (Fig. 6.1). Contrast-enhanced T1-weighted images (T1WI) give important additional information in almost every problem and should be therefore routinely performed [1–6]. However, kidney functions (kreatinine) should be checked before the intravenous application of contrast media. As intravenous MR contrast agent is gadolinium (Gd)-based, thyroid function is therefore not required to be checked. In recent years, diffusion weighted imaging (DWI) gains more and more attention. This imaging technique was designed to depict alterations in thermally induced random (Brownian) motion of water molecules within tissues and the degree of this motion is known as diffusion [7]. DWI can be performed quickly, without the necessity of contrast i.v. The technique yields qualitative and quantitative information about tissue cellularity and cellular membrane integrity. High cellularity and cell membrane integrity restrict water mobility and therefore diffusion, as seen e.g. in tumors. During MR-performance, diffusion sensitivity can easily be varied by changing the *b* value used during image acquisition [7]. Quantitative analysis of diffusion may be performed by obtaining and mapping apparent diffusion coefficient (ADC) values [7].

For the evaluation of inflammation or fistulas, T2WI with fat saturation are helpful, especially with patients where no contrast media application is possible. For the differentiation between hemorrhage or lipid contents, a native T1-weighted sequence without and with fat saturation is helpful. For lymph node detection, a native T1-weighted sequence or proton-weighted (PD) sequence is helpful (Table 6.1) [8].

Computed Tomography (CT)

With a multidetector CT (MDCT) the examination of a region of interest can be performed in axial plane in a short examination time with submillimeter resolution. The row data can be postprocessed in any plane with approximately the same resolution. It should be noticed that intravenous contrast application is essential for soft tissue contrast because even CT in venous phase has less tissue contrast compared to native MRI (Figs. 6.2, 6.3, and 6.4) [9]. Before performing contrast enhanced CT (CECT), kidney function (kreatinine) and thyroid function (TSH, fT3, fT4) should be checked to be with normal values.

Leiomyoma

Leiomyomas have a pseudo-capsule, are almost clearly defined and can be located submucosal (growth intraluminal), intramural or subserous (growth to the outside), yet can also be pedunculated. More localisations are cervical, vaginal or intraligamental [10]. Usually, the diagnosis is based on the clinical-vaginal examination and ultrasound. In case of myomas large in size or number, a high-resolution MRI of the pelvis may be helpful for the planning of an individual therapy (hysterectomy, myomectomy, open versus laparoscopic surgery, uterine artery embolisation, MR guided focused ultrasound) or the distinction between benign or malignant appearance (Fig. 6.5). Depending on their content,

C.D. Alt-Radke, MD
Department of Diagnostic and Interventional Radiology, Medical Faculty, University Duesseldorf, D-40225 Duesseldorf, Germany
e-mail: celine.alt@med.uni-duesseldorf.de

I. Alkatout, L. Mettler (eds.), *Hysterectomy*, DOI 10.1007/978-3-319-22497-8_6

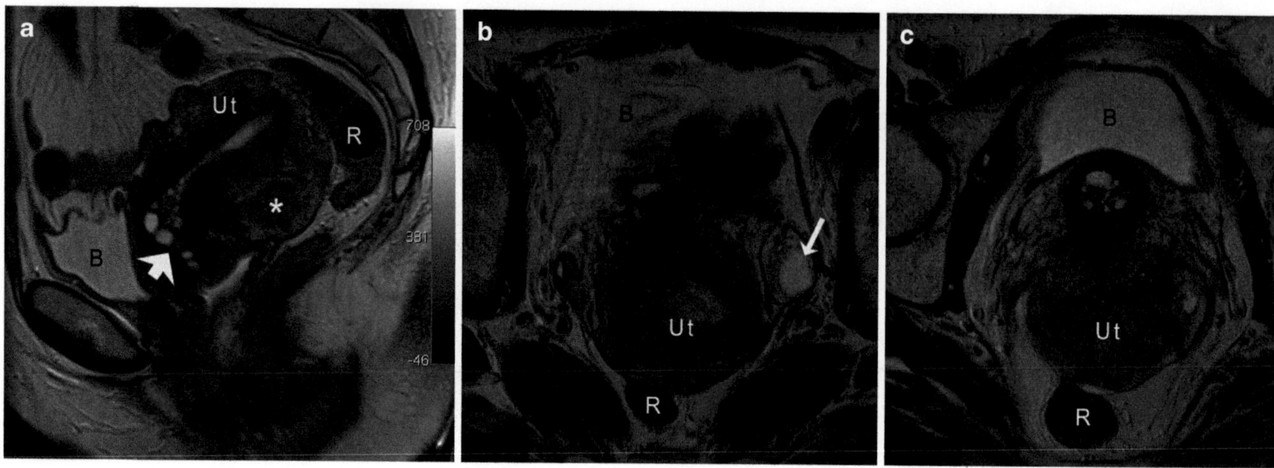

Fig. 6.1 Information given by native T2-weighted MRI of the female pelvis: (**a**) on sagittal plane, the uterus presents retroflected with a normal three-layer appearance and an intramural leiomyoma of the posterior wall (*asterisk*). The cervix contains nabothian cysts (*arrowhead*). (**b**) On T2-weighted transverse oblique plane to the cervix, additional information can be given for the left ovary containing a corpus luteum cyst (*arrow*). (**c**) On T2-weighted transverse plane oblique to the cervix, the hypointense stromal ring of the cervix presents intact, the cervical cavity presents with nabothian cysts. *Ut* uterus, *B* bladder, *R* rectum

Table 6.1 Common MR-sequences used for female pelvic imaging

	Sequence	Specification	Example	
1	High resolution T2WI	Morphology of pelvic organs	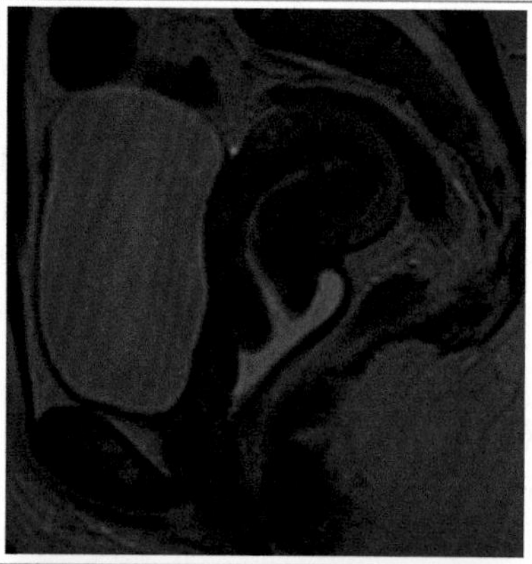	[Table 6.2 image 1]
2	T2WI with fat saturation	Oedema, inflammation, fistula	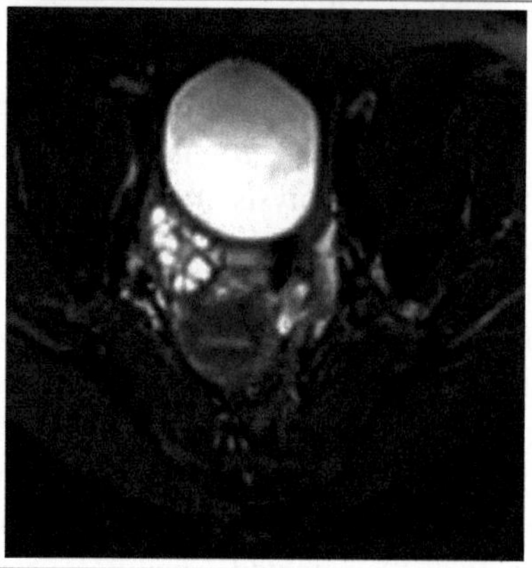	[Table 6.2 image 2]

(continued)

Table 6.1 (continued)

	Sequence	Specification	Example	
3	T1WI native/with fat saturation	Lymph nodes/ differentiation between lipids or hemorrhage	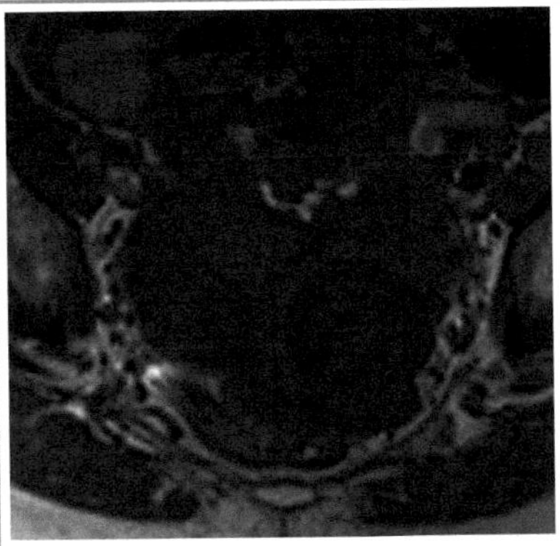	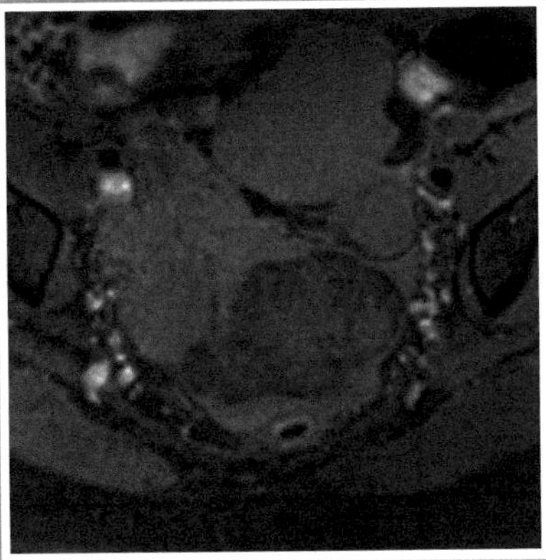
4	DWI (diffusion weighted imaging)	Diffusion restriction in inflammation, differentiation between benign to malignant lesions	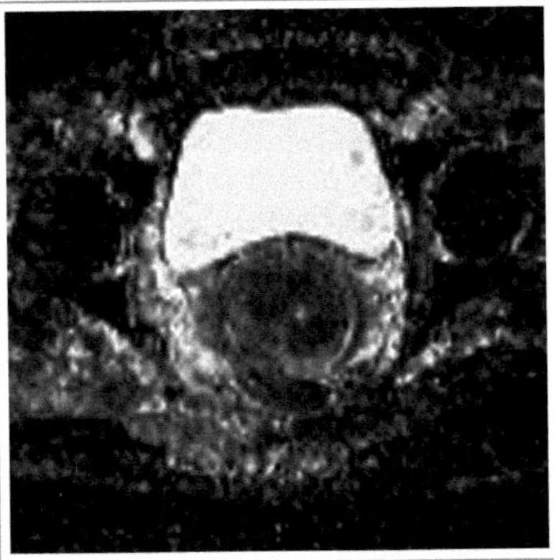	[Table 6.2 image 3.1 and 3.2 are above] [Table 6.2 image 4 here] [Table 6.2 image 5.1 and 5.2 are below]
5	DCE (dynamic contrast enhanced)	Evaluation of tissues in arterial and venous phase, vascularisation, hyperemia	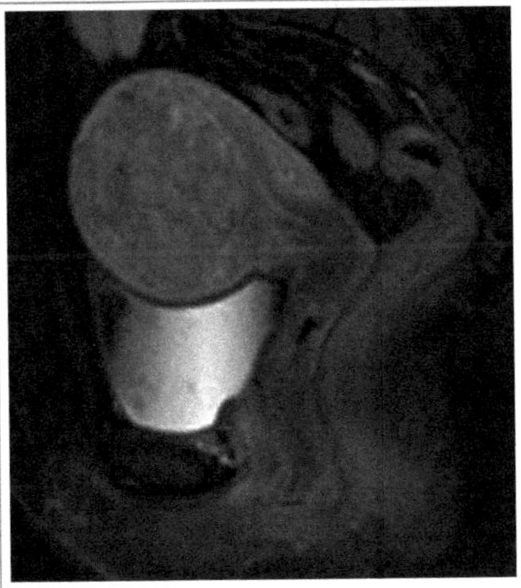	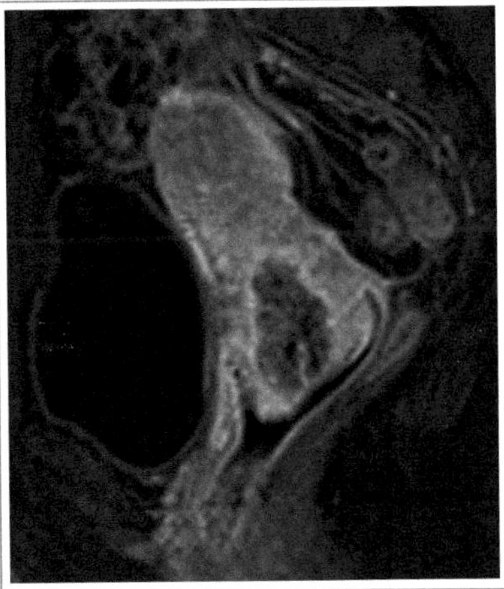

T2WI T2-weighted imaging, *T1WI* T1- weighted imaging

myomas are shown with different signal behaviour in MRI [10]. A non-degeneratively changed (fibrous) leiomyoma is rich in fibrous tissue, round to ovally shaped, clearly defined and circumscribed, and is hypointense in T1WI and highly hypointense in T2WI in comparison to the myometrium. After application of contrast media i.v., signal behaviour tends to be non-homogenous. Often, a pseudo-capsule can be detected [3, 11]. Due to inlaid calcifications or hyaline, fat or liquid contents, degenerated leiomyomas show heterogenous signal behaviour as early in as in native sequences (Figs. 6.6, 6.7, and 6.8) [11]. If myomas are classified as secondary findings in CT-examinations, they commonly show early enhancement in the arterial phase and are more likely to be hypodense in the late phase. Depending on their size, myomas are homogenous (small myomas) or heterogenous (large myomas) (Fig. 6.4). Ring-shaped calcifications, which can be more easily discerned in CT than in MRI, are often part of myomas. Hyperdense foci in CT may point to hemorrhage, whereas hypodense areas may be a sign of necrosis or infection (Figs. 6.8 and 6.9).

Possible differential diagnoses for leiomyomas are polyps (if submucous myoma) (Fig. 6.10), adenomyosis (if intramu-

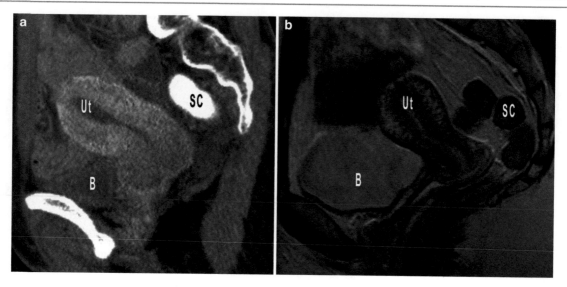

Fig. 6.2 Two patients presenting with sagittal images of the entire pelvis. (**a**) contrast enhanced CT gives an overview of the pelvic organs but lacks of good morphological differentiation. (**b**) High resolution T2 weighted image on MRI presents with a high soft tissue contrast and allows differentiation of different tissues, e.g. the differentiation between endometrium, junctional zone, myometrium and perimetrium. *B* bladder, *Ut* uterus, *SC* sigmoid colon

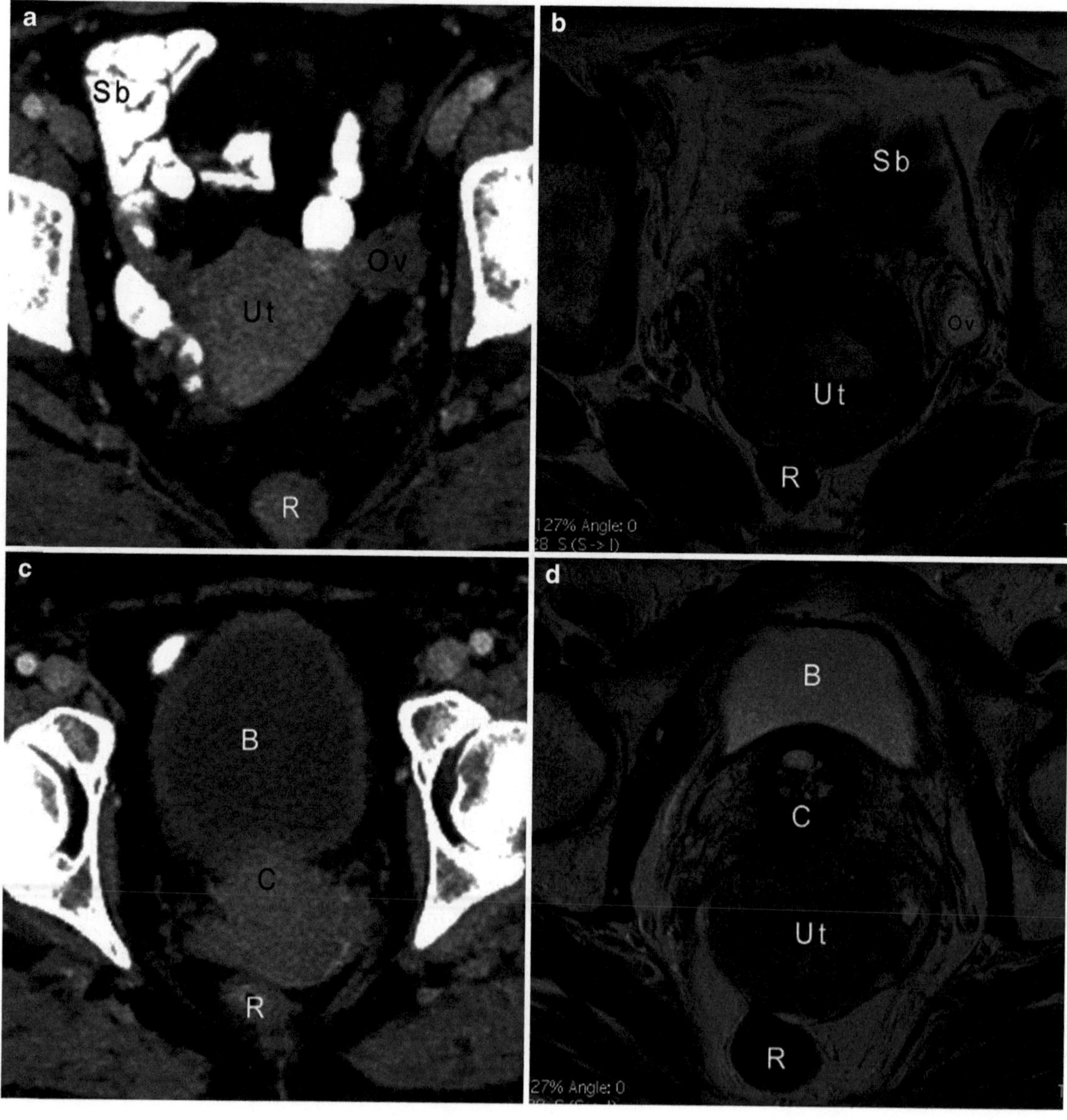

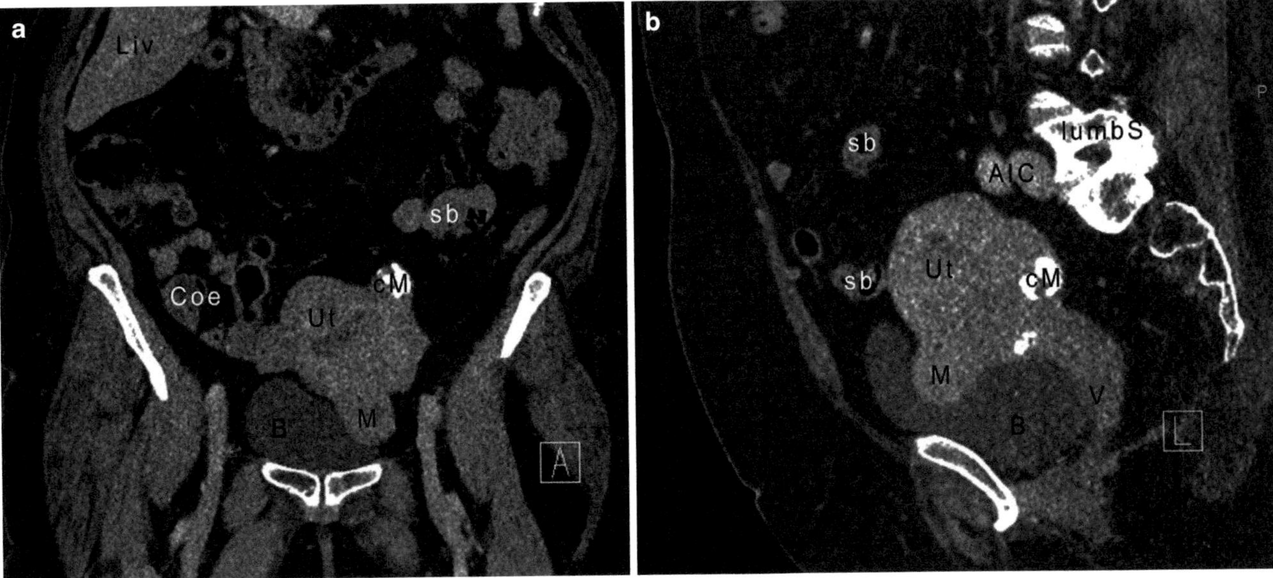

Fig. 6.4 Contrast enhanced CT performed for another indication. As a secondary finding, the woman presents with uterus myomatosus, partially calcified. Image on coronal (**a**) and sagittal (**b**) plane for anatomical landmarks. *Ut* uterus, *M* myoma, *cM* calcified myoma, *V* vagina; *B* bladder, *R* rectum, *Liv* liver, *sb* small bowel, *Coe* coecum, *AIC* common iliac arteries, *lumbS* lumbar spine

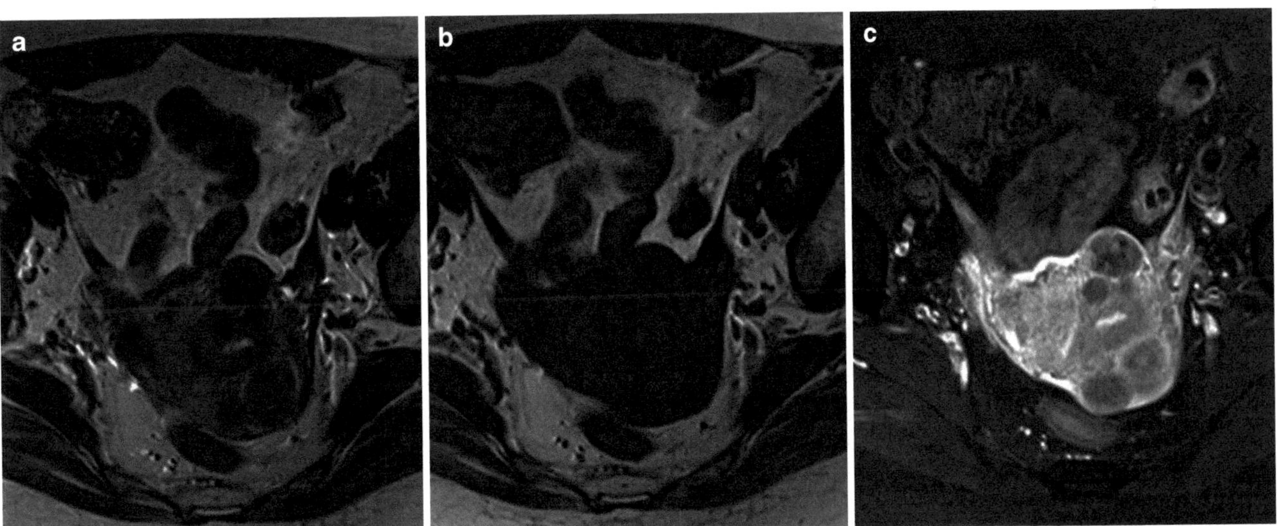

Fig. 6.5 Patient presenting with symptomatic uterus myomatosus. Without cross sectional imaging, the clear differentiation between degenerated/non degenerated leiomyoma, the number and localisation and the differentiation to small bowel loops, respectively, may be challenging with ultrasound alone. These images at transversal plane show the uterus myomatosus with at least 6 leiomyomas at this slice on (**a**) T2WI (**b**) native T1WI and (**c**) after contrast i.v

Fig. 6.3 Comparison of contrast enhanced CT (*left*) to native MRI of the female pelvis (*right*). The excellent soft tissue contrast of MRI without radiation gives more detailed information of the female pelvis as CT is able to. Therefore, whenever possible, MRI with an adopted gyne protocol should be performed instead of CT. *Ut* Uterus, *Ov* ovary; *C* cervix, *B* bladder, *Sb* small bowel, *R* rectum

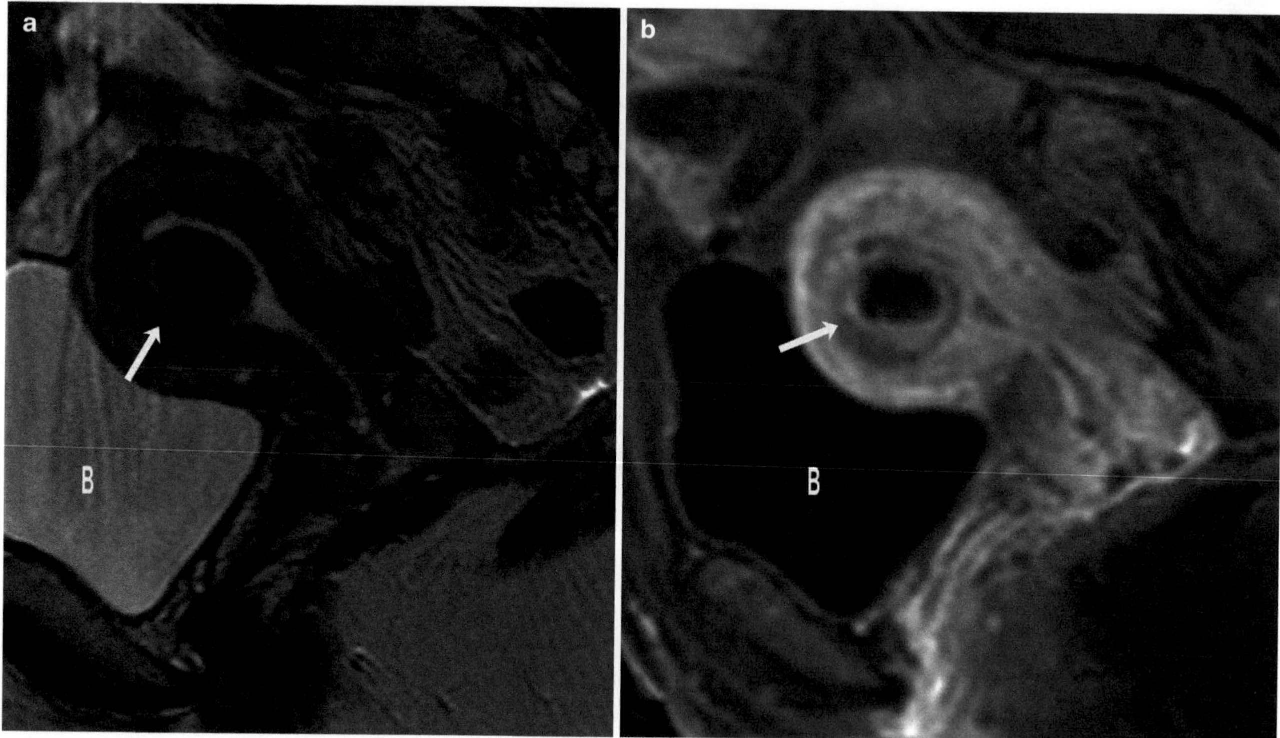

Fig. 6.6 Presentation of a submucous leiomyoma of the anterior wall of the uterine corpus with a wide based connection to the endometrium (*arrow*). (**a**) It presents with a hypointense center with an isointense ring shape on T2WI. (**b**) After application of contrast i.v., the center of the leiomyoma remains hypointense, possibly due to calcifications. *B* bladder

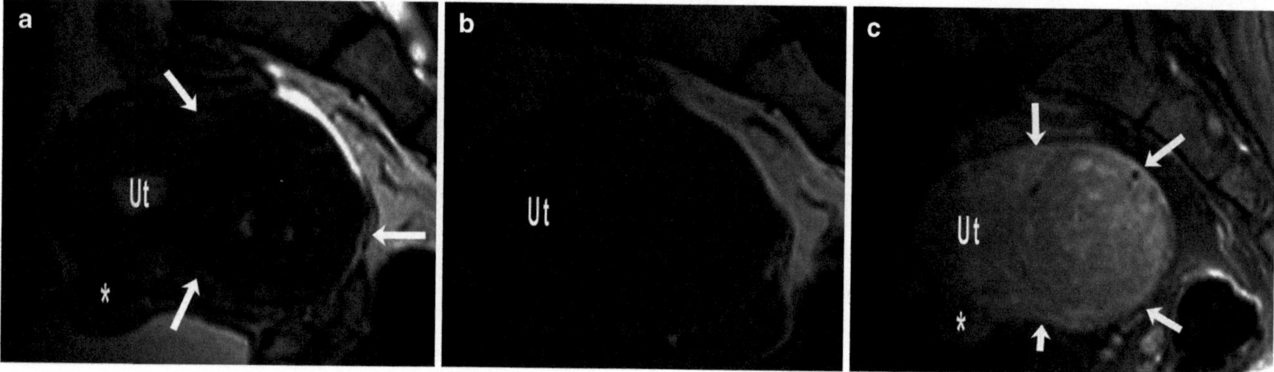

Fig. 6.7 Huge subserous non-degenerated leiomyoma of the uterus (*arrows*). (**a**) The leiomyoma is hypointense with some minor hyperintense spots at T2WI. (**b**) It presents with the same signal intensity as the myometrium at native T1WI. (**c**) It enhances homogenously after contrast i.v., comparable to the myometrium. Additionally, the claw sign is present (the serosa surrounds of the fibroid). There is a small second subserous leiomyoma at the anterior wall (*asterisk*). *Ut* uterus

Fig. 6.10 Presentation of an endometrial polyp on contrast enhanced CT scan (**a**) and MRI (**b**). (**a**) On CT scan, a homogenously enhancing lesion, located at uterine cavity is present (*arrow*). A clear identification cannot be made between submucous myoma, hemorrhage or polyp, histopathologically proven as endometrial polyp. (**b**) T2-weighted MRI presents with a well circumscribed hypointense lesion at the hyperintense uterine cavity with a small peduncle to the endometrium (*arrow*). Clear identification of a polyp can be made, histopathologically proven. Secondary finding is a follicle cyst right sided with partial hemorrhage

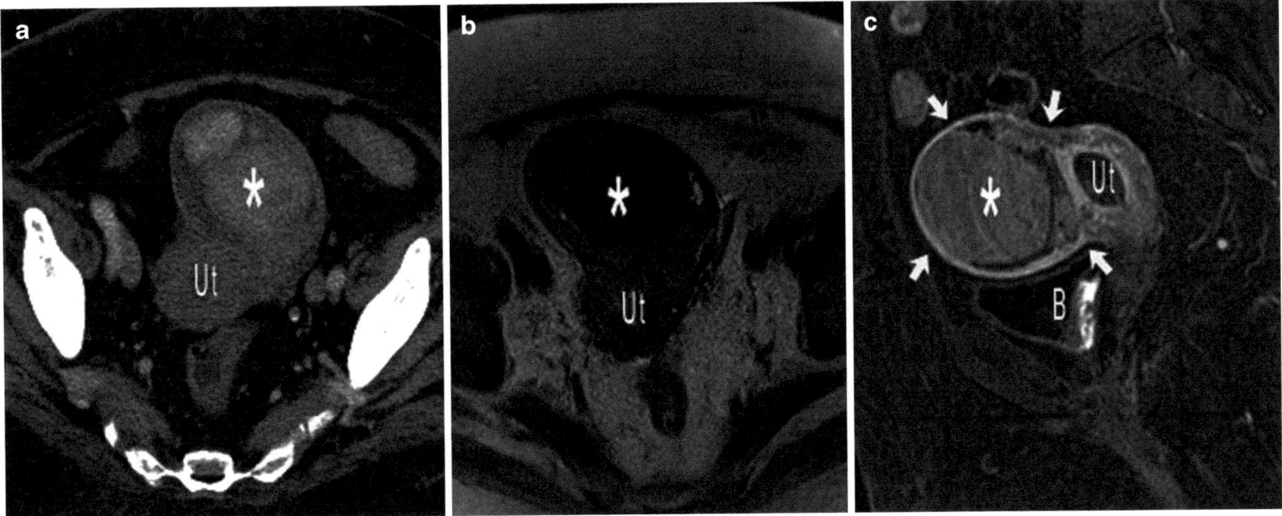

Fig. 6.8 (**a**) CT scan of the pelvis presents with a mass like lesion of the uterus with heterogenous densities (*asterisk*). (**b**) MRI in the same patient shows this mass as hypointense on T2WI associated with the uterus and well defined margins (*asterisk*). (**c**) application of contrast i.v. shows the typical claw-sign for subserous leiomyoma (*arrows*). This result was histopathologically proven. *B* bladder, *Ut* uterus

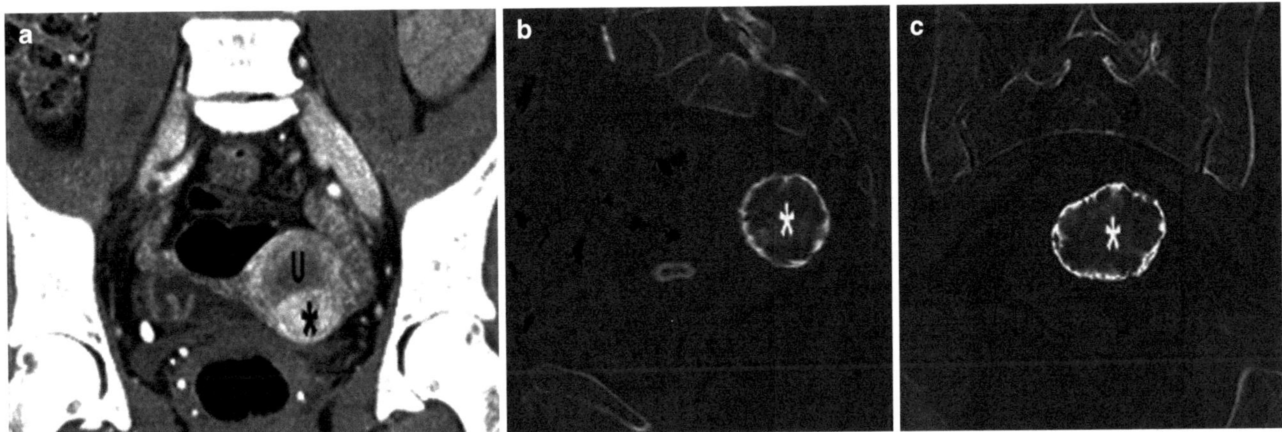

Fig. 6.9 (**a**) Presentation of a subserous non degenerated leiomyoma of the uterus at CT at venous phase (*asterisk*). The lesion is slightly more hyperdense than the myometrium. The uterine cavity presents as hypointense (*U*). Tissue contrast is reduced compared to MRI. (**b**) and (**c**) Degenerated myoma with ring-shape calcifications in another patient as a secondary finding on CT in sagittal and coronal plane (*asterisk*). Using the bone window, calcifications are best seen. This leiomyoma is located directly presacral and may be a cause for unspecific lower lumbar pain

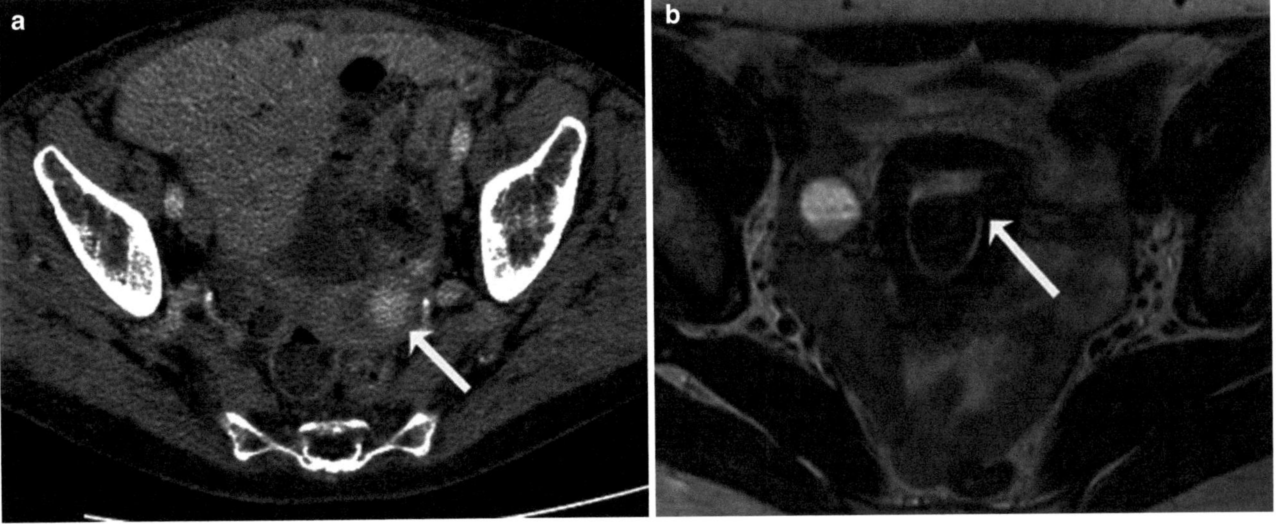

Table 6.2 Cross sectional imaging modalities for female pelvic pathologies

	Native MRI	CE MRI	Native CT	CECT	PET/CT	Specification of disease
1	+	+	–	(+)	–	Localisation, number, morphology, possible suspicious areals (early focal enhancement)
2	+	+	–	–	–	Differentiation and detection of adnexal, uterine or subperitoneal manifestations
3	+	–	–	–	–	Evaluation of entire pelvis with dynamic sequences during valsalva maneuver
4	+	+	–	(+)	–	Visualisation of fistulas and their origin/entry/re-entry better detection with rectal and/or vaginal filling with ultrasound gel MRI modality of choice for fistulas, CECT only if use of MRI is limited due to contraindications
5	+	+	–	+	+	CE MRI of the pelvis including the level of the renal veins for local staging and lymph node detection CECT of the abdomen and thorax for pretreatment staging in advanced stages CECT of the pelvis only if MRI is impossible to perform (e.g. pacemaker, implants) CE MRI for local recurrence PET/CT for diffuse or occult metastases
6	+	+	–	+	+	CE MRI of the pelvis including the level of the renal veins for local staging and lymph node detection CECT of the chest and abdomen for pretreatment staging in advanced stages CECT of the pelvis only if MRI is impossible to perform (e.g. pacemaker, implants) CE MRI for local recurrence PET/CT for diffuse or occult metastases

CE contrast enhanced, *MRI* Magnetic Resonance Imaging, *CECT* Contrast Enhanced Computed Tomography, *PET* Positron Emission Tomography

ral ill-defined myoma), uterine sarcoma (especially in fast growing intramural myoma), leiomyosarcoma of the cervix or vagina, ovarian fibroma or ovarian cancer (if subserous or pedunculated myoma). If local tumor differentiation is required, MRI of the pelvis is the imaging modality of choice (Table 6.2).

Endometriosis

MRI is recommended in cases with suspicion for subperitoneal endometrioses or in cases with unclear dysmenorrhoea and suspicion for adenomyosis [12–14].

Subperitoneal Implants of Endometriosis

Suberitoneal implants from endometriosis may be detected with MRI from at least 7 mm in diameter. Endometrial implants are hypointense in native T1WI and T2WI images. Sometimes T1WI hyperintense spots may be present in between the implant [12, 15]. If endometriosis is implanted in the abdominal wall, detection is made with a T1WI sequence with fat saturation. Angulation of the MR-sequences to the uterine corpus is essential for correct visualisation of the sacrouterine ligament, the torus uterinus and the fornix vaginae. Slice thickness should not exceed 3–4 mm for detection of small implants [16]. There is no indication for CT performance in endometriosis [17].

Adenomyoma/Adenomyosis Uteri

The adenomyoma and the adenomyosis uteri are two special forms of subperitoneal endometriosis and are located in the myometrium or the junctional zone of the uterus. Areas of endometriosis found within a myoma are defined as adenomyoma. The adenomyoma is almost ovally shaped and slightly blurred around its border with the surrounding myometrium when compared to an intramural leiomyoma. The signal intensity is comparable between both forms of myomas (Figs. 6.11 and 6.12) [11].

One distinguishing feature may be the fact that in adenomyoma, the junctional zone is commonly an integral part of the lesion, whereas in leiomyoma, even a small myometrial layer is notable close to the junctional zone.

An adenomyosis uteri is characterised by haphazardly scattered endometrial tissue within the uterus wall (Fig. 6.9). Using ultrasound, the adenomyosis uteri often represents heterogenous and includes microcysts. The accuracy using ultrasound was reported by Bazot et al. with 88 % and a sensitivity of 65 %, a specificity of 97.5 %, a PPV of 93 % and a NPV of 89 % when combining transvaginal and transabdominal ultrasound in patients without

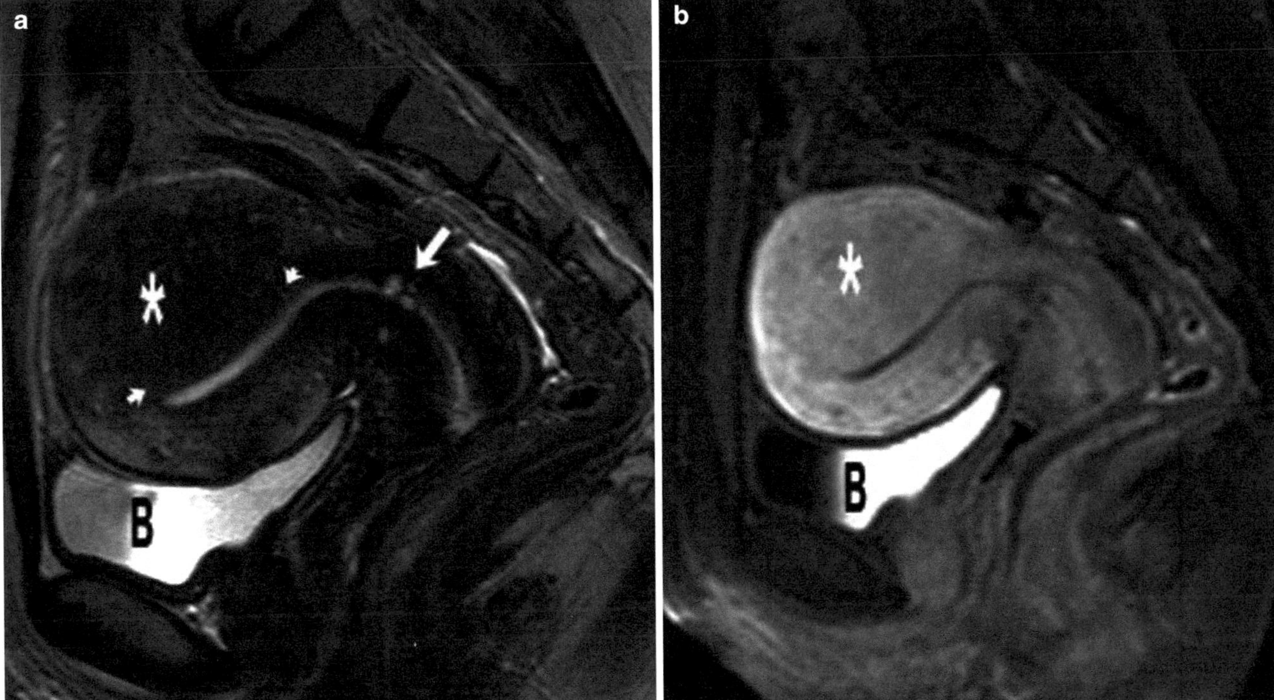

Fig. 6.11 Presentation of an adenomyoma in the posterior uterine wall with slightly blurry margins to surrounding myometrium (*asterisk*). Additionally, the adjacent junctional zone is not well defined (*arrowheads*). In the anterior wall there are several hyperintense spots, which are typical for diffuse adenomyosis. Small nabothian cysts as secondary findings (*arrow*). *B* bladder

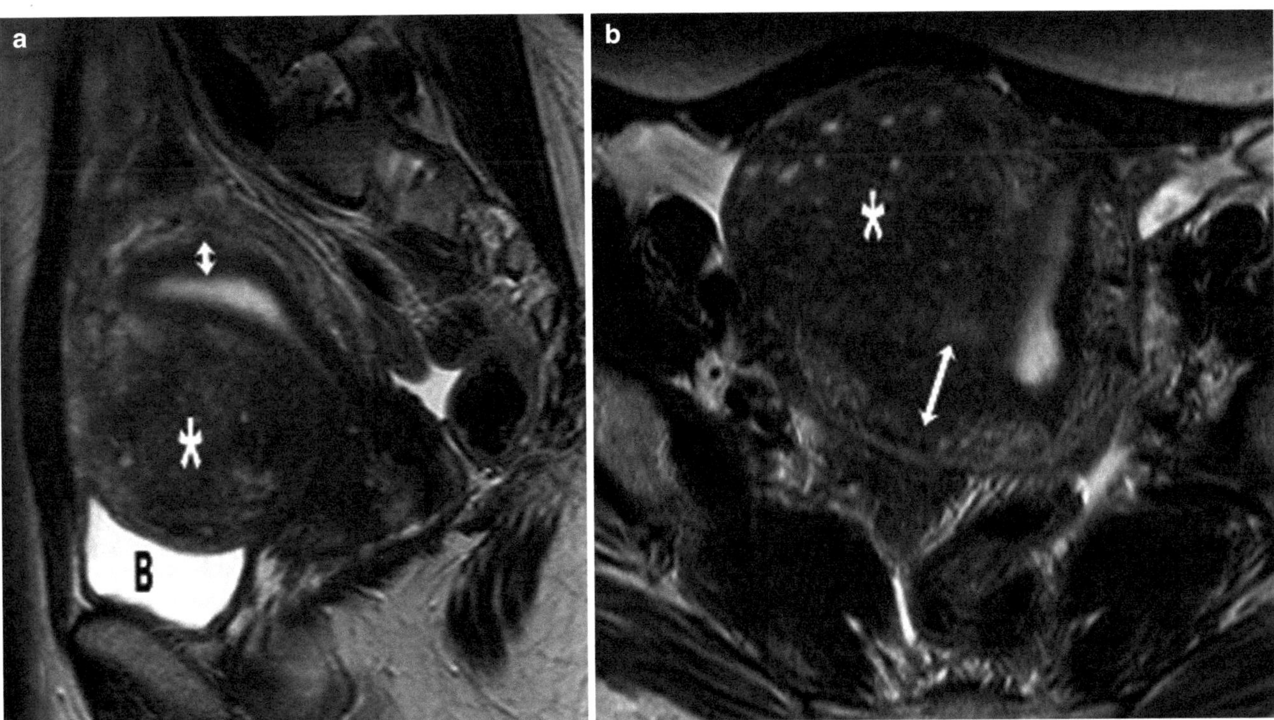

Fig. 6.12 (**a**) Presentation of an adenomyoma in the anterior uterine wall on T2WI on sagittal plane with slightly blurry margins to surrounding myometrium and several hyperintense spots. (**b**) The junctional zone is thin despite of a focal thickening at the posterior wall (*distance arrows*). This finding is typical for focal adenomyosis. *B* bladder

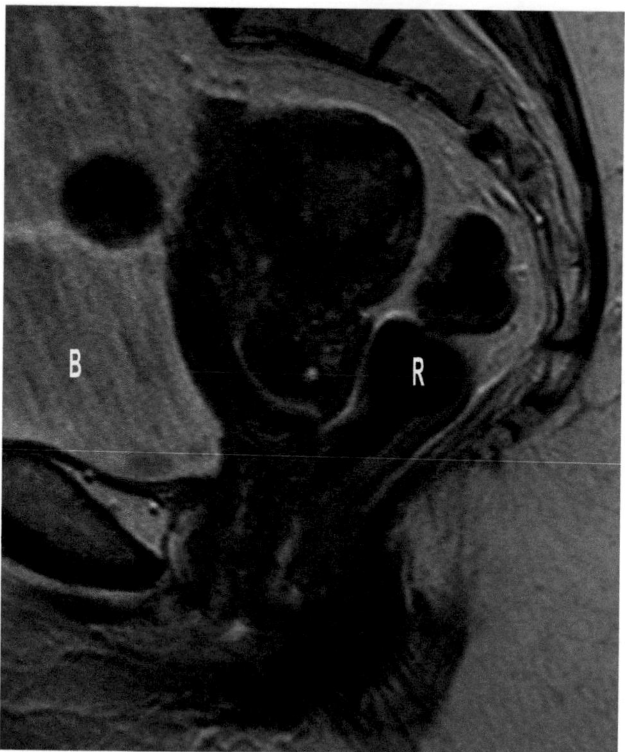

Fig. 6.13 Presentation of diffuse adenomyosis with heterogenous signal intensity of the myometrium and a thickened junctional zone with hyperintense spots on T2WI. Retroflected uterus. *B* bladder, *R* rectum

associated uterine disorders [18]. However, in patients with accompanied uterine disorders, e.g. leiomyomas, or with an enlarged uterus, ultrasound is limited in correct diagnosis of adenomyosis [18]. In those cases, MRI is able to visualize the uterine corpus on its whole extent and free of superimposition [19].

Using MRI, an adenomyosis characteristically shows a thickened junctional zone of more than 12 mm (the norm being max. 5 mm), hyperintense spots on T1WI and microcysts (Fig. 6.13). The accuracy using MRI was reported to be 87.5 % with a sensitivity of 77.5 %, a specificity of 92.5 %, a PPV of 84 % and a NPV of 89 % [18]. Typically, a discrepancy between the anterior and posterior wall of the uterine corpus can also be detected [20]. Differential diagnoses for adenomyoma are leiomyoma or uterine sarcoma. A study by Moghadam et al. evaluated the predictive value of an preoperative MRI in differentiating between leiomyoma and adenomyosis compared with pathologic findings in 153 women, suggesting that pelvic MRI is highly specific in the diagnosis of adenomyosis with 91 % and highly sensitive for leiomyomas with 94 % [19].

Fistulas

Vaginal fistulas may commonly occur after surgery (e.g. hysterectomy), radiation therapy or with the background of (chronic) inflammatory disease. Surgical reconstruction of such fistulas may be challenging, wherefore the detection and exact location of the fistula is crucial for therapy planning. With thin sliced T2-weighted or PD-images with fat saturation angulated to the vaginal cavity, the fistula presents hyperintense and is commonly well delineable to the surrounding tissue (Table 6.1). Patient's preparation with vaginal and rectal filling with ultrasound gel helps to better identify the origin of the fistula (Figs. 6.14 and 6.15). CT is mostly unable to detect small fistulas, why indication is usually not authorized.

Symptomatic Pelvic Floor Dysfunction

The prevalence of pelvic organ prolapse in developing countries is reported to be around 19.7 % [21]. Vaginal childbirth was demonstrated to be a predictor for levator ani trauma and an increased prevalence of pelvic floor dysfunction (PFD) even in younger, parous women [22–26]. Affected women may suffer from an abnormal frequency and urgency of emptying of the bladder, organ protrusion, pelvic pain or from dyspareunia, as well as from urinary or fecal incontinence [27–30]. To evaluate the pelvic floor structures and its integrity, MRI with high resolution T2 weighted images are performed at rest. This is best done in three planes [31–34]. The dynamic MR scans are performed during straining or defecation in the sagittal plane to evaluate pelvic organ prolapse (POP) and concordant PFD. The radiological report should give standardized measurements of pelvic organ prolapse, as well as a quantitative description of the pelvic organ position at rest and during straining or evacuation (Figs. 6.16, 6.17, 6.18, and 6.19) [35]. This precise description gives an impression of an individual woman's pelvic support in addition to an accurate, observer-independend, site-specific observation of the stability or progression of prolapse over time. Similar judgments are made regarding the outcome of surgical repair of prolapse, without interpreting the data using a grading system [36]. It was shown that the visualization of pelvic organ mobility, the detection of all involved structures and the extent of POP, detached from a grading system based on maximal prolapse values, might have more impact for intraindividual evaluation [37].

Dynamic MRI has benefits especially in regard to women suffering from re-prolapse after surgical repair and in the

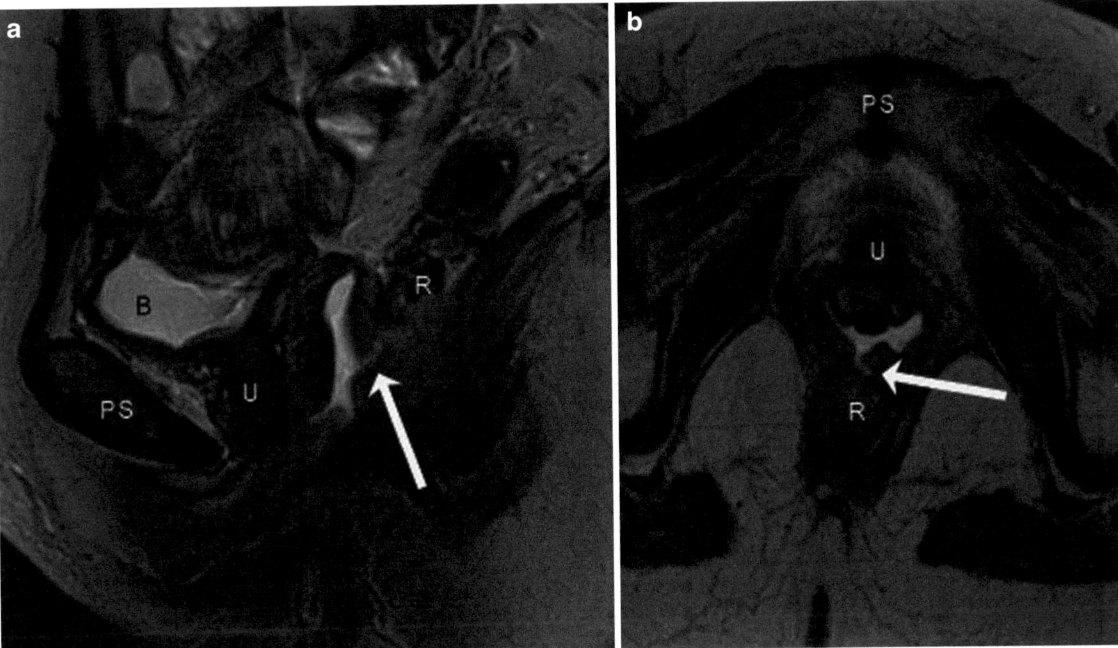

Fig. 6.14 Recto-vaginal fistula on high-resolution T2-weighted images. (**a**) on sagittal plane, the vaginal vault is filled and distended with ultrasonic gel. The fistula to the rectum with its angled form is also filled with gel, why detection is easy (*arrow*). (**b**) On transverse plane, the fistula starts at the posterior vaginal wall at 6 o'clock (*arrow*). At this level, the rectal wall is still intact. The entry to the rectum is located above (see (**a**)). *PS* pubic symphysis, *B* bladder, *U* urethra, *R* rectum

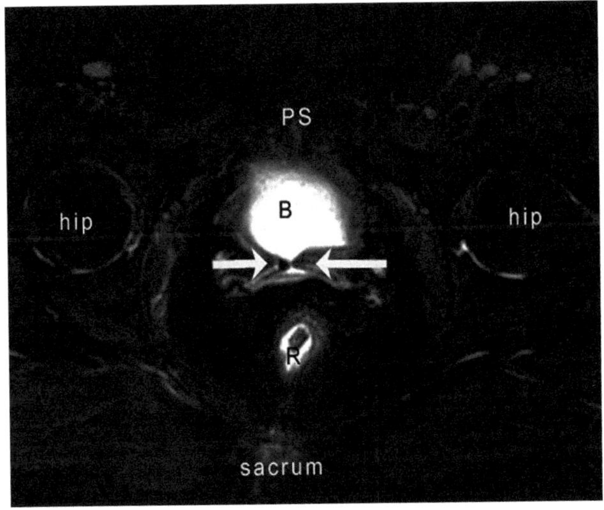

Fig. 6.15 Patient with vesico-vaginal fistula. T2-weighted images on transverse plane with fat saturation easily detect the fistula due to the high contrast of urine in the bladder and the vaginal filling with ultrasonic gel (*arrows*). The rectum was also filled with ultrasonic gel. *PS* pubic symphysis, *B* bladder, *R* rectum

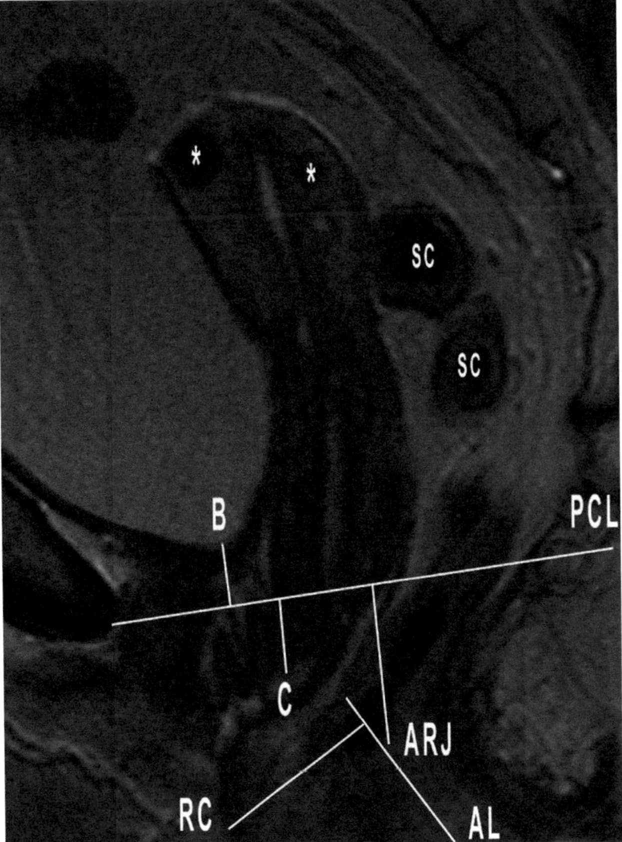

Fig. 6.16 T2WI on sagittal plane at rest in a 62 year old female. Even at rest, a partial uterine prolapse (*C*), a small rectal descent (*ARJ*) and a small rectocele (*RC*) can be noted. The bladder base (*B*) is above the reference line (*PCL*). Two small intramural leiomyomas are seen at T2WI on sagittal plane (*asterisk*). *AL* anal line (reference line for rectoceles), *SC* sigmoid colon, *ARJ* anorectal junction

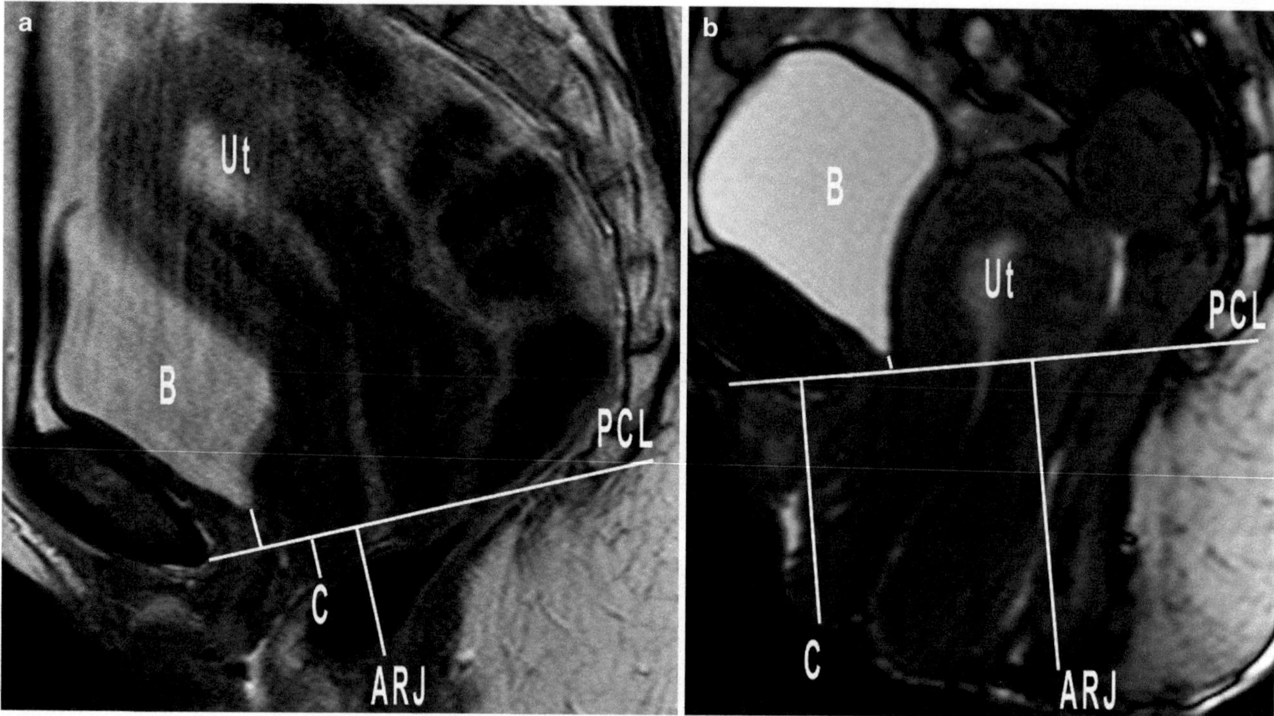

Fig. 6.17 (**a**) T2WI on sagittal plane at rest presenting with small descent of the cervix and a small rectal descent (*ARJ*). (**b**) During maximum strain presentation of a partial uterine prolapse and a severe rectal descent. The bladder is moved ventrally to the pubic symphysis. No bladder descent due to lack of hiatal space. *PCL* pubococcygeal line, *B* bladder, *Ut* uterus, *C* cervix, *ARJ* anorectal junction

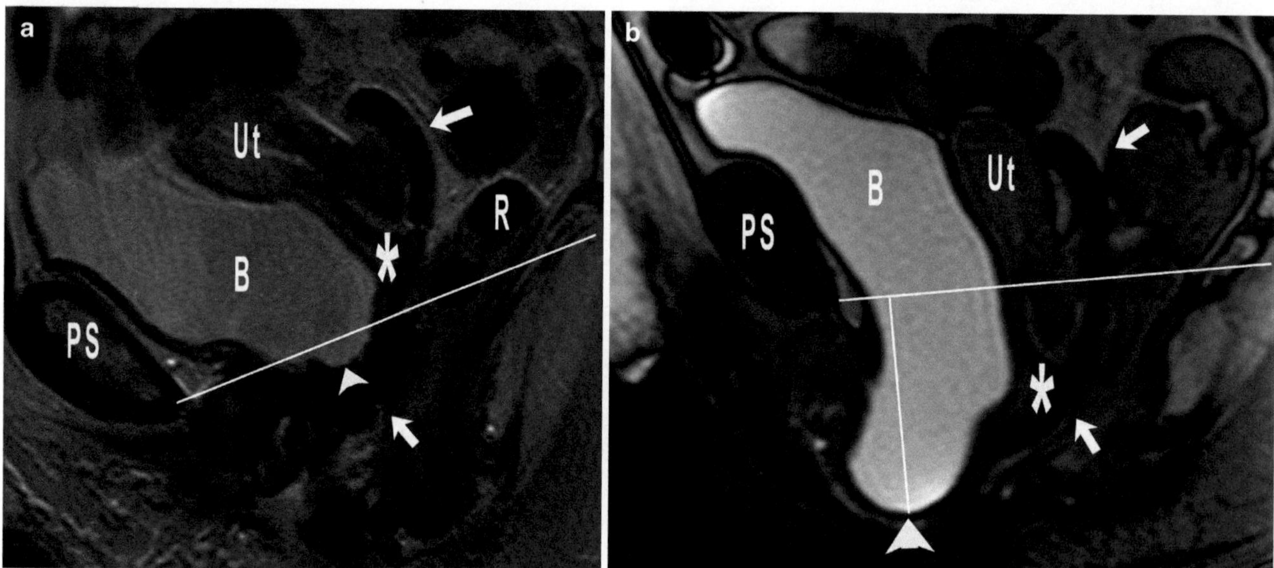

Fig. 6.18 (**a**) T2 W sagittal image at rest showing a moderately filled bladder with the bladder base slightly below the reference line (PCL). The uterus and cervix are also located above the reference line, supported by a pessary (*arrows*). (**b**) During maximum strain, the bladder base, as well as the cervix descent below the reference line, irrespective of the pessary presenting with a distraction cystocele (lateral defect of the endopelvic fascia) (*arrowhead*) and a partial uterine prolapse (*asterisk*). Additionally, hypermobility of the urethra is present (*thin arrows*). *B* bladder, *Ut* uterus, *PS* pubic symphysis

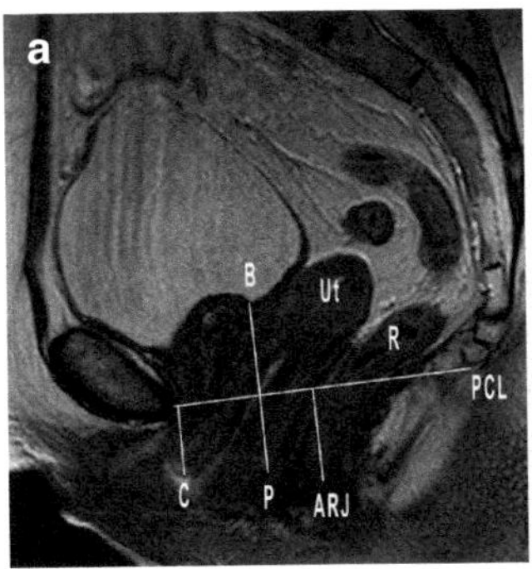

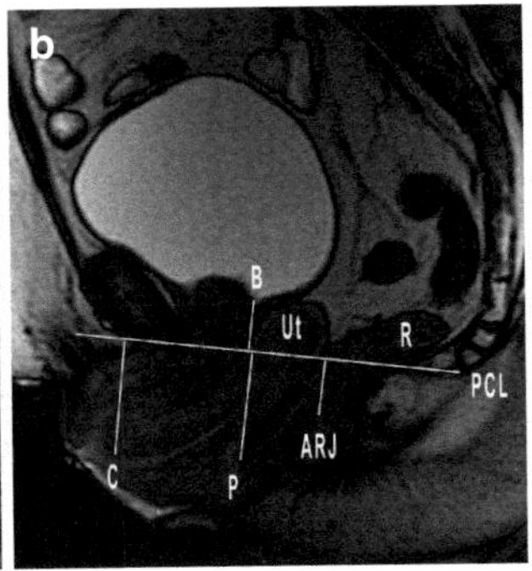

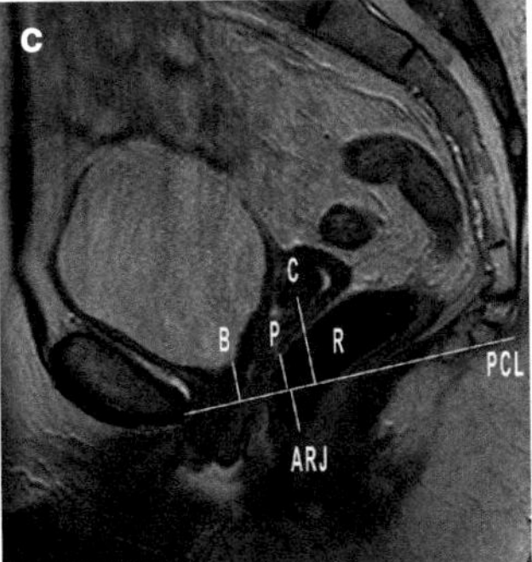

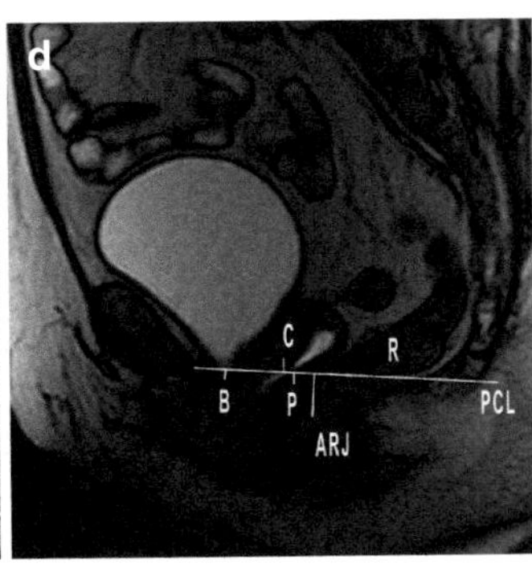

Fig. 6.19 Dynamic MRI of the pelvic floor (**a**) at rest and (**b**) during maximum strain before treatment presenting with partial uterine prolapse (*C*), peritoneocele (*P*) and rectal descent (*R*). Dynamic MRI of the pelvic floor 12 weeks after total mesh repair surgery combined with supracervical hysterectomy (**c**) at rest and (**d**) during maximum strain presenting reconstructed pelvic floor without pelvic organ descent. *B* bladder base, *C* cervix, *P* pouch of Douglas, *ARJ* anorectal angle, *PCL* pubococcygeus line

increasing sensitivity of findings in symptomatic women after surgery without findings during clinical examination [38]. MRI is able to detect the mechanisms responsible for topographic changes, which cannot be fully reached by the POP-Q system only, but are frequently needed to determine the steps necessary for successful surgical repair [39–42]. Therefore, MRI needs more attention before planned surgical repair to identify all involved compartments in POP and to detect incidental pathologic conditions in order. This is done to minimize the risk of incomplete surgical repair or recurrence [26, 27, 43, 44]. CT has no indication in evaluating POP [45].

References

1. Balleyguier C, Sala E, Da Cunha T, et al. Staging of uterine cervical cancer with MRI: guidelines of the European Society of Urogenital Radiology. Eur Radiol. 2011;21:1102–10.
2. Kinkel K, Forstner R, Danza FM, et al. Staging of endometrial cancer with MRI: guidelines of the European Society of Urogenital Imaging. Eur Radiol. 2009;19:1565–74.
3. Kirchhoff S. MR Vagina, Uterus, Adnexe. In: Scheffel H, Alkadhi H, Boss A, Merkle E, editors. Praxisbuch MRT Abdomen und Becken. Berlin: Springer; 2012. p. 181–94.
4. Thomassin-Naggara I, Darai E, Bazot M. Gynecological pelvic infection: what is the role of imaging? Diagn Interv Imaging. 2012;93:491–9.
5. Brocker KA, Alt CD, Eichbaum M, et al. Imaging of female pelvic malignancies regarding MRI, CT, and PET/CT: part 1. Strahlenther Onkol. 2011;187:611–8.
6. Sala E, Rockall AG, Freeman SJ, et al. The added role of MR imaging in treatment stratification of patients with gynecologic malignancies: what the radiologist needs to know. Radiology. 2013;266: 717–40.
7. Pano B, Sebastia C, Bunesch L, et al. Pathways of lymphatic spread in male urogenital pelvic malignancies. Radiographics. 2011;31:135–60.
8. Scheidler J. Bildgebende Diagnostik der inneren weiblichen Genitalorgane – Adnexe. In: Adams S, Nicolas V, Freyschmidt J, editors. Urogenitaltrakt, Retroperitoneum, Mamma. Berlin/Heidelberg: Springer; 2004. p. 221–40.
9. Horton KM, Sheth S, Corl F, et al. Multidetector row CT: principles and clinical applications. Crit Rev Comput Tomogr. 2002;43:143–81.
10. Kröncke T. Benign Uterine Lesions. In: Hamm B, Forstner R, editors. MRI and CT of the Female Pelvis. Berlin/Heidelberg/New York: Springer; 2007. p. 61–100.
11. Alt C, Gebauer G. Uterus. In: Hallscheidt P, Haferkamp A, editors. Urogenitale Bildgebung. Berlin/Heidelberg: Springer; 2011. p. 232–301.
12. Bazot M, Darai E, Hourani R, et al. Deep pelvic endometriosis: MR imaging for diagnosis and prediction of extension of disease. Radiology. 2004;232:379–89.
13. Del Frate C, Girometti R, Pittino M, et al. Deep retroperitoneal pelvic endometriosis: MR imaging appearance with laparoscopic correlation. Radiographics. 2006;26:1705–18.
14. Schindler A. Epidemiologie, Pathogenese und Diagnostik der Endometriose. Journal für Fertilität und Reproduktion. 2007;17:22–7.
15. Bazot M, Gasner A, Ballester M, et al. Value of thin-section oblique axial T2-weighted magnetic resonance images to assess uterosacral ligament endometriosis. Hum Reprod. 2011;26:346–53.
16. Kinkel K, Frei KA, Balleyguier C, et al. Diagnosis of endometriosis with imaging: a review. Eur Radiol. 2006;16:285–98.
17. Radeleff B. Ovarien. In: Hallscheidt P, Haferkamp A, editors. Urogenitale Bildgebung. Berlin/Heidelberg: Springer; 2011. p. 303–46.
18. Bazot M, Cortez A, Darai E, et al. Ultrasonography compared with magnetic resonance imaging for the diagnosis of adenomyosis: correlation with histopathology. Hum Reprod. 2001;16:2427–33.
19. Moghadam R, Lathi RB, Shahmohamady B, et al. Predictive value of magnetic resonance imaging in differentiating between leiomyoma and adenomyosis. JSLS. 2006;10:216–9.
20. CG R. Magnetic resonance imaging of the female pelvis. Fundamentals of body MRI. Philadelphia: Elsevier Saunders; 2012. p. 261–368.
21. Walker GJ, Gunasekera P. Pelvic organ prolapse and incontinence in developing countries: review of prevalence and risk factors. Int Urogynecol J. 2011;22:127–35.
22. DeLancey JO, Kearney R, Chou Q, et al. The appearance of levator ani muscle abnormalities in magnetic resonance images after vaginal delivery. Obstet Gynecol. 2003;101:46–53.
23. Lanzarone V, Dietz HP. Three-dimensional ultrasound imaging of the levator hiatus in late pregnancy and associations with delivery outcomes. Aust N Z J Obstet Gynaecol. 2007;47:176–80.
24. Mant J, Painter R, Vessey M. Epidemiology of genital prolapse: observations from the Oxford Family Planning Association Study. Br J Obstet Gynaecol. 1997;104:579–85.

25. Rortveit G, Subak LL, Thom DH, et al. Urinary incontinence, fecal incontinence and pelvic organ prolapse in a population-based, racially diverse cohort: prevalence and risk factors. Female Pelvic Med Reconstr Surg. 2010;16:278–83.
26. Nygaard I, Barber MD, Burgio KL, et al. Prevalence of symptomatic pelvic floor disorders in US women. JAMA. 2008;300:1311–6.
27. Boyadzhyan L, Raman SS, Raz S. Role of static and dynamic MR imaging in surgical pelvic floor dysfunction. Radiographics. 2008;28:949–67.
28. Harris TA, Bent AE. Genital prolapse with and without urinary incontinence. J Reprod Med. 1990;35:792–8.
29. Petros P. The female pelvic floor : function, dysfunction, and management according to the integral theory:subtitle. 2nd ed. Heidelberg: Springer; 2007.
30. Rush CB, Entman SS. Pelvic organ prolapse and stress urinary incontinence. Med Clin North Am. 1995;79:1473–9.
31. Alt CD, Hampel F, Hallscheidt P, et al. 3 T MRI-based measurements for the integrity of the female pelvic floor in 25 healthy nulliparous women. NeurourolUrodyn. 2014;35(2):218–23.
32. El Sayed RF, El Mashed S, Farag A, et al. Pelvic floor dysfunction: assessment with combined analysis of static and dynamic MR imaging findings. Radiology. 2008;248:518–30.
33. Hoyte L, Schierlitz L, Zou K, et al. Two- and 3-dimensional MRI comparison of levator ani structure, volume, and integrity in women with stress incontinence and prolapse. Am J Obstet Gynecol. 2001;185:11–9.
34. Tunn R, Goldammer K, Neymeyer J, et al. MRI morphology of the levator ani muscle, endopelvic fascia, and urethra in women with stress urinary incontinence. Eur J Obstet Gynecol Reprod Biol. 2006;126:239–45.
35. El Sayed RF, Alt CD, et al. Magnetic resonance imaging of pelvic floor dysfunction - joint recommendations of the ESUR and ESGAR Pelvic Floor Working Group. Eur Radiol. 2016. [Epub ahead of print] DOI:10.1007/s00330-016-4471-7.
36. Bump RC, Mattiasson A, Bo K, et al. The standardization of terminology of female pelvic organ prolapse and pelvic floor dysfunction. Am J Obstet Gynecol. 1996;175:10–7.
37. Alt CD, Brocker KA, Lenz F, et al. MRI findings before and after prolapse surgery. Acta Radiol. 2014;55:495–504.
38. Goodrich MA, Webb MJ, King BF, et al. Magnetic resonance imaging of pelvic floor relaxation: dynamic analysis and evaluation of patients before and after surgical repair. Obstet Gynecol. 1993;82:883–91.
39. Altringer WE, Saclarides TJ, Dominguez JM, et al. Four-contrast defecography: pelvic "floor-oscopy". Dis Colon rectum. 1995;38: 695–9.
40. Broekhuis SR, Futterer JJ, Barentsz JO, et al. A systematic review of clinical studies on dynamic magnetic resonance imaging of pelvic organ prolapse: the use of reference lines and anatomical landmarks. Int Urogynecol J Pelvic Floor Dysfunct. 2009;20:721–9.
41. Hock D, Lombard R, Jehaes C, et al. Colpocystodefecography. Dis Colon rectum. 1993;36:1015–21.
42. Kelvin FM, Maglinte DD, Hornback JA, et al. Pelvic prolapse: assessment with evacuation proctography (defecography). Radiology. 1992;184:547–51.
43. Olsen AL, Smith VJ, Bergstrom JO, et al. Epidemiology of surgically managed pelvic organ prolapse and urinary incontinence. Obstet Gynecol. 1997;89:501–6.
44. Rentsch M, Paetzel C, Lenhart M, et al. Dynamic magnetic resonance imaging defecography: a diagnostic alternative in the assessment of pelvic floor disorders in proctology. Dis Colon rectum. 2001;44:999–1007.
45. Alt C, Lenz F, Haferkamp A. Beckenbodendysfunktion der Frau. In: Hallscheidt P, Haferkamp A, editors. Urogenitale Bildgebung. Berlin/Heidelberg: Springer; 2011. p. 399–441.

Radio-Imaging for Malignant Uterine Disease

7

Céline D. Alt-Radke

Introduction

Magnetic Resonance Imaging (MRI)

Native high-resolution T2-weighted images (T2WI) are essential for morphological differentiation of pelvic organ tissue. Contrast-enhanced T1-weighted images (CE T1WI) give important additional information in almost every problem and should be therefore routinely performed [1, 3, 6–9]. However, kidney functions (kreatinine) should be checked before the intravenous application of contrast media. In recent years, diffusion weighted imaging gains more and more attention. This imaging technique was designed to depict alterations in thermally induced random (Brownian) motion of water molecules within tissues and the degree of this motion is known as diffusion [5]. Diffusion-weighted MR imaging (DWI) can be performed quickly, without the necessity of contrast i.v. The technique yields qualitative and quantitative information about cellularity and cellular membrane integrity. High cellularity and cell membrane integrity restrict water mobility and therefore diffusion, as seen e.g. in tumors. During MR-performance, diffusion sensitivity can easily be varied by changing the *b* value used during image acquisition [5]. For gynecologic malignancies, b-values up to 800–1000 are recommended for local tumor staging and the evaluation of lymph node affection [10–12]. Quantitative analysis of diffusion may be performed by obtaining and mapping apparent diffusion coefficient (ADC) values [5]. This technique can be performed in patients with contraindication for contrast i.v., which is of great benefit for further evaluation in case of tumorous. For lymph node detection, a native T1WI sequence or proton-weighted (PD) sequence is helpful [13].

C.D. Alt-Radke, MD
Department of Diagnostic and Interventional Radiology, Medical Faculty, University Duesseldorf,
D-40225 Duesseldorf, Germany
e-mail: celine.alt@med.uni-duesseldorf.de

Computed Tomography (CT)

With a multidetector CT (MDCT) the examination of a region of interest can be performed in axial plane in a short examination time with submillimeter resolution. The row data can be postprocessed in any plane with approximately the same resolution. It should be noticed that intravenous contrast application is essential for soft tissue contrast because even CT in venous phase has less tissue contrast compared to native MRI (see Fig. 6.1) [14]. Before performing contrast enhanced CT (CECT), kidney function (kreatinine) and thyroid function (TSH, fT3, fT4) should be checked to be with normal values.

Endometrial Cancer

Regardless of hormone status, the normal endometrium is always hyperintense in native T2w images, the junctional zone is hypointense and the outer myometrium is of moderate signal intensity [15]. Endometrial cancer is moderately hyperintense in T2WI. However, small tumors can be isointense in regard to the endometrium and may be therefore difficult to detect. CE T1WI sequence with fat saturation is therefore recommended, as the tumor then represents hypointense compared to the myometrium (best delineation approx. 2 min after contrast media injection i.v.) (Figs. 7.1, 7.2, and 7.3) [1].

Diffusion weighted images may also be helpful for tumor detection, as this shows a stronger signal decrease in ADC map than the surrounding normal myometrium [12]. The lack of the fat layer between organs (best seen in the native T1WI), as well as a thickened bladder or rectal wall, are an indicator for a beginning infiltration of the bladder or the rectal mucosa [1]. Staging is done using UICC-criteria (Union Internationale Contre le Cancer), the most recent version dating to 2010 [2, 16].

A CT-examination is not used for local staging. However, it is used for radiation planning or for complete staging for

I. Alkatout, L. Mettler (eds.), *Hysterectomy*, DOI 10.1007/978-3-319-22497-8_7

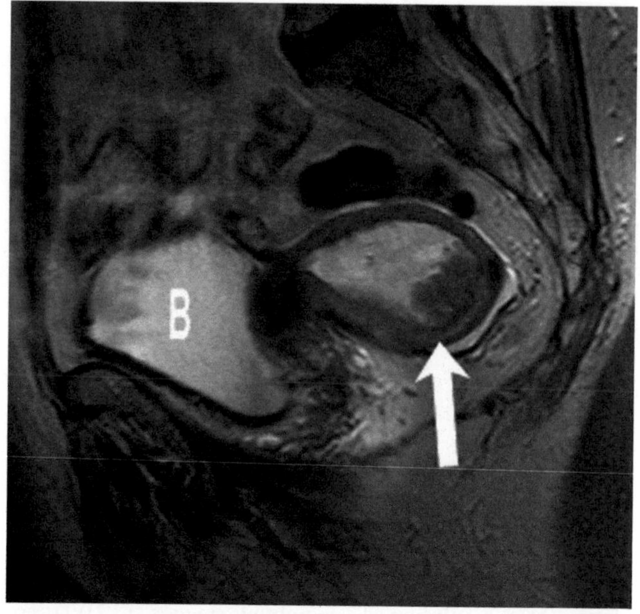

Fig. 7.1 Histopathologically proven early stage endometrial cancer in a retroflected uterus with mucos retention in the uterine cavity. There is no infiltration of the myometrium, as there is a clear demarcation on T2WI of the hypointense junctional zone between the intraluminal endometrial mass and the myometrium (*arrow*). T-Stage T1a. *B* bladder

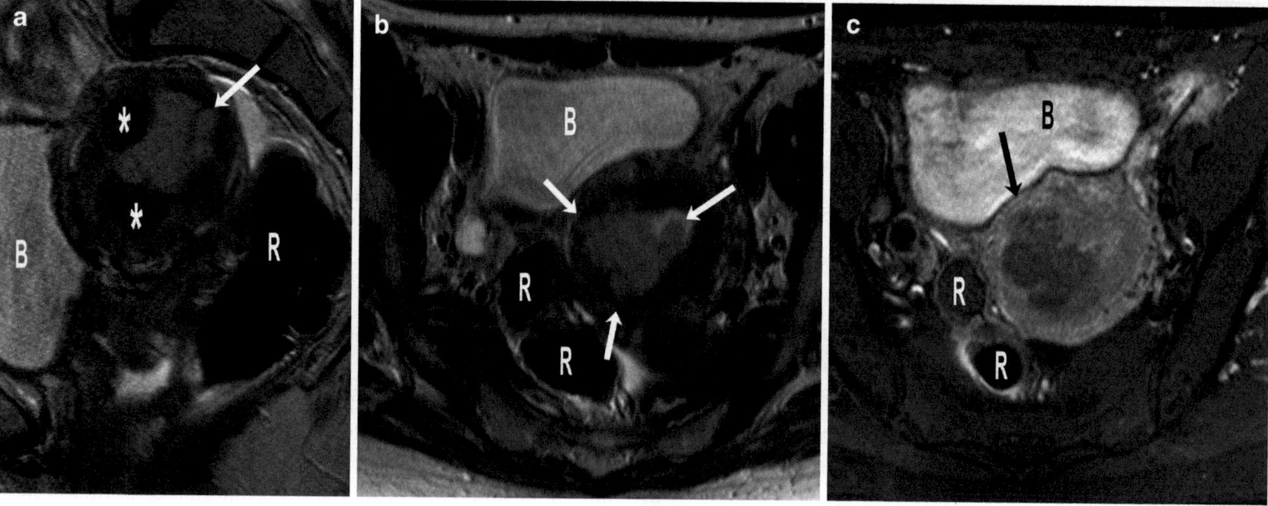

Fig. 7.2 Uterus myomatosus (*asterisk*) with the presence of an hyperintense endometrial mass (*arrow*), biopsy proven endometrial cancer. (**a**) The endometrial cancer is hyperintense on T2WI. (**b**) It presents hypointense after application of contrast i.v. Myometrial invasion is partly more than 50 %, defined on T2WI images on transversal oblique plane and was verified after contrast i.v. with hypointense demarcation of the tumor compared to surrounding myometrium on transversal oblique plane (*arrows*). T-stage T1b. This result was histopathologically proven. *B* bladder, *R* rectum

Fig. 7.3 (**a**) Locally advanced endometrial cancer (*arrows*) with infiltration of the cervix. The serosa is intact. No vaginal infiltration. T-stage T2. (**b**) One lymph node at the right pelvic sidewall is suspicious for metastatic affection (*asterisk*). N-stage N1. This result was histopathologically proven

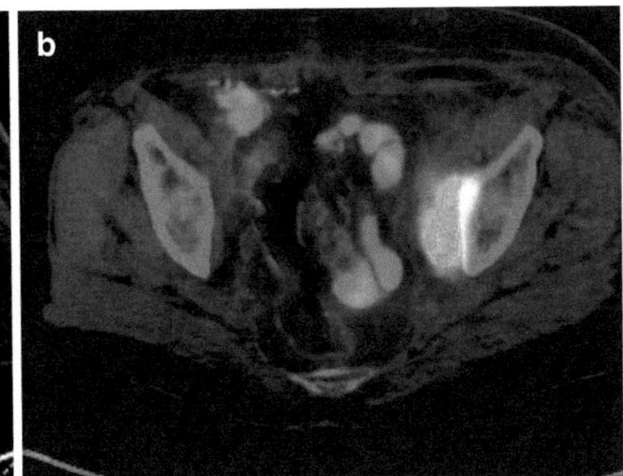

Fig. 7.4 PET/CT scan of a patient with suspected recurrence of endometrial cancer. (**a**) CT scan gives the anatomical overview. (**b**) PET presents with the pathological tracer uptake (*yellow*). Metastasis was found at the left pelvic side wall. Without any other manifestation of occult or visible metastases, the patient underwent radiation therapy

distant metastases (especially pulmonary, hepar, retroperitoneal lymph nodes). If CECT is performed for another indication, an endometrial cancer represents as a hypodense mass in the endometrial cavity. The evaluation of the depth of myometrial infiltration with CECT is made more difficult due to the low contrast of soft tissue as sensitivity is only around 58–61 %. If the cervix is heterogenous and thickened, suspicion of infiltration must be filed. If a tumor expands beyond the serosa a blurred reticular streaking can be expected. A bladder or rectum infiltration is to be presumed when the fat layer is missing. When solid tissue expansions in the lumen can be proven, an infiltration is the case [17]. The PET/CT has a standing in the diagnosis of distal metastases and in the diagnosis of recurrent disease (Fig. 7.4) [1].

Cervical Cancer

The decision for primary surgery or primary combined chemoradiation or brachytherapy, respectively, is based in particular on tumor size and the discovery of an infiltration of the parametrium [6]. With the expansion of cervical cancer along the parametrium to the pelvic wall or to the lower third of the vagina, the probability of positive paraaortal or inguinal lymph nodes grows. Metastases in the liver, the lungs or bones could exist in the advanced tumor stages. For this reason, a complete cross-sectional imaging based staging including MRI of the pelvis and CT of the body and chest is recommended before treatment. Ultrasound is often not sufficient for a complete evaluation of a local finding. However, this technique is used to exclude hydronephrosis or liver metastases.

In MRI, the mucosa of the normal cervix represents hyperintensive in the native T2WI, whereas the cervical stroma is hypointense [15]. Cervical cancer represents hyperintensive in the native T2WI in relation to the hypointense stroma tissue (Fig. 7.5). If the cervical stromal ring appears intact on T2WI on transverse oblique plane, parametrial invasion is present in 0–6 % of cases [20]. In a large meta-analysis by Rigon et al., the authors found an overall sensitivity of 66 % and a specificity of 84 % for detection of parametrial invasion in 1341 patients using 1.5 T MRI [21]. In rare cases, the tumor is isointense to the surrounding tissue in the T2WI or too small in diameter, as this may be residual tumor tissue after curettage. In these cases, DWI or CE T1WI with fat saturation is relevant for tumor detection (Fig. 7.6) [6]. There is a signal decrease on ADC map and a hypointense signal in early phase after application of contrast i.v. in T1WI with fat saturation compared to surrounding tissue. Best delineation will be reached 15–30 s after contrast injection. In late phase, however, the tumor represents hyperintense compared to uterine myometrium. Dynamic contrast enhanced sequences are therefore recommended (Figs. 7.7, 7.8, 7.9, 7.10, 7.11, and 7.12) [18, 19].

The staging for cervical cancer is done according to UICC-criteria (Union Internationale Contre le Cancer), the most recent version dating to 2010 [2, 16].

While the intravenous application of contrast i.v. can be forgone during primary detection as the tumor is easily detectable in the native T2WI in most cases, such an application is compulsive for therapy control after brachytherapy, after combined chemoradiation or after surgery to differentiate between a residual tumor or scar-like changes [6].

The CT is not necessary for primary diagnosis but is used for planning radiation or detecting distal mestastases (lungs, liver, bones) or peripheral lymph node metastases [3]. In case of a contrast media-enhanced CT, cervical cancer usually represents as a thickening of non-centric cervical tissue with a diameter of more than 3.5 cm (Fig. 7.13) [17]. Parametrial involvement is probable if cervical borders are blurry, thickened and spiculated (Fig. 7.14) [19]. An infiltration of the bladder or rectal wall represents in an irregular

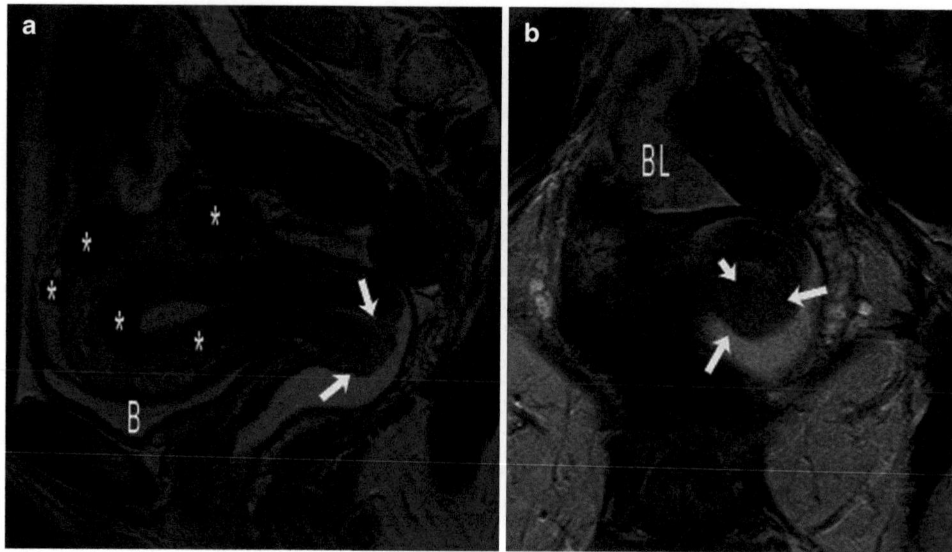

Fig. 7.5 (**a**) T2WI on midsagittal plane. Vaginal filling with ultrasound gel distends the vaginal cavity and gives a better demarcation of the cervical structures and the vaginal fornices. Due to this preparation, the dome-shaped mass of the anterior cervical lip is well visible and tumor extent can be easily detect (*arrows*). As a secondary finding, uterine corpus presents with 5 leiomyomas (submucosal – transmural – subserosal) (*asterisk*). (**b**) Transversal oblique plane of the cervix shows the circumscribed tumor extent (*arrows*). Cervical cancer at T-stage T1b1, histopathologically proven. *B* bladder, *BL* bowel loops

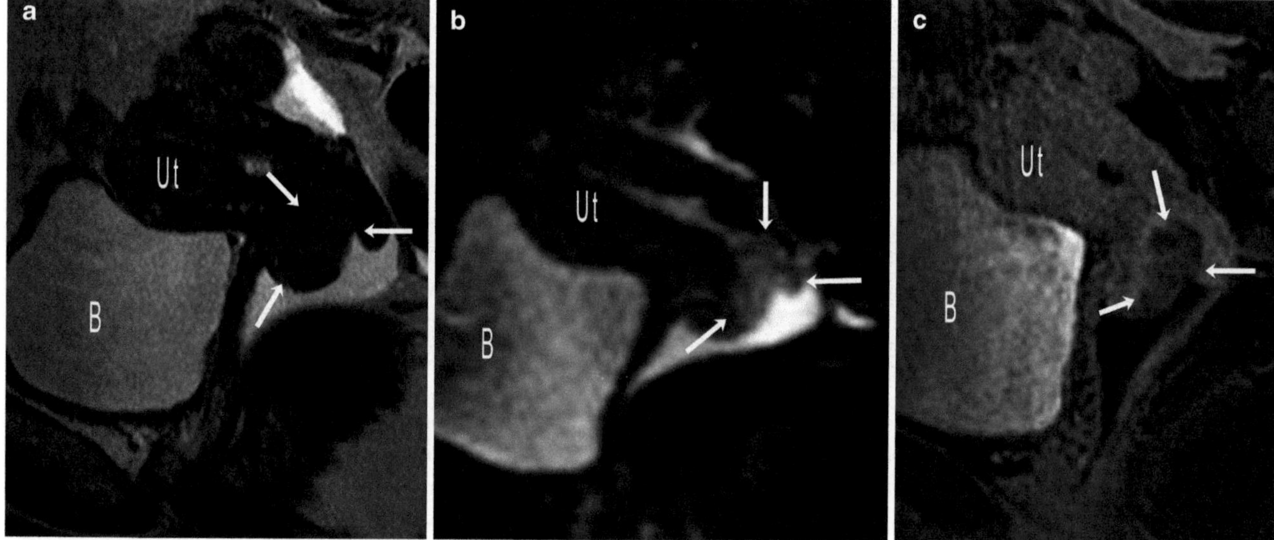

Fig. 7.6 Biopsy proven cervical cancer. MRI performed for pretherapeutic staging. (**a**) T2 WI presents a mass like lesion of the cervix originating from the anterior cervical lip (*arrows*). In this case, the tumor is not well delineated on T2WI and functional imaging techniques like diffusion weighted imaging or dynamic contrast enhanced images are helpful. (**b**) Diffusion weighted imaging with a *b*-value of 800 shows high signal intense tumor, well delineatable from surrounding tissue (*arrows*). (**c**) after application of contrast i.v. the tumor delineates as hypointense compared to surrounding tissue (*arrows*). *B* bladder, *Ut* uterus

thickening of the wall or a solid tumor that extends into the cavity and is probably present, if the fat layer is missing (Fig. 7.15) [17].

The PET/CT has a standing with locally advanced cervical cancer, especially for the detection of morphological, at first glance seemingly harmless lymph node metastases [22].

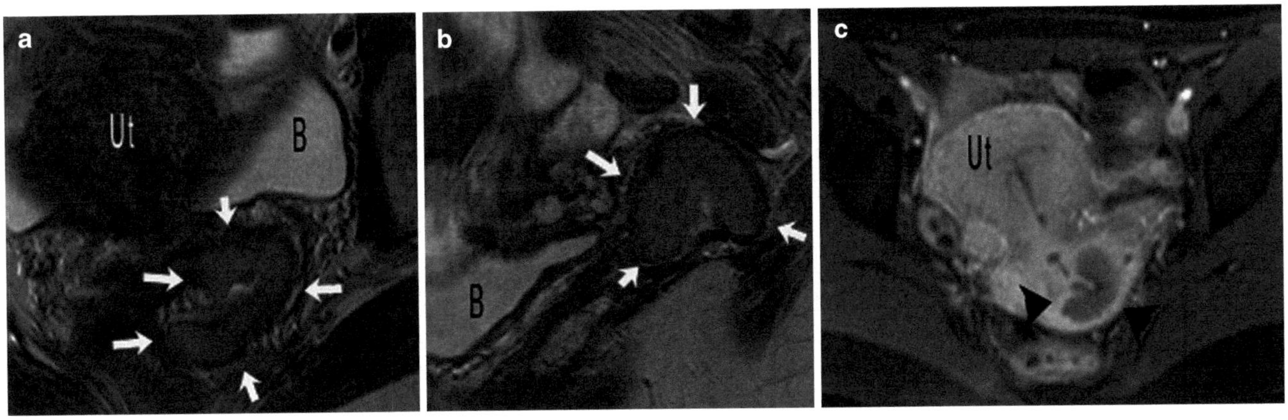

Fig. 7.7 Horseshoe-like mass of the cervix with well defined margins and a maximum diameter of >4 cm presented on (**a**) transversal oblique and (**b**) sagittal plane. (**c**) After application of contrast i.v. the tumor demasks hypointense to the surrounding cervical stroma (*black arrow head*). The cervical stroma ring is not interrupted, no infiltration of adjacent structures. T-stage T1b2, histopathologically proven. *B* bladder, *Ut* uterus

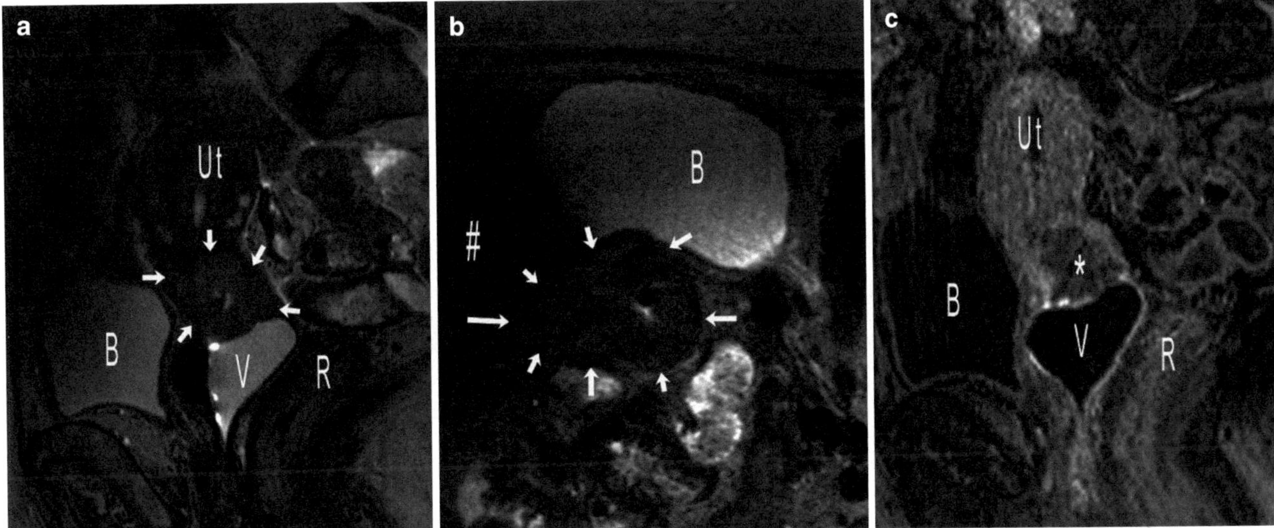

Fig. 7.8 Histopathologically proven cervical cancer. (**a**) T2WI on sagittal plane with vaginal filling with ultrasound gel. This preparation better delineates the cervical cancer with moderate hyperintense signal intensity (*arrows*). The vaginal fornix becomes infiltrated. (**b**) The cervical carcinoma invades the right parametrium, whereas the cervical stroma is still well delineated to the left parametrium on transversal oblique sequences (*arrows*). (**c**) Hypointense demarcation of the carcinoma after application of contrast i.v. (*asterisk*). *B* bladder, *V* vagina, *Ut* uterus, *R* rectum, # artefact due to endoprothesis of the right hip

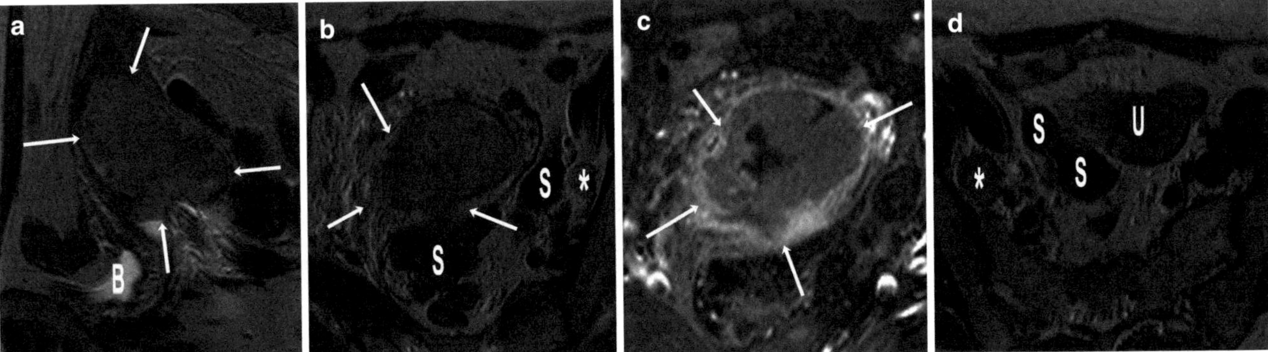

Fig. 7.9 Biopsy proven cervical cancer with invasion into the uterine corpus and the proximal vagina (*arrows*) on T2WI on sagittal plane. (**b**) Invasion into the right parametrium on T2WI on transversal oblique plane. (**c**) After application of contrast i.v. the carcinoma presents hypointense to surrounding tissue with central necrotic parts. T-Stage T2b. (**d**) Additionally, a large lymph node metastasis iliacal right sided is present (*asterisk*). N-stage N1. This result was histopathologically proven. *S* sigmoid colon, *U* uterus

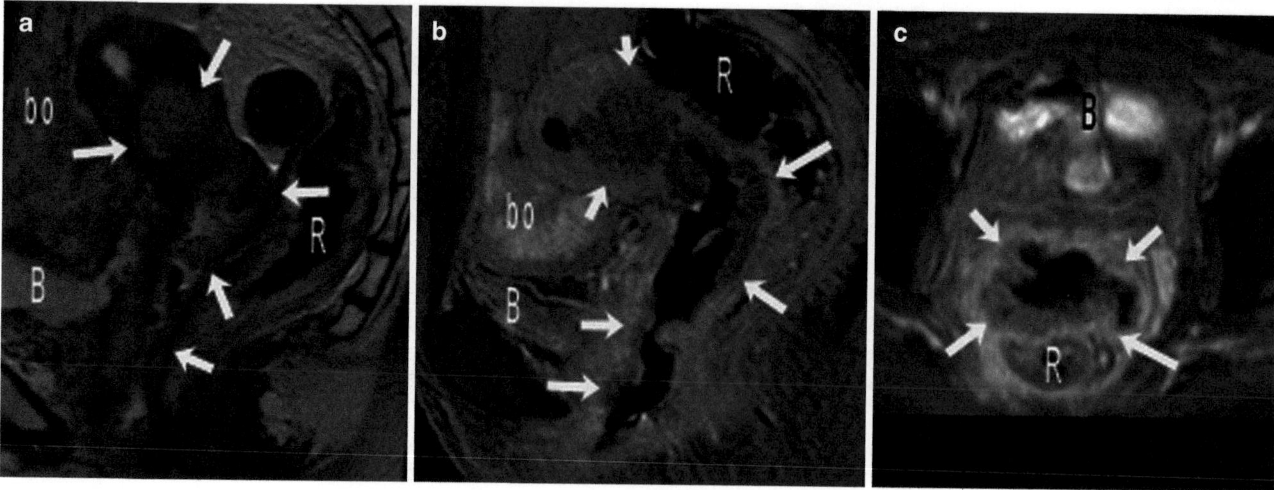

Fig. 7.10 Biopsy proven cervical cancer. (**a**) MRI with T2WI on sagittal plane shows infiltration of the uterine corpus and the vaginal wall until the lower third (*arrows*). (**b**) After contrast i.v. the tumor presents as hypointense (*arrows*). (**c**) CE T1WI on transversal oblique plane shows an intact layer to anterior rectal wall. T-stage T3a. This patient underwent primary chemoreadiation therapy. *B* bladder, *R* rectum, *bo* bowel

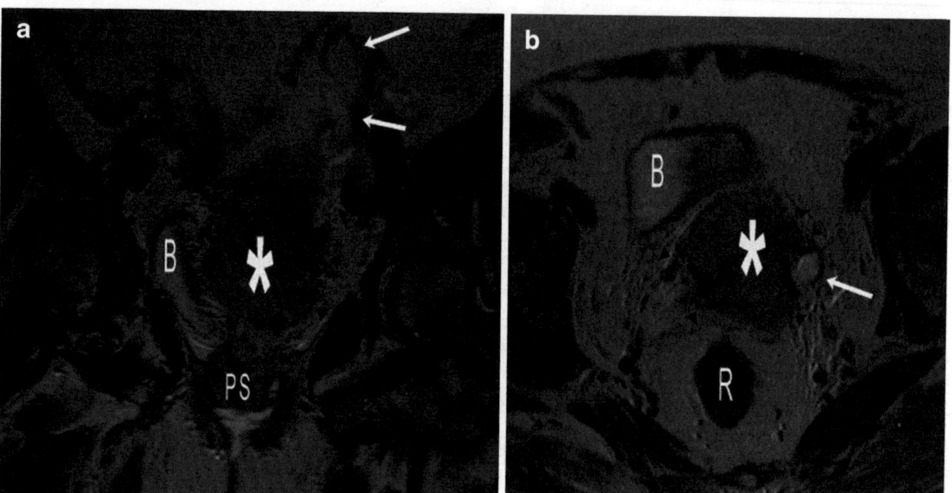

Fig. 7.11 Biopsy proven cervical cancer (*asterisk*). (**a**) The T2WI on coronal oblique plane shows a dilated left ureter (*arrows*). (**b**) On T2WI on transversal oblique plane invasion of the parametrium bilaterally with impression of the left distal ureter is present (*arrow*). T-stage T3b. This patient underwent splint implantation into the ureter bilaterally and underwent primary chemoradiation therapy. *B* bladder, *R* rectum, *PS* pubic symphysis

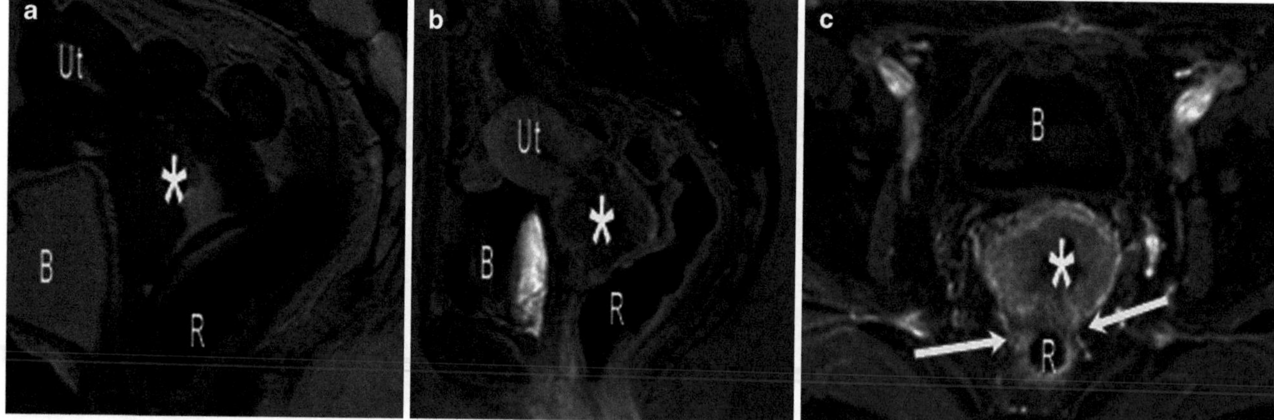

Fig. 7.12 (**a**) Cervical cancer (*asterisk*) on sagittal plane with infiltration of the isthmus uteri. (**b**) Better tumor demarcation after contrast i.v. suggesting local tumor disease. (**c**) On transversal oblique plane, however, the tumor (*asterisk*) invades the anterior rectal wall (*arrows*). T-stage T4. This result was proven by rectoscopy. The patient underwent primary chemoradiation therapy. *B* bladder, *Ut* uterus, *R* rectum

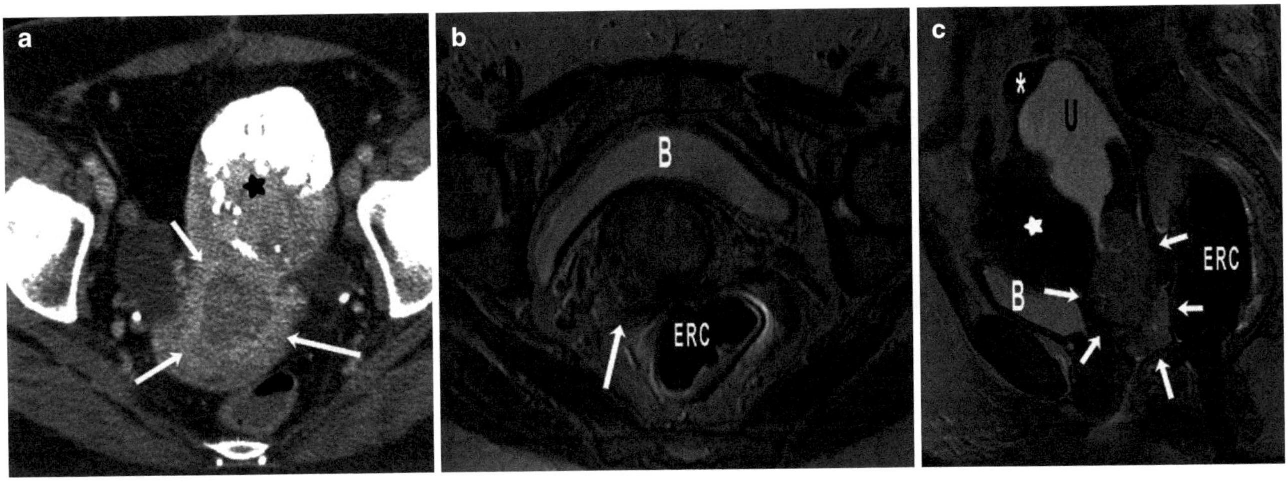

Fig. 7.13 (**a**) Axial CT scan at venous phase shows an enlarged cervix with centrally hypointense area (*arrows*). A subserous leiomyoma with calcifications is located ventrally (*star*). (**b**) MRI of the same patient shows cervical mass with infiltration of the right parametrium on transversal oblique plane (*arrow*). *B* bladder, *ERC* endorectal coil. (**c**) On sagittal plane, invasion of the uterine corpus and the upper third of the vagina is visible (*arrows*). The fat layer between the bladder and the rectum wall is present. Cervical carcinoma at T-stage T2b, histopathologically proven. The calcified leiomyoma presents as hypointense on T2WI (*star*). There is a small subserous leiomyoma at the fundus (*asterisk*). *B* bladder, *ERC* endorectal coil, *U* uterus

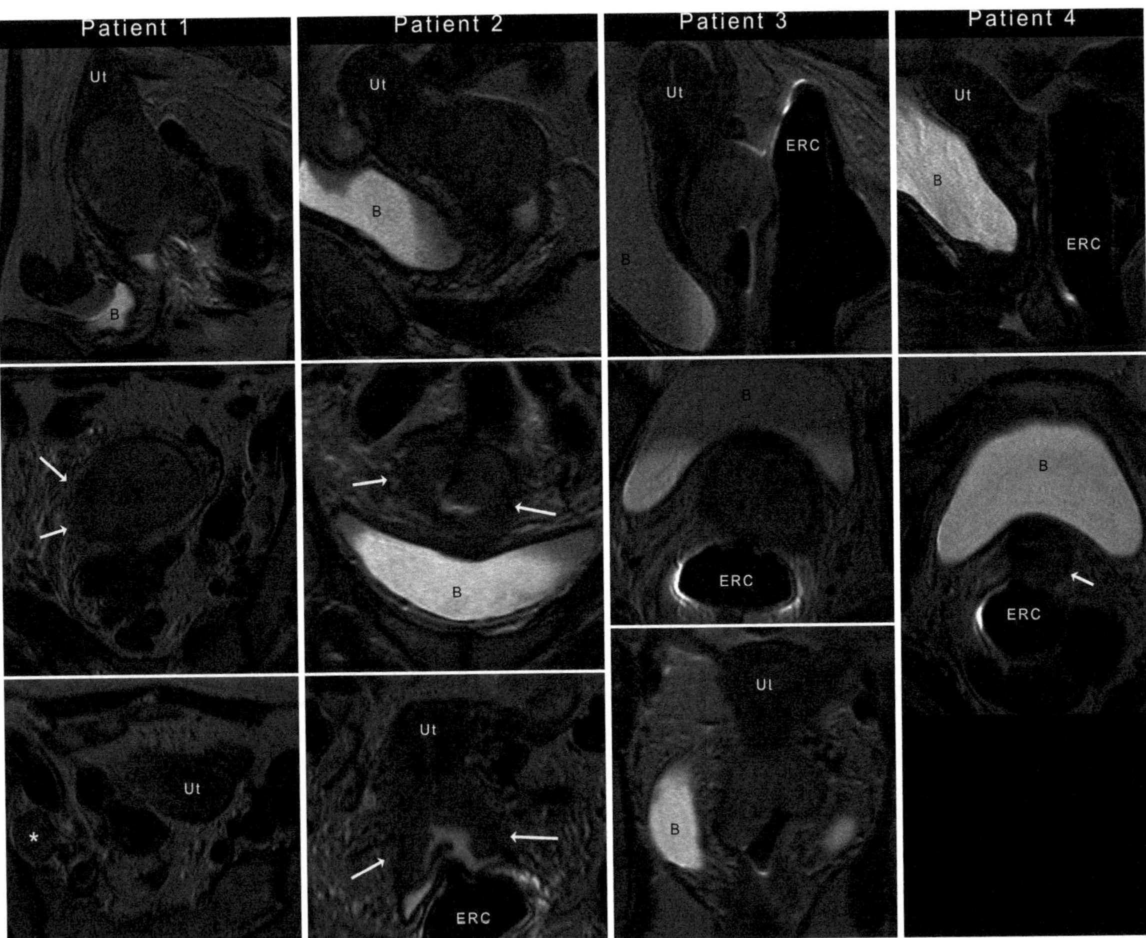

Fig. 7.14 Four patients with histopathologically proven cervical cancer stage T2b. Patient 1: Cervical cancer with infiltration into the uterine corpus, the proximal anterior vaginal fornix and the right parametrium (*arrows*). Patient 2: Cervical cancer with invasion of the vaginal fornix and bilateral parametrial invasion (*arrows*). Patient 3: Cervical cancer originating from the posterior cervical lip. The stromal ring is only intact ventrally, whereas the margins to the parametrium are blurry bilaterall. Patient 4: Cervical cancer with invasion into the left parametrium (*arrow*). The hypointense cervical stromal ring is well delineated at the right side. *B* Bladder; *Ut* uterus; *ERC* endorectal coil

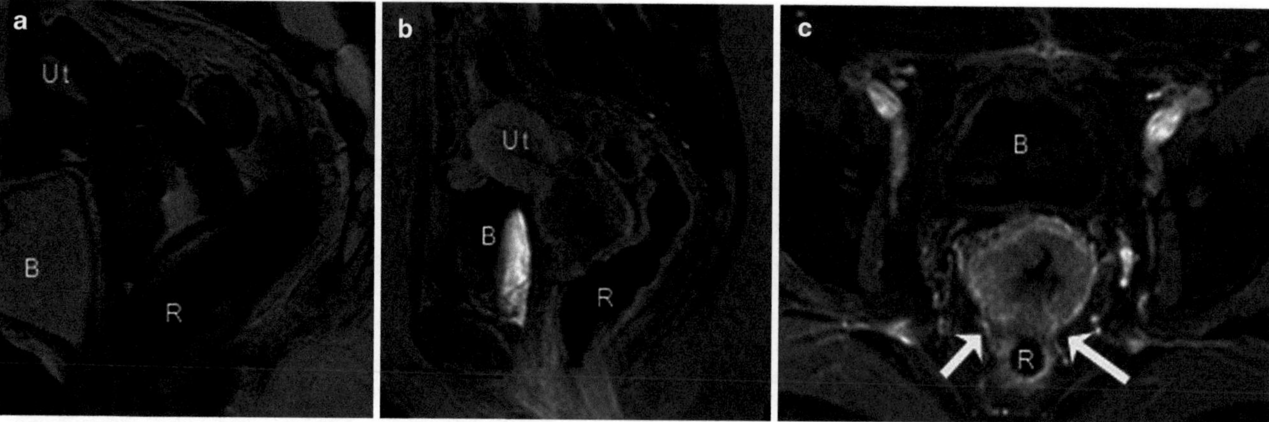

Fig. 7.15 (**a**, **b**) Patient presenting with a pseudo-well described cervical cancer on sagittal plane. (**c**) On transverse oblique plane to the cervical cavity, the wide based invasion of the upper part of the anterior rectal wall is visible (*arrows*). *B* bladder, *R* rectum, *Ut* uterus

Uterine Sarcoma

Uterine sarcoma can be classified into three histological subtypes: leiomyosarcoma (commonly myometrial origin), endometrial stromal sarcoma, *and* adenosarcoma (commonly endometrial origin) [16]. The transvaginal ultrasound is used as the primary standard image modality. In addition to this, MRI offers relevant additional informationen about tumor expansion. The CECT provides an overview of the infiltrated surrounding structures, distant metastases, ascites or peritoneal implants (Figs. 7.16 and 7.17) [23]. The PET/CT offers promising possibilities for staging, grading and therapy control for sarcomas [24]. All in all, differentiating between leiomyoma and leiomyosarcoma is challenging by using MRI. Apart from a fast growth, a large heterogenous tumor, hypervascular foci or central necrotic components can be indicators [25, 26]. Endometrial stromal sarcoma commonly represents an infiltrative mass with cystic parts. The endometrium as well as the myometrium is involved (Figs. 7.18 and 7.19).

Leiomyosarcoma, however, is mostly shown through heterogenous signal intensity with a fuzzy boundary. Commonly, at least 50 % are hyperintense on T2WI, with additional hyperintensities on T1WI (Fig. 7.20). On CECT, the uterus commonly presents as a heterogeneous mass with ill defined boundaries and irregular central zones, commonly due to necrosis (Fig. 7.21).

The adenosarcoma is often defined as a large, multiseptated, cystic mass with heterogenous solid components in the uterine cavity. The solid components are mostly hypointense in the native T2WI, which represent with strong contrast enhancement in CE T1WI [27]. Adenosarcoma may also presents as a large polypoid mass occupying the endometrial cavity, possibly protruding into the vaginal cavity (Fig. 7.22) [28]. Staging is done according to UICC-criteria (Union Internationale Contre le Cancer), the most recent version dating to 2010 [16].

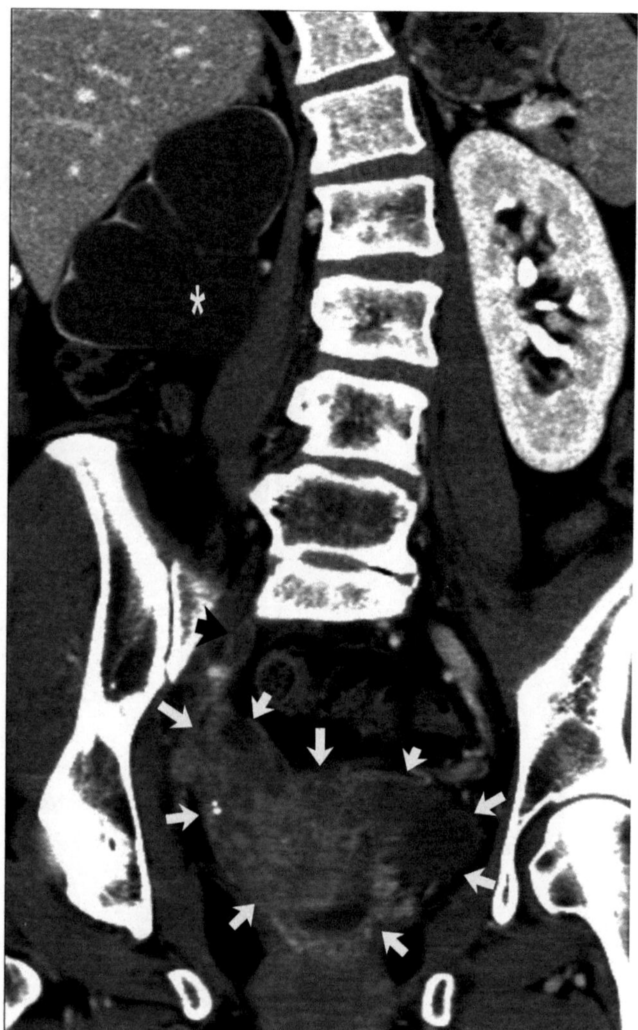

Fig. 7.16 Histopathological proven uterine sarcoma, which can be depict with CECT as a inhomogenous mass with impression of the bladder and the uterine corpus right sided (*white arrows*). The right ureter is dilated (*black arrowhead*) due to tumor impression. The right kidney presents with concecutive hydronephrosis °IV (*asterisk*) with already narrow width of the parenchyma

Fig. 7.17 Contrast enhanced CT with positive contrast of the small bowel loops. (**a**) On axial plane uterine calcifications (*black asterisk*) and a hypodense mass ventrally (*arrows*) is present. (**b**, **c**) On sagittal plane in two different slices presenting the hypodense mass (*arrows*) and the calcifications (*black asterisk*). Histologically proven as uterine sarcoma ventrally and a degenerated leiomyoma with calcifications. *B* bladder

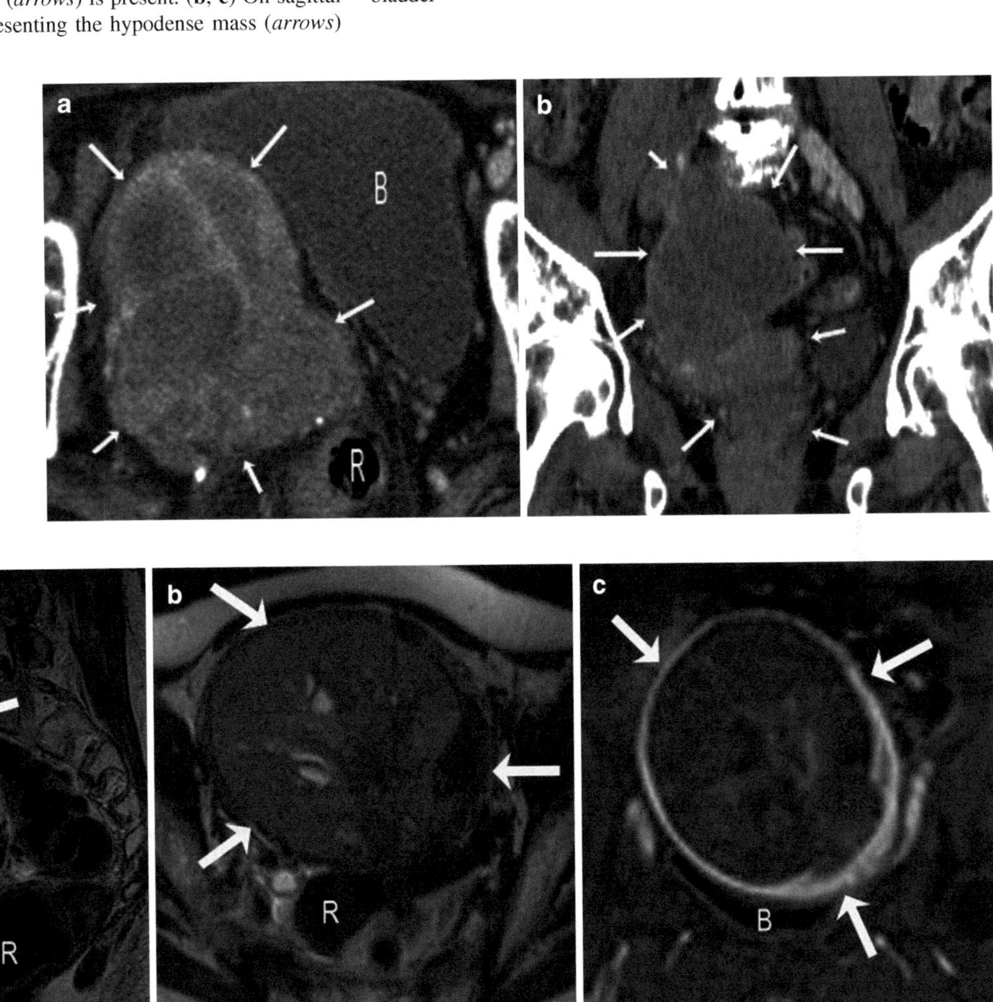

Fig. 7.18 On contrast enhanced CT in venous phase (**a** axial, **b** coronal), the uterus presented as oedematous, with ill defined margins and with a heterogenous density (*arrows*). Histopathological proven as endometrial stromal sarcoma. *B* bladder, *R* rectum

Fig. 7.19 Patient with medical history of uterus myomatosus underwent MRI before planned hysterectomy. (**a**) T2WI image on sagittal plane presents a huge and heterogenous, but well circumscribed, mass in the uterine cavity (*arrows*). (**b**) Even on transverse plane, the mass seems to be well circumscribed with a pseudo-capsule (*arrows*). (**c**) Contrast-enhanced MRI on transverse plane shows the enhanced myometrium (*arrows*) and the heterogenous hypointense mass in the uterine cavity. Histopathological result was endometrial stromal sarcoma. *B* bladder; *R* rectum

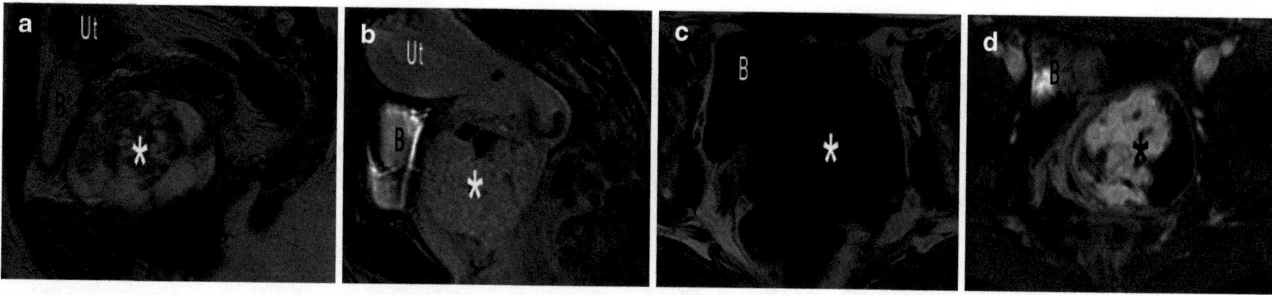

Fig. 7.20 (a) Huge inhomogenous mass in entire pelvis with septa and different signal intensities at T2WI (*asterisk*). (b) CE T1WI on sagittal plane shows homogenous enhancement of the solid parts of the mass (*asterisk*). The vagina is distended. (c) The mass presents as hypointense on native T1WI (*asterisk*). (d) On dynamic contrast enhanced images, the mass presents with hypervascular areas on arterial phase (*asterisk*). Histopathologically proven as leiomyosarcoma of the uterus. *B* bladder, *Ut* uterus

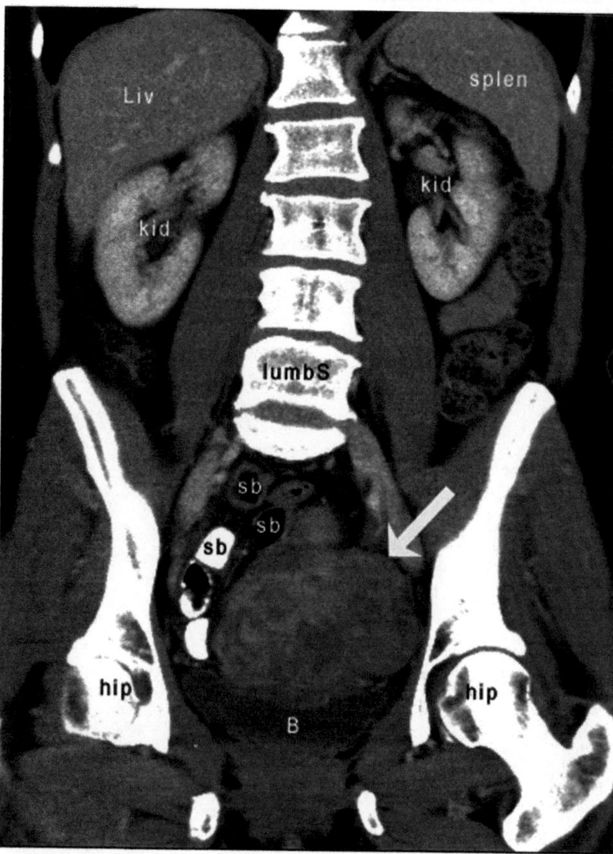

Fig. 7.21 Contrast enhanced CT scan in coronal plane. The entire pelvis presents with a huge heterogeneous mass (*arrow*) impressing the bladder. Hypointense central areas suggest central necrosis. The tumor was histopathologically confirmed as leiomyosarcoma of the uterus. *B* bladder, *sb* small bowel, *Liv* liver, *kid* kidney, *lumbS* lumbar spine

Uterine Lymphoma

Non-Hodgkin-lymphoma of the uterus and the cervix are very rare (<1 %) and may affect women between the ages of 20–80 [29].

Local tumor detection can be undertaken by using ultrasound. However, in some case the entire extent of the lymphoma cannot be depicted, so cross sectional image modality may be useful. If there is already a clinically based suspicion of a tumor extent beyond the small pelvis, a CECT of the abdomen for therapy planning and for follow-up examinations should be initiated (Fig. 7.23) [30]. For the visualisation of local findings, contrast enhanced MRI of the pelvis ought to be the image modality of choice. Using MRI, uterine lymphomas are mostly visible as homogenous, hyperintense masses in native T2WI, without a clear differentiation to the surrounding tissue and with a strong enhancement after contrast application [31].

Recurrent Tumor Disease

Recurrence of endometrial cancer after primary surgery mostly occur within the first 2 years. Metastases can be found as solid mass within the vagina and the parametrium or as lymph node metastases (Fig. 7.24). Recurrence of endometrial cancer after primary radiation therapy can often be found within the uterus or the ovaries [32]. For local recurrence, MRI is the cross sectional imaging modality of choice, however, if there is suspicion for distant metastases, CECT gives a better overview and is commonly performed for the chest and the body in one examination (Fig. 7.25).

Recurrence of a cervical cancer is seen in approx. 10–42 % of primary surgically treated patients. They often show as a solid mass at the vaginal vault, but can also manifest themselves within the vagina, the parametrium, the pelvic wall or the bones (Figs. 7.26, 7.27, and 7.28) [17, 32]. If there is a clinicial suspicion of tumor recurrence in the entire pelvis, contrast enhanced MRI for detection and diagnosis of its extent is relevant. The differentiation to scar tissue is especially important. Scar tissue as well as residual tumor tissue shows as moderately hyperintense in native T2WI. For differentiation, the CE T1WI is used: scar tissue is hypointense due to missing enhancement, inflamed/ tumorous tissue mostly absorbs contrast media and represents hyperintense (Fig. 7.29) [19]. It is to be mentioned however, that differentiation may be challenging in between the first 6 month due to contrast enhancement of fibrous scar tissue [19].

Fig. 7.22 MRI of a women with histopathologically proven adenosarcoma of the uterus. (**a**) On T2WI image on sagittal plane the uterine cavity is filled with a solid mass (*arrows*), the serosa is slightly interrupted at the fundus. Secondary finding is a subserous leiomyoma (*asterisk*). (**b**) On CE T1WI images with fat saturation on transverse oblique plane, the mass presents with a relatively homogeneous contrast enhancement (*arrows*), although the surrounding myometrium presents with a stronger enhancement. *PS* pubic symphysis, *B* bladder, *R* rectum, *sb* small bowel, *sig* sigmoid colon

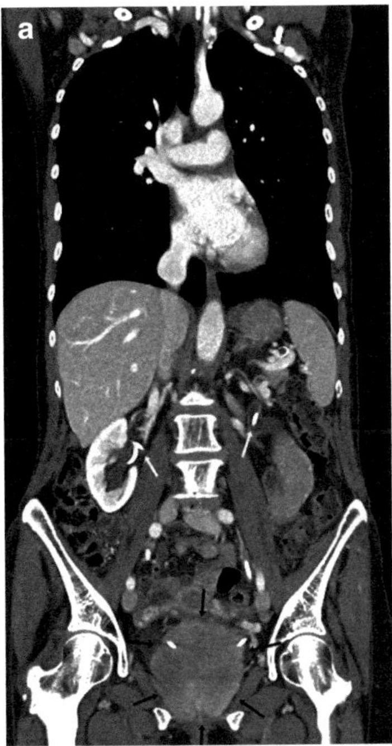

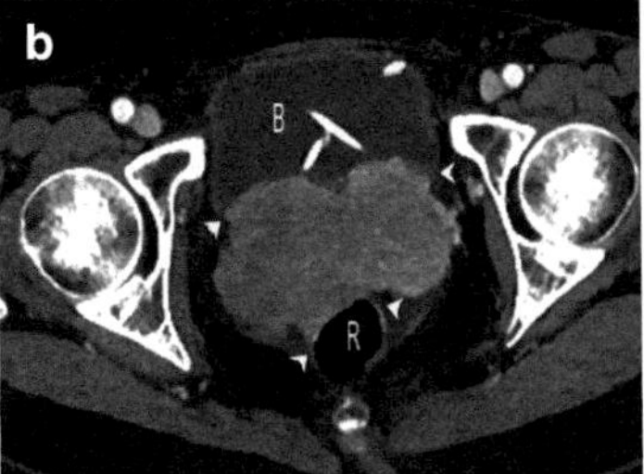

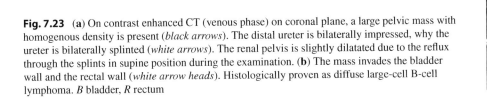

Fig. 7.23 (**a**) On contrast enhanced CT (venous phase) on coronal plane, a large pelvic mass with homogenous density is present (*black arrows*). The distal ureter is bilaterally impressed, why the ureter is bilaterally splinted (*white arrows*). The renal pelvis is slightly dilatated due to the reflux through the splints in supine position during the examination. (**b**) The mass invades the bladder wall and the rectal wall (*white arrow heads*). Histologically proven as diffuse large-cell B-cell lymphoma. *B* bladder, *R* rectum

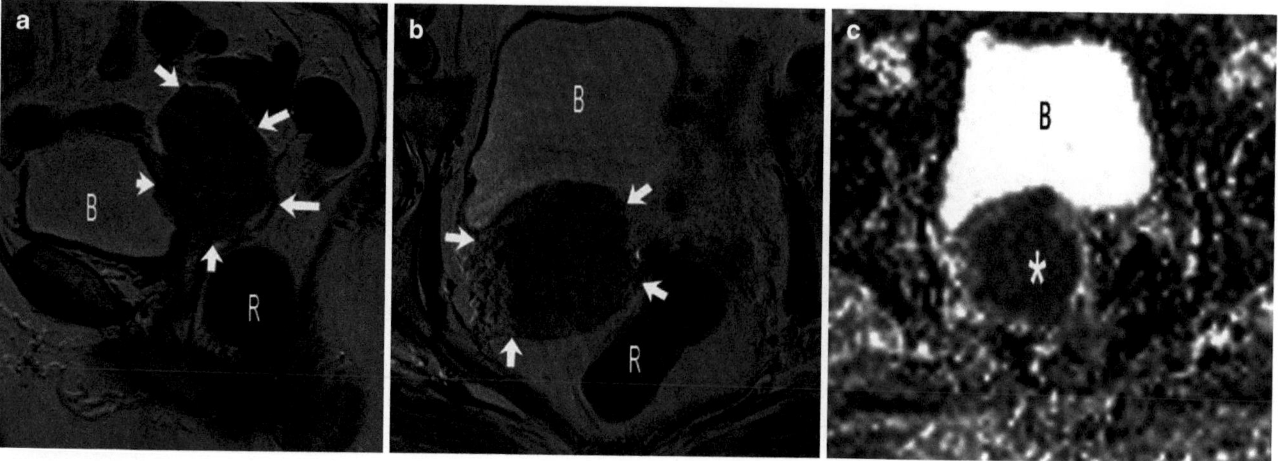

Fig. 7.24 Histologically proven recurrence of endometrial cancer. (**a**) T2WI on sagittal plane presenting with a huge mass at the vaginal vault (*arrows*). (**b**) T2WI on transversal oblique plane presents without infiltration of adjacent structures (*arrows*). (**c**) Diffusion weighted imaging shows restriction in tumor tissue (*asterisk*), delineating well the tumor margins. Tumor is close to the bladder wall, but no transmural invasion. *B* bladder, *R* rectum

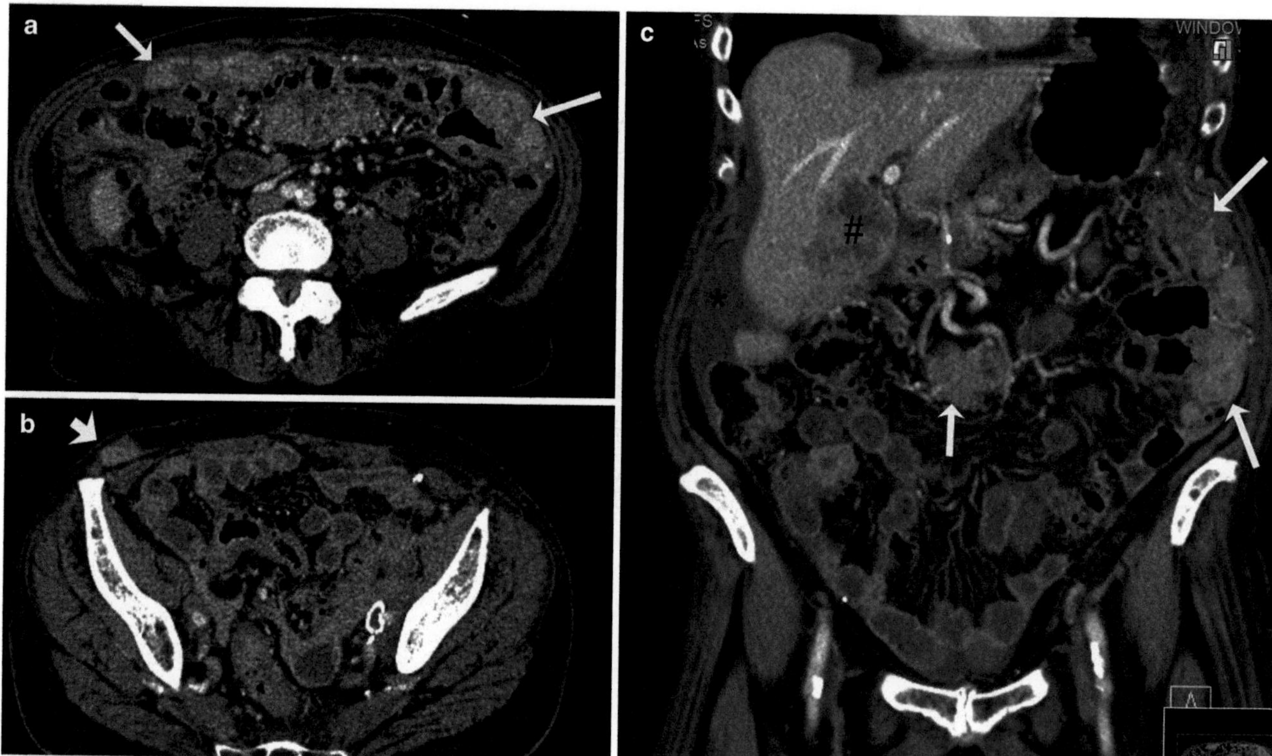

Fig. 7.25 Patient with recurrence of endometrial cancer. (**a, b**) Contrast enhanced CT scan on axial plane in different planes detects multiple peritoneal implants (*arrows*) and a cutaneous metastasis (*arrowhead*). (**c**) The coronal reconstruction of the same patient additionally shows a huge liver metastasis (#) and ascites (*)

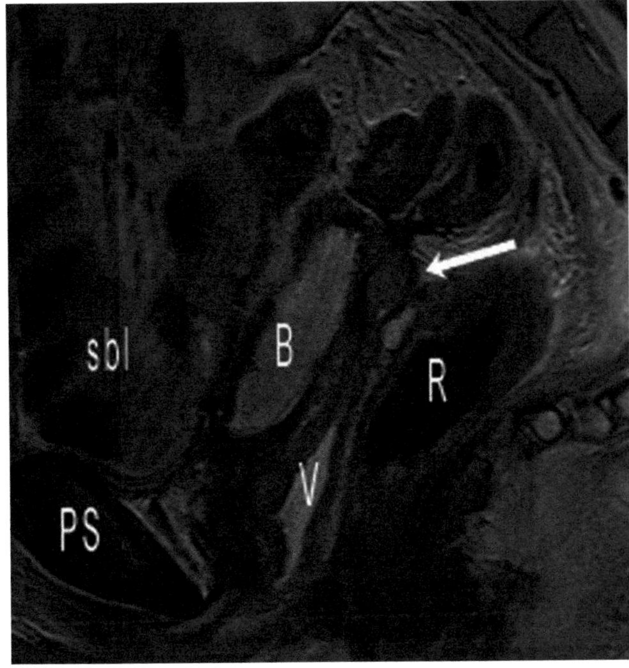

Fig. 7.26 Histologically proven recurrence of cervical cancer after hysterectomy, located between the vaginal vault and the bladder wall (*arrow*). The tumor presents slightly hyperintense on T2WI. *B* bladder, *V* vagina, *R* rectum, *PS* pubic symphysis, *sbl* small bowel loops

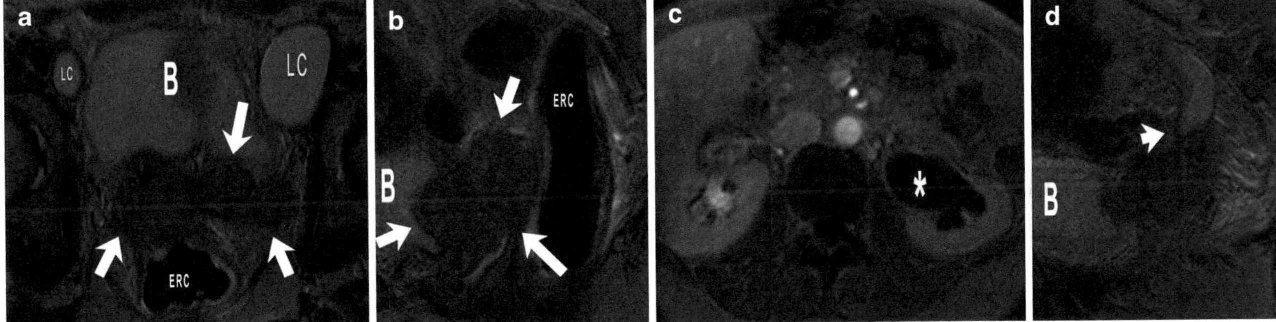

Fig. 7.27 Case of a patient after hysterectomy 4 month ago due to cervical cancer T2b N1 (same patient as in Fig. 7.21). (**a**) In entire pelvis, one solid lesion at the vaginal vault and two solid lesions close by are present, hyperintense on T2WI (*arrows*). The bilaterally inguinal oval cystic-like lesions correspond to lymphoceles (LC). (**b**) The vaginal vault mass is well delineated between the bladder wall and the rectal wall (*arrows*). (**c**) Hydronephrosis of the left kidney (*asterisk*). (**d**) The left distal ureter is compressed by the mass (*arrowhead*). *B* bladder, *ERC* endorectal coil

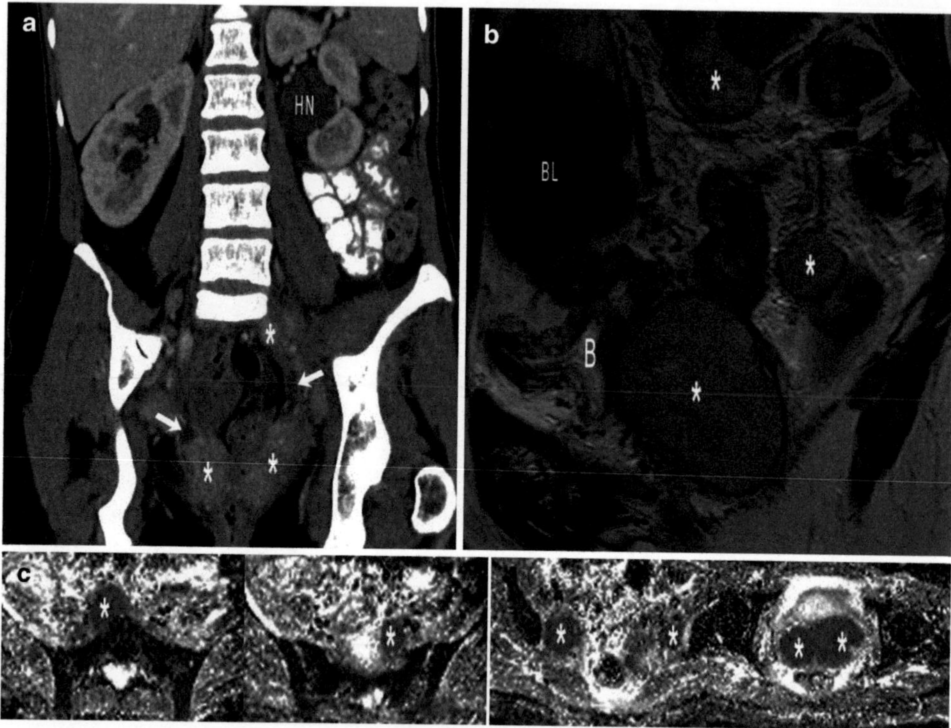

Fig. 7.28 Histologically proven recurrence of cervical cancer. (**a**) On contrast enhanced CT scan in coronal plane, hyperdense masses are present in entire pelvis as well as at the level of the aortal bifurcation (*asterisk*). The ureter is dilatated bilaterally (*arrows*) with concecutive hydronephrosis (HN). (**b**) On T2WI on sagittal plane, the masses are slightly hyperintense and well defined (*asterisk*). (**c**) Diffusion weighted imaging on axial plane on severeal slices present with multiple diffusion restriction tissues, defining tumor recurrence (*asterisk*). *B* bladder

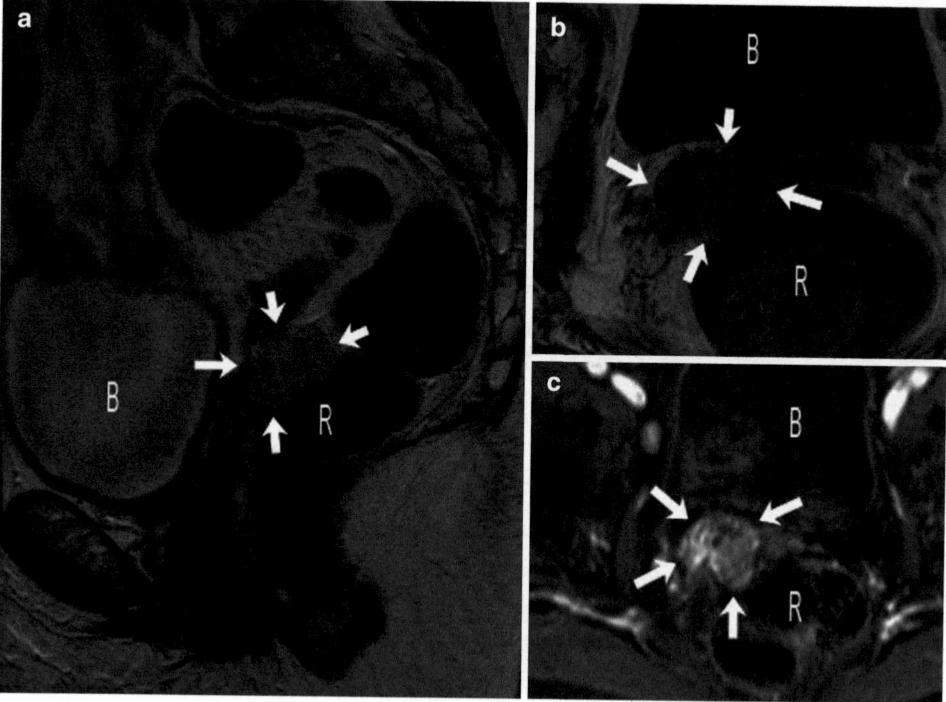

Fig. 7.29 (**a**) On T2WI on sagital plane a hyperintense mass at the vaginal vault is present (*arrows*), histopathologically proven as recurrence from cervical cancer. (**b**) On native T1WI on transversal plane, the mass is hypointense with slightly blurry margins (*arrows*). (**c**) After contrast i.v. the mass shows increased contrast enhancement (*arrows*). No infiltration into surrounding structures. *B* bladder, *R* rectum

References

1. Kinkel K, Forstner R, Danza FM, et al. Staging of endometrial cancer with MRI: guidelines of the European Society of Urogenital Imaging. Eur Radiol. 2009;19:1565–74.
2. Pecorelli S. Revised FIGO staging for carcinoma of the vulva, cervix, and endometrium. Int J Gynaecol Obstet. 2009;105:103–4.
3. Brocker KA, Alt CD, Eichbaum M, et al. Imaging of female pelvic malignancies regarding MRI, CT, and PET/CT: part 1. Strahlenther Onkol. 2011;187:611–8.
4. Colombo N, Van Gorp T, Parma G, et al. Ovarian cancer. Crit Rev Oncol Hematol. 2006;60:159–79.
5. Pano B, Sebastia C, Bunesch L, et al. Pathways of lymphatic spread in male urogenital pelvic malignancies. Radiographics. 2011;31:135–60.
6. Balleyguier C, Sala E, Da Cunha T, et al. Staging of uterine cervical cancer with MRI: guidelines of the European Society of Urogenital Radiology. Eur Radiol. 2011;21:1102–10.
7. Kirchhoff S. MR Vagina, Uterus, Adnexe. In: Scheffel H, Alkadhi H, Boss A, Merkle E, editors. Praxisbuch MRT Abdomen und Becken. Berlin: Springer; 2012. p. 181–94.
8. Thomassin-Naggara I, Darai E, Bazot M. Gynecological pelvic infection: what is the role of imaging? Diagn Interv Imaging. 2012;93:491–9.
9. Sala E, Rockall AG, Freeman SJ, et al. The added role of MR imaging in treatment stratification of patients with gynecologic malignancies: what the radiologist needs to know. Radiology. 2013;266:717–40.
10. Beddy P, Moyle P, Kataoka M, et al. Evaluation of depth of myometrial invasion and overall staging in endometrial cancer: comparison of diffusion-weighted and dynamic contrast-enhanced MR imaging. Radiology. 2012;262:530–7.
11. Forstner R, Sala E, Kinkel K, et al. ESUR guidelines: ovarian cancer staging and follow-up. Eur Radiol. 2010;20:2773–80.
12. Shen SH, Chiou YY, Wang JH, et al. Diffusion-weighted single-shot echo-planar imaging with parallel technique in assessment of endometrial cancer. AJR Am J Roentgenol. 2008;190:481–8.
13. Scheidler J. Bildgebende Diagnostik der inneren weiblichen Genitalorgane – Adnexe. In: Adams S, Nicolas V, Freyschmidt J, editors. Urogenitaltrakt, Retroperitoneum, Mamma. Berlin/Heidelberg: Springer; 2004. p. 221–40.
14. Horton KM, Sheth S, Corl F, et al. Multidetector row CT: principles and clinical applications. Crit Rev Comput Tomogr. 2002;43:143–81.
15. Sala E, Hricak H. Female pelvis. In: Reiser MFHH, Semmler W, editors. Magnetic Resonance Tomography. Berlin/Heidelberg: Springer; 2008. p. 964–97.
16. Wittekind C, Meyer H-J. International Union against Cancer. TNM Klassifikation maligner Tumoren. 7. Aufl. Weinheim: Wiley-Blackwell; 2010.
17. Brant W. Pelvis. In: Webb W, Brant W, Major N, editors. Fundamentals of Body CT. Philadelphia: Saunders; 2006. p. 355–76.
18. Naganawa S, Sato C, Kumada H, et al. Apparent diffusion coefficient in cervical cancer of the uterus: comparison with the normal uterine cervix. Eur Radiol. 2005;15:71–8.
19. Zaspel U, Hamm B. Cervical cancer. In: Hamm B, Forstner R, editors. MRI and CT of the female pelvis. Berlin/Heidelberg: Springer; 2007. p. 121–80.
20. Sala E, Wakely S, Senior E, et al. MRI of malignant neoplasms of the uterine corpus and cervix. AJR Am J Roentgenol. 2007;188:1577–87.
21. Rigon G, Vallone C, Starita A, et al. Diagnostic accuracy of MRI in primary cervical cancer. Open J Radiol. 2012;2:14–21.
22. Pandharipande PV, Choy G, del Carmen MG, et al. MRI and PET/CT for triaging stage IB clinically operable cervical cancer to appropriate therapy: decision analysis to assess patient outcomes. AJR Am J Roentgenol. 2009;192:802–14.
23. Kortmann B, Reimer T, Gerber B, et al. Concurrent radiochemotherapy of locally recurrent or advanced sarcomas of the uterus. Strahlenther Onkol. 2006;182:318–24.
24. Benz MR, Tchekmedyian N, Eilber FC, et al. Utilization of positron emission tomography in the management of patients with sarcoma. Curr Opin Oncol. 2009;21:345–51.
25. Roth CG. Magnetic resonance imaging of the female pelvis. Fundamentals of body MRI. Philadelphia: Elsevier Saunders; 2012. p. 261–368.
26. Sumi A, Terasaki H, Sanada S, et al. Assessment of MR imaging as a tool to differentiate between the major histological types of uterine sarcomas. Magn Reson Med Sci. 2015;14(4):295–304.
27. Nucci MR, Oliva E. Gynecologic pathology. Edinburgh: Churchill Livingstone; 2009.
28. Takeuchi M, Matsuzaki K, Yoshida S, et al. Adenosarcoma of the uterus: magnetic resonance imaging characteristics. Clin Imaging. 2009;33:244–7.
29. Griffin N, Grant LA, Sala E. Magnetic resonance imaging of vaginal and vulval pathology. Eur Radiol. 2008;18:1269–80.
30. Tateishi U, Terauchi T, Inoue T, et al. Nodal status of malignant lymphoma in pelvic and retroperitoneal lymphatic pathways: PET/CT. Abdom Imaging. 2010;35:232–40.
31. Kim YS, Koh BH, Cho OK, et al. MR imaging of primary uterine lymphoma. Abdom Imaging. 1997;22:441–4.
32. Jonat W, Bauerschlag D, Schem C, et al. Gut- und bösartige gynäkologische Tumoren. In: Diedrich K, Holzgreve W, Jonat W, Schneider K-T, Schultze-Mosgau A, Weiss J, editors. Gynäkologie und Geburtshilfe. Berlin/Heidelberg: Springer; 2007. p. 211–98.

Interventional Diagnostics Before Hysterectomy

8

Sergio Haimovich

Office Hysteroscopy

It was in 1980 when Hamou, considered the father of modern hysteroscopy, designed the first microcolpohysteroscope, offering a new combination of hysteroscopy and microscopy. His device allowed for multiple magnifications (X1, X20, X60, and X150) for cellular exploration and it presented new diagnostic opportunities (Fig. 8.1).

Introduction of bipolar system 'Gynecare Versa Point' by Ethicon Inc. in 1997 was the turning point of modern office hysteroscopy. This technology enabled to increase spectrum of intrauterine surgical procedures by means of thin miniaturized instruments without both anesthesia and dilatation of cervix at outpatient clinics. It was de beginning of the "see and treat" concept that is applied in the hysteroscopy units now a day.

The office setting hysteroscopy is becoming prevalent based among others in the convenient and efficiency of the procedure for both the physician and patient. An additional benefit of office-based hysteroscopy has been suggested by Lindheim et al. [1], who more than a decade ago, noted the cost saving per case of at least 50 % when compared with the hospital equivalent. The approach with vaginoscopy or "no touch" technique, without using speculum, tenaculum or even anesthesia is another well tolerated advantage of office hysteroscopy and patients reported just little discomfort [2].

Hysteroscopy is currently considered the best technique for investigating the uterine cavity [3, 4]. Several comparative studies between hysteroscopy and histology have demonstrated that hysteroscopy has a very high diagnostic accuracy for most intrauterine abnormalities [4] and for endometrial cancer [5, 6].

In 2002 Clark and coworkers in a systematic review concluded that diagnostic accuracy of hysteroscopy is high for endometrial cancer but only moderate for endometrial disease (cancer or hyperplasia) [7].

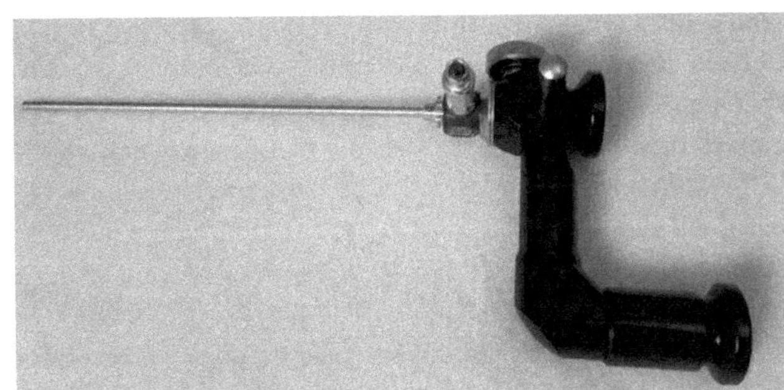

Fig. 8.1 Hamou microcolpohysteroscope

Indication for Office Hysteroscopy

When is a diagnostic hysteroscopy indicated? There are different clinical conditions as abnormal uterine bleeding (AUB). AUB is the most common indication in women over 45 years old.

Based on suspicious images especially by transvaginal ultrasound (TVUS) but also by CT or MRI, the endometrial pathology can be divided to focal (polyps and myoma) or diffuse (hyperplasia with or without cytological atypia and adenocarcinoma) (Table 8.1).

Any image of suspected endometrial cavity occupation by focal or diffused pathology is an indication for performing a diagnostic hysteroscopy.

When diffuse endometrial pathology is suspected (thickened endometrium image) the first choice is to obtain tissue sample by using a Pipelle. It has a low false positive rate but the false negative rate can be over 20 %, for this reason a diagnostic hysteroscopy is indicated after a negative result [8].

The similarity in morphological appearance of endometrial atypia hyperplasia (EAH) and well-differentiated

S. Haimovich, MD, PhD
Head of the Hysteroscopy Unit, Del Mar University Hospital, Barcelona, Spain
e-mail: Sergio@haimovich.net

I. Alkatout, L. Mettler (eds.), *Hysterectomy*, DOI 10.1007/978-3-319-22497-8_8

Table 8.1 Hysteroscopy indications

Clinical features	Images of suspected uterine occupation
Post-menopausal bleeding	Focal (polyp/myoma)
Abnormal Uterine Bleeding	Non Focal – Endometrial Thickness >5 mm (Hyperplasia/ Adenocarcinoma)

endometrial carcinoma represents a major challenge to histopathologists. When a diagnosis of atypical hyperplasia is made, there is a risk of concomitant invasive carcinoma in the uterus. This discrepancy between endometrial specimens and hysterectomy specimens on histopathological examination has been found in several reports, with 7–50 % of women with endometrial hyperplasia with cytological atypia reported to have concomitant carcinoma in subsequent hysterectomy specimens [9–14].

On biopsy specimens, the distinction between well-differentiated carcinomas and atypical hyperplasias, on the basis of distortion of glands architecture and cytologic atypia, is neither simple nor reproducible even by experienced pathologists [15]. On Figs. 8.2 and 8.3, it is possible to see the great difficulty to differentiate between Hyperplasia and Adenocarcinoma.

We define the pathology that will end in a hysterectomy as High Risk Endometrial Pathology, this group includes:

1. Adenocarcinoma on a polyp (AP)
2. Endometrial adenocarcinoma (EA)
3. Endometrial atypical hyperplasia (EAH).

Except in EA were the hysteroscopy has a great grade of accuracy with histopathology, both in AP and EHA many times hysteroscopic images are no so easy to interpret.

The hysteroscopic appearance of an endometrial carcinoma is quite typical, and this visual diagnosis is generally based on the presence of a gross distortion of endometrial cavity, because of focal or extensive nodular, polypoid, papillary or mixed patterns of neoplastic growth. Focal necrosis, friable consistency, and atypical vessels are other features almost invariably associated with endometrial cancer and easily detected by hysteroscopic inspection (Fig. 8.4).

High-risk polyps are presented in postmenopausal women as an image of more than 10 mm and symptomatic (bleeding or spotting). It is important to perform a complete hysteroscopic dissection of the polyp and no to leave any tissue including the pedicle, sometimes adenocarcinoma can be find in the polyp's base.

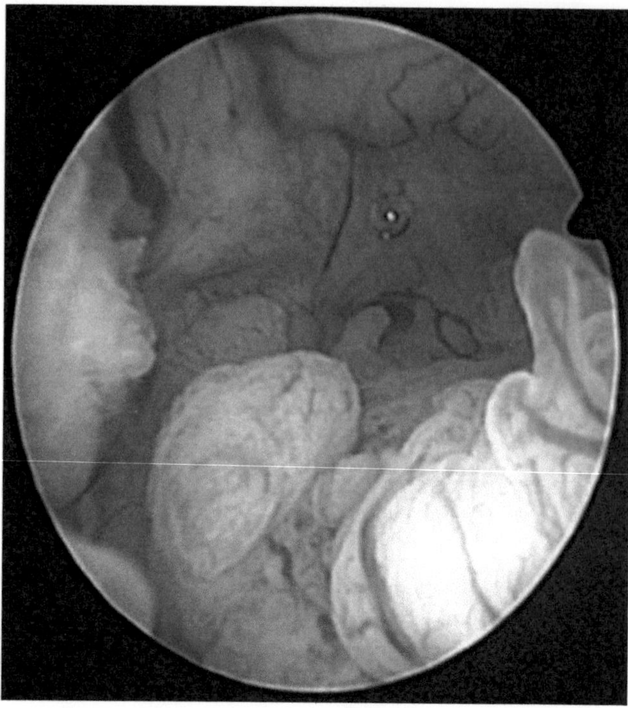

Fig. 8.2 Complex hyperplasia (Courtesy of Dr. Luis Alonso)

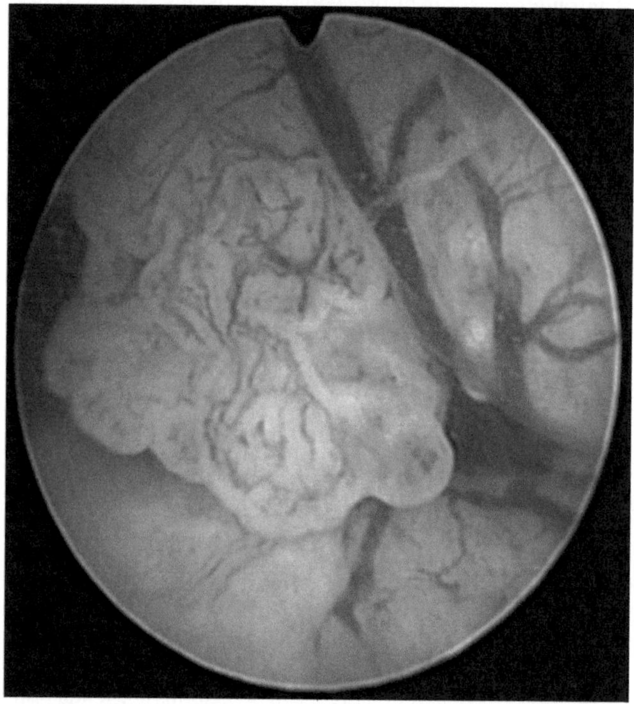

Fig. 8.3 Well-differentiated adenocarcinoma (Courtesy of Dr. Luis Alonso)

Narrow Band Imaging (NBI) and Hysteroscopy

An element that helps in the diagnosis of endometrial high-risk pathology when applied during hysteroscopy is the narrow-band imaging (NBI). This technology is a real-time, on-demand endoscopic imaging technique designed to enhance visualization of the vascular network and surface texture of the mucosa in an effort to improve tissue characterization, differentiation, and diagnosis [16] (Fig. 8.5).

Enhancement of particular mucosal features with NBI is achieved by observation of light transmission at selected wavelengths (or colors) because the interaction of particular tissue structures with light is wavelength dependent.

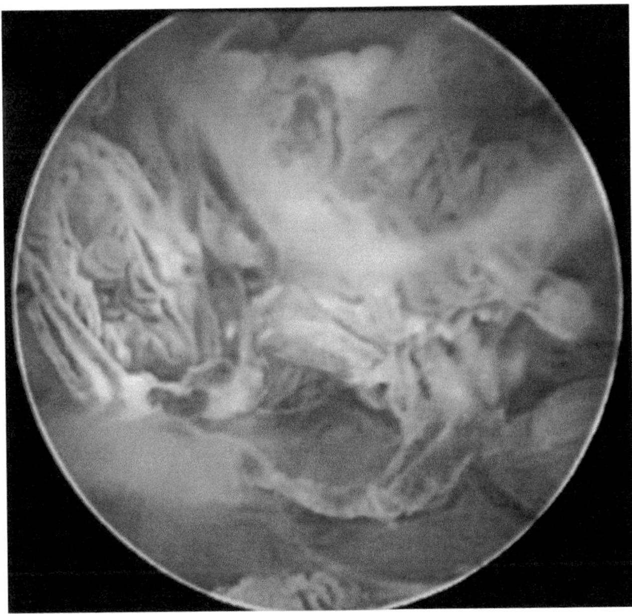

Fig. 8.4 Endometrial adenocarcinoma

Selective light transmittance is accomplished by optical filtering of white light (WL) in NBI. The use of a band of light of 415 nm, blue light, correspond to the peak light absorption of hemoglobin, and this enables NBI to make the organization of blood vessels on the surface of the analyzed structures clearer and sharper with respect to observation with WL. Narrow-band blue light displays superficial capillary networks, offering an extremely high-contrast image of the tissue surface.

NBI has a very good correlation with histology especially in the difficult cases like atypical hyperplasia. Lasmar et al. have reported that the sensitivities of hysteroscopy for endometrial hyperplasia (EMH) and endometrial carcinoma are 56.3 and 80.0 %, respectively [17].

In the last years many authors have published their results in the use of NBI during hysteroscopy showing an improvement in the diagnostic sensitivity for atypical endometrial hyperplasia or endometrial carcinoma, compared with conventional hysteroscopy [18–20]. With NBI helps a variety of atypical blood vessels were observed in the mucosa of endometrial malignant lesions, including vessels with expanded, tortuous, and zigzagged shapes; variable diameter; inflectional, interrupted, papillary shapes; and sea anemone shapes. The visualization of this patterns helps in the orientation of high-risk endometrial pathology [18].

Figure 8.6 shows the enhancement of the capillary vascularization with NBI compared with WL in a case of EHA shows the difference between WL and NBI on a polyp's pedicle.

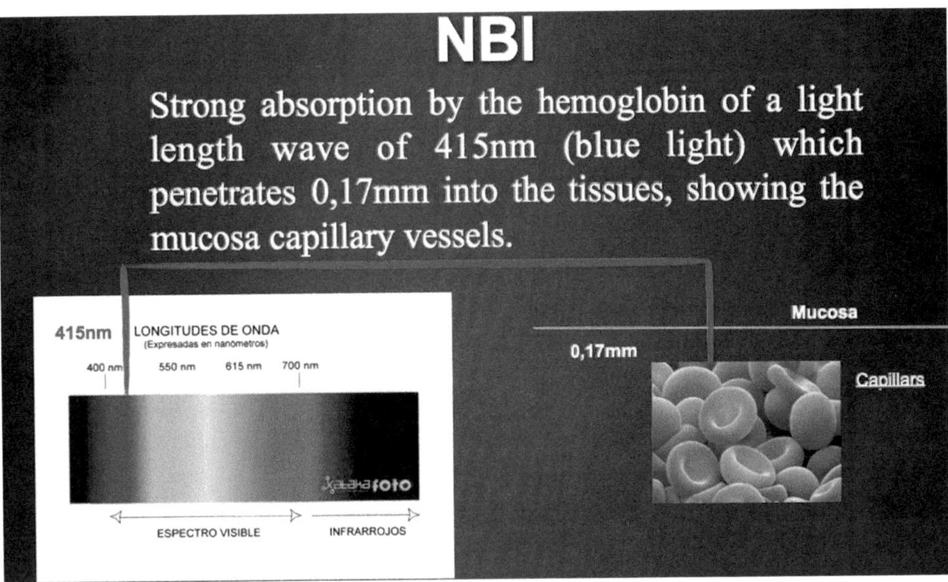

Fig. 8.5 NBI

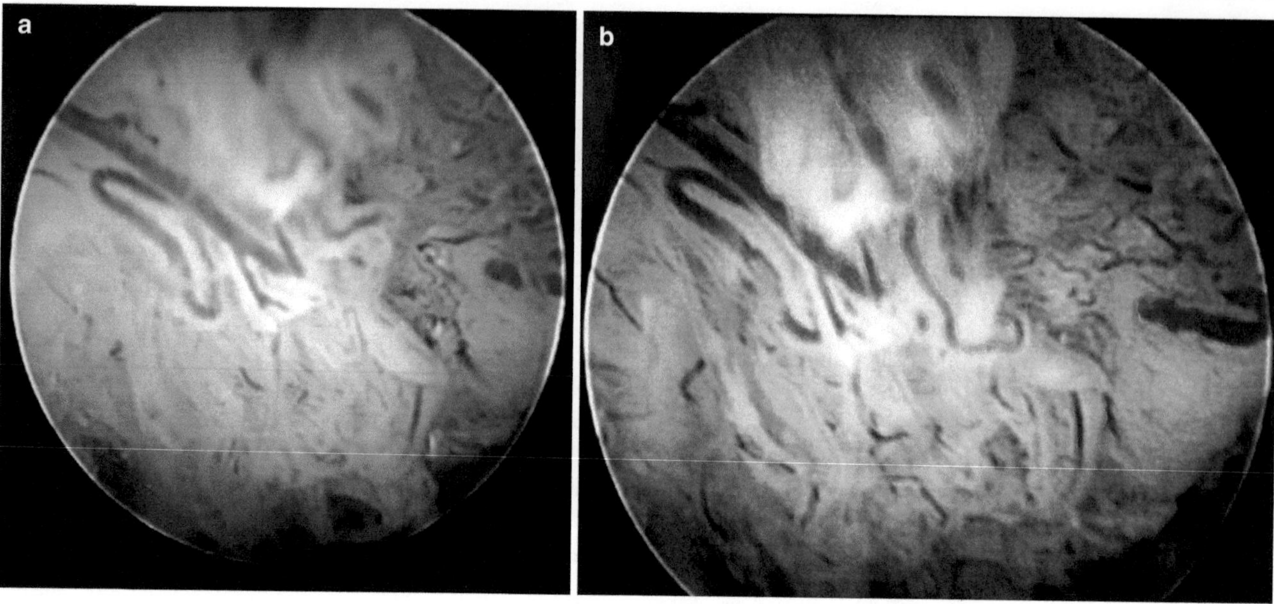

Fig. 8.6 Hyperplasia with atypia: (**a**) WL versus (**b**) NBI

Hysteroscopy and Endometrial Cancer

As seen in this chapter endometrial sampling for histopathology examination is essential to diagnose endometrial cancer. Hysteroscopy provides an accurate evaluation of the endometrial cavity and allows directed sampling of suspected lesion.

However, there have been concerns that endometrial cells could be flushed into the fallopian tubes and the peritoneal cavity. It is a controversial subject with no enough evidence in order to achieve a clear conclusion.

In one study, Vilos at al found that hysteroscopy did not adversely affect the 5-year survival and the long-term prognosis in 14 women with endometrial cancer [21].

Polyzos et al. in a Meta-Analysis [22] estimated the risk for disease upstaging associated with the hysteroscopic procedure before surgery in women with endometrial cancer. The outcomes considered were the incidence of malignant cells in peritoneal washings before hysterectomy, incidence of tumour upstaging due solely to the presence of a positive peritoneal cytological feature in patients with apparent clinical early-stage disease limited to the uterus; overall survival, disease-free survival, and disease recurrence.

The results showed that hysteroscopy in patients with endometrial cancer resulted in statistically significant higher endometrial cancer cell seeding within the peritoneal cavity [OR: 1.78; (95 % CI, 1.13–2.79)]. Sensitivity analysis including only trials in which hysteroscopy with isotonic sodium chloride was used showed a further increased risk [OR, 2.89; (95 % CI, 1.48–5.64)], as well as sensitivity analysis including only trials in which inflated distension medium pressure reached or exerted 100 mmHg [OR 3.23; (95 % CI, 0.94–11.09)].

Also a statistically significant higher tumour upstaging was found when hysteroscopy was performed in patients with disease limited to the uterus compared with no hysteroscopy [OR, 2.61; (95 % CI, 1.47–4.63)]. Data regarding overall survival and disease recurrence supported the notion that no significant difference for the prognostic outcomes tested was observed.

The possible risk of the spreading into the abdominal cavity of neoplasic cells should not limit the use of hysteroscopy in favor of blind techniques (LEVEL OF EVIDENCE II, STRENGH OF THE RECOMMENDATION A).

In order to minimize the small risk of cancer dissemination, hysteroscopy should be performed with an intrauterine pressure of less than 80 mmHg, and the duration of the procedure should be as short as possible.

Prognosis Value of Diagnostic Hysteroscopy

The staging of endometrial cancer by hysteroscopy has not demonstrated its utility. In 1988, Cronjé et al. found no differences between dilatation curettage and hysteroscopy in pre surgical staging of endometrial adenocarcinoma [23].

Cervical involvement may vary between free tumor cells in the endocervical canal and endometrial infiltration of the endocervix. Cervical involvement is important to determinate staging, prognosis, and adjuvant treatment [24].

The prevalence of cervical involvement in endometrial cancer is between 10 and 20 % [25].

Panoramic hysteroscopy is the best procedure for excluding cervical involvement from endometrial cancer [26]. Moreover, as hysteroscopy enables us to estimate the extent of the cancerous spread within the uterine cavity, it could indirectly be predictive of tumoral size.

The cervical spreads is shown by irregularly eroded endocervical lining, well-marked coarse undulation of cervical mucosa, and endocervical exophytic growth of tissue displaying vascular atypia consistent with tumor growth were the hallmarks defining the spread of endometrial neoplasia to the endocervical canal.

In a group of 87 women with endometrial cancer, Villegas et al. found with a predictive positive value of hysteroscopy in the detection of cervical cancer was of 80 %, concluding that Hysteroscopy is a useful method for assessing cervical invasion in endometrial carcinoma, as it allows direct visual inspection of the uterine cavity and guided biopsies [27].

Hysteroscopy is the best and probably the only diagnostic tool for a preoperative estimation of the extent of endometrial lining involvement from endometrial carcinoma [28, 29].

Although unproven, a direct relationship between the extention of endometrial spread detected hysteroscopically and tumor volume appears rational. Morrow and Curtin's suggested in their work [30] that 50 % endocavity tumor spreading assessed by hysteroscopic view can be assumed as a reliable cutoff for selecting patients at high risk of metastatic disease.

References

1. Lindheim SR, Kavic S, Shulman SV, Sauer MV. Operative hysteroscopy in the office setting. J Am Assoc Gynecol Laparosc. 2000;7:65–9.
2. Bettocchi S, Ceci O, Nappi L, et al. Operative hysteroscopy without anesthesia: analysis of 4863 cases performed with mechanical instruments. J Am Assoc Gynecol Laparosc. 2004;11:59–61.
3. Balasch J. Investigation of the infertile couple: investigation of the infertile couple in the era of assisted reproductive technology: a time for reappraisal. Hum Reprod. 2000;15:2251–7.
4. Brand A. Diagnosis of endometrial cancer in women with abnormal uterine bleeding. J SOGC. 2000;86:1–3.
5. Chambers JT, Chambers SK. Endometrial sampling: when? Where? Why? With what? Clin Obstet Gynecol. 1992;35:28–39.
6. Creasman WT. Endometrial cancer: incidence, prognostic factors, diagnosis, and treatment. Semin Oncol. 1997;24 :S1–140–50.
7. Clark TJ, Voit D, Gupta JK, Hyde C, Song F, Khan KS. Accuracy of hysteroscopy in the diagnosis of endometrial cancer and hyperplasia: a systematic quantitative review. JAMA. 2002;288:1610–21.
8. Farrell T, Jones N, Owen P, Baird A. The significance of an "insufficient" Pipelle sample in the investigation of postmenopausal bleeding. Acta Obstet Gynecol Scand. 1999;78:810–2.
9. Valenzuela P, Sanz JM, Keller J. Atypical endometrial hyperplasia: grounds for possible misdiagnosis of endometrial adenocarcinoma. Gynecol Obstet Invest. 2003;56:163–7.
10. Trimble CL, Kauderer J, Zaino R, Silverberg S, Lim PC, Burke JJ, et al. Concurrent endometrial carcinoma in women with a biopsy diagnosis of atypical endometrial hyperplasia: a Gynecologyc Oncology Group study. Cancer. 2006;106:812–9.
11. Schutter J, Wright Jr TC. Prevalence of underlying adenocarcinoma in women with atypical endometrial hyperplasia. Int J Gynecol Pathol. 2005;24:313–8.
12. Garuti G, Mirra M, Luerti M. Hysteroscopic view in atypical endometrial hyperplasias: a correlation with pathologic findings on hysterectomy specimens. J Minim Invasive Gynecol. 2006;13:325–30.
13. Bilgin T, Ozuysal S, Ozan H, Atakan T. Coexisting endometrial cancer in patients with a preoperative diagnosis of atypical endometrial hyperplasia. J Obtet Gynaecol Res. 2004;30:205–9.
14. Daud S, Jalil S, Griffin M, Ewies A. Endometrial hyperplasia – the dilemma of management remains: a retrospective observational study of 280 women. Eur J Obstet Gynecol Repro Biol. 2011;159:172–5.
15. Kendall BS, Ronnett BM, Isacson C, Cho KR, Hedrick L, Diener-West M, et al. Reproducibility of the diagnosis of endometrial hyperplasia, atypical hyperplasia, and well differentiated carcinoma. Am J Surg Pathol. 1998;22:1012–7.
16. Vincent BD, Fraig M. A pilot study of narrow-band imaging compared to white light bronchoscopy for evaluation of normal airways and premalignant and malignant airways disease. Chest. 2007;131:1794–9.
17. Lasmar RB, Barrozo PR, De Oliveira MA, Coutinho ES, Dias R. Validation of hysteroscopic view in cases of endometrial hyperplasia and cancer in patients with abnormal uterine bleeding. J Minim Invasive Gynecol. 2006;13:409–12.
18. Kisu I, Banno K, Kobayashi Y, Ono A, Masuda K, Ueki A, Nomura H, Hirasawa A, Abe T, Kouyama K, Susumo N, Aoki D. Flexible hysteroscopy with narrow band imaging (NBI) for endoscopic diagnosis of malignant endometrial lesions. Int J Oncol. 2011;38:613–8.
19. Surico D, Vigone A, Bonvini D, Tinelli R, Leo L, Surico N. Narrow-band imaging in diagnosis of endometrial cancer and hyperplasia: a new option? J Minim Invasive Gynecol. 2010;17:620–5.
20. Cicinelli E, Tinelli R, Colafiglio G, Pastore A, Mastrolia S, Lepera A, Clevin L. Reliability of narrow-band imaging (NBI) hysteroscopy: a comparative study. Fertil Steril. 2010;94(6):2303–7.
21. Vilos G, Edris F, Al-Mubarak A, Ettler H, Hollett-Caines J, Abu-Rafea B. Hysteroscopic surgery does not adversely affect the long-term prognosis of women with endometrial adenocarcinoma. J Minim Invasive Gynecol. 2007;14(2):205–10.
22. Polyzos NP, Mauri D, Tsioras S, Messini CI, Valachis A, Messinis IE. Intraperitoneal dissemination of endometrial cancer cells after hysteroscopy: a systematic review and meta-analysis. Int J Gynecol Cancer. 2010;20:261–7.
23. Cronje HS, Deale CJC. Staging of endometrial cancer by hysteroscopy. S Afr Med J. 1988;73:716–7.
24. Garuti G, De Giorgi O, Sambruni I, Cellani F, Luerti M. Prognostic significance of hysteroscopic imaging in endometrioid endometrial adenocarcinoma. Gynecol Oncol. 2001;81:408–13.
25. Leminen A, Forss M, Lehtovirta P. Endometrial adenocarcinoma with clinical evidence of cervical involvement: accuracy of diagnostic procedures, clinical course, and prognostic factors. Acta Obstet Gynecol Scand. 1995;74:61–6.
26. Toky T, Oka K, Nakayama K, Oguchi O, Fujii S. A comparative study of pre-operative procedures to assess cervical invasión by endometrial carcinoma. Br J Obstet Gynaecol. 1998;105:512–6.
27. Villegas I, Andía D, Rui-Wamba MJ, De la Rosa JH, Marqués M. Utility of hysteroscopy in the presurgical diagnosis of cervical invasion in endometrial carcinoma. Prog Obstet Ginecol. 2004;47(12):548–53.
28. Sugimoto O. Diagnostic hysteroscopy. In: Coppleson M, Monaghan JM, Morrow CP, Tattersall MHN, editors. Gynecologic oncology, fundamental principles and clinical practice, vol. 1. 2nd ed. New York: Churchill Livingstone; 1992. p. 341–56.
29. Taddei GL, Mancini D, Scarselli G, Tantini C, Bargelli G. Can hysteroscopic evaluation of endometrial carcinoma influence therapeutic treatment? Ann N Y Acad Sci. 1994;734:482–7.
30. Morrow CP, Curtin JP. Management of uterine neoplasia. In: Morrow CP, Curtin JP, De La Osa EL, editors. Gynecologic cancer surgery. New York: Churchill Livingstone; 1996. p. 569–625.

Part IV

Extended Aspects Regarding Indications and Contraindications

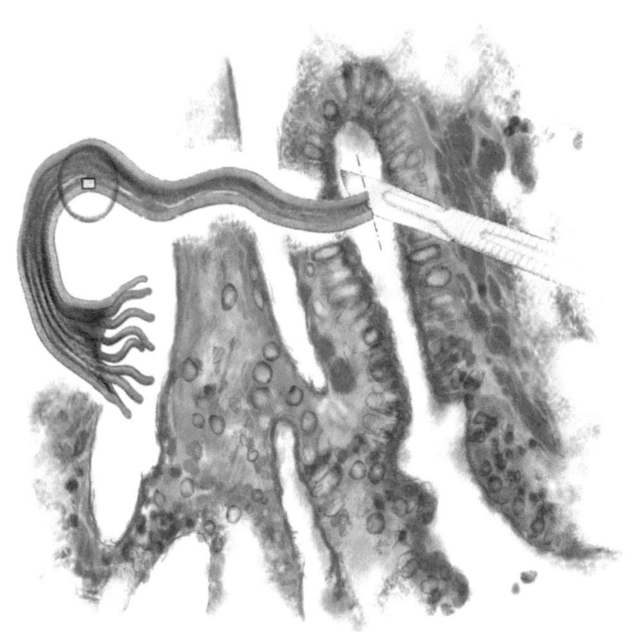

9 Evidence Based Review of Hysterectomy and Sexuality

Farah Lone

Sexuality and Prevalence of Female Sexual Dysfunction

Sexuality, its expression and intimacy remains important throughout the lifespan of a woman, and hence needs to be well understood in health as well as in illness. Sexuality contributes to some of the most complex aspects of human behaviour. Sexual dysfunction is more prevalent in women than men (43 vs 31 %).

Prevalence studies of female sexual dysfunction (FSD) are confounded by a lack of consistent methodology. Classification and determination of FSD are complicated by variability in levels of normal sexual function and the importance of sexual function to individuals and cultural beliefs. Community studies indicate that the prevalence of female sexual dysfunction ranges from 25 to 63 %. An important population-based study, a sub study of the National Health and Social Life Survey, was conducted in 1992 [1]. It provides a probability sample among 1749 women and 1410 men living in the USA, aged 18–59 years, and is based on face-to-face interviews conducted by trained interviewers. The population was matched for age, education level and marital status. Following are the ranges of dysfunctions across the age groups:

- Lack of interest in sex: 27–32 %
- Unable to achieve orgasm: 22–28 %
- Pain during sex: 8–21 %
- Sex not pleasurable: 17–27 %

Comparable prevalence rates were calculated by Hayes et al. from 11 published prevalence studies that included assessment of all FSDs [2]. Similar results have been reported by another population-based telephone survey of women aged 30–70 years to ascertain prevalence of FSD [3] using the validated Profile of Female Sexual Function and Personal Distress Scale instruments [3].

Women's sexuality can be associated with personal, physical, social and cultural factors. Therefore sexual problems may be associated with significant distress including a low self-esteem, a reduction in life satisfaction and a decline in the quality of the relationship with her partner [4, 5].

It is estimated that more than 600,000 hysterectomies (an average of more than one per minute) are performed in the United States per annum [6]. Amongst other concerns with hysterectomy, is the possible effect of the surgery on woman's sexual response. In the United Kingdom 33–46 % of women report decreased sexual response after hysterectomy with oophorectomy. Although sexual problems are highly prevalent, a very small proportion of women consult a physician.

Indications for Hysterectomy

These include benign conditions such as menometrorrhagia, uterine fibroids (leiomyoma), adenomyosis, endometriosis, pelvic pain and for actual and possible malignancies.

Types of Hysterectomy

- Total (i.e., removal of uterus and cervix)
- Subtotal (supracervical i.e., removal of uterus), with or without unilateral or bilateral oophorectomy.

Surgical Routes for Hysterectomy

- Abdominal
- Vaginal
- Endoscopic (including robotic).

F. Lone, MBBS, MRCOG
Obstetrics and Gynaecology, Royal Cornwall Hospital, Truro, Cornwall, UK
e-mail: Farah.lone@rcht.cornwall.nhs.uk

I. Alkatout, L. Mettler (eds.), *Hysterectomy*, DOI 10.1007/978-3-319-22497-8_9

Reasons for Decreased Sexual Response

Various reasons have been described for reduction in sexual response following a hysterectomy, including hormonal changes, psychological factors, and anatomical factors.

Hormonal Changes

Common hormones produced by the ovaries include estrogen, progesterone and testosterone. Women who have had bilateral oophorectomy lose most of their ability to produce the hormones estrogen and progesterone, and lose about half of their ability to produce testosterone, and subsequently enter what is known as "surgical menopause" (as opposed to normal menopause, which occurs naturally in women as part of the aging process). In natural menopause the ovaries generally continue to produce low levels of hormones, especially androgens, even after menopause. These symptoms are commonly addressed through hormone therapy, utilizing various forms of estrogen, testosterone, progesterone or a combination.

There is paucity of consistent evidence to draw a conclusion as to the effect on sexuality of oophorectomy with or without hormone replacement therapy (HRT). Almost half the papers do not specify whether HRT was administered, other papers report that some of the women in their study received oophorectomy, and some received HRT, but contingent relationships are not specified between hysterectomy with or without oophorectomy and its impact on sexuality. However, the available data shows no significant difference in changes in women's perception of their sexual functioning has been reported before and after hysterectomy based on whether the women had their ovaries conserved or removed, with or without receiving hormone replacement therapy [7].

Psychological Factors

A wide range of psychological characteristics influence sexual function after hysterectomy.

Psychological factors with a negative impact on sexuality after hysterectomy [8–11]:

- Preoperative psychiatric morbidity
- Depression
- Unsatisfactory preoperative sexual relations with poor outcome

Psychological factors with a positive impact on sexuality after hysterectomy [9, 11, 12]:

- Frequency of coitus
- Frequency of desire
- Orgasmic response
- A healthy relationship with a partner
- Good general health of both partners
- Being stress free

Therefore those women who retained an overall desire for sexual activity, and were presumably affected by negative symptoms might be expected to experience an improvement in their sexual function after hysterectomy.

Anatomical Factors

Anatomical factors include:

(a) The lack of the uterine contractions which in some women are an important aspect of orgasm.

(b) Scar tissue preventing expansion of vagina, which may make intercourse difficult.

(c) Scarring or nerve damage causing discomfort and interference with feeling sexual pleasure.

(d) Reduced quantity of tissue resulting in diminished vasocongestion may reduce sexual arousal and the probability of multiple orgasms, and also the disruption of vaginal blood flow, local nerve supply and anatomical relationships, which could have a negative effect on overall pelvic floor function [13–16].

In addition to these factors, the pathology for which the hysterectomy is performed may differentially affect sexual response. It has been reported that women who had a hysterectomy due to endometriosis reported more difficulty and less satisfaction with orgasm than women who had a hysterectomy for other reasons. There is considerable evidence that simple abdominal hysterectomy does not have an adverse affect on pelvic organ function (bladder, bowel and sexual) [17].

Evidence-Based Review of Effects of Hysterectomy on Sexuality

Hysterectomy is the most frequently performed gynecological operation. Therefore, the myths regarding hysterectomy need to be dispelled and women requiring hysterectomy should be counseled using the best available evidence.

Simple Hysterectomy {Total Abdominal (TAH), Subtotal Abdominal (STAH) and Vaginal Hysterectomy (VH)}

Farrell and Kieser performed a systematic review of sexuality after hysterectomy and found that research in this area was largely retrospective without the use of validated outcome measures [18]. Most studies showed either no change or enhancement of sexuality following hysterectomy. Theoretically hysterectomy should increase sexual pleasure by removing the fear of pregnancy, relieving dyspareunia and uterine disease particularly cancer. Roussis et al. [19] performed a retrospective study to assess the patient's own appraisal of their sexual responsiveness after hysterectomy (61 TAH, 22 STAH, 42 VH) and found that sexuality did not diminish after any type of hysterectomy. Alexander et al. [20] performed a prospective randomised trial comparing hysterectomy with endometrial ablation using validated measures of psychological and sexual function both pre and postoperatively. They found no difference in post operative sexuality after 12 months. Differences in libido and sexual sensitivity following various types of hysterectomies have been evaluated by Wierrani et al. [21] and found no difference at 12 months follow-up. Galyer et al. compared sexual function in women who had undergone TAH with those who had VH and found no difference in sexual desire postoperatively [22]. Roovers et al. in a prospective study over 6 months, found a reduction in sexual problems VH, TAH or STAH [23]. A large prospective study (the Maryland Women's Health study) which enrolled 1299 women who were interviewed with validated questionnaire preoperatively and at 6, 12, 18 and 24 months after hysterectomy for benign condition and found significant increase in frequency of sexual activity, a decrease in dyspareunia and a reduction in low libido [16]. Overall this study found substantial improvements in sexual function after hysterectomy.

It has been hypothesised that the disturbance of innervation of cervix and upper vagina after total hysterectomy interferes with lubrication and orgasm. Other factors that might contribute to sexual problems include a reduction in cervical mucus and vaginal shortening [24]. However Weber et al. do not agree with these views [25]. Kilkku et al. highlighted the influence of anatomical changes by comparing coital frequency, dyspareunia, libido and frequency of orgasm before and at 6 weeks, 6 months and 1 year in 105 women with TAH and 107 with STAH [26, 27]. Both groups showed an equal but slight reduction in coital frequency and dyspareunia with statistically significant deterioration after STAH. The frequency of orgasm was significantly reduced in TAH group but not in STAH group. However two randomised studies by Thakar et al. [28] and Zobbe et al. [29] found no difference in frequency of intercourse or orgasm between TAH and STAH. However there was a significant increase in frequency of intercourse [30] and decrease in dyspareunia [30, 31] after hysterectomy.

Current evidence suggests that dyspareunia reduces after hysterectomy. Sexual function does not usually deteriorate after a simple hysterectomy although a few women may develop sexual problems. There does not appear to be a difference in sexual function in women who have STAH and TAH.

Radical Hysterectomy (RH)

Women after surgery for genital cancer have to deal with not only the fear and anxiety generated by the diagnosis, treatment and prognosis, but also with the constant fear of recurrence. These women are often unaware of the consequences of the operation on sexual function. Although there is extensive evidence in the literature that shows adverse sexual functioning after treatment for cervical cancer [32–34], most studies report on heterogeneous groups of patients undergoing surgery, radiotherapy or both [35]. Primary or adjuvant radiotherapy has been reported to result in more severe sexual difficulties than hysterectomy alone [33, 36]. Patients treated with radical hysterectomy alone seem to regain their full sexual capacity and satisfaction more frequently [37]. Bergman et al. compared 256 women who had been treated for early cervical cancer and 350 controls [36]. They found that treatment of cervical cancer caused changes in vaginal anatomy and had negative effect on sexual function. These changes included decreased lubrication and reduction in perceived vaginal length and elasticity during intercourse. However the difference in the two groups with respect to frequency of intercourse, orgasmic frequency and pleasure were small. Grumann et al. prospectively compared 18 patients with stage 1B cervical cancer undergoing RH with 20 women undergoing hysterectomy for a benign cause-over 8 months using standardised questionnaires [37]. The cancer patients showed slightly better sexual function preoperatively than the other group but this deteriorated with time. Sexual function among patients with benign disease showed steady improvement indicating that RH for stage 1B cervical cancer is not associated with major disruption in sexual function. However this study had a small sample size so must be interpreted with caution. A large prospective study comparing 173 patients who had RH with age-matched controls indicated that RH had a persistent and negative impact on patients' sexual function, whereas majority of vaginal problems disappear over time [38]. Maas et al. objectively assessed sexual arousal in women who had RH (n = 12), TAH (n = 12) and 17 age-matched controls by measuring vaginal blood flow during sexual arousal using erotic films [39]. The authors suggested that although RH appears to be associated with a disturbed blood flow after sexual response, larger studies are needed for confirmation.

Overall, however, while RH affects some aspects of female sexuality, the majority appears to be transient and may be influenced by other overriding issues related to the diagnosis of cancer.

Laparoscopic Hysterectomy

A prospective case control study found no alteration of sexual function in premenopausal women undergoing either conventional or single port laparoscopically assisted

Table 9.1 Effects of hysterectomy, summary of 40 papers, 1952–2013

Effect	Increase	Decrease	No change	Variable	Undesirable effect on:
Dyspareunia	0	14	4	0	22
Vaginal lubrication	2	1	8	0	10
Libido	5	3	17	0	20
Orgasm frequency	2	4	9	0	12
Orgasm intensity	2	0	5	1	5
Sexual function	4	3	4	0	4
Sexual activity	4	1	18	3	14

vaginal hysterectomy [40]. Serati et al. found that laparoscopic radical hysterectomy did not show any benefit on women's sexuality over the open abdominal surgery for cervical cancer [41].

With recent advances in robotic surgery, this modality has been used for hysterectomy (benign and radical). Laparoscopic robotic-assisted radical hysterectomy with nerve sparing technique for bowel and bladder is proposed to be an attractive surgical approach for early invasive cervical cancer. However, effect on sexuality has not been studied to date and needs further exploration [42].

Kupperman et al. [43] conducted a randomized trial of 135women (67 TAH and 68 STAH) for benign conditions with a 2 year follow up. Sexual functioning and quality of life variables were measured with a telephone and clinic interviews. Both groups reported improvement in most measures of sexual functioning. The study by Thakar et al. [44] of 279 women (146 TAH and 133 STAH) was the only double-blind RCT. Each woman was followed for 1 year. A short-form, previously validated 36-question health survey (SF-36) and psychological outcome measure (GHQ: general health questionnaire) were used preoperatively and at 6 and 12 months postoperatively (0–100 scale). No statistical difference was found between the 2 groups before and after surgery. The frequency of intercourse, desire for intercourse, orgasm, and initiation of intercourse did not differ significantly between the groups. There was also a significant increase in the frequency of intercourse in both groups after surgery ($P = 0.01$). Deep dyspareunia was reduced significantly in both groups (46.2–6.6 % STAH and 39.3–14.3 % TAH) at 12 months ($P < 0.001$), but there was no statistical difference between groups. Zobbe et al. [29] conducted a randomized trial of 319 women (158 TAH and 161 SCH) with a one year follow-up and found no statistical difference between the 2 intervention groups regarding frequency of sexual desire, intercourse, masturbation, and orgasm, as well as quality of orgasm, vaginal lubrication, or satisfaction with sexual life ($P > 0.05$). Dyspareunia decreased significantly in both groups (89 women pre surgery and 22 post surgery $P = 0.009$). A multivariate logistic regression analysis identified preoperative satisfaction with sexual life, good relationship with partner, chronic disease, and use of hormone therapy as significant predictors of postoperative satisfaction with sexual life. Flory et al. [45] conducted a randomized trial of 63 women (32 LAVH and 31 laparoscopic subtotal hysterectomy) with a 7 month follow up. There were no differences in sexual functioning overall ($P > 0.05$).

Table 9.1 gives a summary of findings reported in the papers regarding the variably reported outcomes of hysterectomy. Any individual study reporting on at least some women who experienced deleterious effects after hysterectomy, whether or not statistically significant, was included in the last column of the table – "Undesirable Effects On:" It is important to identify and report incidence of deleterious effects of hysterectomy on any individuals. Since very few papers elaborated on these deleterious effects, we could not distinguish whether the women who, for example, experienced dyspareunia after hysterectomy developed this condition after the surgery or if the condition was present preoperatively but not treated with surgery.

Conclusion

The research on the effect of hysterectomy on sexual function that has been performed to date is not conclusive. There are discrepancies in the literature as to whether hysterectomy improves or attenuates sexuality. Hysterectomy may alleviate the discomfort of pain and bleeding, resulting in positive psychological factors such as elimination of anxiety over unwanted pregnancy and cancer risk. Symptom relief may have led to increased sexual enjoyment and increased orgasm frequency. While women report an improvement of sexual functioning after hysterectomy, this may be the result of the relief of symptoms (such as vaginal bleeding and dyspareunia) from the uterus, some women develop sexual dysfunction as a result of hysterectomy. More research is needed to clarify the issue of the effect of hysterectomy on sexual response.

Tips for the Reader

It is imperative that sexual function/dysfunction should be addressed in counseling women undergoing hysterectomy. The evaluation process for women with sexual dysfunction includes identification of the dysfunction, patient education and modification of reversible factors. The history should include a sexual function history, medical history and psychosocial history. The examination should include both an external and internal physical exam. A multidisciplinary approach with involvement of gynaecologist, vulval pain specialist and a psychosexual counselor should be used, where indicated.

Treatment for physical causes may include the use of vaginal estrogen pessaries especially in presence of vaginal atrophy. Testosterone therapy also converts to estrogen so women in transition from peri-menopause to menopause who have vasomotor symptoms (hot flashes, night sweats) and low androgens may need to take additional estrogen in conjunction with androgens. Other treatments include Dehydroepiandrosterone (DHEA), which may result in enhanced androstenedione and testosterone levels and improvement of sexual symptoms including better Female Sexual Function Index (FSFI) and Sexual Dysfunction Score (SDS). Considering the low incidence of the adverse effect of hysterectomy on sexual function psychosexual counseling and therapy is an integral part of treatment of patients with sexual problems after hysterectomy.

References

1. Laumann EO, Paik A, Rosen RC. Sexual dysfunction in the United States: prevalence and predictors. JAMA. 1999;281(6):537–44.
2. Hayes RD, Bennett CM, Fairley CK, et al. What can prevalence studies tell us about female sexual difficulty and dysfunction? J Sex Med. 2006;3:589–95.
3. West SL, D'Aloisio AA, Agans RP, et al. Prevalence of low sexual desire and hypoactive sexual desire disorder in a nationally representative sample of US women. Arch Intern Med. 2008;168:1441–9.
4. DeRogatis LR, Graziottin A, Bitzer J, et al. Clinically relevant changes in sexual desire, satisfying sexual activity and personal distress as measured by the profile of female sexual function, sexual activity log, and personal distress scale in postmenopausal women with hypoactive sexual desire disorder. J Sex Med. 2009;6:175–83.
5. Dennerstein L, Guthrie JR, Hayes RD, DeRogatis LR, Lehert P. Sexual function, dysfunction, and sexual distress in a prospective, population-based sample of mid-aged, Australian born women. J Sex Med. 2008;5:2291–9.
6. Whiteman MK, Hillis SD, Jamieson DJ, et al. Inpatient hysterectomy surveillance in the United States, 2000–2004. Am J Obstet Gynecol. 2008;198:31–7.
7. Bhattacharya S, Mollison J, Pinion S, et al. A comparison of bladder and ovarian function two years following hysterectomy or endometrial ablation. BJOG. 1996;103:898–903.
8. Lalinec-Michaud M, Engelsmann F. Psychological profile of depressed women undergoing hysterectomy. J Psychosom Obstet Gynecol. 1988;8:53–66.
9. Rhodes JC, Kjerulff K, Langenberg PW, Guzinski GM. Hysterectomy and sexual functioning. JAMA. 1999;282:1934–41.
10. Dennerstein L, Wood C, Burrows GD. Sexual responses following hysterectomy and oophorectomy. Obstet Gynaecol. 1977;49:92–6.
11. Helstorm L, Lundberg PO, Sorborm D, Backstorm T. Sexuality after hysterectomy: factor analysis of women's sexual lives before and after subtotal hysterectomy. Obstet Gynaecol. 1995;74:142–6.
12. Darling CA, McKay-Smith YM. Understanding hysterectomies: sexual satisfaction and quality of life. J Sex Res. 1993;30:324–35.
13. Langer R, Neuman M, Ron-el R, et al. The effect of total abdominal hysterectomy on bladder function in asymptomatic women. Obstet Gynecol. 1989;74:205–7.
14. Carlson KJ, Miller BA, Fowler Jr FJ. The Maine Women's Health Study I. Outcomes of hysterectomy. Obstet Gynecol. 1994;83:556–65.
15. Kjerulff KH, Langenberg PW, Greenaway L, Uman J, Harvey LA. Urinary incontinence and hysterectomy in a large prospective cohort study in American women. J Urol. 2002;167:2088–92.
16. Griffith-Jones MD, Jarvis GJ, McNamara HM. Adverse urinary symptoms after total abdominal hysterectomy—fact or fiction? Br J Urol. 1991;67:295–7.
17. Thakar R. Dispelling the myth-does hysterectomy cause pelvic organ dysfunction. BJOG. 2004;111:20–3.
18. Farrell SA, Kieser K. Sexuality after hysterectomy. Am J Obstet Gynaecol. 2000;95:1045–51.
19. Roussis NP, Waltrous L, Kerr A, et al. Sexual response in the patient after hysterectomy: total abdominal versus supracervical versus vaginal procedure. Am J Obstet Gynaecol. 2004;190:1427–8.
20. Alexander AD, Naji AA, Pinion SB, et al. A randomised trial of hysterectomy versus endometrial ablation for dysfunctional uterine bleeding: psychiatric and psychosocial outcome. Br Med J. 1996;312:280–312.
21. Wierrani F, Huber M, Grin W, et al. Prospective libido and genital sexual sensitivity following various forms of hysterectomy. J Gynecol Surg. 1995;11:127–32.
22. Galyer KT, Conaglen HM, Hare A, Conaglen JV. The effect of gynecological surgery on sexual desire. J Sex Marital Ther. 1999;25:81–8.
23. Roovers JWR, Van der Bom JG, Van der Vaat CH, Heintz PM. Hysterectomy and sexual wellbeing: prospective observational study of vaginal hysterectomy, subtotal abdominal hysterectomy and total abdominal hysterectomy. Br Med J. 2003;327:774–7.
24. Jewett JF. Vaginal length and incidence of dyspareunia following total abdominal hysterectomy. Am J Obstet Gynaecol. 1952;63:400–7.
25. Weber AM, Walters MD, Piedmonte MR. Sexual function and vaginal anatomy in women before and after surgery for pelvic organ prolapse and urinary incontinence. Am J Obstet Gynaecol. 2000;182:1610–5.
26. Kilkku P, Gronoos M, Hirovnen T, Rauramo L. Supravaginal uterine amputation versus hysterectomy: effects on libido and orgasm. Acta Obstet Gynecol Scand. 1983;62:147–52.
27. Kilkku P. Supravaginal uterine amputation versus hysterectomy: effects on coital frequency and dyspareunia. Acta Obstet Gynecol Scand. 1983;62:141–5.
28. Thakar R, Ayers S, Clarkson P, Stanton S, Manyonda I. Outcomes after total versus subtotal abdominal hysterectomy. N Engl J Med. 2002;347:1318–25.
29. Zobbe V, Gimbel H, Anderson BM, et al. Sexuality after total and subtotal hysterectomy. Acta Obstet Gynecol Scand. 2004;83:191–6.
30. Van der Wiel HBM, Weijmar Schultz WCM, Hallensleben A, et al. Sexual functioning following treatment of cervical cancer. Eur J Gynecol Oncol. 1988;9:275–81.
31. Schover LR, Fife M, Gershenson DM. Sexual dysfunction and treatment of early stage cervical cancer. Cancer. 1989;63:204–12.
32. Horton B. Sexual outcomes arising from diagnosis and treatment of cervical cancer and cervical intraepithelial neoplasia: a review of literature. J Sex Marital Ther. 1991;6:29–39.
33. Weijmar Schultz WCM, Bransfield DD, Van der Wiel HBM. Sexual functioning following female genital cancer treatment: a critical

review of methods of investigation and results. J Sex Marital Ther. 1992;7:29–64.
34. Siebel MM, Freeman MG, Graves WL. Carcinoma of the cervix and sexual function. Obstet Gynecol. 1980;55:484–7.
35. Thranov I, Klee M. Sexuality amongst gynaecologic cancer patients–a cross-sectional study. Gynecol Oncol. 1994;52:14–9.
36. Bergmark K, Avall-Lundqvist E, Dickman PW, et al. Vaginal changes and sexuality in women with a history of cervical cancer. N Engl J Med. 1999;340:1383–9.
37. Grumann M, Robertson R, Hacker NF, Sommer G. Sexual functioning in patients following radical hysterectomy for stage 1B cancer of the cervix. Int J Gynecol Cancer. 2001;11:372–80.
38. Jensen PT, Groenvold M, Klee MC, et al. Does radical hysterectomy have an impact on sexual function in early stage cervical cancer patients? Int J Gynecol Cancer. 2003;13:22.
39. Maas CP, ter Kuile MM, Laan E, et al. Objective assessment of sexual arousal in women with a history of hysterectomy. BJOG. 2004;111:456–62.
40. Lee JH, Choi JS, Hong JH, Joo KJ, Kim BY. Does conventional or single port laparoscopically assisted hysterectomy affect female sexual function? Acta Obstet Gynecol Scand. 2011;90(12):1410–5.
41. Serati M, Salvatore S, Uccella S, Laterza RM, Cromi A, Ghezzi F, Bolis P. Sexual function after radical hysterectomy for early-stage cervical cancer: is there a difference between laparoscopy and laparotomy? J Sex Med. 2009;6(9):2516–22.
42. Gil-lbanez B, Diaz-Feijoo B, Perez-Benavente A, Puig-Puig O, Franco-Camps S, Centeno C, Xercavins J, Gil-Moreno A. Nerve sparing technique in robotic-assisted radical hysterectomy: results. Int J Med Robot 2013. doi: 10.1002/rcs 1480. Epub.
43. Kuppermann M, Summitt Jr RL, Varner RE, McNeeley SG, Goodman-Gruen D, Learman LA, et al. and Total or Supracervical Hysterectomy Research GroupSexual functioning after total compared with supracervical hysterectomy: a randomized trial. Obstet Gynecol. 2005;105(6):1309–18.
44. Thakar R, Ayers S, Georgakapolou A, Clarkson P, Stanton S, Manyonda I. Hysterectomy improves quality of life and decreases psychiatric symptoms: a prospective and randomised comparison of total versus subtotal hysterectomy. BJOG. 2004;111(10):1115–20.
45. Flory N, Bissonnette F, Amsel RT, Binik YM. The psychosocial outcomes of total and subtotal hysterectomy: a randomized controlled trial. J Sex Med. 2006;3(3):483–91.

10 Guidelines and Recommendations of Scientific Societies and Associations for Hysterectomy

Klaus Neis and Felix Neis

Hysterectomy represents the second most performed surgery in gynecology after the Cesarean Section. In Germany there are 100,000 hysterectomies performed a year in case of benign indication. 27 % of these are prolapse surgeries. Thus, there remain 75,000 hysterectomies due to benign diagnostic findings in 2012 [1]. Worldwide most of the hysterectomies of this group are performed abdominally. Only in Germany, Austria and Switzerland a lower rate could be found. As in the USA 64 % of the hysterectomies are performed abdominally, in Canada 60 %, Austria 29.6 %, Switzerland 26.0 % and in Germany 17.5 % [2].

At the beginning of the 90s, when the laparoscopic surgery has been introduced for hysterectomy, the aim was to reduce the number of abdominal hysterectomies. In individual hospitals which decided to specialize in this field, this could be realized in an impressive way. [3]. Regarding however the national statistics this development has only lead to moderate adjustments [4]. For example declined the rate of abdominal hysterectomy in the USA from 66.1 % in 2003 [4] to 54.2 % in 2010 [5].

Two Cochrane Analysis, in which the different methods of hysterectomy have been evaluated, showed however that the vaginal hysterectomy is the method of the lowest rate of complications, the lowest blood loss and also the shortest time of surgery. Additionally, cost analyses demonstrate that the vaginal hysterectomy represents the most economical method by far in the whole range of hysterectomies [6, 7].

In Germany the rate of vaginal hysterectomies lies at about 50 %, in Austria at 46.2 %, in Switzerland at 41 %. In the USA the rate of vaginal hysterectomies lies at only 20 % [8–11].

In 2009 this had been the reason for the American College of Obstetricians and Gynecologists (ACOG) to publish a statement, in which the vaginal hysterectomy was recommended as first option. In cases where a vaginal hysterectomy seems not to be viable the possibility of laparoscopic hysterectomy should be investigated. If both options are unviable then there is given an indication for abdominal hysterectomy [12].

Analogously there is also the recommendation of the AAGL (American Association of Gynecologic Laparoscopists) of 2011. In the meantime a working group in the AAGL is established where colleagues with special interests in vaginal surgeries are united [13].

Meanwhile also the insurance companies suggest that the vaginal hysterectomy should be the method of first choice. They justify their suggestion as they want to offer their insurants the method of least complications. The fact, that this method is the most economical one at the same time, may probably be also an important point for an insurance company.

In 2010, a group under the auspices of K.J. Neis and K. Schwerdtfeger has been authorized by the German Society of Gynecology and Obstetrics (Deutsche Gesellschaft für Gynäkologie und Geburtshilfe e.V. ,DGGG) to develop in Germany a guideline for indication and methodology of hysterectomy. The guideline was compiled by 24 scientifically and clinically operating colleagues and was available in 2012. It reflects the situation in Germany, Austria and Switzerland, where the vaginal hysterectomy is preferred traditionally and where today the laparoscopic surgeries are integrated to the greatest possible extent into the range of surgeries for hysterectomy.

When compiling the individual chapters it became more and more clear, that also the alternative methods as hysteroscopy, the systemic und local hormone therapy or Uterine artery embolization (UAE) are all effectible. However, the most satisfied women are to be found in the group of patients who underwent a hysterectomy (Table 10.1).

K. Neis (✉)
Klinik für Frauenheilkunde, Geburtshilfe und Reproduktionsmedizin, der Universität des Saarlandes, Kirrbergstr. 100, 66421 Homburg, Saar, Germany

European Training Center for Gynecologic Endoscopy, Bismarckstr. 39–41, 66121 Saarbrücken, Germany
e-mail: kjneis@gyn-saar.de

F. Neis
Universitätsfrauenklinik Tübingen, Calwer Str.7, 72076 Tübingen, Germany

I. Alkatout, L. Mettler (eds.), *Hysterectomy*, DOI 10.1007/978-3-319-22497-8_10

Table 10.1 Comparison of satisfaction rates of women who underwent hysterectomy, endometrial ablation or the levonorgestrel-releasing intrauterine system (LNG-IUS)

	Hysterectomy	Endometrial ablation	LNG-IUS
Control of bleeding symptoms	+++	++(+)	++
Rate of reinterventions within 5 years	<5 %	10–36 %	42 %
Quality of life	++++	+++(+)	+++
Chance of success Length of uterine cavity >8 cm	+++	+	+

+ = degree of satisfaction

Due to the highly sociopolitical importance the board of DGGG had decided to subordinate these already compiled statements to an evidence analysis. This analysis had been executed by Dr. M. Nothacker, an employee of AWMF (Arbeitsgemeinschaft der Wissenschaftlichen Medizinischen Fachgesellschaften e.V.) especially skilled in this field.

The evidence, which includes the present literature until 12/2014, leads fortunately to the same results and recommendations as the primary 2 k-guideline. Thus, all predications, recommendations and statements are supported objectively. Accordingly, the guideline was upgraded to the highest scientific level S3.

The full text of the German guideline and the report of evidence, inclusive the list of authors, is available at http://www.awmf.org/leitlinien/detail/ll/015-070.html.

The recommendations of this guideline concerning the preference of the methods are:

Evidence Based Recommendations

Evidence Grade **1a**	*Recommendation Grade* **A**	*Consensus Level* +++

If possible the vaginal hysterectomy shall be preferred to the abdominal hysterectomy.

Evidence Grade **1a**	*Recommendation Grade* **B**	*Consensus Level* +++

If the vaginal hysterectomy is not viable, the possibility of a laparoscopic hysterectomy shall be investigated.

Evidence Grade **1a**	Recommendation *Grade* **0**	*Consensus Level* +++

The LASH can be performed alternatively to the abdominal hysterectomy as well as to the vaginal hysterectomy.

Consensus Based Statement

Expert Consensus	*Consensus Level* +++

However, the recorded data does not allow at present to differ exactly between the various laparoscopic techniques.

Consensus Based Recommendation

Expert Consensus	*Consensus Level* +++

The abdominal hysterectomy should only be performed in case of special indication.

Quality of Life

The patient's question, whether the disorders impairing her quality of life will really be improved by hysterectomy, represent a very central point within the medical counseling.

There exist numerous investigations to this question and all of them show the result that quality of life will be considerably improved after hysterectomy [14–16].

Thus, an evidence based recommendation could be compiled:

Evidence Grade **1a**	Recommendation Grade **B**	*Consensus Level* +++

The patients should be informed that they can expect predominantly an improvement of quality of life and sexuality after an indicated hysterectomy compared to their pre-operative situation.

Alternatives to Hysterectomy and Counseling

When evaluating the different operative and non-operative alternatives to hysterectomy it can be stated that all of them are effective at the end. Though, due to the fact that the uterus is conserved, the alternative methods naturally have a risk of recurrence respectively a failure rate which then requires after all in lots of cases still a hysterectomy.

Thus, the hysterectomy is at least the most effective method to eliminate the disorders.

Independent of this, in each individual case it has to be examined whether the medically most reasonable method is also the best method for the patient.

So, the latent desire to have children independent of the age represents always a contra indication against hysterectomy. The same is valid for women who occupied their uterus with very important personal feelings. For those the loss of the uterus may be technically the perfect solution, but emotionally they would suffer.

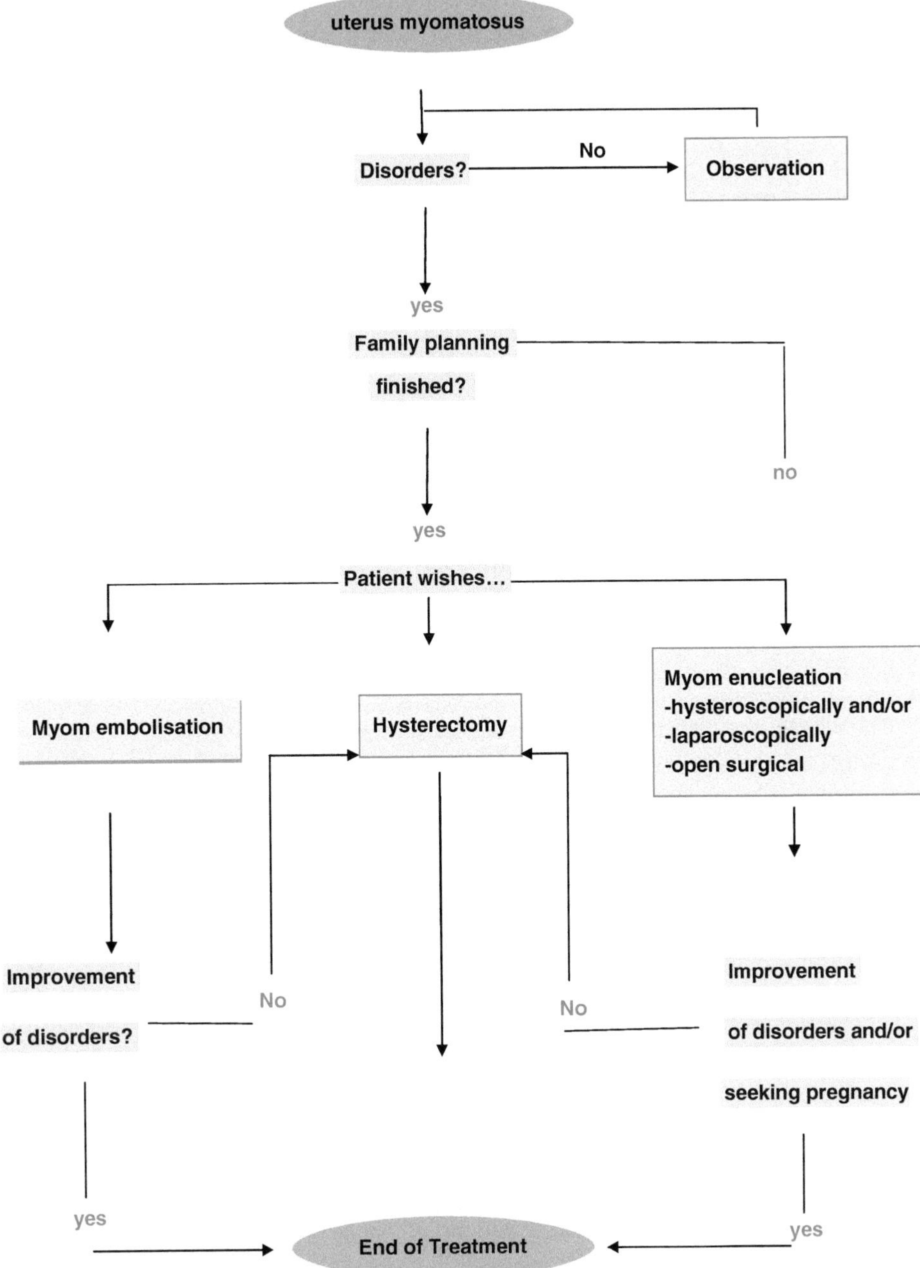

Fig. 10.1 Algorithm: alternatives to hysterectomy

Those women have to be identified and selected within an intensive talk before surgery. In order to guarantee that a complete and highly-qualified counseling is made it is recommended to follow the algorithms compiled by the guideline group (for example, uterus myomatosus shown in Fig. 10.1). That way the patient can realize at a glance the complete range of her possibilities.

The discussion of the individual steps, explaining the advantages and disadvantages of the different possibilities, require however a special education in the field of hysterectomy and its alternatives. As also the alternatives have indications and contra-indications and the probability that the success hoped for is different due to various medical findings and varying anamnesis, the consultant physician should have qualified for this field by advanced training.

It is the aim of the counseling, that on one side transparency is shown, but on the other side, the evidence situation of the individual contemplable methods has to be presented that way that the woman knowing her different possibilities is able to choose that therapy option of which she believes it suits the best to her and her situation of life.

The experience shows that women who are used to take responsibility in their lives are also able to take a decision quickly, or that they already have made a decision for themselves based on their own research before the counseling.

Even in those cases the patient should be informed again in order to assure that really all aspects were considered for the decision making.

Hesitant women are never to be urged in one or another direction. If there is no imminent danger, as e.g. an anemiating bleeding disorder, the woman can take the time to deal in detail with her disorders and her psychological strain.

Frequently, she will seek medical advice also somewhere else, where she hopefully will be advised just as qualified, transparent, evident and impartial.

When comparing the possibilities we have today with those given 100 years before, as the hysterectomy has been a surgery with high mortality and morbidity and which therefore only has been performed in exactly justified individual cases, with the broad range which we have today as well in the field of hysterectomy as in the field of uterus conserving alternatives, so it is possible today to offer each woman an effective method individually specific to her, so that she can regain the lost quality of life.

The woman always should decide by herself which way to go. In our opinion, with a qualified patient information each woman independent of the primary educational level is able to make her own decision at the end with which she is satisfied also years thereafter.

In summary it can be stated that at present there is generated one standard worldwide concerning the method of hysterectomy. The first option is and will be the vaginal hysterectomy. The second option represents the laparoscopic surgeries which differ decreasingly in their complication rate, so that it is recommended here to choose the method which can be performed best by the surgeon. Then, there are only a few indications remaining for the abdominal hysterectomy. In the meantime, the organ conserving alternatives also have a fixed significance. Their presentation is an essential part of the patient information today.

References

1. Institut A. Bundesauswertung 2012. https://www.sqgde/downloads/Bundesauswertungen/2012/bu_Gesamt_15N1-GYN-OP_2012pdf. 2012.
2. Obstetrics GotGSoGa. Indication and technics of hysterectomy for benigne diseases. AWMF Registry No 015/077, March 2015. 2015. http://www.awmf.org/leitlinien/detail/ll/015-070.html.
3. Brandner P, Neis KJ. The significance of laparoscopically-assisted vaginal hysterectomy–LAVH. Zentralbl Gynakol. 1995;117(12):620–4.
4. Wu JM, Wechter ME, Geller EJ, Nguyen TV, Visco AG. Hysterectomy rates in the United States, 2003. Obstet Gynecol. 2007;110(5):1091–5.
5. Wright JD, Herzog TJ, Tsui J, Ananth CV, Lewin SN, Lu YS, et al. Nationwide trends in the performance of inpatient hysterectomy in the United States. Obstet Gynecol. 2013;122(2 Pt 1):233–41.
6. Nieboer TE, Johnson N, Lethaby A, Tavender E, Curr E, Garry R, et al. Surgical approach to hysterectomy for benign gynaecological disease. Cochrane Database Syst Rev. 2009;3:CD003677.
7. Aarts JW, Nieboer TE, Johnson N, Tavender E, Garry R, Mol BW, et al. Surgical approach to hysterectomy for benign gynaecological disease. Cochrane Database Syst Rev. 2015;8:Cd003677.
8. Gesundheit A. http://www.statistik.at/web-de/suchergerniss/index.htlm. Zugriff: 1022012.
9. (ASF) ASF. http://www.sevisa.ch/. Zugriff: 27102014. 2010.
10. Jacobson TZ, Duffy JM, Barlow D, Koninckx PR, Garry R. Laparoscopic surgery for pelvic pain associated with endometriosis. Cochrane Database Syst Rev. 2009;4:CD001300.
11. Merrill RM. Hysterectomy surveillance in de United States, 1997 through 2005. Med Sci Monit Int Med J Exp Clin Res. 2008;14(1):CR24–31.
12. ACOG Committee Opinion No. 444: choosing the route of hysterectomy for benign disease. Obstet Gynecol. 2009;114(5):1156–8.
13. Worldwide AAMIG. AAGL position statement: route of hysterectomy to treat benign uterine disease. J Minim Invasive Gynecol. 2011;18(1):1–3.
14. Kuppermann M, Varner RE, Summitt Jr RL, Learman LA, Ireland C, Vittinghoff E, et al. Effect of hysterectomy vs medical treatment on health-related quality of life and sexual functioning: the medicine or surgery (Ms) randomized trial. JAMA. 2004;291(12):1447–55.
15. Varner RE, Ireland CC, Summitt Jr RL, Richter HE, Learman LA, Vittinghoff E, et al. Medicine or Surgery (Ms): a randomized clinical trial comparing hysterectomy and medical treatment in premenopausal women with abnormal uterine bleeding. Control Clin Trials. 2004;25(1):104–18.
16. Radosa JC, Meyberg-Solomayer G, Kastl C, Radosa CG, Mavrova R, Graber S, et al. Influences of different hysterectomy techniques on patients' postoperative sexual function and quality of life. J Sex Med. 2014;11(9):2342–50.

11 Choosing the Correct Hysterectomy Technique

Linda-Dalal J. Shiber and Resad Pasic

Introduction

In 2009, a systematic review of all randomized control trials comparing surgical approach to hysterectomy for benign disease was published. The objective of this review was to determine the 'most beneficial and least harmful surgical approach to hysterectomy' [1]. The conclusion was that, based on cumulative outcomes of time to recovery, complication rates and length of hospital stay, vaginal hysterectomy should be performed preferentially to abdominal hysterectomy and, when vaginal hysterectomy is not possible, laparoscopic approaches should be considered over the abdominal route.

Existing data clearly indicates that vaginal approach to hysterectomy is associated with fewer complications, faster recovery and lower healthcare costs than abdominal hysterectomy and shorter operative time than laparoscopic hysterectomy (Table 11.1) [1, 2]. Comparisons between vaginal hysterectomy and laparoscopic hysterectomy typically indicate longer operative time with the laparoscopic approach. Some studies have suggested increased complication rates with laparoscopic hysterectomy, namely urinary tract injury [2, 3]. Others have found no significant increase in such complications [4, 5].

Position statements from the American College of Obstetricians and Gynecologists (ACOG) and the American Association of Gynecologic Laparoscopists (AAGL) echo the above recommendations [6, 7]. The concept seems simple-i.e., vaginal hysterectomy is preferable, followed by laparoscopic approach, followed by laparotomy. In reality, however, selecting the route for hysterectomy is a complex task that requires consideration of patient preference, surgical indications, patient characteristics, available resources/procedural costs and surgeon skills and limitations. Perhaps the better way to address this chapter is to ask the question–how do we identify women who are *not* candidates for vaginal hysterectomy? And, of these women, how do we choose who undergoes abdominal hysterectomy over laparoscopic hysterectomy?

Note: For the purpose of this discussion, robotic-assisted laparoscopy will be considered to be within the category of laparoscopic techniques unless otherwise specified.

L.-D. J. Shiber, MD (✉)
Metrohealth Medical Center/Case Western Reserve University
Cleveland, Cuyahoga County, OH, USA
e-mail: lindashiber@gmail.com

R. Pasic, MD, PhD
Minimally Invasive Gynecologic Surgery OB/GYN, University of Louisville, Louisville, Jefferson County, KY, USA
e-mail: Resad.pasic@louisville.edu

Operative Indication

In benign gynecologic practice, the most common indication for hysterectomy is symptomatic uterine fibroids, followed by abnormal uterine bleeding. A plethora of other indications exist, including pelvic organ prolapse, endometriosis, pelvic pain and prophylaxis against reproductive system cancers in high-risk women [8].

Selecting the surgical route for hysterectomy is intimately linked with the indication for surgery (Fig. 11.1). The surgical management of gynecologic malignancies is beyond the scope of this chapter and will be considered separately.

For women who present with pelvic pain symptoms or a definite indication for adnexectomy, it is most reasonable to offer a surgical approach that allows a systematic inspection of the pelvic peritoneum, the abdominal contents and the adnexa. Vaginal hysterectomy does not provide a reliable or global survey of the pelvis in these women and does not consistently allow for identification and resection of disease such as endometriotic lesions, adnexal masses or other abnormalities that may contribute to pelvic pain. Though underpowered, a 2004 study found that despite the inherent advantages of vaginal hysterectomy in many women, laparoscopic route to hysterectomy was associated with a higher incidence of detecting unexpected pathology [9]. Certainly, for women who seek hysterectomy for pain

I. Alkatout, L. Mettler (eds.), *Hysterectomy*, DOI 10.1007/978-3-319-22497-8_11

Table 11.1 Advantages and limitations of surgical approaches to hysterectomy[1, 6]

	Vaginal	Laparoscopic	Robotic	Abdominal
Advantages	Shorter recovery time[a] Shorter operating time[b] Most cost-effective	Shorter recovery time[a] Facilitates global evaluation of pelvis Less blood loss[a] Less infectious morbidity[a]	Improved ergonomics Facilitates ease of suturing Shorter recovery time[a]	Default approach for massive uteri, disseminated malignancy
Limitations	Uteri >12 week size Cannot reliably evaluate for extra-uterine disease	May be associated with higher incidence urinary tract injury[a] Longer operating time[a] Uteri >24 week. size	Least cost-effective	Longer recovery time[c] Higher incidence of febrile morbidity[c] Higher blood loss[b]

[a]As compared with abdominal hysterectomy
[b]As compared with laparoscopic hysterectomy
[c]As compared with laparoscopic and vaginal hysterectomy

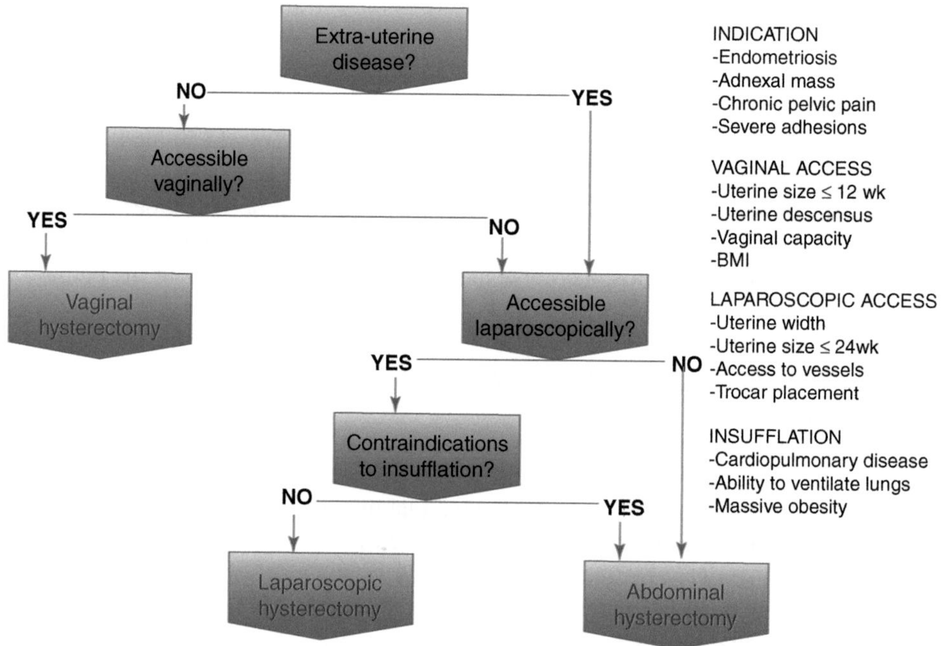

Fig. 11.1 Choosing the route of hysterectomy

symptoms, it is imperative that inspection of the abdomino-pelvic contents occurs. This should preferentially occur via laparoscopy rather than laparotomy. Though salpingo-oophorectomy is often performed at the time of vaginal hysterectomy, there is no guarantee that adnexal structures will be visible or mobilized from below. Again, in a patient who has adnexal pathology or desires risk-reducing BSO, the laparoscopic approach is most reliable and appropriate.

Concomitant, planned procedures must also be considered when selecting the route of hysterectomy. In women with pelvic organ prolapse who are candidates for vaginal repair, the vaginal route to hysterectomy is most logical. However, in women who require sacro-colpopexy, a laparoscopic or robotic route is preferable to laparotomy.

Co-morbid Conditions: Obesity and Cardiopulmonary Disease

As the obese patient population grows, surgical complication rates and post-operative morbidity increase. It is important to offer these high-risk patients a minimally invasive approach to hysterectomy [10, 11]. Obese patients may have poorer wound healing with higher rates of wound infection and postoperative complications such as venous thromboembolic events. Providing surgical options that minimize hospital stay and immobility is key. Abdominal hysterectomy should therefore be avoided in most scenarios. In a parous patient without indication for abdominopelvic survey and with a uterus of feasible size, vaginal hysterectomy is preferable.

Devices such as the vaginal Bookwalter retractor may aid with visualization and completion of surgery.

If vaginal access is not possible, if the patient suffers from pelvic pain or if the uterus is very enlarged, laparoscopic approaches to hysterectomy are ideal and offer equivalent benefits. However, it is important to counsel the super obese patient considering a laparoscopic or robotic hysterectomy that steep Trendelenburg position and abdominal insufflation may not be tolerated, resulting in laparotomy.

The role of robotic-assisted laparoscopic hysterectomy in the obese patient remains unclear. Anecdotally, the robot may aid with minimizing surgeon fatigue and optimizing visualization during minimally invasive hysterectomy and is certainly preferable to laparotomy in terms of decreasing hospital stay [12]. Randomized control trials comparing surgical outcomes for robotic hysterectomy to laparoscopic and vaginal hysterectomy in obese women are not currently available. One study comparing surgical outcomes of robotic hysterectomy in morbidly obese (body mass index (BMI) > 35) patients versus patients with BMI < 35 found equivalent outcomes but increased operative time for these heavier patients [13]. Regarding the general population, a recent Cochrane systematic review found limited evidence that robotic assisted laparoscopy affords benefit in benign disease [14] and it is well accepted that the robotic approach is more costly [15, 16].

Patients with certain types of heart failure or severe pulmonary conditions such as chronic obstructive pulmonary disease and obstructive sleep apnea may not tolerate the increased intra-peritoneal pressures created by carbon dioxide insufflation during laparoscopy. Deep trendelenburg position, necessary for pelvic surgery in these patients, may not be possible either. Depending on the co-morbid condition present, evaluation of pulmonary and cardiac function is necessary prior to surgery. Consultation with cardiology, pulmonology and anesthesia services is of great importance to surgical planning. These patients should be offered vaginal hysterectomy if possible, but unfortunately may require laparotomy for safe completion of surgery (Fig. 11.1).

Surgical History

In women with multiple abdominal surgeries, adhesion formation is common. Levrant et al. found the incidence of adhesions to be 59 % in women with a prior vertical midline incision versus 28 % in women with a prior Pfannenstiel incision [17]. In women with multiple laparotomies or prior pelvic infections, the likelihood of pelvic and anterior abdominal wall adhesions involving bowel increases. This may preclude safe vaginal hysterectomy. In addition, with the increased rates of cesarean sections in the US and certain other countries, severe vesicouterine adhesions may be present, making bladder dissection from below challenging and dangerous. Although one prior cesarean delivery is certainly not a contraindication to vaginal hysterectomy, clinical judgement must be used. In a patient who is high risk for severe pelvic adhesions, the laparoscopic route to hysterectomy is recommended and laparotomy may ultimately be required to complete the procedure safely.

Parity, Pelvis, Uterine Size

The obstetrician within every gynecologic surgeon must consider the anatomic feasibility of removing the uterus vaginally. When considering vaginal hysterectomy, it is important to assess the vaginal capacity, the uterine size and degree of uterine descensus [18]. For experienced vaginal surgeons, the upper limit of uterine size when considering vaginal route to hysterectomy may approach 16–18 week size. However, in an era when the typical OB/GYN resident is finishing training with fewer vaginal hysterectomies, this is neither a safe nor acceptable parameter. Typically, for uteri larger than 10–12 week size, a laparoscopic or robotic approach allows easier visualization of upper pedicles and even the uterine vasculature. For very large uteri or even uteri >12 week size with an inexperienced laparoscopic surgeon, the abdominal route to hysterectomy may be indicated. In women with rapidly growing fibroids or strong suspicion for malignancy, laparotomy is indicated.

In addition to uterine size, consideration of the shape of the uterus and mapping of fibroids is imperative to surgical planning. For women who have large lower uterine segment fibroids precluding peritoneal access from below, vaginal hysterectomy may not be possible.

Nulliparity and limitations posed by the bony pelvis (i.e., narrow pubic arch) are other important considerations when assessing candidacy for vaginal hysterectomy. Vaginal hysterectomy may be challenging in these women as descensus may not be present and visualization may be very difficult. An important point, however, is that if the patient is otherwise an appropriate candidate for TVH, it may be appropriate to attempt vaginal surgery with preoperative counseling that a laparoscopic approach may be necessary if that fails.

Surgeon Skills/Strengths/Limitation

Despite recommendations set forth by professional societies, it is important to critically assess one's surgical skill set prior to consenting a patient for a particular route of hysterectomy. For surgeons who are inexperienced in *any* approach, the rate of complications and intra/post-operative morbidity increases exponentially for that approach despite purported benefits [18–20].

Decreasing surgical numbers during residency training and a paucity of hysterectomy cases per year of practice have contributed to continued, widespread use of the abdominal route for benign hysterectomy, even in women who would be candidates for TVH or TLH in more experienced hands [21–23]. Surgeons who identify a candidate for MIS hysterectomy but who do not possess the skill set to perform such procedures should actively seek consultation from surgical specialists who can provide optimal hysterectomy care for their patients.

Cost Considerations, Resources

With regard to healthcare costs, vaginal hysterectomy is the most cost-effective approach with robotic hysterectomy accruing the highest costs, both in operating room time and equipment/maintenance, etc. [14–16, 24–27]. In a world recognizing the importance of evidence-based, cost-conscious and high-quality healthcare, the use of expensive robotic technology in benign gynecology is not justifiable.

Patient Preference

Ultimately, after clinical considerations have been outlined and the objective risks and benefits of each approach to hysterectomy detailed to the patient, her informed opinion regarding which technique she prefers must be taken into consideration.

With recent debates in the United States on tissue extraction, many women are declining even vaginal morcellation of tissue and requesting laparotomy. Some women concerned for cosmesis allow this to govern their decision regarding surgery. One study surveyed 100 women and found that the majority preferred a suprapubic mini-laparotomy incision or single-site laparoscopy incisions over laparoscopic, pfannenstiel and robotic incisions [28]. In addition, despite data that has suggested supracervical hysterectomy affords no long-term benefit to sexual function or post-operative outcomes and quality of life [29, 30], some women desire to retain the cervix and this request must be honored in the medically appropriate patient.

In conclusion, selecting the route of hysterectomy for benign gynecologic disease is a complex task that requires consideration of patient preference, surgical indications, patient characteristics, available resources/procedural costs and surgeon skills and limitations. As existing data on surgical outcomes, benefits, limitations and costs continues to evolve, it is important to incorporate these new findings in the patient counseling process.

References

1. TE N, Johnson N, Lethaby A, Tavender E, Curr E, Garry R, van Voorst S, BW M, KB K. Surgical approach to hysterectomy for benign disease. Cochrane Database Syst Rev. 2009;3:CD003677. doi:10.1002/14651858.CD003677.pub4.
2. Johnson N, Barlow D, Lethaby A, et al. Methods of hysterectomy: systematic review and meta-analysis of randomized controlled trials. BMJ. 2005;330:1478.
3. Drahonovsky et al. A prospective randomized comparison of vaginal hysterectomy, laparoscopically assisted vaginal hysterectomy and total laparoscopic hysterectomy in women with benign uterine disease. Eur J Obstet Gynecol Reprod Biol. 2010;148(2):172–6. doi:10.1016/j.ejogrb.2009.10.019. Epub 2009 Nov 18
4. Gendy R, Walsh CA, Walsh SR, Karantanis E. Vaginal hysterectomy versus total laparoscopic hysterectomy for benign disease: a metanalysis of randomized controlled trials. Am J Obstet Gynecol. 2011;204(5):388.e1–8. doi:10.1016/j.ajog.2010.12.059. Epub 2011 Mar 4
5. Donnez O, Donnez J. A series of 400 laparoscopic hysterectomies for benign disease: a single centre, single surgeon prospective study of complications confirming previous retrospective study. BJOG. 2010;117:752–5.
6. Choosing the route of hysterectomy for benign disease. ACOG Committee Opinion No. 444. American College of Obstetricians and Gynecologists. Obstet Gynecol. 2009; 114:1156–8.
7. Route of hysterectomy to treat benign uterine disease. AAGL position statement, American Association of Gynecologic Laparoscopists. J Minim Invasive Gynecol. 2011;18: 1–3. doi:10.1016/j.jmig.2010.10.001.
8. Walters M, Barber M. Hysterectomy for benign disease. Philadelphia: Saunders Elsevier ; 2010.http://www.clinicalkey.com.au/dura/browse/bookChapter/3-s2.0-C20090388534
9. Garry et al. EVALUATE hysterectomy trial: a multicentre randomised trial comparing abdominal, vaginal and laparoscopic methods of hysterectomy. Health Technol Assess. 2004;8(26):1–154.
10. Siedhoff MT et al. Effect of extreme obesity on outcomes in laparoscopic hysterectomy. J Minim Invasive Gynecol. 2012;19(6):701–7. doi:10.1016/j.jmig.2012.07.005.
11. Scheib SA et al. Laparoscopy in the morbidly obese: physiologic considerations and surgical techniques to optimize success. J Minim Invasive Gynecol. 2014;21(2):182–95. doi:10.1016/j.jmig.2013.09.009. Epub 2013 Oct 4
12. Silasi DA et al. Robotic versus abdominal hysterectomy for very large uteri. JSLS. 2013;17(3):400–6. doi:10.4293/108680813X13693422521755.
13. Eddib A et al. Influence of morbid obesity on surgical outcomes in robotic-assisted gynecologic surgery. J Gynecol Surg. 2014;30(2):81–6.

14. Liu H et al. WITHDRAWN: Robotic surgery for benign gynecological disease. Cochrane Database Syst Rev 2014;(12):CD008978. [Epub ahead of print]
15. Rosero EB et al. Comparison of robotic and laparoscopic hysterectomy for benign gynecologic disease. Obstet Gynecol. 2013;122(4):778–86. doi:10.1097/AOG.0b013e3182a4ee4d.
16. Wright JD et al. An economic analysis of robotically assisted hysterectomy. Obstet Gynecol. 2014;123(5):1038–48. doi:10.1097/AOG.0000000000000244.
17. Levrant SG et al. Anterior abdominal wall adhesions after laparotomy or laparoscopy. J Am Assoc Gynecol Laparosc. 1997;4(3):353–6.
18. Skinner BD, Delancey JO. Selecting the route for hysterectomy: a structured approach. Contemporary OB/GYN. 2013;58(8):p24.
19. Rogo-Gupta LJ et al. The effect of surgeon volume on outcomes and resource use for vaginal hysterectomy. Obstet Gynecol. 2010;116(6):1341–7. doi:10.1097/AOG.0b013e3181fca8c5.
20. Boyd LR et al. Effect of surgical volume on route of hysterectomy and short-term morbidity. Obstet Gynecol. 2010 Oct;116(4):909–15. doi:10.1097/AOG.0b013e3181f395d9.
21. Burkett D et al. Assessing current trends in resident hysterectomy training. Female Pelvic Med Reconstr Surg. 2011;17(5):210–4. doi:10.1097/SPV.0b013e3182309a22.
22. Kenton K et al. How well are we training residents in female pelvic medicine and reconstructive surgery? Am J Obstet Gynecol. 2008;198(5):567.e1–4. doi:10.1016/j.ajog.2008.01.045. Epub 2008 Mar 20
23. Moen M et al. Considerations to improve the evidence-based use of vaginal hysterectomy in benign gynecology. Obstet Gynecol. 2014;124(3):585–8. doi:10.1097/AOG.0000000000000398.
24. Barbash GI, Glied SA. New technology and health care costs: the case of robot-assisted surgery. N Engl J Med. 2010;363:701–4.
25. Pasic R, Rizzo J, Fang H, et al. Comparing robot-assisted with conventional laparoscopic hysterectomy: Impact on cost and clinical outcomes. J Minim Invasive Gynecol. 2010;6:730–8.
26. Robotic-assisted laparoscopic surgery in benign gynecology. AAGL position statement, American Association of Gynecologic Laparoscopists. J Minim Invasive Gynecol. 2013;20: 2–9.
27. Davaratna S et al. Hospital costs of total vaginal hysterectomy compared with other minimally invasive hysterectomy. Am J Obstet Gynecol. 2014;210(2):120.e1–6. doi:10.1016/j.ajog.2013.09.028. Epub 2013 Sep 20
28. Goebal K, Goldberg JM. Women's preference of cosmetic results after gynecologic surgery. J Minim Invasive Gynecol. 2014;21(1):64–7. doi:10.1016/j.jmig.2013.05.004.
29. Lethaby et al. Total versus subtotal hysterectomy for benign gynaecological conditions. Cochrane Database Syst Rev. 2006;2:CD004993. (Evidence I)
30. AAGL practice report: practice guidelines for laparoscopic subtotal/supracervical hysterectomy(LSH). American Association of Gynecologic Laparoscopists. J Minim Invasive Gynecol. 2014;21(1):9–16. doi: 10.1016/j.jmig.2013.08.001. Epub 2013 Aug 15.

Indications for Salpingectomy

12

Roberta Venturella

Anatomical and Functional Considerations

The uterine tubes (Fallopian Tubes, FT) are two hollow muscle-mucosal organs, about 10–12 cm long, divided into three portions: the intramural, the isthmic and the ampullary ones. This last portion terminates in an enlarged end, called infundibulum, with some protrusions called fimbriae. The ovarian fimbria, in particular, is connected through the meso-salpinx to the ovary. The tubal ostium, laterally, is the site where the tubal canal meets the pelvic cavity, while the uterine opening of the FT is the entrance into the uterine cavity, the utero-tubal junction (Fig. 12.1).

As the cervix and endometrium, also the FT are derived from the müllerian ducts. The wall of the tube has a mucous layer and a muscle one, thicker in the medial part of the tube. The contraction of the muscle bundles allows the tubes having their own peristaltic motility. The mucosal layer is covered with cells, some of which ciliated, that determine a bidirectional internal movement of fluids and cells, both to the uterus and towards the pelvis. The production of cilia on these cells is increased by Estrogens. Scattered between the ciliated cells are secretory cells, which contain apical granules and produce the tubular fluid. The number of these cells is increased by Progesterone, while Estrogens increase their secretory activity. The tubal fluid contains nutrients as lipids and glycogen for spermatozoa, oocytes, and zygotes and also promote capacitation of the sperm.

After ovulation, physiologically, the oocyte is caught by the fimbriated end and travels to the ampulla of the uterine tube where the sperm are met and fertilization occurs. The fertilized ovum, now a zygote, comes towards the uterus thanks to the activity of tubal cilia and muscle. After four to five days the embryo reachs the uterine cavity and on about the sixth day implants on the wall of the fundus of the uterus.

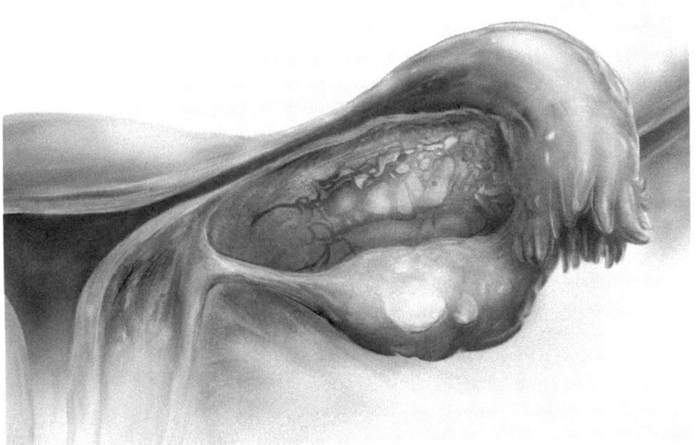

Fig. 12.1 Normal tubal anatomy

Given their bidirectional motility, moreover, the FT are able to let cells, pathogens, blood and substances from the vagina, the cervix and the endometrium to reach the abdomino-pelvic cavity.

Benign Tubal Pathologies as Indication to Salpingectomy

Inflammatory diseases are the most important tubal disorders, due to their frequency and their consequences, sometimes serious [1].

FT indeed, placed between the uterus and ovaries, are frequently infected by one of these two organs. The communication with the peritoneal cavity, moreover, exposes the tube also to any abdominal infection. Appendicitis is a frequent source of descending infection. Rarely, the tubal infection is transmitted by blood, as in the case of tuberculous salpingitis.

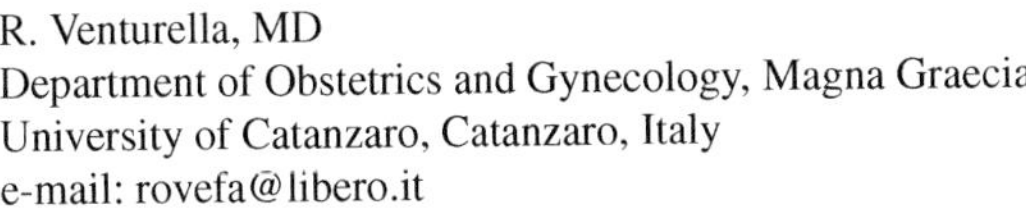

R. Venturella, MD
Department of Obstetrics and Gynecology, Magna Graecia University of Catanzaro, Catanzaro, Italy
e-mail: rovefa@libero.it

I. Alkatout, L. Mettler (eds.), *Hysterectomy*, DOI 10.1007/978-3-319-22497-8_12

More often, the infectious processes ascending from the lower genital tract extend to the tube and reach the peritoneal cavity, leading to Pelvic Inflammatory Disease (PID) [1].

The narrow tubal lumen undergoes important consequences in case of inflammation. The mucosal edema can completely occlude the utero-tubal junction, preventing drainage of inflammatory secretions in the uterine cavity. This causes the onset of acute salpingitis, in which the tube is red, swollen, tortuous, with thickened wall and the lumen filled with pus. The progress of each salpingitis is very slow. Exceptionally acute inflammation can heal spontaneously and the restoration of tubal anatomy and function occurs. Usually, however, the infection becomes chronic and causes permanent tubal occlusion (Fig. 12.2). The tube becomes more dilated, takes the form of a sausage and is filled with pus, leukocytes or plasma-cells (pyosalpinx). The drainage of this infected tube into abdominal cavity can cause the insurgence of peritonitis.

The purulent content may gradually melt turning into a serous or sero-hematic fluid (hydrosalpinx or hematosalpinx). This conditions can remain asymptomatic for a long time, and the diagnosis is often difficult or accidental. When salpingitis becomes chronic, the peritoneal adhesions surrounding the tube and ovaries distort the course of the FT and cause infertility.

In tubal factor infertility, when the cause is bilateral hydrosalpinx, in vitro fertilization (IVF) is now considering the first option rather than attempting to restore tubal function [2]. The hydrosalpinges themselves, however, adversely affect IVF outcomes, reducing the implantation rate and increasing the risk of miscarriage [3]. Among the pathogenic mechanisms proposed, embryotoxic effects, mechanical flushing and changes in endometrial receptivity are the most shared by reproductive gynecologists [3]. The hydrosalpinx fluid, indeed, is able to reach the uterine cavity, in which embryos try to implant, and exerts a toxic effect on this delicate phase of pregnancy.

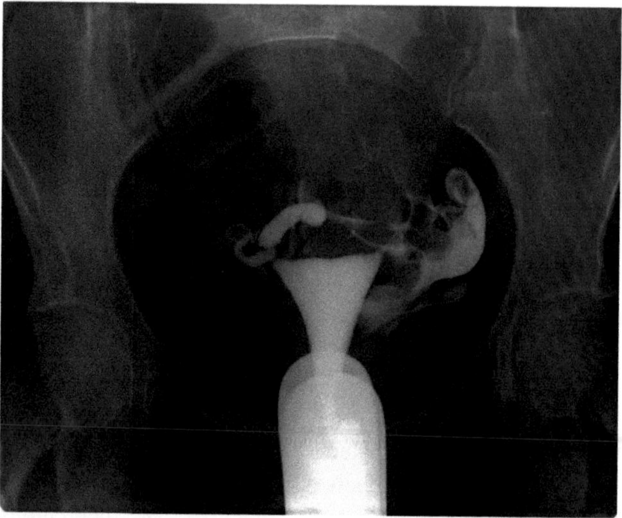

Fig. 12.2 Hysterosalpingografic image suggestive of right hydrosalpinx

Laparoscopic salpingectomy has been demonstrated to be an effective option for avoiding this negative reproductive interference, improving pregnancy rates and removing the risk of PID and ectopic pregnancies. Whenever laparoscopy is not recommended due to the presence of dense pelvic adhesions, hysteroscopic insertion of device seems a very effective option for management of hydrosalpinx before IVF [4].

Recently, a systematic review and meta-analysis of studies comparing the pregnancy outcomes in hydrosalpinx patients treated with salpingectomy versus those treated with proximal tubal occlusion prior to IVF has been published [5]. In this study, comparable responses to controlled ovarian hyperstimulation and pregnancy outcome were observed between groups, demonstrating that salpingectomy does not worsen reproductive prognosis of patients in which excisional surgery is chosen.

Hydrosalpinx is also the most frequent (35.5 %) complication of the blind-ended remnants of the FT in patients undergoing hysterectomy with tubal preservation [6]. Others pathologies that may emerge from retained FT are tube prolapse, torsion, PID, benign and malignant Fallopian Tube tumors.

Other frequent causes of peritoneal adhesions, responsible of anatomical and functional FT alterations, are previous pelvic and abdominal surgeries, especially if performed by laparotomy. Caesarean sections, surgeries for uterine myomas or ovarian cysts, but especially the presence of peritoneal or ovarian endometriosis are well-known risk factors for tubal alterations and occlusion.

Many variables have to be considered when counseling patients with tubal alterations regarding corrective surgery or direct IVF. The chronological and ovarian age of the woman, the site and extent of tubal pathology, the semen analysis of the male partner, the presence of other infertility factors (such as ovarian endometriosis), the experience of the surgeon and the quality and success rate of the referring IVF center are the most important. Given the costs and benefits associated to both surgery and IVF, the ideal candidate for surgical tubal restoration is probably a young woman, with no other infertility factors, a partner with a normal semen analysis and a tubal anatomy amenable to repair. Conversely, patients with extensive omolateral dense peritubal adhesions from endometriosis and/or dilated tubes (>3 cm) with thick fibrotic walls have poor prognosis: in all these cases the tube is usually damaged beyond repair and omolateral salpingectomy is indicated when pregnancy can be achieved by spontaneous attempts. In patients with tubal factor infertility, however, IVF has a higher pregnancy rate per cycle and this information need to be discussed with the patient to provide assistance in her decision making.

The second most frequent benign condition affecting the FT is the ectopic pregnancy (EP). Between 1 and 2 % of live births in developed countries, and as high as 4 % of pregnancies involving assisted reproductive technology [7] are complicated by EP, in which the embryo is implanted outside the uterine cavity.

At least 93 % of ectopic pregnancies are located in a FT (Fig. 12.3) [8]. Of these, 75 % are located in the ampullar portion, 13 % are located in the isthmus, and 12 % in the fimbriae [7] but ectopic implantation can also occur in the cervix, ovaries, and abdomen.

EP can be a life-threatening condition as it is responsible for 6 % of maternal deaths during the first trimester of pregnancy [8].

In a typical tubal pregnancy, the embryo adheres to the lining of the FT and burrows into the tubal wall. Commonly, it invades vessels and causes intratubal bleeding, which may discharges the implanted embryo out of the tube as a tubal abortion. Sometimes this bleeding might be heavy enough to threaten the life of the woman, even if, in developed countries, this event is today luckily rare.

Identified risk factors for EP include: PID, infertility, use of an intrauterine device (IUD), previous exposure to toxicants, tubal or intrauterine surgery (e.g. D&C), smoking, previous EP, and tubal ligation [9].

Fertility following EP is dependent from several factors, the most important of which is a prior history of infertility [10]. The treatment choice seems not to play a great role. A recent randomized study concluded that the rates of intrauterine pregnancy two years after treatment of EP are approximately 64 % with excisional surgery, 67 % with methotrexate, and 70 % with conservative surgery (salpingotomy) [11].

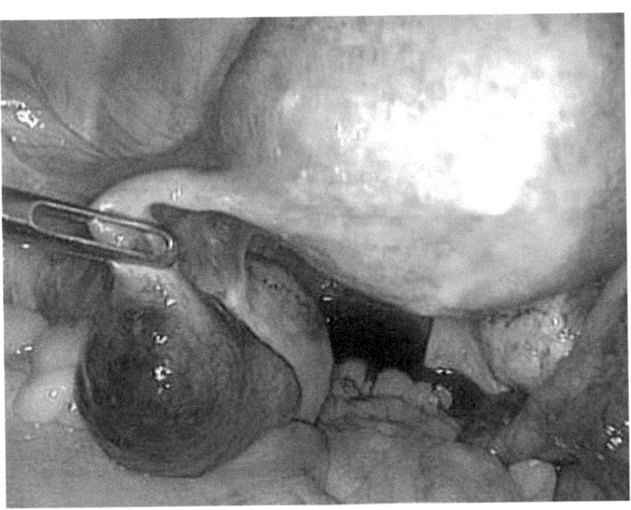

Fig. 12.3 Laparoscopic view of a left tubal ectopic pregnancy

In 2014, in a new open-label, multicentre, international, randomised controlled trial, women aged 18 years and older with a laparoscopically confirmed tubal pregnancy and a healthy contralateral tube were randomly assigned to receive salpingotomy or salpingectomy [12]. In this study, the cumulative ongoing pregnancy rate was 60.7 % after salpingotomy and 56.2 % after salpingectomy (difference not significant between groups). Persistent trophoblast, however, occurred more frequently in the salpingotomy group than in the salpingectomy group (7 % vs < 1 %). Repeat ectopic pregnancy occurred in 8 % of women in the salpingotomy group and 5 % of those in the salpingectomy group. The number of ongoing pregnancies after ovulation induction, intrauterine insemination, or IVF did not differ significantly between the groups.

Meta-analysis of data substantiated the results of the trial so that authors concluded that in women with a tubal EP and a healthy contralateral tube, salpingotomy does not significantly improve fertility prospects compared with salpingectomy.

Malignant and Pre-neoplastic Tubal Pathologies as Indication to Salpingectomy

Historically, primitive tumors of the FT were described as rare [13]. In women with advanced peritoneal carcinoma, the involvement of the ovary usually hides and incorporates the fallopian tube, drawing the attention of surgeons and pathologists and resulting in a diagnosis of ovarian primary carcinoma. In those cases, however, salpingectomy is only a little part of the more radical surgical procedure that is total hysterectomy plus bilateral salpingo-oophorectomy, with pelvic and aortic lymph node dissection when indicated.

Recently, however, morphologic, immune-histochemical and molecular studies [14, 15] have led to the development of a new theory on the pathogenesis of Epithelial Ovarian Carcinomas (EOCs) based on a dualistic model of carcinogenesis [15], which identifies type II neoplasia (high-grade serous (HGSC), high-grade endometrioid, malignant mixed mesodermal tumours and undifferentiated carcinomas) as cancers typically genetically unstable, aggressive and presented in advanced stages [15]. Among these, HGSC is the most common Ovarian Cancer (OC), responsible for the higher death rate among the others types.

Interestingly, the new proposed theory shifts the early events of carcinogenesis to the FT instead of the ovary [15], suggesting that types II tumors derive from the epithelium of the Fallopian tube, whereas clear cell and endometrioid tumors derive from endometrial tissue that migrate to the ovary by retrograde menstruation [14].

These observations have been mainly collected from women carrying BRCA1/2 mutations and undergoing

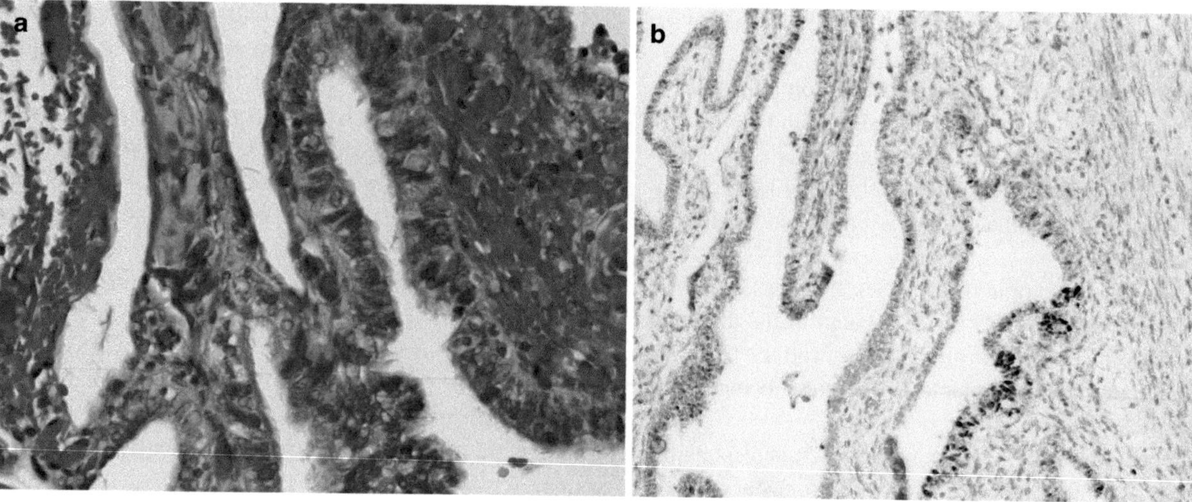

Fig. 12.4 Histologic view of a serous intraepithelial tubal cancer (STIC). In this H&E staining, (**a**) the STIC cells show polymorphic nuclei and a multilayer epithelium, compared with normal tubal epithelium (**b**), in which a distinct transition from normal tubal epithelium to p53 positive STIC (p53 immunohistochemistry) is also shown

prophylactic salpingo-oophorectomy, in which most of the incidentally diagnosed in situ carcinomas or intraepithelial precursors of cancers (STIC) were detected not in the ovary but in the fimbrial end of the FT [16–18] (Fig. 12.4). STIC were also subsequently diagnosed in many women not carrying BRCA mutations, thanks to an extended protocol of pathologic examination of the Fallopian Tubes (SEE-FIM) of patients operated for sporadic HGSC [19–22].

Based on these evidences, prophylactic bilateral salpingectomy (PBS) without ovariectomy has been proposed as a new preventive approach to reduce the risk of sporadic neoplasia [23, 24] in women at population risk of ovarian cancer (i.e. those not carrying BRCA 1/2 mutations) [25], without exposing these patients to the adverse effects of iatrogenic premature menopause.

Even if opinions vary regarding short and long term outcomes of PBS [26, 27], consistent preliminary data demonstrated its safety both in term of ovarian reserve preservation and surgical complication [28, 29]; moreover, several authors have shown a significant reduction in OC risk among women with previous bilateral salpingectomy compared to tubal preservation [30, 31] or unilateral salpingectomy [31].

Therefore, a 2011 position paper by the Society of Gynaecologic Oncology of Canada [25] encouraged physicians to discuss the risks and benefits of PBS at the time of hysterectomy or tubal ligation with women at population risk for OC and this recommendation has been confirmed in 2015 by the American College of Obstetricians and Gynaecologists [32].

The advantage of PBS has been estimated also in term of cost-effectiveness. A recent analysis on PBS (elective salpingectomy at hysterectomy or instead of tubal ligation), showed as salpingectomy with hysterectomy for benign conditions will reduce ovarian cancer risk at acceptable cost and is a cost-effective alternative to tubal ligation for sterilization [33].

Concerning BRCA women, current recommendations include bilateral salpingo- oophorectomy (PBSO) by the age of 40 years or on completion of childbearing to reduce their risk of both ovarian and breast cancers. In these women, indeed, PBS might reduce risk of OC and premature death secondary to cardiovascular disease, but it would not reduce breast cancer risk; conversely, PBSO is able to decrease the risk of OC and breast cancer by approximately 80–90 % and 50 %, respectively.

Permanent Contraception as Indication to Salpingectomy

Surgical sterilization is the most used method worldwide [34] involving 8.1 % of the 15-to 49-year-old married women in developed countries, and 22.3 % of women of reproductive age in less-developed countries [35].

Surgical sterilization it is often achieved by resection (i.e. during a Caesarean section) or laparoscopic coagulation of the isthmic portion of the FT. The remnant segment of the transected tube, however, frequently exhibits histological modifications that let unsuccessful the micro-reanastomotic procedures [36]; the most successful contraception, moreover, is recognized to be obtained by total salpingectomy [37].

For those of women(1–2 %) who revise the previous decision for sterilization for any reason, it was demonstrated that the best method to obtain a pregnancy would be IVF [38], so that bilateral salpingectomy doesn't have any disadvantages

Fig. 12.5 Old and new indication for salpingectomy

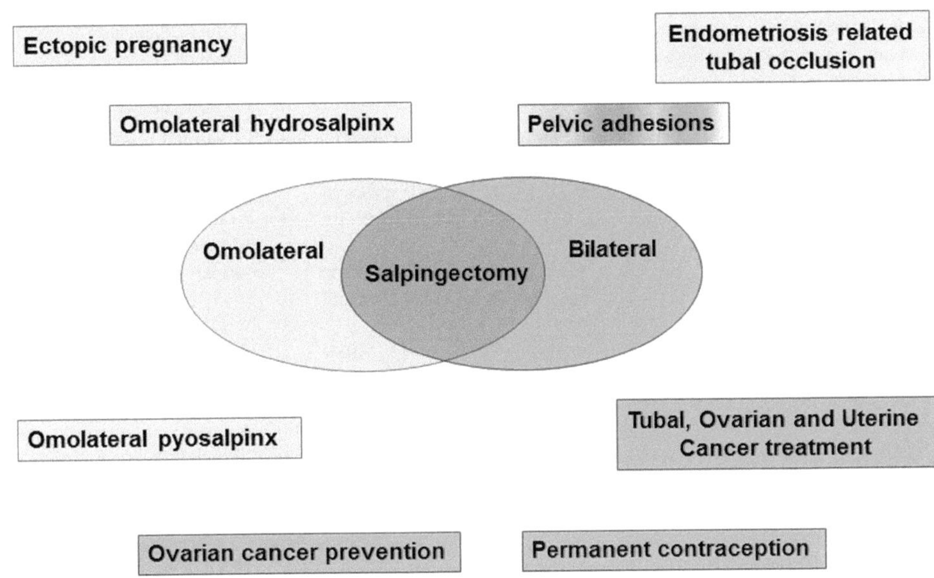

in this population of women, while tubal preservation with subsequent tubal disease, definitively impair the implantation of transferred embryos [39].

Hysteroscopic sterilization was recently introduced as an attempt to provide a less invasive but similarly effective alternative to the abdominal approach. Current methodologies, unfortunately, have limitations that make the procedure less promising than expected [40].

Considering the new theory on OC pathogenesis, even if also tubal ligation seems to reduce the risk of EOC of 33 % both in no-BRCA1 [41] and BRCA1 carriers [42, 43], recent data demonstrated that excisional tubal sterilization confers greater risk reduction (64 %) than other methods [44], thus representing the more advisable sterilization procedure to be adopted in the clinical practice.

Bilateral salpingectomy, indeed, would offer to those women requesting for permanent contraception not only the absolute prevention of intrauterine pregnancies and the almost complete elimination of tubal pregnancies, but also protection against EOCs, further providing the chance to assess, along the years, the efficacy of this risk-reducing procedure [35] (Fig. 12.5).

References

1. RCOG Green-top Guideline No. 32, Management of acute pelvic inflammatory disease. Nov 2008.
2. Johnson N, van Voorst S, Sowter MC, Strandell A, Mol BW. Surgical treatment for tubal disease in women due to undergo in vitro fertilisation. Cochrane Database Syst Rev. 2010:1.
3. Matorras R, Rabanal A, Prieto B, Diez S, Brouard I, Mendoza R, Exposito A. Hysteroscopic hydrosalpinx occlusion with Essure device in IVF patients when salpingectomy or laparoscopy is contraindicated. Eur J Obstet Gynecol Reprod Biol. 2013;169:54–9.
4. D'Arpe S, Franceschetti S, Caccetta J, Pietrangeli D, Muzii L, Panici PB. Management of hydrosalpinx before IVF: a literature review. J Obstet Gynaecol. 2014;1:1–4.
5. Zhang Y, Sun Y, Guo Y, Li TC, Duan H. Salpingectomy and proximal tubal occlusion for hydrosalpinx prior to in vitro fertilization: a meta-analysis of randomized controlled trials. Obstet Gynecol Surv. 2015;70:33–8.
6. Repasy I, Lendvai V, Koppan A, Bodis J, Koppan M. Effect of the removal of the Fallopian tube during hysterectomy on ovarian survival: the orphan ovary syndrome. Eur J Obstet Gynecol Reprod Biol. 2009;144:64–7.
7. Kirk E, Bottomley C, Bourne T. Diagnosing ectopic pregnancy and current concepts in the management of pregnancy of unknown location. Hum Reprod Update. 2014;20:250–61.
8. Crochet JR, Bastian LA, Chireau MV. Does this woman have an ectopic pregnancy?: the rational clinical examination systematic review. JAMA. 2013;309:1722–9.
9. Farquhar CM. Ectopic pregnancy. Lancet. 2005;366:583–91.
10. Tulandi T, Tan SL. Advances in reproductive endocrinology and infertility: current trends and developments. UK: Informa Healthcare; 2002. p. 240.
11. Fernandez H, Capmas P, Lucot JP, Resch B, Panel P, Bouyer J. Fertility after ectopic pregnancy: the DEMETER randomized trial. Hum Reprod. 2013;28:1247–53.
12. Mol F, van Mello NM, Strandell A, Strandell K, Jurkovic D, et al. Salpingotomy versus salpingectomy in women with tubal pregnancy (ESEP study): an open-label, multicentre, randomised controlled trial. Lancet. 2014;383:1483–9.
13. Tone AA, Salvador S, Finlayson SJ, Tinker AV, Kwon JS, Lee CH, et al. The role of the fallopian tube in ovarian cancer. Clin Adv Hematol Oncol. 2012;10:296–306.
14. Kurman RJ, Shih IM. The origin and pathogenesis of epithelial ovarian cancer: a proposed unifying theory. Am J Surg Pathol. 2010;34:433–43.
15. Kurman RJ, Shih IM. Molecular pathogenesis and extraovarian origin of epithelial ovarian cancer–shifting the paradigm. Hum Pathol. 2011;42:918–31.

16. Crum CP, Drapkin R, Kindelberger D, Medeiros F, Miron A, Lee Y. Lessons from BRCA: the tubal fimbria emerges as an origin for pelvic serous cancer. Clin Med Res. 2007;5:35–44.
17. Manchanda R, Abdelraheim A, Johnson M, Rosenthal A, Benjamin E, Brunell C, Burnell M, Side L, Gessler S, Saridogan E, et al. Outcome of risk-reducing salpingo-oophorectomy in BRCA carriers and women of unknown mutation status. BJOG. 2011;118:814–24.
18. Powell CB, Chen LM, McLennan J, Crawford B, Zaloudek C, Rabban JT, et al. Risk-reducing salpingo-oophorectomy (RRSO) in BRCA mutation carriers: experience with a consecutive series of 111 patients using a standardized surgicalpathological protocol. Int J Gynecol Cancer. 2011;21:846–51.
19. Crum CP, McKeon FD, Xian W. BRCA, the oviduct, and the space and time continuum of pelvic serous carcinogenesis. Int J Gynecol Cancer. 2012;22:S29–34.
20. Salvador S, Rempel A, Soslow RA, Gilks B, Hunsman D, Miller D. Chromosomal instability in fallopian tube precursor lesions of serous carcinoma and frequent monoclonality of synchronous ovarian and fallopian tube mucosal serous carcinoma. Gynecol Oncol. 2008;110:408–17.
21. Wiegand KC, Shah SP, Al-Agha OM, Zhao Y, Tse K, Zeng T, et al. ARID1A mutations in endometriosis-associated ovarian carcinomas. N Engl J Med. 2010;363:1532–43.
22. Medeiros F, Muto MG, Lee Y, et al. The tubal fimbria is a preferred site for early adenocarcinoma in women with familial ovarian cancer syndrome. Am J Surg Pathol. 2006;30:230–6.
23. Parker WH, Broder MS, Chang E, Feskanich D, Farquhar C, Liu Z, et al. Ovarian conservation at the time of hysterectomy and long-term health outcomes in the nurses' health study. Obstet Gynecol. 2009;113:1027–37.
24. McAlpine JN, Hanley GE, Woo MM, Tone AA, Rozenberg N, Swenerton KD, et al.; Ovarian Cancer Research Program of British Columbia. Opportunistic salpingectomy: uptake, risks, and complications of a regional initiative for ovarian cancer prevention. Am J Obstet Gynecol 2014;210:471.e1-471.11.
25. The Society of Gynecologic Oncology of Canada. GOC statement regarding salpingectomy and ovarian cancer prevention. Sep 2011.
26. Thiel J. It sounded like a good idea at the time. J Obstet Gynaecol Can. 2012;34:611–2.
27. Tone A, McAlpine J, Finlayson S, Gilks CB, Heywood M, Huntsman D, et al. It sounded like a good idea at the time. J Obstet Gynaecol Can. 2012;34:1127–30.
28. Morelli M, Venturella R, Mocciaro R, Di Cello A, Rania E, Lico D, et al. Prophylactic salpingectomy in premenopausal low-risk women for ovarian cancer: primum non nocere. Gynecol Oncol. 2013;129:448–51.
29. Reade CJ, Finlayson S, McAlpine J, Tone AA, Fung-Kee-Fung M, Ferguson SE. Risk-reducing salpingectomy in Canada: a survey of obstetrician-Gynaecologists. J Obstet Gynaecol Can. 2013;35:627–34.
30. Zhou B, Sun QM, Cong RH, Gu HJ, Tang NP, Yang L, et al. Hormone replacement therapy and ovarian cancer risk: a meta-analysis. Gynecol Oncol. 2008;108:641–51.
31. Falconer H, Yin L, Grönberg H, Altman D. Ovarian cancer risk after salpingectomy: a nationwide population-based study. J Natl Cancer Inst. 2015;27:107.
32. Committee on Gynecologic Practice. ACOG Committee opinion no. 620. Salpingectomy for ovarian cancer prevention. Obstet Gynecol. 2015;125:279–81.
33. Kwon JS, McAlpine JN, Hanley GE, Finlayson SJ, Cohen T, Miller DM, et al. Costs and benefits of opportunistic salpingectomy as an ovarian cancer prevention strategy. Obstet Gynecol. 2015;125:338–45.
34. http://www.un.org/esa/population/publications/contraceptive2005/2005_World_Contraceptive_files/WallChart_WCU2005.pdf.
35. Dietl J, Wischhusen J, Hauslert SFM. The post-reproductive Fallopian tube: better removed? Hum Reprod. 2011;11:2918–24.
36. Stock RJ. Histopathologic changes in fallopian tubes subsequent to sterilization procedures. Int J Gynecol Pathol. 1983;2:13–27.
37. Bartz D, Greenberg JA. Sterilization in the United States. Rev Obstet Gynecol. 2008;1:23–32.
38. Boeckxstaens A, Devroey P, Collins J, et al. Getting pregnant after tubal sterilization: surgical reversal or IVF? Hum Reprod. 2007;22:2660–4.
39. Cakmak H, Taylor HS. Implantation failure: molecular mechanisms and clinical treatment. Hum Reprod Update. 2011;17:242–53.
40. Creinin MD, Zite N. Female tubal sterilization: the time has come to routinely consider removal. Obstet Gynecol. 2014;124:596–9.
41. Cibula D, Widschwendter M, Majek O, Dusek L. Tubal ligation and the risk of ovarian cancer: review and meta-analysis. Hum Reprod Update. 2011;17:55–67.
42. Antoniou AC, Rookus M, Andrieu N, Brohet R, Chang-Claude J, Peock S, et al. Reproductive and hormonal factors, and ovarian cancer risk for BRCA1 and BRCA2 mutation carriers: results from the International BRCA1/2 Carrier Cohort Study. Cancer Epidemiol Biomarkers Prev. 2009;18:601–10.
43. Narod SA, Sun P, Ghadirian P, Lynch H, Isaacs C, Garber J, et al. Tubal ligation and risk of ovarian cancer in carriers of BRCA1 or BRCA2 mutations: a case-control study. Lancet. 2001;357:1467–70.
44. Lessard-Anderson CR, Handlogten KS, Molitor RJ, Dowdy SC, Cliby WA, Weaver AL, et al. Effect of tubal sterilization technique on risk of serous epithelial ovarian and primary peritoneal carcinoma. Gynecol Oncol. 2014;135:423–7.

Indications for Oophorectomy and Adnexectomy

13

William H. Parker

The continued hormonal function of the ovaries after menopause has been well established and the current understanding of the health-related long-term effects of removal of the ovaries has effected a change in the indications for oophorectomy. While adnexectomy is presently indicated for women with an adnexal mass suspicious for cancer, increased risk of ovarian/tubal cancer due to genetic mutations, or for some women with severe symptomatic endometriosis, conservation of the ovaries should be considered for most other women without these conditions.

Benefits of Ovarian Conservation

Prophylactic oophorectomy in order to prevent the subsequent development of ovarian cancer was first proposed in the 1970s. This proposal leads to approximately 250,000 US women having normal ovaries removed at the time of hysterectomy for benign disease every year.

However, endocrine studies first performed in the 1970s and subsequently confirmed, showed that the ovaries continue to produce androgens which are converted to estrone throughout a woman's lifetime [1, 2]. Studies showing the potential benefits of endogenous estrogen exposure on long-term women's health outcomes led to a 2005 Markov model constructed from previously published studies [3]. This model suggested that the health benefits of ovarian conservation outweighed the very small risk of ovarian cancer.

In 2013, an analysis of the Nurses' Health Study cohort examined health outcomes after 28 years of follow-up for 16,873 (56.3 %) women who had a hysterectomy with bilateral oophorectomy for benign disease and 13,113 (43.7 %) women who had a hysterectomy with ovarian conservation [4]. Although oophorectomy was associated with a much lower mortality from ovarian cancer, less than 1 % of the women with ovarian conservation died of ovarian cancer. In contrast, more women who had bilateral oophorectomy died from lung cancer (HR = 1.32), colorectal cancer (HR = 1.56), total cancers (HR = 1.18) and coronary heart disease (HR = 1.26) when compared with women who had ovarian conservation. Importantly, at no age was oophorectomy associated with an increased survival.

Studies from the Mayo Clinic had similar findings ; women who had bilateral oophorectomy before age 45 had a 44 % increased risk of cardiovascular mortality [5]. Other Mayo studies showed higher risks of anxiety/depression, dementia/cognitive impairment and Parkinsonism in women who had their ovaries removed [6]. In addition, after oophorectomy about 90 % of premenopausal women will have vasomotor symptoms and many women will also experience mood changes, a decline in well-being, a decrease in sexual desire, sleep disturbances, and headaches [7, 8]. Additionally, vaginal dryness, painful intercourse, bladder dysfunction, and symptoms of depression may occur [9, 10].

In both the NHS and Mayo studies, these detrimental effects on health outcomes were not seen in women who took estrogen following oophorectomy. Therefore, some gynecologists have suggested that oophorectomy be performed at the time of hysterectomy for benign disease and these women be given prescriptions for menopausal hormone therapy and statins to ward off harmful cardiovascular effects. But studies show that within 5 years of a first prescription, only 17 % of women continue to take estrogen and fewer than 18 % are still taking statins [11]. And, these numbers are overstated since they do not include women who never see a doctor, see a doctor but don't get a prescription or women who get a first prescription but never fill it. Consequently, removing ovaries and prescribing medication to prevent the health consequences is not likely to be effective.

Medical ethics suggests that prophylactic procedures should follow two guidelines: there is a reasonable expectation that the procedure will result in a net benefit to the patient; and, without the intervention the individual would be

W.H. Parker, MD
Obstetrics and Gynecology, UCLA School of Medicine, Santa Monica, CA, USA
e-mail: wparker@ucla.edu

I. Alkatout, L. Mettler (eds.), *Hysterectomy*, DOI 10.1007/978-3-319-22497-8_13

at high risk of developing the disease. Therefore, the evidence suggests that removal of healthy ovaries does not meet the definition of a prophylactic intervention. Therefore, prophylactic oophorectomy, in women at average risk of ovarian cancer, should be approached with caution.

Tubal Cancer and Salpingectomy

Recently, the origin of "epithelial ovarian cancer" has been questioned. Interestingly, the ovary contains no epithelial cells and metaplasia of surface mullerian cells to epithelial cells has been hypothethized to explain the types of epithelial ovarian cancer: serous, mucinous and endometriod. Recently, with careful pathologic analysis of ovaries and tubes removed from BRCA positive women, precursor lesions called serous tubal intra-epithelial cancer (STIC) have been found in the fallopian tubes, but no such precursor lesions have been found in the ovary. STIC lesions have the same p53 mutations found in high-grade serous "ovarian" cancers. The more indolent and treatable Stage I low grade cancers, found rarely inside the ovary do not have these p53 mutations. Astonishingly, the deadly form of ovarian cancer does not come from the ovary; most aggressive "ovarian" cancers are, in fact, tubal cancers [12].

Bilateral salpingectomy has been proposed as an alternative to oophorectomy, as it removes the source of aggressive cancers but conserves functioning ovaries. Interestingly, a recent study found that women having hysterectomy and salpingectomy had similar sonographically measured antral follicle counts, mean ovarian diameters and similar blood levels of AMH and FSH. Therefore, it appears that the ovaries function normally after salpingectomy. Based on all of the evidence, and following the lead of the Society of Gynecologic Oncologists of Canada, the Society of Gynecologic Oncologists recently published practice guidelines suggesting that for women at average risk for ovarian cancer, salpingectomy should be considered at the time of hysterectomy, in lieu of tubal ligation, and also at the time of other pelvic surgery (after completion of childbearing) [13]. This strategy is being closely studied in Canada.

It appears that there is now a convergence of ideas: aggressive "ovarian" cancer appears to be "tubal" cancer and salpingectomy may prevent many of these horrible deaths; oophorectomy has adverse long-term health consequences for women and ovarian conservation should be encouraged.

Oophorectomy Not Indicated for Most Ovarian Cysts

Benign ovarian cysts are a common finding in women. In asymptomatic women aged 25–40, 8 % are found to have ovarian cysts larger than 2.5 cm [1] and a study of women age 50 or older found 18 % had unilocular cysts less than 10 cm. However, most ovarian cysts will resolve, even in post-menopausal women. The University of Kentucky Ovarian Cancer Screening Program monitored 39,337 women with baseline and subsequent transvaginal ultrasonography over 25 years of follow-up [14]. Abnormal sonograms were found in 6807 women (17.3 %) over this time. Ovarian cysts were commonly found: in premenopausal women the prevalence was 34.9 % and the incidence was 15.3 %; in postmenopausal women the prevalence was 17.0 % and the incidence was 8.2 %. For the group having an initial abnormal transvaginal sonogram, 63.2 % resolved on subsequent sonograms. The abnormal findings were classified: unilocular cysts (11.5 %), cysts with septations (9.8 %), cysts with solid areas (7.1 %), and solid masses (1.8 %). Surgery was performed on 557 women with the findings of 472 benign cysts and 85 ovarian malignancies. Serial sonography found that many ovarian abnormalities resolved, even if the initial appearance is complex, solid, or bilateral. Cysts considered low risk for malignancy (unilocular and cysts with septations) had a median time to resolution of 12 months. Interestingly, cysts considered higher risk for malignancy (cysts with solid areas or predominantly solid masses) had a shorter median time to resolution – 2 months. Although many cysts resolved in less than 6–12 months, some cysts took longer and, when documented to be stable, these cysts were then followed on an annual basis. However, after 6–12 weeks, cysts that increased in complexity or size were more likely to be malignant and the authors recommended surgery [15]. Using this strategy of serial sonographic monitoring was associated with a positive predictive value of 25 %. Therefore, the authors recommended avoiding a single sonographic abnormality as the sole indication for surgery and they recommended using serial sonograms to reduce false-positive results and unnecessary surgery.

When evaluating women with an adnexal mass, it is a good idea to view the images yourself. Many radiologists use the descriptive term "complex" to denote any cyst other than entirely clear simple cysts. However, "complex" cysts include many benign etiologies: dermoid cysts, endometriomas, hemorrhagic cysts and cystadenomas. Very young women are at risk for developing germ cell tumors, which may produce BHCG or Alpha feto-protein, so these tumor markers should also be considered. Tumor markers, such as CA-125, are rarely helpful in determining the management of cysts in premenopausal women since the chance of a false positive is about 70 %. Endometriosis, functional cysts, fibroids or adenomyosis, cyclic elevations associated with the menstrual cycle, pelvic infection and pregnancy, all common conditions in premenopausal women, have all been associated with abnormally high CA-125 values. Also, 50 % of women with stage I ovarian cancer will have a negative test. Therefore, this test should be avoided in premenopausal women.

Careful scrutiny of the images and serial sonography will often be indicated and, at times, other imaging studies can often help determine the most likely diagnosis and help guide management. Suspected dermoid cysts can often be confirmed by limited CT scan, when fat (sebaceous material), teeth or bone is seen within the ovary. If a hemorrhagic cyst is present, a follow-up sonogram about two weeks later may show either a smaller cyst or changes in the internal echoes consistent with organizing clot.

One study showed that surgery for adnexal masses found during cancer screening does not decrease the death rate from ovarian cancer and subjects some women to the risks of unnecessary surgery. The Prostate, Lung, Colorectal and Ovarian (PLCO) Cancer Screening Randomized Controlled Trial randomized 78,216 women ages 55–74 to a study group screened with annual CA-125 and transvaginal ultrasonography and a control group who received usual medical care [16]. The women were followed for 11–13 years and managed based on the findings.

In the study group, 212 women were found to have ovarian cancer and 118 women died from ovarian cancer (3.1 per 10,000 person-years); in the usual care group 176 women were found to have ovarian cancer and 100 women died from ovarian cancer (2.6 per 10,000 person-years). The risk of death was statistically no higher in the screened group (mortality RR, 1.18; 95 % CI, 0.82–1.71). However, 3285 women had false-positive screening results and 1080 of these women underwent oophorectomy for the findings. Importantly, 163 of these women (15 %) had at least one serious complication occur as the result of unnecessary surgery for an adnexal mass.

Detorsion Rather than Adnexectomy for Adnexal Torsion

Especially in pre-menopausal women, detorsion of the adnexa even in apparently severely injured ovaries can be accomplished with good recovery of ovarian follicles and hormonal function. The not infrequent black-blue appearance of a torsed adnexa results from venous and lymphatic stasis, but some blood supply continues from the ovarian or uterine artery [17]. Some studies suggest that time from the onset of pain to de-torsion best predicts viability of the ovary. One study found evidence of necrosis on microscopy only after 48 h following the onset of pelvic pain [18]. Eighteen young women, ages 23–35, undergoing in-vitro fertilization and ovarian stimulation, were studied with sonography following detorsion of the adnexa [19]. There was no difference in mean antral follicle counts when the de-torsed ovary was compared with the contra-lateral ovary at 6 months following surgery.

Due to the edema caused by torsion, some authors recommend detorsion of the ovary and postoperative follow-up with serial ultrasounds to determine cyst resolution [20]. Cystectomy at time of detorsion may be difficult due to the edema and loss of tissue planes. Additionally, one study found that in 3 of 4 women treated with cystectomy at the time of de-torsion, loss of ovarian function was found in follow-up sonograms 6 months later [21].

However, if the cyst is not removed, there is risk of re-torsion and need for another operation. One study found higher rates of recurrence among 40 women managed with detorsion or detorsion and cyst aspiration, compared with detorsion with cystectomy or salpingo-oophorectomy [22] Malignancy is present in 2 % of women with adnexal torsion, and oophorectomy should be considered in postmenopausal women. However, in pre- menopausal women, detorsion and ovarian conservation should be strongly considered.

When Adnexectomy Is Warranted

Oophorectomy is indicated when the mass is considered suspicious for a neoplastic lesion. Criteria for suspicious lesions include a high initial morphology index, increasing size or complexity on serial sonography over a 6–12 week time period, or an elevated CA-125 in a postmenopausal woman. The University of Kentucky developed a morphology index (MI) in a cohort of post-menopausal women, which can be helpful in predicting the likelihood of malignancy for ovarian tumors (Fig. 13.1) [15].

The MI calculates a score between 0 and 10, using sonographically determined volume and morphologic complexity, with complexity having twice the weight of volume. A score of 0–4 implies that the cyst is likely benign; 5–10 implies that the cyst is likely malignant. Eighty-five percent of all cancers had a MI score $\geq$ 5. Of the 38,983 women in the study cohort, 472 women had surgery and 74 women were found to have ovarian cancer. The risk of malignancy based on the calculated MI was: MI = 5 (3 %); MI = 6 (3.7 %); MI = 7 (12.6 %); MI = 8 (26.7 %); MI = 9 (27.8 %); and, MI = 10 (33.3 %).

The best predictive values for malignancy were achieved with serial sonographic evaluation at 6–12 week intervals. The mean increase in MI for tumors found to be malignant was 1.6 per month. Women who were found to have benign tumors at surgery had a mean decrease of the MI of −0.3 per month. Tumors that resolved over time had a mean decrease MI of −1.0 compared to tumors subjected to surgery.

This study is very helpful to show that most ovarian tumors, even those with morphologic complexity, resolve over time. However, tumors that have an increase in MI over time should be considered for surgical exploration, oophorectomy, frozen section and surgical staging if malignancy is found.

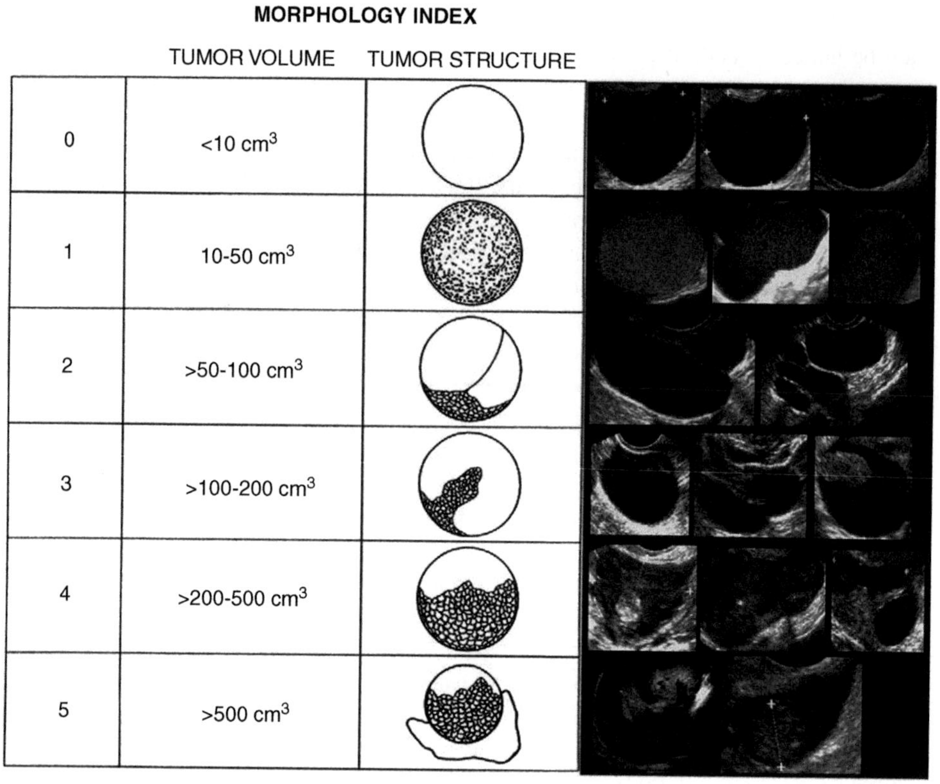

MORPHOLOGY INDEX

	TUMOR VOLUME	TUMOR STRUCTURE
0	<10 cm^3	
1	10-50 cm^3	
2	>50-100 cm^3	
3	>100-200 cm^3	
4	>200-500 cm^3	
5	>500 cm^3	

Fig. 13.1 Morphology index (Reprinted from Elder et al. [15] Copyright 2014, with permission from Elsevier)

Risk-Reducing Adnexectomy for BRCA, Lynch

Women with BRCA 1 have 40 % risk of having ovarian cancer in their lifetime and BRCA 2 confers a 20 % lifetime risk. Women with a BRCA 1 mutation have an increased risk of ovarian/tubal cancer as early as age 35, and 2–3 % of these women will develop ovarian cancer by age 40. The risk of women with the BRCA2 mutation developing ovarian/tubal cancer occurs about one decade later [23]. Women with Lynch Syndrome, especially those with the MSH2 gene, have a lifetime risk of ovarian cancer of 33 % and they also have a 40–60 % risk of developing endometrial cancer.

In a BRCA positive woman, oophorectomy, or more correctly, adnexectomy, reduces the risks of ovarian/tubal cancer to less than 3 %. Current recommendations suggest adnexectomy at the completion of child-bearing or: for BRCA 1, before age 35–40; for BRCA 2, before age 50; for Lynch Syndrome, adnexectomy and hysterectomy before age 40 [24].

Endometriosis and Oophorectomy

For women with severe, symptomatic endometriosis unresponsive to conservative management, bilateral oophorectomy concurrent with hysterectomy may decrease recurrent or persistent symptoms and the need for reoperation [25]. One study of women with symptomatic endometriosis compared outcomes between women who had a hysterectomy with ovarian conservation and women who had a hysterectomy with concurrent bilateral oophorectomy [26]. For the women who had ovarian conservation, 18/29 (62 %) had recurrent pain and 9/29 (31 %) required reoperation. For the women who had both ovaries removed, 11/109 (10 %) had recurrent pain and 4/109 (4 %) required reoperation.

Another study of women with endometriosis found that of the 47 women who had a hysterectomy with ovarian conservation, 9 (19 %) required further surgery over the 7 years of follow-up [27]. Of the 50 women who had a hysterectomy with bilateral oophorectomy, only 4 (8 %) required reoperation. Preservation of both ovaries doubled the risk of reoperation regardless of the patient's age. Nevertheless, given the problems associated with early menopause, the authors recommended that for women younger than 40 years, hysterectomy with ovarian conservation should be considered.

Large Masses

Some women may be symptomatic from larger cysts, or they may not be comfortable with, or available for, close follow-up. For these women, surgery may be indicated. There is some evidence for removal of endometriomas, that ovarian function decreases after removal of cysts >4 cm when compared with cystectomy for cysts smaller than 4 cm [28]. However, a review of the literature found no studies showing loss of ovarian function related to the size of cyst removed. It may be prudent to conserve ovarian tissue even in large cysts clearly thought to be benign.

Summary

Oophorectomy is associated with decreased long-term health outcomes and ovarian conservation should be considered in many woman having pelvic surgery. Salpingectomy may be the procedure of choice for "ovarian/tubal" cancer prophylaxis. Oophorectomy is indicated for women with an adnexal mass that is suspicious for malignancy or for a mass that increases in size or complexity when monitored with serial sonography. Adnexal torsion can usually be treated with detorsion rather than adnexectomy. Oophorectomy decreases the likelihood of repeat surgery in women with severe, symptomatic endometriosis, but ovarian conservation should be considered in those women who are younger than age 40, since conservation avoids early surgical menopause.

References

1. Judd H, Judd G, Lucas W, Yen S. Endocrine function of the postmentopausal ovary: concentration of androgens and estrogens in ovarian and peripheral vein blood. J Clin Endocrinl Metab. 1974;39:1020–4.
2. Fogle R, Stanczyk F, Zhang X, Paulson R. Ovarian androgen production in postmenopausal women. J Clin Endocrinol Metab. 2007;92:3040–3.
3. Parker W, Broder M, Liu Z, Shoupe D, Farquhar C, Berek J. Ovarian conservation at the time of hysterectomy for benign disease. Obstet Gynecol. 2005;106:219–26.
4. Parker WH, Feskanich D, Broder MS, Chang E, Shoupe D, Farquhar CM, Berek JS, Manson JE. Long-term mortality associated with oophorectomy compared with ovarian conservation in the nurses' health study. Obstet Gynecol. 2013;121:709–16.
5. Rocca W, Grossardt B, de Andrade M, Malkasian G, Melton J. Survival patterns after oophorectomy in premenopausal women: a population-based cohort study. Lancet Oncol. 2006;7:821–8.
6. Rocca W, Bower J, Maraganore D, Ahlskog J, Grossardt B, de Andrade M, Melton L. Increased risk of cognitive impairment or dementia in women who underwent oophorectomy before menopause. Neurology. 2007;69:1074–83.
7. Nathorst-Böös J, von Schoultz B, Carlström K. Elective ovarian removal and estrogen replacement therapy–effects on sexual life, psychological well-being and androgen status. J Psychosom Obstet Gynaecol. 1993;14(4):283–93.
8. Elit L, Esplen MJ, Butler K, Narod S. Quality of life and psychosexual adjustment after prophylactic oophorectomy for a family history of ovarian cancer. Fam Cancer. 2001;1(3–4):149–56.
9. Bachmann GA, Nevadunsky NS. Diagnosis and treatment of atrophic vaginitis. Am Fam Physician. 2000;61(10):3090–6.
10. Shifren JL, Avis NE. Surgical menopause: effects on psychological well-being and sexuality. Menopause. 2007;14(3 Pt 2):586–91.
11. Buist DS, Newton KM, Miglioretti DL, Beverly K, Connelly MT, Andrade S, et al. Hormone therapy prescribing patterns in the United States. Obstet Gynecol. 2004;104:1042–50.
12. Kurman RJ, Shih IM. The origin and pathogenesis of epithelial ovarian cancer: a proposed unifying theory. Am J Surg Pathol. 2010;34:433–43.
13. SGO clinical practice statement: salpingectomy for ovarian cancer prevention, November 2013. Available at: https://www.sgo.org/clinical-practice/guidelines/sgo-clinical-practice-statement-salpingectomy-for-ovarian-cancer-prevention. Accessed 3/8/2015.
14. Pavlik EJ, Ueland FR, Miller RW, Ubellacker JM, DeSimone CP, Elder J, Hoff J, Baldwin L, Kryscio RJ, van Nagell Jr JR. Frequency and disposition of ovarian abnormalities followed with serial transvaginal ultrasonography. Obstet Gynecol. 2013;122:210–7.
15. Elder JW, Pavlik EJ, Long A, Miller RW, DeSimone CP, Hoff JT, Ueland WR, Kryscio RJ, van Nagell Jr JR, FR U. Serial ultrasonographic evaluation of ovarian abnormalities with a morphology index. Gynecol Oncol. 2014;135:8–12.
16. SS B, Partridge E, Black A, et al. Effect of screening on ovarian cancer mortality: the Prostate, Lung, Colorectal and Ovarian (PLCO) Cancer Screening Randomized Controlled Trial. JAMA. 2011;305:2295–303.
17. Oelsner G, Shashar D. Adnexal torsion. Clin Obstet Gynecol. 2006;49:459–63.
18. Chen M, Chen CD, Yang YS. Torsion of the previously normal uterine adnexa. Evaluation of the correlation between the pathological changes and the clinical characteristics. Acta Obstet Gynecol Scand. 2001;80:58–61.
19. Bozdag G, Demir B, Calis PT, Zengin D, Dilbaz B. The impact of adnexal torsion on antral follicle count when compared with contralateral ovary. J Minim Invasive Gynecol. 2014;21:632–5.
20. Cohen SB, Wattiez A, Seidman DS, Goldenberg M, Admon D, Mashiach S, Oelsner G. Laparoscopy versus laparotomy for detorsion and sparing of twisted ischemic adnexa. JSLS. 2003;7:295–9.
21. Cohen SB, Oelsner G, Seidman DS, Admon D, Mashiach S, Goldenberg M. Laparoscopic detorsion allows sparing of the twisted ischemic adnexa. J Am Assoc Gynecol Laparosc. 1999;6:139–43.
22. Pansky M, Smorgick N, Herman A, Schneider D, Halperin R. Torsion of normal adnexa in postmenarchal women and risk of recurrence. Obstet Gynecol. 2007;109:355–9.
23. Boyd J, Sonoda Y, Federici MG, et al. Clinicopathologic features of BRCA-linked and sporadic ovarian cancer. JAMA. 2000;283:2260–5.
24. GA MC, EL E. Hereditary cancer syndromes with high risk of endometrial and ovarian cancer: surgical options for personalized care. J Surg Oncol. 2015;111:118–24.
25. Vercellini P, Barbara G, Abbiati A, Somigliana E, Viganò P, Fedele L. Repetitive surgery for recurrent symptomatic endometriosis: what to do? Eur J Obstet Gynecol Reprod Biol. 2009;146:15–21.
26. Namnoum AB, Hickman TN, Goodman SB, Gehlbach DL, Rock JA. Incidence of symptom recurrence after hysterectomy for endometriosis. Fertil Steril. 1995;64(5):898–902.
27. Shakiba K, Bena JF, McGill KM, Minger J, Falcone T. Surgical treatment of endometriosis: a 7-year follow-up on the requirement for further surgery. Obstet Gynecol. 2008;111(6):1285–92.
28. Tang Y, SL C, Chen X, YX H, DS Y, Guo W, HY Z, XH Y. Ovarian damage after laparoscopic endometrioma excision might be related to the size of cyst. Fertil Steril. 2013;100:464–9.

Uterine Sarcomas and Atypical Smooth-Muscle Tumors: Clinic, Diagnostics and Appropriate Surgical Therapy

14

Günter Köhler and Marek T. Zygmunt

Abbreviations

AAGL	American Association of Gynecologic Laparoscopists
AS	Adenosarcoma
BSO	Bilateral salpingo-oophorectomy
CT	Computed tomography
DD	Differential diagnosis
DGGG	Deutsche Gesellschaft für Gynäkologie und Geburtshilfe e. V. (German Society for Gynecology and Obstetrics)
DKSM	Deutsches klinisches Kompetenzzentrum für genitale Sarkome und Mischtumoren (German Clinical Center of Excellence for Genital Sarcomas and Mixed Tumors)
ER	Estrogen receptors
ESN	Endometrial stromal nodule
ESTECLE	Endometrial stromal tumor with sex cord-like elements
GCIG	Gynecologic Cancer InterGroup
HE	Hysterectomy
HR	Hormone receptor
HG-ESS	High-grade endometrial stromal sarcoma
HSC	Hysteroscopy
LG-ESS	Low-grade endometrial stromal sarcoma
LM	Leiomyoma
LMS	Leiomyosarcoma
LN	Lymph node
LNE	Lymphadenectomy
LSC	Laparoscopy
M/10 HPF	Mitoses per 10 high-power fields
MI	Mitotic index
Mo	Months
MRT	Magnetic resonance tomography
NCCN	National Comprehensive Cancer Network
NPV	Negative predictive value
OS	Overall survival
Pat.	Patients
PECom	Perivascular epithelioid cell tumor
RFI	Relapse free interval
PFS	Progression free survival
PPV	Positive predictive value
PR	Progesterone receptor
RI	Resistance index in Doppler sonography
SEER	Surveillance, Epidemiology and End Results
SI	Signal intensity
SO	Sarcomatous overgrowth
STUMP	Smooth muscle tumor of uncertain malignant potential, atypical
T1/T2 W	T1 or T2-weighting in MRT imaging
T1 WC	T1-weighted contrast-MRT
TVS	Transvaginal sonography
TZN	Tumor cell necrosis
UTROSCT	Uterine tumors resembling ovarian sex cord/stromal tumors
UUS	Undifferentiated uterine sarcoma
WOP	Weeks of pregnancy

G. Köhler (✉) • M.T. Zygmunt
Department of Obstetrics and Gynaecology, University Greifswald, Greifswald 17475, Germany
e-mail: koehlerg@uni-greifswald.de

Leiomyosarcoma

Epidemiology, Etiology, Pathogenesis, Staging

In Germany and Norway, LMSs constitute 47 [143] resp. 68 % [2] of all uterine sarcomas. The annual incidence rate is 0.55/100,000 among white women and 0.92/100,000 for black women [283]. In northern Europe, with around 0.4 cases/100,000 women of all age groups, the highest incidence rates could be observed among women aged between 45 and 59 [155]. The median and mean ages of disease onset are 53

I. Alkatout, L. Mettler (eds.), *Hysterectomy*, DOI 10.1007/978-3-319-22497-8_14

Table 14.1 Staging for uterine leiomyosarcomas and stromal sarcomas, according to FIGO and UICC 2009 [291]

TNM	FIGO	Definition
T1	I	Tumor limited to uterus
T1a	IA	Tumor 5 cm or less in largest dimension
T1b	IB	Tumor >5 cm
T2	II	Tumor extends beyond the uterus to the lesser pelvis
T2a	IIA	Adnexal involvement
T2b	IIB	Involvement of other pelvic tissues/structures
T3	III	Tumor invades abdominal tissues
T3a	IIIA	One site
T3b	IIIB	>one site
N1	IIIC	Metastasis to pelvic and/or para-aortic lymph nodes
T4	IVA	Tumor invades bladder and/or rectum
M1	IVB	Distant metastasis

and 54 years, respectively (min. 31, max. 90 years) [143]. Other sources point to a median age of 48–57 years [2, 6, 116, 168, 231, 223, 247]. According to data from the German Clinical Center of Excellence for Genital Sarcomas and Mixed Tumors (Deutsches klinisches Kompetenzzentrum für genitale Sarkome und Mischtumoren, DKSM), 64.9 % of women are postmenopausal and 64.0 % are aged older than 50 [143] (Table 14.8). Only 5 to 13 % of LMSs primarily originate in the cervix, tubal LMS are the exception [23, 124, 143]. Medical histories have increasingly revealed a previous exposure to tamoxifen [298].

LMSs arise primarily in the wall of the uterus. Progression of an LMS from an LM is regarded as the exception, and is in fact widely rejected due to the differing gene expression profiles of LMs and LMSs [230, 290]. On the basis of genetics and morphology, it appears highly probable that a smooth muscle tumor of uncertain malignant potential (STUMP) can progress into an LMS [193, 194]. This is further suggested by the fact that the median and mean ages for STUMPs are 5 years lower [143] and that these tumors can also metastasize as LMS (see subchapter STUMP). LMS-growth is regarded as being estrogen-independent (see also prognostic factors).

New binding FIGO-staging [83, 264] for uterine LMSs and stromal sarcomas was released in 2009 (Table 14.1). Current staging takes tumor size into consideration as well as the fact that LMSs can also primarily develop in the cervix, which need not necessarily imply a higher stage or justify a different course of therapy.

Macroscopical and Microscopical Findings

LMSs are mostly intramural. They initially displace the cavum, then break into it and fill it with tumor masses which can subsequently protrude into the vagina via the cervix. Myometrial invasion can be so comprehensive that the myometrium is only covered by the serosa (Figs. 14.1a–f and 14.3a). It is not uncommon for the serosa to rupture. Tumor size ranges between 0.7 and 30 cm, and in 50 % of cases the tumor is solitary [143]. The presence of multiple "myomas" bears the general risk that an LMS may not be recognized as such. In 94 % of such cases, however, the LMS constitutes the largest "LM" [143]. Gross appearance and the cut surface can be strongly reminiscent of an LM (Fig. 14.2a, b). However, the whorled structure that is typical for LMs is missing in most cases (Figs. 14.3a, b and 14.4a). The tumor usually has a rosy, yellowish or grayish-white, "dirty" color. The macroscopic appearance can be markedly pleomorphous, with numerous haemorrhagia, decomposed greenish-yellowish necrotic tissue, and blood-filled cysts (Figs. 14.1d, 14.3a, b, and 14.4a). What usually results is a noticeably soft consistency. In actual fact, what appear to be "capsules" in fact virtually always consist of compressed tumor tissue (Fig. 14.4a). Thus the margins to surrounding tissue are usually poorly defined. The soft consistency of the tumors and the absence of a capsule frequently result in intraoperative tumor perforations (Fig. 14.4b, c). Accordingly, unlike LMs, LMSs cannot be enucleated or abraded ("shelled-out"). Ultimately, the spectrum of gross macroscopic appearance ranges from myoma-like aspects to almost entirely decomposed tumors. Epithelioid LMSs can barely be differentiated from typical LMSs on gross observation. Myxoid LMSs, by contrast, have a more or less gelatinous, shiny surface (Fig. 14.3a, b).

At the microscopic level, LMSs are categorized into spindle cell, epithelioid, and myxoid types [201]. Spindle cell LMSs are much more common than the other variants. They usually have a high degree of cellularity and consist of intersecting bundles of spindle cells and/or pleomorphic cells with eosinophilic cytoplasm. However, cell count is not relevant when seeking to categorize an LMS as such. Destructive myometrial invasion is common. The presence of vascular invasions is characteristic and can be found in 30–34 % of non-epithelioid and non-myxoid LMSs [2, 61]. The decisive

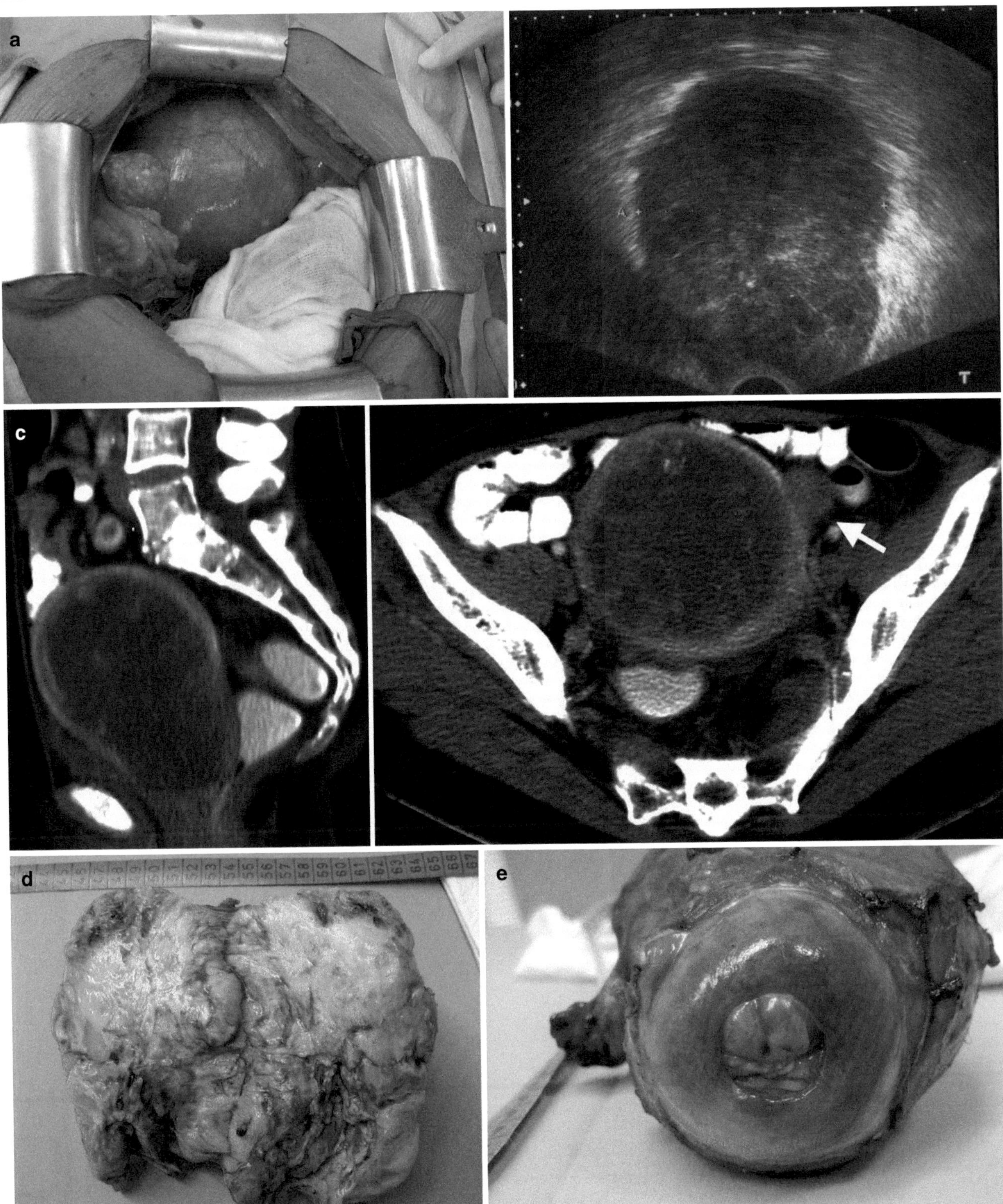

Fig. 14.1 Leiomyosarcoma. (**a**) Looking at the left of the uterine fundus, an LMS has visibly grown into the abdominal cavity, but still remains covered by the serosa; (**b**) in axial sonography, the uterine structures have disappeared and the LMS is practically only surrounded by the serosa; (**c**) both sagittal (*left*) and axial (*right*) CT clearly show that the distinguishability between different tissue layers has been entirely compromised by hypodense tumor masses that are pervaded by enhancing septa. The protrusion of the tumor into the cavity as described under A is clearly visible in the axial CT image (*arrow*); (**d**) macroscopic observation of the opened uterus served to confirm the findings from imaging diagnostics; (**e**) the strong pressure generated by its rapid rate of growth caused the tumor depicted in A–D to protrude through and from the cervix; (**f**) this monstrous cervical LMS appeared to be an LM both clinically and in LSC (With permission of Köhler et al. [145], Fig. 1.2–1a–f)

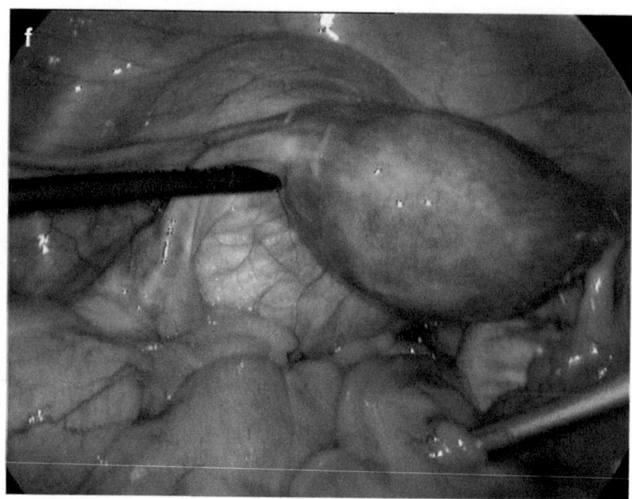

Fig. 14.1 (continued)

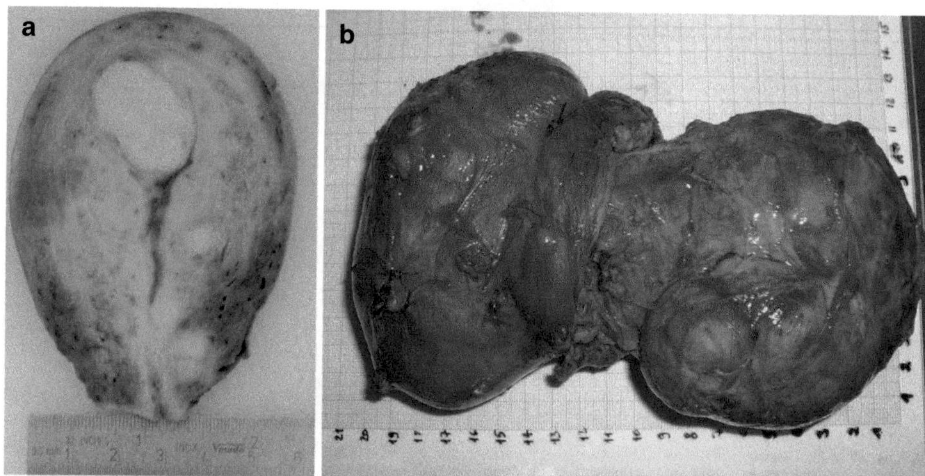

Fig. 14.2 Leiomyosarcoma. (**a**) This LMS, incidentally detected post-operatively following supracervical HE, was the largest of four lesions. The three smaller tumors were ordinary LMs that barely differed from LMS on gross observation; (**b**) even during supracervical HE, this monstrous LMS gave the impression of being an LM (With permission of Köhler et al. [145], Fig. 1.2–2a, b)

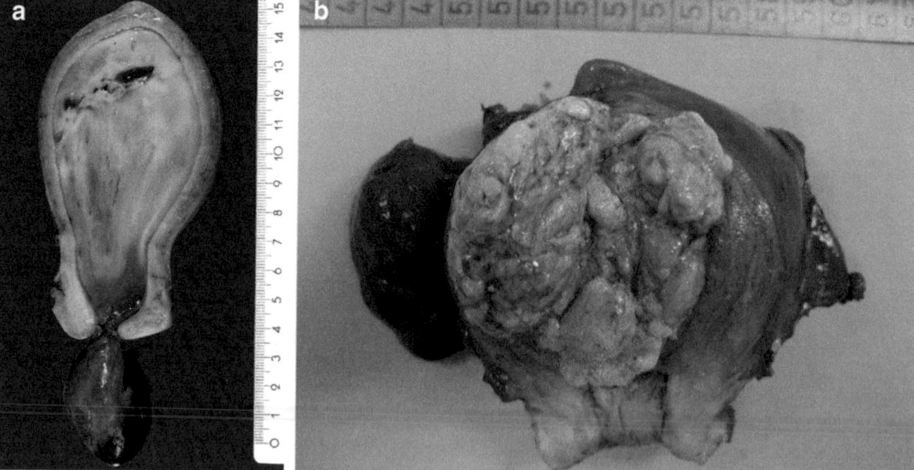

Fig. 14.3 Leiomyosarcoma. (**a**) The very smooth, almost hyaline cut surface, featuring several hemorrhages and cysts, is already a first macroscopic characteristic suggestive of myxoid LMS; (**b**) what is particularly noteworthy about these myxoid LMSs, besides their visible degree of macroscopical pleomorphism, is their hyaline, greasy appearance (With permission of Köhler et al. [145], Fig. 1.2–4a, b)

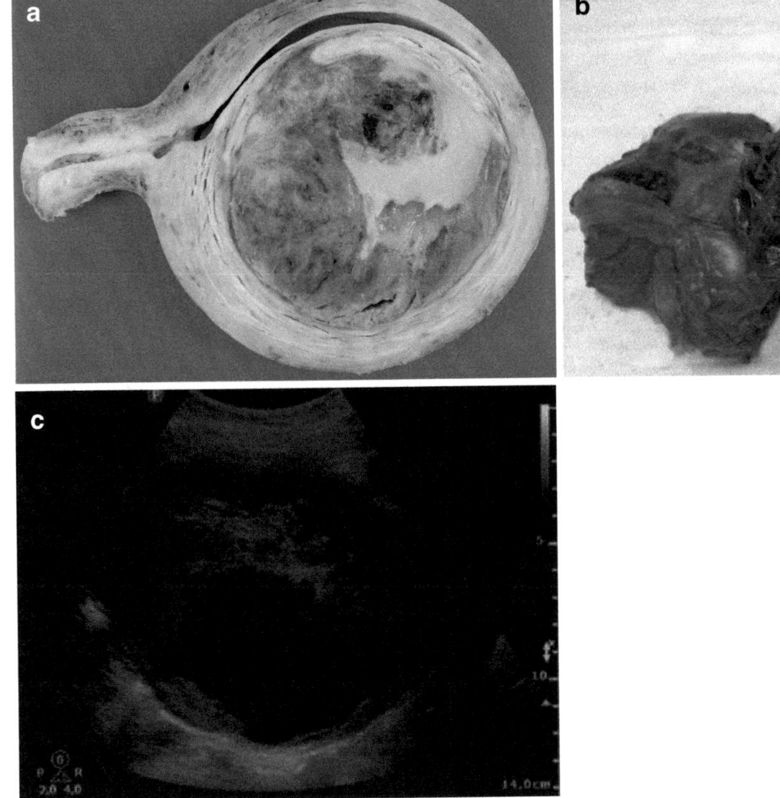

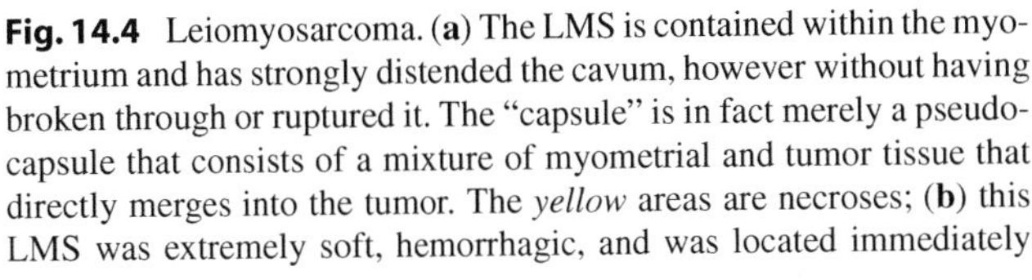

Fig. 14.4 Leiomyosarcoma. (**a**) The LMS is contained within the myometrium and has strongly distended the cavum, however without having broken through or ruptured it. The "capsule" is in fact merely a pseudocapsule that consists of a mixture of myometrial and tumor tissue that directly merges into the tumor. The *yellow* areas are necroses; (**b**) this LMS was extremely soft, hemorrhagic, and was located immediately beneath the serosa. The attempt to lift the uterus from the pelvis by hand was already enough to cause perforation to the tumor; (**c**) sonography of the same tumor clearly shows that the cystic necrotic tumor was covered only by the serosa (With permission of Köhler et al. [145], Fig. 1.2–12, 1.2–2d, e)

3 factors for classifying a lesion as an LMS are: the presence of TCN, mitotic activity, and nuclear and cytologic atypia [28, 57, 207, 282].

TCN (synonyms: geographic or coagulative necrosis) usually occurs multifocally and is characterized by irregular, well-defined margins to surrounding vital tissue. Differentiating TCN from hyaline necrosis, which also frequently occurs in LMSs, can be challenging. Necroses for which such a clear differentiation is not possible are termed uncertain necroses or questionable TCNs.

MI constitutes the second diagnostic pillar and is measured as the mean number of mitoses per 10 HPF. Mitoses usually occur in so-called "hot spots" (i.e. areas with the most mitoses). Only measuring MI in randomly selected areas of the tumor should thus be avoided, a recommendation that can often not be fulfilled when opting for punch biopsy.

Significant diffuse or multifocal moderate-to-severe nuclear and cellular atypia provide the third diagnostic criterion for LMSs. .

In order to come to the diagnosis "LMS", at least 2 of the following characteristics must be fulfilled:

- TCN;
- an MI of ≥10 M/10 HPF (significantly lower in epithelioid and myxoid LMS);
- significant diffuse or multifocal moderate-to-severe atypia.

Where TCNs have been identified beyond doubt and there is any degree of mitotic activity, i. e. any MI, the diagnosis must be LMS, even in the absence of nuclear and cellular atypia. If the typical necroses are absent, then the MI must be ≥10 M/10 HPF and, additionally (!), there must also be diffuse or multifocal moderate-to-severe atypia in order to allow the tumor to be classified as LMS. Even when the diagnosis is already clear on the basis of the necroses and atypia, the MI should nonetheless always be noted so as to be able to determine prognosis according to the overall survival probability prediction tool for LMSs [308].

ER-expression is positive in 63 % of LMS patients, while the PRs are positive in 50 %; 29 % of tumors are negative in terms of both ER and PR-expression [112]. Other sources have measured positive ER and PR-expression in 20–60 % of LMSs. However, receptors were said to be focally localized in the majority of cases [5, 34, 204].

Myogenic markers, such as desmin and H-caldesmon, are normally well-expressed. LMSs show diffuse moderate Ki-67 (or MIB-1) staining and a moderate-to-strong expression of p53 and p16 [50, 61, 213]. The tumor suppressor protein p16 was in fact immunologically substantiated in 100 % of LMSs [50, 190]. The particulars of the very rare epithelioid and myxoid LMSs are described in great detail in the respective specialist literature [145].

No consensually accepted grading for uterine LMSs currently exists. Current UICC-TNM-classification provides no grading for uterine sarcomas [212, 291].

A re-evaluation of LMSs revealed that one third of lesions that had previously been classified as low-grade LMSs were in fact STUMPs [99] (s. a. section on STUMP). In a further study [287], only 31 % of low-grade LMSs actually fulfilled the LMS criteria.

Symptoms, Clinical Presentation, Clinical Diagnostics, Imaging, Differential Diagnosis

Abnormal vaginal bleeding is the most important symptom of LMS, present in 43–53 % of cases. It occurs as abnormal bleeding in form of intermenstrual bleeding and/or heavy, and/or prolonged, and/or irregular and postmenopausal bleeding [143, 168]. Hemorrhaging is observed in 54 % of postmenopausal women [143]. Compared to endometrial carcinoma and AS originating in the endometrium, in LMS and LG-ESS patients, such bleeding only occurs once the tumor has broken into the cavum. Uterine or lower abdominal pains as well as increased urinary urgency without any signs of bladder inflammation have also been observed [143, 168]. Overall, 86 % of patients show symptoms or report complaints of any sort in the course of tumor development. Symptoms that are independent of a patient's menstrual cycle are, in most cases, a result of the high rate of tumor growth. Said growth also causes the cervix to dilate (accompanied by labor-like pains) and tumor masses to protrude out of the cervical canal. An "LM" is particularly suspicious of being sarcoma when the tumor has developed *de novo* or grown during postmenopause, and when such patients' first symptoms or abnormal bleedings occur postmenopausally. Symptoms normally arise relatively late, with the consequence that the tumors have often already grown to a considerable size by the time they are initially diagnosed (see above and Table 14.8).

Continued LM growth or persistently symptomatic LMs within 12 Mo of embolization, high frequency ultrasound therapy, cryoablation, electromyolisis, or treatment with GnRH-analogues are all factors suggestive of an LMS [85, 101, 117, 191, 215, 289]. A lack of regression following embolization and/or the recurrence of vaginal bleeding are first signs for a primary misdiagnosis [43].

Gynecological examination reveals a relatively soft tumor in the majority of cases. This noticeable "softness" is also frequently stated as an intraoperative finding (Tables 14.4 and 14.11). LMSs have median and mean diameters of 8.0 cm and 9.5 cm, respectively [143]. According to other sources, 67–74 % of LMSs are >5 cm and 25–34.3 % are >10 cm in size [2, 234] (s. a. last section). The data from the DKSM [143] are presented in Table 14.8. The true significance of rapid uterine or myometrial growth for properly diagnosing LMSs has long been, and remains, a highly debated issue. One essential facet of this problem is that there are at least four definitions of what actually constitutes "rapid growth" [21, 41, 219, 222]. This overall lack of certainty needs to be borne in mind if one wishes to draw on rapid growth as a factor for discriminating between LMSs and LMs. Ultimately, one will have to rely on the expertise of the attending gynecologist. Rapid uterine growth was observed in 36 % of LMSs in the materials of the DKSM [143]. A recent report states, albeit anecdotally and without providing exact figures, that LMSs are strongly associated with a rapid increase in tumor size [130]. The issue of rapid growth, pertaining in particular to the differentiation between LMSs and LMs, is discussed below under DD.

Performing an HSC in combination with fractional curettage is indicated when patients present with abnormal uterine or postmenopausal bleeding. However, since LMSs remain in the myometrium for a relatively long time, they are correctly recognized as such on the basis of the curettage specimen in only 25 % of cases (i.e. a false-negative rate of 75 %) [143]. Curettage is thus not indicated when there is no abnormal uterine bleeding and where intracavitary sonography yields no suspicious findings – current NCCN-guidelines deem curettage inappropriate in such cases [191]. In postmenopausal patients, or patients who are premenopausal with suspicious clinical and/or sonographic findings, and who complain of uterine bleeding, unsuspicious findings resulting from analysis of curettage tissue specimens should not be blindly trusted or assumed to be correct. Likewise, the results from HSC could lead to an LMS being mistaken for an LM. Dilated, irregular and crossed vessels with diameter fluctuations could be suggestive of a malignancy and thus give rise to performing a deeper hysteroscopical biopsy and/ or more intensive diagnostics.

It often only becomes evident intraoperatively – usually following morcellation – that a removed LM exhibits further unusual or uncharacteristic features, for instance serous or hemorrhagic cysts and/or decomposing or necrotic tissue in the absence of a capsule (Fig. 14.4a–c, Table 14.11).

Diagnoses reached via frozen section are correct in only 19–28 % of cases [251], though it should be pointed out that these data are somewhat dated. The occurrence of mitoses, TCN and atypia in so-called "hot spots" further exacerbates these insecurities. Myomectomies are also known to have yielded misdiagnoses [263]. The difficult DD between benign, semi-malignant and malignant smooth muscle (!) tumors makes pathologico-anatomical diagnostics based on tissue removed via morcellation particularly challenging. The intraoperative findings presented in Table 14.11 however, provide clinicians with important pointers suggestive of a potentially non-ordinary LM.

While there are no specific tumor markers for LMSs, they do produce LDH and its isoenzymes. LDH-levels are known to have been elevated in up to 80 % of LMSs, but also in STUMPs and occasionally in LMs and degenerated LMs [103, 250]. According to DKSM data, even in recurring or metastasized LMSs, the LDH values reach pathological levels in about 50 % of cases [143]. LDH-values are not suitable for screening due to their relatively low sensitivity. Notwithstanding, they can indeed be helpful in the context of differential diagnosis, if clinical assessment and symptoms are unclear or inconclusive and/or imaging reveals suspicious findings [58, 103, 187].

Sonography nearly always reveals findings suggestive of an LMS. What makes sonography so valuable is that it serves to provide results that point to an LMS even when clinical diagnostics do not. Such findings make further diagnostic measures necessary, or at the very least require the therapeutic approach opted for to be re-evaluated. Currently, 47 % of LMSs sonographically present and are subsequently described as unclear tumors (though not LM). A further 30 % appear to be suspicious LMs in sonography, while only 10 % are described as sarcomas [143]. In other sources, 30 % of LMSs are classified as unsuspicious findings following sonography, while 45 % are deemed abnormal [251]. As also applies to morphological diagnostics, in general, the largest mass should always be subjected to particularly close examination. The combination (!) of clear rapid tumor growth between successive sonographic examinations with an age of >45 years or present clinical symptoms is suggestive of a malignant or semi-malignant tumor. Solitary tumors with a diameter of ≥5–8 cm are generally to be suspected to be LMSs (see also flow chart) [143]. LMSs occur as solitary tumors ≥8 cm in 56.5 % of cases, compared to 9.1 % among LMs [143].

Changed echogenicity compared to myometrium is an important factor suggestive of an LMS or a malignant mesenchymal tumor. Furthermore, characteristic sonographic findings include: derounded tumors with, in part, bizarre and poorly defined margins to the myometrium; irregular cystic structures with and without hemorrhagic content; necroses. The septa between the cysts usually differ in thickness. The necroses and/or cystic structures usually have bizarre margins. This also applies to the interfaces between zones of differing echogenicity. In particular, numerous central and peripheral hypoechoic spaces can be observed in the tumor that usually reflect abundant vascularity, but also small cysts and necroses. The vessels can often be identified relatively easily due to their narrow hyperechoic rim. They reflect the presence of central hypervascularity, a typical characteristic of all uterine sarcomas. Tumors are highly suspicious of being malignant if they have ruptured the serosa and protrude through it (Figs. 14.1b, 14.4c, and 14.5c, d). Transvaginal sonography should be supplemented with transabdominal sonography in cases in which the former cannot sufficiently visualize the tumor due to its size.

Suspicious or unclear/ambiguous sonographic findings should be followed up by a Doppler examination, unless a primary total HE is already planned. Doppler- or color Doppler sonography usually reveal elevated levels of peripheral and intratumoral vascularity (Fig. 14.5b) [78, 225]. While LMSs are characterized by irregular or incidental vascularity, in LMs the vessels are predominantly peripheral and in a circular pattern. Vascularization of the septa between the cystic regions is also typical for LMSs [75]. A sensitivity of 88, a specificity of 96 and a PPV of 44 % are achieved when only the presence of marked central vascularity in LMSs is considered. The combination of a solitary intramural lesion, a diameter of >8 cm, central vascularity, and the presence of cystic areas is associated with a specificity of 99 % and a PPV of 57 %, albeit with a low sensitivity of 50 % [75]. Central vascularity can also be absent and thus promote a misdiagnosis as an LM. The RI can provide important information suggestive of sarcoma. The mean RI in cases of LM is 0.58, which is lower than in normal myometrium and in adenomyosis (mean: 0.67). RI in LMSs, with a mean of 0.31, is significantly lower than in LMs [161]. Another study has revealed that the median RIs in LMs (0.59) and LMSs (0.49) do not differ to any degree of statistical significance. The authors, however, go on to state that this could be a consequence of the small number of LMS-cases included in their study [19]. Overall, RI is highest in the myometrium, lower in LMs and at its lowest (relatively) in sarcomas. Setting a cut-off value of 0.4 for the RI is reported as being highly appropriate for distinguishing between benign and malignant lesions, i. e. for diagnosing malignant smooth muscle tumors, with a sensitivity of 90.9 and a specificity of 99.8 % (PPV 71.4 %, NPV 99.96 %) [160, 162, 225]. Applying an RI cut-off value of 0.5 yields a detection rate for LMSs of 67 %, with a false-positive rate of 11.8 % [270]. In principle, it is legitimate to assume that an RI < 0.4 is associated with a malignancy, while an RI > 0.7 is reliably suggestive of a benign condition. Further clarification via

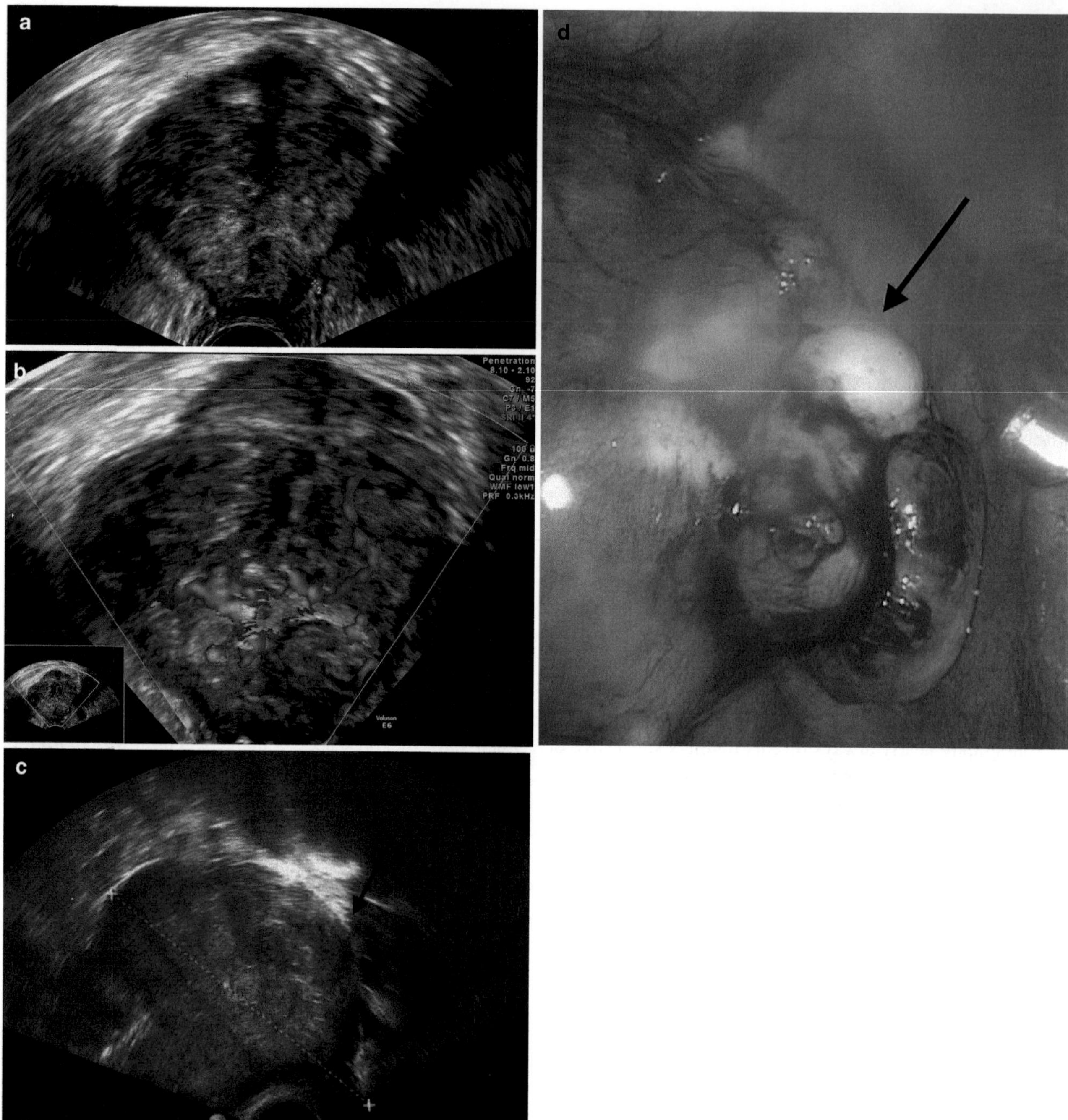

Fig. 14.5 Leiomyosarcoma. (**a**) This ultrasound image bears numerous characteristics that are suggestive of a malignant mesenchymal tumor; (**b**) color Doppler sonography confirmed this suspicion by showing up strong irregular vascularization that in part corresponded to the signal voids; (**c**) tumor with unobtrusively heterogeneous echogenicity that has broken through the serosa in the fundus region; (**d**) endoscopy confirmed that the tumor had broken through the serosa (*arrow*). The visible *yellow* mass was in fact necrotic tissue. The signal voids apparently correspond to the widened atypical vessels that are clearly visible on gross observation (With permission of Köhler et al. [145], Fig. 1.2–8d, e, 1.2–7i, j)

MRT should be sought in doubtful or questionable cases. Typical sonographic characteristics of LMSs are summarized in Table 14.2. The more criteria that are fulfilled, the greater the risk of a malignant mesenchymal tumor or another uterine sarcoma. Even if only one such criterion is fulfilled, diagnostics must be conducted in strict accordance with the flowchart depicted in Fig. 14.22, and/or any planned organ-preserving/sparing surgical procedures or interventional measures should be dispensed with. This equally applies when sonographic findings are unclear or difficult to assess.

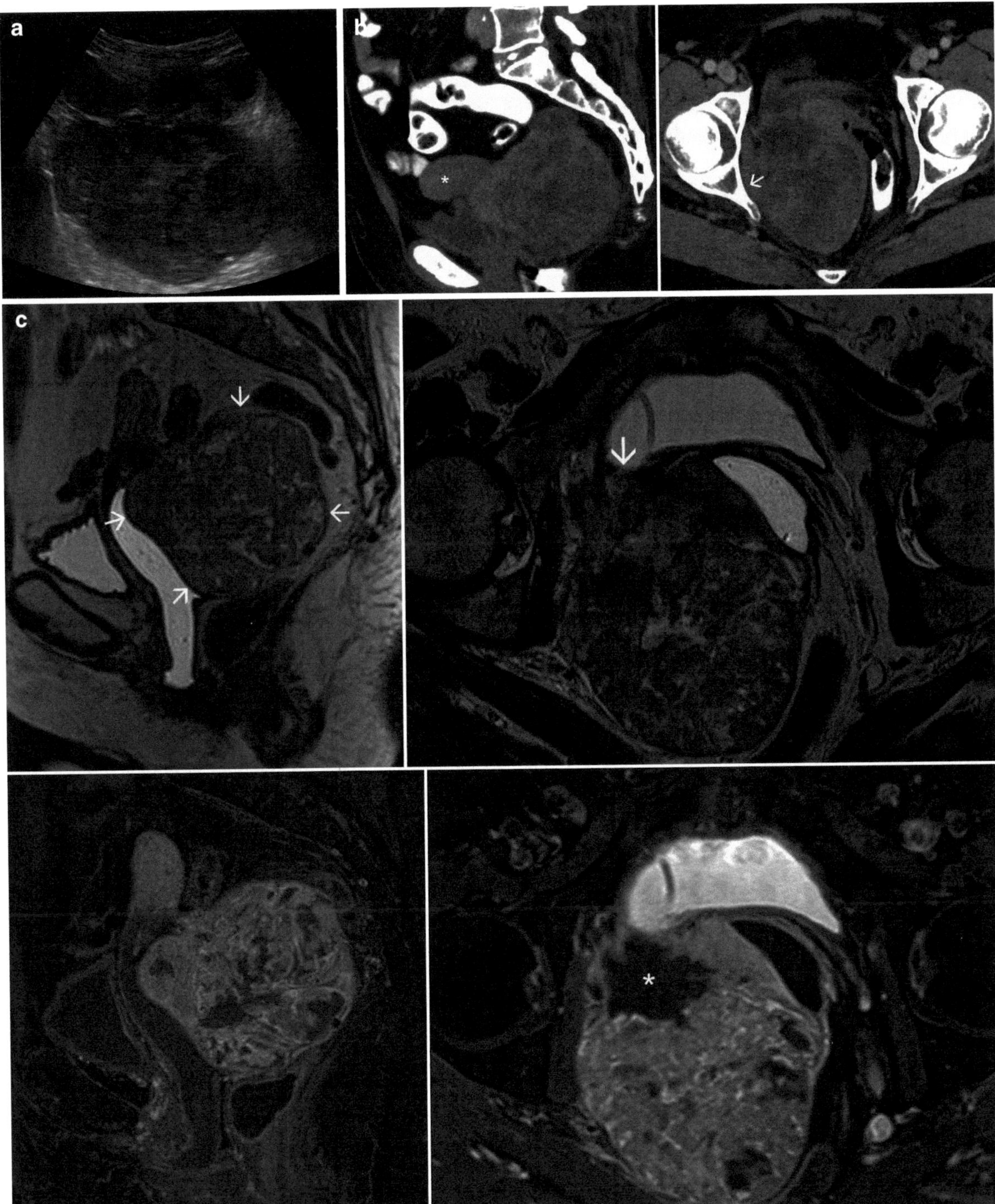

Fig. 14.6 Leiomyosarcoma. Sonographic (**a**), CECT (**b**) and MRT-image (**c**) of a large cervical LMS; (**a**) abdominal sonography shows a tumor with heterogeneous echogenicity that apparently contains numerous necroses with bizarre margins; (**b**) sagittal (*left*) and axial (*right*) CT findings of a large heterogeneously dense tumor in the Douglas that borders the pelvic wall on the patient's right (*arrow*). The corpus uteri (*asterisk*) is anteflected. Most of the hypodense areas are necroses with irregular margins, which corresponds with the findings from sonography and MRI; (**c**) in sagittal and axial T2 W-MRT (*left* and *right*, *top*), the LMS (boundaries marked with *small arrows*) appears as an inhomogeneous hypointense mass that is interspersed with hyperintense areas. A fistula to the bladder (*vertical arrow*) has already developed. Below the *arrow*, a predominantly hyperintense necrosis is recognizable. In sagittal and axial T1 W-MR images (*left* and *right*, *bottom*), upon application of the contrast agent and fat suppression, the LMS shows clearly inhomogeneous enhancement with several non-enhancing tumor necroses (*asterisk*). The latter correspond to the hyperintense mass revealed in T2 W (*top right*) and to the hypodense areas shown in axial CECT (With permission of Köhler et al. [145], Fig. 1.2–10a–c)

Table 14.2 Sonographic characteristics of uterine leiomyosarcomas

Boundaries to the myometrium are poorly defined, derounded, often bizarre or with pointed, tapered extensions
Tumor has clear heterogeneous echogenicity with larger areas of strong hyperechogenicity
Patchy or predominating hypo- to anechoic regions across the entire tumor
Margins between areas of differing echogenicity are derounded, often bizarre or with pointed, tapered extensions
Serosa reached or ruptured
Marked peripheral and irregular central hypervascularity
Central vascularity plus cystic sections plus tumor >8 cm
RI < 0.4

Köhler et al. [145]

Table 14.3 Characteristics of leiomyosarcomas in MRI

T1 W	Tumor with intermediate SI or low (cystic necroses in particular) SI, scattered areas of high SI (hemorrhages in particular)
T2 W	SI primarily intermediate, with heterogeneous hypo- (hemorrhages) and hyperintense SI, some sections with very high SI (necroses, cysts)
T1 WC	Tumor with heterogeneous enhancement
	Weaker enhancement than the homogeneously enhancing myometrium
	Necroses and cysts show no enhancement, often irregular margins

Köhler et al. [145]

Analogous to MRT, determining the LDH-value can be a useful means for further narrowing down the diagnostic options in cases of suspicious sonographic findings as well. It is, therefore, essential that, whenever an LM is suspected, sonography be performed prior to any projected surgical or interventional therapeutic measures – both as a means of preventing inappropriate therapy, and also on grounds of legal certainty.

Expanding imaging diagnostics to include MRT is indicated when sonography and Doppler sonography plus LDH-testing cannot provide sufficient clarification, but organ-sparing surgery and/or morcellation or interventional measures (embolization, high-frequency ultrasound destruction) are planned (see Fig. 14.22). A CT would be inadequate for resolving such issues, but could be a sensible option for determining disease spread when an LMS has been histologically verified (Fig. 14.6b). Taking into consideration that performing an LNE has yet to be scientifically proven as beneficial for almost all types of genital sarcoma, resorting to imaging diagnostics to determine nodal status is generally questionable. One study revealed a sensitivity and specificity of 40–60 % and 80–90 %, respectively, for pelvic LN involvement [296]. The values for para-aortic metastases were 43 % and 91 %, respectively.

MRI (Table 14.3) is better suited than CT for assessing the resectability of locally spread tumors, in particular in relation to neighboring organs, due to its high level of tissue resolution. In terms of LN-involvement, the same statements apply as have already been made regarding CT. 7.5 % of MRT-findings pertaining to LMSs are classified as normal findings, while 30 % are abnormal findings. No clear specification is made for the remaining 62.5 % of LMSs [247].

In T2-weighted MRT images, a high SI, irregular tumor structures, and cystic and necrotic areas (high SI) in combination with ill-defined tumor margins generally are important signs for a malignancy. An SI of >50 % in T2-weighted images together with the mere presence of high SI in T1-weighted MRT images and non-enhancing signal voids in T1 WC are strongly suggestive of a STUMP or an LMS. There have been accounts of LMSs showing homogeneous hypointense SI in T1 W [259, 285]. In T1 WC MRT with gadolinium, LMSs exhibited rapid contrast agent enhancement within 20–90 s, while LMs and the myometrium showed a delayed and gradual enhancement [103]. The necroses and cysts, with their irregular margins, do not enhance (Fig. 14.6c). Degenerated LMs and STUMPs can exhibit similar behavior in MRT [118].

The highest degree of diagnostic accuracy is achieved when there is a combination of the following findings: >50 % high SI on T2 W images plus hyperintense areas on T1 W images and well-defined areas of non-enhancement on T1 WC images [59, 277]. Respective findings also apply to STUMPs, however [277]. Despite the characteristic MRT images with their high specificity, and due to the low sensitivity of all of the findings, no statistically significant objective criteria exist that are associated with the presence or absence of an LMS or a STUMP. Combining the most important criteria [59] with sonography offers a sensitivity of 17–56 % and a specificity of 80–100 % for correctly identifying an LMS, which constitutes a far superior likelihood than can be achieved using purely clinical methods. Performing additional LDH-testing can serve to substantially narrow down the possible diagnoses. Combining MRT findings with elevated LDH-values is said to have a sensitivity of 100 % for diagnosing LMSs. In one study [103], the specificity, PPV, and NPV as well as diagnostic accuracy associated with stand-alone MRI diagnostics were 93.1 %, 52.6 %, 100 % and 93.1 %, respectively. Combining MRI with LDH-testing served to raise all four of these figures to 100 %. It is important to note, however, that, in more than 50 % of LMSs, the LDH-values are within the normal range [143].

Degenerated LMs are the most important diagnostic pitfall, both clinically and in the context of imaging diagnostics. Differentiating between malignant tumors with cystic structures and degenerated LMs is somewhat simplified by the fact that, in the case of the latter, the cysts are located in an otherwise unsuspicious myometrial environment, exceptionally have bizarre margins, and women with degenerated LMs tend to be younger [230]. Cellular LMs can bear marked similarity to LMSs, both in T2 W and T1 WC images [199].

Performing an FDG-PET-CT can be indicated in exceptional cases (f. ex. in the case of an urgent desire to preserve fertility) when uncertain MRT results leave a need for further clarification [70]. PET-CT is said to have a diagnostic accuracy of 100 % when combined with LDH-testing [200]. There is currently no scientific justification for performing primary PET-CT [235].

Currently, the most substantial problem with LMSs lies in the fact that they are frequently not recognized as such, both before and during surgery, and that 51–68 % of LMSs are operated on under the indication of LM [143, 247]. LM is thus the most important and significant DD for LMS. The median age of women with LMs is 35.5 years at the time of initial presentation [38]. Decisively, however, the median age of women at the time at which LM-surgery is indicated is 45 years, according to the results from two DKSM working groups [143]. LMs are thus subjected to surgery 6–8 years earlier than LMSs are. LMs are predominantly associated with cycle-related pains (dysmenorrhea or hypermenorrhea and menorrhagia), while LMS-patients are more likely to complain of cycle-unrelated symptoms. Symptoms like *de novo* urinary urgency without signs of bladder inflammation or sensations of pressure are generally characteristic of larger tumors. Accompanying symptoms are somewhat more common in LMS than in LM patients. These findings notwithstanding, 14–31 % of LMS-patients show no clinical symptoms [143]. For contrast, 4–80 % of women with LMs are symptom-free [64, 199].

LMSs have median and mean diameters of 8.0 cm and 9.5 cm, respectively. A more detailed breakdown reveals that 85.6 % are ≥5 cm, 55.6 % are ≥8 cm, and 38.5 % are ≥10 cm in their largest dimension [143]. By contrast, according to two separate DKSM-analyses, only 55.2 % resp. 16.9 % of LMs have diameters of ≥5 cm to ≥8 cm [143] (Table 14.8). A further study [64] revealed a respective share of 13.5 % for the latter. A tumor size of ≥5 cm, and even more so tumors with a diameter of ≥8 cm, can be regarded as a criterion for differentiating LMSs from LMs.

According to DKSM-data, LMSs occur as solitary tumors in 50 % of cases [143]. Two separate DKSM studies have shown that 40.1 % of LMs are solitary lesions [143]. On its own, the fact that the tumor is solitary is insufficient for safely differentiating an LM from an LMS. When the two differentiation criteria “diameter ≥8 cm” and “solitary tumor” are combined, however, the differences in frequency become more apparent: while 9.1 % of LMs fulfill both criteria, the respective share among LMSs is significantly greater, at 25.5 % [143]. A solitary tumor with a diameter of ≥8 cm should thus be interpreted as being suggestive of LMS. The aforementioned data are considered in the diagnostics flowchart for preventing inappropriate surgery below (Fig. 14.22).

Two DKSM working groups revealed that 13.3 % of ordinary LMs and 26.0 % of LMSs exhibited rapid growth [143]. Other sources have observed rapid growth in up to 31 % of LMs [64]. In one prospective study, 26.7 % of LMs showed volume gains of 30 % within 1 year. In 26 % of those cases, a 30 % increase in volume was observed within just 3 Mo. There were no accounts of an LMS developing in that study. Interestingly, short-term growth spurts were less common or extensive in LMs that had a diameter of 5 cm or more at the time of initial observation [21, 64]. A further DKSM-analysis revealed that 13.3 % of LMs with a diameter of ≥5 cm exhibited rapid growth, compared to 26.0 % of LMSs. In a further prospective study, 34 % of LMs were rapidly growing. The study also revealed that the rapidity of growth declined dramatically as age increased – rapid LM growth in women aged 45 and above was the exception in the study [222]. It is currently contested whether rapid uterus growth in premenopausal women without accompanying symptoms should be regarded as a warning sign [64]. Besides the fact that LMSs exhibit rapid growth twice as frequently as LMs do, the DKSM-results and studies mentioned above [21, 222] also imply, however, that an LMS should be seriously considered in cases in which tumors with an initial diameter of ≥5 cm exhibit rapid growth and/or when there is rapid tumor growth in women aged 45 and above. At least one of the symptoms stated at the beginning of this section was present in 68 % of LMSs that exhibited rapid growth [143]. Reversely, this also implies that 32 % of patients with rapidly growing LMSs do not complain of any symptoms. According to a further study, asymptomatic, rapidly growing LMs up to a size of 16 WOP with and without rapid growth do not require any special measures to be taken – tumors beyond that size should be subjected to more intensive examination [78]. The clinical criteria that can be suggestive of an LMS as well as other uterine sarcomas are presented in Tables 14.4 and 14.8, and are also considered in the diagnostic flowchart (Fig. 14.22) below.

Table 14.4. Risk factors, symptoms, and clinical findings of uterine sarcomas in particular leiomyosarcoma suitable as selection criteria for preventing or excluding inappropriate sarcoma operations under the indication of a leiomyoma

Tamoxifen exposure
Suspicious sonography in particular in combination with elevated LDH-values
Newly occurring or growing "myoma" in women ≥50 years in particular during postmenopause
"Myoma" turns symptomatic postmenopausally (in particular bleeding)
Tumor diameter ≥8 cm in particular in solitary tumors
Myoma growth under medication therapy
Rapid growth from a starting diameter of ≥5 cm and/or with newly arising symptoms and/or aged >45 years
Myoma with abnormal uterine bleeding (beyond menses)
Very soft tumor

Modified from Köhler et al. [145]

Determining the GDF-15 factor and the unspecific N/L--ratio can be helpful in diagnostically differentiating an LMS from an LM [141, 284].

Both during and after surgery, an LMS need not necessarily be macroscopically discernible as such from other LMs alongside which it has developed. In 94.4 % of cases in which LMSs and LMs occur simultaneously, the former constitutes the largest lesion [143], the soft consistency of which is usually another factor strongly suggestive of it being an LMS. LMs are relatively solid and rough, and show a whorled structure on the cut surface. They have well-defined margins compared to LMSs and a discernible pseudo-capsule is present, out of which they can normally be easily enucleated.

STUMPs constitute the biggest challenge for DD at the histological level. They are difficult to discern – clinically, pathoanatomically and in imaging – from both LMSs and LMs. TCN, MI, and atypia are the pivotal histologic differentiation criteria. The particularities in this regard are discussed in the section on STUMPs. For more detail pertaining to histological appearance in the context of DD, reference should be had to the specialist literature [144]. The same applies to information on the diagnostic differentiation of LMSs from PEComs (perivascular epithelioid cell tumors) [152].

If the results from all imaging and laboratory-chemical options as well as curettage and HSC (where necessary due to abnormal uterine bleeding) provide no clarification, and the patient insists on a conservative strategy, a transcervical punch biopsy can be performed under ultrasound guidance. Experiences with this approach have been surprisingly positive. In one study, transcervical punch biopsies were taken from 453 women whose tumors were LMS-suspicious (high SI in T1/2 W MRT and/or high LDH-values and/or rapidly growing tumor with threefold gain in volume within 1 year) [135]. Among 372 eligible cases, only 7 sarcomas were found. In no case in which histologic examination revealed no suspicious findings (atypia, mitoses, TCN, infiltrations, vascular invasions, epithelioid or myxoid components) was an LMS subsequently revealed in the further course. Examinations performed on 312 women showed that a transcervical punch biopsy under ultrasound guidance is in fact less burdensome for/on patients than curettage [136]. Nonetheless, false-negative results need to be reckoned with, for spindle-cell sarcomas in particular [96]. One reason for this is because mitoses, atypia, and necroses can in fact be concentrated in so-called "hot spots". There is a real risk of missing these hot spots using punch biopsy, so that, essentially, only positive findings can be truly relied on. There are reports that measuring the CD34 and Ki-67 indexes can serve to minimize that risk [300]. The authors defined a case as positive when the measured Ki-67 index was ≥ 15 % [300]. Nonetheless, the Ki-67 index does not constitute a histological criterion for correctly diagnosing an LMS as such (!) (see section on STUMP). Due to the stated problems, biopsy should not be performed at the time of definitive surgery. The described problems and pitfalls notwithstanding, in a further study, the results from performing sonography-assisted trans- or intraabdominal needle biopsies (18-gauge needle) on suspicious lesions with high SI in T2-weighted images were greatly beneficial. Malignant tumors were found in 12 of 63 cases (19 %) (11 LMSs, one LG-ESS). Among the remaining 81 % (n = 51) that were classed as benign, surgery revealed only one LG-ESS. The other 50 lesions were LMs, 27 of which were surgically removed. The remaining 23 tumors exhibited no signs of malignancy in a median follow-up period of 32 Mo. The results are a specificity of 100 % and a sensitivity of 91.7 %, with positive and negative predictive values of 100 and 96.2 %, respectively [276]. The positive morphological results notwithstanding, the risks associated with intraabdominal (!) biopsy suffice to regard the procedure as a counter-indication. The high growth-related pressure within the tumor, that, in turn, is thus frequently pressed up against the serosa (Fig. 14.1a–d), can cause tumor cells to ooze out of the puncture point and subsequently disseminate within the abdominal cavity. Furthermore, tumor perforation cannot be ruled out (Fig. 14.4b, c). These risks are knowingly condoned when intraperitoneal biopsy is performed, and can be avoided by instead opting for a transcervical punch biopsy.

Clinical Course and Prognostic Factors Relevant to Therapy

With reference to the current staging system, median OS for stages I, II, III and IV is 75, 66, 34 and 20 Mo, respectively [232], while mean OS is 45.2, 28.1, 37.6 and 34.3 Mo, respectively [176].

Disease stage is regarded as the most significant prognostic factor, independent of patient age [6, 93]. 42.6–55 % of patients have stage I disease, 4–4.3 % have stage II, 11–12.1 % have stage III, and 30–40.9 % have stage IV disease at initial presentation [232, 233]. Tumor size is also a strong independent prognostic factor in multivariate analysis [2, 95, 232]. According to recent data, stage I disease has a 3 and 5 year OS of 64 % and 38 %, respectively, while OS remains stable at around 30 % in patients with stage II–IV disease. The median time to recurrence is 19.7 Mo across all stages [93].

An MI beyond 20 M/10 HPF is related to a significantly shorter RFI [182]. For instance, 5-year OS for patients with an MI of 6–10 is 60 %, and 23 % for an MI of >20/10 HPF [2]. More recent findings suggest that, in multivariate analysis, an MI of 12 M/10 HPF and above is already significantly associated with a higher rate of recurrence [93]. Ki-67 expression is said to have no influence on recurrence, i. e. it is of no predictive value [93].

Overall, the following pathoanatomical characteristics are said to be associated with poorer survival: size ≥5 cm, unclear gross margins, an MI of >20 M/10 HPF, epithelioid or myxoid components, extensive TCNs, diffuse severe atypia, lymphatic invasion, p53 positivity, and an absence of ER and PR-expression [57].

Most recent analyses suggest that the number of M/10 HPF alone (<25 vs. ≥25 M/10 HPF) constitutes the most important predictive factor for OS [233]. MI and tumor size as well as patient age and the presence of extrauterine spread are the most important factors in calculating prognostic scores according to Zivanovic [308]. The lymphocyte/monocyte ratio, a new independent prognostic variable for soft tissue sarcomas, including LMSs, is significantly associated with RFI and tumor-specific OS in both uni- and multivariate analyses. Preoperative values < 2.85 are associated with an inferior prognosis [271].

LMSs predominantly metastasize hematogenously, while lymphogenous spread plays only a subordinate role. LMSs have a propensity to metastasize to the lungs (65 %) and the liver (23 %) [233]. Overall, 56 % of disease recurrences involved hematogenous metastases, while pelvic metastases were found in only 7 % of cases [182]. According to other sources, up to 31 % of recurrences are solely distant metastases; 73 % are distant metastases plus pelvic recurrences [89].

Metastases to the ovaries occur in only 3.5 % of cases of stage I disease [187], and are almost always observed in connection with further extrauterine spread [57, 100, 168]. At the time of primary diagnosis, no metastases could be found in the ovaries of 202 DKSM-cases of LMSs of all stages [143]. It has yet to be proven that not performing a BSO has a negative impact on prognosis [106]. According to a case-control study [98] and a SEER-analysis [134], whether the ovaries are removed or left during premenopause has no effect on prognosis. A further study has shown that performing a BSO in fact has negative effects on disease-specific survival [95, 98]. This is in line with data that suggest that patients aged up to 55 years have a more promising prognosis than older women [95, 123], and that OS progressively worsens from age 55 onwards [6]. Other studies suggest that ER and PR-expression are not correlated with patient age, stage of disease, vascular invasion, and relapse rate, and have no influence on PFI and OS [33, 61, 93].

In a SEER-analysis, all lymph node-positive patients had stage IIIB or stage IV disease [134]. Nodal positivity was observed in 6.6 % of stage I–IV cases; positive LNs without extrauterine spread were observed in only 3.5 % [168, 182]. In a sample of 884 LMSs of all stages, positive LNs were found in only 3.3 % of cases. Similarly, nodal involvement was found in only 4 % of all LMS-cases included in the DKSM material database [143]. In all of these cases, positive LNs were accompanied by simultaneous extrauterine involvement. Positive LNs were not found in any of the cases of cervical LMS [24]. Accordingly, it has yet to be proven that performing an LNE has beneficial effects on RFI and OS [4, 60, 134, 154, 156]. This is in line with the findings that the number of distant metastases clearly exceeds the number of pelvic recurrences, that LN-involvement is usually accompanied by other extrauterine spread, and that recurrences are common despite patients being lymph node-negative.

The increased demand for conservative modes of treatment has been accompanied by parallel rise in the frequency of reports of surgical procedures being performed that are inadequate/inappropriate for LMSs [1, 87, 117, 201, 215, 226, 289]. An analysis of retroperitoneal sarcomas, including LMSs, identified R1/R2 resections and tumor ruptures as significant independent predictors for worsened OS [37]. These data can be regarded as surrogate evidence for the negative impact of tumor injury occurring in the course of surgical procedures that are inappropriate for uterine sarcomas. A negative impact on patient prognosis should always be expected whenever an LMS is subjected to morcellation [72, 223]. First studies have shown that morcellation only results in a slight increase in the rate of disease recurrence without any measurable impact on OS [197]. Three further studies have revealed a significantly shorter RFI for LMS and LG-ESS patients subjected to morcellation, as well as shorter OS among LMS patients, even though the women were younger and the tumors were smaller than in women who underwent appropriate surgery [97, 199, 217, 225, 254]. A recent analysis compared the effects of morcellation and total abdominal HE on patient prognosis [97]. The study revealed a four-fold reduction in RFI when morcellation was performed (10.9 vs. 39.6 Mo for total abdominal HE) accompanied by a doubling of mortality risk. Endoscopic follow-up examinations of LG-ESS, STUMP and LMS patients who underwent morcellation revealed intraperitoneal tumor dissemination in 64 % of cases that occurred within 3 Mo in 43 % of cases, and that had not been present at the time of primary surgery. Follow-ups on 2 LMS patients originally subjected to conservative morcellation revealed that extensive metastasization had occurred within one Mo [104]. 75 % of LMS patients in whom there was peritoneal dissemination following morcellation succumbed to their disease within 8.4–40.3 Mo [210, 254]. The causal connection between morcellation and a shorter RFI is further supported by the fact that, in these cases, locoregional and intraabdominal recurrences were considerably more frequent than in LMS-patients who underwent appropriate surgical procedures [188, 217]. A recent meta-analysis covering morcellated vs. non-morcellated LMSs revealed an odds-ratio of 3.16 for all recurrences, 4.11 for intraabdominal recurrences and 2.42 for the death rate. The cumulative extraabdominal relapse rate was not elevated [35]. The higher relapse risk associated with endoscopic morcellation [217] might be due to changes in pathophysiological conditions during LSC. Experimental studies appear to be supportive of this assumption [221]. Another reason is seen in the use of electric morcellators during LSC that apparently propel tumor cells into the abdominal cavity [68, 247]. That would certainly help to explain why tumor cell dissemination seems to occur less frequently when a scalpel or other cutting instrument is used during open surgery. At 0.16–1.18 %, the very low rate of port-site metastases for endoscopic gynecologic carcinoma surgery [179, 185, 307] thus does not necessarily speak against there being an elevated risk of recurrence in performing endoscopic morcellation or the enucleation of sarcomas. What is more, intraperitoneal tumor implants cannot be equated to port-site metastases and, overall, sarcomas and carcinomas behave differently in general. However, the risk of port-site metastases is nonetheless regarded as also being elevated in cases of gynecologic high-risk neoplasms. In such cases, robot-assisted LSC should be avoided [179]. In the meantime, the AAGL and the FDA have issued warnings against using electric morcellators [1, 80].

Besides morcellation, tumor injury and positive surgical margins <1 mm are further independent risk factors that have been significantly associated with local disease recurrence and poorer OS. According to one study [292], local recurrence was in fact 5.6-fold more likely. For these reasons, tumor enucleation, too, is to be viewed critically from a prognostic perspective. There is generally no indication for performing tumor enucleation on LMS patients [74]. LMSs have no capsule, or rather appear to have a pseudo-capsule consisting of compressed tumor tissue, making it inevitable that only R1 (or at least RX) resection margins can be achieved. A recent study revealed a significant RFI-reduction compared to total abdominal HE (8.2 Mo for myomectomies, vs. 46.6 Mo for total abdominal HE) [130].

There is the risk that intravascular or myometrial infiltrations remain in the uterine stump following laparoscopic and abdominal supracervical HEs. Therefore, from a clinical perspective, even when R0-resection margins have been described, an RX-situation should always be assumed. Early disease recurrences within 3 Mo of such operations have been reported [14]. The situation appears to be similar when the uterus is injured with a sharp instrument. In fact, supracervical HE and other uterus disruptions resulted in a 2.8-fold increase in mortality-risk with simultaneous decreases in RFI and OS [223]. In the DKSM-sample, the rate of relapse after inappropriate operations (any form of tumor and uterus injury) is 28.3 %, compared to 27.7 % among patients subjected to appropriate surgical procedures. It needs to be noted, though, that the women who underwent appropriate surgery (n = 101), with a mean age of 55 years and an average tumor diameter of 9 cm, had a poorer primary prognosis than the patients who were subjected to inadequate surgical procedures (mean age of 47 years, tumor diameter of 6.5 cm) [143].

Two studies [246, 260] have shown that death due to LMS was more common in endoscopic HE with morcellation versus open abdominal HE. However, estimated overall (!) deaths were lower in the former. The authors state that the risk of LMS morcellation is balanced by complications that are associated with laparotomy, including death. Better quality of life and lower costs were further highlighted as advantages of endoscopic procedures. Such statements interfere with efforts to avoid inadequate LMS surgery, and to improve diagnostics for these tumors.

Surgical Therapy and Problems

The prognostic data unambiguously show that uterine sarcomas have to be resected in a manner that doubtlessly leaves R0 resection margins and that causes no injury to the tumor whatsoever. What this implies for uterine LMSs is that such tumors have to be removed together with their compartment "uterus" without injuring or damaging it. Total HE without injuring the uterus is thus to be regarded as the standard surgical procedure for LMSs, too [113, 172]. There is no indication for a primarily vaginal approach due to the risk of causing injury to the uterus that this procedure entails, as well as the lack of possibilities for exploring the abdominal cavity. When opting for laparoscopically assisted vaginal HE or total endoscopic HE, neither the tumor nor the uterus are allowed to sustain injury. There are no data to confirm that performing such surgeries without injuring the uterus leads to less-promising results than would be achieved via open surgery. Intrauterine manipulators should not be used when endoscopic procedures are performed. In the USA and in Germany, 89.4 resp. 64 % of LMS patients undergo total abdominal or total laparoscopic HE [143, 233]. Since supracervical HEs always go hand in hand with injuries to the uterus (potential opening of microscopic invasion routes), they must be classified as inappropriate operations, not least because – as endoscopic procedures – they are virtually always performed in connection with morcellation. The prognostic consequences that could potentially result have been described in the subsection on prognosis. According to the current NCCN-guidelines, the GCIG consensus, the AAGL-recommendations, and the position paper of the German Society for Gynecology and Obstetrics (Deutsche Gesellschaft für Gynäkologie und Geburtshilfe, DGGG), morcellation should always be avoided when an LMS is suspected [1, 27, 113, 202].

Due to the impact that tumor and uterus injuries have on prognosis [204, 217, 223], intraabdominal *in vivo* excisional and punch biopsies as well as tumor enucleation (see prognosis) should not be performed when an LMS is suspected.

Based on the prognostic analyses (see prognosis), there is no indication for performing a BSO on LMSs that are confined to the uterus when the ovaries are unsuspicious from a clinical standpoint. Likewise, a BSO is not necessary according to the ESMO-guidelines [74]. The NCCN-guidelines and the current GCIG consensus [113, 202] state that a BSO can be performed on an individualized, i.e. case-specific basis, bearing in mind the age of the patient. The AAGL [1] recommends a BSO for premenopausal women who do not wish to preserve fertility, albeit without providing any scientific justification. The Japanese guidelines, too, do not back up their recommendation to perform a BSO with any scientific evidence [201]. Whether or not a BSO is indicated is thus dependent on the will of the patient, her menopausal status and the surgical conditions. Overall, in Germany, a BSO is performed on 67 % of LMS patients [143], in the USA this applies to 99.2 % [233]. The fact that at least 50 % of LMS-patients are postmenopausal could also help, at least in part, to explain the high frequency to which BSOs are performed.

According to the current NCCN-, ESMO- and Japanese guidelines as well as the GCIG-consensus, an LNE is not routinely necessary [74, 113, 201]. This takes into consideration that, currently, it has yet to be proven that performing an LNE would have any effect on RFI and OS (see also prognosis) [4, 60, 95, 134, 154, 156]. Furthermore, whether the LNs test positively or negatively does not allow for any further therapeutic consequences to be deduced. There has thus yet been no indication for routinely performing systematic and selective LNEs on patients with LMSs for some time now [91, 134]. Nor is an LNE recommended for cervical LMSs [24]. It remains unproven whether performing a selective LNE on enlarged or suspicious nodes offers any benefits [113], but such course of action can nonetheless be taken according to the GCIG-consensus [113]. Regional LNE does not fall within the surgical spectrum envisaged for retroperitoneal soft tissue sarcomas and LMSs [37, 85, 106]. Nonetheless, LNE in some form is performed in 27–30 % of LMS patients [143, 231, 233].

Omentectomy is not indicated unless there is omental disease involvement [202]. In the DKSM materials, omentectomies accounted for 13 % of 158 LMS-operations, and omental involvement was identified in 15.2 % of those cases. However, in all of those cases, said involvement was accompanied by other extrauterine spread [143]. Cytological smear testing of the abdominal cavity has no implications for therapy, as the resulting findings have not yet been proven to be of prognostic significance.

The poor overall prognosis (!) and the aforementioned risks (see prognosis) associated with certain surgical methods and procedures serve as a counter-indication against performing tumor extirpation on lesions that have been identified as LMSs. The RX-resection as the overriding problem with which tumor extirpation mostly because of the missing capsule (Fig. 14.4a–c) is associated cannot be remedied by using an extraction bag. The same applies to morcellating the tumor inside an extraction bag. A critical review of the literature reveals that a significant share of the conservative operations that resulted in favorable outcomes was in fact performed on so-called low-grade LMSs, that are in fact mainly classified as STUMPs nowadays [170, 248]. The promising courses and outcomes thus need to be treated and interpreted with caution. Should identified LMSs nonetheless be subjected to tumor extirpation in absolutely exceptional cases, the tumor should be no larger than 5 cm and R0 resection margins must be achieved without doubt. Overall, subjecting an LMS to conservative surgery is currently regarded as an inappropriate measure [91]. Should a patient who has been correctly diagnosed with an LMS wish to preserve her fertility and thus insist on conservative surgery, she must be insistently informed that such surgery will further worsen an already very poor overall prognosis, and follow-up LSC (see below) as well as total HE once the desire for fertility-preservation ceases (i.e. upon child birth) should be urgently recommended.

For the risks associated with incidentally inappropriate surgery, see the final section below.

If an LMS is diagnosed post-operatively following conservative primary surgical procedures, including supracervical HE, the residual uterus/cervix as well as all tumor masses should be fully resected in any case [1, 27, 202], notwithstanding that having undergone inappropriate primary surgery will have already increased the risk of recurrence. The possibility of residual tumors remaining in the uterus and/or its lymphatic vessels is the primary motivation behind this course of action. In one study, 15 % of re-operated patients were upstaged [72]. Drawing on the experiences reported by the DKSM and more recent literature [143, 210], in these cases, the tumor stage was not primarily incorrectly assessed – rather, new tumor residuals or occurrences had arisen/developed. In a total of 12 DKSM-cases involving LMSs and LG-ESSs, metastases that had previously not been detectable were identified in the 2–4 weeks following primary surgery [143]. It is thus urgently recommended that patients who undergo morcellations or "myoma enucleations" be subjected to endoscopic follow-up or re-operation/completion surgery within 3 to 6 Mo [202, 210, 254]. The AAGL, too, recommends re-operation or LSC as means for follow-up, and to remove any suspicious tissue [1]. Where the aforementioned measures are not performed, following-up via imaging techniques is strongly advised [177, 202].

The surgical management of advanced LMSs applies to all LMSs that have spread beyond the uterus. Locally advanced LMSs are predominantly accompanied by dissemination to the abdominal cavity. Simultaneous distant metastasization, in particular to the lungs, is also common. If the LMS is confined to the pelvis or the abdominal cavity, and no distant metastatic disease is present, then maximal debulking should be aspired to. Aggressive cytoreduction can apparently serve to prolong survival even when only R1-resection margins have been achieved [66]. It is also possible to perform intra- and extraperitoneal interventions (the latter in the lung in particular) when conditions are favorable [169]. Absence of clinical post-operative residual disease was associated with a significantly improved RFI as well as improved OS. While the benefits for OS were not statistically significant, the median OS in such cases was still a remarkable 31.9 Mo [169]. Currently, in light of the few applicable chemotherapeutic agents available, and their poor response rates and very short PFIs, subjecting patients with advanced disease to remedial surgery should be the therapeutic strategy of choice. Accordingly, the current NCCN-guidelines and the GCIG-consensus [113, 202] both strongly prioritize the surgical resection of all metastases, depending on their resectability and the extent of disease. Where metastasization is extensive, a palliative HE is always indicated if uterine bleeding cannot be controlled by other means [113].

Follow-up and aftercare should entail gynecological and general examinations that are clinically guided by the presenting symptoms. Follow-up examinations should be conducted every 3 Mo for the first 2 years, every 6 Mo in the following 3 years, and every 12 Mo thereafter. The current NCCN-guidelines make a 2A–recommendation to consider running a CT on the thorax, the abdomen, and the pelvis at these follow-up examinations. MRI or PET and further diagnostic procedures should be reserved for when there are suspicious findings or when patients show clinical symptoms [202]. It remains unclear, however, what course of action should be taken when imaging diagnostics yield positive findings in symptom-free patients. Benefits for survival resulting from complex laboratory-chemical and instrument examinations have yet to be scientifically substantiated. Clinical examination should always be combined with vaginal sonography, and abdominal sonography where deemed necessary. This applies in particular to cases in which patients have undergone primary surgical procedures that are associated with increased risk of locoregional disease recurrence.

There are no indications for adjuvant or postoperative chemo- and/or radiation therapy. More detailed information, including data pertaining to the therapeutic approach for metastases, should be taken from the specialist literature [145].

Atypical Smooth Muscle Tumors (Smooth Muscle Tumors with Uncertain Malignant Potential, STUMP)

Epidemiology, Etiology, Pathogenesis

The term "atypical smooth muscle tumor" has come to be increasingly used in place of the term STUMP. Current WHO-classification [212] defines a STUMP as a smooth muscle tumor with characteristics that clearly preclude a diagnosis as an LMS, while at the same time not fulfilling the criteria for being classified as an LM or one of its variants. The common characteristic of these heterogeneous tumors (that are too rare to be able to definitively predict their behavior) is their metastatic potential, which is very low, and much lower than that of an LMS. The current nomenclature "atypical smooth muscle tumor" includes such tumors that had previously been termed 'atypical LM'.

STUMPs are observed in women with a mean age of 35 to 42 years, in an age range from 25 to 77 years [227, 277]. According to DKSM data, the median and mean ages are 46 and 44.9 years, respectively [143]. Thus, they occur roughly 7–9 years earlier than LMSs and can consequently be regarded as a kind of precursor or forerunner. In clear contrast to LMSs, only 20 % of women with STUMPs are postmenopausal and 28 % are ≥ 50 years old. Calculations conducted by two DKSM working groups revealed in summary that STUMPs account for 0.153 % (6 of 3920, 1:653) women who underwent any form of LM surgery (*14334*). Atypical LMs differ from LMs in that they can have proven chromosome-p1-deletions, which are suggestive of an independent etiology [53].

Macroscopic and Microscopic Appearance

According to DKSM data, STUMPs have median and mean diameters of 6 resp. 6.8 cm [143]. STUMPs are occasionally observed side by side with LMSs [164]. Cutting open the surgical specimen often reveals macroscopic characteristics that differ from those of ordinary LMs, for instance the absence of the whorled structure, and a more fleshy gross appearance. Necroses, hemorrhages and cystic sections can be present (Fig. 14.7a, b). It sometimes occurs that final diagnosis as a STUMP is only reached upon specimen re-examination on the occasion of a patient presenting with disease recurrence.

The histological criteria for categorizing an atypical smooth muscle tumor as such are the MI, the presence of cellular and nuclear atypia, and an absence of clear TCN (s. section on LMS). The lack of unambiguous TCN is the most important histological difference to an LMS. TCN needs to be distinguished from so-called hyaline (infarct-like) necrosis, which occurs relatively frequently in normal LMs as a spontaneous regression phenomenon. Necroses that cannot be reliably categorized as either TCN or hyaline necrosis are termed questionable or uncertain necroses, and constitute an important criterion for diagnostically classifying a STUMP as such.

According to the current WHO-classification [212], lesions are to be classified as atypical smooth muscle tumors or STUMPs if they fulfill the following histological characteristics [28, 57, 119, 120, 121, 212]:

- MI of > 15 M/10 HPF without TCNs and without atypia,
- focal/multifocal moderate to severe atypia with an MI of 3–5 M/10 HPF,
- diffuse moderate to severe atypia with an MI of 2–9 M/10 HPF,
- uncertain necroses or isolated/sporadic TCNs without mitoses and without atypia.

Opinion is divided on TCN in this context. While some hold the view that only uncertain necroses are eligible as a criterion [181, 207], others state that it is also sufficient if there are isolated/sporadic necroses coupled with no more than a low MI and mild atypia [62, 212]. The presence of multiple TCNs that have been reliably identified as such, however, is a criterion that clearly points towards LMS. Histologically, around 20 % of STUMPs exhibit hyaline necroses [181]. Hyaline necroses and areas of edema showed more frequently in atypical LMs treated prior with hormonal therapy. Microscopic examination demonstrated that 46 of 51 cases had pushing margins, i.e. margins penetrating the myometrium [181].

In one study, 100 % of atypical LMs exhibited strong PR-expression, and 10 of 13 tumors had moderate to strong ER-expression [269]. In other studies, ER and PR-expression tested positive in around 50 resp. 70–100 % of cases [34, 192, 305]. Measured ER-expression levels closely resemble those of LMSs and differ significantly from levels found in ordinary LMs. By contrast, PR expression is significantly higher than is the case in LMSs. These findings underline the special position that STUMP holds between LM and LMS, and serve to clarify the importance

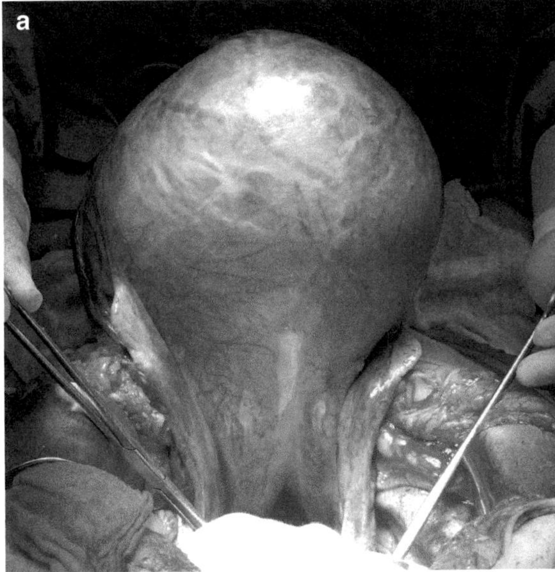

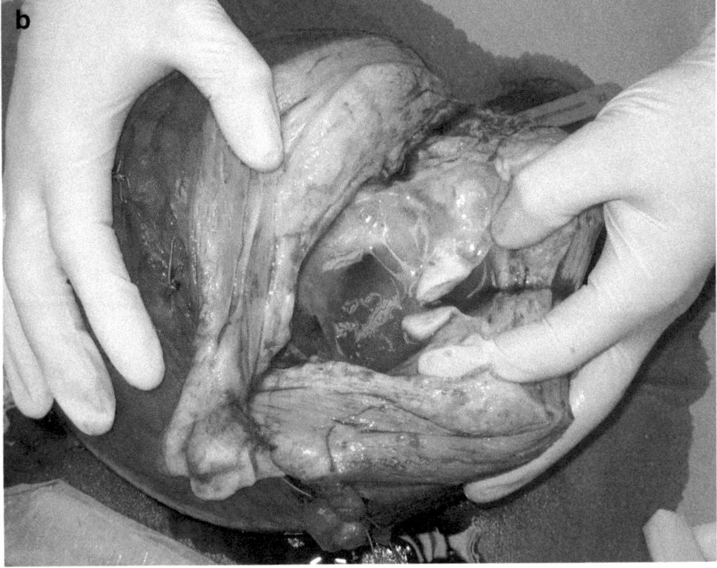

Fig. 14.7 Atypical smooth-muscle tumor (STUMP). AB: this 52 y.o. patient is a prime example for the fact that these tumors have often already grown to quite a size at the time of primary diagnosis. Compared to ordinary LMs, they are usually softer, less fascicular, and often inhomogeneously colored. Additional gelatinous components and cystic structures are not uncommon. (With permission of Köhler et al. [144], Fig. 1.1–15a, b)

of PR-expression as a factor for differentiating a STUMP from an LMS.

The Ki67-index of atypical LMs fluctuates between 0 and 25 % (mean 2 %). Since LMSs have a Ki67-index of between 6 and 50 % (mean: 25 %), said index can only be used with caution as a means for differentiating between LM and LMS. 84.6 resp. 38.5 % of atypical LMs show a strong immune reaction to p16 and p53 [269]. A further study [50] revealed a mediate-to-strong diffuse p16 staining pattern in 100 % of LMSs and STUMPs (WHO-classification pre-2014). STUMPs with diffuse p16 staining and TCN should be classified as LMSs [18, 142]. Diffuse p16 and/or p53 staining is regarded as the most important indicator for an increased risk of recurrence [57]. Overall, drawing a line and differentiating between STUMPs and LMSs is remarkably difficult. For more detailed information, also on the extremely rare myxoid and epithelioid STUMPs, reference should be had to the specialist literature [144].

Symptoms, Clinical Presentation, Diagnostics, Imaging, Differential Diagnosis

The symptomatology associated with STUMPs largely corresponds to that of ordinary LMs, and also that of LMSs, featuring heavy menstrual and prolonged bleeding, menorrhagia, dysmenorrhea, and premenstrual pains. The same can be said of their clinical presentation. STUMPs often exhibit a rapid rate of growth, in young women in particular [143]. Postmenopausal LM-growth points to a STUMP or an LMS. Lack of remission following treatment with GnRH-analogues or UPA, or continued LM-growth, are also suspicious. On palpation, STUMPs often feel softer than ordinary LMs, a finding that is reported almost without exception in surgery reports [143]. During surgery in which the tumor remains *in situ* or is not cut open, the differences to ordinary LMs are often only implied, or are not even visible and discernible at all. In opened tumors, however, hemorrhaging, gross necroses, or cystic areas are not uncommon. When in doubt, a frozen section can be performed. However, such practice can often not provide definitive clarification if not accompanied by immunohistochemical testing. The problems and difficulties that frozen section procedures entail are referred to in the chapters on LMS and LG-ESS. What can be said at this point is that frozen section procedures should only be performed on fully excised tumors (excisional biopsy), since otherwise, as with morcellation, tumor cell conveyance is virtually unavoidable.

STUMPs have a polymorphic sonographic appearance that can be similar to that of ordinary/degenerated LMs and LMSs. Heterogeneous echogenicity and the presence of anechoic regions, in the form of cysts and necroses that are usually an expression of cystic degeneration or hyaline necroses, could be suggestive of a STUMP (Fig. 14.8a) [180]. Narrow anechogenic areas usually correspond to dilated vessels. STUMPs thus cannot be differentiated from ordinary, degenerated and cellular LMs or from LMSs solely on the basis of cystic structures being present. However, the presence of bizarre margins between the individual echogenic and anechoic regions constitutes an important criterion for differentiating STUMPs from LMs. Doppler sonography reveals that STUMPs have a significantly higher degree of central vascularity than both cellular LMs and ordinary LMs (Fig. 14.8b) [75]. STUMPs have an RI between those of

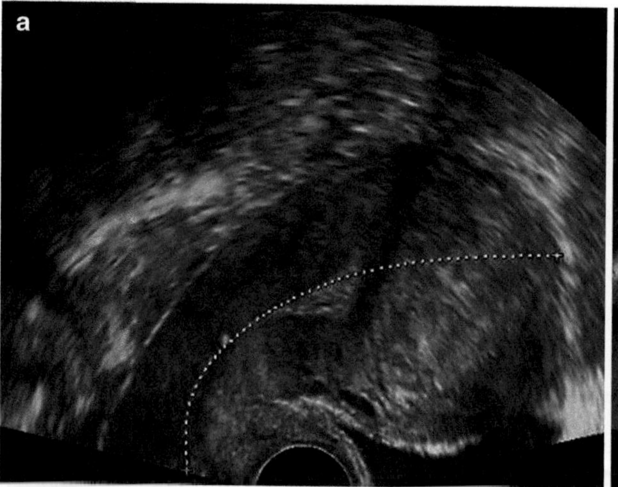

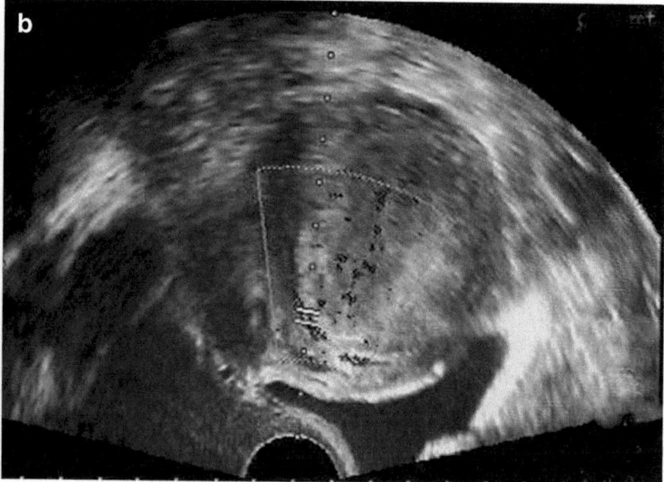

Fig. 14.8 Atypical smooth-muscle tumor (STUMP). (**a**) Closer observation of this predominantly hyperechoic tumor shows margins between the different echogenicities that are bizarre in part. The anechoic voids just above the bladder, with their hyperechoic margins, correspond to dilated vessels, as confirmed in Doppler sonography (B); (**b**) color Doppler sonography of the same tumor also reveals the tumor's central but weak vascularization that in turn speaks less likely for an LMS. The RI of 0.58 lies between those of ordinary LMs and LMSs (With permission of Köhler et al. [144], Fig. 1.1–18a, b)

Table 14.5 Variants of leiomyomas and smooth muscle tumors of uncertain malignant potential

Variant	Tumor cell necroses	Mitotic rate/10 HPF	Atypia or other criteria
Cellular leiomyoma[a]	Missing	<4	Missing or light, but cellular
Leiomyoma with bizarre nuclei	Missing	Missing or low	Bizarre cells and nuclei diffuse p16 and/or p53 staining possible [2]
Mitotically active leiomyoma	Missing	≥ 5 (10) and ≤ 15	Missing
Atypical smooth muscle tumor (STUMP [4])	Few present or questionable [3]	none	None
	Missing	>15	Missing
	Missing	3–5	Moderate to severe, focal or multifocal
	Missing	2–9	Moderate to severe, diffuse

Modified from Köhler et al. [144]

[a]Particularly when chromosome p1-deletions are positive, cellular leiomyomas exhibit the prognostic behavior of STUMPs [2], classification as STUMP when there is diffuse p16 and/or p53 staining [3], when hyaline necroses and TCN cannot be clearly discerned from one another [4], elevated risk of recurrence for all STUMPs in case of diffuse p16 and p53 expression

LMs and LMSs in most cases (0.4–0.7). More detailed particularities are described in the chapter on LMSs.

CT does not allow for a specific diagnosis to be reached. As is also the case with LMs, for STUMPs, in many cases T2 W MRI reveals a homogeneous hypointense mass [257, 277]. Differentiation from an ordinary LM is not possible in such cases. However, as is the case with LMS, T2 Ws can also reveal hyperintense tumor sections or cysts. The non-enhancing cystic regions and necroses within the enhancing tumor are easily discernible in T1 WC images. A clear differentiation from an LMS is often not possible [257, 277]. Despite remaining uncertainties, the probability of identifying an LMS or a STUMP is very high (with an accuracy of 87 %, a sensitivity of 72.7 %, and a specificity of 100 %), if >50 % of the tumor has a high SI in T2 W images, smaller sections have a high SI in T1 W images, and several non-enhancing pockets are recognizable in T1 WC images.

In terms of DD, the greatest histological challenges are posed by cases that are borderline between STUMP and LMS. Due to the frequent localization of mitoses, atypia, and necroses in so-called 'hot spots', results from frozen section examinations that are suggestive of a STUMP are to be deemed uncertain unless there is a clear and unambiguous LMS-diagnosis. Moreover, MI is elevated during progestin therapy and pregnancy. The pathologist must be provided with such information where present, so as to prevent false diagnoses that otherwise have been avoidable. Analyzing mast cell count in the tumor can be helpful for differentiating between a STUMP and an LMS. Mast cell counts are significantly lower in LMSs than in cellular and atypical LMs [214, 297]. The cut-off value is 16 mast cells per HPF [214], with a sensitivity of 100 % and a specificity of 96 % [214]. In uncertain cases, p16 expression should be taken into account – where p16 expression is diffuse, then a diagnosis of LMS should rather be opted for [18]. According to a different source, immunohistochemically determining p16, p53, and Ki67-indexes is not suitable for differentiating between LMSs and STUMPs. It should be borne in mind that p16-expression does not constitute an independent diagnostic criterion for LMSs. Histologically differentiating STUMPs from mitotically active LMs, from LMs with bizarre nuclei, as well as from cellular LMs can be challenging (Table 14.5). Differentiating the very rare epithelioid and myxoid STUMPs from the respective LM and LMS variants is particularly difficult. For more detail, reference should be had to the specialist literature [144].

Clinical Course, Prognostic Factors Relevant for Therapy

As a general rule, the different STUMP variants are all benign lesions. Recurrence and metastasis usually occur within the uterus, the pelvis, the abdominal cavity, the retroperitoneal region, the lung, the liver, in the bones, and the LNs. Distant metastases usually occur in the lungs [31, 108, 227]. There have also been accounts of metastasis in the deep soft tissue of the neck, the posterior mediastinum, and the paravertebral region [51, 245]. Interestingly, with a mean age of 34 years, women with recurring disease are roughly 10 years younger than women without recurrence [108, 119]. There are only few morphological criteria that serve to predict the risk of disease recurrence and the sites of recurrence and metastasis. There have been accounts of recurrences of atypical LMs with entirely absent MI or an MI < 2 M/10 HPF. From an immunohistochemical and molecular genetic perspective, diffuse immunoreactivity for p16 and/or p53 is regarded as a strong predictive factor for recurrence or metastasis in STUMPs [18, 50, 119, 121]. Even the presence of only minimal TCN is apparently associated with an elevated risk of disease recurrence [10], though it should be noted that, in these cases, the differences to LMSs are not stark or overly blatant. Estrogen and progesterone receptor expression are of no prognostic significance [31, 34].

According to different sources, the rate of recurrence in STUMPs is between 7.7 and 26.7 % [108, 121, 224, 270], and thus markedly lower than for LMSs. Another study comes to the conclusion that recurrences and metastases occur after a mean period of 46.9 Mo (15–108 Mo). Median OS in these cases was 63.9 Mo (40–108 Mo) [121]. Even after 20 years, the risk of recurrence cannot be entirely ruled out. The majority of disease-specific deaths occur 6–11 years after diagnosis [99]. Accordingly, the disease-specific 5, 10, and 15-year survival rates are 100, 88, and 81 %, respectively [99]. A considerable share of STUMPs also recurs and metastasizes as LMSs [10, 107, 108, 227, 258]. Of the 12 STUMPs in the DKSM material that developed metastases, 42 % did so as STUMP, while in the remaining 58 % disease metastasized as LMS [143]. Given the current data situation, the transformation of a STUMP into an LMS should be deemed a serious possibility, not least because STUMPs generally provide the necessary genetic and microbiological preconditions.

Recurrences and metastases only seem to occur following conservative "myoma therapies" and abdominal or endoscopic supracervical HE (Fig. 14.9) [3, 31, 258, 269]. It cannot be safely deduced from the merely occasional accounts of recurrences occurring following total HE that a morcellation was not performed in those cases [108, 181]. Performing morcellation on smooth muscle tumors has increasingly come to constitute a special risk factor, not least due to the danger of spreading cellular tumor material. There have been accounts of STUMP-recurrences occurring within only a few weeks [143]. The problems associated with morcellation are addressed in detail in the chapter on LMSs. In order to prevent morcellation being performed on the wrong object, when clinical and sonographic findings are suspicious, more intensive diagnostics should be conducted, in particular prior to organ-sparing surgery. Due to the numerous clinical and sonographic commonalities between STUMPs and LMSs, the diagnostics-flow chart (Fig. 14.22) presented in the chapter "risk and prevention of inadequate surgery" should be consulted as a decision-making aid.

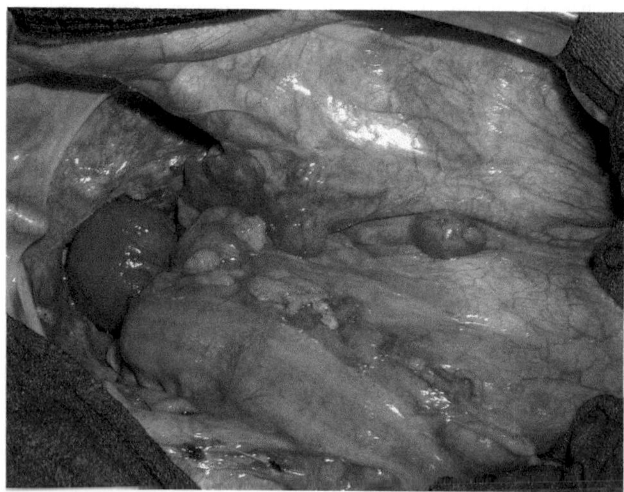

Fig. 14.9 Atypical smooth-muscle tumor (STUMP). Peritoneal metastases of an atypical smooth muscle tumor that was incidentally discovered post-operatively following endoscopic supracervical HE with morcellation, 22 months after primary surgery (With permission of Köhler et al. [144], Fig. 1.1–20a)

Overall, total HE without injuring the tumor is the best method for preventing recurrence. In 3 of 51 cases (34 HE, 17 myomectomies), subsequent HE resp. Myomectomy revealed two atypical LMs in the residual uterus and one atypical LM in the retroperitoneum. Interestingly, in the latter case, the recurrent tumor had been preceded by a total HE, probably in combination with laparoscopic morcellation [181]. It in fact currently remains difficult to assess whether performing laparoscopic myomectomy on STUMPs results in more intrauterine recurrent disease than in ordinary LMs [181]. The cumulative risk of intrauterine recurrence following laparoscopic myomectomy of ordinary LMs is at around 51 % [203]. This rate is possibly no lower than that for recurrence following myomectomies performed on STUMP patients. What is decisive, though, is that recurring tumors and metastases of STUMPs need to be assessed differently than LMs in terms of whether or not they are malignant, and that transformation into an LMS is a possibility that should be reckoned with.

Surgical Therapy and Problems

According to the current literature, total HE is the standard surgical procedure for STUMPs [181]. Surgery should be performed without injuring the tumor (morcellation, sharp clamping). There is no indication for a systematic and/or selective LNE. Recurrences are known to occur both in cases in which a BSO has been performed, as well as in such in which it has not [31]. One analysis found that having undergone BSO has no influence on the rate of disease recurrence [108]. Data pertaining to LMSs suggest that a BSO has no influence on the further course of disease [134]. A case has been reported in which a STUMP patient developed LMS metastases following a supracervical abdominal HE with BSO [258]. BSO can thus be indicated on the basis of the patient's wishes, her menopausal status, or other circumstances that give rise to an independent indication for such surgery. There is no indication for performing a BSO *ex post*.

Where a STUMP has been diagnosed, in exceptional cases – for instance where the patient has an urgent and pressing desire to have children [121] – conservative uterus-sparing surgery can be considered [181]. In doing so, the tumor must not be injured during resection, and the cut must be made outside the pseudocapsule in tissue that is definitely disease-free. Since disease recurrences and metastases almost exclusively occur after conservative procedures, patients must be insistently informed of the increased risk of recurrence and the danger of a possible transformation into an LMS. It is strongly recommended that patients undergo a total HE once their desire to have children has been fulfilled, i.e. following pregnancy and childbirth [121].

Whether or not a subsequent HE should be recommended upon the incidental finding of an R0-enucleated STUMP can be decided based on the immune reaction to p16 and p53, as well as the presence of coagulative or questionable necroses. From a pathological-anatomical perspective, it is urgently advised to perform the HE in all cases in which there is no certainty of tumor benignity (f. ex. questionable necroses, size, atypia, the presence of any mitotic activity) [207]. Whether or not performing a gasless endoscopic myomectomy in STUMP patients, as is recommended by some authors [274], should indeed be regarded as innocuous in terms of recurrence risk, remains unproven and rather unlikely. R1/2 resections should be followed by a follow-up resection, or even better by HE.

Cases of very early post-surgery tumor dissemination following morcellation of a STUMP have been reported [210]. The recent literature [198, 210, 254] recommends a follow-up LSC within 3–6 months of performed myomectomy, morcellation/tumor injury, and unclear resection margins, unless a subsequent total HE is planned [210, 254]. Possible tumor deposits should be R0 resected in the course of these procedures. Total HE is indicated for cases in which patients have no desire to preserve fertility.

Due to the problems associated with determining and specifying the MI, as well as the possibility of overlooking a STUMP or (in the worst case) an LMS as a consequence thereof, conservative surgery should rather not be considered for lesions classified as myxoid or epithelioid LMs or STUMPs. For more detail, reference should be had to the specialist literature [144].

Clinical aftercare should be designed according to the symptoms shown and can be roughly adapted to aftercare for LMS patients. There are no indications for post-operative chemo, hormone, or radiation therapy. There are no known contraindications for hormone replacement therapy.

Low-Grade Endometrial Stromal Sarcomas (LG-ESS)

Epidemiology, Etiology, Pathogenesis, Staging

In Germany and Norway, LG-ESSs account for 26.9 resp. 20 % of all uterine sarcomas, excluding carcinosarcomas [2, 143]. Incidence of LG-ESSs in Southern and Northern Europe is at around 0.23 resp. 0.3 cases/100,000 women [155, 186]. According to various sources, the age of affected women ranges from 15 to 96 years. Median age is 42–52 years; 50 % to 88 % of LG-ESSs arise prior to menopause [20, 47, 299]. The age range in Germany is 18–80 years according to DKSM-data [143], median age is 46 years, and only 18 % of presenting women are postmenopausal.

LG-ESSs exhibit t(7;17) translocations and consecutive fusions of the JAZF1- and SUZ12- (previously: JJAZ1) genes as well as t(6;7) translocations (JAZF1/SUZ12-gene fusion), which are typical genetic abnormalities [206]. t(7;17)(p15;q21) translocation is an early genetic aberration in the development of LG-ESSs. Interestingly, this translocation can also be observed in LG-ESSs that exhibit a focal smooth-muscle differentiation, which allows the conclusion that such tumors originate from a pluripotential mesenchymal precursor cell (progenitor cell) [32, 206, 211]. Identical genetic aberrations are also found in so-called endometrial stromal nodules (ESN), which are regarded as a precursor of LG-ESSs [157].

ER, PR, and aromatase expression as well as association with pregnancy and endometriosis allow the assumption that estrogens are involved in the etiology, pathogenesis, and progression of LG-ESSs [236–241]. Previous or ongoing tamoxifen or toremifen therapy is regarded as another etiological factor [15, 111, 115].

Since 2009, FIGO-staging and UICC-TNM-classification for stromal sarcomas and LMSs have applied (Table 14.1) [83, 217, 264].

Macroscopic and Microscopic Findings

LG-ESSs predominantly have the appearance of an intramural nodulated tumor with strong similarities to an LM or the rare ESNs. LG-ESSs can expand into the cavum and protrude through the cervix when growth persists (Fig. 14.10a–c). They have a median size of 5.5 to 5–8 cm [94, 143]. Compared to LMs, LG-ESSs almost always have a softer consistency. Like with LMs, the cut surface may exhibit whorled structures, but is usually significantly smoother. Like ESNs, the opened tumor often has a yellowish to tan-yellow, sometimes light reddish appearance. On gross examination, intramural tumors can appear well circumscribed and can displace the surrounding myometrium and endometrium. Compressed tumor and surrounding tissue can form a kind of pseudocapsule (Fig. 14.11). Macroscopically visible finger-, worm- or tongue-like infiltrations, when present, are a typical gross characteristic.

Cystic structures, necroses, and focal hemorrhages are present to varying degrees (Fig. 14.13a). LG-ESSs can also exhibit a less common growth pattern in which diffuse myometrial infiltration forces the myometrium apart/separates it. In such cases, the wall of the uterus appears enlarged and

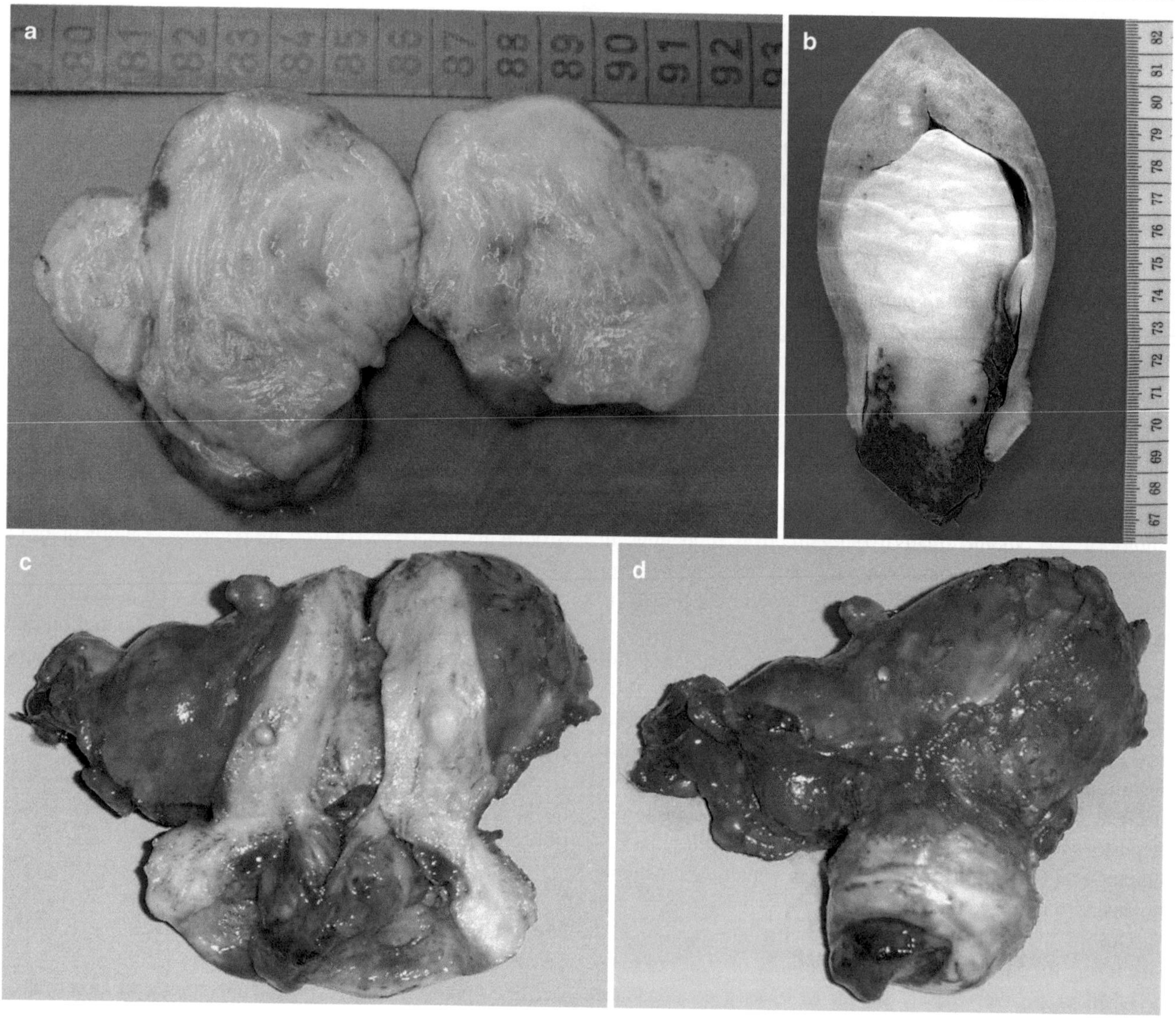

Fig. 14.10 Low-grade endometrial stromal sarcoma. (**a**) Knotty tumor that can barely be macroscopically discerned from an LM; (**b**) large smooth formalin-fixated LG-ESS that had filled out the entire cavum uteri; (**c, d**): pedunculated tumor macroscopically similar to an LM that is protruding from and through the cervix (With permission of Köhler et al. [147], Fig. 2.2–1a–d)

thickened, with a certain degree of nodulation. LG-ESSs occasionally also originate primarily in the cervix.

Overall, an LG-ESS consists of cells that are reminiscent of endometrial stroma in the proliferation phase. The cells cannot be morphologically discerned from ESNs. Microscopically, LG-ESSs are characterized by opulent small uniform cells with oval nuclei, small or absent nucleoli, scant cytoplasm, and poorly defined cytoplasm boundaries. Significant atypia are absent by definition [195]. Accordingly, the microscopic appearance is monotonous and bland. Necroses and hemorrhages also occur in LG-ESSs [286]. The MI does not correlate with diagnosis and prognosis, and is usually measured at around <5 M/10 HPF, but can also exceed 10 M/10 HPF. Atypical mitoses are rare, and true TCNs hardly ever occur. The vessels most closely resemble uniformly distributed endometrial spiral arteries. Lymphatic and blood vessel invasion are observed in 19.1–26.6 [20, 143] resp. 30.8 % of cases [143].

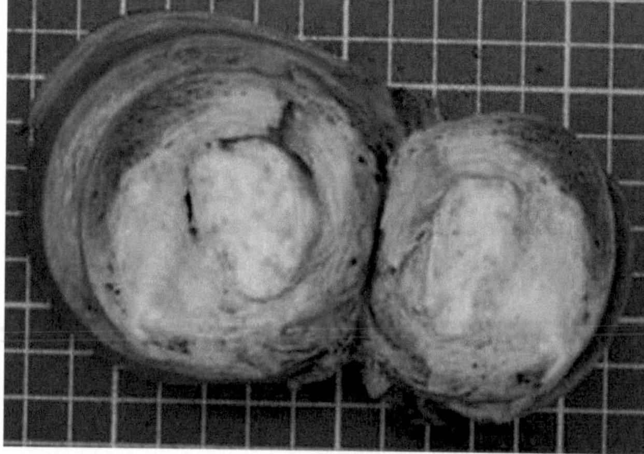

Fig. 14.11 Low-grade endometrial stromal sarcoma. Cut-open LG-ESS specimen with what appears to be a capsule – in the left of the image – that gradually diminishes (or fades) towards the cut base and crosses over into infiltration on the opposite side that is clearly visible on gross observation (With permission of Köhler et al. [147])

LG-ESSs typically have a strong expression of ER and PR (in 71–95 % of cases) [22, 54, 118, 237]. Missing ER and PR-expressions have been reported, albeit with ER being negative more frequently than PR [286, 299]. LG-ESSs can contain aromatases and can thus synthesize estrogens themselves [237]. CD10 expression is characteristical of LG-ESSs, though not specific to them.

Symptoms, Clinical Presentation, Diagnostics, Imaging, Differential Diagnosis

In about 70 % of cases, LG-ESS is an incidental finding during or after HE that is performed on the basis of an LM diagnosis [20, 143, 247, 299]. Forty-eight to seventy-two percent of all patients present with abnormal uterine bleeding in form of intermenstral bleeding and/or heavy und prolonged menstrual, or postmenopausal bleeding. Abnormal uterine bleeding, while it may be absent in some patients, thus constitutes the most common symptom [20, 143, 299]. Tumor growth causes diffuse enlargement of the uterus and is linked with lower abdominal pains in around 20 % of cases. Feelings of satiation and pressure are also occasionally reported [143, 299]. Palpation reveals a noticeably soft, fleshy consistency and/or a lumpy surface on the (usually enlarged) uterus or the palpated "LM". A soft consistency is generally to be taken as suggestive of a malignant or semi-malignant mesenchymal tumor. On average, LG-ESSs are said not to be larger than ordinary LMs [59]. Among the DKSM materials [143], and according to a further source, the median size of LG-ESSs is 5.5 resp. 5.8 cm [94, 143]. Data from a further study revealed a mean tumor size of 6.2 cm (0.3–18 cm), with 58.8 % being ≤5 cm [20]. Rapid growth of an "LM" or a rapidly growing uterus during pubescence is not a common clinical finding in women with LG-ESSs, and is observed in only 6.5 % of cases [20]. By contrast, 30 % of all ordinary LMs occurring during pubescence are rapidly growing tumors [64]. Compared to LMSs and UUSs, symptoms associated with rapid tumor growth, like lower abdominal pains and uresiesthesis, are rather less common in LG-ESS patients. Nonetheless, uterine growth or "myoma growth", especially when postmenopausal, is to be regarded as strongly suggestive of a malignant or semi-malignant mesenchymal uterine tumor.

It is essential that conventional clinico-gynecological examination be accompanied by sonographic examination. Abnormal and postmenopausal uterine bleeding most commonly suggest that the LG-ESS has developed into the cavum of the uterus. Hysteroscopy and fractional curettage are always indicated in such cases. The hysteroscopic appearance shall bear similarity either to a pedunculated LM or a polypoid tumor. Since LG-ESSs are frequently located intramurally, curettage will yield unsuspicious findings or a wrong diagnosis in 50–59 % of cases [23, 143, 269]. It is thus unavoidable that hysteroscopy and/or curettage result in misdiagnoses, a typical diagnostic pitfall.

Analogous to gross appearance, sonography, too, predominantly reveals LG-ESSs within the myometrium. Depending on the extent and depth of infiltration, the tumor margins appear either well-defined or poorly defined/irregular in sonography. According to the literature, solid lesions are generally homogeneously or heterogeneously hypoechoic or intermediately echoic [139, 165, 281]. Hypoechogenicity can correspond to that found in LMs and can apply to the entire tumor. There are also accounts of masses being isoechogenic to the myometrium [44]. Differentiation from an LM can be particularly difficult in such cases. A heterogeneous echogenicity, with anechoic regions and strongly hypoechogenic sections separated by washy or bizarre margins, is most commonly encountered, as is also confirmed by DKSM research [143]. LG-ESSs usually clearly displace the hyperechoic endometrium. Growth of the tumor into the cavum usually interrupts the endometrial layer [165]. It is often the case that anechoic clefts or small cysts are visible, either solitary or spread across the entire tumor, that in part correspond to dilated vessels [122], cystic areas, or necroses. The vessels usually have very small hyperechoic edges (Figs. 14.12a, and 14.13b). A diffuse heterogeneous echogenic thickening of the myometrium with partially nodular components is not an uncommon sonographic correlate for diffusely growing LG-ESSs [139, 242].

Between 68 % and 71 % of cases, sonography yields a diagnosis of LM [143, 265], with substantial consequences for surgery indication and surgical procedure (see also the section on risk and prevention of inadequate surgery). Only 18 % of findings are described as malignant tumors, and overall, 17.9 % are classified as suspicious tumors [143].

In Doppler sonography, LG-ESSs show a strong degree of irregularly and focally distributed vascularity in combination with a low RI of 0.21–0.42 and a PI of 0.2–0.49 [46, 49, 126, 139, 162, 242]. The RI cut-off value of 0.4, with a sensitivity of 90.9 % and a specificity of 99.8 %, is largely adequate for differentiating between benign and malignant lesions, or for classifying a tumor as highly suspicious. In Doppler sonography, visible cysts are surrounded by numerous vessels (Fig. 14.12b) [259]. These findings, however, are by no means unique or specific to LG-ESSs, and in fact also apply to other sarcomas. Nonetheless, they serve as a useful criterion for distinguishing malignant lesions from LMs [153]. It can occasionally so occur that color Doppler sonography provides a visual appearance typical of an LM. Should the suspicion of a malignant mesenchymal tumor prevail in light of the patient's medical history and the clinical findings, and should the patient desire organ-preserving/sparing surgery, then adherence to the diagnostic flowchart (Fig. 14.22) (sec-

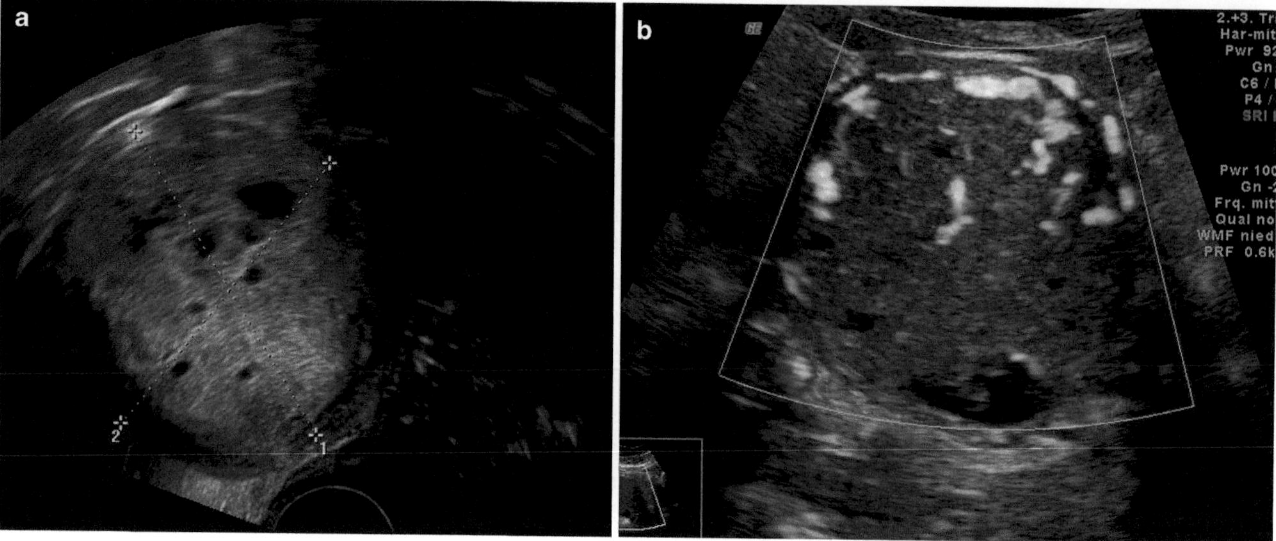

Fig. 14.12 Low-grade endometrial stromal sarcoma. (**a**) Gray scale sonography showing a tumor with heterogeneous echogenicity containing numerous anechoic spaces and gaps. The larger anechoic spaces most likely correspond to necroses with bizarre margins; (**b**) color Doppler sonography revealed that many of the anechoic gaps corresponded to vessels. The strong degree of irregular central vascularity is suggestive of a malignancy (With permission of Köhler et al. [147], Fig. 2.2–9c, d)

tion: risk and prevention of inadequate surgery) is strongly indicated.

Regarding CT, the same applies as previously described for LMSs.

In the majority of cases, MRT images show LG-ESSs as lesions within the myometrium (Fig. 14.13c, d). T1-weighted images typically show a predominantly heterogeneous SI that is hypo- to isointense (and occasionally hyperintense) compared to the myometrium. Signal-free regions are usually necroses or cystic areas that show no enhancement in T1 WC images, but strong hyperintense enhancement in T2 W images. In T1 and T2-weighted images, the tumor is delimited from the surrounding areas by a hypointense layer or rim that can be interrupted by tumor infiltrations. Enhancement in T1 WC-images is predominantly intense (occasionally mild) and heterogeneous (occasionally also homogeneous). Here, too, there is a recognizable band of enhancement that is weaker compared to the rest of the tumor and the myometrium, and that corresponds to the hypointense margin visualized in T1/2 W MRI images. T2-weighted images show a recognizably homogeneous or heterogeneous, sometimes intermediate SI that is higher than that of the myometrium and the skeletal muscles. Cystic structures that appear hypointense in T1 W imaging, but show no enhancement in T1 WC images, are strongly hyperintense in T2 W [88, 259]. In tumors with myometrial involvement, i. e. muscle infiltration/invasion, preserved bundles of muscle fibers are recognizable as bands of low signal intensity (hypointense) within the myometrium in T2-weighted images. This imaging feature is regarded as one of the most important criteria suggestive of an LG-ESS (Table 14.6) [138, 158, 242, 257, 259, 281].

The definitively benign ESN is the most important macroscopic and microscopic DD for LG-ESSs. ESNs and LG-ESSs have identical cytological pictures, so that they only really differ in that, in case of the former, there is no lymphovascular, vascular, or myometrial invasion [268]. Differentiating between ESNs and LG-ESSs on the basis of the tissue specimens gathered via curettage or morcellation without bordering neighboring tissue can thus be very difficult, or even impossible. The attending clinician must be aware of this problem and, where such cases arise, bear the real possibility of an LG-ESS in mind and inform the patient of that possibility and what it implies.

Since LG-ESSs bear great similarity to LMs, both clinically and macroscopically, and predominantly occur prior to menopause, successfully differentiating them from LMs is of particular importance. Accordingly, LG-ESSs are operated under the indication of an LM in 69–78 % of cases [20, 143, 216, 247, 299]. Thus, the majority of LG-ESSs are incidentally diagnosed as such either during or post-surgery. The risk of encountering an LMS or an LG-ESS during HE, regardless of the indication on the basis of which it is performed, is addressed in detail in the section on the risk and prevention of inadequate surgery.

Successfully histologically differentiating LG-ESSs from cellular LMs is by far the greatest differential diagnostic challenge, since both tumors express ER and PR as well as SMA and desmin (the latter albeit rarely among LG-ESSs). Measuring CD10 expression (which, unfortunately, is not seldom positive in LMs and LMSs), especially in combination with H-Caldesmon-expression, can be helpful in this regard [178, 306]. The attending clinician must be aware of the fact that successfully differentiating

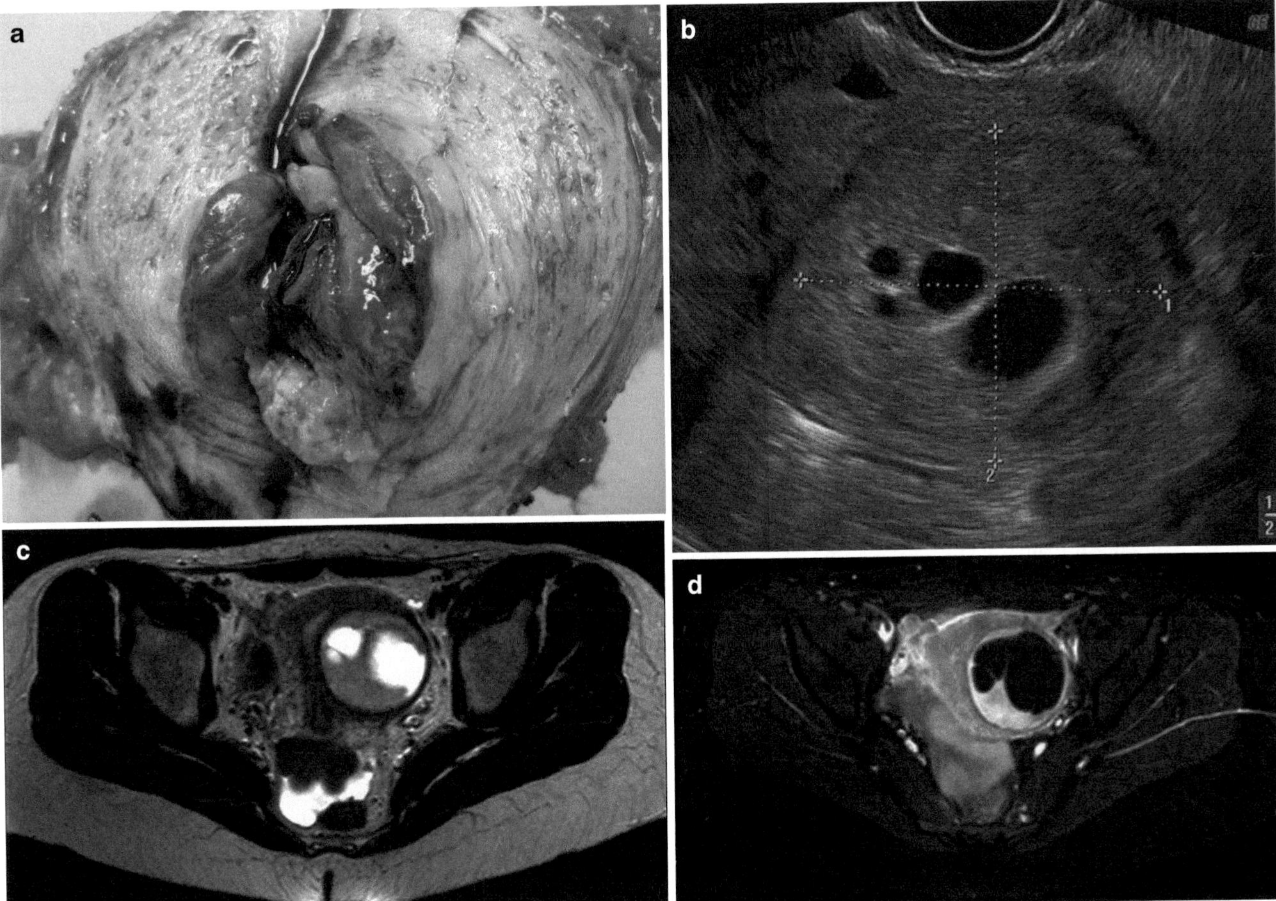

Fig. 14.13 Low-grade endometrial stromal sarcoma. (**a**) Intramurally located LG-ESS with predominantly necrotic (*yellow color*) and cystic components; (**b**) the necrotic and cystic regions of the same tumor showed as anechoic areas in abdominal sonography; (**c**) results from axial T2 W MRI correlated very well to the sonographic findings. The necroses showed typically high levels of signal intensity. The LG-ESS is intramurally located and has visibly displaced the endometrium and the cavum. The typical intratumoral hypointense bands are only barely discernible; (**d**) T1 W contrast-MRI with fat suppression confirmed the necroses as such – they showed no enhancement and showed up as signal free sections. The hypodense rim at the margins is recognizable in all of these images (With permission of Köhler et al. [147], Fig. 2.2–3a, 2.2–11a, c, e)

Table 14.6 Characteristics of low-grade endometrial stromal sarcomas in MRI

T1 W	Tumor with intermediate SI and low (necroses, cysts) SI, scattered areas with high SI (hemorrhages in particular), hypointense rim
T2 W	Predominantly intermediate to hyperintense SI with intratumoral hypointense bands, in part sections with very high SI (necroses, cysts), hypointense rim
T1 WC	intensive homogeneous enhancement, up to heterogeneous enhancement compared to the homogeneously enhancing myometrium
	Rim with weaker enhancement compared to tumor and myometrium
	hyperintense necroses and cysts show no enhancement in T2 W

From Köhler et al. [147]

LG-ESSs from cellular LMs on the basis of frozen section specimens without accompanying immunohistochemical testing can be difficult to impossible. Any diagnosis of a cellular LM that is based solely on photo-optical observation of the biopsy or curettage specimen, and without immunohistochemical testing, should be subjected to critical scrutiny.

Clinical Course and Prognostic Factors Relevant to Therapy

Stage of disease is also the most important prognostic factor for LG-ESSs [6, 94]. Prognosis for tumors >10 cm is apparently no worse than for such that are 5.1–10 cm in size [2, 94]. Prognosis worsens as age progresses [20, 47, 94, 256]

and is significantly less promising in postmenopausal than in premenopausal women. Drawing on numerous accounts, the median time to first recurrence is 36–130 Mo for Stage I, 3 years for Stage I/II and only 9 Mo for stages III/IV (FIGO pre 2009) [7, 48, 129, 140]. Nonetheless, the occurrence of late relapses after more than 10–30 years is distinctive. SEER-data (FIGO pre-2009), calculated for a sample of 356 cases, have revealed a 5-year OS of 96 % for stages I and II, 89 % for stages III and IV, and 92 % for stages I–IV [256]. Two larger retrospective studies measured a 10-year-OS of 87.1–95.8 % and a 10-year RFI of 49.6–52.1 % [20, 299]. LG-ESSs can thus be considered tumors with a relatively promising prognosis. Even relapsed LG-ESSs remain local for a long time and only develop distant metastases relatively late.

Positive pelvic and/or para-aortic LNs are found in 2.6–17 % of women with stage I-IV disease [143, 162, 299] and in 10 % [69] of cases in which the LG-ESS is confined to the uterus. According to SEER-data [256], LNs test positive in 7 % of cases (mean number of removed LNs: 12; 63 % of stage I/II tumors, acc. to FIGO pre-2009). It is thus apparent that positive LNs do not correlate to distant metastasis and disease recurrence in the context of LG-ESSs that are confined to the uterus, while, however, being linked to simultaneous extrauterine spread in the majority of cases [69]. Whether performing an LNE has any effect on prognosis remains unproven. A SEER-analysis compared 100 women who underwent an LNE with 283 patients who did not, and revealed no differences in terms of OS [256]. Benefits could not even be identified for cases in which LNs tested positive. Further SEER-analyses covering 310 and 1010 LG-ESSs, respectively, as well as a smaller and a larger retrospective study, all came to the unanimous conclusion that undergoing an LNE effects no change in OS [11, 20, 25, 94, 261, 299]. Recurrences occurred entirely locoregionally in 40–42 % of cases, albeit without any marked preference for the draining lymphovascular spaces or nodes [20, 143]. The remaining 60 % of cases were comprised of intraabdominal recurrences, distant metastases, or a combination of all forms of dissemination [140]. Distant metastasization occurs to the lungs in particular, though bone metastases have also been reported in isolated cases [20, 299].

Metastatic dissemination to the ovaries is known to occur – in the DKSM-materials, such spread, without involvement of other organs, occurs in 2.4 % of cases [143, 302]. Adnexal involvement has been observed in 9.5 % of cases, and almost uniformly goes hand in hand with further extrauterine dissemination [69]. Despite the fact that HRs usually test positive, the benefits of performing a BSO for both OS and disease-free survival are highly contested. Retrospective studies suggest that sparing the ovaries in premenopausal women increases the risk of recurrence without having any effect on OS [11, 20, 26, 29, 129, 174, 299]. One study determined a median RFI of 5 years for patients who did not undergo BSO, compared to 2 years when the ovaries were left *in situ* [73]. A more recent study concludes that ovarian preservation constitutes a "high-level risk factor" for recurrence [82]. What stands out in this study, besides the relatively small sample size (61 with vs. 7 without BSO), is the relatively low median age of women who did (35.4 years) or did not (43 years) undergo a BSO. Since the surgical methods applied are not described anywhere in the study, it is rather likely that organ-sparing surgical techniques were performed in these cases that in turn are associated with an increased risk of recurrence. In two further studies, leaving the ovaries *in situ* was associated with an increased rate of recurrence (87.5–95.5 resp. 27.4–59.6 %) and a shorter RFI however without being statistically significant [20, 299]. In one of these studies, however, almost without exception, the women on whom BSO was not performed underwent a myomectomy [20]. In practice, the ovaries remain *in situ* significantly more often when conservative surgery is performed [20, 143, 216]. The actual effects of a BSO on RFI thus remain unclear. However, in all analyses stated, myomectomy and sparing the ovaries, notwithstanding the shorter RFI had no influence on OS [20]. Other studies observed identical OS and RFI both with and without BSO being performed [140, 174, 218]. The relatively extensive SEER-data also suggest that leaving the ovaries *in situ* in premenopausal women has no negative effects on OS [122, 256]. Despite their inherent bias, all larger retrospective studies [140, 174, 256] allude that retaining the ovaries is relatively unobjectionable. However, the ovaries are still removed in 46.5–49.4 % of all cases [143, 299]. Overall, and in summary, to date, evidence has yet to be presented that leaving the ovaries *in situ* has a negative effect on patients' OS. However, a potentially elevated risk of recurrence cannot be ruled out entirely.

The surgical techniques applied have a crucial influence on prognosis. The fact that 69–78 % of LS-ESSs are operated under the primary diagnosis of an LM [20, 143, 216, 247, 299] subsequently results in a large number of inadequate surgical procedures being performed. At present, in Germany, 23 % of all women with an LG-ESS undergo tumor enucleation, and laparoscopic or abdominal supracervical HE is performed in 13.2 % of cases. 42 % of the different surgical procedures include morcellation [143]. Other sources report that myomectomies are performed in 12.4 % of cases, all of which are connected with foregoing a BSO [20]. In 0.28 % of cases in which morcellation was performed under the diagnosis of an LM, an LG-ESS was revealed as an incidental finding [71]. Since LG-ESSs, like LMSs, do not have a capsule or pseudocapsule, every enucleation poses a high risk of achieving only R1-resection margins (at the very least RX-resection margins). Accordingly, tumor extirpation bears a significantly higher risk of recurrence (78.9 %) than total HE (25.4 %). Resection margins that are not definitely tumor free are equally associated with increased rates of recurrence. Not one patient remained relapse-free within the five years following tumor enucleation, however without differences in terms of OS [20]. There have been multiple accounts of (sometimes extensive) intraperitoneal deposits being observed within 1–3 Mo of endoscopic morcellation or tumor enucleation [65, 143, 221, 223]. A further study compared outcomes of LG-ESS patients who underwent morcellation during abdominal tumor enucleation, total abdominal HE, or a laparoscopy-assisted vaginal HE with outcomes of patients on whom total abdominal HE was performed without morcellation [216]. The results show that both 5-year PFS and abdominopelvic PFS were significantly poorer in the group of morcellation patients, of whom the majority had undergone endoscopic procedures. The problems pertaining to elevated risk of recurrence following morcellation are elaborated in greater detail in the chapter on LMSs.

Generally, laparoscopic or abdominal supracervical HE bears the danger of residual intravascular or myometrial infiltrations in the uterine stump. Moreover, in practice, supracervical laparoscopic HE is virtually always performed in connection with morcellation. Even if an R1-resection cannot be observed, from a clinical perspective, an RX-situation should be assumed. There have been accounts of early tumor deposits occurring within three months of such procedures being performed (Fig. 14.14a, b) [143]. Any form of supracervical HE should thus be classified as inadequate procedure until proven otherwise. An increased risk of tumor cell spillage should apparently also be assumed even if the uterus has only been damaged with a sharp instrument. Therefore, the uterus must not be subjected to any clawing with sharp instruments whenever an LG-ESS has been unambiguously identified as such or is even suspected. DKSM-data reveal a median time to first recurrence of 17 and 7 Mo following adequate and inadequate operations, respectively [143].

In summary, tumor enucleation and/or R1-resection are regarded as independent risk factors for locoregional and intraabdominal disease recurrence, but have no influence on OS. The fact that OS remains unaffected, in contrast to the encountered reduction in RFI, can evidently be accounted for by the good level of surgical tumor control achieved in 63.6 % of LG-ESS recurrences [20] and can help to explain the high response rates to HT that have been known to last for several years in some cases. To date, no cases have been reported in which LG-ESS patients with local recurrence have succumbed to their disease [20].

The negative prognostic impact of BSOs performed during adequate (!) surgical procedures, as is claimed by some authors (see above), remains highly questionable.

No valid, reliable RFI or OS-related data exist to date that militate against operating LG-ESSs endoscopically, so long as tumors and/or the uterus remain uninjured in the process.

Surgical Therapy and Problems

Total HE and BSO without causing injury to the tumor and/or the uterus is the generally accepted standard for patients with LG-ESSs. Opting for a primarily vaginal approach is

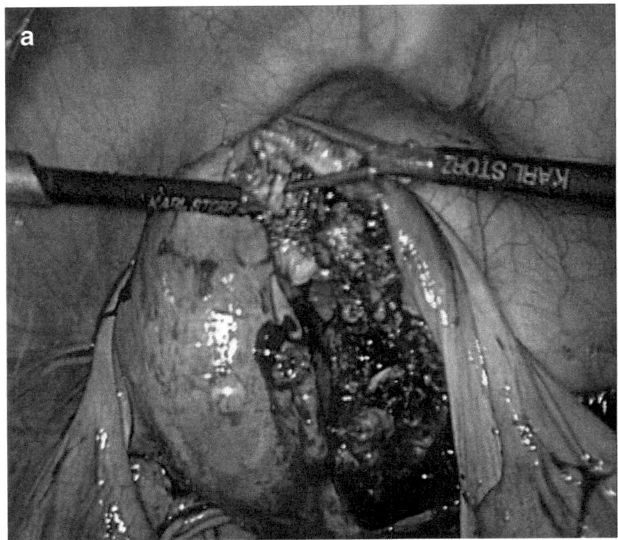

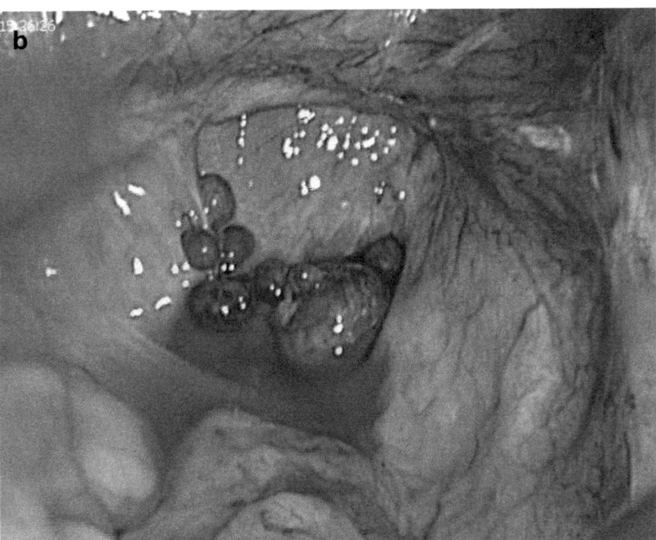

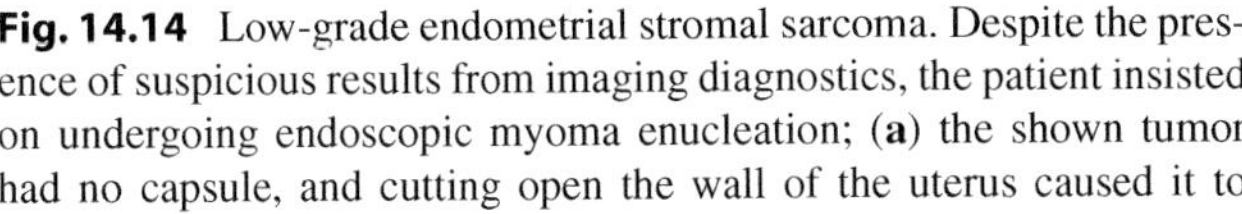

Fig. 14.14 Low-grade endometrial stromal sarcoma. Despite the presence of suspicious results from imaging diagnostics, the patient insisted on undergoing endoscopic myoma enucleation; (**a**) the shown tumor had no capsule, and cutting open the wall of the uterus caused it to immediately expand (or virtually "jump") out of its "bed"; (**b**) despite having undergone subsequent HE with BSO, within a short period of time the patient developed comprehensive local recurrence (With permission of Köhler et al. [147], Fig. 2.2–12a, d)

not indicated due to the risk of damaging the uterus and the lack of possibilities for abdominal exploration. Laparoscopy-assisted vaginal HE must be performed without injuring the tumor or the uterus. Subjecting an intact uterus retrieved via laparoscopy-assisted HE to vaginal morcellation inside a vaginally inserted protective pouch/endobag can be an acceptable solution for achieving this [79].

The benefits of a BSO are contested and have been described in great detail in the subchapter on prognosis. In light of the rarity of isolated ovarian metastases, a respective surgical procedure need not be necessarily justified when the ovaries are unsuspicious on gross examination. According to the current NCCN-recommendations and the GCIG-consensus, decisions for or against a BSO can be made on a case-specific basis dependent on the patient's reproductive age and/or desire to preserve fertility [12, 202]. The ESMO-guidelines – while not making a respective recommendation – merely draw attention to the fact that BSOs are performed in practice *per se* [74]. Taking all data pertaining to prognostic consequences together, preserving the ovaries cannot be deemed erroneous practice, and subsequent i.e. later extirpation can be foregone if the LG-ESS was subjected to adequate primary surgery. Patients should be informed of the potentially increased risk of recurrence, albeit without any consequences for OS, when deciding whether or not the ovaries should be preserved. The consensus [11, 29, 81, 82, 91, 174] that had existed previously, namely that a BSO is indicated for premenopausal women due to the high levels of HR-expression found in LG-ESSs, can no longer be sustained. A BSO is nonetheless performed in 71.2–78.4 % of cases [20, 94]. In Germany, the respective rate is 47 % [143].

There are recommendations for performing at least selective pelvic and para-aortic LNE in patients with enlarged LNs so long as such course of action can reasonably be expected of them [196]. Such a recommendation, however, cannot be made on the basis of the recurrence and metastasization patterns described in the subsection on prognosis above. The NCCN-guidelines no longer make any mention of performing LNE alongside total HE with or without BSO [202]. Likewise, the ESMO-guidelines and the GCIG-consensus do not recommend systematic LNE, as such course of action has yet to be proven to be beneficial [12, 74]. The aforementioned publications do, however, suggest that LNs that appear enlarged, either clinically or via imaging diagnostics, be subjected to cytoreductive resection (debulking). The NCCN-recommendation is somewhat confusing, since it assumes in its commentary that surgical staging be performed in accordance with staging for endometrial carcinoma. A holistic observation of all the available data reveals that, currently, the scientific basis is insufficient to support an indication for conducting systematic LNE. Accordingly, systematic LNE cannot be defined as standard practice. Moreover, the findings currently have no ramifications for the further course of therapy, even when the LNs are positive. This does not mandatorily preclude that clinically suspicious LNs can be resected in the absence of evidence that doing so bears any benefits. However, an LNE is nonetheless performed in 26.4–39.5 % of cases [20, 94, 143, 299].

There is no indication for an omentectomy if the omentum appears tumor-free, i.e. there is no omental involvement, on gross examination.

Taking all available data into account, there is no indication that patients with LG-ESSs should undergo an organ-preserving extirpation. One exception could be cases in which young women, upon extensive elucidation, wish to preserve fertility and their physical ability to have children [67, 267]. In such cases, the tumor must be R0-resected. As the pseudo-capsule usually consists of compressed tumor material (Fig. 14.14a), it not seldom occurs that the tumor is damaged or injured during surgery.

A subsequent pregnancy will obviously have a negative impact on prognosis and further exacerbate the risk of recurrence that is already elevated due to having undergone inadequate primary surgery. Patients must be unequivocally informed of these circumstances. Reference should be had to the respective specialist literature [309] for more detailed information.

The problem of inadequate surgery and means of preventing it, which apply in equal measure to both LG-ESSs and LMSs, are discussed at length in the chapter "risk and prevention of inadequate surgery", together with the diagnostic flow-chart (Fig. 14.22).

As is also the case for LMSs, surgical procedures that preserve or spare organs either wholly or partially should be followed up by total HE or a resection of the residual uterus. Additional BSO is recommended in these cases. Such course of action also corresponds to current recommendations of the AAGL, the DGGG and the NCCN [1, 27, 72, 202, 254]. Should the patient decline such course of action, then at the very least an endoscopic follow-up examination/counter-check should be sought within 3–6 months [198] (see also section on LMS), and postoperative hormone therapy should be given serious consideration [1, 254].

Taking the patient's general state of health and overall condition into account, maximal debulking should be performed in cases of LG-ESSs that have spread in the pelvis and abdominal cavity. Systematic LNE is not indicated and thus not deemed sensible [91, 202]. No data are available to underline that performing a selective LNE on enlarged LNs when an intraabdominal R0-resection has been achieved is in fact beneficial. Overall, as is also the case for soft tissue sarcomas, having 'no macroscopic tumor-burden' and 'clear resection margins' are regarded as the most important prognostic factors [13, 114, 205]. Even for LG-ESS patients who have undergone surgery on metastases and/or disease recurrences with or without gross residual tumor burden, the 5-year PFS rates were 65 % and 100 %, respectively [20]. The available data, therefore, suggest that maximal debulking is the gold standard to be aspired to in cases of advanced disease. The same results might also be achieved with HT. Since recurrences remain in the abdomen for a long time and remissions are known to occur years later, even after an R1-resection with subsequent HT [20, 143], surgical intervention should always be prioritized.

Aftercare corresponds to what has been described for LMSs. Regarding indications for a thorax CT in the context of LG-ESS, both the implications of radiation exposure and the relative rarity of lung metastases need to be taken into consideration. There are no indications for adjuvant or postoperative chemo- and/or radiation therapy. Particularities in this regard, as well as more details pertaining to the necessity for postoperative hormone therapy following inadequate operations, can be found in the specialist literature [147].

High-Grade Endometrial Stromal Sarcoma and Undifferentiated Uterine Sarcoma

Epidemiology, Etiology, Pathogenesis, Staging

HG-ESSs and UUSs need to be clearly pathogenetically, morphologically, clinically, and prognostically distinguished from LG-ESSs. The data situation pertaining to HG-ESSs and UUSs is extremely poor, particularly in terms of the therapeutic approach to be followed. Recommendations are mainly based on individual case reports and retrospective studies with relatively small sample sizes and often include all stages of disease. HG-ESSs and UUSs account for 10.1 % and 3.7 %, respectively, of all uterine sarcomas [143]. Women with HG-ESSs and UUSs have a median age of 58 and 63 years, respectively, and are thus noticeably older than LG-ESS patients [143]. These tumors thus occur in postmenopausal women in the majority of cases.

HG-ESSs and LG-ESSs both derive from the endometrial stroma [57, 163, 212]. This commonality notwithstanding, they are nonetheless pathogenetically independent of one another. A fusion of the YWHAE and NUTM2 genes (YWHAE-FAM22), a result of chromosomal translocation of t(10;17) (q22;p13), can be found in HG-ESSs. In LG-ESSs, by contrast, JAZF1-SUZ12 is the most characteristic gene fusion (see the section on LG-ESS) [105, 166, 167]. The fact that HG-ESSs and LG-ESSs exhibit differing fusion genes suggests that an HG-ESS does not usually develop from an LG-ESS [252]. The principal difference between HG-ESSs and UUSs lies in the fact that the cytological criteria of the former resemble endometrial stroma *to any degree* [252]. These cytological criteria as well as the fusion genes found in LG-ESSs and HG-ESSs are absent in UUSs [105, 160, 163, 166]. In contrast, UUSs exhibit complex chromosomal aberrations, with gains on 2q, 4q, 6q, 7p, 9q, and 20q, and losses/deletions on 3q, 10p, 14q [109]. UUSs generally exhibit no specific type of differentiation, and their histogenesis remains unclear [212]. UUSs thus constitute an independent type of neoplasm. There have been accounts of cases in which HG-ESSs and UUSs have developed from or alongside an LG-ESS [90, 133, 160, 212]. Significant associations between HG-ESSs/UUSs and tamoxifen therapy are considerably rarer than is the case for LG-ESSs and LMSs [111, 255].

FIGO-staging and UICC-TNM-classification correspond to those provided for LMSs (Table 14.1).

Macroscopic and Microscopic Appearance

Gross examination of HG-ESSs/UUSs often reveals polypous fleshy masses in the cavity of the uterus that are yellowish, yellowish-gray, or grayish-white in color, and which are characterized by hemorrhages and necroses as well as extensive myometrial invasion in some cases. Decomposed necrotic masses can make up up to 90 % of the tumor. HG-ESSs/UUSs generally exhibit rapid growth, quickly fill the entire uterine cavity, and are associated with a rapid increase in the size of the uterus. The borders of the uterus are often exceeded within a very short period of time (Figs. 14.15a–c, 14.16a, and 14.17a). Due to their rapid growth rate, HG-ESSs already have mean and median diameters of 8.0 cm and 7.5 cm, respectively, at the time of initial diagnosis (min.: 1.7 cm; max.: 15 cm) [143]. UUSs have mean and median sizes of 12.2 cm and 11 cm (min.: 2.6 cm; max.: 24 cm), respectively [143]. The fact that UUSs are generally larger at the time of initial diagnosis strongly underlines their higher degree of malignancy compared to HG-ESSs. The low-grade component of HG-ESSs can sometimes be easy to discern on gross observation, and bears resemblance to the low-grade component found in LG-ESS [252].

HG-ESSs and UUSs are highly pleomorphic and thus can already be clearly discerned from the more knotty, nodal, and uniform LG-ESSs on the basis of gross macroscopic appearance.

Within HG-ESSs, there is a coexistence of areas of low-grade structures with a close resemblance to LG-ESS on the one hand, and (usually predominating) high-grade areas on the other. The low-grade component is characterized by uniform low-grade spindle cells with visible cytological connections to the endometrial stroma, and finger or worm-like (permeative) myometrial infiltrations. The high-grade areas, in contrast, exhibit higher degrees of nuclear atypia, ample TCNs, a usually clearly elevated MI (>10 M/10 HPF), lymphovascular invasions, and destruc-

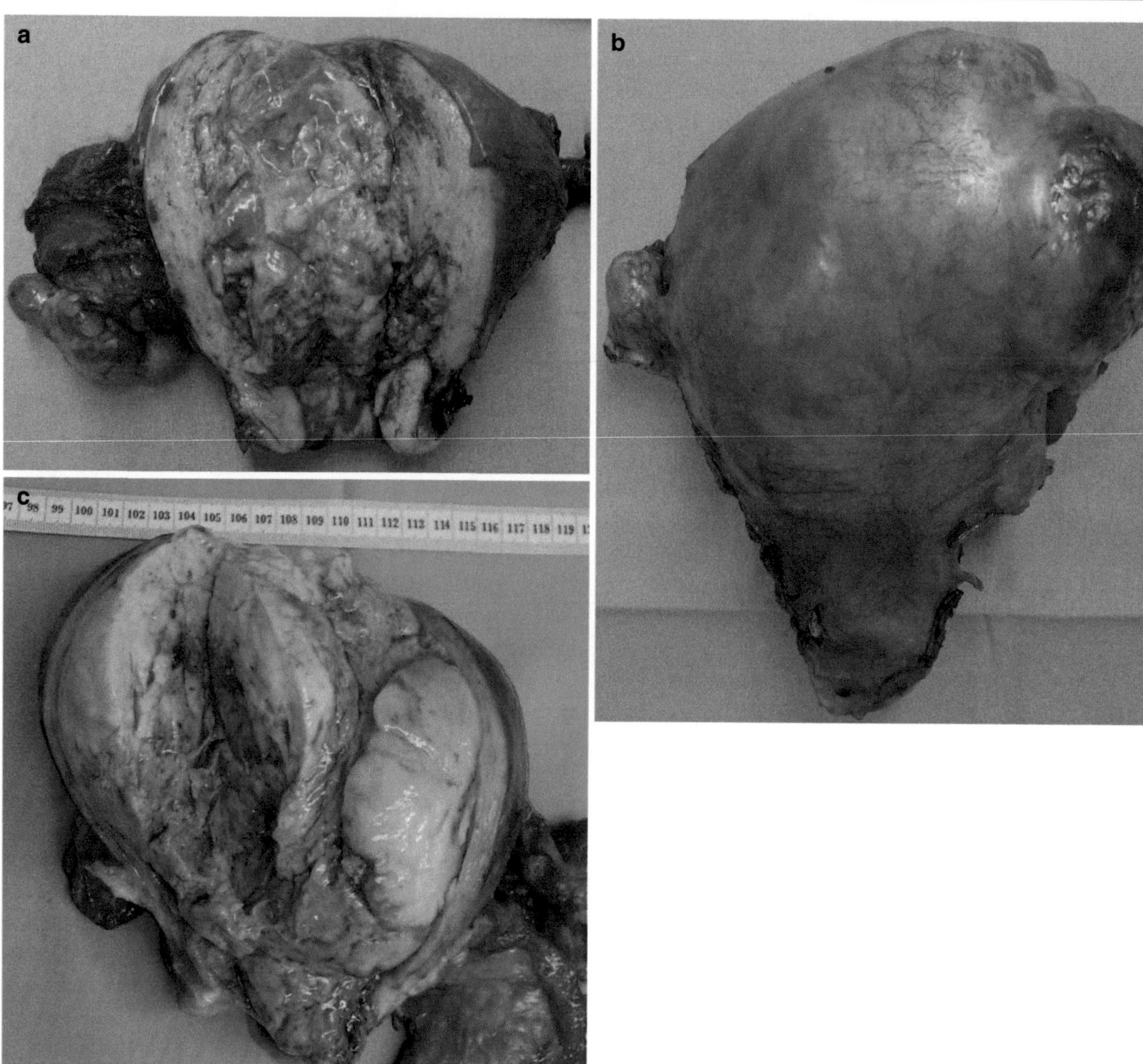

Fig. 14.15 Undifferentiated uterine sarcoma. (**a**) Necrotic tissue accounts for almost 90 % of the depicted UUS. The immense pressure generated by strong tumor growth has distended the cervix; (**b**) in this case, the uterine cavity is completely filled by a predominantly necrotic UUS that has prolapsed through the cervix. Moreover, metastases were found on the peritoneum of the bladder and in the left adnex; (**c**) due to their extremely rapid rate of growth, UUSs are often found to have perforated the wall of the uterus (With permission of Köhler et al. [148], Fig. 2.3–1a–c)

tive myometrial invasions. This coexistence of differing cytological criteria is also associated with variations in CD10-, ER-, and PR-expressions within the tumor [160, 207, 212, 252]. Diffuse and strong CD10-, ER-, and PR-expression can be found in the low-grade component in particular. It is thus by all means appropriate to conduct HR testing at least in HG-ESSs with a view to potential HT. By contrast, the high-grade component is characterized by ER-, PR-, and CD10-negativity [252]. These findings correlate with diffuse and strong cyclin D1-positivity. Cyclin D1 is regarded as a marker for the fusion gene YWHAE-FAM22 [163, 166] that is only found in the high-grade component of HG-ESSs. While this fusion gene may not be traceable in some cases, it nonetheless remains an important characteristic of HG-ESSs that does not or only in a few exceptions occur in LG-ESSs or UUSs. Overall, the simultaneous presence of positive, negative or hetero geneous ER-, PR-, CD10-, and cyclin D1-expression, and of the YWHAE-FAM22 and JAZF1 and JJAZ1 fusion genes shows that both HG-ESSs and LG-ESSs derive from

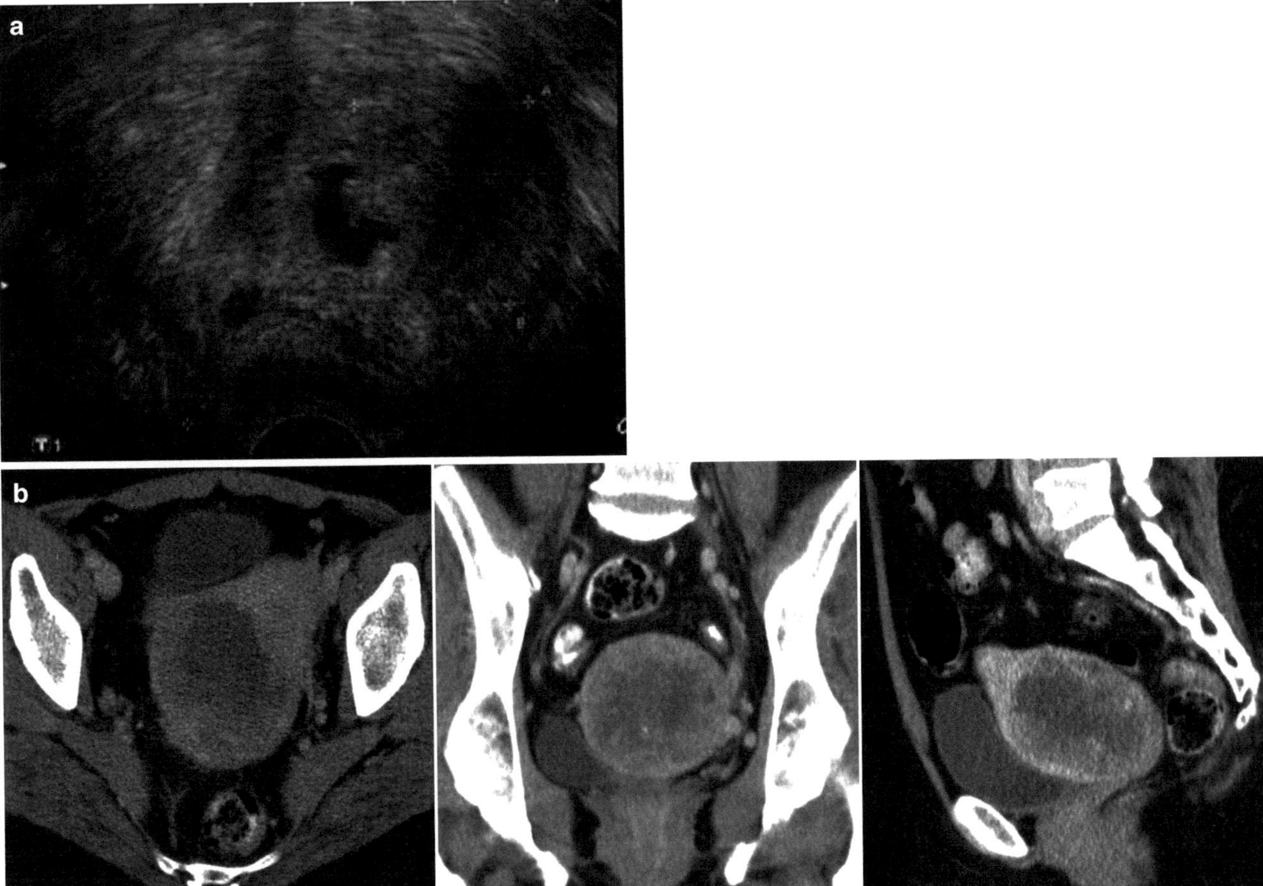

Fig. 14.16 Undifferentiated uterine sarcoma. (**a**) This UUS shows heterogeneous echogenicity in axial sonography, with the exception of some signal voids that correspond to necroses. The tumor fills out the entire cavum. The narrow hyerechoic endometrial rim that is primarily indicated in the right half of the image serves to visibly delimit the UUS from its surroundings there. Said demarcation decreases and is gradually lost as we move to the opposite side of the image; (**b**) the tumor enhances homogeneously in the axial CECT image (*left*) which, analogous to the sonographic findings, recognizably shows that the tumor margins are not clear and sharp throughout. The extent to which the notably enlarged uterus has been infiltrated becomes clear in the coronal (*center*) and sagittal (*right*) planes. Enhancement was heterogeneous in these images. The remainder of the myometrium has been compressed and reduced to a narrow seam (With permission of Köhler et al. [148], Fig. 2.3–6a, b)

the endometrial stroma. The observation that an HG-ESS is reminiscent of or bears resemblance to the endometrial stroma in any way is a decisive diagnostic factor that clearly delineates such neoplasms from UUSs [252].

UUSs exhibit such extensive dedifferentiation that it can often no longer be discerned that (or whether) they originated from the endometrial stroma or the myometrium. The cells are characterized by clear aneuploidy, marked cellular and nuclear pleomorphism including prominent nucleoli and bizarre polynuclear giant cells, and no specific type of differentiation. Expansive foci of coagulative necrosis and high rates of often atypical mitoses are typical characteristics of UUSs [160, 212, 304]. The MI usually clearly exceeds 10 M/10 HPF. Destructive myometrial invasion is already visible on gross observation. Furthermore, early and extensive lymphovascular and blood vessel invasion is observed in 47 % and 48 % of cases, respectively [143]. UUSs exhibit no (or occasionally weak) HR- and CD10-expression [61, 125, 160, 212]. Desmin, SMA, or cytokeratins have also been traced in UUSs in some cases [160, 278]. P53-positivity is detected in 57 % of UUSs [125]. Ultimately, immunohistochemical analyses of UUSs are very unreliable, as these dedifferentiated tumors have already lost their reactivity to numerous antigens [295]. Taken together, the evidence underlines that, unlike LG-ESSs and HG-ESSs, and bar a few exceptional cases, UUSs do not derive from the endometrial stroma.

The most evident commonality between UUSs and HG-ESSs is the fact that both are highly aggressive neoplasms.

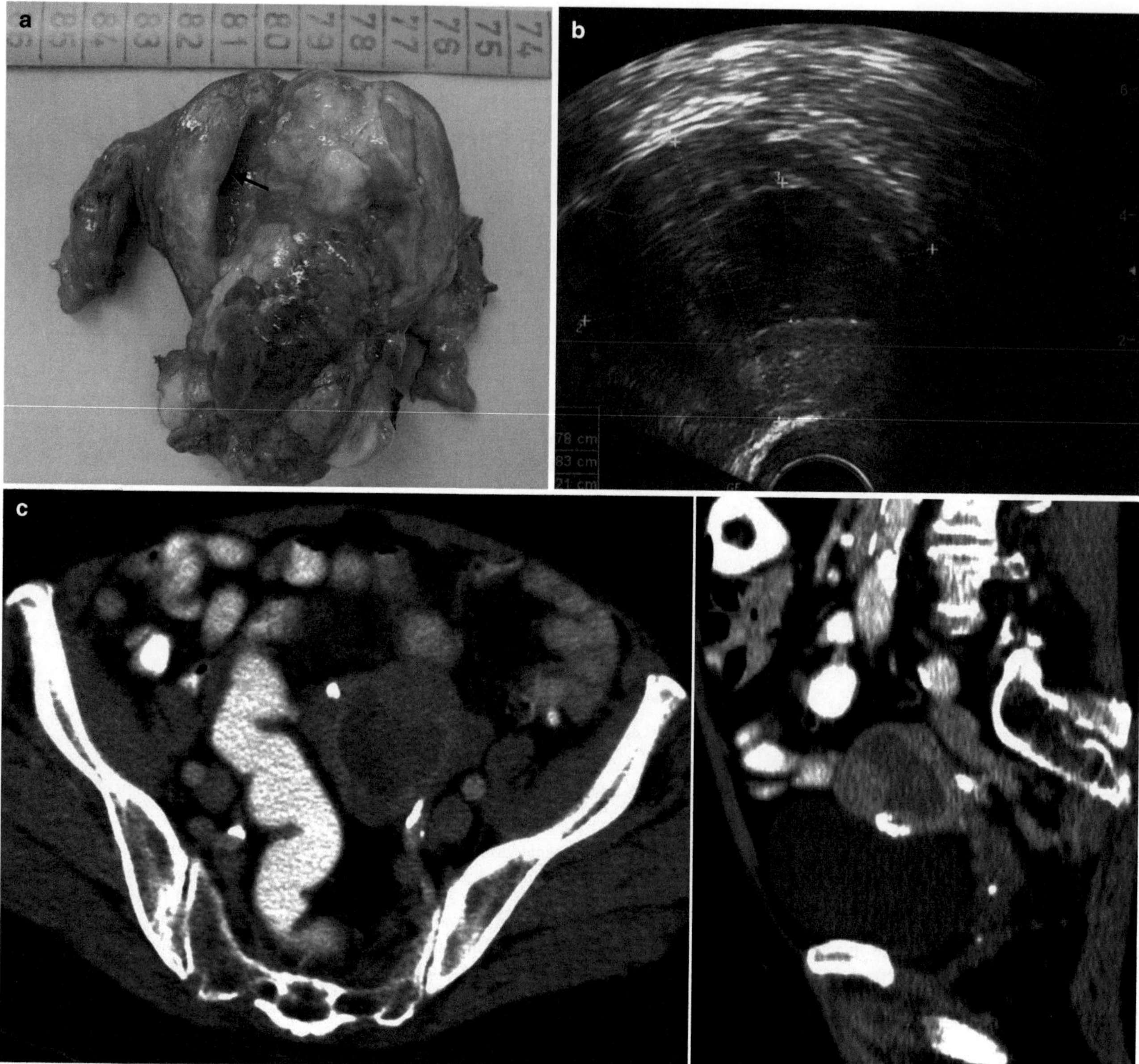

Fig. 14.17 High-grade endometrial stromal sarcoma. (**a**) Macroscopic appearance of an HG-ESS that originated in the anterior wall of the fundus and subsequently filled out the entire cavum. The endometrium is still visibly intact (*arrow*); (**b**) in sonography, the heterogeneous, predominantly hypoechoic HG-ESS is recognizably located within the endometrial hyperechoic band. The image also shows that the tumor interupts the endometrial band towards the fundus (*left side* of the image). The visible round finding with an echogenicity even lower than that of the surrounding tumor tissue, with dull interior echoes, most likely corresponds to a pathological-anatomically verified necrosis; (**c**) axial and sagittal CECT images show that the HG-ESS – with an enhancement weaker than that of the endometrium and the myometrium – is mostly located in the distended cavum of the uterus. As a secondary finding, an LM can be seen in the anterior wall of the uterus. This LM is also clearly visible when observing the macroscopic specimen (With permission of Köhler et al. [148], Fig. 2.3–17a, b, d)

Symptoms, Clinical Presentation, Clinical Diagnostics, Imaging, Differential Diagnosis

Postmenopausal bleeding is the pivotal symptom of HG-ESSs/USSs. Premenopausal women usually present with abnormal uterine or irregular menstrual bleeding. Rapid tumor growth results in marked, usually irregular enlargement of the uterus, and is usually associated with lower abdominal pains and uresiesthesis. Postmenopausal growth of the uterus is generally an observation that serves to arouse suspicion of sarcoma. HG-ESSs/USSs have a predominantly soft consistency. The rapid growth of the tumor can cause tumor masses to protrude from the cervix at a very early stage (Fig. 14.15a, b). Distant metastatic disease occurs very early. It is thus not seldom the case that HG-ESSs/UUSs are primarily discovered upon detection of their metastases.

Diagnostics largely correspond to the procedure followed for LMSs. Since up to 90 % of the tumor can consist of necrotic tissue, it can so occur that performing multiple curettages still fails to yield any actual tumor tissue. HG-ESSs/UUSs or malignant neoplasms are correctly diagnosed as such on the basis of curettage specimen analysis in only 35–65 % of cases [143, 278]. As metastatic spread to the abdominal cavity and the lungs is already present in up to 52 % of cases at the time of primary diagnosis [278], the pelvis, the abdomen, and the thorax should be subjected to imaging-based staging using CT or MRI after receipt of the histological diagnosis.

The sonographic picture correlates with the tumor's polymorphous gross appearance, characterized by decomposing tumor tissue, necroses, cysts, and dilated vessels alongside solid areas with high cell counts. Sonography, too, shows that the tumor usually fills the entire cavity of the uterus with clearly discernible myometrial invasion. As long as the tumor is predominantly located in the cavum, the endometrium is usually recognizable as a thin hyperechoic layer or band. It can be punctured or interrupted by the tumor in one or numerous locations, and is known to have been entirely consumed in some cases. Both HG-ESSs and UUSs are almost exclusively heterogeneously echogenic and are predominated by areas of hypoechoicity in the majority of cases. Tumors can also be predominantly hyperechoic in some cases. Anechoic areas, resembling larger cysts or wide seams/clefts, can be found in both the hypoechoic and the hyperechoic areas of virtually all such tumors. Narrow seams or signal voids often resemble vessels, while large hypoechoic areas resemble necroses or cystic structures. The borders between the hyperechoic and hypoechoic areas are virtually always derounded, with, in part, bizarrely frayed, ragged margins (Figs. 14.16a and 14.17b).

As is also the case for the other types of uterine sarcoma, Doppler sonography shows a highly hypervascular tumor, with an RI of 0.27 [208]. Despite noticeable conspicuous features, 56 % of HG-ESSs are assessed in sonography as being LMs, and 34.6 % are also subjected to surgery under that indication [143]. While 26.1 % of UUSs are operated on under the indication of an LM, to date, no UUSs are reported to have been sonographically classified as an LM [143].

CT is not suitable for precisely diagnosing or classifying HG-ESSs/UUSs, but is a useful method for staging diagnostics (Figs. 14.16b and 14.17c). Only very few data are available pertaining to the MRI-characteristics of these tumors. The absence of low SI in T2-weighted images (100 %), an inhomogeneous SI in T1-weighted images (88 %), and the presence of necroses (69 %) have the highest sensitivities in this regard, with respective specificities of 26, 42, and 98 %. There have been accounts in which adjacent regions of both high and low SI within the same tumor have been described [259]. Necroses and hemorrhagic areas are more common than in LG-ESSs, and the hypointense bands with low SI, that are typical of LG-ESSs, are absent in T2-weighted images [111, 158, 234]. Numerous signal voids can be observed within the areas of myometrial involvement that reflect the hypervascular nature of the tumors [158, 259]. There are accounts of normal myometrium having a clearly stronger enhancement than tumor tissue in T1C-weighted images [272]. There are also reports of iso- or hyperintense contrast enhancement compared with normal myometrium that can help in differentiating from endometrial carcinomas [249].

While both LG-ESSs and LMSs are primarily intramurally localised, clinical and imaging diagnostics usually reveal that HG-ESSs/UUSs are predominantly located within the cavity. In contrast to LG-ESSs, HG-ESSs/UUSs have a noticeably pleomorphic macroscopic appearance, with numerous necroses and hemorrhages that are not seldom accompanied by a pyometra.

HG-ESSs and UUSs do differ in terms of their microscopic appearance. In contrast to HG-ESSs, most UUSs exhibit no specific type of differentiation, both cytologically and immunohistochemically. HG-ESSs can be differentiated from UUSs by measuring cyclin-D1, CD10, and possibly ER- and PR-expression, all of which are negative in UUSs. Histologically discerning HG-ESSs/UUSs from LG-ESSs is usually unproblematic. Complications can arise when doing so solely on the basis of tissue specimens gathered via curettage or biopsy, since HG-ESSs can contain focal areas consisting of LG-ESS. Special attention needs to be devoted to identifying possible epithelial structures during microscopic examination so as not to overlook an AS or a carcinosarcoma.

Clinical Course, Prognostic Factors Relevant for Therapy

Both HG-ESSs and UUSs have a substantially poorer prognosis than LG-ESSs [163, 166]. Prognosis for HG-ESS/UUS worsens as patient age increases, and is especially unfavorable for women of particularly advanced aged [6, 47, 94]. Stage of disease is the most important prognostic factor [6]. Fifty-two to seventy-two percent of cases already exhibit primary involvement of the abdominal cavity [183, 278]. Overall, UUSs have an even worse prognosis than HG-ESSs [105, 160, 228]. Twenty percent of HG-ESS patients present with stage IA disease at the time of initial diagnosis, compared to only 12 % of UUS patients [143]. Moreover, among UUS patients, 32 resp. 28 % presented with FIGO-stage IVa resp. IVb disease at the time of initial diagnosis. For HG-ESS patients, the rate was 10 % both for stage IVa and stage IVb.

Metastases predominantly occur in the lung, the abdomen, the liver, and sometimes in the bones [183, 278]. There is significant variation in the data pertaining to regional LN involvement. An analysis of stage I-IV primary HG-ESSs and UUSs revealed positive pelvic and para-aortic LNs in 18 % resp. 15 % of cases [163]. A further study revealed an incidence of pelvic and/or para-aortic LN involvement of 44.4 % [183]. SEER-data [47], covering 143 patients with stage I-IV disease, revealed positive LNs in 18 % of cases, with a mean number of 12 removed LNs. Within the DKSM sample, positive LNs were found in 25 % of UUSs and only 7.7 % of HG-ESSs [143]. Positive LNs are a clear sign of a particularly poor prognosis. This evidently has to do with the fact that positive LNs are virtually always found in patients in whom disease has also spread to other extrauterine sites [183]. In light of research findings, according to which extrapelvic metastases with simultaneous pelvic disease recurrence are found in 75 % of cases [91], and isolated distant metastases occur in 67 % of cases [143], survival appears to be mainly determined by extrapelvic sites of recurrence or metastasization [183]. The ineffectiveness of LNE is thus primarily footed in the fact that disease is frequently already so extensive at the time of primary diagnosis. Accordingly, despite their intrinsic bias, the few available retrospective studies, including the SEER-data, have been unable to verify that performing an LNE on HG-ESS/UUS patients has any beneficial effects on survival [94, 154, 185, 256].

Removing or preserving the ovaries has no influence on survival, neither for HG-ESSs nor for UUSs [94, 257].

Median RFI and OS for all cases is 5–11 resp. 11.8 Mo [129, 143, 163]. Among other factors, the median RFI is strongly dependent on the type of surgery performed – 8 Mo for cases of adequate surgery, and 3 Mo for inadequate operations [143]. In contrast to LG-ESS, R2-resection margins, in particular, are associated with an extremely negative prognosis [163, 183]. It more than seldom occurs that recurrences become clinically evident within only a few weeks of primary diagnosis [278].

Surgical Therapy and Problems

Total abdominal HE with BSO is regarded as the generally accepted surgical standard for HG-ESSs/UUSs. Since steroid receptor expression is nearly always negative in UUSs, resection of the adnexa is not absolutely necessary in premenopausal women. Given that HG-ESSs and UUSs are said to metastasize to the ovaries rather frequently [302], performing a BSO by all means seems to be appropriate. However, it remains scientifically unproven that performing such surgery offers any benefits in cases in which the ovaries are clinically tumor-free. The current NCCN-guidelines, accordingly, state that decisions to leave the ovaries *in situ* should be made on an individualized case-by-case basis that takes reproductive age into account [202]. Clinically tumor-free ovaries need not be removed, according to the ESMO-guidelines [74]. HG-ESSs that express ER- and/or PR-positivity should be subjected to surgical therapy as described for LG-ESSs.

Since the number of extrapelvic recurrences and distant metastases clearly exceeds the incidence of local disease recurrence, the degree to which performing a systematic LNE can be deemed appropriate is both questionable and strongly debated (see prognosis for details). Isolated LN-metastases only rarely occur postoperatively [183, 278]. LNE has not been included as a surgical measure in the current NCCN-guidelines [202], and well-researched reviews [91] as well as the current ESMO-guidelines do not recommend it [74]. The Japanese guidelines state that pelvic and para-aortic LNE can nonetheless be considered, but simultaneously draw attention to the absence of scientifically proven therapeutic benefits [201]. The aforementioned guidelines go on to state that LNs can be resected in order to reduce tumor burden when they are radiologically or clinically suspicious. The GCIG-consensus does not recommend performing a systematic LNE unless there is a radiological or clinical suspicion of nodal involvement [220]. However, no statement is made in the guidelines as to the benefits of such practice.

Overall, all forms of LNE currently lack an adequate and sufficing scientific evidence base and thus cannot be defined as standard practice. Where this procedure is nonetheless opted for, it must be borne in mind that no therapeutic consequences can be deduced from the findings resulting from said course of action, even in cases of LN-positivity.

The risks associated with tumor enucleation, supracervical HE, and injuring the uterus or the tumor are addressed in detail in the sections on LMSs and LG-ESSs. 35.7 % of HG-ESSs and 36.4 % of UUSs are subjected to inadequate surgical procedures. While these rates are lower than those measured for LG-ESSs, from a prognostic perspective, they are still too high [143]. Adhering to the diagnostics flowchart (Fig. 14.22) presented in the section "risks and prevention of inadequate surgery" can contribute significantly to preventing inadequate operations being performed, as the criteria described there equally apply to HG-ESSs/UUSs.

HG-ESSs/UUSs that have invaded the abdominal cavity (stage III) should be subjected to maximal cytoreductive surgery. According to retrospective studies pertaining to all uterine sarcomas, and a retrospective study on HG-ESSs/UUSs [163], maximal debulking is evidently associated with improved survival. Complete macroscopic resection was achieved in 60–86 % of patients, though it should be noted that these figures also include intestinal resections [183, 272]. However, due to the fact that these tumors are highly malignant, rapid progression is still identified in 61 % of cases despite having achieved complete gross (R0) resection [278]. Overall, free resection margins are regarded as the most important prognostic factor [205]. Compared to incomplete macroscopic resection, maximal cytoreduction is associated with significantly improved OS [183]. Some studies suggest that cytoreductive surgery generally has no influence on OS [280]. According to the current NCCN-2A-recommendations and the Japanese guidelines, the decision to surgically resect all tumor tissue can be made on an individualized i.e. case-specific basis, depending on symptoms, extent of disease, and resectability [201, 202]. The GCIG-consensus [220] points out that debulking apparently (though not significantly) improves OS, albeit without making a formal recommendation to that end. An LNE is deemed inappropriate when there is evidence of extrauterine disease [202]. Selective resection of affected enlarged LNs could be appropriate, if it has also been achieved that the patient is intrabdominally tumor free. Overall, the available data pertaining to such cases are very slim at best.

Regarding aftercare, reference should be had to what is stated for LMSs. There is no indication for adjuvant/postoperative chemo- and/or radiotherapy. For more detailed information, reference should be had to the specialist literature [148].

Adenosarcoma

Epidemiology, Etiology, Pathogenesis, Staging

AS is a mixed tumor that consists of a benign epithelial and a malignant mesenchymal (stromal) component. ASs occur with and without SO (sarcomatous overgrowth, see below). Due to the rarity of this variety of tumor, there are currently no "evidence based" therapeutic strategies. The NCCN-guidelines for uterine sarcomas make no reference to ASs. Studies that are devoted solely to ASs are, without exception, retrospective case studies with relatively small sample sizes on average.

When carcinosarcomas are excluded, ASs account for 8.9 % of all uterine sarcomas [143]. More detailed information pertaining to AS prevalence rates are generally non-existent. The majority of AS-patients are aged 50–70 years, with a median age of 54–58 years [45]. Patients covered in the DKSM material database are aged between 22 and 82 years (mean: 55.6, median: 56 years) [143]. There are clear age differences between AS-patients with and without SO: according to the literature, the median age of patients without SO is 58 years (29–87 years), compared to 67 years [38–94] among patients with SO [24]. According to DKSM-data, the median ages are 56 and 55 years, respectively [143]. ASs thus occur in postmenopausal women in the majority of cases.

Uterine ASs develop in the endometrium in more than 90 % of cases. ASs that originate in the myometrium are likely to have developed from an adenomyosis [102, 209]. There are accounts of ASs primarily originating in the cervix [24, 184]. Likewise, cases in which ASs have developed from adenofibromas are long known to exist. AS-patients often exhibit a previous medical history of cervical or corporal polyps. It is likely that ASs or adenofibromas were not primarily recognized as such in these cases. There are multiple reports pertaining to the existence of a connection between AS and tamoxifen exposure [17, 52, 56, 77, 127].

Since 2009, new binding FIGO-staging and UICC-classifications [83, 264] have been in place for ASs that differ from those provided for pure uterine sarcomas (Table 14.7), and that take into consideration the fact that ASs generally originate in the endometrium in 90 % of cases.

Macroscopic and Microscopic Appearance

ASs are usually polypoid or papillary, often broad-based pedunculated masses that frequently fill the endometrial cavity (Figs. 14.18a, b and 14.21a, c, e). ASs can grow to a considerable size. Diameters of up to 20 cm have been described in the literature [92]. In most cases, the tumor forces the myometrium apart. Myometrial infiltration only rarely occurs in cases of ASs without SO. ASs contain epithelial

Table 14.7 FIGO staging for adenosarcomas [291]

I	**Tumor limited to uterus**
IA	Tumor limited to endometrium/endocervix with no myometrial invasion
IB	Less than or equal to half myometrial invasion
IC	More than half myometrial invasion
II	**Tumor extends to the pelvis**
IIA	Adnexal involvement
IIB	Tumor extends to extrauterine pelvic tissue
III	**Tumor invades abdominal tissues**
IIIA	One site/organ
IIIB	> one site/organ
IIIC	Metastasis to pelvic and/or para-aortic lymph nodes
IV	**Tumor invades bladder and/or rectum and/or distant metastasis**
IVA	Tumor invades bladder and/or rectum
IVB	Distant metastasis

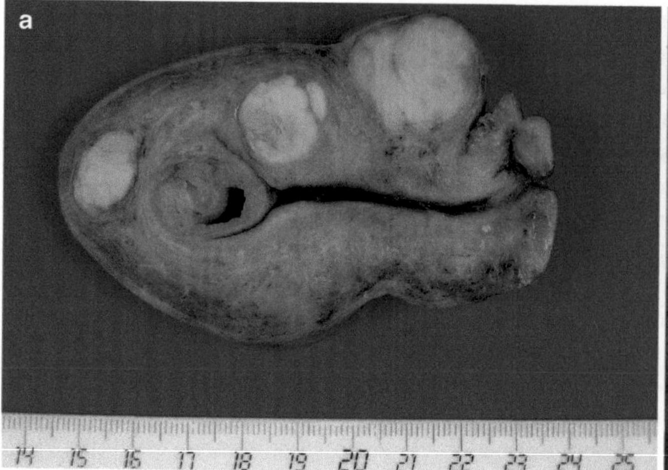

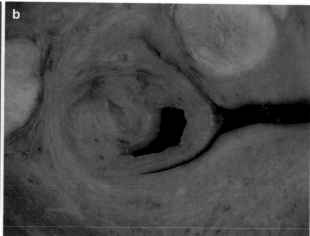

Fig. 14.18 Adenosarcoma. (**a**) An AS alongside several LMs in the fundus of the uterus; (**b**) it becomes apparent upon magnification that the AS developed from the endometrium and subsequently advanced into the cavum like a broad-based polyp. Numerous smaller and larger cysts are recognizable within tumor. They usually correspond to dilated endometrial glands and can be easily visualized via imaging diagnostics (With permission of Köhler et al. [153], Fig. 3.2–1a, b)

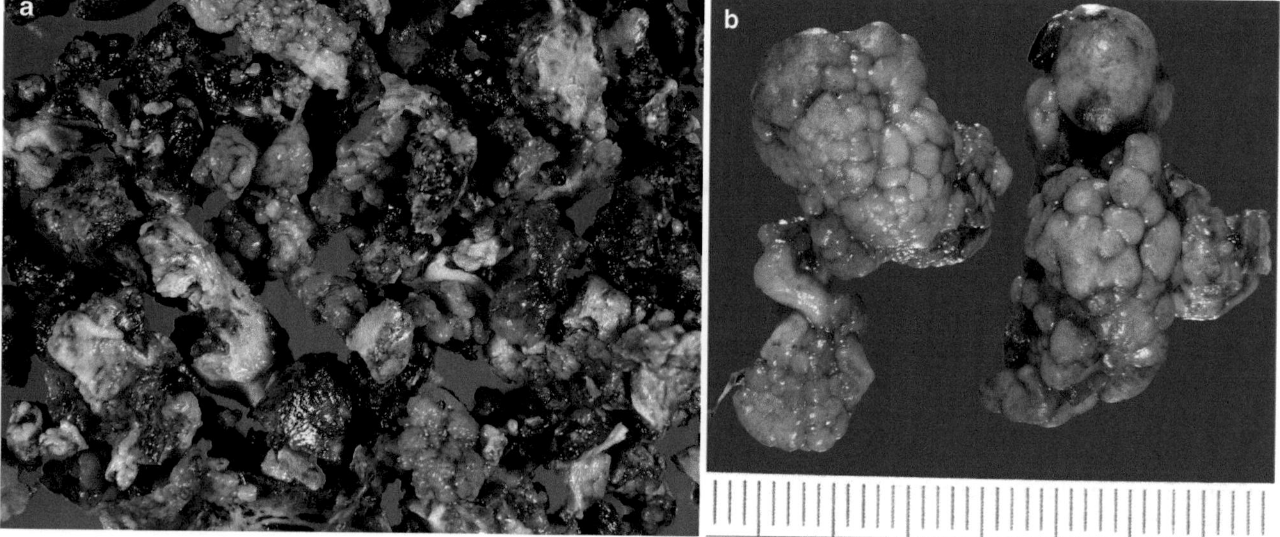

Fig. 14.19 Adenosarcoma without sarcomatous overgrowth. (**a, b**) The AS specimens obtained via curettage have a noticeable grape-like appearance that becomes even more apparent when magnified (**b**) (With permission of Köhler et al. [153], Fig. 3.2–2a, b)

cysts that vary in size and that effect a spongy appearance on the cut surface. Grape-shaped tumor masses are also typical in this context (Fig. 14.19a, b). The yellowish to brownish, pink or white to gray tumor is usually also macroscopically well differentiated from the myometrium. Outside the cystic areas, the tumor can be of a solid or fleshy, but also a soft and gelatinous consistency. Grossly visible necroses and hemorrhages can be observed in roughly one quarter of all cases.

An AS is classified as homologous when the sarcomatous component is of uterine origin (endometrial stroma, myometrium, connective tissue, vessels). Said component is comprised of an LG-ESS, an HG-ESS, a UUS, or an LMS in the vast majority of such cases. Roughly 75–80 % of ASs are homologous tumors [55, 92]. By contrast, an AS is heterologous if the sarcomatous component derives from extrauterine tissue. In those cases, the mesenchymal component usually consists of rhabdomyosarcoma or chondrosarcoma, or osteosarcoma, liposarcoma, or another form of sarcoma in rarer cases.

Classification of ASs into tumors with or without SO is of considerable clinical and prognostic importance. An AS is classified as having SO when more than 25 % of the tumor volume is composed of pure (i. e. epithelium-free) sarcoma [178]. AS without SO is regarded as the “classical” or “typical” variant of AS. Unfortunately, numerous studies and publications make no precise distinction between these two

AS-variants. A look at the histological appearance of ASs reveals an eye-catching phylloid, leaf-like, or papillary growth pattern. Epithelium-lined clefts and cysts of varying size, combined with papillary protrusions of cellular stroma into these cysts, serve to generate this appearance.

The epithelium is distributed across the entire tumor, usually in the form of benign glandular isles, however without fostering an impression of infiltration. In most cases, the epithelium is atrophic/inactive or resembles the normal phase of proliferation. The presence of malignant epithelial cells is indicative of carcinosarcoma.

The characteristic abounding, collar-like growth of stroma cells around the benign glands has resulted in the coining of the term "cuffing", a phenomenon that is strongly suggestive of an AS both in diagnostics and DD. The fact that ASs are closely related to adenofibromas is also more than apparent at the microscopic level. Prime criteria for distinguishing ASs from adenofibromas are: an MI $\geq$ 2 M/10 HPF, marked stromal hypercellularity with periglandular or subepithelial stroma cell congestions (collar, cuff), and significant stromal cell atypia. The mitotic rate is usually between 2–4 M/10 HPF. However, the mean mitotic rate across the whole tumor is only 2.2 M/10 HPF [266]. Nuclear atypia are predominantly mild-to-moderate. The majority of ASs without SO are confined to the cavity of the uterus or to the endometrium. Myometrial invasions are rare and non-destructive. They occurre in roughly 20 % (16–42 %) of cases, and usually reach only a few millimeters deep [55, 92]. Lymphovascular invasion is reported in only 7 % of cases [131]. Analogous to LG-ESSs, ASs without SO are characterized by high levels of HR-expression: in one study, ER- resp. PR-positivity were measured in the epithelial component of 85 resp. 65 %, while the stromal component was ER- resp. PR-positive in 80 resp. 60 % of cases. Both ER- and PR-positivity were detected in 90 % of cases [8]. Analogous to LG-ESSs, CD10 expression tests positively in 81–100 % of ASs without SO. Moreover, immunohistochemical testing has verified a smooth muscle differentiation in numerous cases (smooth muscle actin, desmin) [8, 189, 266]. Overall, ASs without SO and LG-ESSs share numerous morphological and immunophenotypical commonalities.

ASs with SO differ from the aforementioned typical or classic ASs in numerous aspects. The literature suggests a rather wide range of frequency, from 8 to 60 % of all ASs. The majority of studies narrow their share down to 20 to 48 % [45, 55, 92, 131, 178, 253, 266, 279]. 35.1 % of all ASs in the DKSM-materials exhibited SO [143]. While no significant differences between ASs with and without SO are discernible in the epithelial component of the tumor, the sarcomatous component of ASs with SO usually consists of an HG-ESS, a UUS, or another high-grade sarcoma, for instance rhabdomyosarcoma or angiosarcoma. With an MI of up to 115 M/10 HPF and a mean MI of 13.5 M/10 HPF, the number of mitoses is significantly higher in ASs with SO compared to ASs without SO [55, 92, 266]. Myometrial invasion is observed in 53–60 % of cases [92, 159] and often borders on the serosa. Lymphovascular invasion is verified in up to 24 % of cases. Hemorrhaging, necroses, and heterologous components are much more frequent in this neoplasm than in its counterpart without SO [131]. Analogous to HG-ESSs and UUSs, and in contrast to LG-ESSs, ER- and PR-expression are very low or non-existent. The epithelial component has shown ER- and PR-positivity in 50 % resp. 25 %, while the stromal component has shown ER-positivity in 0 % and PR-positivity in only 0–12 % of cases [9, 92]. CD10-expression is positively measured in the sarcomatous component of no more than 28 % of ASs with SO [8, 92, 255].

Symptoms, Clinical Presentation, Clinical Diagnostics, Imaging, Differential Diagnosis

Since ASs originate in the endometrium or the cervix, abnormal vaginal bleeding or postmenopausal bleeding are the most commonly presenting symptoms. Overall, the symptoms correspond to those of endometrial carcinomas. Like for the other uterine sarcomas, a broad-based, usually polypoid tumor protruding from the cervix is a commonly reported finding (Fig. 14.20a–c). Especially in very young patients, such tumors usually turn out to be cervical ASs. Lower abdominal pain is a frequent symptom resulting from rapid tumor growth, which in turn causes the uterus to expand and/or the cervix to dilate. Performing an HSC and/or fractional curettage is indicated when patients present with abnormal/postmenopausal bleeding (Fig. 14.20c, d). ASs can primarily originate in the myometrium; however, this is only rarely known to have occurred. Notwithstanding, in such cases, the AS might not be traceable in tissue specimens retrieved via curettage.

Since ASs originate in the endometrium in more than 90 % of cases, in contrast to both LG-ESSs and LMSs, sonography, too, shows that they are limited to the endometrium or primarily centrally located. The tumor often fills the endometrial cavity. In contrast to polyps, which constitute an important DD for ASs, sonography reveals a broad-based connection to the endometrium almost without exception.

The AS has a higher echogenicity than the surrounding myometrium and is thus well differentiated from it. ASs are heterogeneously echogenic in the majority of cases [273] and thus essentially correspond the echogenic texture of the endometrium [52]. Analogous to the macroscopic and microscopic appearance that is characterized by cystically dilated glands, sonography, too, reveals an internal structure that comprises numerous anechoic areas that represent said

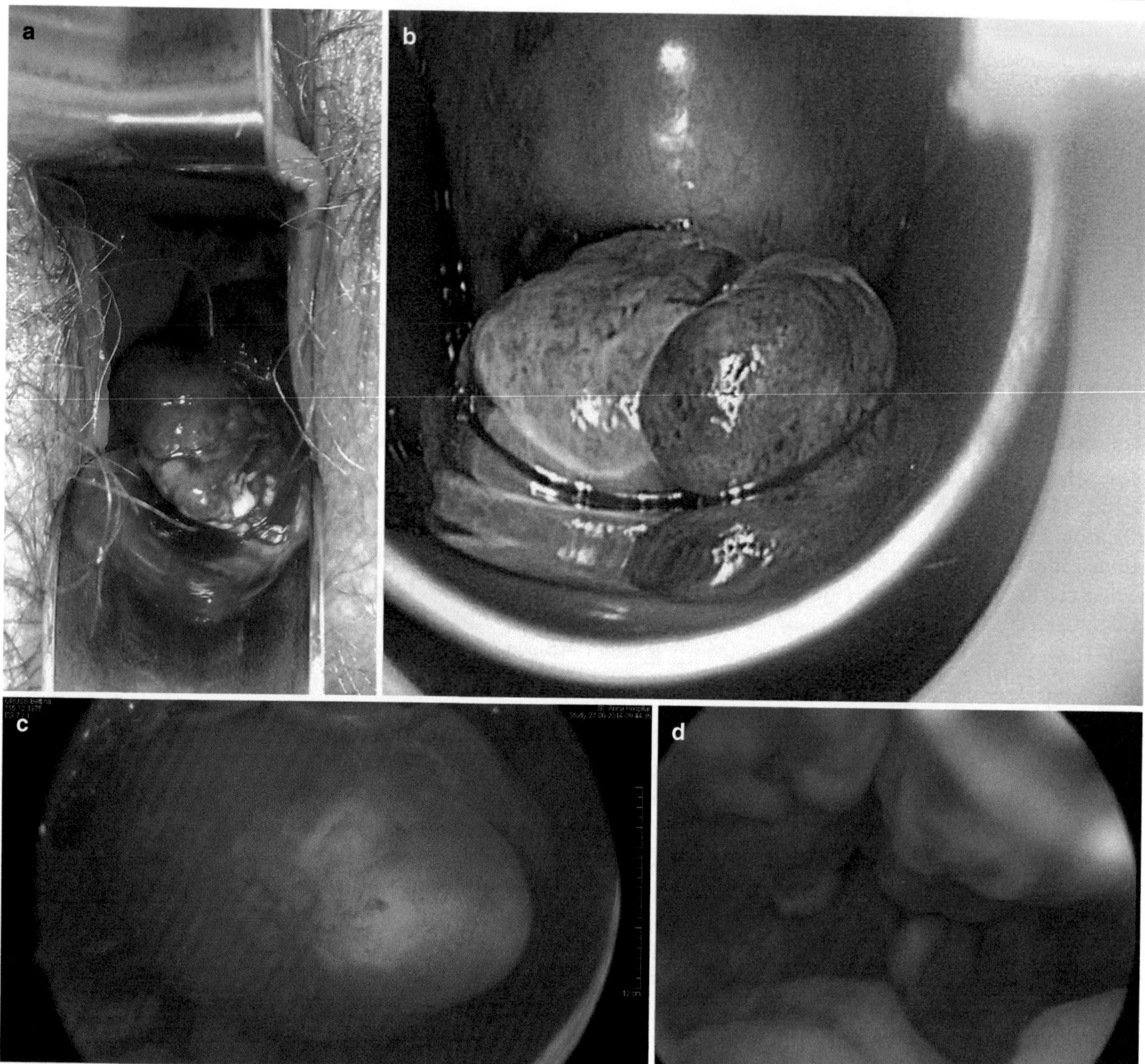

Fig. 14.20 Adenosarcoma with and without sarcomatous overgrowth. (**a**) AS without SO that has prolapsed into the vagina, the cystic-polypoid structure is clearly recognizable on close observation; (**b**) two polyps removed via hysteroscopic resection that turned out to be AS with SO. The presence of only very few barely discernible cysts is a typical feature; (**c**) hysteroscopic finding of a relatively smooth intracavitary tumor the macroscopic observation of which yielded no suspicions of AS; (**d**) typical HSC-image depicting grape-like AS without SO in a 21 y.o. patient (With permission of Köhler et al. [153], Fig. 3.2–6a–d)

glands [52]. The resulting respective visual appearance is of seminal importance for arriving at the proper diagnosis. The phylloid growth pattern can also be clearly recognizable in fortunate cases (Fig. 14.21a). Nonetheless, the location of these tumors within the cavity and their predominantly hyperechogenic texture make them difficult to differentiate from carcinosarcomas and endometrial carcinomas.

Doppler-sonographic criteria correspond to those for LG-ESSs and LMSs, characterized in particular by strong irregular central vascularity. One marked difference, however, lies in the fact that, in ASs, the numerous differently sized cysts are easily recognizable alongside the visible vessels (Fig. 14.21b).

CT is not suitable for precisely diagnosing or classifying tumors, but is a useful method for spread-related diagnostics and staging. However, the presence of numerous intratumoral cysts with a density equal to that of water (Hounsfield-unit 0) could be suggestive of an AS (Fig. 14.21c). T1 W MR-images reveal a heterogeneous tumor with intermediate SI that is usually isointense to the myometrium. Hemorrhagic areas are characterized by areas of high SI, while the (usually numerous) cystic areas of varying size have low SI on

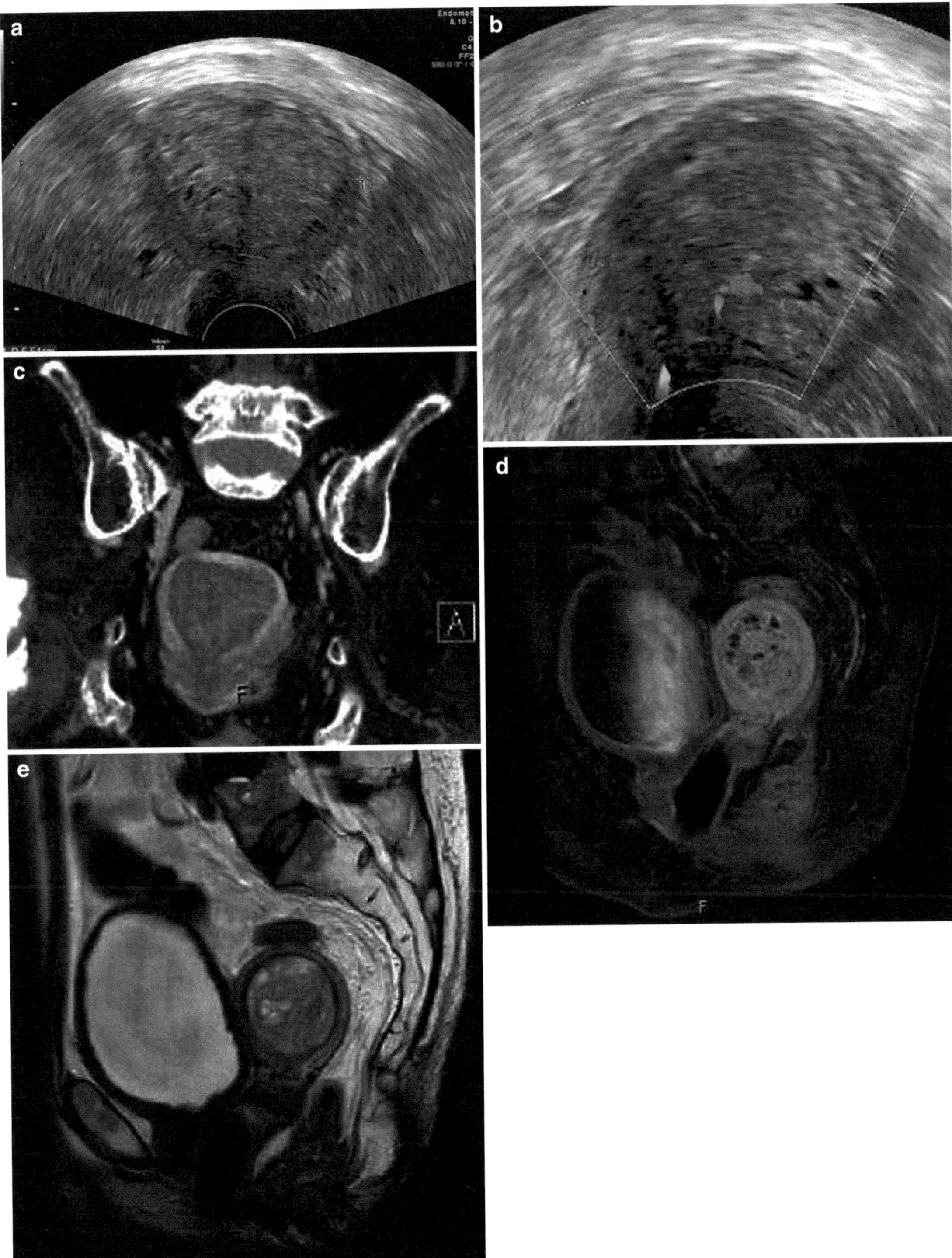

Fig. 14.21 Adenosarcoma without sarcomatous overgrowth. (**a**) Grayscale sonography of an AS without SO with a mesenchymal component resembling LG-ESS shows a tumor with irregular bizarre margins that is hyperechoic to normal myometrium, that fills the entire cavum, and that has inflitrated the myometrium in multiple locations. Numerous anechoic areas are visible that correspond to vessels and dilated endometrial glands; (**b**) color Doppler sonography reveals some of these anechoic spaces to be dilated vessels; (**c**) the findings from CECT correspond to those from sonography, the non-enhancing areas correspond to dilated glands; infiltrations of the more hyperdense myometrium are clearly recognizable; (**d**) AS shows a similar enhancement to normal myometrium in T1 W-contrast MRT with fat suppression. As is also the case in T2 W, here, too, there is a discernible margin (albeit with a lesser degree of hypointensity at the bottom of the tumor) that is interrupted in several places (as is also recognizable in **e**). The non-enhancing hypointense sections correspond to the hyperintense areas in T2 W; (**e**) analogous to LG-ESS, this T2 W images show a clear hypointense rim or margin that is breached in the lower part of the uterus, where it most likely corresponds to myometrial infiltration. The strongly hyperintense sections predominantly correspond to the greatly dilated, fluid-filled glands (With permission of Köhler et al. [153], Fig. 6–8a–d, f)

T1-weighted images [52, 301]. ASs have heterogeneous SI on T2 W-images with hypointense, intermediate, and hyperintense areas. The multitudinous hyperintense regions represent the cystic components, while the areas of low-to-intermediate SI correspond to the solid components of the tumor [272, 273, 275, 281]. Clustered cystic components with strong SI are regarded as a key finding. The tumor components that are hypointense in T2 W-images show a strong enhancement in T1 WC images [272]. There are accounts of cases in which the myometrium has a stronger enhancement than the tumor, which makes tumor invasions easy to recognize, as well as of SIs that appear isointense compared to the myometrium [301]. The enhancing solid tumor components, as well as the enhancing septa between the non-enhancing cystic areas, often generate a lattice- or truss-like overall visual impression [52, 275, 301] (Fig. 14.21d, e).

It is barely possible to grossly differentiate an AS from endometrial carcinoma, carcinosarcoma, adenofibroma, stromal sarcomas as well as from large necrotic endometrial polyps solely on the basis of macroscopic observation of the resected and opened uterus. Real polyps usually have a tapered, gradually narrowing stem and a generally smooth appearance. ASs, by contrast, usually have a broad-based connection to the corpus or the cervix. Multitudinous cystic structures or a grape-like appearance are suggestive of an AS, but are also characteristics of botryoid rhabdomyosarcoma.

Adenofibroma constitutes the most difficult and challenging DD, since the histological transition from adenofibroma to adenosarcoma is a continuous, gradual one [55, 92]. ASs without SO are generally difficult to differentiate from LG-ESSs, since these two tumor types are largely identical in terms of their morphology and immunophenotypic profiles [266]. In particular, basing diagnostic decisions and conclusions on a relatively small amount of tissue, for example such stemming from a frozen section or curettage, bears numerous trap doors and much room for potential misinterpretation. In such cases, the specimens might omit the epithelial components or facilitate them being overlooked, thus making misdiagnoses as pure sarcomas more likely. Within the DKSM-materials, on the basis of the curettage specimens alone, 17.6 % of all ASs were primarily diagnosed as purely homologous or heterologous sarcomas (LG-ESS, HG-ESS, UUS, LMS, rhabdomyosarcoma) [143]. Final diagnosis is thus frequently only reached upon examination of the surgical specimen.

Clinical Course, Prognostic Factors Relevant for Therapy

Generally speaking, stage of disease is the most important prognostic factor for both AS-types [2]. There is apparently no correlation between MI-levels and rates of recurrence [131]. Deep myometrial invasion and lymphovascular invasion are regarded as predictors of recurrence and metastasis [92, 131].

According to DKSM findings and the majority of other studies, metastatic spread to the ovaries is not observed at the time of primary diagnosis [16, 30, 143, 279]. One further study reported ovarian involvement at the time of primary therapy in 8 % of cases. Metastases were not visible on gross observation in 2 of 5 cases [45].

Only limited data are available pertaining to the rate to which LNs test positive in cases of AS with and without SO. According to one study covering 262 cases of AS, nodal metastases were found in only 3.1 % of cases of AS (all stages) with and without SO [16]. A further study [45] identified positive LNs in only one case of AS with SO, accompanied by further extrauterine spread. Within the DKSM materials, LN-metastases could be verified for 33 % of ASs with SO and 11 % of ASs without SO. Interestingly, recurrences only occurred in patients with negative LNs. 25 % of distant metastases occurred in patients with positive LNs, while the LNs of the remaining 75 % of patients who developed distant metastatic disease tested negative [143]. Accordingly, the prognostic value of positive LNs is indeed questionable. Data stemming from some smaller research series suggest that performing an LNE may well serve to reduce the number of pelvic recurrences [244, 280]. These findings notwithstanding, according to SEER-data, performing an LNE does not seem to affect OS beneficially, even in cases of positive lymph node metastasis [256]. Further retrospective studies, too, have confirmed that, to date, performing an LNE apparently serves to provide no benefits in terms of OS [30, 154].

The typical (classical) AS-variant – AS without SO – is associated with a relatively favorable prognosis (analogous to LG-ESS) and is often cited as a tumor with low malignant potential [92, 131, 228, 293]. In actual fact, up to 96 % of AS patients initially present with stage I disease [30]. Tumor growth is relatively slow and recurrences usually occur in the form of late recurrences in the vagina, the lesser pelvis, and the abdomen. Reported rates of recurrence range from 7–14 % [30, 55, 131, 279]. Distant metastasis has been described in up to 50 % of cases [30], with a median time to recurrence of 21.3 Mo (10.4–60.9 Mo) [30].

Presence of SO is significantly statistically associated with less favorable OS and is regarded as an independent prognostic determinant *per se* [42, 92, 288]. Thirty to forty percent of ASs with OS are already at an advanced stage of disease at the time of initial diagnosis [30, 159]. Overall, rapid tumor growth and early recurrence and/or metastasization should be expected when SO is present. Recurrence rates for ASs with SO have been measured at 44–80 % [30, 55, 131, 279] and distant metastases occur in up to 90 % of cases [30]. In 30 % of cases overall, lung metastases arise without local recurrences or metastases in the abdominal cavity [30]. The risk of recurrence is roughly 3.2 times higher than for classic ASs [131]. The median period of time until the occurrence of first tumor recurrence is 21.3 Mo (2.1–87.8 Mo) [30]. Overall, the presence of SO and/or predominantly myometrial invasion as well as lymphovascular invasion are regarded as the most reliable histological predictors for recurrence of AS [45, 110, 266].

Taking both AS variants together, the time period until first recurrence is around 3.4–5 years; 38–40 % of first recurrences occur after 5 years or more. There are accounts of dramatic courses in which tumors recurred within just 2 weeks [76]. Isolated recurrences in the vagina and the pelvis are observed in 33 % and 28 % of cases, respectively. Roughly 38 % of recurrences occur in the abdomen and the pelvis with and without distant metastases. By contrast, isolated (!) distant metastases are observed in only 5–9 % of all AS patients. Hematogenous metastatic spread is rather the exception and practically only occurs in AS-patients with SO [55, 303]. A recent analysis [45] measured a median RFI and a median OS of 29.4 resp. 55.4 Mo for ASs with SO, compared to 105.9 resp. 112.4 Mo for ASs without SO. Among stage I disease patients, 77 % with SO and 22 % of patients without SO showed recurrence. The difference was statistically significant.

Thus, ASs with SO and ASs without SO differ significantly in terms of their prognosis. The former exhibits clinical and prognostic behavior and characteristics more reminiscent of HG-ESSs and other high-grade sarcomas, while the latter more closely resembles LG-ESSs from a clinical and prognostic perspective.

Surgical Therapy and Problems

Since ASs are rare malignancies, there are currently no therapeutic studies that are devoted solely to this form of tumor. Accordingly, there are no recommendations that fulfill the criteria for "evidence based medicine". The NCCN-guidelines [202] contain no provisions pertaining to ASs. The situation is even more unsatisfactory if one differentiates between ASs with and without SO. Therapeutic decision-making is made somewhat easier, however, by the fact that ASs and stromal sarcomas share certain clinical, microscopic, biochemical, and prognostic commonalities [266]: AS without SO is more reminiscent of LG-ESS, while AS with SO more closely resembles HG-ESS or other high-grade sarcomas, not least because, in ASs, prognosis is primarily influenced by or dependent on the mesenchymal component. Procedure should or can thus be guided by the procedure applied to the sarcomas to which the different AS variants bear close resemblance [86, 266, 288]. One exception is when the sarcomatous component consists of a rhabdomyosarcoma, in which case the tumor should not be approached as if it were a rhabdomyosarcoma, but instead analogous to the other high-grade sarcomas.

In accordance with the current NCCN-guidelines for LG-ESSs and HG-ESSs and the GCIG-consensus [86, 202], total HE without injuring the uterus with accompanying BSO is regarded as the adequate surgical approach to be applied, and thus as accepted standard practice. There is no indication for performing total vaginal HE when an AS has been diagnosed, due to the risk of injuring the uterus and the fact that this procedure does not allow for abdominal exploration. Laparoscopically assisted vaginal HE or total laparoscopic HE, when opted for, must be performed without causing injury to the uterus.

The SEER-analyses and the lack of scientific evidence notwithstanding, there is nonetheless consensus among several studies that a BSO is more likely indicated when the tumor expresses HR positivity [11, 29, 91, 174]. The data, when taken together, suggest that preserving the adnexa is at least a possibility, i.e. that a subsequent extirpation can be forgone. According to the NCCN-guidelines, in referring to LG-ESS, decisions for or against performing a BSO can be made on an individualized basis under consideration of patients' reproductive age or desire for fertility preservation [202]. This statement is supported by the current GCIG-consensus [86]. Patients with HR-positive ASs should, however, be informed of the potentially elevated risk of recurrence that is associated with ovarian preservation. Said risk obviously only applies to uterus-preserving surgical procedures. This issue is discussed in more detail in the section on LG-ESSs. Since ASs with SO are usually HR-negative, a BSO is not indicated when the ovaries are unsuspicious.

It is currently contested whether or not performing an LNE is necessary [131], not least because the share of cases with nodal involvement is low (see prognosis). In the current NCCN-guidelines, LNE has been removed from the recommendations for all uterine sarcomas [202]. Likewise, according to the current GCIG-consensus, the benefits of an LNE have yet to be scientifically proven. Routinely performing a systematic LNE is thus not recommended [86]. However, the guidelines do indeed recommend the removal of all metastatic masses, which can be interpreted as a recommendation for performing selective LNE on enlarged LNs on an individualized basis. It needs to be reiterated that the preceding statement is not supported by evidence-based data, and that it has yet to be scientifically proven to any degree that performing any form of LNE is beneficial for prognosis.

In summary, systematic LNE or LN-sampling currently lack a sufficing and adequate scientific basis, and can thus not be defined as standard practice [45, 86, 91, 256]. Sampling enlarged LNs is currently deemed a justifiable compromise. If an LNE of any type is opted for, it must be borne in mind that no therapeutic consequences can be deduced from the findings resulting from said course of action, even when the LNs test positive. Overall, therefore, not performing an LNE cannot be regarded as erroneous practice.

Stand-alone tumor extirpation, any form of morcellation, and any form of supracervical HE all constitute inadequate surgical procedures for ASs. As also applies for LG-ESSs, HG-ESSs, UUSs, and LMSs, a negative impact on the prognosis has to be expected when such procedures are performed [72]. However, 19 % of all ASs are still operated on under the indication of an LM [143]. The problems connected with and arising from inadequate surgical procedures, including morcellation in particular, are elaborated in detail in the section on LMS, while strategies for preventing inadequate surgery are discussed in the section on "risk and prevention of inadequate surgery" using a diagnostic flowchart (Fig. 14.22).

Local resection appears to be an option in exceptional cases of young women who urgently desire fertility-preservation and in whom the AS without SO is conveniently located within and confined to the uterus [55, 110, 184, 267]. It is necessary that R0-resection margins are achieved beyond doubt. One study revealed that one patient who underwent curettage alone, and two patients who underwent supracervical HE, had no recurrences [30]. According to two further studies [42, 84], among 7 adolescents who underwent organ-sparing surgery for cervical ASs, 5 developed recurrences. Conservative procedures are best suited for pedunculated tumors confined to the endometrium, under the condition that R0-resection is achieved [110]. In general, organ-sparing surgery, including supracervical HE, should nonetheless be classified as inadequate procedure and should thus not be recommended by physicians. Should the patient insist on such surgery, she must be thoroughly informed of the implications of such course of action, not least because preserving the ovaries when an HR-positive AS has been subjected to inadequate surgery could potentially promote recurrence (as also applies to LG-ESSs). A case has been reported in which adnexal preservation was not accompanied by recurrence in the follow-up period [184].

ASs that have spread within the pelvis and the abdominal cavity should be subjected to maximal cytoreductive surgery. Retrospective studies, albeit referring to all uterine sarcomas, suggest that such procedure is associated with improved OS [91]. There is an account of a patient with an AS with SO that had spread to and within the pelvis, who underwent a total of three cytoreductive operations following total HE with BSO plus cytoreduction plus hyperthermic intraperitoneal CHT with 50 mg/m^2 melphalan. The patient was still alive with disease after 55 months [128]. However, it remains unclear in this case whether hyperthermic CHT actually had any effects. Drawing on findings relating to LG-ESSs, it can be assumed that performing maximal cytoreductive surgery in cases of ASs without SO allows improvements in OS to be expected [280]. "Removal of all tumor" and "free resection margins" are deemed the most important prognostic factors [205]. For ASs with SO, analogous to HG-ESSs, due to the absence of effective alternatives, maximal cytoreductive surgery should also be considered. According to the current NCCN-2A-recommendations (that refer to all uterine sarcomas), the decision to surgically resect all tumor tissue can be made on an individualized i.e. case-specific basis, depending on symptoms, extent of disease, and resectability. LNE is deemed inadequate where there is extrauterine spread [202]. There are currently no data available pertaining to the potential benefits of performing a selective LNE, even when R0 resection margins have been achieved.

More extensive surgical procedures, for example exenterations, are generally rejected on the grounds of the substantial complications that can arise and in light of the poor prognosis with which sarcomas with exception of LG-ESS are generally associated. Pelvic exenteration should only be considered in exceptional cases, in which R0-resection (i.e. resection with clear margins) can be achieved and the patient is young and in a good general state of health [137].

Aftercare should be managed in accordance to what has been stated for LMSs and LG-ESSs. There is no indication for adjuvant/postoperative chemo- and/or radiotherapy. For detailed information in this regard, as well as for information pertaining to potential postoperative HT in cases of HR-positive ASs that have been subjected to inadequate surgical procedures, reference should be had to the specialist literature [153].

Other Uterine Sarcomas and Rare Mesenchymal Tumors

Angiosarcomas and liposarcomas also occasionally occur in the uterus. Regarding the different variants of liposarcoma, only the dedifferentiated, myxoid-round cell, and pleomorphic variants are known to occur in the uterus, while well-differentiated liposarcoma does not. Liposarcomas stand out for their imaging characteristics in particular. The tumor component containing adipocytes is typically hyperechoic in sonography. The lipogenic components show hyperintense SI in T1 and T2-weighted MR images. By contrast, fat suppression results in a complete loss of signal intensity. Combining the findings from these two imaging methods is expedient for diagnosing liposarcomas or lipogenic tumors. Analogous to LMSs, angiosarcomas and liposarcomas are treated with total HE without injuring the uterus. No adjuvant therapeutic measures have yet been established in practice.

There are also occasional accounts of embryonic, alveolar, and pleomorphic rhabdomyosarcomas occurring in the uterus in adult women (1.8 % of DKSM cases, 143). While the surgical management of pleomorphic rhabdomyosarcomas resembles that of LMSs, performing surgical therapy with and without LNE on the other two variants constitutes only one aspect of a multimodal therapeutic strategy that – depending on which of the pre-defined risk groups is at hand in the individual case – usually includes radiotherapy and chemotherapy. Particularities pertaining to PEComs (perivascular epithelioid cell tumors), endometrial stromal tumors with sex cord-like elements (ESTSCLEs), and uterine tumors resembling ovarian sex cord/stromal tumors (UTROSCTs) can be found in the specialist literature [146, 149–152].

Risk and Prevention of Inadequate Surgery

The central problem for diagnosing and adequately treating uterine sarcomas is that, in many cases, they are incidental or unexpected diagnoses that are reached intra- or postoperatively. Due to the frequent absence of specific symptoms, but also due to clinical, sonographic, and anamnestic clues or risk factors being overlooked, 68 % of all LG-ESSs and 51 % of all LMSs in the DKSM-materials were operated under the indication of an LM [143]. Unfortunately, the same applies to 19 %, 26 %, and 35 % of ASs, UUSs, and HG-ESSs, respectively (Table 14.8) [143].

The likelihood of encountering an LMS or an LG-ESS in the course of or following HE, regardless of the indication under which it was performed, is 0.14 % (LMS: 0.07 %; LG-ESS: 0.07 %) [132]. Among patients operated on under the indication of an LM, the risk is 0.23 % (LMS 0.08, LG-ESS 0.15 %) [171, 219]. Other studies have reported likelihoods of 0.09 % [263] and 0.39 % [262] for encountering unexpected LMSs during or following sole LM-enucleation. In 1.2 % of cases, LM-morcellation (1091 instances) reveals unexpected LMSs (0.09 %), LG-ESSs (0.09 %), or STUMPSs [243]. However, the risk of incidentally diagnosing an LMS in patients subjected to HE for symptomatic LMs is substantially higher, at 0.49 %, and increases from 0.2 % at age 36 to 1.4 % beyond the age of 50, and 1.7 % from the age of 62 [172]. Further analyses report a 0.22 % likelihood of discovering an occult LMS or LG-ESS on morcellated specimens taken under any indication [104]. The aforementioned data are, however, all based on relatively small samples. A more recent and extensive study of 41,777 women who underwent a myomectomy with or without power morcellation revealed an 0.18 % chance of encountering occult uterine sarcomas and (!) endometrial carcinomas (codified as ICD-9-codes 179 and 182). This corresponds to 1 tumor per 550 cases. The ratio changes to 1 tumor per 161 cases in women aged 50 and older. The rate for patients who underwent power morcellation was 0.09 % [294].

In a recent German analysis, the rate of all occult sarcoma (LMS and LG-ESS) among 10,731 women who underwent supracervical laparoscopic HE was 1:1788 (LMS 1:5365, LG-ESS 1:2683) [36]. Two separate analyses were conducted by cooperation partners of the DKSM [143] in 2015. The first (143) revealed an 0.22 % chance (1:455) of incidental uterine sarcoma (1 LMS, 6 LG-ESS, 1 AS), but only an 0.027 chance (1:3703) of LMS in 3717 women who underwent any form of LM surgery. The second study (143) revealed a risk of 0.06 % (1:1666) of finding occult uterine sarcomas (LMS, LG-ESS, carcinosarcoma) among 31,227 patients who were subjected to LM-surgery. This risk was significantly higher among postmenopausal women (1:100). The risk for LMS and LG-ESS was 0.05 % (1:2000) and 0,006 % (1:16,666), respectively. A review of the available literature suggests that the prevalence of unexpected sarcomas in cases of suspected LM is roughly 0.14 % (1:700) [40]. Taking the more recent German studies with their larger respective cohorts into consideration, it is justifiable to assume that the prevalence rate is closer to 1:1000 for all uterine sarcomas and from 1300 up to 1:5000 for LMS. In an up-to date meta-analysis [229], 134 studies (without the German analysis (31)) were analyzed, covering 30,193 women in whom fibroid related indications were the primary reason for an HE or a myomectomy. The analyses of 64 prospective studies revealed an estimated prevalence of LMS of 0.12 per 1000 surgeries (1:8300). When restricted to the retrospective analyses, the estimated prevalence was 0.57 per 1000 surgeries (1:1700). Meta-analyses of all 134 studies estimated prevalence to be 0.57 per 1000 surgeries (approximately 1 LMS for every 2000 procedures). The latter is similar to the results of the DKSM-study [143].

In the DKSM database [143], of the LMS patients who were operated on under the indication of an LM, 5 % were subjected to myoma enucleation, 27 % underwent morcellation, and a total of 66 % received inadequate surgery (all techniques that cause injury to the tumor and/or the uterus, including supracervical abdominal or endoscopic HE). The figures are significantly higher for LG-ESSs, at 23 %, 41 %, and 70 %, respectively. What this implies in terms of patient prognosis has already been elaborated in detail in the respective subsections. The situation is similar for uterine ASs, HG-ESSs, and UUSs, albeit with significantly smaller shares of these tumors being operated on under the indication of an LM (Table 14.8). Pre-therapeutic and intraoperative selection thus requires vast improvement, and more thought and consideration need to be devoted to indications for surgery. The fact that the risk of 1 sarcoma per 1000 LM-operations is rather low by comparison should not serve to distract from that need.

The AAGL [1] recommends that morcellation should only be considered when appropriate examinations of the myome-

Table 14.8 Epidemiological and clinical characteristics and primary indication for surgery of 1132 uterine sarcomas and 3920 leiomyomas covered by the Doctoral Research Group (Promotions- und Forschungsgruppe) of the DKSM [143]

	Med. age years	≥50 years %	Postmeno-pause %	Med. tumor Ø cm	Tumor Ø ≥5 cm %	Tumor Ø ≥8 cm %	OP-indication LM %
LM	44	16.1	3.4	5.0	55.2	16.9	100
STUMP	46	28,0	20.0	6	68.4	36.8	92
LG-ESS	46	25.0	17.9	5.5	64.5	24.2	68
AS	56	64.3	61.9	5.5	54.3	27.8	19
LMS	53	66.1	62.5	8.0	85.6	60.2	51
HG-ESS	58	80.4	73.3	7.5	90.0	36.6	35
UUS	63	84.0	80.7	11	83.3	72.2	26

Table 14.9 Clinical criteria and differences between Leiomyoma (n = 3920) and leiomyosarcoma (n = 224) according to the data from the DKSM, all criteria $p < 0.001$ [143]

Clinical criteria	Myoma %	Leiomyosarcoma %
age ≥50 years	15.9	66.1
Postmenopause	3,3	62.5
Additional bleeding in premenopause	4,3	41.6
Bleeding in postmenopause	22	45
Suspicious sonography	5.3	88.4
Suspicious sonography in tumor ≥5 cm	3.6	40.5
Rapid growth	16.9	42.2
Rapid growth with symptoms	8.7	17.3
Rapid growth in tumor ≥5 cm	13.4	26.7
Rapid growth ≥45 years	9.4	24
Diameter ≥8 cm	16.7	60.2
Diameter ≥8 cm and solitary	9,1	28.0

trium, the cervix, and the endometrium have revealed no suspicious findings. When the pre-operative findings are suggestive of a malignancy and/or the patient is postmenopausal, alternative measures, including laparotomy, should be opted for. At the same time, morcellation should not be performed when examinations have revealed malignant or premalignant findings. This view is also reflected in the most recent recommendations of the DGGG as well as the current NCCN-guidelines [27, 202]. Whenever electric morcellation is being seriously considered, the specific risks associated with performing the procedure on benign (!) LMs (for instance provocation of a disseminated peritoneal leiomyomatosis or benign metastasizing LM) need to be explicitly discussed with the patient. Particularities pertaining to these clinical situations should be sought in the specialist literature [145].

Consistently having regard to the anamnestic, clinical, and sonographic criteria and risk factors that are suggestive of uterine sarcoma (Tables 14.2, 14.4, 14.8, and 14.9), while consistently adhering to a respective diagnostic flowchart (Fig. 14.22) prior to every LM-operation, can rather easily serve to protect uterine sarcoma patients from being subjected to inappropriate therapeutic procedures in the majority of cases.

In women aged 50 and older, the chance of encountering unexpected uterine sarcomas during LM-surgery is 0.62 % (1:116). The risk increases to 3.4 % in patients aged ≥60 years (1:29). In contrast, for women aged <40 years, the likelihood is only 0.04 % [293]. Overall, about 66 % of LMSs occur in women aged 50 and above, and about 62 % are found in postmenopausal patients [8, 9] [143]. Currently, 64.2 % of all LMSs are subjected to inappropriate surgical treatment [143]. If one were to exclude all women aged 50 and above as well as all postmenopausal patients from inappropriate surgery or advise against undergoing such surgery, as is recommended by the AAGL [1], then such inappropriate surgery would be prevented in well more than 50 % of LMS-cases. For ASs, HG-ESSs, and UUSs, the proportion of patients aged ≥50 is 64.3 %, 80.4 %, and 84 % (!), respectively (see Table 14.8). In order to better protect LG-ESS patients from being subjected to inadequate surgery, it is sensible to set the upper age threshold for organ-sparing surgery to 50 years, not least because LG-ESS patients have a median age of 46 years and only 18 % of these tumors occur postmenopausally (see also the section on LG-ESS).

For premenopausal patients (even better, patients aged <50) who desire organ sparing surgery (including supracervical HE), following anamnesis and clinical examination, selection must be based on the results from sonographic examination (and from curettage and HSC in cases of abnormal bleeding). Should gray-scale sonography reveal findings that are suspicious of sarcoma (Table 14.2) or other suggestive findings (Tables 14.4, 14.8, and 14.9), then total HE without injuring the uterus should be the primary surgical course of action. Otherwise, further diagnostic measures are necessary.

According to the data from the DKSM [143] factors (Table 14.9) suggestive of sarcoma are, in particular, rapid tumor growth in women aged ≥45 years (24 % in LMS and 9.4 % in LM) and/or in combination with newly arising symptoms (17.3 % in LMS and 8.7 % in LM). Of all LMs ≥5 cm 13.4 % exhibit rapid growth, compared to 26.7 % of LMSs of the same size. Tumors with a diameter of ≥8 cm (60.2 % in LMS, 16.7 % in LMs) are particularly suspicious of being sarcomas, especially when they are solitary tumors or are noticeably soft. Only 9.1 % of ordinary LMs are solitary tumors with a diameter of ≥8 cm, while 28.0 % of LMSs fulfill these criteria. So the fact that LMSs have a median diameter of 8.0 cm would in itself serve to avoid inadequate surgery for at least 50 % of all LMSs, regardless of patient age, symptoms and rapid growth (Table 14.9).

Lowering the threshold for critical tumor size from 8 to 5 cm would be particularly helpful from the perspective of advanced diagnostics. Doing so would bring more than 50 % of all LG-ESSs and ASs within the remit of the selection criteria, bearing in mind that LG-ESSs and ASs have a median diameter of 5.5 cm at the time of initial presentation. The share of LMSs that would thus be covered by the criteria would be 85.6 %. Moreover, in the DKSM database, 69.2 % of LG-ESSs that were described as LMs in clinical examination and/or sonography and that were subsequently operated on as such were ≥5 cm in diameter, and 87.5 % of them were morcellated [143]. Expanding the diagnostic criteria to include all tumors with diameters of ≥5 cm would have been extraordinarily helpful in these cases. While changing the diagnostic criteria to this end would indeed entail that a larger proportion of

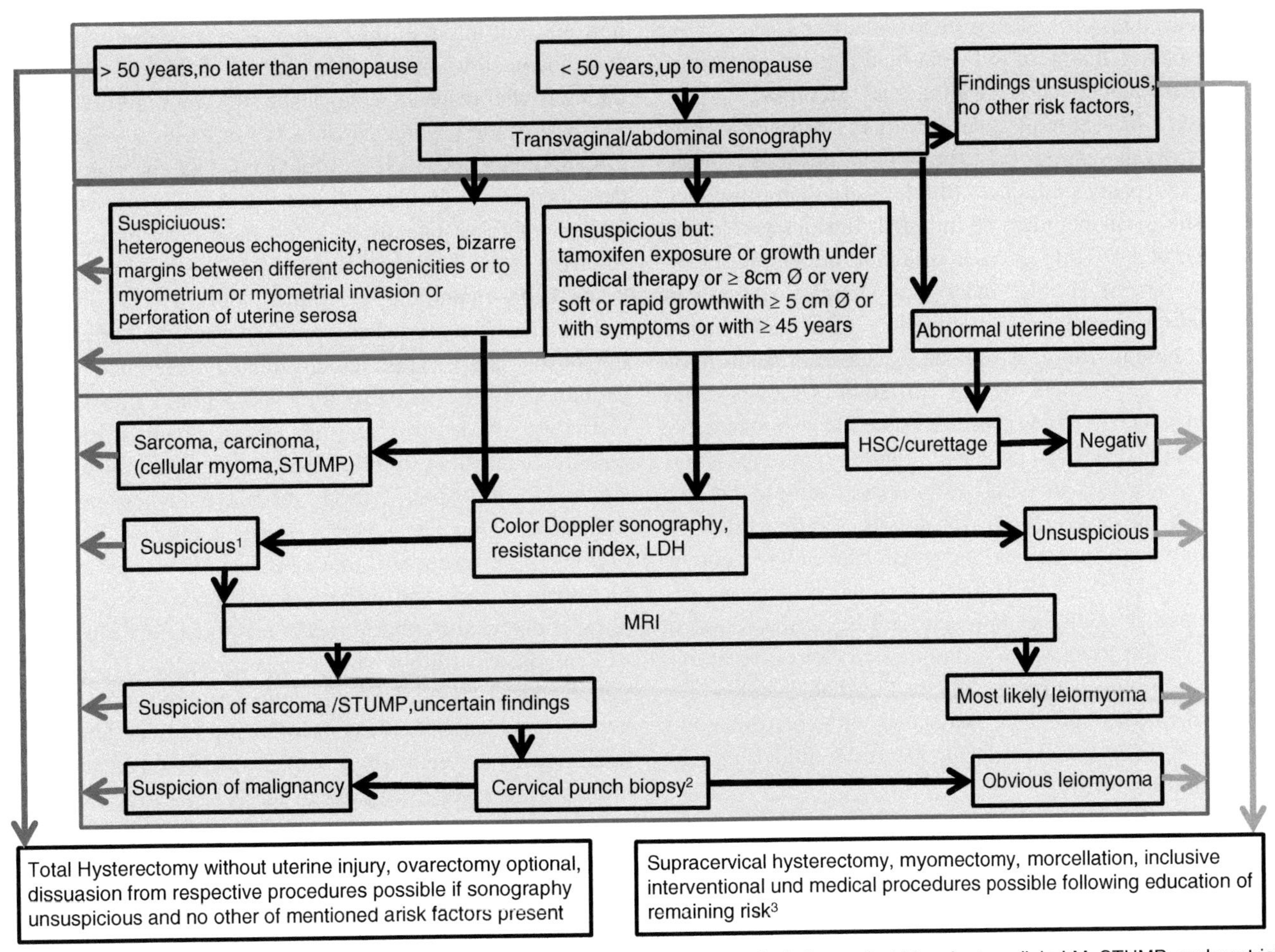

Fig. 14.22 Flowchart for preventing inappropriate surgery being performed on uterine sarcomas operated on under the assumption of a leiomyoma (With permission of Köhler et al. [144], Fig. 1.2–13)

Table 14.10 Results of the flowchart, if used prior to surgical procedure according to the data from the DKSM [143]

Surgical procedure	LMS	Proven risk factors	
	n	n	%
Inadequate surgery	129	122	94.6
Adequate surgery	72	71	98.6

patients would be subjected to Doppler sonography, at the same time, it would also imply that inappropriate surgical procedures could be prevented for up to 85.6 % of LMS, 83.3 %, of UUS and 90 % of HG-ESS patients. However, adapting the diagnostic criteria in the flowchart below to include tumors with a diameter of ≥5 cm with (apparently) unsuspicious results from gray-scale sonography inevitably has a negative impact on sensitivity, as 55.2 % of regular LMs and have a diameter of ≥5 (LMS in 85.6 %) (Table 14.8) [143].

The resulting decrease in sensitivity notwithstanding, tumors with a diameter of ≥5 cm should be included in the scope of expanded diagnostic criteria so as to improve diagnostic security and accuracy.

A medical history of exposure to tamoxifen is also among the risk factors that need to be clarified prior to performing surgery (see pathogenesis for all uterine sarcomas).

Should a patient request surgery that is either entirely or partially organ-sparing, even though one or more risk factors for a sarcoma are fulfilled (Table 14.4), then subsequent diagnostic measures must be initiated. Besides performing curettage and/or HSC in cases of abnormal vaginal bleeding, the patient should undergo a Doppler sonography examination, ideally in combination with LDH-testing. Both of these measures have been discussed in detail in the respective subchapters on the different sarcoma types. Where results from these procedures are likewise suspicious or pathological, and the patient continues (!) to request conservative surgery, an MRT examination should be performed. If the MRT results (for details, see the respective subsections) are suspicious or unclear, especially in combination with elevated LDH-levels (reference value × 1.2), and the patient continues to reject total HE in the course of which the uterus would not sustain injury, then performing a transcervical punch biopsy is the last available option. The potential pitfalls and risks associated with this procedure have been elaborated in detail in the differential diagnosis subsection for LMSs.

Overall, the diagnostic flowchart (Fig. 14.22) generally implies that sonographic examination has been performed prior to any LM-operation. Routinely subjecting patients with anamnestically, clinically, and sonographically unsuspicious LMs to curettage and/or HSC, color Doppler sonography, and/or MRT is not necessary according to the current state of information. Nonetheless, even when the flowchart is applied, incidental discoveries of uterine sarcomas and STUMPs cannot be entirely ruled out. Patients must be informed of this remaining risk.

Even in cases with ordinary LM patients must be informed of the fact that performing enucleation or morcellation can increase the risk of disseminated peritoneal leiomyomatosis and benign metastasizing LM.

When considering interventional therapy (embolization, ultrasound-guided destruction) for LM-patients, it must be borne in mind that the object on which such therapy is to be performed might well be inappropriate for such course of action [226]. However, in the DKSM-sample, embolizations accounted for only 1.2 % of all primary LMS-operations [143]. In contrast to older publications [63], more recent analyses and meta-analyses on LM-embolization lack any reference to potential sarcoma risk. Attending physicians should, however, not interpret this state of affairs as absolving them from the need to inform their patients of this risk, nor from taking further respective diagnostic steps to minimize it.

5.4 % of the 129 inadequate LMS surgeries covered in the DKSM materials [143] exhibited none of the risk factors described above (Table 14.9 and Fig. 14.22). Consequently, 94.6 % of these operations could have been prevented by referring to the flow chart (Table 14.10). Among the 72 adequate LMS operations performed, only 1.4 % of LMSs would have been missed as a consequence of adhering to the diagnostic chart. This (albeit minor) difference can be explained by the fact that total HE without injury to the uterus was often performed in cases in which an LMS had already been primarily diagnosed or suspected. In a further study [175] 4791 patients were referred to surgery under the indication of an LM. Among them, a total of 26 LMSs (1:183) were discovered. 20 LMSs could be successfully identified as such and referred to adequate surgery on the basis of diagnostics (curettage) or arising clinical suspicions of malignancy (tumor size). Only 6 cases (1:799) thus remained undetected. Ultimately, the share of LMSs that are detected incidentally during or following LM operations can be decreased dramatically if suspected LMs are subjected to more critical assessment prior to surgery.

This notwithstanding, an analysis conducted by the cooperation partners of the DKSM [143] revealed that, among 3920 ordinary LMs, 1739 (44.4 %) exhibited at least one of the risk factors stated above. However, only those patients who decline primary total HE need to be subjected to further diagnostics (yes when HSC/curettage and/or color Doppler sonography yield findings).

Therefore, seeking to prevent subjecting uterine sarcomas to inadequate surgery under the indication of an LM would not entail much effort, not least because, in its flow chart, the

Table 14.11 Descriptive accounts of uterine sarcomas, rendered either intraoperatively or immediately following surgery, based on 804 DKSM-surgical reports [143]

Intraoperative
Tumor very soft
Tumor primarily ruptured
Tumor extremely fragile (ruptures upon slight pressure)
Protrusion/outpour of hemorrhagic, marrowy, cauliflower-like, degrading or liquefied material upon cutting/dissection
Resected, opened tumor
If present, pseudo-capsule consists mostly of compressed tumor tissue
Hemorrhagic tumor, cystic structures, necrotic components
Entirely or partially gray, greenish-gray, dirty, intense yellow color
Very smooth cut surface, either partially or overall

ESGE [40] already regards color Doppler sonography as a precondition for conservative myoma surgery.

The performance of inappropriate modes of surgery on patients with sarcoma types not covered in the flowchart can nonetheless be prevented, if the attending physicians bear the factors suggestive of sarcomas (Table 14.11) in mind both during and immediately after surgery. The surgical approach should be reconsidered and/or a frozen section should be performed in respectively appropriate cases. The problems and pitfalls associated with frozen section procedures have to be taken into consideration (see LMS).

When findings are deemed unsuspicious according to the flowchart, and no intraoperative suspicions arise, there is currently no sound reason to deviate from tried and tested interventional and conservative surgical procedures for LMs, or to refrain from performing endoscopic procedures or morcellation where necessary. Notwithstanding, the patient must nonetheless be informed of the risks associated with morcellation (disseminated peritoneal leiomyomatosis and benign metastasizing LM). Electric morcellation should currently not be resorted to due to the large number of unresolved questions pertaining to the procedure. In their flowchart, the European Society of Gynaecological Endoscopy prioritizes performing a Doppler sonography examination as the primary method for verifying indications for surgery, a demand that is currently unrealistic context. The aforementioned chart [40] also demonstrates a number of other weaknesses and unclear, in part ambiguous wordings.

A real LMS risk score will be published soon by the DKSM.

Conclusions

LMs shall not be subjected to surgery without prior sonographic examination

Consistent application of the diagnostics flowchart

Consistent consideration of suspicious findings arising intraoperatively

Patients to be informed that, despite appropriate diagnostics, additional surgical procedures could be necessary if a finding of a malignancy arises

Patients to be informed that performing enucleation or morcellation on unsuspicious, ordinary LMs can result in disseminated peritoneal leiomyomatosis or a benign metastasizing LM.

References

1. AAGL Advancing Minimally Invasive Gynecology Worldwide. AAGL practice report: morcellation during uterine tissue extraction. J Minim Invasive Gynecol. 2014;21:517–30.
2. Abeler VM, Røyne O, Thoresen S, Danielsen HE, Nesland JM, Kristensen GB. Uterine sarcomas in Norway. A histopathological and prognostic survey of a total population from 1970 to 2000 including 419 patients. Histopathology. 2009;54:355–564.
3. Abu-Rustum N, Curtin JP, Burt M, Jones WB. Regression of uterine low-grade smooth-muscle tumors metastatic to the lung after oophorectomy. Obstet Gynecol. 1997;89:850–2.
4. Akahira J, Tokunaga H, Toyoshima M, Takano T, Nagase S, Yoshinaga K, Tase T, Wada Y, Ito K, Niikura H, Yamada H, Sato A, Sasano H, Yaegashi N. Prognosis and prognostic factors of carcinosarcoma, endometrial stromal sarcoma and uterine leiomyosarcoma: a comparison with uterine endometrial adenocarcinoma. Oncology. 2006;71:333–40.
5. Akhan SE, Yavuz E, Tecer A, Iyibozkurt CA, Topuz S, Tuzlali S, Bengisu E, Berkman S. The expression of Ki-67, p53, estrogen and progesterone receptors affecting survival in uterine leiomyosarcomas. A clinicopathologic study. Gynecol Oncol. 2005;99:36–42.
6. Albrektsen G, Heuch I, Wik E, Salvesen HB. Prognostic impact of parity in 493 uterine sarcoma patients. Int J Gynecol Cancer. 2009;19:1062–7.
7. Amant F, Moerman P, Cadron I, Neven P, Berteloot P, Vergote I. The diagnostic problem of endometrial stromal sarcoma: report on 6 cases. Gynecol Oncol. 2003;90:37–43.
8. Amant F, Steenkiste E, Schurmans K, Verbist L, Abeler VM, Tulunay G, Jonge E de, Massuger L, Moermann P, Vergote I. Immunhistochemical expression of CD10 antigen in uterine adenosarcoma. Int J Gynecol Cancer 2004; 14: 1118–1121
9. Amant F, Schurmans K, Steenkiste E, Verbist L, Abeler VM, Tulunay G, Jonge E de, Massuger L, Moermann P, Vergote I. Immunhistochemical determination of estrogen and progesterone receptor positivity in uterine adenosarcoma. Gynecol Oncol 2004; 93: 680–685
10. Amant F, Moerman P, Vergote I. Report of an unusual problematic uterine smooth muscle neoplasm, emphasizing the prognostic

importance of coagulative tumor cell necrosis. Int J Gynecol Cancer. 2005;15:1210–2.

11. Amant F, De Knijf A, Van Calster B, Leunen K, Neven P, Berteloot P, Vergote I, Van Huffel S, Moerman P. Clinical study investigating the role of lymphadenectomy, surgical castration, and adjuvant hormonal treatment in endometrial stromal sarcoma. Br J Cancer. 2007;97:1194–9.
12. Amant F, Floquet A, Friedlander M, Kristensen G, Mahner S, Nam EJ, Powell MA, Ray-Coquard I, Siddiqui N, Sykes P, Westermann AM, Seddon B. Gynecological Cancer InterGroup consensus review for endometrial stromal sarcoma. Int J Gynecol Cancer. 2014;24(Suppl 3):S67–72.
13. Anaya DA, Lev DC, Pollock RE. The role of surgical margin status in retroperitoneal sarcoma. J Surg Oncol. 2008;98:607–10.
14. Anderson TM, McMahon JJ, Nwogu CE, Pombo MW, Urschel JD, Driscoll DL, Lele SB. Pulmonary resection in metastatic uterine and cervical malignancies. Gynecol Oncol. 2001;83:472–6.
15. Arenas M, Rovirosa A, Hernández V, Ordi J, Jorcano S, Mellado B, Biete A. Uterine sarcomas in breast cancer patients treated with tamoxifen. Int J Gynecol Cancer. 2006;16:861–5.
16. Arend R, Bagaria M, Lewin SN, Sun X, Deutsch I, Burke WM, Herzog TJ, Wright JD. Long-term outcome and natural history of uterine adenosarcomas. Gynecol Oncol. 2010;119:305–8.
17. Arici DS, Aker H, Yildiz E, Tasyurt A. Mullerian adenosarcoma of the uterus associated with tamoxifen therapy. Arch Gynecol Obstet. 2000;164:105–7.
18. Atkins KA, Arronte N, Darus CJ, Rice LW. The Use of p16 in enhancing the histologic classification of uterine smooth muscle tumors. Am J Surg Pathol. 2008;32:98–102.
19. Aviram R, Ochshorn Y, Markovitch O, Fishman A, Cohen I, Altaras MM, Tepper R. Uterine sarcomas versus leiomyomas: gray-scale and Doppler sonographic findings. J Clin Ultrasound. 2005;33:10–3.
20. Bai H, Yang J, Cao D, Huang H, Xiang Y, Wu M, Cui Q, Chen J, Lang J, Shen K. Ovary and uterus-sparing procedures for low-grade endometrial stromal sarcoma: a retrospective study of 153 cases. Gynecol Oncol Gynecol Oncol. 2014;132:654–60.
21. Baird DD, Garrett TA, Laughlin SK, Davis B, Semelka RC, Peddada SD. Short-term change in growth of uterine leiomyoma: tumor growth spurts. Fertil Steril. 2011;95:242–6.
22. Balleine RL, Earls PJ, Webster LR, Mote PA, deFazio A, Harnett PR, Clarke CL. Expression of progesterone receptor A and B isoforms in low-grade endometrial stromal sarcoma. Int J Gynecol Pathol. 2004;23:138–44.
23. Bansal N, Herzog TJ, Burke W, Cohen CJ, Wright JD. The utility of preoperative endometrial sampling for the detection of uterine sarcomas. Gynecol Oncol. 2008;110:43–8.
24. Bansal S, Lewin SN, Burke WM, Deutsch I, Sun X, Herzog TJ, Wright JD. Sarcoma of the cervix: natural history and outcomes. Gynecol Oncol. 2010;118:134–8.
25. Barney B, Tward JD, Skidmore T, Gaffney DK. Does radiotherapy or lymphadenectomy improve survival in endometrial stromal sarcoma? Int J Gynecol Cancer. 2009;19:1232–8.
26. Beck TL, Singhal PK, Ehrenberg HM, Rose PG, Lele SB, Krivak TC, McBee Jr WC. Endometrial stromal sarcoma: analysis of recurrence following adjuvant treatment. Gynecol Oncol. 2012;125:141–4.
27. Beckmann MW, Juhasz-Böss I, Denschlag D, Gaß P, Dimpfl T, Harter P, Mallmann P, Renner SP, Rimbach S, Runnebaum I, Untch M, Brucker SY, Wallwiener D. Surgical methods for the treatment of uterine fibroids – risk of uterine sarcoma and problems of morcellation: position paper of the DGGG. Geburtshilfe Frauenheilkd. 2015;75:148–64.
28. Bell SW, Kempson RL, Hendrickson MR. Problematic uterine smooth muscle neoplasms. a clinicopathologic study of 213 cases. Am J Surg Pathol. 1994;18:535–58.
29. Berchuk A, Rubin SC, Hoskins WJ, Saigo PE, Pierce VK, JL Jr L. Treatment of endometrial stromal tumors. Gynecol Oncol. 1990;71:60–5.
30. Bernard B, Clarke BA, Malowany JI, McAlpine J, Lee CH, Atenafu EG, Ferguson S, Mackay H. Uterine adenosarcomas: a dual-institution update on staging, prognosis and survival. Gynecol Oncol. 2013;131:634–9.
31. Berretta R, Rolla M, Merisio C, Goirdano G, Nardelli GB. Uterine smooth muscle tumor of uncertain malignant potential: a three-case report. Int J Gynecol Cancer. 2007;18:1108–31.
32. Blom R, Malmström H, Guerrieri C. Endometrial stromal sarcoma of the uterus: a clinicopathologic, DNA flow cytometric, p53, and mdm-2 analysis of 17 cases. Int J Gynecol Cancer. 1999;9:98–104.
33. Bodner K, Bodner-Adler B, Kimberger O, Czerwenka K, Leodolter S, Mayerhofer K. Estrogen and progesterone receptor expression in patients with uterine leiomyosarcoma and correlation with different clinicopathological parameters. Anticancer Res. 2003;23:729–32.
34. Bodner K, Bodner-Adler B, Kimberger O, Czerwenka K, Mayerhofer K. Estrogen and progesterone receptor expression in patients with uterine smooth muscle tumors. Fertil Steril. 2004;81:1062–6.
35. Bogani G, Cliby WA, Aletti GD. Impact of morcellation on survival outcomes of patients with unexpected uterine leiomyosarcoma: a systematic review and meta-analysis. Gynecol Oncol. 2015;137:167–72.
36. Bojahr B, De Wilde RL, Tchartchian G. Malignancy rate of 10,731 uteri morcellated during laparoscopic supracervical hysterectomy (LASH). Arch Gynecol Obstet. 2015; doi:10.1007/s00404-015-3696-z.
37. Bonvalot S, Rivoire M, Castaing M, Stoeckle E, Le Cesne A, Blay JY, Laplanche A. Primary retroperitoneal sarcomas: a multivariate analysis of surgical factors associated with local control. J Clin Oncol. 2009;27:31–7.
38. Borah BJ, Nicholson WK, Bradley L, Stewart EA. The impact of uterine leiomyomas: a national survey of affected women. Am J Obstet Gynecol. 2013;209:319.e1–319.
39. Bradley LD. Uterine fibroid embolization: a viable alternative to hysterectomy. Am J Obstet Gynecol. 2009;201:127–35.
40. Brölmann H, Tanos V, Grimbizis G, Ind T, Philips K, van den Bosch T, Sawalhe T, van den Haak L, Jansen FW, Pijnenborg J, Taran FA, Brucker S, Wattiez A, Campo R, O'Donovan P, de Wilde RL, On behalf of the European Society of Gynaecological Endoscopy (ESGE) Steering Committee on Fibroid Morcellation. Options on fibroid morcellation: a literature review. Gynecol Surg. 2015;12:3–15.
41. Buttram V, Reiter R. Uterine leiomyomata: etiology, symptomatology, and management. Fertil Steril. 1981;36:433–45.
42. Buyukkurt S, Guzel AB, Gumurdulu D, Vardar MA, Zeren H, Sucu M. Mullerian adenosarcoma of the uterine cervix in an adolescent girl. J Pediatr Adolesc Gynecol. 2010;23:e13–5.
43. Buzaglo K, Bruchim I, Lau SK, Ferenczy A, Tulandi T, Gotlieb WH. Sarcoma post-embolization for presumed uterine fibrosis. Gynecol Oncol. 2008;108:244–7.
44. Cacciatore B, Lehtovirta P, Wahlström T, Ylöstalo P. Ultrasound findings in uterine mixed müllerian sarcomas and endometrial stromal sarcomas. Gynecol Oncol. 1989;35:290–3.
45. Carroll A, Ramirez PT, Westin SN, Soliman PT, Munsell MF, Nick AM, Schmeler KM, Klopp AH, Fleming ND. Uterine adenosarcoma: an analysis on management, outcomes, and risk factors for recurrence. Gynecol Oncol. 2014;135:455–61.

46. Carter J, Perrone T, Carson LF, Carlson J, Twiggs LB. Uterine malignancy predicted by transvaginal sonography and color flow Doppler ultrasonography. J Clin Ultrasound. 1993;21:405–8.
47. Chan JK, Kawar NM, Shin JY, Osann K, Chen L, Powell C, Kapp S. Endometrial stromal sarcoma: a population based analysis. Br J Cancer. 2008;99:1210–5.
48. Chang KL, Crabtree GS, Lim-Tan SK, Kempson RL, Hendrickson R. Primary uterine endometrial stromal neoplasms. A clinicopathologic study of 117 cases. Am J Surg Pathol. 1990;14:415–38.
49. Chen CD, Huang CC, Wu CC, Tseng GC, Lee CN, Lin GJ, Hsieh CY, Hsieh FJ. Sonographic characteristics in low-grade endometrial stromal sarcoma: a report of two cases. J Ultrasound Med. 1995;14:165–8.
50. Chen L, Yang B. Immunohistochemical analysis of p16, p53, and Ki-67 expression in uterine smooth muscle tumors. Int J Gynecol Pathol. 2008;27:326–32.
51. Cho KR, Woodruff JD, Epstein JI. Leiomyoma of the uterus with multiple extrauterine smooth muscle tumors: a case report suggesting multifocal origin. Hum Pathol. 1989;20:80–3.
52. Chourmouzi D, Boulogianni G, Zarampoukas T, Drevelengas A. Sonography and MRI of tamoxifen-associated müllerian adenosarcoma of the uterus. AJR Am J Roentgenol. 2003;181:1673–5.
53. Christacos NC, Quade BJ, Dal Cin P, Morton CC. Uterine leiomyomata with deletions of Ip represent a distinct cytogenetic subgroup associated with unusual histologic features. Genes Chromosom Cancer. 2006;45:304–12.
54. Chu MC, Mor G, Lim C, Zheng W, Parkash V, Schwartz PE. Low-grade endometrial stroma sarcoma: hormonal aspects. Gynecol Oncol. 2003;90:170–6.
55. Clement P, Scully R. Mullerian adenosarcoma of the uterus: a clinico-pathologic analysis of 100 cases with areview of the literature. Hum Pathol. 1990;21:363–81.
56. Clement PB, Oliva E, Young RH. Mullerian adenosarcoma of the uterine corpus associated with tamoxifen therapy: a report of six cases and a review of tamoxifen-associated endometrial lesions. Int J Gynecol Pathol. 1996;15:222–9.
57. Clement PB, Young RH. Atlas of gynecologic surgical pathology. 3rd ed. Saunders Elsevier; 2014.
58. Coley HM, Lewandowicz G, Sargent JM, Verrill MW. Chemosensitivity testing of fresh and continuous tumor cell cultures using lactate dehydrogenase. Anticancer Res. 1997;17:231–6.
59. Cornfeld D, Israel G, Martel M, Weinreb J, Schwartz P, McCarthy S. MRI appearance of mesenchymal tumors of the uterus. Eur J Radiol. 2010;74:241–9.
60. Dafopoulos A, Tsikouras P, Dimitraki M, Galazios G, Liberis V, Maroulis G, Teichmann AT. The role of lymphadenectomy in uterine leiomyosarcoma: review of the literature and recommendations for the standard surgical procedure. Arch Gynecol Obstet. 2010;282:293–300.
61. D'Angelo E, Spagnoli LG, Prat J. Comparative clinicopathologic and immunohistochemical analysis of uterine sarcomas diagnosed using the World Health Organization classification system. Hum Pathol. 2009;40:1571–85.
62. D'Angelo E, Quade BJ, Prat J. Uterine smooth muscle tumors. In: Mutter GL, Prat J, editors. Pathology of the female reproductive tract. 3rd ed. Churchill-Livingstone Elsevier; 2014. p. 402–24.
63. David M, Warschewske G, Hengst S, Ehrenstein T. Die uteruserhaltende Myombehandlung. Frauenarzt. 2003;44:1164–76.
64. David M, Krätschell R, Stupin JH. Welches Myomwachstum ist normal? Frauenarzt. 2013;54:1162–7.
65. Della Badia C, Karini H. Endometrial stromal sarcoma diagnosed after uterine morcellation in laparoscopic supracervical hysterectomy. Minim Invasive Gynecol. 2010;17:791–3.
66. Dinh TA, Oliva EA, Fuller Jr AF, Lee H, Goodman A. The treatment of uterine leiomyosarcoma. Results from a 10-year experience (1990–1999) at the Massachusetts General Hospital. Gynecol Oncol. 2004;92:648–65.
67. Dong R, Mao H, Zhang P. Conservative management of endometrial stromal sarcoma at stage III: a case report. Oncol Lett. 2014;8:1234–6.
68. Donnez O, Squifflet J, Leconte I, Jadoul P, Donnez J. Posthysterectomy pelvic adenomyotic masses observed in 8 cases out of a series of 1405 laparoscopic subtotal hysterectomies. J Minim Invasive Gynecol. 2007;14:156–60.
69. Dos Santos L, Garg K, Diaz JP, Soslow RA, Hensley ML, Alektiar KM, Barakat RR, Leitao MM. Incidence of adnexal and lymph node metastases in endometrial stromal sarcoma. J Clin Oncol. 2009;27(Suppl):Abstr. 5589.
70. Eary JF, Conrad EU. Imaging in sarcoma. J Nucl Med. 2011;52:1903–13.
71. Ehdaivand S, Simon RA, Sung CJ, Steinhoff MM, Lawrence WD, Quddus MR. Incidental gynecologic neoplasms in morcellated uterine specimens: a case series with follow-up. Hum Pathol. 2014;45:2311–7.
72. Einstein MH, Barakat RR, Chi DS, Sonoda Y, Alektiar KM, Hensley ML, Abu-Rustum NR. Management of uterine malignancy found incidentally after supracervical hysterectomy or uterine morcellation for presumed benign disease. Int J Gynecol Cancer. 2008;10:1065–70.
73. El Maalouf G, Duvillard P, Rey A, Morice P, Haie-Meder C, Lhommé C, Pautier P. Clinical features, recurrence patterns and treatment in endometrial stromal sarcomas: a thirty-year single-institution experience. J Clin Oncol. 2008;26(Suppl 15):Abstr 10574.
74. ESMO/European Sarcoma Network Working Group. Soft tissue and visceral sarcomas: ESMO Clinical Practice Guidelines for diagnosis, treatment and follow-up. Ann Oncol. 2012;23(Suppl 7):vii 92–9.
75. Exacoustos C, Romanini ME, Amadio A, Amoroso C, Szabolcs B, Zupi E, Arduini D. Can gray-scale and color Doppler sonography differentiate between uterine leiomyosarcoma and leiomyoma? J Clin Ultrasound. 2007;35:449–57.
76. Farhat MH, Hobeika EM, Moumneh G, Nassar AH. Uterine mullerian adenosarcoma with sarcomatous overgrowth fatal recurrence within two weeks of diagnosis: a case report. Med Case Reports. 2007;25:103.
77. Farhat F, Fakhruddine NA. A case of synchronous relapse of breast cancer and uterine müllerian adenosarcoma post tamoxifen in a premenopausal woman. Eur J Gynaecol Oncol. 2008;29:95–7.
78. Farquhar C, Arroll B, Ekeroma A, Fentiman G, Lethaby A, Rademaker L, Roberts H, Sadler L, Strid J, Working Party of the New Zealand Guidelines Group. An evidence-based guideline for the management of uterine fibroids. Aust N Z J Obstet Gynaecol. 2001;41:125–40.
79. Favero G, Anton C, Silva e Silva A, Ribeiro A, MP A, Miglino G, EC B, JP C. Vaginal morcellation: a new strategy for large gynecological malignant tumor extraction: a pilot study. Gynecol Oncol. 2012;126:443–7.
80. FDA – SOURCES: April 17, 2014, U.S. Food and Drug Administration news briefing with William Maisel, M.D., M.P.H., deputy director for science and chief scientist, Center for Devices and Radiological Health; March 17, 2014, The New York Times; Dec. 24, 2013, Wall Street Journal.
81. Feng W, Hua K, Malpica A, Zhou X, Baak JP. Stages I to II WHO 2003-defined low-grade endometrial stromal sarcoma: how much primary therapy is needed and how little is enough? Int J Gynecol Cancer. 2013;23:488–93.

82. Feng W, Hua K, Gudlaugsson E, Yu Y, Zhou X, Baak JP. Prognostic indicators in WHO 2003 low-grade endometrial stromal sarcoma. Histopathology. 2013;62:675–87.
83. FIGO Committee on Gynecologic Oncology: FIGO staging for uterine sarcomas. Int J Gynecol Obstet. 2009;104:179.
84. Fleming NA, Hopkins L, de Nanassy J, Senterman M, Black AY. Mullerian adenosarcoma of the cervix in a 10-year-old girl: case report and review of the literature. J Pediatr Adolesc Gynecol. 2009;22:45–51.
85. Fong Y, Coit DG, Woodruff JM, Brennan MF. Lymph node metastasis from soft tissue sarcoma in adults. Analysis of data from a prospective database of 1772 sarcoma patients. Ann Surg. 1993;217:72–7.
86. Friedlander ML, Covens A, Glasspool RM, Hilpert F, Kristensen G, Kwon S, Selle F, Small W, Witteveen E, Russell P. Gynecologic Cancer InterGroup (GCIG) consensus review for mullerian adenosarcoma of the female genital tract. Int J Gynecol Cancer. 2014;24(9 Suppl 3):S78–82.
87. Fukunishi H, Funaki K, Ikuma K, Kaji Y, Sugimura K, Kitazawa R, Kitazawa S. Unsuspected uterine leiomyosarcoma: magnetic resonance imaging findings before and after focused ultrasound surgery. Int J Gynecol Cancer. 2007;17:724–8.
88. Furukawa R, Akahane M, Yamada H, Kiryu S, Sato J, Komatsu S, Inoh S, Yoshioka N, Maeda E, Takazawa Y, Ohtomo K. Endometrial stromal sarcoma located in the myometrium with a low-intensity rim on T2-weighted images: report of three cases and literature review. J Magn Reson Imaging. 2010;31:975–9.
89. Gadducci A, Landoni F, Sartori E, Zola P, Maggino T, Lissoni A, Bazzurini L, Arisio R, Romagnolo C, Cristofani R. Uterine leiomyosarcoma: analysis of treatment failures and survival. Gynecol Oncol. 1996;62:25–32.
90. Gadducci A, Sartori E, Landoni F, Zola P, Maggino T, Urgesi A, Lissoni A, Losa G, Fanucchi A. Endometrial stromal sarcoma: analysis of treatment failures and survival. Gynecol Oncol. 1996;63:247–53.
91. Gadducci A, Cosio S, Romanini A, Genazzani AR. The management of patients with uterine sarcoma: a debated clinical challenge. Crit Rev Oncol Hematol. 2008;65:129–42.
92. Gallardo A, Prat J. Mullerian adenosarcoma: a clinicopathologic and immunohistochemical study of 55 cases challenging the existence of adenofibroma. Am J Surg Pathol. 2009;33:278–88.
93. Garcia C, Kubat JS, Fulton RS, Anthony AT, Combs M, Powell CB, Littell RD. Clinical outcomes and prognostic markers in uterine leiomyosarcoma: a population-based cohort. Int J Gynecol Cancer. 2015;25:622–8.
94. Garg G, Shah JP, Toy EP, Bryant CS, Kumar S, Morris RT. Stage IA vs. IB endometrial stromal sarcoma: does the new staging system predict survival? Gynecol Oncol. 2010;118:8–13.
95. Garg G, Shah JP, Liu JR, Bryant CS, Kumar S, Munkarah A, Morris RT. Validation of tumor size as staging variable in the revised International Federation of Gynecology and Obstetrics stage I leiomyosarcoma: a population-based study. Int J Gynecol Cancer. 2010;20:1201–6.
96. Geisinger, K. R., Abdul-Karim, F. W. Fine needle aspiration bopsy of soft tissue tumors. In: Weiss SW, Goldblum JR, editors. Enzinger and Weiss's soft tissue tumors. 5th ed. Philadelphia: Mosby Elsevier; 2008. p. 103–117.
97. George S, Barysauskas C, Serrano C, et al. Retrospective cohort study evaluating the impact of intraperitoneal morcellation on outcomes of localized uterine leiomyosarcoma. Cancer. 2014;120:3154–8.
98. Giuntoli RL, Metzinger DS, DiMarco CS, Cha SS, Sloan JA, Keeney GL, Gostout BS. Retrospective review of 208 patients with leiomyosarcoma of the uterus: prognostic indicators, surgical management, and adjuvant therapy. Gynecol Oncol. 2003;89:460–9.
99. Giuntoli RL, Gostout BS, DiMarco CS, Metzinger DS, Keeney GL. Diagnostic criteria for uterine smooth muscle tumors: leiomyoma variants associated with malignant behavior. J Reprod Med. 2007;52:1001–10.
100. Goff BA, Rice LW, Fleischhacker D, Muntz HG, Falkenberry SS, Nikrui N, Fuller AF. Uterine leiomyosarcoma and endometrial stromal sarcoma: lymph node metastases and sites of recurrences. Gynecol Oncol. 1993;50:105–9.
101. Goldberg J, Burd I, Price FV, Worthington-Kirsch R. Leiomyosarcoma in a premenopausal patient after uterine artery embolization. Am J Obstet Gynecol. 2004;191:1733–5.
102. Gollard R, Kosty M, Bordin G, Wax A, Lacey C. Two unusual presentations of müllerian adenosarcoma: case reports, literature review, and treatment considerations. Gynecol Oncol. 1995;59:412–22.
103. Goto A, Takeuchi S, Sugimura K, Maruo T. Usefulness of Gd-DTPA contrast-enhanced dynamic MRI and serum determination of LDH and its isozymes in the differential diagnosis of leiomyosarcoma from degenerated leiomyoma of the uterus. Int J Gynecol Cancer. 2002;12:354–61.
104. Graebe K, Garcia-Soto A, Aziz M, Valarezo V, Heller PB, Tchabo N, Tobias DH, Salamon C, Ramieri J, Dise C, Slomovitz BM. Incidental power morcellation of malignancy: a retrospective cohort study. Gynecol Oncol. 2015;136:274–7.
105. Gremel G, Liew M, Hamzei F, Hardell E, Selling J, Ghaderi M, Stemme S, Pontén F, Carlson JW. A prognosis based classification of undifferentiated uterine sarcomas: identification of mitotic index, hormone receptors and YWHAE-FAM22 translocation status as predictors of survival. Int J Cancer. 2014; doi:10.1002/ijc.29141.
106. Gronchi A, Lo Vullo S, Fiore M, Mussi C, Stacchiotti S, Collini P, Lozza L, Pennacchioli E, Mariani L, Casali PG. Aggressive surgical policies in a retrospectively reviewed single-institution case series of retroperitoneal soft tissue sarcoma patients. J Clin Oncol. 2009;27:24–30.
107. Guntupalli SR, Anderson ML, Milam MR, Bodurka D, Ramirez PT. Clinical outcomes of smooth muscle tumors of uncertain malignant potential. Gynecol Oncol. 2008;108:94–5.
108. Guntupalli SR, Ramirez PT, Anderson ML, Milam MR, Bodurka DC, Malpica A. Uterine smooth muscle tumor of uncertain malignant potential: a retrospective analysis. Gynecol Oncol. 2009;11:324–6.
109. Halbwedl I, Ullmann R, Kremser ML, Man YG, Isadi-Moud N, Lax S, Denk H, Popper HH, Tavassoli FA, Moinfar F. Chromosomal alterations in low-grade endometrial stromal sarcoma and undifferentiated endometrial sarcoma as detected by comparative genomic hybridization. Gynecol Oncol. 2005;97:582–7.
110. Han XY, Xiang Y, Guo LN, Shen K, Wan XR, Huang HF, Pan LY. Clinicopathological analysis of mullerian adenosarcoma of the uterus. Chin Med J. 2010;123:756–9.
111. Hayasaka K, Morita K, Saitoh T, Tanaka Y. Uterine adenofibroma and endometrial stromal sarcoma associated with tamoxifen therapy: MR findings. Comput Med Imaging Graph. 2006;30:315–8.
112. Hensley ML, Wathen JK, Maki RG, Araujo DM, Sutton G, Priebat DA, George S, Soslow RA, Baker LH. Adjuvant therapy for high-grade, uterus-limited leiomyosarcoma: results of a phase 2 trial (SARC005). Cancer. 2013;119:1555–61.
113. Hensley ML, Barrette BA, Baumann K, Gaffney D, Hamilton AL, Kim JW, Maenpaa JU, Pautier P, Siddiqui NA, Westermann AM, Ray-Coquard I. Gynecologic Cancer InterGroup (GCIG) consensus review: uterine and ovarian leiomyosarcomas. Int J Gynecol Cancer. 2014;24(9 Suppl 3):S61–6.
114. Hohenberger P, Kasper B, Ahrar K. Surgical management and minimally invasive approaches for the treatment of metastatic sarcoma. Am Soc Clin Oncol Educ Book. 2013;33:457–64.

115. Homer L, Muller M, Dupré PF, Lucas B, Pradier OJ. Uterine sarcoma associated with tamoxifen use after breast cancer: review of the pathogenesis. Gynecol Obstet Biol Reprod. 2009;38:629–33.
116. Iasonos A, Keung EZ, Zivanovic O, Mancari R, Peiretti M, Nucci M, George S, Colombo N, Carinelli S, Hensley ML, Raut CP. External validation of a prognostic nomogram for overall survival in women with uterine leiomyosarcoma. Cancer. 2013;119:1816–22.
117. Iihara K, Hirano K, Fujioka Y, Sakamoto A. Leiomyosarcoma with dedifferentiation in a premenopausal patient discovered after uterine artery embolization. Pathol Int. 2007;57:681–7.
118. Ioffe YJ, Li AJ, Walsh CS, Karlan BY, Leuchter R, Forscher C, Cass I. Hormone receptor expression in uterine sarcomas: prognostic and therapeutic roles. Gynecol Oncol. 2009;115:466–71.
119. Ip PP, Cheung AN, Clement PB. Uterine smooth muscle tumors of uncertain malignant potential (STUMP): a clinicopathologic analysis of 16 cases. Am J Surg Pathol. 2009;33:992–1005.
120. Ip PP, Tse KY, Tam KF. Uterine smooth muscle tumors other than the ordinary leiomyomas and leiomyosarcomas: a review of selected variants with emphasis on recent advances and unusual morphology that may cause concern for malignancy. Adv Anat Pathol. 2010;17:91–112.
121. Ip PP, Cheung AN. Pathology of uterine leiomyosarcomas and smooth muscle tumours of uncertain malignant potential. Best Pract Res Clin Obstet Gynaecol. 2011;25:691–704.
122. Jaakkola S, Lyytinen HK, Pukkala E, Ylikorkala O. Use of estradiol-progestin therapy associates with increased risk for uterine sarcomas. Gynecol Oncol. 2011;122:260–3.
123. Jacobs VR, Zemzoum I, Kremer M, Gottschalk N, Baumgärtner AK, Krol J, Kiechle M. Primary metastatic leiomyosarcoma of the fallopian tube: a rare case report. Onkologie. 2010;33:49–52.
124. Jacoby AF, Fuller AF Jr, Thor AD, Muntz HG. Primary leiomyosarcoma of the fallopian tube. Gynecol Oncol. 1993;51:404–7.
125. Jakate K, Azimi F, Ali RH, Lee CH, Clarke BA, Rasty G, Shaw PA, Melnyk N, Huntsman DG, Laframboise S, Rouzbahman M. Endometrial sarcomas: an immunohistochemical and JAZF1 re-arrangement study in low-grade and undifferentiated tumors. Mod Pathol. 2013;26:95–105.
126. Jayakrishnan K, Koshy AK, Manjula P, Nair AM, Ramachandran A, Kattoor J. Endometrial stromal sarcoma mimicking a myoma. Fertil Steril. 2009;92:1744–6.
127. Jessop FA, Roberts PF. Müllerian adenosarcoma of the uterus in association with tamoxifen therapy. Histopathology. 2000;36:91–2.
128. Jimenez WA, Sardi A, Nieroda C, Gushchin V. Cytoreductive surgery and hyperthermic intraperitoneal chemotherapy in the management of recurrent high-grade uterine sarcoma with peritoneal dissemination. Am J Obstet Gynecol. 2014;210:259.e1–8. doi:10.1016/j.ajog.2013.11.002.
129. Jin Y, Pan L, Wang X, Dai Z, Huang H, Guo L, Shen K, Lian L. Clinical characteristics of endometrial stromal sarcoma from an academic medical hospital in China. Int J Gynecol Cancer. 2010;20:1535–9.
130. Judson IR, Miah AB. Uterine sarcoma dissemination during myomectomy: if not "acceptable collateral damage," is it possible to mitigate the risk? Cancer. 2014;120(20):3100–2. doi:10.1002/cncr.28841.
131. Kaku T, Silverberg SG, Major FJ, Miller A, Fetter B, Brady MF. Adenosarcoma of the uterus: a Gynecologic Oncology Group clinicopathologic study of 31 cases. Int J Gynecol Pathol. 1992;11:75–88.
132. Kamikabeya TS, Etchebehere RM, Nomelini RS, Murta EF. Gynecological malignant neoplasias diagnosed after hysterectomy performed for leiomyoma in a university hospital. Eur J Gynaecol Oncol. 2010;31:651–3.
133. Kanda M, Sonoyama A, Hirano H, Kizaki T, Ohara N. Transition of low-grade to high-grade endometrial stromal sarcoma: a case report. Eur J Gynaecol Oncol. 2013;34:358–61.
134. Kapp DS, Shin JY, Chan JK. Prognostic factors and survival in 1396 patients with uterine leiomyosarcomas. Emphasis on impact of lymphadenectomy and oophorectomy. Cancer. 2008;112:820–30.
135. Kawamura N, Ichimura T, Ito F, Shibata S, Takahashi K, Tsujimura A, Ishiko O, Haba T, Wakasa K, Ogita S. Transcervical needle biopsy for the differential diagnosis between uterine sarcoma and leiomyoma. Cancer. 2002;94:1713–20.
136. Kawamura N, Ichimura T, Takahashi K, Tsujimura A, Ishiko O, Ogita S. Transcervical needle biopsy of uterine myoma-like tumors using an automatic biopsy gun. Fertil Steril. 2002;77:1060–4.
137. Khoury-Collado F, Einstein MH, Bochner BH, Alektiar KM, Sonoda Y, Abu-Rustum NR, Brown CL, Gardner GJ, Barakat RR, Chi DS. Pelvic exenteration with curative intent for recurrent uterine malignancies. Gynecol Oncol. 2012;124:42–7.
138. Kido A, Togashi K, Koyama T, Yamaoka T, Fujiwara T, Fujii S. Diffusely enlarged uterus: evaluation with MR imaging. Radiographics. 2003;23:1423–39.
139. Kim JA, Lee MS, Choi JS. Sonographic findings of uterine endometrial stromal sarcoma. Korean J Radiol. 2006;7:281–6.
140. Kim WY, Lee JW, Choi CH, Kang H, Kim TJ, Kim GB, Lee JH, Bae DS. Low grade endometrial stromal sarcoma: a single center's experience with 22 cases. Int J Gynecol Cancer. 2008;18:1084–9.
141. Kim HS, Han KH, Chung HH, Kim JW, Park NH, Song YS, Kang SB. Neutrophil to lymphocyte ratio for preoperative diagnosis of uterine sarcomas: a case-matched comparison. Eur J Surg Oncol. 2010;36:691–8.
142. Kobayashi H, Uekuri C, Akasaka J, Ito F, Shigemitsu A, Koike N, Shigetomi H. The biology of uterine sarcomas: A review and update. Mol Clin Oncol. 2013;1:599–609.
143. Köhler G, Belau, A, Dennis K, Evert K, Evert M, Hesse J, Hegenscheid K, Lehnhoff H, Krichbaum J, Kühnast M, Lehr A, Linke L, Marcinek A, Müller S, Schalitz S, Simon J, Spring P, Ständer C, Trojnarska S, Witte N, Zygmunt M. Deutsches klinisches Kompetenzzentrum für genitale Sarkome und Mischtumoren an der Universitätsmedizin Greifswald (DKSM) und Kooperationspartner – Institut für Pathologie Univ.-Klinikum Greifswald/Regensburg, VAAO Deutschland und Frauenklinik Frankfurt/Sachsenhausen. Datenbank und Promotions- und Forschungsgruppe genitale Sarkome, Greifswald 2016, http://www2.medizin.uni-greifswald.de/gyn/forschung/dksm/.
144. Köhler G, Evert K, Zygmunt M, Evert M. Glattmuskuläre Tumoren – Varianten des Leiomyoms (Angio- u. Lipoleiomyom, kotyledonoides u. zellreiches Leiomyom, Leiomyom mit bizarren Kernen, mitotisch aktives, epitheloides u. myxoides Leiomyom), glattmuskuläre Tumoren mit unsicherem malignem Potential (atypische glattmuskuläre Tumoren), disseminierte peritoneale Leiomyomatose, benignes metastasierendes Leiomyom, intravenöse Leiomyomatose. In: Köhler G, Evert M, Evert K, Zygmunt M, editors. Sarkome des weiblichen Genitale, Bd. 1 Glattmuskuläre und stromale Tumoren. Berlin/Boston: Walter de Gruyter GmbH; 2016. p. 1–114.
145. Köhler G, Evert K, Zygmunt M, Evert M. Das Leiomyosarkom. In: Köhler G, Evert M, Evert K, Zygmunt M, editors. Sarkome des weiblichen Genitale, Bd. 1 Glattmuskuläre und stromale Tumoren. Berlin/Boston: Walter de Gruyter GmbH; 2016. p. 115–225.
146. Köhler G, Evert K, Zygmunt M, Evert M. Stromale Tumoren – Endometriale Stromatumoren – Endometrialer Stromaknoten, endometrialer Stromatumor mit keimstrangähnlichen Elementen (ESTSCLE), uterine tumor resembling ovarian sex-cord tumor (UTROSCT) und ähnliche Tumoren. In: Köhler G, Evert M, Evert

K, Zygmunt M, editors. Sarkome des weiblichen Genitale, Bd. 1 Glattmuskuläre und stromale Tumoren. Berlin/Boston: Walter de Gruyter GmbH; 2016. p. 226–49.
147. Köhler G, Evert K, Zygmunt M, Evert M. Low-grade endometriales Stromasarkom. In: Köhler G, Evert M, Evert K, Zygmunt M, editors. Sarkome des weiblichen Genitale, Bd. 1 Glattmuskuläre und stromale Tumoren. Berlin/Boston: Walter de Gruyter GmbH; 2016. p. 250–313.
148. Köhler G, Evert K, Zygmunt M, Evert M. High-grade endometriales Stromasarkom und undifferenziertes uterines Sarkom. In: Köhler G, Evert M, Evert K, Zygmunt M, editors. Sarkome des weiblichen Genitale, Bd. 1 Glattmuskuläre und stromale Tumoren. Berlin/Boston: Walter de Gruyter GmbH; 2016. p. 314–53.
149. Köhler G, Evert K, Zygmunt M, Evert M. Angiosarkom. In: Köhler G, Evert M, Evert K, Zygmunt M, editors. Sarkome des weiblichen Genitale, Bd. 2 Andere seltene Sarkome, Mischtumoren, genitale Sarkome und Schwangerschaft. Berlin/Boston: Walter de Gruyter GmbH; 2016. p. 1–27.
150. Köhler G, Evert K, Zygmunt M, Evert M. Liposarkome. In: Köhler G, Evert M, Evert K, Zygmunt M, editors. Sarkome des weiblichen Genitale, Bd. 2 Andere seltene Sarkome, Mischtumoren, genitale Sarkome und Schwangerschaft. Berlin/Boston: Walter de Gruyter GmbH; 2016. p. 28–60.
151. Köhler G, Evert K, Zygmunt M, Evert M. Rhabdomyosarkome. In: Köhler G, Evert M, Evert K, Zygmunt M, editors. Sarkome des weiblichen Genitale, Bd. 2 Andere seltene Sarkome, Mischtumoren, genitale Sarkome und Schwangerschaft. Berlin/Boston: Walter de Gruyter GmbH; 2016. p. 61–112.
152. Köhler G, Evert K, Zygmunt M, Evert M. Perivaskulärer Epitheloidzelltumor (PECom). In: Köhler G, Evert M, Evert K, Zygmunt M, editors. Sarkome des weiblichen Genitale, Bd. 2 Andere seltene Sarkome, Mischtumoren, genitale Sarkome und Schwangerschaft. Berlin/Boston: Walter de Gruyter GmbH; 2016. p. 113–38.
153. Köhler G, Evert K, Zygmunt M, Evert M. Adenosarkom. In: Köhler G, Evert M, Evert K, Zygmunt M. Sarkome des weiblichen Genitale, Bd. 2 Andere seltene Sarkome, Mischtumoren, genitale Sarkome und Schwangerschaft. Berlin/Boston: Walter de Gruyter GmbH; 2016. p. 151–212. (a) Köhler G, Evert K, Zygmunt M, Evert M. Adenosarcoma. In: Köhler G, Evert M, Evert K, Zygmunt M. Sarcoma of the female genitalia, Volume 2: Other rare sarcomas, mixed tumors, genital sarcomas and pregnancy. Berlin/Boston: Walter de Gruyter GmbH; 2016 (in press).
154. Koivisto-Korander R, Butzow R, Koivisto AM, Leminen A. Clinical outcome and prognostic factors in 100 cases of uterine sarcoma: experience in Helsinki University Central Hospital 1990–2001. Gynecol Oncol. 2008;11:74–81.
155. Koivisto-Korander R, Martinsen JI, Weiderpass E, Leminen A, Pukkala E. Incidence of uterine leiomyosarcoma and endometrial stromal sarcoma in Nordic countries: results from NORDCAN and NOCCA databases. Maturitas. 2012;72:56–60.
156. Kokawa K, Nishiyama K, Ikeuchi M, Ihara Y, Akamatsu N, Enomoto T, Ishiko O, Motoyama S, Fujii S, Umesaki N. Clinical outcomes of uterine sarcomas: results from 14 years worth of experience in the kinki district in Japan (1990–2003). Int J Gynecol Cancer. 2006;16:1358–63.
157. Koontz JI, Soreng AL, Nucci M, Kuo FC, Pauwels P, van Den Berghe H, Dal Cin P, Fletcher JA, Sklar J. Frequent fusion of the JAZF1 and JJAZ1 genes in endometrial stromal tumors. Proc Natl Acad Sci U S A. 2001;98:6348–53.
158. Koyama T, Togashi K, Konishi I, Kobayashi H, Ueda H, Kataoka ML, Kobayashi H, Itoh T, Higuchi T, Fujii S, Konishi J. MR imaging of endometrial stromal sarcoma: correlation with pathologic findings. Am J Roentgenol. 1999;173:767–72.
159. Krivak TC, Seidman JD, McBroom JW, MacKoul PJ, Aye LM, Rose GS. Uterine adenosarcoma with sarcomatous overgrowth versus uterine carcinosarcoma: comparison of treatment and survival. Gynecol Oncol. 2001;83:89–94.
160. Kurihara S, Oda Y, Ohishi Y, Iwasa A, Takahira T, Kaneki E, Kobayashi H, Wake N, Tsuneyoshi M. Endometrial stromal sarcomas and related high-grade sarcomas: immunohistochemical and molecular genetic study of 31 cases. Am J Surg Pathol. 2008;32:1228–38.
161. Kurjak A, Zalud I. The characterization of uterine tumors by transvaginal color Doppler. Ultrasound Obstet Gynecol. 1991;1:50–2.
162. Kurjak A, Kupesic S, Shalan H, Jukic S, Kosuta D, Ilijas M. Uterine sarcoma: a report of 10 cases studied by transvaginal color and pulsed Doppler sonography. Gynecol Oncol. 1995;59:342–6.
163. Leath III CA, Huh WK, Hyde Jr J, Cohn DE, Resnick KE, Taylor NP, Powell MA, Mutch DG, Bradley WH, Geller MA, Argenta PA, Gold MA. A multi-institutional review of outcomes of endometrial stromal sarcoma. Gynecol Oncol. 2007;105:630–4.
164. Lee WY, Tzeng CC, Chou CY. Uterine leiomyosarcomas coexistent with cellular and atypical leiomyomata in a young woman during the treatment with luteinizing hormone-releasing hormone agonist. Gynecol Oncol. 1994;52:74–9.
165. Lee J. Sonohysterography. In: Kim SH, editor. Radiology illustrated gynecologic imaging. 2nd ed. Berlin/Heidelberg: Springer; 2012. p. 1149–81.
166. Lee CH, Mariño-Enriquez A, Ou W, Zhu M, Ali RH, Chiang S, Amant F, Gilks CB, van de Rijn M, Oliva E, Debiec-Rychter M, Dal Cin P, Fletcher JA, Nucci MR. The clinicopathologic features of YWHAE-FAM22 endometrial stromal sarcomas: a histologically high-grade and clinically aggressive tumor. Am J Surg Pathol. 2012;36:641–53.
167. Lee CH, Ali RH, Rouzbahman M, Marino-Enriquez A, Zhu M, Guo X, Brunner AL, Chiang S, Leung S, Nelnyk N, Huntsman DG, Blake Gilks C, Nielsen TO, Dal Cin P, van de Rijn M, Oliva E, Fletcher JA, Nucci MR. Cyclin D1 as a diagnostic immunomarker for endometrial stromal sarcoma with YWHAE-FAM22 rearrangement. Am J Surg Pathol. 2012;36:1562–70.
168. Leitao MM, Sonoda Y, Brennan MF, Barakat RR, Chi DS. Incidence of lymph node and ovarian metastases in leiomyosarcoma of the uterus. Gynecol Oncol. 2003;91:209–12.
169. Leitao Jr MM, Zivanovic O, Chi DS, Hensley ML, O'Cearbhaill R, Soslow RA, Barakat RR. Surgical cytoreduction in patients with metastatic uterine leiomyosarcoma at the time of initial diagnosis. Gynecol Oncol. 2012;125:409–13.
170. Lerman H, Bar-On S, Helpman L, Even-Sapir E, Grisaru D. Estrogen-dependent variations in 18F-fluorodeoxyglucose uptake in uterine leiomyomas. Int J Gynecol Cancer. 2012;22:1187–91.
171. Leung F, Terzibachian JJ, Gay C, Chung Fat B, Aouar Z, Lassabe C, Maillet R, Riethmuller D. Hysterectomies performed for presumed leiomyomas: should the fear of leiomyosarcoma make us apprehend non laparotomic surgical routes? Gynecol Obstet Fertil. 2009;37:109–14.
172. Leung F, Terzibachian JJ. Re: "The impact of tumor morcellation during surgery on the prognosis of patients with apparently early uterine leiomyosarcoma". Gynecol Oncol. 2012;124:172–3.
173. Li A, Giuntoli R, Drake RSY, Rojas F, Barbuto D, Klipfel N, Edmonds P, Miller D, Karlan B. Ovarian preservation in stage I low-grade endometrial stromal sarcoma. Obstet Gynecol. 2005;106:1304–8.
174. Li N, Wu LY, Zhang HT, An JS, Li XG, Ma SK. Treatment options in stage I endometrial stromal sarcoma: a retrospective analysis of 53 cases. Gynecol Oncol. 2008;108:306–11.
175. Lieng M, Berner E, Busund B. Risk of morcellation of uterine leiomyosarcomas in laparoscopic supracervical hysterectomy and laparoscopic myomectomy, a retrospective trial including 4791 women. J Minim Invasive Gynecol. 2015;22:410–4. doi:10.1016/j.jmig.2014.10.022.

176. Lim D, Wang WL, Lee CH, Dodge T, Gilks B, Oliva E. Old versus new FIGO staging systems in predicting overall survival in patients with uterine leiomyosarcoma: a study of 86 cases. Gynecol Oncol. 2013;128:322–6.
177. Lissoni A, Cormio G, Bonazzi C, Perego P, Lomonocio S, Gabriele A, Bratina G. Fertility sparing surgery in uterine leiomyosarcoma. Gynecol Oncol. 1998;70:348–50.
178. Löning T. Funktionelle Morphologie und Pathologie des Myometriums. In: Löning T, Riethdorf L, Hrsg. Pathologie der weiblichen Genitalorgane III – Pathologie des Uterus der Vagina und Vulva. Berlin/Heidelberg/New York: Springer; 2001. p. 652–704.
179. Lönnerfors C, Bossmar T, Persson J. Port-site metastases following robot-assisted laparoscopic surgery for gynecological malignancies. Acta Obstet Gynecol Scand. 2013;92:1361–8.
180. Lousse JC, Jourct M, Marbaix E, Fellah L, Squifflet J, Donne J. Suspicious myometrial mass on ultrasonography and MRIdoes not necessarily mean a sarcoma on histology. Gynecol Surg. 2010;7:263–5.
181. Ly A, Mills AM, McKenney JK, Balzer BL, Kempson RL, Hendrickson MR, Longacre TA. Atypical leiomyomas of the uterus: a clinicopathologic study of 51 cases. Am J Surg Pathol. 2013;37:643–9.
182. Major F, Blessing J, Silverberg S, Morrow P, Creasman W, Curry JL, Yordan E, Brady MF. Prognostic factors in early stage uterine sarcoma: a Gynecologic Oncology study. Cancer. 1993;71:1702–9.
183. Malouf GG, Lhommé C, Duvillard P, Morice P, Haie-Meder C, Pautier P. Prognostic factors and outcome of undifferentiated endometrial sarcoma treated by multimodal therapy. Int J Gynaecol Obstet. 2013;122:57–61.
184. Manoharan M, Azmi MA, Soosay G, Mould T, Weekes AR. Mullerian adenosarcoma of uterine cervix: report of three cases and review of literature. Gynecol Oncol. 2007;105:256–60.
185. Martínez A, Querleu D, Leblanc E, Narducci F, Ferron G. Low incidence of port-site metastases after laparoscopic staging of uterine cancer. Gynecol Oncol. 2010;118:145–50.
186. Mastrangelo G, Coindre JM, Ducimetière F, Dei Tos AP, Fadda E, Blay JY, Buja A, Fedeli U, Cegolon L, Frasson A, Anchère-Vince D, Montesco C, Ray-Coquard I, Riccardo RC. Incidence of soft tissue sarcoma and beyond. A population-based prospective study in 3 European regions. Cancer. 2012;118:5339–48.
187. Matsuda M, Ichimura T, Kasai M, Murakami M, Kawamura N, Hayashi T, Sumi T. Preoperative diagnosis of usual leiomyoma, atypical leiomyoma, and leiomyosarcoma. Sarcoma. 2014;2014:498682. doi:10.1155/2014/498682.
188. Menge F, Hartmann E, Mathew M, Kasper B, Hohenberger P. The impact of operative techniques to the onset of peritoneal tumor dissemination in parients with uterine Leiomyosarcomas. 18th Annual Meeting of Connective Tissue Oncology Society 2013; Paper 010.
189. Mikami Y, Hata S, Kiyokawa T, Manabe T. Expression of CD10 in malignant müllerian mixed tumors and adenosarcomas: an immunohistochemical study. Mod Pathol. 2002;15:923–30.
190. Mills AM, Ly A, Balzer BL, Hendrickson MR, Kempson RL, McKenney JK, Longacre TA. Cell cycle regulatory markers in uterine atypical leiomyoma and leiomyosarcoma: immunohistochemical study of 68 cases with clinical follow-up. Am J Surg Pathol. 2013;37:634–42.
191. Milman D, Zalel Y, Biran H, Open M, Caspi B, Hagay Z, Dgani R. Unsuspected uterine leiomyosarcoma discovered during treatment with a gonadotropin-releasing hormone analogue: a case report and literature review. Eur J Obstet Gynecol Reprod Biol. 1998;76:237–40.
192. Mittal K, Demopoulos RI. MIB-1 (Ki-67), p53, estrogen receptor, and progesterone receptor expression in uterine smooth muscle tumors. Hum Pathol. 2001;32:984–7.
193. Mittal K, Joutovsky A. Areas with benign morphologic and immunohistochemical features are associated with some uterine leiomyosarcomas. Gynecol Oncol. 2007;104:362–5.
194. Mittal KR, Chen F, Wei JJ, Rijhvani K, Kurvathi R, Streck D, Dermody J, Toruner GA. Molecular and immunohistochemical evidence for the origin of uterine leiomyosarcomas from associated leiomyoma and symplastic leiomyoma-like areas. Mod Pathol. 2009;22:1303–11.
195. Moinfar F, Azodi M, Tavassoli FA. Uterine sarcomas. Pathology. 2007;39:55–71.
196. Morice P, Rodrigues A, Pautier P, Rey A, Camatte S, Atallah D, Pomel C, Lhommé C, Haie-Meder C, Duvillard P, Castaigne D. Chirurgie des sarcomas utérins: revue de la littérature et recommandations sur la prise en charge chirurgicale. Surgical procedures for uterine sarcoma. Gynecol Obstet Fertil. 2003;31:147–50.
197. Morice P, Rodriguez A, Rey A, Pautier P, Atallah D, Genestie C, Pomel C, Lhommé C, Haie-Meder C, Duvillard P, Castaigne D. Prognostic value of initial surgical procedure for patients with uterine sarcoma: analysis of 123 patients. Eur J Gynaecol Oncol. 2003;24:237–40.
198. Mowers EL, Skinner B, McLean K, Reynolds RK. Effects of morcellation of uterine smooth muscle tumor of uncertain malignant potential and endometrial stromal sarcoma: case series and recommendations for clinical practice. J Minim Invasive Gynecol. 2015;22:601–6. doi:10.1016/j.jmig.2015.01.007.
199. Murase E, Siegelman ES, Outwater EK, Perez-Jaffe LA, Tureck RW. Uterine leiomyomas: histopathologic features, MR imaging findings, differential diagnosis, and treatment. Radiographics. 1999;19:1179–97.
200. Naqamatsu A, Umesaki N, Li L, Tanaka T. Use of 18F-fluorodeoxyglucose positron emission tomography for diagnosis of uterine sarcomas. Oncol Rep. 2010;23:1069–76.
201. Nagase S, Katabuchi H, Hiura M, Sakuragi N, Aoki Y, Kigawa J, Saito T, Hachisuga T, Ito K, Uno T, Katsumata N, Komiyama S, Susumu N, Emoto M, Kobayashi H, Metoki H, Konishi I, Ochiai K, Mikami M, Sugiyama T, Mukai M, Sagae S, Hoshiai H, Aoki D, Ohmichi M, Yoshikawa H, Iwasaka T, Udagawa Y, Yaegashi N, Japan Society of Gynecologic Oncology. Evidence-based guidelines for treatment of uterine body neoplasm in Japan: Japan Society of Gynecologic Oncology (JSGO) 2009 edition. Int J Clin Oncol. 2010;15:531–42.
202. National Comprehensive Cancer Network: NCCN Practice Guidelines in Oncology – Uterine neoplasms – Version 1.2016. www.nccn.org.
203. Nezhat FR, Roemisch M, Nezhat CH, et al. Recurrence rate after laparoscopic myomectomy. J Am Assoc Gynecol Laparosc. 1998;5:237–40.
204. Ngan HY, Fisher C, Blake P, Shepherd JH. Vaginal sarcoma: the Royal Marsden experience. Int J Gynecol Cancer. 1994;4:337–41.
205. Nordal R, Kristensen GB, Kaern J, Stenwig A, Pettersen EO, Tropé CG. The prognostic significance of surgery, tumor size, malignancy grade, menopausal status, and DNA ploidy in endometrial stromal sarcoma. Gynecol Oncol. 1996;62:254–9.
206. Nucci MR, Harburger D, Koontz J, Dal Cin P, Sklar J. Molecular analysis of the JAZF1-JJAZ1 gene fusion by RT-PCR and fluorescence in situ hybridization in endometrial stromal neoplasms. Am J Surg Pathol. 2007;31:65–70.
207. Nucci MR, Quade BJ. Uterine mesenchymal tumors. In: Crum CP, Nucci MR, Lee KR, editors. Diagnostic gynecologic and obstetric pathology. 2nd ed. Philadelphia: Elsevier Saunders; 2011. p. 582–639.
208. Numa F, Umayahara K, Ogata H, Nawata S, Sakaguchi Y, Emoto T, Kawasaki K, Hirakawa H, Sase M, Oga A, Kato H. De novo uterine sarcoma with good response to neo-adjuvant chemotherapy. Int J Gynecol Cancer. 2003;13:364–7.

209. Oda Y, Nakanishi I, Tateiwa T. Intramural müllerian adenosarcoma of the uterus with adenomyosis. Arch Pathol Lab Med. 1984;108:798–801.
210. Oduyebo T, Rauh-Hain AJ, Meserve EE, Seidman MA, Hinchcliff E, George S, Quade B, Nucci MR, Del Carmen MG, Muto MG. The value of re-exploration in patients with inadvertently morcellated uterine sarcoma. Gynecol Oncol. 2014;132:360–5.
211. Oliva E, de Leval L, Soslow RA, Herens C. High frequency of JAZF1-JJAZ1 gene fusion in endometrial stromal tumors with smooth muscle differentiation by interphase FISH detection. Am J Surg Pathol. 2007;31:277–84.
212. Oliva E, Caracangiu ML, Carinelli SG, Ip P, Loening T, Longacre TA, Nucci MR, Prat J, Zaloudek CJ. Tumours of the uterine corpus. Mesenchymal tumors. In: Kurman RJ, Carcangiu ML, Herrington CS, Young RH, editors. WHO classification of tumors of female reproductive organs. 4th ed. Lyon: IARC; 2014. p. 135–52.
213. O'Neill CJO, McBride HA, Connolly LE, McCluggage WG. Uterine leiomyosarcomas are characterized by high p16, p53 and MIB1 expression in comparison with usual leiomyomas, leiomyoma variants and smooth muscle tumours of uncertain malignant potential. Histopathology. 2007;50:851–8.
214. Orii A, Mori A, Zhai YL, Toki T, Nikaido T, Fujii S. Mast cells in smooth muscle tumors of the uterus. Int J Gynecol Pathol. 1998;17:336–42.
215. Papadia A, Salom EM, Fulcheri E, Ragni N. Uterine sarcoma occurring in a premenopausal patient after uterine artery embolization: a case report and review of the literature. Gynecol Oncol. 2007;104:260–3.
216. Park JY, Kim DY, Kim JH, Kim YM, Kim YT, Nam JH. The impact of tumor morcellation during surgery on the outcomes of patients with apparently early low-grade endometrial stromal sarcoma of the uterus. Ann Surg Oncol. 2011;18:3453–61.
217. Park JY, Park SK, Kim DY, Kim JH, Kim YM, Kim YT, Nam JH. The impact of tumor morcellation during surgery on the prognosis of patients with apparently early uterine leiomyosarcoma. Gynecol Oncol. 2011;122:255–9.
218. Park JY, Kim KR, Nam JH. Immunohistochemical analysis for therapeutic targets and prognostic markers in low-grade endometrial stromal sarcoma. Int J Gynecol Cancer. 2013;23:81–9.
219. Parker WH, Fu YS, Berek JS. Uterine sarcomas in patients operated for presumed leiomyoma and rapidly growing leiomyoma. Obstet Gynecol. 1994;83:414–8.
220. Pautier P, Nam EJ, Provencher DM, Hamilton AL, Mangili G, Siddiqui NA, Westermann AM, Reed NS, Harter P, Ray-Coquard I. Gynecologic Cancer InterGroup (GCIG) consensus review for high-grade undifferentiated sarcomas of the uterus. Int J Gynecol Cancer. 2014;24(9 Suppl 3):S73–7.
221. Pavlakis K, Messini I, Papadimitriou CA, Zagouri F, Yiannou P, Mavrelos D, Panoskaltis T. Tumor dissemination after laparoscopic surgery for an unsuspected endometrial stromal tumor. Eur J Gynaecol Oncol. 2011;32:362–3.
222. Peddada SD, Laughlin SK, Miner K, Guyon JP, Haneke K, Vahdat HL, Semelka RC, Kowalik A, Armao D, Davis B, Baird DD. Growth of uterine leiomyomata among premenopausal black and white women. Proc Natl Acad Sci U S A. 2008;105:19887–92.
223. Perri T, Korach J, Sadetzki S, Oberman B, Fridman E, Ben-Baruch G. Uterine leiomyosarcoma: does the primary surgical procedure matter? Int J Gynecol Cancer. 2009;19:257–60.
224. Peters 3rd WA, Howard DR, Andersen WA, Figge DC. Uterine smooth-muscle tumors of uncertain malignant potential. Obstet Gynecol. 1994;83:1015–20.
225. Plasvsic SK, Patham B, Honemeyer U, Kurjak A. Uterine lesions: advances in ultrasound diagnosis. In. Kurjak A, Chervenak FA, editors. Donald School Textbook of ultrasound in obstetrics and gynecology. 3rd ed. New Delhi/Panama City/London: Jaypee Brothers Medical Publishers LTD; 2011. p. 770–787.
226. Posy HE, Elkas JC, Yemelyanova AV, Diaz-Montes TP, Bristow RE, Giuntoli RL. Metastatic leiomyosarcoma diagnosed after uterine artery embolization. Eur J Gynaecol Oncol. 2009;30:199–202.
227. Pothuri B, Kehoe M, Wright T, Herzog T. Clinical outcome of atypical uterine smooth muscle tumors. ASCO Annual Meeting 2006; Abstr. 15028.
228. Prat J. FIGO staging for uterine sarcomas. Int J Gynecol Obstet. 2009;104:177–8.
229. Pritts EA, Vanness DJ, Berek JS, Parker W, Feinberg R, Feinberg J, Olive DL. The prevalence of occult leiomyosarcoma at surgery for presumed uterine fibroids: a meta-analysis. Gynecol Surg. 2015;12:165–77.
230. Protopapas A, Milingos S, Markaki S, Loutradis D, Haidopoulos D, Sotiropoulou M, Antsaklis A. Cystic uterine tumors. Gynecol Obstet Investig. 2008;65:275–80.
231. Quade BJ, Wang TY, Sornberger K, Dal Cin P, Mutter GL, Morton CC. Molecular pathogenesis of uterine smooth muscle tumors from transcriptional profiling. Genes Chromosom Cancer. 2004;40:97–108.
232. Rauh-Hain JA, Oduyebo T, Diver EJ, Guseh SH, George S, Muto MG, del Carmen MG. Uterine leiomyosarcoma: an updated series. Int J Gynecol Cancer. 2013;23:1036–43.
233. Rauh-Hain JA, Hinchcliff EM, Oduyebo T, Worley Jr MJ, Andrade CA, Schorge JO, George S, Muto MG, Del Carmen MG. Clinical outcomes of women with recurrent or persistent uterine leiomyosarcoma. Int J Gynecol Cancer. 2014;24:1434–40.
234. Raut CP, Nucci MR, Wang Q, Manola J, Bertagnolli MM, Demetri GD, Morgan JA, Muto MG, Fletcher CD, George S. Predictive value of FIGO and AJCC staging systems in patients with uterine leiomyosarcoma. Eur J Cancer. 2009;45:2818–24.
235. Reed NS. The management of uterine sarcomas. Clin Oncol. 2008;20:470–8.
236. Reich O, Regauer S, Urdl W, Lahousen M, Winter R. Expression of oestrogen and progesterone receptors in low-grade endometrial stromal sarcomas. Br J Cancer. 2000;82:1030–4.
237. Reich O, Regauer S. Aromatase expression in low-grade endometrial stromal sarcoma. An immunohistochemical study. Mod Pathol. 2004;17:104–8.
238. Reich O, Regauer S. Survey of adjuvant hormone therapy in patients after endometrial stromal sarcoma. Eur J Gynaecol Oncol. 2006;27:150–2.
239. Reich O, Regauer S. Hormonal therapy in endometrial stromale sarcoma. Curr Opin Oncol. 2007;19:347–52.
240. Reich O, Regauer S, Scharf S. High levels of xenoestrogens in patients with low-grade endometrial stromal sarcoma–report of two cases. Eur J Gynaecol Oncol. 2010;31:105–6.
241. Reich O, Regauer S, Tempfer C, Schneeberger C, Huber J. Polymorphism 1558 C > T in the aromatase gene (CYP19A1) in low-grade endometrial stromal sarcoma. Eur J Gynaecol Oncol. 2011;32:626–7.
242. Reinhold C, Zand KR. Endometrial stromal sarcoma. In: Hricak HH, Akin O, Sala E, Ascher SM, Levine D, Reinhold C, editors. Diagnostic imaging gynecology. Amyrsis; 2007. p. 2–162–6.
243. Rha SE, Byun JY, Jung SE, Lee SL, Cho SM, Hwang SS, Lee HG, Namkoong SE, Lee JM. CT and MRI of uterine sarcomas and their mimickers. Am J Roentgenol. 2003;181:1369–74.
244. Riopel J, Plante M, Renaud MC, Roy M, Têtu B. Lymph node metastases in low-grade endometrial stromal sarcoma. Gynecol Oncol. 2005;96:402–6.
245. Rivera JA, Christopoulos S, Small D, Trifiro M. Hormonal manipulation of benign metastasizing leiomyomas: report of two cases and review of the literature. J Clin Endocrinol Metab. 2004;89:3183–8.

246. Rutstein SE, Siedhoff MT, Geller EJ, Doll KM, Wu JM, Clarke-Pearson DL, Wheeler SB. Cost-effectiveness of laparoscopic hysterectomy with morcellation compared to abdominal hysterectomy for presumed fibroids. J Minim Invasive Gynecol. 2015;13. pii: S1553–4650(15)01618–0. doi:10.1016/j.jmig.2015.09.025.
247. Sagae S, Yamashita K, Ishioka S, Nishioka Y, Terasawa K, Mori M, Yamashiro K, Kanemoto T, Kudo R. Preoperative diagnosis and treatment results in 106 patients with uterine sarcoma in Hokkaido, Japan. Oncology. 2004;67:33–9.
248. Salman MC, Guler OT, Kucukali T, Karaman N, Ayhan A. Fertility-saving surgery for low-grade uterine leiomyosarcoma with subsequent pregnancy. Int J Gynaecol Obstet. 2007;98:160–1.
249. Santos P, Cunha TM. Uterine sarcomas: clinical presentation and MRI features. Diagn Interv Radiol. 2015;21:4–9. doi:10.5152/dir.2014.14053.
250. Sato K, Yuasa N, Fujita M, Fukushima Y. Clinical application of diffusion-weighted imaging for preoperative differentiation between uterine leiomyoma and leiomyosarcoma. Am J Obstet Gynecol. 2014;210:368.e1–8.
251. Schwartz LB, Diamond MP, Schwartz PE. Leiomyosarcomas: clinical presentation. Am J Obstet Gynecol. 1993;168:180–3.
252. Sciallis AP, Bedroske PP, Schoolmeester JK, Sukov WR, Keeney GL, Hodge JC, Bell DA. High-grade Endometrial Stromal Sarcomas: a clinicopathologic study of a group of tumors with heterogenous morphologic and genetic features. Am J Surg Pathol. 2014;38:1161–72.
253. Seidman JD, Wasserman CS, Aye LM, MacKoul PJ, O'Leary TJ. Cluster of uterine mullerian adenosarcoma in the Washington, DC metropolitan area with high incidence of sarcomatous overgrowth. Am J Surg Pathol. 1999;23:809–14.
254. Seidman MA, Oduyebo T, Muto MG, Crum CP, Nucci MR, Quade BJ. Peritoneal dissemination complicating morcellation of uterine mesenchymal neoplasms. PLoS One. 2012;7(11):e50058. doi:10.1371/journal.pone.0050058.
255. Sesti F, Patrizi L, Ermini B, Palmieri G, Orlandi A, Piccione E. High-grade endometrial stromal sarcoma after tamoxifen therapy for breast cancer. Gynecol Obstet Investig. 2005;60:117–20.
256. Shah JP, Bryant CS, Kumar S, Ali-Fehmi R, Malone JM, Morris RT. Lymphadenectomy and ovarian preservation in low grade endometrial stromal sarcoma. Obstet Gynecol. 2008;112:1102–8.
257. Shah SH, Jagannathan JP, Krajewski K, O'Regan KN, George S, Ramaiya NH. Uterine sarcomas: then and now. Am J Roentgenol. 2012;199:213–23.
258. Shapiro A, Ferenczy A, Turcotte R, Bruchim I, Gotlieb WH. Uterine smooth-muscle tumor of uncertain malignant potential metastasizing to the humerus as a high-grade leiomyosarcoma. Gynecol Oncol. 2004;94:818–20.
259. Shin YR, Rha SE. Miscellaneous tumors of the uterus. In: Kim SH, editor. Radiology illustrated gynecologic imaging. 2nd ed. Berlin/Heidelberg; Springer; 2012. p. 249–97.
260. Siedhoff MT, Wheeler SB, Rutstein SE, Geller EJ, Doll KM, Wu JM, Clarke-Pearson DL. Laparoscopic hysterectomy with morcellation vs abdominal hysterectomy for presumed fibroid tumors in premenopausal women: a decision analysis. Am J Obstet Gynecol. 2015;212:591.e1–8. doi:10.1016/j.ajog.2015.03.006.
261. Signorelli M, Fruscio R, Dell'Anna T, Buda A, Giuliani D, Ceppi L, Milani R. Lymphadenectomy in uterine low-grade endometrial stromal sarcoma: an analysis of 19 cases and a literature review. Int J Gynecol Cancer. 2010;20:1363–6.
262. Sinha R, Hegde A, Mahajan C, Dubey N, Sundaram MJ. Laparoscopic myomectomy: do size, number, and location of the myomas form limiting factors for laparoscopic myomectomy? J Minim Invasive Gynecol. 2008;15:292–300.
263. Sizzi O, Rossetti A, Malzoni M, Minelli L, La Grotta F, Soranna L, Panunzi S, Spagnolo R, Imperato F, Landi S, Fiaccamento A, Stola E. Italian multicenter study on complications of laparoscopic myomectomy. J Minim Invasive Gynecol. 2007;14:453–62.
264. Sobin LH, Gospadarowicz MK, Wittekind CH, editors. TMN classification of malignant tumours. 7th ed. Weinheim: Wiley; 2010.
265. Somoye G, Lawton H, Havenga S. Endometrial stromal sarcoma: experience from a district hospital and literature review. Eur J Gynaecol Oncol. 2009;30:664–7.
266. Soslow RA, Ali A, Oliva E. Mullerian adenosarcomas: an immunophenotypic analysis of 35 cases. Am J Surg Pathol. 2008;32:1013–21.
267. Stadsvold JL, Molpus KL, Baker JJ, Michael K, Remmenga SW. Conservative management of a myxoid endometrial stromal sarcoma in a 16-year old nulliparous woman. Gynecol Oncol. 2005;99:243–5.
268. Stemme S, Ghaderi M, Carlson JW. Diagnosis of endometrial stromal tumors: a clinicopathologic study of 25 biopsy specimens with identification of problematic areas. Am J Clin Pathol. 2014;141:133–9.
269. Sung CO, Ahn G, Song SY, Choi YL, Bae DS. Atypical leiomyomas of the uterus with long-term follow-up after myomectomy with immunohistochemical analysis for pl6, INK4A, p53, Ki-67, estrogen receptors, and progesterone receptors. Int J Gynecol Pathol. 2009;280:529–34.
270. Szabó I, Szánthó A, Csabay L, Csapó Z, Szirmai K, Papp Z. Color Doppler ultrasonography in the differentiation of uterine sarcomas from uterine leiomyomas. Eur J Gynaecol Oncol. 2002;23:29–4.
271. Szkandera J, Gerger A, Liegl-Atzwanger B, Absenger G, Stotz M, Friesenbichler J, Trajanoski S, Stojakovic T, Eberhard K, Leithner A, Pichler M. The lymphocyte/monocyte ratio predicts poor clinical outcome and improves the predictive accuracy in patients with soft tissue sarcomas. Int J Cancer. 2014;135:362–70.
272. Szklaruk J, Tamm EP, Choi H, Varavithya V. MR imaging of common and uncommon large pelvic masses. Radiographics. 2003;23:403–24.
273. Taga S, Sawada M, Nagai A, Yamamoto D, Hayase R. A case of adenosarcoma of the uterus. Case Rep Obstet Gynecol. 2014;Article ID 342187:4. http://dx.doi.org/10.1155/2014/J42187.
274. Takeda A, Imoto S, Mori M, Nakamura H. Successful pregnancy outcome after laparoscopic-assisted excision of a bizarre leiomyoma: a case report. J Med Case Rep. 2011;5:344.
275. Takeuchi M, Matsuzaki K, Yoshida S, Kudo E, Bando Y, Hasebe H, Kamada M, Nishitani H. Adenosarcoma of the uterus: magnetic resonance imaging characteristics. Clin Imaging. 2009;33:244–7.
276. Tamura R, Kashima K, Asatani M, Nishino K, Nishikawa N, Sekine M, Serikawa T, Enomoto T. Preoperative ultrasound-guided needle biopsy of 63 uterine tumors having high signal intensity upon T2-weighted magnetic resonance imaging. Int J Gynecol Cancer. 2014;24:1042–7.
277. Tanaka YO, Nishida M, Tsunoda H, Okamoto Y, Yoshikawa H. Smooth muscle tumors of uncertain malignant potential and leiomyosarcomas of the uterus: MR findings. J Magn Reson Imaging. 2004;20:998–1007.
278. Tanner EJ, Garg K, Leitao Jr MM, Soslow RA, Hensley ML. High grade undifferentiated uterine sarcoma: surgery, treatment, and survival outcomes. Gynecol Oncol. 2012;127:27–31.
279. Tanner EJ, Toussaint T, Leitao Jr MM, Hensley ML, Soslow RA, Gardner GJ, Jewell EL. Management of uterine adenosarcomas with and without sarcomatous overgrowth. Gynecol Oncol. 2013;129:140–4.
280. Thomas MB, Keeney GL, Podratz KC, Dowdy SC. Endometrial stromal sarcoma: treatment and patterns of recurrence. Int J Gynecol Cancer. 2009;19:253–6.

281. Tirumani SH, Ojili V, Shanbhogue AK, Fasih N, Ryan JG, Reinhold C. Current concepts in the imaging of uterine sarcoma. Abdom Imaging. 2013;38:397–411.
282. Toledo G, Oliva E. Smooth muscle tumors of the uterus. Arch Pathol Lab Med. 2008;132:595–605.
283. Toro JR, Travis LB, Wu HJ, Zhu K, Fletcher CD, Devesa SS. Incidence patterns of soft tissue sarcomas, regardless of primary site, in the surveillance, epidemiology and end results program, 1978-2001: an analysis of 26,758 cases. Int J Cancer. 2006;119:2922–30.
284. Trovik J, Salvesen HB, Cuppens T, Amant F, Staff AC. Growth differentiation factor-15 as biomarker in uterine sarcomas. Int J Gynecol Cancer. 2014;24:252–9.
285. Umesaki N, Tanaka T, Miyama M, Ogita S, Kawabe J, Okamura T, Koyama K, Ochi H. Positron emission tomography using 2-[(18)F] fluoro-2-deoxy-D-glucose in the diagnosis of uterine leiomyosarcoma: a case report. Clin Imaging. 2001;25:203–5.
286. Vera AA, Guadarrama MB. Endometrial stromal sarcoma: clinicopathological and immunophenotype study of 18 cases. Ann Diagn Pathol. 2011;15:312–7.
287. Veras E, Zivanovic O, Jacks L, Chiappetta D, Hensley M, Soslow R. "Low-grade leiomyosarcoma" and late-recurring smooth muscle tumors of the uterus: a heterogenous collection of frequently misdiagnosed tumors associated with an overall favorable prognosis relative to conventional uterine leiomyosarcomas. Am J Surg Pathol. 2011;35:1626–37.
288. Verschraegen CF, Vasuratna A, Edwards C, Freedman R, Kudelka AP, Tornos C, Kavanagh JJ. Clinicopathologic analysis of mullerian adenosarcoma: the M.D. Anderson Cancer Center experience. Oncol Rep. 1998;5:939–44.
289. Vilos GA, Hollett-Caines J, Abu-Rafea B, Allen HH, Inculet R, Kirk ME. Leiomyosarcoma diagnosed six years after laparoscopic electromyolysis. J Obstet Gynaecol Can. 2008;30:500–4.
290. Walker CL, Stewart EA. Uterine fibroids: the elephant in the room. Science. 2005;308:1589–92.
291. Wittekind C, Comptom CC, Brierley J, Sobin LH. TNM-supplement – a commentary on uniform use. 4th ed. Genf: UICC and Wiley; 2012.
292. Wong P, Han K, Sykes J, Catton C, Laframboise S, Fyles A, Manchul L, Levin W, Milosevic M. Postoperative radiotherapy improves local control and survival in patients with uterine leiomyosarcomas. Radiat Oncol. 2013;8:128.
293. Wright JD, Seshan VE, Shah M, Schiff PB, Burke WM, Cohen CJ, Herzog TJ. The role of radiation in improving survival for early-stage carcinosarcoma and leiomyosarcoma. Am J Obstet Gynecol. 2008;199:536.e1–8.
294. Wright JD, Tergas AI, Cui R, Burke WM, Hou JY, Ananth CV, Chen L, Richards C, Neugut AI, Hershman DL. Use of electric power morcellation and prevalence of underlying cancer in women who undergo myomectomy. JAMA Oncol. doi:10.1001/jamaoncol.2014.206, Published online February 19, 2015.
295. Xue WC, Cheung AN. Endometrial stromal sarcoma of uterus. Best Pract Res Clin Obstet Gynaecol. 2011;25:719–32.
296. Yang WT, Lam WW, Yu MY, Cheung TH, Metreweli C. Comparison of dynamic helical CT and dynamic MR imaging in the evaluation of pelvic lymph nodes in cervical carcinoma. Am J Roentgenol. 2000;75:759–66.
297. Yavuz E, Güllüoğlu MG, Akbaş N, Tuzlali S, Ilhan R, Iplikçi A, Akhan SE. The values of intratumoral mast cell count and Ki-67 immunoreactivity index in differential diagnosis of uterine smooth muscle neoplasms. Pathol Int. 2001;51:938–41.
298. Yildirim Y, Inal MM, Sanci M, Yildirim YK, Mit T, Polat M, Tinar S. Development of uterine sarcoma after tamoxifen treatment for breast cancer: report of four cases. Int J Gynecol Cancer. 2005;15:1239–42.
299. Yoon A, Park JY, Park JY, Lee YY, Kim TJ, Choi CH, Bae DS, Kim BG, Lee JW, Nam JH. Prognostic factors and outcomes in endometrial stromal sarcoma with the 2009 FIGO staging system: a multicenter review of 114 cases. Gynecol Oncol. 2014;132:70–5.
300. Yoshida C, Ichimura T, Kawamura N, Nakano A, Kasai M, Sumi T, Ishiko O. A scoring system for histopathologic and immunohistochemical evaluations of uterine leiomyosarcomas. Oncol Rep. 2009;22:725–31.
301. Yoshizako T, Wada A, Kitagaki H, Ishikawa N, Miyazaki K. MR imaging of uterine adenosarcoma: case report and literature review. Magn Reson Med Sci. 2011;10:251–4.
302. Young RH, Scully RE. Sarcomas metastatic to the ovary: a report of 21 cases. Int J Gynecol Pathol. 1990;9:231–51.
303. Zaloudek CJ, Norris HJ. Adenofibroma and adenosarcoma of the uterus: a clinicopathologic study of 35 cases. Cancer. 1981;15:354–66.
304. Zaloudek C, Hendrickson MR, Soslow RA. Mesenchymal tumors of the uterus. In: Kurman RJ, Ellenson RH, Ronnett M, editors. Blaustein's pathology of the female tract. 6th ed. New York/Dodrecht/Heidelberg/London: Springer; 2011. p. 453–527.
305. Zhai YL, Kobayashi Y, Mori A, Orii A, Nikaido T, Konishi I, Fujii S. Expression of steroid receptors, Ki-67, and p53 in uterine leiomyosarcomas. Int J Gynecol Pathol. 1999;18:20–8.
306. Zhu XQ, Shi YF, Cheng XD, Zhao CL, Wu YZ. Immunohistochemical markers in differential diagnosis of endometrial stromal sarcoma and cellular leiomyoma. Gynecol Oncol. 2004;92:71–9.
307. Zivanovic O, Sonoda Y, Diaz JP, Levine DA, Brown CL, Chi DS, Barakat RR, Abu-Rustum NR. The rate of port-site metastases after 2251 laparoscopic procedures in women with underlying malignant disease. Gynecol Oncol. 2008;111:431–7.
308. Zivanovic O, Jacks LM, Iasonos A, Leitao Jr MM, Soslow RA, Veras E, Chi DS, Abu-Rustum NR, Barakat RR, Brennan MF, Hensley ML. A nomogram to predict postresection 5-year overall survival for patients with uterine leiomyosarcoma. Cancer. 2012;118:660–9.
309. Zygmunt M, Evert M, Evert K, Köhler G. Fertilität und Schwangerschaft bei Varianten des Leiomyoms, glattmuskulären Tumoren mit unsicherem malignen Potential, stromalen Tumoren, genitalen Sarkomen, PEComen und Mischtumoren. In: Köhler G, Evert M, Evert K, Zygmunt M, editors. Sarkome des weiblichen Genitale, Bd. 2 Andere seltene Sarkome, Mischtumoren, genitale Sarkome und Schwangerschaft. Berlin/Boston: Walter de Gruyter GmbH; 2016. p. 286–327.

List of Image Sources

Amberger M et al. Röntgenpraxis Trier, Trier 13CD.

Erler MA. GMP für Pathologie Krech/Christians Osnabrück/Rheine, Rheine. 2A.

Evert M, Evert K. Universitätsmedizin Greifswald, Institut für Pathologie, Greifswald. 3A, 4A, 10B, 18AB, 19AB.

Göttsching H. Universitätsklinikum Schleswig-Holstein – Campus Lübeck, Klinik für Frauenheilkunde und Geburtshilfe, Lübeck. 12AB.

Gürtler F. Kreiskrankenhaus Wolgast, Abt. Gynäkologie u. Geburtshilfe, Wolgast. 1B.

Hegenscheid K. Universitätsmedizin Greifswald, Institut für Diagnostische Radiologie und Neuroradiologie, Greifswald. 1C, 6ABC, 17C.

Heidkamp L. Albertinen Krankenhaus Hamburg, Albertinen Frauenkliniken, Hamburg. 4 BC.

Hessler PA, Kuhfus S, Dennis K. Krankenhaus Sachsenhausen, operative Gynäkologie, Frankfurt/Main. 1F, 14AB, 20B.

Karl M. DRK Krankenhaus Kirchen, gynäkologisch-geburtshilfliche Abteilung, Kirchen. 11.

Kärner Ch, Leinen K. Gemeinschaftspraxis – Frauenärztinnen, Konz. 13B.

Klee M. St. Vincenz Krankenhaus Paderborn, Klinik für Frauenheilkunde und Geburtshilfe, Paderborn. 16A.

Köhler G, Zygmunt M. Universitätsmedizin Greifswald, Klinik Frauenheilkunde und Geburtshilfe, Greifswald. 1ADE, 3B, 7AB, 10ACD, 13A, 15ABC, 17AB, 22.

Krings W. St. Vincenz Krankenhaus Paderborn, Klinik für Diagnostische und InterventionelleRadiologie/Neuroradiologie, Paderborn. 16B.

Krentel H. St. Anna Hospital Herne, Klinik für Frauenheilkunde und Geburtshilfe, Herne. 20C.

Krystek E: St. Josefskrankenhaus Heidelberg, Gynäkologie und Geburtshilfe, Heidelberg. 2B.

Kürzl R, Hutter S. LMU München, Campus Innenstadt, Klinik und Poliklinik für Frauenheilkunde und Geburtshilfe, München. 9.

Lederer A. Abt. f. Gynäkologie, Krankenhaus der barmherzigen Brüder Salzburg, Abt. f. Gynäkologie, Salzburg. 21AB.

Quakernack J. Gynmünster -Gynvelen, operative Gynäkologie, Münster. 8AB.

Ruhwedel W. St. Vinzenz-Hospital Köln, Klinik für Gynäkologie und Geburtshilfe, Köln. 20A.

Schaffler G. Krankenhaus der barmherzigen Brüder Salzburg, Abt. f. Radiologie u. Nuklearmedizin, Salzburg. 21CDE.

Schwärzler P. Asklepios Klinik Barmbek, Gynäkologie und Geburtshilfe, Hamburg. 5AB.

Stibora M. Marienhospital Gelsenkirchen, Klinik für Gynäkologie und Geburtshilfe, Gelsenkirchen. 20D.

Widschwendter P. Rotkreuzklinikum München, Gynäkologie, München 5CD.

Uterine Morcellation

15

Courtney J. Steller and Charles E. Miller

Minimally invasive surgical techniques have been proven to lead to decreased post operative pain, decreased morbidity, and faster recovery times when compared to open abdominal procedures [1]. According to committee opinions from ACOG and the AAGL, the preferred route for hysterectomy is a minimally invasive approach, including a laparoscopic or vaginal approach when feasible [2]. Fibroids are the most common indication for a hysterectomy (40.7 %) [3] which in turn makes specimen removal difficult as the specimen size is often larger than the abdominal or vaginal incisions made during surgery. As stated by Wright et al., patients who are nulliparous or have a large uterine size are at higher risk of requiring alternate methods of specimen removal such as morcellation [4]. Morcellation is defined as "division and removal in small pieces" in the Merriam-Webster dictionary. In addition, a similar challenge arises when removing tissue in the absence of a colpotomy, as in a supracervical hysterectomy or myomectomy.

History

Dr. Kurt Semm in Kiel, Germany originally developed a solution to the problem of specimen removal when he introduced a hand held manual morcellator in 1973. This hand-activated morcellator was produced by WISAP and resulted in a procedure that was very time consuming, arduous and painful for the surgeon. In order to avoid these issues, he developed a battery driven power morcellator in 1984 which was called the S.E.M.M. (serrated-edge macro morcellator). Then, in 1991 this was replaced by a completely electrically driven power morcellator [5]. This new S.E.M.M. worked by punching out tissue cylinders up to 1.5 cm in diameter. If used together with a myoma drill, large holes could be punched into the specimen, making them easily removable [6].

Dr. Rolf A. Steiner out of Zurich, Switzerland developed the first power morcellator, which was FDA approved in 1995. Utilizing a rotating knife driven by an electric micro-engine and controlled via foot pedal, the function was, again, to cut tissue in cylinder-shaped pieces. The cutting cylinder, which was 13 mm in diameter and 25 cm long, was placed in a 14 mm trocar sleeve and protruded a few millimeters past the sleeve of the trocar into the abdomen. Outside the abdomen was a gearbox, by which the electrical micro-engine produced the turning motion. A 10 mm grasping forceps was used through the cutting cylinder to grasp the tissue and a rubber ring ensured an air-tight seal. In his paper, Steiner stated that the transmission of power was sufficient to cut almost any type of tissue. He originally performed this technique with uterine fibroids or ovaries, reporting 11 successful cases with mean specimen removal times of 6.5 min for fibroids and 4.5 min for ovaries, as compared to the "conventional technique" which he reported at 30 min [7].

Carter JE, et al. published a time and cost analysis of power vs. manual morcellation in 1997. He demonstrated that electromechanical morcellation reduced the average time for extraction of specimen <100 g by 15 min and of specimen weighing 401–500 g by 150 min. This also led to a significant cost reduction despite the more expensive nature of the electromechanical morcellators [8]. Electromechanical ("power") morcellators began to gain significant popularity and several new developments and models were created.

C.J. Steller, DO (✉)
Minimally Invasive Gynecologic Surgery, Obstetrics and Gynecology, Advocate Lutheran General Hospital, 1775 Dempster St, Park Ridge, IL 6006, USA
e-mail: Courtney.steller@gmail.com

C.E. Miller, MD, FACOG
Department of Obstetrics & Gynecology, University of Illinois at Chicago, Chicago, IL, USA

Minimally Invasive Gynecologic Surgery, Advocate Lutheran General Hospital, Park Ridge, IL, USA

The Advanced Gynecologic Surgery Institute, 120 Osler Dr, Suite 100, Naperville, IL 60540, USA

I. Alkatout, L. Mettler (eds.), *Hysterectomy*, DOI 10.1007/978-3-319-22497-8_15

Modern Morcellators

The general engineering of the modern electromechanical morcellator is similar to that described by Steiner. The ideal morcellator is easy to handle, ergonomic, maintains pneumoperitoneum, and enables constant visualization of the rotating knife with minimal operator effort [9].

The Morcellator Knife was developed in 2000. It was a classic lancet with an interchangeable blade that was inserted through at 10 mm trocar and used to cut a specimen as it was held between two forceps. A posterior culdotomy was made to remove the small pieces of the specimen [10]. The Sawalhe morcellator, developed by Karl Storz, modified the Steiner model and enabled removal morcellated tissue from the abdominal cavity via the sleeve, obviating the need for a posterior culdotomy that was necessary with the Morcellator Knife [9].

Karl Storz then developed an even more competitive morcellator in 2007 called the Rotocut G1 morcellator (Fig. 15.1). In comparison to the existing Sawalhe model in a study published in 2007, the Rotocut G1 device accomplished significantly shorter morcellation time, operative time and duration of anesthesia. It also created fewer and longer pieces of tissue due to a more effective power output and drive transmission. In this model, the generator is located in the hand piece and is activated by a foot pedal.

The Gynecare Morcellex tissue morcellator developed by Ethicon, Inc. is another popular power morcellator (Fig. 15.2). Unlike the Rotocut G1, the Gynecare Morcellex does not require a foot pedal. In 2009, a randomized controlled trial was initiated to compare the two popular models, the Gynecare Morcellex and the Rotocut G1. There was no statistical difference between the two groups in regards to operative time, morcellation time, weight of excised pieces, blood loss/blood transfusion, intra or post operative complications, post operative pain, hospitalization or time to return to full activity. The two morcellators were evaluated by the surgeon using a VAS score ranging from 0 (low handling, easy) to 10 (high handling, difficult). There was a significant difference in ease of use, with the Gynecare Morcellex having a higher handling score (average 7.0 for supracervical hysterectomy and 7.2 for myomectomy). Also noted in this study, since the Rotocut G1 morcellator is reusable, it was more cost effective in large volume hospitals where laparoscopy is performed routinely. However, in hospitals where laparoscopy is not performed routinely, the Gynecare Morcellex was more cost-effective since more than 30 laparoscopic procedures requiring morcellation are needed to reach the cost of the Rotocut G1 [11]. The Gynecare Morcellex was voluntarily withdrawn from the market by Johnson and Johnson in late July, 2014 after a statement discouraging the use of power morcellators was released by the FDA. See "Updated FDA Recommendations under Complications" for further details.

There is also a morcellator currently on the market developed by Olympus Gyrus that uses purely bipolar technology and does not have a bladed system. The device, known as the PKS PlasmaSORD (Solid Organ Removal Device), utilizes bipolar energy to morcellate the tissue instead of sharp blades (Fig. 15.3). Theoretically, this creates fewer tissue fragments. It connects to a standard bipolar generator (Fig. 15.4), requires minimal set up, is lightweight and is ergonomical. There have been reports of successful morcellation

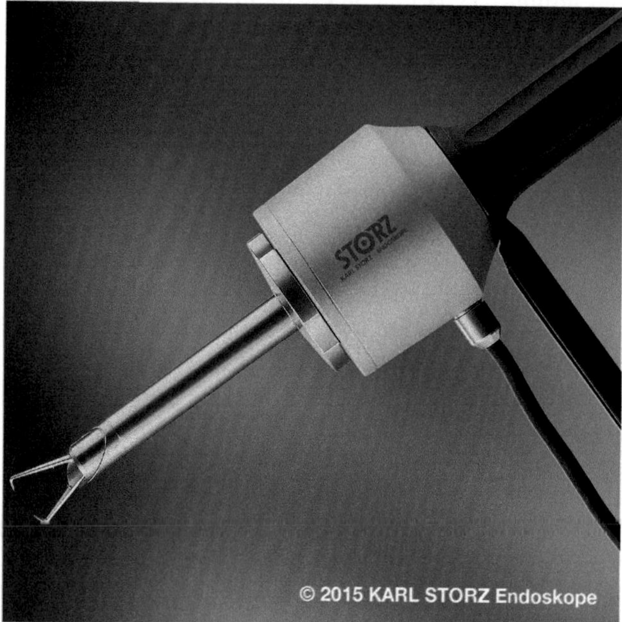

Fig. 15.1 Rotocut G1 Morcellator by Karl Storz (©2015 Photo Courtesy of KARL STORZ Endoscopy-America, Inc.)

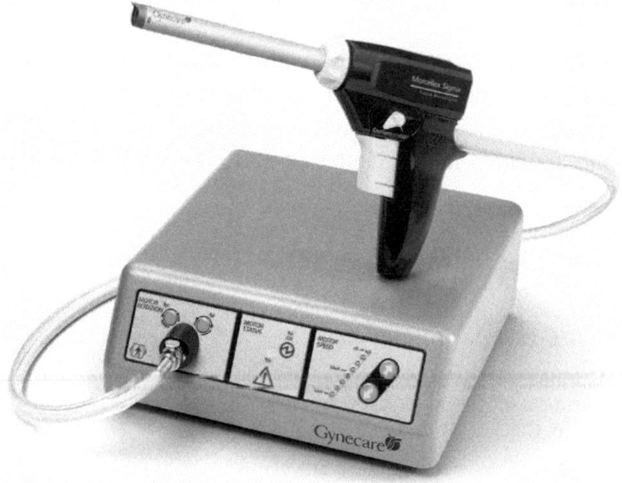

Fig. 15.2 MORCELLEX SIGMA™ Tissue Morcellator System, manufactured by Ethicon US, LLC

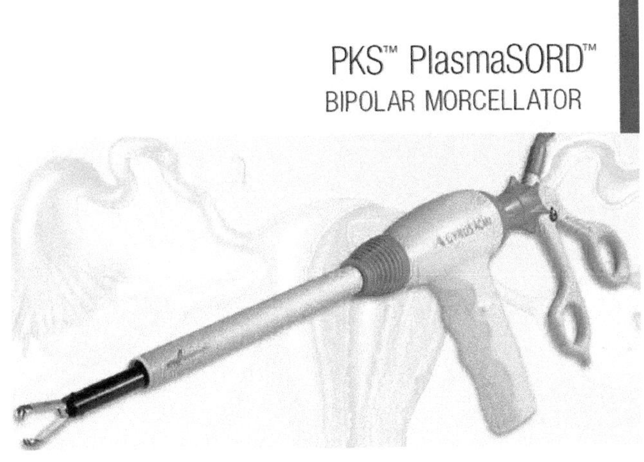

Fig. 15.3 PKS PlasmaSORD Bipolar Morcellator by Olympus

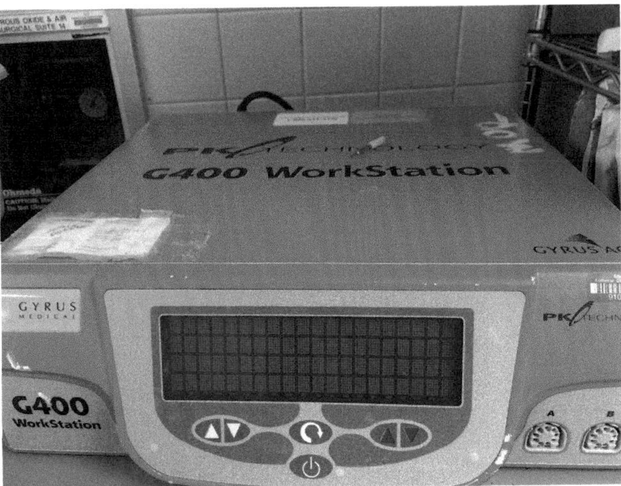

Fig. 15.4 Bipolar Generator Box used with the PKS PlasmaSORD Morcellator

Table 15.1 Types of morcellators

Date introduced	Date discontinued	Manufacturer	Make	Diameter (mm)	Blade speed (rpm)	Disposable/Reusable	Motor	Activation
Feb-00	Jul-14	Ethicon, Inc.	Gynecare X-Tract	12	125–1000	Disposable	Generator box	Foot
Jul-06	2013	Ethicon, Inc.	Gynecare Morcellex	15	125–1000	Disposable	Generator box	Hand or foot
2013	Jul-14	Ethicon, Inc.	Morcellex Sigma	15	125–1000	Disposable	Generator box	Hand
Jul-06	n/a	Karl Storz	Rotocut G1	12 or 15	0–1200	Disposable blade	Hand piece	Foot
May-08	n/a	Olympus	PKS Plasma SORD	15	n/a	Disposable	**Bipolar generator box	Foot
Jun-09	n/a	Richard Wolf	Morce Power Plus	12, 15, 20	100–1000	Reusable	Generator box	Foot
Mar-11	n/a	Blue Endo	MOREsolution	12.5, 15, 20	100–800	Reusable	Generator box	Hand or foot
Mar-11	n/a	LiNA Medical	Xcise	15	1000	Completely disposable	Hand piece, cordless	Hand

of large uteri using this device [12] but few studies have been performed comparing this bipolar technology with the standard bladed technique. Reported injuries have been related to limited visualization due to electrosurgical smoke and skin burns due to the bipolar system [13].

A comparison of these and other current models of morcellators is listed in Table 15.1.

Use

The use of most power morcellators is similar amongst manufacturers. Figure 15.5 shows the various pieces of the Storz Rotocut G1 Morcellator. The technique is historically done with the power morcellator placed in the abdominal wall. First, the largest trocar is removed from the abdominal wall. The incision is extended to the appropriate diameter, usually by dilators, under direct visualization. Once the appropriate diameter is reached, the morcellator cannula with obturator is inserted through this incision under direct visualization (Fig. 15.6). The obturator is removed and the blade is placed into the cannula (Fig. 15.7). A grasper, usually a 10 mm-diameter tenaculum or spoon, is then inserted through this cannula/blade and the tissue to be morcellated is grasped (Fig. 15.8). The cannula should contain a seal in order to maintain pneumoperitoneum. The tissue is brought up flush with the morcellator blade. Care should be taken to bring the specimen to the morcellator, not the morcellator to the specimen. The motor is then activated and the blade rotates while an upward force is exerted by the surgeon to allow the blade

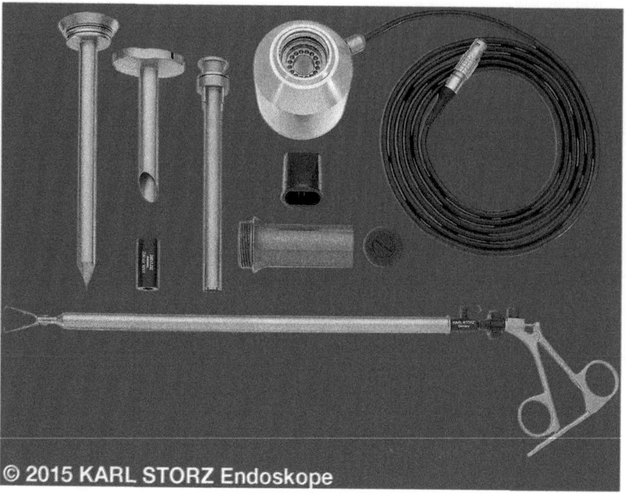

Fig. 15.5 Separate pieces of the Rotocut G1 Morcellator. Pieces include (from left to right): obturator, sleeve (12 or 15 mm), blade, motor with power cord, motor valve, blade handle, sealing cap, and tenaculum (©2015 Photo Courtesy of KARL STORZ Endoscopy-America, Inc.)

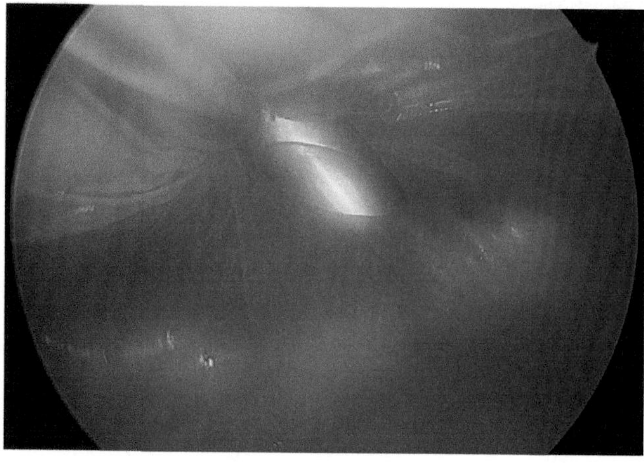

Fig. 15.6 The morcellator cannula inside the abdomen. Dilate the incision to the appropriate size prior to placement. Take care to have the long arm of the cannula bevel anterior

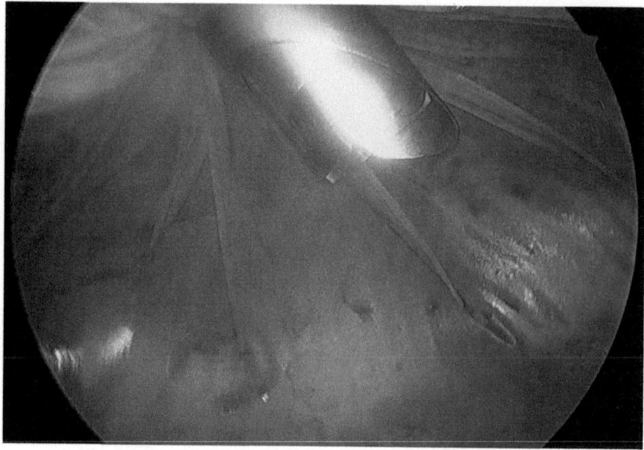

Fig. 15.7 The morcellator blade is now inserted through the cannula. Always aim towards the pelvis

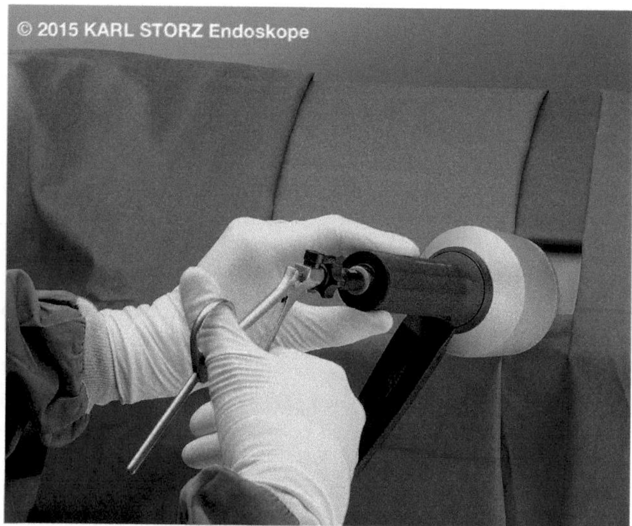

Fig. 15.8 Using the Rotocut G1 Morcellator: one hand holds the morcellator steady while the other hand uses the tenaculum to grasp the tissue. This hand then pulls the tissue against the blade, the blade is activated, and morcellation ensues (©2015 Photo Courtesy of KARL STORZ Endoscopy-America, Inc.)

to cut through the tissue. This action cuts the tissue into cylindrical strips and allows for its removal through the cannula. The long arm of the bevel of the cannula should be anterior to allow a "coring" of the tissue, like peeling an apple [14]. The blade should be pointed away from the abdominal organs toward the pelvis with the cannula close to the abdominal wall (Fig. 15.9). When the tissue breaks, the activation of the morcellator should be stopped until a new piece of tissue is grasped. This is repeated until the entire specimen is able to be removed. Visualization should be maintained throughout the entire procedure and the end of the blade should be constantly seen by the surgeon. During this process, small pieces of the tissue may be separated from the specimen and dispersed throughout the abdominal cavity (Fig. 15.10). Careful inspection of the cavity should be performed and all small pieces removed prior to terminating the morcellation procedure. Small pieces should be removed by a spoon rather than a tenaculum [14].

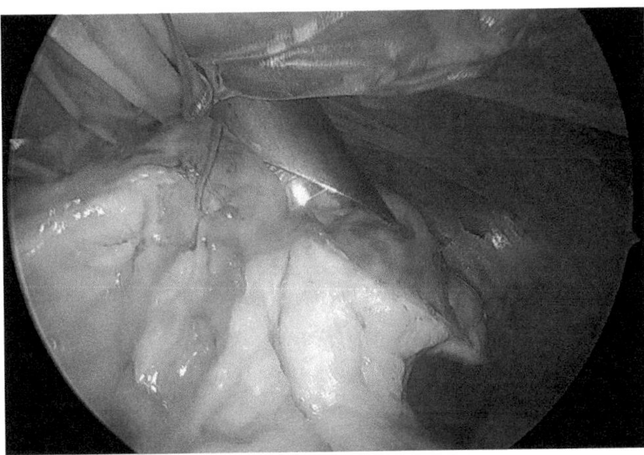

Fig. 15.9 Morcellating the specimen. Grasp specimen with a tenaculum or spoon and pull towards the morcellator until flush against morcellator. Point morcellator towards the pelvis. Pull back on the specimen while activating the blade. Use a "coring" technique to morcellate

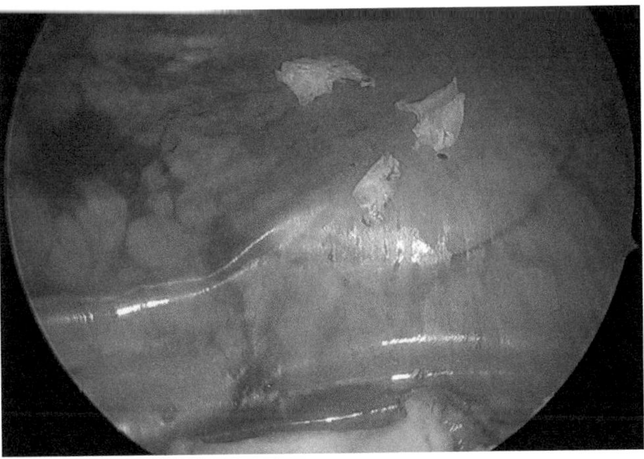

Fig. 15.10 Small fragments of tissue that may be dispersed after morcellation. Take care to remove all small pieces

Transcervical Morcellation

Morcellation has also been described using a transcervical approach after a supracervical hysterectomy. The steps are essentially the same; however, instead of extending an abdominal wall incision by dilation, the cervical canal is dilated until the morcellator cannula can be inserted. A longer cannula and blade must be used to traverse the vaginal canal. Morcellation is then completed in the same manner and the dilated cervical so may be closed using a single stitch laparoscopically. This technique allows the surgeon to avoid making a large abdominal wall incision and thus decreases the risk of future herniation. This technique was first reported in the literature by Rosenblatt et al. in 2010 [15].

At our institution, we have successfully performed transcervical morcellation after supracervical hysterectomy in several patients. We utilize the 12 mm Rotocut G1 Morcellator with the extra-long cannula. However, we have recently abandoned this method in order to routinely utilize contained in-bag morcellation which, at this time, can only be performed trans-abdominally and trans-vaginally. See "Updated FDA Recommendations under Complications" and "Contained Morcellation" for more details.

Manual Morcellation

An alternative form of morcellation can be performed by hand. This historically is performed vaginally, using a scalpel or scissors to cut a large specimen into smaller, retrievable pieces. It can also be performed abdominally through a small incision. In a study published in 2006 by Wang, et al., extraction of uterine myomas by culdotomy with hand morcellation vs. power morcellation was compared. The time for specimen removal with power morcellation was significantly less and there were no differences in myoma weight, size, number removed, blood loss or post-operative stay and no major complications occurred [16].

Complications

As morcellators have become more common place in laparoscopic surgery, morcellator-related injuries have also increased. These injuries range from direct surgical risks resulting in immediate complications to sequelae of morcellated tissue fragments and morcellation of undiagnosed malignancy resulting in more long term complications.

Immediate Complications

Immediate complications inherent in morcellation are generally caused by the sharp blade that is placed in the abdomen. Several advances have been made to decrease the incidence of these injuries, such as improved visualization of the blade due to a beveled trocar, completely covered blades and improved maintenance of pneumoperitonum. Some morcellators, such as Xcise, have different settings allowing the blade to protrude by different lengths. Despite these advances, adverse events can still occur. Milad et al. performed a systematic review using a literature search and a search of the FDA Medical Device Reporting (MDR) and Manufacturer and User Facility Device Experience (MAUDE) databases to determine the frequency of immediate morcellator injuries from 1992 to 2012 [13]. This study examined morcellation after hysterectomy, myomectomy, nephrectomy, splenectomy, and "other." He found a total of 55 complications, specifically including injuries to the small and large bowels (n = 31), vascular system (n = 27), kidney (n = 3), ureter (n = 3), bladder (n = 1) and diaphragm (n = 1). Most (66 %) of these injuries were identified intraoperatively. Six patients died of morcellator related complications. No single manufacturer was solely associated with visceral or vascular injuries. The most common contributing factor for the injuries was lack of surgeon experience (n = 16) followed by lack of visualization (n = 4) and device malfunction (n = 4). Therefore, it is imperative that surgeons planning on performing power morcellation undergo training to gain experience and understand how to use, put together, operate and troubleshoot the device they plan to use. Other tips to reduce the surgical risk of morcellator use include:

1. Use the beveled tip of the morcellator anteriorly to allow an "apple peeling" technique.
2. Make sure, prior to activating the morcellator, that only the specimen is grasped and that the specimen is away from underlying bowel which may incidentally be grasped.
3. Only morcellate when the blade tip is visible
4. Never bring the morcellator to the specimen; instead, bring the specimen to the morcellator.
5. Always ensure adequate visualization is obtained prior to morcellation.

Long-Term Complications

Long term complications of morcellation include retained or parasitic tissue, leiomyomatosis or dissemination of undiagnosed malignancy. The term "iatrogenic parasitic myoma" has been developed to describe the formation of new myomas that are not attached to the uterus presenting after uterine or myoma morcellation. This is thought to occur when fragments of myomas are left behind following morcellation and become implanted in normal tissue in the abdominal cavity. The morcellated fragments are then able to grow via neovasculariazation from the peritoneum or adjacent tissue. Although Donnez et al. estimated the incidence to be 0.57 % of subtotal hysterectomies, the true incidence of retained uterine fragments is unknown. There are several case reports and literature reviews documenting the development of iatrogenic parasitic myomas but the numbers are too low to justify any substantial conclusions or to determine the incidence. In 2010, Larrain et al. reported a series of four cases of parasitic myomas diagnosed after prior morcellation at their institution. They also reviewed the literature, revealing 14 different reported cases or series of iatrogenic parasitic myomas at that time [17]. In 2011, Cucinella et al. reviewed four cases of parasitic myomas over a three year study period, giving an incidence of 0.9 % in their institution [18]. Finally, in 2012, a review out of Scandinavia reported three cases of parasitic myomas between 2004–2011, making their reported incidence of parasitic myomas only 0.12 % [19]. These lesions are usually confined to the pelvis, especially in the paravesical, pararectal, and rectovaginal spaces [18, 20, 21] however, reports exist of parasitic myomas found in the upper abdomen, anterior abdominal wall and port sites as well [9, 22–25]. Symptoms of parasitic myomas are not specific and patients are often asymptomatic. Palpable masses have also been described, as well as pelvic pain dyspareunia and abnormal vaginal bleeding [17, 26]. Treatment is surgical removal.

Disseminated peritoneal leiomyomatosis is another condition that has been reported after morcellation of leiomyoma. It is a rare hormonally dependent condition in which multiple nodules stud the pelvic and peritoneal surfaces, often giving the appearance of metastatic ovarian or peritoneal carcinoma [27]. There are approximately 150 cases reported in the literature since the first report in 1952 [28, 29]. Complete or partial smooth muscle differentiation in the absence of cytologic atypia is seen on morphologic, immunohistochemical evaluation. It is generally a benign condition but there are rare reports of malignant transformation. Patients can be asymptomatic and therefore, the condition is often diagnosed incidentally. However, abdominopelvic pain or palpable masses, dysmenorrhea, menorrhagia and intestinal obstruction have all been reported as presenting symptoms. If suspected, surgical exploration is indicated for diagnostic and therapeutic purposes with removal of the masses. This has been successfully reported by the laparoscopic approach [30]. Recent reports of successful treatment with GnRH agonists [31] or aromatase inhibitors [32] are documented as well.

Iatrogenic endometriosis has been reported to occur after uterine morcellation, but not all of the literature is consistent. A case report by Sepilian demonstrated widespread endometriosis and symptoms of cyclic pelvic pain six months following morcellation after a supracervical hysterectomy performed for uterine fibroids with an absence of endometriosis [33]. Implants have also been reported in the abdomen, pelvis and port sites [33–35]. One proposed theory is that viable endometrial tissue can seed the pelvis and peritoneum during hysterectomy and uterine morcellation. This would lead to implantation and proliferation of this endometrial tissue, leading to endometriosis formation. Other possible causes include retrograde flow from remaining endometrial tissue in a cervical stump or the presence of endometriosis that was not visualized on initial procedure [33, 36]. However, a case control study reported by Schuster et al. showed no difference (p = 0.998, n = 464) in new-onset endometriosis in patients after hysterectomy with morcellation compared to hysterectomy without morcellation [36]. Therefore, despite some case reports, uterine morcellation does not seem to increase the risk of a subsequent diagnosis of endometriosis.

In a systematic review analyzing 66 patients between 1990 and 2014 who underwent reoperation after morcellation during laparoscopic hysterectomy or myomectomy, the most common reason for reoperation was parasitic leiomyomata (33.3 %). The majority of the reoperations were due to new clinical symptoms, 60 % in the myomectomy group and 60 % in the hysterectomy group. The remaining reoperations were performed due to unsuspected malignancy, and the majority of these malignancies were leiomyosarcomas (24 %) [37].

Disseminated Malignancy

The biggest concern in regards to dissemination of tissue during morcellation is the inadvertent dissemination of malignancy.

Endometrial Adenocarcinoma

Morcellation of endometrial adenocarcinoma can cause cancerous tissue to be spread throughout the abdomen and lead to possible upstaging of an existing malignancy. Morcellation of endometrial adenocarcinoma can usually be avoided by appropriate pre-operative evaluation with endometrial biopsy or dilation and curettage; however, this is not always accurate. In symptomatic patients with confirmed endometrial malignancies, cancer detection rates are as high as 95 % with office based endometrial biopsy. However, in women undergoing hysterectomy without these symptoms, office sampling is much less effective [38]. In addition, curettage may be preferred over biopsy for endometrial sampling in certain situations. Studies have shown a discrepancy of 10–16 % in histologic diagnosis with endometrial biopsy or curettage when compared to hysterectomy [39]. A recent study out of Europe showed a concordance rate of only 62 % and 67 % of endometrial biopsy and curettage (respectively) when compared to hysterectomy [40].

Although the exact guidelines vary by source, it is always necessary to undergo appropriate preoperative evaluation. In patients with abnormal uterine bleeding, endometrial evaluation with ultrasound and endometrial biopsy should always be performed. If the endometrial lining is thickened, sonohysterogram should be considered to evaluate for polyps or intracavitary fibroids. Abnormally thickened endometrium is defined as thickness > 4 mm in post-menopausal women or >5 mm on days 3–5 of the menstrual cycle of a pre-menopausal women. If, after sonohysterogram and biopsy, there is no evidence of intracavatary pathology and the biopsy is negative, uterine curettage may be warranted. In patients without abnormal uterine bleeding, ultrasound should still be performed for operative planning. Although there are no strict guidelines, it may be beneficial to proceed with endometrial sampling for abnormally thickened endometrium in these patients as well, especially when morcellation is anticipated. In our practice, we perform a routine hysterosonogram and endometrial biopsy prior to any case that may undergo uterine or fibroid morcellation regardless of their presenting symptoms.

Yet, even with appropriate pre-operative evaluation, an endometrial cancer can remain undetected and inadvertent morcellation and dissemination of malignancy can, rarely, occur. In a study evaluating 708 women undergoing hysterectomy for pelvic organ prolapse (i.e. benign disease), five patients had pathologic diagnosis of endometrial cancer (0.6 %) and 4/5 of these cases had normal preoperative screening [41]. Finally, a case report out of Duke University Medical Center in 2013 describes a case where laparoscopic hysterectomy was performed with morcellation after an endometrial curettage with frozen section was negative for malignancy. The morcellated specimen was evaluated by pathology and was also found to be negative for malignancy. Fourteen months later, the patient had left lower quadrant pain and a persistent cough and was found to have evidence of metastatic disease on PET-CT. Biopsy showed grade three endometrioid adenocarcinoma. The differential included unrecognized malignancy at the time of initial hysterectomy or malignant transformation of retained endometrial tissue or endometriosis after morcellation [42]. Despite these anecdotal examples, it is imperative to undergo strict and standardized pre-operative evaluation with all patients, especially when uterine morcellation is planned.

Other Tumors

Case reports of rare undiagnosed tumors that were morcellated have been reported as well. Upstaging of these tumors is possible, but due to low number, no incidence can be determined. In a case series out of the University of Pennsylvania, a series of 101 patients undergoing laparoscopic hysterectomy with morcellation was reviewed. In this series, one case was noted to have an atypical trophoblastic nodule with necrosis and myometrial infiltration, suspected to represent epithelioid trophoblastic tumor [43]. A case reported out of Drexel University revealed morcellation of a low-grade endometrial stromal sarcoma after laparoscopic supracervical hysterectomy for abnormal uterine bleeding. This patient had a benign pre-operative dilation and curettage. She was transferred to a gynecologic oncologist who performed a laparotomy, bilateral salpingo-oophorectomy and removal of the cervical stump as well as debulking of extensive sarcoma throughout the pelvis that was not seen on initial laparoscopy. The authors concluded that morcellation of the tissue likely accelerated the spread of the disease [44]. It must be recognized that these are anecdotal cases. While in discussion with patients, the risks must be noted but it should be recognized that the likelihood of morcellation of these tumors is rare, especially if age stratification is recognized and the patient is properly evaluated.

Leiomyosarcoma

Of greatest concern is the inadvertent morcellation of a leiomyosarcoma. Leiomyosarcoma is the most common malignant nonepithelial tumor of the uterus [45] representing 1–2 % of all uterine malignancies [46]. It is an aggressive malignancy with 5-year survival rate of 18.8–65 %. It typically affects women in the perimenopausal years with a median age of 52 years and is very rare in women below the age of 40. Leiomyosarcoma presents as a solitary, fleshy and necrotic intramural tumor [47] in patients noting uterine enlargement, pain, a sensation of pressure, abnormal uterine bleeding or a lower abdominal mass. The classic sign of this malignancy is a rapidly growing uterus; however, because it is uncommon, only 0.23 % of patients with this finding will have leiomyosarcoma [48]. Preoperative diagnosis is challenging because the symptoms and the clinical appearance associated with leiomyosarcoma are nearly identical to benign leiomyoma. MRI with diffusion-weighted imaging and PET/CT with F-FDG have both been evaluated in the pre-operative diagnosis of leiomyosarcoma [49, 50]; however, neither has been sufficiently proven to offer accurate diagnosis. Utilizing serum lactate dehydrogenase (LDH) and its isoenzymes, especially isozyme type 3, has also been utilized to distinguish leiomyosarcoma from benign leiomyoma and is a promising technique. The correlation was first seen in a series of 1886 patients who underwent hysterectomy for uterine myomas, 7 of which were found to have leiomyosarcoma. Three of these 7 patients had an elevated LDH and these 3 patients had tumors with worse prognostic factors [51]. In a follow up study evaluating 10 patients with leiomyosarcoma and 130 patients with degenerated leiomyoma, all patients with leiomyosarcoma had elevated total LDH and LDH isozyme type 3. When LDH was combined with MRI, the specificity, positive predictive value and negative predictive value were all 100 % in this particular study [52].

Despite these findings, there is no formal recommendation to use specific labs or imaging to pre-operatively diagnose leiomyosarcoma. At this time the only way to accurately distinguish a leiomyosarcoma from a benign leiomyoma is through histologic evaluation with leiomyosarcomas revealing coagulative tumor cell necrosis, moderate to severe cytologic atypia and numerous mitotic figures [47]. However, in our practice we will utilize serum LDH and/or MRI based on individual patient findings. We do not obtain them on all patients with fibroids; however, if a patient is at an increased risk for a leiomyosarcoma, we may consider using these diagnostic modalities. High risk patients include perimenopausal patients with any sized fibroid, a fibroid that is rapidly growing or has been present for an unknown amount of time, or a fibroid that looks suspicious on ultrasonography. Of note, in the few patients in our practice that had elevated LDH and LDH3 levels pre-operatively, the final pathology was benign.

An updated series on uterine leiomyosarcomas was published in 2013. In 198 patients with leiomyosarcomas over 10 years the presenting symptoms varied. Eight percent were incidental, 29 % of patients had menorrhagia or abnormal uterine bleeding, 25 % had pelvic pain, 17 % had postmenopausal bleeding, 19 % had abdominal fullness and 4 % had an unknown presenting symptom. Of the patients who had preoperative endometrial sampling, only 46 % were suggestive of leiomyosarcoma. The mean tumor size was 10 cm. The median disease free survival and median overall survival for women with stage 1 were 37 and 75 months, stage 2 were 23 and 66 months, stage 3 were 10 and 34 months and stage 4 were 3 and 20 months respectively [46].

There are currently nine studies in the literature on unsuspected leiomyosarcomas in patients who had a hysterectomy or myomectomy for presumed benign disease [52]. The rate of leiomyosarcoma in these studies ranges from 0 to 0.49 % with the average being 0.18 % [53]. The FDA recently released a statement quoting the incidence to be 1 per 350 or 0.29 % [54]. This incidence has been challenged by Elizabeth Pritts, et al. at the FDA meeting. Her more extensive evaluation of the literature was correlated to a much lower risk of leiomyosarcoma.

Morcellating these unsuspected malignancies can result in upstaging and a worse prognosis [55, 56]. In a comparison of 56 patients with LMS, 25 with and 31 without morcellation, tumor morcellation was significantly associated with poorer disease free survival ($p = 0.043$), higher stage (I vs. II, $p = 0.037$) and poorer overall survival (0.040). It was also found that the percentage of patients with abdominopelvic dissemination was significantly greater in patients with tumor morcellation (44 % vs. 12.9 %) [55]. Of course, one must always question whether the patients were originally staged adequately. In a review out of Sloan Kettering, four patients who underwent completion operations after laparoscopic morcellation of an unknown malignancy were evaluated. One patient had uterine endometrioid cancer and three had uterine leiomyosarcomas. Two of the three leiomyosarcoma patients were upstaged from stage one to stage three. The patient with uterine endometrioid cancer with stage 1B disease was not upstaged at reoperation [56]. Another retrospective study of 58 patients, 19 of whom underwent morcellation, showed a significant increase in the risk of abdominal/pelvic recurrences and shorter median recurrence-free survival in patients with unsuspected leiomyosarcomas who underwent intraperitoneal morcellation [57]. Oduyebo et al. reviewed 21 patients with the diagnosis of leiomyosarcoma or uterine smooth muscle tumors of uncertain malignant potential (STUMP) after morcellation. Twelve of these patients had re-exploration surgery and 28.5 % of the leiomyosarcoma patients and 25 % of the STUMP patients had findings of disseminated intraperitoneal disease [58]. Yet, despite these reports, this data is still limited and controversial. In a systematic review of six studies, data seemed to be highly biased and of poor quality, resulting in the author's conclusion that there is no reliable evidence that morcellation significantly results in tumor upstaging or in poorer patient outcome. There is also no evidence from these studies that power morcellation affects patient outcomes differently than any other type of morcellation, or even simple myomectomy [59]. Finally, in a decision-tree analysis using base-case estimates, a lower overall mortality rate is seen with laparoscopic hysterectomy with morcellation versus abdominal hysterectomy for the treatment of presumed fibroid uterus in premenopausal women. Although there were more deaths from leiomyosarcoma after laparoscopic hysterectomy, there were more hysterectomy-related deaths with abdominal hysterectomy as well as higher rates of transfusion, infection, thromboembolism and hernia [60].

Updated FDA Recommendations

Due to these controversial findings and reports, the FDA put out a statement discouraging the use of power morcellators, citing safety concerns, mostly the inadvertent dissemination for occult uterine cancer in patients undergoing hysterectomy and myomectomy for presumed leiomyomata. They state that morcellation is contraindicated in peri- or postmenopausal women or in anyone where an alternative form of specimen removal can be performed [54]. According to the SGO, morcellation is contraindicated in the presence of a documented or highly suspected malignancy and may be inadvisable in premalignant conditions or risk-reducing surgery. They quote other options to intracorporeal morcellation including removing the uterus through a mini-laparotomy or morcellating the uterus inside a laparoscopic bag [61]. The AAGL states that when comparing the risks involved in open hysterectomy versus those of power morcellation, gynecologists should improve but not abandon power morcellation, and that power morcellation with appropriate informed consent should remain available to appropriately screened, low risk women [62].

Contained Morcellation

Due to these recent reports, the method of morcellating in a laparoscopic specimen retrieval bag has been proposed. Cohen et al. released a feasibility study in September 2014 reporting 73 successful cases of morcellation of uteri or myomas with and insufflated bag. There were no complications in this report and no visual evidence of tissue dissemination outside of the isolation bag. The bag used in this case was developed by one of the authors specifically for this use [63].

At our institution, we have performed contained in-bag morcellation since May 2014. We use the EcoSac230 bag made by Espiner (Fig. 15.11). Our standard technique is as follows: the bag is inserted through the umbilical port (Fig. 15.12) and the specimen placed inside (Fig. 15.13). The cinched bag edge is pulled out through a 15 mm umbilical incision (Fig. 15.14) and a 12–15 mm trocar is replaced into the bag through the pulled-up bag edge (Fig. 15.15). The bag is insufflated to 25 mmHg allowing a bladed lateral trocar to be placed through the bag (Fig. 15.17). Ideally, this trocar should have balloon on the end, which is then inflated and pulled against the abdominal wall to prevent leakage of insufflation or tissue (Fig. 15.16). The 5 mm laparoscope is used through the lateral port for visualization. The umbilical trocar is removed and the morcellator is placed through this incision into the bag under direct visualization (Fig. 15.18).

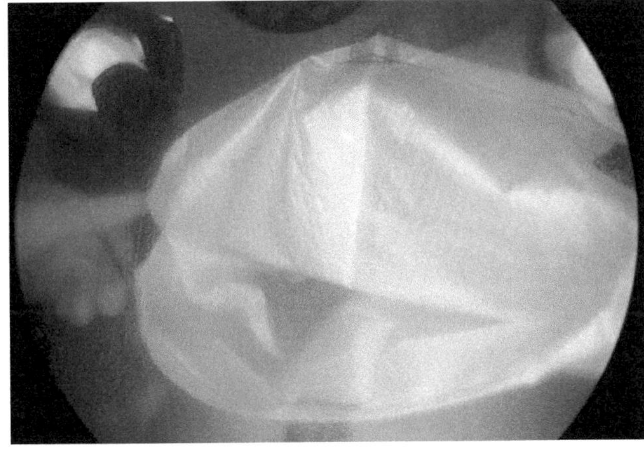

Fig. 15.11 The Espiner EcoSac230 bag

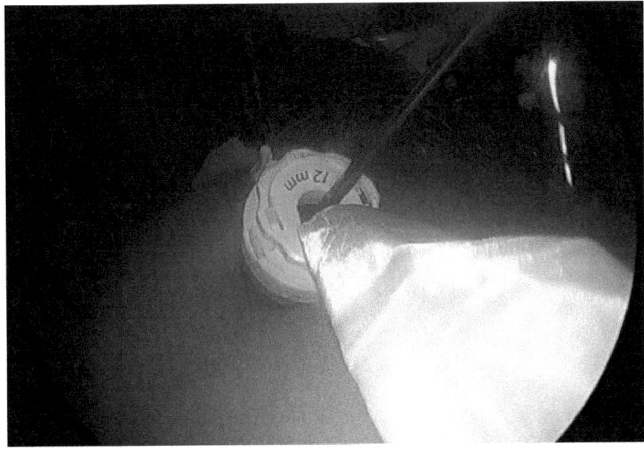

Fig. 15.12 Inserting the Espiner EcoSac 230 bag through the umbilical port

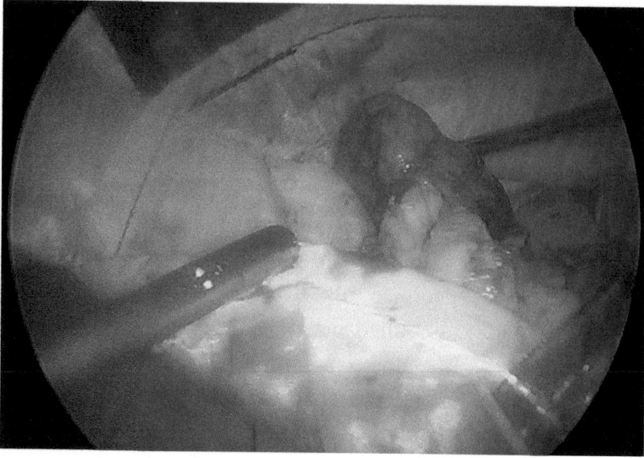

Fig. 15.13 Specimen placed inside Espiner EcoSac230 bag. The bag is ultimately cinched closed and pulled up through the umbilical incision

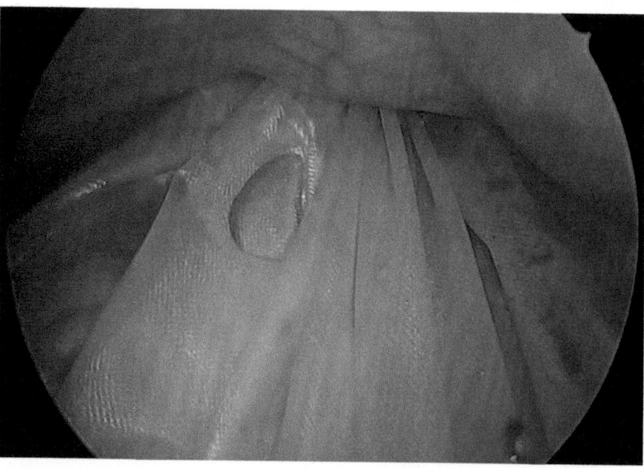

Fig. 15.14 The bag is cinched closed and pulled up through the umbilical incision

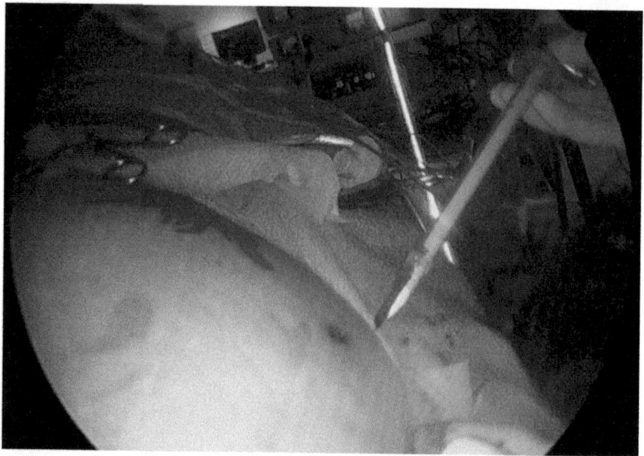

Fig. 15.16 A lateral trocar is placed inside EcoSac230 bag after bag is insufflated to 25 mmHg. This trocar should be bladed to allow adequate puncture of the bag. This is inserted under direct visualization through the umbilical trocar prior to placement of the morcellator

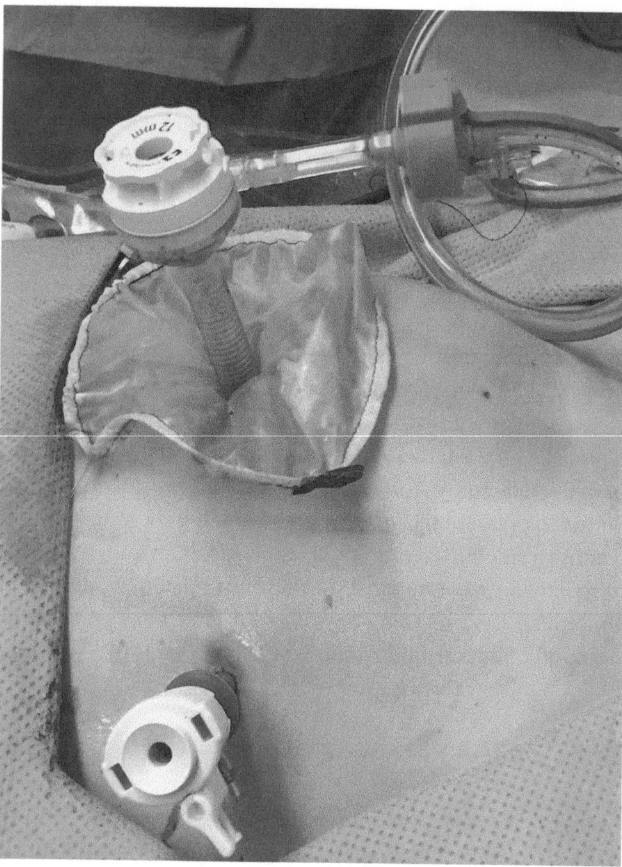

Fig. 15.15 The umbilical trocar is replaced into the bag through the pulled-up bag edge. Insufflation is then attached to this trocar and the bag is insufflated to 15 mmHg

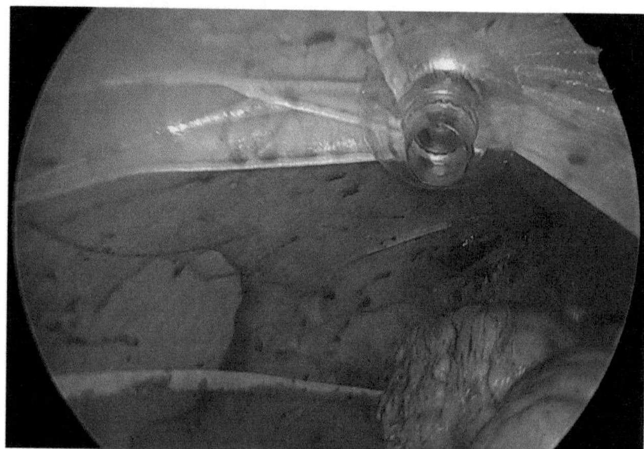

Fig. 15.17 The lateral trocar seen through the bag. The balloon on the end of the lateral trocar is inflated and pulled against the abdominal wall to prevent leakage. This trocar is now used for the laparoscope

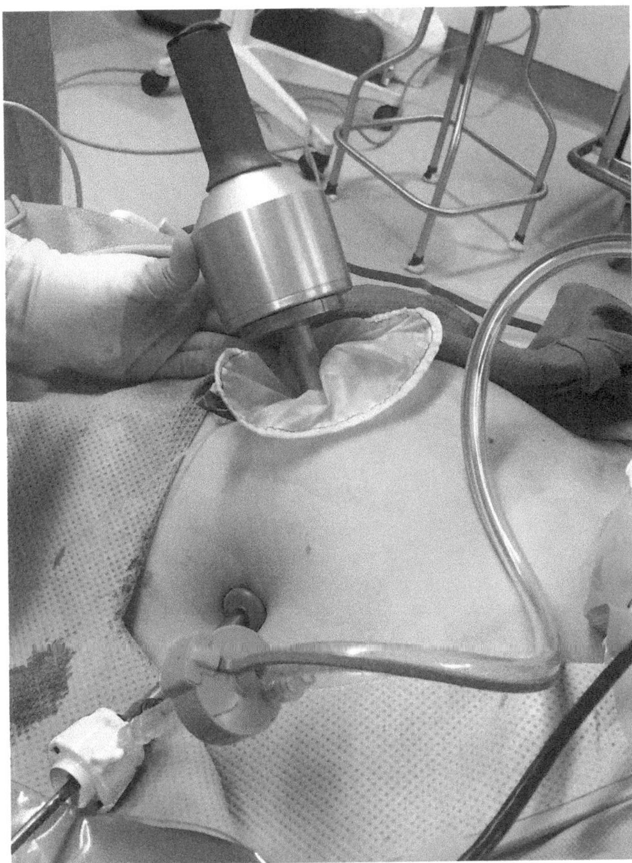

Fig. 15.18 The umbilical trocar is removed and replaced with the morcellator. The morcellator is placed through the umbilical incision into the bag. This is done under direct visualization using the laparoscope in the lateral port

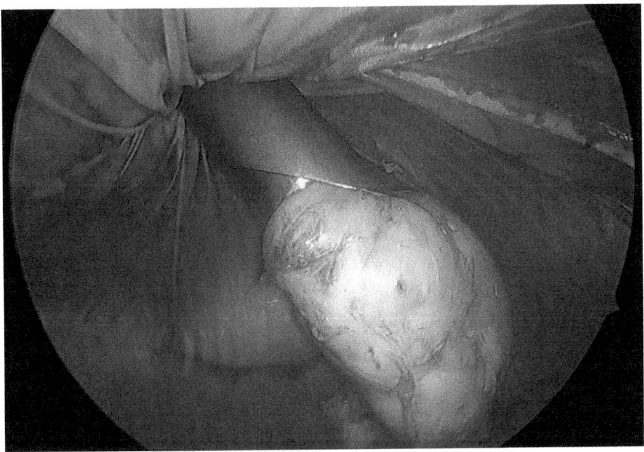

Fig. 15.19 Morcellation occurring with the Storz Rotocut G1 Morcellator. The 5 mm laparoscope is utilized for visualization from the lateral trocar

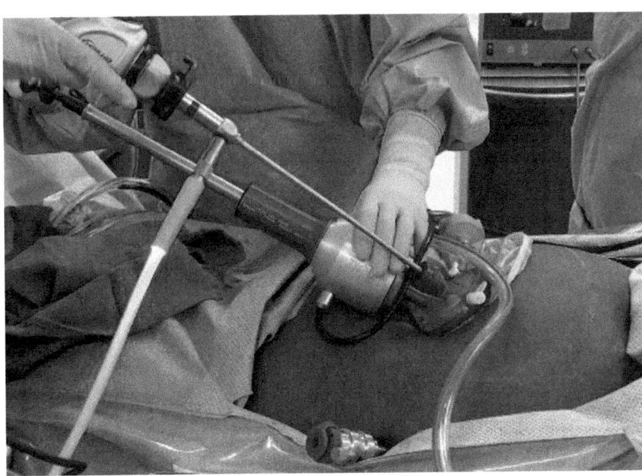

Fig. 15.20 Abdominal set-up of the GelPOINT Mini Advanced Access Platform with the 5 mm laparoscope and the Storz Rotocut G1 Morcellator

Morcellation is then performed through the umbilical incision (Fig. 15.19). We have successfully used this technique in over 90 patients, 27 % of which have been hysterectomies. Our average specimen weight was 288 g, with the largest specimen weighing 2134 g, proving the efficacy of this technique even with larger specimen.

In order to avoid puncturing the bag with a lateral trocar, we have developed another technique of contained in-bag morcellation utilizing the GelPOINT Mini Advanced Access Platform made by Applied Medical. This technique allows the EcoSac230 bag and the laparoscope to both be inserted through the GelPOINT platform simultaneously. It necessitates a slightly larger umbilical incision of 25 mm to allow insertion of the Platform, but prevents the creation of an extra hole in the bag for laparoscopic visualization (Fig. 15.20).

Other institutions are using previously manufactured specimen retrieval bags with insufflation for morcellation under direct visualization. Many studies regarding this new method of morcellation are currently in progress across the country. There are also new specimen bags being developed specifically for this purpose which are under investigation. No FDA approval on the use of specimen retrieval bags for morcellation has been obtained at this point.

Patient Counseling/Informed Consent

When considering morcellation in conjunction with hysterectomy, it is prudent to provide adequate patient counseling. The discussion with the patient should be open, honest and all questions should be answered. The technique of morcellation should be described as well as the reason for performing morcellation. It is important to discuss the risk of underlying malignancy tailored to the individual patient. In appropriate patients, the reasoning behind pre-operative evaluation can be reviewed. It is imperative to include the risk of leiomyosarcoma in this discussion. It should be noted that the precise incidence of this malignancy is unknown but a risk estimate of 1/350 is quoted by the FDA [54]. The aggressive nature of the tumor as well as the possibility of upstaging due to morcellation leading to a worse prognosis should be reviewed. It may also be beneficial to discuss the recent decision-tree analysis concluding that there are fewer predicted overall deaths with laparoscopic hysterectomy with morcellation compared with abdominal hysterectomy [60]. The possibility of dissemination of benign tissue to should be included in the discussion as well. Once this discussion is complete, any methods to avoid complications involving uterine malignancy should be reviewed. This includes the possibility of morcellation in a bag. The patient should be aware that there is no literature proving the efficacy of contained morcellation at this time, but there are many studies in progress. If vaginal morcellation is feasible, this can be offered to the patient as well. The patient should also be offered an alternative to morcellation, which would be to create a mini-laparotomy, laparotomy or colpotomy to remove the specimen. The size the incision can vary based on the size of the specimen. With any larger incision, the patient should be aware that her recovery time will be longer, pain will be greater, and she will have a higher risk of infection and other morbidities. Once this discussion is complete, specific consent forms allowing for uterine morcellation should be reviewed and signed with the patient [64].

Conclusion and Recommendations

In conclusion, morcellation is an effective way of removing a large specimen via a minimally invasive approach. Manual morcellation can be performed vaginally, through a culdotomy or abdominally but is often time consuming and laborious for the surgeon. Power morcellation may improve surgeon ergonomics and spare time; however, it has controversial complications. Proper visualization of the blade and surrounding tissues should be employed at all times. Care should be taken to remove all morcellated fragments from the abdomen. When possible, the use of a laparoscopic bag may be beneficial during power morcellation to avoid dissemination of tissue. Other techniques to reduce complications include handing the tissue to the tenaculum as opposed to reaching with the tenaculum, using an atraumatic "spoon" forceps when retrieving small fragments, keeping the longer portion of the beveled sleeve more anterior and being sure to consistently maintain sufficient pneumoperitoneum [13]. Appropriate pre-operative work up is essential when planning on potential morcellation in order to exclude pre-existing uterine malignancy. If malignancy is found incidentally after morcellation, the patient should be immediately referred to a gynecologic oncologist [52]. Finally, patient counseling and education is prudent when planning on utilizing the benefits of morcellation. Informed consent should always be addressed and any patient concerns or questions should be attended to in detail. Most importantly, surgeons should always have proper training and sufficient surgical experience prior to entering a case with the potential need for power morcellation.

References

1. Nieboer TE, Johnson N, Lethaby A, Tavender E, Curr E, Garry R, et al. Surgical approach to hysterectomy for benign gynaecological disease. Cochrane Database Syst Rev. 2009;3:CD003677.
2. American College of Obstetrics and Gynecology. Choosing the route of hysterectomy for benign disease. ACOG Committee Opinion Number 444, Nov 2009.
3. Whiteman MK, Hillis SD, Jamieson DJ, et al. Inpatient hysterectomy surveillance in the United States, 2000–2004. Am J Obstet Gynecol. 2008;198:34.e1–7.
4. Wright JD, Herzog TJ, Tsui J, et al. Nationwide trends in the performance of inpatient hysterectomy in the United States. Obstet Gynecol. 2013;122(2 pt 1):233–41.
5. Mettler, Liselotte. Letter to the author. 14 May 2015 TS.
6. Semm K. Morcellement and suturing using pelviscopy: not a problem any more [in German]. Geburtshilfe Frauenheilkd. 1991;51:843–6.
7. Steiner RA, Wight E, Tadir Y, Haller U. Electrical cutting device for laparoscopic removal of tissue from the abdominal cavity. Obstet Gynecol. 1993;81:471–4.
8. Carter JE, McCarus SD. Laparoscopic myomectomy. time and cost analysis of power vs. manual morcellation. J Reprod Med. 1997;42:383–8.
9. Brucker S, Solomayer E, Zubke W, et al. A newly developed morcellator creates a new dimension in minimally invasive surgery. J Minim Invasive Gynecol. 2007;14:233–9.
10. De Grandi P, Chardonnens E, Gerber S. The morcellator knife: a new laparoscopic instrument for supracervical hysterectomy and morcellation. Obstet Gynecol. 2000;95(5):777–8.
11. Zullo F, Falbo A, Iuliano A, et al. Randomized controlled study comparing the Gynecare Morcellex and Rotocut G1 tissue morcellators. J Minim Invasive Gynecol. 2010;17(2):192–9.
12. Walid MS, Heaton RL. A large fibroid uterus removed with a bipolar morcellator. Proc Obstet Gynecol. 2011;1(3):11.
13. Milad MP, Milad EA. Laparoscopic morcellator-related complications. J Minim Invasive Gynecol. 2014;21:486–91.
14. Streicher L. A gynecologist's guide to laparoscopic morcellation. Female Patient. 2010;35:26–35.
15. Rosenblatt PL, Makai G, DiSciullo AJ. Laparoscopic supracervical hysterectomy with transcervical morcellation. J Minim Invasive Gynecol. 2010;17:331–6.
16. Wang CJ, Yuen LT, Lee CL, Kay N, Soong YK. A prospective comparison of morcellator and culdotomy for extracting of uterine myomas laparoscopically in nullipara. J Minim Invasive Gynecol. 2006;13(5):463–6.
17. Larrain D, Rabischong B, Khoo CK, et al. "Iatrogenic" parasitic myomas: unusual late complication of laparoscopic morcellation procedures. J Minim Invasive Gynecol. 2010;17(6):719–24.
18. Cucinella G, Granese R, Calagna G, Somigliana E, Perino A. Parasitic myomas after laparoscopic surgery: an emerging

complication in the use of morcellator? Description of four cases. Fertil Steril. 2011;96:e90–6.
19. Leren V, Langebrekke A, Qvigstad E. Parasitic leiomyomas after laparoscopic surgery with morcellation. Acta Obstet Gynecol Scand. 2012;91:1233–6.
20. Donnez O, Squifflet J, Leconte I, Jadoul P, Donnez J. Posthysterectomy pelvic adenomyotic masses observed in 8 cases out of a series of 1405 laparoscopic subtotal hysterectomies. J Minim Invasive Gynecol. 2007;14(2):156–60.
21. Kho KA, Nezhat C. Parasitic myomas. Obstet Gyencol. 2009;114:611–5.
22. Moon HS, Koo JS, Park SH, et al. Parasitic leiomyoma in the abdominal wall after laparoscopic myomectomy. Fertil Steril. 2008;90:e1–2.
23. Hutchins Jr FL, Reinoehl EM. Retained myoma after laparoscopic supracervical hysterectomy with morcellation. J Am Assoc Gynecol Laparosc. 1998;5:293–5.
24. Paul PG, Koshy AK. Multiple peritoneal parasitic myomas after laparoscopic myomectomy and morcellation. Fertil Steril. 2006;85:492–3.
25. Ostrzenski A. Uterine leiomyoma particle growing in an abdominal wall incision after laparoscopic retrieval. Obstet Gynecol. 1997;89:853–4.
26. Takeda A, Mori M, Sakai K, et al. Parasitic peritoneal leiomyomatosis diagnosed 6 years after laparoscopic myomectomy with electric tissue morcellation: report of a case and review of the literature. J Minim Invasive Gynecol. 2007;14(6):770–5.
27. Hardman 3rd WJ, Majmudar B. Leiomyomatosis peritonealis disseminate: clinicopathologic analysis of five cases. South Med J. 1996;89(3):291–4.
28. Bisceglia M, Galliani C, Pizzolitto S, et al. Selected case from the Arkadi M. Rywlin International Pathology Slide Series: Leiomyomatosis peritonealis disseminata: report of 3 cases with extensive review of the literature. Adv Anat Pathol. 2014;21(3):201–15.
29. Al-Talib A, Tulandi T. Pathophysiology and possible iatrogenic cause of leiomyomatosis peritonealis disseminate. Gynecol Obstet Invest. 2010;69(4):239–44.
30. Takeda A, Mori M, Sakai K. Parasitic peritoneal leiomyomatosis diagnosed 6 years after laparoscopic myomectomy with electric tissue morcellation: report of a case and review of the literature. J Minim Invasive Gynecol. 2007;14:770–5.
31. Hales HA, Peterson CM, Jones KP, et al. Leiomyomatosis peritonealis disseminate treated with a gonadotropin-releasing hormone agonist. a case report. Am J Obstet Gynecol. 1992;167:515–6.
32. Takeda T, Masuhara K, Kamiura S. Successful management of a leiomyomatosis peritonealis disseminate with an aromatase inhibitor. Obstet Gynecol. 2008;112(2 pt2):491–3.
33. Sepilian V, Della BC. Iatrogenic endometriosis caused by uterine morcellation during a supracervical hysterectomy. Obstet Gynecol. 2003;102:1125–7.
34. Brown RL. Iatrogenic endometriosis caused by uterine morcellation during a supracervical hysterectomy. Obstet Gynecol. 2004;103:583. , author reply 583–84.
35. Decenzo JA. Iatrogenic endometriosis caused by uterine morcellation during a supracervical hysterectomy. Obstet Gynecol. 2004;103:583.
36. Schuster MW, Wheller TL, Richter HE. Endometriosis after laparoscopic supracervical hysterectomy with uterine morcellation: a case control study. J Minim Invasive Gynecol. 2012;19(2):183–7.
37. Pereira N, Buchanan T, Wishall K, et al. Electric morcellation-related reoperations after laparoscopic myomectomy and nonmyomectomy procedures. J Minim Invasive Gynecol. 2014;S1553-4650(14):01292–8.
38. American Association of Gynecologic Laparoscopists. AAGL practice report: Morcellation during uterine tissue extraction. J Minim Invasive Gynecol. 2014;21(4):517–30.
39. Katz VL, Lentz GM, Lobo RA, Gershenson DM. Comprehensive gynecology. 5th ed. Philadelphia: Mosby; 2007.
40. Gungorduk K, Asicioglu O, Ertas IE, et al. Comparison of the histopathological diagnoses of preoperative dilation and curettage and Pipelle biopsy. Eur J Gynaecol Oncol. 2014;35(5):539–43.
41. Ramm O, Gleason JL, Segal S, Antosh DD, Kenton KS. Utility of preoperative endometrial assessment in asymptomatic women undergoing hysterectomy for pelvic floor dysfunction. In Urogynecol J. 2012;23(7):913–7.
42. Turner T, Secord AA, Lowery WJ, Sfakianos G, Lee PS. Metastatic adenocarcinoma after laparoscopic supracervical hysterectomy with morcellation: a case report. Gynecol Oncol Case Rep. 2013;5:19–21.
43. Hagemann IS, Hagemann AR, LiVolsi VA, Montone KT, Chu CS. Risk of occult malignancy in morcellated hysterectomy: a case series. Int J Gynecol Pathol. 2011;30:476–83.
44. Della Badia C, Karini H. Endometrial stromal sarcoma diagnosed after uterine morcellation in laparoscopic supracervical hysterectomy. J Minim Invasive Gynecol. 2010;17:791–3.
45. Silverberg SG. Leiomyosarcoma of the uterus. a clinicopathologic study. Obstet Gynecol. 1971 Oct;38(4):613–28.
46. Rauh-Hain JA, Oduyebo T, Diver E, et al. Uterine Leiomyosarcoma: an updated series. Int J Gyencol Cancer. 2013;23(6):1036–43.
47. Berek JS, Hacker NF. Gynecologic oncology. 5th ed. Philadelphia: Lippincott Williams & Wilkens; 2010.
48. Rose PG. Cancer of the uterine corpus. Precis: an update in obstetrics and gynecology. Oncology. 3rd ed. Washington, DC: The American College of Obstetricians and Gynecologists; 2008.
49. Sato K, Yuasa N, Fujita M, et al. Clinical application of diffusion-weighted imaging for preoperative differentiation between uterine leiomyoma and leiomyosarcoma. Am J Obstet Gynecol. 2014;210(4):368.e1–8.
50. Kitajima K, Murakami K, Kaji Y, et al. Spectrum of FDG PET/CT findings of uterine tumors. AJR Am J Roentgenol. 2010;195(30):737–43.
51. Seki K, Hoshihara T, Nagata I. Leiomyosarcoma of the uterus: ultrasonography and serum lactate dehydrogenase level. Gynecol Obstet Invest. 1992;33:114–8.
52. Goto A, Takeuchi S, Sugimura K, Maruo T. Usefulness of Gd-DTPA contrast-enhanced dynamic MRI and serus determination of LDH and its isozymes in the differential diagnosis of leiomyosarcoma from degenerated leiomyoma of the uterus. Int J Gynecol Cancer. 2002;12(4):354–61.
53. Stine JE, Clarke-Pearson DL, Gehrig PA. Uterine morcellation at the time of hysterectomy: techniques, risks, and recommendations. Obstet and Gynecol Surv. 2014;69(7):415–25.
54. US Food and Drug Administration. Laparoscopic uterine power morcellation in hysterectomy and myomectomy: FDA safety communication. Nov 2014.
55. Park JY, Park SK, Kim DY, Kim JH, Kim YM, Kim YT, et al. The impact of tumor morcellation during surgery on the prognosis of patients with apparently early uterine leiomyosarcoma. Gynecol Oncol. 2011;122:255–9.
56. Einstein MH, Barakat RR, Chi DS, Sonoda Y, Alektiar KM, Hensley ML, et al. Management of uterine malignancy found incidentally after supracervical hysterectomy or uterine morcellation for presumed benign disease. Int J Gynecol Cancer. 2008;18:1065–70.
57. George S, Barysauskas C, Serrano C, Oduyebo T, JA R-H, et al. Retrospective cohort study evaluating the impact of intraperitoneal morcellation on outcomes of localized uterine leiomyosarcoma. Cancer. 2014;120(20):3154–8. [Epub ahead of print].

58. Oduyebo T, Rauh-Hain AJ, Meserve EE, et al. The value of re-exploration in patients with inadvertently morcellated uterine sarcoma. Gynecol Oncol. 2014;132:360–5.
59. Pritts EA, Parker WH, Brown J, Ollive DL. Outcome of occult uterine leiomyosarcoma after surgery for presumed uterine fibroids: a systematic review. J Minim Invasive Gynecol. 2014;2 [epub ahead of print].
60. Siedhoff MT, Wheeler SB, Rutstein SE, et al. Laparoscopic hysterectomy with morcellation vs abdominal hysterectomy for presumed fibroid tumors in premenopausal women: a decision analysis. Am J Obstet Gynecol. 2015;212:591.
61. SGO Position Statement: Morcellation. Dec 2013. https://www.sgo.org/newsroom/position-statements-2/morcellation. Accessed 10/2014.
62. Brown, Jubilee and board of trustees. AAGL statement to the FDA on power morcellation. 2014. www.aagl.org.
63. Cohen SL, Einarsson JI, Wang KC, Brown D, Boruta D, Scheib SA, Fader AN, Shibley T. Contained power morcellation within an insufflated isolation bag. Obstet Gynecol. 2014 Sep;124(3):491–7.
64. American College of Obstetricians and Gynecologists. Power morcellation and occult malignancy in gynecologic surgery. A Special Report. May 2014.

Part V

Surgical Education and Training

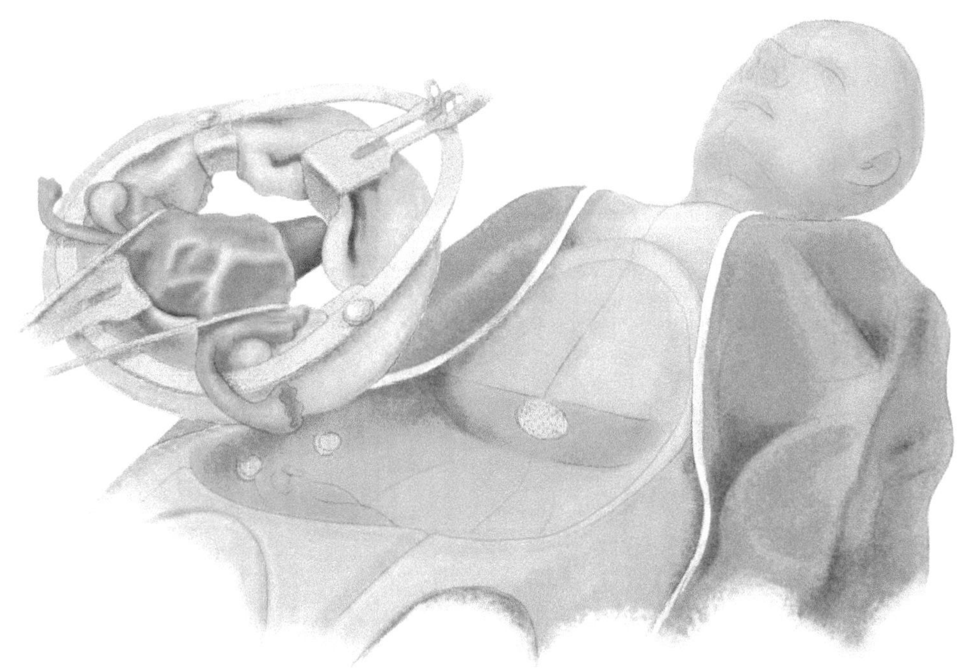

Learning by Doing: How to Teach Hysterectomy

16

Carolin Spüntrup, Marc Banerjee, and Elmar Spüntrup

The Hippocratic oath reminds since more than 2000 years to heal patients to the best of knowledge and to impart knowledge to the next generation. Over centuries history showed that individual ethically and morally understanding as well as motivation for education are adapted to external factors – advantaged by base motives as personal professional advancement or the uncritical acceptance of specific ideologies. Dreadful experiments using living human being were performed and legitimated by the pretended scientific benefit.

Following the ideals medicines should hold for: Medical knowledge is common knowledge – it should be denied neither patients nor younger colleagues. Medical education of younger colleagues must be carried out in an ethically and morally acceptable way and always with the focus on the benefit of patients.

Introduction

For century's surgical education based on a learning-by-doing apprenticeship model using a high patient volume to teach the residency step by step certain surgical skills under various levels of supervision. Mistakes and costs resulting from the trainee's learning curve were accepted by the society [1].

Today a couple of factors limit this traditional model: surgical procedures have become more complex and specified resulting in a reduced patient volume for certain operation morally and ethical aspects came into focus, the acceptance of the society concerning medical mistakes has changed and finally financial aspects especially concerning operation time, complication rate as well as time and costs for a surgical education came more into focus of both, society as well as surgeons (Fig. 16.1) [1].

Several studies analysed the influence of repetition of specific interventions to iatrogenic injury and found an association between number of repetitions and declining injury rate (Fig. 16.2). But also other associations were found correlating to repetition such as operative time, operative result etc. This indicates that repetition is a central factor for the surgeons learning curve and how complex and multifactorial the process of operative learning is.

Considering these factors it seemed likely to establish a new surgical education system which includes a repetitive step by step education of complex operations under ethical, morally and financially more acceptable conditions.

Educational Concepts

The idea to update the traditional apprenticeship-model is not new. Over the past century several proposals were reported how to innovate the traditional system [2]. The American Bord of surgeons complained in 1916 that the traditional apprenticeship model does not result in a broad and well-grounded surgical education respectively the operative quality [3]. To improve surgical education, some American universities introduced surgical education programs including refresher courses in anatomy, pathology, biochemistry and skill training using cadavers and animals before residents performed operations in real patients [3].

C. Spüntrup, MD (✉)
University of Witten/Herdecke, Alfred-Herrhausen-Str. 50, 58448 Witten, Germany

University of Witten/Herdecke, Endoscopic Gynecology, Pelvic School Saarbrücken, Hohe Wacht 77, Saarbrücken, Saarland 66119, Germany
e-mail: pelvicschoolsaarbruecken@gmx.de

M. Banerjee, MD
University of Witten/Herdecke, Alfred-Herrhausen-Str. 50, 58448 Witten, Germany

University of Witten/Herdecke, Praxis für Orthopädie und Unfallchirurgie, Media Park Klinik, Im Media Park 3, Cologne 50670, Germany
e-mail: marc.banerjee@gmx.de

E. Spüntrup, MD
Department of Radiology, Klinikum Saarbrücken, Winterberg 1, Saarbrücken, Saarland 66119, Germany
e-mail: espuentrup@klinikum-saarbruecken.de

I. Alkatout, L. Mettler (eds.), *Hysterectomy*, DOI 10.1007/978-3-319-22497-8_16

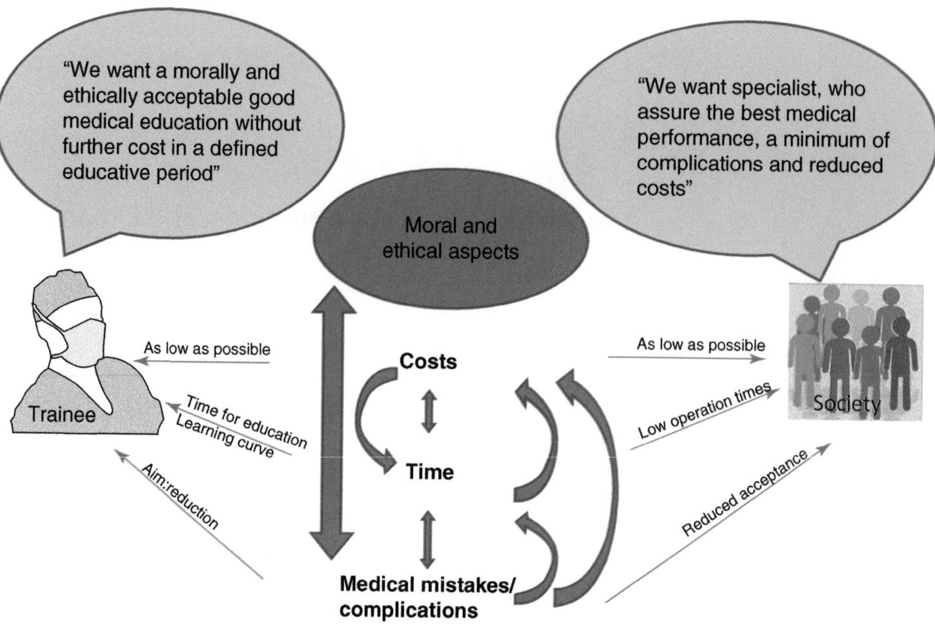

Fig. 16.1 The dilemma of surgical education

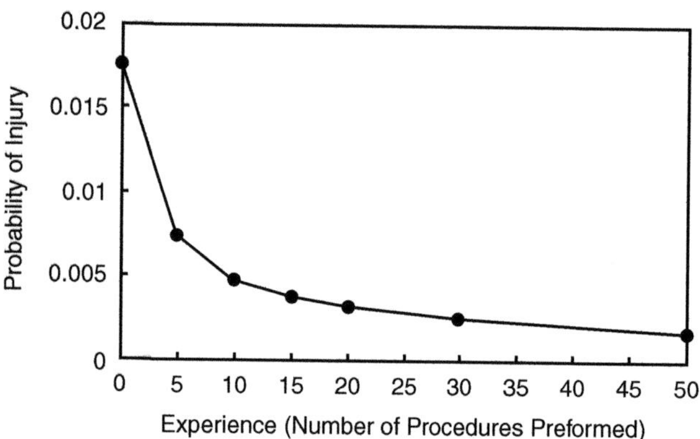

Fig. 16.2 Typical example for the decline of a learning curve. Instead of probability of injury also time for the performance of a specific task could be chosen (compare Fig. 16.4a) (From Rogers et al. [25])

With regard to the success of simulated training for pilots, surgical training in a simulated environment came more into focus and is meanwhile one of the central parts of innovative surgical trainings-models [4, 5]. In pilot trainings difficult situations, e.g. a clear defined storm of certain intensity hits the airplane and induces some damages. The pilot trainee learns how to handle this situation in a simulated, not life threatening environment. By repetition he will develop mental schemes and he will also increase psychic stability to manage these extreme situations in case of real occurrence. Modern findings of behavioral cognitive sciences describe a couple of modifications which can be used as variances to reach specific aims in such pilot trainings-schedules [6]. Theoretically similar schemes could be adopted for a surgeon to handle different situations e.g. the step-by-step training of a routine hysterectomy or a complication occurring during a hysterectomy. Technically it is already possible to simulate a couple of difficult intraoperative situations with some of the existing trainers presented later. In reality for a resident it is still not a routine to train such situations on a simulator [4, 5]. The main difference between education of pilots and surgeons is that pilots *must* undergo trainings units while surgeons do it optional. This is reflected in the fact that airlines bear the expenses for pilot training while surgeons often have to come up themselves for the costs. Surgical admission boards mostly do not demand a participation in simulated training to reach a certain educational level. The associated high costs for the trainees as well as the volunteer status of simulator training are probably reasons why still no widespread educational concept has been accomplished.

Behavioral Sciences and Surgical Training

Behavioral sciences analyzed the complexity of learning in several fields and defined specific terms for learning processes [7]. From a behavioral point of view experts are characterized by cognition in a certain field. Cognition itself is composed of several factors: perception, attention, information processing, information storage (including organization), and then retrieval from long-term memory at the appropriate time as "knowledge" which helps the individual make their decision [5, 8].

Gallagher emphasizes the value of attention for surgical learning [5]. Attention of an experienced surgeon will focus the intraoperative progress searching the best way of operation to minimize the individual patients risks and possible complications while the novices attention is focused –depending on his educational level- on basics, such as anatomical orientation or guiding his instruments etc. [5]. It has been proposed that simulators can help to reach the point where many of the psychomotor skills (e.g. hand-eye coordination) and spatial orientation have been automated. This process is called "shaping" in a behavioral sciences sense. It generates new resources of attention for the trainee [5] and allows the trainee to focus more on learning of the operation steps itself or the management of complications [4, 5]. Figure 16.3 outlines behavioral aspects focusing the aims of surgical learning, the pathways of internalizing and mediums to optimize the processes.

Manual Dexterity

Teachers often subjectively report on talented surgical trainees and it must be contributed that even in the eyes of experienced surgeons some colleagues stick out by performing difficult procedures with a phenomenal ease. Talent in its usual sense meaning a pre-existing manual dexterity seems to be useful but not a precondition to become a good surgeon [4, 5]. For endoscopic knotting and suture techniques it was found that the influence of concomitant factors which might influence the talent of manual dexterity is of less importance (Fig. 16.4a, b) [9]. Only during the first five procedures individuals, who trained their bimanual dexterity before (e.g. by playing guitar, knitting or former endoscopic experience for more than 10 h) but were novices concerning self-performed endoscopic operations, had a significant advantage concerning knotting times. Learning curve improved most remarkably during the first five procedures. Afterwards a kind of steady state is reached without a further significant improvement of knotting time for the individual surgeon and an adaption of knotting times between all individuals is found (Fig. 16.4a, b) [9]. Thus it is proposed

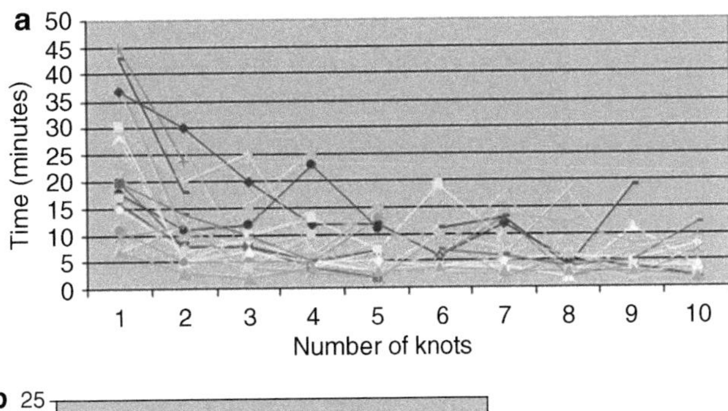

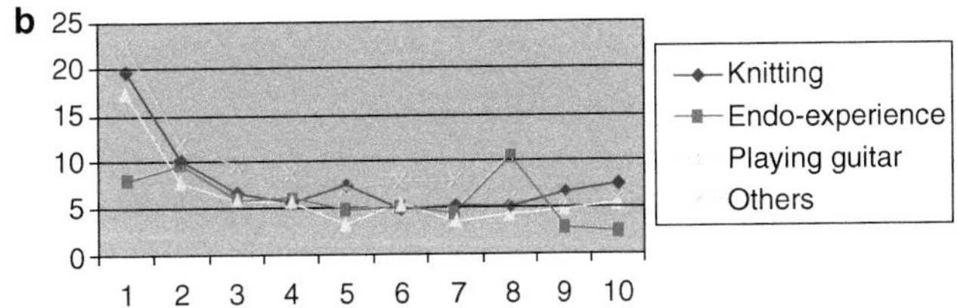

Fig. 16.4 (**a**) Repetions and times of the first 10 knots of novices (each *color lines* one novice). (**b**) Novices, who played guitar, had experience in endoscopic assistance or knitted started on a faster niveau of time for each knot. These findings adapted after 5 knots

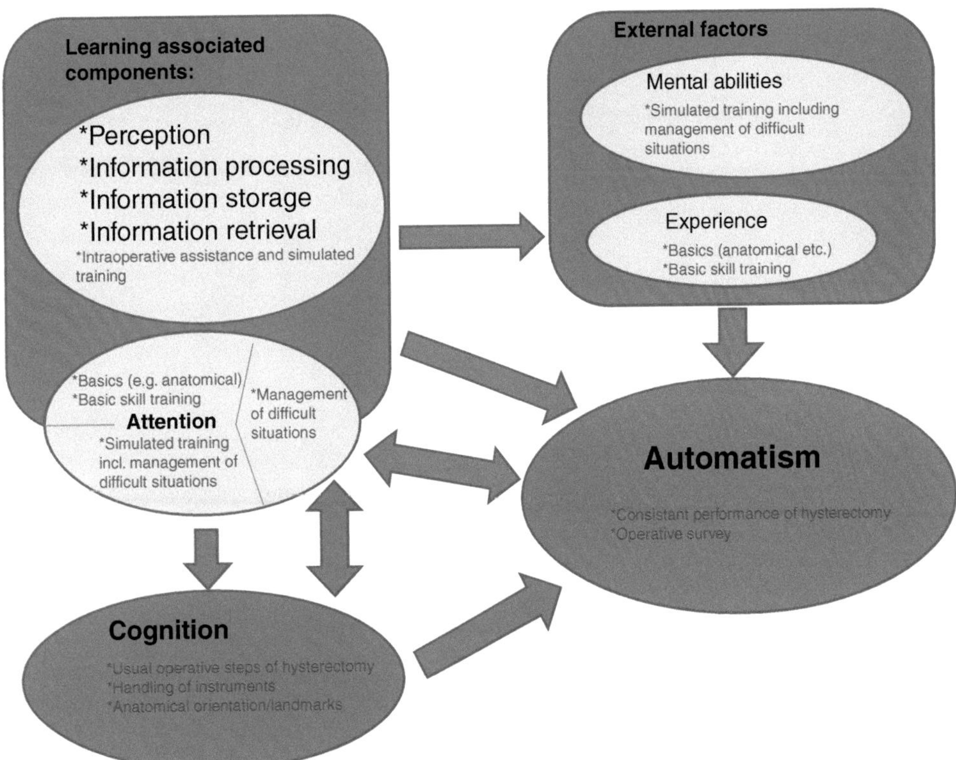

Fig. 16.3 Behavioral aspects of endoscopic learning. In a behavioral sense of learning, automatisms for a specific tasks are the designated learning aim. Several components influence the generation of automatisms. The graphic summarizes the influence of superior components (*black, bold face*), subitems (*black*) and related endocsopical trainings levels (*red*). Attention is a central point for developing automatisms and the focus of attention changes in correlation to the trainees educative level

that surgical manual dexterity concerning knotting is not a specific talent. It can be improved after a few repetitions and interindividual differences will adapt over time.

Gallager and Satana [10] reported about three trials on a virtual reality trainer comparing the surgical skills of novices (no experiences), juniors (10–100 operations) and experts (more than 100 operations). Also in this study surgical basic skills adapted after three trials, but novices and experts showed a very different behavior concerning the instrumental activity: while the experts used electrocoagulation rather conservative and situate adapted, the novices ignored alerts concerning thermic damages and did not change their behavior during the trials. Juniors tried to reduce the use of electrocoagulation after repeated alert [10].

Surgical Trainings-Aims

In accordance to these findings it has been estimated that the performance of a skillfull operation depends in 75 % percent in decision making and only in 25 % in manual dexterity [11]. Correct decisions require a good intraoperative survey and are compound by an excellent fact knowledge and other factors which are summarized under the behavioral scientific term "cognition". This weighting of the factor "decision making" changes former concepts of surgical skill training. Former concepts separated theoretical knowledge and practical skill training depending on individual trainings level. Theoretical knowledge included the theoretical knowledge of anatomic landmark, operative steps etc. The education of practical skills concentrated in exercises for the hand-eye coordination. Not before the performance of operations in living patients both components were united. Newer trainings programs allow focusing on the togetherness of components, fact knowledge and practical training [4, 5, 11, 12]. They respect the complete field that influences intraoperative decisions. Theoretical and practical aspects of operations are thus more joined even on an early educative level (Fig. 16.5).

Accordingly new trainings aims base on a entirety concept focusing both, operation specific practical knowledge (manual dexterity, guidance of instruments, intraoperative details etc.) and theoretical knowledge (anatomical, pathological, bio-

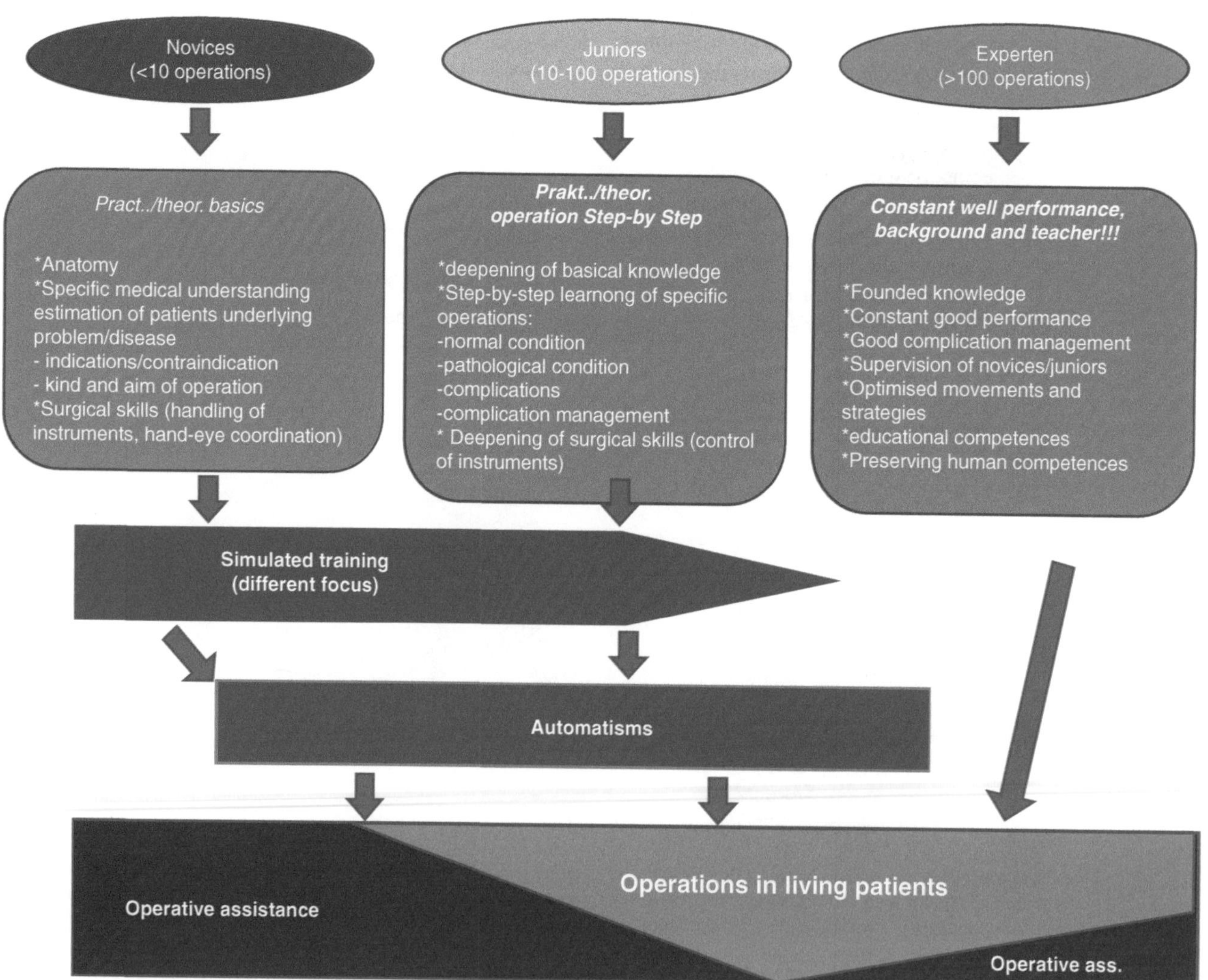

Fig. 16.5 Learning aims of novices, juniors and experts. Simulated training (with different trainings aims) decreases with rising trainings level and generation of automatisms

chemisty, theoretical knowledge on procedure etc). Trainings aims are correlated to the individual trainings level [2, 12–14]. The tripartitude into novices, juniors and experts is a recurrent classification in literature and seems suitable to summarize trainings aims for an entirety concept (Fig. 16.5) [5, 10, 13].

Novices are unexperienced in all respects. For novices trainings aims are the implementation of automatisms concerning basics: anatomical basics, intraoperative anatomical orientation, handling of the surgical instruments, understanding of the aim of the surgical procedure (that means why is the procedure done, how is it done and what is the final aim) [5, 10, 13].

Juniors are low experienced with a beginning survey on operative procedures. Defined subordinated targets can be accomplished. The trainings aims of juniors are the implementation of automatisms concerning the single steps of a certain operative procedure, internalizing specific subordinate targets and the control of instruments. With an increasing experience on the way to become an expert, juniors will also learn automatisms concerning pathological situation, complications and other difficult intraoperative situations [5, 10, 13].

Experts (more than 100 procedures) featured automatisms for operative basics, have a founded knowledge and internalized pathways for many intraoperative situations. Intraoperative movements and activities are optimized, with a clear defined final aim and several sub-ordinate targets, knowing and respecting the consequences of each movement and activity. In case of complications the expert acts more calm and stringent in order to return to the "normal" operative pathway. For the definition of trainings aim the priority aim should be to reach this expert level with optimized and constant performance as well as a reduction of errors [4, 5]. The aims of experts are finally to optimize the education of novices and juniors as well as to supervise operation in real patients and help in case of problems (Figs. 16.5 and 16.6) [4, 5, 12, 13].

Associated Factors for an Optimized Training and Opportunities for Efficiency Control

Concerning an optimized trainings scheme for the ideal implementation of trainings aims the distributed short interval training has been described as more effective than single long sessions. According to behavioral sciences the cognitively implementation of surgical skills is better consolidated, if an interval between training is realized [5, 15]. In practice this means that e.g. a splitted overnight training (afternoon session on one day and morning session on the next day) is more effective than a complete one day training (morning session and afternoon session on the same day).

Feedback mechanisms and similar control respectively test tools visualizing the success of simulated training seem to be useful. The trainee gets information whether he has reached the accomplished trainings aims. Depending on the system mistakes are pointed instantly and can be reduced by repeated training [8, 11].

Test systems additionally provide a good tool for the trainers to assess whether the trainee is able to reach the next level. This can be also used for the award of a certificate. Trainees who verify their ability of successful performance of a specific operation before they start performing supervised operations in real patients will reduce operation time and complication rate in an ethical acceptable way [1, 4, 5, 15]. For the daily routine this could ease the disposition of operators and maybe also benefits the mutual trust between patient and surgeon.

Several predictors have been tested as control systems for the estimation of learning success in simulated trainers. Time is not only influenced by experience but also by quality and is therefore as a single item not a good predictor [5, 16]. The number of required repetitions for a specific task is also not a good predictor. Basically surgical skills are reproductive acceptable after about three repetitions. Concerning more

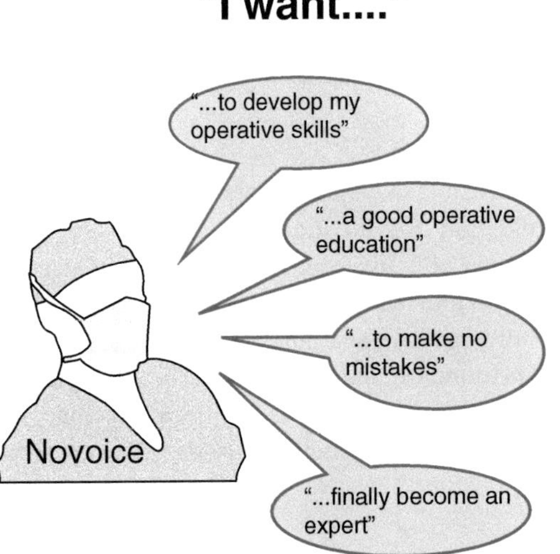
"I want...."
"...to develop my operative skills"
"...a good operative education"
"...to make no mistakes"
"...finally become an expert"
Novoice

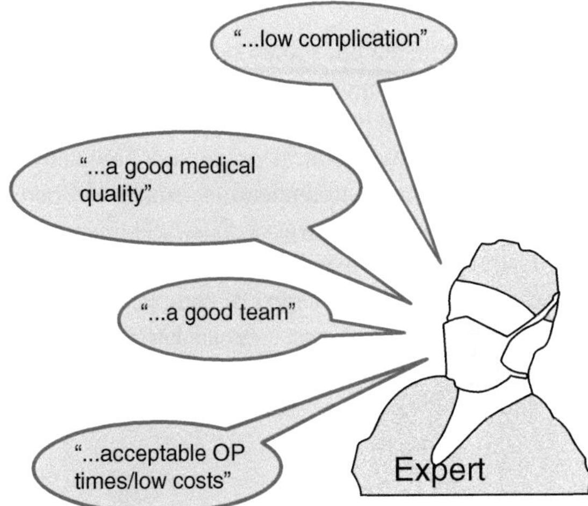

Fig. 16.6 Claims on surgical education from different points of view (pict.: pixabay)

complex tasks (e.g. a complete operative procedure with the need of a more distinguished efficiency control) the number of necessary repetitions depends on the individual trainee and does not reflect the quality of performance in detail. For those complex tasks the achievement of a certain degree of proficiency including a constantly well performance or the evaluation of relevant single items including mistakes is provided to be more useful [5, 13, 17]. Several factors such as the relation between time and accuracy or knowledge and manual dexterity influence the operative result. These factors are difficult to estimate objectively. For that reason predictors ideally should be measurable in any way. For the objective assessment of technical skills performance the economy of hand movements using an electromagnetically tracking system (ICSAD) [18] seems to be appropriate to differ between very experienced surgeons and less experienced surgeons. The system can be also used for open approaches. Other control instruments use more metric systems to objectify the trainee's performance, e.g. measuring the difference between the ideal puncture of a suture and the actual puncture. In combination with other factors (time etc.) a points-based system can be used for evaluation.

Trainings Concepts for Hysterectomy

In accordance to former surgical training systems and respecting behavioral findings concerning cognition, the adoption of an educational system with three levels (surgical basics, practical training on simulators and final education schedules in real patients) seems suitable [5]. The three levels are overlapping and respect the different start levels of trainees [novice, juniors (non-experienced and experienced), expert].

In detail the implementation of levels for a structured hysterectomy education comprises:

Surgical Basics

This educational stadium should be hallmarked by the aims of deepening anatomical, topographical and pathological knowledge of the pelvis minor and adjacent structures, an understanding of biochemical processes, knowledge about correct indications/contraindication for a hysterectomy including judicial consequences, basically management of complications (kind of possible complications, perception of complications, adequate therapy of complications, strategies to avoid complications) and a broad knowledge about the postoperative sequence in general. This stadium should be more than only a recapitulation of students-knowledge. Especially anatomical and topographical knowledge should be specifically considered under the operative aspect, e.g. using certain structures as landmarks, acquire a 3-dimensional idea of the course of the ureter and other structures etc. These aims can be reached by practical assistance and hospitation during operations and indications, refreshing the literature including modern opportunities such as videos, video animations etc. and participation in special courses. Hand eye-coordination and first steps in instruments handling can be improved by the use of simulators.

The stadium of *surgical basics* will have its maximum learning effect during the first years of residency but in fact learning effect of this stadium will attend throughout a doctor's life with a lower intensity and changing focus than during the first few years of surgical education.

Simulated Hysterectomy

Modern surgical simulators can be used to achieve more or less the following trainings aims:

- improvement of manual dexterity (also concerning single steps, e.g. suture of the vagina)
- continuing enlarging experience and fact knowledge (active use of the basic knowledge of stadium I, e.g. concerning the course of the ureter or identification of leading structures)
- induction of schemes and strategies for the solution of difficult situations by repeated hysterectomies in a not life threatening surrounding (e.g. how to handle intraligamental myoma etc.)
- accomplishing the steady state of the learning curve concerning hysterectomy before continuing stadium three
- improvement of operative survey including the knowledge to make quick and correct decisions
- making correct valuations of intraoperative findings (e.g. the valuation of endometriosis)
- finding strategies concerning prevention respectively management of iatrogenic complications
- performing examinations to verify certain levels of certification

It becomes feasible that the differentiation into novice and junior is important for the trainings aims of this level. Simulators are an effective tool for both group, but with a different focus. While the novice can improve his knowledge concerning intraoperative anatomical orientation, control on the surgical instruments, understanding of the aim of the surgical procedure (that means why is the procedure done, how is it done and what is the final aim), juniors will deepen their skills concerning the implementation of automatisms concerning the single steps of a certain operative procedure, pathological situation, complications and other difficult intraoperative situations.

Most hospitals possess on box trainers so trainees have the opportunity to learn certain steps such as knotting/ suturing as well as the handling in general. Anatomical models of the pelvis are also often available and partly even integrated in the box- trainers. These trainings tools allow an advanced anatomical and topographical education. The complete imitation of hysterectomies, ideally with a simulated sick uterus (e.g. uterus myomatosus), will be more a subject of courses in specialized training centers, but at present the costs of such courses must be mostly beared by the trainee himself. It is of high importance, that – according to the pilot training-these specified courses focus on clear defined education aims which can be realistically achieved by the trainee during the course. Otherwise courses will only lead to a certificate-without a real surgical use to the trainee or finally to the patient!

The participation of courses in such institutions should be integrated part of this stadium. Several courses concerning hysterectomy are available focusing on different educational aims, e.g. deepening hysterectomy-specific anatomical and topographical knowledge (human cadaver courses), training of hysterectomy steps in general (hysterectomy of living porcs), advanced training of hysterectomy with simulation of different uterine diseases (intraligamental myoma, large uterus myomatosus, endometriosis etc.; Realsimulator), test instruments for estimation of surgical skill level (computer assisted systems). The different trainings systems will be précised later.

Training in Patients

In this educational stadium the trainee will continue his surgical hysterectomy education in real patients. In contrast to the traditional system the trainee will start making hysterectomies on a higher education level. That means that he has reached already a certain steady state of his learning curve and his attention can be focused on the essentials of hysterectomy. Combined with the supervision of an experienced surgeon a preferably simple hysterectomy (normal weighted patients without expected adhesions or complications) can be chosen. In case of any complication the experienced surgeon can either guide the trainee throughout the operation or can take over the hysterectomy. According to trainings-degree supervision by an experienced surgeon can be reduced step by step and degree of difficulty of the sick uterus can be elevated step by step until the trainee has reached a level to take the full responsibility even for expected difficult hysterectomies.

Training Systems

Several training modules are available today and it is difficult to get an overview about all existing systems. According to Munro et al., the division into organic (that means human cadavers or animals) and inorganic trainers (others) is adopted here and complemented by combined organic/inorganic trainers [1].

Most trainings systems have been developed for unspecific surgical intervention such as hand-eye- coordination or suturing techniques. With a new focus on surgical survey and the induction of automatisms for intraoperative decision making as trainings aims, the simulation of complete operations seems useful. Such high complex training systems have been developed for open abdominal, vaginal or endoscopical approach opportunities and offer theoretically a couple of interventional possibilities [19, 20]. These training systems partly allow the performance of "complete" operative procedures, such as access to operative field, specific operations and reconstruction of abdominal/vaginal wall. In practice these simulators are very expensive and most of the patented simulators obviously have not been produced in a broad mass.

Other simulators consist on vessels as well as on nerve simulations, so even defined complications are possible. The operative procedure itself is mostly simulated by the use of animal organs. For the simulation of surgical operations porcine gall bladder or porcine intestine are common used trainings-objects [1, 4, 5]. Porcine gall bladder and adjacent structures allow a realistic simulation of gall bladder extirpation including preparation of bile duct etc. Porcine guts system is favorited as trainings –tool for a couple of surgical interventions (resections, enteroanastomosis, use of staplers, suturing and knotting, endoscopic resections etc.) [1, 4, 5]. Simulators which allow the use of animal organs offer special equipment for fixation of the focused structures.

As the organic simulators are associated with some disadvantages (unpleasant odor, explanation of organs, no planned pathologies) during the last decades inorganic trainings moduls came more into focus. Concerning hysterectomy such simulators are still rare.

In the following section we give an overview over the existing training systems, which can be used to improve surgical skills regarding hysterectomy. Also a short interpretation is given for which purpose or trainings aim the presented systems are fitting (Table 16.1).

Table 16.1 Characteristics of different endoscopic trainings and education levels

	Anatomical/pathological details	HE simulation	Hand eye coordination	Infectious	Ethical vote	costs	Proportion HE: trainee	Planned Pathologies	Tests for certificates
Human Cadavers	Very good	+ (o,e,v)	+	Risk	(Agreement of patient)	++	1:3	Not planned	No
Living pigs	Partly comparable	+ (o,e)	+	Low risk	Yes	+++	1:3	Not planned	No
Box trainers	Not at all	–	+	Low risk	No	(+)	–	–	Yes
Advanced Trainers	Partly comparable - good	+ (o,e)	+	No	No	++	1:1	Partly yes	Partly yes
VRT	Very good if programmed	+ (e)	+	No	No	++++	1:1	Yes	Yes
Real Simulator	Good	+ (o,e)	+	Very low risk	No	++	1:1	Yes	Yes

Organic Trainers

Organic simulators are in common human cadavers or animals.

Human cadavers have been used as a teaching tool for centuries. Learning aims of hysterectomy courses using human cadavers are focusing on a recapitulation and deepening of anatomical and topographical details around the operated field on the one hand and the possibility of performing the steps of a hysterectomy on the other hand. The simulation of a hysterectomy is possible in all variations (vaginal, open abdominal, endoscopical, supracervical or complete etc.). Operative access is comparable to living patients. In general two to three persons learn on one human cadaver. Therefor not all trainees will perform a complete hysterectomy during the courses. A vascular perfusion of the cadaver to imitate blood flow is in most cases not realized. Nevertheless coagulation, ligation, sutures, morcellations , incisions and other steps, which are important during hysterectomy are similar to a real hysterectomy. Pathologies in the operative field can be used as a welcome special challenge during the course, but they cannot be planned.

Formaldehyde-based fixation techniques are not appropriate due to the rigid consistency of pelvic organs and abdominal wall and, thus, have to be replaced either by alternative fixation methods or the use of fresh frozen cadavers. Fixation procedures providing good conditions to perform open abdominal or laparoscopic procedures include embalming techniques based on ethanol-glycerin or Thiel fixation [21, 22]. Although the tissue properties (e.g. color, water content, consistency, mobility) still differ from the in-vivo situation, virtually all surgical procedures including the use of electrocautery and ultrasound devices are feasible applying these alternative fixation methods. Decision making, acquire operative survey, guidance of assistance as well as single steps (appropriate use of coagulation, preparation, sutures, hand eye-coordination etc.) are trainings aims which can be learned using this setting. Disadvantages of the use of human cadavers are the risk of transferring certain infections during the procedure and the partly unpleasant odor. The transvaginal access is sometimes limited either by natural factors as the higher age at the time of death (associated with narrow and thin walled vagina) or by a certain disgust of the trainees.

Simulation on Animals

Animals, either living or death, were used for medical learning and education purposes since antiquity. Claudius Galenus performed a couple of sections in different animals (e.g. neurolysis in pigs, study of organs in elephants).

For hysterectomy trainings the uterus of pigs seems to be most qualified, as the size and adjacent structures are tolerably comparable to real patients. Operations on living pigs allow a perfusion of the uterus, which makes the operation more realistic. Haptic, color, admittance (at least open abdominal or endoscopic) are similar to operations in real patients. All intraoperative steps including admittance, complete steps of hysterectomy and closing the admittance are possible.

Decision making, acquire operative survey, guidance of assistance as well as single steps (appropriate use of coagulation, preparation, sutures, hand eye-coordination etc.) are trainings aims which can be learned using this system. In living pigs the trainee gets a comparable intraoperative feedback concerning his operative behavior (e.g. via the anesthesist etc).

Limiting factors are the necessity of a positive ethical votum for each course and the high costs of each pig. In living pigs for ethical reasons pigs must get a general anesthesia. In most courses two to three trainees will operate one pig, so not all participants will operate a complete hysterectomy themselves. In general, animals will die after operation. Pathologies cannot be planned. Anatomic and topographic details are only partly comparable to human beings. The risk of zoonosis exists, but is small.

Inorganic Trainers

Inorganic trainers can be divided into classical box trainers, advanced trainers and virtual reality systems (VRT) with the subgroup of robotic assisted VRT's. Most inorganic trainers refer more to the endoscopic approach, but also allow at least an open abdominal access. Some trainers are even equipped with a vagina.

Box Trainers (Fig. 16.7)

Classical box trainers are characterized by a kind of box covered by an exchangeable layer, which simulates the abdominal wall. The box includes possibilities for fixation of artificial layers, structures or even simulated organs. Box trainers are widespread trainings tool and are available in most hospitals. In general they are not associated to a certain operative field. Thus trainee can learn basic steps such as admittance, hand-eye coordination, instrument handling or knotting and suture techniques.

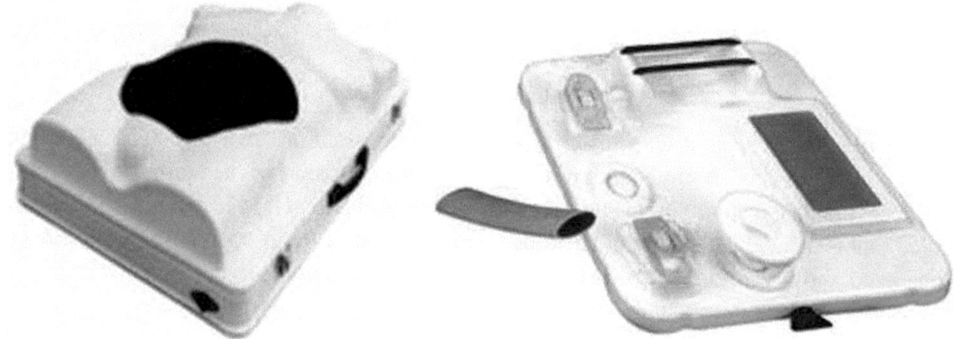

Fig. 16.7 Box Trainer and fitting inlay for hand-eye coordination and suture -knitting skills (By courtesy of Erler-Zimmer)

Advanced Trainers

Advanced (endoscopic) trainers allow the fixation of operative inlays for specific operations. Some endoscopic advanced trainers are additionally equipped with USB connections to overcome the problem of optical system. Genuine endoscopes are no longer necessary to learn on the simulator but it is possible to adapt the integrated camera e.g. to the own computer or laptop. Often a mannequin form is chosen with openings on the upper or lower abdomen. Access ports are either determined or can be chosen free on a complete flexible abdominal wall. Operative inlays consist on all important structures and landmarks which are necessary for specific operations. Inlays are rather expensive, but often two or three organs with pathologies (uterus, ovarian cyst, ectopic tubal pregnancy) are simulated. After operation(s) inlays must be rejected. They can be changed easily and are fixed by a kind of click-in system. They are made completely from inorganic material. This lightens storage.

Concerning hysterectomy very less simulators have been described using artificial tissue (e.g. a kind of special foam) to simulate organs and structures. Hysterectomy steps including preparation, cutting, sutures etc. are realistically possible to a certain degree. Some systems allow even the simulation of pathologies such as myoma etc.

Decision making, acquire operative survey, guidance of assistance as well as single steps (preparation, sutures, hand eye-coordination etc.) are trainings aims which can be learned using this system. The use of additional training success tool gives the trainee feedback concerning his operative behavior and allows also evaluating the success of learning.

Disadvantage of the systems is that they are not aligned for electrocoagulation or HF surgery. No coagulation of prefunded vessels or electric surgery procedures on tissue (monopolar cutting, sealing etc.) is possible. Additionally the systems are rather expensive for the daily clinical use and therefor more useful in courses.

Virtual Reality Trainers (Fig. 16.8)

During the last decade for endoscopic procedures a new generation of computed based simulator has been introduced. Simplified virtual reality trainers are comparable to a wii system, using detectors and microprocessors to convert the surgeon instruments movement into an imaginative movement on the monitor. The underlying imaginative computerized matrix is very realistic and bases on real happened cases.

In first systems sometimes leaps in time or mistakes in converting the surgeons movements occurred which were meanwhile reduced.

Virtual reality trainers have a large potential, as already every operation and complication can be simulated. Additionally operations can be performed only by the trainee without the need of assistance. Additionally specific hand eye coordination tools are available.

All procedures which are necessary during hysterectomy such as preparation, cutting, sutures, electrocoagulation, monopolar cutting, sealing etc. are theoretically possible, but must be implemented by the codes.

Decision making, acquire operative survey and single steps (appropriate use of coagulation, preparation, sutures, hand eye-coordination etc.) are trainings aims which can be learned using this system. The use of additional training success tool gives the trainee feedback concerning his operative behavior and allows also evaluating the success of learning.

A great problem is the lack of haptic. The development of a haptical feeling is a relevant factor for a trainee. Newer systems implemented codes for a kind of haptical feeling but there is still no solution to copy the original feeling in all situations during the operation.

A further disadvantage is that the coded systems only allow defined steps of the trainee. That means, that the system answers with a programmed displacement activity in

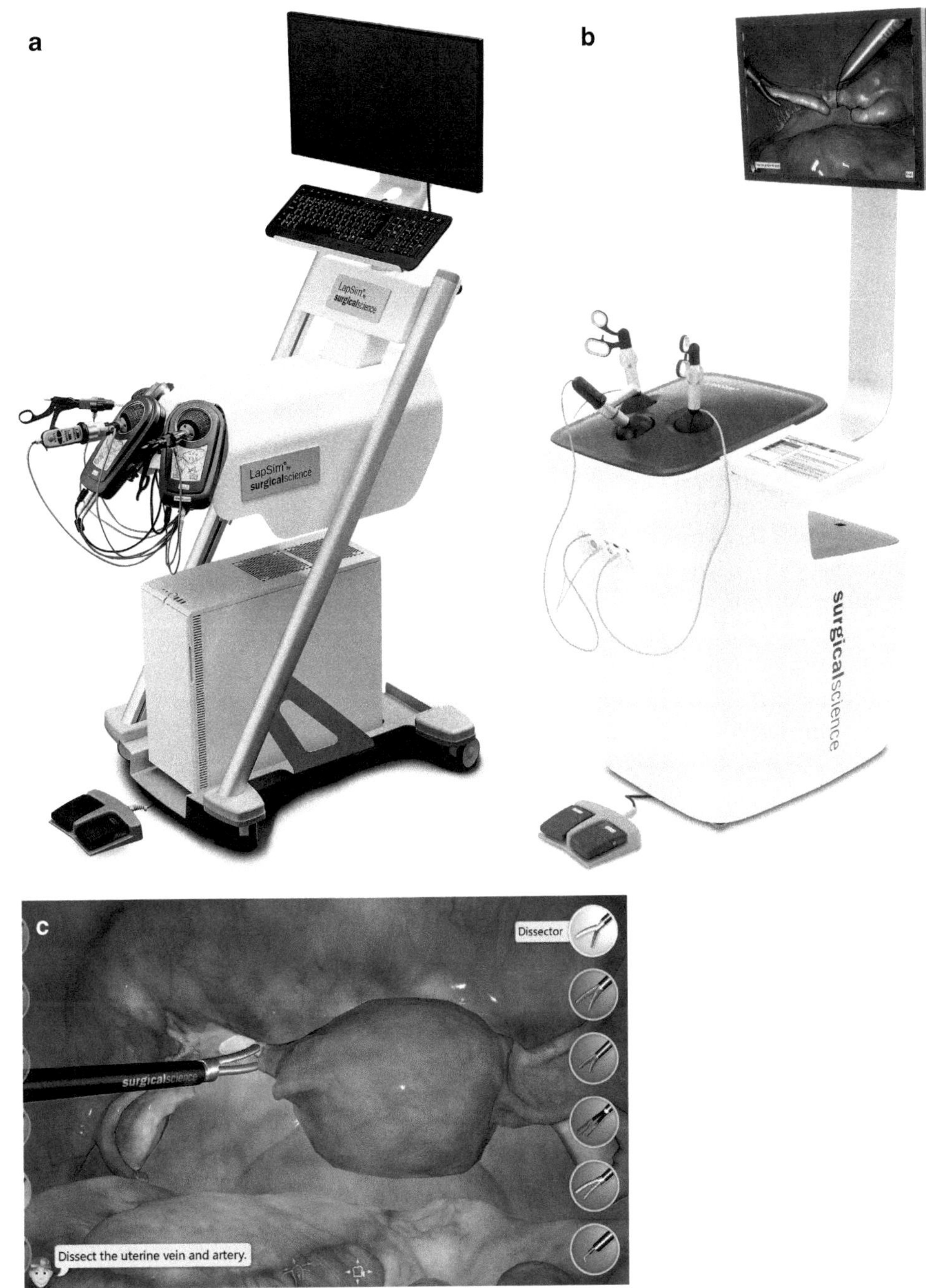

Fig. 16.8 Virtual Reality Systems: (**a**) LapSim® Haptic System, (**b**) LapSim® Non-Haptic System, (**c**) LapSim® virtual hysterectomy., LapSim® Laparoscopic Trainer (Source: LapSim®)

case of movements of the trainee, which have not been programmed. So an accidental injury of a gut during a hysterectomy is not possible and the gut evades, if the simulated operation has not been coded for the complication "injury of guts".

The fact that in some systems no further assistance is necessary seems to be positive on the first sight. Regarding the trainings aim of intraoperative survey it must be contributed that also the guidance of an intraoperative assistance is a relevant factor and should be trained.

Further disadvantages are the high costs for the systems, which are reasoned in the developing cost for the different tools.

Summarizing virtual reality trainers are at present not seen in the first line of simulated training for novices. They are rather used as control instruments of trainings success in specialized courses. If all "teething troubles" including the lack of haptic will be overcome and a really broad spectrum of intraoperative courses including spontaneous induced complications can be realistically simulated, this system could be the surgical counterpart of simulators for pilots.

Integrated Virtual Reality Trainers in Robotic Assisted Surgical Systems

During the last decade robotic assisted surgical systems have been introduced also for hysterectomy. The robotic assisted surgical systems are in general featured with an integrated virtual reality trainer. These "robotic" VRT's focus on the one hand in general skill training and on the other hand on a training to optimize the use of all function which are provided by the robotic system.

Moglia et al. published in 2015 a review comparing the different VRT's of robotic systems concerning general skill training and skill transfer to robotic operation.

They found in all analysed systems a realistic simulation, which made the tool usable and useful for the trainee, but trainings tools are not standardized at all [23]. Robotic VRT's are a useful tool for bimanual wristed manipulation, camera control, master clutching to manage hand position, use of third instrument arm, activating energy sources, appropriate depth perception, and awareness of forces applied by instruments for surgeons who intend to use robotic systems [24].

Concerning the items of general skill training and especially on simulated hysterectomy no additional facts than those of VRT's have been reported.

Combined Organic/Inorganic Trainers (Fig. 16.9)

Combined trainers are characterized by the combination of advantages of organic trainers such as the possibility of electrocoagulation or perfusion with advantages of inorganic trainers such as reproducible simulation of pathological conditions. By the combination of both components the realistic simulation of a couple of operative steps is optimized and l a realistic haptic is given [15]. Additional hand-eye-coordination tools are available.

In a certain way box trainers with the fixation possibility for organic parts of animals can be considered as precursor of combined trainers but the characteristic difference is that pathologies cannot be planned and that they are not exactly reproducible. In a real combined trainer organic structures are not used in its entity but only components of organic origin are processed to create reproducible artificial pathological organs. According to bionic sciences characteristics of organic material is analysed and useful components for each operative step are composed until a fully functional simulation of a certain operation is created. The organic parts are often by-products of vegetable, meat or fish processing.

The Gynecological Real Simulator (GRS) system is a combined trainings tool for frequent gynecological operations (hysterectomy, ovarian surgery, endoscopic descensus surgery and anti-incontinence procedures). The unit consists of three parts:

1. The Gynecological Real Simulator
2. Pelvic models
3. Operation-specific inlays

The Real Simulator imitates a female torso. It consists of a closable opening on the lower abdomen, a vaginal opening and smaller holes for connection of equipment (e.g. perfusion). Endoscopic equipment is introduced via four defined areas on the classical introduction places. The pelvic models are scaled to the GRS and are fixed by bolted connections. Pelvic models are specific for the simulation of defined operations so different pelvic models are available (hysterectomy model, ovarian cyst model, descensus model, anterior compartment model). An additional basic-skills model is available, using classical tools for hand eye-coordination and handling of instruments .

Pelvic models consist of all structures which are important landmarks for the specific operations. Depending on the trainings aim learning success tools as well as perfusion or the possibility for the use of electrocoagulative instruments are possible.

The operative area of the pelvic models is recessed for the according inlays and provides fixation mechanisms for the inlays. The inlays are the centerpiece of the simulated operations. They simulate specific operations as realistic as possible, can be changed easily by a click-in system and are thrown away after operation.

For a simulation of a hysterectomy using the GRS system additional to the GRS a hysterectomy model and appendant inlays are necessary. The hysterectomy model consists on the pelvic bone ring, a flexible pelvic floor, sigma and rectum, bladder, ovaries, tubes, Ligg. Suspensorium, ureters, fatty tissue and peritoneum. All structures are hardly inflammable and are resistant to a certain level of transmitted heat resulting by the use of common electrosurgical instruments. The model itself can be cleaned with water and a mild cleaning agent.

The hysterectomy inlays can be fixed easily by a click-in system. Perfusion lines must be connected. If monopolar instruments are intended to use, a neutral electrode must be fixed on the inlay. Different hysterectomy inlays with an increasing degree of difficulty are available (normal uterus, uterus with intraligamental myoma, large uterus myomatosus, attached gut/endometriosis). All inlays of one category (e.g. large uterus myomatosus) are exact reproducable. Hysterectomy inlays allow all relevant operative steps including preparation, coagulation, monopolar cuts, use of slings, sealing, morcellation, sutures etc. and are thrown away after operation. Decision making, acquire operative survey, guidance of assistance as well as single steps

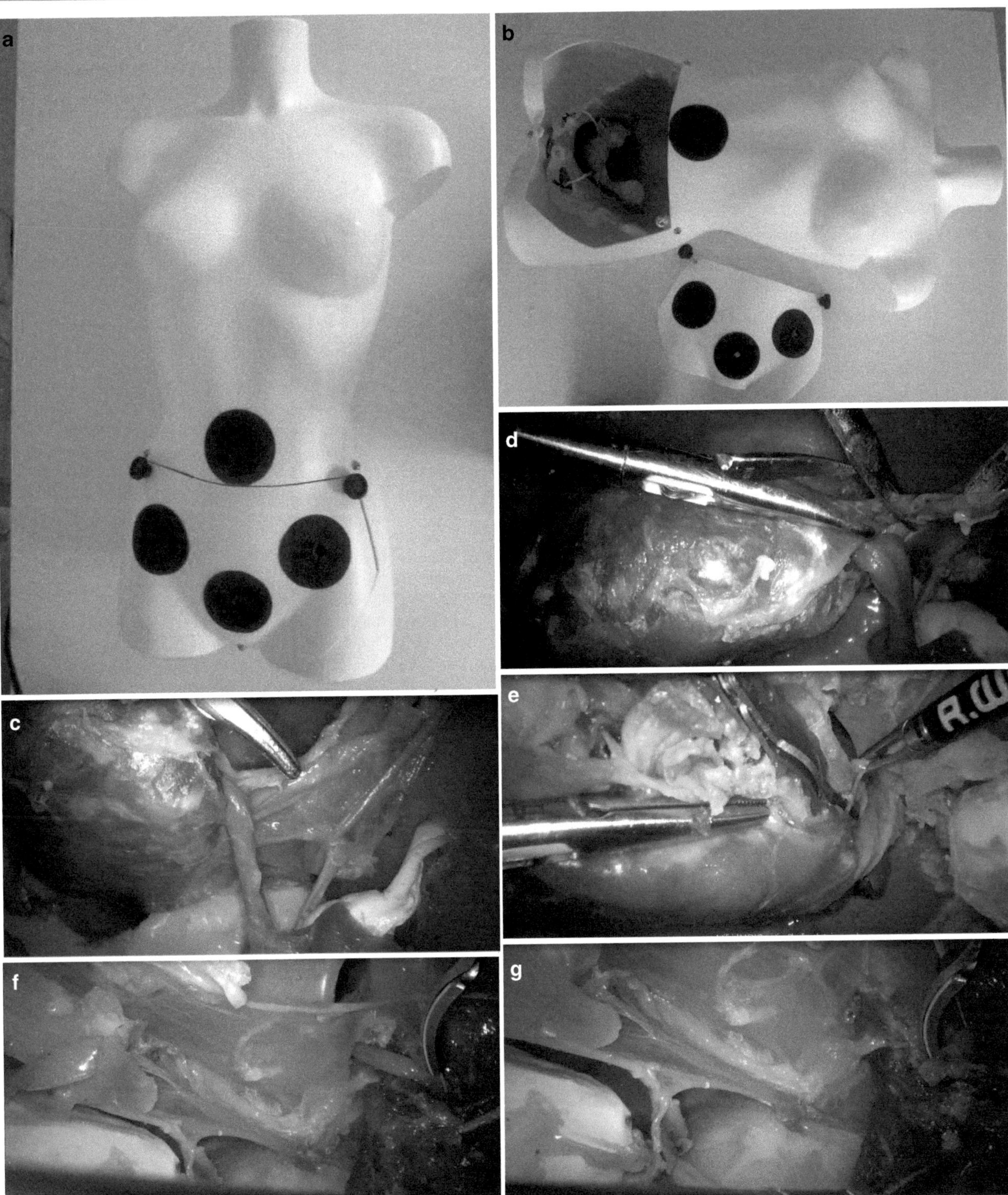

Fig. 16.9 Combined System, Real Simulator (GRS): (**a**) Closed Real Simulator System; (**b**) Opened Real Simulator System with adapted pelvic model; (**c–g**) Hysterectomy inlay during a trainings session. (**c**) artificial hysterectomy trainings inlay, (**d**) dissection of round ligament, (**e**) separation of broad ligament layers and preparation, (**f**) exposure of uterine vessels, (**g**) dissected uterine vessels (after coagulation, not shown) (Courtesy of Pelvic School Saaarbuecken)

(appropriate use of coagulation, preparation, sutures, hand eye-coordination etc.) are trainings aims which can be learned using this system. The use of additional training success tool gives the trainee feedback concerning his operative behavior and allows also evaluating the success of learning.

Disadvantages are the necessity of unfreezing inlays before use. Connection of vessels, neutral etc. is associated with a lead time of about 15 min.

Outlook

An educational concept for hysterectomy basing on three levels (surgical basics-simulated training-hysterectomy in patients) seems suitable and complies ethical and morally requirements. It allows trainees to graduate their individual educational niveau and helps defining trainings aims which should be focused next. Concerning simulated training, trainings aims should be clearly defined in order to choose the optimal simulated trainer for the focused aim. The financial aspect of simulated training cannot be resolved finally. The costs of simulated training are high and correlate to the technical and scientifically effort. A structured education, at least for the second level, in trainings-centers seems more appropriate than an individual, self-ministered training in each hospital. Maybe the wide spread implementation of structured trainings-programs will help to come closer to a conceptual medical counterpart of pilot training.

Tools for learning success as a basis e.g. for a hysterectomy certificate are an interesting vision. A certificate verifying a defined trainings level as precondition for operation in real patients would give patients who undergo hysterectomy the feeling of security and could simplify the clinical daily routine for trainees and trainers.

References

1. Munro MG. Surgical simulation: where have we come from? Where are we now? Where are we going? J Minim Invasive Gynecol. 2012;19(3):272–83.
2. Fried GM, Feldmann LS, Vassiliou MC, Fraser SA, Stanbridge D, Ghitulescu G, Andrew CG. Proving the value of simulation in laparoscopic surgery. Ann Surg. 2004;240:518–25.
3. Smyth CM. Graduate surgical training in America. Ann Surg. 1945;121(6):793–802.
4. Gallagher AG, Lederman AB, McGlade K, Satava RM, Smith CD. Discriminative validity of the Minimally Invasive Surgical Trainer in Virtual Reality (MIST-VR) using criteria levels based on expert performance. Surg Endosc. 2004;18(4):660–5.
5. Gallagher AG, Ritter EM, Champion H, Higgins G, Fried MP, Moses G, Smith CD, Satava RM. Virtual reality simulation for the operating room: proficiency-based training as a paradigm shift in surgical skill training. Ann Surg. 2005;241(2):364–72.
6. www.faa.gov/regulations_policies/handbooks_manuals/aviation/risk_management_handbook/media/rmh_ch02.pdf
7. Fitts FM, Posner MI. Human performance. Belmont: Brooks/Cole Publishing Co; 1967.
8. Esysenck M, Keane M. Cognitive psychology: a student handbook. Hove: Erlbaum; 1995.
9. Banerjee C, Cosentino M, Hatzmann W, Noé KG. Endoscopic intracorporal knotting and suture techniques: talent or experience? Gyn Surg. 2010;7:16_4.
10. Gallagher A, Satava R. Virtual reality as a metric for the assessment of laparoscopic psychomotor skills: learning curves and reliability measures. Surg Endosc. 2002;16:1746–52.
11. Spencer F. Teaching and measuring surgical techniques: the technical evaluation of competence. Bull Am Coll Surg. 1978:9–12.
12. Hier und heute Reportage 2010 ("nähkurs für ärzte").
13. Ritter E, McClusky D, Gallagher A, et al. Objective psychomotor skills assessment of experienced and novice flexible endoscopists with a virtual reality simulator. J Gastrointest Surg. 2003;7:871–8.
14. Club TSS. The learning curve for laparoscopic cholecystectomy. Am J Surg. 1995;170:55–9.
15. Spüntrup C, Noé GK, Spüntrup E. Lernprogramme in der Gynäkologie: learning by doing – aber bitte erst am Modell. Der Frauenarzt. 2012;53(10):952–7.
16. Hanna G, Frank T, Cuschieri A. Objective assessment of endoscopic knot quality. Am J Surg. 1997;174:410–3.
17. Gallagher A, Richie K, McClure N, et al. Objective psychomotor skills assessment of experienced, junior, and novice laparoscopists with virtual reality. World J Surg. 2001;25:1478–83.
18. Darzi A, Smith S, Taffinder N. Assessing operative skill. BMJ. 1999;318:887.
19. Patent Henrickson D. Bellezzo F. US 2014/0072941 A1, Mar 13, 2014.
20. Patent WO 2011/046606 A1 (MIYAZAKI DOUGLAS W US) 21. Apr 2011 (2011-04-21).
21. Hammer N, Löffler S, Feja C, Sandrock M, Schmidt W, Bechmann I, Steinke H. Ethanol-glycerin fixation with thymol conservation: a potential alternative to formaldehyde and phenol embalming. Anat Sci Educ. 2012;5(4):225–33.
22. Hammer N, Löffler S, Bechmann I, Steinke H, Hädrich C, Feja C. Comparison of modified thiel embalming and ethanol-glycerin fixation in an anatomy environment: potentials and limitations of two complementary techniques. Anat Sci Educ. 2015;8(1):74–85.
23. Moglia A, Ferrari V, Morelli L, Ferrari M, Mosca F, Cuschieri A. A systematic review of virtual reality simulators for robot-assisted surgery. Eur Urol. 2015;69(6):1065–80. doi:10.1016/j.eururo.2015.09.021. S0302-2838(15)00929-X. [Epub ahead of print].
24. Liu M, Curet M. A review of training research and virtual reality simulators for the da Vinci surgical system. Teach Learn Med. 2015;27(1):12–26.
25. Rogers DA, Elstein AS, Bordage G. Improving continuing medical education for surgical techniques: applying the lessons learned in the first decade of minimal access surgery. Ann Surg. 2001;233:159–66.

17 Communicative and Ethical Aspects of the Doctor-Patient Relationship in Extreme Situations

Ibrahim Alkatout

Introduction

A doctor's actions constitute the very core of the medical profession. A doctor's actions are, by their very nature, unique, unrepeatable, and irrevocable. The element of irreversibility and constant contact with the patient's biological existence impose an enormous burden of responsibility on the doctor's actions [1]. The residual lack of safety and uncertainty, which cannot be eliminated despite most recent discoveries in medical science and technology, still make it almost impossible for the doctor to guarantee the success he/she intends to achieve [2]. The general purpose of a doctor's actions is to cure an ill person. This includes the prevention of disease as well as its cure, the patient's rehabilitation, palliation, the diagnostic procedures required for these measures, and their consequence, which is the treatment [2]. In order to ensure that the treatment addresses the specific disease as well as the patient's right to individual care, the patient must be viewed in his/her entirety at all times. A successful doctor-patient relationship can be learned and applied in all fields of medicine.

The Doctor-Patient Relationship Is the Basis of All Fields of Interaction

A positively perceived and productive relationship between the doctor and the patient is primarily based on the following three basic attitudes: *empathy* (sensitivity), *congruence* (authenticity) and absolute (unconditional) *esteem* [3].

Assuming that the diseased patient is a self-determined individual, his/her autonomy is in no way reduced by the loss of his/her physical integrity. The doctor and the patient are partners with equal rights; each of them has specific competences and responsibilities.

Empathy

Empathy may be defined as understanding the emotional and cognitive processes of another, the ability to recognize a person's conflicts, feelings and attitudes, and be able to experience the emotions of another [4].

The doctor should, in lieu of the patient, be able to put the latter's feelings into words and determine the patient's needs, which the patient himself/herself may not yet be fully aware of. These processes occur at the emotional and intuitive level in the form of empathy, as well as the cognitive level in the form of comprehension. The therapist's ability to identify himself/herself with the patient for a limited period of time enables the therapist to share the patient's experience. Gestures, facial expression, body posture, the speed of talking, the tone of voice, and other features of non-verbal communication trigger empathy in the interacting partner [5]. Thus, empathy is also an attempt to understand the reasons for another's actions and opinions, based on the latter's view of the world and horizon of experience (Fig. 17.1) [6].

I. Alkatout
Gynecology and Obstetrics,
University Hospitals Schleswig-Holstein,
Campus Kiel, Kiel, Germany
e-mail: ibrahim.alkatout@uksh.de

I. Alkatout, L. Mettler (eds.), *Hysterectomy*, DOI 10.1007/978-3-319-22497-8_17

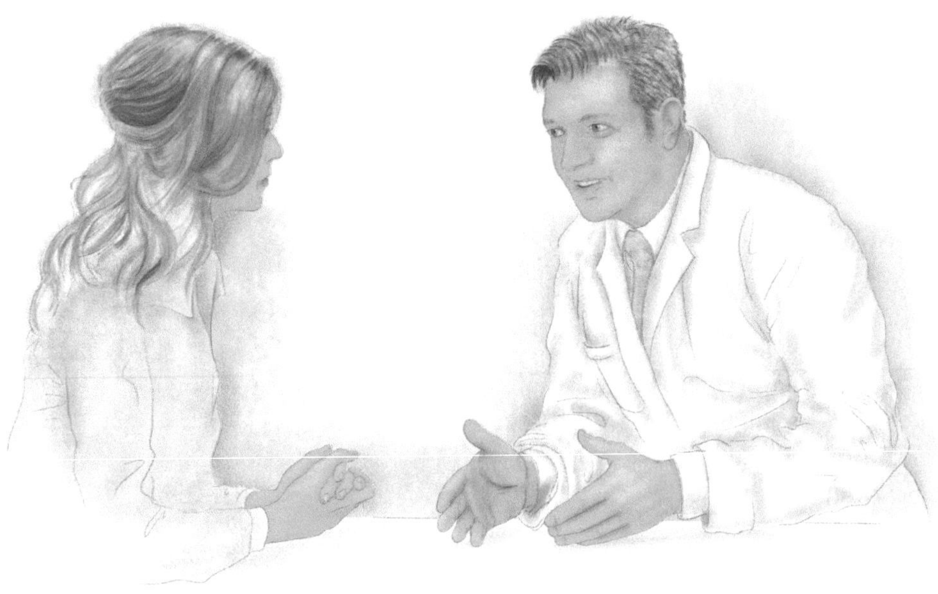

Fig. 17.1 Authentic empathic setting in preoperative counseling based on congruence and esteem

Congruence (Authenticity)

Congruence (authenticity) refers to the therapist's attitude: he/she is entirely sincere towards the patient, without any deception of himself/herself or the patient. The doctor is aware of his feelings at all times and can communicate these to the patient if necessary [4].

Thus, the doctor-patient relationship incorporates the therapist's authentic communication towards the patient. Authenticity refers to everything the doctor feels and experiences, those parts of his/her feelings and experiences he/she is aware of, and those parts he/she eventually communicates. Thus the therapist is able to access his own thoughts and feelings towards the client and the therapy situation [7]. The therapy principle of authenticity makes it necessary for the doctor to render his identity (which differs from that of the patient) transparent to the patient, answer questions sincerely, and seek opportunities to face the patient and communicate with him/her [7, 8].

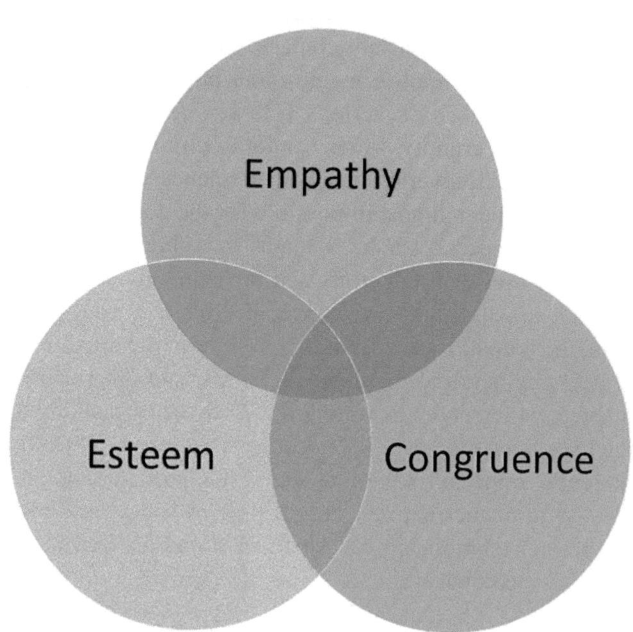

Fig. 17.2 The doctor-patient relationship is the basis of all fields of interaction. It is founded on the three cornerstones of empathy (sensitivity), congruence (authenticity), and absolute (unconditional) esteem

Unconditional Positive Esteem (Unreserved Acceptance)

A relationship of unconditional positive esteem is marked by trust, appreciation and respect; these qualities form the foundation of the doctor-patient relationship [8].

The patient is welcomed and accepted, independent of what he/she says and how he/she behaves at the present time. This unrestricted acceptance is incompatible with an attitude expressing judgment, dislike or disapproval, or even a selectively expressed esteem of another (depending on the contents of the conversation). Unconditional acceptance consolidates the therapeutic relationship, promotes one's experience of self-respect, and mobilizes the patient's own resources. The doctor focuses his entire attention on the patient and confirms the patient's ambitions by acknowledgement, encouragement, and expressions of solidarity and concern. The patient's communication is accepted exactly as expressed by the patient, and is not questioned further [8]. This gives the patient the certainty he/she needs in order to fully experience his/her feelings at the moment, although the therapist is still obliged to align his/her experience to his/her values [5] (Fig. 17.2).

Creating the Doctor-Patient Relationship

The doctor's professional rule of conduct has existed since the antique ages of medicine: *primum non nocere* (above all, you should do no harm).[1] The principle of *Nonmaleficience* or prevention of damage is, in addition to the *patient's autonomy*, the *patient's wellbeing* and *justice*, one of the four ethical guiding principles of decision-making by a doctor. The art of ethical judgement is derived from a balance of these four basic principles: dispensing with harmful interventions (*primum non nocere*), respecting the patient's self-determined decision (*voluntas aegroti*), ensuring that any medical measures serve the preservation and improvement of the patient's mental and physical health (*benevolence*); and being just in one's actions (*fairness*) [9, 10]. The four principles incorporate a number of explicit, implicit and potential standards, which may contradict each other in many ways but result in a coherentistic approach in terms of application [9, 11, 12].

Self-Determined Decision (The Patient's Autonomy)

The term autonomy is derived from the Greek words *autos* (self) and *nomos* (law, rule), and means self-legislation or self-determination. It was initially used to express the self-determination and self-government of independent city states of the antique period. Kant regarded the autonomy of practical reason as the commitment of human will – driven by the legitimate categorical imperative – to assign greater importance to unconditional obligation than to primordial intentions.

Preconditions for autonomous decisions are the following:

1. *Awareness*: Being able to understand the issue in question
2. *Competence*: The ability to inspect, judge, and make decisions; in other words, to be competent
3. *Freedom*: To make one's decision without the controlling influence of another, and also implement one's decision.

In the medical context, autonomy is the ability to act freely in regard of one's own mental and physical matters. The contrary term *heteronomy* refers to dependence and external determination. Promotion and restoration of one's ability to exercise self-determinism is one of the major goals of medical action [13]. Respect for autonomy, in its minimal form, is expressed as respect for the basic rights of the patient. The relationship between the doctor and the patient must ensure asymmetry between action and suffering on the one hand, and symmetry of self-determinism and freedom of action on the other [14]. The doctor-patient relationship is outlined in three basic models: (1) *Paternalistic model*, (2) *Contractual or Client Model*, and (3) *Partnership model*. External influences exist due to secularization, economization, and technological developments in medicine on the one hand, and the changing values of our pluralistic society on the other. The diverse and variable *models of relationship* differ especially in regard of the criterion of trust and the actual degree of patient autonomy in the respective interaction. We are concerned with the communication requirements to be fulfilled by the doctor [15, 16].

[1] The dictum is attributed to the Roman physician Scribonius Largus, court physician of the emperor Tiberius Claudius Nero Caesar Drusus who ruled Rome around 50 A.D. A similar phrase is also found in the Corpus Hippocraticum (Epidemics, Book I, Section XI).

Techniques of Conducting a Doctor's Conversation with the Patient from the Viewpoint of Autonomy

The core aspects of a successful conversation conducted by the doctor with the patient include, above all, active listening, determining the structure of the conversation, as well as identifying and resolving difficult patterns of interaction.

1. Active listening. Techniques of active listening are summarized in Table 17.1.
2. Determining the structure of the conversation. *Transparency* is a basic instrument for structuring the conversation and adhering to the time frame. This includes transparency of the elements of the conversation, such as providing information about the steps of the treatment, the necessary medical informatioin, and informing the patient as to why a step is being performed. The transparency of basic conditions includes informing the patient about potential disorders and the time frame of the conversation. Transparency concerning the individual phases of the conversation enables the patient to differentiate between doctor-centered and patient-centered sections of the conversation.

The conversation can be reflected on and corrected through *metacommunicative statements*. Metacommunicative statements concern the content of the conversation, the style of conversation, the positions of those conducting the conversation, and problems in the doctor-patient relationship.

3. Identifying and resolving complex patterns of interaction. Harmonious communication patterns are oriented to the anticipated reactions of one's counterpart. This calls for a

Table 17.1 Techniques of active listening

Active listening	
Let the patient finish speaking	The first few minutes form the basis of the relationship. Active listening is encouraging and delivers valuable information
Ask open questions	Open questions yield comprehensive information, clarify associations, and provide background data beyond the actual facts of the case
Inquire	Problems of comprehension can be addressed immediately
Balance pros and cons	Helps to determine the patient's priorities or encourages him to think about them. Especially by explaining why a step is being given preferences
Pause	Short pauses (about 3 s) have a relieving effect. The patient thinks of data he/she had ignored until now
Encourage the patient to speak further	Echoing or nonverbal communication (nodding, eye contact, body facing the patient) signalizes one's presence
Paraphrase (repeat)	Focus on those parts of the patient's statements that are most significant (verbal accompaniment) and thus open new perspectives
Summarize what has been said	Agreement between the doctor and the patient by expressing longer portions of the conversation in one's own words
Reflect emotions	Address emotions verbally in the form of a suggestion

high degree of flexibility and thorough knowledge of role expectations. Interaction may be disrupted by inadequate social competence, fixation on oneself, or distorted perception of social behavior.

Individual Requirements of the Doctor in a Patient-Centered Doctor-Patient Relationship

A successful doctor-patient relationship is the foundation of any successful treatment and the breeding ground for sustained satisfaction in the professional existence of a doctor.

The action-guiding *obligations of a doctor* include the willingness to take responsibility, confidentiality, and authenticity. Action-guiding *virtues of a doctor* are patience, empathy, compassion, and the willingness to help. Finally, one needs to work out what the various optional decisions mean in terms of obligations towards third parties. In this context one needs to consider the patient's family members and close friends, as well as the entire community of the insured person [17].

Very urgent decisions and chronic diseases are the easiest to handle from the ethical point of view. In highly acute situations, such as emergencies, the responsibility of decisions is still handed over to the doctor without considering the patient's opinion (accepted paternalism). In this setting the patient is informed of the bare essentials, without disregarding the his/her right of self-determination. Even when the patient's ability to help himself/herself is on the decline and the patient needs help and care to an increasing extent, as in old age frailty and/or cognitive impairment, his/her modified autonomy should be accompanied by a high degree of empathy on the part of the doctor concerning the putative will of the patient. Chronic diseases differ from this approach in that a satisfactory outcome of care and the required degree of compliance can only be achieved cooperatively by the doctor and the patient. The less urgent the decision is, the more responsibility one may assign to the patient; in this setting decisions can be made in accordance with the *shared decision-making model* (Fig. 17.3) [18]. The degree of autonomy depends on the momentary and general condition of the individual patient (such as the patient's mental condition, degree of intellectual differentiation, severity of symptoms, severity of disease), and must be adapted to the current situation. The patient's values (estimation of the disease, will, concept of life) should be viewed along with the values of his environment (the patient's living environment, the treatment team) and the values of society (implicit values, institutionalized values). Even if the patient's living values are clear, there may be ambiguity concerning what is meaningful, appropriate, and beneficial for the patient.

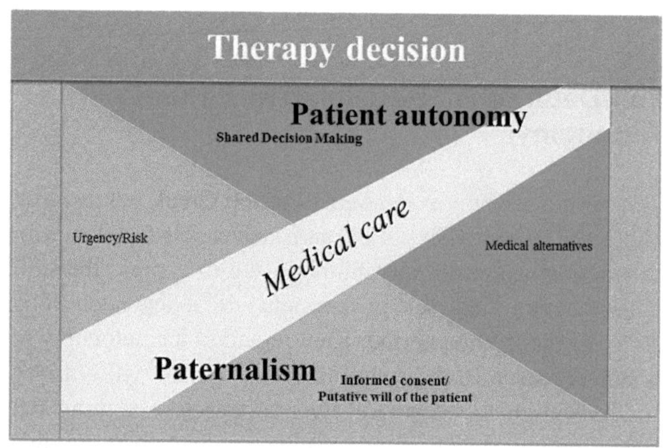

Fig. 17.3 Reciprocal flow diagram of paternalism and Informed Consent on the one hand, and patient autonomy and Shared Decision Making on the other. Dependent variables are medically equivalent alternatives and the medical urgency or risk for the patient. Medical care should respect the patient's wellbeing as well as his/her will

In many medical situations, the relationship between the doctor and the patient remains no more than an idealized behavior pattern. Many situations are rendered complex by the indefinite prognosis of acute diseases, especially when the initiated maximal therapy has not been successful and the doctor contemplates a change in the goals of treatment. However, particularly such extreme situations call for mastery over, and the application of, medico- ethical principles.

Borderline Situations in Dealing with Aged Patients and Those with Cognitive Impairment (Dementia)

The rising number of aged patients and those with cognitive impairment (dementia) permits complete patient autonomy in a very small number of cases. However, demographic developments necessitate the establishment of applicable concepts that will do justice to the altered spectrum of morbidity, which includes a rise in chronic diseases and multimorbid conditions. When coordinating the medical reports and other collected data with the individual patient's value system and also when considering the available resources in a specific case, the treatment team needs to employ a high degree of empathy and respect for the patient's autonomy. Again, it may be necessary to re-check and ensure congruency between the medical approach and the patient's concept of living, and make the respective putative decisions anew [19, 20].

Borderline Situations in Dealing with Psychiatric Patients, Young Children, and Mentally Challenged Persons

According to the principle of autonomy, young children, psychiatric patients and less gifted persons also have the right to be informed comprehensively. On the other hand, a comprehensive explanation may involve potential harm or delay in all three groups. Therefore, in the patient's interest many decisions about him/her are made on his/her behalf. When making serious decisions one must integrate the patient to the greatest possible degree. Consulting and including family members and caregivers is especially relevant in these situations. Showing empathy and sympathy for the patient and the family, answering questions, and explaining the medical treatment are highly valued aspects in this setting [21].

The Doctor-Patient Relationship in Oncology

Tumor patients are typical candidates for patient-centered doctor-patient communication. Cancer patients need a great deal of information about their disease, its consequences, and the available options. In many cases, the treating doctor and the patient share an intensive and long-term relationship. Therapy decisions are of long duration and have far-reaching consequences on the patient's quality of life and the prognosis of his/her disease. The doctor's task and responsibilities in providing medical assistance for cancer patients involves, to a much greater extent now than ever before, inviting the patient's active participation in decisions regarding treatment [22].

In 1819 Goethe wrote in *West-Östlichen Diwan (West-Eastern Divan)*: "What I thank Allah most for? That he has made a division between suffering and knowing. Any ill person would be desperate if he knew the disease as thoroughly as the doctor does".[2]

Slevin et al. were able to show that, in apparently hopeless situations, cancer patients are much more willing to undergo stressful chemotherapy with minimal chances of cure than the medical personnel in charge of their treatment would be willing to subject them to such treatment. Also with regard to the prolongation of overall survival and the improvement of quality of life, the acceptance threshold of severe side effects is highly underestimated (Table 17.2) [23]. Although many ill persons will accept a stressful treatment that prolongs their lives by a few months or provides brief symptomatic relief, some patients refuse to undergo a stressful therapy although the prognosis of their disease may be quite favorable [24]. Achievement of the goals of therapy, in this case, is not dependent on the effects or the efficacy of therapeutic measures alone, but is subject to a positive evaluation of the treatment by the patient [25].

Patient-centered medicine includes the ability to deliver bad news. Communications about impending death and statements about the significance of a disease or death are major challenges for the doctor and the patient. Empathy, congruence, and unrestrained respect for the patient when delivering bad news have culminated, for instance, in the SPIKES protocol described by Baile (Table 17.3) [26].

Questions to establish one's estimation of the patient's perception include, for instance, "What do you know about your medical situation so far?" or "What is your understanding of the reasons we wish to do the investigation?"

Table 17.2 The threshold likelihood (in percentage) of cure, prolongation of life, or symptomatic relief: the point from which patients are willing to accept chemotherapy associated with severe side effects and complications. This survey was conducted among cancer patients as well as a group of doctors and nursing staff [23]

	Patient	Therapist
Chances of cure	1 %	10–50 %
Prolongation of life	12 months	12–60 months
Alleviation of symptoms	10 %	50–70 %

[2]In: Johann Wolfgang von Goethe: *West-Östlicher Diwan*, Frankfurt am Main 1999, page 47.

Table 17.3 The SPIKES model. A six-step protocol for delivering bad news. This is a tool for obtaining information about the patient's current level of knowledge. He/she can also be informed about medical facts, depending on his/her need for information, support can be expressed, and suitable options can be rendered accessible. Finally, a treatment plan can be drafted in cooperation with the patient

SPIKES	Steps	Contents
S	1. Setting up the interview	Arrange for some privacy Involve significant others Sit down Avoid interruptions
P	2. Assessing the patient's perception	Open questions to assess the patient's current perception (avoid misunderstandings early)
I	3. Obtaining the patient's invitation	Assess the patient's willingness to receive bad news Mention that the patient can speak to the doctor at a later point in time
K	4. Giving knowledge and information	Warning before delivering bad news Optimizing communication
E	5. Addressing the patient's emotions with empathic responses	Empathic statements express support
S	6. Strategy and Summary	Depends on level of wellbeing Discuss the next steps

To better estimate the ability of one's counterpart to receive bad news, it may be useful to ask questions like "How would you like me to give the information about the test results? Would you like me to give you all the information or sketch out the results and spend more time discussing the treatment plan?" To warn the patient before delivering bad news, one could try to steer the conversation, "Unfortunately I've got some bad news to tell you…" or "I'm sorry to tell you that …". While speaking to the patient, it would be advisable to make repeated and active attempts to optimize the conversation. This includes alignment of one's language to the patient's vocabulary and omitting specialized medical terms. Excessive directness should be avoided, and the required or desired information should be given in small units. The level of communication can be further improved by avoiding phrases like "There's nothing more we can do for you." Empathic statements in these exceptional situations express support. Specifically, the patient is helped when emotions are registered, named, and identified (such as grief, anger or shock). The patient is also helped when the doctor signalizes that the patient may express himself/herself. Agreeing upon a plan of treatment simultaneously makes the patient feel that his/her wishes are being taken into account; it also avoids misunderstanding, uncertainty and anxiety (Fig. 17.4).

The Doctor-Patient Relationship in Obstetrics from the Invasive Point of View

Obstetrics and prenatal medicine constitute an equally important part of our spectrum of activities. In contrast to gynecology, the doctor is called upon to bear responsibilities beyond the patient's scope of action. High-risk pregnancies have risen greatly in the last few years because of improved procedures in reproduction medicine. Maternal diseases may become consolidated or be exacerbated during pregnancy. The increasing complexity of this subject calls for interdisciplinary management and imposes the highest medico-ethical demands on our specialty.

In addition to the medico-ethical questions of the mother, the demands of the unborn child also must be taken into account. A crucial aspect of decision-making when dealing with the unborn child is the moral status an embryo must achieve in order to be granted specific rights – such as the right to live – as a practical subject. The fundamental rights granted to nascent life and the consequent legal protection that goes with these can be described in different ways [27].

1. *The species argument*: All members of the biological species known as *Homo sapiens* and, in fact, only this species, are entitled to human dignity and the comprehensive legal and moral protection that go with it.
2. *Potentiality argument*: The potential of entire human development is present in the primary cells. An embryo, which normally develops into a human being, is therefore worthy of protection and possesses the same moral characteristics as the fully developed human being.
3. *Identity argument*: The human embryo/fetus has the same rights as the persons they will become in the normal course of life, because the two are basically identical. The identity of the developed individual results from the composite of cells he/she evolves from.
4. *Continuity argument*: The process of development that starts with nidation is a continuous process with no sharp divisions and therefore does not permit any specific demarcation of the stages of development. Despite the

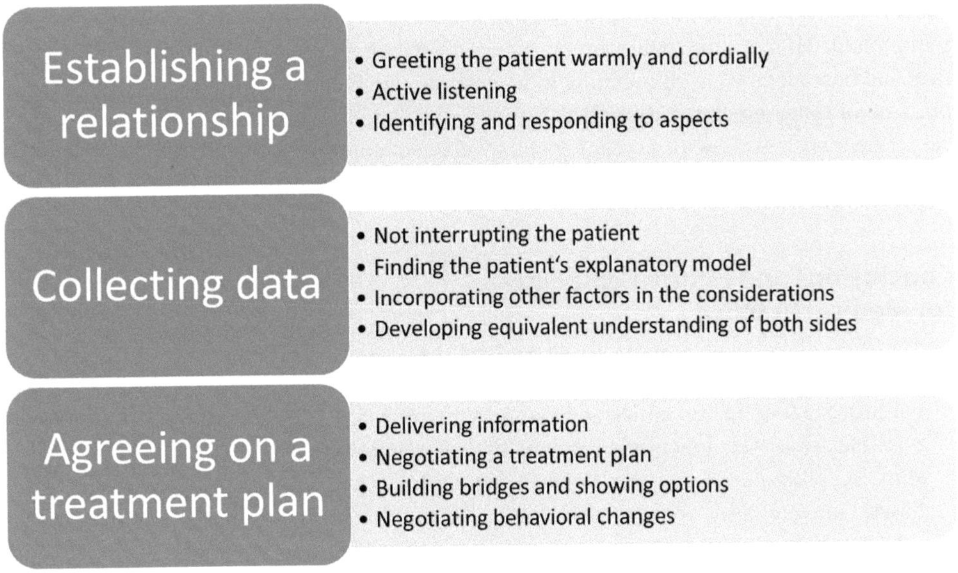

Fig. 17.4 Three functions of a doctor's consultation

Establishing a relationship	• Greeting the patient warmly and cordially • Active listening • Identifying and responding to aspects
Collecting data	• Not interrupting the patient • Finding the patient's explanatory model • Incorporating other factors in the considerations • Developing equivalent understanding of both sides
Agreeing on a treatment plan	• Delivering information • Negotiating a treatment plan • Building bridges and showing options • Negotiating behavioral changes

continuity of human development from the very start, one can identifiy various stages of development whose demarcations, however, are blurred.

Fetomaternal conflicts result from the need to set priorities regarding the wellbeing of the expectant mother or the future child. Once the moral and ethical status of both parents and their right of self-determination have been established, it will be necessary to register the moral and ethical status of the unborn child. Any decision in favor of one would be accompanied by neglect of the other. Equal treatment of the interests and possessions of the unborn child and the future parents is practically impossible. Once the individuality of the embryo starts to take shape – which would be at the time of insemination or later – the individual possesses complete human dignity and must be protected accordingly. From this time on, the existence of the human being and his/her individuality is determined by the uniqueness of his/her genetic material. Based on the ethical principle of autonomy, one is obliged to justify any hindrance to self-determined life and protect the value of freedom. However, embryos and fetuses are unable to make competent decisions and are therefore incapable of moral, independent, and autonomous action or decisions – which, however, are essential for the self-determined decision-making process. Therefore, *competent representatives* have to make decisions on their behalf. The representative also has to align the child's value system with general ethical considerations in order to make appropriate decisions in keeping with the presumed life concept of the unborn child. Thus, a person who makes decisions for others is especially obliged to adhere to ethical principles, standards and criteria.

Given these facts, many prenatal diagnostic and obstetric situations pose a dilemma because it is impossible to act in the interests of the embryo or fetus as well as the expectant mother, not do them any harm, preserve their autonomy, and behave in a just manner. The options of action from the medico-ethical point of view would be quite clear if the unborn child's right to live would be ranked secondary to the expectant mother's. These questions are not, by any means, conclusively clarified at the present time.

Since parents are those who have to live with their decisions in favor of one of the courses of action and its respective dramatic consequences, they should be given all of the tools that enable them to make a sustainable decision. These include, in addition to the medical information provided by an interdisciplinary team of doctors (obstetrics, human genetics, prenatal diagnosis, neonatology, pediatrics), information about further decision-making aids and about tools for coping with the conflict-ridden situation.

Endangerment of the Doctor-Patient Relationship

The atmosphere of trust created by both of these parties is currently at risk of being lost forever. Three factors are worthy of mention in this regard. *Increasing anonymity* is a result of increasingly complex infrastructures. The patient is compelled to surrender his relationship with his treating physician and share his existence as an ill person as well as his doctor (a confidant) with the entire institution. *Juridification*, by which the doctor-patient relationship is subject to an increasing degree of legal control. The third source of uncertainty is *probabilization*. Statements about the disease process can only be made with certain degrees of probability.

Industrialization and the enhancement of efficiency in the health care system through measurable performance have, in many instances, reduced non-measurable medical services to a minimum. Higher-level optimization processes, technocracy and bureaucracy are culminating in an unsurmountable pressure of time, which is partly offset by specialized medical services such as those of psychologists, specialized nursing staff, or social workers.

Conclusions and Future Perspectives for Medical Practice

Decision-making in medical treatment is an individual process founded on ethics and can only be rendered possible by a well-functioning doctor-patient relationship. A prerequisite for the latter is communication based on empathy, congruence, and unconditional esteem. With a foundation of this nature, the patient and the doctor will be able to strive for the patient's wellbeing while preserving the patient's autonomy, avoid damage or injustice, and tread a common pathway, ideally as partners, which would lead to sustained satisfaction – also from the doctor's point of view – and render the two extremes of paternalism and contractual action unnecessary. In the majority of situations, the basic demands of the two parties must be weighed against each other and may not be achieved simultaneously. In the joint process of decision-making, it will be necessary to strike a compromise between the respective non-negotiable principles.

References

1. Wieland W. Strukturwandel der Medizin und ärztliche Ethik – philosophische Überlegungen zu Grundfragen einer praktischen Wissenschaft. Heidelberg: Universitätsverlag; 1986.
2. Gethmann CF. Gesundheit nach Maß? Eine transdisziplinäre Studie zu den Grundlagen eines dauerhaften Gesundheitssystems. Berlin: Akademie Verlag GmbH; 2004.
3. Rogers CR. Therapeut und Klient: Grundlagen der Gesprächspsychotherapie. 20th ed. Frankfurt: Fischer Verlag; 1983.
4. Mittelstraß J. Enzyklopädie: Philosophie und Wissenschaftstheorie . Stuttgart: J.B. Metzler Verlag; 2004.Special Edition ed
5. Argyle M. Körpersprache und Kommunikation: Das Handbuch zur nonverbalen Kommunikation. 9th ed. Junfermann Verlag: Paderborn; 2005.
6. Geisler LS. Patient autonomy–a critical concept analysis. Dtsch Med Wochenschr. 2004;129(9):453–6.
7. Rogers CR. Entwicklung der Persönlichkeit. 13 th ed. Stuttgart: Klett-Cotta; 1996.
8. Finke J. Gesprächspychotherapie – Grundlagen und spezifische Anwendungen. 3rd ed. Stuttgart: Georg Thieme Verlag; 2004.
9. Beauchamp TL, Childress JF. Principles of Biomedical Ethics. 6th ed. New York, Oxford: Oxford University Press; 2009.
10. Smith CM. Origin and uses of primum non nocere–above all, do no harm! J Clin Pharmacol. 2005;45(4):371–7.
11. Schöne-Seifert B. Medizinethik. In: Nida-Rümelin J, editor. Angewandte Ethik. Die Bereichsethiken und ihre theoretische Fundierung. Ein Handbuch. 2nd ed. Stuttgart: Alfred Kröner Verlag; 2005. p. 690–803.
12. Alkatout I, Rummer A. Intrauterines Lebensrecht von Zwillingen mit ungleichen Überlebenschancen – Kommentar zum Fall. Ethik in der Medizin. 2011;23(3):233–4.
13. Gabl C, Jox RJ. Paternalism and autonomy–no contradiction. Wien Med Wochenschr. 2008;158(23–24):642–9.
14. Marckmann G, Bormuth M. Arzt-Patient-Verhältnis und Informiertes Einverständnis. In: Wiesing U, editor. Ethik in der Medizin. Ein Reader. Stuttgart: Philipp Reclam; 2000. p. 76–85.
15. Krones T, Richter G. Physicians' responsibility: doctor-patient relationship. Bundesgesundheitsblatt Gesundheitsforschung Gesundheitsschutz. 2008;51(8):818–26.
16. von Engelhardt D. Ethik in der Onkologie – Dem kranken Menschen gerecht werden. Im Focus Onkologie. 2006;09:65–8.
17. Marckmann G, Mayer F. Ethische Fallbesprechungen in der Onkologie – Grundlagen einer prinzipienorientierten Falldiskussion. Der Onkologe. 2009;10(15):980–8.
18. Krones T, Richter G. Die Arzt-Patient-Beziehung. In: Schulz S, Seigleder K, Fangerau H, NW P, editors. Geschichte, Theorie und Ethik der Medizin. Frankfurt am Main: Suhrkamp Verlag; 2006. p. 94–117.
19. Wolf E, Lahrmann H. The seriously affected stroke patient who is not able to communicate – treatment to the best of one's knowledge and ethical principles. Wien Med Wochenschr. 2014;164(9–10):195–200.
20. Meran JG. Palliative care and quality of life as therapy goal. Wien Med Wochenschr. 2012;162(1–2):1–2.
21. Espinel AG, Shah RK, Beach MC, Boss EF. What parents say about their child's surgeon: parent-reported experiences with pediatric surgical physicians. JAMA Otolaryngol Head Neck Surg. 2014;140(5):397–402.
22. Hahn J, Mandraka F, Fröhlich G. Ethische Aspekte in der Therapie kritisch kranker Tumorpatienten. Intensivmedizin und Notfallmedizin. 2007;44(7):416–28.
23. Slevin ML, Stubbs L, Plant HJ, Wilson P, Gregory WM, Armes PJ, et al. Attitudes to chemotherapy: comparing views of patients with cancer with those of doctors, nurses, and general public. BMJ. 1990;300(6737):1458–60.
24. Silvestri G, Pritchard R, Welch HG. Preferences for chemotherapy in patients with advanced non-small cell lung cancer: descriptive study based on scripted interviews. BMJ. 1998;317(7161):771–5.
25. Krones CJ, Willis S, Steinau G, Schumpelick V. Current patient perceptions of the physician. Chirurg. 2006;77(8):718–24.
26. Baile WF, Buckman R, Lenzi R, Glober G, Beale EA, Kudelka AP. SPIKES-A six-step protocol for delivering bad news: application to the patient with cancer. Oncologist. 2000;5(4):302–11.
27. Schulz S. Person oder Keim? Der moralische Status des Ungeborenen in der Geschichte der Abtreibungsdiskussion. In: Schulz S, Seigleder K, Fangerau H, NW P, editors. Geschichte, Theorie und Ethik der Medizin. Frankfurt am Main: Suhrkamp Verlag; 2006. p. 303–15.

Part VI

Macroscopic and Microscopic Pathological Aspects

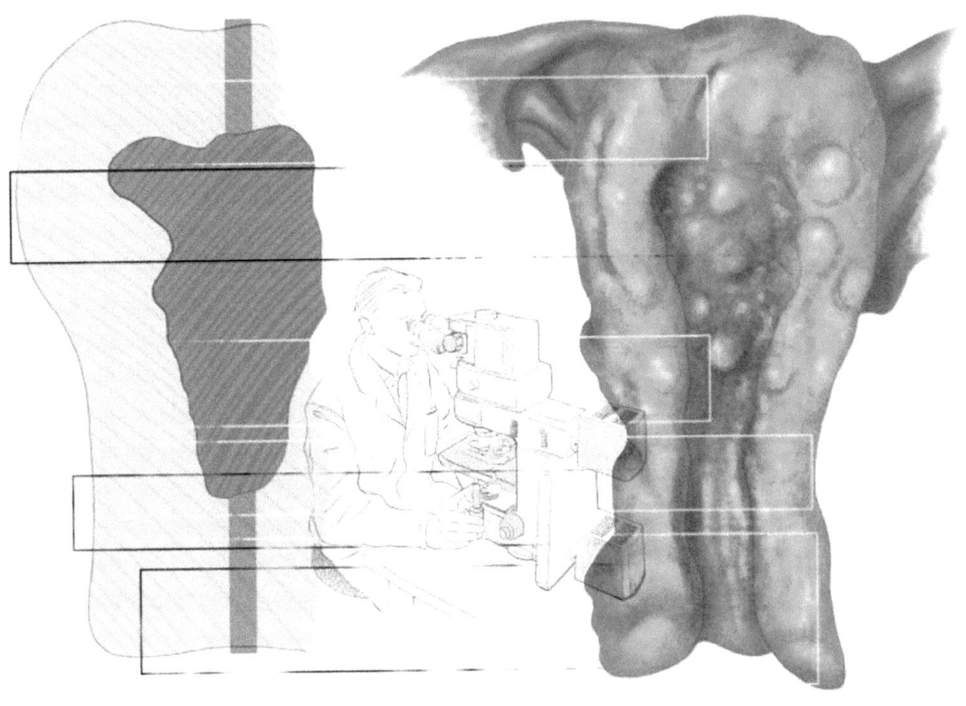

Processing and Histopathological Workup of Hysterectomy Specimens

18

Lars-Christian Horn and Anne K. Höhn

Introduction

The challenges of histopathology have been changed dramatically during the last years. The pathologist nowadays is a diagnostic oncologist and in the majority of the cases the management of patients is influenced by the histopathology report so, the surgical pathologist performs a "background treatment" of the patient.

The histopathologic report is one cornerstone and within the majority of cases the basement of quality control and decision making for adjuvant treatment and guides the selection of appropriate approach in additional treatment, especially in patients suffering malignant disease.

The gross description of a resection specimen is one important, if not the most important, part in several cases of the entire surgical pathology report.

The following chapter describes an approach of gross examination and the method of reporting the pathologic findings for benign and malignant gynaecologic diseases within hysterectomies, guided by the clinical principles of patient management, focussing on a concise report to guide the decision makings in multidisciplinary meetings.

Crosstalk Between Clinicians and Treating Pathologists

The surgical pathology report gives the final diagnosis and includes specific information about the success of surgical treatment and just in case about prognosis and treatment. So, the "treating pathologist" must have sufficient familiarity with the management of obstetric and gynaecologic disorders to assure that the report, as its major focus, communicates the clinically relevant information [143].

But, the quality of the histopathological report is mainly influenced by the available clinical information. Some important points of interaction between the clinicians and the surgical pathologist should be addressed.

The gynaecologic surgeon has seen the situation and the disease in vivo in conjunction with several anatomic landmarks. These landmarks cannot be reconstructed by the pathologist within the laboratory. So, it is absolutely necessary that the gynaecologist communicates important intraoperative findings on the requisition sheet. For proper orientation of the specimen in the lab, a marking of relevant structures/landmarks/resection margins on focus on the resection specimen (e.g. by sutures) is mandatory. Especially in complex resection specimens, special requirements of the gynaecologic surgeon, special intraoperative findings and a proper orientation of the specimen will directly influence how the pathologist will handle and process the specimen postoperatively at the cutting room. This is also the case during intraoperative frozen section analysis.

Intraoperative frozen section examination of a specimen should guide the operation procedure by evaluation the status of resection margins and the extent of the disease. Unnecessary frozen sections should be avoided to cut the costs and save manpower. It should be recognised that frozen section analysis present a preliminary method and is not as good as permanent sections from any tissue [37, 47]. The overall accuracy of frozen section analysis has tested and proved on numerous occasions, both in university and community hospitals with good results [121, 144]. A review, sponsored by the College of American Pathologists covering over 90,000 frozen sections, performed at 461 institutions showed a concordance rate with permanent sections of 98.6 % [144]. Given limited sampling, frequent paucity of clinical information and the various artifacts introduced by the freezing process, the technique is remarkable accurate but not perfect. So, the diagnosis of frozen section examina-

L.-C. Horn (✉) • A.K. Höhn
Division of Breast, Perinatal & Gynecologic Pathology, Institute of Pathology, University Hospital of Leipzig, Leipzig 04103, Germany
e-mail: hornl@medizin.uni-leipzig.de; Annekathrin.hoehn@medizin.uni-leipzig.de

I. Alkatout, L. Mettler (eds.), *Hysterectomy*, DOI 10.1007/978-3-319-22497-8_18

tion might be changed after examination of the whole specimen by permanent slides.

The surgical specimen will be examined and described at the cutting room. For frozen section analyses and the selection of tissue blocks for the histopathologic examination the tissue will be sliced and dissected. During the cutting of the specimen it will be distorted and a complete reconstruction in context with all structures removed will be impossible.

The examined tissue will be stored for several weeks. Then, the tissue will be discarded under the line of legal regulations. So, there is no way to return to the specimen for re-examination and/or additional embedding of tissue after that time. This means for the clinician to contact your pathologist as early as possible if there are any questions regarding the specimen and its histopathological report.

Proper fixation of surgical specimens is an absolutely prerequisite for adequate handling and processing of the tissue. Improper fixation causes problems in cutting the paraffin blocks, sadly influences the quality of H&E-staining (Fig. 18.1a, b) and may cause false-negative or false-positive results in immunohistochemical staining (Fig. 18.1d, e; [98, 140]). Improper fixation may also cause problems in moleculapathologic analyses [98, 120]. Formalin-based fixatives are most commonly used today. For proper fixation 10 % buffered formalin should be used. The relationship between specimen size and the amount of formalin used should be 1:10.

In therapeutic resections a larger amount of tissue will be resected within each individual specimen. The formalin-based fixation works by the penetration of the formalin in the tissue from the periphery to its centre with a speed of ~0.1 cm per hour [29]. So, a minimum of about 12 h for medium sized specimens (simple hysterectomy) and a minimum of 24 h for larger specimens (e.g. radical hysterectomies, exenteration specimens) will be needed for proper fixation. The processing of the specimen and its histopathological interpretation (without additional immunohistochemical stains) needs about 24–48 h. This timeline (Fig. 18.2) should be kept in mind by the clinician for proper information of the patient. In complex therapeutic resections, some information will be available earlier as the result from frozen section examination (e.g. status of the resection margins, dignity of the lesion). Additionally, some patients will need intensive or intermediate-care after operation procedure. So, in almost all cases with extended gynaecologic surgery there will be no need to rush up the pathologist. The major points of the crosstalk between pathologists and clinicians are summarised in Table 18.1.

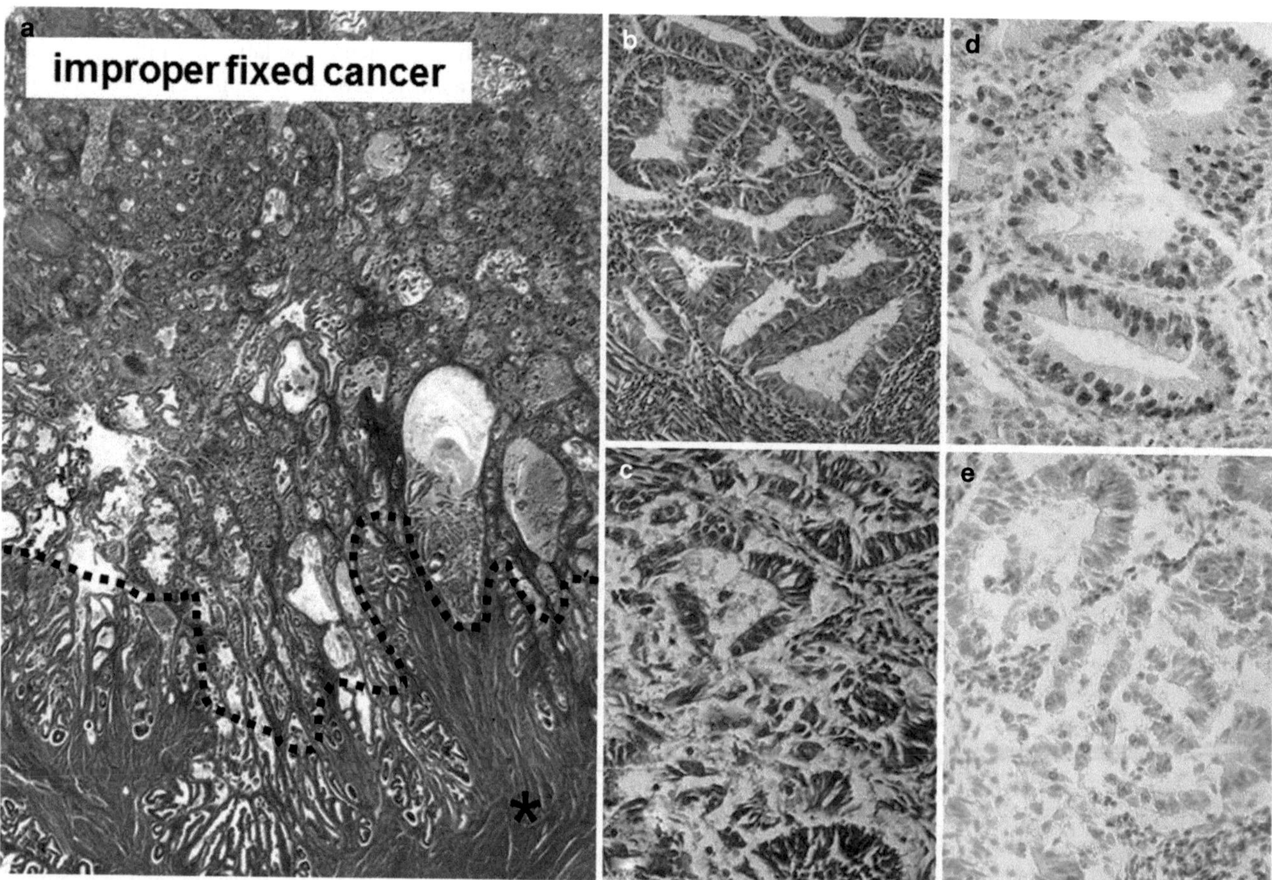

Fig. 18.1 Impact of fixation on morphology. (**a**) Poorly fixed endometrioid adenocarcinoma within a hysterectomy specimen above the dotted line. The cancer below the *dotted line* in proximity to myometrium (*asterix*) is well fixed. (**b**, **c**) Well fixed cancer and improper fixed cancer; the latter one represents with fragmented glands. (**d**, **e**) well defined immunohistochemical staining of the proper fixed cancer cell nuclei (**d**) and invalid staining for estrogen receptor within the poorly fixed tumor cells (**e**)

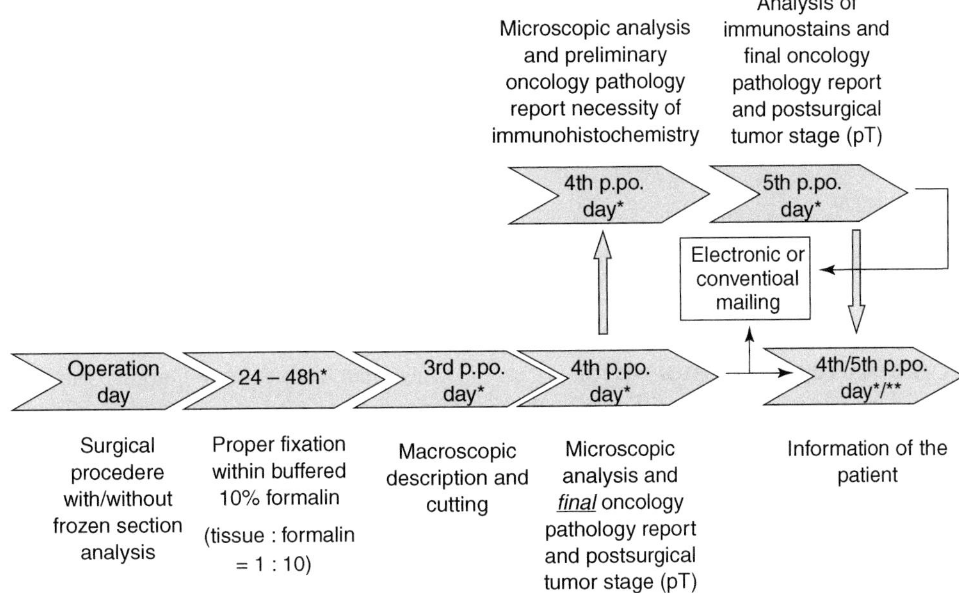

Fig. 18.2 Approximative timeline for building the final pathology oncology report for hysterectomy specimens

Table 18.1 Major points within the dialog between the gynaecologic surgeon and the gynaecologic surgical pathologist (for details see text)

Needs from the clinician	Why needed by the pathologist
1. **Anamnestic/clinical data**	
Anamnestic data about malignancies	Proper interpretation of the findings,
	Proper selection of immunohistochemical stains
If available, tumor markers should be given on the requisition sheet	Proper interpretation of the findings,
	Proper selection of immunohistochemical stains
Technique used in surgical approach	Proper interpretation and description of the specimen, quality control of surgical management and pathological workup
Special intraoperative findings should be communicated on the requisition sheet	Proper orientation and handling of the specimen
Relevant structures/landmarks/resection margins should be marked by sutures	Proper orientation and handling of the specimen
Contact your pathologist as early as possible in case of questions or re-orders	In-time re-examination and re-cutting, before the tissue is discarded
2. **Frozen section (FS) examination**	
Prevent "unnecessary" frozen sections	Prevention of tissue destruction
	Prevent loss of diagnostic relevant tissue
Guide FS analyses by marking the relevant resection margins by sutures and ask clear questions on requisition sheet	Reducing the stress level of the pathologist
	Reducing the time necessary for FS
	Reducing the number of FS-blocks
3. **Pre-analytic variables**	
Use of 10 % buffered formalin for fixation	Improved quality of (immuno-) stains and moleculas analyser
Adequate relation between tissue and formaline 1:10	Improved quality of (immuno-) stains and moleculas analyser
Give adequate time-line for the fixation, processing and histopathologic interpretation of complex surgical specimens	Proper quality of staining and interpretation

Table 18.2 Issues for frozen section examination in endometrial cancer and its relative risk for lymph node involvement [5, 147, 183]

Feature	Relative increase for lymph node involvement
Invasion of the outer half of the myometrium	5×
Involvement of the cervical stroma	4×
Ovarian/adnexal involvement	4×
Grade 3 endometrioid carcinoma	3×
Serous/clear cell histology	3×

General Aspects of Cutup for Pathologists

The techniques of the cutup of resection specimens, i.e. its gross description and cutting and processing, should be guided by the needs of the clinician for patients management and recommendation of national guidelines and recommendations of several societies ([7, 17, 38, 88, 96, 107]; see Table 18.2).

A good gross description enables the examining/re-examining pathologist but also the gynaecologic surgeon to reconstruct an image which corresponds to the treated lesion. Several general key points can be determined for good medical practice in surgical pathology [17, 63, 143]:

- appropriate gross description and selection of paraffin blocks for histopathology requires a full understanding of what should be in the final report for each specimen type and why,
- opening sentence of gross description should indicate how the tissue is received (fresh or inadequate/adequate fixed),
- it should be mentioned if the specimen received intact or if there are some incisions made by the gynaecologic surgeon,
- sutures for marking the specimens should be mentioned,
- the weight and three dimensional measurement should be given,
- gross description should be given in an orderly fashion, focussing on the primary lesion,
- descriptions should be full but economical in words and space,
- elaborate descriptions of normal anatomy of adjacent, uninvolved anatomy should be avoided,
- obvious lesions should be described using diagnostic terms, not by prosaic texts,
- gross description should focus on the site and the extent of the lesion,
- the main lesion should be described in detail by giving its three-dimensional size, the presence of its borders to adjacent tissue (its contour) and organs, its consistency and colour, the presence/absence of necroses and haemorrhage, its presence of the cutting surface,
- application of ink is useful for the identification of margins that lack natural margins (i.e. surgical resection margins),
- inking should be sparingly and blot-dry to prevent spill-over or running,
- the reporting of the status of the resection margins is mandatory,
- the reporting of the metric distance between the infiltrating edge of the tumor and adjacent resection margin is mandatory,
- in complex cases or specimens with inadequate orientation drawings or photographs may be helpful for adequate interpretation,
- photographic documentation of complex specimens or those with rare disease is helpful and mandatory in our digital world,
- the number of blocks embedded should be given to document how many tissue has been processed
- the use of adequate section codes is mandatory.

Resection Margins and Inking

The determination of resection margins is mandatory for the management of the patients, for prognostic evaluation and for quality control of gynaecologic surgical treatment.

The status of all resection margins of a lesion should be given in the gross description with the metric distance between the lesion and the margin. All close margins (e.g., margins <1 cm) should be examined histologically.

Application of ink is necessary to identify surgical resection margins on histological slides (Fig. 18.3). The use of multiple colours may be helpful, but it is also adequate to use only one colour. At the authors department we have good experiences to use writing correction fluid if only one colour is needed for inking. In our opinion it represents a good practicable, cheap and easiely handling tool. The correction fluid appears white on macroscopy but black on histology Fig. 18.3a–g). Sometime it is helpful to dry up the specimen before inking using a tissue towel. The application of the ink should avoid a spill-over of the ink and an inadvertently covering of the lesion. The use of perpendicular sections is favoured by the authors rather than the use of

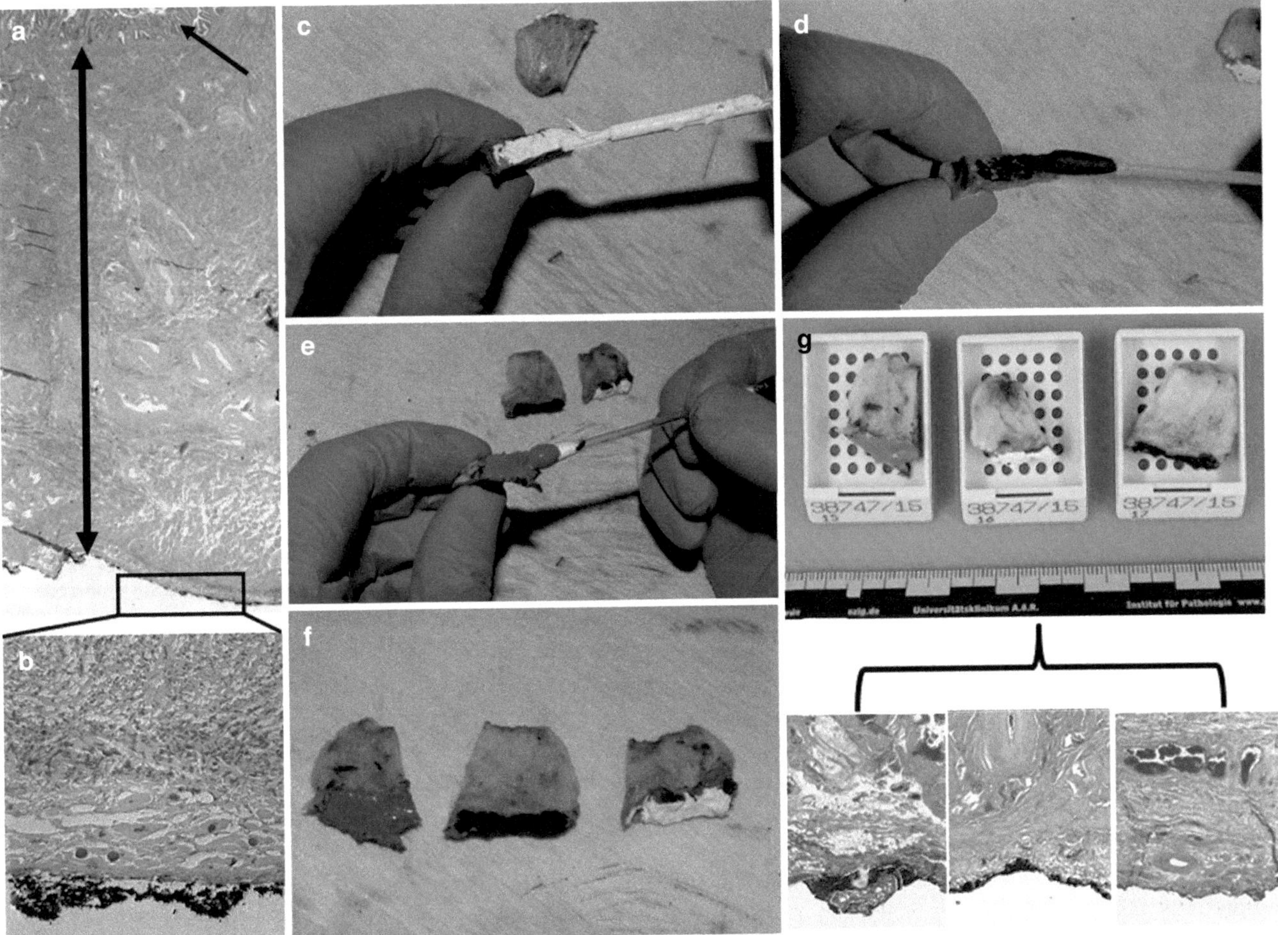

Fig. 18.3 Inking of hysterectomy specimens. (**a**, **b**) Inking of the serosal surface with correction fluid of a hysterectomy specimen with endometrioid endometrial cancer (*arrow*) indicating the distance from the serosal surface (*double headed arrow*). The serosal surface appears black inkend on the microscope. (**b**–**g**) Inking of the anterior resection margin of radical hysterectomy specimens by different colours (for details please see text)

sections parallel to the margins. But in special cases transverse sections fits. Although the number of blocks might be higher, the use of perpendicular sections allows the exact measurement of the distance to the margin.

During frozen section examination but also on permanent sections, the interpretation of the resection margins may be difficult because of cautering artifacts.

Frozen Section Analyses

Frozen section examination of a specimen may be necessary to evaluate the dignity of a uterine lesion (rarely), the extent of a lesion, its relation to the resection margins or to guide the extension of the surgical approach intraoperatively.

For adequate evaluation of the specimens the requirements and questions of the gynaecologic surgeon directly guide the pathologist how to handle the specimen [37, 47]. It is very helpful to contact the surgeon by phone call if there are missing/unclear marking sutures within the specimen or if it is unclear why the specimen was sent for frozen section analyses *before* any cutting of the tissue. To avoid misinterpretation of histological findings the pathologist should get in dialogue with the surgeon, rather than with the anaesthesiologist and/or the operation room nurses or technicians.

For special issues regarding the handling and reporting of hysterectomy specimens sent for frozen section, see Chap. starting at line 312.

Fixation of the Specimen

Well fixed specimens allow an easier handling and cutting of the tissue and produce better results in H&E-staining and immunohistochemical examination (Fig. 18.1).

Especially in exenteration specimens a complete or partial opening of resected bladder or bowel followed by tamponation using tissue towels (preferred by the authors, because of easier handling) or cellulose may be helpful. At the authors experiences a minimum fixation time of (radical) hysterectomies is about 24 h and of exenteration specimens 48 h. Large specimens might be cross-sectioned at intervals of about 1–2 cm. If there is a need to speed up the examination, the specimen may be fixed in an adequate amount of formalin and heating it up (at ~40 °C) in an incubator. The time depends of the size from the specimen. In the author opinion, (radical) hysterectomy specimen may heated up for about 6–8 h without any damage of the tissue.

Number of Sections Required

Judging what number of blocks required to optimally examine a specimen is one of the more controversial subjects in gynaecological pathology [143].

In the authors opinion, each resection margin and each resected structure should be documented by histologic slides. In case of smaller anatomic structures resected two identical ones (i.e. anterior and posterior vaginal margin) can be blocked into one cassette and one of the tissue slices (e.g. the anterior one) can be marked by ink. The relationship of a lesion to its adjacent structures as well as its resection margins should be documented. During the cutting of the specimen it should be determined which cut brings the most information on the histologic slide within one block. In lesions with known difficulties in histologic diagnosis and/or high intratumoral heterogeneity (e.g. MMMTs, leiomyosarcomas, endometrial stromal sarcomas, carcinomas after previous radio-(chemo-)therapy), a more extensive embedding is recommended.

Definition Relevant Parameters for Tumor Staging

The diagnosis of *lymphovascular space involvement (LVSI)* requires the demonstration of tumor cells (single cells or groups) within channels that are unequivocal lined with endothelium (Fig. 18.4a, e; [182]). It has been stated within the TNM-supplement of the UICC that if spaces around tumor cell nests caused by shrinkage during tissue processing and spaces which cannot clearly defined as lymphatic vessels should be classified as no LVSI (i.e. L0; [182]). The use of immunohistochemical stains (e.g. D2-40) to indentify LVSI is not being recommended for routine use.

The most recent TNM-supplement has defined (venous) *vessel invasion* if there is a tumor invasion within the vessels wall. It is not necessarily require demonstration of tumor cells in the lumen of the vessels (Fig. 18.3b; [182]).

Perineural involvement (PNI) has been defined as the detection of malignant cells in the perineural space of nerves, regardless if the nerve itself is infiltrated by the tumor and regardless of the extension of the involvement of the perineural tissue (Fig. 18.4c, d; [68, 72, 101, 116]).

Isolated tumor cells (ITC) are single tumor cells or small clusters of cells not more than 0.2 mm in greatest extent that can be detected by routine H&E-staining or immunohistochemically (Fig. 18.4f; [182]). ITC do not typically show evidence of metastatic activity (e.g. proliferation or stromal reaction) or penetration of lymphatic sinus walls [182]. The use of immunistochemistry to detect ITC cannot be recommended in routine workup. The presence of ITC within lymph nodes should not categorised as pN1 but as pN0(i+) if the ITC were morphologically identified (H&E or by immunohistochemistry) and as pN0(mol+) if they were diagnoses by non-morphologic techniques (e.g. DNA-cytometry or molecular techniques; [182]).

Micrometastases within lymph nodes are defined as tumor cell deposits larger than or equal 0.2 mm but not larger than 0.2 cm (Fig. 18.4g; [182]). The TNM/UICC suggest the use of pN1(mi) within the tumor classification [159, 182]. For easier communication, the authors prefer the use of pN1mic for the designation of micrometastases within lymph nodes according to the earlier TNM-classification in breast cancer.

Frozen Section Analyses of Hysterectomy Specimens

Frozen section diagnosis (FS) will guide the gynaecologic surgeon to perform lymph node dissection, the removal of additional tissue to complete the resection of possibly tumor burden tissue or to perform other surgical staging procedures (e.g. peritoneal biopsies, omentectomy etc.).

There are different approaches and indications for intraoperative frozen section analyses for hysterectomy specimens [26]. Some of them are dependent from the surgical philosophy and individual experience of the surgeon [190]. Within the authors institution there is a wide range of intraoperative treatment of the patient by the pathologist. The distribution of FS-examination during a 5-year period is illustrated in Fig. 18.5.

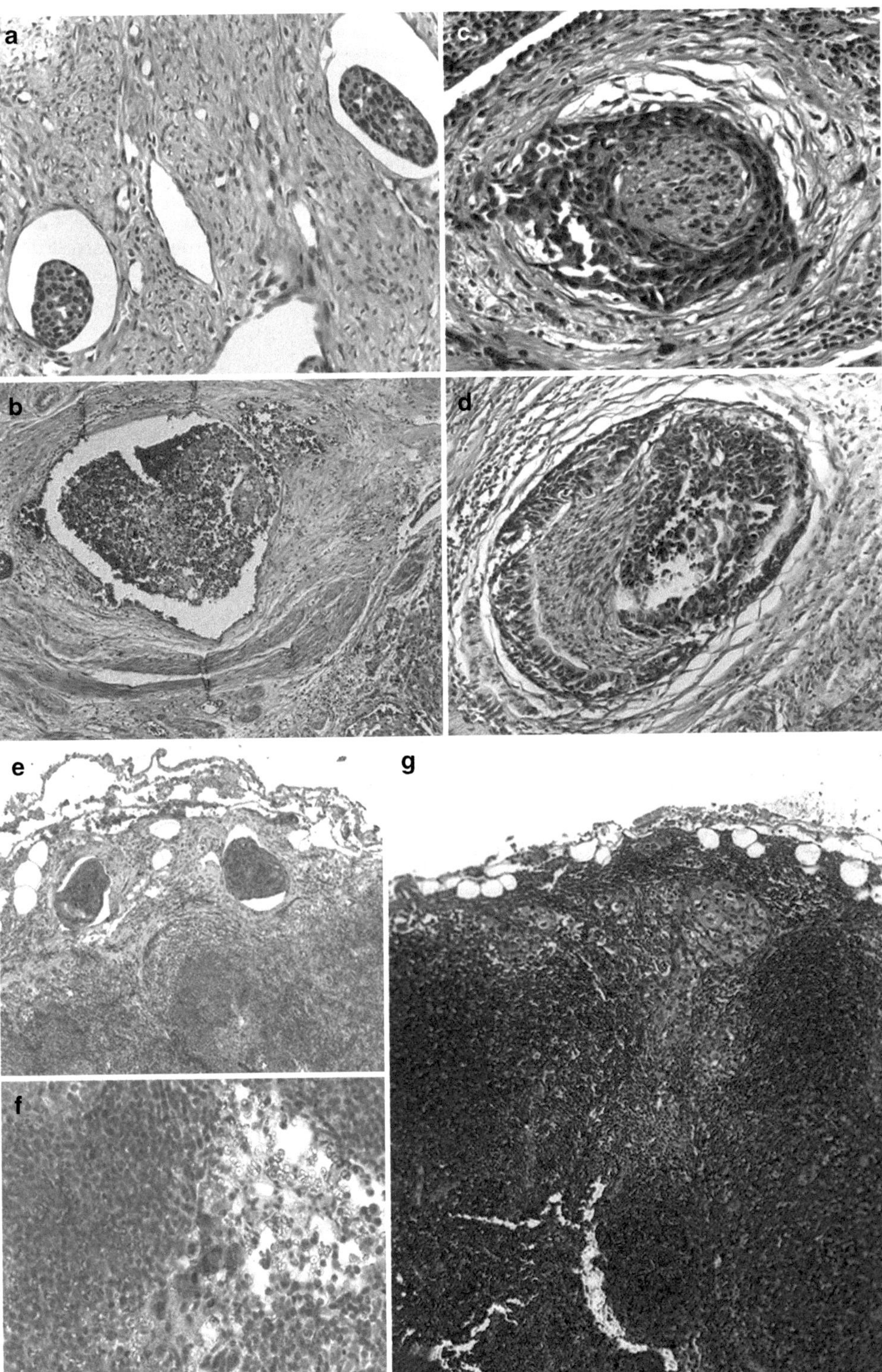

Fig. 18.4 Histopathologic parameters for staging of uterine cancers. (**a**) Lymphovascular space involvement by a squamous cell carcinoma within lymphatic vessels, lined by a single layer of endothelial cells (H&E staining). (**b**) Venous infiltration by a squamous cell carcinoma, note the erythrocytes admixed with tumor cells (H&E staining). (**c**, **d**) Perineural involvement by a squamous cell (**c**) and poorly differentiated adenocarcinoma of the uterine cervix (**d**). (**e**) lymphovascular space involvement within the capsule of a pelvic lymph node by squamous cell carcinoma which will categorised as L1 and not as lymph node metastasis (immunostain for cytokeratines; AE 1/3). (**f**) Isolated tumor cells of a squamous cell carcinoma within a pelvic lymph node (immunostain for p16). (**g**) Micrometastasis of a squamous cell carcinoma within a pelvic lymph node (H&E staining)

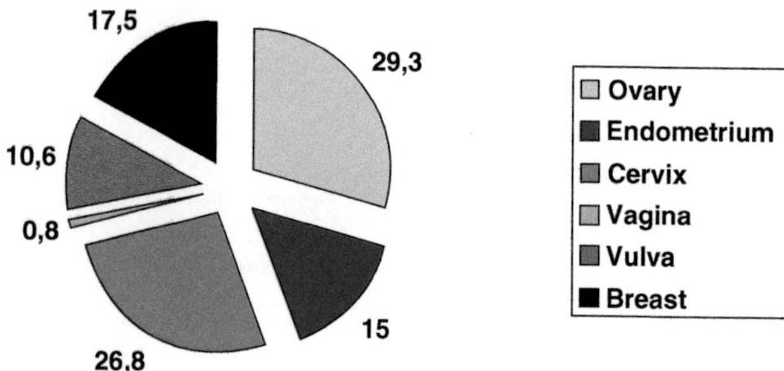

Fig. 18.5 Percentage of requested frozen section analysis from gynaecologic oncology during a 5-year period [74]. Within 7,921 frozen sections, 17.5 % (N = 1.368) were requested by gynecologic oncologic surgeons

Frozen Section in Endometrial Cancer, Malignant Mixed Müllerian Tumors (MMMT) and Atypical Endometrial Hyperplasia

FS-examination in hysterectomies is done to document the extent of the tumor which will directly impact patient's surgical management. The issues for FS-examination in endometrial cancer and its relative risk for lymph node involvement is summarised in Table 18.2.

Within the majority of cases the assessment of the depth of invasion represents the leading question [5, 42, 83, 146, 162] in endometrial cancer surgery. If the involvement of endocervical stroma represents a prognostic factor is still under discussion [132, 187], but its recognition mandatory for staging.

To determine the extent of the endometrial cancer the serosal surface and adnexal tissue should inspected. The ovaries should be incised along its long axis and all suspicious findings should be examined by histology. The uterus should be opened (by scissor at 12-o'clock position or bivalved at 3-o'clock and 9-o'clock position). Then the tumor and its adjacent myometrium should be sliced and the deepest point of infiltration should be frozen, ideally as full thickness or in a manner to preserve the overall depth and total thickness measurements [143, 183]. The macroscopic only evaluation of the depth of invasion may be problematic [33, 50, 97, 138]. Within the authors opinion macroscopic only evaluation may result in an underestimation of the depth of invasion especially in cases of endometrioid cancer representing microcystic, elongated, fragmented glands (MELF) pattern of invasion [40, 125], in case of endometrioid carcinoma with minimal deviation growth pattern [2, 76, 79, 92, 104, 126] as well as in cases of serous endometrial cancer with glandular pattern [11, 76] where the diagnosis was not made on the curetting. So, the depth of invasion should be proofed by histologic examination of FS in all cases [138]. One example of minimal deviation carcinoma is illustrated in Fig. 18.6.

The gross assessment of myometrial invasion is no better than 70 % [44, 50] and increases up to 90 % by histologic examination [86, 134, 146, 162, 173].

The differentiation between myometrial invasion and involvement of an endometriosis by endometrial adenocarcinoma may be challenging [5, 55, 83]. Helpful features distinguishing involvement of an endometriosis versus true myometrial invasion are discussed in the paragraps of cut-up of hysterectomies with uterine cancer and MMMT at page 1021.

Areas for suspicion of endocervical involvement should also be frozen to determine endocervical stromal invasion. The involvement of endocervical glands has no longer impact for staging. Although, there is still a debate about the necessity of radical hysterectomy in endometrial cancer with endocervical stromal invasion (stage pT2; [132, 167]), this feature should be examined and reported during frozen section examination also [112, 187].

The evaluation of the tumor grade by intraoperative biopsy has a reported sensitivity and a specificity of 40 % and 98 %, respectively [86, 134, 146]. A recommendation may be to report the grade at frozen section if there is an upgrade of the tumor [162].

The determination of the histologic subtype, mainly the distinction between type 1 and type 2 endometrial cancers should base on the histology of the curetting specimen, if there is a previously undiagnosed serous/clear cell cancer on frozen section the diagnosis should be given to the clinician [162].

Malignant mixed Müllerian tumors (MMMT) represent high grade carcinomas of the uterus [61] and will be treated by hysterectomy with bilateral salpingo-oophorectomy and pelvic and para-aortic lymphonodectomy [157]. So, intraoperative evaluation is of no impact.

A significant number of women diagnosed with atypical endometrial hyperplasia on endometrial curetting will be diagnosed with endometrial cancer on the hysterectomy specimen [71]. So, in individual cases there may be an indication for frozen section on hysterectomies with previously diagnosed endometrial hyperplasia [169, 171]. There may be some challenges within the diagnosis of low grade endometrioid endometrial cancers [141], high risk cancers are efficiently identified in frozen section [123, 141].

Frozen section analysis of lymph nodes in endometrial cancer may result in a discrepancy betwenn frozen and permanent section in 7–13 % [87, 175].

Frozen Section Radical Hysterectomies for Cervical Cancer

Frozen section analyses may be indicated in radical trachelectomy to determine the status of endocervical margins [20, 49, 122].

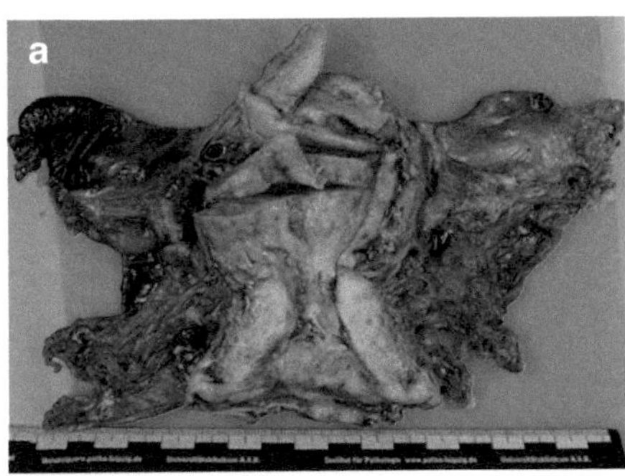

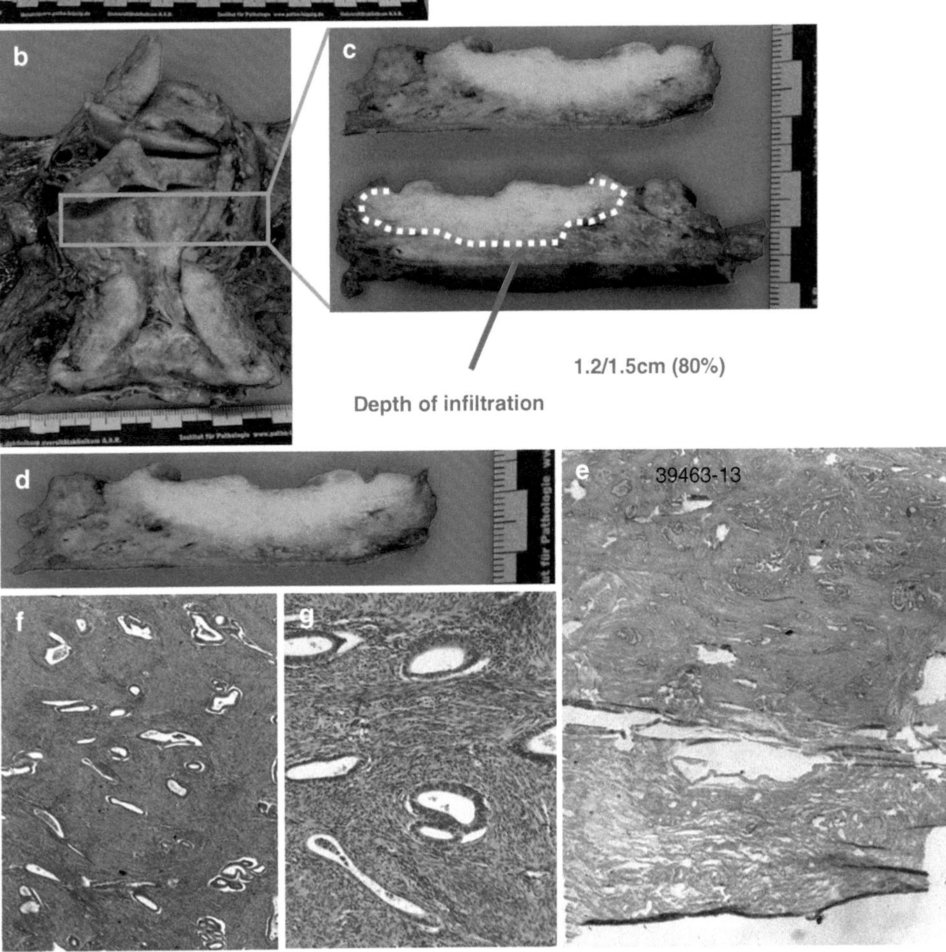

Initial gross description
• Right wall of the cavum uteri representing 0.9 x 0.7 x 0.5 exophytic lesion
• Endometrium atrophic
• Corpus uteri with multinodular appearance of 4.5 x 3.5 x 1.1 cm
• Myometrial thickness 1.5cm
1.2/1.5cm (80%)
Depth of infiltration
39463-13
Final Report
• PMMR-specimen representing well differentiated endometrioid adenocarcinoma of 4.5 x 3.5 x 1.2 cm (G1) with minimal deviation growth pattern and exophytic part of 0.9 x 0.7 cm
• Maximum depth of invasion 1.2/1.5cm with some lymphovascular invasions
• pT1b pN0 (0/56) M0 L1 V0 Pn0, R0

Fig. 18.6 PMMR specimen of endometrial cancer with well differentiated endometrioid adenocarcinoma with minimal deviation growth pattern. The initial gross description indicated a 0.9 cm exophytic tumor in maximal dimension. But frozen section analysis revealed a deeply invasive tumor with maximal depth of invasion of 1.2 into the myometrium which represented a maximal thickness of 1.5 cm. Final tumor size of 4.5 × 3.5 × 1.2 cm

But intraoperative examination of radical hysterectomy for cervical cancer is rarely requested within most institutions [9]. At the authors institution, that procedure was requested in all cases representing 26.8 % of all frozen section analyses for gynaecologic malignancies [73]. Routinely, the vaginal resection margin was examined by tangential sections. In cases with close posterior or anterior resection margins (i.e. in direction to the mesorectum and urinary bladder) and in cases with close margins at mesometrial (parametrial) infiltration the margins are examined using perpendicular sectioning. Recognising the concept of ontogenetic anatomy of the female genital tract [58] and the concept of therapeutic lymphonodectomy [56], routinely we examine the hysterectomy specimen for corpus involvement by the cervical tumor macroscopically. In suspicious cases the leading edge of the cervical tumor in direction to the uterine corpus will be examined by frozen section histologically. In case of corpus involvement the lymph node dissection will be expanded to the para-aortic nodes, even in cases in which the first-line pelvic nodes were without metastatic deposits on previous frozen section examination.

The examination of lymph nodes in cervical cancer may be challenging and an inaccuracy up to 33 % has been reported [12, 41, 48]. These numbers are very high in the authors opinion. But these high rates are caused by the examination of sentinel nodes and under recognition of micrometastases. In case of macrometastases the accuracy rates will be higher.

Frozen Section Hysterectomies for Mesenchymal Tumors of the Uterus

Frozen section for mesenchymal tumors of the uterus is rarely requested [5, 9, 49, 97, 122, 183]. So, here is limited information in the literature addressing the practical issues commonly encountered regarding intraoperative frozen section of uterine mesenchymal lesions [10].

The depth of myometrial involvement of endometrial stromal sarcoma may be determined by frozen section analysis but has no direct impact of surgical procedure. Some leiomyosarcoma may be diagnosed by frozen section but it is impossible to separate between low grade spindle cell leimoysarcomas from smooth muscle tumors of uncertain malignant potential (STUMP) or highly cellular leiomyomas with mitotic activity [77] as well as between myxoid leiomyomas and myxoid leiomyosarcomas. The same diagnostic dilemma exists within the differential diagnosis of endometrial stromal nodules and low-grade endometrial stromal sarcomas (LG-ESS) as well as for the differential between high-grade endometrial stromal sarcomas (HG-ESS) and undifferentiated uterine sarcomas (UUS). Because of the limitations of the diagnostic safety and its impact on surgery frozen section examination of uterine sarcomas is not indicated within the majority of cases [46, 135].

There are case reports about frozen section examination of biopsies obtained from mesenchymal uterine lesions before laparoscopic morcellation procedure [172].

Handling of Hysterectomy Specimens for Final Cutup

Hysterectomy in Benign Diseases (Figs. 18.7 and 18.8)

There are several causes for hysterectomy in benign diseases. Cutting and examination of uteri removed for functional diseases is one of the most performed procedures in gynaecologic surgery [160]. This includes hysterectomy for decensus uteri, leiomyomas, pelvic discomfort in case of endometriosis/adenomyosis, persistent dysfunctional and/or postmenopausal bleeding and endometrial hyperplasia. A special indication is the risk-reducing (elective or prophylactic) hysterectomy in women at risk of hereditary endometrial cancer [89]. For a detailed description, see page 612.

Hysterectomy in Uterine Prolapse, Persistent Dysfunctional Bleeding and Pelvic Dyscomfort

There are some general aspects of the gross description of any hysterectomy specimen, regardless of the background disease for surgery which are summarised in Tables 18.3 and 18.4.

For normal appearing cervix one section of the anterior and one of the posterior lips fits. The sections are adequate if the squamo-columnar junction (transition zone) is included, because it represents the preferred location of CIN or ACIS [54, 119]. If the uterus is small, both sections can be embedded in one block and one lip (e.g., the anterior one) may be inked.

For examination of the endometrium in premenopausal women two sections, one of the anterior and one of the posterior parts of the fundus uteri is adequate. If the endometrium is atrophic and the woman is postmenopausal, one section is adequate. The section of the endometrium should represent a full thickness section, including the endometrium, adjacent myometrium and the uterine serosa, if not too thick.

The number of sections should be increased if there is a dysfunctional bleeding up to four. Alternatively, wedge sections can be performed by cutting small peaces of the endometrium and the immediately adjoining myometrium putting them in one cassette [143].

From any suspicious lesion within the uterine serosa and the myometrium, one block should be embedded.

The details of histopathology report are listed in Table 18.4.

Hysterectomy in Endometrial Hyperplasia

General aspects of gross description and parameters of the histopathology report are summarised in Table 18.3.

Uteri removed with the previous histopathology of endometrial hyperplasia require more extensive sampling of the myometrium to state residual disease and to exclude / diagnose endometrial carcinoma.

About six sections, three of the anterior and three of the posterior parts of the fundus uteri is have been recommended [143] to detect small well differentiated endometrial cancer [154]. The section of the endometrium should represent a full thickness section. Alternatively, wedge sections can be performed by cutting small peaces of the endometrium and the immediately adjoining myometrium putting them in one cassette [143]. The preferred site of embedding is the macroscopically thickened endometrium.

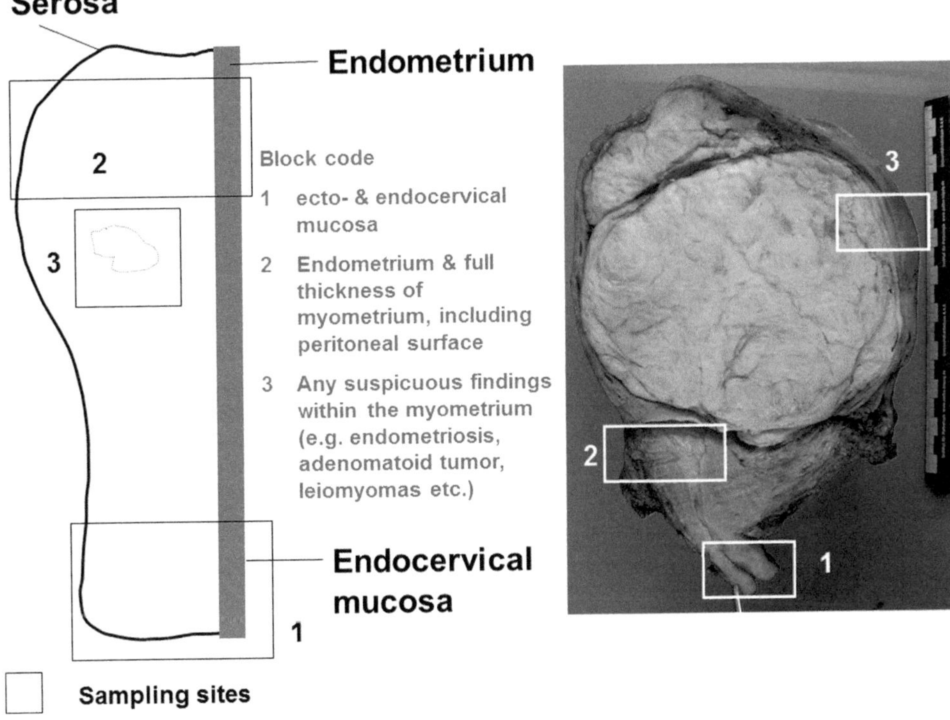

Fig. 18.7 Handling of a hysterectomy specimen for benign disease (see text)

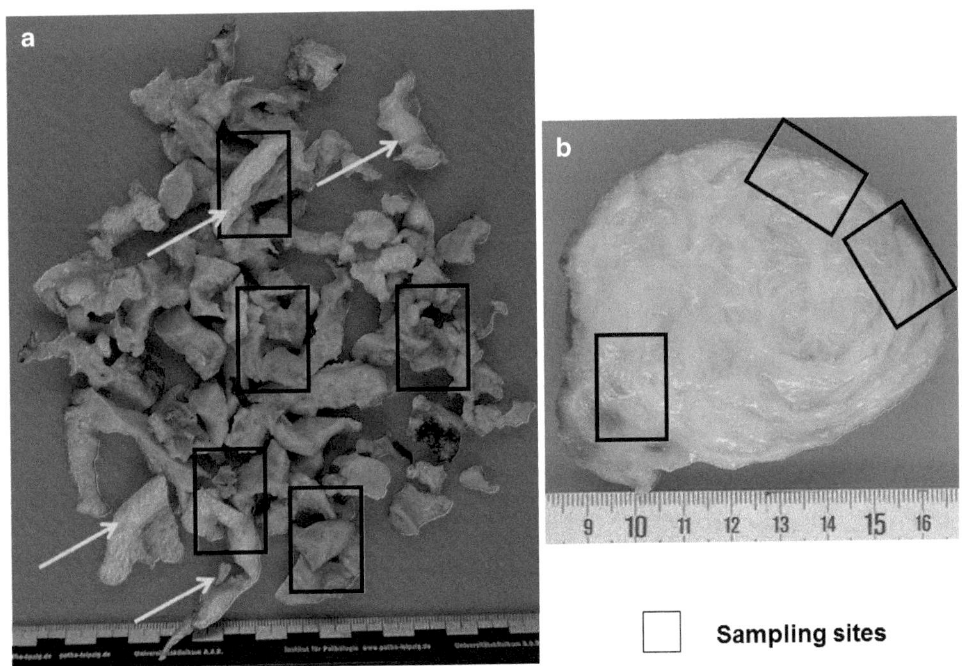

Fig. 18.8 Morcellated uterus and myomectomy. (**a**) Fragments resulted from morcellation during LASH-procedure with fragments of a leimoyma (*arrow*). (**b**) Myomectomy specimen with smooth outline of the leiomyoma with fasciculas (whirled) cutting surface, no necroses, no hemorrhage. Quadrats indicate embedding sites

Table 18.3 General aspects for the cutup of hysterectomy specimens [17, 62, 69, 88, 95, 143, 145]

List which specimens received (uterus alone, with one/two adnexae, tubes only etc.)
Indicate, how the tissue is received (fresh or inadequate/adequate fixed)
Note if the specimen is received intact or in parts or if it is morcellated
Note any defects on the uterine surface
Note if there are sutures made by the clinician to reconstruct the specimen
Make a proper orientation of the uterus
If the adnexae are present: the ovaries lay posteriorily to the Fallopian tubes
The posterior surface of the uterus is covered by a larger area of the peritoneum and extends farther down (in direction of cul-de-sac)
Give the appearance of the uterine surface (serosa)
The posterior part is of special interest
state if the surface is smooth or if there are peritoneal adhesions
State if there is rough surface or some discolorations
Look for small cysts (peritoneal cysts or endosalpingiosis) or probably implants of ovarian borderline tumor
State if there is a vaginal cuff present or not
State if mesometrial/parametrial tissue is present
State if ovarian ligament and/or infundibulum pelvicum is present
Weight the specimen
Give the size of each resected structure in three dimensions
State the performance of the ectocervical surface
Measure the thickness of the normal appearing myometrium
State if the cutting surface of the myometrium is abnormal
Irregular thickening, whirled appearance, cysts, haemorrhages
State the appearance of the endometrium and measure it
State if the endometrium is atrophic, polypoid, irregularly shaped or haemorrhagic
Record the location, shape (sessile or polypoid) and size of any polyps
State if there are abnormal findings within the myometrium (leiomyomata, endometriosis etc.)

Table 18.4 Details of the histopathology report within a hysterectomyspecimen without previously determined malignant disease [62, 69, 95, 143]

List the findings of ecto- and endocervix
List the findings of the endometrium
Atrophic/cyst-atrophic endometrium
Different phases of proliferation and secretion of the endometrium
Changes caused by hormones (oral contraceptives, HRT, selective progesterone receptor modulators, IUD etc.)
Any inflammatory changes
Presence of disordered proliferation/endometrial hyperplasia
List the findings of the myometrium
Leiomyomas, endometriosis/adenomyosis etc.

In case of atypical endometrial hyperplasia a careful examination is required to exclude well differentiated endometrioid adenocarcinoma.

The histopathologic report should give the kind of endometrial hyperplasia according to the most recent WHO-classification [186].

Hysterectomy in Precancerous Lesions or Microinvasive Carcinoma of the Cervix

Precancerous lesion of the cervix includes those deriving from the squamous epithelium (CIN-lesions, [165]) and from the endocervical columnar epithelium (adenocarcinoma in situ; AIS; [179]), some proceed to microinvasive carcinomas.

In the majority of cases there is a history of previous conisation. In hysterectomy specimens with the previous diagnosis of precancerous lesion of the cervix the transformation zone should be embedded completely.

The cervix should be amputated about 1.5 cm above the external os and should be processed similarly to a cone. Radial sectioning in a clockwise manner is the preferred method [17, 61, 62, 69, 88, 143]. Serially blocks should be submitted. Some authors prefer the submission of one sliced specimen within one cassette (e.g. cassette with number 1 indicates 1:00 o'clock). But, in the authors opinion and of others [143] it is also possible to put three sliced specimen in one cassette (e.g. cassette with number 1 indicates 1:00 to 3:00 o'clock and so on). Especially in case of previously diagnosed AIS one additional block of the endocervical mucosa immediate to the complete embedded transition zone is required.

The complete embedding of the transition zone is recommended if previous conisation was performed within the last six months. If it was up to 12 months previously, the embedding of the transition zone performing one block from the 12:00; 3:00; 6:00 and 9:00 o'clock position may be adequate. Perhaps the slices from 12:00 and 6:00 as well as from 3:00 and 6:00 may be processed together and one slice (e.g. 12:00) may be inked. Is there a history of previous CIN/AIS or conisation of >12 months, the cervix should be handled as described in the chapter Hysterectomy in Benign disease at page 435.

The performance of step sectioning (three sections with an interval of 200 μm; [7]) will be required in cases in which the diagnosis was made only be colposcopic guided biopsy or endocervical curetting without previous conisation to exclude microinvasive carcinoma and to document the extension of the lesion. (Secondary) step sectioning is also required when a precancerous lesion is microscopically suspicious for microinvasion. In all other cases up-front step sectioning is not indicated.

General aspects of gross description and parameters of the histopathology report are summarised in Tables 18.3 and 18.4.

The histopathologic report should state the precancerous/micro-invasive lesion according to the most recent WHO-classification [165, 179] and the status (perhaps distance) to the distal (ectocervical/vaginal/ circumferential) resection margin should be given.

Risk-Reducing Hysterectomy in Hereditary Cancer Syndromes

A special condition is the risk-reducing (elective or prophylactic) hysterectomy in women with hereditary cancer syndromes or familial history of endometrial cancer [15, 89, 90, 102, 148].

In those cases the endometrium should carefully examined [27, 80]. As in endometrial hyperplasia, embedding of about six sections, three of the anterior and three of the posterior parts of the fundus uteri is recommended. In some cases complete examination of the endometrium, especially of the lower uterine segment may be required [34]. The section of the endometrium in any grossly visible tumor should represent a full thickness section. Without grossly evident tumor, wedge sections can be performed by cutting small peaces of the endometrium and the immediately adjoining myometrium putting them in one cassette [143].

Some endometrial malignancy in women with HNPCC-(Lynch-) syndrome, occur within the isthmus uteri (lower uterine segment; [11, 27, 139]), so about three additional blocks are recommended to cover the isthmic endometrium. Some authors recommend complete embedding [34].

Colonic adenocarcinoma is the most common malignancy in hereditary nonpolyposis colon cancer (HNPCC; Lynch syndrome). However, endometrial carcinoma may develop before colon carcinoma in ~50 % of women with HNPCC [18, 177, 178]. There may be some features associated with HNPCC-related endometrial carcinoma i.e. age 50 year or younger, personal/family cancer pedigree that meets Bethesda guideline criteria, presence of MMR-associated tumor morphology (poorly differentiated endometrioid carcinoma, presence of high peri-/intratumoral lymphocytes; i.e. ≥40/10 HPF; [27, 152]), or location in the lower uterine segment [11]. In these cases, testing for defective DNA mismatch repair genes (MSH1, MLH2, MLH6, and PMS2) may be performed by immunohistochemistry [27]. Loss of MSH2 expression indicates Lynch syndrome and MSH6 is related to MSH2. HNPCC-related endometrial carcinoma is predominantly associated with MSH2 mutations, and MLH6 mutations in particular [18, 177, 178]. PMS2 loss is often associated with loss of MLH1 and is only independently meaningful if MLH1 is intact. More recently, a first-line testing for defective MMR-genes, followed by methylation testing was suggested for all endometrial cancer patients younger than 60-years of age [14, 43, 139] and by some authors for all newly diagnosed endometrial cancers [118].

The histopathologic report should give the endometrial pathology according to the most recent WHO-classification [186].

Hysterectomy for Leiomyomas and Endometriosis/Adenomyosis (Figs. 18.7 and 18.9)

In *uteri removed for leiomyomas*, the number and its location of the leiomyomas should be recorded. Their minimal and maximal size should be given. It should be stated if the myoma distorts the endometrium or protrudes into the isthmus uteri. These conditions may represent the cause for dysfunctional bleeding or may mimic endometrial polyp clinically and on ultrasound.

Each leiomyoma should be sectioned and examined grossly. If the cutting surface obtaining represents a white, fasciculas, well circumscribed appearance, obtaining one block with the surrounding myometrium will be adequate. If the lesion is >5 cm in largest dimension or represents some necroses or haemorrhagic foci or a softening of its consistence, one block per 1–2 cm largest diameter should be taken in context with the surrounding myometrium.

General aspects of gross description and parameters of the histopathology report are summarised in Tables 18.3 and 18.4.

Two conditions may clinically simulate uterine leiomyomas. For endometriosis/adenomyosis see the paragraph below. Another smooth muscle proliferation with unusual growth pattern represents the (diffuse) myometrial hypertrophia. *Myometrial hypertrophy* is a condition in which the myometrium is thickened and the uterus is (in the majority of cases) symmetrically enlarged without any microscopically abnormalities and without present and most recent pregnancy. This condition is not well defined. The weight of an uterus decreases after menopause and is influenced by the number of previous pregnancies. A weight of >130 g for nulliparous women, >210 g for parity 1–3 and >250 g for parity for and above 4 has been defined as myometrial hypertrophia [93]. Another, less plausible, definition indicates a weight of >200 g with a myometrial thickness of >2 cm [170].

Sometimes the clinicians perform a *myomectomy*. The tissue received should be weighted and measured in three dimensions. Each tissue should be transacted and examined grossly. The embedding of multiple slices in one cassette, altogether of two cassettes fits. Sometimes tiny surrounding tissue is grossly visible and the cuts should cover the transition of the lesion to its surrounding tissue (Fig. 18.8b). If the lesion is >5 cm or present with suspicious findings (see above), additional embedding is required.

The histopathologic report should recognise the criteria for the diagnostic of mesenchymal lesions of the uterus and their terminology of most recent WHO-classification [129].

Within the English literature the *endometriosis uteri* is termed adenomyosis. It is defined as the ectopic presence of endometrial glands surrounded by stroma within the myometrium beyond the histological interface with the endometrium (Fig. 18.9a). No commonly accepted diagnostic criteria of uterine endometriosis exist. On practical purpose the endometriosis should represent more than the field width of an intermediate magnification (i.e. deeper than the microscopic field seen using 10× objective and 10× ocular lenses, within a conventionally configured microscope, or 0.2–0.3 cm below the endometrial (myometrial interface) [128]. Consequently the diagnosis of uterine endometriosis is made on a hysterectomy specimen and not on currettings. Endometriosis uteri may provoke some diagnostic challenges within the clinicians because it may be associated with non-specific signs, may be asymptomatic or may mimic uterine tumors. On histology the endometriotic glands and its surrounding stroma may display the same range of changes seen within the endometrium. Especially on postmenopausal women the glands may disappear (so called gland poor or stromal endometriosis; Fig. 18.9b). Larger foci of stromal endometriosis must be separated from uterine stromal nodule and low-grade endometrial stromal sarcomas [21].

Within a serious number of cases the diagnosin of endometriosis uteri is incidental on microscopy. By careful examination a circumscribed whirling of the myometrium may occur (Fig. 18.9c). Some uterine endometrioses may be tumorlike and may clinically as well as macroscopically mimic leiomyomas (e.g. provoking pelvic discomfort, tumorlike appearance, bleeding disorders). On histology the endometriotic foci are surrounded by a reactive proliferation of the myometrium (Fig. 18.9d, e; representing a "real" adenomyosis of the uterus). Tumorlike uterine endometriosis may mimic low-grade endometrial stromal sarcomas with glandular features [111].

Hysterectomy with Morcellated Uterus

There may be an increased frequency of operation procedures resulting in the fragmentation and morcellation of the uterus (as laparoscopic assisted supracervical hysterectomy; LASH) especially in heavily adipose women [13, 52].

In a serious number of cases it is difficult to get an orientation within the fragmented tissue to identify the endometrium. The preoperative use of methylene blue [136] may simplify macroscopic identification of the endometrium.

The risk of incident malignancies after morcellated hysterectomy ranges between 0.2 and 1 % [36, 51, 53, 149] but may increase with increasing age of the women treated [184].

The tissue received should be weighted and measured in three dimensions as well as examined carefully. From any suspicious findings/discolorations tissue should be processed. Four cassettes, containing two to three tissue slices may be submitted for histopathologic examination. Other authors prefer the embedding of one block per cm largest dimension of the fragmented tissue (D. Mayr, personal communication 2015). From all tissue with any discoloration or different consistency additional embedding is required. The endometrium should be identified. In case of lesions suspicious for leiomyoma, the lesion and the adjacent myometrium should be embedded (Fig. 18.8a). In case of incident malignancies, unclear smooth muscle proliferations or missing endometrium, additional embedding is required.

Hysterectomy with Macroinvasive Cervical Cancer

Trachelectomy (Fig. 18.10)

The specimen should be weighted and measured in three dimensions. The presence and its size of adjacent mesome-

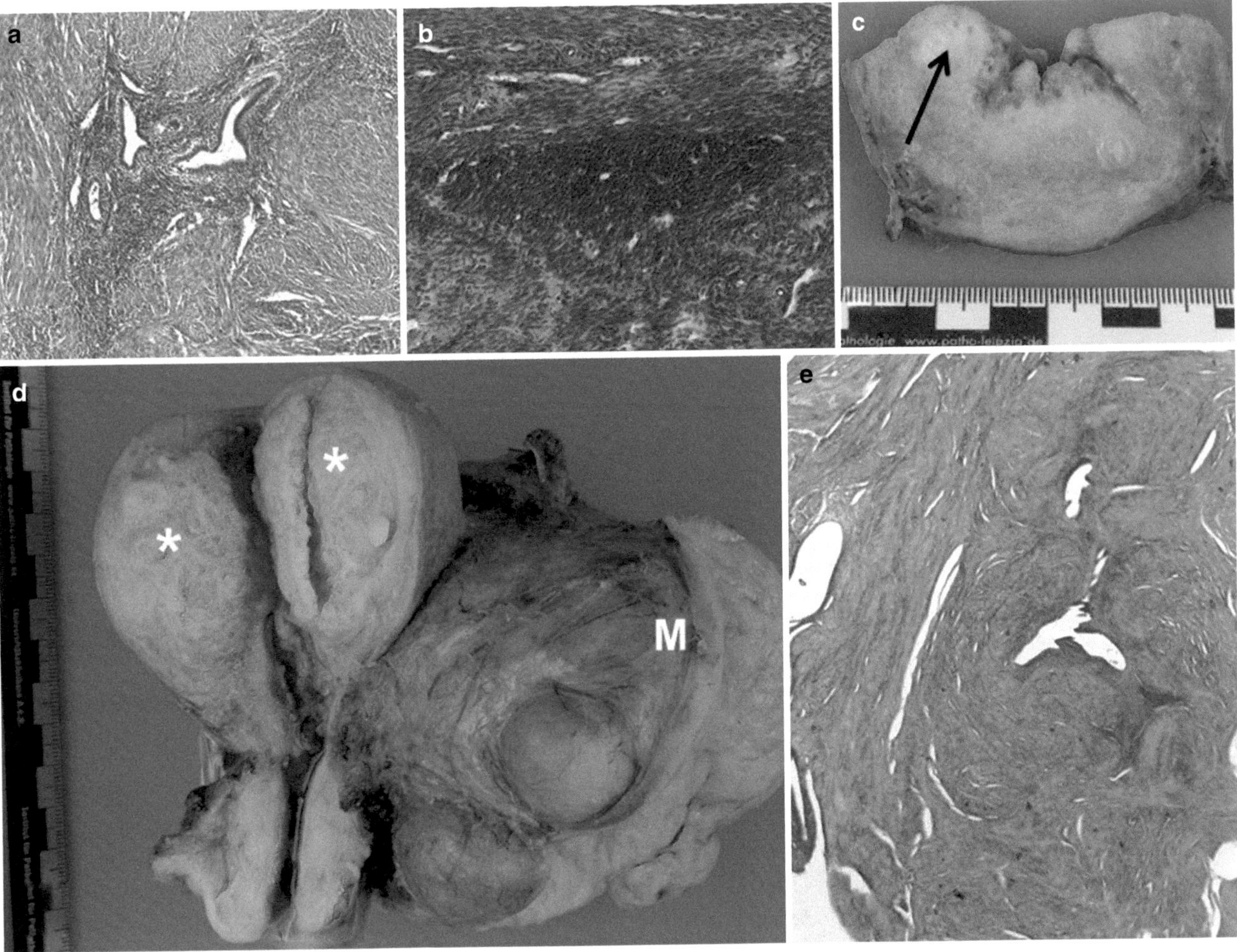

Fig. 18.9 Endometriosis affecting hysterectomy specimen. (**a**) Typical histologic appearance of uterine endometriosis representing endometrial glands and surrounding stroma within the myometrium. (**b**) So called gland poor (or stromal) endometriosis representing solely endometrial stroma without glands within uterine myometrium. (**c**) Macroscopic appearance of small endometriosis (*arrow*). (**d**, **e**) Tumorlike endometriosis within uterine corpus (*stars*), the endometrial glands are surrounded by circular reactive proliferation of smooth muscle fibers of the myometrium, representing an adenomyosis uteri. *M* uterine leiomyoma

trial/parametrial tissue should be given. The length of the vaginal cuff, if present, should be given, separately for its anterior and posterior part. The appearance of the ectocervix and external os should be stated (smooth, erosions, ulcerated, funnel-shaped etc.). The presence of lymph nodes within mesometrial/parametrial tissue should be stated and its size given.

The distal vaginal resection margin should be embedded separately or inked. The proximal endocervical resection margin should be examined separately as well. If present and not removed by previous conisation, the size of the cervical tumor should be given in three dimensions. Its distance to the resection margins (distal/ectocervical, proximal/endocervical, anterior and posterior) should be stated as the involvement of mesometrial/parametrial tissue.

The transformation zone should be embedded completely. Radial sectioning in a clockwise manner is the preferred method. Serially blocks should be submitted preferring the submission of one sliced specimen within one cassette (e.g. cassette with number 1 indicates 1:00 o'clock). The adjacent endocervical tissue should be processed completely as is for the mesometrial/parametrial tissue. The resection margin of the mesometrial/parametrial tissue may be inked.

A synopsis of histopathologic oncology report is summarised in Table 18.5.

The tumor typing and staging should be performed according to the most recent WHO- and TNM-classification [159, 165, 179].

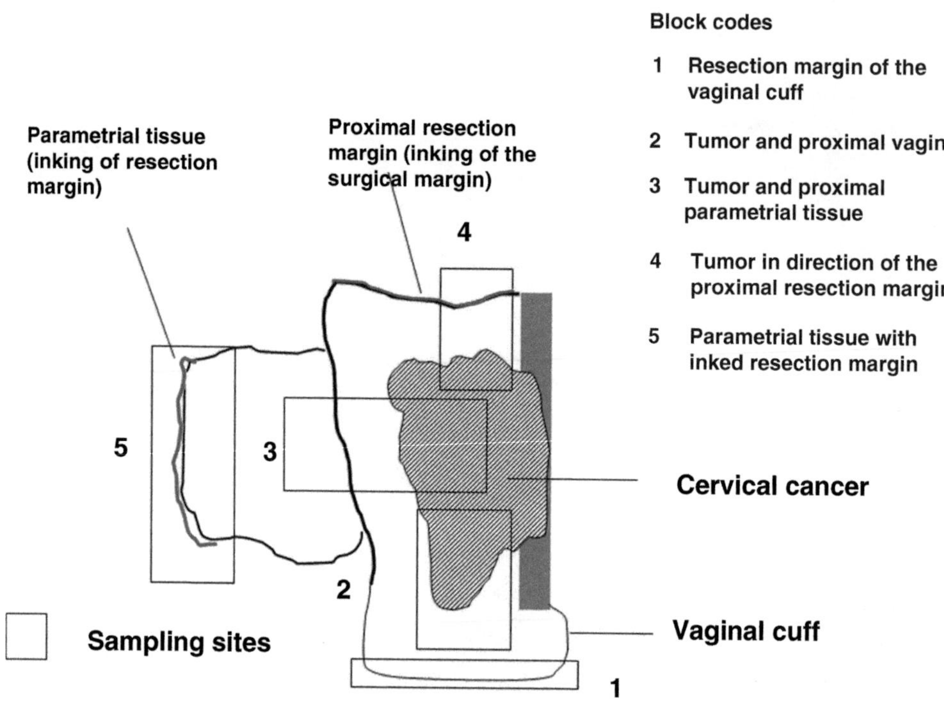

Fig. 18.10 Schematic sectioning of a radical trachelectomy specimen with cervical carcinoma and block codes (for details see text; adopted from Horn et al. 60)

Radical Hysterectomy (Figs. 18.11, 18.12, and 18.13)

Radical hysterectomy will be performed for macroinvasive cervical carcinoma [142, 176] or in some cases with endometrial carcinoma/MMMT with cervical stromal involvement.

General aspects of gross description and parameters of the histopathology report are summarised in Table 18.3.

The final oncology pathology report should recognise the most recent WHO-classification [165, 179] for tumor typing the TNM-classification [159] for staging.

The gross description in radical hysterectomy needs the documentation of the location of the tumor, its three dimensional measurement and its relation to the vaginal cuff (if present) and the resected mesometrial/parametrial tissue as well as the involvement of the corpus uteri. The exact anatomic location of the cervical tumor should be stated (e.g. anterior or posterior lip, ecto- or endocervix; the authors prefer to give an "o'clock location" on localised tumors or to state circular involvement of the transition zone).

The three dimensional size of the resected mesometrial/parametrial tissue should be given. Within specimens resulted from the surgical TMMR-technique the macroscopic description should be separate between the ligamental and vascular part of the mesometrial tissue (Figs. 18.11 and 18.13). By the way, almost all lymph nodes within the mesometrial tissue are located within its vascular part (Fig. 18.11).

The circumferential distal vaginal margin should be embedded separately, one block covering the margin between 9:00 and 3:00 (anterior margin) and one covering the margin between 3:00 and 9:00 (posterior margin) in a tangential manner. Sections of the tumor need to demonstrate the depth of invasion into the cervical stroma, its relationship to the vaginal cuff, the mesometrial/parametrial tissue and the distance to the resection margins. Each section should be perpendicular (if possible) and full thickness and should include the maximum amount of tissue that will fit into the cassette. One block should document the distance to the anterior and posterior resection margin of the cervix uteri.

Since there is a low intratumoral heterogeneity in cervical carcinomas [8, 109], two blocks each from the anterior and posterior part of the cervical stroma is adequate. Especially in larger tumors and/or deep cervical stromal invasion, careful embedding of the transition zone between the cervical stroma and the adjacent mesometrial/parametrial tissue is mandatory. After transecting the resected mesometrial/parametrial tissue, the transition zone to the endocervical stroma should be embedded using perpendicular sections. In the authors institution, in small tumors where there is macroscopically no evidence for mesometrial/parametrial invasion one block from the right and left side will be embedded. In larger tumors or grossly suspicion of mesometrial/parametrial involvement two blocks from each side will be processed.

The transected mesometrial/parametrial tissue will be processed completely to evaluate lymphovascular space or perineural involvement, discontinuity of tumor spread and the detection of small lymph nodes. The mesometrial/para-

Table 18.5 Synopsis of the features within the final oncologic histopathology report of cancer of the cervix uteri [7, 17, 62, 69, 88, 95, 143, 145]

Histopathologic tumor type (WHO)[a]
Grading (WHO)
Tumor regression after previous radio (chemo-) therapy
Absence/presence of lymphovascular and blood vessel (venous) involvement (L- and V-status)
Absence/presence of perineural invasion (Pn-status)
Tumor stage (TNM)
Tumor size and depth of invasion in microinvasive disease (pT1a1 and pT1a2)
Tumor size in three dimensions in macroinvasive disease (≥pT1b1)
Relative depth of invasion within (endo-) cervical stroma (pT1b and pT2a)
Presence/localisation and extension of vaginal invasion
Presence/localisation and extension of mesometrial/parametrial invasion
Minimal distance to the resection margins
R-classification (UICC)
Status of the adnexae

[a]it is important to note that (small cell) neuroendocrine carcinomas of the uterine cervix represent a poor prognosis [6, 185] and that up to 33% of these tumors represent a non-neuroendocrine component [64]. Because mixed neuroendocrine/non-neuroendocrine carcinomas represent decreased survival [64], the percentage of the neuroendocrine component of the whole tumor should be stated within the report [7]

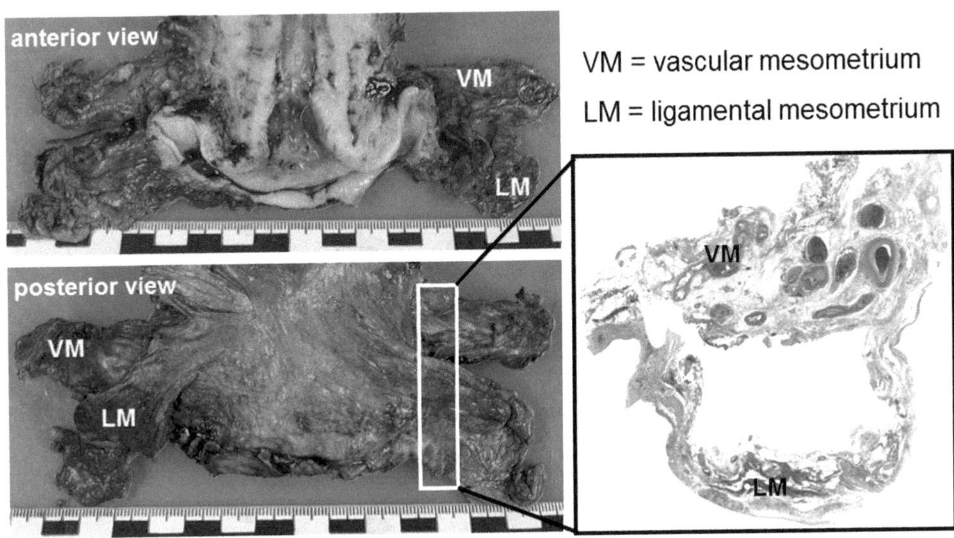

Fig. 18.11 TMMR-specimen (previously opened by scissor at 12 o'clock) representing vascular and ligamental mesometrium using perpendicular section for embedding (see text). Within the vascular mesometrium small lymph nodes are present

metrial tissue will be virtually separated in its proximal (near the uterus), medial and distal third and processed each within one (ore more) cassette. If small lymph nodes are grossly visible, step sections (three sections with an interval of 200 μm) are performed.

Because there may be an increased risk of (para-aortic) lymph node spread [117] and higher frequency of ovarian metastases [81] in cases representing invasion of the uterine corpus this feature should be documented. In each case of macroscopically suspected corpus infiltration (especially in larger tumors), one or two blocks from the cranial end of the tumor into the direction to the corpus uteri should be embedded. Although, involvement of the corpus uteri has no impact on staging at time, that feature should be given within the pathology report, perhaps stating if the infiltration occurs at endometrial or myometrial level or both.

In cases with previous conisation and grossly no visible tumor within the radical hysterectomy specimen, the distal part of the cervix should be embedded completely as described in the chapter about Hysterectomy in Precancerous Lesions or Microinvasive Carcinoma of the Cervix at page 560. The transition zone between the endocervical stroma and the mesometrial/parametrial tissue should be handled as described above.

Based on ontogenetic rather than functional anatomy, new surgical approaches of radical hysterectomy in uterine cervical cancer, known as TMMR-technique [56, 57], has been described. A more radical approach represents the extended mesometrial resection (EMMR; [56]). In EMMR additional

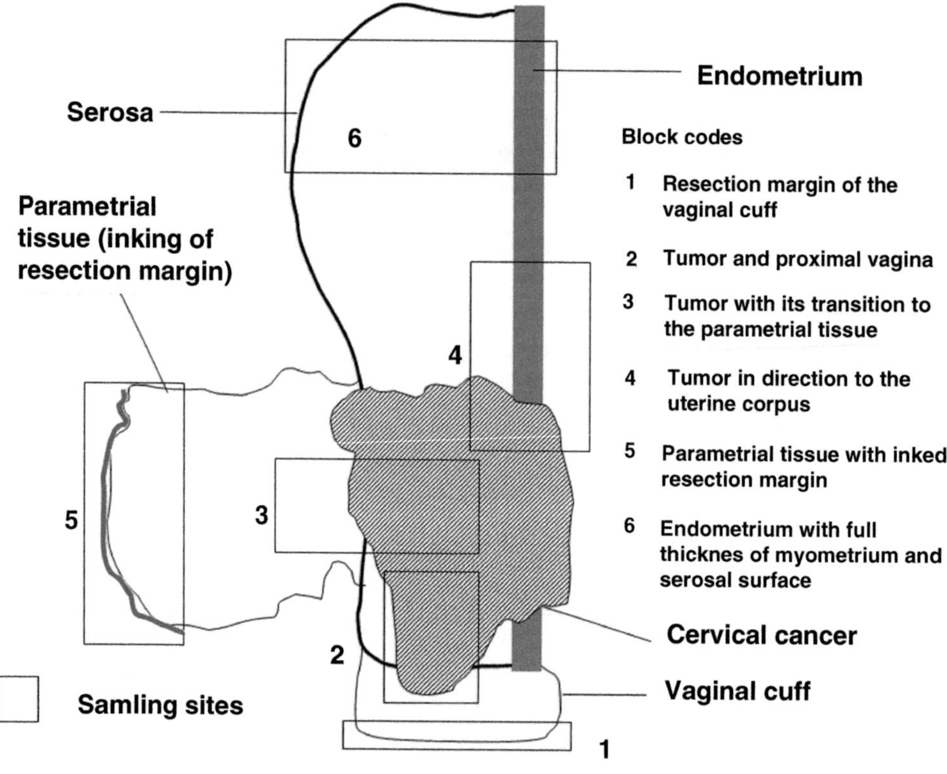

Fig. 18.12 Schematic sectioning of a radical hysterectomy specimen with cervical carcinoma and block codes (for details see text and Table 18.5)

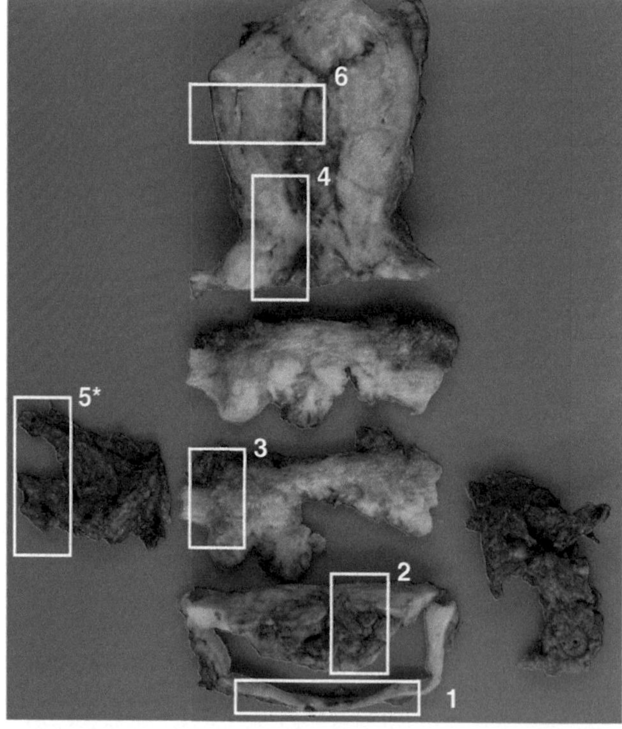

Fig. 18.13 Sectioning of a TMMR-specimen with cervical cancer. For more information please see text (*For detailed handling of the mesometrial tissue please see Fig. 18.11)

pelvic tissue, suspected to be involved by the tumor clinically or on radiologic findings will be removed (Fig. 18.14). This includes for example lipo-fibrous tissue surrounding the ureter (mesoureter) or the resection of the ureter itself and/or the dorso-lateral parts of the urinary bladder (meso of the urinary bladder). This tissue is sometimes incorporated within the mesometrial tissue and may be hard to be identified on macroscopic description and dissection. So, detailed information from the gynaecologic surgeon is mandatory which tissue was removed during EMMR-operation

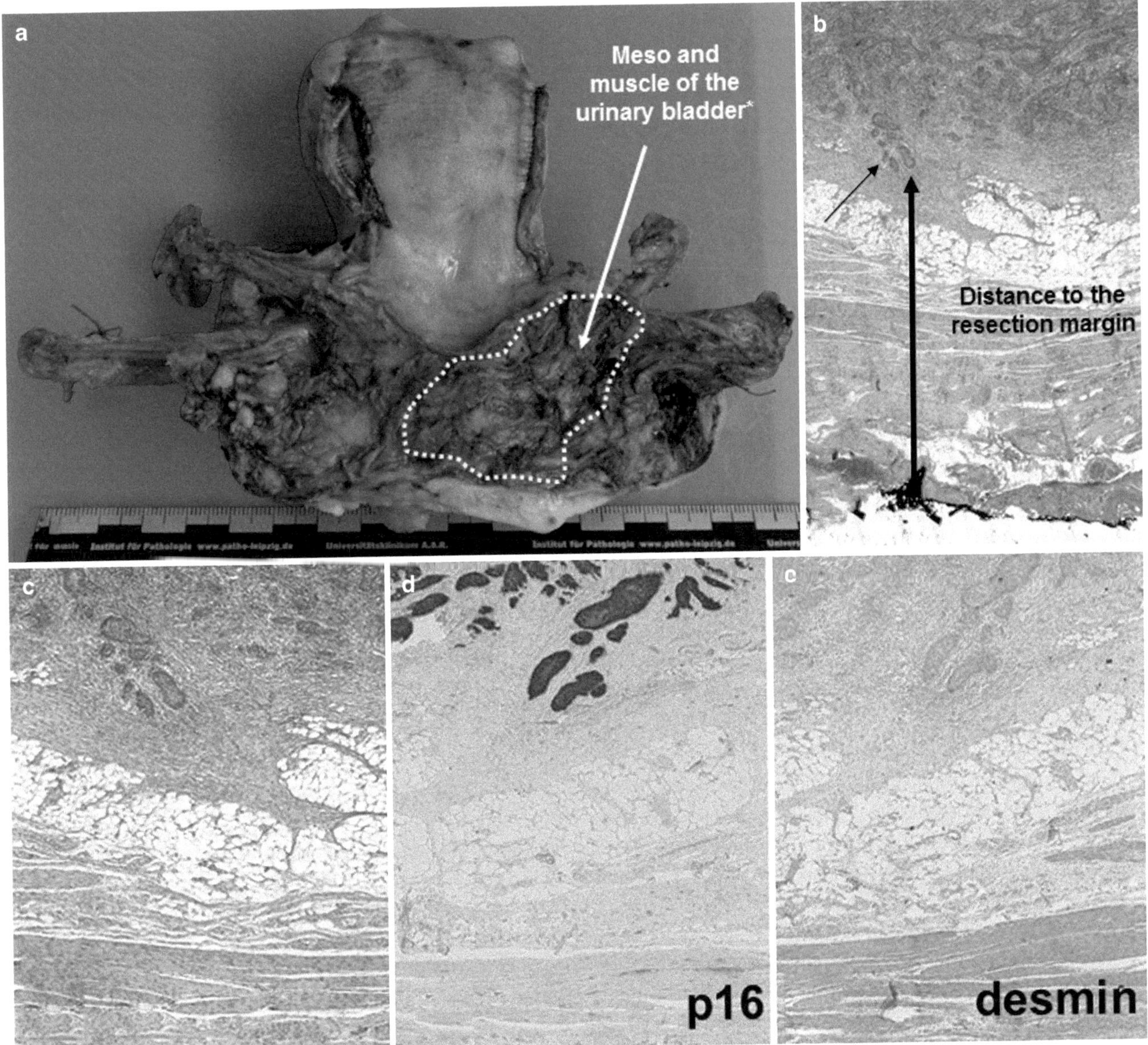

Fig. 18.14 Extended mesometrial resection (EMMR). (**a**) Anterior view of EMMR specimen, encircled the additional removed tissue containing the fatty tissue surrounding the dorsal part of the urinary bladder (bladder's meso) and some outer lines of smooth muscle of the bladders wall, (**b**) microscopic view representing squamous cell carcinoma infiltrating the bladder's meso (*small arrow*), note the peritumoral desmoplastic stromal response surrounding the leading edge of the tumor. *The thick double headed arrow* indicates the distance to the inked resection margin, (**c**–**e**) higher magnification from (**b**) featuring the infiltration of the bladder's meso by the tumor which stained positive for p16, no infiltration of the bladder's muscle which is stained positive for desmin in (**e**)

procedure. The size of that additionally resected tissue should be incorporated in the measurement at gross description and its resection margins should carefully be examined. Sometimes individual components are only detected by histologic examination (Fig. 18.14c–e). The presence or absence of tumor infiltration and its distances should be given in the oncologic pathology report to exactly document the tumor spread within the pelvis and to correlate the pathologic findings with the clinical and radiologic ones.

In cases with radical hysterectomy after neoadjuvant radio- (chemo-) therapy, and grossly no visible tumor within the radical hysterectomy specimen, the distal part of the cervix should be embedded completely as described in the chapter about Hysterectomy in Precancerous Lesions or Microinvasive Carcinoma of the Cervix at page 560. The transition zone between the endocervical stroma and the mesometrial/parametrial tissue should be handled as described above.

The tumor typing and staging should be performed according to the most resent WHO- and TNM-classification [159, 165, 179].

A synopsis of histopathologic oncology report is summarised in Table 18.5.

There may be a prognostic effect of the distance to the anterior and posterior resection margins in patients with were treated by radical hysterectomy using the Wertheim-Meigs-technique [39, 106], but not in patients who were treated by TMMR-technique [59]. Regardless of the used surgical approach, the (metric) distance to the margins should be given in the pathology report. In small tumors the distance can be determined macroscopically, but in large tumors or close resection margins it should be determined histologically using a liner after marking on the slide or in even much more closer margins using an ocular micrometre (Fig. 18.15).

Despite there is no established regression grading system in cervical carcinomas [189] after neoadjuvant radio-(chemo-) therapy, the histopathological report should state if there are any therapeutic effects or not.

Regardless if there is a mesometrial/parametrial involvement, infiltration of the vaginal cuff should be given in the final report with its extension, localisation and distance to the resection margin.

Microscopically, there is no clear transition between the endocervical stroma and the mesometrial/parametrial tissue [94, 131]. But, if tumor is seen outside the endocervical stroma with infiltrative growth within the fibrous paracervical tissue, mesometrial/parametrial involvement should be diagnosed (Fig. 18.16). There is no doubt that the presence of tumor between large vessels and/or fatty tissue it represents stage pT2b. Some authors suggest that the infiltration of paracervical (fibrous) tissue and that of mesometrial tissue with invasion of fatty tissue represents two different ontogenetic tumor stages (oT-stage; [56]).

Metastatic involvement of mesometrial/parametrial lymph nodes represent lymph node involvement and should be staged as pN1 and not as stage pT2b.

There is no doubt that deep cervical stromal invasion represents a prognostic factor but, different studies have used different cut-off points for defining deep infiltrative growth, ranging from >25 to >75 % [28, 84, 91, 191]. Within the German guidelines for the diagnosis and treatment of carcinoma of the uterine cervix, deep stromal invasion was defined very recently as infiltration of >66 % [7]. Depth of invasion is measured from the level of the cervical mucosa up to the deepest point of invasion. The relative depth on invasion is calculated by the relationship between the deepest point of invasion and the full thickness of the cervical wall (see Fig. 18.17). The presence of lymphovascular space involvement outside the deepest point of tumor stromal infiltration will not alter the depth of invasion and should be diagnosed as L1.

There may be a prognostic impact of different patterns of invasion in squamous cell carcinoma of the uterine cervix ([64, 67]; Fig. 18.18). For adenocarcinomas a prognostic relevant 3-tired pattern of invasion has been described [31]. Pattern A represents an infiltrative growth of well-demarced well or moderate differentiated glands with rounded contours, frequently forming groups of glands or cribriform pattern, without lymphovascular space involvement, desmoplastic stromal reaction and without single cell invasion. Pattern B is characterised by early destructive stromal invasion arising from glands with pattern A-like features, with or without lymphovascular space involvement, whereas pattern C shows destructive invasion. It may be recommended to add the pattern of invasion within the histology report.

In case of radical hysterectomy after previous conisation and availability of the histopathology report of the conisation a final (maximal) tumor size should be calculated by summarising both sizes [7].

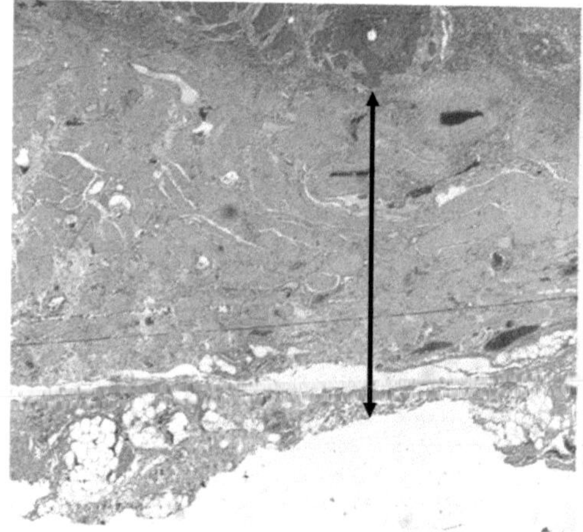

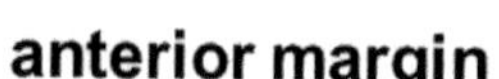

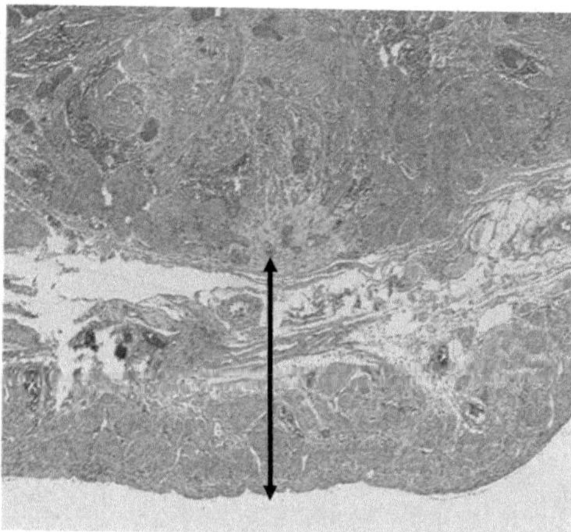

Fig. 18.15 Distances to the anterior and posterior resection margin of a TMMR-specimen with squamous cell carcinoma

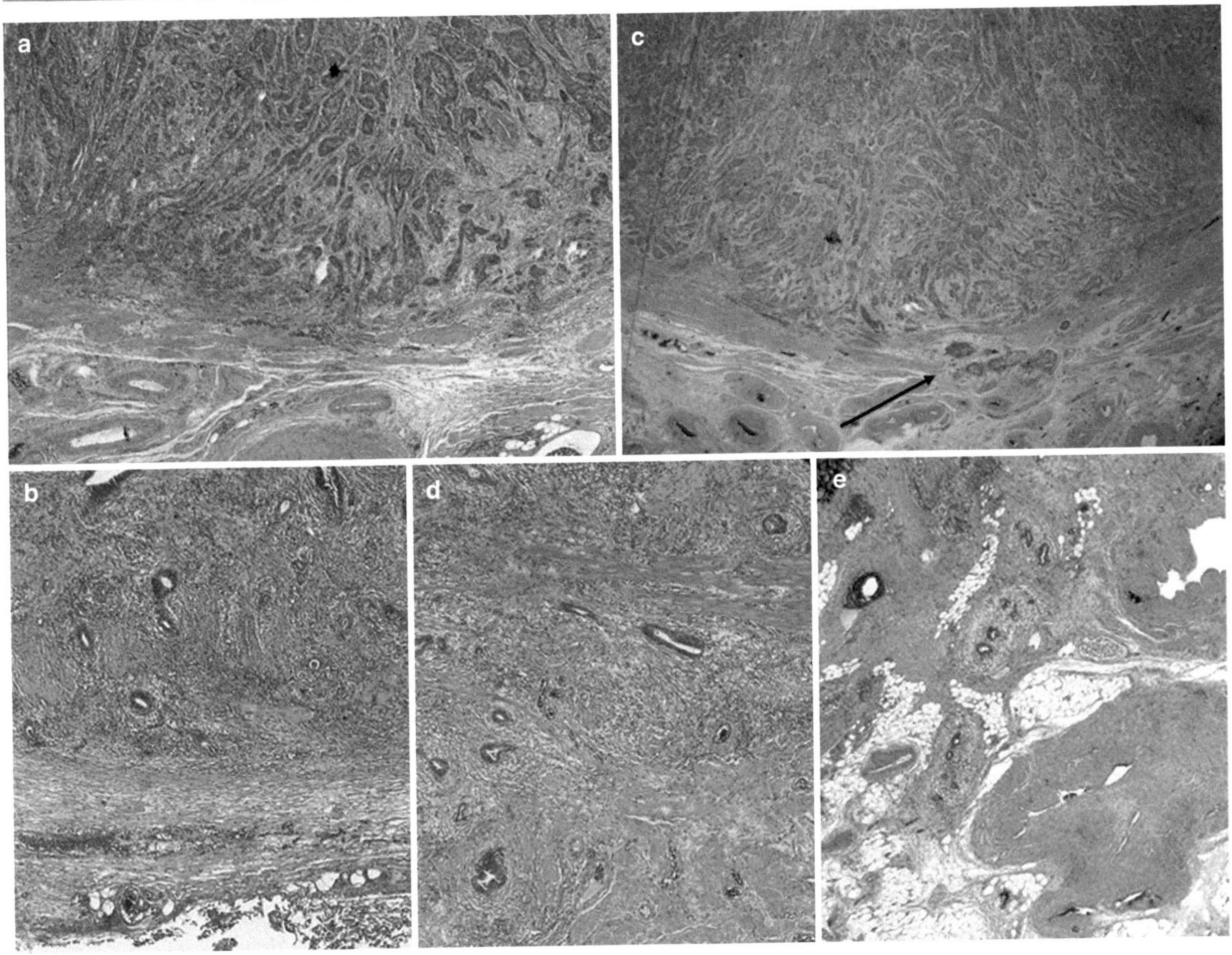

Fig. 18.16 Different patterns of parametrial (mesometrial) invasion by squamous cell carcinoma, indicating pT2b tumors. (**a**, **b**) complete infiltration of the cervical stroma (deep stromal invasion), tumor confined to the cervix, indicating pT1b tumor. (**c**) Very early infiltration outside the endocervical stroma, representing early pT2b tumor. (**d**) Infiltration of the fibrous tissue very close to the endocervical stroma, so called paracervical tissue (Höckel et al. 2014), which represents a part of parametrial (meosmetrial) tissue. (**e**) Infiltration of the fatty tissue of the parametrium (mesometrium)

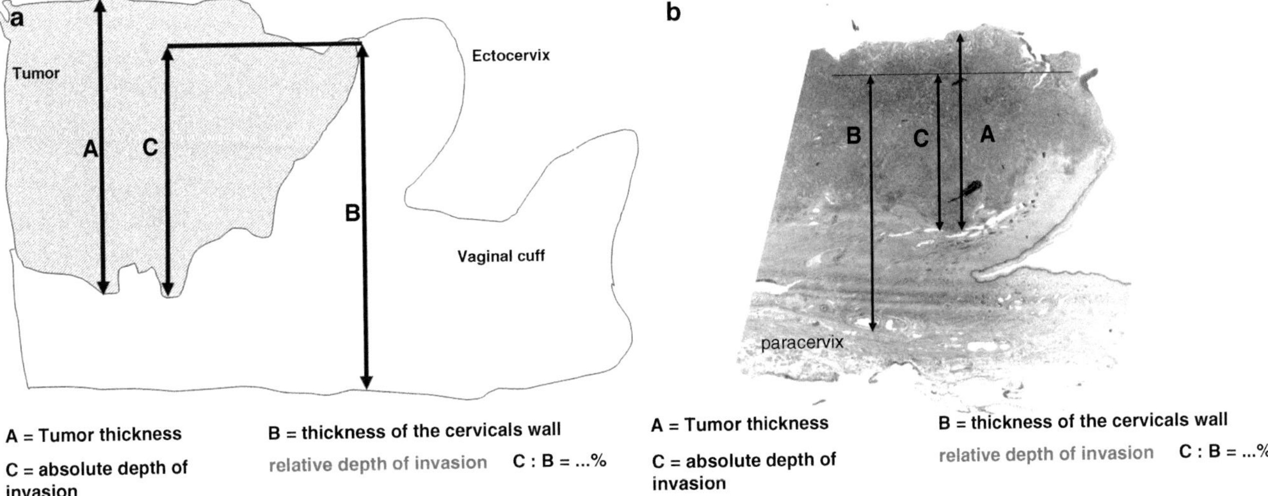

Fig. 18.17 Measurement of the depth of invasion for cervical carcinoma. Deep stromal invasion has been defined by the German guidelines as infiltration of >66 % of the endocervical stroma [7]. (**a**) Scheme for the measurement of absolute and relative depth of invasion. (**b**) Histologic scan containing the proximal part of the vaginal cuff, endo- and ectocervical transition (i.e. transformation zone) and full thickness of tumor and cervical wall

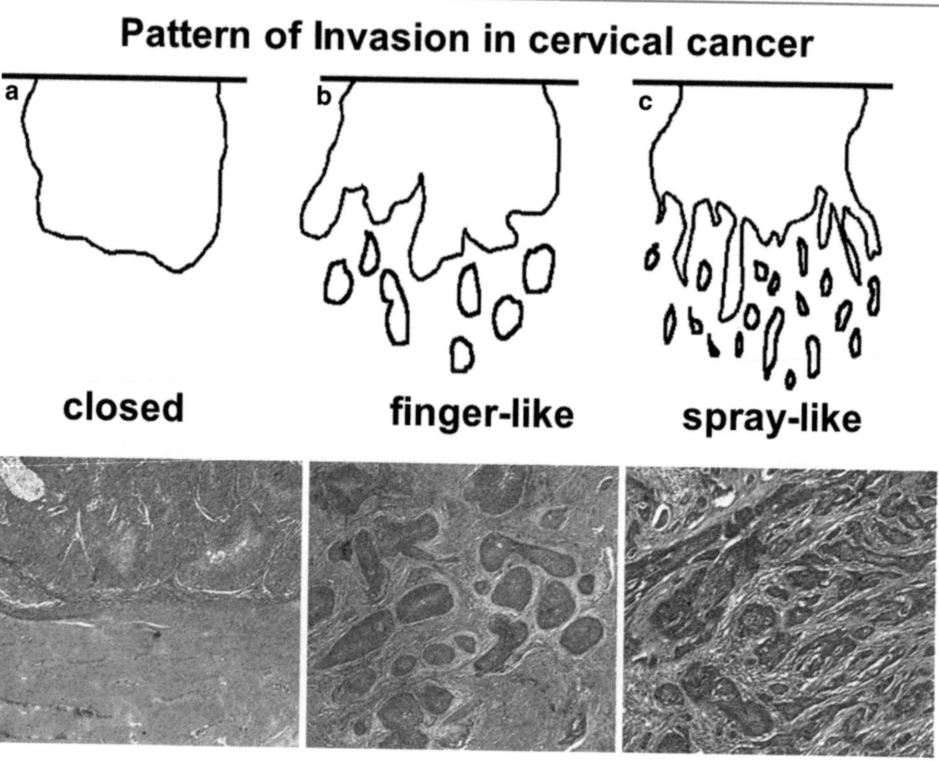

Fig. 18.18 Pattern of invasion of squamous cell carcinoma of the uterine cervix: Schematic description of the modified three-level scoring system for the description of the different types of infiltrative growth [64]. Histologic pictures of the different types of infiltrative growth: (**a**) closed pattern of invasion with cohesive tumor growth with well-delineated infiltrating borders and "pushing" margins, (**b**) finger-like pattern of invasion with trabecular tumor growth in solid cords and tumor cell nests, (**c**) spray-like pattern of invasion with tumor growth in small groups of infiltrating cells and high tumor cell dissociation

There is one major unclear topic within the staging of uterine cervical cancer [55]. The involvement of the Fallopian tube, ovary or adjacent mesoadnexal tissue ("adnexal involvement") is not recognised within the TNM-/FIGO-system [70, 159]. There are only limited studies dealing with the prognostic impact of that topic [78, 81, 153]. So, the impact of "adnexal involvement" is quite unclear at time. In the authors opinion, adnexal involvement represents a feature of local advanced disease and poor prognostic outcome [81] within uterine cervical carcinoma and should be stated as distant metastatic disease, categorised as pM1 OTH.

Hysterectomy with Endometrial Carcinoma and Malignant Mixed Müllerian Tumors (MMMT) (Figs. 18.19, 18.20, 18.21, 18.22, 18.23, and 18.24)

The term *endometrial* designs a lesion which is located within the endometrium. It says nothing about a special histopathological type and its clinical behaviour. Whereas the term *endometrioid* defines a lesion which is histopathologically similar to the morphology of endometrial glands (of the proliferative endometrium). So, an endometrioid endometrial adenocarcinoma means an adenocarcinoma within the endometrium representing a glandular morphology which is similar to the non-neoplastic glands of the endometrium (the adenocarcinoma looks alike normal glands of the endometrium).

According to recent research results MMMTs represent a special morphologic type of endometrial cancer [103, 114]. Consequently, the staging should be performed according to endometrial cancer [159].

The gross description of the endometrial tumor must include the exact anatomic location of the tumor (isthmus uteri (lower uterine segment), or where it is located within the corpus (anterior, posterior wall, dome), its three dimensional measurement and its relation to the cervix uteri as well as its shape (polypoid, sessile, diffuse). Sometimes the length of the vaginal cuff will be important. So, the length (or its absence) of the vaginal cuff should be given, separately for its anterior and posterior part. Some authors state the distance of the tumor to the internal/external cervical os.

For prognostic purposes, staging and adjuvant treatment, the size of the lesion, its depth of invasion within the myometrium and cervical involvement is very important [15, 16].

The cervix uteri should be sampled by one block from anterior and one from the posterior lip [127]. Regardless of macroscopic involvement of the cervix uteri or not, the endocervix should be sampled by (one) perpendicular section (Fig. 18.19). For adequate sampling some authors recommend embedding of several blocks [166]. In some cases,

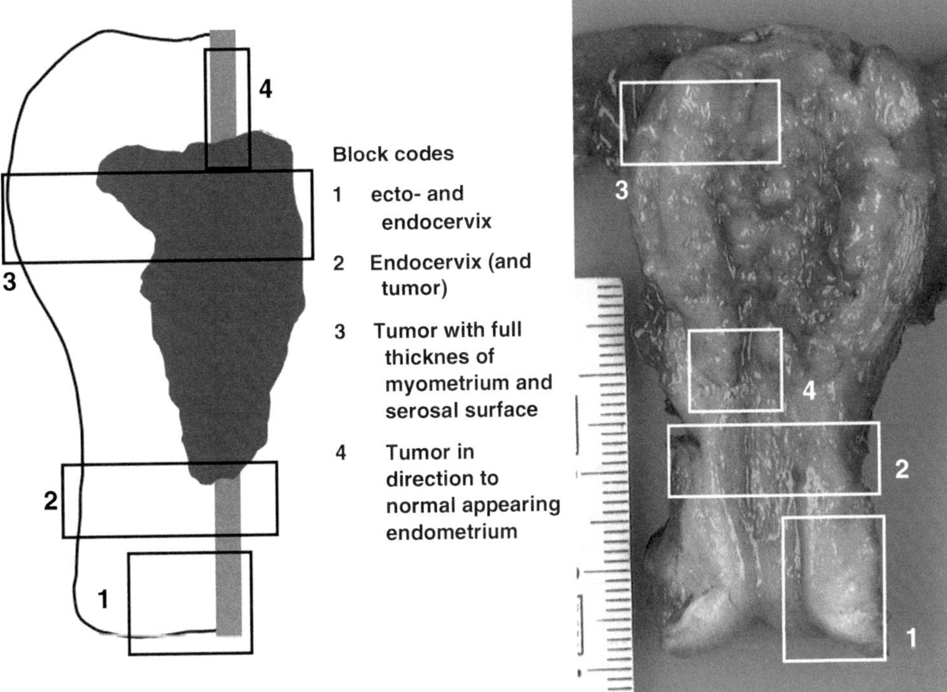

Fig. 18.19 Schematic sectioning of a hysterectomy specimen with endometrial carcinoma and block codes (for details see text and Tables 18.6 and 18.7)

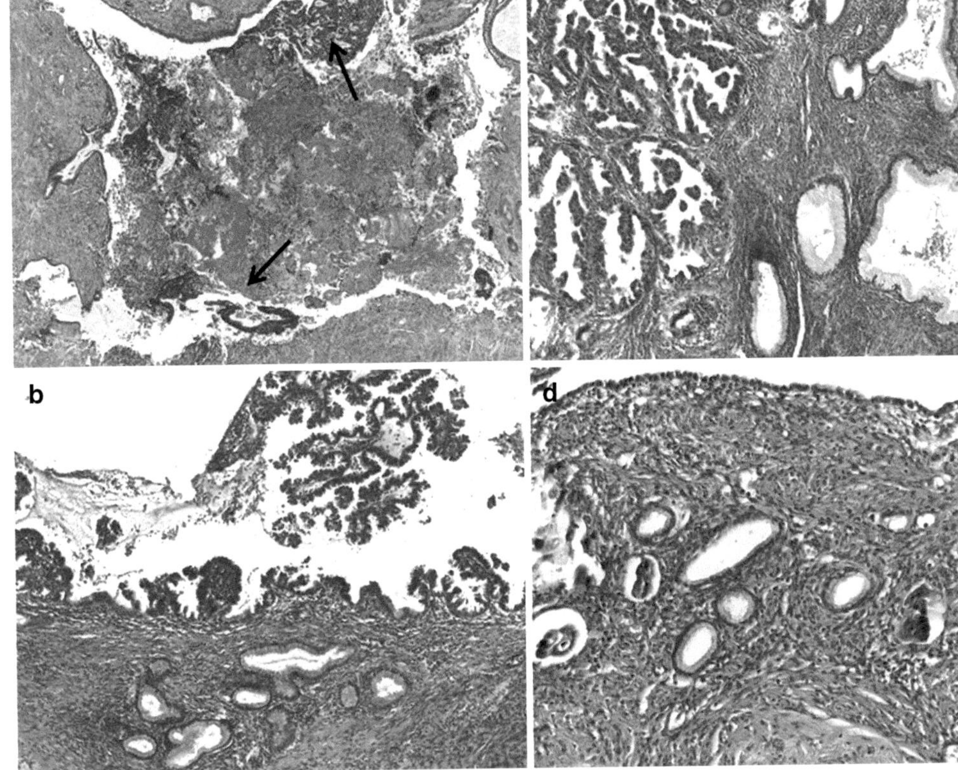

Fig. 18.20 Different patterns of cervical involvement by an endometrial carcinoma (**a–c** adopted from: Horn et al. 2011 [70]): (**a**) dislocated tissue of a well differentiated endometrioid ECX (*arrows*) within the cervical channel during irregular bleeding. (**b**) Involvement of endocervical glands by a serous endometrial carcinoma. Note the dislocated glands within the cervical channel (*arrows*) (**c**) infiltration of the cervical stroma by a serous endometrial carcinoma. (**d**) Lymphovascular space involvement of the endocervical stroma by a serous endometrial carcinoma

especially in those with serous endometrial carcinoma, lymphovascular space involvement (LVSI) or occult (microscopic) involvement of the endocervical stroma may occur (Fig. 18.20d). The presence of LVSI represents no "invasion" of the endocervical stroma and should not stated as pT2-tumor, but should be separately mentioned within the report and categorised as L1 [159]. Involvement of the endocervical glands (Fig. 18.20b) by the endometrial carcinoma has no longer impact on staging, whereas the invasion of the endocervical stroma has [132, 159]. The assessment of cervical involvement in endometrial carcinoma may cause some diagnostic problems but there is at most a fair-to-good agreement among specialist gynaecologic pathologists [112]. The determination and reporting of the depth of cervical stromal involvement is facultative at time (but may be asked by the clinicians), because it has no impact on treatment decisions and prognosis.

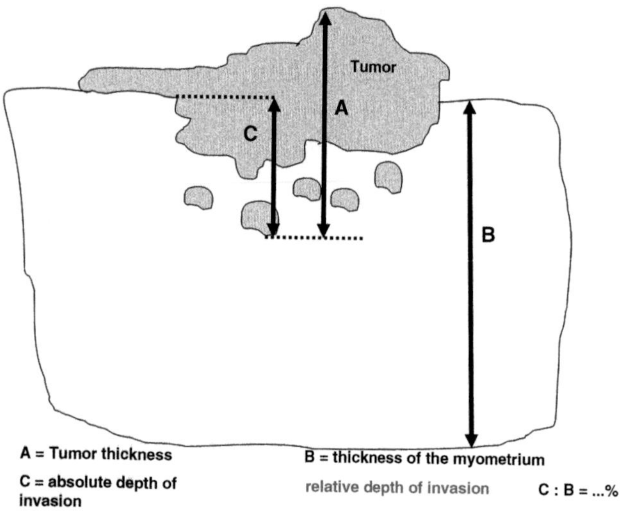

Fig. 18.21 Scheme for the measurement of the depth of invasion for endometrial cancer (Adopted from Robboy et al. [143]).

Within previously diagnosed pure endometrioid or serous endometrial cancer on fractional curetting one block per 2 cm largest tumor dimension is adequate. In mixed endometrioid/serous cancer (or other mixed histologic types, e.g. neuroendocrine carcinoma) and in MMMTs one block per 1 cm largest tumor dimension is recommended.

If there is no grossly visible tumor at the hysterectomy specimen extensive embedding as described for endometrial hyperplasia with embedding of about six sections, three of the anterior and three of the posterior parts of the fundus uteri [143] is recommended. Alternatively, wedge sections

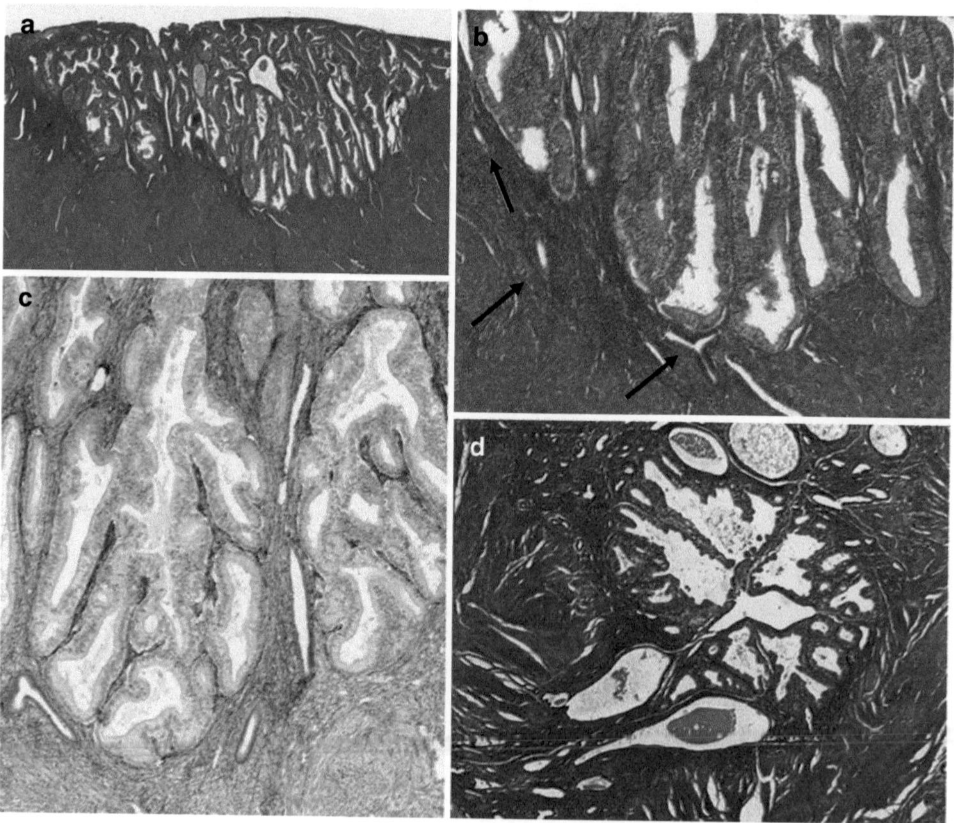

Fig. 18.22 Endometrioid endometrial adenocarcinoma. (**a**) Small well differentiated carcinoma within hysterectomy specimen. (**b**) Tumor glands protruding in direction to the myometrium. Note benign glands at the base of the tumor (*arrows*) as an morphologic feature that the carcinoma is confined to the endometrium. (**c**) Tumor glands are surrounded by a small rim of endometrial stroma cells, highlighted by CD 10 immunostaining (*brown colour*). (**d**) Endometrioid adenocarcinoma involving an endometriosis (see text)

Fig. 18.23 Hysterectomy specimens with endometrial carcinoma. (**a**) Simple hysterectomy with bilateral salpingo-oophorectomy with an endometrial cancer within the corpus uteri representing myometrial infiltration up to the outer third of the myometrium. (**b**, **c**) Anterior and posterior view of a endometrial carcinoma at the right tubal insertion within the uterine corpus (*arrow*) in a PMMR-Specimen (please see text)

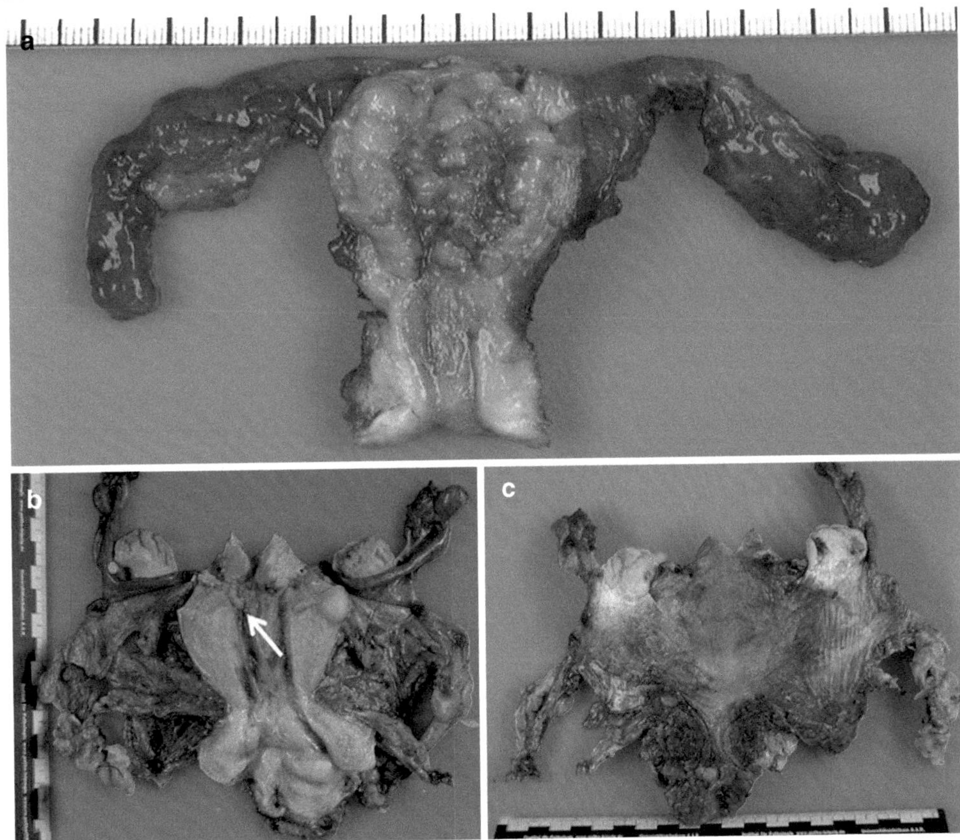

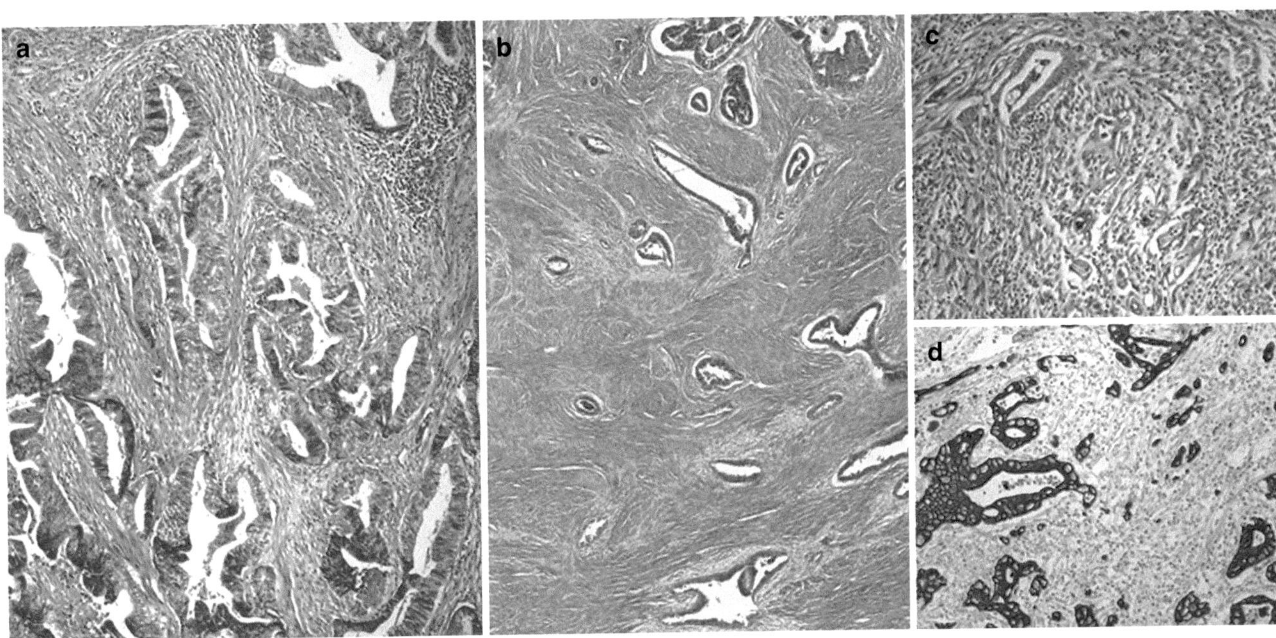

Fig. 18.24 Different patterns of invasion of endometrial adenocarcinoma. (**a**) Conventional pattern of myometrial invasion by a well differentiated endometrioid adenocarcinoma. (**b**) Minimal deviation pattern of myometrial invasion [62, 69]. (**c**, **d**) MELF-pattern of invasion, representing infiltrative growth of microcystic, elongated, fragmented glands (MELF), fragmented glands; highlighted in (**d**) by CK 18 immunostaining

can be performed by cutting small peaces of the endometrium and the immediately adjoining myometrium putting them in one cassette [143]. If there is no residual tumor seen (i.e. *vanishing endometrial cancer*; [3, 35]), complete embedding of the endometrium is recommended using wedge sections.

According to the WHO-classification [186], the term mixed carcinoma should only be used when two or more distinctive subtypes of endometrial carcinoma are identified, each representing more than 5 % of the tumor. When a carcinoma is classified as "mixed," the major and minor types and their relative proportions should be specified and the different percentages should be given in the pathology report.

It should be noted that for mixed endometrioid and serous carcinomas, studies have found variable results regarding tumor behaviour based on percentage of the serous component. Some studies have found that tumors with >25 % serous component behave like pure serous carcinomas [181], whereas other studies have shown that tumors with <10 % serous component also behave like pure serous carcinomas [100].

The depth of invasion should be noted grossly and the embedded tissue should document the area with maximal tumor invasion. The final depth on invasion should be calculated using the histological slides. The depth of invasion should be measured from the level of the adjacent endometrium up to the deepest point of tumor infiltration. If there is an exophytic growth of the tumor, the adjacent endometrium should be identified and an imaginary line should be drawn from that level through the tumor [143]. The distance below that line up to the deepest point of direct tumor infiltration represents the depth on invasion. This distance plus the distance above that line up to the surface of the tumor represent its thickness (Fig. 18.21). Any lymphovascular invasion below the infiltrating tumor front does not alter the depth of invasion and should be categorised as L1. The fact of LVSI below the infiltrating tumor edge should be transferred to the clinician.

Very rarely, *endometrial carcinoma* arises *within an uterine endometriosis* [85]. There, the depth of invasion should be calculated from the most superficial endometrial gland of that endometriosis up to the most distant tumor edge.

Determination of depth of invasion may be challenging [4]. There is no sharp border between the normal endometrium and myometrium, rather than a serrating/interdigitating appearance [55]. Infiltrating glands of endometrial cancer represent in a direct contact to the myometrium, sometimes surrounded by a tiny desmoplastic change (sometimes highlighted by van Gieson stain), but are not surrounded by normal endometrial ands and/or endometrial stroma. The latter one may be highlighted by CD 10-immunohistochemistry (Fig. 18.22a–c).

Involvement of endometriosis by endometrioid adenocarcinoma (Fig. 18.22d) is a known mimicker of myometrial infiltration and may occur in ~25 % of the cases. There is no adverse prognostic impact of that feature. The following features may be useful distinguishing involvement of an endometriosis versus true myometrial invasion [5, 55]:

- presence of benign and endometrial glands adjacent to the carcinoma,
- benign endometrial glands admixed within the carcinoma
- lack of desmoplastic stromal response,
- lack of inflammatory response,
- rounded appearance of the lesion with smooth border on low power.

It has been reported that there is the same thickness of the anterior and posterior wall of the uterus [180] so, the uninvolved myometrium from the opposite wall can be used as reference value determining myometrial thickness.

In contrast to simple hysterectomy for endometrial cancer (or radical hysterectomy in FIGO-stage II disease), women may be treated by peritoneal mesometrial resection (PMMR; Fig. 18.23b, c; [82]; in the chapter about Hysterectomy in Precancerous Lesions or Microinvasive Carcinoma of the Cervix at page 560).

There are some different patterns of invasion within endometrial carcinomas (Fig. 18.24). Beside the classic pattern of growth, an adenoma malignum-like pattern has been described [79].

The so called MELF-pattern of invasion, representing infiltrative growth of microcystic, elongated, fragmented glands (MELF), surrounded by peritumoral desmoplastic stromal response [125] may represent an indicator for high epithelial-mesenchymal transition [164] and has recently been discussed as prognostic factor [40]. So, the different types of invasive growth should be stated within the histopathological report.

There is one major unclear topic within the staging of endometrial cancer and MMMTs, which has been discussed previously [55, 68, 72, 137, 188].

Within the current issue of FIGO/TNM-classification, stage pT3a disease is defined as "tumor invades uterine serous and/or adnexa (direct extension or metastasis) and/or cancer cells in ascites or peritoneal washings" [70, 159]. There is no clear statement how the term adnexal involvement is defined. Tumor deposits within the Fallopian tube and the ovary with histologically proven stromal invasion represents adnexal involvement as is in case of adnexal meso-infiltration (see Fig. 18.25).

The recently recognised intramucosal spread of endometrial and non-gynaecologic cancers to the Fallopians tubal mucosa [163] also represents adnexal involvement (Fig. 18.25e). But, what is about the presence of LVSI within the meso-salpinx, mes-ovarium, the Fallopian tube and the ovarian stroma?

In our opinion LVSI at that location represents biologically stage pT3a-disease [68, 72]. But under staging purposes, LVSI within the adnexal structures must be categorised as L1 rather than as stage pT3a-disease [159, 182]. The histopathologic report should give the clinician detailed information about the localisation of LVSI and the patterns in case of adnexal involvement.

Because the adnexal involvement may be grossly not evident in a serious number of cases [68, 72], careful examination of adnexal tissue is recommended. The majority of patients with ECX are postmenopausal and the ovaries are usually small and atrophic, so extensive/complete embedding may not be time and/or cost consuming. As suggested by others [156], and under recognition of our above mentioned results, we would recommend complete processing of macroscopic inconspicuous adnexae, regardless of the histologic type of ECX. Within the cutting of the ovary we prefer sectioning along the short axis of the ovary with embedding of the adjacent mesovarian tissue [62, 69] and for handling of the Fallopian tube we adopted the protocol which is currently used for the handling of the tubes in prophylactic adnexectomies from women with BRCA mutations (so called SEE-FIM-protocol; [115, 151]).

A direct invasion or metastatic spread into the parametrial tissue and/or vagina will be staged as pT3b [159]. The presence of LVSI represents no "metastatic spread" and should

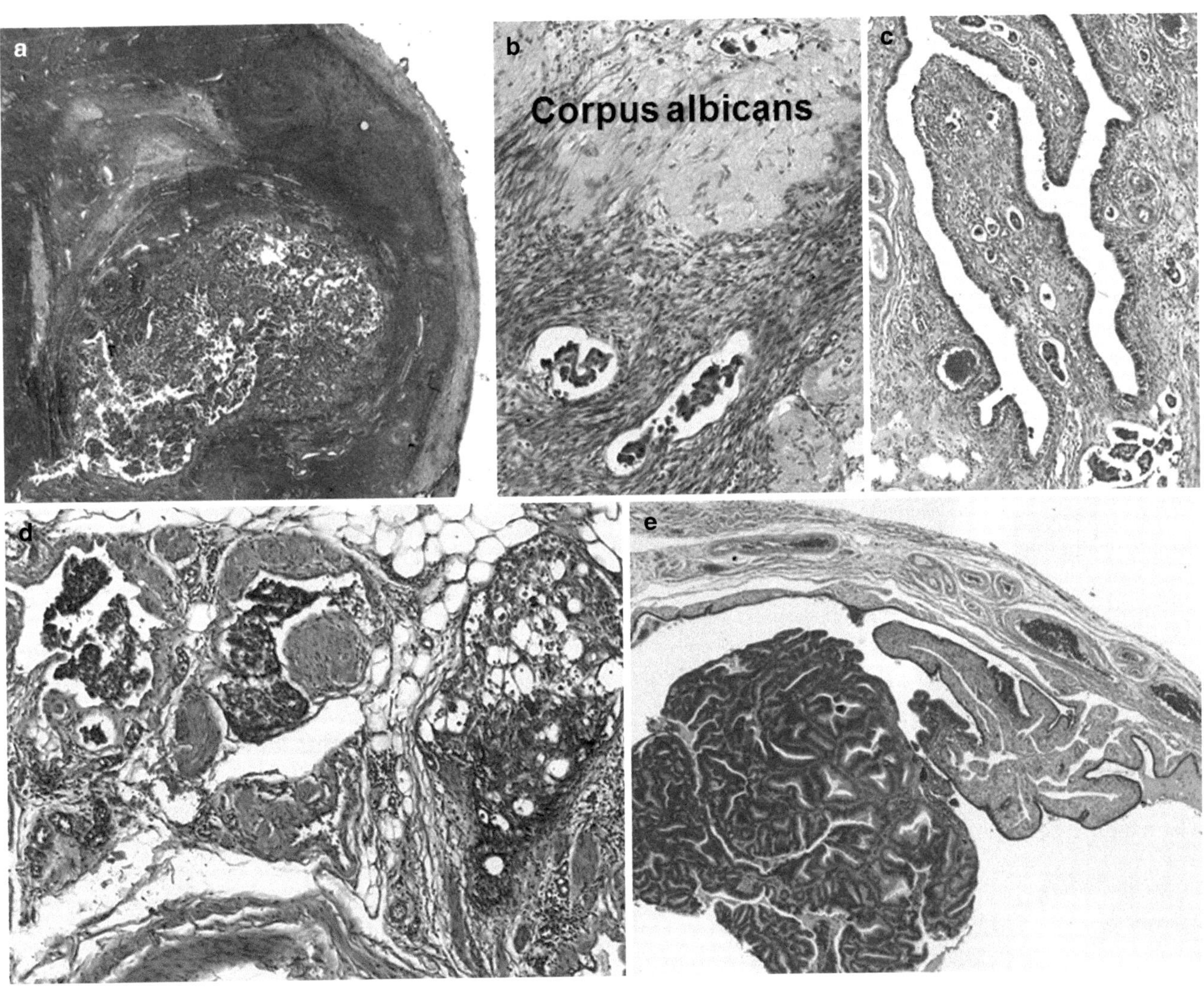

Fig. 18.25 Different patterns of adnexal involvement by endometrial carcinoma [70]. (**a**) Metastasis to the ovarian stroma of an adenosquamous carcinoma of the endometrium. (**b**) lymphovascular space involvement of the ovarian stroma by a serous endometrial carcinoma. (**c**) lymphovascular space involvement of the Fallopian's tubal mucosa by a serous endometrial cancer. (**d**) lymphovascular space involvement of mesoadnexal tissue by a poorly differentiated endometrioid cancer. (**e**) Intramucosal spread to the Fallopina stube mucosa by an endometrioid endometrial adenocarcinoma

Table 18.6 Synopsis of the features within the final oncologic histopathology report of endometrial cancer and malignant Müllerian mixed tumors (MMMT) of the uterus [17, 62, 69, 110, 124, 145, 155]

Histopathologic tumor type (WHO)[a]
Grading (WHO/FIGO)
Absence/presence of lymphovascular and blood vessel (venous) involvement (L- and V-status)
Absence/presence of perineural invasion (Pn-status)
Tumor stage (TNM)
Tumor size and depth of invasion into the myometrium
Tumor size in three dimensions in macroinvasive disease
Presence of (endo-) cervical stromal invasion
Presence/localisation and extension of mesometrial/parametrial invasion
Minimal distance to the resection margins
R-classification (UICC)
Status of the adnexae

[a]the WHO-classification [186] defines mixed carcinomas as tumors where two or more distinctive subtypes are identified, each representing more than 5 % of the tumor. Some studies have found that mixed serous cancer with even >10 % or >25 % of serous component represent adverse outcome [100, 181]. So, each percentage of serous component should be given within the pathology report

not be stated as pT3b-tumor, but should be separately mentioned within the pathology report and categorised as L1 [159].

An unclear issue by definition is the categorisation of the presence of lymph node metastases within the parametrial tissue in endometrial cancer. Lymph node metastases at that location represent metastatic involvement and according to the TNM-classification it represents a pT3b tumor. But, parametrial lymph nodes are defined as regional lymph nodes in endometrial cancer. So, the question appears, if the parametrial nodes are involved should they counted as pN1 as well? Uninvolved parametrial nodes should be counted within the overall number of resected regional nodes.

General aspects of gross description and parameters of the histopathology report are summarised in Tables 18.3 and 18.6.

The final oncology pathology report should recognise the most recent WHO-classification [186] for tumor typing the TNM-classification for staging [159].

Hysterectomy with Uterine Sarcomas

The majority of uterine sarcomas occur within the corpus uteri.

So, the cervix uteri should be sampled by one block from anterior and one from the posterior lip. In case of gross involvement of the endocervix, it should be sampled by perpendicular section(s). To ensure correct diagnosis, extensive sampling i.e. one paraffine block per 1 cm largest tumor dimension should be performed [110, 133, 168]. To cover different morphologic features within the tumor it is helpful to obtain different blocks from different locations with embedding the edges of hemorrhagic and necrotic foci or those with different colours and edges of the lesion protruding in the adjacent myometrium [110, 130, 133].

At time, there is no grading for leimoysarcomas in the WHO classification [129]. Some clinical oncologists urge their pathologist to give a grading for these tumors. In those cases the grading system of the Fédération Nationale des Centres de Lutte Contre le Cancer [23, 24, 30] i.e. FNCLCC-grading system should be adopted.

General aspects of gross description and parameters of the histopathology report are summarised in Tables 18.3 and 18.7.

The final oncology pathology report should recognise the most recent WHO-classification [129] for tumor typing the TNM-classification for staging [159].

Handling of Lymphonodectomy Specimens in Uterine Malignancies (Figs. 18.3 and 18.26)

In uterine cancer and MMMT regional lymph node involvement represents the locoregional spread.

It should be documented (three dimensional measuring) how many tissue was sent for each defined location of lymph node resection. Careful dissection of the specimen is necessary with submission of all visible and palpable lymph nodes. The embedding of the whole lymph node up a maxi-

Table 18.7 Synopsis of the features within the final oncologic histopathology report of uterine sarcomas [22, 26, 77, 110, 133, 168]

Histopathologic tumor type (WHO)
Grading (WHO) of endometrial stromal sarcomas[a]
Tumor regression after previous treatment (including hormonal treatment)
Absence/presence of lymphovascular and blood vessel (venous) involvement (L- and V-status)
Absence/presence of perineural invasion (Pn-status)
Tumor stage (TNM)
Tumor size in three dimensions
Depth of invasion within the myometrium
Presence/localisation and extension of extrauterine infiltration
Minimal distance to the resection margins
R-classification (UICC)

[a]The WHO-classification separate endometrial stromal tumor in low-grade and high-grade enodmetrial stromal tumors and separate them from undifferentiated uterine sarcomas (UUS)

mum dimension of 0.3 cm without slicing has been recommended [63]. Larger nodes should be bivalved along its longest axis and processed completely as well [63, 75, 96, 145].

If the gross lymph node number is small and the remaining soft tissue is small, it may be worthwhile to entirely submit the tissue from that special location for histopathologic analysis [143]. Extensive or complete embedding of the soft tissue resulting from lymph node resection may reassure the clinician that a thorough examination of the tissue has been performed. The use of so called clearing techniques may increase the number of detected nodes [1]. But in case of careful handling of the removed tissue during lymph node resection, clearing techniques cannot being recommended by the authors and others [145] for gynaecologic malignancies.

The performance of step sections (e.g. three step sections with an interval of 200 μm) may increase the detection of small metastases [75, 96].

Isolated tumor cells (ITC) within a lymph node are single tumor cells or small tumor cell clusters not more than 0.2 mm in greatest dimension that can be detected on routine H&E-staining or using immunohistochemistry [182]. To the best of our knowledge, there are no studies regarding prognostic impact of ITC for cervical and endometrial cancer at time. Two reports are dealing with "low volume lymphe node involvement" in patients with cervical carcinoma [19, 161]. In these studies there are no definitions of ITC and micrometastases according to the UICC and AJCC definitions and cases with ITC and micrometastases were not seprated within statistical evaluation. So the question of the prognostic impact of ITC in cervical carcinoma is still unanswered. In the author opinion, the presence of ITC should be reported to the clinician, because that feature indicates the capability for lymphovascuar spread of the given tumor.

The same issues must be stated for the presence of lymphovascular involvement within the fatty tissue surrounding the lymph nodes and within the Vasa afferentia of the lymph nodes in the lymph nodes capsule (Fig. 18.26a, e). Both features are categorised within the L-category of the TNM-system but not as lymph node involvement (N-category).

Micrometastases within lymph nodes are defined by the UICC as the presence of tumor cell deposits larger than 0.2 mm, but not exceeding 0.2 cm ([182]; Figs. 18.4g and 18.26b). This definition was adopted for cervical carcinoma by the last version of the German National guidelines for the diagnosis and treatment of cervical cancer [7] and will be adopted within the next issue of the guidelines for endometrial cancer.

There are some studies which reported the prognostic impact of micrometastases (pN1mic) for cervical carcinomas [45, 65, 66, 99, 105]. Within one study patients with pN1mic have had a poor prognostic outcome than node negative patients but an improved one when it was compared to those with macrometastatic disease [65, 66].

Extracapsular extension of the metastatic deposits into the perinodal fatty tissue (i.e. extracapsular extension; ECS; Fig. 18.26f, g) is an established prognostic factor for vulvar cancer and that feature is included in the N-categorisation within the TNM-system. For carcinoma of the uterine cervix it has been reported that ECS may be of prognostic impact as well [62, 69, 108]. So, that feature may be included within the pathology report of removed lymph nodes representing with metastases of any gynecologic malignancy.

A synopsis of histopathologic report of lymphonodectomy specimens is summarised in Table 18.8.

Block codes

1 Ectocervix

2 Endocervix (and placenta)

3 Myometrium and chorionis membrane

4 Umbilical cord#

5 Amnion membrane

6 Placenta and implatation site within the myometrium

7 Placenta and implantation site with thinned myometrium

8 Placenta and thinned uterine wall within the lower uterine segment

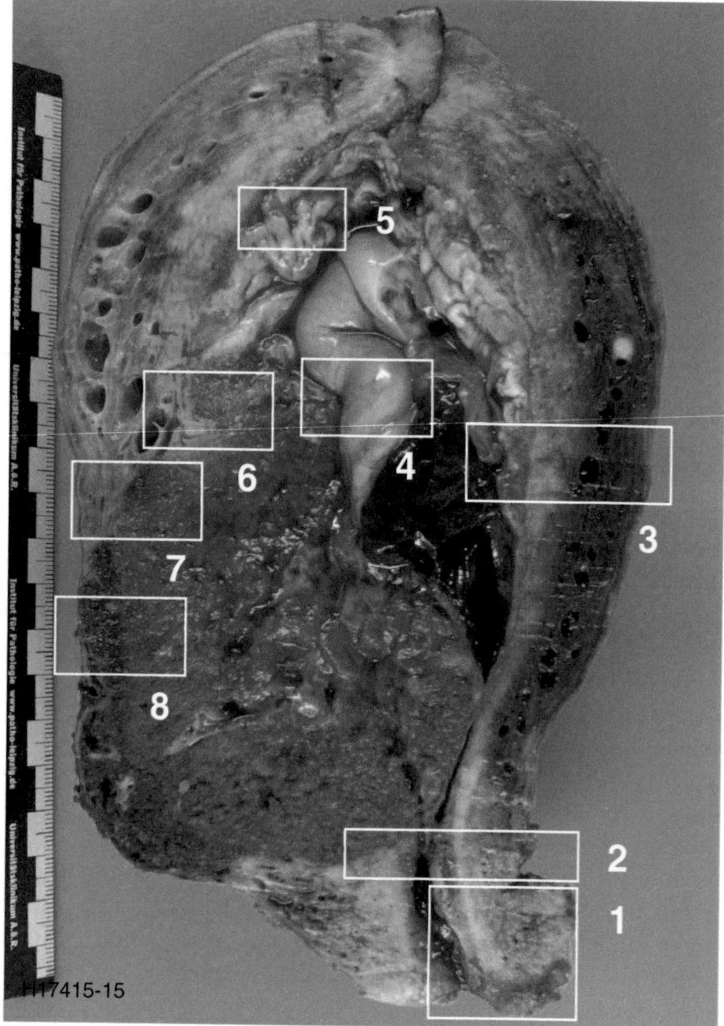

Fig. 18.26 Frontal cut of an hysterectomy with placenta praevia with block code for tissue embedding

Table 18.8 Synopsis of the features within the final histopathology report for removed lymph nodes [63, 96, 143, 145]

Give the location and the dimension of the removed tissue for lymphonodectomy
Give the number of removed/examined nodes per location
Give the number of positive nodes in relation to the number of removed/examined nodes (e.g. 4/13 right pelvic nodes or 0/15 para-aortic nodes)
Largest dimension of nodal metastatic deposit per location
Absence of presence of extracapsular spread of the metastatic deposits per location
Presence or absence of lymphovascular space involvement within the fatty tissue surrounding the lymph node
After pre-operative chemotherapy and/or radiotherapy, regressive changes should be roprted

Handling Omentectomy Specimens

Omentectomy represents a routine part of staging surgery in type 2 endometrial carcinomas (serous and clear-cell carcinomas) and in some cases of malignant mixed Müllerian tumors as well as in selected cases of endometrioid adenocarcinoma.

Macroscopically three dimensions of the omentum should be provided in the pathology report to document the size. This may be useful in certain scenarios to direct the need for further surgery. Additionally, the size may be also helpful to determine the extent of sampling for histologic examination. Any unusual gross findings should be noted and proofed by tissue embedding.

At time, there are no standardized guidelines for sampling omental specimens in gynecologic malignancies. Interestingly, omental sampling is not mentioned within the recommendations of the College of American Pathologists (CAP) and the International Collaboration on Cancer Reporting (ICCR) within their protocols for endometrial malignancies.

The following suggestions are based mainly on studies of ovarian malignancies.

In a *grossly involved omentum*, submitting 1 block for histologic examination is probably sufficient [32, 174].

For *grossly negative omental specimens* the sampling methods vary within different studies.

For ovarian borderline tumors, a meticulously gross examination with an embedding of at least 1 section per 2 cm of maximum dimension was suggested [150]. Usubütün et al. [174] recommended one section per 2–3 cm of maximum omental diameter in cases with ovarian or endometrial cancer. Another studie suggest 1 block for every 67 mm of maximal dimension of omentum in ovarian neoplasms [32]. A recent study reported an estimated sensitivity of 82 % by an examination of 5 blocks and of 95 % by 10 blocks performing a theoretical model ("*in silico*")for optimal sampling of grossly normal omentum in various gynecologic malignancies [158]. In real life studies, the examination of 3–5 blocks was suggested as representative in cases with gynecologic malignancies [158, 174]. The CAP-protocol for ovarian neoplasms generally recommend to take 5–10 sections (a section means a tissue sample transferred to the embedding cassette) from the omentum [25] which may blocked in about 5 paraffine blocks.

For practical purposes in the author opinion, the recommendation for omental sampling of the ICCR for primary ovarian, Fallopian tube and peritoneal cancer [113] should be adopted for endometrial cancer. There, the embedding of 4–6 blocks in cases where the omentum is grossly negative is recommended.

Within pathology report, the size of the largest tumour deposit should be recorded. It should also be reported the presence of omental lymph nodes with or without metastatic deposits. Omental lymph nodes represent not regional lymph nodes in endometrial cancer by the definition of the TNM. So, omental lymph node involvement represents stage T3/FIGO III disease. Any additional findings (e.g. inflammatory change, mesothelial hyperplasia, scaring) should be noted as well.

References

1. Abassi-Ghadi N, Boshier PR, Goldin R, Hanna GB. Techniques to increase lymph node harvest from gastrointestinal cancer specimens: a systematic review and meta-analysis. Histopathology. 2012;61(4):531–42.
2. Abiko K, Baba T, Ogawa M, Mikami Y, Koyama T, Mandai M, Konishi I. Minimal deviation mucinous adenocarcinoma ('adenoma malignum') of the uterine corpus. Pathol Int. 2010;60(1):42–7.
3. Ahmed QF, Gattoc L, Al-Wahab Z, Abdulfatah E, Ruterbusch JJ, Cote M, Bandyopadhyay S, Morris RT, Ali-Fehmi R. Vanishing endometrial cancer in hysterectomy specimens: a myth or a fact. Am J Surg Pathol. 2015;39(2):221–6.
4. Ali A, Black D, Soslow RA. Difficulties in assessing the depth of myometrial invasion in endometrial carcinoma. Int J Gynecol Pathol. 2007;26:115–23.
5. Argani P, Cimino-Mathews A. Intraoperative frozen sections. Diagnostic pitfalls. New York: demosMedical; 2014. p. 255–8.
6. Atienza-Amores M, Guerini-Rocco E, Soslow RA, Park KJ, Weigelt B. Small cell carcinoma of the gynecologic tract: a multifaceted spectrum of lesions. Gynecol Oncol. 2014;134(2):410–8.
7. AWMF. S3-Leitlinie Diagnostik, Therapie und Nachsorge der Patientin mit Zervixkarzinom. Langversion; 2014. http://www.awmf.org/uploads/tx_szleitlinien/032-033OL1_S3_Zervixkarzinom_2014-10.pdf.
8. Bachtiary B, Boutros PC, Pintilie M, Shi W, Bastianutto C, Li JH, Schwock J, Zhang W, Penn LZ, Jurisica I, Fyles A, Liu FF. Gene expression profiling in cervical cancer: an exploration of intratumor heterogeneity. Clin Cancer Res. 2006;12(19):5632–40.

9. Baker P, Oliva E. A practical approach to intraoperative consultation in gynecological pathology. Int J Gynecol Pathol. 2008;27(3):353–65.
10. Bartosch C, Exposito MI, Lopes JM. Low-grade endometrial stromal sarcoma and undifferentiated endometrial sarcoma: a comparative analysis emphasizing the importance of distinguishing between these two groups. Int J Surg Pathol. 2010; 18(4):286–91.
11. Bartosch C, Manuel Lopes J, Oliva E. Endometrial carcinomas: a review emphasizing overlapping and distinctive morphological and immunohistochemical features. Adv Anat Pathol. 2011;18(6):415–37.
12. Bjornsson BL, Nelson BE, Reale FR, Rose PG. Accuracy of frozen section for lymph node metastasis in patients undergoing radical hysterectomy for carcinoma of the cervix. Gynecol Oncol. 1993;51(1):50–3.
13. Bojahr B, Tchartchian G, Ohlinger R. Laparoscopic supracervical hysterectomy: a retrospective analysis of 1000 cases. JSLS. 2009;13(2):129–34.
14. Buchanan DD, Tan YY, Walsh MD, Clendenning M, Metcalf AM, Ferguson K, Arnold ST, Thompson BA, Lose FA, Parsons MT, Walters RJ, Pearson SA, Cummings M, Oehler MK, Blomfield PB, Quinn MA, Kirk JA, Stewart CJ, Obermair A, Young JP, Webb PM, Spurdle AB. Tumor mismatch repair immunohistochemistry and DNA MLH1 methylation testing of patients with endometrial cancer diagnosed at age younger than 60 years optimizes triage for population-level germline mismatch repair gene mutation testing. J Clin Oncol. 2014;32(2):90–100.
15. Burke WM, SGO Clinical Practice Endometrial Cancer Working Group, Orr J, Leitao M, Salom E, Gehrig P, Olawaiye AB, Brewer M, Boruta D, Villella J, Herzog T, Abu Shahin F, Society of Gynecologic Oncology Clinical Practice Committee. Endmetrial cancer: a review and current management strategies: part I. Gynecol Oncol. 2014;134(2):385–92.
16. Burke WM, SGO Clinical Practice Endometrial Cancer Working Group, Orr J, Leitao M, Salom E, Gehrig P, Olawaiye AB, Brewer M, Boruta D, Herzog TJ, Shahin FA, Society of Gynecologic Oncology Clinical Practice Committee. Endometrial cancer: a review and current management strategies: part II. Gynecol Oncol. 2014 Aug;134(2):393–402.
17. CAP. College of American Pathologists. 2011. http://www.cap.org/apps/docs/committees/cancer/cancer_protocols/2011/Cervix_11protocol.pdf.
18. Charames GS, Millar AL, Pal T, Narod S, Bapat B. Do MSH6 mutations contribute to double primary cancers of the colorectum and endometrium? Hum Genet. 2000;107:623–9.
19. Cibula D, Abu-Rustum NR, Dusek L, Zikán M, Zaal A, Sevcik L, Kenter GG, Querleu D, Jach R, Bats AS, Dyduch G, Graf P, Klat J, Lacheta J, Meijer CJ, Mery E, Verheijen R, Zweemer RP. Prognostic significance of low volume sentinel lymph node disease in early-stage cervical cancer. Gynecol Oncol. 2012;124(3):496–501.
20. Cibula D, Sláma J, Svárovský J, Fischerova D, Freitag P, Zikán M, Pinkavová I, Pavlista D, Dundr P, Hill M. Abdominal radical trachelectomy in fertility-sparing treatment of early-stage cervical cancer. Int J Gynecol Cancer. 2009;19(8):1407–11.
21. Clement PB. The pathology of endometriosis: a survey of the many faces of a common disease emphasizing diagnostic pitfalls and unusual and newly appreciated aspects. Adv Anat Pathol. 2007;14(4):241–60.
22. Clement PB. The pathology of uterine smooth muscle tumors and mixed endometrial stromal-smooth muscle tumors: a selective review with emphasis on recent advances. Int J Gynecol Pathol. 2000;19:39–55.
23. Coindre JM. Grading and staging of sarcoma. In: CDM F, Bridge JA, PCW H, Mertens F, editors. WHO classification of tumours of soft tissue and bone. Lyon: IARC Press; 2013. p. 17–8.
24. Coindre JM. Grading of soft tissue sarcomas: review and update. Arch Pathol Lab Med. 2006;130(10):1448–53.
25. CAP: College of American Pathologists. Protocol for the examination of specimens from patients with carcinoma of the ovary. 2015. http://www.cap.org/web/oracle/webcenter/portalapp/pages/search-results.jspx?searchTerms=hysterectomy+omentectomy+peritoneal+biopsies+specify&_adf.ctrl-state=263oqd8k1_21&_afrLoop=629838432981632.
26. Coffey D, Kaplan AL, Ramzy I. Intraoperative consultation in gynecologic pathology. Arch Pathol Lab Med. 2005;129:1544–57.
27. Conklin CMJ, Longacre TA. Lynch syndrome in endometrial carcinoma: a sentinel diagnosis. Pathol Case Rev. 2014;19:78–84.
28. Delgado G, Bundy B, Zaino R, Sevin BU, Creasman WT, Major F. Prospective surgical-pathological study of disease-free interval in patients with stage IB squamous cell carcinoma of the cervix: a Gynecologic Oncology Group study. Gynecol Oncol. 1990;38(3):352–7.
29. Dempster WT. Rates of penetration of fixing fluids. Am J Anat. 1960;107:59–72.
30. Deyrup AT, Weiss SW. Grading of soft tissue sarcomas: the challenge of providing precise information in an imprecise world. Histopathology. 2006;48(1):42–50.
31. Diaz De Vivar A, Roma AA, Park KJ, Alvarado-Cabrero I, Rasty G, Chanona-Vilchis JG, Mikami Y, Hong SR, Arville B, Teramoto N, Ali-Fehmi R, Rutgers JK, Tabassum F, Barbuto D, Aguilera-Barrantes I, Shaye-Brown A, Daya D, Silva EG. Invasive endocervical adenocarcinoma: proposal for a new pattern-based classification system with significant clinical implications: a multi-institutional study. Int J Gynecol Pathol. 2013;32(6):592–601.
32. Doig T, Monaghan H. Sampling the omentum in ovarian neoplasia: when one block is enough. Int J Gynecol Cancer. 2006;16:36–40.
33. Doering DL, Barnhill DR, Weiser EB, et al. Intraoperative evaluation of depth of myometrial invasion in stage I endometrial adenocarcinoma. Obstet Gynecol. 1989;74:930–3.
34. Downes MR, Allo G, McCluggage WG, Sy K, Ferguson SE, Aronson M, Pollett A, Gallinger S, Bilbily E, Shaw P, Clarke BA. Review of findings in prophylactic gynaecological specimens in Lynch syndrome with literature review and recommendations for grossing. Histopathology. 2014;65(2):228–39.
35. Dubé V, Macdonald D, Allingham-Hawkins DJ, Kamel-Reid S, Colgan TJ. Vanishing endometrial carcinoma. Int J Gynecol Pathol. 2007;26(3):271–7.
36. Ehdaivand S, Simon RA, Sung CJ, Steinhoff MM, Lawrence WD, Quddus MR. Incidental gynecologic neoplasms in morcellated uterine specimens: a case series with follow-up. Hum Pathol. 2014;45(11):2311–7.
37. El-Bahrawy M, Ganesan R. Frozen section in gynaecology: uses and limitations. Arch Gynecol Obstet. 2014;289(6):1165–70.
38. Emons G, Mallmann P, members of the Uterus Commission of AGO. Recommendations for the diagnosis and treatment of endometrial caner, update 2013. Geburtshilfe Frauenheilk. 2014;74:244–7.
39. Estape RE, Angioli R, Madrigal M, Janicek M, Gomez C, Penalver M, Averette H. Close vaginal margins as a prognostic factor after radical hysterectomy. Gynecol Oncol. 1998;68(3):229–32.
40. Euscher E, Fox P, Bassett R, Al-Ghawi H, Ali-Fehmi R, Barbuto D, Djordjevic B, Frauenhoffer E, Kim I, Hong SR, Montiel D, Moschiano E, Roma A, Silva E, Malpica A. The pattern of myometrial invasion as a predictor of lymph node metastasis or extrauterine disease in low-grade endometrial carcinoma. Am J Surg Pathol. 2013;37(11):1728–36.
41. Fader AN, Edwards RP, Cost M, Kanbour-Shakir A, Kelley JL, Schwartz B, Sukumvanich P, Comerci J, Sumkin J, Elishaev E, Rohan LC. Sentinel lymph node biopsy in early-stage cervical cancer: utility of intraoperative versus postoperative assessment. Gynecol Oncol. 2008;111(1):13–7.

42. Fanning J, Tsukada Y, Piver MS. Intraoperative frozen section diagnosis of depth of myometrial invasion in endometrial adenocarcinoma. Gynecol Oncol. 1990;37:47–50.
43. Ferguson SE, Aronson M, Pollett A, Eiriksson LR, Oza AM, Gallinger S, Lerner-Ellis J, Alvandi Z, Bernardini MQ, MacKay HJ, Mojtahedi G, Tone AA, Massey C, Clarke BA. Performance characteristics of screening strategies for Lynch syndrome in unselected women with newly diagnosed endometrial cancer who have undergone universal germline mutation testing. Cancer. 2014; 120(24):3932–9.
44. Franchi M, Ghezzi F, Melpignano M, Cherchi PL, Scarabelli C, Apolloni C, Zanaboni F. Clinical value of intraoperative gross examination in endometrial cancer. Gynecol Oncol. 2000;76(3): 357–61.
45. Fregnani JH, Latorre MR, Novik PR, Lopes A, Soares FA. Assessment of pelvic lymph node micrometastatic disease in stages IB and IIA of carcinoma of the uterine cervix. Int J Gynecol Cancer. 2006;16:1188–94.
46. Friedlander ML, Covens A, Glasspool RM, Hilpert F, Kristensen G, Kwon S, Selle F, Small W, Witteveen E, Russell P. Gynecologic Cancer InterGroup (GCIG) consensus review for mullerian adenosarcoma of the female genital tract. Int J Gynecol Cancer. 2014;24(9 Suppl 3):S78–82.
47. Ganesan R, Brown LJ, Kehoe S, McCluggage WG, El-Bahrawy MA. The role of frozen sections in gynaecological oncology: survey of practice in the United Kingdom. Eur J Obstet Gynecol Reprod Biol. 2013;166(2):204–8.
48. Garg G, Shah JP, Toy EP, Field JB, Bryant CS, Liu JR, Morris RT. Intra-operative detection of nodal metastasis in early stage cervical cancer: a survey of the practice patterns of SGO members. Gynecol Oncol. 2011;121(1):143–7.
49. Ghaemmaghami F, Behnamfar F, Ensani F. Intraoperative frozen sections for assessment of female cancers. Asian Pac J Cancer Prev. 2007;8(4):635–9.
50. Goff BA, Rice LW. Assessment of depth of myometrial invasion in endometrial adenocarcinoma. Gynecol Oncol. 1990;38(1):46–8.
51. Graebe K, Garcia-Soto A, Aziz M, Valarezo V, Heller PB, Tchabo N, Tobias DH, Salamon C, Ramieri J, Dise C, Slomovitz BM. Incidental power morcellation of malignancy: a retrospective cohort study. Gynecol Oncol. 2015;136(2):274–7.
52. Grosse-Drieling D, Schlutius JC, Altgassen C, Kelling K, Theben J. Laparoscopic supracervical hysterectomy (LASH), a retrospective study of 1,584 cases regarding intra- and perioperative complications. Arch Gynecol Obstet. 2012;285(5):1391–6.
53. Hagemann IS, Hagemann AR, LiVolsi VA, Montone KT, Chu CS. Risk of occult malignancy in morcellated hysterectomy: a case series. Int J Gynecol Pathol. 2011;30(5):476–83.
54. Herfs M, Yamamoto Y, Laury A, Wang X, Nucci MR, McLaughlin-Drubin ME, Münger K, Feldman S, McKeon FD, Xian W, Crum CP. A discrete population of squamocolumnar junction cells implicated in the pathogenesis of cervical cancer. Proc Natl Acad Sci U S A. 2012;109(26):10516–21.
55. Hirschowitz L, Nucci M, Zaino RJ. Problematic issues in the staging of endometrial, cervical and vulval carcinomas. Histopathology. 2013;62(1):176–202.
56. Höckel M, Hentschel B, Horn LC. Association between developmental steps in the organogenesis of the uterine cervix and locoregional progression of cervical cancer: a prospective clinicopathological analysis. Lancet Oncol. 2014;15(4):445–56.
57. Höckel M, Horn LC, Hentschel B, Höckel S, Naumann G. Total mesometrial resection: high resolution nerve-sparing radical hysterectomy based on developmentally defined surgical anatomy. Int J Gynecol Cancer. 2003;13(6):791–803.
58. Höckel M, Horn LC, Illig R, Dornhöfer N, Fritsch H. Ontogenetic anatomy of the distal vagina: relevance for local tumor spread and implications for cancer surgery. Gynecol Oncol. 2011;122(2):313–8.
59. Höckel M, Horn LC. The puzzle of close surgical margins is not puzzling. Gynecol Oncol. 2013;130(1):224–5.
60. Horn LC, Beckmann MW, Follmann M, Koch MC, Mallmann P, Marnitz S, Schmidt D. 3-Leitlinie Diagnostik und Therapie des Zervixkarzinoms – Anforderungen an die Pathologie. Pathologe. 2015, im Druck.
61. Horn LC, Dallacker M, Bilek K. Carcinosarcomas (malignant mixed Mullerian tumors) of the uterus. Morphology, pathogenetic aspects and prognostic factors. Pathologe. 2009;30(4):292–301.
62. Horn LC, Einenkel J, Höckel M, Kölbl H, Kommoss F, Lax SF, Reich O, Riethdorf L, Schmidt D. Pathoanatomical preparation and reporting for dysplasias and cancers of the cervix uteri: cervical biopsy, conization, radical hysterectomy and exenteration. Pathologe. 2007;28(4):249–60.
63. Horn LC, Einenkel J, Höckel M, Kölbl H, Kommoss F, Lax SF, Riethdorf L, Schnürch HG, Schmidt D. Recommendations for the handling and oncologic pathology report of lymph node specimens submitted for evaluation of metastatic disease in gynecologic malignancies. Pathologe. 2005;26(4):266–72.
64. Horn LC, Fischer U, Raptis G, Bilek K, Hentschel B, Richter CE, Braumann UD, Einenkel J. Pattern of invasion is of prognostic value in surgically treated cervical cancer patients. Gynecol Oncol. 2006;103(3):906–11.
65. Horn LC, Hentschel B, Fischer U, Peter D, Bilek K. Detection of micrometastases in pelvic lymph nodes in patients with carcinoma of the cervix uteri using step sectioning: Frequency, topographic distribution and prognostic impact. Gynecol Oncol. 2008;111(2):276–81.
66. Horn LC, Hentschel B, Galle D, Bilek K. Extracapsular extension of pelvic lymph node metastases is of prognostic value in carcinoma of the cervix uteri. Gynecol Oncol. 2008;108(1):63–7.
67. Horn LC, Hommel N, Roschlau U, Bilek K, Hentschel B, Einenkel J. Peritumoral stromal remodeling, pattern of invasion and expression of c-met/HGF in advanced squamous cell carcinoma of the cervix uteri, FIGO stages III and IV. Eur J Obstet Gynecol Reprod Biol. 2012;163(1):76–80.
68. Horn LC, Meinel A, Fischer U, Bilek K, Hentschel B. Perineural invasion in carcinoma of the cervix uteri–prognostic impact. J Cancer Res Clin Oncol. 2010;136(10):1557–62.
69. Horn LC, Meinel A, Handzel R, Einenkel J. Histopathology of endometrial hyperplasia and endometrial carcinoma: an update. Ann Diagn Pathol. 2007;11:297–311.
70. Horn LC, Schierle K, Schmidt D, Ulrich U, Liebmann A, Wittekind C. Current TNM/FIGO classification for cervical and endometrial cancer as well as malignant mixed müllerian tumors. Facts and background. Pathologe. 2011;32(3):239–43.
71. Horn LC, Schnurrbusch U, Bilek K, Hentschel B, Einenkel J. Risk of progression in complex and atypical endometrial hyperplasia: clinicopathologic analysis in cases with and without progestogen treatment. Int J Gynecol Cancer. 2004;14(2):348–53.
72. Horn LC, Trost M, Bilek K. Staging of endometrial carcinoma: aspects of ovarian and cervical involvement. Int J Gynecol Pathol. 2010;29(1):63–6.
73. Horn LC, Wagner S. Frozen section analysis of vulvectomy specimens: results of a 5-year study period. Int J Gynecol Pathol. 2010;29(2):165–72.
74. Horn LC, Klostermann K. Precancerous lesions of the uterine cervix: morphology and molecular pathology. Pathologe. 2011;32(Suppl 2):242–54.
75. Hunt JL, Baloch ZW, LiVolsi VA. Sentinel lymph node evaluation for tumor metastasis. Semin Diagn Pathol. 2002;19(4):263–77.
76. Ioffe OB. Recent developments and selected diagnostic problems in carcinomas of the endometrium. Am J Clin Pathol. 2005;124(Suppl):S42–51.
77. Ip PP, Cheung AN. Pathology of uterine leiomyosarcomas and smooth muscle tumours of uncertain malignant potential. Best Pract Res Clin Abstet Gynaecol. 2011;25(6):691–704.

78. Jaiman S, Surampudi K, Gundabattula SR, Garg D. Bilateral ovarian metastatic squamous cell carcinoma arising from the uterine cervix and eluding the Mullerian mucosa. Diagn Pathol. 2014; 9:109.
79. Kalyanasundaram K, Ganesan R, Perunovic B, McCluggage WG. Diffusely infiltrating endometrial carcinomas with no stromal response: report of a series, including cases with cervical and ovarian involvement and emphasis on the potential for misdiagnosis. Int J Surg Pathol. 2010;18(2):138–43.
80. Karamurzin Y, Soslow RA, Garg K. Histologic evaluation of prophylactic hysterectomy and oophorectomy in Lynch syndrome. Am J Surg Pathol. 2013;37(4):579–85.
81. Kato T, Watari H, Takeda M, Hosaka M, Mitamura T, Kobayashi N, Sudo S, Kaneuchi M, Kudo M, Sakuragi N. Multivariate prognostic analysis of adenocarcinoma of the uterine cervix treated with radical hysterectomy and systematic lymphadenectomy. J Gynecol Oncol. 2013;24(3):222–8.
82. Kimmig R, Aktas B, Buderath P, Wimberger P, Iannaccone A, Heubner M. Definition of compartment-based radical surgery in uterine cancer: modified radical hysterectomy in intermediate/high-risk endometrial cancer using peritoneal mesometrial resection (PMMR) by M Höckel translated to robotic surgery. World J Surg Oncol. 2013;11:198.
83. Kir G, Kir M, Cetiner H, Karateke A, Gurbuz A. Diagnostic problems on frozen section examination of myometrial invasion in patients with endometrial carcinoma with special emphasis on the pitfalls of deep adenomyosis with carcinomatous involvement. Eur J Gynaecol Oncol. 2004;25(2):211–4.
84. Kodama J, Kusumoto T, Nakamura K, Seki N, Hongo A, Hiramatsu Y. Factors associated with parametrial involvement in stage IB1 cervical cancer and identification of patients suitable for less radical surgery. Gynecol Oncol. 2011;122(3):491–4.
85. Koshiyama M, Suzuki A, Ozawa M, Fujita K, Sakakibara A, Kawamura M, Takahashi S, Fujii H, Hirano T, Okagaki A, Nagano T, Ban C. Adenocarcinomas arising from uterine adenomyosis: a report of four cases. Int J Gynecol Pathol. 2002;21(3): 239–45.
86. Kucera E, Kainz C, Reinthaller A, Sliutz G, Leodolter S, Kucera H, Breitenecker G. Accuracy of intraoperative frozen-section diagnosis in stage I endometrial adenocarcinoma. Gynecol Obstst Invest. 2000;49(1):62–6.
87. Kumar S, Bandyopadhyay S, Semaan A, Shah JP, Mahdi H, Morris R, Munkarah A, Ali-Fehmi R. The role of frozen section in surgical staging of low risk endometrial cancer. PLoS One. 2011;6(9): e21912.
88. Kurman RJ, Amin MB, Members of the Cancer Committee, College of American Pathologists. Protocol for the examination of specimens from patients with carcinomas of the cervix. A basis for checklists. Arch Pathol Lab Med. 1999;123:55–61.
89. Lachiewicz MP, Kravochuck SE, O'Malley MM, Heald B, Church JM, Kalady MF, Drake RD. Prevalence of occult gynecologic malignancy at the time of risk reducing and nonprophylactic surgery in patients with Lynch syndrome. Gynecol Oncol. 2014;132(2):434–7.
90. Lancaster JM, Powell CB, Chen LM, Richardson DL, SGO Clinical Practice Committee. Society of Gynecologic Oncology statement on risk assessment for inherited gynecologic cancer predispositions. Gynecol Oncol. 2015;136(1):3–7.
91. Landoni F, Maneo A, Colombo A, Placa F, Milani R, Perego P, Favini G, Ferri L, Mangioni C. Randomised study of radical surgery versus radiotherapy for stage IB-IIA cervical cancer. Lancet. 1997;350:535–40.
92. Landry D, Mai KT, Senterman MK, Perkins DG, Yazdi HM, Veinot JP, Thomas J. Endometrioid adenocarcinoma of the uterus with a minimal deviation invasive pattern. Histopathology. 2003;42(1):77–82.
93. Langlois PL. The size of the normal uterus. J Reprod Med. 1970;4(6):220–8.
94. Langreder W. Das Parametrium. In: Schröder R (Hrsg). Zwanglose Abhandlungen auf dem Gebiete der Frauenheilkunde. Band 18, Leipzig: Thieme; 1955.
95. Lawrence WD, Abdul-Karim FW, Crum C, Fu YS for the Association of Directors of Anatomic and Surgical Pathology. Recommendations for the reporting of surgical specimens containing uterine cervical neoplasms. Hum Pathol. 2000;31:1194–8.
96. Lawrence WD, Association of Directors of Anatomic and Surgical Pathology. ADASP recommendations for processing and reporting of lymph node specimens submitted for evaluation of metastatic disease. Virchows Arch. 2001;439(5):601–3.
97. Lax S, Tamussino K, Prein K, Lang P. Intraoperative frozen sections in diseases of the female genital tract. Pathologe. 2012;33(5):430–40.
98. Lee AH, Key HP, Bell JA, Kumah P, Hodi Z, Ellis IO. The effect of delay in fixation on HER2 expression in invasive carcinoma of the breast assessed with immunohistochemistry and in situ hybridisation. J Clin Pathol. 2014;67:573–5.
99. Lentz SE, Muderspach LI, Felix JC, Ye W, Groshen S, Amezuca CA. Identification of mircometastases in histologically negative nodes of early-stage cervical cancer patients. Obstet Gynecol. 2004;103:1204–10.
100. Lim P, Al Kushi A, Gilks B, Wong F, Aquino-Parsons C. Early stage papillary serous carcinoma of the endometrium: effect of adjuvant whole abdominal radiotherapy and pathologic parameters on outcome. Cancer. 2001;91:752–7.
101. Liebig C, Ayala G, Wilks JA, Berger DH, Albo D. Perineural invasion in cancer: a review of the literature. Cancer. 2009;115: 3379–91.
102. Lindor NM, Petersen GM, Hadley DW, Kinney AY, Miesfeldt S, Lu KH, Lynch P, Burke W, Press N. Recommendations for the care of individuals with an inherited predisposition to Lynch syndrome: a systematic review. JAMA. 2006;296(12):1507–17.
103. Lopez-Garcia MA, Palacios J. Pathologic and molecular features of uterine carcinosarcomas. Semin Diagn Pathol. 2010;27(4):274–86.
104. Mai KT, Perkins DG, Yazdi HM, Thomas J. Endometrioid carcinoma of the endometrium with an invasive component of minimal deviation carcinoma. Hum Pathol. 2002;33(8):856–8.
105. Marchiole P, Buenerd A, Benchaib M, Nezhat K, Dargent D, Mathevet P. Clinical significance of lympho vascular space involvement and lymph node micrometastases in early-stage cervical cancer: a retrospective case-control surgico-pathological study. Gynecol Oncol. 2005;97:727–32.
106. McCann GA, Taege SK, Boutsicaris CE, Phillips GS, Eisenhauer EL, Fowler JM, O'Malley DM, Copeland LJ, Cohn DE, Salani R. The impact of close surgical margins after radical hysterectomy for early-stage cervical cancer. Gynecol Oncol. 2013;128(1):44–8.
107. McCluggage WG, Colgan T, Duggan M, Hacker NF, Mulvany N, Otis C, Wilkinson N, Zaino RJ, Hirschowitz L. Dataset for reporting of endometrial carcinomas: recommendations from the International Collaboration on Cancer Reporting (ICCR) between United Kingdom, United States, Canada, and Australasia. Int J Gynaecol Pathol. 2012;32:45–65.
108. Metindir J, Bilir Dilek G. Evaluation of prognostic significance in extracapsular spread of pelvic lymph node metastasis in patients with cervical cancer. Eur J Gynaecol Oncol. 2008;29(5):476–8.
109. Kidd EA, Grigsby PW. Intratumoral metabolic heterogeneity of cervical cancer. Clin Cancer Res. 2008;14(16):5236–41.
110. McCluggage WG, Fisher C, Hirschowitz L for the Roayl College of Pathologists. Dataset for histological reporting of uterine sarcomas. 2014. http://www.rcpath.org/publications-media/publications/datasets/uterine-sarcomas.

111. McCluggage WG, Ganesan R, Herrington CS. Endometrial stromal sarcomas with extensive endometrioid glandular differentiation: report of a series with emphasis on the potential for misdiagnosis and discussion of the differential diagnosis. Histopathology. 2009;54(3):365–73.
112. McCluggage WG, Hirschowitz L, Wilson GE, Oliva E, Soslow RA, Zaino RJ. Significant variation in the assessment of cervical involvement in endometrial carcinoma: an interobserver variation study. Am J Surg Pathol. 2011;35(2):289–94.
113. McCluggage WG, Judge MJ, Clarke BA, Davidson B, Gilks CB, Hollema H, Ledermann JA, Matias-Guiu X, Mikami Y, Stewart CJR, Vang R, Hirschowitz L. Dataset for reporting of ovary, fallopian tube and primary peritoneal carcinoma: recommendations from the International Collaboration on Cancer Reporting (ICCR). Mod Pathol. 2015;28(8):1101–22.
114. McCluggage WG. Malignant biphasic uterine tumours: carcinosarcomas or metaplastic carcinomas? J Clin Pathol. 2002;55(5):321–5.
115. Medeiros F, Muto MG, Lee Y, Elvin JA, Callahan MJ, Feltmate C, Garber JE, Cramer DW, Crum CP. The tubal fimbria is a preferred site for early adenocarcinoma in women with familial ovarian cancer syndrome. Am J Surg Pathol. 2006;30:230–6.
116. Meinel A, Fischer U, Bilek K, Hentschel B, Horn LC. Morphological parameters associated with perineural invasion (PNI) in carcinoma of the cervix uteri. Int J Surg Pathol. 2011;19(2):159–63.
117. Mileshkin L, Paramanathan A, Kondalsamy-Chennakesavan S, Bernshaw D, Khaw P, Narayan K. Smokers with cervix cancer have more uterine corpus invasive disease and an increased risk of recurrence after treatment with chemoradiation. Int J Gynecol Cancer. 2014;24(7):1286–91.
118. Mills AM, Liou S, Ford JM, Berek JS, Pai RK, Longacre TA. Lynch syndrome screening should be considered for all patients with newly diagnosed endometrial cancer. Am J Surg Pathol. 2014;38(11):1501–9.
119. Mirkovic J, Howitt BE, Roncarati P, Demoulin S, Suarez-Carmona M, Hubert P, McKeon FD, Xian W, Li A, Delvenne P, Crum CP, Herfs M. Carcinogenic HPV infection in the cervical squamo-columnar junction. J Pathol. 2015;236(3):265–71.
120. Moatamed NA, Nanjangud G, Pucci R, Lowe A, Shintaku IP, Shapourifar-Tehrani S, Rao N, Lu DY, Apple SK. Effect of ischemic time, fixation time, and fixative type on HER2/neu immunohistochemical and fluorescence in situ hybridization results in breast cancer. Am J Clin Pathol. 2011;136(5):754–61.
121. Montag AG. The frozen section: historical background, technique and quality assurance. In: Taxy JB, Husain AN, Montag AG, editors. Biopsy interpretation: the frozen section. Philadelphia/Baltimore/New York/London/Buenos Aires/Hong Kong/Sydney/Tokyo: Wolters Kluwer/Lippincott Williams & Wilkin; 2014. p. 1–15.
122. Moodley M, Bramdev A. Frozen section: its role in gynaecological oncology. J Obstet Gynaecol. 2005;25(7):629–34.
123. Morotti M, Menada MV, Moioli M, Sala P, Maffeo I, Abete L, Fulcheri E, Menoni S, Venturini P, Papadia A. Frozen section pathology at time of hysterectomy accurately predicts endometrial cancer in patients with preoperative diagnosis of atypical endometrial hyperplasia. Gynecol Oncol. 2012;125(3):536–40.
124. Movahedi-Lankarani S, Gilks CB, Soslow R, Oliva E, Members of the Cancer Committee, College of American Pathologists. Protocol for the examination of specimens from patients with carcinoma of the endometrium. http://www.cap.org/apps/docs/committees/cancer/cancer_protocols/2011/Endometrium_11protocol.doc.
125. Murray SK, Young RH, Scully RE. Unusual epithelial and stromal changes in myoinvasive endometrioid adenocarcinoma: a study of their frequency, associated diagnostic problems, and prognostic significance. Int J Gynecol Pathol. 2003;22(4):324–33.
126. Nakao Y, Yamasaki F, Yokoyama M, Aihara S, Yasunaga M, Iwasaka T. Minimal deviation endometrioid adenocarcinoma of the endometrium and its MRI findings. Eur J Gynaecol Oncol. 2014;35(2):185–7.
127. Nayar AG, Cross PA, Bulmer JN, Deen S, El-Sherif A. Comparison of examination of the entire uterine cervix with routine cervical sampling in hysterectomy specimens from women with endometrial cancer. J Clin Pathol. 2008;61(5):621–2.
128. Nucci MR, Quade BJ. Uterine mesenchymal tumors. In: Crum CP, Lee KR, editors. Diagnostic gynecologic and obstetric pathology. Philadelphia: Elsevier; 2006. p. 655–7.
129. Oliva E, Carcangiu ML, Carinelli SG, Ip P, Loening T, Longacre TA, Nucci MR, Prat J, Zaloudek CJ. Mesenchymal tumors of the uterine corpus. In: Kurman RJ, Carcangiou ML, Herrington S, Young RH, editors. WHO classification of tumours of femal reproductive organs. Lyon: IARC Press; 2014. p. 135–48.
130. Oliva E. Cellar mesenchymal tumors of the uterus: a review emphasizing recent observations. Int J Gynecol Pathol. 2014;33(4):374–84.
131. Ober KG, Huhn FO. Die Ausbreitung des Cervixkrebses auf die Parametrien und die Lymphknoten der Beckenwand. Arch Gynäkol. 1962;197:262–90.
132. Orezzoli JP, Sioletic S, Olawaiye A, Oliva E, del Carmen MG. Stage II endometrioid adenocarcinoma of the endometrium: clinical implications of cervical stromal invasion. Gynecol Oncol. 2009;113(3):316–23.
133. Otis CN, Ocampo AC, Nucci MR, McCluggage WG, For the Members of the Cancer Committee, College of American Pathologists. Protocol for the examination of specimens from patients with sarcoma of the uterus. http://www.cap.org/apps/docs/committees/cancer/cancer_protocols/2013/UterineSarcomaProtocol_3000.pdf.
134. Ozturk E, Dikensoy E, Balat O, Ugur MG, Aydin A. Intraoperative frozen section is essential for assessment of myometrial invasion but not for histologic grade confirmation in endometrial cancer: a ten-year experience. Arch Gynaecol Obstet. 2012;285(5):1415–9.
135. Pautier P, Nam EJ, Provencher DM, Hamilton AL, Mangili G, Siddiqui NA, Westermann AM, Reed NS, Harter P, Ray-Coquard I. Gynecologic Cancer InterGroup (GCIG) consensus review for high-grade undifferentiated sarcomas of the uterus. Int J Gynecol Cancer. 2014;24(9 Suppl 3):S73–7.
136. Pavlakis K, Vrekoussis T, Pistofidis G, Gavresea T, Panoskaltsis T. Methylene blue: how to visualize the endometrium in uterine morcellation material. Int J Gynecol Pathol. 2014;33(2):135–9.
137. Prat J. Prognostic parameters of endometrial carcinoma. Hum Pathol. 2004;35:649–62.
138. Quinlivan JA, Petersen RW, Nicklin JL. Accuracy of frozen section for the operative management of endometrial cancer. BJOG. 2001;108(8):798–803.
139. Rabban JT, Calkins SM, Karnezis AN, Grenert JP, Blanco A, Crawford B, Chen LM. Association of tumor morphology with mismatch-repair protein status in older endometrial cancer patients: implications for universal versus selective screening strategies for Lynch syndrome. Am J Surg Pathol. 2014;38(6):793–800.
140. Rakha EA, Pinder SE, Bartlett JM, Ibrahim M, Starczynski J, Carder PJ, Provenzano E, Hanby A, Hales S, Lee AH, Ellis IO, National Coordinating Committee for Breast Pathology. Updated UK Recommendations for HER2 assessment in breast cancer. J Clin Pathol. 2015;68(2):93–9.
141. Rakha E, Wong SC, Soomro I, Chaudry Z, Sharma A, Deen S, Chan S, Abu J, Nunns D, Williamson K, McGregor A, Hammond R, Brown L. Clinical outcome of atypical endometrial hyperplasia diagnosed on an endometrial biopsy: institutional experience and review of literature. Am J Surg Pathol. 2012;36(11):1683–90.

142. Rob L, Robova H, Chmel R, Komar M, Halaska M, Skapa P. Surgical options in early cervical cancer. Int J Hyperthermia. 2012;28:489–500.
143. Robboy SJ, Mutter GL, Shako-Levy R, Bean SM, Prat J, Bentley RC, Russel P. Cutup – gross description and processing of specimens. In: Robboy SJ, Mutter GL, Prat J, Bentley RC, Russel P, Anderson MC, editors. Robboy's pathology of the female reproductive tract. Edinburgh/London/New York/Oxford/Philadelphia/St. Louis/Sydney/Toronto: Elsevier; 2009. p. 979–91.
144. Rosai J. Foreword. In: Argani P, Cimino-Mathews A, editors. Intraoperative frozen sections. Diagnostic pitfalls. New York: demosMedical; 2014. p. XIII–XV.
145. Rosai J, editor. Rosai and Ackerman's surgical pathology. Edinburgh/London/New York/Oxford/Philadelphia/St. Louis/Sydney/Toronto: Elsevier; 2011. p. 2553–4, 2579–83, 2633–6.
146. Sanjuán A, Cobo T, Pahisa J, Escaramís G, Ordi J, Ayuso JR, Garcia S, Hernández S, Torné A, Martínez Román S, Lejárcegui JA, Vanrell JA. Preoperative and intraoperative assessment of myometrial invasion and histologic grade in endometrial cancer: role of magnetic resonance imaging and frozen section. Int J Gynecol Cancer. 2006;16(1):385–90.
147. Savelli L, Testa AC, Mabrouk M, Zannoni L, Ludovisi M, Seracchioli R, Scambia G, De Iaco P. A prospective blinded comparison of the accuracy of transvaginal sonography and frozen section in the assessment of myometrial invasion in endometrial cancer. Gynecol Oncol. 2012;124(3):549–52.
148. Schmeler KM, Lynch HT, Chen LM, Munsell MF, Soliman PT, Clark MB, Daniels MS, White KG, Boyd-Rogers SG, Conrad PG, Yang KY, Rubin MM, Sun CC, Slomovitz BM, Gershenson DM, Lu KH. Prophylactic surgery to reduce the risk of gynecologic cancers in the Lynch syndrome. N Engl J Med. 2006;354(3):261–9.
149. Seidman MA, Oduyebo T, Muto MG, Crum CP, Nucci MR, Quade BJ. Peritoneal dissemination complicating morcellation of uterine mesenchymal neoplasms. PLoS One. 2012;7(11):e50058.
150. Seidman JD, Soslow RA, Vang R, Berman JJ, Stoler MH, Sherman ME, Oliva E, Kajdacsy-Balla A, Berman DM, Copeland LJ. Borderline ovarian tumors: diverse contemporary viewpoints on terminology and diagnostic criteria with illustrative images. Hum Pathol. 2004;35(8):918–33.
151. SGO. Society of Gynecologic Oncologists Clinical Practice Committee statement on prohpylactic Salpingo-oophorectomy. Gynecol Oncol. 2005;98:179–81.
152. Shia J, Black D, Hummer AJ, Boyd J, Soslow RA. Routinely assessed morphological features correlate with microsatellite instability status in endometrial cancer. Hum Pathol. 2008;39(1):116–25.
153. Shimada M, Kigawa J, Nishimura R, Yamaguchi S, Kuzuya K, Nakanishi T, Suzuki M, Kita T, Iwasaka T, Terakawa N. Ovarian metastasis in carcinoma of the uterine cervix. Gynecol Oncol. 2006;101(2):234–7.
154. Shutter J, Wright TC Jr. Prevalence of underlying adenocarcinoma in women with atypical endometrial hyperplasia. Int J Gynecol Pathol. 2005;24(4):313–8.
155. Silverberg SG. Protocol for the examination of specimens from patients with carcinomas of the endometrium: a basis for checklists. Cancer Committee, College of American Pathologists. Arch Pathol Lab Med. 1999;123(1):28–32.
156. Silverberg SG. The endometrium. Pathologic principles and pitfalls. Arch Pathol Lab Med. 2007;131:372–82.
157. Singh R. Review literature on uterine carcinosarcoma. J Cancer Res Ther. 2014;10(3):461–8.
158. Skala SL, Hagemann IS. Optimal sampling of grossly normal omentum in staging of gynecologic malignancies. Int J Gynecol Pathol. 2015;34(3):281–7.
159. Sobin LH, Gospodarowicz MK, Wittekind C. TNM-classification of malignant tumors. 7th ed. London: Wiley-Blackwell; 2009.
160. Stang A, Merrill RM, Kuss O. Hysterectomy in Germany: a DRG-based nationwide analysis, 2005–2006. Dtsch Arztebl Int. 2011;108(30):508–14.
161. Stany MP, Stone PJ, Felix JC, Amezcua CA, Groshen S, Ye W, Kyser KL, Howard RS, Zahn CM, Muderspach LI, Lentz SE, Chernofsky MR. Lymph node micrometastases in early-stage cervical cancer are not predictive of survival. Int J Gynecol Pathol. 2015;34(4):379–84.
162. Stephan JM, Hansen J, Samuelson M, McDonald M, Chin Y, Bender D, Reyes HD, Button A, Goodheart MJ. Intra-operative frozen section results reliably predict final pathology in endometrial cancer. Gynecol Oncol. 2014;133(3):499–505.
163. Stewart CJ, Leung YC, Whitehouse A. Fallopian tube metastases of non-gynaecological origin: a series of 20 cases emphasizing patterns of involvement including intra-epithelial spread. Histopathology. 2012;60(6B):E106–14.
164. Stewart CJ, Little L. Immunophenotypic features of MELF pattern invasion in endometrial adenocarcinoma: evidence for epithelial-mesenchymal transition. Histopathology. 2009;55(1):91–101.
165. Stoler M, Bergeron C, Colgan TJ, Ferency AS, Herrington CS, Kim KR, Loening T, Schneider A, Sherman ME, Wilbur DC, Wright T. In: Kurman RJ, Carcangiou ML, Herrington S, Young RH, editors. WHO classification of tumours of femal reproductive organs. Lyon: IARC Press; 2014. p.172–82.
166. Syed S, Reed N, Millan D. Adequacy of cervical sampling in hysterectomy specimens for endometrial cancer. Ann Diagn Pathol. 2015;19(2):43–4.
167. Takano M, Ochi H, Takei Y, Miyamoto M, Hasumi Y, Kaneta Y, Nakamura K, Kurosaki A, Satoh T, Fujiwara H, Nagao S, Furuya K, Yokota H, Ito K, Minegishi T, Yoshikawa H, Fujiwara K, Suzuki M. Surgery for endometrial cancers with suspected cervical involvement: is radical hysterectomy needed (a GOTIC study)? Br J Cancer. 2013;109(7):1760–5.
168. Toledo G, Oliva E. Smooth muscle tumors of the uterus: a practical approach. Arch Pathol Lab Med. 2008;132(4):595–605.
169. Torres ML, Weaver AL, Kumar S, Uccella S, Famuyide AO, Cliby WA, Dowdy SC, Gostout BS, Mariani A. Risk factors for developing endometrial cancer after benign endometrial sampling. Obstet Gynecol. 2012;120(5):998–1004.
170. Traiman P, Saldiva P, Haiashi A, Franco M. Criteria for the diagnosis of diffuse uterine myohypertrophy. Int J Gynaecol Obstet. 1996;54(1):31–6.
171. Trimble CL, Method M, Leitao M, Lu K, Ioffe O, Hampton M, Higgins R, Zaino R, Mutter GL, Society of Gynecologic Oncology Clinical Practice Committee. Management of endometrial precancers. Obstet Gynecol. 2012;120(5):1160–75.
172. Tulandi T, Ferenczy A. Biopsy of uterine leiomyomata and frozen sections before laparoscopic morcellation. J Minim Invasive Gynecol. 2014;21(5):963–6.
173. Turan T, Oguz E, Unlubilgin E, Tulunay G, Boran N, Demir OF, Kose MF. Accuracy of frozen-section examination for myometrial invasion and grade in endometrial cancer. Eur J Obstet Gynecol Reprod Biol. 2013;167(1):90–5.
174. Usubütün A, Ozseker HS, Himmetoglu C, Balci S, Ayhan A. Omentectomy for gynecologic cancer: how much sampling is adequate for microscopic examination? Arch Pathol Lab Med. 2007;131(10):1578–81.
175. Vidal F, Rafii A. Lymph node assessment in endometrial cancer: towards personalized medicine. Obstet Gynecol Int. 2013;2013:892465.
176. Wagner AE, Pappas L, Ghia AJ, Gaffney DK. Impact of tumor size on survival in cancer of the cervix and validation of stage IIA1 and IIA2 subdivisions. Gynecol Oncol. 2013;129:517–21.

177. Watson P, Vasen HF, Mecklin JP, Järvinen H, Lynch HT. The risk of endometrial cancer in hereditary nonpolyposis colorectal cancer. Am J Med. 1994;96:516–20.
178. Wijnen J, de Leeuw W, Vasen H, et al. Familial endometrial cancer in female carriers of MSH6 germline mutations. Nat Genet. 1999;23:142–4.
179. Wilbur DC, Colgan TJ, Ferenczy AS, Hisrchowitz L, Loening T, McCluggage WG, Mikami Y, Park KJ, Ronnett BM, Schneider A, Soslow R, Wells M, Wright T. In: Kurman RJ, Carcangiou ML, Herrington S, Young RH, editors. WHO classification of tumours of femal reproductive organs. Lyon: IARC Press; 2014. p. 183–94.
180. Williams JW, Hirschowitz L. Assessment of uterine wall thickness and position of the vascular plexus in the deep myometrium: implications for the measurement of depth of myometrial invasion of endometrial carcinomas. Int J Gynecol Pathol. 2006; 25(1):59–64.
181. Williams KE, Waters ED, Woolas RP, Hammond IG, McCartney AJ. Mixed serous endometrioid carcinoma of the uterus: pathologic and cytopathologic analysis of a high-risk endometrial carcinoma. Int J Gynecol Cancer. 1994;4:7–18.
182. Wittekind C, Compton CC, Brierley J, Sobin LH. TNM-supplement. A commentary on uniform use. Oxford: Wiley-Blackwell; 2012. p. 9–11, 21–2.
183. Wolsky RJ, Montag AG. Female genital tract. In: Taxy JB, Husain AN, Montag AG, editors. Biopsy interpretation: the frozen section. Philadelphia/Baltimore/New York/London/Buenos Aires/Hong Kong/Sydney/Tokyo: Wolters Kluwer/Lippincott Williams & Wilkin; 2014. p. 69–88.
184. Wright JD, Tergas AI, Burke WM, Cui RR, Ananth CV, Chen L, Hershman DL. Uterine pathology in women undergoing minimally invasive hysterectomy using morcellation. JAMA. 2014;312(12):1253–5.
185. Yin ZM, Yu AJ, Wu MJ, Zhu JQ, Zhang X, Chen JH, Yuan SH, Yu H. Prognostic factors and treatment comparison in small cell neuroendocrine cervical carcinoma. Eur J Gynaecol Oncol. 2014;35(3):259–63.
186. Zaino R, Carinellei SG, Ellenson LH, Eng C, Katabuchi H, Konishi I, Lax S, Matis-Guiu X, Mutter GL, Peters WA, Sherman ME, Shih IM, Soslow R. Stewart CJR. In: Kurman RJ, Carcangiou ML, Herrington S, Young RH, editors. WHO classification of tumours of femal reproductive organs. Lyon: IARC Press; 2014. p. 121–34.
187. Zaino RJ, Abendroth C, Yemelyanova A, Oliva E, Lim D, Soslow R, Delair D, Hagemann IS, Montone K, Zhu J. Endocervical involvement in endometrial adenocarcinoma is not prognostically significant and the pathologic assessment of the pattern of involvement is not reproducible. Gynecol Oncol. 2013;128(1):83–7.
188. Zaino RJ. FIGO staging of endometrial adenocarcinoma: a critical review and proposal. Int J Gynecol Pathol. 2009;28:1–9.
189. Zannoni GF, Vellone VG, Carbone A. Morphological effects of radiochemotherapy on cervical carcinoma: a morphological study of 50 cases of hysterectomy specimens after neoadjuvant treatment. Int J Gynecol Pathol. 2008;27(2):274–81.
190. Zarbo RJ, Schmidt WA, Bachner P, Howanitz PJ, Meier FA, Schifman RB, Boone DJ, Herron RM Jr. Indications and immediate patient outcomes of pathology intraoperative consultations. College of American Pathologists/Centers for Disease Control and Prevention Outcomes Working Group Study. Arch Pathol Lab Med. 1996;120(1):19–25.
191. Zaino RJ, Ward S, Delgado G, Bungy B, Gore H, Fetter G, Ganjei P, Frauenhoffer E. Histopathological predictors of the behavior of surgically treated stage Ib squamous cell carcinoma of the cervix. Cancer. 1992;69:1750–8.

Part VII

Specific Hematological and Anesthesiological Aspects

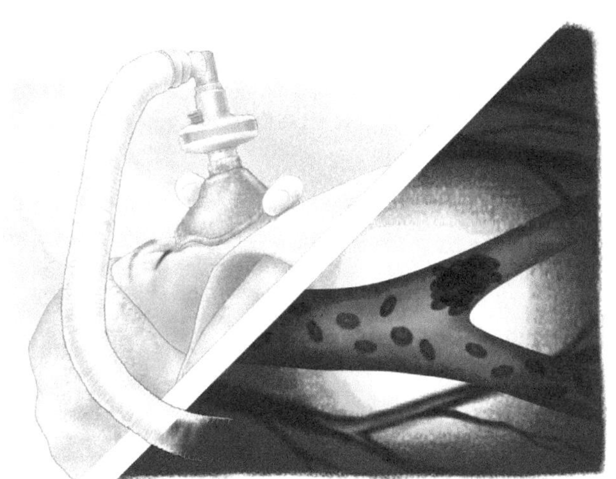

Perioperative Management of Antithrombotic Therapy in the Periprocedural Period of Patients Undergoing Hysterectomy

19

Verena Limperger, Florian Langer, Rolf Mesters, Ralf Ulrich Trappe, and Ulrike Nowak-Göttl

Introduction

The use of oral anticoagulants (OAC) especially Vitamin-K-antagonists (VKA) and antiplatelet agents (AA) (ASA, Clopidogrel, Prasugrel, Ticagrelor) alone or combined is necessary to prevent or treat thromboembolic diseases. Patients with the indication for a long-term therapy with OAC, for example with chronic atrial fibrillation, artificial cardiac valve or after thromboembolic events, or patients with the indication for treatment with AA for example after a stroke, TIA, myocardial infarct, implantation of a bare-metal-stent (BMS) or drug-eluting-stent (DES), need in case of surgical interventions a bridging with medication with a short half-time [1, 3, 5–9, 14, 21, 23, 25].

This review covers the recent published recommendations and guidelines related to elective hysterectomies in patients taking an OAC or AA. These recommendations are based on a few randomized trials with limited data only [8, 9, 34, 35]; therefore is the evidence level of these recommendations grade "2C" [1, 3, 5–9, 12, 14, 18, 21, 23, 25, 38]: In contrast with recommendation grade "1" are these [7]; it is comparable with "we suggest, that". The impact of study quality is divided into A, B and C, where as "C" is weaker than "A" or "B".

V. Limperger (✉)
Institute of Clinical Chemistry, University Hospital Schleswig Holstein, Kiel 24105, Germany
e-mail: Verena.limperger@uksh.de

F. Langer
II. Medizinische Klinik und Poliklinik, Universitätskliniken Eppendorf, Hamburg 22453, Germany
e-mail: langer@uke.de

R. Mesters
Medizinische Klinik und Poliklinik A, University Hospital Münster, Münster 48149, Germany
e-mail: Rolf.Mesters@ukmuenster.de

R.U. Trappe
Hematology and Oncology, Ev. Diakonie-Krankenhaus gemeinnützige GmbH, Bremen 28239, Germany
e-mail: r.trappe@diako-bremen.de

U. Nowak-Göttl
University Hospital Schleswig-Holstein, Institute of Clinical Chemistry, Thrombosis and Haemostatsis Treatment Unit, Kiel 24105, Germany

Preoperative Evaluation

In every patient taking an oral anticoagulant (Table 19.1) or antiplatelet agent (Table 19.2) the risk of the bleeding versus the risk for thromboembolic events must be evaluated at least two to three weeks prior to an elective surgical intervention: The risk of bleeding in terms of hysterectomy is fairly low but stays in contrast to the medium risk for thromboembolic events [7, 21]. Table 19.3 shows the yearly risk for thromboembolic recurrence after withdrawal of the oral anticoagulant or antiplatelet agent therapy.

The risk of bleeding is a summary of the patients inherited and acquired risk factors. A standardized bleeding questionnaire is the best way to identify the individual bleeding risk [16, 18, 26, 27]. This includes the record of the oral anticoagulant or antiplatelet agent taken as well as the documentation of potentially taken co-medication and of acquired diseases which can affect the hemostasis [13]: This includes the liver as the most important organ for the synthesis of coagulation factors, the kidneys as organs for the elimination of heparin and the direct oral anticoagulants [DOACs] und possibly hemostatic changes due to hemato-oncological diseases. In addition to that is it possible that for example cardiac diseases can lead to an acquired von Willebrand's disease [42].

Drugs, that for example can increase the effect of OACs, are androgen steroids, anabolic drugs, antacids, antibiotics, antidepressants, ß-inhibitors, gout medication, insulin, cholesterol lowering medication and thyroid hormones.

Conclusion: in every patient using an anticoagulant the risk of bleeding versus the risk for thromboembolism has to be evaluated.

The risk for thromboembolism in patients with inherited thrombophilia depends on the risk factor (Tables 19.4 and 19.5).

I. Alkatout, L. Mettler (eds.), *Hysterectomy*, DOI 10.1007/978-3-319-22497-8_19

Table 19.1 Oral or parenteral anticoagulant agents

Agent	Half-time	Target enzyme	Antidote
VKA: Phenprocoumon Warfarin Acenocoumarol	6 days 35–45 h 6,6 h	VK-depending y-carboxylation	Vitamin K1 oral/iv PPSB
Heparins: UFH LMWH Fondaparinux	30–60 min 3–7 h 17–21 h	AT-depending serine proteinase	Protamine –[a]
Dabigatran	11–14 h	Thrombin	Idarucizumab –[a]
Rivaroxaban	7–13 h	Factor Xa	Andexanet alfa & Ciraparantag –[a]
Apixaban	8–18 h	Factor Xa	Andexanet alfa & Ciraparantag –[a]
Edoxaban	10–14 h	Factor Xa	Andexanet alfa & Ciraparantag –[a]

Abbreviations: *AT* Antithrombin, *LMWH* low molecular weight Heparin, *UFH* unfractionated Heparin, *VK* Vitamin K, *VKA* Vitamin-K-Antagonist, *PPSB* Prothrombin complex concentrate

[a]General procedures for hemostasis: mechanical compression/ sealing the source of bleeding, volume replacement, if necessary infusion of erythrocyte concentrates, platelet concentrate, plasma, PPSB, rFVIIa, tranexamic acid [20 mg/kg body weight: 31,39]. The use of dialysis (Dabigatran) or the administration of active coal may be useful in case of overdose of DOACs

Table 19.2 Antiplatelet agents

Agent	Half-time	Target enzyme	Antidote
Acetylsalicylic acid [ASA]	15–30 min	COX-1; COX-2	–[a]
Clopidogrel	8 h [with loading-dose shorter]	$P2Y_{12}$ ADP receptor-irreversible	–[a]
Ticlopidin [is rarely used]	24–36 h	$P2Y_{12}$ ADP receptor-irreversible	–[a]
Prasugrel	7 h	$P2Y_{12}$ ADP receptor -irreversible	–[a]
Ticagrelor	7 h	$P2Y_{12}$ ADP receptor-reversible	–[a]
Cangrelor	2–5 min	$P2Y_{12}$ ADP receptor-reversible	
GPIIb-IIIa antagonists: Abciximab[b] Eptifibatide Tirofiban	10–30 min 150 min 1,8 h	Fibrinogen- receptor (GPIIb-IIIa)	platelet concentrate[a] Hemodialysis

[a]General procedures for hemostasis: mechanical compression/sealing the source of bleeding, volume replacement, if necessary infusion of erythrocyte concentrates, platelet concentrate, plasma, PPSB, rFVIIa, tranexamic acid [16–18, 20–22, 31, 39]. In case of platelet disorders due to ASA platelet concentrates can be combined with DDAVP i.v. [20, 22, 32, 38]

[b]Caution: not eligible for "bridging", because the effect on the receptor is too long

Table 19.3 Risk of arterial / venous thromboembolism in case of interruption of the OAC/AA therapy

High risk of thrombosis [circa 10 % per year]	Medium risk of thrombosis [4–10 % per year]	Low risk of thrombosis [<4 % per year]
Artificial heart valves	Biological heart valves [first 3 months]	Biological heart valves [>3 months]
Atrial fibrillation with fresh stroke/TIA or CHADS2 score[a]> 5	Atrial fibrillation & CHADS2 score[a] 3–4 without stroke / TIA	Atrial Fibrillation & CHADS2 score [a] 0–2 without stroke/TIA
BMS [<4 weeks]	BMS [4 weeks; – 12 months][b]	BMS [>12 months][b]
DES [<6 months]	DES [6–24 months][b]	DES [>24 months][b]
MI [<6 weeks] rheumatic valvular disease	MI [6 weeks – 12 months]	MI [>12 months]
Venous thromboembolism [<3 months]	Venous thromboembolism [3–12 months]	Venous thromboembolism [>12 months]
Severe thrombophilia[antiphospholipid syndrome, antithrombin, protein C- / S- deficiency]	Recurrent venous thromboembolism	
	Active malignancy	

Abbreviations: *BMS* Bare-metal-Stent, *DES* Drug-eluting-Stent; *MI* heart attack, *TIA* transient ischemic attack

[a]$CHADS_2$: heart failure, hypertension, age > 75 years, diabetes mellitus, stroke or TIA

[b]Recent studies come to the conclusion that the antiplatelet therapy can be discontinued in case of BMS the dual after 3 months and in case of new DES often already after 6 weeks [11, 16]

Table 19.4 Risk of thromboembolism in various interventions

High risk of thrombosis	Medium risk of thrombosis	Low risk of thrombosis
Arthroplasty	Upper limb & other interventions lower extremity	Visceral surgery, **gynecology**, urology [<30 min]
Hip fractures	visceral surgery, **gynecology**, urology [>30 min]	Metal removal
Large abdominal surgery	surgery of lung, chest wall, mediastinum	juxtaarticular surgeries without immobilization
Tumor surgery	Varicosis surgery	
	Vascular surgery	

Table 19.5 Relative risk [RR] of inherited thrombophilia on venous thromboembolism in family studies [43]

Risk factor	Prevalence [%]	RR of first venous thrombosis
Antithrombin deficiency	0.02	5–10
Protein C deficiency	0.2	4–6.5
Protein S deficiency	0.03–0.13	1–10
Faktor V Leiden/APC-Resistance	3.0–7.0	3–5
Prothrombin G20210A	0.7–4.0	2–3
High factor VIII	10	5

Venous thromboembolism is a multifactorial disorder. Antithrombin-, protein C- protein S- deficiency are high risk factors for the onset of venous thromboembolism. In contrast, factor V Leiden, the prothrombin mutation G20210A and elevated factor VIII levels are discussed as common but mild risk factors of thromboembolism. Combinations between established prothrombotic risk factors increase the risk of thrombosis [19, 43].

In patients with or without a history a venous thromboembolism and inherited thrombophilia the updated Chest guidelines and the German AWMF Guidelines suggest a prophylaxis in risk situations for thrombosis. The dosage has to be determined on an individual basis, inter alia depending on the body weight [7, 33].

Perioperative Management: Vitamin K-Antagonists

The median risk for thromboembolism is the most common situation in the daily praxis, so is the risk of hysterectomy for thromboembolism: the current guidelines for the perioperative management focus the expecting bleeding tendency in this case. In case of intervention with a high risk for bleeding an interruption of the OAC can be taken place without a bridging, in case of a low bleeding tendency a bridging with UFH or LMWH can be taken place depending the half-time of the OAC [1, 3, 5–7, 9, 14, 21, 23, 25, 40].

(i). low bleeding risk & median thromboembolic risk: is there a minor bleeding risk due to the scheduled intervention, in most cases the oral anticoagulation can be taken unmodified or can be reduced in its intensity.

(ii). medium to high bleeding risk & medium thromboembolic risk: when the intervention causes a medium to high bleeding risk the anticoagulant therapy can be paused for a short period.

(iii). high bleeding risk & high thromboembolic risk: when the intervention causes a high bleeding und thromboembolic risk the change of a vitamin K antagonist to UFH [limited renal function] or LMWH is necessary. In this cases the VKA is paused approximately 7 days [Phenprocoumon] respectively 5 days [Warfarin] prior to the scheduled intervention or if the INR is below its therapeutic level [INR < 2] and UFH or LMWH is used for bridging. If there will be high thromboembolic risk a therapeutic heparin use should be aimed: For UFH an aPTT prolongation of 1.5–2 times the standard is intended, for LMWH the dose which is recommended by their manufacturers for the acute treatment of deep vein thrombosis or pulmonary embolism should be selected.

There are only a few comparative studies for UHF and LMWH for bridging therapy [9, 9]. These show no difference in bleeding and the occurrence of thromboembolic complications, however, the length of hospital stay was significantly shorter with LMWH and hence more cost-effective.

For (iii) applies, in cases of severe renal insufficiency [creatinine clearance <30 ml/min] the heparin therapy should be carried out with UFH [7, 21], in other cases, LMWH can be used. In the current 9th guideline of the "American College of Chest Physicians" it is recommended, that stop UFH 6–8 h and LMWH 24 h before the procedure and to start the therapy again after 24–48 h depending on postoperative bleeding tendency [7]. In early resuming heparin therapy a reduced dose of LMWH or a heparin is discussed without a bolus of UFH.

The reuptake of OAC depends on the risk of bleeding of the performed surgery and should be done at the earliest from 1 to 2 days post-surgery, the parallel heparinization should be continued up to a reproducible INR > 2 [7, 21, 25].

Unlike in elective surgeries the management in emergency cases cannot be planned: The effect of the OAC must be lifted as soon as possible. To do this the administration of vitamin K1 10 mg iv [effectiveness within 24 h] or the substitution of vitamin K-dependent coagulation factors [PPSB: 4-factor concentrate] which work within minutes can be performed. If there is a life-threatening bleeding under OAC vitamin K1 and PPSB ca be administered simultaneously.

When bridging with a parenteral anticoagulant the INR, aPTT and anti-Factor Xa activity should be measured in addition to the clinical evaluation of the bleeding preoperatively. During the postoperative period the blood count, prothrombin time according to thromboplastin time and aPTT should be determined to evaluate the bleeding tendency before reuptake.

To summarize: the current recommendations for the perioperative management are based on the expected risk of bleeding. For planned interventions with high risk of bleeding the interruption of OAC without bridging may be considered. At a low risk of bleeding a bridging therapy with UFH or LMWH can be applied after discontinuation of OAC.

Perioperative Management: Platelet Inhibition Therapy

The use of medication with reversible and irreversible inhibition of platelets (Table 19.2) is indicated for primary and secondary prevention of atherothrombosis-related cerebrovascular and cardiovascular diseases. This includes for example stroke, TIA, myocardial infarction, interventional radiological procedures such as PTCA with or without implantation of bare-metal stents [BMS] or drug-eluting stents [DES], radiofrequency ablation, and peripheral arterial thromboembolic diseases. Platelet-inhibitory substances are used either as monotherapy [primary prophylaxis or long-term therapy] or as a temporary combination therapy for example in high risk patients after stenting. In this group of patients is the annual recurrence risk of atherothrombotic occlusion or stent thrombosis after discontinuation of a AA therapy within 6 months after a implantation of a BMS and up to 12 months after using a DES is high to very high. According to the current guidelines elective procedures should not carried out or planned in this period, vice versa, a stent implantation should be performed only after an urgent surgical intervention has taken place [7, 16–18, 20–22, 32]. Recent publications show a broad consensus that the dual platelet inhibition may be often finished after 3 months when using a BMS and when using a novel DES already after 6 weeks [12, 17].

The assessment of periprocedural bleeding risk (Table 19.3) is similar to the assessment taking an OAC [35]. At medium to high risk of bleeding the cardiovascular risk determines the procedures for non cardiosurgical necessary interventions [5, 7, 21].

(i). *Low risk of bleeding and high cardiovascular risk: Is the risk of bleeding through the planned intervention low, the AA therapy can be continued unchanged in most cases.*

(ii). *Medium to high risk of bleeding and high cardiovascular risk: aspirin in these patients should not be paused but continued [if the intervention cannot be moved].*

(iii). High risk of bleeding and high cardiovascular risk: if a surgery is urgent and not unmovable, the short-term interruption of the AA therapy by administration of platelet concentrates and the use of a short-acting GPIIb-IIIa antagonists iv can be performed.

(iv). *Medium to high risk of bleeding and low cardiovascular risk: an interruption of the AA medication is justifiable.*

ASA, [common dose 100 mg per day] can be discontinued 5 days before the planned intervention, clopidogrel or ticagrelor should be paused 5 days and prasugrel 7 days in advance [16–18].

In aspirin-induced bleeding, DDAVP can be administered i.v. [0.3–0.4 mg/kg] in consideration of the contraindications for DDAVP in combination of platelet concentrates administration [18, 20, 22, 32, 38]: in 2014 the EMA approval has been extended in this indication for DDAVP administration.

After interruption of an AA therapy to the procedure can be applied in analogy for OAC, approximately 24 h following surgery the reuptake of the AA therapy can be scheduled. ASA is effective within minutes; Clopidogrel reaches its full effect without saturation after about 7 days.

For high-risk patients who have to undergo a necessary intervention, a bridging with a short-acting GPIIb-IIIa antagonists iv [Eptifibatide, Tirofiban: 29] is possible in addition to the short-term interruption of AA therapy with platelet concentrates.

In patients with renal impairment Eptifibatide is the GPIIb-IIIa inhibitor of choice. First experiences on the short-term bridging therapy with reversible direct P2Y12 inhibitor Cangrelor are available [1], but this substance is not yet approved in Germany.

When bridging an AA therapy in addition to the clinical evaluation of the bleeding measurements of blood count, thromboplastin time and aPTT should be performed preoperatively and postoperative. In addition, preoperative and possibly in the inpatient period of time the measurement of the residual platelet function by appropriate test methods might be helpful.

To summarize: the risk of recurrence of stent thrombosis after (too) early discontinuation of AA therapy after implantation of a BMS or DES is high [–please consider manufacturer's instructions and current guidelines-]. Generally, elective surgery should not be performed during this period. ASA may be discontinued 5 days before the planned intervention, Clopidogrel or Ticagrelor should be discontinued 5 days and Prasugrel should be paused 7 days in advance.

Perioperative Management: Direct Oral Anticoagulants

Among the class of DOACs the class of thrombin inhibitors and factor Xa inhibitors are combined [2, 15, 31]. Dabigatran is a thrombin inhibitor, Rivaroxaban, Apixaban and Edoxaban are factor Xa inhibitors. Both classes are used in fixed dosage without laboratory control both for primary prevention as well as in therapeutic indications.

The audited dosage for the treatment of deep vein thrombosis will be for Dabigatran 2 × 150 mg daily after the initial use of UFH, LMWH or Fondaparinux for at least 5 days, for Rivaroxaban in the first three weeks 2 × 15 mg followed by 1 × 20 mg daily, for Apixaban initial 2 × 10 mg daily for 7 days and then 2 × 5 mg and 60 mg once daily for Edoxaban after initial administration of UFH, LMWH or Fondaparinux for at least 5 days. In atrial fibrillation, the standard dose of Dabigatran is 150 mg 2 × daily, 1 × 20 mg daily of Rivaroxaban, 2 × 5 mg per day for Apixaban and 60 mg once daily for Edoxaban (regarding dosage recommendations, for example in renal impairment, we refer to the prescribing information respectively) [4, 31].

For DOACs no bridging therapy in the perioperative period is usually required due to the short half-lives because the necessary treatment interruption can be achieved by simply omitting before surgery [23, 24]. Peak levels are reached after oral administration of Dabigatran after 1.5–2 h, for Rivaroxaban 2–4 h, for Apixaban after 3–4 h and for Edoxaban after 1–2 h [2, 4, 25].

For Dabigatran discontinuation is recommended 2 days before a standard intervention in normal renal function, mild and moderate renal impairment a break of 3–4 days should be discussed [21]. For Rivaroxaban a break usually ranges from of at least 24 h before planned surgery, Apixaban and Edoxaban should be discontinued 24–48 h before the planned surgery [4, 21].

If the time of last intake is unclear and urgently required intervention with high bleeding tendency is a determination by modified thrombin time possible for Dabigatran and an anti-factor Xa determination for Rivaroxaban, Apixaban and Edoxaban possible [11, 15, 28, 41]: It this context it should be noted that the respective anti-factor Xa test for the DOAC-substance must be calibrated. In addition, it should be mentioned that a Rivaroxaban-sensitive thromboplastin time (for example Neoplastin reagent) for detecting the effect of Rivaroxaban is also suitable [15].

In contrast to therapy with OAC the DOACs achieve at point of restart with DOACs in the original dose an immediate anticoagulant effect, it is recommended to start these drug classes again only after a secure clinical exclusion of postoperative bleeding tendency or to reduce the starting dose of both agents [21]. If necessary, the administration of UFH or LMWH should post-operatively initially carried out (in the first 48–72 h), as there is no experience for the postoperative administration of DOACs outside of VTE prophylaxis in hip and knee replacement surgery. If oral drug absorption should not be possible for a long time postoperatively a thromboembolic prophylaxis is to be ensured with for example UFH or LMWH.

Finally, we have to point out that DOACs do not represent a medication to bridge a therapy with OAC or AA.

To summarize: Dabigatran is discontinued in normal renal function 2 days before a standard procedure, Rivaroxaban should be discontinued at least 24 h in advance and Apixaban and Edoxaban 24–48 h before. DOACs are no medication for a bridging therapy with OAC or AA.

Future Prospects

Further prospective and randomized trials and meta-analyzes of randomized studies are needed to be able to pronounce recommendations on a higher evidence level in the future. These studies should be based on a harmonized definition and evaluation criteria for study endpoints and bridging therapies [10, 29, 30, 36, 37].

Conclusions for Clinical Practice

Current recommendations for bridging a chronic OAK or AA-therapy are still based on not sufficient data and therefore are subject to uncertainty, so that in each patient the bleeding and thromboembolic risk must be weighed against each other.

With a medium risk of thromboembolism, such as during the hysterectomy, the individual bleeding risk of the planned intervention determines the bridging therapy:

Is the risk of bleeding due to the planned intervention low, the OAK / AA therapy can be continued unchanged or be slightly reduced in intensity in most cases.

Is risk of thrombosis low in case of a medium to high risk of bleeding, antiplatelet therapy can be paused temporarily.

At high risk of bleeding and thromboembolism, a change of OAC to UFH [impaired renal function] or LMWH is required.

The AA-therapy can be bridged with cases of a high risk of bleeding and thromboembolism with platelet concentrates and short-acting GPIIb-IIIa antagonists [Eptifibatide, Tirofiban].

Patients using a direct oral anticoagulant [Dabigatran, Rivaroxaban, Apixaban, Edoxaban] need an intermission of therapy prior to the planned intervention depending the individual half-time of the specific medication and the individually renal function. These patients do not need a bridging with heparins.

Modified with permission from Nowak-Göttl U, Langer F, Limperger V, Mesters R, et al. [bridging: perioperative management of chronic anticoagulation or antiplatelet therapy]. Dtsch. Med. Wochenschr. 2014; 139: 1301–7. © Georg Thieme Verlag KG.

References

1. Angiolillo DJ, Firstenberg MS, Price MJ, et al. Bridging antiplatelet therapy with cangrelor in patients undergoing cardiac surgery. A randomized controlled trial. JAMA. 2012;307:265–74.
2. Baglin T. Clinical use of new oral anticoagulant drugs: dabigatran and rivaroxaban. Br J Haematol. 2013;163:160–7.
3. BRIDGE study investigators. Bridging anticoagulation. Is it needed when warfarin is interrupted around the time of a surgery or procedure – cardiology patient page. Circulation. 2012;125:e496–8.
4. Chan L, Pisano M. Edoxaban (savaysa): a factor xa inhibitor. P T. 2015;40:651–95.
5. Dimitrova G, Tulman DB, Bergese SD. Perioperative management of antiplatelet therapy in patients with drug-eluting stents. HSR Proc Intensive Care Cardiovas Anesth. 2012;4:153–67.
6. Douketis JD. Perioperative management of patients who are receiving warfarin therapy: an evidence-based and practical approach. Blood. 2011;117:5044–9.
7. Douketis JD, Spyropoulos AC, Spencer FA, American College of Chest Surgeons, et al. Perioperative management of anticoagulant therapy: Antithrombotic Therapy and Prevention of Thrombosis, 9th ed: American College of Chest Physicians Evidence-Based Clinical Practice Guidelines [erratum appears in Chest 2012;141(4):1129]. Chest. 2012;141(Suppl 2):e326S–50S.
8. Hammerstingl C, Schmitz A, Fimmers R, Omran H. Bridging of chronic oral anticoagulation with enoxaparin in patients with atrial fibrillation: results from the prospective BRAVE registry. Cardiovasc Ther. 2009;27:230–8.
9. Halbritter KM, Wawer A, Beyer J, Oettler W, Schellong SM. Bridging anticoagulation for patients on long-term vitamin-K-antagonists. A prospective registry of 311 episodes. J Thromb Haemost. 2005;3:2823–5.
10. Healey J, Eiklboom J, Douketis J, et al. Periprocedural bleeding and thromboembolic events with dabigatran compared with warfarin – results from the randomised evaluation of long-term anticoagulation therapy (RE-LY) randomised trial. Circulation. 2012;126:343–8.
11. Hillarp A, Baghaei F, Fagerberg BI, et al. Effects of the oral, direct factor Xa inhibitor rivaroxaban on commonly used coagulation assays. J Thromb Haemost. 2011;9:133–9.
12. Lip GY, Huber K, Andreotti F, et al. Management of antithrombotic therapy in atrial fibrillation patients presenting with acute coronary syndrome and/or undergoing percutaneous coronary intervention/stenting. Thromb Haemost. 2010;103:13–28.
13. Joist JH, George JN. Hemostatic abnormalities in liver and renal disease. In: RW C, Hirsh J, VJ M, et al., editors. Hemostasis and thrombosis. Basic principals and clinical practice. Philadelphia: Lippincott, Williams & Wilkins; 2004. p. 955–73.
14. Kearon C, Hirsh J. Management of anticoagulation before and after elective surgery. N Engl J Med. 1997;336:1506–11.
15. Koscielny J, Beyer-Westendorf J, von Heymann C, et al. Risk of bleeding and haemorrhagic complication with rivaroxaban-periprocedural management of haemostasis – Konsensus. Hamostaseologie. 2012;32(4):287–93.
16. Koscielny J, Rutkauskaite E. Preinterventional change in the clotting medication. Viszeralmedizin (Gastrointestinal Medicine and Surgery). 2013;29:1–13.
17. Korte W, Cattaneo M, PG C, et al. Perioperative management of antiplatelet therapy in patients with coronary artery disease: joint position paper by members of the working group on Perioperative Haemostasis of the Society on Thrombosis and Haemostasis Research (GTH), the working group on Perioperative Coagulation of the Austrian Society for Anesthesiology, Resuscitation and Intensive Care (ÖGARI) and the Working Group Thrombosis of the European Society for Cardiology (ESC). Thromb Haemost. 2011;105(5):743–9.
18. Kozek-Langenecker S, Afshari A, Albaladejo P, et al. Management of severe perioperative bleeding: guidelines from the European Society of Anaesthesiology. Eur J Anaesthesiol. 2013;30:270–382.
19. Lijfering WM, J.-L B, Veeger N, et al. Selective testing for thrombophilia in patients with first venous thrombosis: results from a retrospective family cohort study on absolute thrombotic risk for currently known thrombophilic defects in 2479 relatives. Blood. 2009;113(21):5314–22.
20. Mannucci PM. Desmopressin (DDAVP) in the treatment of bleeding disorders: the first 20 years. Blood. 1997;90:2515–21.
21. Ortel TL. Perioperative management of patients on chronic antithrombotic therapy. Hematology. 2012;529-535
22. Levi M, Eerenberg E, Kamphuisen PW. Bleeding risk and reversal strategies for old and new anticoagulants and antiplatelet agents. J Thromb Haemost. 2011;9:1705–12.
23. Levy JH, Faraoni D, Spring JL, Douketis JD, Samama CM. Managing new oral anticoagulants in the perioperative and intensive care unit setting. Anesthesiology. 2013;118:1466–74.
24. Patel M, Mahaffey K, Garg J, et al. Rivaroxaban versus warfarin in nonvalvular atrial fibrillation. N Engl J Med. 2011;365:883–91.
25. Patel JP, Arya R. The current status of bridging anticoagulation. Br J Haematol. 2013; doi:10.1111/bjh.12644.
26. Pfanner G, Koscielny J, Pernerstorfer T, et al. Die präoperative Blutungsanamnese. Empfehlungen der Arbeitsgruppe perioperative Gerinnung (AGPG) der Österreichischen Gesellschaft für Anästhesiologie, Reanimation und Intensivmedizin (ÖGARI). Anaesthesist. 2007;56(6):604–11. [in German]
27. Rodeghiero F, Tosetto A, Abshire T, Arnold DM, Coller B, James P, Neunert C, Lillicrap D. ISTH/SSC bleeding assessment tool: a standardized questionnaire and a proposal for a new bleeding score for inherited bleeding disorders. J Thromb Haemost. 2010;8:2063–5. on behalf of the ISTH/SSC Joint VWF and Perinatal/ Pediatric Haemostasis Subcommittees Working Group: http://www.wfh.org/en/resources/bleeding-assessment-tool-isth-batt
28. Samama MM, Contant G, Spiro TE, et al. Evaluation of the anti-factor Xa chromogenic assay for the measurement of rivaroxaban plasma concentrations using calibrators and controls. Thromb Haemost. 2012;107:379–87.
29. Savonitto S, D'Urbano M, Caracciolo M, et al. Urgent surgery in patients with a recently implanted coronary drug-eluting stent: a phase II study of 'bridging' antiplatelet therapy with tirofiban during temporary withdrawal of clopidogrel. Br J Anaesth. 2010;104:285–91.
30. Schulman S, Kearon C, on behalf of the subcommittee on control of anticoagulation of the Scientific and Standardization committee of the International Society on Thrombosis and Haemostasis. Definition of major bleeding in clinical investigations of antihemostatic medicinal products in non-surgical patients. Scientific and Standardization Committee Communication. J Thromb Haemost. 2005;3:692–4.
31. Schellong SM, Haas S. Perioperative Thromboseprophylaxe – Neue orale Antikoagulanzien und ihre Anwendung. Anästhesiol Intensivmed Notfallmed Schmerzther. 2012;47:266–72. [in German]
32. S3 – Leitlinie Polytrauma/Schwerverletzten-Behandlung. Deutsche Gesellschaft für Unfallchirurgie. AWMF (Arbeitskreis wissen-

schaftlicher medizinischer Fachgesellschaften) – Register Nr. 012/019: 1–445. [in German].
33. S3 – Leitlinie Prophylaxe der venösen Thromboembolie (VTE). AWMF (Arbeitskreis wissenschaftlicher medizinischer Fachgesellschaften) – Register Nr. 003/001: 1–243. [in German].
34. Siegal D, Yudin J, Kaatz S, Douketis J, Lim W, Spyropoulos AC. Periprocedural heparin bridging in patients receiving vitamin K antagonists: systematic review and meta-analysis of bleeding and thromboembolic rates. Circulation. 2012;126:1630–9.
35. Sørensen R, Hansen ML, Abildstrom SZ, et al. Risk of bleeding in patients with acute myocardial infarction treated with different combinations of aspirin, clopidogrel, and vitamin K antagonists in Denmark: a retrospective analysis of nationwide registry data. Lancet. 2009;374(9706):1967–74.
36. Spyropoulos AC, Albaladejo P, Godier A, et al. Periprocedural antiplatelet therapy: recommendations for standardized reporting in patients on antiplatelet therapy: communication from the SSC of the ISTH. J Thromb Haemost. 2013 Aug;11(8): 1593–156.
37. Spyropoulos A, Douketis JD, Gerotziafas G, Kaatz S, Ortel TL, Schulman S, on behalf of the subcommittee on control of anticoagulation of the SSC of the ISTH. Periprocedural antithrombotic and bridging therapy: recommendations for standardized reporting in patients with arterial indications for chronic oral anticoagulant therapy. J Thromb Haemost. 2012;10:692–4.
38. The Society of Thoracic Surgeons Blood Conservation Guideline Task Force, The Society of Cardiovascular Anesthesiologists Special Task Force on Blood Transfusion. Perioperative blood transfusion and blood conservation in cardiac surgery: the Society of Thoracic Surgeons and The Society of Cardiovascular Anesthesiologists clinical practice guideline. Ann Thorac Surg. 2007;83(Suppl):S27–86.
39. Thiele T, Sumnig A, Hron G, et al. Platelet transfusion for reversal of dual antiplatelet therapy in patients requiring urgent surgery: a pilot study. J Thromb Haemost. 2012;10:968–71.
40. Ufer M. Comparative pharmacokinetics of vitamin K antagonists: warfarin, phenprocoumon and acenocoumarol. Clin Pharmacokinet. 2005;4412:1227–46.
41. van Ryn J, Tangier J, Haertter S, et al. Dabigatran etexilate—a novel, reversible, oral direct thrombin inhibitor: Interpretation of coagulation assays and reversal of anticoagulant activity. Thromb Haemost. 2010;103:1116–27.
42. Vincentelli A, Susen S, le Turneau E, et al. Acquired von Willebrand syndrome in aortic stenosis. N Engl J Med. 2003;349:343–49.
43. Vossen CY, Conard J, Fontcuberta J, et al. Familial thrombophilia and lifetime risk of venous thrombosis. J Thromb Haemost. 2004;2;1526–32.

Anaesthesia in Gynaecology

20

Michael Sonntagbauer

Abbreviations

5HT3	5-hydroxytriptamine
ATP	Adenosine triphosphate
CO	Cardiac output
CO_2	Carbon dioxide
COPD	Chronic obstructive pulmonary disease
CS	Compartment syndrome
FRC	Functional residual capacity
GnRH	Gonadotropin-releasing hormone
HSC	Hysteroscopy
IAP	Intra-abdominal pressure
IOH	Intra-operative hypotension
IUP	Intra-uterine pressure
K+	Potassium
MAP	Mean arterial pressure
MOV	Multiple organ failure
MV	Minute volume
NK1	Neurokinin 1
Na+	Sodium
PACU	Post anaesthesia care unit
Pinsp	Pressure, inspiratoric
PONV	Postoperative nausea and vomiting
RAAS	Renin-angiotensin-aldosterone system
RR	Respiratory rate
SIRS	Systemic inflammatory response syndrome
TUR	Trans-urethral resection
VC	Vital capacity

Gynaecologists and anaesthesiologists are both at the patient's service when performing gynaecological procedures.

In order to achieve the best possible outcome concerning patient safety and comfort and to establish a smooth course in the operating theatre and a good environment for performing surgery it is necessary to maintain an on-going communication and teamwork between gynaecologists and anaesthesiologists. Both sides have to be aware of each other's specific needs and problems.

Therefore this book, which is addressed to operating gynaecologists includes a chapter emphasizing on anaesthesiological difficulties of vaginal procedures, laparotomy, laparoscopy and robotic assisted gynaecological surgery.

General Considerations of Gynaecological Anaesthesia

Gynaecological procedures are often perceived as mutilating by patients. Therefore a high level of fear has to be expected and considered by all involved disciplines. The first contact between anaesthesiologist and patient usually takes place at the pre-operative assessment. The main objective here is the evaluation of cardiopulmonary risk factors and the completion of additionally necessary diagnostic investigations. Especially when dealing with multimorbid patients or invasive surgery an interdisciplinary perioperative risk evaluation is important. By taking account of the patient's wishes the anaesthesiologist chooses a certain technique. The pre--operative assessment needs to be discussed with the patient. All information as well as the patient's consent are documented. The patient is informed about fasting times and administration of her own medication. Furthermore the anaesthesiologist should try to reduce the patient's fears during the conversation. The pre-operative administration of anxiolytic medication is an integral component for achieving this goal.

An outpatient surgical procedure is only permitted if the procedural and patient-related requirements are fulfilled. The patient's status should be passed on to the anaesthesiological

Translation revised by
Victoria Loise Ellerbroek
Anne Caroline Queisser

M. Sonntagbauer
Department of Anaesthesia, Intensive Care Medicine and Pain Therapy, Frankfurt University Hospital, Theodor Stern-Kai 7, Frankfurt 60590, Germany
e-mail: michael.sonntagbauer@kgu.de

I. Alkatout, L. Mettler (eds.), *Hysterectomy*, DOI 10.1007/978-3-319-22497-8_20

department prior to their assessment. Thereby possible contraindications can be detected and an inpatient treatment can be planned if necessary.

Postoperative Nausea and Vomiting

One of the most common complications after anaesthesia is the occurrence of PONV. The general incidence is about 30 % [1–3]. In gynaecological surgery the incidence is even two to three times higher and lies at ca. 80 % [4]. Even though the exact pathogenesis of PONV remains unknown it was possible to identify numerous significant independent risk factors by analysis of large cohort studies. In addition to patient-specific risk factors anaesthesia- and surgery-related risk factors should be determined (Table 20.1). Surgical risk factors include "gynaecological surgery "as well as" laparoscopy" [3, 5] underlining the gynaecology-specific relevance of PONV for the anaesthesiological care. The patient's discomfort due to PONV is one of the most common reasons for poor patient satisfaction rating in the postoperative period [6]. Given the possibility to allocate a certain amount of money to prevent all postoperative complications, patients would spend one third and also the largest amount to avoid PONV [7]. Persistent PONV can lead to a prolonged stay in the postoperative care unit [3] and unanticipated hospital admission which results in a significant increase of overall health care costs [8, 9]. To address these findings risk scores are used to objectify the patient's individual baseline risk for PONV. Simplified PONV risk scores with a sensitivity and specificity of about 70 % [1, 2, 10] are equally precise in predicting PONV as compared to more complex approaches and may significantly reduce the rate of PONV (Fig. 20.1); Nowadays they are part of everyday practice at most institutions. Prevention and treatment of PONV may be achieved by altering the anaesthesiological approach and by applicating antiemetic drugs (Table 20.1).

Positioning

Lithotomy position is commonly used during gynaecological interventions. It allows the best access to the perineum. An additional advantage is the extra space between the patient's legs for an assistant surgeon during abdominal procedures without restricting the operator's mobility.

When placing patients in lithotomy position awareness for nerve injuries caused by intraoperative positioning is crucial.

Femoral neuropathy may occur due to distinctive angulation of the femoral nerve beneath the unyielding inguinal ligament. Sciatic nerve function may be compromised since

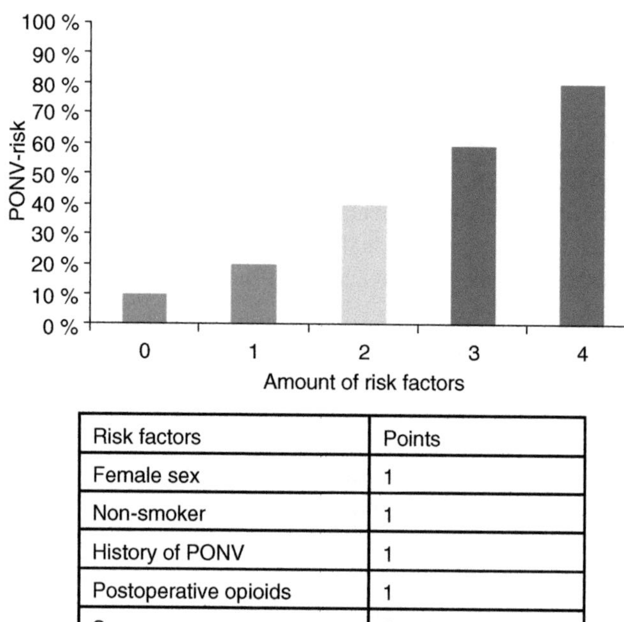

Risk factors	Points
Female sex	1
Non-smoker	1
History of PONV	1
Postoperative opioids	1
Sum =	0 ... 4

Fig. 20.1 Risk score for PONV in adults. Simplified risk score from Apfel et al. [1] to predict the patient's risk for PONV. *PONV* postoperative nausea and vomiting

Table 20.1 Risk factors for PONV as well as options for prophylaxis and treatment of PONV in adults [1]

Risk factors for PONV in adults	Options for prophylaxis/treatment of PONV in adults
Female sex	Propofol anaesthesia
History of PONV or motion sickness	Regional anaesthesia
Nonsmoking	Dexamethasone
Younger age	$5HT_3$ antagonists
General versus regional anaesthesia	Dimenhydrinate
Use of volatile anaesthetics and nitrous oxide	NK_1 receptor antagonists
Postoperative opioids	Propofol subhypnotic dose infusion or Propofol in PACU (rescue-only)
Duration of anaesthesia	Scopolamine
Type of surgery (cholecystectomy, laparoscopic, gynaecological)	Non pharmacological: acupuncture
	Perphenazine
	Droperidol/Haloperidol

PONV postoperative nausea and vomiting, *PACU* post-anaesthesia care unit, *5HT3* 5-hydroxytryptamine, *NK1* neurokinin-1

it is fixed at the sciatic notch and extreme positioning, especially external rotation may lead to stretch injury. The common peroneal nerve is susceptible to compression injury due to its superficial course near the lateral fibular head.

Excessive hip flexion (>90°), abduction (>45°) and external hip rotation should be avoided. Maximum abduction is reached when the contralateral shoulder is in line with thigh, knee and heel of the patient.

Special care must be taken if the patient's mobility in the knee and hip joint is limited (e.g. condition after hip replacement). In these cases it is advisable to perform positioning while the patient is still awake.

Nerve injury of the brachial plexus may occur when shoulder padding is used during Trendelenburg position to prevent sliding of the patient. The neural structures of the brachial plexus pass the cervical intervertebral foramina, the interscalene triangle and run between the clavicle and the first rib to the axilla. Potential compression along the way can be caused by soft tissue as well as bony structures when pressure is applied. The contact point of shoulder padding should be at the acromioclavicular joint. Abduction of the arm increases the risk of nerve injury and should never exceed 90° [11].

Less common is the development of a compartment syndrome (CS) during lithotomy position. The incidence of CS lies around 1:3500 during gynaecological procedures. Since delayed diagnosis and treatment may result in catastrophic consequences for the patient this rather rare complication will be further discussed in this chapter. The occurrence of CS in a previously healthy leg is also described as "well-leg-compartment-syndrome".

The arterio-venous pressure gradient theory is the most accepted theory today for description of the pathophysiology of CS [12]. This hypothesis states that capillary perfusion is only assured when the arterial pressure transcends the venous pressure.

During lithotomy position increased external pressure on the calf, the weight of the calf itself in the positioning devise and venous obstruction due to kinking of the veins will increase venous pressure.

Arterial pressure may be decreased by elevation of the lower extremity, anaesthesia-related hypotension or hypovolemia due to haemorrhage [13]. This constellation especially during long-lasting lithotomy position can result in a reduction of capillary perfusion beyond tissue viability. Ischemia itself and post ischemia reperfusion injury can cause increased endothelial permeability due to liberation of inflammatory mediators with a leakage of fluid into the interstitial space. The resulting edema within the non-expandable compartment causes further reduction of arterial and increase of venous pressure and is ultimately the start of a vicious circle (Fig. 20.2).

If necrosis occurs the function of the extremity can be compromised and amputation may be the only option. In the case of cell death rhabdomyolisis, kidney failure, hyperkalaemia and acidosis can lead to multiple organ failure and death.

So far it was not possible to identify any independent risk factors for CS. However, increased body mass index (BMI) and peripheral arterial disease have been considered to predispose an individual to be affected by CS. From what is known duration and extent of lithotomy position seems to be

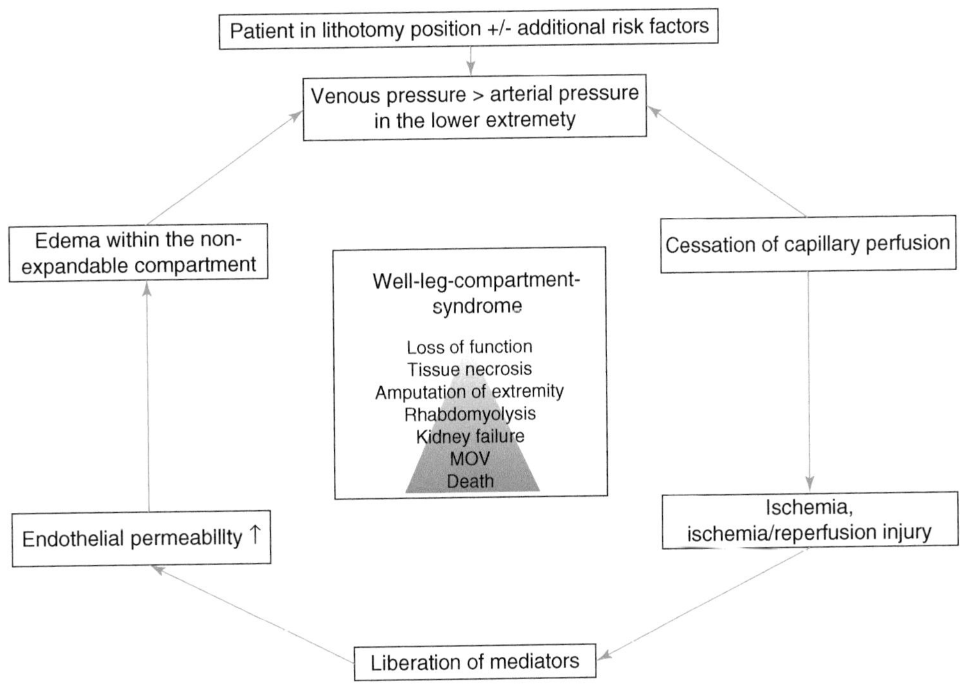

Fig. 20.2 Vicious cycle of the development of well-leg-compartment-syndrome. *MOV* Multiple organ failure

the major cornerstone in the development of CS [14]. Seventy percent of CS occur after more than 5 h [15] spent in lithotomy position (which also means that 30 % occur before that). So far evidence-based recommendations for preventing CS have not been established [15].

At some institutions preventive measures have been implemented. It remains unclear whether one of these measures or their combination can achieve the desired impact (Table 20.2).

Treatment of CS is achieved by pressure release through fasciotomy of the affected compartment [16]. To reduce edema and ischemia/reperfusion injury intravenous mannitol can be considered as a treatment option [17].

CS is primarily a clinical diagnosis. Leg pain, that is not otherwise explainable and is intensified by passive stretch and paraesthesia have to be interpreted as alarming symptoms and should be recognized.

Although large reviews could find no correlation it has been controversially discussed if diagnosis of CS may be delayed due to the use of epidural anaesthesia [18, 19]. Strong breakthrough pain has to be expected even if sufficient epidural anaesthesia is in place [20–22].

Vaginal (Access-) Surgery

The majority of vaginal procedures are less invasive. Due to short duration and limited tissue trauma many of these interventions are performed as outpatient surgery. For the anaesthesiological management the use of short-acting substances is preferred to ensure a prompt dismissal while the patient is objectively and subjectively at comfort. Postoperative nausea and vomiting can lead to prolonged observation time in the post anaesthesia care unit and unexpected admissions. Therefore adequate prophylaxis and treatment of PONV is advised.

If lack of contraindications is assured (e.g. gastro--oesophageal reflux) the airway can be secured with supraglottic devices. Thereby the use of muscle relaxants can be avoided and the risk of prolonged respiratory assistance due to overdosing or overhang can be minimized.

During short procedures an on-going communication between gynaecologist and anaesthesiologist is necessary to assure a well scheduled and adequate depth of anaesthesia. Hereby a smooth process in the operating theatre with little delay can be achieved.

Possible complications during vaginal procedures can develop when surgical manipulation leads to vagal reaction. In most cases interruption of that manipulation is sufficient as a causal treatment although cardiac arrest may occur [23].

For surgical procedures with a duration of 1–2 h or patient-specific factors (e.g. COPD) spinal anaesthesia may be an alternative technique if steep Trendelenburg position is not required. Respectful and considerate interaction with the conscious patient and an appropriate conversation and noise level need to be regarded. Spinal anaesthesia per se is not a contraindication for outpatient surgery.

Fluid Overload Syndrome

Diagnosis and treatment of intra-uterine pathologies requires distension of the uterus. Today fluid distending media are predominantly used. Distension of the endometrial cavity is only feasible if the distending media is applied with a certain pressure. Systemic absorption may cause "fluid overload syndrome". Heart failure and lung edema can develop due to sudden exposure to additional preload. Pathogenesis and clinical appearance are similar to TUR-syndrome known from urological surgery.

In diagnostic hysteroscopy the anticipated risk for systemic absorption is low due to the lack of vessel transection since media has no opportunity to enter systemic circulation. Consequently the risk increases if resection (e.g. of a myoma) is performed and tissue is traumatised.

While mechanical instruments may be an alternative for resection in some cases, most hysteroscopic resectoscopies are performed using monopolar or bipolar electrosurgical instru-

Table 20.2 Potential risk factors of CS and potential strategies for preventing CS during lithotomy position

Potential risk factors of CS during lithotomy position	Potential strategies for preventing CS during lithotomy position
Extreme lithotomy position	Avoidance of lithotomy position whenever there is no need for perineal and vaginal access
Trendelenburg position	Intraoperative modification of position of lower extremity
Long duration of lithotomy position and head down tilt	Intraoperative warming of lower extremity
Intraoperative hypotension/hypovolemia	Avoidance of hypotension
Hypothermia	Minimization of time in lithotomy–/Trendelenburg position
High extent of flexion in knee- and hip joints	Avoidance of high degree of lithotomy–/Trendelenburg position
External pressure due to positioning support material	Adequate substitution of fluid loss
Patient-specific risk factors	Intermittent compression of lower extremity
Misinterpretation of clinical symptoms	Awareness of clinical symptoms

CS compartment syndrome

ments. Monopolar cauterisation requires completion of an electrical circuit between the surgical instrument and the remotely located dispersive electrode to achieve a thermal effect. If such instruments are used in the presence of conductive particles (e.g. ions in saline) dispersion prevents the completion of the electrical circuit and therefore the surgical effect.

This explains the requirement of electrolyte-free and hypotonic distension media if monopolar electrocauterisation is used. If these hypotonic fluids find their way into the systemic circulation of the patient not only fluid overload may occur, but also hypotonic haemodilution. Resulting hyponatremia and osmotic imbalances can lead to cerebral edema with symptoms as seizures, coma or death [24, 25].

Premenopausal women are at increased risk of neurological complications due to sodium-potassium adenosine triphosphatase (NA^+/K^+- ATPase) "pump"-inhibition by female sex steroids, most likely oestrogens [26]. Preoperative GnRH-agonist administration may therefore be considered [27].

The risk of neurological complication using electrolyte-free distending media has led to the development of bipolar electrosurgical instruments that can be used even in complex hysteroscopic surgery [28, 29]. The electrical circuit is completed at the tip of the instrument. The presence of charged particles is therefore required and electrolyte-containing media (e.g. normal saline) is used.

To prevent neurological complications during hysteroscopy it is recommended to avoid hypotonic distending media whenever possible. The uterine cavity distension pressure should be the lowest pressure necessary to distend the uterine cavity and ideally should be maintained below the mean arterial pressure (MAP) especially with regard to long-lasting procedures.

Input and output of distending solution should be accurately monitored, since differences may indicate increased absorption or fluid loss due to accidental uterus perforation.

When using hypotonic distending media not more than 1000 mL should be absorbed. For elderly patients and others with comorbid conditions including compromised cardiovascular systems, a maximum fluid deficit of 750 mL is recommended.

In case of use of high-viscosity distending media, the maximum infused volume should be maintained below 500 mL in healthy patients, and below 300 mL if risk factors are present.

The maximum limit for isotonic media remains unclear, but absorption volumes of more than 2500 mL even in healthy patients should be prevented.

Preoperatively gynaecologist and anaesthesiologist should agree upon a maximum deficit volume with respect to the distending media used, the planned procedure and patient-specific risk factors. If that limit is exceeded during surgery termination has to be considered. If absorption of hypotonic solution is suspected, immediate measurement of plasma electrolytes and osmolality is indicated [30].

Some authors propagate intra-cervical injection of a dilute vasopressin solution to reduce distending media absorption during resectoscopy [31, 32]. This approach should be communicated with the anaesthesiologist, since absorption of large systemic doses have resulted in cardiovascular collapse, myocardial infarction and death [33].

Treatment options for manifest fluid overload syndrome include supportive intensive care, use of diuretics and substitution with sodium-containing solution. Special care must be taken when correcting severe hyponatremia, since pontine myelinolysis can occur (Fig. 20.3).

Laparoscopy

In recent centuries laparoscopy has become the standard technique for numerous gynaecological procedures. Advantageous for the anaesthesiologist are less haemorrhage, less postoperative pain and an improved lung function that results in a shorter hospital stay [34]. Especially overweight patients and patients with significant cardiopulmonary comorbidities benefit from laparoscopy.

However insufflation of carbon dioxide (CO_2) in order to establish and maintain pneumoperitoneum causes relevant changes in haemodynamics, lung function and the acid-base balance. Other organ systems like liver and kidney function may be altered as well.

Pulmonary Difficulties During Laparoscopy

CO_2 best satisfies the characteristics demanded from a gas used for pneumoperitoneum insufflation. It is non-flammable, inexpensive and easily expelled from the body, the latter because CO_2 is readily soluble. Therefore the risk for embolism is low but insufflation of CO_2 into the peritoneal cavity causes increased blood levels. To prevent development of hypercarbia and following acidosis the anaesthesiologist needs to alter ventilator settings. An increased respiratory rate (RR) and inspiratory pressures (P_{insp}) generate the necessary elevation of respiratory minute volume (MV).

$$\text{Pneumoperitoneum} \rightarrow CO_2\uparrow \rightarrow MV\uparrow \left(RR\uparrow \text{ and } P_{insp}\uparrow\right)$$

Increased inspiratory pressures are also required due to the pneumoperitoneum itself. Increased intra-abdominal pressure will shift the diaphragm cranial. Therefore higher pressure settings are required to maintain a certain tidal volume. Thus pulmonary compliance decreases. Also functional residual capacity and vital capacity decline following pneumoperitoneum. The use of Trendelenburg

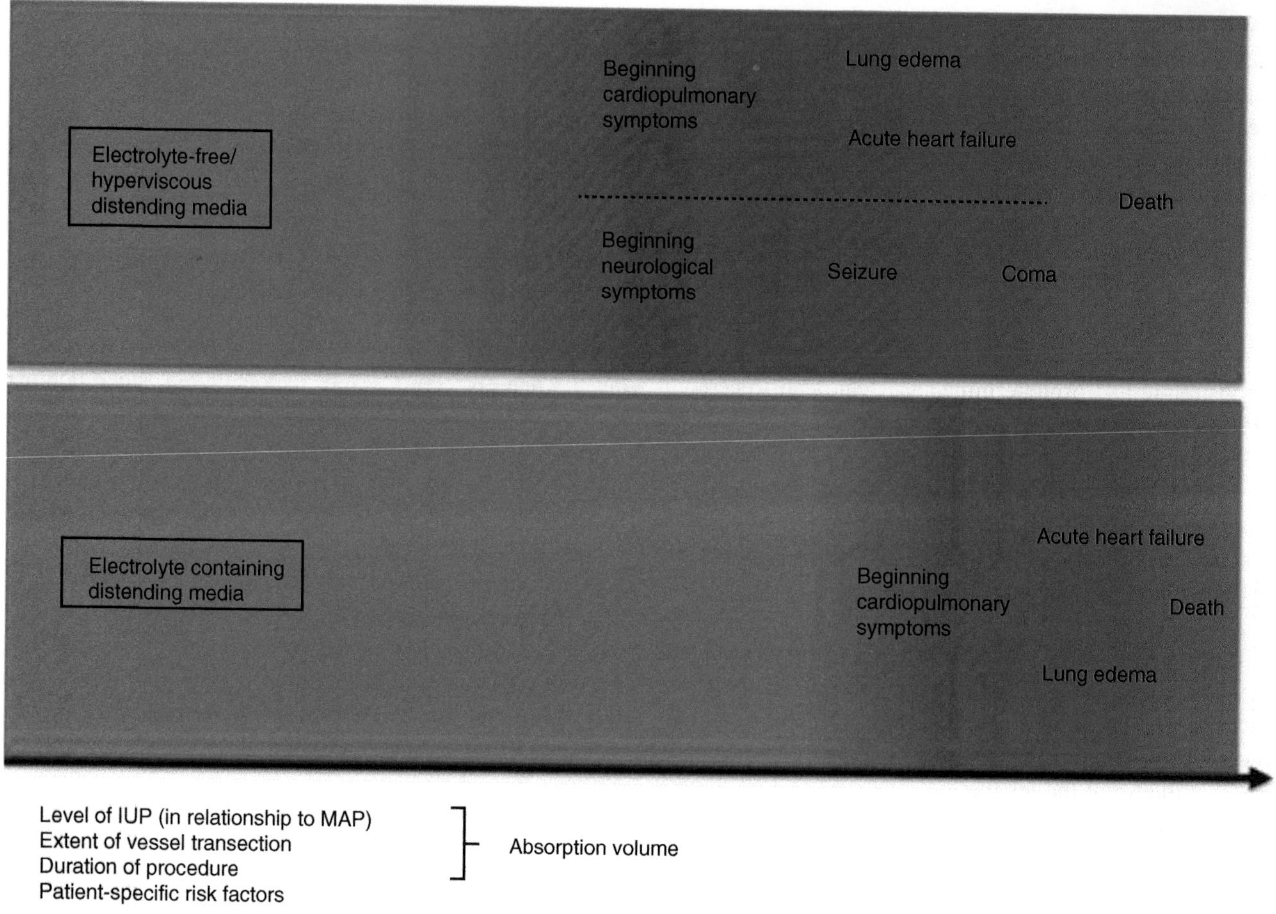

Fig. 20.3 Risk for complications using electrolyte-containing and electrolyte-free/hyperviscous distending media in hysteroscopic procedures. *IUP* intra-uterine pressure, *MAP* mean arterial pressure

position intensifies diaphragm transfer with its pulmonary consequences.

$$\text{Pneumoperitoneum} \rightarrow \text{cranial shift of the diaphragm} \rightarrow \text{compliance} \downarrow \rightarrow P_{insp} \uparrow$$

Increased inspiratory pressure leads to increased intra--thoracic pressure that directly affect the vessels of the pulmonary circuit resulting in decreased lung perfusion. Additionally the development of atelectasis leads to a reduction of lung tissue taking part in gas exchange. Consequently ventilation/perfusion ratio will be decreased inducing a deterioration of CO_2 elimination and an oxygenation deficiency.

$$P_{insp} \uparrow \rightarrow \text{intra-thoracic pressure} \uparrow \rightarrow \text{ventilation / perfusion mismatch} \uparrow \leftarrow \text{atelectasis} \uparrow$$

Summarizing, pneumoperitoneum results in increased levels of CO_2 in the blood. At the same time decreasing pulmonary compliance and an increasing ventilation/perfusion mismatch lead to reduced performance of the pulmonary system, which is supposed to eliminate CO_2. It needs to be kept in mind that the anaesthesiologist can hardly improve the pulmonary system itself during laparoscopy/Trendelenburg position. To avoid acidosis the invasiveness of ventilator settings needs to be increased which may eventually harm the patient.

For the patient's safety the gynaecologist therefore needs to be informed by the anaesthesiologist if excessive acidosis and/or oxygenation deficiency develop. Since pneumoperitoneum is the main cornerstone for pulmonary exacerbation during laparoscopic surgery reduction of intra-abdominal pressure and Trendelenburg position is the adequate de-escalation strategy. If the pulmonary status remains critical the termination of the procedure has to be taken into account.

Subcutaneous Emphysema During Laparoscopy

In rare cases the insufflation gas extends beyond the peritoneum causing subcutaneous emphysema. Extension of insufflated gas may directly harm the patient if extravasation occurs within the mediastinum. Swelling of the larynx region may result in dyspnoea and stridor after extubation.

Pneumothorax caused by extension of insufflated gas through diaphragmatic congenital channels into the pleural cavities has been reported [35–37].

While minor extravasations of gas can only be detected by radiological imaging distinctive manifestations may be palpated as crepitations.

CO_2 extension beyond peritoneal cavity
→ direct harm due to gas expansion

Extension of CO_2 beyond the peritoneal cavity impairs integrity of pneumoperitoneum required by the operator. To maintain the predetermined pressure set point the insufflator increases the gas flow rate resulting in an increased overall exposure with CO_2. CO_2 is therefore not only absorbed from the peritoneal cavity but also the surrounding tissue. Severe, long-lasting acidosis may develop.

Excessive hypercarbia requires invasive respirator settings with high tidal volumes and inspiratory pressures that may also harm the patient.

Hypercarbia beyond extubation requires increased work of breathing. Exhaustion may result in CO_2 narcosis and possible reintubation.

It is therefore recommended to not only monitor pressure and flow rate but also the total CO_2 volume during laparoscopy in order to detect loss of gas [38].

CO_2 extension beyond peritoneal cavity → pressure of pneumoperitoneum ↓→ flow rate of insufflator ↑→ total exposition to CO_2 ↑→ absorption ↑→ acidosis ↑→ escalation of ventilatory support

The incidence of subcutaneous emphysema varies with regard to the extent of extravasation. Grossly detectable subcutaneous emphysema can be found in 0.43–2.3% [38]. Postoperative computed tomography scans showed subcutaneous emphysema in 56 % 24 h after laparoscopy [39]. Mediastinal emphysema was detectable in 20 % after laparoscopy using x-ray imaging [40–43].

High intra-abdominal pressure leads to increased incidence of subcutaneous emphysema, especially during long-lasting procedures. Each increase in pressure is transmitted against the inner abdominal wall and transmitted to tissues, resulting in decreased perfusion, hypoxia, increased gas absorption, and increased likelihood of tissue dissection and subcutaneous emphysema. Even though intra-abdominal pressures between 0 and 20 mmHg are considered as safe, the use of pressures between 12 and 14 mmHg is recommended.

Locations of increased vulnerability of CO_2 escape are the insertion sites of the trocars. Gas extension beyond the peritoneal cavity increases with the amount and size of the trocars used. Due to their length surgical instruments act as lever arms and the force applied is multiplied at the fulcrum, which in case of laparoscopy is the boundary between the trocars and the tissue surrounding it. Shear forces may cause trauma and eventually lead to dissection of tissue and loss of CO_2. Knowledge of this fact is particularly crucial when performing robotic assisted surgery since the surgeon lacks haptic feedback from the tissue [38].

Cardiocirculatory Difficulties During Laparoscopy

Prediction of cardiocirculatory reactions during laparoscopy is difficult due to complex processes, since both, pneumoperitoneum and Trendelenburg position cause a cardiocirculatory response.

Pneumoperitoneum affects circulation through increased intra-abdominal pressure and acidosis resulting from CO_2 absorption.

IAP < 15 mmHg causes mobilization of pooled venous blood and increases cardiac preload and cardiac output. If IAP exceeds 15 mmHg the contrary has to be expected. Increased pressure is directly transmitted to the vessel walls and causes compression resulting in reduced venous return. At the same time the arterial system is affected and systemic vascular resistance increases. Decreased CO and elevated MAP may be witnessed [44].

Mesenterial and renal perfusion decreases during pneumoperitoneum, causing activation of renin-angiotensin-aldosterone system (RAAS) and thus liberation of catecholamines.

Acidosis resulting from hypercarbia causes sympathetic activation while severe acidosis decreases left ventricular function [45].

As mentioned above pneumoperitoneum is associated with increased inspiratory pressures that compromise venous return. Trendelenburg position may partly revoke these effects due to orthostatic effects. Possible tachycardia and hypertension due to a lack of analgesia as well as cardiocirculatory effective medication taken by the patient may alter cardiocirculatory response as well.

Therefore implementation of pneumoperitoneum and changes in patient position should occur gently, especially in patients with cardiopulmonary comorbidities, to allow circulation to adapt.

Introduction of the veress-needle, trocars and establishing pneumoperitoneum may cause vagal reactions that can lead to bradycardia and asystole even in healthy individuals [44].

Similar symptoms can occur through manipulation on uterus and adnexa [23].

Additional Considerations During Laparoscopic Surgery

CO_2 absorption and Trendelenburg position may cause an increase in cerebral blood flow, which can result in cerebral edema and increased intracranial pressure especially during long-lasting procedures. If cerebral edema is suspected prolonged ventilatory support in anti-Trendelenburg position and treatment with mannitol should be considered. Pre-existing increased intracranial pressure is a contraindication for laparoscopy [46].

Intra-ocular pressure may also increase during pneumoperitoneum. Vision loss after long-lasting laparoscopy in steep Trendelenburg position is a rare but catastrophic complication [47, 48]. In patients with glaucoma ophthalmologic assessment is advised.

Elevated intra-abdominal pressure during laparoscopy increases the risk for aspiration. The airway is therefore secured via endotracheal tube. Intra-gastric pressure is resolved using a gastric tube.

The anaesthesiologist must be aware that inadvertent one-sided intubation and consequent hypoxemia is a distinct possibility during laparoscopic surgery because of the Trendelenburg position, which with the raised IAP, lifts the diaphragm and carina, while the endotracheal tube remains fixed at its proximal end. This complication can easily be detected by auscultating the patient and then resolved.

Restricted Access in emergency situations to the patient's airway, intravenous lines and thorax for possible resuscitation during laparoscopy has to be considered.

Gas Embolism

With implementation of pneumoperitoneum, immediate gas embolism may occur, and in very rare cases it may lead to severe cardiovascular failure, decreased pulmonary blood flow, and death. Since CO_2 is readily soluble this complication is extremely rare during laparoscopy. Contamination of the abdominal cavity with room air needs to be prevented because the contained oxygen can maintain combustion and nitrogen could cause embolism due to its poor solubility. If embolism occurs pulmonary circulation is generally affected causing an increased vascular resistance. Sudden elevation of right hearted afterload may cause right heart failure. Transfer to arterial circulation (patent foramen ovale) can result in end organ failure, especially stroke. The clinical manifestations of embolism generally include a sudden increase followed by a rapid reduction in end-tidal CO_2, tachycardia and hypotension. If suspected the patient should be brought in head down/left-side tilt (durant maneuver) to prevent further embolism of the pulmonary circulation. Gas embolism can be detected sonographically and a central venous line can be used to evacuate emboli via aspiration (Fig. 20.4).

Robotic Surgery

Improved precision and three-dimensional display allows execution of even complex gynaecological procedures in minimal invasive technique. Further dissemination of robotic assisted surgery in the years to come can be expected.

For anaesthesiologists the evolution of laparoscopy to robotic assisted surgery can be a challenge.

The considerations for laparoscopy are even more valid for the robotic approach. Essential problems include patient positioning, duration of the procedures and limited access to the patient.

Patient positioning is crucial in robotic assisted surgery since after docking of the robot no further movement of the patient is permitted. Patient movement while the robot is docked can cause serious injury at the insertion site of the trocars, which is why adequate muscle relaxation is critical for success. To achieve optimal circumstances to perform surgery the patient is positioned in steep (up to 45°) Trendelenburg position. Especially in overweight patients undesired sliding and intraoperative neuropathic injury can only be prevented if positioning is performed meticulously prior to robot docking using shoulder braces, antiskid foam material and vacuum mattresses etc.

The creation of pneumoperitoneum is associated with the earlier mentioned problems as hypercarbia, decreased pulmonary compliance, ventilation/perfusion mismatch and interference with venous return and systemic vascular resistance.

Intravenous lines should be introduced on both sides of the upper extremity to compensate for loss since access (for further puncturing) after robot docking may be restricted. Preoperative communication between gynaecologist and anaesthesiologist is essential to plan anaesthesiological management with regard to extent and duration of the procedure [49, 50]. Moreover the anaesthesiologist evaluates the indication for arterial line and central venous catheter considering the patient's comorbidities.

If the bulky robot is draped and docked access to the patient's thorax is limited. In emergency situation chest compressions or cardiac defibrillation can only be executed once the robotic arms have been removed. That way the resuscitation can be initiated immediately. Removal of the trocars and the robot itself has to be done subsequently to allow access to the entire patient. Reaction time in emergency situations during robotic assisted surgery can be improved with simulator training [51].

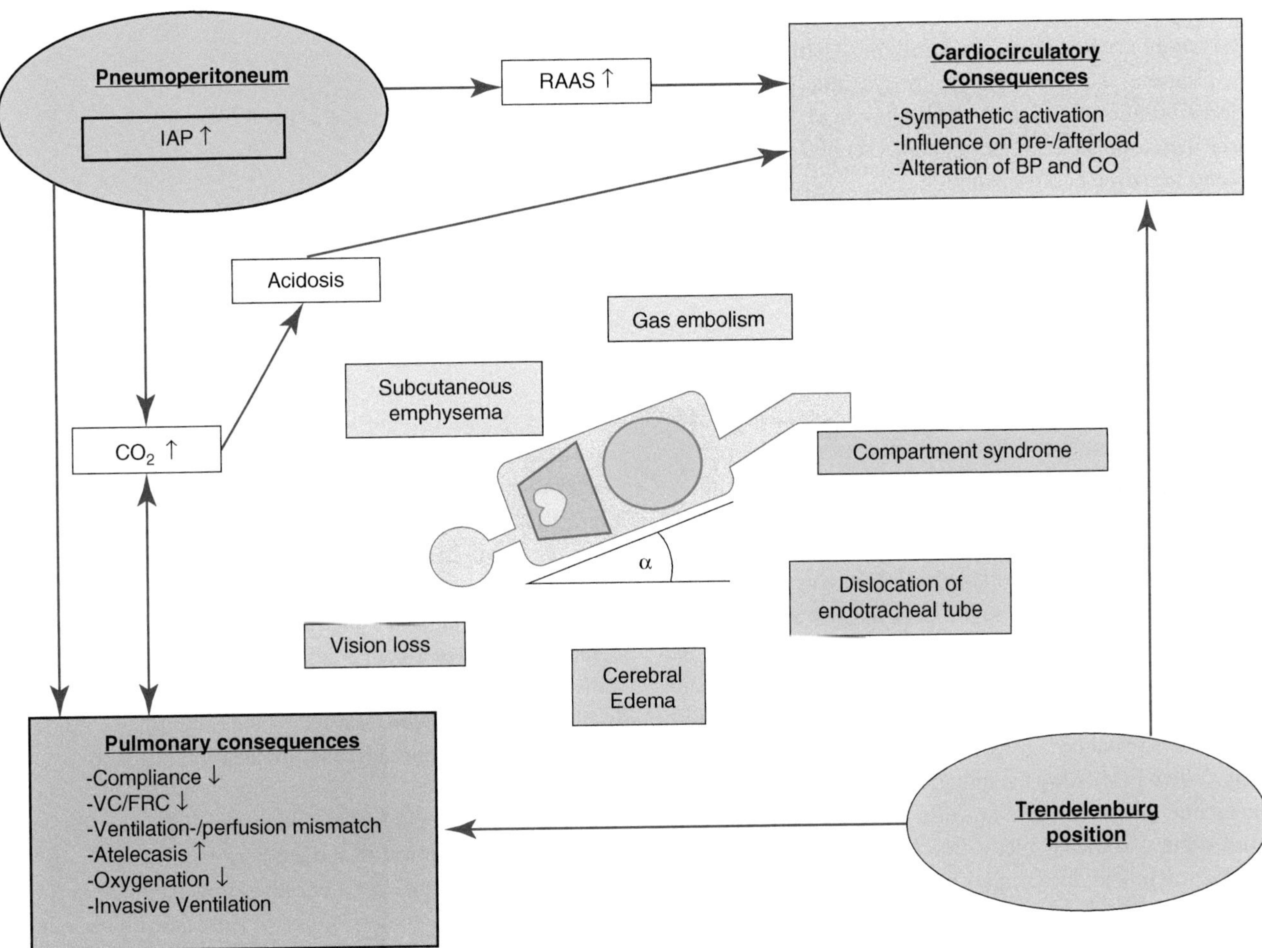

Fig. 20.4 (Patho-) Physiological alterations and complications during laparoscopy/robotic assisted surgery. The complications are coloured corresponding to the leading risk factor. *CO_2* Carbon dioxide, *CO* Cardiac output, *IAP* intra-abdominal pressure, *FRC* Functional residual capacity, *RAAS* Renin-angiotensin-aldosterone system, *BP* Blood pressure, *VC* Vital capacity, *α* angle (extent) of Trendelenburg position

Resuscitation

Remove the arms of the robot → start chest compressions / defibrillation → remove all trocars from the robot → remove the robot

The long duration of most robotic assisted procedures intensifies the effects of pneumoperitoneum and patient position (also see Fig. 20.4). Therefore all issues discussed above concerning laparoscopy need to be considered during robotic assisted surgery in particular. That includes:

- Pulmonary difficulties (including risk of subcutaneous emphysema)
- Cardiocirculatory difficulties
- Risk of cerebral edema and increased intra-ocular pressure
- Risk of nerve injuries and compartment syndrome
- Risk of aspiration due to increased intra-abdominal pressure
- Risk of one-sided intubation
- Restricted access

Also general factors of long-lasting surgery as fluid loss, hypothermia and haemorrhage need to be anticipated by the anaesthesiologist.

Laparotomy

Despite the advances in laparoscopic techniques oncologic surgery in gynaecology is today mostly performed via laparotomy.

Oncologic patients more often present in poor general condition and are older than the usual gynaecologic cohort. Preoperative tumor-associated anaemia is common. Large intra-abdominal masses and the presence of ascites may increase intra-abdominal pressure and risk for aspiration.

Compared to laparoscopy tissue trauma during laparotomy is more severe. Therefore vast, long-lasting procedures may promote the development of systemic inflammatory response syndrome (SIRS). The liberation of mediators causes increased capillary permeability, endothelial dysfunction and impaired cardiac function.

The anaesthesiological management relies on the knowledge of anticipated blood loss, duration and patient-specific risk factors. Particularly for the operative setting it has to be considered if vasopressors or postoperative parenteral nutrition are required. Extravasation of vasopressors (e.g. norepinephrine and epinephrine) can propagate cell damage by inducing venous and arterial vasospasms and causing disruption to vein wall integrity. Parenteral nutrition is a hypertonic agent that can cause tissue damage by shifting the equilibrium between intracellular and extracellular fluid. Intracellular fluid is forced out of cells and into the interstitial space, causing direct cell damage. Extravasation of these substances may lead to significant tissue damage, skin sloughing, and dermal necrosis with following infection and even amputation [52–54]. Therefore central venous line placement is advisable whenever there is a high probability that these substances need to be administered perioperatively. When evaluating the indication for central venous line placement possible adverse effects like pneumothorax, central-line associated bloodstream infections, thrombosis, misplacement and arrhythmias need to be considered.

While measurement of central venous pressure is no longer recommended for controlling volume management, central venous oxygenation may pose essential information regarding the patient's circulation [55].

Introduction of an arterial line should be performed for vast, long-lasting surgery or in patients with cardiopulmonary comorbidities. It allows the continuous and exact monitoring of blood pressure and the analysis of the arterial blood gases may give additional information on the patient's volume and respiratory status.

To decrease the risk of hypothermia the patient's temperature is monitored and convective warming systems and preheated infusion solution are used. In the case of severe hypothermia adapting the room temperature in the operating theatre can be considered.

Adequate muscle relaxation during abdominal surgery improves conditions to perform surgery by decreasing tone of skeletal muscle of the abdominal wall and the diaphragm. Muscle relaxants decrease transmission of nerve impulses at the site of neuromuscular junction. Therefore the muscle itself will be susceptible to direct electrical stimulation even after a muscle relaxant has been administered. The clinical effect of muscle relaxants is commonly monitored by acceleromyography (quality of muscle response after repeated nerve stimulation). Smooth muscle cell function and therefore intestinal motility is not affected by muscle relaxants.

The introduction of an epidural catheter is an important tool to shorten the time of recovery, manage pain and improve postoperative lung function. Nevertheless epidural haematoma with the risk of persisting paraplegia has an incidence between 1:3000 and 1:6000 [56–58] and therefore is far more common than previously suspected. The placement is performed prior to the operation while the patient is still awake in order to detect paraesthesia during catheter introduction and possible misplacement of the catheter into the subarachnoid space. The patient's wish, pre-existing anti--coagulant medication and possible patient-specific risk factors need to be evaluated in a risk benefit assessment prior to operation. The recent implementation of newer anticoagulants has to be considered with regard to timing of puncture and removal of epidural catheters (Table 20.3). A monotherapy with acetylsalicylic acid is not a contraindication for epidural puncture. While the epidural catheter is in place an anaesthesiologist and/or pain nurse will consult the patient at least once daily to asses adequate pain relieve and to detect signs for infection or neurological abnormalities. Usually the catheter is removed once sufficient analgesia without epidural infusion has been assured. When removing an epidural catheter intake of anticoagulant medication needs to be considered (Table 20.3).

For abdominal surgery intravenous lidocaine infusion poses a possible option to reduce perioperative pain and to improve recovery of postoperative bowel function [59]. Analgesic [60], anti-hyperalgesic [61] and anti-inflammatory effects [60, 62] characterize intravenous lidocaine. Increased postoperative sedation and the occurrence of cardiac arrhythmias may be possible side effects [63].

Vast oncologic surgery is associated with a high risk for haemorrhage and distinctive fluid shifts. Thus compatible erythrocyte concentrate needs to be provided. It has to be considered that transfusion of erythrocyte concentrate poses an independent risk factor for infection and sepsis [64], multiple organ failure [65] and death [66]. This reflects in more restrictive transfusion recommendations. Due to early presentation prior to surgery existing anaemia can be detected and possibly treated. Hereby the patient's red blood cell count and haemoglobin concentration can be optimized and mortality may be decreased [67–69].

If acute profuse bleeding (e.g. due to vessel transection) occurs during surgery basic physiology (Ohm's law) teaches that during hypertension will cause an increased blood loss due to an increased pressure gradient (pressure within the vessel vs. surrounding (atmospheric) pressure). Not only because the bleeding itself is stronger but also because haemostasis may be impeded due to clot disruption [70].

Therefore lower blood pressure via intraoperative controlled hypotension may be advantageous during acute bleeding and possibly reduce transfusion rate and blood loss. However intraoperative hypotension (IOH) is one of the

Table 20.3 Recommended time intervals prior to and after epidural catheter placement and removal [78]

Substance	Half-life period	Interval prior to placement/removal	Interval after placement/removal
Heparin, unfractionated (prophylaxis)	1, 5–2 h	4 h	1 h
Heparin, unfractionated (therapeutic)	2–3 h	i.v. 4–6 h s.c. 8–12 h	1 h
Low molecular weight heparin (prophylaxis)	4–6 h[a]	12 h	4 h
Low molecular weight heparin (therapeutic)		24 h	4 h
Fondaparinux (1 × 2.5 mg/day)	15–20 h[a]	36–42 h	6–12 h
Danaparaoid (2 × 750 I.E./day)	22–24 h[a]	48 h	3–4 h
Hirudinea Desirudin Bivalirudin	120 min[a] 25 min[a]	8–10 h 4 h	6 h 8 h
Argatroban (prophylaxis)[b]	35–45 min	4 h	5–7 h
Dabigatran (max. 1 × 150–220 mg/day)	14–17 h[a]	28–34 h	6 h
Dabigatran (max. 2 × 150 mg/day)	14–17 h[a]	56–85 h	6 h
Rivaroxaban (1 × 10 mg/day)	11–13 h[a]	22–26 h	4–5.5 h
Rivaroxaban (2 × 15 mg/day, 1 × 20 mg/day)	11–13 h[a]	44–65 h	4–5.5 h
Apixaban (2 × 2.5 mg/day)	10–15 h[a]	26–30 h	5–7 h
Apixaban (2 × 5 mg/day)	10–15 h[a]	40–75 h	5–7 h
Vitamin k antagonists	Days	INR < 1.4	After removal
Acetylsalicylic acid (100 mg/day)[c]	Life span of thrombocytes	None	None
Clopidogrel Ticlopidin	Life span of thrombocytes	7–10 days	After removal
Prasugrel	Life span of thrombocytes	7–10 days	6 h
Ticagrelor	7–8.5 h	5 days	6 h
Abciximab	12–24 h	Contraindication for puncture/48 h prior to removal	8 h

[a]Half-life period depends on renal function
[b]Half-life period depends on liver function
[c]Treatment with acetylsalicylic acid requires disruption of other anticoagulants for 4–5 half-life periods, while acetylsalicylic acid may be continued

most important concerns associated with the occurrence of postoperative myocardial ischemia and infarction, acute kidney failure and stroke (watershed infarcts) [71, 72].

IOH still lacks exact definition and needs to be considered a dynamic phenomenon depending on patient specific risk factors such as comorbidity, age and surgical factors. Therefore intraoperative controlled hypotension should not be based on fixed, arbitrarily chosen thresholds but needs to be adapted (extent and duration of IOH) according to the clinical setting [71–73].

Perioperative coagulopathy may occur during gynaecologic surgery and necessitate substitution of coagulant factors. Coagulopathy in the operative setting often is initiated due to blood loss and dilution but remains a multifactorial disorder involving:

- Abnormalities of basic physiological conditions (e.g. temperature, pH, ionized calcium),
- Disorders of primary haemostasis (pre-existing or acquired),
- Abnormalities of blood plasma (clotting-factor deficits) or
- Complex coagulopathies (hyperfibrinolysis, disseminated intravascular coagulation).

Detection of perioperative coagulopathies and the monitoring of their treatment are difficult tasks and an on-going field of research [74–77].

While "classical" routine testing of blood coagulation (INR, aPTT) is limited in terms reflecting the complexity of bleeding disorders, point-of-care (POC) testing (e.g. aggregometric or viscoelastic testing) may potentially reveal additional information on the underlying coagulopathy and help guide the use of allogeneic blood products, clotting-factor concentrates and other hemotherapeutic agents.

References

1. Apfel CC, Laara E, Koivuranta M, Greim CA, Roewer N. A simplified risk score for predicting postoperative nausea and vomiting: conclusions from cross-validations between two centers. Anesthesiology. 1999;91:693–700.
2. Koivuranta M, Laara E, Snare L, Alahuhta S. A survey of postoperative nausea and vomiting. Anaesthesia. 1997;52:443–9.
3. Sinclair DR, Chung F, Mezei G. Can postoperative nausea and vomiting be predicted? Anesthesiology. 1999;91:109–18.
4. Apfel CC, Heidrich FM, Jukar-Rao S, Jalota L, Hornuss C, Whelan RP, et al. Evidence-based analysis of risk factors for postoperative nausea and vomiting. Br J Anaesth. 2012;109:742–53.
5. Apfel CC, Kranke P, Eberhart LH. Comparison of surgical site and patient's history with a simplified risk score for the prediction of postoperative nausea and vomiting. Anaesthesia. 2004;59:1078–82.
6. Myles PS, Williams DL, Hendrata M, Anderson H, Weeks AM. Patient satisfaction after anaesthesia and surgery: results of a prospective survey of 10,811 patients. Br J Anaesth. 2000;84:6–10.
7. Macario A, Weinger M, Carney S, Kim A. Which clinical anesthesia outcomes are important to avoid? The perspective of patients. Anesth Analg. 1999;89:652–8.
8. Fortier J, Chung F, Su J. Unanticipated admission after ambulatory surgery–a prospective study. Can J Anaesth. 1998;45:612–9.
9. Hill RP, Lubarsky DA, Phillips-Bute B, Fortney JT, Creed MR, Glass PS, et al. Cost-effectiveness of prophylactic antiemetic therapy with ondansetron, droperidol, or placebo. Anesthesiology. 2000;92:958–67.
10. Eberhart LH, Geldner G, Kranke P, Morin AM, Schauffelen A, Treiber H, et al. The development and validation of a risk score to predict the probability of postoperative vomiting in pediatric patients. Anesth Analg. 2004;99:1630–7. table of contents.
11. Recommendations for the prevention of positioning injuries during gynecologic operations. Guideline of the German Society of Gynecology and Obstetrics (AWMF Registry No. 015/077) [Internet]. 2015. Available from: http://www.awmf.org/leitlinien/detail/ll/015-077.html.
12. Vollmar B, Westermann S, Menger MD. Microvascular response to compartment syndrome-like external pressure elevation: an in vivo fluorescence microscopic study in the hamster striated muscle. J Trauma. 1999;46:91–6.
13. Matsen FA, Krugmire RB, King RV. Nicolas Andry Award. Increased tissue pressure and its effects on muscle oxygenation in level and elevated human limbs. Clin Orthop Relat Res. 1979;144:311–20.
14. Anema JG, Morey AF, McAninch JW, Mario LA, Wessells H. Complications related to the high lithotomy position during urethral reconstruction. J Urol. 2000;164:360–3.
15. Bauer EC, Koch N, Janni W, Bender HG, Fleisch MC. Compartment syndrome after gynecologic operations: evidence from case reports and reviews. Eur J Obstet Gynecol Reprod Biol. 2014;173:7–12.
16. Matsen FA, Winquist RA, Krugmire RB. Diagnosis and management of compartmental syndromes. J Bone Joint Surg Am. 1980;62:286–91.
17. Shah DM, Bock DE, Darling RC, Chang BB, Kupinski AM, Leather RP. Beneficial effects of hypertonic mannitol in acute ischemia–reperfusion injuries in humans. Cardiovasc Surg. 1996;4:97–100.
18. Johnson DJ, Chalkiadis GA. Does epidural analgesia delay the diagnosis of lower limb compartment syndrome in children? Paediatr Anaesth. 2009;19:83–91.
19. Mar GJ, Barrington MJ, McGuirk BR. Acute compartment syndrome of the lower limb and the effect of postoperative analgesia on diagnosis. Br J Anaesth. 2009;102:3–11.
20. Cohen SA, Hurt WG. Compartment syndrome associated with lithotomy position and intermittent compression stockings. Obstet Gynecol. 2001;97:832–3.
21. Montgomery CJ, Ready LB. Epidural opioid analgesia does not obscure diagnosis of compartment syndrome resulting from prolonged lithotomy position. Anesthesiology. 1991;75:541–3.
22. Radosa JC, Radosa MP, Sutterlin M. Acute lower limb compartment syndrome after Cesarean section: a case report. J Med Case Reports. 2011;5:161.
23. Sprung J, Abdelmalak B, Schoenwald PK. Recurrent complete heart block in a healthy patient during laparoscopic electrocauterization of the fallopian tube. Anesthesiology. 1998;88:1401–3.
24. Arieff AI. Hyponatremia associated with permanent brain damage. Adv Intern Med. 1987;32:325–44.
25. Istre O, Bjoennes J, Naess R, Hornbaek K, Forman A. Postoperative cerebral oedema after transcervical endometrial resection and uterine irrigation with 1.5 % glycine. Lancet. 1994;344:1187–9.
26. Ayus JC, Wheeler JM, Arieff AI. Postoperative hyponatremic encephalopathy in menstruant women. Ann Intern Med. 1992;117:891–7.
27. Taskin O, Buhur A, Birincioglu M, Burak F, Atmaca R, Yilmaz I, et al. Endometrial Na+, K + –ATPase pump function and vasopressin levels during hysteroscopic surgery in patients pretreated with GnRH agonist. J Am Assoc Gynecol Laparosc. 1998;5:119–24.
28. Berg A, Sandvik L, Langebrekke A, Istre O. A randomized trial comparing monopolar electrodes using glycine 1.5 % with two different types of bipolar electrodes (TCRis, Versapoint) using saline, in hysteroscopic surgery. Fertil Steril. 2009;91:1273–8.
29. Darwish AM, Hassan ZZ, Attia AM, Abdelraheem SS, Ahmed YM. Biological effects of distension media in bipolar versus monopolar resectoscopic myomectomy: a randomized trial. J Obstet Gynaecol Res. 2010;36:810–7.
30. Munro MG, Storz K, Abbott JA, Falcone T, Jacobs VR, Muzii L, et al. AAGL Practice Report: Practice Guidelines for the Management of Hysteroscopic Distending Media: (Replaces Hysteroscopic Fluid Monitoring Guidelines. J Am Assoc Gynecol Laparosc. 2000;7:167–168.). J Minim Invasive Gynecol. 2013;20:137–48.
31. Corson SL, Brooks PG, Serden SP, Batzer FR, Gocial B. Effects of vasopressin administration during hysteroscopic surgery. J Reprod Med. 1994;39:419–23.
32. Phillips DR, Nathanson HG, Milim SJ, Haselkorn JS, Khapra A, Ross PL. The effect of dilute vasopressin solution on blood loss during operative hysteroscopy: a randomized controlled trial. Obstet Gynecol. 1996;88:761–6.
33. Martin JD, Shenk LG. Intraoperative myocardial infarction after paracervical vasopressin infiltration. Anesth Analg. 1994;79:1201–2.
34. Gonzalez R, Smith CD, McClusky DA, Ramaswamy A, Branum GD, Hunter JG, et al. Laparoscopic approach reduces likelihood of perioperative complications in patients undergoing adrenalectomy. Am Surg. 2004;70:668–74.
35. Batra MS, Driscoll JJ, Coburn WA, Marks WM. Evanescent nitrous oxide pneumothorax after laparoscopy. Anesth Analg. 1983;62:1121–3.
36. Fitzgerald SD, Andrus CH, Baudendistel LJ, Dahms TE, Kaminski DL. Hypercarbia during carbon dioxide pneumoperitoneum. Am J Surg. 1992;163:186–90.
37. Sharma KC, Kabinoff G, Ducheine Y, Tierney J, Brandstetter RD. Laparoscopic surgery and its potential for medical complications. Heart Lung. 1997;26:52–64. quiz 65–7.
38. Ott DE. Subcutaneous emphysema–beyond the pneumoperitoneum. JSLS. 2014;18:1–7.
39. McAllister JD, D'Altorio RA, Snyder A. CT findings after uncomplicated percutaneous laparoscopic cholecystectomy. J Comput Assist Tomogr. 1991;15:770–2.
40. Celik H, Cremins A, Jones KA, Harmanli O. Massive subcutaneous emphysema in robotic sacrocolpopexy. JSLS. 2013;17:245–8.

41. Herati AS, Andonian S, Rais-Bahrami S, Atalla MA, Srinivasan AK, Richstone L, et al. Use of the valveless trocar system reduces carbon dioxide absorption during laparoscopy when compared with standard trocars. Urology. 2011;77:1126–32.
42. Waisbren SJ, Herz BL, Ducheine Y, Yang HK, Karanfilian RG. Iatrogenic "respiratory acidosis" during laparoscopic preperitoneal hernia repair. J Laparoendosc Surg. 1996;6:181–3.
43. Wolf JS, Monk TG, McDougall EM, McClennan BL, Clayman RV. The extraperitoneal approach and subcutaneous emphysema are associated with greater absorption of carbon dioxide during laparoscopic renal surgery. J Urol. 1995;154:959–63.
44. Gerges FJ, Kanazi GE, Jabbour-Khoury SI. Anesthesia for laparoscopy: a review. J Clin Anesth. 2006;18:67–78.
45. Rasmussen JP, Dauchot PJ, DePalma RG, Sorensen B, Regula G, Anton AH, et al. Cardiac function and hypercarbia. Arch Surg. 1978;113:1196–200.
46. Bloomfield GL, Ridings PC, Blocher CR, Marmarou A, Sugerman HJ. Effects of increased intra-abdominal pressure upon intracranial and cerebral perfusion pressure before and after volume expansion. J Trauma. 1996;40:936–41. discussion 941–3.
47. Awad H, Santilli S, Ohr M, Roth A, Yan W, Fernandez S, et al. The effects of steep Trendelenburg positioning on intraocular pressure during robotic radical prostatectomy. Anesth Analg. 2009;109:473–8.
48. Molloy BL. Implications for postoperative visual loss: steep trendelenburg position and effects on intraocular pressure. AANA J. 2011;79:115–21.
49. Kaye AD, Vadivelu N, Ahuja N, Mitra S, Silasi D, Urman RD. Anesthetic considerations in robotic-assisted gynecologic surgery. Ochsner J. 2013;13:517–24.
50. Lee JR. Anesthetic considerations for robotic surgery. Korean J Anesthesiol. 2014;66:3–11.
51. Huser AS, Muller D, Brunkhorst V, Kannisto P, Musch M, Kropfl D, et al. Simulated life-threatening emergency during robot-assisted surgery. J Endourol. 2014;28:717–21.
52. Overgaard CB, Dzavik V. Inotropes and vasopressors: review of physiology and clinical use in cardiovascular disease. Circulation. 2008;118:1047–56.
53. Tran DQH, Finlayson RJ. Use of stellate ganglion block to salvage an ischemic hand caused by the extravasation of vasopressors. Reg Anesth Pain Med. 2005;30:405–8.
54. Le A, Patel S. Extravasation of noncytotoxic drugs: a review of the literature. Ann Pharmacother. 2014;48(7):870–86.
55. Marik PE, Cavallazzi R. Does the central venous pressure predict fluid responsiveness? An updated meta-analysis and a plea for some common sense. Crit Care Med. 2013;41:1774–81.
56. Cook TM, Counsell D, Wildsmith JA. Major complications of central neuraxial block: report on the Third National Audit Project of the Royal College of Anaesthetists. Br J Anaesth. 2009;102:179–90.
57. Moen V, Dahlgren N, Irestedt L. Severe neurological complications after central neuraxial blockades in Sweden 1990–1999. Anesthesiology. 2004;101:950–9.
58. Volk T, Wolf A, Van Aken H, Burkle H, Wiebalck A, Steinfeldt T. Incidence of spinal haematoma after epidural puncture: analysis from the German network for safety in regional anaesthesia. Eur J Anaesthesiol. 2012;29:170–6.
59. Vigneault L, Turgeon AF, Cote D, Lauzier F, Zarychanski R, Moore L, et al. Perioperative intravenous lidocaine infusion for postoperative pain control: a meta-analysis of randomized controlled trials. Can J Anaesth. 2011;58:22–37.
60. Lauretti GR. Mechanisms of analgesia of intravenous lidocaine. Rev Bras Anestesiol. 2008;58:280–6.
61. Koppert W, Ostermeier N, Sittl R, Weidner C, Schmelz M. Low--dose lidocaine reduces secondary hyperalgesia by a central mode of action. Pain. 2000;85:217–24.
62. Hollmann MW, Durieux ME. Local anesthetics and the inflammatory response: a new therapeutic indication? Anesthesiology. 2000;93:858–75.
63. McCarthy GC, Megalla SA, Habib AS. Impact of intravenous lidocaine infusion on postoperative analgesia and recovery from surgery: a systematic review of randomized controlled trials. Drugs. 2010;70:1149–63.
64. Bernard AC, Davenport DL, Chang PK, Vaughan TB, Zwischenberger JB. Intraoperative transfusion of 1 U to 2 U packed red blood cells is associated with increased 30-day mortality, surgical-site infection, pneumonia, and sepsis in general surgery patients. J Am Coll Surg. 2009;208:931–7. 937.e1–2; discussion 938–9.
65. Vincent JL, Baron JF, Reinhart K, Gattinoni L, Thijs L, Webb A, et al. Anemia and blood transfusion in critically ill patients. JAMA. 2002;288:1499–507.
66. Musallam KM, Tamim HM, Richards T, Spahn DR, Rosendaal FR, Habbal A, et al. Preoperative anaemia and postoperative outcomes in non-cardiac surgery: a retrospective cohort study. Lancet. 2011;378:1396–407.
67. Gombotz H, Hofmann A. Patient Blood Management : three pillar strategy to improve outcome through avoidance of allogeneic blood products. Anaesthesist. 2013;62:519–27.
68. Goodnough LT, Maniatis A, Earnshaw P, Benoni G, Beris P, Bisbe E, et al. Detection, evaluation, and management of preoperative anaemia in the elective orthopaedic surgical patient: NATA guidelines. Br J Anaesth. 2011;106:13–22.
69. Fischer DP, Zacharowski KD, Meybohm P. Savoring every drop – vampire or mosquito? Crit Care. 2014;18:306.
70. Sondeen JL, Coppes VG, Holcomb JB. Blood pressure at which rebleeding occurs after resuscitation in swine with aortic injury. J Trauma. 2003;54:S110–7.
71. Bijker JB, Gelb AW. Review article: the role of hypotension in perioperative stroke. Can J Anaesth. 2013;60:159–67.
72. Bijker JB, van Klei WA, Kappen TH, van Wolfswinkel L, Moons KGM, Kalkman CJ. Incidence of intraoperative hypotension as a function of the chosen definition: literature definitions applied to a retrospective cohort using automated data collection. Anesthesiology. 2007;107:213–20.
73. Walsh M, Devereaux PJ, Garg AX, Kurz A, Turan A, Rodseth RN, et al. Relationship between intraoperative mean arterial pressure and clinical outcomes after noncardiac surgery: toward an empirical definition of hypotension. Anesthesiology. 2013;119:507–15.
74. Weber CF, Zacharowski K, Meybohm P, Adam EH, Hofer S, Brun K, et al. Hemotherapy algorithms for coagulopathic cardiac surgery patients. Clin Lab. 2014;60:1059–63.
75. Weber CF, Zacharowski K. Perioperative point of care coagulation testing. Dtsch Arztebl Int. 2012;109:369–75.
76. Kozek-Langenecker S. Management of massive operative blood loss. Minerva Anestesiol. 2007;73:401–15.
77. Ganter MT, Hofer CK. Coagulation monitoring: current techniques and clinical use of viscoelastic point-of-care coagulation devices. Anesth Analg. 2008;106:1366–75.
78. Waurik K, Riess H, Van Aken H, Kessler P, Gogarten W, Volk T. Regional anaesthesia and thromboembolism prophylaxis/anticoagulation 3. Revised recommendations of the German Society of Anaesthesiology and Intensive Care Medicine [Internet]. 2014. Available from: http://www.awmf.org/uploads/tx_szleitlinien/001-005l_S1_R%C3%BCckenmarksnahe_Regionalan%C3%A4sthesie_Thromboembolieprophylaxe_2015-01.pdf.

Part VIII

Laparoscopic Hysterectomy and Extended Procedures for Benign and Malignant Indications

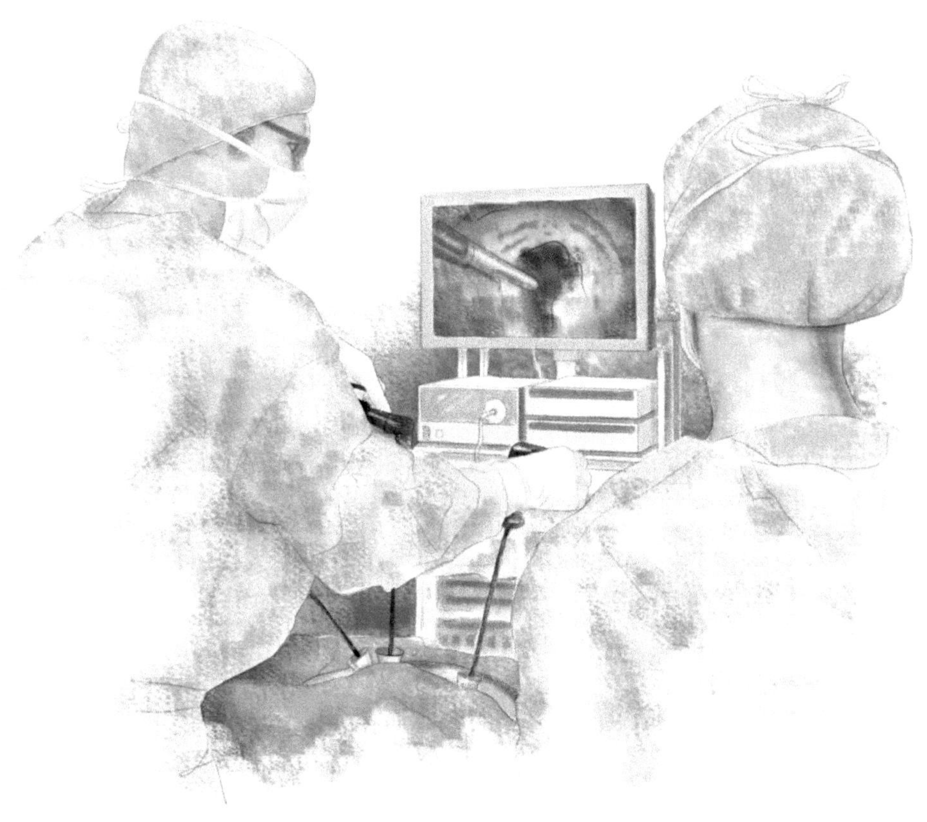

Indications and Contraindications for Laparoscopic Hysterectomy

21

Helder Ferreira and António Braga

Introduction

Hysterectomy is one of the most common surgical procedures performed worldwide. Laparoscopic hysterectomy (LH) ultimate aim is to reduce morbidity and mortality of abdominal hysterectomy (AH) to the levels seen with vaginal hysterectomy (VH) and minimise the rate of AH. Many advantages are referred to laparoscopy like the image magnification offering better visualization of anatomical structures and disease identification. It allows improved access to retroperitoneal spaces due to CO_2 pneumo-dissection. The vessels, ureter, and nerves can be better recognized. When LH is compared with AH, the laparoscopic approach is associated with less blood loss, fewer transfusions, less post-operative pain, shorter hospital stay, decrease risk of wound infection, better quality of life and lower levels of disability [1–12] (Table 21.1).

In 2015, Cochrane published a meta-analysis of 47 randomizes controlled trials with the aim to determine the most appropriate type of hysterectomy for gynaecologic nonmalignant conditions [13]. This study concluded that there are no differences between laparoscopic and vaginal hysterectomies in time to return to normal activities, duration of hospital stay and the rate of conversion to laparotomy. This study also concluded that the incidence of pelvic hematoma, vaginal cuff infection, urinary tract or respiratory infections, and venous thromboembolism were similar for these two types of hysterectomies [13]. There was a higher rate of bladder and ureteral injuries in total laparoscopic hysterectomy (TLH) in comparison with total abdominal hysterectomy (TAH), but similar to total vaginal hysterectomy (TVH) [13].

Classically, the operative time is higher with TLH when compared with TAH or TVH. However, with an increment of surgical experience and expertise, the operative time, as well as the conversion rate to laparotomy or the incidence of major complications is significantly reduced [14, 15].

In spite of these, according to the American College of Obstetricians and Gynaecologists 2009 Committee Opinion[16] and American Association of Gynecologic Laparoscopists [17] TVH is the overall preferred approach when feasible. Factors that influence the surgical approach in hysterectomy include vagina and uterus size and shape, the mobility and accessibility of uterus, the extension of extra uterine disease when present, the need for concurrent procedures and the surgical team experience.

Table 21.1 Advantages of laparoscopic hysterectomy *versus* abdominal hysterectomy

Less blood loss
Fewer transfusions
Less post-operative pain
Shorter hospital stay
Decreased risk of wound infection
Better quality of life
Lower levels of disability

H. Ferreira (✉)
Department of Gynecology, Centro Materno-Infantil do Norte/Centro Hospitalar do Porto, Largo da Maternidade Júlio Dinis, Porto 4050-371, Portugal
e-mail: helferreira@hotmail.com

A. Braga
Department of Obstetrics and Gynaecology, Centro Materno-Infantil do Norte/Centro Hospitalar do Porto, Largo da Maternidade Júlio Dinis, Porto 4050-371, Portugal
e-mail: ajcbraga@gmail.com

I. Alkatout, L. Mettler (eds.), *Hysterectomy*, DOI 10.1007/978-3-319-22497-8_21

Indications

TLH indications are similar to those for TAH. Usual indications include leiomyomata (Figs. 21.1 and 21.2), pelvic organ prolapse, abnormal uterine bleeding, adnexal pathology (Fig. 21.3), chronic pelvic pain and endometriosis (Fig. 21.4) [18]. TLH may also be indicated for resection and debulking of both malignant and premalignant disease, especially endometrial and cervical cancer, as noted by extensive case series in the gynaecologic oncologic literature (Table 21.2).

Laparoscopic approach to hysterectomy may be indicated when vaginal access is complicated by a narrow subpubic arch, a nulliparous pelvis, a large uterus (16-week size is usually the upper limit for a TVH) [19] when uterine mobilization is compromised by adhesions or by multiple or large leiomyomas [18].

In case of a very large uterus, it is more feasible to perform transitory uterine arteries clamping using a laparoscopic approach than a vaginal or abdominal access. The need of concomitant procedures and the necessity to explore the pelvis is also an indication for the laparoscopic approach (e.g. endometriosis, pelvic inflammatory disease).

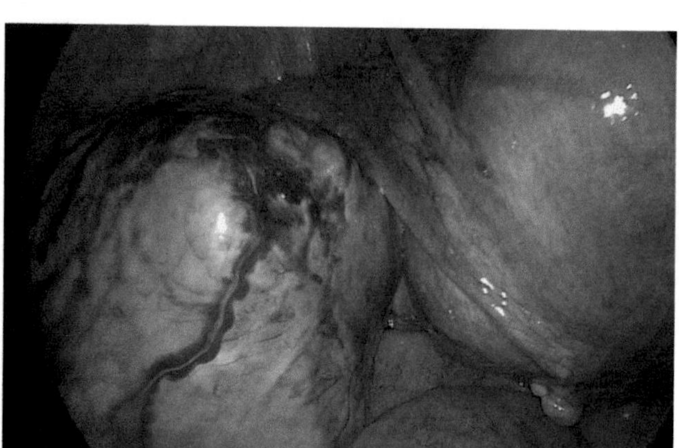

Fig. 21.1 Uterine leiomyomas

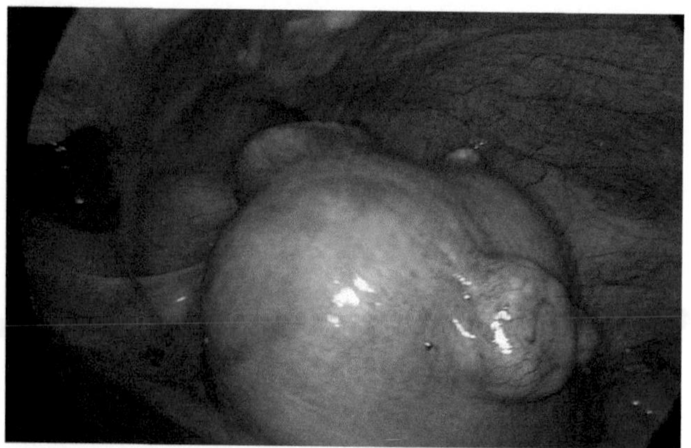

Fig. 21.2 Uterine leiomyomas

An old argument against the use of TLH was the procedure cost. A meta-analysis of 12 randomized controlled studies compared the cost of TLH against the TAH. The total direct costs for the laparoscopic approach were slightly higher, whereas the total indirect cost for TLH was half of TAH. This study concluded that the shorter hospital stay and decreased morbidity in the laparoscopic group compensates for the increased operating cost compared to the laparotomic route [20] (Fig. 21.5).

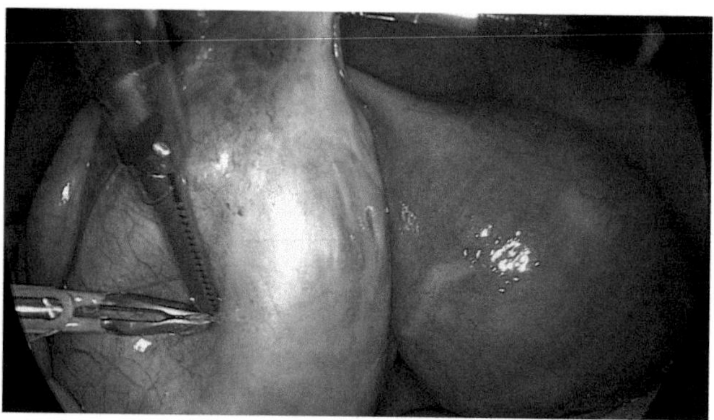

Fig. 21.3 Adnexal cystic mass

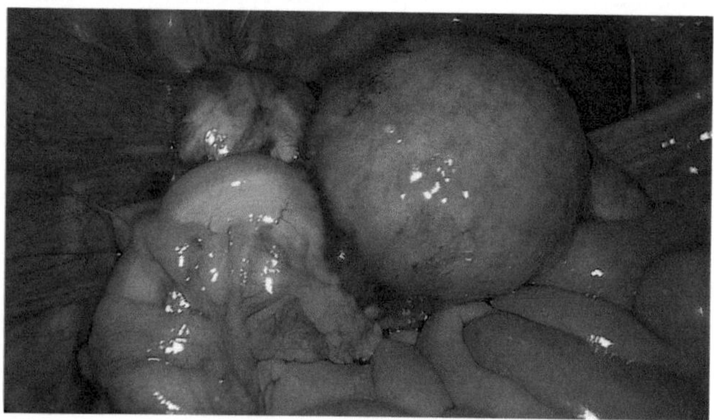

Fig. 21.4 Pelvic endometriosis

Table 21.2 Indications for total laparoscopic hysterectomy

Benign indications	Adenomyosis
	Chronic pelvic pain
	Dysfunctional uterine bleeding
	Endometriosis
	Leiomyoma
	Pelvic organ prolapse
Premalignant indications	Adnexial mass
	Cervical intraepithelial neoplasia
	Endometrial hyperplasia
Malignant indications	Cervical cancer
	Endometrial Cancer

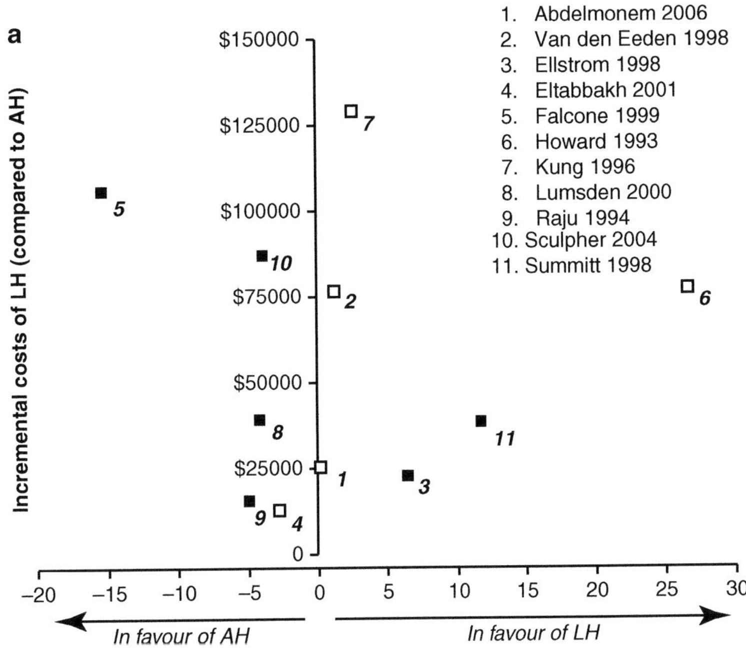

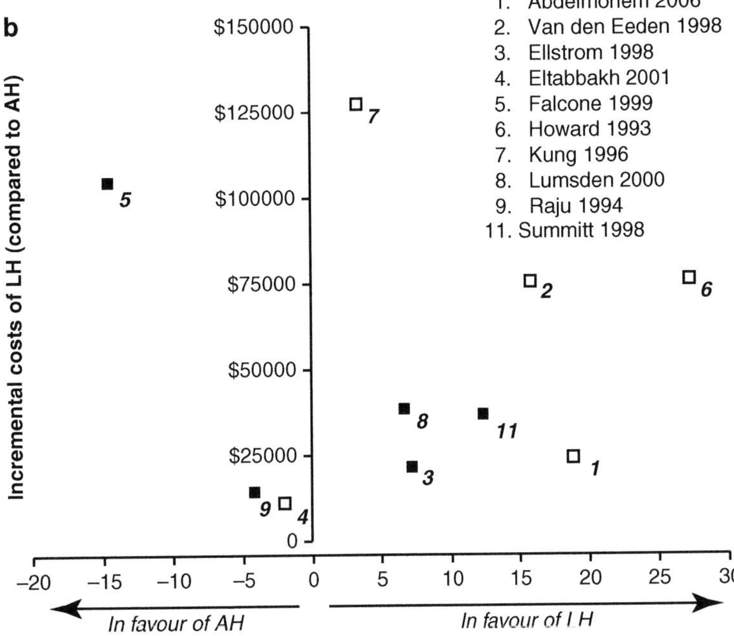

Fig. 21.5 Incremental costs and effects for patients with major complications (**a**) and all complications (**b**) per 100 patients. ■ RC T, □ CCT (From Bijen et al. [20])

Contraindications

There are no absolute contraindications for laparoscopic hysterectomy with the exception to the anaesthetic contraindication to perform the pneumoperitoneum. The experience of the surgical team and the patient's pelvic anatomy are the most important factors. The presence of severe adhesive disease, obstructive uterus or leiomyoma or any other anatomic limitation that prevent a safe entry or adequate working space remain the leading contraindication for the laparoscopic route. LH is also not advised for the diagnosis and treatment of a suspicious pelvic mass that cannot be removed intact through, for example, a culdotomy incision or into an impermeable sack. This is important because, in the presence of a malignant lesion, spillage may change the surgical stage of an ovarian cancer or an uterine sarcoma [21].

Risk factors for conversion to laparotomy include an elevated body mass index, increased uterine width greater than 10 cm, lateral or lower uterine segment fibroids over 5 cm, and previous adhesion-forming abdominopelvic surgery [14]. Previous abdominal scars, especially midline incisions, increase the risk of abdominal adhesions. This can make abdominal entry and surgery more difficult, leading to a major incidence of bowel lesions and conversion to a laparotomic approach [14] (Table 21.3).

Considerations

Remarkably, the most relevant contraindication for laparoscopic hysterectomy is the lack of expertise of the surgical team. In some countries, the rate of TLH increased very quickly at the beginning but, because many surgeons have not received a proper education, many complications happened and the number of minimally invasive procedures decreased. Fortunately, in the recent years, more and better educational programs have allowed a significant increase in TLH offering much superior outcomes in comparison to classic laparotomic approach.

If the surgeon respects the rules, the risk of complications is really low. The placement of the patient in a correct position (Fig. 21.6), the use of correct instrumentation (Figs. 21.7 and 21.8) and trocars positioning (Fig. 21.9) are factors of paramount importance. The key of the success to perform a laparoscopic hysterectomy is to follow the standard steps (Figs. 21.10, 21.11, 21.12, 21.13, 21.14, 21.15, 21.16, 21.17, 21.18, 21.19, 21.20, 21.21, 21.22, 21.23, 21.24, 21.25, and 21.26).

Table 21.3 Contraindications for total laparoscopic hysterectomy

Absolute	Anaesthetic contraindication for pneumoperitoneum confection
	Lack of laparoscopic surgery experience
	Lack of adequate equipment
Relative	Obstructive uterus or leiomyoma
	Severe adhesive disease
	Suspicious pelvic mass that cannot be removed intact

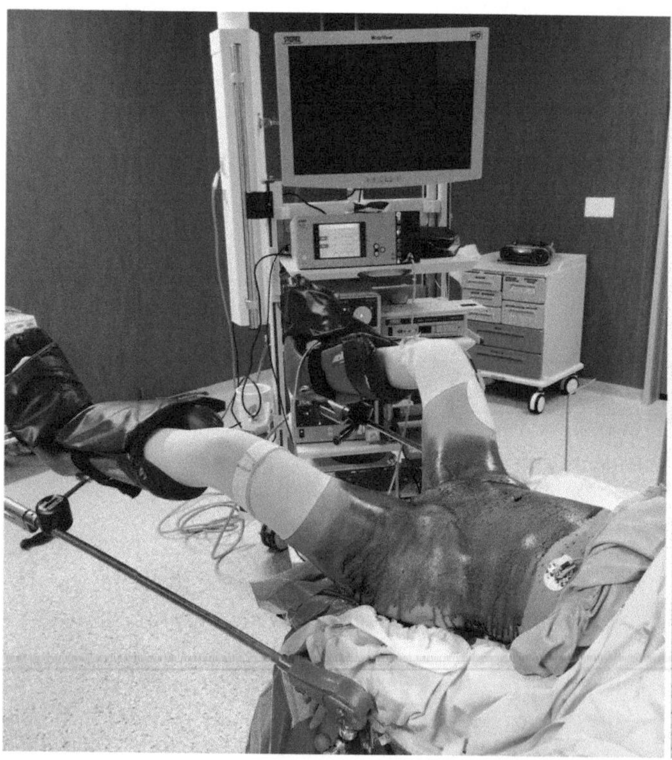

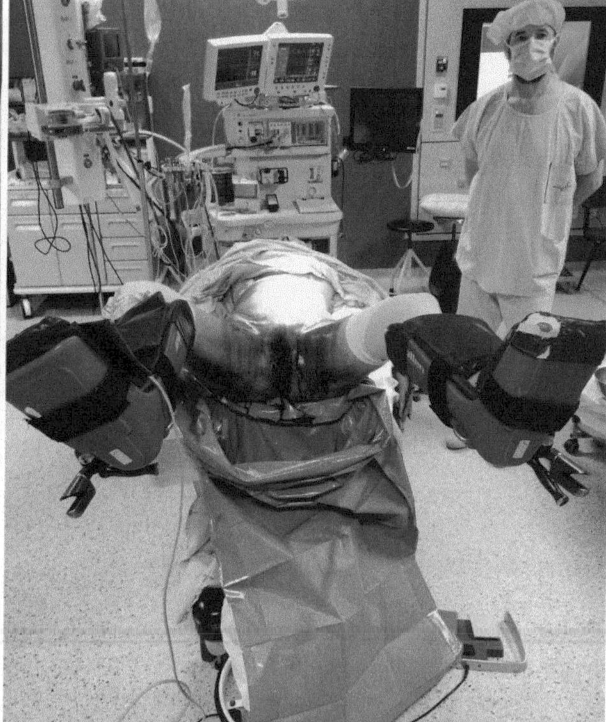

Fig. 21.6 Patient correct positioning

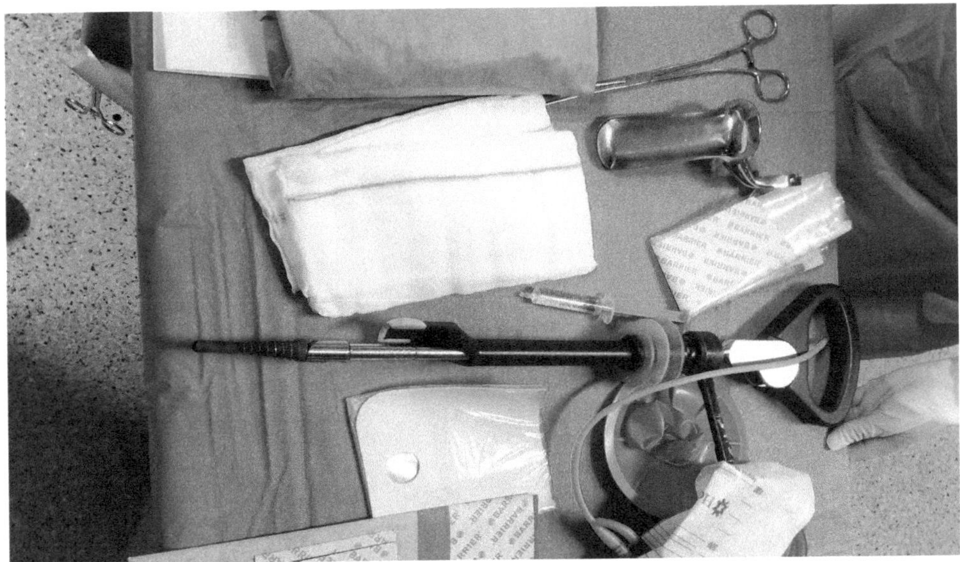

Fig. 21.7 Uterine manipulator

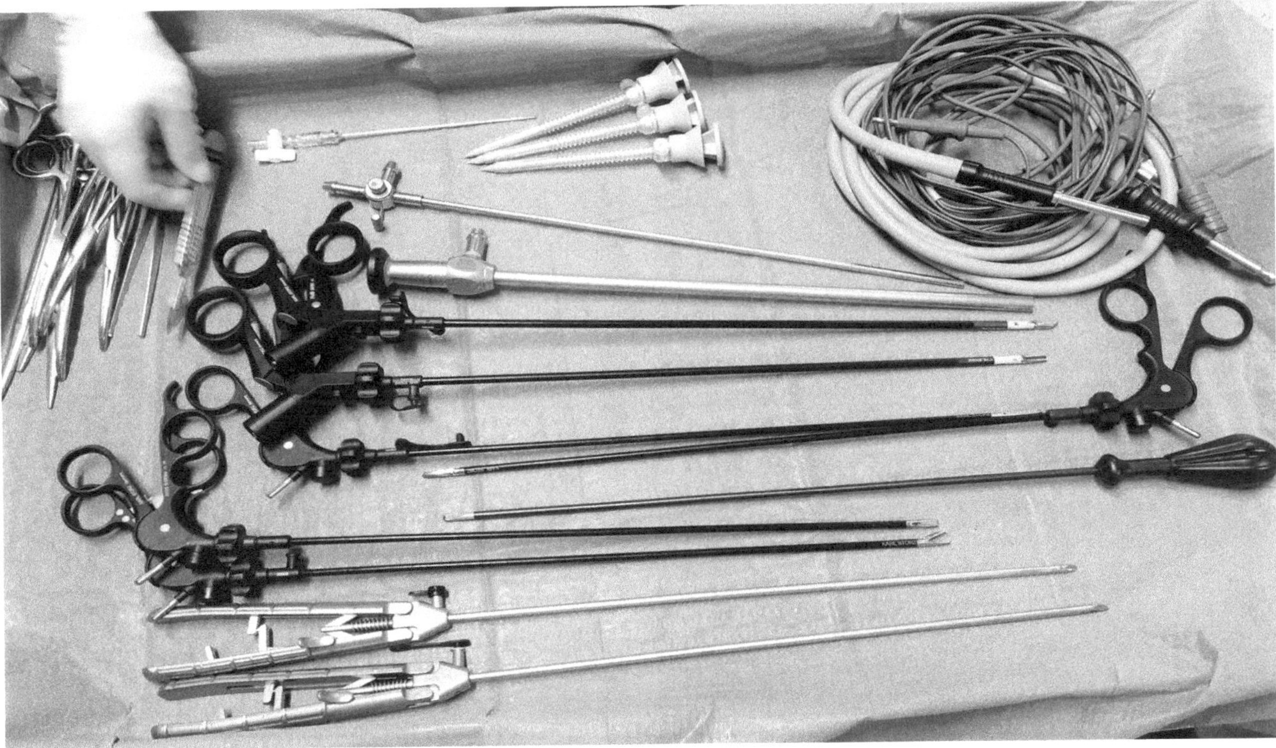

Fig. 21.8 Instruments set for laparoscopic hysterectomy

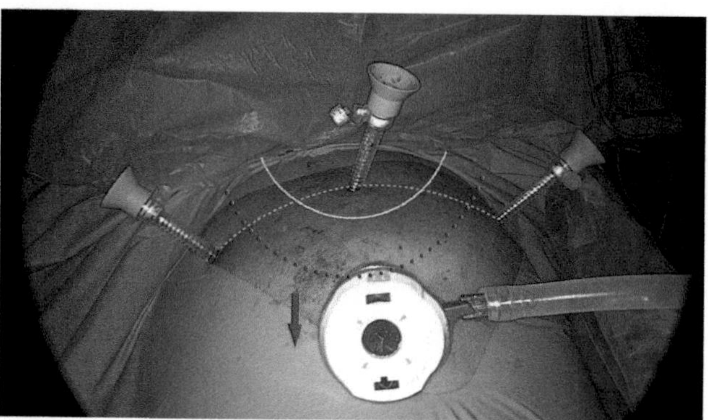

Fig. 21.9 Trocars positioning: in case of a big uterus (*red line*), optical trocar should be placed upwards (*arrow*) and the supra pubic ancillary trocar should be placed on the umbilical area

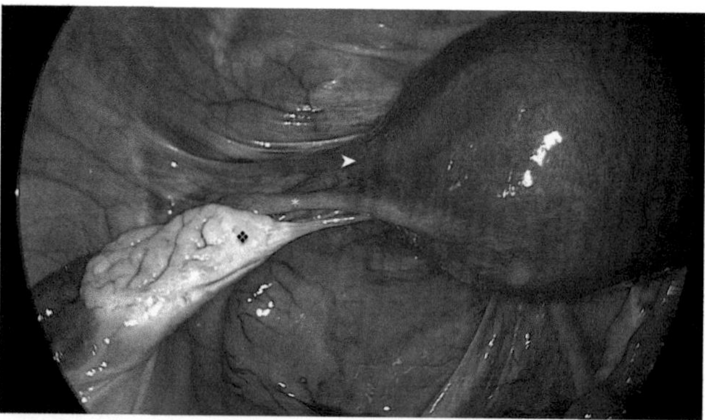

Fig. 21.10 ➤Round ligament, * fallopium tube, ❖ ovary

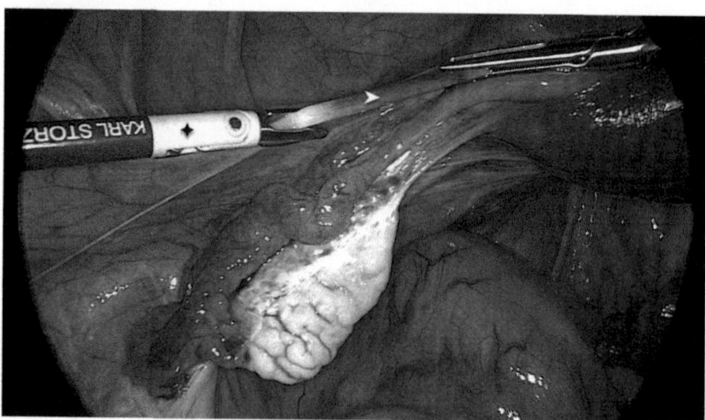

Fig. 21.11 ➤Round ligament

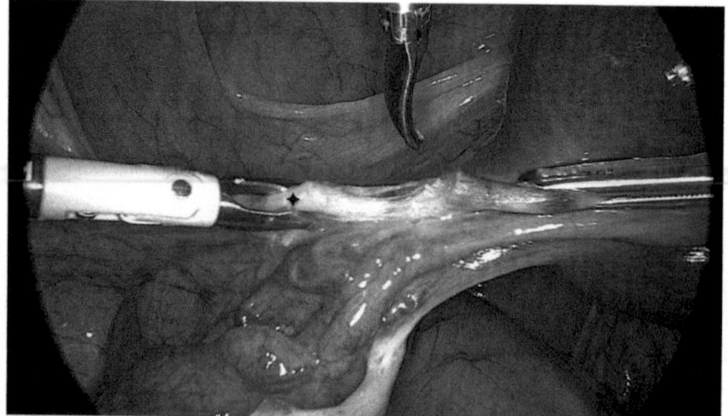

Fig. 21.12 ✦ Rotating bipolar grasper

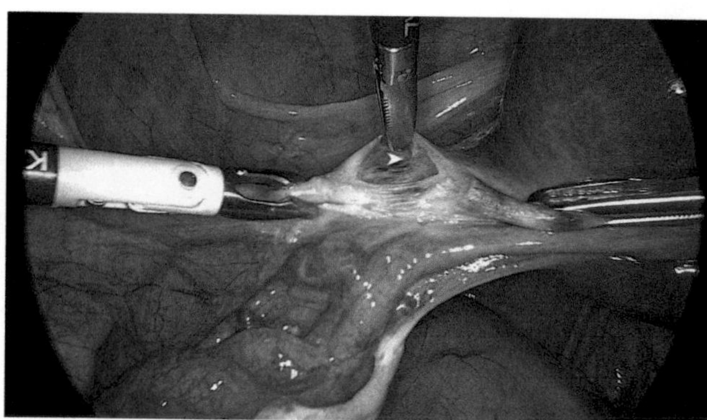

Fig. 21.13 ➤ Opening the broad ligament

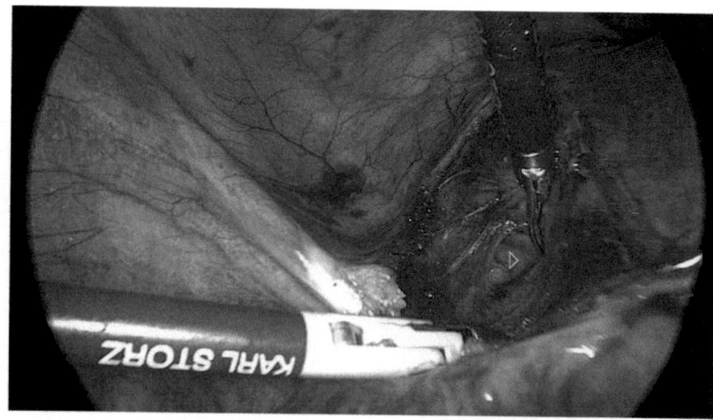

Fig. 21.14 ▹ Fenestration of broad ligament

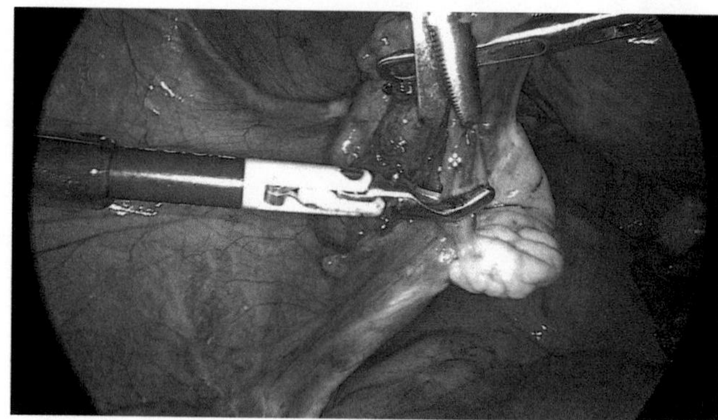

Fig. 21.15 ✣ Coagulation and section of salpingo-ovarian ligament

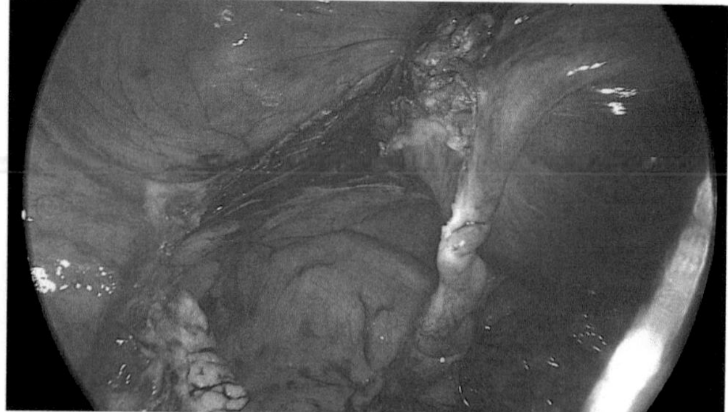

Fig. 21.16 Uterus with left salpinx

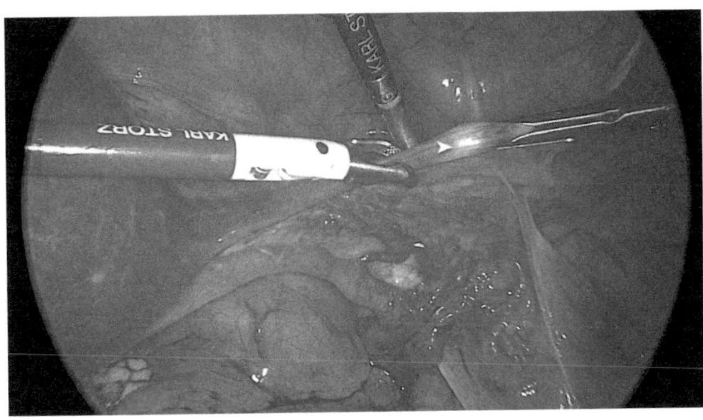

Fig. 21.17 ➤ Right round ligament

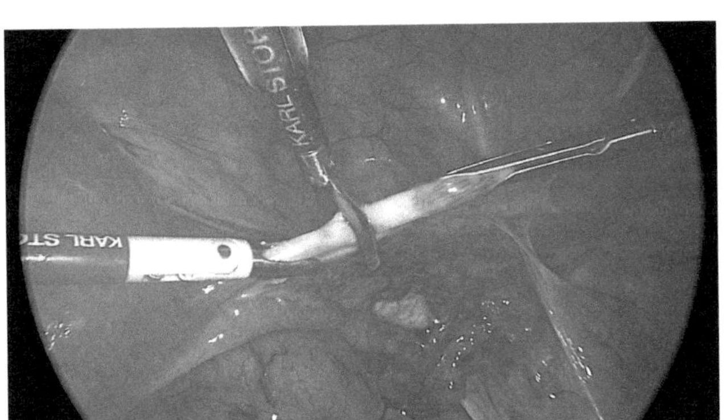

Fig. 21.18 Coagulation and section of right round ligament

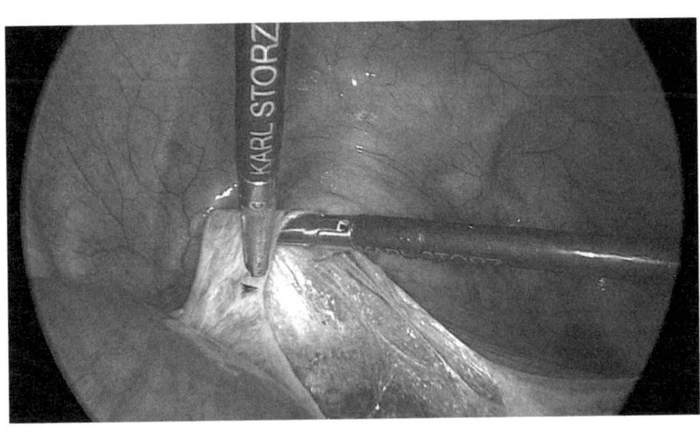

Fig. 21.19 Cutting the peritoneum over the vesico-uterine space

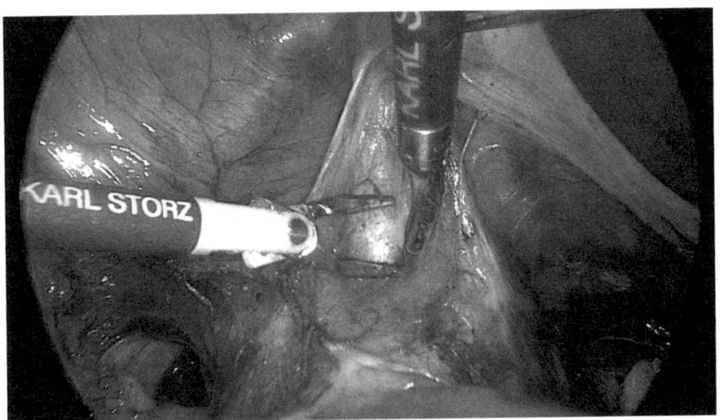

Fig. 21.20 Dissection of vesico-vaginal space

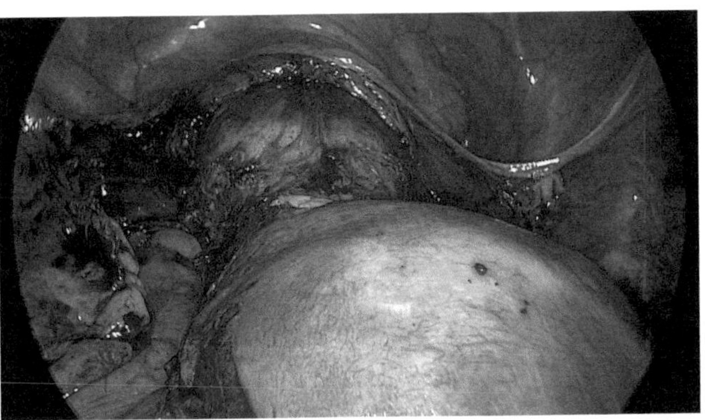

Fig. 21.21 Uterine artery coagulation using a bipolar rotating grasper

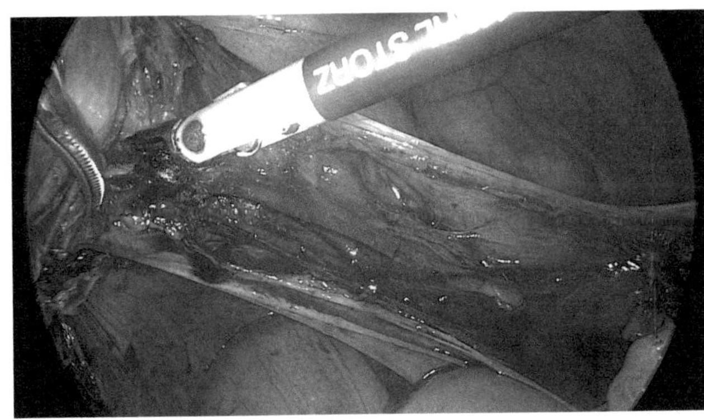

Fig. 21.22 Dissection of the bladder away from the anterior vagina along the vesicovaginal space

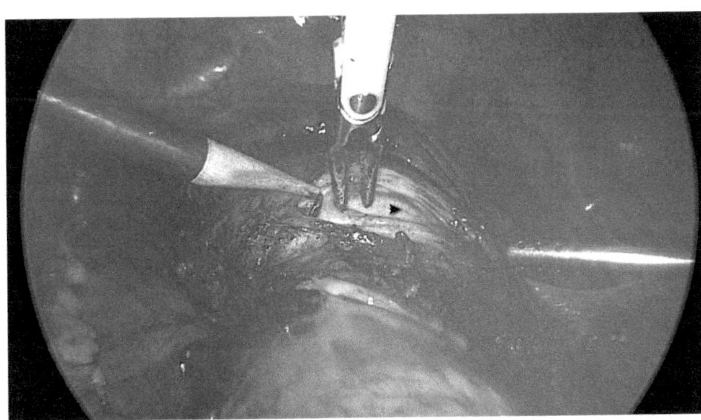

Fig. 21.23 Opcning the vaginal cuff using a monopolar hook and a bipolar grasper

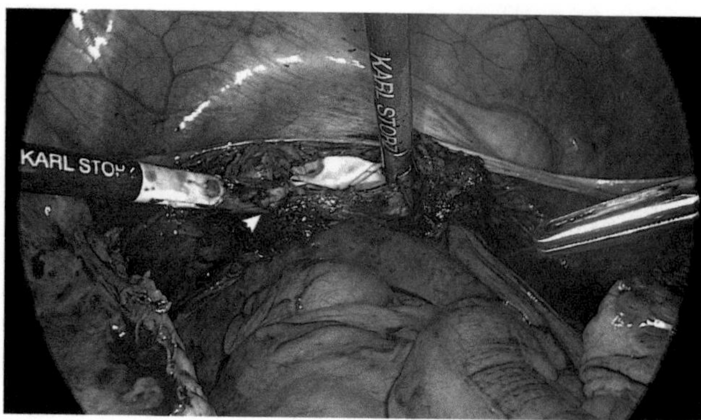

Fig. 21.24 Coagulation of vaginal cuff using a bipolar grasper (ROBI® WATTIEZ Grasping Forceps)

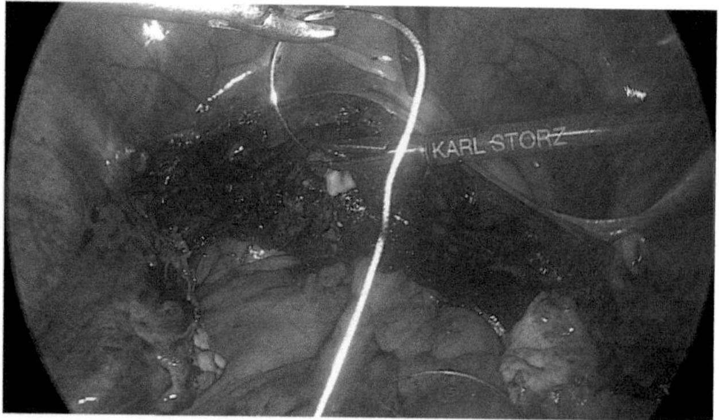

Fig. 21.25 Vaginal cuff closure using an intra-corporeal absorbable suture

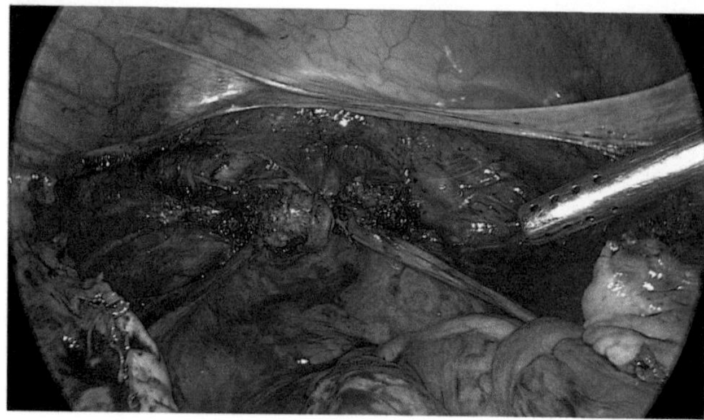

Fig. 21.26 Vaginal cuff closure approximating both uterosacral ligaments and pubocervical fascia

Conclusion

Surely, the old paradigm "big surgeon means big incisions" has absolutely changed. Laparoscopic hysterectomy is noticeably favorable for patients in whom vaginal surgery is contraindicated or cannot be done. We go towards a concept that the best surgeon performs the smallest incisions.

References

1. Garry R et al. The eVALuate study: two parallel randomised trials, one comparing laparoscopic with abdominal hysterectomy, the other comparing laparoscopic with vaginal hysterectomy. BMJ. 2004;328(7432):129.
2. Nezhat F et al. Laparoscopic versus abdominal hysterectomy. J Reprod Med. 1992;37(3):247–50.
3. Phipps JH, John M, Nayak S. Comparison of laparoscopically assisted vaginal hysterectomy and bilateral salpingo-oophorectomy with conventional abdominal hysterectomy and bilateral salpingo-oophorectomy. Br J Obstet Gynaecol. 1993;100(7):698–700.
4. Raju KS, Auld BJ. A randomised prospective study of laparoscopic vaginal hysterectomy versus abdominal hysterectomy each with bilateral salpingo-oophorectomy. Br J Obstet Gynaecol. 1994; 101(12):1068–71.
5. Olsson JH, Ellstrom M, Hahlin M. A randomised prospective trial comparing laparoscopic and abdominal hysterectomy. Br J Obstet Gynaecol. 1996;103(4):345–50.
6. Langebrekke A et al. Abdominal hysterectomy should not be considered as a primary method for uterine removal. A prospective randomised study of 100 patients referred to hysterectomy. Acta Obstet Gynecol Scand. 1996;75(4):404–7.
7. Marana R et al. Laparoscopically assisted vaginal hysterectomy versus total abdominal hysterectomy: a prospective, randomized, multicenter study. Am J Obstet Gynecol. 1999;180(2 Pt 1):270–5.
8. Falcone T, Paraiso MF, Mascha E. Prospective randomized clinical trial of laparoscopically assisted vaginal hysterectomy versus total abdominal hysterectomy. Am J Obstet Gynecol. 1999;180(4): 955–62.
9. Ferrari MM et al. Identifying the indications for laparoscopically assisted vaginal hysterectomy: a prospective, randomised comparison with abdominal hysterectomy in patients with symptomatic uterine fibroids. BJOG. 2000;107(5):620–5.
10. Lumsden MA et al. A randomised comparison and economic evaluation of laparoscopic-assisted hysterectomy and abdominal hysterectomy. BJOG. 2000;107(11):1386–91.
11. Schutz K et al. Prospective randomized comparison of laparoscopic-assisted vaginal hysterectomy (LAVH) with abdominal hysterectomy (AH) for the treatment of the uterus weighing >200 g. Surg Endosc. 2002;16(1):121–5.
12. Walsh CA et al. Total abdominal hysterectomy versus total laparoscopic hysterectomy for benign disease: a meta-analysis. Eur J Obstet Gynecol Reprod Biol. 2009;144(1):3–7.
13. Aarts JW et al. Surgical approach to hysterectomy for benign gynaecological disease. Cochrane Database Syst Rev. 2015;12(8):CD003677. doi: 10.1002/14651858.CD003677.pub5.
14. Wattiez A, Cohen SB, Selvaggi L. Laparoscopic hysterectomy. Curr Opin Obstet Gynecol. 2002;14(4):417–22.
15. Ghezzi F et al. Postoperative pain after laparoscopic and vaginal hysterectomy for benign gynecologic disease: a randomized trial. Am J Obstet Gynecol. 2010;203(2):118 e1–8.
16. ACOG Committee Opinion No. 444: choosing the route of hysterectomy for benign disease. Obstet Gynecol. 2009;114(5):1156–8.
17. A.A.M.I.G. Worldwide. AAGL position statement: route of hysterectomy to treat benign uterine disease. J Minim Invasive Gynecol. 2011;18(1):1–3.
18. Walters MD. Choosing a route of hysterectomy for benign disease. Uptodate. 2015.
19. Shiota M et al. Indication for laparoscopically assisted vaginal hysterectomy. JSLS. 2011;15(3):343–5.
20. Bijen CB et al. Costs and effects of abdominal versus laparoscopic hysterectomy: systematic review of controlled trials. PLoS One. 2009;4(10):e7340.
21. Reich H. Laparoscopic hysterectomy. Surg Laparosc Endosc. 1992; 2(1):85–8.

22 Preparation (Medical History, Surgical Set-Up, Antibiotics, Anticoagulants)

Magdalena Zalewski and Mohamed Elessawy

Introduction

Hysterectomy is the most frequently performed major gynaecologic surgical procedure [1, 2]. The overall rate of hysterectomy in Germany in the period 2005–2006 was 362.9 (295.0 for benign diseases of the genital tract and 44.0 for primary malignant tumors of the genital tract) per 100,000 person-years. Hysterectomy rates varied considerably across federal states: the rate for benign disease was lowest in Hamburg (213.8 per 100,000 women per year) and highest in Mecklenburg–West Pomerania (361.9 per 100,000 women per year) [3]. The CDC (Centers for Disease Control and Prevention) reported that in the USA the hysterectomy rate in 2000–2004 was 5.4/1000 per year [4].

Hysterectomies are preformed abdominally, vaginally, or with laparoscopic or robotic assistance. When choosing the route of hysterectomy, the physician should take into consideration the safest and most cost-effective route to fulfil all needs of the patient. The surgeon's decision is based on the patient's wishes and the route preferred by the surgeon. The art of surgery has developed and changed with the advancement of technology so that nowadays hysterectomy nowadays is mostly performed as a minimal invasive operation, accounting for nearly 60 % of all hysterectomy operations [5].

The preparation of the patient is a crucial factor towards obtaining the best surgical results. It should include the preparation of the tissues to encourage healing and bowel preparation to optimize the endoscopic space. In this chapter we will discuss our experience in preparing patients for laparoscopic hysterectomy.

M. Zalewski
Klinik für Gynäkologie und Geburtsmedizin,
Uniklinik RWTH Aachen, Aachen 52062, Germany
e-mail: mzalewski@ukaachen.de

M. Elessawy (✉)
OB/GYN, University Hospitals Schleswig-Holstein,
Campus Kiel, Germany, Kiel 24105, Germany
e-mail: Mohamed.Elessawy@uksh.de

Medical History

Taking a detailed medical history is the first step towards planning and successfully achieving a safe surgery.

Our patients complete a standardized questionnaire sheet covering their personal data and medical history. A Pap smear test is important before deciding to perform a supracervical hysterectomy.

Special consideration is given to patients with an oncological history in their families. Ongoing treatment for a breast cancer patient or a high-risk tumour patient might influence our decision to perform prophylactic adnectomy during the hysterectomy procedure.

Additional consideration must be given to prolapse and incontinence, which account for up to 14 % of indications for hysterectomy, in order to plan the best operative route for hysterectomy with corrective fixation surgery [5].

A detailed surgical history revealing the number of vaginal deliveries, laparotomies and cesarean section is important for deciding the route and the preparation for the hysterectomy operation.

Cesarean section is the most commonly performed surgery in obstetrics, and its incidence is increasing with rates as high as 17–31 % in some countries [6]. Estimates of the prevalence of cesarean delivery on maternal request range from 1–18 % of all caesarean deliveries worldwide, and <–1 to 3 % of all cesarean deliveries in the United States [7]. In certain cases, resulting scar formation may lead to adhesions and pain in many patients and possible difficulties at a later hysterectomy operation. In addition, cesarean scar dehiscence can be a risk for perforation during insertion of the uterine manipulator at total laparoscopic hysterectomy (Fig. 22.1).

I. Alkatout, L. Mettler (eds.), *Hysterectomy*, DOI 10.1007/978-3-319-22497-8_22

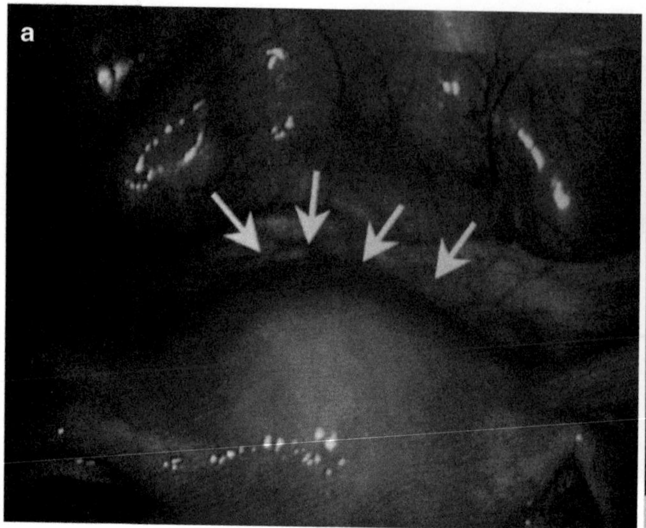

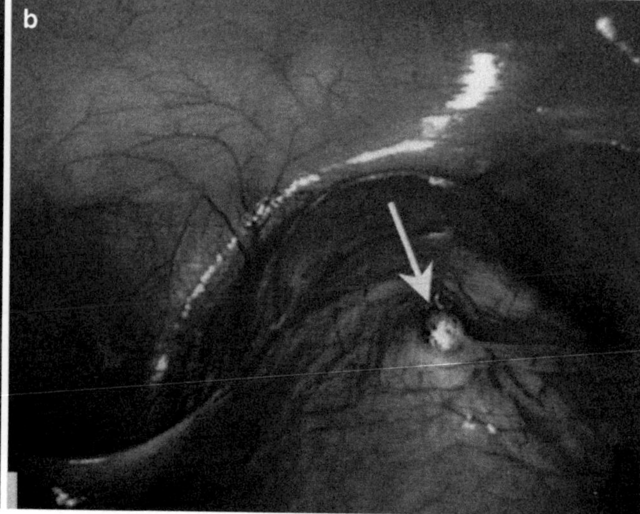

Fig. 22.1 Shows that cesarean scar dehiscence can be a risk for perforation during insertion of the uterine manipulator at total laparoscopic hysterectomy (**a**). Shows that the inseration of utrine manipulator should be carefully inserted to avoid perforation of the thin uterine wall by cesarean scar dehiscence (**b**)

In the literature, there is little information on the ability of MRI findings to detect cesarean scar dehiscence. Ultrasonographic evaluation of the anterior uterine wall is mandatory to evaluate the thickness of the lower uterine segment in the case of previous cesarean section.

It is well known that previous operations can result in the development of postoperative adhesions, which are a natural consequence of tissue trauma. This leads to an inclusion entity of adhesiolysis which is usually associated with a higher risk of complications. A review of the PubMed library shows that the correlation between a preoperative risk score and the complication incidence at the time of hysterectomy has not been sufficiently examined. At the Kiel University Department of Obstetrics and Gynecology, Germany, the estimated risk has been examined in comparison with the incidence of the intraoperative and post-operative complications. The data were statistically evaluated to investigate the relationship between the occurrence of the complication and the preoperative score at the time of the hysterectomy. For the preoperative score, patients who had undergone a previous laparoscopy were assigned 1 point; those who had undergone a previous Pfannenstiel laparotomy were assigned 2 points; those who had undergone 1 cesarean delivery were assigned 3 points; those who had undergone 2 cesarean deliveries were assigned 4 points; those who had undergone 3 cesarean deliveries were assigned 5 points; and those with no previous operations were assigned 0 points.

Of the intraoperative complications recorded 28.6 % of patients had a preoperative score more than 1, of the major postoperative complications recorded 33.3 % had a preoperative score more than 1 and of the minor postoperative complications recorded 25 % of patients had a preoperative score more than 1 [8]. Patients with a history of previous operations have to be informed of the risk of adhesions which can lead to a prolongation of the operative procedure to achieve a sufficient adhesiolysis and a longer hospital stay.

Gilmour et al. found from studies without routine cystoscopy that combined ureter and bladder injury rates varied according to the complexity of the surgery, ranging from less than 1 injury per 1000 for subtotal hysterectomy with or without bilateral salpingo-oophorectomy to as many as 13 injuries per 1000 surgeries for laparoscopic hysterectomy with or without bilateral salpingo-oophorectomy and for other gynecologic and urogynecologic surgeries [9].

Preoperative Evaluation and Treatment

Preoperative detection and evaluation differs according to the symptoms, needs of the patient and the indication for hysterectomy. The six most common reasons for performing a hysterectomy in the period 2002–2010 at the Kiel university hospital were uterine myoma (65.19 %), adenomyosis (11.21 %), dysfunctional uterine bleeding (12.99 %), endometriosis (5.03 %), hyperplasia of the endometrium of the cervix (1.99 %) and total uterine prolapse (14.79 %) [5].

This data is comparable to national data. In Germany the main reasons for performing a hysterectomy were uterine myoma (60.7 %), uterine prolapse (27.9 %), bleeding disorders (25.2 %), hyperplasia (2.9 %) and endometriosis (15.1 %).

The preoperative work-up should include: the measurement of preoperative haemoglobin levels and an abdominal and transvaginal ultrasonography. A blood count and serum ferritin test provide information on the necessity of administering oral iron, particularly in patients with menometrorrhagia. The correction of sideropenic anemia by giving oral iron is essential to reduce the risk of a blood transfusion.

Ultrasonography should include the measurement of the entire uterus (length, depth and width) and the number, size and location of myomas. Such information may play an important role in the determination of the operative strategy.

Magnetic resonance imaging is mandatory when the ultrasound examination is difficult to analyse and in cases of associated adnexal pathology. We follow the concept of obtaining the required information with minimum exploration for both psychological and economic reasons.

Ulipristal acetate (UPA) significantly reduces uterine fibroid volume, reduces menstrual blood loss and improves quality of life without serious adverse events. UPA is a selective progesterone receptor modulator (SPRM) blocking most progestational effects with a reduced antiglucocorticoid activity [10]. Gonadotropin-releasing hormone agonists (GnRH) cause myoma shrinkage by reducing the circulating oestrogen levels [11].

A vaginal preparation with 0.05 mg oestrogen is the standard dose recommended for regeneration of the vagina; however, preparations with 0.03 mg are currently in use and are usually administered for one to three weeks. With the absence of sufficient feedback a vaginal oestrogen preparation is sometimes prescribed for at least one month prior to surgery to improve the vaginal cell regeneration and proliferation of tissues. This enables a better healing in the case of additional vaginal corrective surgery for prolapse patients. Recent studies suggest that hormone replacement therapy decreases the risk of recurrence of breast cancer [12].

Informed Consent

No intervention can be undertaken without the patient's voluntary consent. For consent to be valid, the patient must be considered competent. In the setting of informed consent, competence or capacity means that the patient has the mental ability to understand problems and make decisions about accepting or rejecting medical treatments that are offered (Table 22.1).

Table 22.1 Informed consent – important topics

Personal discussion about the recommended therapy and the alternatives
Making clear the necessity and the urgency
Possible risks
Making sure the patient understands everything (especially foreign patients)
Provision of sufficient time for an informed decision (day before surgery)
Consent must be voluntary

Bowel Preparation

We aim to empty the bowel to facilitate pushing the loops of the bowel out of the way and flattening them so as to enlarge the operating space. Preparation starts with a standard low residue diet which the patient is required to follow for 5 days prior to the operation. Two days before the operation, the bowel is emptied by administering a laxative solution such as Xprep. Finally, the day before the operation, the lower bowel should be cleaned with an enema. It is important to follow this chronological order to avoid any loss from the anus onto the table, which would give rise to a high risk infection.

Antibiotics

The United States Centers for Disease Control and Prevention (CDC) has published an internationally accepted definition of surgical site infection (SSI). The term SSI is defined as an infection of the skin or the subcutaneous tissue of the incision within 30 days of an operative procedure. Antimicrobial prophylaxis can help to avoid SSI.

The decision for an antimicrobial prophylaxis in a surgical procedure is based on risk stratification for the onset of SSI. The stratification of wounds (clean, clean-contaminated, contaminated, dirty wounds) is the most important factor in this decision. The hysterectomy is defined as a surgery with a clean-contaminated wound and therefore there is a risk of infection during the performed surgery.

However, several additional risk-factors are known to increase the risk of SSI (AWMF-Leitlinie: Perioperative Antibiotikaprophylaxe; Recommendations of the "Paul-Ehrlich-Gesellschaft für Chemotherapie e.V."):

- patient age,
- comorbidities (especially diabetes and immunosuppression),
- obesity,
- nicotine or drug abuse,

Table 22.2 The effect of perioperative antibiotic prophylaxis in different kinds of hysterectomy

Kind of hysterectomy and antibiotic prophylaxis	Number of patients [n]	Number of infections [n (%)]
Abdominal hysterectomy		
Combination	532	31 (5.8)
Cefuroxime	405	28 (6.9)
Metronidazole	178	27 (15.2)
Laparoscopic hysterectomy		
Combination	806	50 (6.2)
Cefuroxime	645	37 (5.7)
Metronidazole	90	13 (14.4)
Vaginal hysterectomy		
Combination	914	35 (3.8)
Cefuroxime	969	38 (3.9)
Metronidazole	250	31 (12.4)

- preoperative infections,
- length of surgery (more than 2 h),
- blood transfusion,
- hypothermia,
- previous radiotherapy,
- previous surgery.

In general SSI occurs less often in laparoscopic surgery than in abdominal surgery [13]. We expect any SSI in abdominal hysterectomy in 10.5 %, and in laparoscopic hysterectomy in 9.0 % of patients.

Nevertheless, a hysterectomy is an indication for an antibiotic prophylaxis, independent of the surgical approach used (abdominal, vaginal, laparoscopic or robotic). The preferred regimen is a single intravenous dose of a second-generation cephalosporin, possibly combined with metronidazole.

In 2013 a prospective study from Finland with 5279 patients compared the effect of perioperative antibiotic prophylaxis in different kinds of hysterectomy. Data on 1115 abdominal hysterectomies (AH), 1541 laparoscopic hysterectomies (LH), and 2133 vaginal hysterectomies (VH) were analysed. The patients received cefuroxime alone, metronidazole alone or a combination of both (Table 22.2).

The results revealed that adding metronidazole to a prophylaxis with cefuroxime did not show any statistically significant additional advantage. A prophylaxis with metronidazole alone led to more infections after surgery [14].

The correct timing of antimicrobial prophylaxis plays a crucial role for an effective prophylaxis. The ideal moment for the first application is 30–60 min before incision. An application more than 60 min before incision significantly increases the risk of SSI. For surgical procedures shorter than 2 h a single shot therapy is sufficient. Longer procedures require a repetition of the prophylaxis. Timing of repeated administration depends on the half-life of the chosen antimicrobial agent. A repetition is needed after 2 half-life periods (half-life of cefuroxime: 70 min; half-life of metronidazole: 7 h). In general, there is no need for continuing the prophylaxis after the end of the procedure.

Anticoagulants

In case of a permanent therapy with anticoagulants some considerations should be made before planning a hysterectomy. Coumarin derivatives should be paused for an operation. A bridging with low molecular weight heparin is recommended. A normalisation of the INR is expected four to seven days later. Rivaroxaban should be paused 24 h before starting the operation. A monitoring is possible by measuring anti-Factor Xa activity. The taking of acetylsalicylic acid should be continued if it is taken for secondary prevention and can be paused if taken for primary prevention. In these cases an interval of seven days is necessary until the platelet aggregation is no longer affected.

Installation and Disinfection

After the induction of anaesthesia, the patient is placed on her back with legs apart and half bent. The buttocks must protrude a few centimetres from the edge of the table to allow uterine manipulation. This position creates three operating spaces: one occupied by the surgeon, another one on the right occupied by the first assistant and a third one between the legs for the second assistant (Fig. 22.2).

The patient's arm is placed alongside her body to avoid any brachial injury.

A warming system can be used to avoid any chilling of the patient. The abdomen, perineum and vagina are prepared with a suitable bactericidal solution and a Foley catheter is inserted.

Conclusion

A laparoscopic hysterectomy can be a long and difficult operation; therefore, the optimal preparation of the patient is of prime ergonomic and economic importance (Table 22.3).

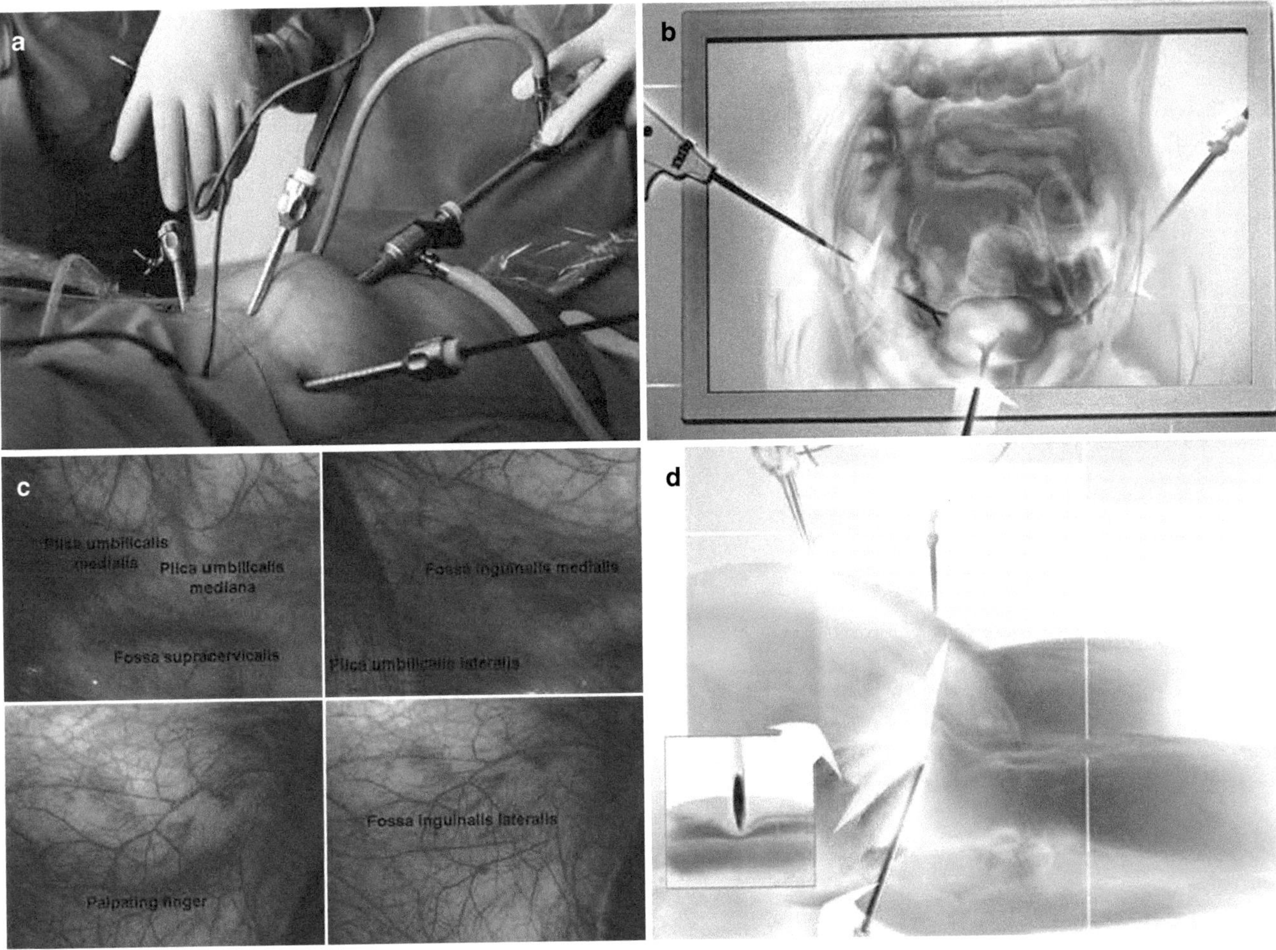

Fig. 22.2 Position of trocars and positions occupied by operating team

Table 22.3 Summary – preparation of a hysterectomy via laparoscopy

Medical history, previous cancers in family medical history
Gynecological examination and ultrasonography
Pap smear
→Indication for hysterectomy via laparoscopy
Informed consent
Anesthesiological preparation
Blood test (haemoglobin, pregnancy test (if patient is fertile)
Bowel preparation
Perioperative antimicrobial prophylaxis (cefuroxime ± metronidazole)

References

1. Altgassen C, Michels W, Schneider A. Learning laparoscopic-assisted hysterectomy. Obstet Gynecol. 2004;104(2):308–13.
2. Briese V., Ulfig N., and Mylonas I., Die vaginale Hysterektomie, in Gynäkologe. 2002. p. 116–124.
3. Stang A, Merrill RM, Kuss O. Prevalence-corrected hysterectomy rates by age and indication in Germany 2005–2006. Arch Gynecol Obstet. 2012;286(5):1193–200.
4. Whiteman MK et al. Inpatient hysterectomy surveillance in the United States, 2000–2004. Am J Obstet Gynecol. 2008;198(1):34 e1–7.
5. Schollmeyer T et al. Hysterectomy trends over a 9-year period in an endoscopic teaching center. Int J Gynaecol Obstet(The Official Organ of the International Federation of Gynaecology and Obstetrics). 2014;126(1):45–9.
6. Seffah JD. Re-laparotomy after Cesarean section. Int J Gynaecol Obstet(The Official Organ of the International Federation of Gynaecology and Obstetrics). 2005;88(3):253–7.
7. MacDorman MF, Menacker F, Declercq E. Cesarean birth in the United States: epidemiology, trends, and outcomes. Clin Perinatol. 2008;35(2):293–307.
8. Elessawy M et al. Arch Gynecol Obstet 2015;292:127. doi:10.1007/s00404-014-3594-9
9. Gilmour DT, Das S, Flowerdew G. Rates of urinary tract injury from gynecologic surgery and the role of intraoperative cystoscopy. Obstet Gynecol. 2006;107(6):1366–72.
10. Zalewski MM, Felix Z, Joseph N. Update of conservative systemic treatment of uterine fibroids. Curr Obstet Gynekol Rep. 2014;3:191–5.

11. Friedman AJ et al. A randomized, placebo-controlled, double-blind study evaluating the efficacy of leuprolide acetate depot in the treatment of uterine leiomyomata. Fertil Steril. 1989;51(2):251–6.
12. Fahlen M et al. Hormone replacement therapy after breast cancer: 10 year follow up of the Stockholm randomised trial. Eur J Cancer. 2013;49(1):52–9.
13. Mahdi H et al. Predictors of surgical site infection in women undergoing hysterectomy for benign gynecologic disease: a multicenter analysis using the national surgical quality improvement program data. J Minim Invasive Gynecol. 2014;21(5):901–9.
14. Brummer TH et al. Antibiotic prophylaxis for hysterectomy, a prospective cohort study: cefuroxime, metronidazole, or both? BJOG. 2013;120(10):1269–76.

23 Instrumentation Systems, Apparatus and Materials in Hysterectomy

Liselotte Mettler, Ibrahim Alkatout, and Artin Ternamian

Introduction

Instruments and apparatus for laparoscopic hysterectomy have been developed over the last 30 years for interventions with multiple ports as well as for single port surgery. Different set of instruments are necessary for subtotal and total laparoscopic hysterectomy and radical hysterectomies. This chapter is divided into.

1. History.
2. General systems for adhesion prevention, mesh, sutures, stables, glue, drains, rinsing solutions and suction.
3. Instrument systems and apparatus for laparoscopic hysterectomies.

All equipment as used in gynecological and general laparoscopic surgery is assembled on instrument trolleys, so called smart carts, which are available as rolling carts or on special platforms hanging down from the ceiling. Panoramic operating room endoscopic settings such as OR1 TM Neo (Karl Storz GmbH, Tuttlingen) or the Endoalpha by Olympus (Olympus Europa SE & CO.KG, Hamburg) or the Stryker unit with SDC Ultra as digital documentation system form the basis to position the necessary equipment for easy use of the surgeon.

L. Mettler (✉) • I. Alkatout
Gynecology and Obstetrics,
University Hospitals Schleswig-Holstein,
Campus Kiel, Kiel, Germany
e-mail: lmettler@email.uni-kiel.de

A. Ternamian
Department of Obstetrics and Gynecology, Faculty of Medicine,
University of Toronto, St Joseph's Health Center Toronto,
Toronto, Canada
e-mail: Artin.ternamian@utoronto.ca

The idea of warming and humidifying the CO_2 gas to avoid damage to the peritoneum has been propagated by Douglas Ott and Philippe Koninckx. The HumiGard TM of Fisher & Paykel Healthcare (Auckland, New Zealand) provides heated, humidified and filtered gas to a patient at a predetermined temperature.

Today, every CO_2 pneu automatic provides up to 37 °C heated CO_2, gas which is controlled by a pressure regulator and within the machine by applying the Quadro-test. In the Quadro-test, the volume of gas flowing through the Veress needle during insufflation, intra-abdominal pressure, total volume and preset filling pressure are measured. Cold light is provided by xenon lamps. The video camera systems are equipped with three-chip camera or HD-cameras and can be used for laparoscopy as well as hysteroscopy. High-resolution video monitors guarantee optimal picture quality. The technological development allows the use of larger monitors in HD quality that facilitate a relaxed working atmosphere for the surgeon.

A realistic, true to life 3D picture is possible due to various technological elements such as digital simulation, a second camera system or the use of shutter lens. Digital devices for the video camera control the picture quality and facilitate automatic white balancing. The Karl Storz company already offers the TRICAM 3D imaging system that allows the surgeon to view crisp, dear image through a pair of lightweight polarizing glasses. Their ENDOCAMELEON laparoscope provides a viewing angle that can be adjusted continuously between 0 and 120° (Fig. 23.1a).

The Olympus 3D system allows a direct vision through the ENDOEYE FLEX 3D, a deflectable tip 3D laparoscope. This tool allows for 100° angulation in 4 directions while the image on the screen is maintaining a fixed horizon. The dual-lens design of the ENOEYE FLEX 3D and the high-density image sensors for high-definition 3D images give a focus-free view (Fig. 23.1b).

I. Alkatout, L. Mettler (eds.), *Hysterectomy*, DOI 10.1007/978-3-319-22497-8_23

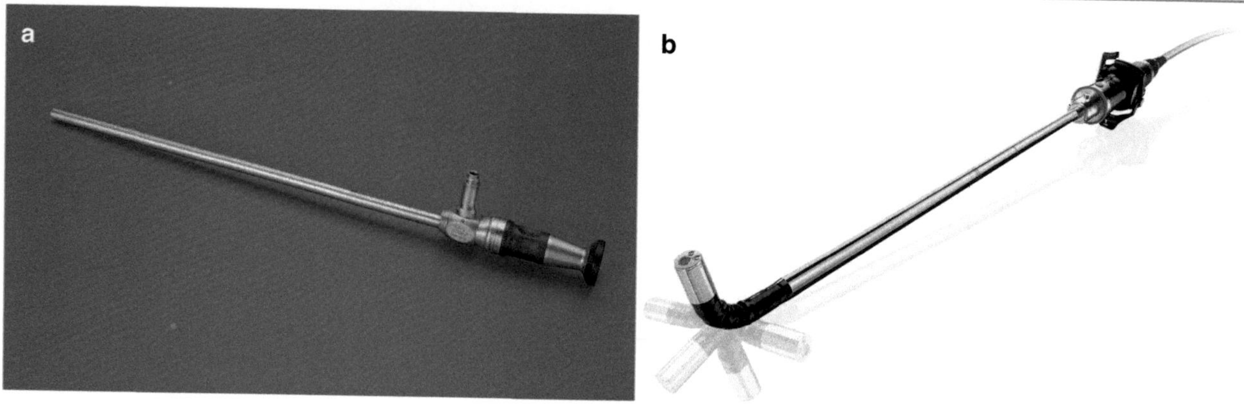

Fig. 23.1 (**a**) Endocameleon laparoscope 0–120° angle (**b**) Endoeye Flex 3 D laparoscope system

History

Although the origin of endoscopy can be found already in a reference of the Babylonian Talmud. Endoscopic surgery has mainly be developed by the use of Bozzini's light guide and the rigid optic system developed by Max Nizze as cystoscope. We consider Georg Kelling, (1866–1945) of Dresden, who added his experience in oral air insufflation as the father of endoscopic surgery. The knowledge of gastric and esophageal endoscopy of air insufflation where the foundation of future trials for the diagnostic and therapeutic examination of enclosed body cavities.

Subtotal hysterectomy by laparotomy, total hysterectomy by laparotomy and vaginal hysterectomy dominated till 1980 the field for this gynecologic surgical procedure. In relation to the development of save instruments and apparatus to be used in endoscopic surgical procedures the desire to perform laparoscopic hysterectomy was noticed worldwide in the groups of many gynecologic endoscopic surgeons. In Kiel we applied laparoscopic assistance to vaginal hysterectomy, first published by Kurt Semm in 1984, routinely in difficult vaginal hysterectomies [1]. In those days the aggression towards laparoscopy as surgical procedure was still very pronounced. We did not dare in Kiel to even talk about laparoscopic hysterectomy in our own department although we freed the uterus from the pelvic side wall in many occasions and then extracted the uterus through the vagina, because everybody already blamed us as irresponsible surgeons. This procedure was later described as laparoscopic vaginal hysterectomy (LAVH). We did not dissect the uterine vessels laparoscopically in those early years.

As worldwide accepted, however, the first laparoscopic hysterectomy was performed by Harry Reich in the 1989 in the William Nesbitt Memorial Hospital in Kingston, Pennsylvania, U.S.A. [2]. Simultaneously Kurt Semm developed the laparoscopic subtotal hysterectomy and performed on Sept.07, 1989 on a Saturday afternoon in Kiel the first then called "Classic Intrafascial Subtotal Hysterectomy" (CISH), which was first published in 1993 [3]. In the same years Jaques Donnez, 1993 and Thomas Lyons, 1993 published their approaches of laparoscopic subtotal hysterectomy. Over the consecutive years till today various modifications and classifications of laparoscopic hysterectomies for benign indications have been described. Radical hysterectomies using laparoscopy date back to the early experience of Daniel Dargent 1986 [4] and have only been performed worldwide on a larger scale in the twenty first century.

General Systems, Adhesion Prevention, Mesh, Sutures, Staples, Glue, Drains, Rising Solutions and Suction)

Generators and Set-Ups

All essential equipment for laparoscopic hysterectomy is assembled on equipment trolleys which are integrated into the panoramic operating rooms. Panoramic viewing possibilities and integrating commanding functions for all operating procedures and documentation are given today by many companies set-ups. An equipment trolley always contains the following apparatus: CO_2 insufflation unit with the possibility of producing heated and humidified gas, endoscopic camera, light sources (cold light is provided by Xenon lamps), suction and irrigation pumps, electrical energy systems, documentation systems. These systems are compatible with third party devices such as operating room lights, energy units, lasers and thermofusion systems. Higher solution video monitors guarantee optimal picture quality. The technical development allows the use of larger monitors in HD quality on flexible arms that fascilitate to position them into a relaxed working atmosphere for the surgeon. A realistic, nearly true to live 3D picuture, various technical elements such as digital simulation, a second camera system or the use of shutter lenses, are engaged. Digital devices for the video camera control the picture quality and facilitate automatic white balancing.

Adhesion Prevention

Adhesions during surgery are primarily defined as a condition in which bodily tissues that are normally separate grow together.

A fibrous band of scar tissue that binds together normally separates anatomical structures (Fig. 23.2). In this chapter, we want to stress the impact of adhesions as defined above as the most common post-surgical complication.

Adhesion formation is influenced by various factors. It starts with a trauma to the peritoneum or any other body site when rapidly fibrin de-position occurs. In peritoneal healing for example there is a balance between fibrin deposition and fibrinolysis. Any impairment of this process leads to increased fibrin deposition, the formation of fibrin strands and stable adhesions may be formed. The incidence of intraperitoneal adhesions in patients following general abdominal or gynecological surgery ranges from 63 to 97 % [5, 6]. The overall risk of hospital readmission related to adhesions following either laparoscopic or open surgery is similar [7]. Although the majority of patients remain asymptomatic, a considerable number experience serious complications, including bowel obstruction [8], female secondary infertility [9] and re-operative complications [10]. The presence of adhesions from previous surgery significantly increases the length of time required in subsequent surgical procedures, adversely affecting the workloads of surgical teams [11]. Certain surgical procedures carry a greater risk of adhesion-related complications. Surgical procedures on the ovary and fallopian tube were shown to have the highest risk of adhesion-related readmission (48.1 % and 41.2 % of women readmitted, respectively) [12]. For laparoscopic myomectomy this increases to 41 in every 100 procedures [13]. In one study, the number of adhesion-related readmissions increased steadily over a ten-year period, with 16 % occurring within the first year after the initial surgical procedure [12]. Some studies have also shown that adhesion-related complications can occur ten years after the initial surgical procedure [6].

Let us introduce into this discussion first an overview on the most common anti adhesion agents, which can be divided into two groups: "Site specific Agents" and compare them with the "broad coverage fluid agents".

Site-Specific Agents: Membranes

Mechanical barriers Interceed® (Gynecare, Ethicon, a Johnson & Johnson Company, Sommerville, NJ, USA): Interceed® is an oxidized regenerated cellulose membrane placed over a suture or a deperitonealised area. No sutures are required to keep Interceed® in place; slight moistening after positioning a single layer will make it adhere to the injured site, where it is absorbed within 4 weeks. Interceed® has been shown to be effective in various studies, and significantly reduces adhesion formation even in severe endometriosis [14].

Seprafilm® (Genzyme, Cambridge, MA, USA) Seprafilm®: is a hyaluronate-carboxymethyl cellulose membrane, which is placed over a suture or an injured area without stitches and remains in place for 7 days. In contrast to Interceed® no loss of efficacy in the presence of blood has

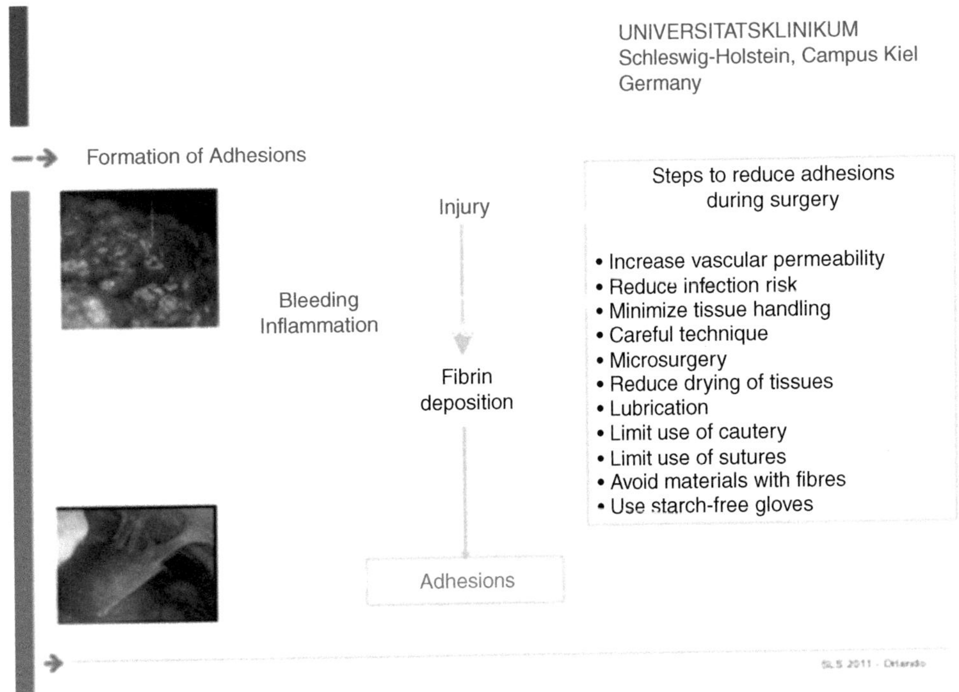

UNIVERSITATSKLINIKUM
Schleswig-Holstein, Campus Kiel
Germany
Formation of Adhesions
Injury
Bleeding
Inflammation
Fibrin
deposition
Adhesions
Steps to reduce adhesions
during surgery
• Increase vascular permeability
• Reduce infection risk
• Minimize tissue handling
• Careful technique
• Microsurgery
• Reduce drying of tissues
• Lubrication
• Limit use of cautery
• Limit use of sutures
• Avoid materials with fibres
• Use starch-free gloves

Fig. 23.2 Formation of adhesions from injury to adhesions

been reported. Several studies have demonstrated the efficacy of Seprafilm® mainly in general surgery, especially bowel surgery [15].

Gel barriers:SprayShield/Spray Gel® (Covidien Bio-Surgery, Waltham, MA, USA): SprayShield® is a synthetic polyethylene glycol solution which is sprayed over the affected area where it remains for approximately 5–7 days. After that period, it is degraded and absorbed. It consists of two components that react immediately on contact with the tissue to form an adherent layer. One of the components contains a blue food colourant, so there is an intraoperative visualization of where SprayShield® was used [16, 17]. In the case of myomectomy a reduction of adhesion formation was demonstrated for SprayGel® in a multi-center randomized controlled trial.

Intercoat®/Oxiplex/AP (FzioMed, Inc., San Luis Ob-ispo, CA, USA): Intercoat® is an absorbable gel composed of polyethylene oxide and sodium carboxymethyl cellulose. Functioning as a mechanical barrier during the healing process, Intercoat® is applied as a single layer at the end of the procedures.

HYA CORP ENDOGEL (BIO SCIENCE, GERMANY) is an absorbable sterile, transparent, high viscous gel produced by condensation of hyaluronic acid, which is one of the main components of human connective tissue. It adheres to tissue surfaces and to the abdominal wall and is effective as an anti-adhesion barrier substance on the local level. The development of Hyacorp Endogel is based on a composition of a substance that already exists for treating and filling tissue defects (Hyacorp Body Con-touring MLF 1).

Hyalobarrier Gel® (Fidia Advanced Biopolymers, Abano Terme, Italy): Hyalobarrier gel is a highly viscous auto-crosslinked hyaluronate used to separate organs and tissues after surgery. The use of hyaluronic acid agents may decrease adhesion formation and prevent the deterioration of preexisting adhesions [18]. CoSeal® (Baxter Healthcare Corporation, Deerfield, IL, USA).

CoSeal® is a resorbable hydrogel consisting of two polyethylene glycol polymer solutions which are mixed together when applied during surgery. The technology is similar to that seen with SprayShield® but in CoSeal® the polyethylene glycol esters have a different isomer structure. CoSeal® is long available for preventing adhesions in cardiac surgery where its efficacy has already been proved. First researches in women undergoing myomectomy demonstrated safety and efficacy of CoSeal® in abdominopelvic surgery [19].

Broad-Coverage Fluid Agents

Adept® (Icodextrin 4 % solution; Baxter Healthcare, Deerfield, Il, USA): Adept® is a clear solution containing icodextrin at a concentration of 4 %. Icodextrin is an a 1–4-linked glucose polymer and is responsible for the longer absorption time of Adept® compared to the previously used crystalloid instillates like saline solution or lactated Ringer's solution, which is rapidly resorbed by the peritoneum and therefore not suitable for adhesion prevention. At the end of a procedure, 1.000 ml of Adept® is instilled into the abdominal cavity. Instillates separate the injured tissue by hydroflotation and should stay in the abdominal cavity during the first days after surgery.

In laparoscopic hysterectomies out of the available pellet of adhesion prevention strategies we advise at present time the application of a site specific barrier either on hyaluronic acid basis (HyaCorp Endo Gel – Bioscience or Hyalobarrier – Nordic Pharma) and in case a large peritoneal defect results as broad liquid barrier Icodextrine – 4 % – adept – Baxter.

Meshes

There are many new kits on the market that involve the placement of the same nylon-like mesh in the TVT but instead used in large sheets between the bladder and the vagina and the rectum and the vagina to reinforce prolapse repair. There is no long term information on these techniques. Therefore we will hold off promoting or criticizing these techniques until there is adequate information available. As these materials are permanent, there is always a benefit in waiting to see the long term complications before jumping on the bandwagon of laparoscopic mesh application in sacro colpopexy or the new technique of prolapse surgery pectopexy after laparoscopic hysterectomy, as the long term complications may include mesh erosion into the vagina, bladder or rectum, painful intercourse, infection or bleeding etc.

Sutures

Ligatures and suturing techniques are besides all the modern coagulation advances many times still necessary for safe surgery in hysterectomy. Therefore we would like to give some basic ideas on hemostasis by loop ligatures, endosutures with extra corporeal knotting technique and endosutures with intra corporeal knotting technique.

Haemostasis by Endosuture with Extra Corporal Knot Tying

In many cases, it is convenient to ligate vascular bundles, adhesion bundles and similar structures with sling ligatures. Timewise it is worthwhile to tie the vascular omental and intestinal adhesions before cutting because searching for bleeders later can be time consuming and associated with much blood loss. Primarily, an 80 cm long Ethi-Endoligature® with a plastic knot pusher by Ethicon is used as a ligature. As an endosuture, it has a 3 cm long and 0,8 mm thick needle. The endosuture with extracorporeal knotting has a 2.5 and 3.5 cm long sharp needle as well as a 2.5 cm round needle. It is supplied with a suture applicator and a 3 mm trocar by Autosuture. After taking a purse string suture, the needle is cut; extracorporeal knots are formed and pushed down in the usual way with the plastic pusher (Figs. 23.3, 23.4, 23.5, 23.6 and 23.7). To push the knot, the applicator is pulled up. When it is pushed again into the 5 mm trocar, the plastic tube pushes the knot into the abdominal cavity. The loop is tightened under vision and the wound edges are adapted, e.g. the wound edges of the vaginal cuff. Cutting scissors are inserted in place of the 5 mm needle holder to cut the thread. The thread must be long enough to be able to form extracorporeal knots outside.

Roeder Knot

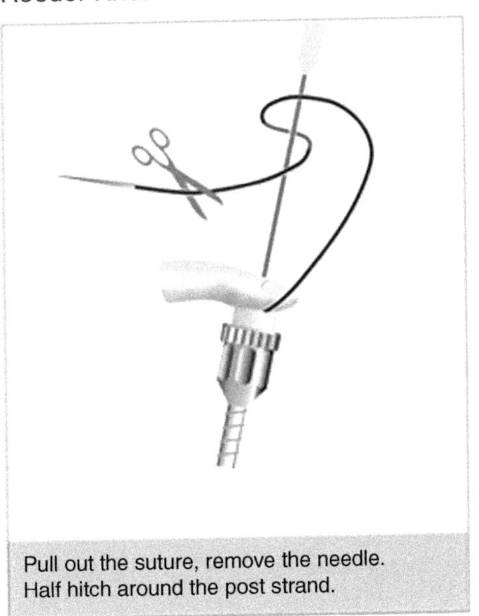

Pull out the suture, remove the needle.
Half hitch around the post strand.

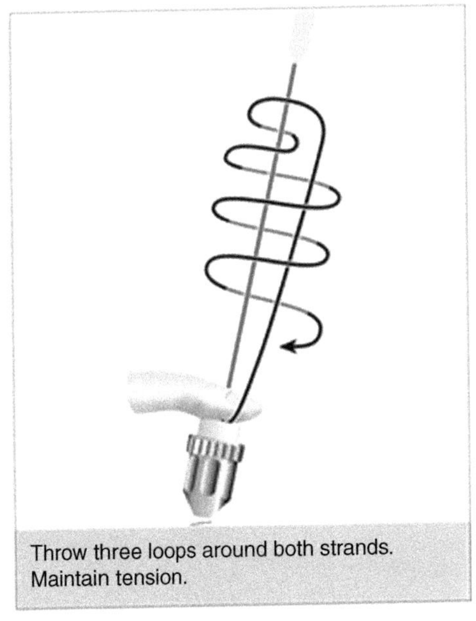

Throw three loops around both strands.
Maintain tension.

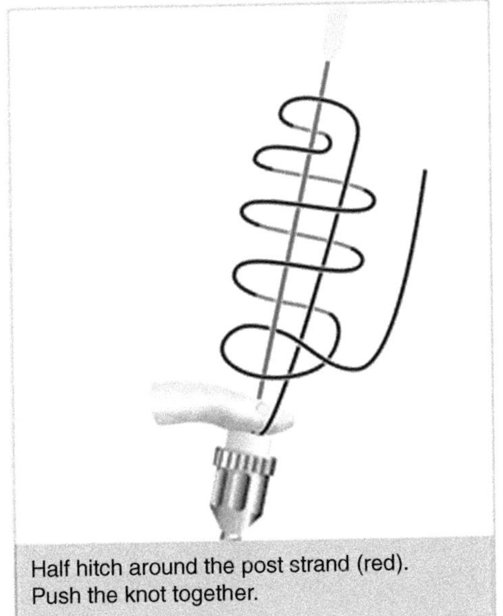

Half hitch around the post strand (red).
Push the knot together.

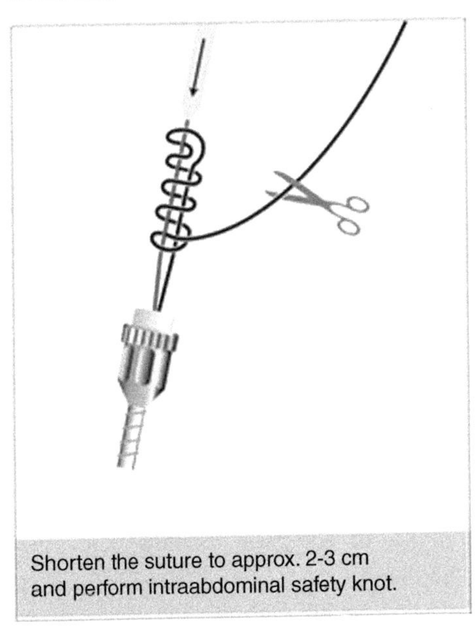

Shorten the suture to approx. 2-3 cm
and perform intraabdominal safety knot.

Fig. 23.3 Roeder Knot

Fig. 23.4 von Leffern Knot

von Leffern Knot

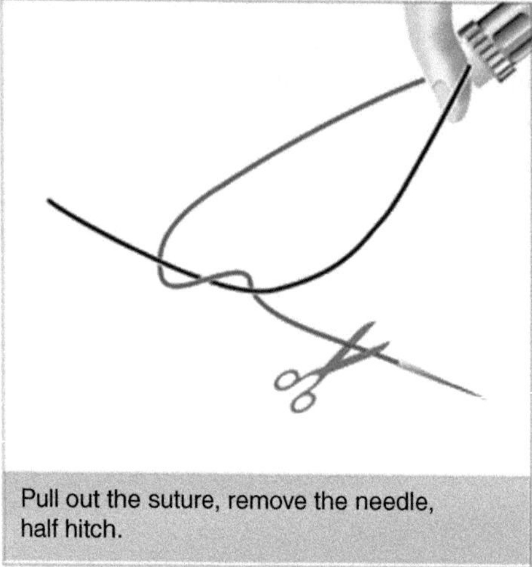
Pull out the suture, remove the needle,
half hitch.

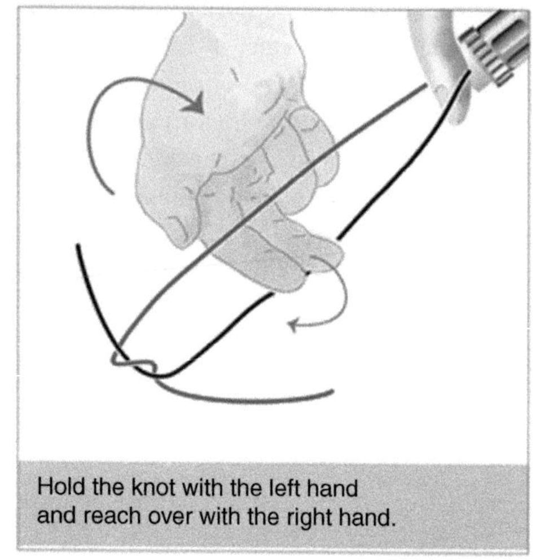
Hold the knot with the left hand
and reach over with the right hand.

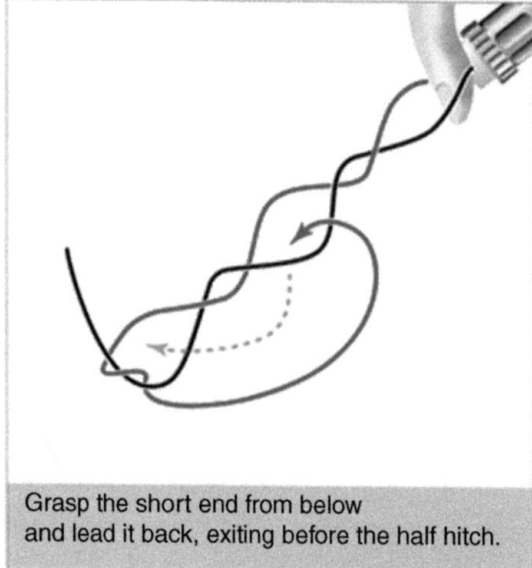
Grasp the short end from below
and lead it back, exiting before the half hitch.

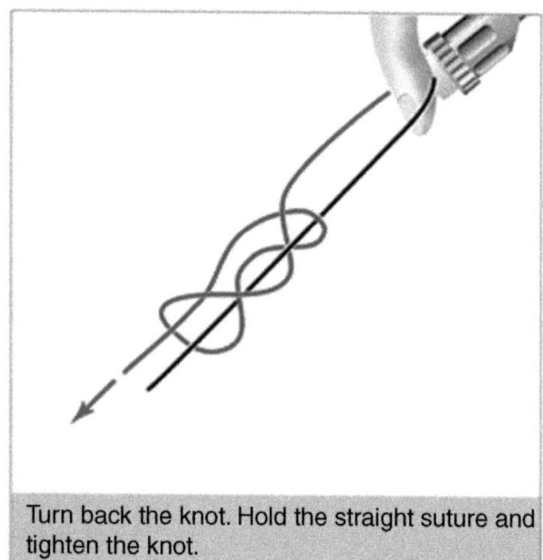
Turn back the knot. Hold the straight suture and
tighten the knot.

Hemostasis by Endosuture with Intracorporeal Knotting

For intracorporeal knotting, a straight or curved needle with different suture calibers is used. For microsurgical interventions, such as end-to-end anastomosis of the tube, 4–0 to 6–0 sutures are used otherwise 1–0 is adequate for vaginal cuff suture. The long-end of a thread, originally knotted extracorporeally, is wrapped around the needle holder twice while the needle holder is aiming for the short-end of the tread to perform an additional, intracorporeal safety knot (Fig. 23.8). Among many other intracorporeal suturings, the baseball suture is specially suitable to compress wounds, e.g. after enucleation of myomas.

Due to this technique of suturing, the size of the wound is minimized and along with it the risk of immediate and later bleeding. In addition, the occurrence of adhesions is reduced since the wound is closed toward the surrounding tissue. Stitching and tying of the whole uterine vessel bundle requires good knowledge of anatomy.

Hemostasis by Suture and Tying Knot with Half Hitch

The Clark knot pusher is used for this procedure. With the extracorporeal thread, a half-hitch is formed and the knot is then pushed down with the knot pusher.

Fig. 23.5 Vaginal closure for descent prevention

Vaginal closure for descent prevention
Te Linde adapted by van Herendael

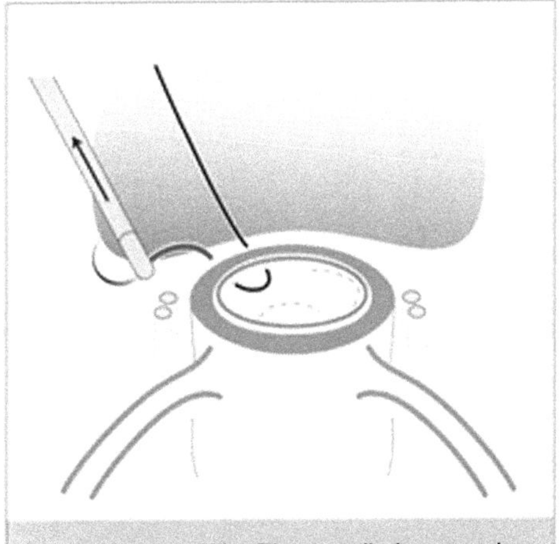

A vicryl suture CT 1 Plus needle is passed through the endopelvic fascia and 1 cm below the cephaled edge of the vaginal epithelium.

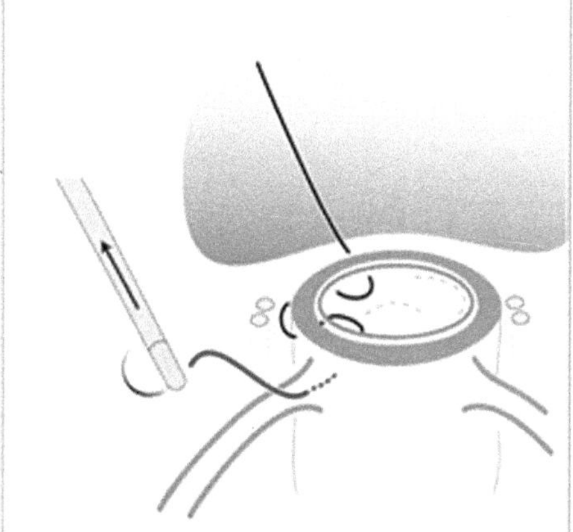

The needle is pushed from the vaginal lumen through the vaginal wall, passed between the uterine vessels (median part of the broad ligament) and brought back through the vaginal lumen.

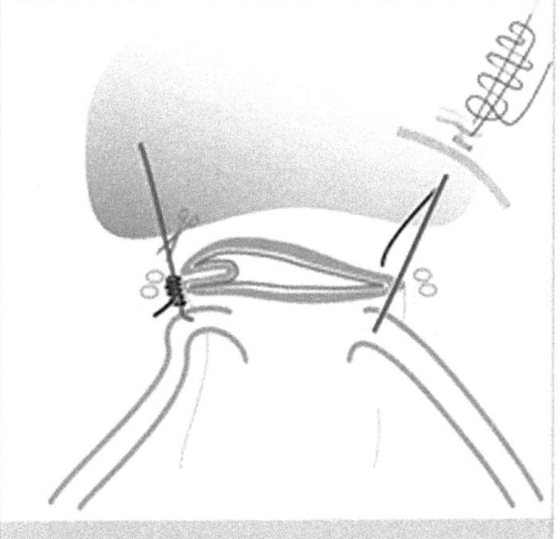

The sacrouterine lig. is identified before the suture is passed through. The needle is pushed from the vaginal lumen through the vaginal wall, rectovaginal septum and transpierces the sacrouterine ligament.

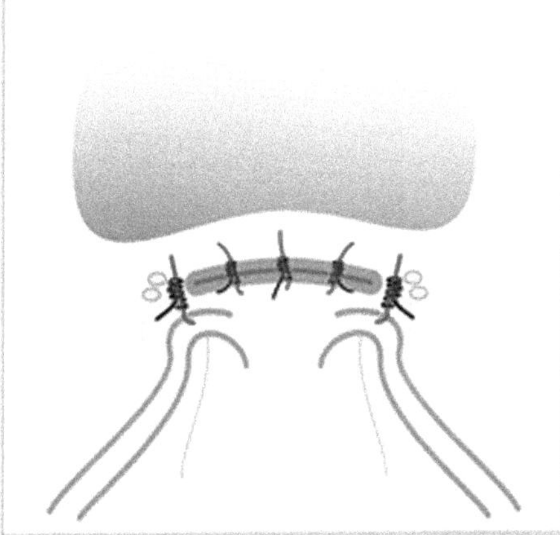

Closure of the vaginal vault with single stitches. Again, the stitch is drawn through the endopelvic fascia - vaginal wall - vaginal wall - rectovaginal septum.

Staples and Stapling Instruments

A safe way for vessel occlusion at laparoscopic hysterectomies is provided by "ENDO GIA" These ENDO GIA's are available with straight and curved tips. The unique Endo GIA™ Curved Tip Reload with Tri-Staple™ Technology of COVIDIEN is a stapler designed with a curved tip at the distal end of the anvil to provide enhanced visibility and maneuverability around target tissues and vessels.

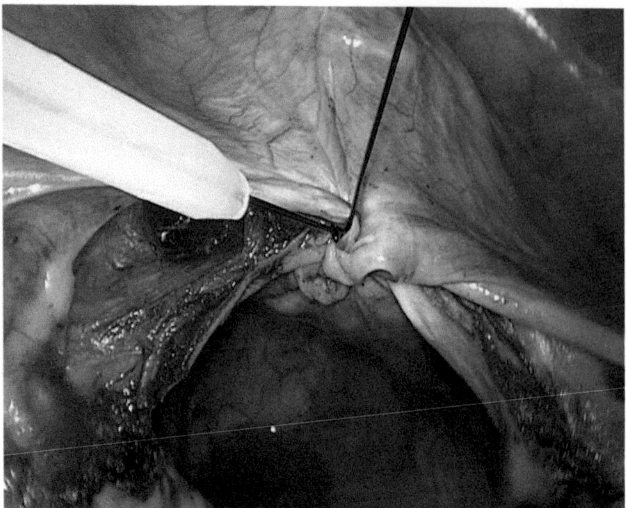

Fig. 23.6 After having formed the knot extracorporally, it is pushed down with the plastic knot pusher

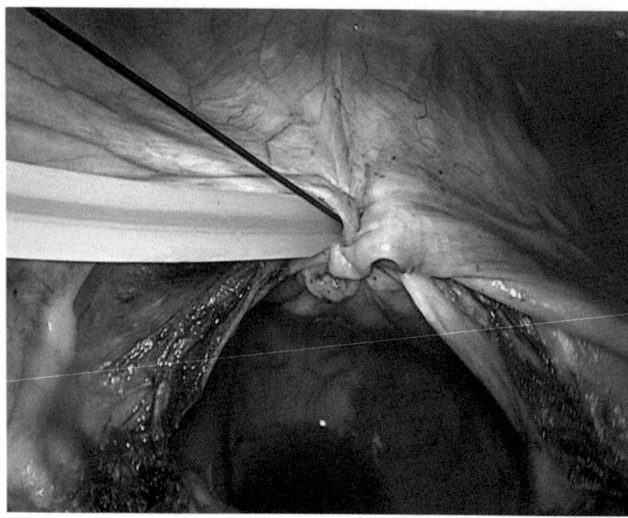

Fig. 23.7 To tighten the knot, the other end of the thread is held with some tension while the knot pusher is pressed onto the knot firmly

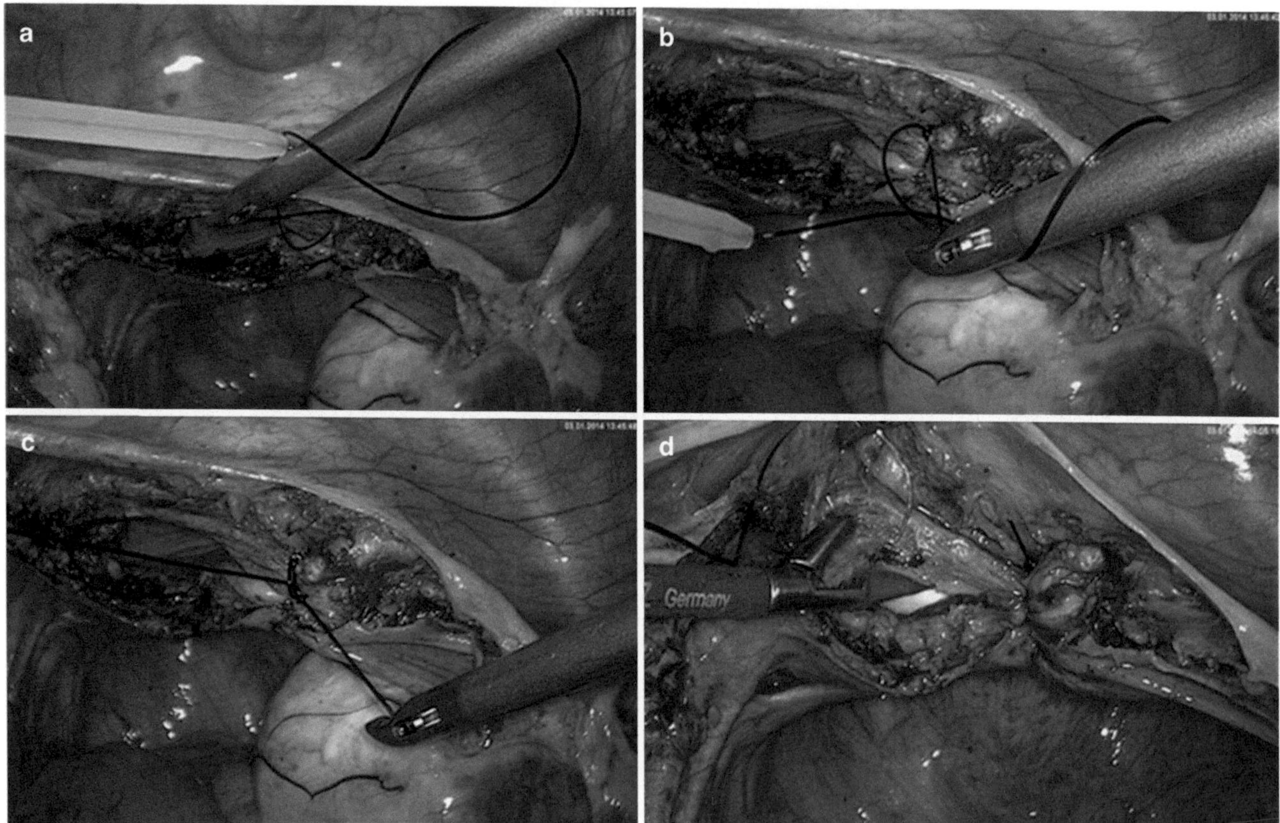

Fig. 23.8 Intracorporal knot to give final tension

Tissue Glues

A variety of adhesive substances can be applied locally during laparoscopic hysterectomy for hemostasis or wound closure. The main classes of tissue adhesives are cyanoacrylate glues, fibrin glue, and thrombin. Cyanoacrylate glues are widely used in GI endoscopy for control of bleeding from gastric varices and, to a much lesser degree, for hemostasis of bleeding peptic ulceration and for closure of fistulas and anastomotic leaks. Fibrin glue (fibrinogen and thrombin) and thrombin have been used extensively in all surgical disciplines for tissue adhesion; suture support; hemostasis; wound care; and the sealing of body cavities, including the subarachnoid space;

Biosurgical agents designed to promote tissue adhesion and hemostasis are being increasingly employed also in hysterectomies. Fibrin sealant is the most widely utilized biosurgical product. Gelatin matrix thrombin has proven to be an efficacious hemostatic agent. Bovine serum albumin-glutaraldehyde is a new promising tissue glue.

TachoSil of Takeda represents a new fibrine sealant with excellent thermostatic possibilities. It contains fibrinogen and thrombin as a dried coating on the surface of a collagen matrix. In contactwith physiological fluids, e.g. blood, lymph or physiological saline solution the components of the coating dissolve and partly diffuse into the wound surface. This is followed by the fibrinogen-thrombin reaction.

which initiates the last phase of physiological blood coagulation.

Instrument Systems and Apparatus for Laparoscopic Hysterectomies

Conventional Laparoscopy

Of the multitude of laparoscopic instruments known today for hysterectomies, we describe here only a selected few which are absolutely necessary and which should be available in duplicate or triplicate on the instrument trolley. Multiple use instruments for cutting, grasping, dissection, pushing, traction, coagulation, irrigation and suction are very helpful.

Instruments for Perforation

- The **Veress needle** is blindly introduced into the abdomen after lifting the anterior abdomen wall [20]. Trocars of 3 mm, 7 mm, 10 mm, 12 mm, 15 mm, 20 mm, 24 mm diameter are used for guiding the endoscopes and operative instruments, irrigation, coagulation and during employment of needle holders and morcellators.
- The simple **automatic flap valves** can leak because of soiling with blood or tissue particles. Therefore they are to be used for single use only. **Trumpet valves** are stable, but must be always opened and closed. They hinder the introduction of needles and thread.
- **Endoscopic lenses** must be frequently washed and removed because of soiling during the operation. Therefore, for such trocars we reluctantly use automatic valve, but prefer trumpet valve.
- **Primary trocars** can be inserted by the Z-puncture technique to prevent dehiscence of aponeurosis and late prolapse of the omentum. The decision, however, depends on the surgeon. We recommend conical and pyramidal trocars. Pyramidal trocars carry the advantage of a sharp cutting edge Optiview^R by Ethicon (Ethicon Endo-Surgery, Cincinnati, USA) , Visiport^R by Covidien (Mansfield, MA, USA) and XCel by Ethicon (Fig. 23.9) offer **insertion under vision**. At present, only 10–11 mm trocars are available through which the 10 mm laparoscope can be passed under direct vision.
- **Optical Veress needles** can be inserted under vision but one looks still through a plastic layer. The insertion under vision can be done below left costal margin also; a suitable trocar can inserted through the umbilicus under vision.
- The linear **expansion trocars** help controlled widening of a narrow canal by serial dilatation
- The **Endo-Tip** is the only trocar to be inserted under direct vision (Fig. 23.10)

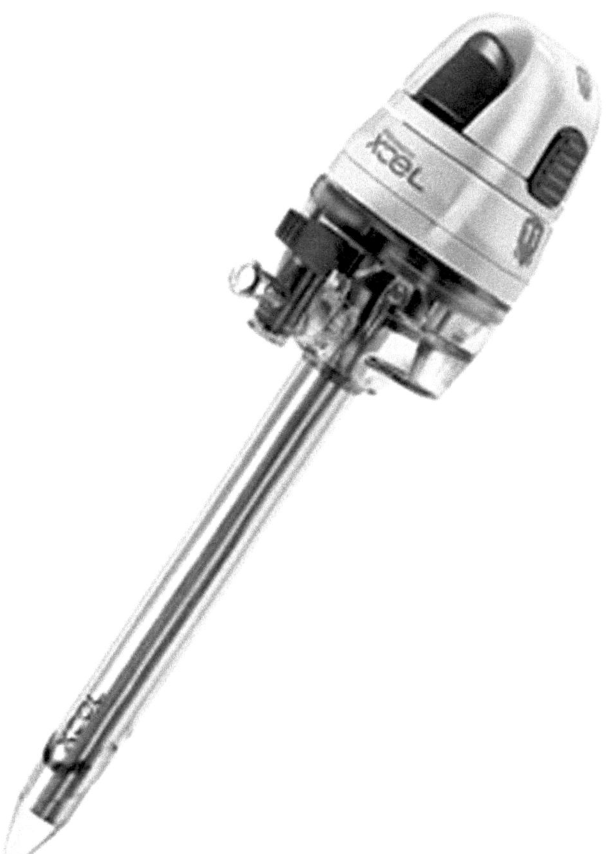

Fig. 23.9 XCeltrocar by Ethicon for entry under vision

Dilatation Instruments

It is possible to dilate up to 10 mm, 12 mm, 15 mm and 20 mm through an introduced rod and a suitable 5 mm threaded trocar.

Holding, Grasping Instruments and Screws

Various types of traumatic and atraumatic forceps are used as endoscopic grasping tools for laparoscopic hysterectomies. They are in 5–20 mm sizes. In 10 mm size we recommend the big toothed forceps and lymph node holding forceps to hold the tissues firmly. The 10 mm swab holding forceps are suitable for holding tissues lightly and for pushing. The 5 and 10 mm swab holders are used in tissue dissection. The 5 and 10 mm myoma screw may be used for traction of the uterus. The handles of the Robi instruments of the Karl Storz company are easier and more ergonomic to use than older roundgrip handle versions. Olympus offers with its HICURA line (Fig. 23.11) a new generation of laparoscopic hand instruments consisting of a wide range of product offerings of different lengths, shafts, handles, and jaws to accommodate surgeon's needs. The adapted handle design for grasping and dissection forceps has new ergonomic handles availbale in two sizes, developed with the goal to improve handling and safety of the instruments).

Cutting Instruments

Five millimeter curved scissors and the 5 mm and the 11 mm saw-toothed scissors as well as different micro knives with changeable disposable blades are available. Mostly, curved scissors are used, but round scissors with electric connection are frequently employed because of their extreme safety. The latter one is often used as a disposable instrument.

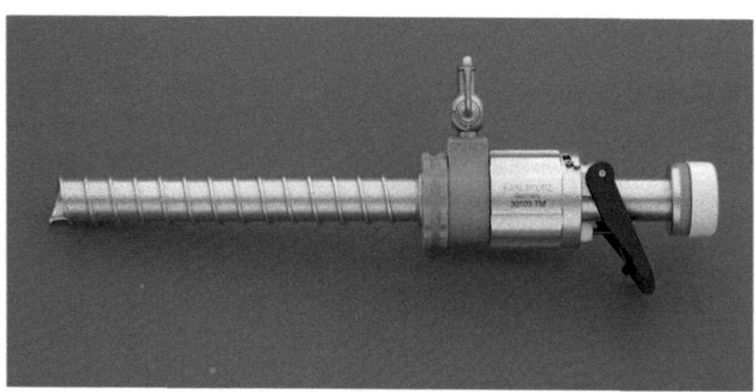

Fig. 23.10 Endo-tip by Ternamian (Karl Storz) for smooth laparoscopic entry under direct vision

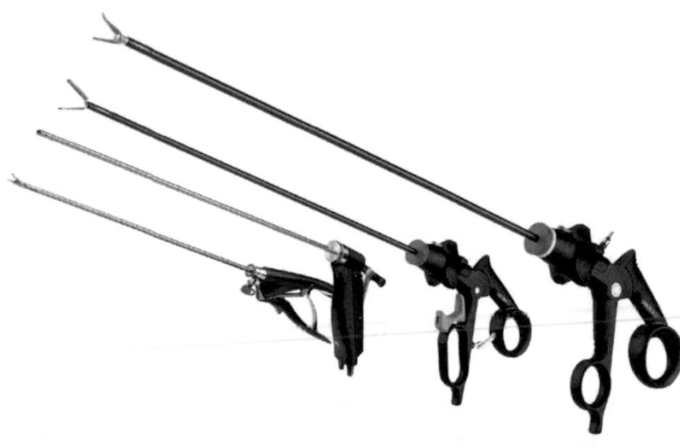

Fig. 23.11 HICURA line laparoscopic instruments

Suction and Irrigation Instruments

The suction irrigation devices of Karl Storz, Olympus, Wolf etc. are well known.

The suction cannula is used either with an open tip or with a perforated tip. Large volumes of fluids are aspirated with these suction irrigation cannulas (Fig. 23.12). They are set at an irrigation pressure of up to 300 mmHg and an aspiration force of up to 1 bar. The normal suction force is maximum 800 mbar; irrigation pressure is 300 mmHg. With extra-long (50 cm) suction irrigation tubes, it is possible to suck even under the dome of diaphragm from the pelvic region. Many disposable systems are also available.

Morcellation Instruments

The development of morcellation instruments was slow. In ovarian resection and enucleation of myoma, the tissue was cut with scissors and knives, depending on the size. The specimen can be removed either with big toothed forceps or a big sponge holding forceps directly through the 11 or 15 mm trocar with conical end. However, the so-called motor drive morcellators in 10 mm, 15 mm and 20 mm diameters are electrically powered and function well. The tissue is slowly cut electrically, nearly shaved from the surface, and pulled into the trocar sleeve. It is particularly suitable for horizontal operations as in vertical use a laceration of bowel or vessels can easily occur. Karl Storz produces the Steiner morcellator®, the Rotocut and a new development, the Sawalhe II Supercut morcellator, all with a tissue protection shield (Figs. 23.13 and 23.14). Single-use devices are available from various companies such as the PKS PlasmaSORD by Olympus. In bag morcellation is more and more being developed to prevent tissue particles being left in the abdominal cavity. Sarcomas should, of course, not be morcelllated and be recognized prior to hysterectomy and morcellation.

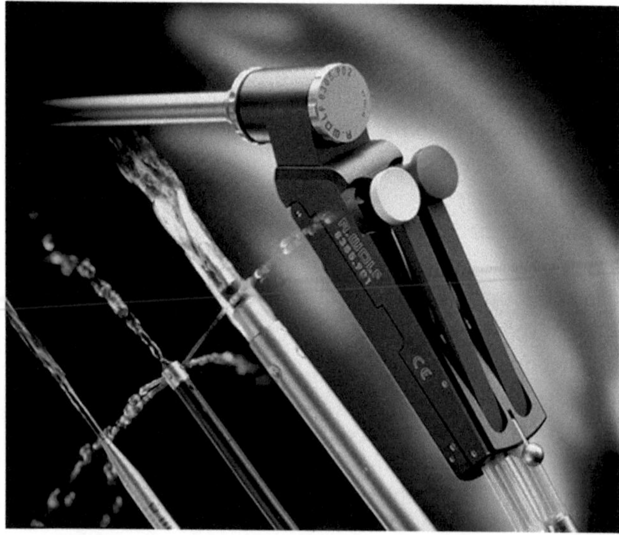

Fig. 23.12 Suction irrigation system (R. Wolf, Knittlingen, Germany)

Many companies have disposable morcellators. The WISAP electric morcellator was the first on the international market. Alternatively, the surgical specimen from the abdominal cavity is put in an endobag (small plastic bags) with forceps. Morcellation is only advised at present for benign specimens. However, I foresee the transformation of fibroid-like material into powder, which can then be aspirated and examined by the molecular geneticist- pathologist for malignancy. In case of uterine tissue this would mean to detect mutations in these carcinosarcomas that are found in about 1–4 per thousand in myomas. Of course any hysterectomy is preceded by careful imaging with ultrasound and often MRI, where bulky polyploid masses with heterogeneous appearance and increased vascularity, lacking calcifications would lead the surgeon to avoid morcellation.

However, after the Boston case of a non-recognition of a sarcoma at morcellation, was published over all public media everyone became more careful not to spread tissue at morcellation. Morcellation in bags became available and some companies have retracted their morcellation devices.

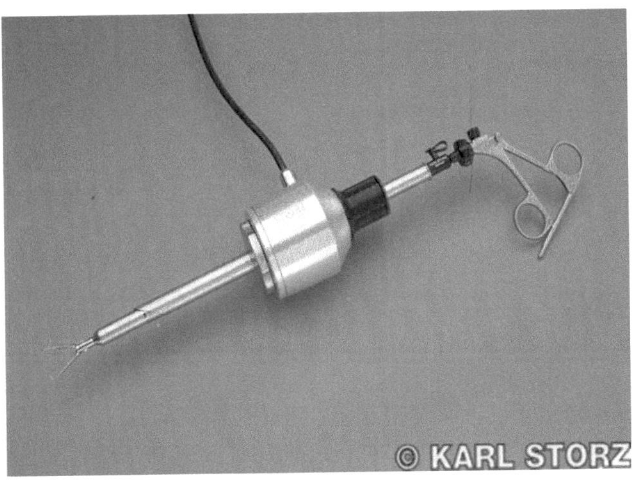

Fig. 23.13 ROTOCUT GI (Karl Storz), morcellation tool with protectivshield, available in 2 sizes (12 and 15 mm)

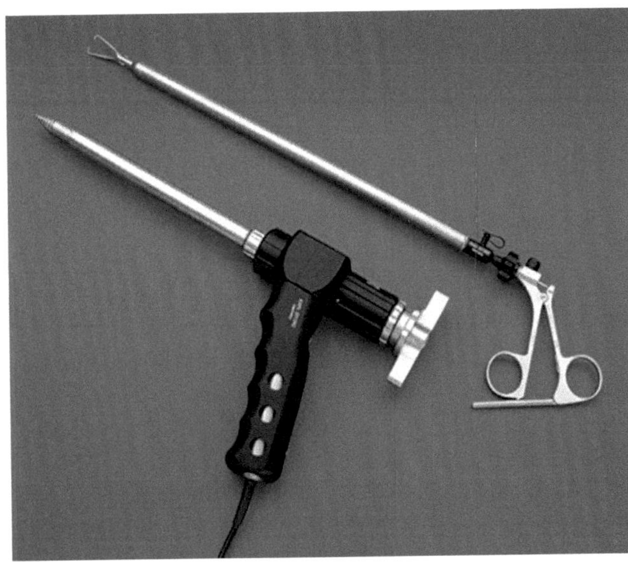

Fig. 23.14 SAWALHE II SUPERCUT Morcellator (Karl Storz)

Instruments for Hemostasis

Instruments for tying the blood vessels such as the Roeder loop, the endoligature or the endosutures with extra or intracorporeal knotting are widely known. Needle holders for straight, curved or Ski needles must be available in different variations.

For hemostasis, endocoagulation, heat denaturation at 100–120 °C, bipolar coagulation in various forms (see section on energy sources in this chapter) and monopolar needle, melting hook, high frequency scissors or other instruments are suitable [21]. For localized ischemia a vasopressin derivative in a dilution of 1–100 is injected subcapsular with an applicator.

Gynaecologists prefer suturing and coagulation devices. However, clips and stapling devices, which are more frequently used by general surgeons, are also used for fixing meshes, for pelvic floor surgery, lymphadenectomy and hysterectomy in our field. Both Ethicon, a Johnson & Johnson company (New Bunswick, NJ, USA), and Covidien have fascinating devices on the market. Let me just mention here Covidien's new Endo Clip Applicator III (5 mm) with easy to be situated clips and a digital clip counter as well as the Ultra Handle Group (Fig. 23.15a, b) and the Endo GIA™ Stapler (Fig. 23.16).

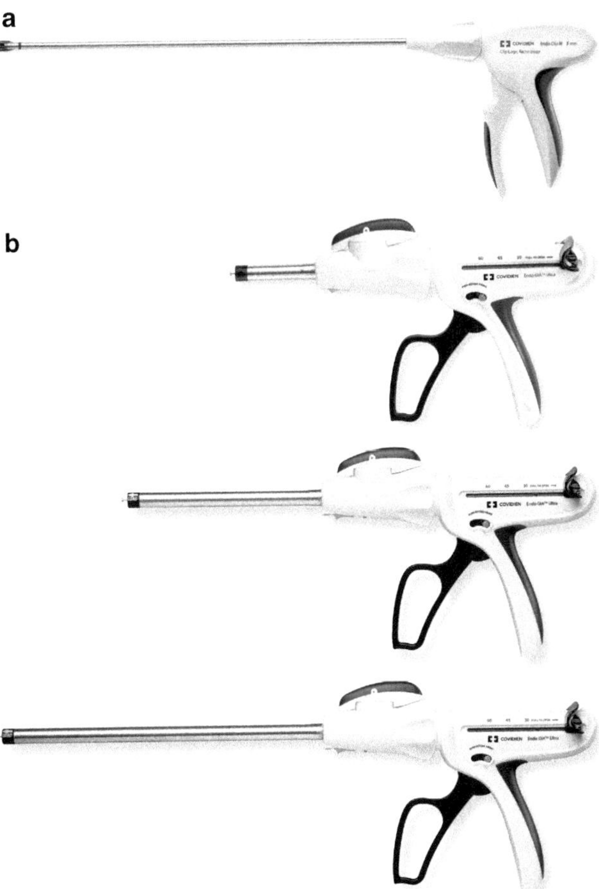

Fig. 23.15 (**a**) Endo-Clip (Covidien) (**b**) Handle Group (Covidien)

Endo GIA™ Reloads with Tri-Staple™ Technology

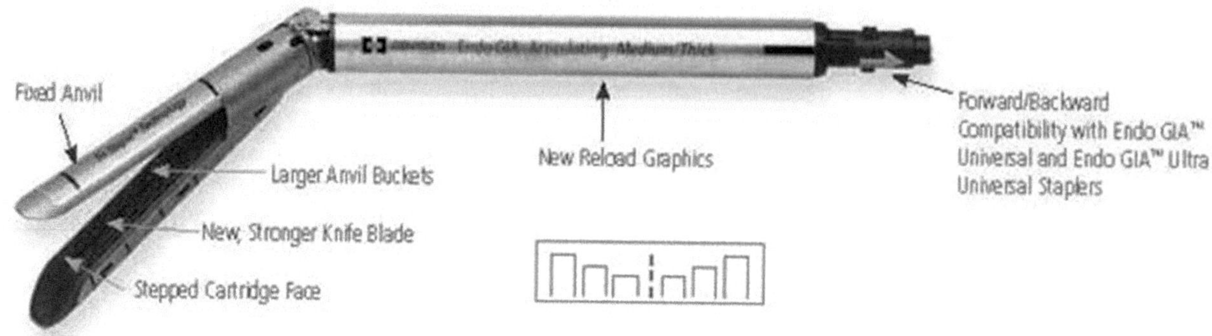

Varied-height Staples and Stepped Cartridge Face

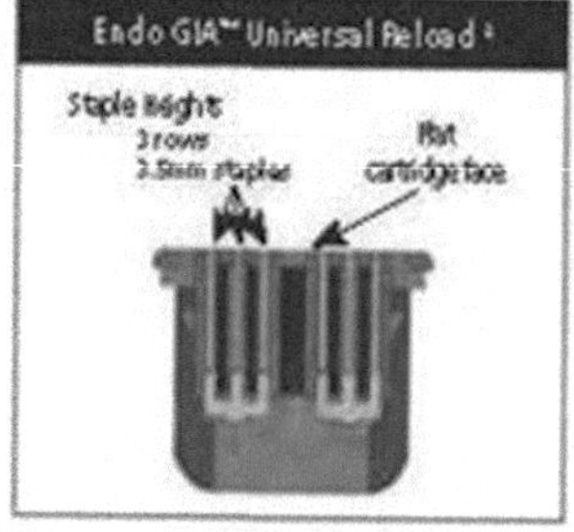

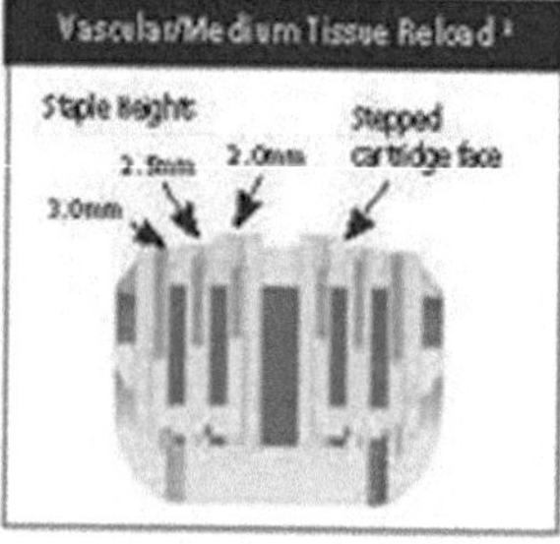

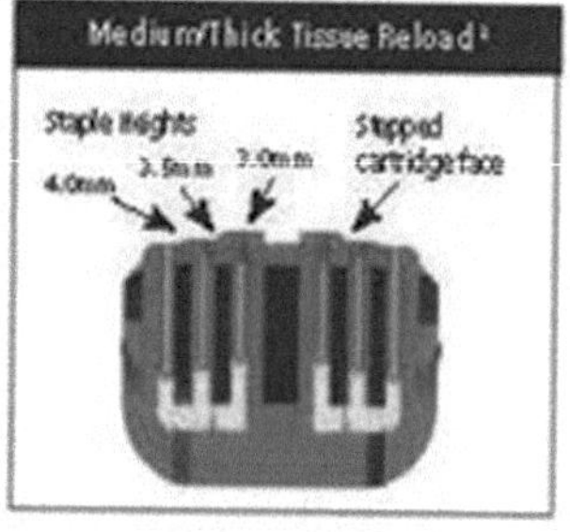

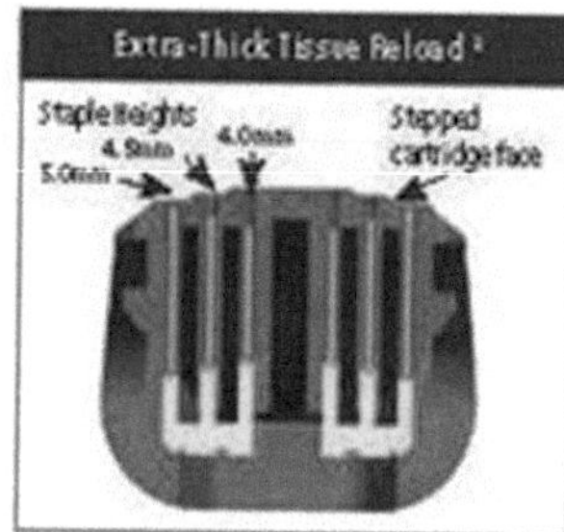

Products depicted are not actual size.

Fig. 23.16 Endo GIA™ Reloads with Tri-Staple™ Technology (Covidien)

Instruments for Clamping Large Vessels, Emergency Needle

Emergency instruments and usual clamps used in routine gynecological operations should not be used for clamping the vessels. Vascular clamps must be readily available. Large vessel injury must be immediately explored by laparotomy and the bleeding vessel clamped. If a vessel in the anterior abdominal wall is injured (epigastric artery), it is advisable to ligate it at an appropriate place with a large emergency needle.

Instruments for Drainage

The Robinson drainage is suitable for abdominal drainage. It works on a gravity basis and as a rule can be left in situ over 24 h.

Instruments for Uterine Manipulation

Vacuum intracervical probes in the standard three sizes allow only partial movement of the uterus and facilitate tubal chrompertubation.

Various instruments for intra uterine manipulation make it possible to move the uterus in side-to-side, ante and retroflexion as well as rotation movements and sometimes allow the possibility of chromopertubation. Uterine manipulation is required in endometriosis of the pouch of Douglas, for hysterectomies, in bladder dome endometriosis and for enucleation of myoma. The ACE (Abdominal Cavity Expander) serves to elevate the anterior abdominal wall in cases with adhesions. Further versions of this principle are used in the gasless laparoscopy, e.g. as Laparolift®.

The Hohl, the Mangeshikar and the Donnez intra–uterine manipulators or mobilizers as well as the Konincxk uterine twister are all produced by Karl Storz and have a cup with a well palpable and visible border to visualize the resection level between vagina and cervix for all cases of TLH (Total Laparoscopic Hysterectomy) (Fig. 23.17). This facilitates the intracervical approach of TLH; however, they are not to be used for the extracervical approach and in oncologic cases of hysterectomy. Many companies have disposable manipulators.

Lenses and Endoscopes

Scopes are available in rigid and flexible systems (Figs. 23.18 and 23.19). The rigid system is based on Hopkins's experience with a rod lens system, which results in good resolution and depth of focus ratio [22]. Flexible endoscopes are based on the use of optical fibre bundles. The rigid laparoscopes are in 3–11 mm sizes, e.g. the arthroscope with a 14° angle. Most of the rigid endoscopes are directly connected to the telescope through the camera coupling system. The picture is enlarged so that it looks even bigger on the monitor. In flexible endoscopes, the bundle of fibres is also enlarged. The standard laparoscopes are rigid instruments

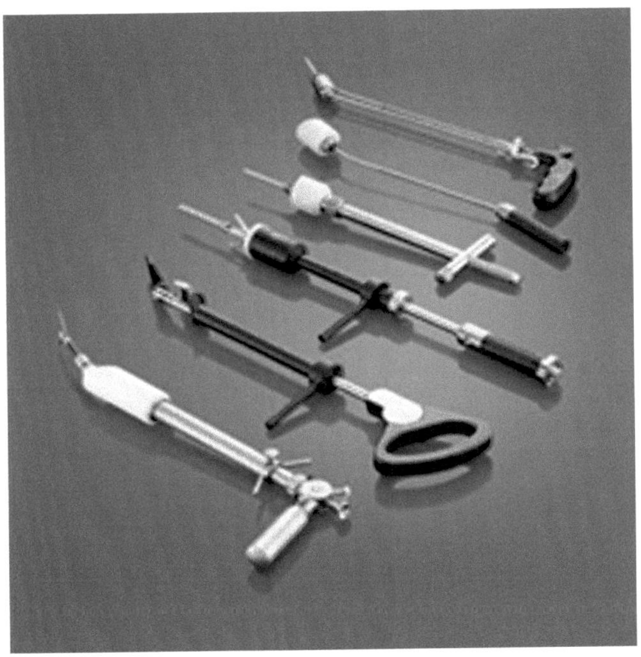

Fig. 23.17 Intrauterine manipulators produced by Karl Storz according to Koninckx, Clermont-Ferrand, Mangeshikar, Hohl, Donnez and Tintara

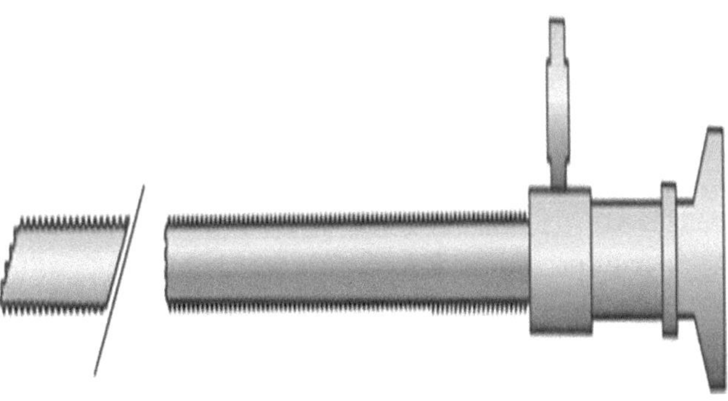

Fig. 23.18 Rigid standard laparoscope (10 mm) with 0° and 30° optic

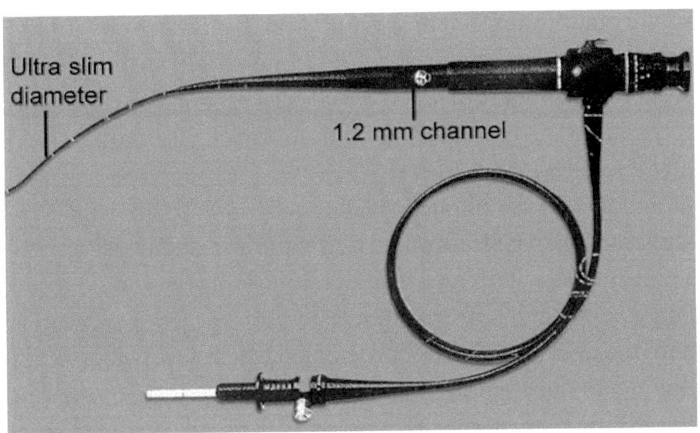

Fig. 23.19 Flexible endoscope

with a 0° lens. The 30° lens has the advantage of a wide panoramic view. With the Endo-Cameleon (Karl Storz) a 120° panoramic view is possible (Fig. 23.1).

Each camera has two components: head and control. A 35 mm coupling system yields a much more enlarged picture than a 28 mm coupler. A direct coupling transmits the picture directly to the camera.

Olympus offers different endoscopes with the chip on the tip of the optic the observation light passes through fewer lenses than on a rigid scope. This allows brighter and sharper images than when the camera is attached to the head of the optic. The ENDOEYE concept includes a range of 5 mm and 10 mmm scopes with advanced optical design that expands the clinical possibilities laparoscopic surgery. The images are smooth and clear, with reproduction so accurate that details and colours remain sharp and true to life. The ENDOEYE FLEX has a flexible tip which can be bend up to 100° in four directions. This means the relevant organs and tissues can be thoroughly examined head-on, from above and from behind (Fig. 23.20).

Energy Systems for Laparoscopic Subtotal, Total and Radical hysterectomies (Electrosurgery and Thermofusion)

Electro section, i.e. cutting of tissue between the active electrode and the tissue where an electrical arc is generated, takes place above 200 °C. During coagulation and desiccation the tissue is heated slowly. It results in denaturation, evaporation of water and secondary hemostasis. The argon beam coagulator is a monopolar electrosurgical instrument. In principle, non-combustible argon gas (4 L/min) across an electrode cannula acts as a bridge for electrical current to burn the tissue superficially (up to 5 mm depth) [23]. As the gas is easier to ionize than air, electrical arcs develop up to 1 cm above the tissue surface. In monopolar electrosurgery, high-density current is used at the active electrode that is conducted to the patient on touching. In bipolar electro surgery, two small electrodes of same size are used which lie close to each other and function as active passive electrodes.

While the use of thermal hemostasis goes back to the glowing iron, according to Paquelin, the development of safe high frequency current techniques took 40 years. The application of the laser technique, ultrasonic cutting and coagulation techniques and the local thermal effects, such as thermocoagulation, take place in the range of 80–120 °C. Suturing and clip techniques are handled in next chapter.

We differentiate between fulguration and coagulation in high frequency hemostasis. In fulguration, electromagnetic oscillations across an air bridge produce radio frequency between the tip of the electrode and the surface of the organ, i.e. they come in direct contact. The generated heat is limited to tissue surface, i.e. the area visible through the scope. By coagulation we mean the heating of the tissues until intracellular water boils under the influence of high frequency current.

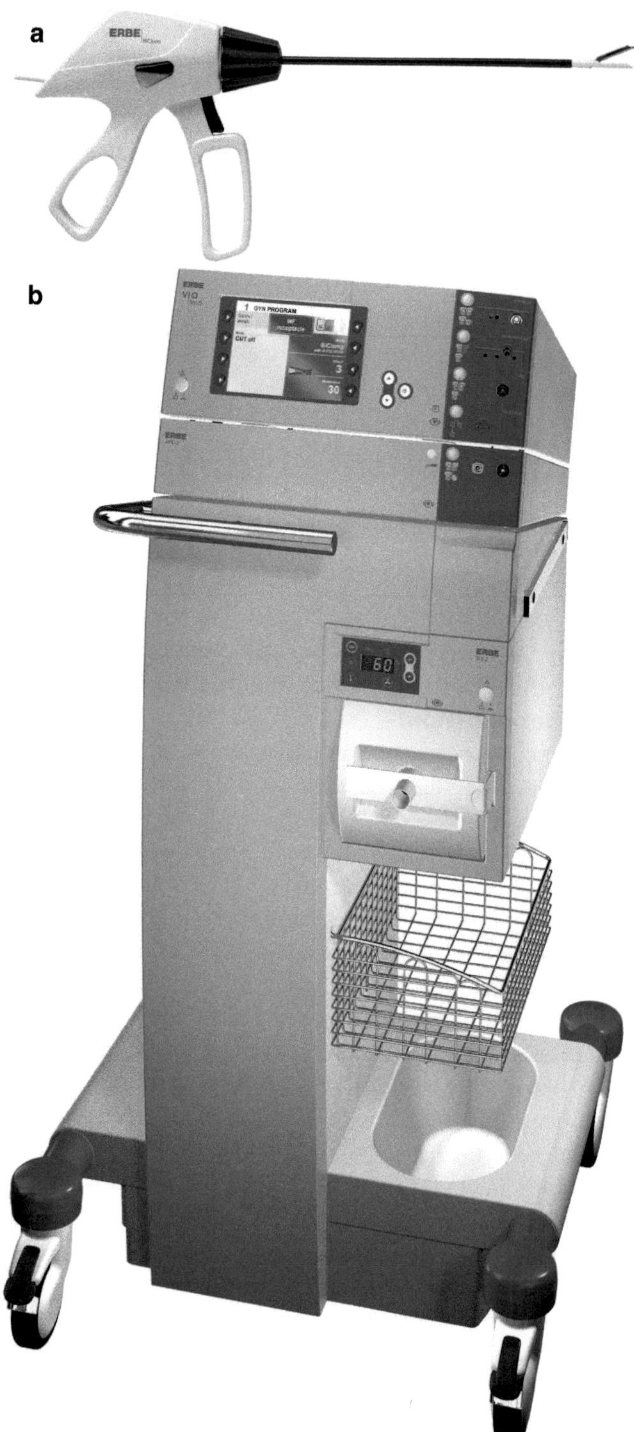

Fig. 23.20 (**a**) EndoEYE video laparoscopes (Olympus) as Endoeyerigid (**b**) EndoEye video laparoscopes (Olympus) as Endoeyeflex

In addition to the technique used for fulguration and for coagulation, the most important technique in medicine and endoscopic surgery is the **electrotomy,** the cutting of tissue with the so-called electrical knife or the electrical loop.

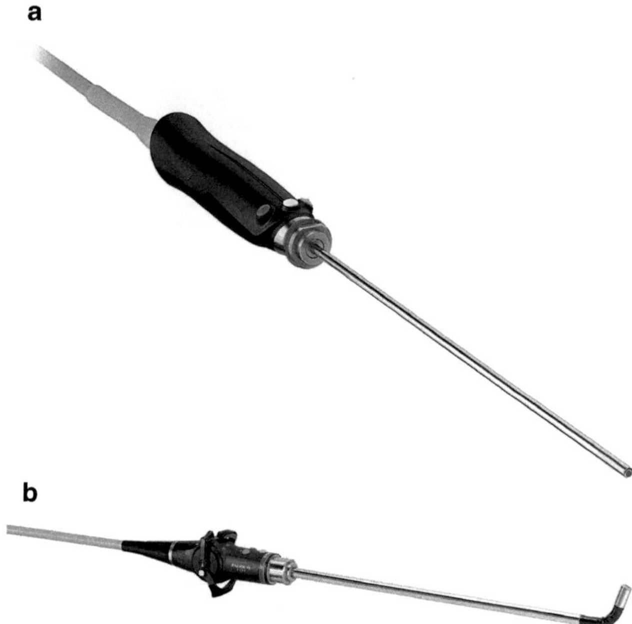

Fig. 23.21 (**a**) BiCision coagulation and cutting forceps (Erbe) (**b**) Erbe Gynaecological Workstation VIO 300 D

At present even with high frequency instruments there is no blind and uncontrolled burning because of the electrical system control. Therefore, we use monopolar current for cutting and bipolar instruments when coagulation is required before cutting big vessels in endoscopic surgery. Most of the systems have an autostop, so that only the required tissue is denatured. It is not set for a very big coagulation zone. Bi-Clamp for vaginal and open surgery and BiCision (Fig. 23.21a) for laparoscopic surgery are the thermofusion devices of Erbe Elektromedizin GmbH (Tübingen, Germany). Their effect is electronically controlled thermofusion and the mechanical separation of tissue.

The electrocoagulation system of Erbe (Fig. 23.21) uses an additional argon beamer, controlled by a foot switch, which facilitates linear coagulation by switching on the argon gas. This gynecological workstation with the high frequency module VIO 300 D can be connected to any monopolar or bipolar coagulation device. It contains several modules, such as the argon plasma coagulation (APC 2) and the smoke plume evacuator (IES 2). The Erbe electro surgical unit (ESU) has a color monitor display that provides the user with an on-screen tutorial as well as settings and operational information. The unit has various cutting and coagulation modes with defined effect levels to provide the physician flexibility in interventional applications (i.e. its ability to generate HF current). The system has automatic start and stop features. The equipment is programmable and various accessories (e.g. footswitches, hand instruments, etc.) as well as modes may be assigned to perform specific functions. Upon activation, the energy

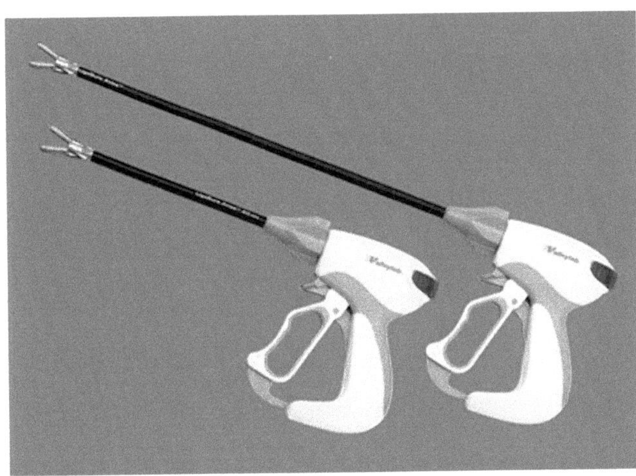

Fig. 23.22 LigaSure (Covidien), bipolar vessel sealing system, 10 mm (Atlas) and 5 mm

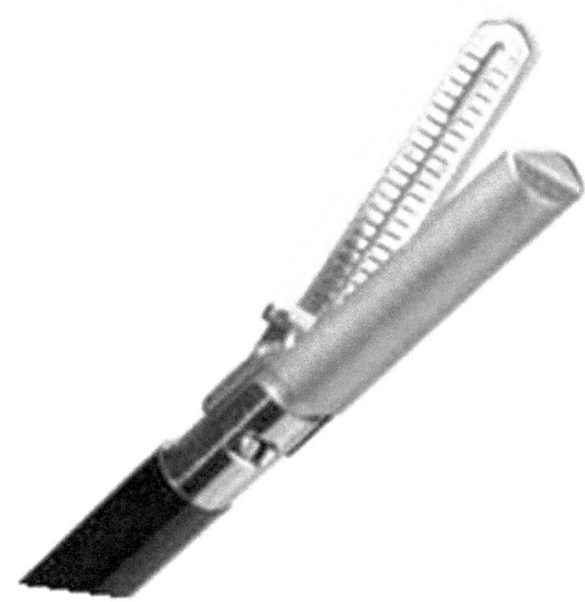

Fig. 23.23 LigaSure (Covidien) jaw providing a combination of pressure and energy to create vessel fusion

delivered (in watts) from the ESU to the tissue is displayed on the display screen.

Bipolar vessel sealing, also described as thermofusion, combined with pressure between the branches of the instruments, is a new, easy to use technique that has been picked up by many companies in the production of disposable instruments with integrated cutting devices such as LigaSure (Covidien) (Figs. 23.22 and 23.23).

The BOWA ARC 400 electrosurgical unit is a multifunctional generator for all surgical specialities. Two monopolar and three bipolar instruments can be used with the generator, and, ARC 400 offers specific setting for gynaecology as for every other supported speciality. Monopolar and bipolar resections for hysteroscopic treatments:

- Laparoscopic interventions

LIGATION and Coagulation: Permanent sealing of vessels and tissue bundles with BOWA LIGATION instruments for laparoscopic procedures with BOWA ERGO 310D and NightKNIFE instruments and open surgical applications with BOWA TissueSeal PLUS.

The Nightknife (BOWA-electronic GmbH, Gomaringen, Germany) (Fig. 23.24) is a bipolar vessel sealing device. The instrument incorporates atraumatic tips for secure dissecting and sealing. The integrated cutting system saves changing instruments for tissue separation. The Ergo 310 D knife 5 mm in diameter integrates the sealing and cutting function likewise

- A special mode for BOWA MetraLOOP, a special laparoscopic instrument for the fast and secure removal of the uterus (LSH surgeries). SimCoag mode offers the possibility for two surgeons to activate monopolar or bipolar instruments simultaneously.
- In combination with the ARC PLUS argon unit, electrosurgical system offers Argon plasma coagulation and argon enhanced cutting. The ionized Argon beam offers homogeneous superficial coagulations which is perfectly suitable for e.g. endometriosis treatments.

To support the surgeon's work, the ARC 400 has a very user-friendly design concept.

- COMFORT instruments are automatically detected during insertion by the Plug'n Cut COMFORT function of the generator. The specific settings of the instrument are preselected and the operation can be carried out immediately.
- The intuitive touch display makes settings easy and the layout of the interface allows the user to always know which socket is being set at the moment.
- The EASY neutral electrode monitoring system increases patient safety in monopolar applications by deactivation and alarm in case of insufficient contact between the neutral electrode and the patient.

Additionally, the system can be equipped with the SHE SHA smoke evacuation system, which helps to protect health of the OR-team by evacuating surgical smoke.

The PKS HALO Cutting Forceps by Olympus are ergonomically designed forceps that allow easy operator use, serrated jaws enable strong grasping, better dissecting, reliable coagulation and cutting. PK Technology is an impedance feedback controlled, advanced bipolar vessel

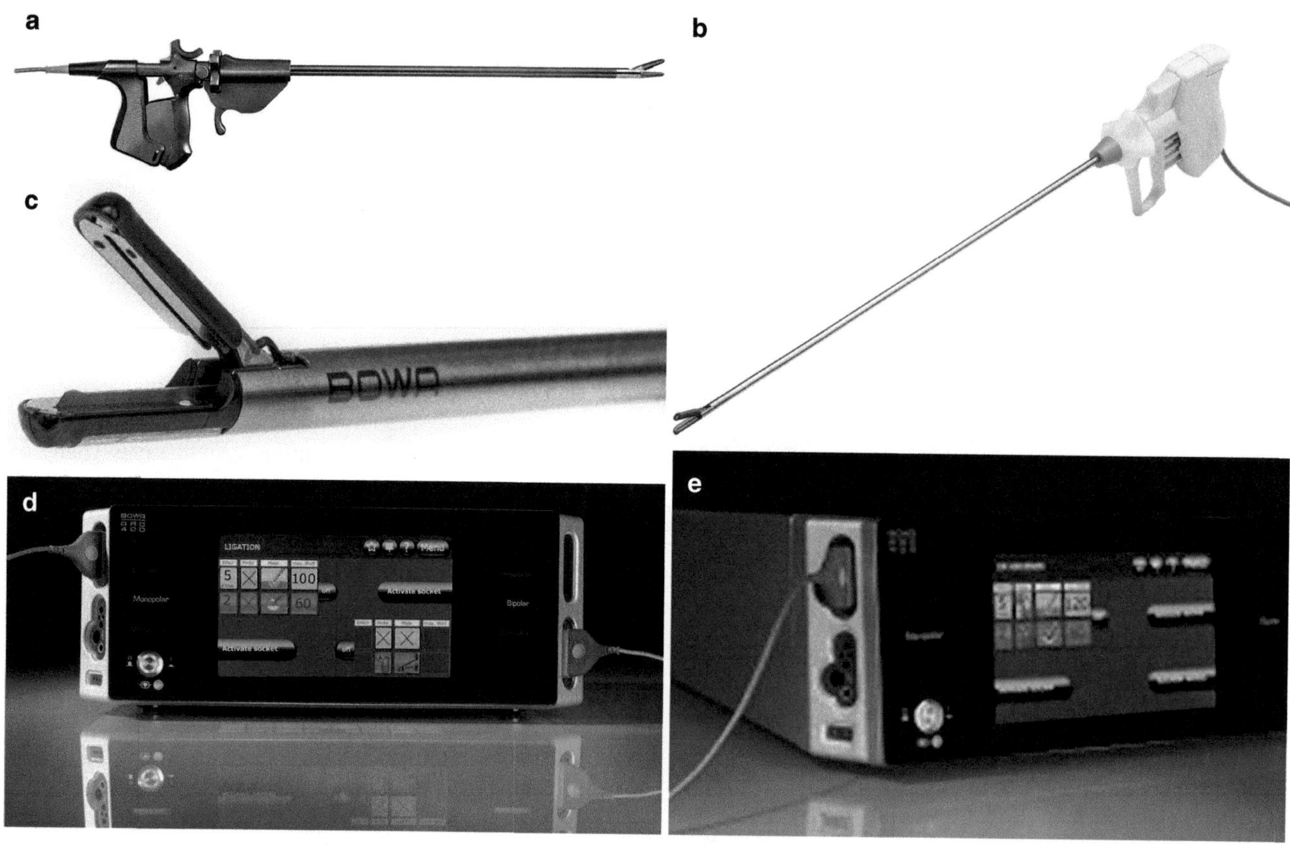

Fig. 23.24 Nightknife (BOWA-electronic) in 5 and 10 mm versions (**a**)Ergo 310 D knife, (**b**) Ergo 310 D, (**c**) open jaws, (**d**) ARC 400 Gynecology/ligation monitor, (**e**) ARC 400 Gynecology plugncut.

sealing system that allows tissue and device tip to cool during the 'energy off' phase, minimizing sticking and charring (Fig. 23.25).

By means of the smart electrode technology, the ENSEAL sealing instrument (Ethicon Endo-Surgery,) permits simultaneous sealing and the possibility of tissue separation, including vessels up to 7 mm (Fig. 23.26). The tip of the instrument has either a 5 mm round tip or a 3 mm slightly curved tip enabling tissue preparation and sealing.

Laser

Laser beam is often described as "light that heals." Laser is acronym for **L**ight **A**mplification by **S**timulated **E**mission of **R**adiation. Fox established the first surgical laser in 1960. Bruhat and his colleagues in 1979 and Tadir and colleagues in 1996 introduced CO_2 laser in laparoscopy. Today, there are enthusiasts of laser surgery and enthusiasts of electro surgery. Light energy is amplified to generate increased coherent electromagnetic radiation. Here we mention the three forms of laser used in endoscopic surgery:

- CO_2-laser
- Nd: YAG-laser
- KTP-lasers

The Neodymium: Yttrium-Aluminium-Garnet (Nd: YAG-) laser, the Argon laser and KTP- (Potassium-Titanium-phosphate-) laser are used for cutting and coagulation. All the tissue effects are produced because of the continuous or pulsing thermodynamic conversion of light in thermal energy. Because of the 15° refraction of the laser beam after arising from the fiber bundle, the effect can be achieved only up to 2 cm from the tip of the fibers. In 1996 Wallwiener et al. introduced laser treatment in the reproductive surgery [24].

Harmonic Scalpel – Ultrasonic Energy

The harmonic scalpel is an ultrasonically activated laparoscopic instrument that uses mechanical energy to cut and coagulate tissues. Today, the harmonic scalpel can be used as 5–10 mm cutting blades and scissors. Activation of the titanium blade takes place by a piezoelectric crystal with a frequency of 55,500/s in the hand set. The cutting and coagulation effects are comparable to that of the CO_2-laser [25]. The lateral thermal damage is less than by high frequency coagulation. Burning and carbonization of tissues are not observed.

The advantages of ultrasound energy in surgical endoscopic instruments produced by Ethicon Endo-Surgery

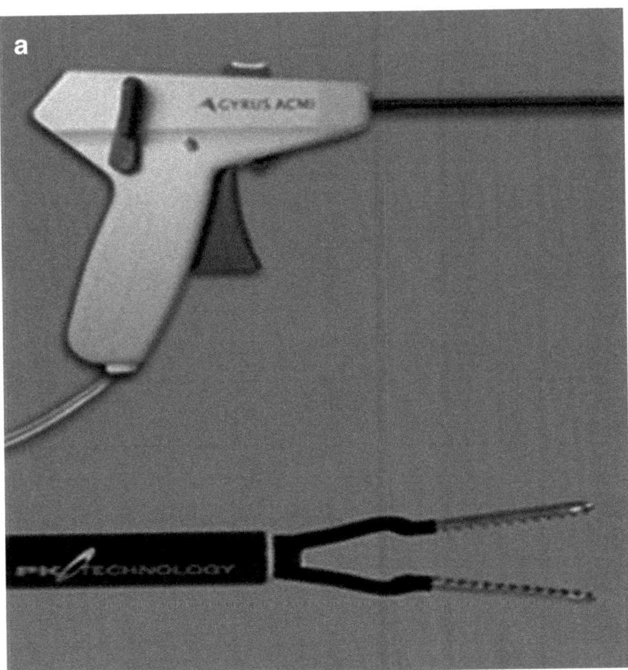

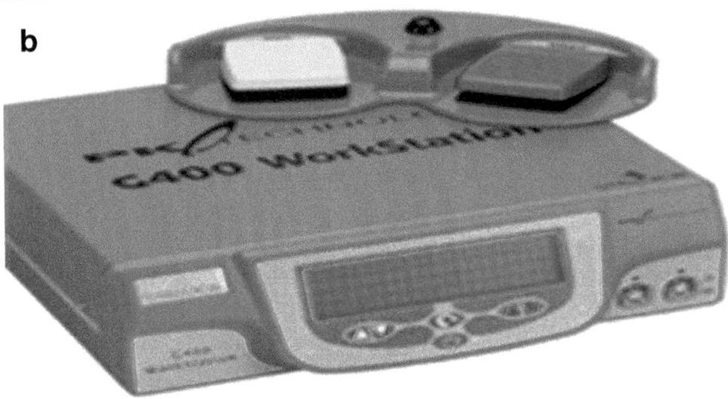

Fig. 23.25 (**a**) Gyrus PK integrated vessel sealing and cutting system (Olympus) (**b**) Gyrus PK control unit (Olympus)

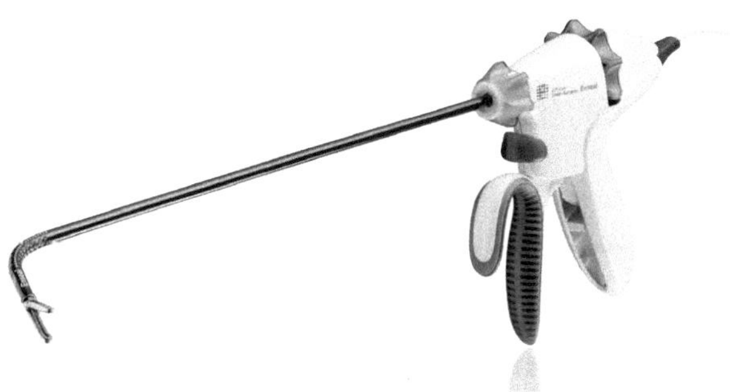

Fig. 23.26 ENSEAL sealing instrument (Ethicon Endo-Surgery)

and Olympus are well known today and highly appreciated. As an example let us focus on the harmonic ace of Ethicon (Fig. 23.27) which with its specific control unit (Fig. 23.28) allows a shorter and a longer effect of sealing and cutting. The mechanical energy works with low temperatures, small lateral damage and minimal desiccation of the tissue.

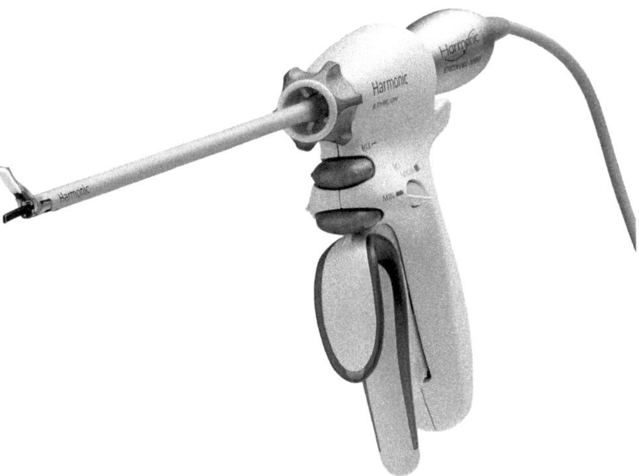

Fig. 23.27 Harmonic Ace forceps (Ethicon)

The THUNDERBEAT by Olympus is the world's first integrated hand instrument that delivers the benefits of both advanced bipolar and ultrasonic energy in a single device. This unique integration of energy modalities combines proven safety of secure haemostasis from advanced bipolar energy with the speed and precision of ultrasonic dissection (Fig. 23.29).

The different harmonic instruments on the market today, such as harmonic shears, forceps and cutting rings, are applied for adhesiolysis as well as any type of adenexectomy, ovarectomy and hysterectomy. It remains up to the surgeon whether he uses them in combination with other sealing instruments or bipolar coagulation.

Summary of Specific Instruments to Be Used in Total Laparoscopic Hysterectomies (TLH)

All the above mentioned instruments are excellent tools to be used for TLH. There are 2 ways of applying traction and contra-traction for the operative field either by using an intrauterine manipulator in uteri up to a certain size or using traction with a myoma screw, introduced from the lateral ports, a principle widely applied in "Radical hysterectomies" in cases of malignancies. The absolutely necessary instruments for TLH, with or without adnexectomies are detailed in Fig. 23.30.

Summary of Specific Instruments to Be Used in Subtotal Hysterectomies (SLH)

Subtotal hysterectomy, as CISH (Classic Intrafascial Supracervical Hysterectomy) or LSH (Laparoscopic Assisted Supracervical Hysterectomy), is facilitated by the use of an electric loop produced by LiNA Medical ApS, Glostrup,

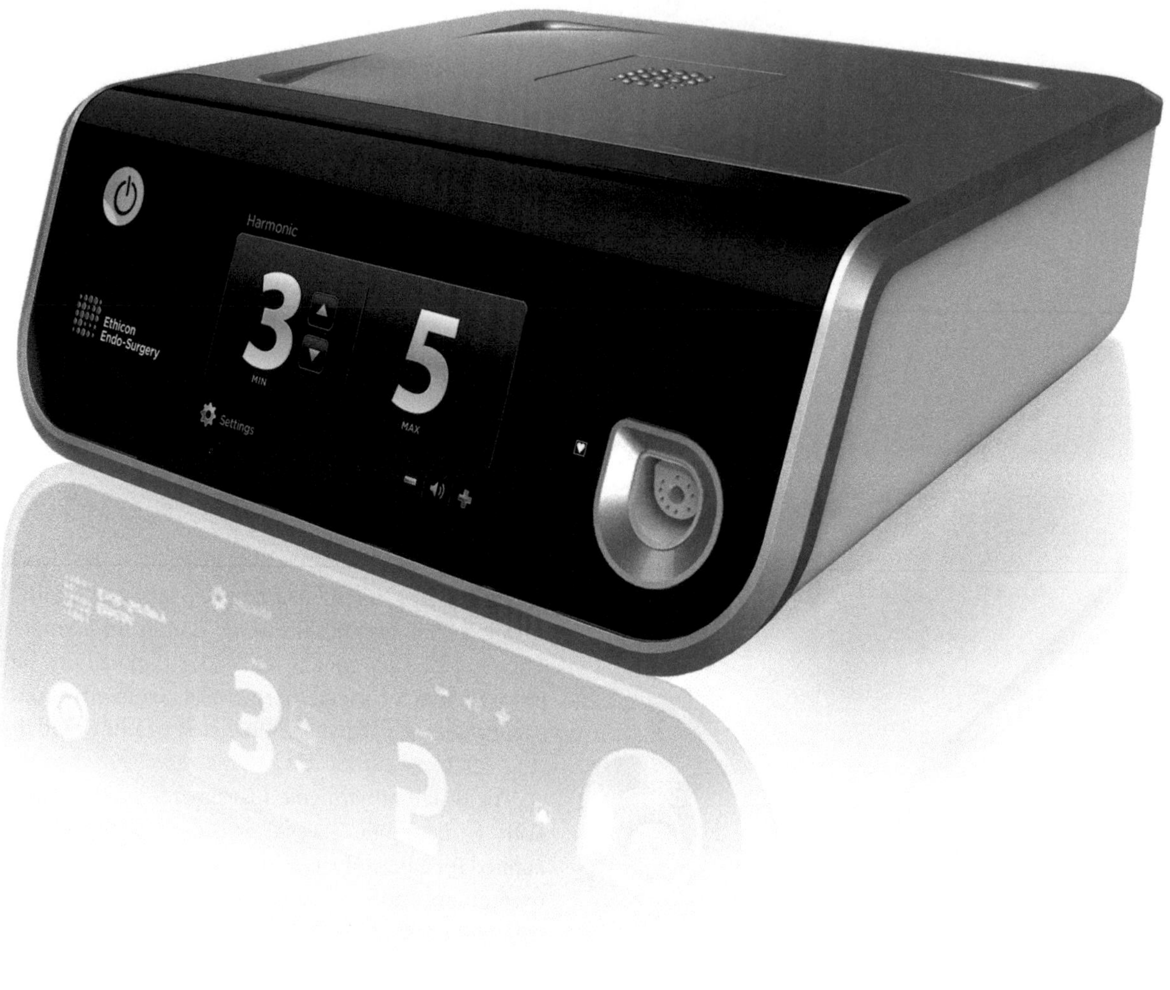

Fig. 23.28 Harmonic Ace control unit (Ethicon)

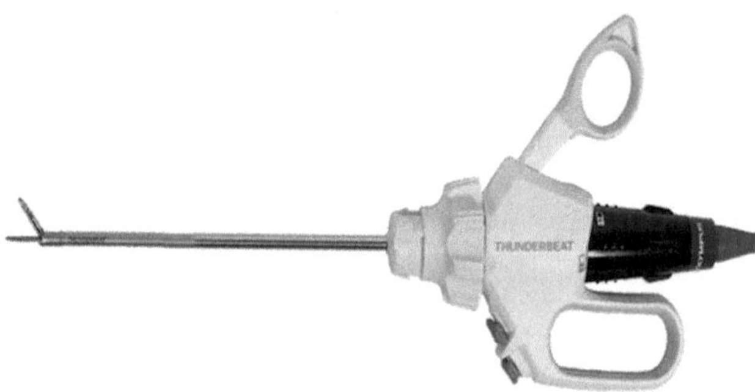

Fig. 23.29 Thunderbeat (Olmypus)

Denmark (Fig. 23.31) as the LiNA Loop and the Storz Loop. With this electric cutting look the cervix is separated from the uterine body. It is of utmost importance not to touch any bowel loops during the activation of the cutting part of the loop.

The PKS BiLL by Olympus is currently the only available bipolar loop for more safety for your patients and fast cutting of the uterus during LSH procedures. With immediate ignition and dry and fast cutting, the PKS BiLL allows for shorter procedure times. The big diamond-shaped loop opens up automatically in the abdomen and is easy and convenient for the surgeon to place even in enlarged uteri (Fig. 23.32). Figure 23.33 details the most necessary instruments for SLH today.

Micro Endoscopy

By rigorously following the concept of minimally invasive access for hysteroscopy and laparoscopy through advances in instrument designing, today optic systems measuring only about 1.8–2 mm including the trocar surrounding

Fig. 23.30 Instrument set for Total Laparoscopic Hysterectomy (TLH)

TLH – Tools

- 1 Trocar 11-5 mm
- 1-2 VERSAPORT* 12-5 mm Trocars (left and right side)
- 1 Bipolare Instrument 5mm or EnSeal or LigaSure
- 1 Scissor 5 mm
- 1 Grasper 10mm (huge uterus)
- Uterus manipulator (Hohl)
- 1 monopolar hook 5 mm
- 1 suture
- 1 needle holder

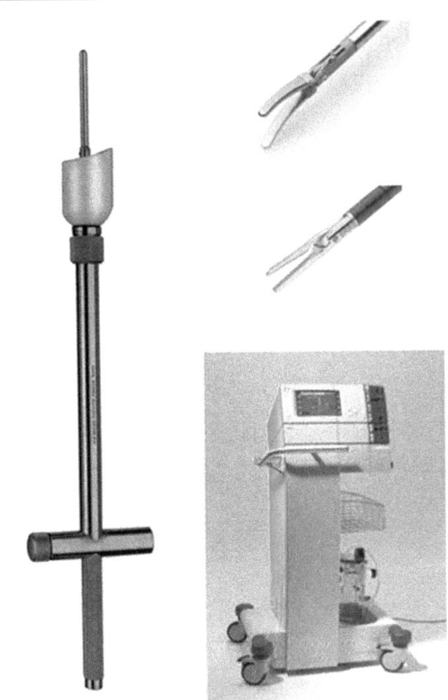

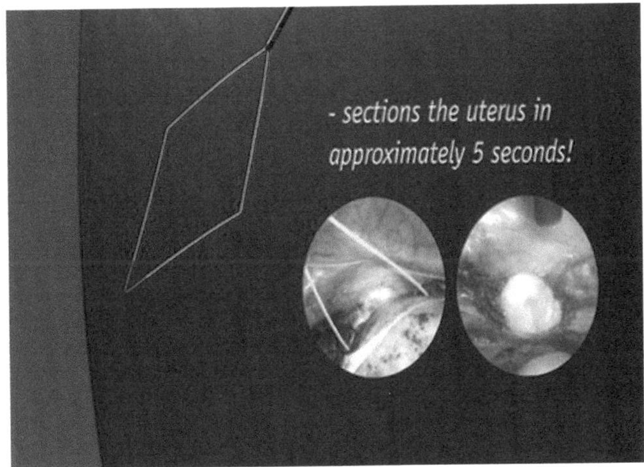
- sections the uterus in
approximately 5 seconds!

Fig. 23.31 LiNA Loop at Subtotal Hysterectomy (SLH)

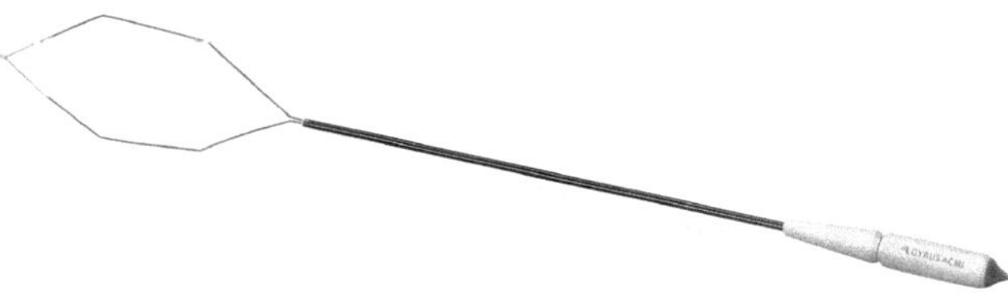

Fig. 23.32 Bipolar cutting loop for SLH (Billbipolar)

them are available. Phase optic and lens optic system with diameter between 1.2 and 2 mm are offered by instrument manufacturers. Common to both of them is that the laparoscope can be passed through the Veress needle or the sleeve. Additional trocar insertion after gas insufflation is therefore superfluous. However, compared to the standard 5 and 10 mm optics, even the most satisfactory of the mini-systems shows deficient lighting efficiency. The instrument trocars are also available in correspondingly small diameters.

The merits of minimal operative trauma and the avoidance of umbilical trocar insertion done by inserting the laparoscope through the Veress cannula in minilaparoscopies used to have disadvantages, such as the mechanical fragility of the minilaparoscopes and difficult operative sites with a restricted view. Today new optics and stabile instruments have virtually eliminated these disadvantages. Therefore, a set of minilaparoscopic instruments must always be available for use in certain surgical interventions. The small diameter of the mini-instruments contributes towards reducing trauma and pain in children and in smaller surgical procedures.

For TLH and SLH in small uteri microendoscopic instruments can be used. However, there should be no limitation to combine the procedure by using conventional laparoscopic instruments, as well.

Single Port or Single Entry Laparoscopy (SEL)

Laparoscopy in the 1940s started with the angled laparoscope (optic and one working channel) of Raoul Palmer in France as SEL. Laparoscopy at that time was mainly used for diagnostic purposes and for sterilizations. Kurt Semm in Germany further developed the procedure into operative laparoscopy by using multiple entries and instruments.

Fig. 23.33 Instrument set for Subtotal Laparoscopic Hysterectomy (SLH)

SLH – Tools

- 1 Trocar 11-5 mm for 0/30° Laproscope
- 1 Versaport 12-5 mm Trocar (left)
  1 Trocar 5 mm (right side)
- 1 Bipolare Instrument 5mm
  or EnSeal or LigaSure
- 1 Scissor 5 mm
- 1 Grasper 10mm (only huge ute
- 1 Monopolar hook or
  1 LiNA Loop or STORZ loop
  1 Dissecting Hook (harmonic)
- 1 Rotocut G1 morcellator system , in bag morcellation
- 1 suture
- 1 needle holder

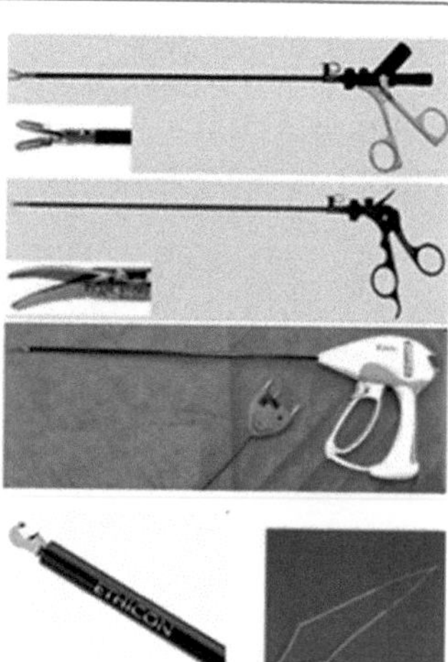

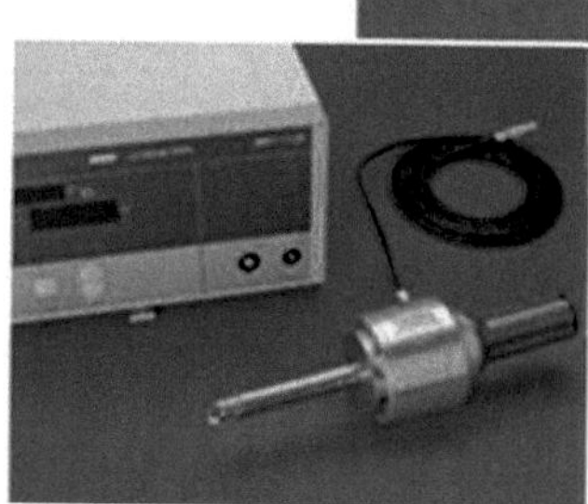

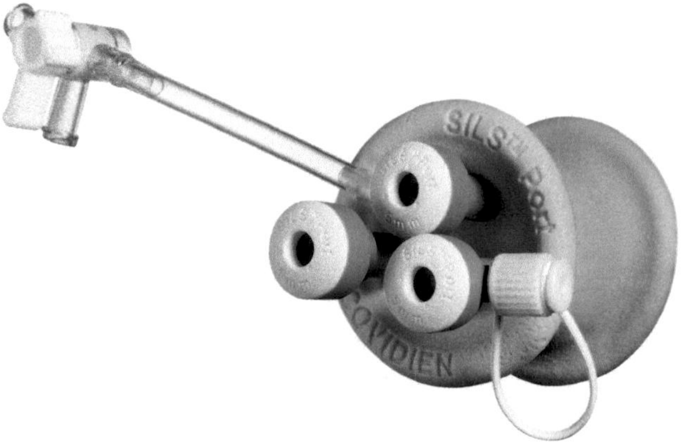

Fig. 23.34 SILS (Covidien) Port New

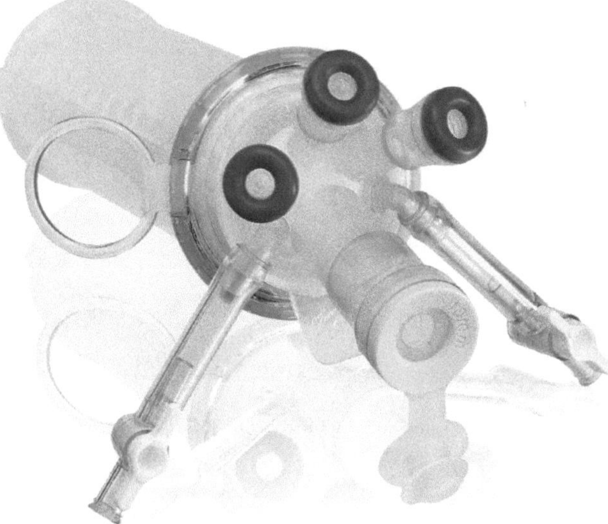

Fig. 23.35 LESS - Laparo-Endoscopic Single-Site Tri-Port Surgery (Olympus)

With the improved technology of today, SEL takes the idea of the early laparoscopy to new horizons. Of the multitude of SEL ports available, let us mention two disposable and one reusable:

1. The SILS port (Covidien) (Fig. 23.34) is a disposable port. Here a silicone port is introduced into the abdominal cavity using a classical curved grasper with a beak of 5–6 cm. The surgeon has the choice of two ports of five mm and one allowing for a large barrel instrument of 10–12 mm or one with four 5 mm ports. The SILS, with the possibility to introduce larger instruments, is suitable for hysterectomies.
2. Another disposable port is the LESS QuadPort + (Fig. 23.35) of Olympus which contains duckbill valves and requires no gel for insertion. Instruments of 5, 10, 12 and 15 mm can be introduced easily for ergonomic surgery. The 5 mm LESS EndoEYE video-laparoscopes provide excellent visualization and help to avoid instrument clashing. Specialized curved HiQ+ LESS instruments allow internal triangulation and mimic traditional laparoscopy

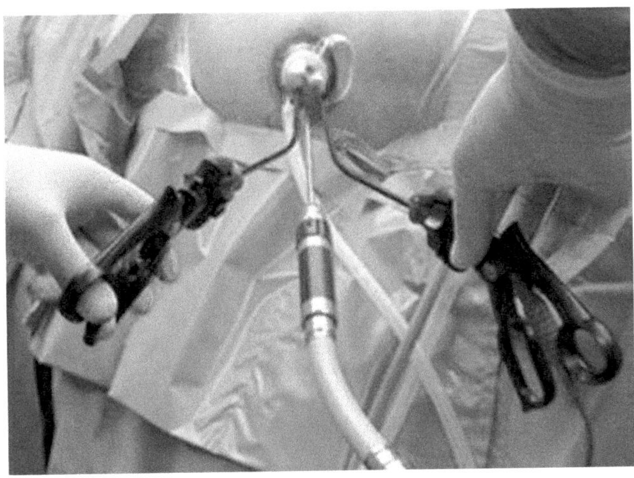

Fig. 23.36 LESS System with EndoEYE and curved instruments (Olympus)

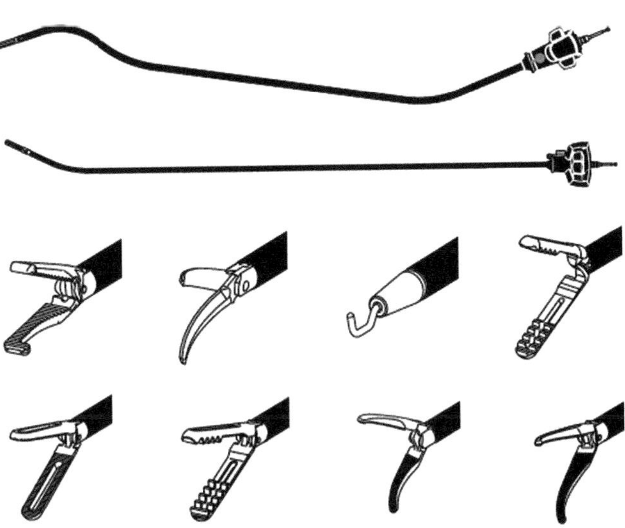

Fig. 23.37 Seven variations of LESS curved instruments (Olympus)

(Figs. 23.36 and 23.37). As a reusable port we use the XCONE (Fig. 23.38) of Karl Storz. This system is operational in the abdomen with 3–5 entry channels, one allowing large barrel instruments. Usually the 3 or 5 mm optic is placed into the middle entry and at least one curved instrument on the left or right side. The ENDOCONE® (Fig. 23.39) is a special access system developed by the general surgeon Cuschieri in which seven instruments can be introduced simultaneously.

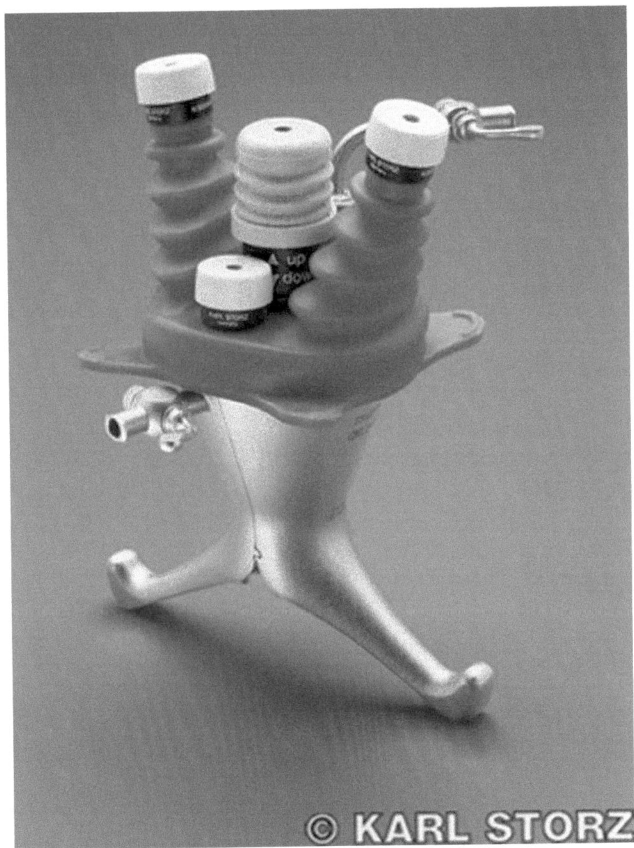

Fig. 23.38 XCONE (Karl Storz)

Developments are ongoing as can be seen by the ETHOS Surgical Platform™ (Ethos Surgical, Beaverton, USA), on which the surgeon is postured over the midline of the patient with optimal port triangulation options. New instruments and apparatus are continuously being appraised. They assist the surgeon but do not replace his knowledge and have always to be critically evaluated and studied before they are applied.

For TLH and SLH at Single Port Laparoscopy an intrauterine manipulator is essential to be used in combination with the following necessary instruments: Graspers, coagulation devices, scissors, electro loop and morcellator.

In summary conventional laparoscopic hysterectomies with single and multiple port entries are easy to be performed with modern gyne-endoscopic instrument and apparatus.

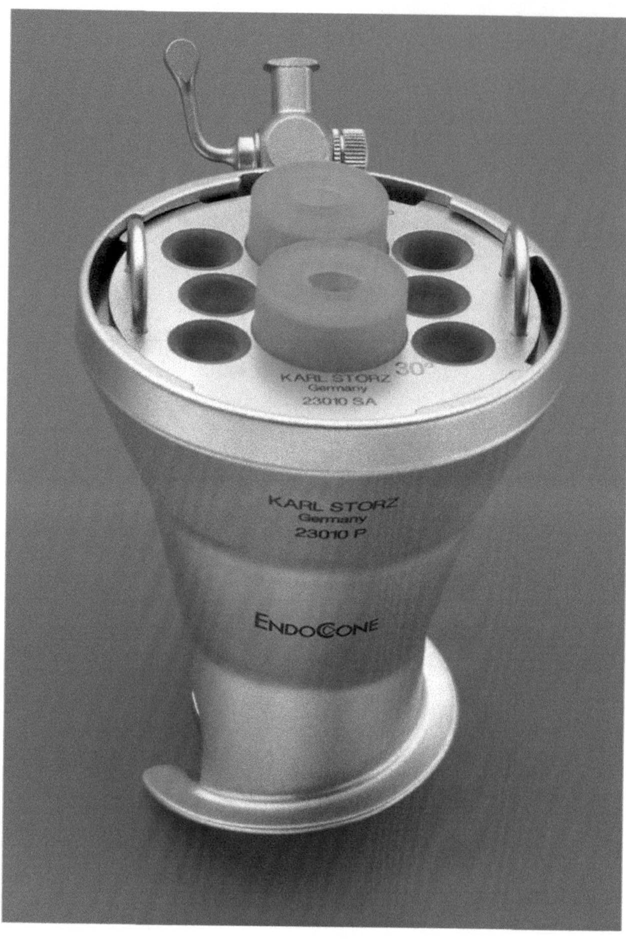

Fig. 23.39 ENDOCONE® (Karl Storz) according to CUSCHIERI

References

1. Semm K, editor. Operationslehre für endoskopische Abdominal-Chirurgie. Stuttgart, New York: Schattauer; 1984.
2. Reich H, De Caprio J, F. MG. Laparoscopic hysterectomy. J Gynecol Surg. 1989;5:213–6.
3. Semm K. CISH (pelviscopic intrafascial hysterectomy–without colpotomy), TUMA (total uterine mucosa ablation) and IVH (intra-fascial vaginal hysterectomy). Gynakologe. 1993;26(6):378–84.
4. Dargent D, Audra P, Miellet CC. Better use of POR 8. Presse Med. 1986;15(23):1106.
5. Weibel MA, Majno G. Peritoneal adhesions and their relation to abdominal surgery. A postmortem study. Am J Surg. 1973;126(3):345–53.
6. Menzies D, Ellis H. Intestinal obstruction from adhesions–how big is the problem? Ann R Coll Surg Engl. 1990;72(1):60–3.
7. Hawthorn RJS, Lower A, Clark D, Knight AD, Crowe AM. Adhesion-related readmissions following gynaecological laparoscopy in Scotland, an epidemiological study of 24,046 patients. Reviews in Gynaecological Practice. 2003;3:1.
8. Beck DE, Opelka FG, Bailey HR, Rauh SM, Pashos CL. Incidence of small-bowel obstruction and adhesiolysis after open colorectal and general surgery. Dis Colon rectum. 1999;42(2):241–8.
9. Hershlag A, Diamond MP, DeCherney AH. Adhesiolysis. Clin Obstet Gynecol. 1991;34(2):395–402.
10. Holmdahl L, Risberg B. Adhesions: prevention and complications in general surgery. Eur J Surg. 1997;163(3):169–74.
11. Beck DE, Ferguson MA, Opelka FG, Fleshman JW, Gervaz P, Wexner SD. Effect of previous surgery on abdominal opening time. Dis Colon rectum. 2000;43(12):1749–53.
12. Lower AM, Hawthorn RJ, Ellis H, O'Brien F, Buchan S, Crowe AM. The impact of adhesions on hospital readmissions over ten years after 8849 open gynaecological operations: an assessment from the Surgical and Clinical Adhesions Research Study. BJOG. 2000;107(7):855–62.
13. Dubuisson JB, Fauconnier A, Chapron C, Kreiker G, Norgaard C. Second look after laparoscopic myomectomy. Hum Reprod. 1998;13(8):2102–6.
14. Sekiba K. Use of Interceed(TC7) absorbable adhesion barrier to reduce postoperative adhesion reformation in infertility and endometriosis surgery. The Obstetrics and Gynecology Adhesion Prevention Committee. Obstet Gynecol. 1992;79(4):518–22.
15. Vrijland WW, Tseng LN, Eijkman HJ, Hop WC, Jakimowicz JJ, Leguit P, et al. Fewer intraperitoneal adhesions with use of hyaluronic acid-carboxymethylcellulose membrane: a randomized clinical trial. Ann Surg. 2002;235(2):193–9.
16. Mettler L, Audebert A, Lehmann-Willenbrock E, Schive-Peterhansl K, Jacobs VR. A randomized, prospective, controlled, multicenter clinical trial of a sprayable, site-specific adhesion barrier system in patients undergoing myomectomy. Fertil Steril. 2004 Aug;82(2):398–404.
17. Ferland R, Campbell PK. Pre-clinical evaluation of a next-generation spray adhesion barrier for multiple site adhesion protection. Surg Technol Int. 2009;18:137–43.
18. Metwally M, Watson A, Lilford R, Vandekerckhove P. Fluid and pharmacological agents for adhesion prevention after gynaecological surgery. Cochrane Database Syst Rev. 2006;2:CD001298.
19. Mettler L, Hucke J, Bojahr B, Tinneberg HR, Leyland N, Avelar R. A safety and efficacy study of a resorbable hydrogel for reduction of post-operative adhesions following myomectomy. Hum Reprod. 2008 May;23(5):1093–100.
20. Veress J. Neues Instrument zur Ausführung von Brust oder Bauchpunktionen und Pneumothoraxbehandlung. Dtsch Med Wschr. 1938;41:1480.
21. Semm K. Die moderne Endoskopie in der Frauenheilkunde. Frauenarzt. 1972;13:300–7.
22. Hopkins HH. On the diffraction theory of optical images. Proc Roy Soc A. 1953;217:408–15.
23. Brill AI. Energy systems for operative laparoscopy. J Am Assoc Gynecol Laparosc. 1998;5(4):333–45. quiz 47–9
24. Wallwiener D, Maleika A, Rimbach S, Homann G, Rabe T, Gauwerky J, et al. The value of laparoscopic and laser-assisted techniques in reconstruction of distal fallopian tube pathology. Zentralbl Gynakol. 1996;118(2):66–72.
25. Schemmel M, Haefner HK, Selvaggi SM, Warren JS, Termin CS, Hurd WW. Comparison of the ultrasonic scalpel to CO2 laser and electrosurgery in terms of tissue injury and adhesion formation in a rabbit model. Fertil Steril. 1997;67(2):382–6.

24 Uterine Manipulators for Total Laparoscopic Hysterectomy

Prashant Mangeshikar and Abhishek P. Mangeshikar

Introduction

With the advent of development of laparoscopic hysterectomy, improving the ease by which the surgery is done, the need to develop the ideal uterine manipulator became necessary. Each new uterine manipulator improved the shortcomings of its predecessor. This chapter will address the significant benefits and shortcomings of the manipulators invented thus far.

Laparoscopic Hysterectomy is in present time, the standard practice of hysterectomy in experienced hands for diseased uteri where vaginal hysterectomy is not possible. Described by Harry Reich, initially as a LAVH procedure (Laparoscopic Assisted Vaginal Hysterectomy) and later as a Total Laparoscopic Hysterectomy (TLH) operation, the operation like all laparoscopic surgeries requires good and optimal surgical exposure. Optimal exposure of the operative field is of prime importance during Laparoscopic Hysterectomy. Despite the advent of high definition cameras, superior optics and newer light sources, complications can occur if optimal exposure is not available at laparoscopy.

Manipulation of the uterus during LH is essential to provide maximal exposure with minimal access. Though manipulation of the uterus is possible by using a laparoscopic myoma screw, it is not as effective in comparison to the multiple functions provided by the uterine manipulator. In addition, the use of the myoma screw blocks an accessory portal, immobilizing one instrument and one hand which is no longer available for help. The use of the myoma screw may not be able to provide uterine access in all the possible views. This would require shifting the fixation of the myoma screw in the uterus in multiple positions. Bleeding can ensue as a result of screwing and unscrewing the myoma screw from the uterus necessitating arrest of bleeding from the fixation sites in the body of the uterus.

The role of uterine manipulators at Laparoscopic Hysterectomy has been well described and established by numerous studies as a safe and effective way to handle the uterus during laparoscopic hysterectomy. This enables the surgeon to develop spaces along the lines of cleavage, facilitating safe dissection and avoiding unnecessary complications.

The ideal uterine manipulator should have the following characteristics:

1. Inexpensive
2. Safe and nonconductive of electricity
3. Quick assembly and disassembly
4. Reusable
5. Have a wide range of movement and mobilize the uterus in different axis.
6. Easy placement and removal within the uterus
7. No complications arising from its use.
8. Maintain the pneumoperitoneum following the circumcision of the vagina.
9. Should not break down into pieces or fragment during surgery
10. Special functions

According to Gamal Eltabbakh [1], a uterine manipulator should perform the following functions:

1. Raise the uterus cephalad bringing it closer to the laparoscopic instruments.
2. Manipulating the uterus, thereby keep the side to be operated upon, on a stretch.
3. Increase the distance between the uterus and the ureters, bladder and rectum preventing any injury or damage to these vital organs

P. Mangeshikar • A.P. Mangeshikar (✉)
Mangeshikar Minimal Access Gynecology Infertility Clinic for Women, 8 Laburnum Road, Gamdevi, Mumbai 400007, India
e-mail: abhishek@mangeshikar.com

I. Alkatout, L. Mettler (eds.), *Hysterectomy*, DOI 10.1007/978-3-319-22497-8_24

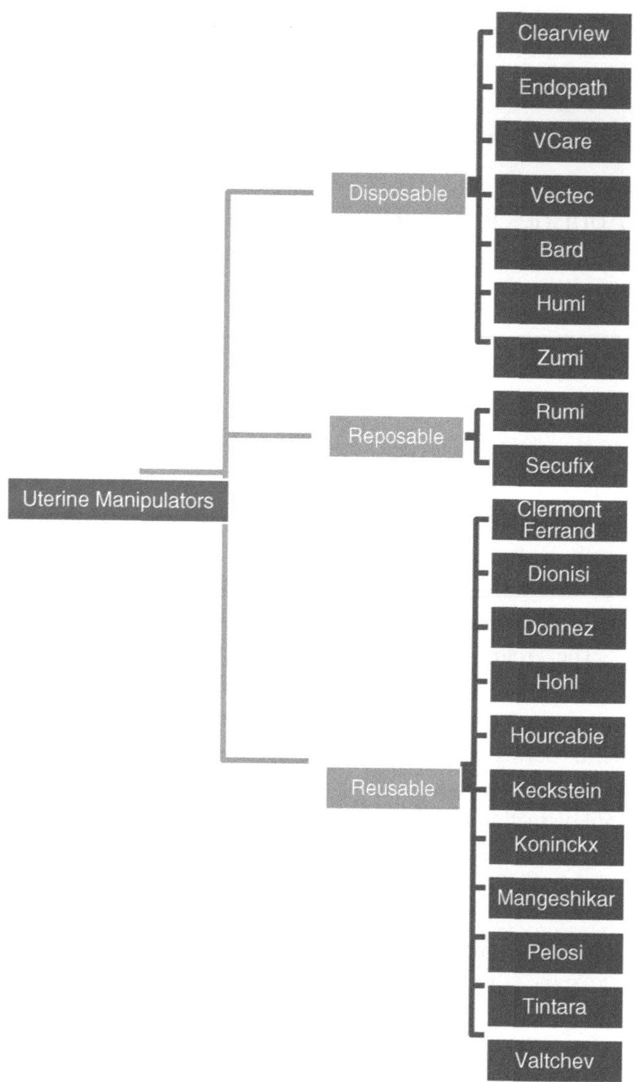

Fig. 24.1 List of Uterine manipulators for Total Laparoscopic Hysterectomy

4. Facilitate identification of the utero-vesical fold of peritoneum, cul-de-sac, and the vaginal cuff at the cervico-vaginal junction.
5. Enable the delivery of the uterus via the vagina once it is free.
6. Maintain the pneumoperitoneum following the circumcision of the vagina.

The uterine manipulator is termed as "The FIFTH Hand in the Pelvis" where in the vaginal assistant is manipulating the uterus via the indwelling instrument: the uterine manipulator. Numerous uterine manipulators have been designed by different authors across the world with the aim to facilitate maximal access during LH as shown in Fig. 24.1.

Clearview Manipulator

The Clearview Manipulator previously known as the Endopath uterine manipulator is a disposable device with ease of handling and assembly with the following characteristics:

1. Allows the uterine manipulation with an inbuilt inflatable balloon in the AP and lateral axis and elevation without the need of a vaginal assistant.
2. In view of the fact that even though it allows 210° of movement in the AP axis, it is not suitable for the TLH operation since it does not allow dextro- and laevo-rotation of the uterus, does not delineate the vagina and also does not maintain the pneumoperitoneum.
3. Two cases of uterine perforation during dilation of cervix due to cervical stenosis reported. Two cases of the Clearview manipulator breaking down into small pieces retained within the patient were reported.

VCare Uterine Manipulator

The VCare Uterine Manipulator is a disposable lightweight device with the following characteristics:

1. It has a wide range of motion (AP, lateral and elevation).
2. It allows easy handling and assembly with an inflatable intrauterine balloon device.
3. Though it offers good vaginal delineation and well maintains the pneumoperitoneum, it is not suitable for TLH in large uteri.
4. Disintegration of the VCare and laceration of the vaginal have been reported as also one case of melting of the cervical cup.

Vectec Manipulator

The Vectec manipulator is an ultra light, inexpensive disposable instrument available either with suction or a screw device to hold the uterus during manipulation.

Rumi Manipulator

The RUMI system consist of the Rumi Manipulator, the Koh cervical cup, and the Koh Colpo-pneumo–occluder, that facilitates 140° degree movement in the AP axis, lateral movements and elevation in the cephaled direction. The indwelling balloon facilitates the manipulation. The injury rate for 0.2 % for ureter and 0.4 % for bladder, and 1 % for the vagina. Two patients had uterine rupture due to hyperinflation of the intra uterine balloon of the Rumi. In another series the Koh cup was found 14 months after the operative procedure. Following other reports of the disintegration of the instruments, parts being left behind, and vaginal wall laceration, the RUMI has been updated to the RUMI II system.

Clermont Ferrand Manipulator

The Clermont Ferrand Manipulator is a reusable device offering movements in the AP axis, lateral movements and elevation in the cephalad direction (Fig. 24.2). Though it is versatile, it is considered difficult to assemble.

However it does not allow levo –and dextro rotation unlike the Mangeshikar uterine manipulator.

Donnez Uterine Manipulator

The Donnez Uterine Manipulator is a reusable device, lightweight in design. It is not a self retaining instrument (Fig. 24.3). The working insert at the distal end of the manipulator facilitate the positioning of the cervix and is available in three sizes as also the caps which delineate the vagina and seal the gas during opening of the vagina. However, though the inherent design is good for small to moderately enlarged uteri, it has limitations in the range of movement as also with variations in the length of the cervix and associated vaginal prolapse.

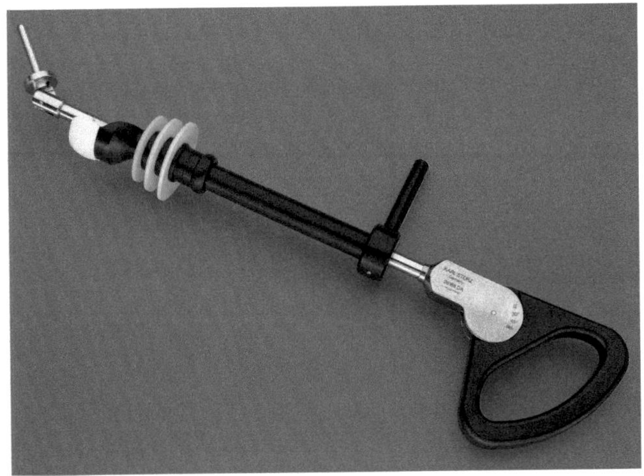

Fig. 24.2 Clermont Ferrand Manipulator

Dionisi Uterine Manipulator

The Dionisi uterine manipulator is a reusable device, which is inserted into the uterine cavity: the distal insert being in a closed position (Fig. 24.4). The rotatory wheel at the proximal end is rotated to open up the distal working insert once in proper position. The distal working inserts are available in three different sizes depending upon the size of the uterus for the hysterectomy. The inherent design does not allow the various ranges of movement unlike the Mangeshikar Uterine manipulator. Further there are no vaginal delineating caps available with this instrument.

Hohl Uterine Manipulator

The Hohl uterine manipulator is a reusable device, which is tightly screwed into the cervical canal using spiral inserts (Fig. 24.5). The working inserts, available in different lengths (60 mm, 80 mm, 100 mm) allows this device to be used for uteri of varying sizes. The ceramic caps in varying sizes are available to match the size of the portio. The caps provide optimal presentation over the fornix during circumcision of

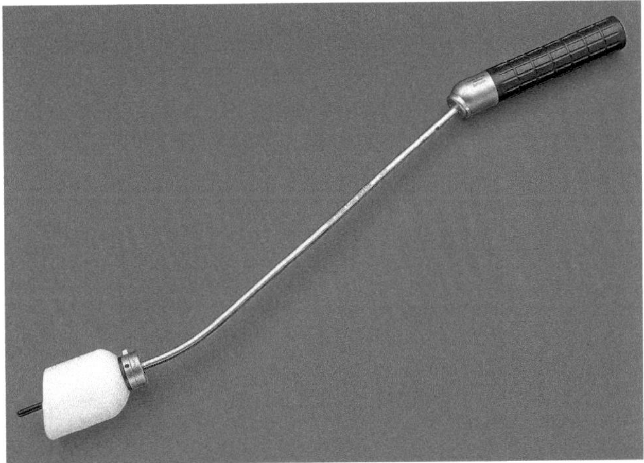

Fig. 24.3 Donnez Uterine Manipulator

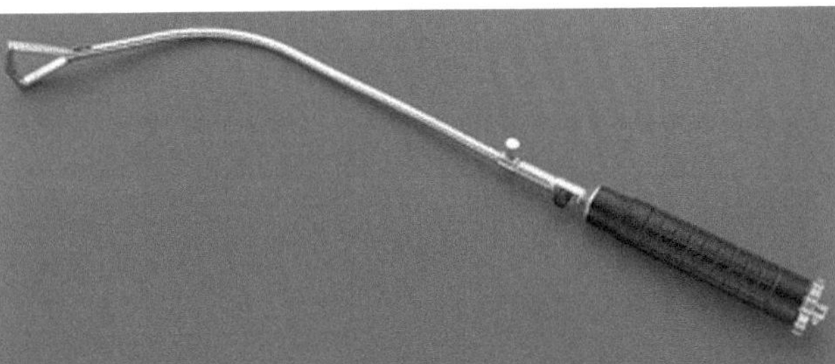

Fig. 24.4 Dionisi Uterine Manipulator

the vagina. Whilst the manipulator provides a wide range of movement of the uterus rotation of the uterus around its axis is not possible.

Keckstein Uterine Manipulator

The Keckstein uterine manipulator is a reusable lightweight device that enables the uterus to be manipulated with maximum mobility: 95° anteflexion and 30° retroflexion (Fig. 24.6). The movable spiral insert facilitates the movement of the uterus whilst the screw mechanism into the cervix fixes the manipulator. Whilst the Keckstein manipulator allows dorsal, ventral and lateral movements, it cannot rotate the uterus around its axis. This versatile device is provided with caps to present the vagina during the hysterectomy procedure and also to prevent loss of pneumoperitoneum. The shallow fixed height of the cap could be a limiting factor for the identification of the cervico-vaginal junction unlike the Mangeshikar Uterine mobilisar, considering the length of the cervix and associated vaginal descent.

Mangeshikar Uterine Mobilizar

The Mangeshikar Uterine Mobilizar was developed by the primary author with the idea of maximizing uterine manipulation in multiple axis or directions to facilitate excellent exposure for surgical dissection during the total lapaoscopic hysterectomy and colpotomy (Fig. 24.7).

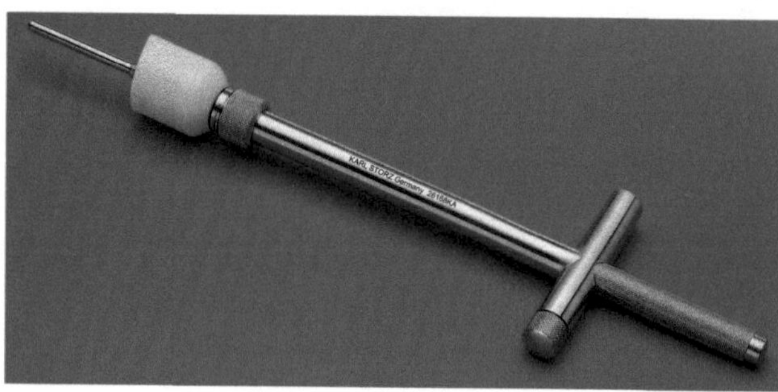

Fig. 24.5 Hohl Uterine Manipulator

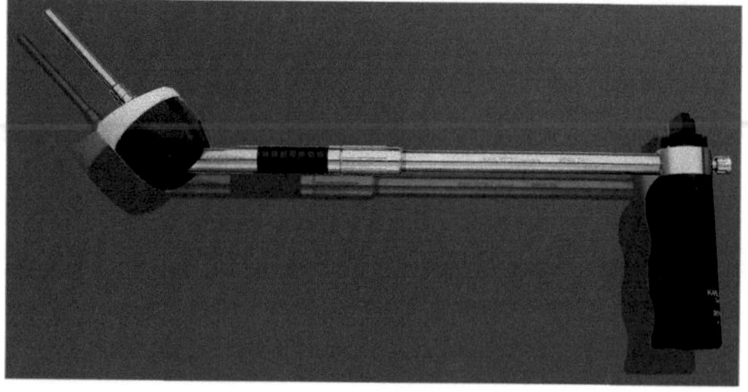

Fig. 24.6 Keckstein Uterine Manipulator

The Mangeshikar Uterine Mobilizar consists of two main components (Fig. 24.8):

1. The central assembly
2. Vaginal Fornix Presenter

The central assembly comprises of:

1. A reusable insert, which is housed in an outer stainless steel tube, has at its distal central end a fixation device for the intrauterine steel element (IUE) (Fig. 24.9) and two built in single toothed tenaculum (Fig. 24.10). At its

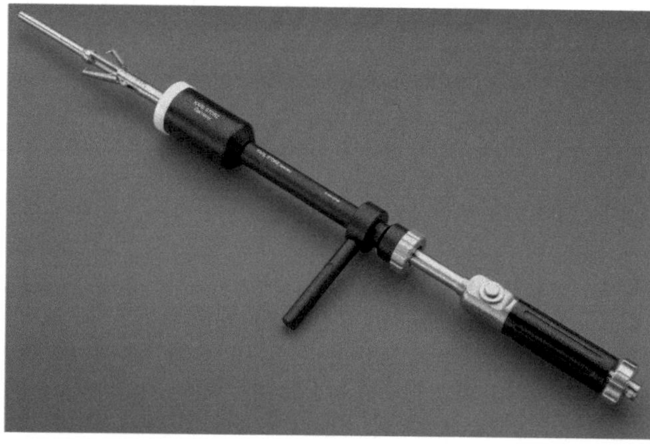

Fig. 24.7 Mangeshikar Uterine Mobilizar

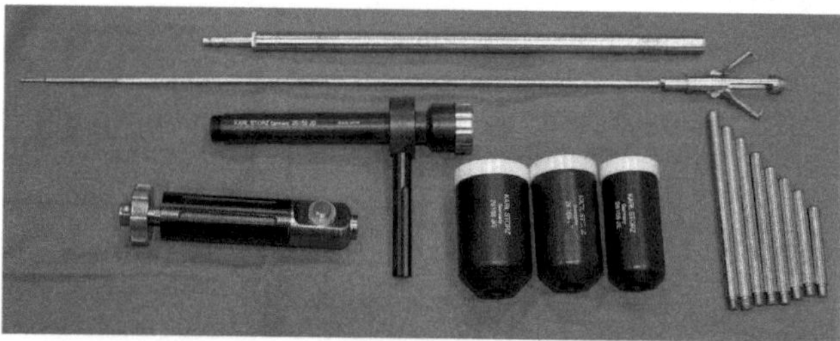

Fig. 24.8 Different parts of Mangeshikar Uterine Mobilizar

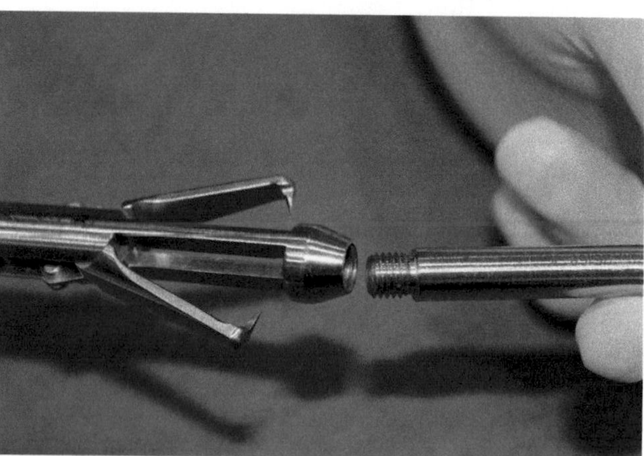

Fig. 24.9 Distal end of MUM with Intrauterine element (IUE)

proximal end, the insert fits snugly into the handle of the manipulator that has a locking device to fix the tenacula into the cervix.

2. The Vaginal Delineating Cup / Vaginal Fornix Presenter (VDC) is made of reusable medical grade PVC (Fig. 24.11). The VDC has a cup at its distal end and houses a tricuspid valve apparatus at the proximal end. It has a locking device within its handle. Once positioned inside the vagina to expose the cervicovaginal junction, it can be locked in place with the inbuilt handle so that the assistant does not have to be concerned with the persistent pushing and handing of the VFP. The cup has a ceramic lip and is flat and not beveled. The standard supplied cup is available in three fixed sizes 30, 35 and 40 mms. Outer diameter.

The Mangeshikar Uterine Mobilizar has no disposable elements and is made up of stainless steel and medical grade PVC that is steam autoclavable.

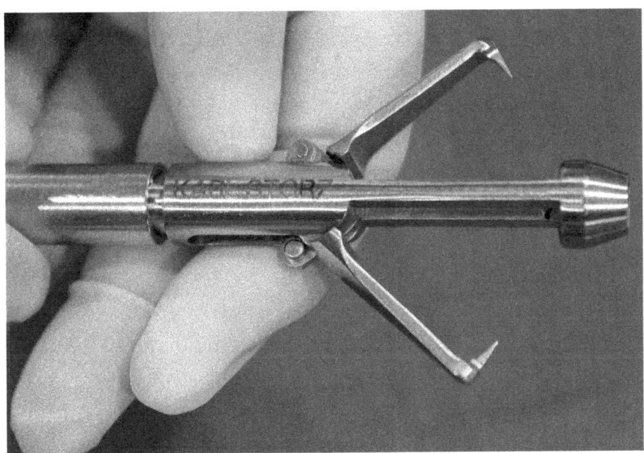

Fig. 24.10 Distal end of MUM showing inbuilt tenaculum

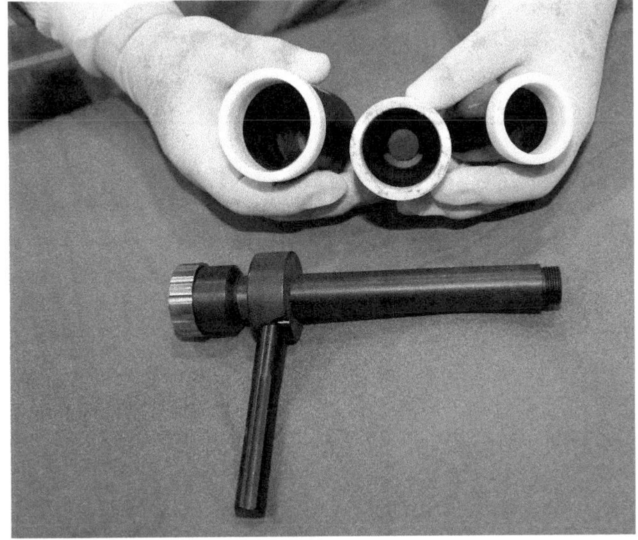

Fig. 24.11 Vaginal Delineating cups with Handle

Operative Steps:

1. With the patient positioned in a modified lithotomy position under general anesthesia, with an indwelling catheter in the Bladder after draping under aseptic precautions, an Assessment is made under anesthesia to determine the uterine size, mobility and the Utero-cervical Length.
2. The cervix is held with a vulsellum at the anterior lip and dilated to 10 Hegar.
3. The uterocervical length (UCL) is determined in cms. With the hysterometer / uterine sound and the appropriate intrauterine element is selected. The length of the element in cms. Is etched at its base as a Number e.g. 8, 9 etc. The correct IUE chosen reduces the risk of uterine perforation and trauma.
4. The MUM is assembled with the appropriate IUE and the vaginal tube Fig. 24.12). The VDC is selected depending upon the width of the vagina and the diameter of the cervix.

After removing the Mangeshikar Uterine Mobilisar from its sterilizing box, the instrument is assembled choosing the appropriate:

A. Intra Uterine Element according to the Utero-cervical length in cms. The appropriate IUE is identified by a Numeral etched at its base e.g. 8, 9, 10 etc.
B. Vaginal Delineating Cup, which is selected depending upon the width of the vagina and the diameter of the cervix (Fig. 24.13).

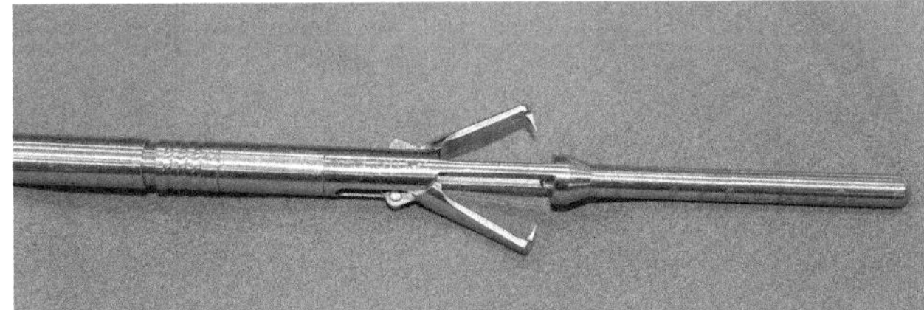

Fig. 24.12 MUM is assembled with the appropriate IUE

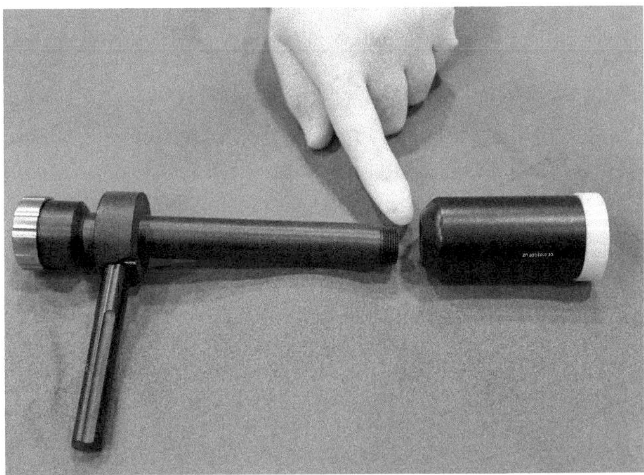

Fig. 24.13 Fixing the Vaginal Delineating Cup to the Handle

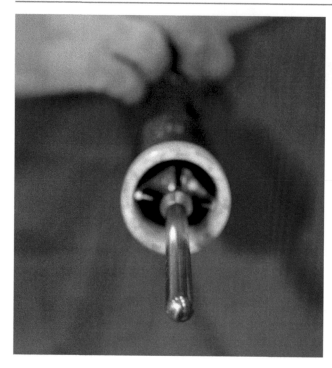

Fig. 24.14 Close-up view of the final assembly of MUM at the distal end

5. Holding the anterior lip of the cervix with vulsellum, the MUM is introduced safely into the uterus with the appropriate IUE and VDC and the two in-built tenacula grasp the cervix securely at 3 and 9 o'clock position (Fig. 24.14). Rotating the proximal knob on the handle in an anti-clockwise manner opens the tenacula.

Precautions are taken to ensure that the vagina is not included in the grip. The steel rotating knob on the handle is rotated in a clockwise direction to secure the grip of the tenacula of the MUM on the cervix avoiding any injury to the vagina or the bladder. The vulsellum on the ant lip of the cervix is now removed.

6. The MUM is now ready for use. Traditionally, the vaginal tube is not inserted into the vagina at the beginning of the TLH. In cases of previous C-section, one may insert the tube at the very beginning of the operation to facilitate bladder dissection as the tube acts as a platform on which safe dissection of the bladder fascia and the adhesions can be performed.

Note:

1. The MUM Mobilizes the Uterus in FOUR directions:
   a. Cephalad
   b. Lateral
   c. Anterior and posterior

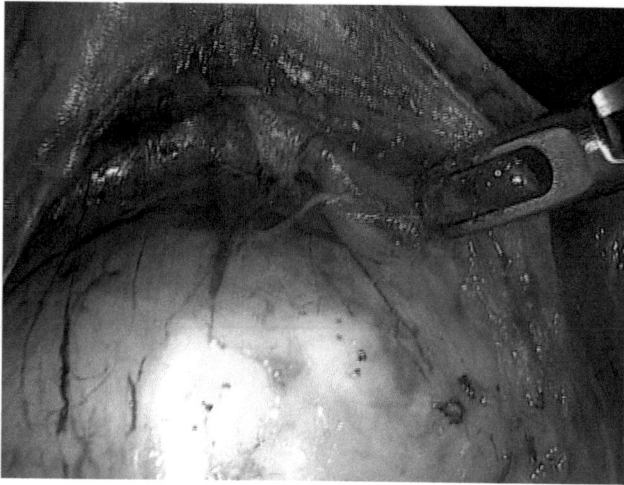

Fig. 24.15 Exposure of Vagina and Bladder dissection

   d. Levo-rotation and Dextro-rotation on the shaft of MUM
2. By pushing the uterus cephalad, the MUM lifts the uterus out of the pelvis into the abdomen and increases the space between the uterus and the lateral wall of the pelvis.
3. The lateral movements of the uterus by the MUM provide maximal exposure and access to the round ligament, the tube and ovary as well as the broad ligament with all its structures. Further, with the lateral push provided by the MUM, maximal access is available for dealing with the uterine vessels and the ureter (Fig. 24.15). The lateral mobilization by the Mum increases the distance between the uterine vessels and the ureter providing safety to the ureter from injury.
4. The MUM can antevert and retrovert the uterus to gain access to the lower part of the uterus in cases of fibroids blocking straight vision. In addition, the cul-de-sac can be well identified with the MUM and the vaginal tube being pushed deep into the depth of the vagina.
5. The secure grip by the tenacula on the cervix enables the MUM to rotate the uterus around its axis thus bringing the uterine vessels anteriorly at 1 and 11 o'clock position while the ureters remain at their normal 3 and 9 o'clock positions. This provides a safe and clear view of the uterine vessels and the ureter Fig. 24.16). The tenacula grip the cervix and this in addition ensures that uterine perforation due to the instrument will not occur during introduction and surgery.

The Mangeshikar Uterine Manipulator aims to be the IDEAL Uterine Manipulator due to its characteristics (Figs. 24.17, 24.18, 24.19, 24.20, 24.21 and 24.22):

1. Lightweight
2. Reusable

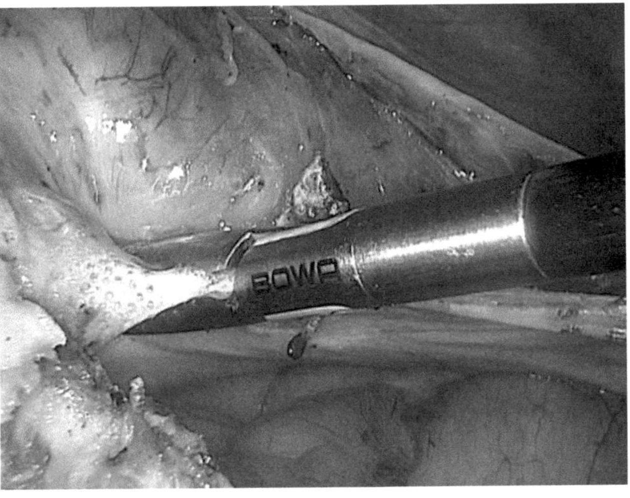

Fig. 24.16 Exposure of Uterine vessels using MUM

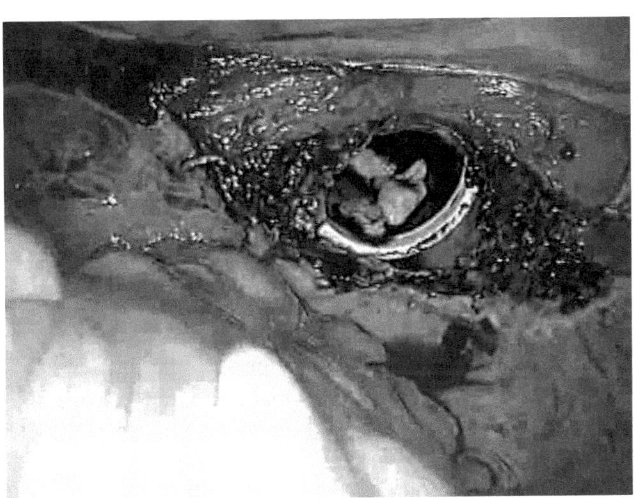

Fig. 24.17 Easy Retrieval of Morcellated tissue via Vaginal Cup

3. Multifunctional
4. Robust
5. For varying uterine sizes
6. Safe
7. Easy to Assemble and Disassemble
8. Easy to Clean and Sterilize
9. Vehicle for Sutures and Needles and Passover Clip
10. Displaces Cervix away from ureters
11. Displaces Bladder Anteriorly and Rectum posteriorly
12. Defines Dissecting plane for Colpotomy
13. Receptacle for sterile gauze pieces
14. Exposes the vaginal edges during laparoscopic closure of the vagina
15. Receptacle for the morcellated tissue remnants, uterine tissue, tubes and ovaries.

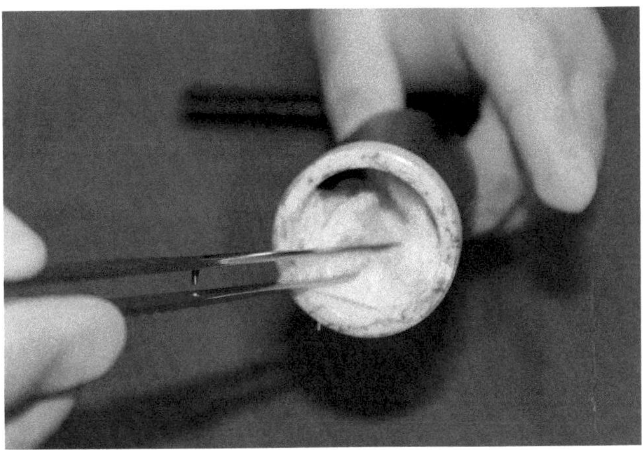

Fig. 24.18 Vaginal Delineating Cup: Storage of gauze piece for mopping the surgical area

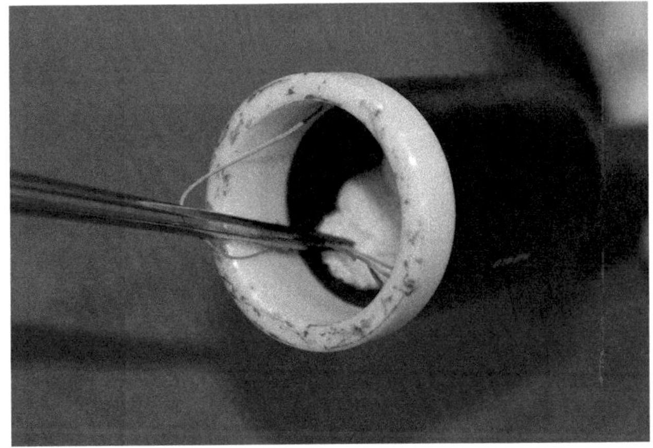

Fig. 24.19 Vaginal Delineating Cup: Storage of Needle with Suture

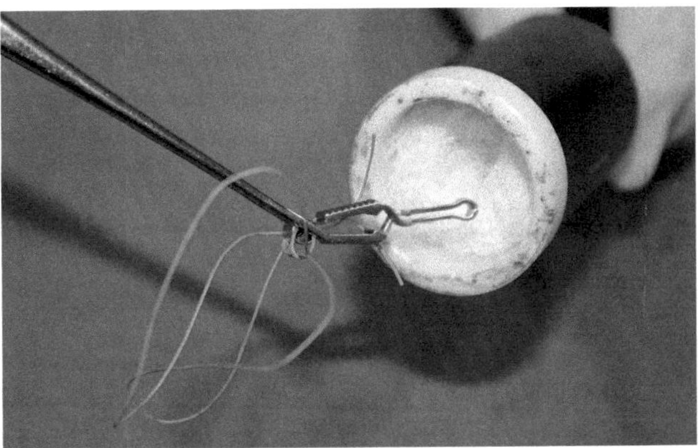

Fig. 24.20 Vaginal Delineating Cup: Storage of Possover Clip

16. Prevents loss and Maintains pneumoperitoneum during circumcision of the vagina as well as during laparoscopic closure of the vagina.

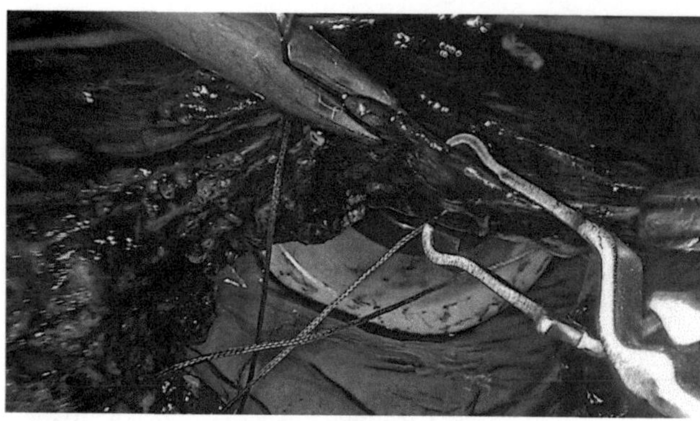

Fig. 24.21 Possover Clip being applied laparoscopically on anterior vaginal wall

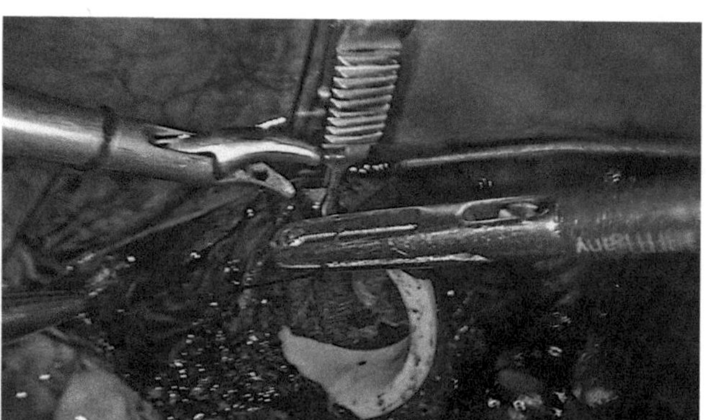

Fig. 24.22 Possover Clip holding anterior vaginal wall providing optimal exposure for easy closure of vagina

Tintara Uterine Manipulator

The Tintara Uterine Manipulator is a lightweight reusable device (Fig. 24.23). It is held in position with the vulsellum on the cervix and allows elevation of the uterus in a cephalad direction and anteflexion upto 90°. It is suitable for LASH (Laparoscopic Supracervical Hysterectomy) and not for Total Laparoscopic Hysterectomy.

Complications

Complications with the use of Uterine Manipulators at Laparoscopic Hysterectomy include:

1. Cervical Tears and Lacerations
2. Vaginal Lacerations
3. Perforation of the uterus during introduction and usage
4. Laceration of Uterine vessels and colporrhexis
5. Bleeding: Intraperitoneal or retroperitoneal.
6. Perforation of Bladder/Bowel/Rectum
7. Breakdown of the Uterine manipulator within the uterus

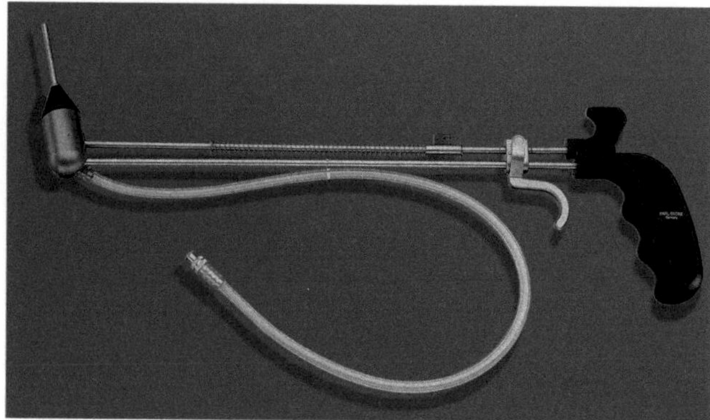

Fig. 24.23 Tintara Uterine Manipulator

Complications are more likely to occur in postmenopausal women or nulliparous women or women who have had no vaginal delivery. The stenotic cervix and the retroverted uterus predispose to complications. Complications can be avoided by proper insertion of the manipulator under laparoscopic visualization.

Ali Akdemir and Teksin Cirpan [2] reported a case of iatrogenic uterine perforation and sigmoid colon penetration caused by the Hohl uterine manipulator during TLH, which required conversion to laparotomy. A prospective study involving 1432 patients undergoing TLH using the Hohl manipulator reported 1 ureter and 8 bladder injuries [3].

The use of uterine manipulators during laparoscopic hysterectomy for endometrial cancer has been a cause of concern that the instrument may push the malignant cells intraperitoneally upstaging the cancer as a retrospective study by Sonoda etal [4] (2001) suggested a higher incidence of 1988 FIGO Stage IIIa (positive peritoneal cytology) among women treated by LAVH. However a prospective study by Eltabbakh and Mount [5] found no such difference in a prospective study in 42 women with endometrial carcinoma who underwent Laparoscopic Hysterectomy using uterine manipulators.

A relatively higher positive peritoneal cytology was found in women who had laparotomy compared to laparoscopy in a study by Walker et al. involving 2616 women with endometrial cancer [6]. These patients were randomly selected for surgery either by laparotomy or by laparoscopy involving different uterine manipulators.

References

1. Eltabbakh GH. Uterine manipulation in laparoscopic hysterectomy. The Female Patient. 2010;35:18–23.
2. Akdemir A, Cirpan T. Iatrogenic uterine perforation and bowel penetration using a Hohlmanipulator: a case report. Int J Surg Case Rep. 2014;5:271–3.

3. Hohl MK, Hauser N. Safe total intrafascial laparoscopic (TAIL) hysterectomy: a prospective cohort study. Gynecol Surg. 2010;7: 231–9.
4. Sonoda Y, Zerbe M, Smith A, Lin O, Barakat RR, Hoskins WJ. High incidence of positive peritoneal cytology in low-risk endometrial cancer treated by laparoscopically assisted vaginal hysterectomy. Gynecol Oncol. 2001;80(3):378–82.
5. Eltabbakh GH, Mount SL. Laparoscopic surgery does not increase the positive peritoneal cytology among women with endometrial carcinoma. Gynecol Oncol. 2006;100(2):361–4.
6. Walker JL, Piedmonte MR, Spirtos NM, et al. Laparoscopy compared with laparotomy for comprehensive surgical staging of uterine cancer. Gynecologic Oncology Group Study LAP2. J Clin Oncol. 2009;27(32):5331–6.

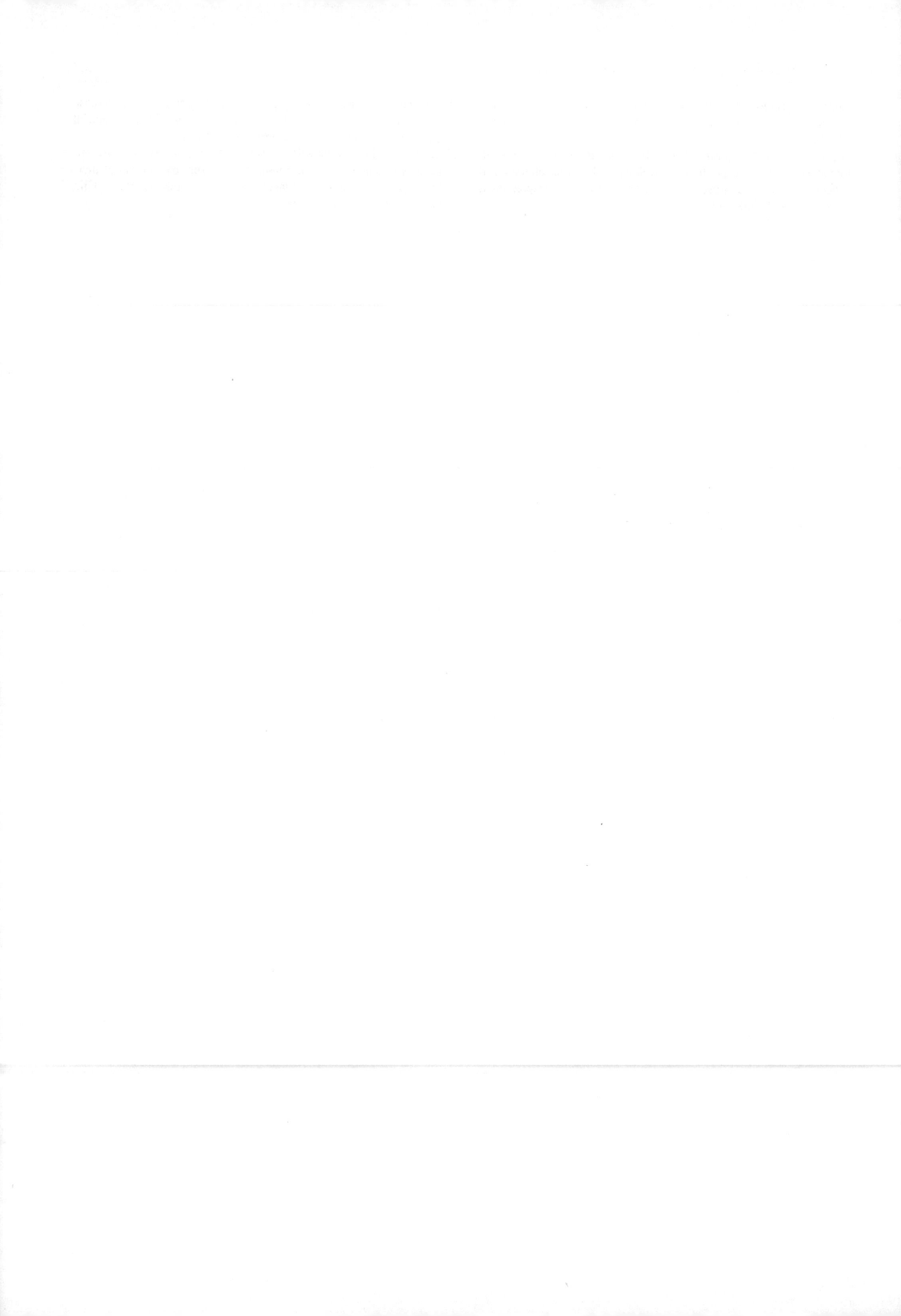

Diagnostic Laparoscopy and Final Site Recognition

25

Julia Serno

With diagnostic or exploratory laparoscopy a direct inspection of intraabdominal organs is possible. Primary access to the intraperitoneal cavity is usually accomplished through the umbilicus, either by direct trocar insertion (open laparoscopy) or by Veress needle placement. This is the most worrisome step in laparoscopic surgery as the surgeon has at this point no knowledge of intraperitoneal adhesions. There is no clear consensus as to the optimal method of entry into the peritoneal cavity [1]. In the open technique, a small subumbilical laparotomy is performed. Skin, rectus sheath, and peritoneum are then incised under direct vision followed by the insertion of a blunt trocar. After that a pneumoperitoneum is created [2]. The closed laparoscopic entry with the use of a Veress needle for insufflation followed by the blind insertion of a trocar is the most common approach used by gynecologists worldwide [3]. A nasogastric or orogastric tube should be placed in order to decompress the stomach prior to insertion of the Veress needle [4]. During the insertion of the needle two "clicks" can be felt, the first corresponds to the piercing of the anterior rectus sheath, the second to the piercing of the posterior rectus sheath and the peritoneum. An intraabdominal pressure of 20–25 mmHg should be administered to elevate the anterior abdominal wall for safety before inserting the first trocar. After the insertion of the first trocar, a scope is introduced to confirm the correct entry into the abdomen without CO_2 insufflation. Once safe entry into the peritoneal cavity is obtained, the pressure can be reduced to the working pressure (10–12 mmHg). All secondary ports should be introduced under vision. Transillumination of the abdominal wall with the endoscope can help identify superficial abdominal wall vessels. Moreover, the anterior surface of the peritoneal cavity should be inspected to locate and avoid injury to the epigastric vessels.

Patients who have had abdominal incisions which extended to or through the umbilicus have a higher risk for bowel adhesions to the anterior abdominal wall area. In this case it is recommended to place the Veress needle in the left upper quadrant (Palmer's Point). Raoul Palmer described this point as being "3 cm below the middle of the left costal margin" [5]. Thus, the risk of bowl injuries can be reduced [6].

The trocar placement depends on surgical indications, organ pathology, adhesions and adipose tissue distribution. A traditional trocar placement for many benign gynecologic surgeries is demonstrated in Fig. 25.1. Two 5 mm ports are inserted on the right and left side of the lower abdomen. In non-obese women with a normal sized uterus, hysterectomy can be performed using this trocar placement.

In more difficult cases additional trocars can be added for example on the right and left side of the umbilicus. With

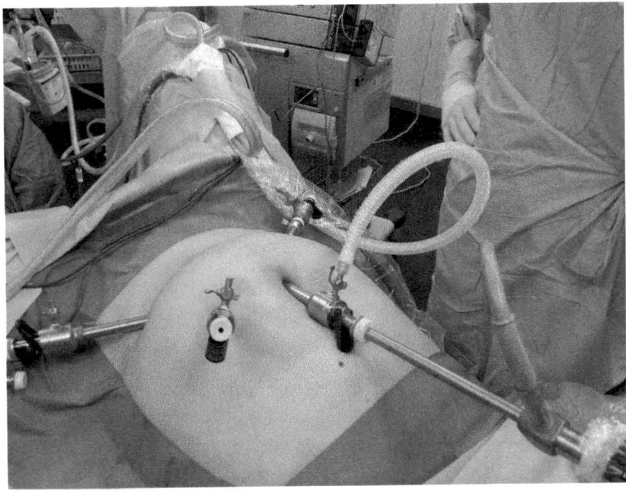

Fig. 25.1 The traditional trocar placement with two trocars on the right and left side of the lower abdomen is complemented by a trocar in the paraumbilical region

J. Serno
Obstetrics and Gynecology, University Hospital RWTH Aachen, Aachen 52074, Germany
e-mail: jserno@ukaachen.ae

I. Alkatout, L. Mettler (eds.), *Hysterectomy*, DOI 10.1007/978-3-319-22497-8_25

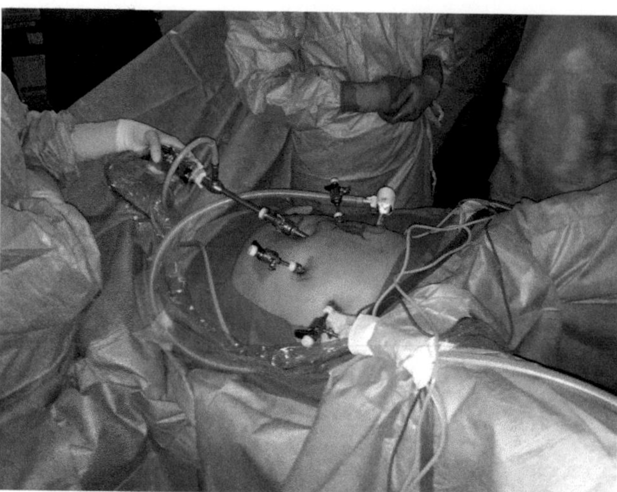

Fig. 25.2 Trocar placement for laparoscopic radical hysterectomy

large uteri or in oncological hysterectomies trocars are generally placed more superior (see Fig. 25.2).

During the course of diagnostic laparoscopy all visible peritoneal surfaces are inspected. The first step is to rule out any injuries that might have been caused by the Veress needle or by the blind insertion of the first trocar. After that the laparoscope can be turned and the upper abdominal organs are displayed (liver, stomach, spleen). After moving the patient in Trendelenburg position two graspers can be used to move the small bowel in the upper abdomen. Thus, a good vision of the pelvic organs is obtained. In case of suspected malignancy any free fluid should be aspirated or normal saline is instilled and then aspirated for cytologic examination [7]. In case of lower abdominal pain it is essential to check the appendix and sigma for signs of inflammation. To rule out unknown endometriosis the most common sites of involvement should be inspected, including the ovaries, the posterior cul-de-sac, the broad ligaments, the uterosacral ligaments, the recto sigmoid colon, the bladder and the distal ureters.

Final Site Recognition

At the end of every laparoscopic surgery the most common complications of laparoscopic surgery should be checked and ruled out (see Table 25.1). Gastrointestinal trauma may occur during the creation of the pneumoperitoneum or during the operative portion of laparoscopy [8]. Both types of injuries are more frequent in cases of previous surgery with present adhesions of the bowel [9]. One simple step to prevent delay in diagnosis is to view the initial trocar site through an alternative port if there is concern about anterior wall adhesions. The bowel close to the operating site should be checked for thermal injuries. Superficial thermal injuries to the bowel can often be repaired by a laparoscopic guided purse-string suture placed beyond the thermally affected

Table 25.1 Checklist final site recognition

Check for thermal injuries (bowel, bladder, ureter)
Check for pneumaturia or hematuria
Consider bladder installation of indigo carmine or methylene blue dye
Remove trocars under vision
Reduce the intra-abdominal pressure and check for (venous) bleeding

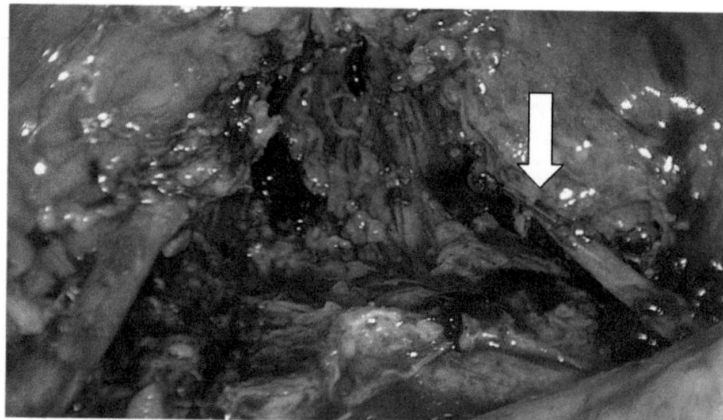

Fig. 25.3 Final site after radical hysterectomy. The veins in the uretric tunnel have been clipped (*arrow*) to avoid thermal damage

tissues. Thus, late onset perforation of the bowel with the risk of sepsis, multi-organ failure and even death can be prevented.

Significant bladder injuries usually result from the placement of a lower midline trocar. The surgeon should check the urine catheter for pneumaturia or hematuria which is a sign for potential bladder injury If a bladder injury is suspected, installation of indigo carmine or methylene blue dye into the bladder may help identify the site of injury. When an injury is noted, laparoscopic suture repair can be used to close the defect ([8], [10]).

Ureteral injury is a serious complication of laparoscopy and unfortunately, in most patients may not be diagnosed at the time of surgery. If injury is identified or suspected intraoperative ureteral stenting may be considered. For intraoperative prevention of ureteral injuries a thorough knowledge of the anatomy is mandatory. Using cautery or any kind of energy source close to the ureter should be avoided. Control of hemorrhage in the area of the ureters should be performed with surgical clips whenever possible (see Fig. 25.3).

All trocars should be removed under vision and it is good practice to inspect all secondary trocar sites for active bleeding before the laparoscope is finally withdrawn. The inspection should be carried out when the intra-abdominal pressure has been lowered, because the pneumoperitoneum can tamponade venous bleeding and by lowering the pressure, these vessels can be identified. In case of injuries to the epigastric vessels blood can be seen dripping down the trocar into the abdomen or haematoma formation can be detected around the trocar site. Minimal bleeding can often be controlled by coagulation of the parietal peritoneum above and below the trocar. A Foley catheter can be passed through the trocar site and used as a tamponade. For moderate to severe bleeding, full thickness abdominal wall sutures can be placed under laparoscopic control both above and below the trocar site using a long and straight needle.

In case of minimal bleeding close to the rectum or the ureter the use of topical haemostatic agents can be considered. Several topical haemostatic agents are currently available in a range of configurations. They improve primary haemostasis, stimulate fibrin formation or inhibit fibrinolysis. Sometimes the procoagulant substance is combined with a vehicle such as collagen matrix.

References

1. Ahmad G, O'Flynn H, Duffy JM, Phillips K, Watson A. Laparoscopic entry techniques. Cochrane Database Syst Rev. 2012;2:CD006583.
2. Pierre F, Chapron C. Complications of laparoscopy: an inquiry about closed versus open-entry technique. Am J Obstet Gynecol. 2005;192(4):1352–3.
3. Jansen FW, Kolkman W, Bakkum EA, de Kroon CD, Trimbos-Kemper TC, Trimbos JB. Complications of laparoscopy: an inquiry about closed- versus open-entry technique. Am J Obstet Gynecol. 2004;190(3):634–8.
4. Agarwala N, Liu CY. Safe entry techniques during laparoscopy: left upper quadrant entry using the ninth intercostal space–a review of 918 procedures. J Minim Invasive Gynecol. 2005;12(1):55–61.
5. Palmer R. Safety in laparoscopy. J Reprod Med. 1974;13(1):1–5.
6. Childers JM, Brzechffa PR, Surwit EA. Laparoscopy using the left upper quadrant as the primary trocar site. Gynecol Oncol. 1993;50(2):221–5.
7. Mettler L, Jacobs V, Brandenburg K, Jonat W, Semm K. Laparoscopic management of 641 adnexal tumors in Kiel, Germany. J Am Assoc Gynecol Laparosc. 2001;8(1):74–82.
8. Ulker K, Anuk T, Bozkurt M, Karasu Y. Large bowel injuries during gynecological laparoscopy. World J Clin Cases. 2014;2(12):846–51.
9. van Goor H. Consequences and complications of peritoneal adhesions. Colorectal Dis. 2007;9(Suppl 2):25–34.
10. Worley MJ, Slomovitz BM, Ramirez PT. Complications of laparoscopy in benign and oncologic gynecological surgery. Rev Obstet Gynecol. 2009;2(3):169–75.

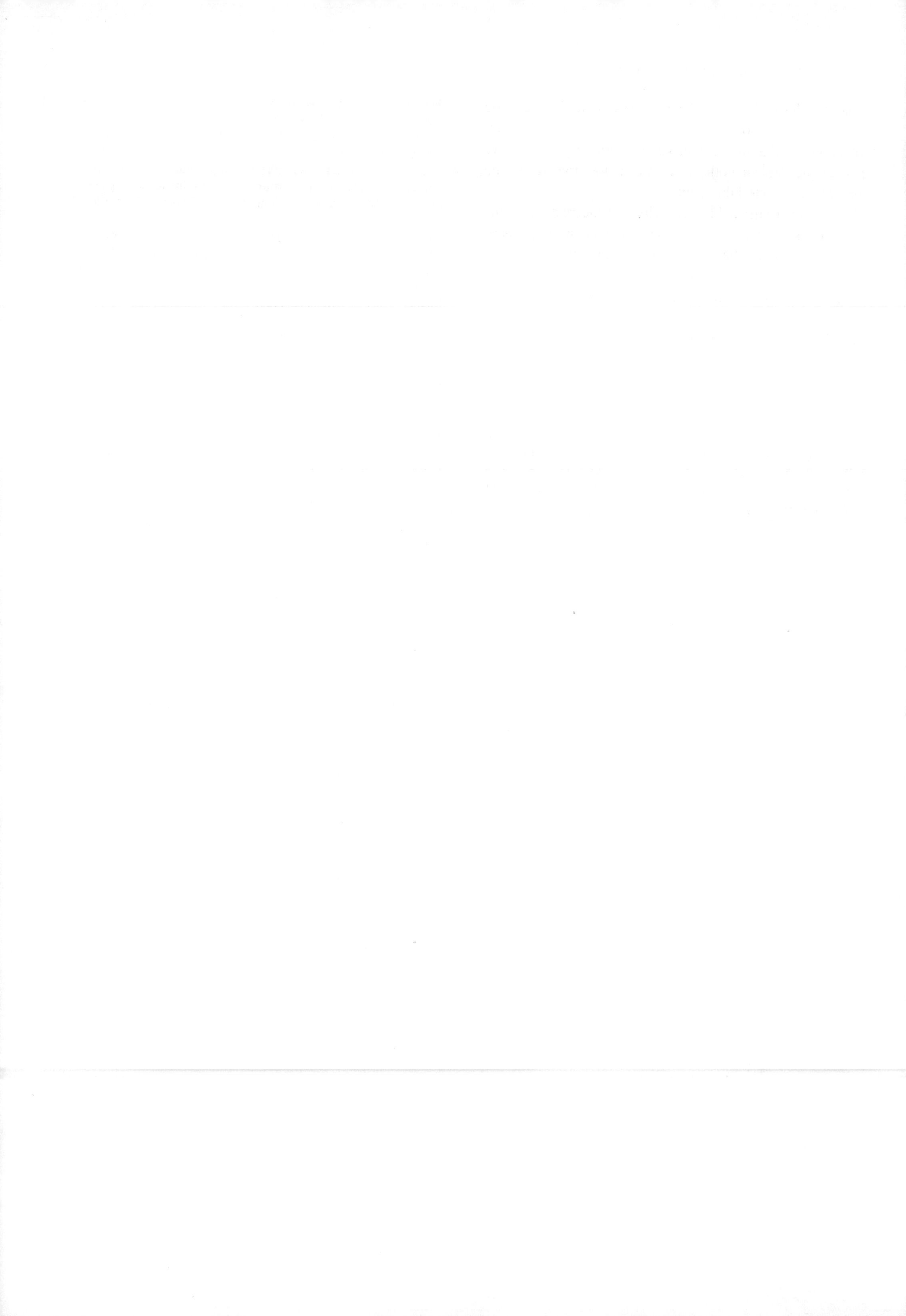

26 General Aspects and Their Handling: Adhesions

Andreas Hackethal, Jörg Engel, Hans-Rudolf Tinneberg, and Sebastian F.M. Häusler

Introduction

Intraabdominal adhesions severely increase the risk of injuries to bladder, omentum, ureter or vessels followed by major blood loss. An enterotomie occurs in 20 % of cases followed by an impaired patient outcome [1]. Elis found, that one third of patients with intraperitoneal operations are readmitted an average of 2.1 times for a disorder directly or possibly related to adhesions, or for repeat surgery that could potentially be complicated by adhesions [2]. Additionally, adhesions are responsible for 65–75 % of small bowel obstructions which could be life threatening and evoke further need of subsequent surgical intervention [2–7]. Therefore, intraabdominal adhesions have a severe impact on the quality of life of many patients. Nevertheless, social and healthcare system associated impacts as well as the increasing burden of medicolegal claims linked to intraperitoneal adhesions and their consequences are often underestimated.

Adhesions result from wound healing processes after peritoneal injury (Fig. 26.1). Since early publications over 100 years ago, a variety of factors influencing mesothelial healing and adhesion formation as well as factors preventing adhesion formation have been discussed and identified [8–13].

A. Hackethal (✉)
Gynecology and Obstetrics, University Clinic Wuerzburg, Wuerzburg 97080, Germany
e-mail: hackvalley@me.com

J. Engel
Department of OB/Gyn, Klinikum Aschaffenburg, Aschaffenburg 63739, Germany
e-mail: joergbengel@hotmail.com

H.-R. Tinneberg
University Clinic Giessen, Department of Gynecology and Obstetrics, Giessen, Germany

S.F.M. Häusler
Universitätsfrauenklinik Würzburg, Universitätsklinikum Würzburg, Würzburg 97080, Germany
e-mail: Haeusler_s@ukw.de

I. Alkatout, L. Mettler (eds.), *Hysterectomy*, DOI 10.1007/978-3-319 22497 8_26

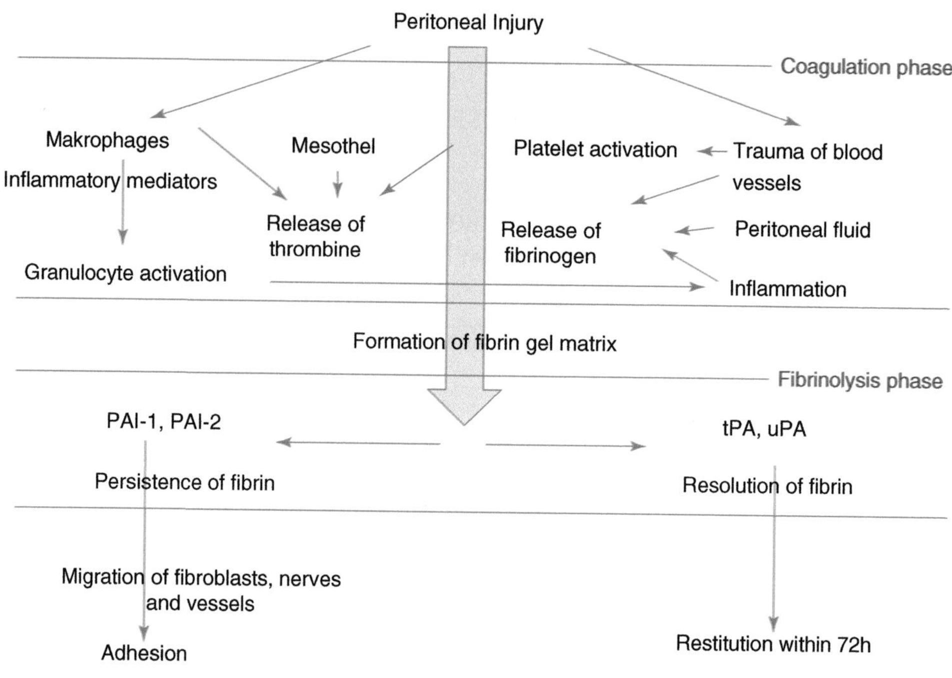

Fig. 26.1 Summary of cellular and humoral responses after peritoneal injury (With permission from Brüggmann et al. [14])

Anticipation, Diagnosis and Considerations of Preoperative Intraabdominal Adhesions

To minimize the risk of adhesion related complications during abdominal entry, one of the key steps is awareness of adhesions and identification of patients with potential intraabdominal adhesions preoperatively. Hence, patients with previous abdominal trauma, histories of pelvic inflammatory or other chronic diseases warrant special attention.

Epidemiologic studies describe postoperative adhesion formation in 50–100 % of surgical patients [4, 15]. The adhesion prevention in gynecological surgery guideline by the Society of Obstetricians and Gynecologists of Canada (SOGC) summarizes in a statement that the risk of adhesion increases with the total number of abdominal and pelvic surgeries performed on one patient [16]. It is well known, that operative laparotomies result in more adhesions than operative laparoscopic approaches [17]. Additionally, adhesions were found more frequently after vertical midline incisions than after transverse suprapubic incisions (59 % vs. 29 %) [17]. Sepilian et al. identified umbilical adhesions after previous laparoscopy in 21 % [18].

The incidence of intraabdominal adhesions after gynecological surgeries is difficult to estimate. Apart from surgeons' experiences, studies with evaluation of adhesion-related complications might help to delineate the incidence.

Within three surveys amongst German, British and European gynecologists regarding their awareness and perceptions of adhesions and adhesion-related consequences, the respondents thought surgeries for endometriosis, adhesiolysis and myomectomy to highest likely be associated with adhesion formation [19–21]. However, the highest rate of readmission to hospital after open gynecological surgery was found after prior adnexal surgery [22]. Additionally, adhesion-related small bowel obstruction after hysterectomy was found to be a significant cause of re-admission to hospital within a Canadian retrospective study [23]. Muffly et al. found 17 small bowel obstructions (SBO) in 3229 hysterectomies within a retrospective analysis. SBOs were identified after abdominal hysterectomy in 9 of 17 (53 %), vaginal hysterectomies in 5/17 (29.4 %) and laparoscopic hysterectomies in 3/17 (17.6 %). The authors claim, that despite the clinical tendency there were no statistical significant differences within the surgical approaches [24].

It is a well-established fact that intra-abdominal adhesions and intra-operative complications increase with successive number of cesarean sections [25, 26]. In regards to adhesion prevention, a recent Cochrane analysis reviewed closure of the peritoneum versus non-closure of the peritoneum [27]. Data of 17,276 women does not support the additional operative time and suture material to close the peritoneum, since the evidence on adhesion formation was limited and inconsistent [27].

Furthermore, intraabdominal adhesions are often found in women with previous pelvic inflammatory disease and suspected or diagnosed endometriosis. Intraabdominal adhesions cause 15–20 % of female infertility and the most common morphologic changes seen in women with chronic abdominal pain are pelvic adhesions [28–30].

Additional to patient history and symptoms, the per vaginal examination might raise the suspicion for pelvic adhesions. Palpation of a fixed pelvic organs or a frozen pelvis, in absence of other causes, may reflect pelvic adhesions. Demco analyzed pain scores of nature and location of adhesion during awake laparoscopy in 30 women. On a visual analogue scale, the highest pain was associated with filmy adhesions that allowed movement between two structures. Fixed adhesions that did not allow movement had the lowest pain scores [31].

To date, only sparse data exist on non-invasive imaging techniques to identify intraabdominal adhesions. However, certain real-time or functional imaging modalities can delineate intraabdominal adhesions. A literature review published in 2010 found 16 studies on transabdominal ultrasonography and cine-MRI which identified adhesions using visceral slide with accuracy of 76 % and 92 %, respectively [32]. The authors conclude that all but one study were biased by not being blinded and they suggest further double-blinded comparative studies to validate the results [32]. Seow and colleagues found a sensitivity of 90 and specificity of 100 % using three-dimensional transvaginal ultrasonography and level of CA12–5 to detect pelvic adhesions preoperatively [33]. More recently, Reid et al. reported on the transvaginal sonographic sliding sign and Kikuchi et al. evaluated the usefulness of the MRI jelly method to predict obliteration of the pouch of Douglas [34, 35]. A positive sign, signalizing no pouch of Douglas obliteration, is shown by gentle pressure with the transvaginal ultrasonography probe. In this case, the anterior rectum glides over the posterior vaginal wall and part of the cervix and the rectosigmoid glides over the posterior uterine wall [34]. Kikuchi et al. used ultrasonography jelly within vagina and rectum during MRI and found an increased sensitivity and specificity in identifying an obliterated pouch of Douglas [35]. However, both imaging modalities could not visualize filmy adhesions and adnexal adhesions.

As stated above, intraabdominal adhesions are a common finding during surgery and lead to a significant higher complications rate. In light of this, an adequate preoperative consent about possible adhesions and their consequences should be mandatory. Rajab et al. evaluated 200 surgical consent forms from 6 hospitals for the documented risk of adhesions related complications, which was only stated in 8.5 % of consent forms [36]. Similar results were found in two nationwide Dutch surveys. Only 5.2 % of Gynecologists and 9.8 % of General Surgeons reported to routinely include adhesion-related morbidity in the informed consent [37, 38]. In spite of the implications of adhesion-related complications, a standardized consent form was developed to educate patients adequately and document this process [39].

Apart from adequate preoperative patient consent, different presurgical measures have been examined to reduce potential adhesion related complications. Seow et al. suggested mechanical bowel preparation to decrease intraabdominal bowel volume and surgical complications [33]. More important are surgical steps during abdominal entry. Here, the site of entry should be adopted if previous laparotomies or laparoscopies have been performed or large pelvic masses are present. The Palmers point entry, 2 cm below the costal margin at midclavicular line left upper quadrant, can be considered as a safe entry approach, if no left upper quadrant abdominal surgery was performed previously [40, 41]. Additionally, a direct optical entry (DOE) was less time consuming and associated with less blood loss compared to an open entry [42]. Though the authors claim no statistical significance, the number of bowel and vascular injuries was 1/86 (1,2 %) in the DOE group compared to 10/82 (12,2 %) in the open entry group [42].

Surgical Management of Intraabdominal Adhesions

As intraabdominal adhesions result from wound healing, every attempt to lyse or dissect adhesions will likely re-form new adhesions. Data suggests the de novo-formation or reformation in 55–100 % of patients [43, 44]. Consequently, it is a valid question whether performing a full adhesiolysis during surgery should be mandatory, or whether exclusively the lysis of symptomatic or potentially symptomatic adhesions should be recommended. Studies from surveys underline, that Gynecologists agree, adhesiolysis should be performed in symptomatic patients [19, 21].

If patients lack symptoms and have no impairment of their quality of life, adhesions should not be treated [5]. However, in symptomatic patients, it is debatable whether to perform an adhesiolysis during diagnostic laparoscopy or not, as the impact of adhesiolysis cannot be predicted confidently. A well-recognized randomized controlled multicenter trial of laparoscopic adhesiolysis in chronic abdominal pain patients showed no significant differences in follow-up pain scores for patients with only diagnostic laparoscopy and those with performed adhesiolysis [45]. It is noteworthy, that patients with bowel obstructing adhesions were excluded in this study. In contrast, other studies have shown chronic abdominopelvic pain improvement rates after laparoscopic adhesiolysis of up to 84 % [46, 47].

Additionally, infertile patients with adnexal adhesions benefit from adhesiolysis. The pregnancy rate were 32 % after 12 month and 45 % after 24 month in the treated group compared with 15 % after 12 month and 16 % after 24 month in women left untreated [48].

It remains common sense that not the question of how many adhesions have been lysed, but rather, which adhesions have been lysed impacts on patients well-being.

Surgical adhesiolysis can be performed in various ways: sharp dissection with scissors with or without bipolar diathermy, with monopolar diathermy, with laser dissection or blunt by traction and counter traction. In general, the latter is the most important step in adhesiolysis. Especially in laparoscopic surgery it is of outmost importance to define the adhesions and involved structures to minimize the risk of organ injury before dissection. We usually use traction and counter traction with a 3D movement of the adhesion to better define the involved structures and define the starting point of adhesiolysis. Studies evaluating the impact on the tissue and reformation of adhesions using these different approaches are lacking.

Strategies to Reduce Adhesions Reformation

The medical professional's awareness of intraabdominal adhesion formation is the key for adhesion reduction or prophylaxis. Therefore, numerous articles and statements concerning the burden of adhesions and strategies for prevention have been published especially within the last few years. The Practice Committee of the American Society for Reproductive Medicine (ASRM) with the Society of Reproductive Surgeons (SRS) published a committee statement concerning pathogenesis, consequences and control of peritoneal adhesions in gynecologic surgery [49]. The Society of Obstetricians and Gynecologists Canada (SOGC) summarized recommendations of adhesion prevention in Gynecology in a guideline published in 2010 [16]. On behalf of the European Society for Gynecological Endoscopy (ESGE), a consensus paper has been published to guide gynecologists in "state of the art" handling of adhesions and to fulfill their duty of patient care [50, 51].

Additionally, a recent Cochrane review analyzed Cochrane data on adhesion prevention agents for gynecological surgery [13].

Apart from individual patient characteristics and the impact of surgical procedures on adhesion formation, the main focus of adhesion prophylaxis comprises surgical technique and barrier methods.

Recognizing that no prevention of adhesions is possible, most authors agree that their formation can be reduced with good surgical practice to minimize tissue trauma and diminished placement of foreign materials in the peritoneal cavity [14, 15, 49, 50, 52, 53]. It is understood, that good surgical technique comprises gentle tissue handling, meticulous hemostasis, excision of necrotic tissue, minimizing ischemia and desiccation, the use of fine, nonreactive suture materials and prevention of foreign body reaction and infection (Table 26.1) [14, 16, 49].

An experimental study by Kraemer et al. analyzed different surgical trauma and their impact on inducing peritoneal adhesions in rats [54]. Brushing of the parietal peritoneum and bipolar coagulation of the peritoneum were the least adhesiogenic trauma. Highest rates of adhesions were found after traumatizing with electrocoagulation of the peritoneum and defect closure with Vicryl sutures [54].

Table 26.1 Good surgical practice [14]

Gentle tissue handling
Meticulous hemostasis
Excision of necrotic tissue
Minimizing ischemia and desiccation
Use of fine, non-reactive sutures
Prevention of foreign body reaction
Prevention of infection

Surgical separation of wound sites, i.e., transient ovariopexy in surgical excision of severe endometriosis, is helpful in reducing adhesion formation and improving fertility outcomes [55, 56]. Interestingly, a recent systematic review and meta-analysis concludes however, that the two main adhesion-related outcomes, small bowel obstruction and infertility, are not reduced by less-invasive techniques or introducing less foreign bodies [57].

Reducing peritoneal adhesions is attempted by various strategies. Pharmacological, mechanical and other adhesion prevention strategies are summarized in Table 26.2.

In recent decades, the armamentarium of commercially available anti-adhesion products has increased. Generally, anti-adhesion agents aim to either reduce the inflammatory response after surgery or act as direct or indirect physical barrier on surgical sites. Reduction of inflammatory response, as example, might be achieved by Non-steroidal antirheumatics or steroids, physical barrier by modified hyaluronic acid or modified cellulose.

Surveys examining the awareness for intraabdominal adhesions in health care practitioners underline that there is uncertainty in the treatment and prophylactic strategies in dealing with adhesions [10, 19, 55].

The American Society for Reproductive Medicine concludes that FDA-approved surgical barriers have been demonstrated effective for reducing postoperative adhesions, but not having an impact on clinical symptoms [49]. The European field guideline for gynecological surgery states, that the implementation of good surgical practice, together with the adoption of adhesion-reduction agents, is paramount to reduce adhesion formation [12]. The Society of Gynecologists and Obstetricians Canada recommends that surgeons could consider using an adhesion barrier for patients who are at high risk of forming clinically significant adhesions [16].

A recent Cochrane review analyzed previous Cochrane reviews on adhesion prevention agents for gynaecological surgery and concludes that there is insufficient evidence to draw any conclusions about the effectiveness and safety of anti-adhesion agents in gynaecological surgery, due to the lack of data on pelvic pain, fertility outcomes, quality of life or safety [13].

Table 26.2 Different pharmacological, mechanical, and other adhesion prevention strategies [10, 56, 57]

Pharmacologic	Ileus prophylactics	*Exogenic tissue*
Anticoagulation	Plication of the intestines (Noble)	Amnotic membrane
Dicumarol	Plication of the mesentery	Fish bladder
Heparin	Intestinal catheter	Gel Photopolymerization
Hirudin	**Suface isolation**	Gore Tex
Oxalate	*Insufflation*	Rubber- and Plastic film
Citrate	Pneumoperitoneum	Bowine peritoneum
Fibrinolysis	*Instillation*	Polytetrafluoroethylene membrane
Actase	Agar	Silk
Chymotrysin	Albumin	Silver- and Gold films
Hyaluronidase	Amnotic fluid	Cellulose and Gelatine films
Calcium antagonists	Chymus	Oxygenized cellulose
Papain	Dextran	*Others*
Pepsin	Ironhyaluronidase gel Intergel	Allopurinol
Plasminogen activator	Electrolyt fluids	Aprotinin
Protoporphyrin	Gelatine	Chinese herbs
Streptokinase	Vitreous body fluid	Fibrin glue
Trypsin	Glycol	Infrasound
Urokinase	Honey	Moor mud wrap
Reduction of fibrosis	Sodium Hyaluronate/ Carboxymethylcellulose	Peristaltics
Anti histaminics	Hydroxyethylstark	Progesterone
Cochicin	Lanoline	Prostacycline
Non steroidal antirheumatics	Olive oile	Superoxiddismutase
Steroids	Paraffine	Tetrachlorodecaoxide
Vitamin E	Phosphatdicholine	**Others**
Cytostatics	Polysiloxan	Ultrasound to stimulate motility
Antibiotics	Polyvinylpyrrolidon	Iron turnings to stimulate bowel motility by external magnets
Antiseptics	Silicone	
Procinetics	Vaseline	
Cisapride	*Autolouge tissue*	
Neostigmine	Bladder	
	Omentum	
	Peritoneum	
	Mesenchymal stem cells	

Conclusion

Intraabdominal adhesions are the most common complication of abdominopelvic surgery. Surgeons' awareness is crucial and should include an adequate preoperative patient counsel. Apart from good surgical practice and continuous education on new surgical strategies to reduce adhesions, results of anti-adhesion products in randomized trials are difficult to obtain and interpretation may be influenced by various factors. It is understood, that not the number of adhesions within the abdomen but rather the clinical impact of adhesions on the patients well-being plays the important role. Though the scientific results of adhesion reduction are promising, the regular use of these agents in clinical practice is mostly uncommon and health care providers mostly do not refund the cost of anti-adhesion products adequately.

Strategies to identify adhesions with clinical impact and classifications of adhesions at the beginning and the end of surgery could eventually help to generate more robust data to define useful adhesion reduction strategies with and without agents.

References

1. Van Der Krabben AA, Dijkstra FR, Nieuwenhuijzen M, et al. Morbidity and mortality of inadvertent enterotomy during adhesiotomy. Br J Surg. 2000;87:467–71.
2. Ellis H, Moran BJ, Thompson JN, et al. Adhesion-related readmissions after abdominal pelvic surgery: a retrospective cohort study. Lancet. 1999;353:1476–80.
3. Mavros MN, Velmahos GC, Lee J, et al. Morbidity related to concomitant adhesions in abdominal surgery. J Surg Res. 2014;192: 286–92.

4. GS dZ. Contemporary adhesion prevention. Fertil Steril. 1994;61: 219–35.
5. Menzies D, Ellis H. Intestinal obstruction from adhesions: How big is the problem? Ann R Coll Surg Engl. 1990;72:60–3.
6. Operative Laparoscopy Study Group. Postoperative adhesion development after operative laparoscopy: evaluation at early second-look procedures. Fertil Steril. 1991;55:700–4.
7. Monk BJ, Berman ML, Monitz FJ. Adhesions after extensive gynecologic surgery: clinical significance, etiology and prevention. Am J Obstet Gynecol. 1994;170:1396–403.
8. Dembowski T. Über die Ursachen der peritonealen Adhäsionen nach chirurgischen Eingriffen mit Rücksicht auf die Frage des Ileus nach Laparotomien. Langenbecks Arch Chir. 1889;37:745.
9. Uhlmann C. Ueber das Auftreten peritonealer Adhäsionen nach Laparotomien, mit besonderer Berücksichtigung des Verhaätnisses zwischen trockener und feuchter Asepsis. Arch Gynecol Obstet. 1897;54:384–411.
10. Grund D. Neue Möglichkeiten zur Reduzierung von postoperativen Adhäsionen. Eine vergleichende tierexperimentelle Studie mit abriebarmen Bauchtüchern und Perfluorcarvon PF 5080. 2004, Promotion Charite – Universitätsmedizin Berlin.
11. Durron JJ. Postoperative intraperitoneal adhesion pathophysiology. Colorectal Dis. 2007;9(Suppl 2):14–24.
12. DeWilde RL, Brölmann H, Koninckx PR, The Anti-Adhesions in Gynecology Expert Panel (ANGEL), et al. Prevention of adhesions in gynaecological surgery: the 2012 European field guideline. Gynecol Surg. 2012;9:365–8.
13. Hindocha A, Beere L, Dias S, et al. Adhesion prevention agents for gynaecological surgery: an overview of Cochrane reviews. Cochrane Database Syst Rev. 2015;1:CD011254.
14. Brüggmann D, Tchartchian G, Wallwiener M, Münstedt K, Tinneberg H-R, Hackethal A. Intra-abdominal adhesions: definition, origin, significance in surgical practice, and treatment options. Dtsch Arztebl Int. 2010;107:769–75.
15. Liakakos T, Thomakos N, Fine PM, Dervenis C, Young RL. Peritoneal adhesions: etiology, pathophysiology, and clinical significance. Dig Surg. 2001;18:260–73.
16. Robertson D, Lefebvre G, Leyland N, et al. Adhesion prevention in gynaecological surgery. J Obstet Gynaecol Can. 2010;32:598–608.
17. Levrant SG, Bieber EJ, Barnes RB. Anterior abdominal wall adhesions after laparotomy or laparoscopy. J Am Assoc Gynecol Laparosc. 1997;4:353–6.
18. Sepilian V, Ku L, Wong H, et al. Prevalence of intraabdominal ahdesions in women with previous laparoscopy. JSLS. 2007;11:| 41–4.
19. Hackethal A, Sick C, Brueggmann D, et al. Awareness and perception of intraabdominal adhesions and related consequences. Survey of gynaecologists in German hospitals. Eur J Obstet Gynecol Reprod Biol. 2010;150:180–9.
20. Trew G, Cooke I, Lower A, McVeigh E. Post-operative abdominal adhesions – awareness of UK gynaecologists – a survey of members of the Royal College of Obstetricians and Gynaecologists. Gynecol Surg. 2009;6:25–37.
21. Wallwiener M, Koninckx PR, Hackethal A, for The Anti-Adhesions in Gynecology Expert Panel (ANGEL), et al. A European survey on awareness of post-surgical adhesions among gynaecological surgeons. Gynecol Surg. 2014;11:105–12.
22. Lower AM, Hawthorn RJ, Ellis H, et al. The impact of adhesions on hospital readmissions over ten years after 8849 open gynaecological operations: an assessment from the Surgical and Clinical Adhesions Research Study. BJOG. 2000;107:855–62.
23. Al-Sunaidi M, Tulandi T. Adhesion-related bowel obstruction after hysterectomy for benign conditions. Obstet Gynecol. 2006;108: 1162–6.
24. Muffly TM, Ridgeway B, Abbott S, et al. Small bowel obstruction after hysterectomy to treat benign disease. J Minim Invasive Gynecol. 2012;19:615–9.
25. Zia S, Rafique M. Intra-operative domplications increase with successive number of cesarean sections: myth or fact? Obstet Gynecol Sci. 2014;57:187–92.
26. Özcan S, Karayalcin R, Kanat PM. Multiple repeat cesarean delivery is associated with increase maternal morbidity irrespective of placenta accreta. Eur Rev Med Pharmacol Sci. 2015;19:1959–63.
27. Bamigboye AA, Hofmeyr GJ. Closure versus non-closure of the peritoneum at caesarean section: short- and long-term outcomes. Cochrane Database Syst Rev. 2014;8:CD000163.
28. Aziz. Laparoscopic evaluation of female factors in infertility. J Coll Physicians Surg Pak. 2010;20:649–52.
29. Luijendijk RW, de Lange DC, Wauters CC, et al. Foreign material in postoperative adhesions. Ann Surg. 1996;223:242–8.
30. Duffy DM, GS dZ. Adhesion controversies: pelvic pain as a cause of adhesions, crystalloids in preventing them. J Reprod Med. 1996;41:19–26.
31. Demco L. Pain mapping of adhesions. J Am Assoc Gynecol Laparosc. 2004;11:181–3.
32. Zinther NB, Fedder J, Friis-Andersen H. Noninvasive detection and mapping of intraabdominal adhesions: a review of the current literature. Surg Endosc. 2010;24:2681–6.
33. Seow KM, Lin YH, Hsieh BC, et al. Transvaginal three-dimensional ultrasonography combined with serum CA 125 level for the diagnosis of pelvic adhesions before laparoscopic surgery. J Am Assoc Gynecol Laparosc. 2003;10:320–6.
34. Reid S, Lu C, Hardy N, et al. Office gel sonovaginography for the prediction of posterior deep infiltrating endometriosis: a multicenter prospective observational study. Ultrasound Obstet Gynecol. 2014;44:710–8.
35. Kikuchi I, Kuwatsuru R, Yamazaki K, et al. Evaluation of the usefulness of the MRI jelly method for diagnosing complete cul-de-sac obliteration. Biomed Res Int. 2014;2014 Article ID 437962, 7 pages
36. Rajab TK, Wallwiener M, Talukdar S, Kraemer B. Adhesion-related complications are common, but rarely discussed in preoperative consent: a multicenter study. World J Surg. 2009;33:748–50.
37. Meuleman T, Schreinemacher MH, van Goor H. Adhesion awareness: a nationwide survey of gynaecologists. Eur J Obstet Gynecol Reprod Biol. 2013;169:353–9.
38. Schreinemacher MH, ten Broek RP, Bakkum EA, et al. Adhesion awareness: a national survey of surgeons. World J Surg. 2010;34: 2805–12.
39. Hirschelmann A, Wallwiender CW, Wallwiender M, et al. Is patient education about adhesions a requirement in abdominopelvic surgery? Geburtshilfe Frauenheilkd. 2012;72:299–304.
40. Granata M, Tsimpanakos I, Moeity F, Magos A. Are we underutilizing Palmer's point entry in gynecologic laparoscopy? Fertil Steril. 2010;94:2716–9.
41. Aust TR, Salma IK, Rowlands DJ. Direct optical entry through Palmer's point: a new technique for those at risk of entry-related trauma at laparoscopy. General Surg. 2009;7:315–7.
42. Tinelli A, Malvasi A, Guido M, et al. Laparoscopy entry in patients with previous abdominal and pelvic surgery. Surg Innov. 2011;18: 201–5.
43. Diamond MP, Daniell JF, Feste J, et al. Adhesion reformation and de novo adhesion formation after reproductive pelvic surgery. Fertil Steril. 1987;47:864–6.
44. Diamond MP, Freeman ML. Clinical implications of postsurgical adhesions. Hum Reprod Update. 2001;7:567–76.
45. Swank DJ, Swank-Bordewijk SC, Hop WC, et al. Laparoscopic adhesiolysis in patients with chronic abdominal pain: a blinded randomised controlled multi- centre trial. Lancet. 2003;361:1247–51.
46. YC C, Reading I, Bailey S, Sadek K, Ledger W, TC L. Should women with chronic pelvic pain have adhesiolysis? BMC Womens Health. 2014;14:36.
47. Schietroma M, Carlei F, Altilia F, et al. The role of laparoscopic adhesiolysis in chronic abdominal pain. Minerva Chir. 2001;56:461–5.

48. Tulandi T, Collins JA, Burrows E, et al. Treatment-dependent and treatment- independent pregnancy among women with periadnexal adhesions. Am J Obstet Gynecol. 1990;162:354–7.
49. Practice Committee of American Society for Reproductive Medicine with Society of Reproductive Surgeons. Pathogenesis, consequences, and control of peritoneal adhesions in gynecologic surgery: a committee opinion. Fertil Steril. 2013;99:1550–5.
50. DeWilde RL, Bakkum EA, Brölmann H, et al. Consensus recommendations on adhesions (version 2014) for the ESGE Adhesions Research Working Group (European Society for Gynecological Endoscopy): an expert opinion. Arch Gynecol Obstet. 2014;290: 581–2.
51. DeWilde RL, Trew G, on behalf of the Expert Adhesions Working Party of the European Society of Gynaecological Endoscopy (ESGE). Postoperative abdom- inal adhesions and their prevention in gynaecological surgery. Expert consen- sus position. Gynecol Surg. 2007;4:161–8.
52. Brochhausen C, Schmitt VH, Planck CN, et al. Current strategies and future perspectives for intraperitoneal adhesion prevention. J Gastrointest Surg. 2012;16:1256–74.
53. Hellebrekers BW, Kooistra T. Pathogenesis of postoperative adhesion formation. Br J Surg. 2011;98:1503–16.
54. Kraemer B, Wallwiener C, Rajab TK, et al. Standardised models for inducing experimental peritoneal adhesions in female rats. Biomed Res Int. 2014;2014:435056. doi:10.1155/2014/435056. Epub 2014 Apr 8
55. Carbonnel M et al. Efficacy of transient abdominal ovariopexy in patients with severe endometriosis. Euro J Obstet Gyneco Reprod Biol. 2011;155:183–7.
56. Ouahba J, Madelenat P, Poncelet C. Transient abdominal ovariopexy for adhesion prevention in patients who underwent surgery for severe pelvic endometriosis. Fertil Steril. 2004;82: 1407–11.
57. Ten Broek RP, Issa Y, van Santbrink EJ, et al. Burden of adhesions in abdominal and pelvic surgery: systematic review and met-analysis. BMJ. 2013;347:f5588.
58. Hackethal A, Sick C, Szalay G, et al. Intra-abdominal adhesion formation: does surgical approach matter? Questionnaire survey of South Asian surgeons and literature review. J Obstet Gynaecol Res. 2011;37:1382–90.
59. Risberg B. Adhesions: preventive strategies. Eur J Surg Suppl. 1997;577:32–9.
60. Treutner KH, Schumpelick V. Adhäsionsprophylaxe. Wunsch und Wirklichkeit Chirurg. 2000;71:510–7.

Comorbidities

27

Ralf Rothmund

Clinical Comorbidity

It can generally be said that a laparoscopic or vaginal approach should be chosen where possible in the presence of serious concomitant disorders, since the intraoperative and postoperative stresses especially are relatively minor compared to those of open surgery. Convalescence usually proves to be correspondingly quick and straightforward.

The duration of surgery, as well as the intra- and postoperative complication rates, increase in obese patients compared to groups of patients of normal weight [1, 2]. The duration of surgery increases further in cases of extreme obesity, as does the risk of severe complications. It is these patients who particularly benefit from a laparoscopic approach [3] when a vaginal hysterectomy is not technically feasible [4, 5].

The technique of the surgical intervention itself remains unchanged in patients with severe obesity; however, the placement of the first trocar is extremely important in these patients. The risk of preperitoneal insufflation is higher in obese patients especially if a Veress-needle is used for insufflation. Therefore, the use of a trocar that enables the insertion of the optic device before CO_2 insufflation is recommended (see Table 27.1). While the surgical technique of hysterectomy in patients with obesity unchanged remains compared to normal weight patients, the surgeon is often constrained to operate with a reduced insufflational pressure and consequently a limited view of the neighbouring structures. In patients with severe obesity the combination of Trendelenburg-positioning and high intraabdominal pressure leads to a higher ventilation pressure. The surgeon is thus forced to work with lower intrabdominal pressure (10–12 mmHg) in order to enable a sufficient ventilation pressure (see Table 27.1). If the respiratory capacity of the patient is further limited by additional factors (e.g. COPD) a laparoscopic approach becomes impossible in some cases [6]. Hence, a COPD might become a limiting factor for the laparoscopic hysterectomy if sufficient intraoperative ventilation is not possible. In contrast, the presence of hypertension, a diagnose that often confounds with obesity, is managed perioperatively by the anaesthesiologist and has no direct implications for laparoscopic hysterectomy (see Table 27.1).

Obesity and diabetes are important risk factors for the development of postoperative infections and sepsis after abdominal hysterectomy. However, the risk of developing postoperative infection or sepsis after a laparoscopic hysterectomy is not increased for obese patients compared to patients of normal weight [7–10].

Table 27.1 Appropriate risk and management

Risk Factor	Intraoperative management	Postoperative management
Obesity	Adaption of the entrance technique (e.g. go without Veress-needle) Lower insufflational pressure	Venous thromboembolism prophylaxis
Chronic obstructive pulmonary disease	Lower insufflational pressure	Monitoring of the lung function
Hypertension	Regulation of blood pressure	Regulation of blood pressure
Diabetes	Monitoring of blood sugar	Monitoring of blood sugar Possible antibiotic prophylaxis in case of coexisting obesity
Deep infiltrating endometriosis	Adaption of preparation technique (e.g. retroperitoneal entrance in analogy to radical hysterectomy; nerve sparing technique) Surgery in dedicated centres	Monitoring of bladder and bowel function

R. Rothmund
Universitäts-Frauenklinik, Tübingen 72076, Germany
e-mail: Ralf.rothmund@med.uni-tuebingen.de

I. Alkatout, L. Mettler (eds.), *Hysterectomy*, DOI 10.1007/978-3-319-22497-8_27

In several studies, obesity was associated with a longer duration of surgery; however the intra- and postoperative complication rates were not increased [11–15].

Thromboembolism occurs less commonly after laparoscopic hysterectomy than after abdominal hysterectomy. It can therefore be concluded that a laparoscopic approach should be chosen where possible if there are risk factors for the development of thromboembolism, naturally in accordance with thromboprophylaxis guidelines [16].

Comorbidities such as obesity, smoking and diabetes do not increase the risk of vaginal cuff dehiscence [17].

Coexistence of Deep Infiltrating Endometriosis or Frozen Pelvis (See Figs. 27.1, 27.2 and 27.3)

Vaginal cuff dehiscence occurs more commonly where there is coexisting deep infiltrating endometriosis [18]. The presence of deep infiltrating endometriosis, especially in the retrovaginal fascia or the parametrial area, makes laparoscopic hysterectomy considerably more difficult. It is then necessary to adapt surgical dissection along the lines of a radical hysterectomy (see Table 27.1). Careful dissection of the ureters and distancing of the rectum from the posterior vaginal wall to avoid injury to the ureters or minimise the risk of fistula development between the rectum and vagina are particularly important in these cases. These procedures, with their significantly increased level of complexity, should only be performed in suitably qualified centres wherever possible.

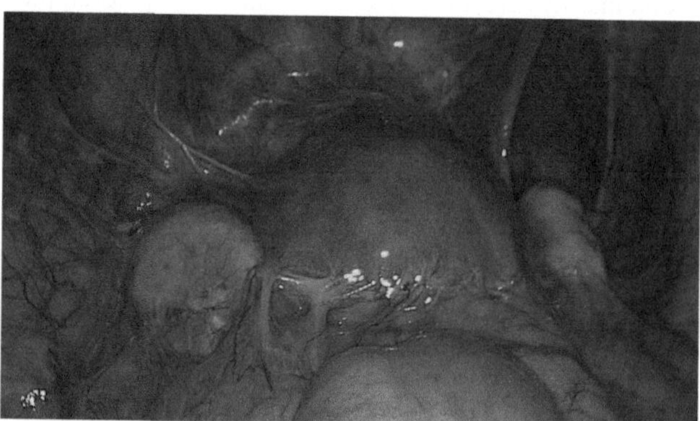

Fig. 27.1 Patient with frozen pelvis and deep infiltrating endometriosis in the rectovaginal fascia with severe dysmenorrhoea undergoing TLH

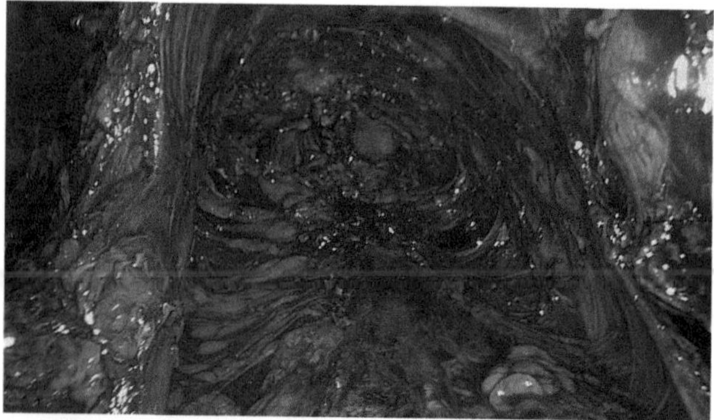

Fig. 27.2 Surgical dissection and excision of the endometriosis in the rectovaginal fascia before displacement of the uterus

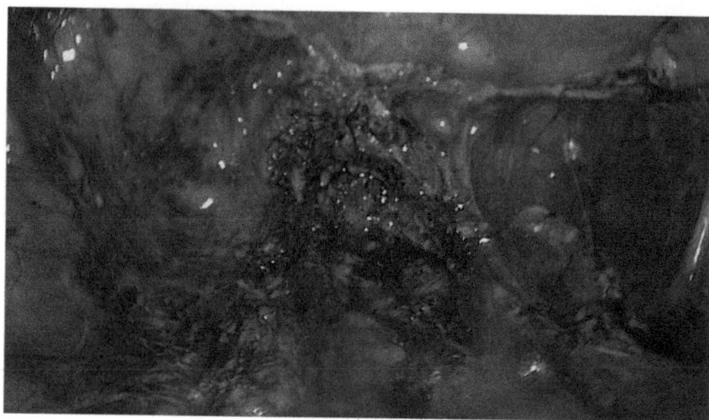

Fig. 27.3 End result: Rectum clearly distanced from the vaginal cuff to avoid fistula development

References

1. Morgan-Ortiz F, Soto-Pineda JM, López-Zepeda MA, Peraza-Garay FJ. Effect of body mass index on clinical outcomes of patients undergoing total laparoscopic hysterectomy. Int J Gynaecol Obstet. 2013;120(1):61–4.
2. McMahon MD, Scott DM, Saks E, Tower A, Raker CA, Matteson KA. Impact of obesity on outcomes of hysterectomy. J Minim Invasive Gynecol. 2014;21(2):259–65.
3. Siedhoff MT, Carey ET, Findley AD, Riggins LE, Garrett JM, Steege JF. Effect of extreme obesity on outcomes in laparoscopic hysterectomy. J Minim Invasive Gynecol. 2012;19(6):701–7.
4. Matthews KJ, Brock E, Cohen SA, Chelmow D. Hysterectomy in obese patients: special considerations. Clin Obstet Gynecol. 2014;57(1):106–14.
5. Committee on Gynecologic Practice. Committee opinion no. 619: gynecologic surgery in the obese woman. Obstet Gynecol. 2015; 125(1):274–8.
6. Afors K, Centini G, Murtada R, Castellano J, Meza C, Wattiez A. Obesity in laparoscopic surgery. Best Pract Res Clin Obstet Gynaecol. 2015;29(4):554–64.
7. Mahdi H, Goodrich S, Lockhart D, DeBernardo R, Moslemi-Kebria M. Predictors of surgical site infection in women undergoing hysterectomy for benign gynecologic disease: a multicenter analysis using the national surgical quality improvement program data. J Minim Invasive Gynecol. 2014;21(5):901–9.
8. Mikhail E, Miladinovic B, Finan M. The relationship between obesity and trends of the routes of hysterectomy for benign indications. Obstet Gynecol. 2014;123(Suppl 1):126S.
9. Mikhail E, Scott L, Imudia AN, Hart S. Total laparoscopic hysterectomy in the obese patient. Surg Technol Int. 2014;25:167–74.
10. Shah DK, Vitonis AF, Missmer SA. Association of body mass index and morbidity after abdominal, vaginal, and laparoscopic hysterectomy. Obstet Gynecol. 2015;125(3):589–98.

11. Hanwright PJ, Mioton LM, Thomassee MS, Bilimoria KY, Van Arsdale J, Brill E, Kim JY. Risk profiles and outcomes of total laparoscopic hysterectomy compared with laparoscopically assisted vaginalhysterectomy. Obstet Gynecol. 2013;121(4):781–7.
12. Kondo W, Bourdel N, Marengo F, Botchorishvili R, Pouly JL, Jardon K, Rabischong B, Mage G, Canis M. What's the impact of the obesity on the safety of laparoscopic hysterectomy techniques? J Laparoendosc Adv Surg Tech A. 2012;22(10): 949–53.
13. Mueller A, Thiel F, Lermann J, Oppelt P, Beckmann MW, Renner SP. Feasibility and safety of total laparoscopic hysterectomy (TLH) using the Hohl instrument in nonobese and obesewomen. J Obstet Gynaecol Res. 2010;36(1):159–64.
14. Guraslan H, Senturk MB, Dogan K, Guraslan B, Babaoglu B, L. Y. Total Laparoscopic Hysterectomy in Obese and Morbidly Obese Women. Gynecol Obstet Invest. 2015;79(3):184–8. [Epub ahead of print]
15. Wallwiener M, Taran FA, Rothmund R, Kasperkowiak A, Auwärter G, Ganz A, Kraemer B, Abele H, Schönfisch B, Isaacson KB, et al. Laparoscopic supracervical hysterectomy (LSH) versus total laparoscopic hysterectomy (TLH): an implementation study in 1,952 patients with an analysis of risk factors for conversion to laparotomy and complications, and of procedure-specific re-operations. Arch Gynecol Obstet. 2013;288(6):1329–39.
16. Barber EL, Neubauer NL, Gossett DR. Risk of venous thromboembolism in abdominal versus minimally invasive hysterectomy for benign conditions. Am J Obstet Gynecol. 2014;212(5):609.e1–7. pii: S0002-9378(14)02407-7
17. Leggieri C, Bertin M, Dalla Toffola A, Fagherazzi S, Vitagliano A, Conte L. Laparoscopic hysterectomy: really so risky to a vaginal cuff dehiscence? Clin Exp Obstet Gynecol. 2014;41(3):300–3.
18. Patzkowsky KE, As-Sanie S, Smorgick N, Song AH, Advincula AP. Perioperative outcomes of robotic versus laparoscopic hysterectomy for benign disease. JSLS. 2013;17(1):100–6.

28 General Surgery Conditions and Techniques for Gyne-Endoscopic Surgeons

John E. Morrison

Abdominal and Pelvic Wall: Hernias

The abdominal wall from the umbilicus superiorly to the symphysis pubis inferiorly and laterally to the iliac crests is an area that can be the site of abnormalities that are encountered either upon entering the abdominal cavity or be identified during the performance of laparoscopic procedures. The different techniques used to enter the abdomen are not within the scope of this chapter, but some of these abnormalities when encountered in the abdominal wall may make safe access a challenge.

The most commonly performed surgical procedure by general surgeons is hernia repair. Approximately 800,000 inguinal hernia repairs and over 200,000 incisional hernia repairs are performed yearly in the US. Primary hernias occur most commonly in the anterior abdominal wall either at the umbilicus or in the inguinal canal. They also may be present lateral to the rectus sheath at the linea semicircularis, the Spigelian Hernia however this is an uncommon type of defect.

The diagnosis of small incisional or inguinal hernias may be difficult preoperatively particularly if the patient is obese or the defect is small, and their presence may not be certain until insufflation is achieved.

Large hernias on the other hand are usually diagnosed preoperatively through a thorough physical exam, or by preoperative imaging, however in the morbidly obese patients this can be a difficult task. When an incisional hernia is suspected, CT scan of the abdomen and pelvis without contrast is the most sensitive imaging exam for hernia defects and is routinely performed to assess the size and number of defects in order to better plan operative repair and safe access into the abdomen.

The treatment of hernias differs depending on the symptoms, location, size and etiology so their diagnosis, location and size are crucial to planning appropriate care.

Umbilical Hernias

Primary umbilical hernias are usually diagnosed preoperatively and may be symptomatic particularly when small. If abdominal entry is planned through the umbilicus, an open (Hasson) technique is preferred because the fascial defect is already present and can be easily closed when exiting the abdominal cavity. Direct entry through the umbilicus when a hernia defect is present can be a very dangerous task, as omentum or bowel can easily be included in the hernia defect and as such can be injured with the Veress needle or visual port entry device. It is not uncommon for adhesions to form at the hernia site even without prior surgery so caution is advised. See Fig. 28.1.

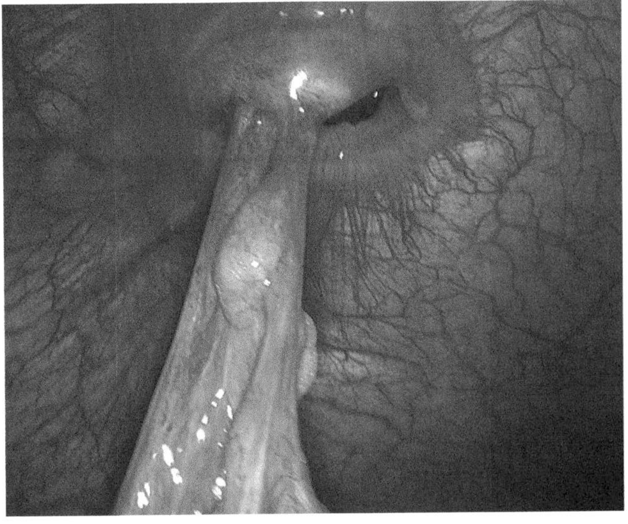

Fig. 28.1 Primary umbilical hernia with adhesions in a patient that has not had previous surgery

Electronic supplementary material The online version of this chapter (doi:10.1007/978-3-319-22497-8_28) contains supplementary material, which is available to authorized users.

J.E. Morrison, MD FACS
LSUHSC Department of Surgery, New Orleans, LA, USA
e-mail: Jmorr3@lsuhsc.edu

I. Alkatout, L. Mettler (eds.), *Hysterectomy*, DOI 10.1007/978-3-319-22497-8_28

Defects 2 cm or less in diameter are closed primarily with permanent suture and do not require mesh reinforcement. The suture chosen is usually a permanent material, polypropylene, or polyester, size 0, and the fascial edges approximated using simple or mattress suture techniques.

If the patient has had an umbilical hernia repaired previously and it is recurrent, then the defect is usually closed utilizing a reinforcing synthetic mesh material. There are several devices available which are designed specifically for these repairs. One such design is C-QUR V-Patch manufactured by Atrium corp. (Fig. 28.2) which is a circular polypropylene mesh coated with omega 3 fatty acid and is placed in the defect then sutured lateral to the fascial edges making certain that the mesh extends at least 3 cm from the fascial edge in all directions. The defect is then closed primarily over the reinforcing mesh.

Any mesh placed intrabdominally should have a barrier substance on the surface of the mesh coming in contact with the underlying bowel in order to reduce adhesions to these structures. Several products exist that have absorbable material incorporated onto the mesh to provide this barrier. If the reinforcing mesh is placed extraperitoneally then barrier material is not necessary.

Tips

Primary umbilical hernias 2 cm or less, close primarily with permanent suture.

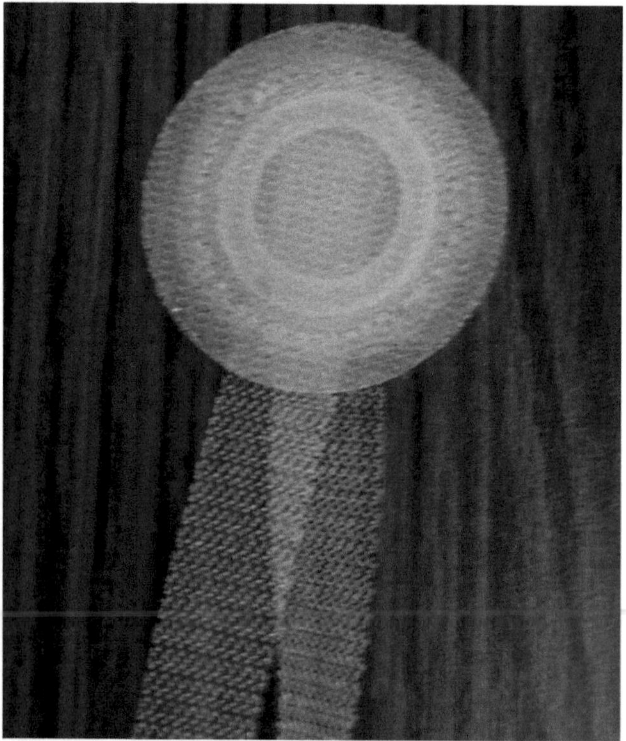

Fig. 28.2 Circular polypropylene mesh with barrier coating manufactured by Atrium Corp

Recurrent umbilical hernias or larger than 2 cm: repair with mesh reinforcement.

Mesh should extend at least 3–5 cm from the fascial edge.

Entry into abdomen through umbilical hernia: open technique is safest.

Incisional Hernias

Patients that have had any prior abdominal surgery are potential candidates for incisional hernias. There are approximately 250,000 incisional hernia repairs performed in the US yearly [1]. If the patient is found to have an incisional hernia, then the surgeon can usually anticipate more than one defect being present in the incision. The majority of incisional hernia defects are asymptomatic when they are small <1 cm Defects between 2 cm and 6 cm usually are symptomatic, and are repaired using a reinforcing synthetic material when they are encountered. There is no difference in treatment of incisional hernias with regards to their location in the abdominal wall whether above or below the umbilicus.

Large defects in the fascia are most often identified on physical exam but the most sensitive method again for diagnosis and measurement of the defect is a CT scan of the abdomen and pelvis.

Primary repair of incisional hernias without reinforcement of mesh has an unacceptably high recurrence rate [2]. The choices for reinforcement material are either synthetic or biologic. There are certain conditions where the biologic grafts have distinct advantages over synthetic materials but discussion of this topic is out of the scope of this chapter.

Most 2–8 cm incisional hernia defects currently are repaired using the laparoscopic approach. The repair most commonly utilized is referred to as a "bridge" repair where the defect is covered by mesh and the fascial edges are not reapproximated. The fascial defect may be primarily approximated and then covered with mesh but this technique is used less commonly. In both instances a reinforcing material is used.

When an incisional hernia defect is encountered during an "open" procedure, the fascia is closed primarily with suture, either permanent or long lasting absorbable suture, with synthetic mesh reinforcement. The synthetic mesh can be placed either (1) under the abdominal wall on the peritoneal surface in which instance the material should have an adhesive barrier, or (2) Between the posterior rectus fascia and anterior rectus muscle and fascia (retro rectus) or (3) as an onlay where the mesh is simply anchored to the abdominal wall covering the reapproximated midline incision and extending laterally at least 5–8 cm from the midline. The onlay method is the easiest and safest approach. See Fig. 28.3.

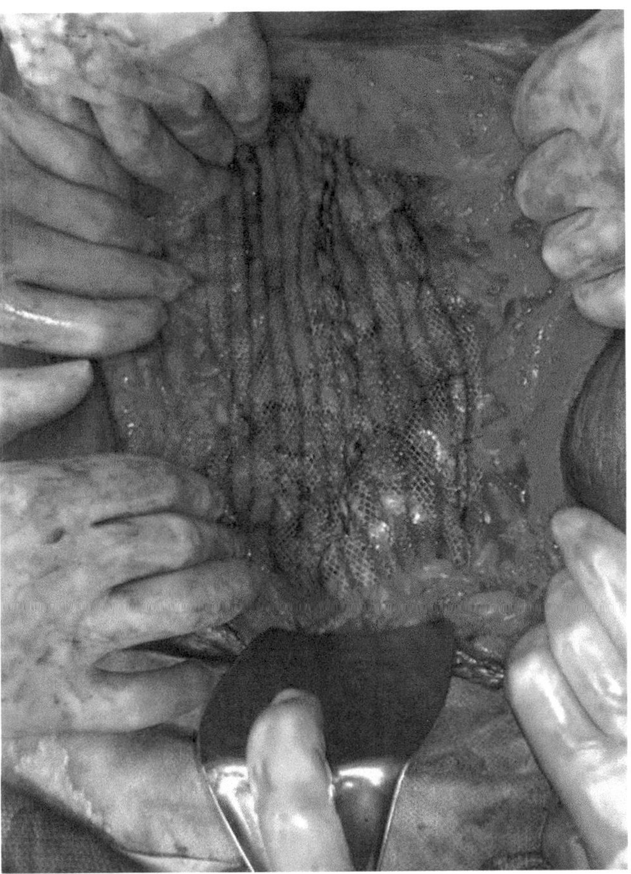

Fig. 28.3 Light weight polypropylene mesh lying over fascial closure

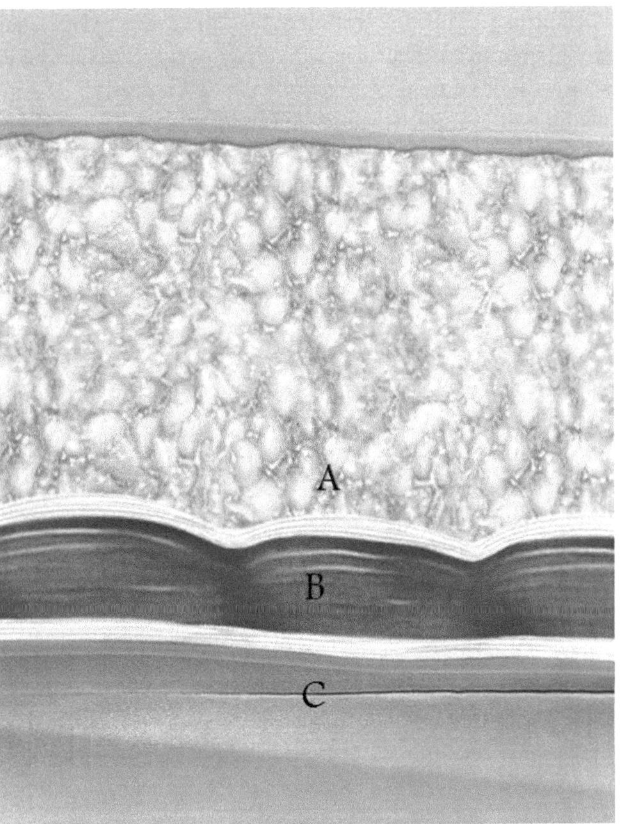

Fig. 28.4 Diagram of abdominal wall: (**A**) area where onlay graft is placed (**B**) area where retrorectus mesh placement occurs (**C**) area where underlay mesh placed and laparoscopic mesh placed

Figure 28.4 demonstrates commonly used sites for mesh placement. A: is where an onlay graft is placed. B: is where an inlay graft is placed. It usually lies between the fascia and muscle layers of the abdominal wall. C: is an underlay. Site C is the site where placement of laparoscopic mesh is usually performed.

Synthetic Materials Used for Repair

The materials used in these repairs must have certain properties:

First: the material must have the strength to tolerate pressures that are generated in the abdominal and pelvic cavity.

There are several studies currently ongoing that are addressing the most accurate way of determining the actual pressures generated in the abdominal and pelvic cavities and thus what strength characteristics the synthetic material must have in order to maintain an adequate repair. Over the past several years the density and structure of the synthetic mesh material used has undergone significant change. The main change is one of thinner, lighter weight materials with large pore structure for flexibility and easy incorporation into the abdominal wall tissues.

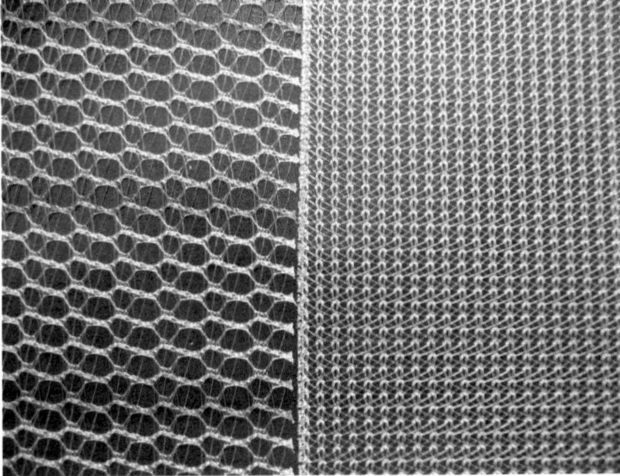

Fig. 28.5 Lightweight polypropylene mesh on left. Medium weight polypropylene mesh on right

Figure 28.5 demonstrates the two most commonly used polypropylene mesh types. The mesh on the left is a light weight mesh and the material on the right of the figure is a medium weight material. The differences are a combination of pore size and weight of the material used. The trend now is to utilize lighter weight materials however in large incisional hernia repairs tearing of this lightweight mesh is being seen with more frequency and there may be a return to using medium or heavier weight materials.

Second characteristic is that the material must adhere securely to the abdominal wall. The material is anchored either with suture or tacking devices or a combination of the two. The anchoring devices assist in preventing slippage of the material while it is being incorporated onto the abdominal wall. Depending on the physical properties of the material used, the mesh elicits a reaction that results in scar formation around the material that also assists in incorporation of the material into the abdominal wall and adding to the strength of the repair.

Third characteristic and one of the most important characteristics is that the material must possess a property that reduces adherence to the bowel and any underlying structures. The mesh must have secured onto it a barrier device that helps reduce adherence to the underlying bowel if it is placed intraperitoneally. Synthetic mesh placed into the abdominal cavity without any barrier carries a risk of erosion into the bowel or any other structure it comes in contact with and thus fistula formation. If this does occur then the synthetic mesh must be removed and the fistula closed. Replacement of the mesh by synthetic materials in this situation is not recommended and a biologic material is usually needed.

Fourth characterisitc is that the material should elicit a minimal inflammatory or immunologic response. Research is ongoing in this area and materials are constantly being tested and refined to reduce this reaction.

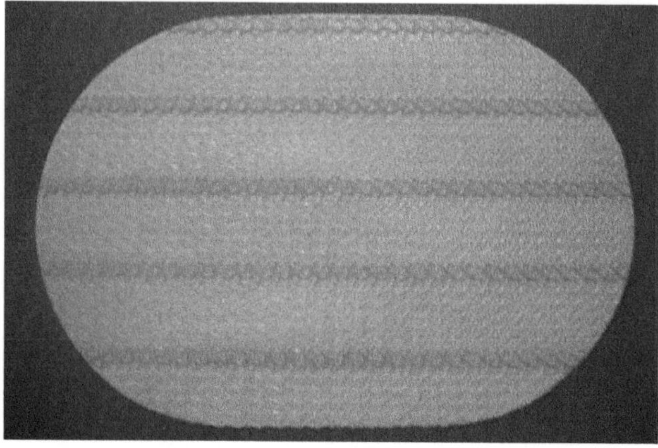

Fig. 28.6 Polypropylene mesh with barrier incorporated onto mesh for intraabdominal placement

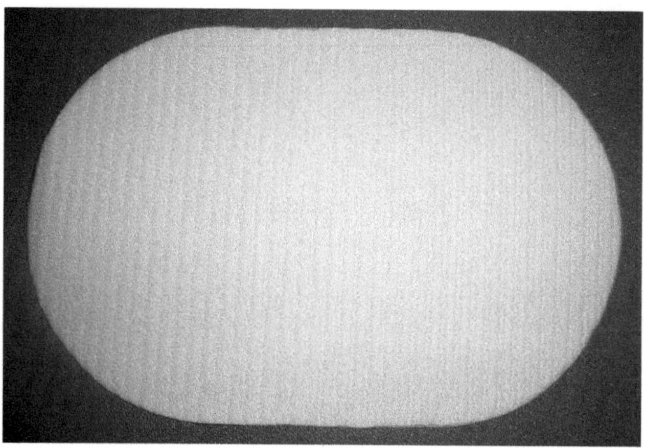

Fig. 28.7 Microporous PTFE mesh for intraabdominal repair

Materials for Repair

The most frequently utilized synthetic material in hernia repairs is polypropylene mesh. Figure 28.6 is an example of a coated polypropylene mesh used for hernia repair when the mesh is placed intraabdominally.

Polypropylene has been used for decades and because surgeons have a long experience and great familiarity with it, it is the preferred mesh material. Because of the hydrophilic nature of the material it does result in the formation of a fibrous capsule which can become firm over time and a source for pain but with reduction of polypropylene mesh weight, this phenomenon is becoming less of a problem.

PTFE (polytetrafluorethylene) is another material utilized in hernia repair in the abdomen. It has properties of minimal adherence to surrounding tissues, and flexibility, but because of its propensity for nonadherance, other materials must be incorporated into the mesh in order to make it adhere to the anterior abdominal wall. Otherwise the material is not incorporated and the repair not secured. Figure 28.7 is an example of a PTFE mesh used for hernia repair.

The PTFE mesh is a micro porous material, so seroma formation above the mesh and below the overlying skin and subcutaneous tissue after bridge repair is not uncommon. These seromas usually are asymptomatic and over time resolve, however if they become infected or symptomatic they can be drained percutaneousely or if mature excised after adequate incorporation of the underlying mesh has occurred. Seroma formation is not uncommon after any bridge type repair regardless of the material used. See Fig. 28.8.

When PTFE material is used for repair if an overlying seroma or the material itself becomes infected, it must be removed. The pore size is such that bacteria are able to enter the mesh but neutrophils cannot so the resulting infection cannot be cleared without mesh removal.

All grafts contract over time, but PTFE grafts do contract the most when compared to other synthetic materials, so this characteristic must be taken into consideration when placing the material and ensuring adequate overlapping of the defect [3].

Polyester mesh is also utilized for hernia repair but less frequently. The material is a woven braided polyester fiber that incorporates into the surrounding tissues well. This material has been used for decades in the manufacture of vascular grafts, so its use has a long history in surgery and thus experience with this material is large. It is a hydrophilic material so

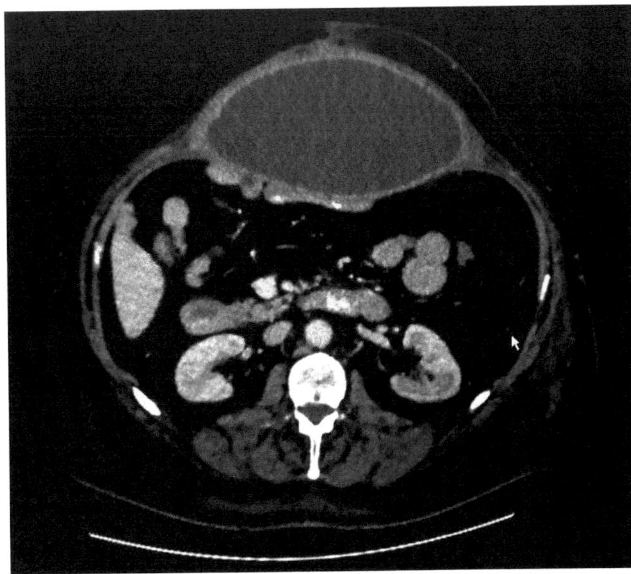

Fig. 28.8 Seroma over mesh under skin of abdominal wall

it does not elicit the intense fibrotic reaction that polypropylene does, but as with any braided material if it does become contaminated with bacteria or infected, it is difficult to clear of bacteria so it may require excision if this does occur.

When and How for Incisional Hernia Repairs?

Defects 2 cm or less may be repaired primarily with permanent suture material as in umbilical hernia repair.

Hernia defects >8 cm may require mobilization of anterior abdominal wall fascial layers with reinforcement by synthetic or biologic material in order to reapproximate the midline fascial edges and restore a dynamic abdominal wall.

To accomplish this there are a number of options which include relaxing incisions in the external oblique muscle bilaterally or in the posterior rectus fascia and transverse abdominal muscle layers in order to mobilize the fascia to get the midline fascial edges together. Discussion of this type of repair is out of the scope of this chapter and these large defects should be **referred** for definitive repair either before gynecologic procedures are performed or preferably repaired at the time of gynecologic surgery by a General Surgeon or Plastic Surgeon familiar with these type of repairs.

The treatment of choice for repair of incisional hernia defects from 2 cm to 6 cm currently is via laparoscopy and is usually performed at the end of other surgical procedures. The mesh should overlap the defect by at least 3 cm preferably up to 5 cm or more on all edges and be anchored to the abdominal wall. If during the primary operative procedure the bowel is entered, gross contamination with infected material is encountered or the vagina or bladder are entered, and an incisional hernia repair is considered, then the use of synthetic mesh is discouraged and biologic graft used in its place. Biologic grafts may be used in a bridge repair or as a reinforcing material to primary closure but there are no good studies to gauge its long-term success and these materials are very expensive.

Procedure for Repair of Incisional Hernia

All contents in the hernia defect must be reduced into the abdominal cavity and the surrounding fascial edges cleared of overlying tissue, bowel and fat in order to ensure adequate incorporation of mesh into the abdominal wall fascia. Figure 28.9 demonstrates a defect prepared for repair.

The material chosen for repair must have an adequate size in order to overlap all aspects of the defect by 5 cm or more and have a barrier for reduction of adhesions.

If the defect is large and a large piece of mesh is needed for coverage, sutures are placed at the four quadrants of the mesh; the sutures are retrieved through the abdominal wall to align the mesh adequately over the defect for final anchoring of the mesh. These sutures can be used to primarily anchor the mesh to the abdominal wall. Figures 28.10 and 28.11 demonstrate the mesh with anchoring sutures and retrieval of the sutures through the abdominal wall.

The mesh is then anchored to the abdominal wall with either suture, or tacking devices or a combination of the two. Particular attention is addressed to the edges of the mesh in order to ensure that adequate anchoring of the mesh has taken place and the possibility of bowel herniation between the mesh and abdominal wall tacks does not take place. Figure 28.12 demonstrates anchoring of the mesh with a permanent tacking device.

Abdominal binders are usually placed on the patient immediately postoperatively to give support to the abdominal wall and reduce pain. It is recommended that the patients wear such devices for 6 weeks or more after surgery.

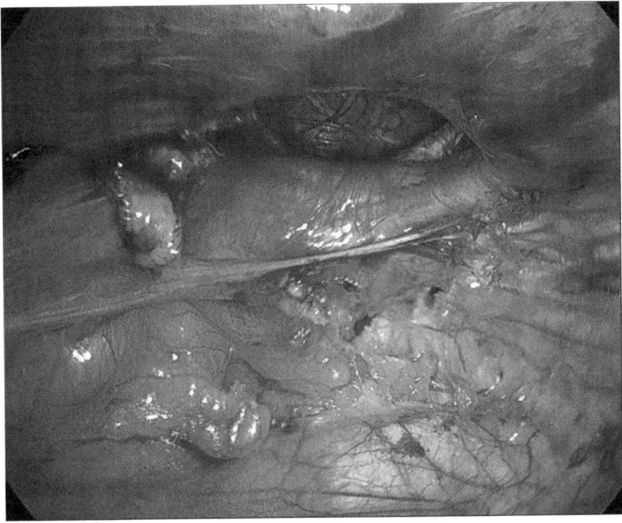

Fig. 28.9 Incisional hernia with adhesions, bowel and fat cleared for placement of mesh on fascia and peritoneum

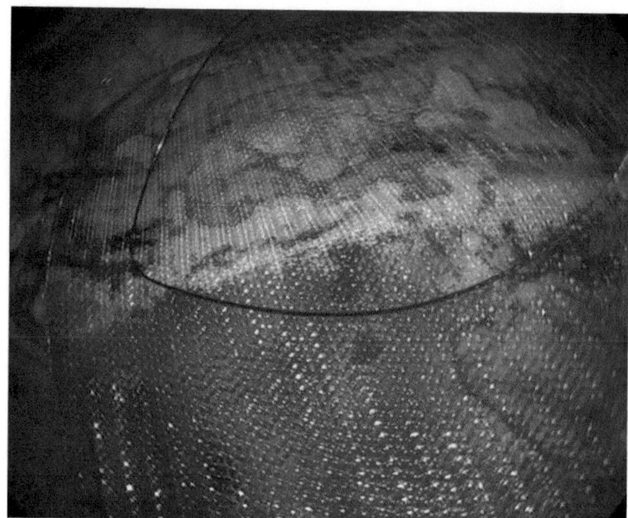

Fig. 28.10 Mesh intraabdominally with suture loop for placement

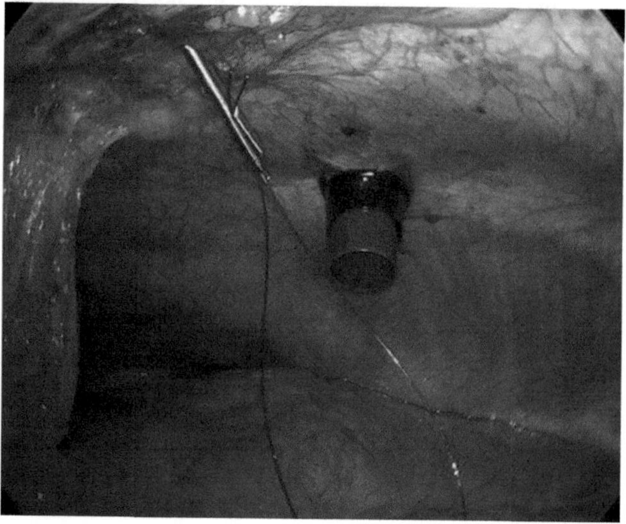

Fig. 28.11 Grasping suture loop to bring mesh under hernia defect for anchoring

Results with laparoscopic bridge repair of incisional hernias have been very good with comparable low recurrence rates when compared to open repair, but with higher major intraoperative complication rates when compared to open repair. Patients do return to normal activities sooner, have less pain and hospital stay is shorter [4].

Special Considerations After Hernia Repair

If a patient has had prior hernia repair utilizing mesh, then special consideration must be given for safe entry into the abdomen. Despite the application and incorporation of adhesive barriers into the mesh, or even if the mesh is completely covered by peritoneum, the presence of adherent bowel or omentum to the mesh and particularly to the edge of the mesh should be expected.

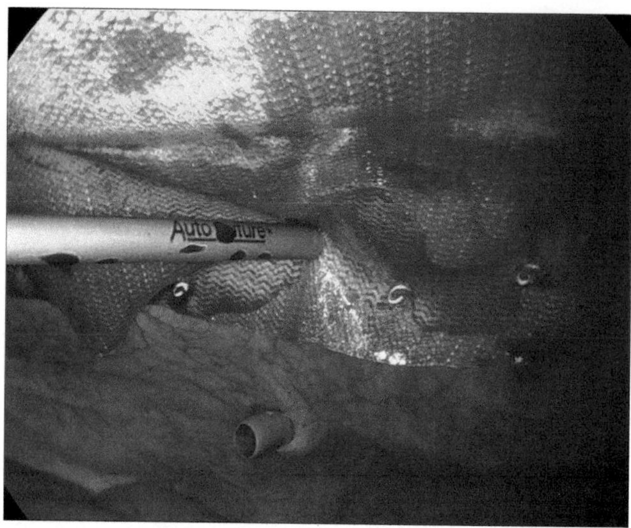

Fig. 28.12 Permanent tacking device securing mesh to fascia

Entry into the abdominal cavity can be accomplished in these instances either by remote entry i.e. Palmer's Point in the left upper quadrant or other sites outside of the prior surgical field. Entry can also be accomplished through the mesh itself. If a laparoscopic procedure is planned, then open (Hasson) technique is recommended either directly through the mesh utilizing careful blunt dissection of adherent bowel and omentum away from the mesh as the abdominal cavity is entered or at a remote site lateral to the prior incision. Extreme care must be taken around the edges of the mesh as this is the area most involved with adhesion formation. Figure 28.13 demonstrates adhesions at the edge of a previously placed mesh.

Once the procedure is completed, upon closure of the incision if it was made through the mesh, the closure should be accomplished with permanent suture.

Repair of complex incisional wall hernia defects may involve the use of biologic grafts intraabdominally or with an onlay over the anterior fascia. The biologic materials used currently consist of an acellular matrix of collagen and come in a variety of substances. The matrix is infiltrated with fibroblasts over time and the hosts' native collagen incorporated into the matrix resulting in a thick scar. In complex hernia repairs, if a biologic graft is used internally, opening directly through the material is recommended with the same considerations and precautions being taken as recommended with opening through synthetic material for abdominal entry.

As discussed above, complex hernia repairs are being performed with primary closure and with combinations of onlay mesh, inlay (between the layers of the abdominal wall) and underlay mesh. It is strongly recommended that the surgeon obtain prior operative notes in order to be familiar with the repair performed so entry into the abdomen can be accomplished safely. A prior knowledge of where the mesh was placed helps makes this possible.

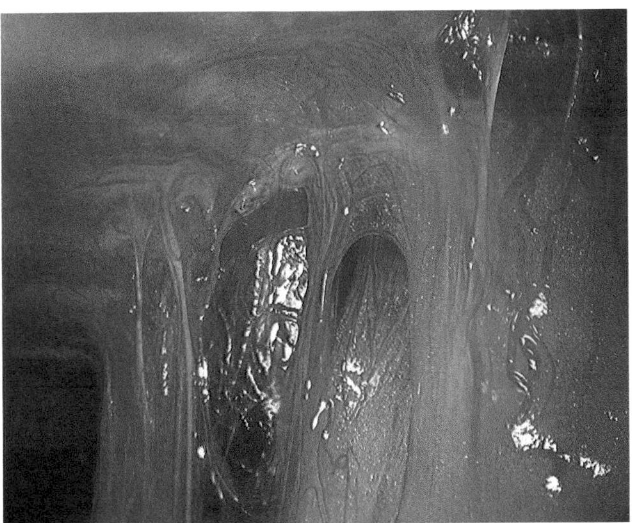

Fig. 28.13 Dense vascular adhesions seen at the lateral border of previously placed mesh

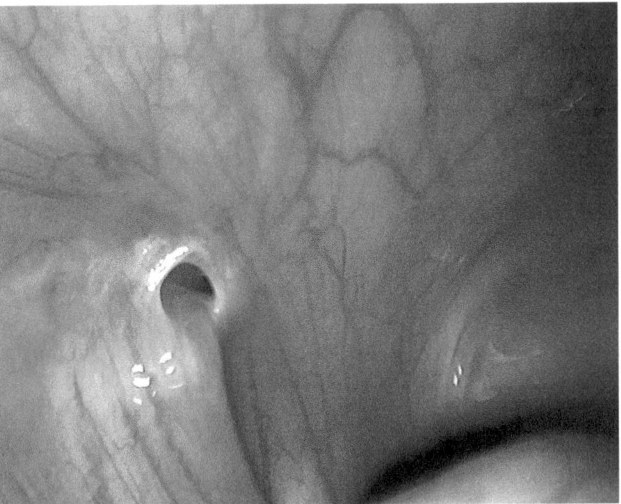

Fig. 28.14 Small indirect hernia on the left inguinal area with round ligament in defect

Tips

2 cm or less defects: close primarily with nonabsorbable suture.

2–8 cm defects: Laparoscopic bridge repair with synthetic material with adhesive barrier. Anchor to the abdominal wall with tacking device and overlap fascial edges 5 cm.

2–8 cm defects: Open repair, reapproximate the fascial edges and incorporate synthetic mesh reinforcement either intrabdominally, subfascial or overlay the midline closure.

Defects larger than 8 cm usually require a more complex repair for closure of the midline fascia and should be performed in conjunction with surgeons familiar with these repair techniques.

When entering the abdomen after prior incisional hernia repair with mesh, enter either through the center of the mesh with caution or at distant point and avoid the edges.

Know beforehand what type of repair was performed on the patient prior to entry to help anticipate when the mesh will be encountered in opening.

Inguinal Hernias

Inguinal hernia defects, when seen during laparoscopy are located in the pelvic side walls lateral to the obliterated umbilical veins. The two most common types of inguinal defects are direct and indirect hernias. Direct defects are medial to the inferior epigastric vessels and indirect defects are lateral to these vessels. The indirect defects can also be identified by the presence of the round ligament in or medial to the defect. Figure 28.14 is an example of a small asymptomatic indirect inguinal hernia and does not require repair.

Symptoms of inguinal hernia include: swelling or bulge in the inguinal floor usually superior to the inguinal ligament. It may or may not be associated with pain. Pain in the area of the inguinal ligament may be the only symptom or sign of a hernia. Inguinal hernias are more difficult to diagnose in females as compared to males. The dilemma is when the hernia is identified at the time of surgery what needs to be done?

Tip

If an inguinal defect is identified and the patient is asymptomatic i.e. the patient does not have inguinal pain, then the defect is noted, the patient is informed but repair is not necessary.

When a single symptomatic inguinal hernia defect is discovered, the choice of repair technique is controversial among surgeons. Patients with a single inguinal hernia are still most commonly repaired using standard open technique. In single surgeon series, the recurrence rate with laparoscopic repair is comparable to open repair and pain scores much better [5]. In large studies, results with laparoscopic repair show slightly higher recurrence rate, but pain scores and return to normal activity was better in the laparoscopic group versus open [6, 7].

Cost must be taken into consideration when choosing a repair, but when evaluated, there is little difference in operating room costs but there can be large differences in facility reimbursement [8].

The laparoscopic repair of inguinal hernias can be either performed entirely preperitoneal or transperitoneal. The principles of the repair and results are similar for both techniques. The anatomy of the inguinal canal and pelvic floor is constant, predictable and familiar to the gynecologic surgeon that performs anterior vaginal wall repairs or vesico-urethral neck suspensions such as Burch procedure. This is the same space routinely dissected and entered in a laparoscopic inguinal hernia repair (Video 28.1).

In either repair, the peritoneum is dissected from the lower pelvic and inguinal floor exposing the inguinal canal, iliac vessels, pubic tubercle, femoral canal and lateral inguinal side wall. It is important to completely reduce the hernia contents into the preperitoneal space. Simply closing the peritoneal defect is inadequate for repair; the inguinal floor must be reinforced with synthetic materials.

The mesh dimensions should be 10 cm by 15 cm in order to adequately cover, the inguinal floor and all potential defects. If polypropylene mesh is used, then this material should be anchored to the inguinal floor. Care must be taken when anchoring the mesh to avoid the major vascular and neural structures that are in the dissection site as injury to these structures is possible.

Anchoring of mesh should only be performed medial to the inferior epigastric vessels on the anterior lower abdominal wall and into the symphysis pubis and Cooper's ligament. Tacking devices should not be utilized in the lateral pelvic side wall as the genitofemoral and ilioinguinal nerves are present and can be easily trapped causing significant postoperative pain.

If polyester mesh is used for repair, because of the hydrophilic nature of the material, the mesh adheres to the underlying tissues well and does not need to be tacked if the repair is performed in a preperitoneal fashion. Results with this type of repair are very good and as such problems with tacking are avoided. Figure 28.15 demonstrates coverage of the inguinal floor with mesh at the end of a repair.

Femoral hernias are more common in females than males and may be a source of chronic pelvic or lower abdominal pain.

Femoral hernia is difficult to diagnose preoperatively. Symptoms usually include pain radiating down the inner aspect of the thigh and or under the inguinal ligament with no palpable mass or bulge. Frequently the first sign that a femoral hernia is present is acute incarceration. The repair of femoral hernia defects can be accomplished either by open or laparoscopic techniques, but the laparoscopic approach affords excellent exposure and allows accurate placement of a single layer of mesh that adequately covers the femoral and inguinal canals creating a very good repair.

The contents of a femoral hernia must be carefully reduced into the preperitoneal space in order to adequately identify the femoral canal structures and complete the repair. Again, if polypropylene mesh is utilized it should be anchored to the pelvis taking precautions as noted previously to avoid major vascular or neural injuries (Video 28.2).

Special Considerations in Inguinal Hernias

Techniques for laparoscopic inguinal hernia repair have evolved over the past 15 years. In the 1990's plug type repair was common, where a mesh plug usually consisting of polypropylene material was simply placed into the defect. This type of repair resulted in significant pain at the repair site because of scarring and contraction of the material, and as a result, this procedure currently is rarely used. Patients that have had this type of repair may present with significant pain with no external palpable "mass" and removal of the mesh plug is usually required for relief. Figure 28.16 is an example of a plug type repair in a patient that presented with pain several years later.

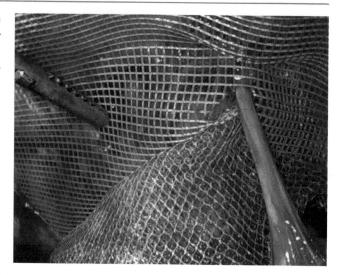

Fig. 28.15 Mesh placed over inguinal floor encircling the round ligament and covering the hernia defect

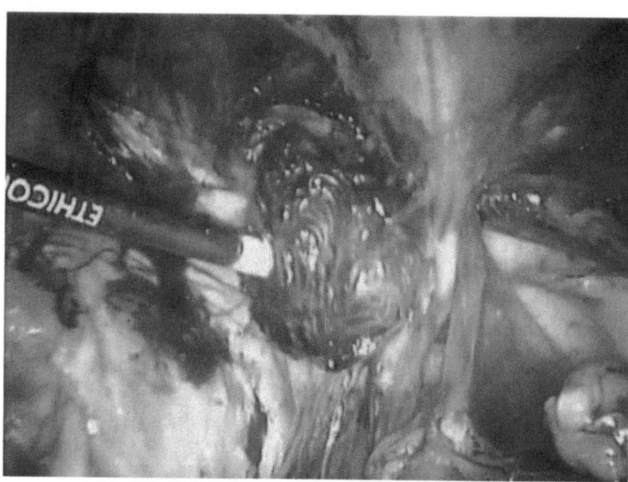

Fig. 28.16 Previously placed mesh plug in inguinal hernia defect

The plug repairs when performed currently utilize an absorbable material primarily or are in combination with open repair systems that utilize lower weight permanent synthetic materials. Figure 28.17 is an example of an absorbable material currently used in plug repairs. The material is Bio-A; manufactured by Gore corporation. This material provides a substrate for collagen deposition by the host resulting in an adequate support for the repair.

Tips

Asymptomatic inguinal hernias found at the time of surgery: Note and inform the patient of their presence but they do not require repair.

Femoral hernias may be a source of pelvic pain: symptoms are: radiating pain to the inner thigh and pain

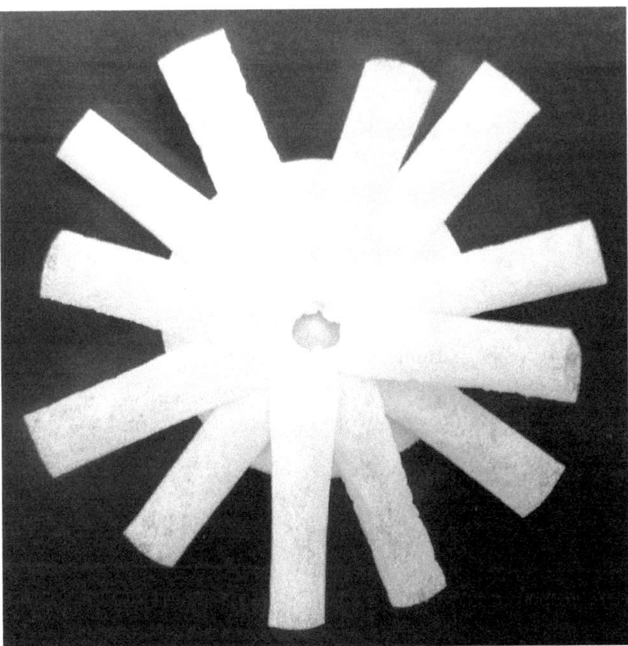

Fig. 28.17 Bio-A absorbable hernia plug manufactured by Gore Corp. used in plug hernia repair

in the groin below the inguinal ligament. If a femoral hernia is found it should be repaired as incarceration is common.

Previous repairs with plug type materials may be a source of chronic pain: diagnosis can be made by prior history of surgery and imaging of the inguinal floor. Resolution of pain usually requires removal of the material.

Single symptomatic inguinal hernias are usually repaired with open technique.

Bilateral or recurrent inguinal hernias usually are repaired with laparoscopic technique.

In patients who have had a prior laparoscopic inguinal hernia repair, the retropubic space will be very difficult to enter due to adherence of the mesh material to the underlying structures.

Internal Hernias

An internal hernia is an opening between any two adjacent structures in the abdominal cavity that has the potential for abdominal contents to protrude through creating a site for obstruction. These hernias are very difficult to diagnose preoperatively and can also be a source of chronic lower abdominal or pelvic pain. They most commonly present with incarceration and bowel obstruction as the first presenting symptom.

Internal hernias are usually the result of prior surgery and adhesive disease. When bowel resection with anastomosis or gastric bypass is performed and the mesenteric defect is not sufficiently closed then this site may be the location of an internal hernia.

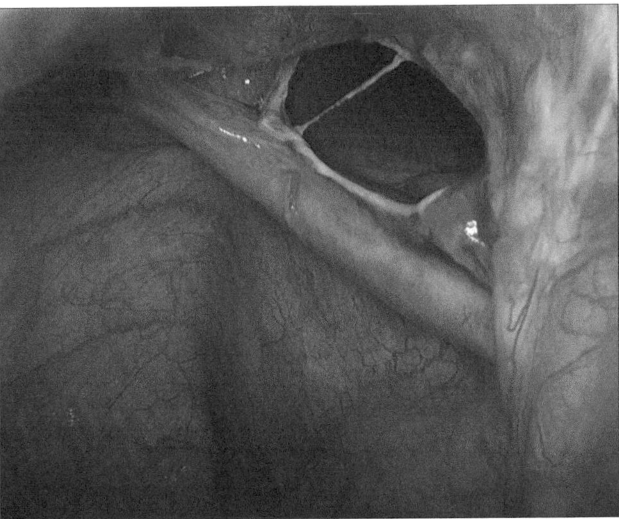

Fig. 28.18 Reduced internal hernia defect in left pelvic side wall

Figure 28.18 demonstrates such an internal hernia where adhesions created a small defect and bowel became entrapped and obstructed. The prior operation that resulted in this defect was a caesarian section with scarring between the uterus, anterior abdominal wall and lateral pelvic side wall.

When an internal hernia is diagnosed it needs to be either fixed by primary closure of the defect or the defect opened widely so the bowel cannot become incarcerated because the potential for complications is high.

Tips

When an internal hernia defect is encountered, it should be either closed completely or opened completely to prevent incarceration of bowel.

Visceral Pathologies

In the true pelvis, the rectosigmoid and the appendix are common sources of pathology. It is important to be able to recognize common conditions affecting these structures that may mimic gynecologic conditions, and be aware of the treatment for these processes. The small bowel also visits the pelvis and conditions that involve this organ may also mimic gynecologic pathologies.

Colon

The most common condition involving the colon in the West that may mimic gynecologic pathology is diverticular disease. Patients with acute hemorrhage or perforation as a result of their diverticular disease usually are referred directly to General Surgery for care; however chronic pain from diverticulosis or low grade diverticulitis may be difficult to distinguish from a gynecologic etiology.

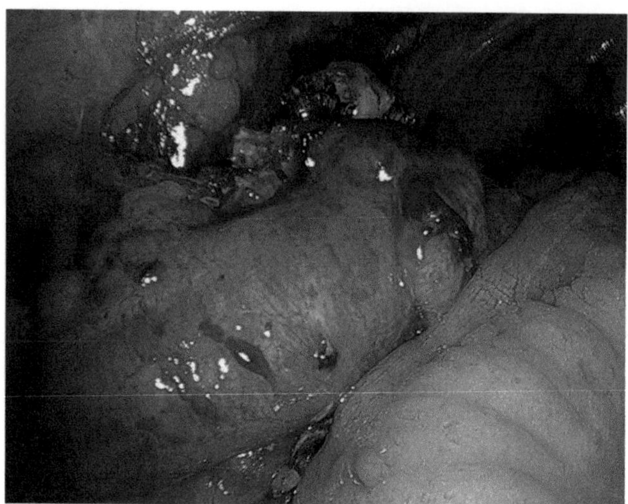

Fig. 28.19 Acute sigmoid diverticulitis with normal appearing bowel in the right lower aspect of the picture

The sigmoid colon is the region of the colon that is most commonly involved with symptomatic diverticuli and the pain is usually present in the left lower quadrant, but may be suprapubic or even in the right lower quadrant.

On inspection and manipulation of the involved colon during laparoscopy, the bowel wall is usually thickened and has lost its normal pliability. In patients that have chronic diverticular disease there are usually adhesions adjacent to the involved segment as a result of repeated bouts of inflammation. See Fig. 28.19.

Diverticuli may actually be seen protruding through the muscular wall of the colon aiding in diagnosis.

Once the GYN surgeon has ruled out any gynecologic pathology and the findings suggest diverticular disease whether it be chronic or acute, no further surgical intervention is necessary. Treatment consists of dietary fiber increase with or without intravenous or oral antibiotics depending on whether an acute process is present or not.

When a patient is explored for pelvic inflammatory disease or presumed tuboovarian abscess, one of the differentials is a contained diverticular perforation with abscess formation. When this is encountered, the segment of involved colon **does not require resection** (except in free perforation and peritonitis where a resection and diverting colostomy may be necessary). The abscess can be drained laparoscopically and a drain left in the abscess cavity.

Malignancies may also perforate however this is less common than in diverticular disease and these patients commonly manifest symptoms of bowel obstruction and as such are usually seen by General Surgeons prior to this happening.

Frequently when operating in the pelvis, congenital "adhesions" are encountered between the sigmoid colon, cecum and the abdominal wall or pelvic side wall. When these structures are noted, if they do not interfere with the planned procedure they are usually left in place and not taken down. The potential problem with mobilizing these structures (sigmoid and cecum) too vigorously is the possibility of volvulus, or twisting of the bowel. So as a rule of thumb, if it is not interfering with the planned procedure leave these support bands in place.

Tips

Diverticular disease of the sigmoid whether it is chronic or acute without perforation; does not require resection. Note and inform the patient.

Perforation with abscess formation: drain the abscess; leave a drain in the cavity, no resection is required.

Appendix

The use of pelvic ultrasound and or CT scan to accurately diagnose appendicitis has been on the rise recently but these have sometimes been unreliable tools to include or exclude the diagnosis, so the use of laparoscopy particularly in the female patient is becoming more frequent when the diagnosis is uncertain. The benefits of laparoscopic appendectomy when compared to open appendectomy are still being hotly debated in the General surgery literature [9]. The majority of appendectomies performed in the US are currently being done laparoscopically. The main advantage being reduction in wound infection rate when compared to open techniques.

The surgical technique used by GI Surgeons for appendectomy most commonly involves utilizing a linear stapling device. These instruments provide a quick simple technique for removal of the appendix; however they are expensive, and may not be readily available so other methods for dissection and removal should be in the surgeons' armamentarium. The technique for appendectomy will be described in stepwise detail.

Procedure Appendectomy

First the appendix must be mobilized from any retroperitoneal or lateral pelvic attachments. This step is important in order to have adequate access to the mesentery of the appendix and avoid injury to retroperitoneal structures, cecum or the ileocecal valve during removal.

Next, a small window is created in the mesoappendix at the base of the appendix. This can be done bluntly using dissectors or energy sources.

Once this is accomplished, the third step is either ligation of the mesoappendix or appendix base. The choice of which one of these structures is to be ligated first is dependent on the anatomy and ease of visualization. Control can also be accomplished using a linear stapling device. The appendix base is usually transected using the 3.5 or 2.8 mm staple depth. The choice depends on whether the base of the appen-

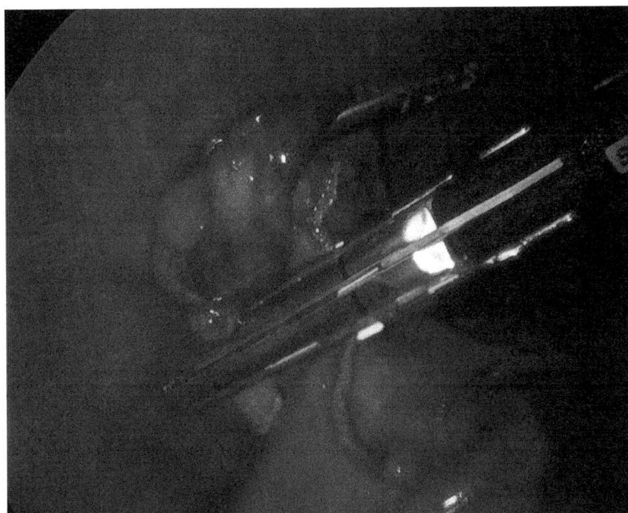

Fig. 28.20 Stapler being applied to the base of the appendix

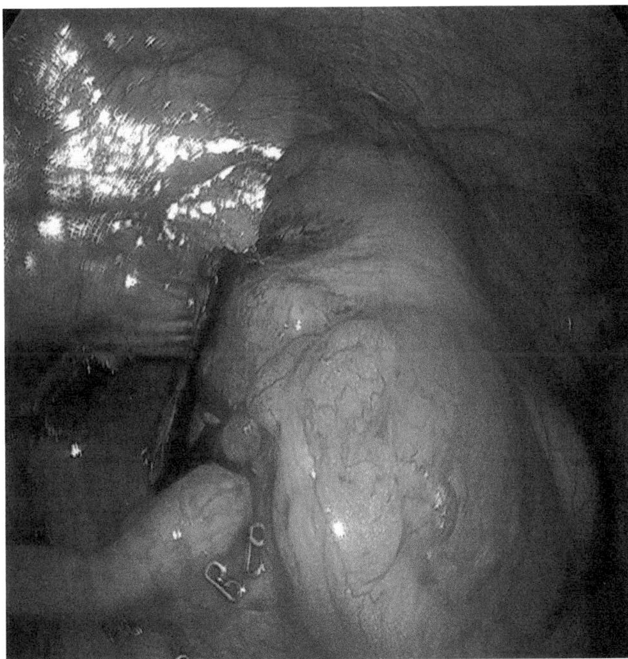

Fig. 28.21 Stapled appendix base to the left and normal cecum to the right of the picture

dix is inflamed or normal. The vascular pedicle is divided using the 2.8 mm staple load. Figure 28.20 shows placement of the stapling device and Fig. 28.21 shows the appendix base after stapling.

Simple ligation of the appendix base or its vascular pedicle using 0-silk or other suture offers good control prior to transection of these structures. This method is much more cost effective when compared to stapling devices. Video 28.3 demonstrates ligation of the appendix base with suture.

After the base of the appendix or mesoappendix is ligated and transected, an Endoloop may be applied for extra security. Video 28.4 shows the transaction of the appendix base after ligation.

In instances where the appendix is necrotic at its base, the stapler has its best utility. The proximal staple line should cross normal cecal wall in order to insure viable tissue is left in the staple line. Stapling across a necrotic appendix can result in delayed perforation and peritonitis since there is no viable tissue left in the staple line.

When the primary ligation method is utilized, and the base of the appendix is necrotic, the appendix base should be inverted into the cecum utilizing either a Z stitch or purse string seromuscular stitch of 2-0 or 3-0 suture. Historically silk suture has been used however an absorbable suture may be utilized but the crucial point is that the tissue in question be closed and inverted with normal viable tissue overlying it.

Special Considerations

In instances where the appendix has perforated and an abscess is encountered which may be the case in exploration for suspected tuboovarian abscess, then just as for diverticular abscess, the surgeon should drain the abscess, leave a drain in the abscess cavity and end the procedure. The appendix does not need to be removed at that time but this can be done at a later date usually several months later if indicated.

In patients with chronic lower abdominal or pelvic pain who are undergoing laparoscopy and the appendix is still present, it is recommended that the appendix be removed. In several studies, relief of pain after appendectomy even without obvious gross pathology shows benefit [10, 11].

Tips

Appendectomy should be performed in patients with pelvic pain when the organ is still present and appears grossly normal.

Appendectomy can easily be accomplished utilizing a stapling device, 3.5 or 2.8 mm load for the appendix base and 2.8 mm size for the mesentery.

Suture ligation using 0-silk or other suture material is as effective as stapling and more cost effective. Pretied loops can also be used to control the appendix base and mesentery base.

In perforation and abscess formation, drain the abscess, do not remove the appendix and leave a drain in the cavity.

Small Bowel

Small bowel pathology is much less common than either colon or appendix pathology, however conditions do exist that may be found during exploration that mimic pelvic pathology.

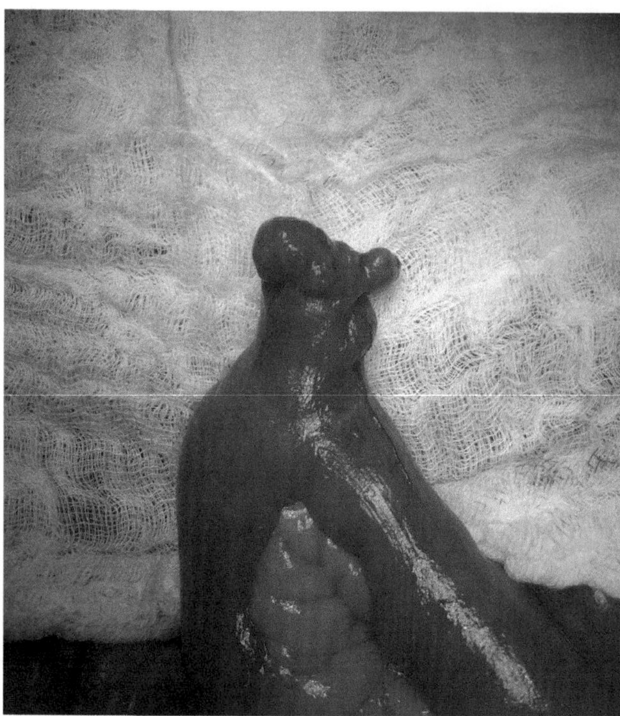

Fig. 28.22 Meckel's diverticulum

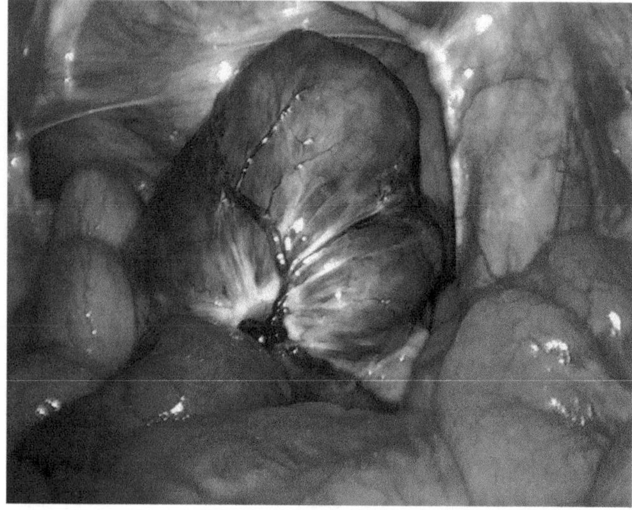

Fig. 28.23 Pedunculated GIST tumor of the small bowel resembling leiomyoma

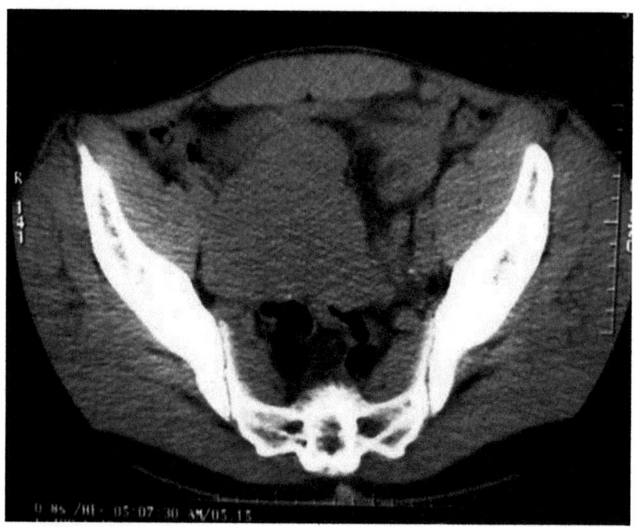

Fig. 28.24 CT scan of the pelvis demonstrating the GIST tumor in Fig. 28.23

Meckel's diverticulum is a true diverticulum that classically is located 2 ft from the ileocecal valve and can be a source of chronic pain. The appearance is typically that of an antimesenteric diverticulum with its own blood supply originating from the mesentery.

Figure 28.22 shows a typical Meckel's diverticulum.

The diverticulum can harbor gastric mucosa that can lead to GI bleeding and also perforation. Bowel obstruction from intussusception also has been described. So when these structures are encountered they are usually removed.

Resection with a linear stapling device 3.5 mm size staple load, placed at the base of the Meckel's diverticulum so as not to compromise the remaining bowel lumen is recommended. Resection utilizing simple excision with two layer suture closure may be used if the surgeon is adept with laparoscopic resection and suturing techniques.

Tips

When Meckel's Diverticulum is found it should be removed.

GIST or gastrointestinal stromal tumors can be found in the small bowel and have the same gross appearance as leiomyomas. Figure 28.23 is that of a small bowel GIST preoperatively mimicking a leiomyoma.

GIST tumors are most commonly found in the stomach 60% with 30% incidence in the large and small bowel. They can be intraluminal or extraluminal with a pedunculated base which can lead to misdiagnosis via imaging as originating from the uterus or ovary. Figure 28.24 shows the appearance on CT of the lesion in Fig. 28.23.

These tumors do have a malignant potential and so when encountered they should be removed. Despite their malignant potential, removal of GIST lesions requires only clear resection margins and a formal nodal dissection is not necessary. Lesions greater than 5 cm or with >5 mitoses per high power field should be referred for consideration for adjuvant chemotherapy.

Because these tumors resemble leiomyomas the urge to morcellate should be avoided when they are removed. They should be removed from the abdomen intact by extending the incision or utilizing a specimen retrieval bag device.

Tips

GIST tumors grossly resemble leiomyomas and as such may be mistaken for gynecologic pathology. When found, they should be removed intact, not morcellated, and no formal cancer nodal dissection is necessary. The bowel margins should be clear.

Regional enteritis or Crohn's Disease can also cause pelvic or lower abdominal pain. The gross appearance is similar to that seen with chronic diverticular disease with marked thickening of the bowel wall, loss of pliability and the characteristic mesenteric creeping fat may be present.

Without any acute problems or complications of the patient's disease (perforation, obstruction), the involved segment does not need to be removed and in fact it is recommended that the involved bowel be left in place. Medical therapy is the mainstay of treatment with surgery being left only for complications such as perforation, stricture, obstruction or fistula formation.

Tips
Crohn's disease when encountered should be noted with no resection recommended except only for complications such as perforation, obstruction, stricture or fistula formation.

Special Considerations in Encountering Bowel, Injuries

In the course of dissection particularly when adhesive disease is encountered, occasionally injury to the bowel wall is noted. Avoidance of injury is the key. The use of any energy source to release bowel from the abdominal wall is to be discouraged and when used, should be performed only with extreme caution.

Use of scissors without cautery is the preferred method. When very loose adhesions are encountered, the bowel may be gently pushed from the abdominal wall with the convex side of the instrument. Figure 28.25 demonstrates the recommended position of the scissors.

This helps reduce chance of an unseen injury by the tip of the scissors on the bowel.

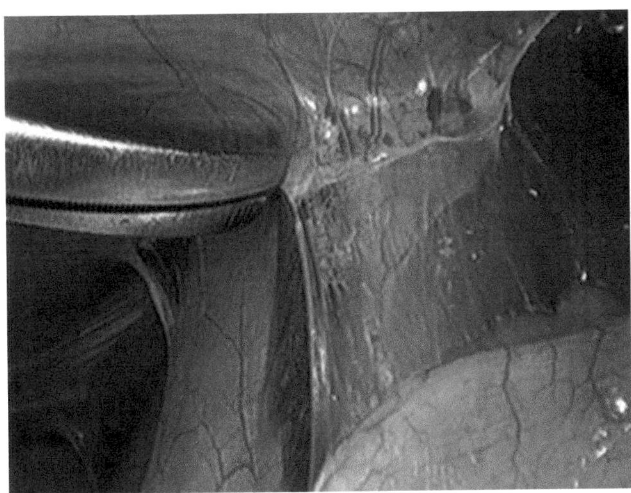

Fig. 28.25 Fibrinous adhesions between the bowel and anterior abdominal wall

Small bowel and colon are encountered frequently in the pelvis during surgery, despite placing the patient in Trendelenberg position. These structures must be mobilized from the pelvis in order to achieve adequate visualization. When grasping the bowel, a method recommended to help reduce the possibility of injury, is that the bowel be grasped gently with an instrument with a large surface area and at an angle parallel to the mesentery (Fig. 28.26) or grasp the mesentery directly (Fig. 28.27).

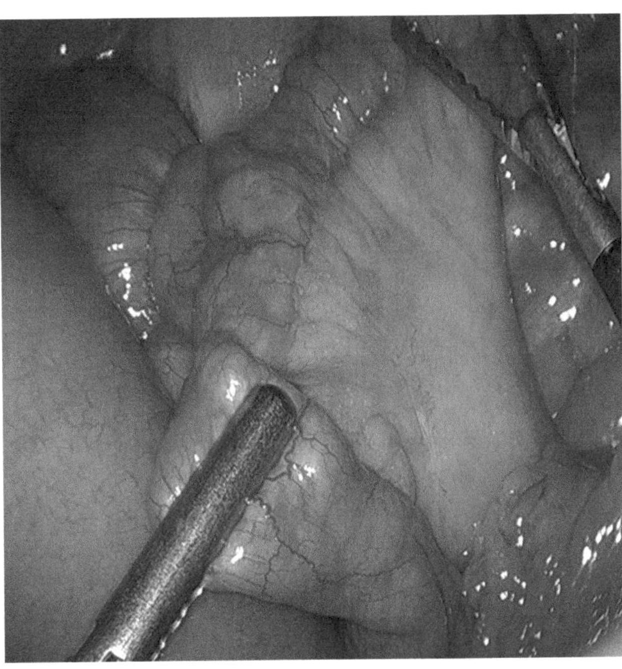

Fig. 28.26 Grasping the bowel with broad based instrument at a 0 degree angle

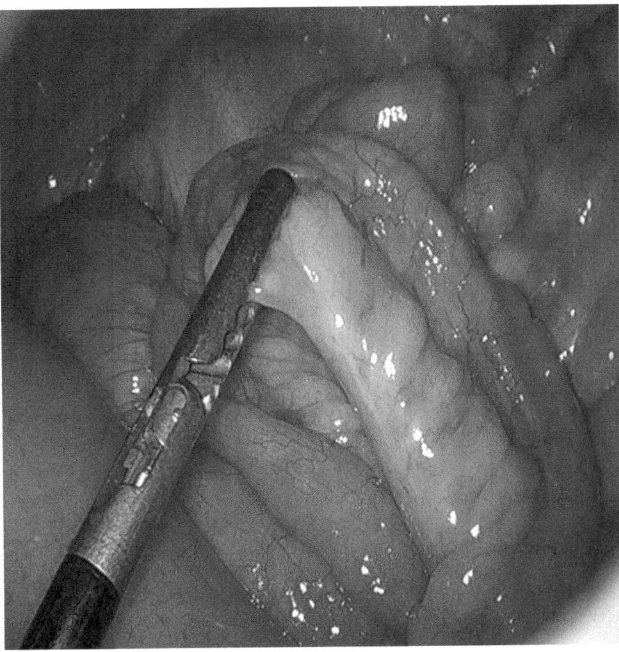

Fig. 28.27 Grasping the mesentery of the bowel avoiding the bowel wall complctely

The larger surfaced area grasper disperses the force generated by the grasper and by grasping the mesentery the bowel itself is avoided thus reducing the risk of injury. The amount of force generated at the tip of laparoscopic instruments has been measured at up to 1500 kPa which is equal to a human bite so excessive force on the instrument can be transferred to the bowel and must be avoided [12].

Extra care must be taken when the bowel is inflamed or diseased as this makes the possibility of injury more likely.

When to Repair Bowel Wall Injuries?

1. If the mucosa is entered or visible, then primary repair is mandatory. Repair is accomplished either in one or two layers. Suture size used may be 4–0 or 3–0 and may be permanent or absorbable suture. The critical aspect of the repair is that the mucosa be completely inverted.
2. When the muscular wall is damaged and mucosa is visible but not injured, see Fig. 28.28, it is still recommended that the bowel wall be repaired. Again either a two or one layer closure is used.
3. When muscular wall is damaged and no mucosa is visible, depending on the length of injury, the bowel wall may not need to be repaired. The decision is surgeon dependant but any injury over 1 cm in size should be reinforced.
4. Serosal injuries do not need to be repaired. See Fig. 28.29

Tips

Full thickness bowel wall injuries need to be repaired either with two layer or one layer technique making certain that mucosa is adequately inverted and or covered with viable tissue.

Muscular wall injury should be repaired depending on degree and size. When in doubt: repair.

Serosal injuries do not require repair.

Grasp bowel carefully with large surface area instruments.

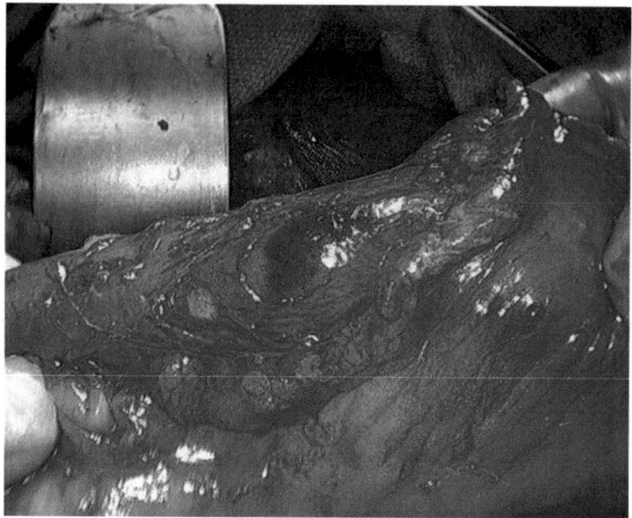

Fig. 28.28 Bowel wall injury with intact mucosa, disrupted serosa and both muscular walls requiring repair

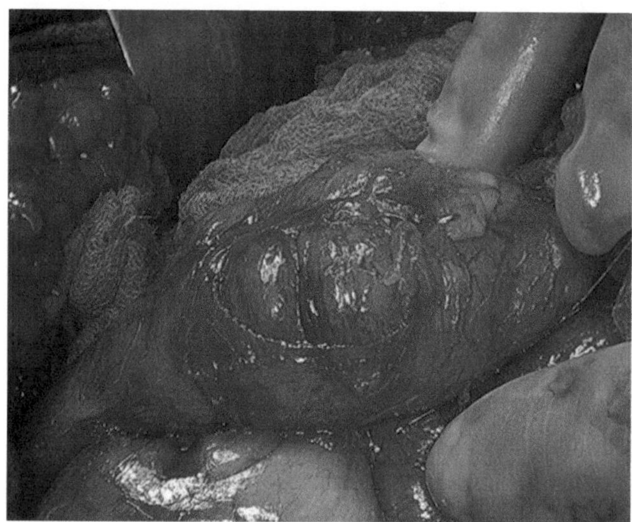

Fig. 28.29 Serosal injury with intact muscular layers not requiring repair

Other Topics

Endometriosis may involve organs other than the uterus or ovaries and this can include bowel particularly the rectosigmoid. Figure 28.30 demonstrates an endometriotic plaque in the Pouch of Douglas.

In order to adequately treat and relieve the patient from their symptoms, complete resection of the involved area is usually required.

When endometriosis involves the colon or rectum, the endometriotic nodule can usually be completely resected without having to perform a formal segmental resection [13]. Anticipation of the need to resect part of the large bowel is usually noted preoperatively and if necessary a general surgeon can be called to assist, however a well trained laparoscopic surgeon competent in suturing can also treat the involved bowel.

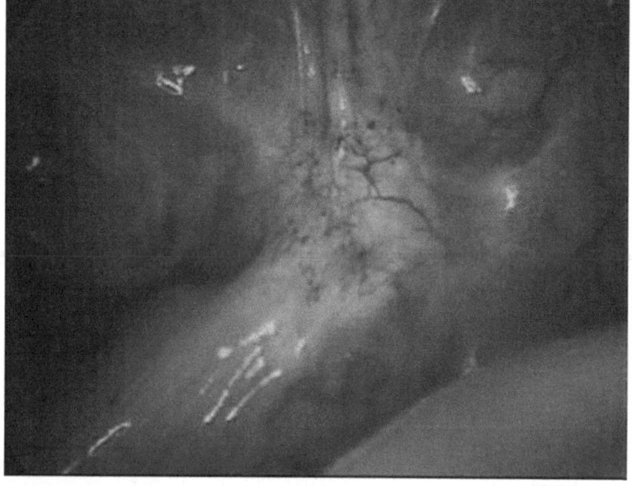

Fig. 28.30 Endometriosis involving the anterior wall of the rectum and posterior wall of the vagina

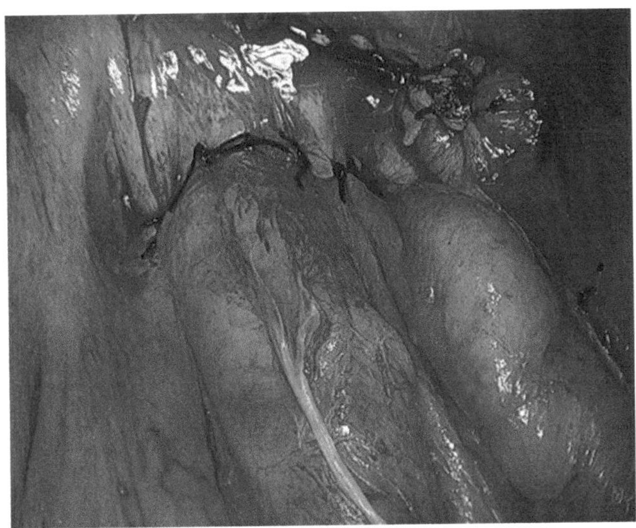

Fig. 28.31 Repair of the rectal wall closed in transverse fashion

If the nodule requires full thickness resection of the bowel wall and closure would not result in compromise of bowel lumen, (usually 50% or less of the bowel wall circumference) then primary repair in a two layer manner is appropriate. The first inverting layer is usually an absorbable suture (chromic or polyglactin) 4-0 or 3-0 size. The injury should be closed so as not to compromise the lumen of the bowel so closure in a transverse fashion rather than longitudinal with interrupted suture is best. See Fig. 28.31.

The second layer may be either absorbable or permanent and is usually either 4-0 or 3-0 size.

The ultimate success of closure depends on standard well recognized principals of general surgery. The first being a tension-free repair and the second being adequate blood supply.

If the rectum and not the sigmoid colon is involved, because of the lack of serosa, the anastomosis is at higher risk of leak since there is no serosa to aid in sealing of the anastomosis, so it is recommended that in these instances, the use of anti-adhesive agents be avoided. The successful scaling of an anastomosis in this circumstance is very dependent on adherence from surrounding tissues, so adhesions in this instance are crucial to good outcome.

Tips

When endometriosis is encountered involving the bowel, it usually can be removed by local excision and primary closure.

Two layer closure without tension and adequate blood supply to the remaining tissues is standard.

When rectum is involved, antiadhesive barrier products should be avoided.

The same management principles apply in a situation where the distal colon or rectum is injured during surgery or entry. The injury is usually repaired in a two layer fashion. If the defect is small, then a one layer closure is adequate as long as the bowel mucosa is inverted. The need for creation of a colostomy is extremely rare when the injury is recognized early and closed primarily.

When bowel resection is anticipated preoperatively, usually the patients are placed on mechanical bowel prep. There is good evidence that when patients have not had bowel prep and subsequently underwent resection when compared to patients that did have a bowel prep and underwent resection with anastomosis, there was no difference in leak rate, abscess formation or complication such as wound infection [14]. The long held notion that all patients that are to undergo bowel surgery need to be on a mechanical prep is now questioned.

In special cases where an entire segment of bowel needs to be removed, the availability of circular staplers has made creation of a low colonic anastomosis simpler. There are certain principles that need to be understood when using these devices. First is that there should be no tension on the anastomosis and staple line. The proximal bowel should easily reach into the pelvis without tension. The descending colon or splenic flexure may need to be mobilized in order to reach the distal sigmoid or rectal stump; if this is needed then care must be taken that the blood supply is not compromised in the process as this is the second important factor in a successful anastomosis.

Choosing staple size is very important. Lower colon anastamosis using a circular stapler should be performed with a 28 mm diameter stapler or larger. Figure 28.32 shows a stapling device manufactured by Covidien Corporation. The anvil and stapler are demonstrated.

Using a stapler smaller than 28 mm usually will lead to stricture. If the proximal bowel lumen is small the staple anvil may be placed in a side fashion forming an end-to-side anastamosis and thus creating an adequately large lumen.

In placing the anvil in the proximal bowel, the bowel should be closed firmly around the anvil post so that when the stapler is closed and fired no bowel wall is extruded from the side of the stapler resulting in a compromised anastomosis.

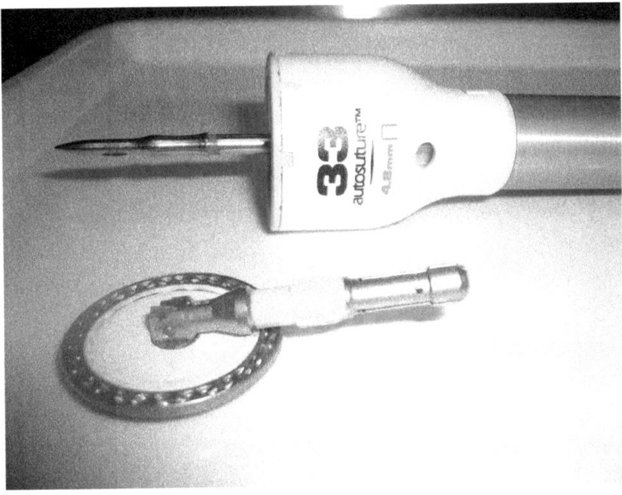

Fig. 28.32 EEA stapler manufactured by Covidien Corp. showing the anvil and stapler

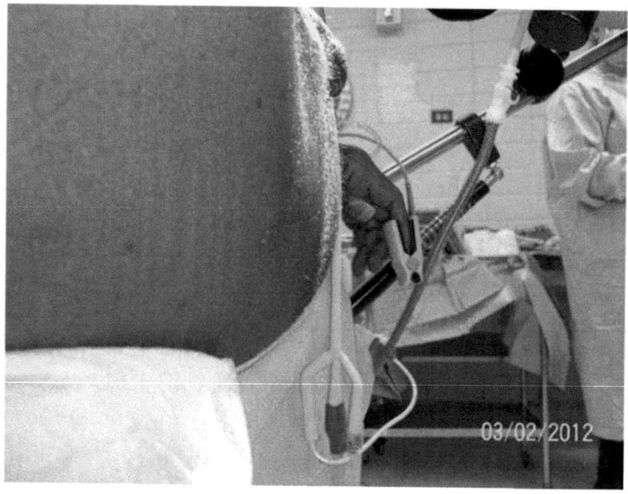

Fig. 28.33 The patient's buttocks extending past the end of the operating table

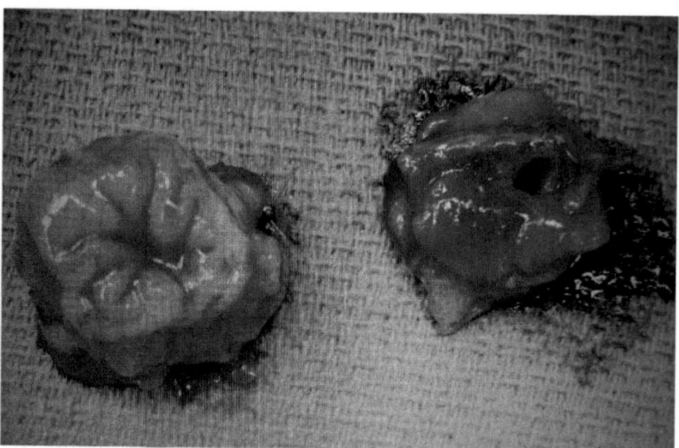

Fig. 28.34 Circular staple tissue donuts from the proximal and distal bowel

In placing the stapling device transanaly, it is very important that the patient's lower buttocks and perineum extend past the edge of the operating table. This allows adequate angling of the stapler into the rectum and first part of the sigmoid. This is absolutely crucial to successful docking and firing of the stapler. See Fig. 28.33.

Once the stapler and anvil are docked, the stapler fired, and removed, the confirmation of two intact tissue "doughnuts" (see Fig. 28.34) and a secure anastomosis via colonoscopy or insufflation using proctoscopy or other device with submersion leak testing should be performed. In the instance of a questionable staple line, the anastomosis site can be reinforced with an inverting stitch or redone. Drains are not usually placed.

Tips

Mechanical bowel prep is not mandatory in colon surgery.

Closure of colon after partial resection or injury should be in two layer fashion.

Circular stapling devices should be 28 mm or greater in diameter when used for anastomosis after segmental resection.

In closure of rectal injury or resection, avoid anti-adhesive materials.

Colostomies are rarely needed when the bowel is injured during surgery; primary repair is preferred.

General surgical conditions can mimic gynecologic disease and may be encountered in the course of surgery for GYN conditions. It is important to be able to recognize, diagnose and have knowledge of treatment for these conditions in order to have good surgical outcomes.

References

1. Millennium Research Group. U.S. markets for soft tissue repair 2009. Toronto: Millennium Research Group, Inc; 2008.
2. Luijendijk RW, Hop WK, van den Tol MP, de Lange DC, Braaksma MM, Ijzermans JN, et al. A comparison of suture repair with mesh repair of incisional hernia. N Engl J Med. 2000;343:392–8.
3. Jonas J. The problem with mesh shrinkage in laparoscopic incisional hernia repair. Zentralbl Chir. 2009;134(3):209–13.
4. Olmi S, Scaini A, Cesana GC, Erba L, Croce E. Laparoscopic versus open incisional hernia repair: an open randomized controlled study. Surg Endosc. 2007;21(4):555–9.
5. Morrison J, Jacobs V. Laparoscopic preperitoneal inguinal hernia repair using preformed polyester mesh without fixation: prospective study with one year follow up results in a rural setting. Surg Laparosc Endosc Percutan Tech. 2008;18(1):33–9.
6. McCormack K, Scott NW, Go PM, Ross S, Grant AM; EU Hernia Trialists Collaboration. Laparoscopic techniques versus open techniques for inguinal hernia repairs. Cochrane Database Syst Rev. 2003;(1):CD001785.
7. Neumayn L, Giobbie-Hurder MS, Jonasson O, Fitzgibbons R, et al. Open mesh versus laparoscopic mesh repair of inguinal hernia. N Engl J Med. 2004;350(18):1819–27.
8. Jacobs V, Morrison J. Comparison of institutional costs for laparoscopic preperitoneal inguinal hernia versus open repair and its reimbursement in an ambulatory surgery center. Surg Laparosc Endosc Percutan Tech. 2008;18(1):70–4.
9. Kathkouda N, Mason R, Towfigh S. Laparoscopic versus open appendectomy a prospective randomized double-blind study. Ann Surg. 2005;242(3):439–50.
10. Lyons T, Winer WK, Woo A. Appendectomy in patients undergoing laparoscopic surgery for pelvic pain. J Am Assoc Gynecol Laparosc. 2001;8(4):542–4.
11. Agarwala N, Liu CY. Laparoscopic appendectomy. J Am Assoc Gynecol Laparosc. 2003;10(2):166–8.
12. Cartmill JA, Shakeshaft AJ, Walsh WR, Martin CJ. High pressures are generated at the tip of laparoscopic graspers. Aust N Z J Surg. 1999;69(2):127–30.
13. Roman H, Rozsnayi F, Puscasiu L, Resch B, Belhiba H, Lefebure B, Scotte M, et al. Complications associated with two laparoscopic procedures used in management of rectal endometriosis. JSLS. 2010;14:169–77.
14. Zmora O, Mahajna A, Bar-Zakai B, Rosin D, Hershko D. Colon and rectal surgery without mechanical bowel preparation a randomized prospective trial. Ann Surg. 2003;237(3):363–7.

29 Fibroids in Laparoscopic Hysterectomy

Xiaofeng Zhao, Lu Huang, and Sheng Xu

Abbreviations

B	Bladder
C	Cervix
CL	Cardinal ligament
CVG	Cervico-vesical gap
FT	Fallopian tube
O	Ovary
OV	Ovarian vessels
R	Rectum
RL	Round ligament
SV	small venae
U	Uterus
UA	Uterine artery
UL	Uterosacral ligament
UOL	Utero-ovarian ligament
UOV	Utero-ovarian vessels
UUL	Umbilicourethralligament
UV	Uterine veins
UVB	Uterine veins bleeding
UVF	Utero-vesical fold
UVS	Uterinevessels
V	Vagina
VCL	Vesico-cervical ligament
VIE	Vena iliaca externa

Uterine fibroids are the most common gynecologic benign tumors. Depending on different symptoms, options for management of uterine fibroids include follow-up observation, medication, surgery or embolization.

Laparoscopic hysterectomy is the most frequently performed minimally invasive procedure for treatment of fibroids. It is applied to patients with indications of surgery but with no desire for fertility or reservation of uterus. It is divided into complete laparoscopic hysterectomy and laparoscopic-assisted vaginal hysterectomy. According to resection range, hysterectomy can be total or supracervical.

With the development of laparoscopic technology and accumulation of surgical experiences, almost all the laparoscopic hysterectomy due to fibroids can be performed successfully, including conditions of large uterus, severe adhesion or specially located fibroids [1–5]. But supracervical hysterectomy or hysterectomy of a large uterus requires power morcellation to facilitate removal, which links to an increased risk of disseminating occult malignancy into the abdominal and peritoneal cavities, and it has become a main concern and reason for restriction of laparoscopic hysterectomy [6–10].

Most of hysterectomies for fibroids can be completed safely by laparoscopy. The crucial part of laparoscopic hysterectomy is safely processing the uterine vessels [11]. The vessels supplied the uterus mainly come from two sources, one is the uterine artery and vein, the other is the anastomoses branch of utero-ovary vessels. The uterus becomes ischemic after devascularization of the two sites and then resection won't be difficult. Core of the whole procedure is to reveal the two groups of vessels precisely and bloodlessly, followed by transfixion or electro-coagulation. Large uteri, cervical fibroids or fibroids located in the lower segment of the uterus may greatly increase the difficulty of devascularization [12]. We will analyze the procedure of laparoscopic hysterectomy step by step.

Appropriate exposure and operating space are the precondition for laparoscopic hysterectomy. To achieve better exposure and operating space, the use of a uterine manipulator and placement of trocars are important. A uterine manipulator should push up the uterus to expose cervico-vesical fold, and provide a good motion range. The placement of trocars is one of the most critical factors for a successful operation. On the basis of anatomical characteristics, the cervix is a relatively fixed point, while the uterus is a partially free

X. Zhao (✉) • L. Huang • S. Xu
Department of Gynecology, Zhejiang Provincial People's Hospital, Hangzhou, Zhejiang Province 310000, China
e-mail: sfzchx@aliyun.com; Yezidegushi1122@163.com; zoe_xs@126.com

I. Alkatout, L. Mettler (eds.), *Hysterectomy*, DOI 10.1007/978-3-319-22497-8_29

organ with relatively bilateral mobility, so three trocars are generally most favorable for hysterectomy. More trocars make no contribution to exposure of anatomic and operative view. The first port-site is for laparoscopic lens. For uteri smaller than the size of 18 weeks gestation, the first port-site is usually at umbilicus point. For bigger uteri, upper umbilicus point is chosen, but often lower than the umbilico-xiphoid midpoint. The left and right port-sites are operating sites, commonly near the anterior axillary line, 2 cm higher than the utero-ovarian ligaments. One side of port-site is for operating and the other side is to help exposure during the procedure. Proper rotation of the uterus helps exposure. Rotate the uterus clockwise when deal with the left side. Rotate anti-clockwise when go to the right.

We first deal with the anastomoses branch of utero-ovarian vessels, which are surrounded by the round ligament, utero-ovarian ligament and fallopian tube (see Fig. 29.1). For uteri that are not too large, a uterine manipulator can help exposure. For large uteri, the effect of uterine manipulator is limited, and grasping forceps are needed to grasp the point where the round ligament connects the uterus, pull and rotate the uterus to one side so that the operative side can be exposed. For patients whose ligaments are thick, transection of fallopian tube, round ligament and utero-ovarian ligament is done before devascularization. For patients with thin ligaments, do the devascularization directly. Transection of these structures should be done 1 cm away from the uterus to avoid injury of vessels on the lateral uterine wall. Then open the broad ligament, dissect the anterior and posterior leaf (see Fig. 29.2). Usually there are only small vessels and loose connective tissue within the broad ligament. Be careful not to injury the uterine vessels which are closed to the lateral uterine wall. Now a uterine manipulator is necessary to push the uterus up to help expose, meanwhile the contra-lateral grasping forceps continue pulling and assist rotation. Open the anterior leaf of the broad ligament up to the cervix, continue to open the utero-vesical fold. Open the posterior leaf of the broad ligament to where the utero-sacral ligament attaches to the cervix. Avoid tear and bleeding of the small veins, electro-coagulate timely to keep the wound bloodless and the operative view clear.

The contra-lateral side is done with the same rule.

With the broad ligaments done, we need to push up the uterus as far as possible, and pin the anterior uterine wall by forceps, thus reveal the cervico-vesical gap, and open the utero-vesical fold and bilateral vesico-cervical ligaments (see Fig. 29.3). Find the correct cervico-vesical gap, reflect the bladder downwards carefully not to cause any bleeding. For supracervical hysterectomy, reflect the ladder just enough to do the devascularization. For total hysterectomy, the bladder has to be reflected down to 1 cm below the upper end of the vagina. It is crucial to reflect the bladder downwards before devascularization, so that the vessels can be processed successfully without injury of the bladder and ureters.

Continue to dissect the peripheral structure of cervical vessels after the bladder is reflected down (see Fig. 29.4). There is often one uterine artery surrounded by several uterine veins. Uterine veins are wide and thin-walled, easy to be damaged, and not easy to electro-coagulate. Once big uterine vein bleeding occurs, clamp the bleeding point and push away the bladder with caution to make space for transfixion. When cervical vessels are dissected, suture the uterine vessels below the isthmus, or electro-coagulate and transect. Desiccation of a vessel should be of a certain width in order to avoid bleeding after transection and blurring of the operative view.

After devascularization, go further to next steps according to total or supracervical hysterectomy.

For supracervical hysterectomy, withdraw the uterine manipulator and remove the uterus by morcellation (see Fig. 29.5). The cervix stump is scissored into a wedge shape, coagulated by electrotome and interruptedly sutured, usually by three stitches. The middle stitch must be deep to the base of the wedge, upper end of the cervical canal, in case of possible postoperative bleeding.

For total hysterectomy, after devascularization, transect the cardinal ligament to the cervico-vaginal fornix junction through the space between uterine vessels and the cervix, then resect the uterus circumferentially off the vaginal fornix, aided by the cup of uterine manipulator , extract the uterine corpus through vagina(see Fig. 29.6). To find the space between uterine vessels and the cervix correctly is vital to prevent bleeding.

Close the vaginal cuff after hysterectomy by interrupted or running suture. Pay special attention to the suture of bilateral utero-sacral ends.

At last, irrigate the pelvic cavity, stanch thoroughly, and examine the ureters, bladder, rectum and other pelvic organs, finish the operation.

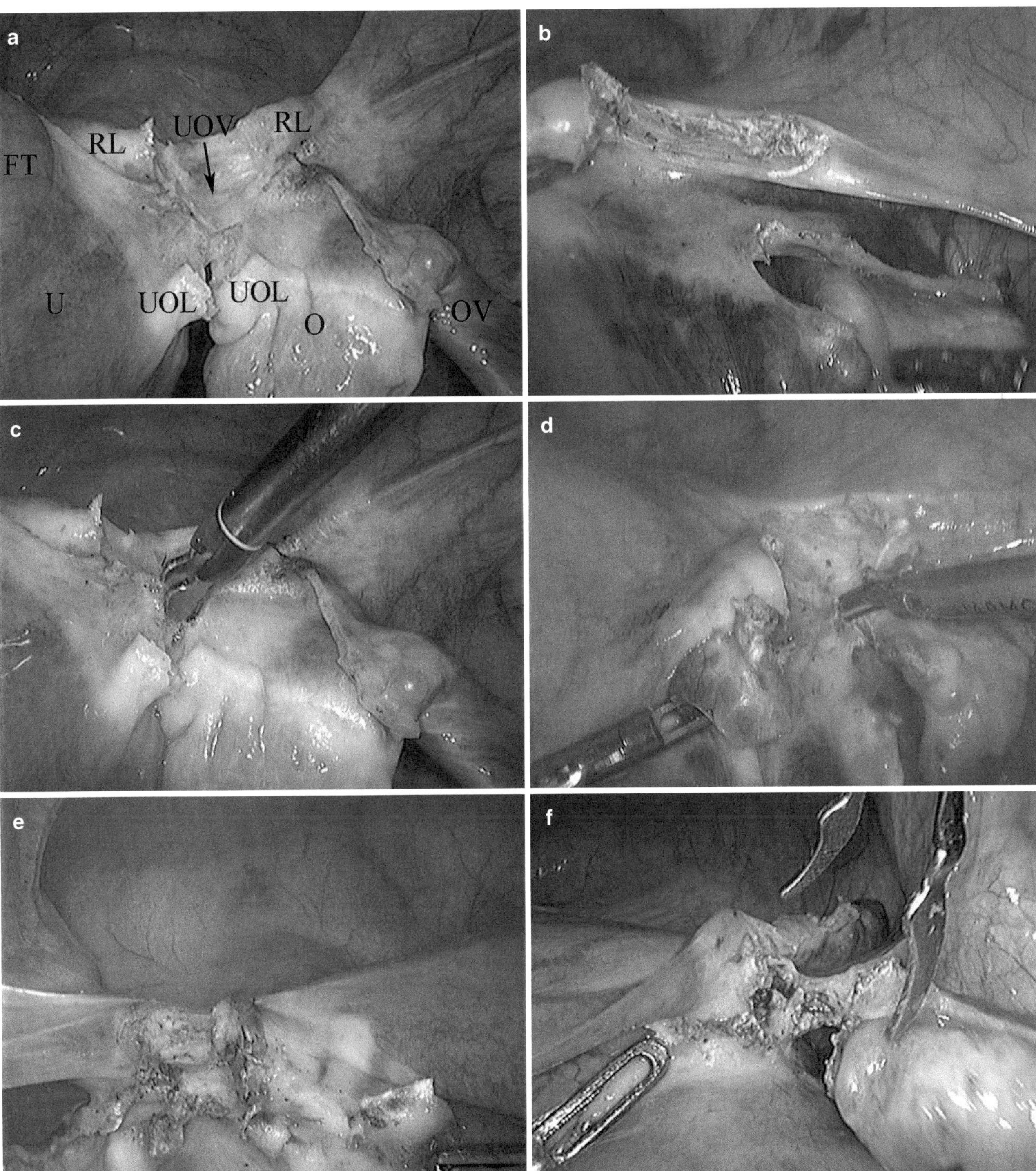

Fig. 29.1 Utero-ovarian vessels and surrounded structures. The anastomoses branch of utero-ovarian vessels, which are surrounded by the round ligament, utero-ovarian ligament and fallopian tube. Round ligament, utero-ovarian ligament and fallopian tube are usually done before devascularization. For patients with thin ligaments, do the devascularization directly. Transection of these structures should be done 1 cm away from the uterus to avoid injury of vessels on the lateral uterine wall. (**a**) Divide the surrounding structure and expose the anastomoses branch of utero-ovarian vessels. (**b**) The round ligament is transected 1 cm away from the uterus. (**c**) electrocoagulation of the anastomoses branch of utero-ovarian vessels. (**d**) Transection of the anastomoses branch of utero-ovarian vessels by ultrasound knife. (**e**) Transect the surrounding structure and expose the anastomoses branch of left ovarian vessel. (**f**) The round ligament and utero-ovarian ligament that surround the anastomoses branch of utero-ovarian vessels are thin, so directly electro-coagulate them. **Abbreviations**: *FT* FallopianTube, *RL* Round Ligament, *UOV* Utero-ovarian Vessels, *OV* Ovarian Vessels, *U* Uterus, *O* Ovary, *UOL* Utero-ovarian Ligament

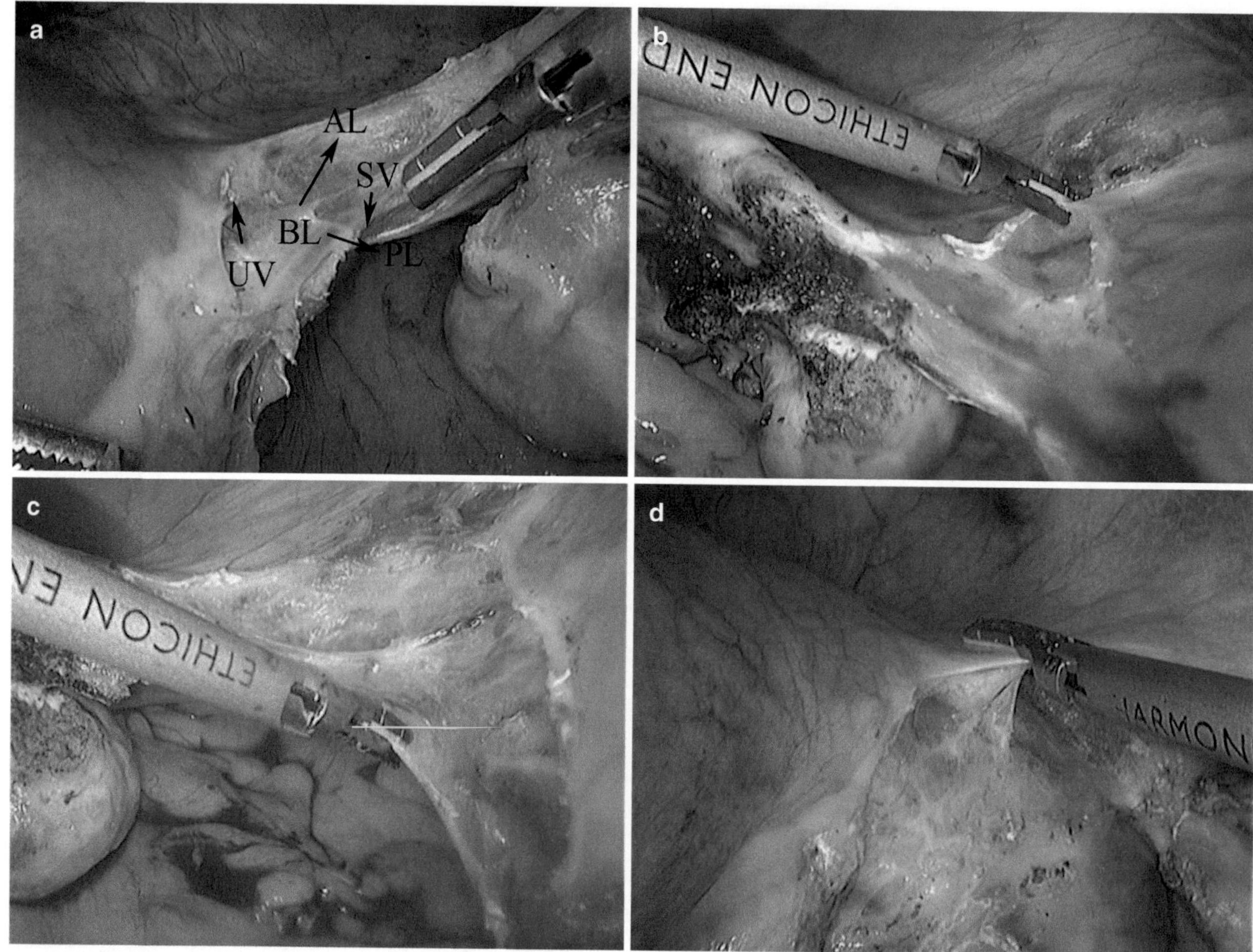

Fig. 29.2 To dissect the broad ligament. To open the broad ligament, dissect the anterior and posterior leaf respectively. Usually there are only small vessels and loose connective tissue within the broad ligament. Be careful not to injure the uterine vessels which are close to the lateral uterine wall. Now a uterine manipulator is necessary to push the uterus up to help expose, meanwhile the contra-lateral grasping forceps continue pulling and assist rotation. (**a**) Open the anterior and posterior leaf of the broad ligament, and small veins can be seen. (**b**) Open the anterior leaf of the left broad ligament to where the utero-vesical fold is, (**c**) Open the anterior and posterior leaf of the left broad ligament;2–4 a uterine with the lower segment enlarged. (**d**) Carefully open the anterior leaf of the broad ligament close to the uterus. (**e**) A uterine with the lower segment enlarged. Carefully open the posterior leaf of the broad ligament close to the uterus. (**f**) Open the anterior and posterior leaf of the broad ligament in a large uterus, and umbilico-vesical ligament, external iliac vein and thick uterine veins can be seen. (**g**) Myoma of the left lower segment of uterine wall. Pull it to right and rotate clockwise, and open the anterior leaf of the broad ligament to the front of the cervix. (**h**) Myoma of the left lower segment of uterine wall. Pull it to right and rotate clockwise, and open the posterior leaf of the broad ligament to the utero-sacral ligaments. **Abbreviations**: *U* Uterus, *UV* Uterine Veins, *VIE* Vena Iliaca Externa, *UUL* Umbilicourethralligament, *AF* Anterior Feaf, *PF* Posterior Feaf, *SV* Small Venae

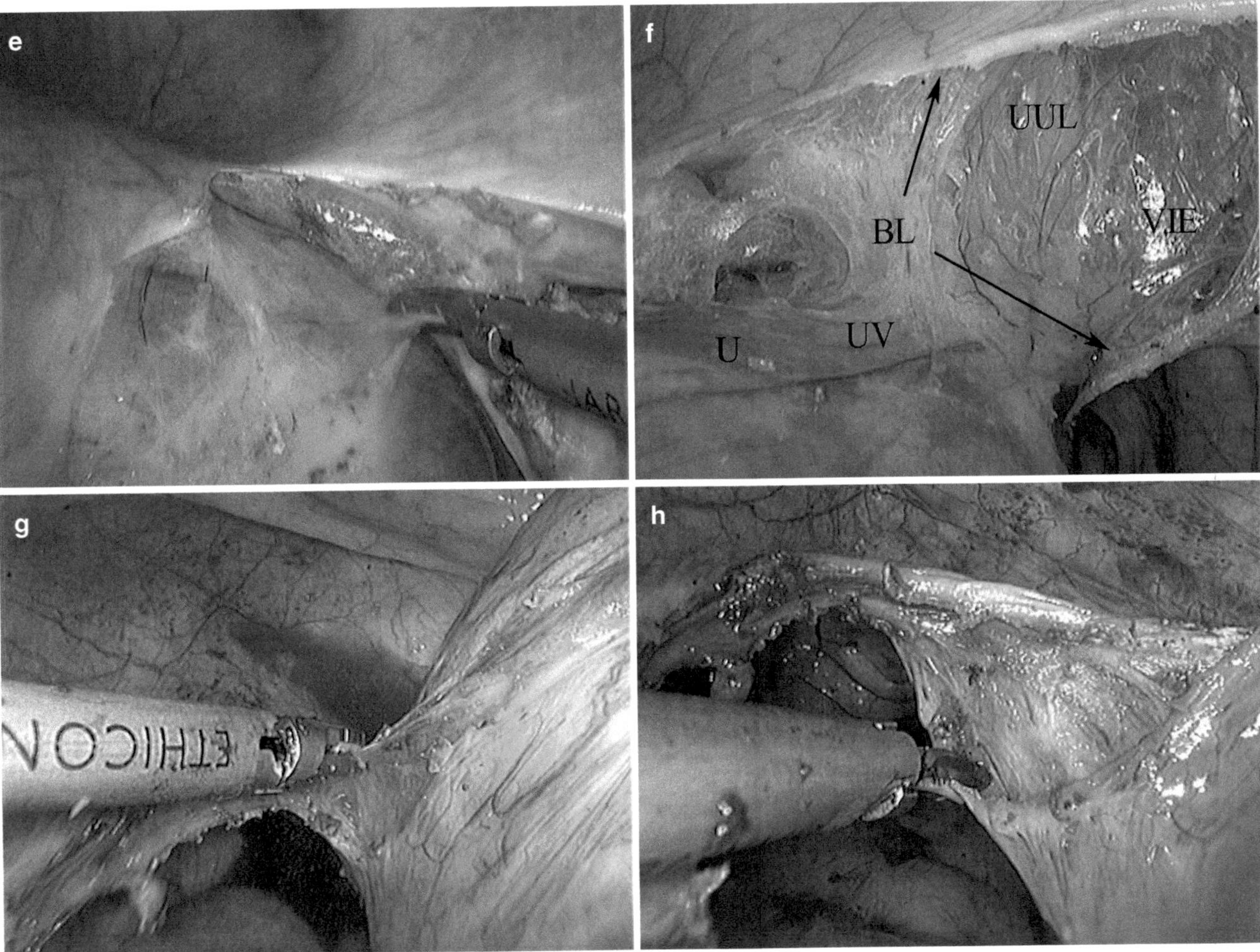

Fig. 29.2 (continued)

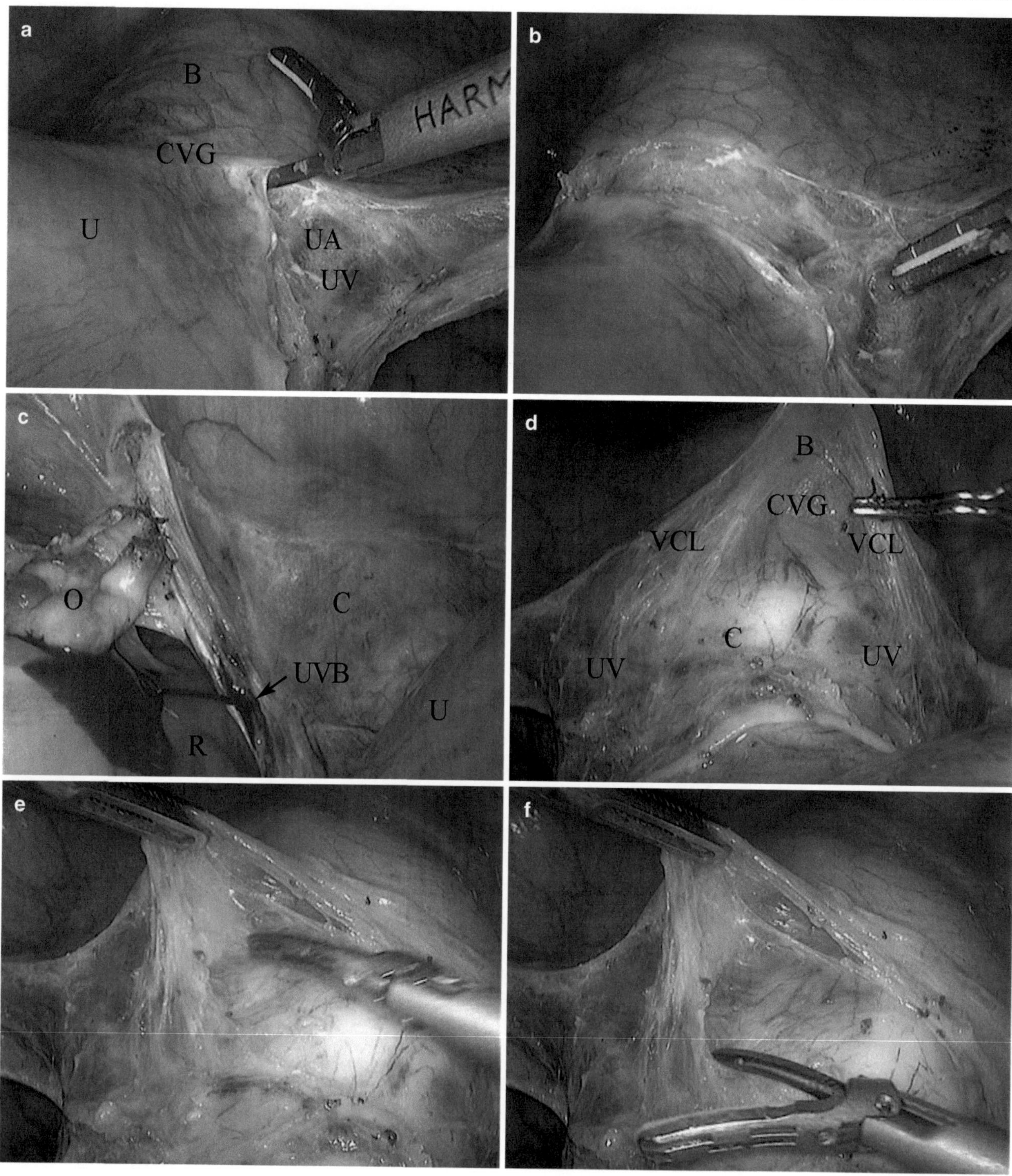

Fig. 29.3 To open the utero-vesical fold and reflect the bladder downwards. Open the anterior leaf of the broad ligament up to cervix; continue to open the utero-vesical fold. Open the posterior leaf of the broad ligament to where the utero-sacral ligament attaches to the cervix. Avoid tear and bleeding of the small veins, electro-coagulate timely to keep the wound bloodless and the operative view clear. The contralateral side is done with the same rule. With the broad ligaments done, we need to push up the uterus as far as possible, and pin the anterior uterine wall by forceps, thus reveal the cervico-vesical gap, and open the utero-vesical fold and bilateral vesico-cervical ligaments. Find the correct cervico-vesical gap, reflect the bladder downwards carefully not to cause any bleeding. For supracervical hysterectomy, reflect the ladder just enough to do the devascularization. For total hysterectomy, the bladder has to be reflected down to 1 cm below the upper end of the vagina. It is crucial to reflect the bladder downwards before devascularization, so that the vessels can be processed successfully without injury of the bladder and ureters. (**a**–**b**) Open the utero-vesical fold. (**c**) Small veins are torn and bleeding during uterine manipulation. (**d**–**f**) Reflect the bladder downwards and transect the vesico-cervical ligaments. (**g**–**h**) Open the utero-vesical fold of a large uterus. (**i**–**j**) Open the utero-vesical fold and reflect the bladder downwards in a patient who used to receive a caesarean section. Pay attention to find the correct cervico-vesical gap.*U* Uterus, *UV* UterineVeins, *UA* Uterine Artery, *UVS* Uterine Vessels, *VIE* Vena Iliaca Externa, *B* Bladder, *C* Cervix, *R* Rectum, *UVB* Uterine Veins Bleeding, *CVG* Cervico-vesical Gap, *VCL* Vesico-cervical Ligament, *SV* Small Venae

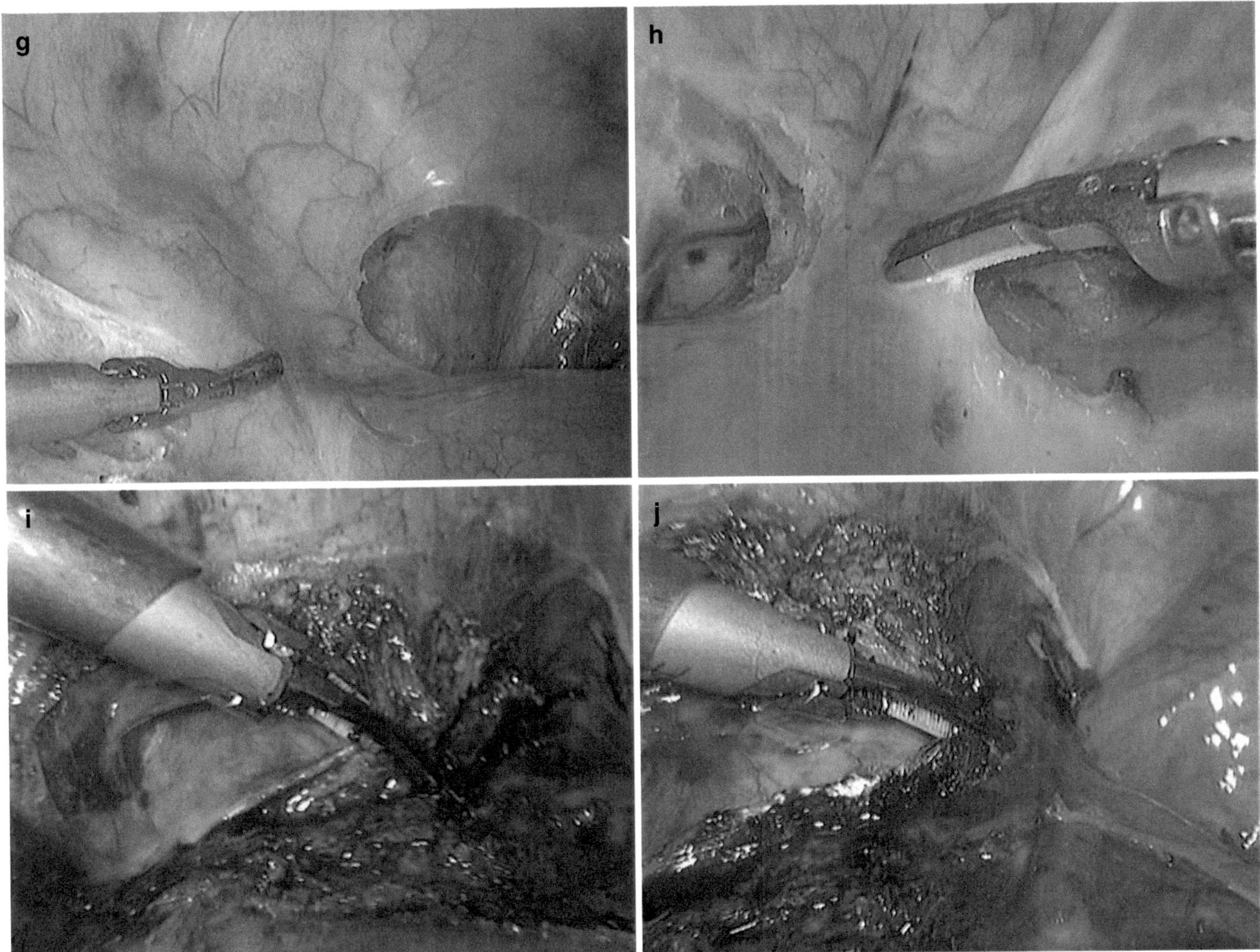

Fig. 29.3 (continued)

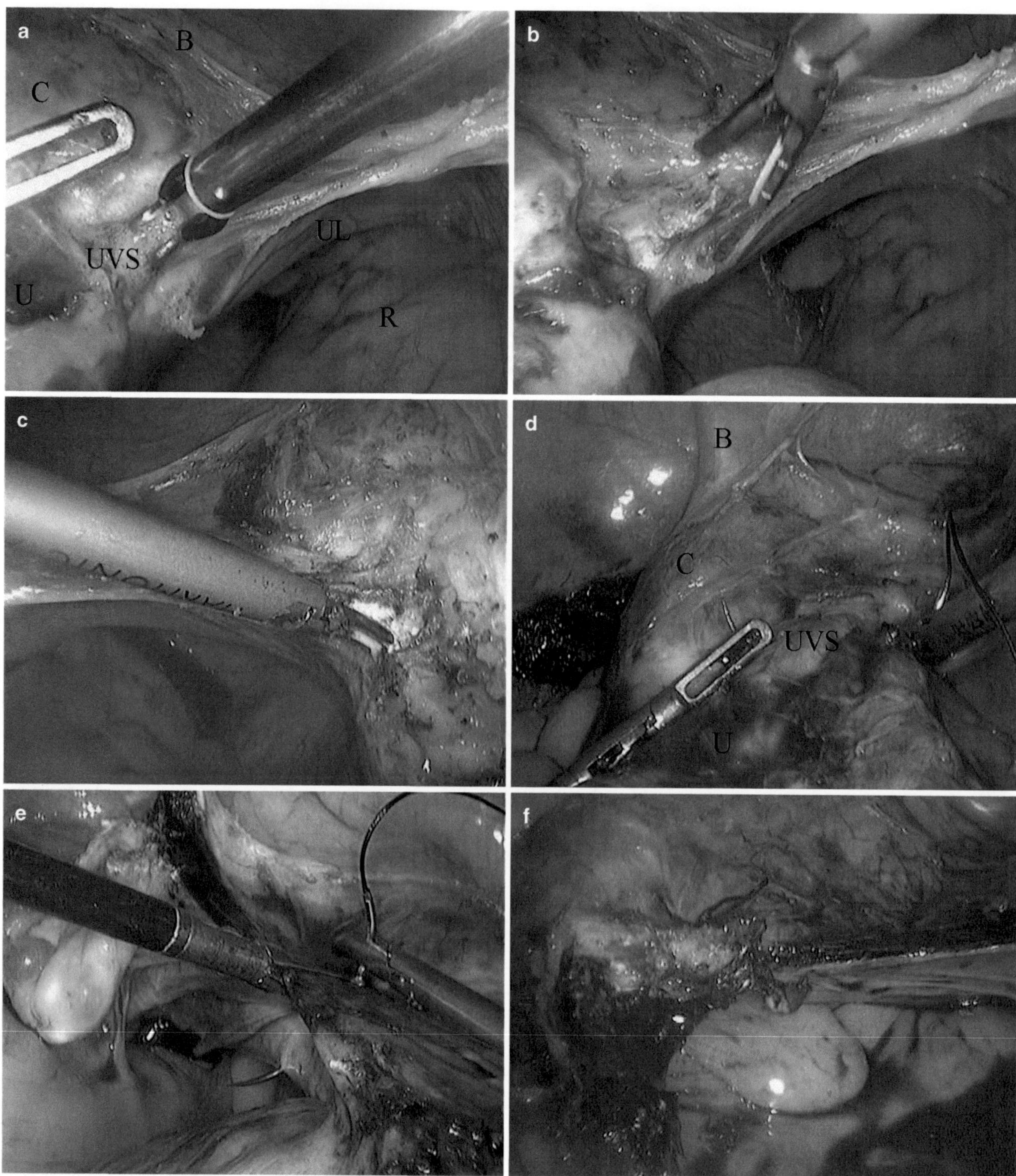

Fig. 29.4 To dissect the uterine vessels and devascularization. Continue to dissect the peripheral structure of cervical vessels after the bladder is reflected down. There is often one uterine artery surrounded by several uterine veins. Uterine veins are wide and thin-walled, easy to be damaged, and not easy to electro-coagulate. Once big uterine vein bleeding occurs, clamp the bleeding point and push away the bladder with caution to make space for transfixion. When cervical vessels are dissected, suture the uterine vessels below the isthmus, or electro-coagulate and transect. Desiccation of a vessel should be of a certain width in order to avoid bleeding after transection and blurring of the operative view. (**a**) Open the anterior and posterior leaf of the broad ligament and the utero vesical fold, reflect the bladder downwards and electro-coagulate the right uterine vessel. (**b**) Transection of the right uterine vessel by ultrasound knife. (**c**) The left uterine vessel is done by the same way. (**d**) Transfixion of the right uterine vessel. (**e**) Transfixion of the left uterine vessel. (**f**) Electro-coagulate and transect the uterine vessel 1–2 cm above the transfixion point. **Abbreviation**: *U* Uterus, *UVS* Uterinevessels, *UL* Uterosacral ligament, *B* Bladder, *C* Cervix, *R* Rectum

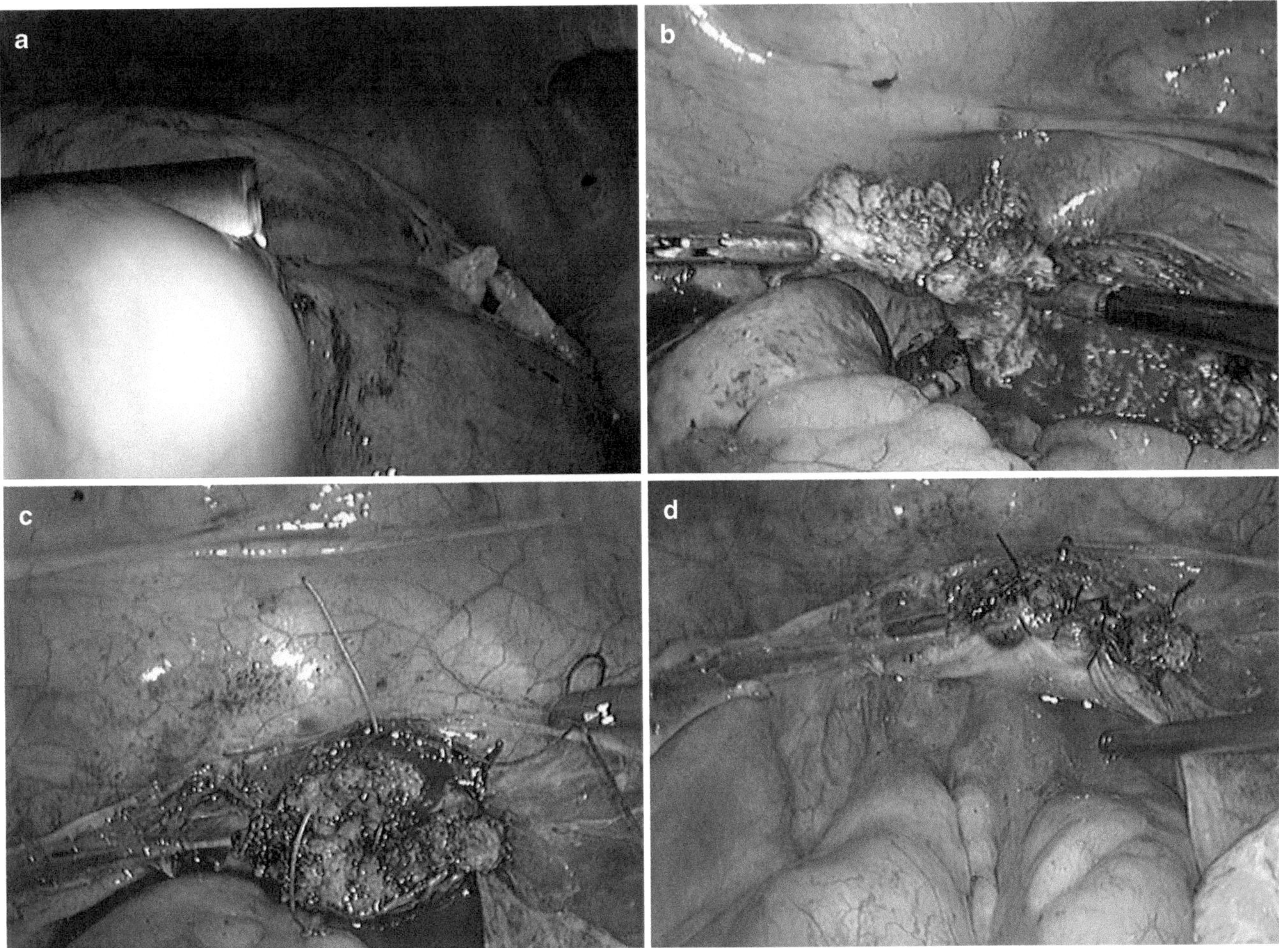

Fig. 29.5 Morcellation and closing cervix stump for supracervical hysterectomy. After devascularization, go further to next steps according to total or supracervical hysterectomy. For supracervical hysterectomy, withdraw the uterine manipulator and remove the uterus by morcellation. The cervix stump is scissored into a wedge shape, coagulated by electrotome and interruptedly sutured, usually by three stitches. The middle stitch must be deep to the base of the wedge, upper end of the cervical canal, in case of possible postoperative bleeding. (**a**) After devascularization, remove the uterus by morcellation. (**b**) Scissoring of The cervix stump in supracervical hysterectomy. (**c**) Coagulate by electrotome and interruptedly suture the cervix stump with 1–0 absorbable line. (**d**) Suture of the cervix stump is done

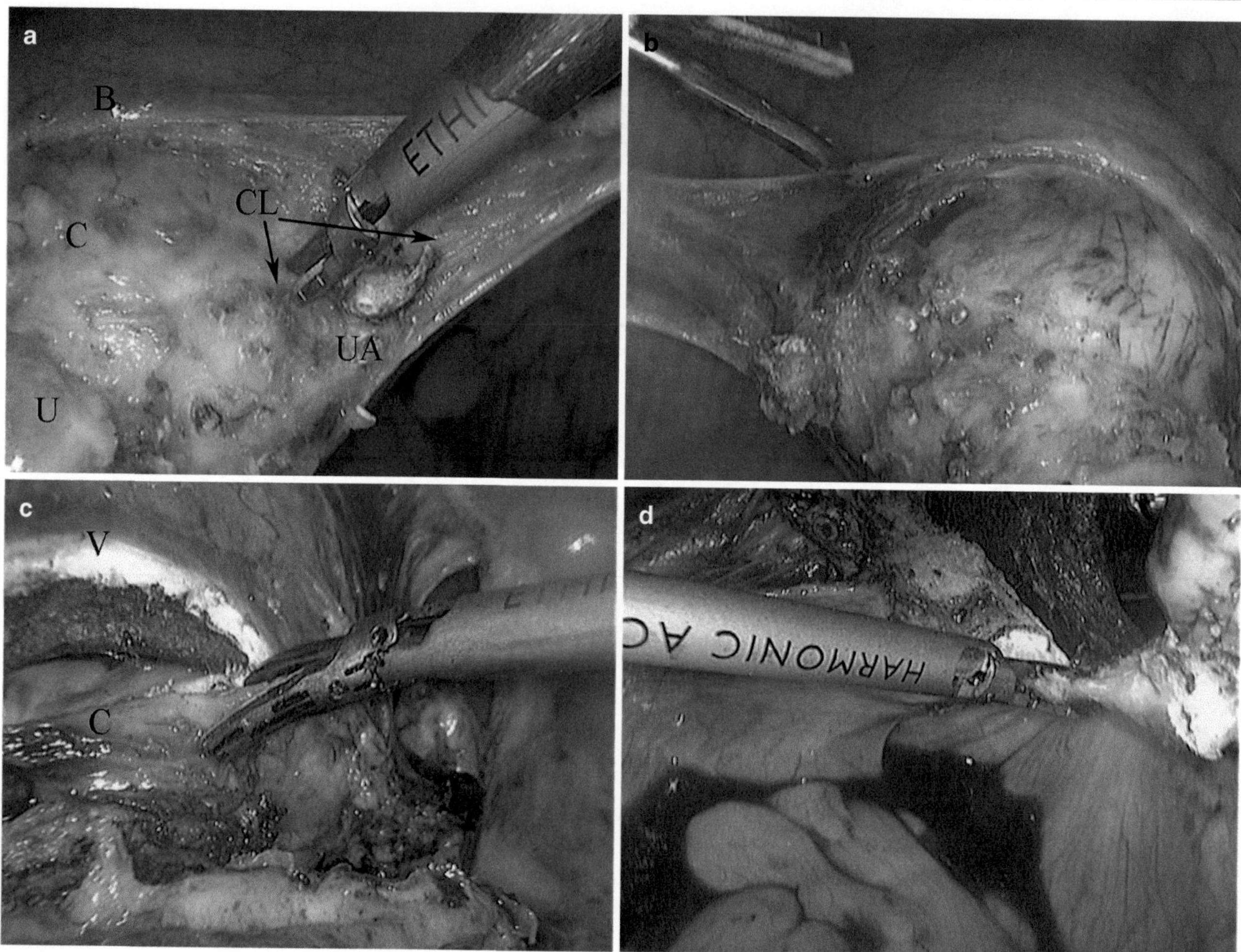

Fig. 29.6 Total hysterectomy. For total hysterectomy, after devascularization, transect the cardinal ligament to the cervico-vaginal fornix junction through the space between uterine vessels and the cervix, then resect the uterus circumferentially off the vaginal fornix, aided by the cup of uterine manipulator, extract the uterine corpus through vagina. To find the space between uterine vessels and the cervix correctly is vital to prevent bleeding. Close the vaginal cuff after hysterectomy by interrupted or running suture. Pay special attention to the suture of bilateral utero-sacral ends. (**a**, **b**) For total hysterectomy, after devascularization, transect the cardinal ligament by ultrasound knife to the cervico-vaginal fornix junction through the space between uterine vessels and the cervix; (**c**, **d**) use a ultrasound knife or unipolar electrotome to resect the uterus circumferentially off the vaginal fornix, aided by the cup of uterine manipulator, and remove through the vagina; (**e**) the vaginal cuff after hysterectomy; (**f**) Close the vaginal cuff by running suture, and Pay attention to the suture of bilateral utero-sacral ends. (**g**) The hysterectomy and closure of the vaginal cuff is done. **Abbreviations**: *U* Uterus, *UL* Uterosacral ligament, *B* Bladder, *C* Cervix, *R* Rectum, *V* Vagina, *CL* Cardinal ligament, *UA* Uterine artery, *UVS* Uterine vessels

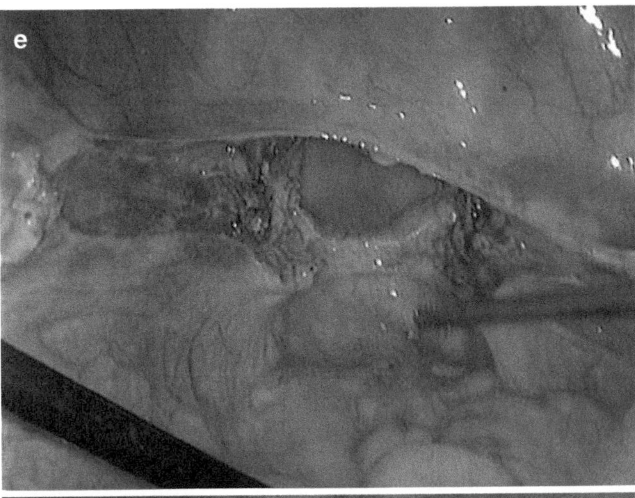

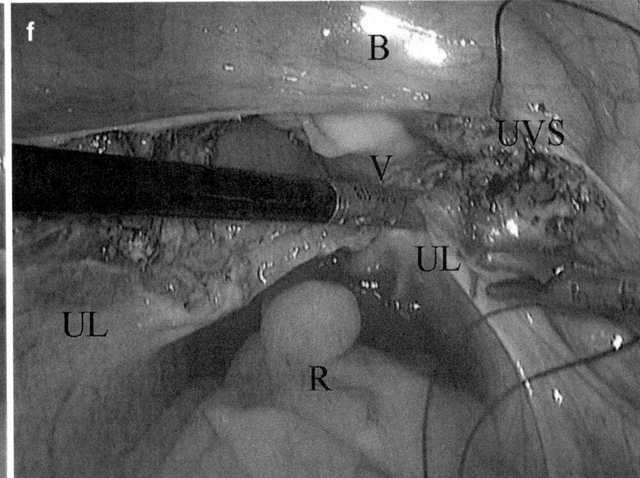

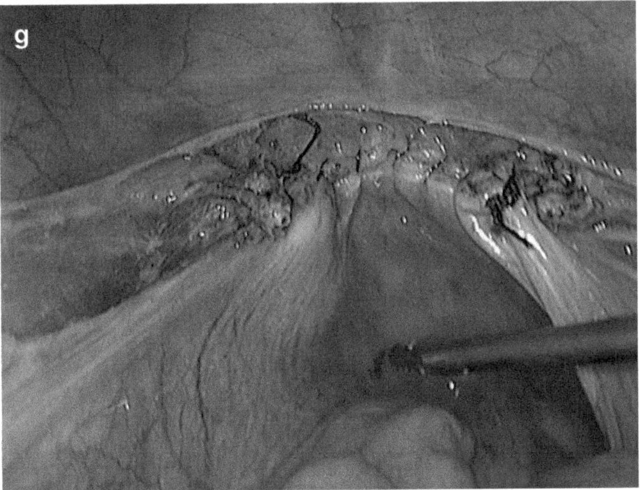

Fig. 29.6 (continued)

References

1. McPherson K, Metcalfe MA, Herbert A, et al. Severe complications of hysterectomy: the VALUE study. BJOG. 2004;111(7):688–94.
2. O'Hanlan KA, McCutcheon SP, McCutcheon JG. Laparoscopic hysterectomy: impact of uterine size. J Minim Invasive Gynecol. 2011;18(1):85–91.
3. Demir RH, Marchand GJ. Safe laparoscopic removal of a 3200 gram fibroid uterus. JSLS (Journal of the Society of Laparoendoscopic Surgeons/Society of Laparoendoscopic Surgeons). 2010;14(4):600–2.
4. Walid MS, Heaton RL. Total laparoscopic hysterectomy for uteri over one kilogram. JSLS (Journal of the Society of Laparoendoscopic Surgeons/Society of Laparoendoscopic Surgeons). 2010;14(2):178–82.
5. Zeng W, Chen L, Du W, Hu J, Fang X, Zhao X. Laparoscopic hysterectomy of large uteri using three-trocar technique. Int J Clin Exp Med. 2015;8(4):6319–26.
6. AAGL Advancing Minimally Invasive Gynecology Worldwide. AAGL practice report: Morcellation during uterine tissue extraction. J Minim Invasive Gynecol. 2014;21(4):517–30.
7. Brown J. AAGL advancing minimally invasive gynecology worldwide: statement to the FDA on power morcellation. J Minim Invasive Gynecol. 2014;21(6):970–1.
8. Senapati S, Tu FF, Magrina JF. Power morcellators: a review of current practice and assessment of risk. Am J Obstet Gynecol. 2015;212(1):18–23.
9. Hampton T. Use of morcellation to remove fibroids scrutinized at FDA hearings. JAMA. 2014;312(6):588.
10. Stephenson J. FDA warns against procedure used in removing fibroids. JAMA. 2014;311(19):1956.
11. Aust T, Reyftmann L, Rosen D, Cario G, Chou D. Anterior approach to laparoscopic uterine artery ligation. J Minim Invasive Gynecol. 2011;18(6):792–5.
12. Manoucheri E, Cohen SL, Sandberg EM, Kibel AS, Einarsson J. Ureteral injury in laparoscopic gynecologic surgery. Rev Obstet Gynecol. 2012;5(2):106–11.

Symptomatic Fibroids as Main Indication for Laparoscopic Hysterectomy and Their Handling

30

Liselotte Mettler and Ibrahim Alkatout

Introduction

One of the multiple treatment possibilities for myomas considering all laparoscopic surgical, medical or interventional techniques is total laparoscopic hysterectomy (TLH) or subtotal laparoscopic hysterectomy (SLH). As SLH is a much less invasive procedure, a good number of patients with myomas can consider a subtotal approach. However, only a total laparoscopic hysterectomy (TLH) can offer 100 % protection from new fibroid formation, later sarcoma formation, uncontrolled bleedings, cervical and endometrial cancer or any other problems arising from the uterus.

In spite of numerous theories, the etiology of fibroid formation remains unclear. While a genetic disposition must be given, as Africans have a much higher frequency of multiple myomas than Caucasians certain up- and down-regulations in the genes of patients with and without myomas have been described. However, as yet no clear guidelines for the prevention of fibroids are available. Hereditary leioyomatosis and renal cell carcinoma syndrome is a rare syndrome involving fibroids. Individuals with the gene that leads to both fibroids and skin leiomyomas have an increased risk of developing a rare case of kidney cell cancer (papillary renal cell carcinoma).

Understanding which genes are involved in fibroids does not automatically tell us why fibroids develop or how to control them. From our understanding of fibroid behavior, we would guess that genes involved in estrogen or progesterone production, metabolism or action are involved. Unfortunately, science is seldom that straightforward. Most guesses regarding these "candidate genes" turn out to be wrong and much research is still required to find out how these genes lead to disease. There are also small variations, called polymorphisms, in genes that may play a role in influencing the risk of fibroids. Both polymorphisms and mutations are changes in the sequence of genes, but the difference is in the degree of change. A mutation makes a major change in the gene that leads to a change in the protein the gene is coding for. For example, it can change the amino acid from alanine to glycine or cause the protein to be prematurely cut off.

L. Mettler • I. Alkatout (✉)
Gynecology and Obstetrics,
University Hospitals Schleswig-Holstein,
Campus Kiel, Kiel, Germany
e-mail: lmettler@email.uni-kiel.de; ibrahim.alkatout@uksh.de

The Genetics of Fibroids, Genotype, Phenotype

The discovery of the structure of DNA (desoxyribonucleic acid) by Watson and Crick revolutionized biology and medicine. They discovered that DNA carries the code for life in a ladder-like structure. Today, it is known that the genes from a single person take up the space of 400,000 times the distance from the earth to the moon or 1000 times the distance from the earth to the sun = 150 billion kilometers [1–3].

Before going further, it is important to define the terms genotype and phenotype. The genotype is the pattern of genes that you inherit. For example, with eye color, brown is a dominant color and is represented by a "B". Blue is a recessive trait and represented by a "b". Therefore, a person can have "BB", "bb", or "Bb" as genotypes for eye color. Each person gets two copies of the gene, one originally from his or her mother and the other from his or her father. The dominant gene will always dominate; it has the power to trump a recessive trait. Phenotype is the physical manifestation, or end result, of the genotype. Although there are three different genotypes (BB, bb, or Bb), there are only two phenotypes: brown eyes and blue eyes. People with the "BB" or the "Bb" genotype have brown eyes because brown is the dominant trait; only the people with the "bb" genotype have blue eyes.

We believe that fibroids are a common phenotype that represents many different underlying genotypes. In other words, in our view, fibroids can arise through multiple

I. Alkatout, L. Mettler (eds.), *Hysterectomy*, DOI 10.1007/978-3-319-22497-8_30

different pathways. In this case, "Bb" might represent two different genes that code for the estrogen receptor beta which influences the action of estrogen on fibroid tissue. A "B" gene may make the fibroid more sensitive to this hormone and therefore more likely to grow. In addition, probably multiple genes influence fibroids so that in addition to "Bb" we may also have "Pp" for progesterone receptors, "Ff" for fibrotic factors, and so on. This information would be most helpful in advancing treatment as women who carry a high risk of recurrent fibroids and have completed their family planning might choose to have a hysterectomy because of the higher chance of their having an additional surgery. We currently have some clinical information (based on physicians' clinical experience with many patients) to predict prognosis for recurrence after myomectomy, but our clinical information for alternative forms of treatment options is limited.

Evidence for the Role of Genes in Fibroid Development and Growth

Studies of women with fibroids suggest several reasons to suspect that genes play a role in fibroid formation. The first is that both women in a pair of identical twins are twice as likely to have had a fibroid-related hysterectomy as both women in a pair of fraternal (non identical) twins. Identical twins share 100 % of their genes, while fraternal twins share only 50 % of their genes. This suggests that the genes that identical twins share make them more likely to form fibroids, since both are identical and non identical twins have equal exposure to environmental factors. This difference between identical and fraternal twins has been observed in a general population of women undergoing hysterectomy and a population of women with fibroids leading to hysterectomy [4, 5].

There is also evidence that women who have close relatives, such as a mother or sister, with fibroids are much more likely to have fibroids themselves [6, 7]. This propensity is called familial aggregation. Just as with breast cancer, if you have many relatives affected by fibroids, your risk of disease is likely to be increased.

Molecular Genetics and Genome-Wide Scan for Fibroid Genes

Finally, in the age of molecular genetics, we can scan markers across the complete sets of DNA, or genomes, of many people to find genetic variations associated with a particular disease. This process is called a genome-wide scan. This is a common approach to finding genes in complex diseases, such as diabetes, asthma and heart disease. With a genome-wide scan, women who are sisters and both have fibroids (an affected sibling pair) are recruited to participate in the study. Their DNA is studied for common genes. If hundreds of women are studied, each region of every chromosome can be examined, and it can be determined which genes are shared by the sisters who share the fibroid phenotype but are different in many other respects. This approach often produces novel genes that were not previously thought to be involved in the disease process [8–11].

Microscopic Facts and Fibroid Viability

Fibroids are composed primarily of smooth muscle cells. The uterus, stomach and bladder are all organs made of smooth muscle. Smooth muscles cells are arranged so that the organ can stretch, instead of being arranged in rigid units like the cells in skeletal muscle in arms and legs that are designed to "pull" in a particular direction. In women with fibroids, tissue from the endometrium typically looks normal under the microscope. Sometimes, however, in submucosal fibroids there is an unusual type of uterine lining that does not have the normal glandular structure. The presence of this abnormality, called aglandular functionalis (functional endometrium with no glands), in women having bleeding disorders is sometimes a clinical clue for their doctors to look more closely for a submucosal fibroid [12]. A second pattern of endometrium, termed chronic endometritis, can also suggest that there may be a submucosal fibroid, although this pattern can also be associated with other problems, such as retained products of conception and various infections of the uterus. Hysterectomy is not the only solution for treating fibroids; distinctions in size, position, and appearance have to be taken into account when deciding upon the best treatment option. If we understand these issues, we may be able to tell why some women have severe bleeding and other women with a similarly sized fibroid have no problem.

Costs of Fibroids

In fact, accurately capturing all the costs attributable to uterine fibroids will help us move toward more, and more effective, innovative therapies. When deciding whether or not to launch a new concept, companies typically look at the amount currently spent for other treatments. The economics of fibroids has chiefly been discussed in terms of the health care costs of hysterectomy. This in itself is a huge amount of money. According to a recent estimate, in the United States, more than $2 billion dollars are spent every year on hospitalization costs due to uterine fibroids alone [13]. Additionally, one study estimates that the health care costs due to uterine fibroids are more than $ 4600 per woman per year [14].

When you incorporate all the costs of fibroids, however, the way of treatment becomes even more significant. Let us consider what costs arise

- The costs of myomectomy, uterine artery embolization (UAE), and other minimally invasive therapies
- The costs of birth control pills and other hormonal treatments to control bleeding
- The costs of tampons, pads, and the adult diapers many women require to contain the bleeding
- The costs of alternative and complementary therapies
- The cost of doing nothing (for many women this means missing work or working less productively during their period).

Reasons for Hysterectomies in Fibroid Patients

Why should a patient have a hysterectomy today when so many alterative treatment possibilities are available? Firstly, up to a certain size of the enlarged uterus, laparoscopic subtotal hysterectomy completely solves the problem and if women want to eliminate every risk of recurrent fibroids, hysterectomy is their only choice. Hysterectomy also solves coexisting problems, such as adenomyosis, endometriosis and endometrial polyps or cervical dysplasia, and there is no danger of ever leaving a sarcoma or carcinoma behind.

Review of All Uterine-Preserving Treatment Possibilities for Fibroids

The surgical treatment of fibroids can be differentiated between less invasive and more invasive surgical techniques. Time and type of treatment have to be chosen individually and are dependent on the patient and the treating gynecologist (Tables 30.1 and 30.2).

Table 30.1 Uterine fibroids or myomatous uterus

Asymptomatic	Symptomatic
Conservative treatment	Operative treatment
No acute need for action	Acute need for action
Medical therapy	Primary operative treatment
Expectant management	Delayed operative treatment with medical pre-treatment

Expectant Management

Wait-and-see is a possibility if patients are asymptomatic, decline medical or surgical treatment or have contraindications to any kind of treatment. However, existing data describe the possibility that fibroids can shrink substantially either by optimizing endocrinological disorders, such as hypothyroidism, or during the postpartum period [15, 16].

To pursue the idea of expectant management, the pelvic mass must definitely be classified as a fibroid and differentiated from an ovarian mass. The complete blood count (CBC) should be normal, especially in patients with severe symptoms, such as menorrhagia or hypermenorrhea. The women must also be informed that the risk of miscarriage, premature labor and delivery, abnormal fetal position and placental abruption is increased during pregnancies with uterine fibroids [17].

Medical Therapy

The benefit of medical treatment in the management of women with symptomatic fibroids is still difficult to prove. Medical therapy can provide adequate symptom relief, especially in cases where hypermenorrhea is the leading problem. The benefit of symptom improvement decreases in long-term treatment periods so that more than 50 % undergo surgery within two years [18].

Nevertheless, there has been a shift in traditional thinking that medical treatment of fibroids is solely based on the manipulation of steroid hormones. A deeper analysis and understanding of specific genes or pathways associated with leiomyomatosis may open new possibilities for prevention and medical treatment [19].

Primarily as a preoperative treatment to decrease heavy bleedings in patients with fibroids, hormonal treatment with selective progesterone modulators, such as ulipristal acetate 5–10 mg daily, have become widely used over the last 2 years [20–22].

Alternative Treatment Methods

If the patient does not want to undergo surgery or there are contraindications to surgery, there are alternative procedures:

Table 30.2 Treatment options for uterine fibroids

Alternative	Surgical						
Uterine artery	Myomectomy				Hysterectomy		
Embolization							
High intensity focused ultrasound	Hysteroscopic	Laparoscopic	Abdomical	Robotic assisted	Vaginal	Laparoscopic	Abdominal
Miscellaneous methods (myoma coagulation, myolysis)						Supracervical	
						Total	

Uterine Artery Embolization (UAE): This minimally invasive therapeutical option allows an occlusion of the specific arteries supplying blood to the fibroids. A catheter is introduced via the femoral artery under local anesthesia and particles are injected to block the blood flow to the fibroid. This can be an effective treatment option if the uterus should not be removed, surgery is contraindicated and family planning is completed. It results in myoma shrinkage of up to 46 %. Nevertheless, there is still a significant rate of postinterventional complications [23, 24].

Magnetic Resonance-guided focused UltraSound (MgRf-US): This is a more recent treatment method for uterine fibroids in premenopausal women. Again, the patients should have completed their family planning. In this noninvasive thermo ablative technique multiple waves of ultrasound energy are converged on a small volume of tissue, resulting in maximal thermal destruction. The limiting factors are size, vascularity and access [25, 26].

Uterine-Preserving Surgical Treatment of Fibroids

The surgical removal of fibroids is still the main pillar in the treatment of leiomyomas. Hysterectomy is the only definitive solution and can be performed as supracervical or total hysterectomy. Myomectomy performed by hysteroscopy, conventional laparoscopy or laparoscopy with robotic assistance and by the open or vaginal approach are alternative surgical methods.

Indications for surgical therapy of uterine fibroids are:

1. Abnormal uterine bleeding disorders (hypermenorrhea, dysmenorrhea, menorrhagia- and metrorrhagia)
2. Bulk-related symptoms
3. Primary or secondary infertility and recurrent pregnancy loss.

Counseling and Informed Consent

Patients undergoing an operative procedure have to be informed of the risks and potential complications as well as alternative operating methods. Counseling before surgery should include discussion of the entry technique and the associated risks: injury of the bowel, urinary tract, blood vessels, omentum and other surrounding organs and, at a later date, wound infection, adhesion-associated pain and hernia formation.

Counseling needs to integrate the individual risk dependent on the BMI of the patient. Depending on the medical history, it is important to consider anatomical malformations, number of vaginal births, midline abdominal incisions, a history of peritonitis or inflammatory bowel disease [27].

Myomectomy

Myomectomy is a surgical treatment option for women who have not completed their family planning or who wish to retain their uterus for any other reasons. The enucleation of fibroids by any method is an effective therapy for bleeding disorders or displacement pressure in the pelvis. Nevertheless, the risk of recurrence remains after myomectomy. Furthermore, if any other pathologies might be causative or only co-causative for the symptoms (such as adenomyosis uteri), these problems will persist [28]. Complications arising at myoma enucleations and pregnancy-related complications have been investigated extensively. All operating possibilities, especially laparoscopic versus laparotomic, but recently also laparoscopic versus robotic-assisted myomectomy have been evaluated. Uterine rupture or uterine dehiscence is rare and occurs in less than 1 % of laparoscopic cases and even less seldom in robotic-assisted and laparotomic cases. Careful patient selection and preparation, as well as suture techniques, appear to be the most important variables for myomectomy in women of reproductive age [29, 30]. Uteri with multiple fibroids have an increased number of uterine arterioles and venules. Therefore, myomectomy can lead to a significant blood loss and corresponding arrangements should be made [31].

Hysteroscopic Myomectomy

Submucosal fibroids have their origin in myometrial cells underneath the endometrium and represent about 15–20 % of all fibroids. Before the establishment of hysteroscopy as a minimally invasive and effective treatment method, these myomas were removed by hysterotomy or even hysterectomy. Increased surgical training, improvement of technology and the widespread use of hysteroscopic myomectomy have made it a safe, fast, effective and cheap method of fibroid resection while preserving the uterus [32].

Patient selection concentrates on intracavitary submucous and some intramural fibroids. More than 50 % of the fibroid circumference needs to be protruding into the uterine cavity. Deep myometrial leiomyomas require advanced operative skills and have an increased risk for perioperative complications and incomplete resection. The depth of myometrial penetration correlates with the volume of distension fluid absorbed [33, 34]. Few data are available on the size of myoma that prevents the use of the hysteroscopic approach. The European Society of Hysteroscopy suggests to limit the myoma size to 4 cm but the few existing data report a significant increase of complications in fibroids that are >3 cm. Surgical skills determine the size and number of myomas that can be resected [35].

Prior to hysteroscopy, knowledge of the patient's medical history is important e.g. history of caesarean section or any other reason to expect an anatomical disorder. A vaginal ultrasound scan must be performed to precisely determine the uterus location, size and all cervical and uterine pathologies [36]. If available and feasible, fluid hystero-sonography should be performed to better differentiate the relationship of leiomyoma to the endometrial cavity and the myometrium. No prophylactic antibiotic is required to prevent surgical site infection.

The first step is the dilation of the cervical channel with Hegar dilators up to Hegar 9. The most commonly used instrument for fibroid resection is the monopolar or bipolar wire loop. Using a monopolar device the fluid medium must be non-electrolytic, using a bipolar device the fluid medium is isotonic [37]. A continuous flow allows the clearance of blood out of the uterine cavity to improve visualization. Furthermore, the resected pieces can be retracted. Nevertheless, the surface of the myoma and the time needed for resection increase the risk of excessive fluid absorption [38].

The resectoscope is inserted through the cervix into the uterine cavity and after distension with fluid the uterine cavity is carefully inspected. The monopolar resectoscope requires a cutting current of 60–120 W. Bipolar resectoscopes offer the possibility of simultaneous cut and coagulation. The wire loop passes easily through the tissue. The incision starts at the highest point of the myoma. Only in pedunculated fibroids might the incision cut the peduncle first. The loop is then moved towards the surgeon using the spring mechanism and simultaneously the entire resectoscope is gently pulled backwards. The wire loop must be in view of the surgeon during the whole procedure. This motion is repeated until the whole myoma has been resected and the surrounding myometrium (depth) and endometrium (side) can be differentiated. All resected specimen is sent to the pathologist. In cases of heavy bleeding and reduced vision the endometrium and the cutting surface have to be reinspected. These areas can be desiccated with the coagulating current.

The resected area will be recovered by the surrounding endometrium during the following weeks. The complication rate is low (0.8–2.6 %) [38, 39]. Complications that can occur, especially after extensive resection, are uterine perforation or excessive fluid absorption. Absorption of distension fluid might result in hyponatremia or volume overload [40]. The recurrence rate is about 20 % in a follow-up period of more than 3 years [35] .

Laparoscopic Myomectomy

With the improvement of laparoscopic techniques and skills myomectomy can be performed laparoscopically in most women. The laparoscopic approach is usually used for intramural or subserosal fibroids. The main advantage compared to abdominal myomectomy is decreased morbidity and a shorter recovery period. Nevertheless, laparoscopic myomectomy is limited by surgical expertise and especially laparoscopic suturing skills [41, 42]. Selection criteria for laparoscopic myomectomy are location, size and number of fibroids. Nevertheless, these characteristics are variable in relation to the surgical expertise. Preoperative imaging is performed by vaginal ultrasound to assess the precise features of the leiomyomas [31, 36, 43, 44].

Laparoscopic myomectomy starts with the usual placement of ports and trocars. After placement of the initial port in the umbilicus or higher up in the midline, depending on the size of the fibroids, 2–3 ancillary trocars are placed in the lower abdomen about 2 cm medial of each iliac crest and possibly in the midline [31, 45, 46]. Myomectomy can lead to severe bleeding that will complicate the procedure due to reduced vision. Vessel bleeding is controlled by bipolar electrosurgical power tools. Intraoperative bleeding can be reduced using vasopressin or other vasoconstrictors. Vasopressin is diluted (e.g. 20 units in 100 ml of saline) and injected into the planned uterine incision site. Vasopressin constricts the smooth muscle in the walls of capillaries, small arterioles and venules. Nevertheless, due to side effects the surgeon should pull back the plunger of the syringe before insertion to check that the needle is not inserted intravascularly [47–49]. Alternatively, misoprostol can be administered vaginally about one hour before surgery to reduce blood loss [50].

The uterine incision is preferably made vertically as this allows a more ergonomic suturing of the defect. The incision is performed with a monopolar hook directly over the fibroid and carried through deeply until the entire myoma tissue has been reached (Figs. 30.1, 30.2, 30.3, 30.4, 30.5 and 30.6).

After exposure of the myoma, it is grasped with a tenaculum or sharp forceps and traction and countertraction are applied. The removal of the myoma can easily be performed with blunt and sharp dissecting devices. Capsular vessels should be coagulated before complete removal of the myoma as coagulation becomes more difficult if traction is unsuccessful and bipolar coagulation occurs in the remaining myometrium wall. Subsequent to removal, the myoma is morcellated with an electromechanical device under direct vision and at a safe distance to all structures, such as the small bowel, to avoid inadvertent injury. The myoma tissue is removed and sent for pathologic evaluation. The uterine defect is closed with delayed absorbable sutures in one or two layers, depending upon the depth of the myometrial defect. It is important that the suture starts at the deepest point to avoid any cavity that might lead to a weak uterine wall. Furthermore, we tie the knot extracorporally so that the knot can be pushed into the deep layers with full strength (Fig. 30.7).

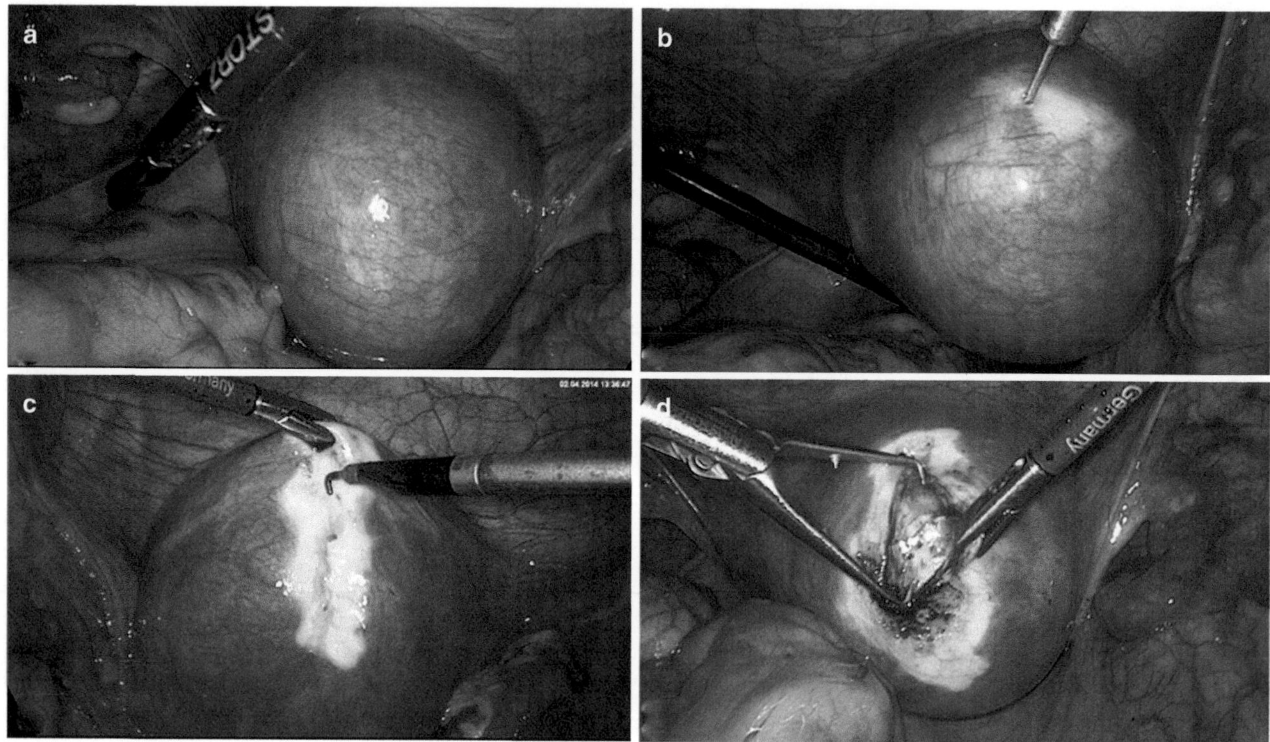

Fig. 30.1 Laparoscopic myoma enucleation. (**a**) Situs of a fundal/anterior wall fibroid. (**b**) Prophylactic hemostasis with 1:100 diluted vasopressin solution (Gylcilpressin) in separate wells. The injection intends to separate the pseudocapsule from the fibroid and reduces bleedings. (**c**) Bipolar superficial coagulation of the longitudinal incision strip and opening of the uterine wall with the monopolar hook or needle up to the fibroid surface. (**d**) Grasping of the fibroid and beginning of the enucleation. The pseudocapsule remains within the uterine wall and is pushed off bluntly

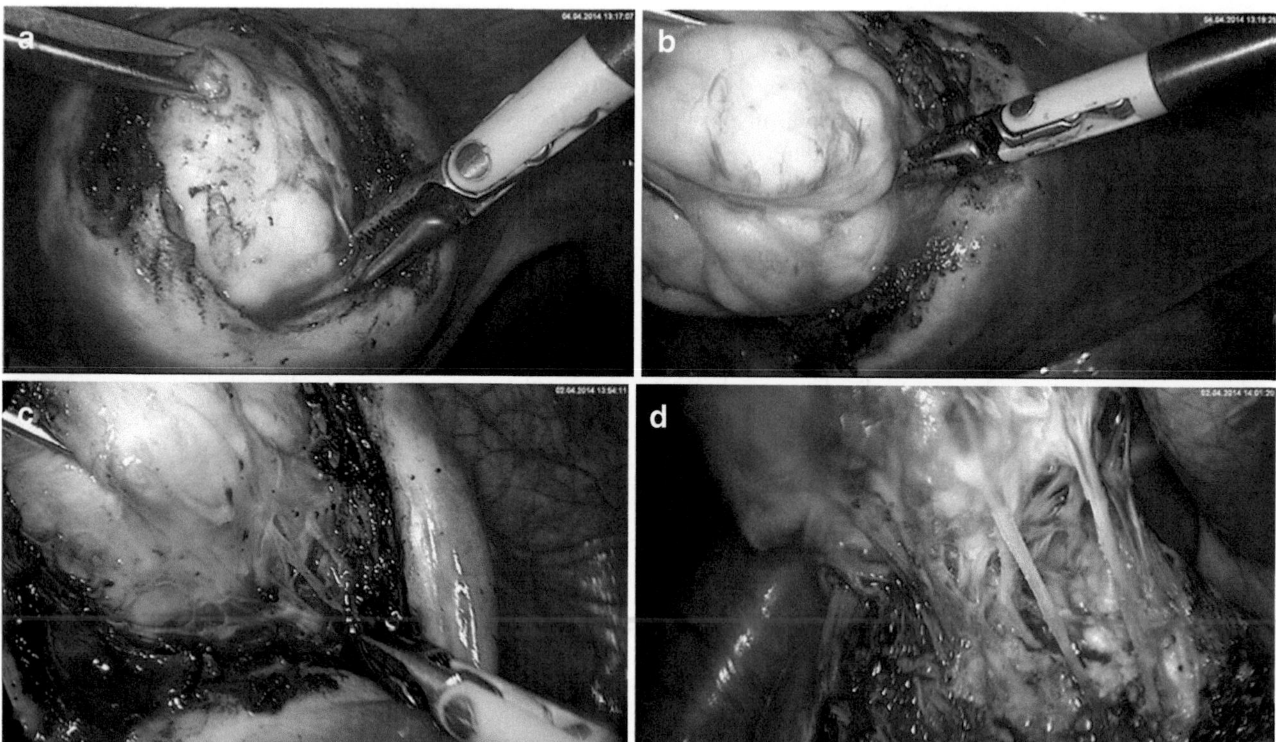

Fig. 30.2 Laparoscopic myoma enucleation. (**a**) Traction of the fibroid with a tenaculum and blunt delineation from the capsule. (**b**) Focal bipolar coagulation of basic vessels. (**c**) Continuous enucleation of the fibroid under traction and specific coagulation of capsule vessels containing fibers. (**d**) Magnification of remaining capsule fibers to be coagulated and cut

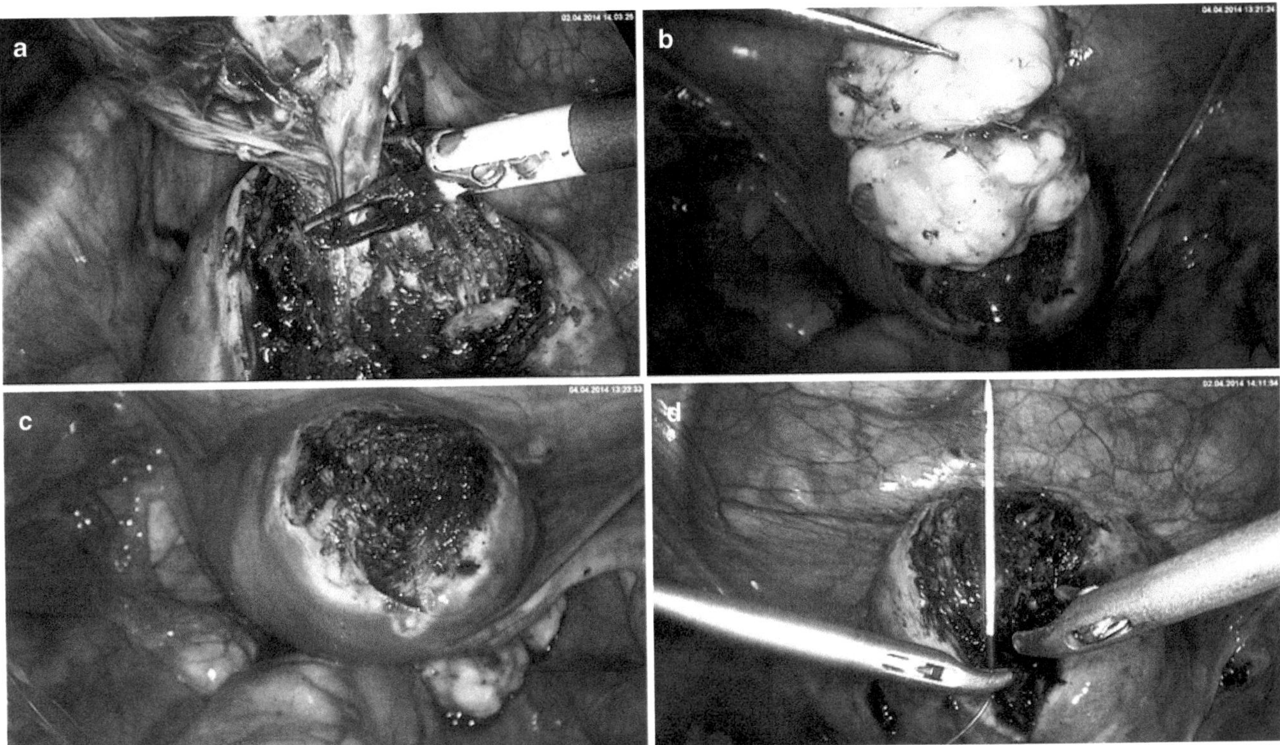

Fig. 30.3 Laparoscopic myoma enucleation. (**a**) Final coagulation of the capsule vessels. (**b**) Double belly fibroid after complete enucleation. (**c**) Minimal coagulation of bleeding vessels under suction and irrigation. (**d**) Approximation of wound edges with either straight or round, sharp needle and a monofilar late-absorbable suture

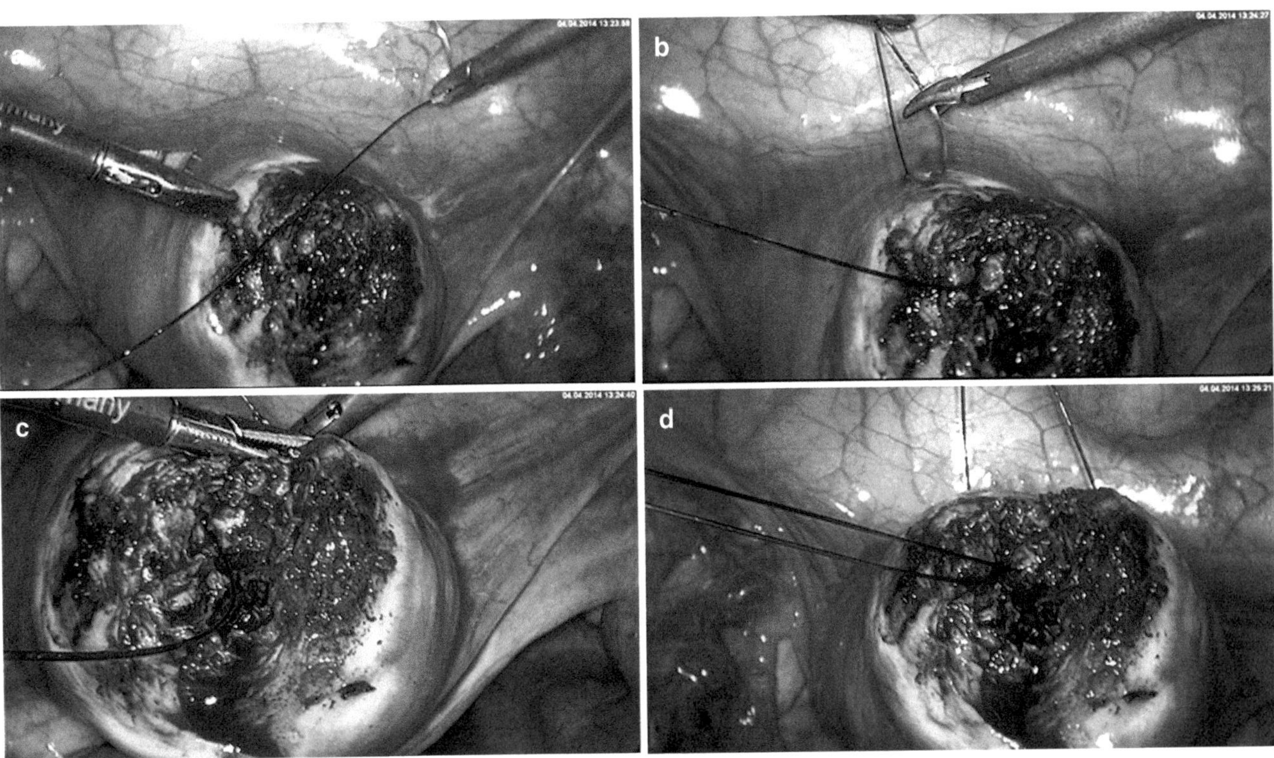

Fig. 30.4 Laparoscopic myoma enucleation. (**a**) Advantage of round needle stitch. The wound angle is elevated safely and completely by elevation with a Manhes forceps. Deeper layers of the myometrium can be grasped more easily using a round needle. (**b**) Needle exit and simplified regrasping with the right needle holder. (**c**) Final stitch to invert the knot. (**d**) Extirpation of the needle and completion of the extracorporeal knot and preparation to push down the extracorporeal knot

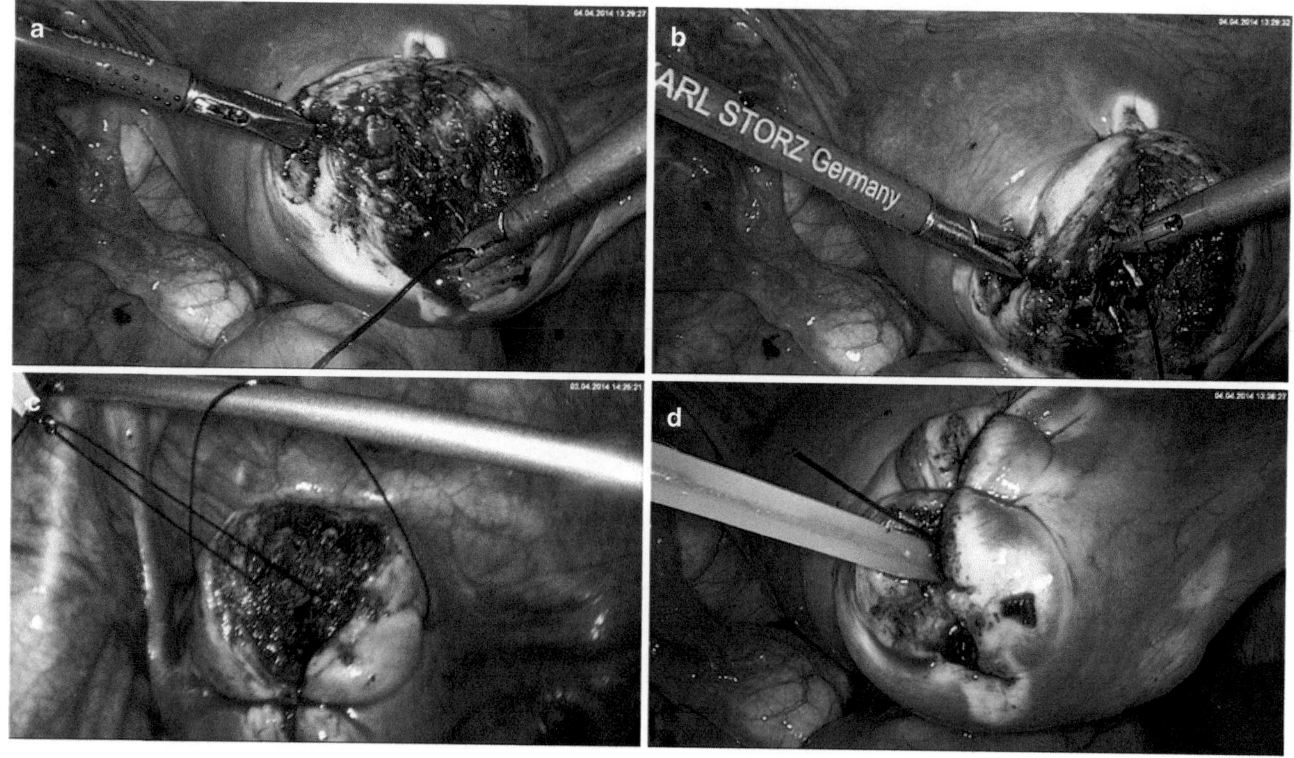

Fig. 30.5 Performance of the extracorporeal "von Leffern" knot. (**a**) Pulling out the suture, removing the needle, half hitch. (**b**) Holding the knot with the left hand and reaching over with the right hand. (**c**) Grasping the short end from below and leading it back, exiting before the half hitch. (**d**) Turning back the knot. Holding the straight suture and tightening the knot

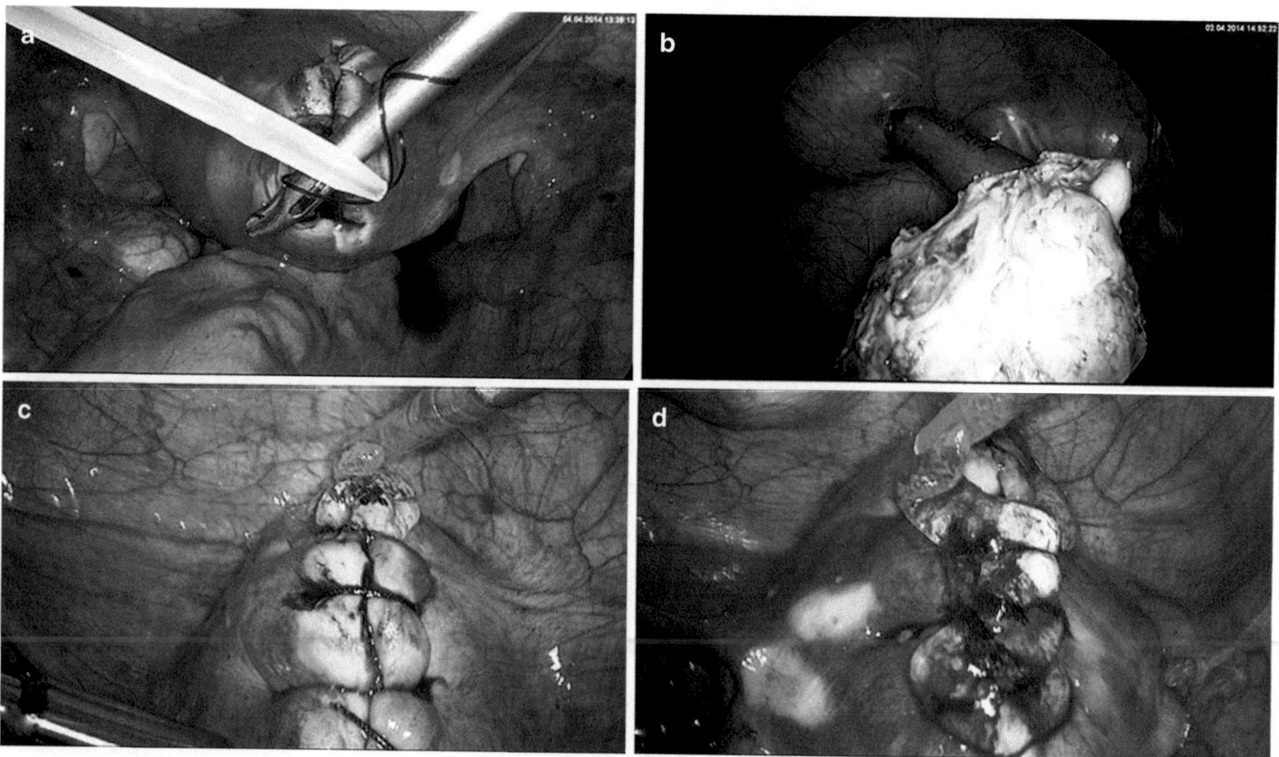

Fig. 30.6 Laparoscopic myoma enucleation. (**a**) Second single stitch starting as deep as possible in the uterine wound. (**b**) Exit of the needle on the left wound margin (just next to the Manhes forceps). (**c**) Completion of the stitch and preparation of the extracorporeal von Leffern knot. The needle holder elevates the thread to avoid tearing of the uterine wall while pulling through the monofilar thread (PDS). (**d**) The extracorporeal knot is pushed down with a plastic push-rod and deposited deep in the wound minimizing the external suture part

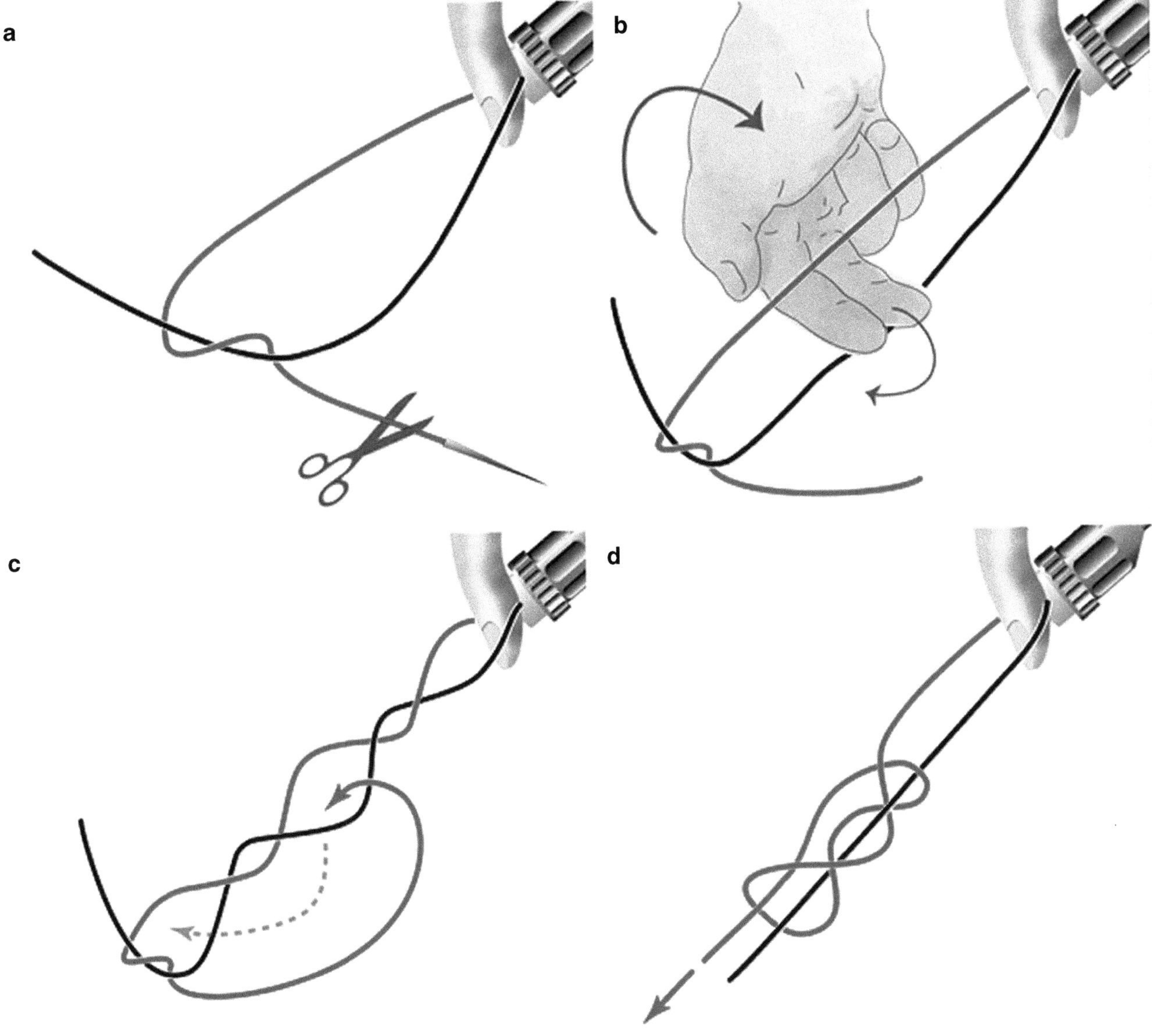

Fig. 30.7 Laparoscopic myoma enucleation. (**a**) Intracorporeal safety knot of the knot performed extracorporeally. (**b**) Morcellation of the fibroid with the Rotocut morcellator (Storz) in an apple-peeling manner. (**c**) Final situs showing the extracorporeal sutures to adapt the uterine wound edges. (**d**) Application of Hyalo Barrier (Nordic Pharma) for adhesion prevention

Alternatively, barbed sutures, such as V-lock, can be used to tighten the tissue or a third ancillary trocar can be inserted to hold the suture tight. The security of the uterine closure has bearing on the risk of uterine rupture in subsequent pregnancy. Different kinds of adhesion prevention barriers can be applied (Fig. 30.8) [51–53]. Women should wait at least 4–6 months before attempting to conceive [54].

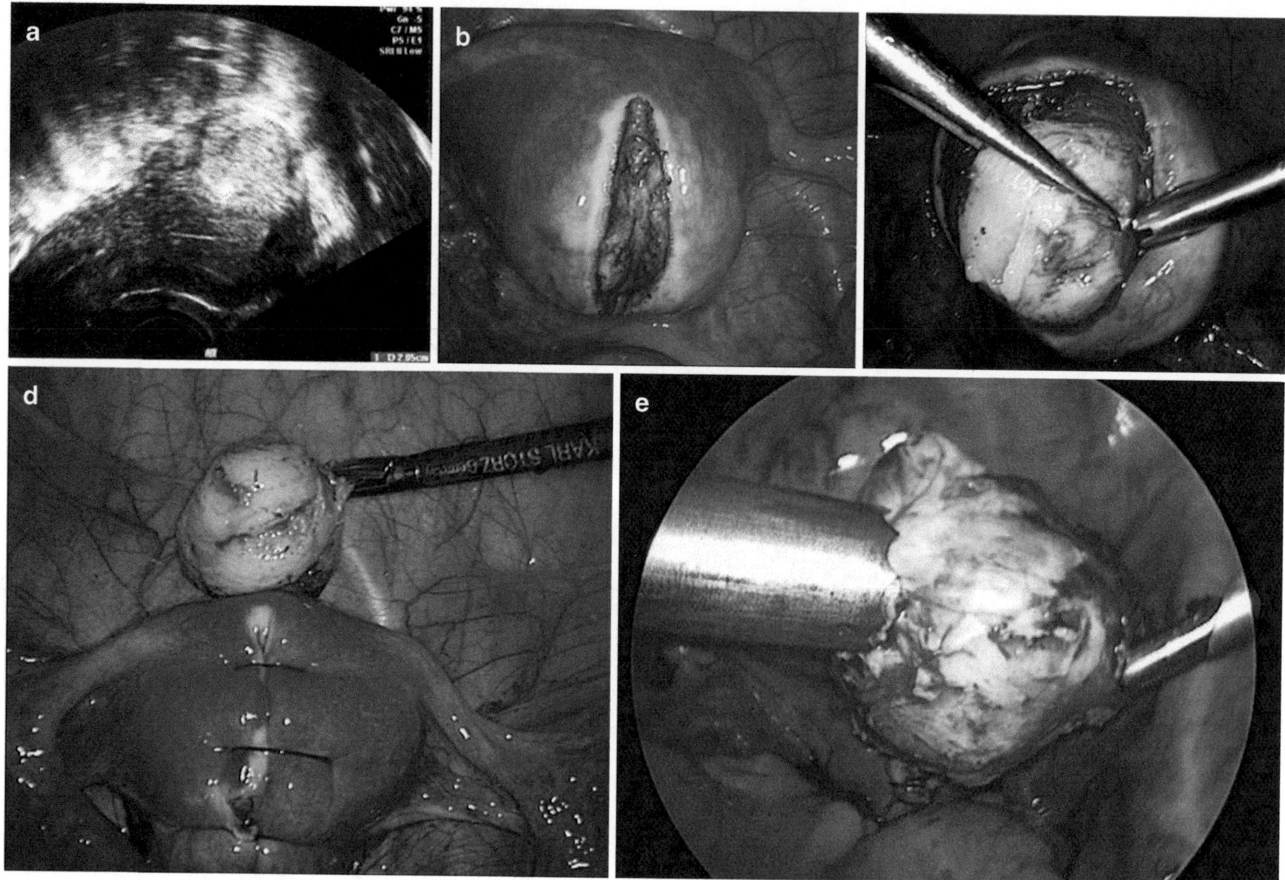

Fig. 30.8 (**a**) Transvaginal ultrasound shows a 3.5 cm intramural myoma in the back wall of the uterus. (**b**) Intraoperative uterotomy just above the myoma after injection of vasopressin. The uterotomy includes the myometrium and the myoma capsule and is done with a monopolar needle. All different tissue layers can be differentiated (**c**) Intraoperative sight of the myoma and its surrounding vascularized capsule. (**d**) Reconstruction of the uterine wall after excision of the tumor. (**e**) Removal of the myoma by morcellation

Abdominal Myomectomy

Abdominal or open myomectomy has its origin in the early 1900s as a uterus-preserving procedure. Today, it is mostly performed for women with intramural or subserosal myomas and less frequently for submucosal localization. Since the introduction of endoscopic procedures, the indication for abdominal myomectomy has become rare. It becomes an option if hysteroscopic or laparoscopic myomectomy is not feasible or if a laparotomy is required for any other reason. The indication to exclude uterine sarcomas has to be taken very strictly; however, uterine sarcoma is a very rare malignancy and the rate of sarcoma after clinical diagnosis of myoma is very low. The risk of severe complications in association with open surgery is higher than with hysteroscopic or laparoscopic moymectomy. Prophylactic antibiotics should be given for any abdominal fibroid operation [55, 56]. After the Pfannenstil incision either a vertical or transverse uterine incision is performed [57]. The myoma enucleation is performed by traction on the myometrial edges, e.g. with Allis clamps. After exposure of the fibroid it can be extirpated. The pseudocapsule is typically dissected bluntly. The uterine defects are closed with sutures in in several layers to reapproximate the tissue and achieve haemostasis without excessive bipolar coagulation.

Robotic Myomectomy

Robot-assisted laparoscopic myomectomy is a relatively new approach. The advantages of robotic surgery are three-dimensional imaging, mechanical improvement, including 7 ° of freedom for each instrument, stabilization of the instruments within the surgical field and improved ergonomics for the surgeon. Technical difficulties are decreased as suturing is easier than during conventional laparoscopy; however, there are few data comparing robot-assisted with conventional laparoscopic myomectomy [58–60]. The advantages compared to abdominal myomectomy are decreased blood loss and shorter recovery time. Nevertheless, operation duration and operating costs are much higher than for conventional procedures. Furthermore, robotic devices are large and bulky. Robotic surgery is limited by the lack of tactile feedback and additional team training is necessary to minimize the risk of mechanical failure [61]. To date, no advantage compared to conventional laparoscopy could be demonstrated regarding blood loss or operative duration. A more secure myometrial closure has not yet been proven [59]. In obese patients robot-assisted surgery might be beneficial [62].

Hysterectomy as Treatment for Myomas

As fibroids are also the most common indication for hysterectomy (30 % of hysterectomies in white and 50 % of hysterectomies in black women), specific focus is given to hysterectomies within this chapter. The decision for a hysterectomy in a multifibroid uterus depends on the wish of the patient, her health status, whether childbearing has been completed and on the combined decision with the doctor. Only if the patient suffers from metrorrhagia does the disorder need to be examined pre-operatively in more detail as this may be a sign of endometrial cancer or sarcoma. Nevertheless, the combined evaluation of MRI and tumor makers pre-operatively leads to a more specific diagnosis of rapidly growing uterine masses or adnexas in the case of a leiomyomatous uterus or adnexal tumors. Only in cases where malignancy is not suspected is a simple TLH or SLH recommended, otherwise an oncological approach has to be selected. Hysterectomy as TLH or SLH is recommended for the following indications:

- Acute hemorrhage with non-response to other therapies
- Completion of family planning and current or increased future risk of other diseases, such as cervical intraepithelial neoplasia, endometrial hyperplasia or an increased risk of uterine or ovarian cancer. Precondition for the indication for hysterectomy is that these risks can be eliminated or decreased by hysterectomy.
- Failure of previous treatment.
- Completion of family planning and significant symptoms (e.g. multiple fibroids or adenomyosis) and the desire for a definitive solution.

The main advantage of hysterectomy over all other therapeutical possibilities is the definitive solution in eliminating all existing symptoms and the risk of recurrence. Nevertheless, the advantage of a definitive solution that allows freedom from future problems can be an obstacle if family planning has not been completed or the patient has a personal inhibition against the removal of the central genital female organ [63]. These issues must be discussed in advance with the patient before the decision for a hysterectomy is taken. Furthermore, for a solitary submucous, subserous, pedunculated or intramural myoma, the complication rate of a hysterectomy has to be compared with the complication rate of a myomectomy. The operational risks have to be compared to the operational risks of hysteroscopy, laparoscopic fibroid enucleation or conservative management. With the advances in cervical cancer screening the prevention of future cervical or uterine pathologies is no longer a relevant indication for hysterectomy. The decision must be tailored to meet the needs of each individual patient.

Laparoscopic hysterectomy was first introduced in 1989 with the aim of reducing the morbidity and mortality of abdominal hysterectomy to the level reached with vaginal hysterectomy. Laparoscopic assistance for vaginal hysterectomy can be of advantage if there is a need for adhesiolysis, a need to treat endometriosis simultaneously, a need to treat large leiomyomas and to ensure an easier and safer adnexectomy. If feasible, vaginal hysterectomy allows a more rapid and less painful recovery than open or laparoscopic surgery and is much cheaper [64].

Should Ovaries and/or Fallopian Tubes Be Removed or Left in Place at Hysterectomy?

Ovaries

Generally, the ovaries are not removed when a hysterectomy is performed for uterine fibroids. Removing the uterus alone will cure the bleeding and the size-related symptoms caused by the fibroids. When treating fibroids it is not necessary to remove the ovaries or fallopian tubes as is sometimes the case when treating other diseases, such as endometriosis or gynecologic cancers.

Many physicians were taught that at a set age (which varies between 35 and 50) women should be told that removal of the ovaries is recommended as part of the surgery, with the speculation of "while we are there, we may as well." The general teaching has been that ovaries do not have any function after menopause and the risk of ovarian cancer increases with increasing age, so removing the ovaries near the time of menopause was a no-lose proposition. This was especially true if hormone replacement therapy could be used to help younger women transition to the time when they would naturally go through menopause.

However, more recent research suggests that although after menopause the ovaries produce little estradiol (the major estrogen in premenopausal women), they produce a tremendous amount of androgens (usually thought of as male hormones) [65]. It is thought that these androgens may be important in maintaining mood and sex drive [66–68]. In addition, the risks of hormone replacement have become clearer, and many women choose to use hormones following menopause [69, 70]. Most women are aware of the research from the Women's Health Initiative demonstrating significant complications with postmenopausal hormone replacement therapy. However, it is not widely known that the risks are lower for women without a uterus, who are able to take estrogen alone [70]. Recently the association of premature loss of ovarian function and the increasing risk of heart disease has also been investigated [71].

Considering all these factors, there are good reasons to retain the ovaries if possible. The major reason to remove them at the time of fibroid surgery is if the woman has a high risk of ovarian cancer.

Fallopian Tubes

According to new research presented at the Annual Clinical Meeting of The American College of Obstetricians and Gynecologists in 2013, bilateral salpingectomy at hysterectomy, with preservation of the ovaries, is considered a safe way of potentially reducing the development of ovarian serous carcinoma, the most common type of ovarian cancer. Increasing evidence points toward the fallopian tubes as the origin of this type of cancer. Removing the fallopian tubes does not cause the onset of menopause, as does the removal of the ovaries.

Prophylactic removal of the fallopian tubes during hysterectomy or sterilization would rule out any subsequent tubal pathology, such as hydrosalpinx, which is observed in up to 30 % of women after hysterectomy. Moreover, this intervention is likely to offer considerable protection against later tumor development, even if the ovaries are retained. Thus, we recommend that any hysterectomy should be combined with salpingectomy. Women undergoing hysterectomy with retained fallopian tubes or sterilization have at least a doubled risk of subsequent salpingectomy. Removal of the fallopian tubes at hysterectomy should therefore be recommended [72, 73].

For this reason, once the reproductive function is completed the tubes of a female of reproductive age should be removed while the ovaries should remain to support the female wellbeing. Beyond the reproductive age, tubes should always be removed with the uterus while ovaries, as previously discussed, are routinely removed only above the age of 65 years.

Abdominal Hysterectomy

As the indication for abdominal hysterectomy in benign diseases has become very rare, it is not discussed in this article [74].

Vaginal Hysterectomy

Before beginning a vaginal hysterectomy, a bimanual pelvic examination is performed to assess uterine mobility and descent and to exclude unsuspected pathology of the adnexa. Only then can a final decision be made whether to proceed with a vaginal or abdominal approach. The operation starts with entry into the cul-de-sac or the vesico vaginal fold. Here we describe the posterior peritoneal opening. The uterosacral ligaments are identified and clamped, including the lower portion of the cardinal ligaments. In the next step the vesicovaginal space is opened and after identification of the peritoneal fold it is cut and the cardinal ligaments are ligated, including the uterine vessels. Most adnexa can be removed by grasping the ovary and clamping the infundibulopelvic ligament. The uterus can then be enucleated stepwise from the remaining peritoneal fold at a safe distance from the bladder. The peritoneum can either be closed or left open and the vaginal epithelium is reapproximated in either a vertical or a horizontal manner. A myomatous uterus has to be morcellated in a circular manner. Sometimes it is necessary to enucleate large solitary myomas or perform intramyometrial coring, especially in cases of diffusely enlarged uteri [75, 76].

Subtotal Laparoscopic Hysterectomy (SLH)

The supracervical (subtotal) hysterectomy was first described by Semm in 1990 and in another technique by Lyons. The operative technique is similar to the total laparoscopic hysterectomy. Only after occluding the ascending branch of the uterine artery is the uterine corpus resected as a reverse conus down to the endocervical canal [77]. For SLH and TLH the trocar placements are the same as for laparoscopic myomectomy and depend on the size of the uterus (see above). There is no need to perform ureterolysis at the beginning of the operation as the ureter is at a safe distance if the suturing line is kept strictly at the uterine wall. The infundibulopelvic ligament and the round ligament are divided from the pelvic side wall and, if the adnexa are to remain in situ, division of the adnexa from the uterus is performed. The broad ligament is then opened, dissected and each leaf separately coagulated. The bladder is separated from the uterus by opening the vesicouterine ligament and pushing the bladder downwards for about 1–2 cm. This is followed by presentation of the ramus ascendens of the uterine artery and division of the uterine pedicles with the same stepwise dissection of the left adnexa. A thorough inspection of the cervix then takes place. The cervix is separated from the uterus with the help of the electric cutting loop or any other cutting instrument. This is followed by coagulation of the cervical canal and closure of the peritoneum over the remaining cervical stump for infection and adhesion prevention. However, the peritoneum can also be left open, according to surgeon preference. Afterwards, morcellation of the uterine body is performed and, if the adnexa are also resected, they should be put into an endo bag for extraction.

As morcellation techniques are described in detail in other chapters of the book, the importance of this technique is not dealt with here.

Total Laparoscopic Hysterectomy (TLH)

LSH should be avoided if adenomyosis uteri is suspected because part of the endometrial glands remain in the cervical and paracervical channel. These can cause an early recurrence or persistence of the symptoms although the few existing data offer no direct confirmation of this view [78, 79].

The surgical steps are identical to the LSH, the only difference being that a uterine manipulator is placed in the vagina before the operation. After separation of the bladder from the uterus, the bladder is pushed and dissected down 2–3 cm to clearly visualize the rim of the cervical cup. In cases of post-caesarean section, a gentle, blunt and intermediate sharp dissection has to be carried out. After the uterus has been lateralized by pushing up the manipulator, the uterine artery and vein with collateral vessels are completely coagulated near the cervix and dissected. The vagina is resected from the cervix with the monopolar hook by firmly stretching the manipulator cranially and carefully performing an intrafascial dissection leaving the sacrouterine ligaments almost completely in place. This is in accordance with the CISH technique introduced by Kurt Semm [80]. The uterus is then retracted through the vagina while still fixed to the manipulator. If the uterus is too large, it has to be morcellated either intraabdominally or transvaginally. The vagina is closed with 2 corner sutures and 1 or 2 sutures in between the corner sutures. The sacrouterine ligaments and the middle portion of the vagina are stitched and elevated by the corner sutures to prevent vaginal prolapse or enterocele formation at a later time. Peritonealization and drainage are not required.

With the improvement of endoscopic surgery and above all the improvement in endoscopic suturing laparoscopic-assisted vaginal hysterectomy has become obsolete, especially as this technique does not include a suspension of the cardinal and sacrouterine ligaments.

Conclusions

Treatment options for uterine leiomyomas vary. The choice of treatment should be made on an individual basis taking into account the following factors: the patient's level of suffering due to bleeding disorders or displacement-caused pain, the status of family planning and the patient's preferences regarding the different treatment options.

In *asymptomatic women* expectant management is suggested except for hydronephrosis caused by displacement or hysteroscopically resectable submucous fibroids in women who pursue pregnancy.

In *postmenopausal women* without hormonal therapy fibroids usually shrink and become asymptomatic. Therefore, expectant management is the method of choice. However, sarcoma should be excluded if a new or an enlarging pelvic mass occurs in a postmenopausal woman. Surgical treatment is the option of choice if the leiomyomas are symptomatic. If there are contraindications to operative procedures or hysterectomy is declined by the patient for personal reasons, any of the alternative treatment options can be considered (medical, embolization or guided ultrasound).

In *premenopausal women* appropriate submucosal leiomyomas should be resected hysteroscopically if the women wish to preserve their childbearing potential and/or they are symptomatic (e.g. bleeding, miscarriage). Intramural and subserosal leiomyomas in women who wish to preserve their fertility can be removed laparoscopically. Nevertheless, an appropriate surgical technique and advanced laparoscopic skills are necessary. If this cannot be guaranteed, abdominal myomectomy has to be recommended or referral to a laparoscopic center to maximize the possibility and safety of pregnancy after uterine reconstruction. The risk of uterine rupture in pregnancy following myomectomy needs to be discussed with the patient.

Robotic assistance makes laparoscopic suturing easier and offers surgery with 3 dimensional vision; however, costs are still high. Further developments in robotic assistance, including force feedback, will catch more of our attention in the future.

For *women who have completed their family planning,* hysterectomy is the definitive procedure for relief of symptoms and prevention of recurrence of fibroid-related problems. With increasing experience in laparoscopic hysterectomies, the risk of side effects has become manageable. In relation to the compliance and individuality of the patient, a suitable solution can be either laparoscopic supracervical or total laparoscopic hysterectomy.

Acknowledgement The authors thank Nicole Guckelsberger and Dawn Rüther for editing the manuscript.

References

1. Watson JD, Crick FH. Molecular structure of nucleic acids; a structure for deoxyribose nucleic acid. Nature. 1953;171(4356):737–8.
2. Watson JD, Crick FH. Genetical implications of the structure of deoxyribonucleic acid. Nature. 1953;171(4361):964–7.
3. Spektrum der Wissenschaft.

4. Treloar SA et al. Pathways to hysterectomy: insights from longitudinal twin research. Am J Obstet Gynecol. 1992;167(1):82–8.
5. Snieder H, MacGregor AJ, Spector TD. Genes control the cessation of a woman's reproductive life: a twin study of hysterectomy and age at menopause. J Clin Endocrinol Metab. 1998;83(6):1875–80.
6. Vikhlyaeva EM, Khodzhaeva ZS, Fantschenko ND. Familial predisposition to uterine leiomyomas. Int J Gynaecol Obstet. 1995;51(2):127–31.
7. Van Voorhis BJ, Romitti PA, Jones MP. Family history as a risk factor for development of uterine leiomyomas. Results of a pilot study. J Reprod Med. 2002;47(8):663–9.
8. Al-Hendy A, Salama SA. Catechol-O-methyltransferase polymorphism is associated with increased uterine leiomyoma risk in different ethnic groups. J Soc Gynecol Investig. 2006;13(2):136–44.
9. Tsibris JC et al. Insights from gene arrays on the development and growth regulation of uterine leiomyomata. Fertil Steril. 2002;78(1):114–21.
10. Wang H et al. Distinctive proliferative phase differences in gene expression in human myometrium and leiomyomata. Fertil Steril. 2003;80(2):266–76.
11. Gross K, Morton C, Stewart E. Finding genes for uterine fibroids. Obstet Gynecol. 2000;95(4 Suppl 1):60.
12. Patterson-Keels LM et al. Morphologic assessment of endometrium overlying submucosal leiomyomas. J Reprod Med. 1994;39(8):579–84.
13. Flynn M et al. Health care resource use for uterine fibroid tumors in the United States. Am J Obstet Gynecol. 2006;195(4):955–64.
14. Hartmann KE et al. Annual costs associated with diagnosis of uterine leiomyomata. Obstet Gynecol. 2006;108(4):930–7.
15. Peddada SD et al. Growth of uterine leiomyomata among premenopausal black and white women. Proc Natl Acad Sci U S A. 2008;105(50):19887–92.
16. Laughlin SK, Hartmann KE, Baird DD. Postpartum factors and natural fibroid regression. Am J Obstet Gynecol. 2011;204(6):496 e1–6.
17. Zaima A, Ash A. Fibroid in pregnancy: characteristics, complications, and management. Postgrad Med J. 2011;87(1034):819–28.
18. Marjoribanks J, Lethaby A, Farquhar C. Surgery versus medical therapy for heavy menstrual bleeding. Cochrane Database Syst Rev. 2006;2:CD003855.
19. Al-Hendy A et al. Gene therapy of uterine leiomyomas: adenovirus-mediated expression of dominant negative estrogen receptor inhibits tumor growth in nude mice. Am J Obstet Gynecol. 2004;191(5):1621–31.
20. Donnez J et al. Ulipristal acetate versus placebo for fibroid treatment before surgery. N Engl J Med. 2012;366(5):409–20.
21. Donnez J et al. Long-term treatment of uterine fibroids with ulipristal acetate. Fertil Steril. 2014;101(6):1565–73. e1–18.
22. Donnez J et al. Efficacy and safety of repeated use of ulipristal acetate in uterine fibroids. Fertil Steril. 2015;103(2):519–27. e3.
23. Edwards RD et al. Uterine-artery embolization versus surgery for symptomatic uterine fibroids. N Engl J Med. 2007;356(4):360–70.
24. van der Kooij SM et al. Uterine artery embolization versus surgery in the treatment of symptomatic fibroids: a systematic review and metaanalysis. Am J Obstet Gynecol. 2011;205(4):317 e1–18.
25. Kim HS et al. MR-guided high-intensity focused ultrasound treatment for symptomatic uterine leiomyomata: long-term outcomes. Acad Radiol. 2011;18(8):970–6.
26. Funaki K, Fukunishi H, Sawada K. Clinical outcomes of magnetic resonance-guided focused ultrasound surgery for uterine myomas: 24-month follow-up. Ultrasound Obstet Gynecol. 2009;34(5):584–9.
27. RCoOa G. Preventing entry-related gynaecological laparoscopic injuries. RCOG Green-top Guideline. 2008;49:1–10.
28. Wallach EE, Vlahos NF. Uterine myomas: an overview of development, clinical features, and management. Obstet Gynecol. 2004;104(2):393–406.
29. Kim MS et al. Obstetric outcomes after uterine myomectomy: laparoscopic versus laparotomic approach. Obstet Gynecol Sci. 2013;56(6):375–81.
30. Lonnerfors C, Persson J. Pregnancy following robot-assisted laparoscopic myomectomy in women with deep intramural myomas. Acta Obstet Gynecol Scand. 2011;90(9):972–7.
31. Mettler L et al. Complications of uterine fibroids and their management, surgical management of fibroids, laparoscopy and hysteroscopy versus hysterectomy, haemorrhage, adhesions, and complications. Obstet Gynecol Int. 2012;2012:791248.
32. Di Spiezio Sardo A et al. Hysteroscopic myomectomy: a comprehensive review of surgical techniques. Hum Reprod Update. 2008;14(2):101–19.
33. Emanuel MH et al. An analysis of fluid loss during transcervical resection of submucous myomas. Fertil Steril. 1997;68(5):881–6.
34. Wamsteker K, Emanuel MH, de Kruif JH. Transcervical hysteroscopic resection of submucous fibroids for abnormal uterine bleeding: results regarding the degree of intramural extension. Obstet Gynecol. 1993;82(5):736–40.
35. Hart R, Molnar BG, Magos A. Long term follow up of hysteroscopic myomectomy assessed by survival analysis. Br J Obstet Gynaecol. 1999;106(7):700–5.
36. Mettler L et al. Imaging in gynecologic surgery. Womens Health (Lond Engl). 2011;7(2):239–48. quiz 249–50.
37. Varma R et al. Hysteroscopic myomectomy for menorrhagia using Versascope bipolar system: efficacy and prognostic factors at a minimum of one year follow up. Eur J Obstet Gynecol Reprod Biol. 2009;142(2):154–9.
38. Loffer FD et al. Hysteroscopic fluid monitoring guidelines. The ad hoc committee on hysteroscopic training guidelines of the American Association of Gynecologic Laparoscopists. J Am Assoc Gynecol Laparosc. 2000;7(1):167–8.
39. Jansen FW et al. Complications of hysteroscopy: a prospective, multicenter study. Obstet Gynecol. 2000;96(2):266–70.
40. Propst AM et al. Complications of hysteroscopic surgery: predicting patients at risk. Obstet Gynecol. 2000;96(4):517–20.
41. Parker WH, Rodi IA. Patient selection for laparoscopic myomectomy. J Am Assoc Gynecol Laparosc. 1994;2(1):23–6.
42. Lefebvre G et al. The management of uterine leiomyomas. J Obstet Gynaecol Can. 2003;25(5):396–418. quiz 419–22.
43. Alkatout I et al. Precarious preoperative diagnostics and hints for the laparoscopic excision of uterine adenomatoid tumors: two exemplary cases and literature review. Fertil Steril. 2011;95(3):1119 e5–8.
44. Dueholm M et al. Accuracy of magnetic resonance imaging and transvaginal ultrasonography in the diagnosis, mapping, and measurement of uterine myomas. Am J Obstet Gynecol. 2002;186(3):409–15.
45. Alkatout I et al. Principles and safety measures of electrosurgery in laparoscopy. JSLS. 2012;16(1):130–9.
46. Alkatout I et al. Organ-preserving management of ovarian pregnancies by laparoscopic approach. Fertil Steril. 2011;95(8):2467–70. e1–2.
47. Kongnyuy EJ, Wiysonge CS. Interventions to reduce haemorrhage during myomectomy for fibroids. Cochrane Database Syst Rev. 2011;11:CD005355.
48. Zhao F et al. Evaluation of loop ligation of larger myoma pseudocapsule combined with vasopressin on laparoscopic myomectomy. Fertil Steril. 2010;95(2):762–6.
49. Tinelli A et al. Impact of surgical approach on blood loss during intracapsular myomectomy. Minim Invasive Ther Allied Technol. 2013;23(2):87–95.
50. Celik H, Sapmaz E. Use of a single preoperative dose of misoprostol is efficacious for patients who undergo abdominal myomectomy. Fertil Steril. 2003;79(5):1207–10.
51. Mettler L et al. Cross-linked sodium hyaluronate, an anti-adhesion barrier gel in gynaecological endoscopic surgery. Minim Invasive Ther Allied Technol. 2013;22(5):260–5.

52. Mettler L, Schollmeyer T, Alkatout I. Adhesions during and after surgical procedures, their prevention and impact on women's health. Womens Health (Lond Engl). 2012;8(5):495–8.
53. Tulandi T, Murray C, Guralnick M. Adhesion formation and reproductive outcome after myomectomy and second-look laparoscopy. Obstet Gynecol. 1993;82(2):213–5.
54. Tsuji S et al. MRI evaluation of the uterine structure after myomectomy. Gynecol Obstet Invest. 2006;61(2):106–10.
55. D'Angelo E, Prat J. Uterine sarcomas: a review. Gynecol Oncol. 2009;116(1):131–9.
56. Mukhopadhaya N, De Silva C, Manyonda IT. Conventional myomectomy. Best Pract Res Clin Obstet Gynaecol. 2008;22(4): 677–705.
57. Discepola F et al. Analysis of arterial blood vessels surrounding the myoma: relevance to myomectomy. Obstet Gynecol. 2007;110(6): 1301–3.
58. Pundir J et al. Robotic-assisted laparoscopic vs abdominal and laparoscopic myomectomy: systematic review and meta-analysis. J Minim Invasive Gynecol. 2013;20(3):335–45.
59. Barakat EE et al. Robotic-assisted, laparoscopic, and abdominal myomectomy: a comparison of surgical outcomes. Obstet Gynecol. 2011;117(2 Pt 1):256–65.
60. Mettler L et al. The past, present and future of minimally invasive endoscopy in gynecology: a review and speculative outlook. Minim Invasive Ther Allied Technol. 2013;22(4):210–26.
61. Schollmeyer T et al. Roboterchirurgie in der Gynäkologie. Gynakologe. 2011;44(3):196–201.
62. George A, Eisenstein D, Wegienka G. Analysis of the impact of body mass index on the surgical outcomes after robot-assisted laparoscopic myomectomy. J Minim Invasive Gynecol. 2009;16(6):730–3.
63. Falcone T, Parker WH. Surgical management of leiomyomas for fertility or uterine preservation. Obstet Gynecol. 2013;121(4): 856–68.
64. Garry R et al. EVALUATE hysterectomy trial: a multicentre randomised trial comparing abdominal, vaginal and laparoscopic methods of hysterectomy. Health Technol Assess. 2004;8(26): 1–154.
65. Adashi EY. The climacteric ovary as a functional gonadotropin-driven androgen-producing gland. Fertil Steril. 1994;62(1):20–7.
66. Shifren JL. The role of androgens in female sexual dysfunction. Mayo Clin Proc. 2004;79(4 Suppl):S19–24.
67. Buster JE et al. Testosterone patch for low sexual desire in surgically menopausal women: a randomized trial. Obstet Gynecol. 2005;105(5 Pt 1):944–52.
68. Nyunt A et al. Androgen status in healthy premenopausal women with loss of libido. J Sex Marital Ther. 2005;31(1):73–80.
69. Manson JE et al. Estrogen plus progestin and the risk of coronary heart disease. N Engl J Med. 2003;349(6):523–34.
70. Anderson GL et al. Effects of conjugated equine estrogen in postmenopausal women with hysterectomy: the Women's Health Initiative randomized controlled trial. JAMA. 2004;291(14): 1701–12.
71. Parker WH et al. Ovarian conservation at the time of hysterectomy for benign disease. Obstet Gynecol. 2005;106(2):219–26.
72. Dietl J, Wischhusen J, Hausler SF. The post-reproductive Fallopian tube: better removed? Hum Reprod. 2011;26(11):2918–24.
73. Guldberg R et al. Salpingectomy as standard at hysterectomy? A Danish cohort study, 1977–2010. BMJ Open. 2013;3(6):e002845.
74. AAMIG W. AAGL position statement: Robotic-assisted laparoscopic surgery in benign gynecology. J Minim Invasive Gynecol. 2013;20(1):2–9.
75. Meeks GR, Harris RL. Surgical approach to hysterectomy: abdominal, laparoscopy-assisted, or vaginal. Clin Obstet Gynecol. 1997; 40(4):886–94.
76. Mazdisnian F et al. Vaginal hysterectomy by uterine morcellation: an efficient, non-morbid procedure. Obstet Gynecol. 1995;86(1): 60–4.
77. Jenkins TR. Laparoscopic supracervical hysterectomy. Am J Obstet Gynecol. 2004;191(6):1875–84.
78. Berner E et al. Pelvic pain and patient satisfaction after laparoscopic supracervical hysterectomy: prospective trial. J Minim Invasive Gynecol. 2013;21(3):406–11.
79. Alkatout I et al. Combined surgical and hormone therapy for endometriosis is the most effective treatment: prospective, randomized, controlled trial. J Minim Invasive Gynecol. 2013;20(4):473–81.
80. Semm K. Hysterectomy via laparotomy or pelviscopy. A new CASH method without colpotomy. Geburtshilfe Frauenheilkd. 1991;51(12):996–1003.

Uterine-Preserving Operative Therapy of Uterus Myomatosus

31

Andrea Tinelli, Ospan A. Mynbaev, Daniele Vergara, Silvia Di Tommaso, Sandro Gerli, Alessandro Favilli, Ivan Mazzon, Radmila Sparic, Marina Eliseeva, Sergei S. Simakov, Alexander A. Danilov, and Antonio Malvasi

Introduction

Uterine fibroids (also known as leiomyomas or myomas) (Fig. 31.1) are the most common benign tumors of the genital organs in women of childbearing age. They could have negative impact on reproductive system and can be single, but are more often multiple, causing significant morbidity, and impairment of the quality of life [1, 2]. According to the literature, 40–60 % of all hysterectomies are performed for the presence of myomas. Myomas are the most common indication for hysterectomy in the USA and Australia [3, 4]. The first who described myomas was Matthew Baille in 1793 [5]. Myomas consist mainly of smooth muscle cells containing different amounts of fibrous tissue [5].

During its growth, myoma determines compression on the surrounding structures (myometrium and endometrium),

A. Tinelli, MD, Prof, PhD (✉)
Department of Gynecology and Obstetrics, Division of Experimental Endoscopic Surgery, Imaging, Minimally Invasive Therapy and Technology, Vito Fazzi Hospital, Lecce, Italy

Laboratory of Human Physiology, Moscow Institute of Physics and Technology (State university), Dolgoprudny, Moscow region, Russia
e-mail: andreatinelli@gmail.com

O.A. Mynbaev, MD, Prof, PhD
The Department of Obstetrics, Gynecology and Reproductive Medicine, Peoples' Friendship University of Russia, Moscow, Russia
e-mail: ospanmynbaev@hotmail.com

D. Vergara, PhD
Department of Biological and Environmental Sciences and Technologies, University of Salento, Via Monteroni, Lecce, Italy

S. Di Tommaso, PhD
Division of Medical Genetics, Department of Biomedical Sciences and Human Oncology, Università "AldoMoro", Bari, Italy
e-mail: slv.ditommaso@gmail.com

S. Gerli, MD, Prof, PhD • A. Favilli, MD, PhD
Department of Obstetrics and Gynecology, University of Perugia, Perugia, Italy
e-mail: sandro.gerli@unipg.it; alessandrofavilli.mail@gmail.com

I. Mazzon, MD
Unit of Gynecology and Obstetrics, "Arbor Vitae" Centre, Clinica Nuova Villa Claudia, Rome, Italy
e-mail: i.mazzon@arborvitae.it

R. Sparic, MD
Clinic of Gynecology and Obstetrics, Clinical Center of Serbia, Belgrade, Serbia

School of Medicine, University of Belgrade, Belgrade, Serbia
e-mail: radmila@rcub.bg.ac.rs

M. Eliseeva, MD, Prof
Department of Obstetrics and Gynecology, Peoples' Friendship University of Russia, Moscow, Russia
e-mail: marinaeliseeva@hotmail.com

S.S. Simakov, Eng, PhD, Prof
Department of Applied Mathematics, International Translational Medicine and Biomodelling Research Group, Moscow Institute of Physics and Technology (MIPT), Moscow, Russia
e-mail: simakovss@ya.ru

A.A. Danilov, Eng, PhD
Institute of Numerical Mathematics, Russian Academy of Sciences, Moscow, Russia

Moscow Institute of Physics and Technology (MIPT), Moscow, Russia
e-mail: a.a.danilov@gmail.com

A. Malvasi, MD, Prof
Department of Gynecology and Obstetrics, Santa Maria Hospital, GVM Care and Research, Bari, Italy
e-mail: antoniomalvasi@gmail.com

I. Alkatout, L. Mettler (eds.), *Hysterectomy*, DOI 10.1007/978-3-319-22497-8_31

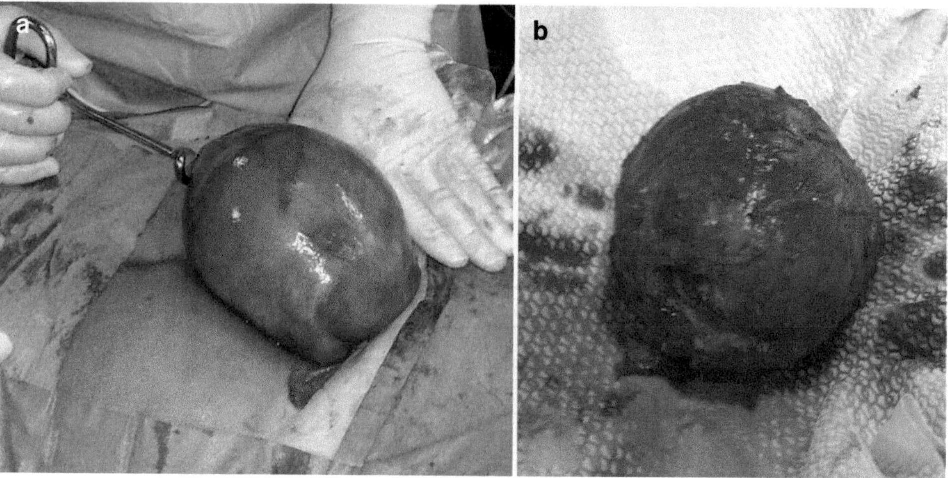

Fig. 31.1 To the left, a uterus removed from the abdomen by suprapubic transverse laparotomy; the uterus is deformed by large intramural myoma of the fundal-body of about 12 cm of diameter (*H*). On the right shows the enucleated myoma myomectomy by laparotomy (**b**)

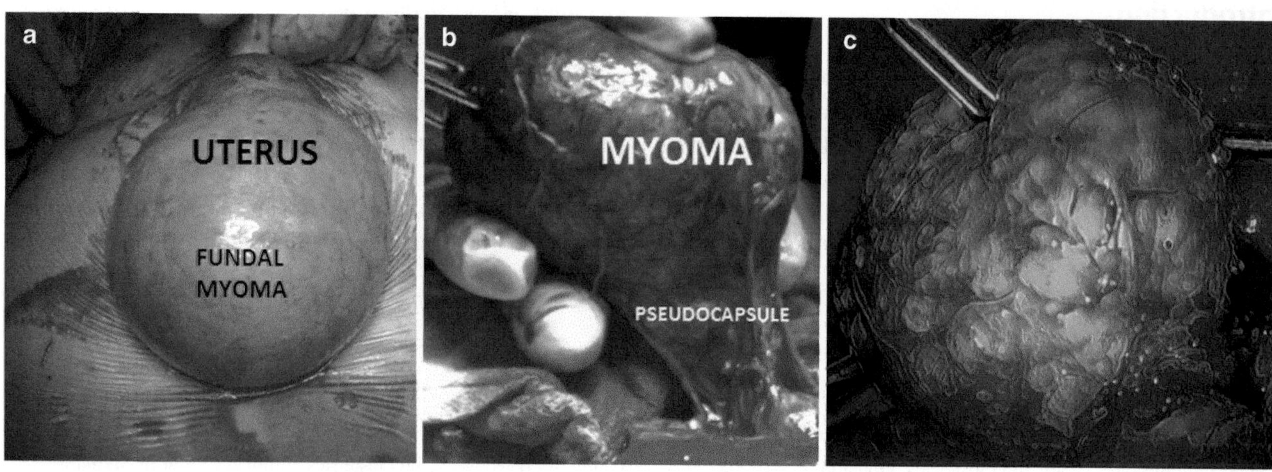

Fig. 31.2 On the left, the picture shows a uterus removed by laparotomy, deformed by a fundal fibroid 7 cm in diameter (**a**); at the center, the image shows a laparotomic myomectomy, with fibroid extraction and highlighting myoma pseudocapsule (**b**); to the right, a myoma with overhanging trace of the myoma pseudocapsule on the fibroid surface (**c**)

causing the progressive formation of a sort of pseudocapsule, rich of collagen fibers, neurofibers and blood vessels (Fig. 31.2).

Occasionally, the pseudocapsule surface is interrupted by bridges of collagen fibers and vessels that anchor the myoma to the myometrium. This causes the formation of a clear cleavage plane between myoma and pseudocapsule, and between pseudocapsule and the surrounding myometrium. This pseudocapsule causes a displacement and not destructive action on the myometrium, maintaining the integrity and contractility of uterine structure [6, 7].

Literature data has show that between 5.4 and 77 % of women have myomas; this wide range depends on the study population or on the diagnostic techniques applied to myoma detection [8].

Ultrasound studies documented that myoma prevalence is lower in Europe than in the United States, probably because of racial differences [9, 10]. In 65–70 % of cases, fibroids are multiple and can be found in various uterine locations. Most frequently they are within the wall of the uterus (Fig. 31.3) where they can expand in the myometrium (intramural leiomyoma), beneath the endometrium, simulating a polyp (submucosal leiomyoma), beneath the serosal surface (subserosal leiomyoma), within the broad ligament, simulating an adnexal neoplasia (intraligamentous leiomyoma) or under the uterine isthmus, called cervical leiomyoma (Fig. 31.4) [8].

The compression of the endometrium causes atrophy and erosion with bleeding. Subserosal leiomyomata (Fig. 31.5) can be pedunculated (Fig. 31.5) and in some cases can separate from the uterus and create a new vascular peduncle with another nearby organ (parasitic leiomyoma) [6–8].

They are well circumscribed, firm, and grey-white and with a whorled cut surface (Fig. 31.6). They may degenerate, especially in pregnancy, and become soft with a yellowish hue in necrosis or a reddish color due to hemorrhaging [8].

Myomas have been in 70 % of cases after hysterectomy, and multiple myomas have been present in more than 80 % of cases [11].

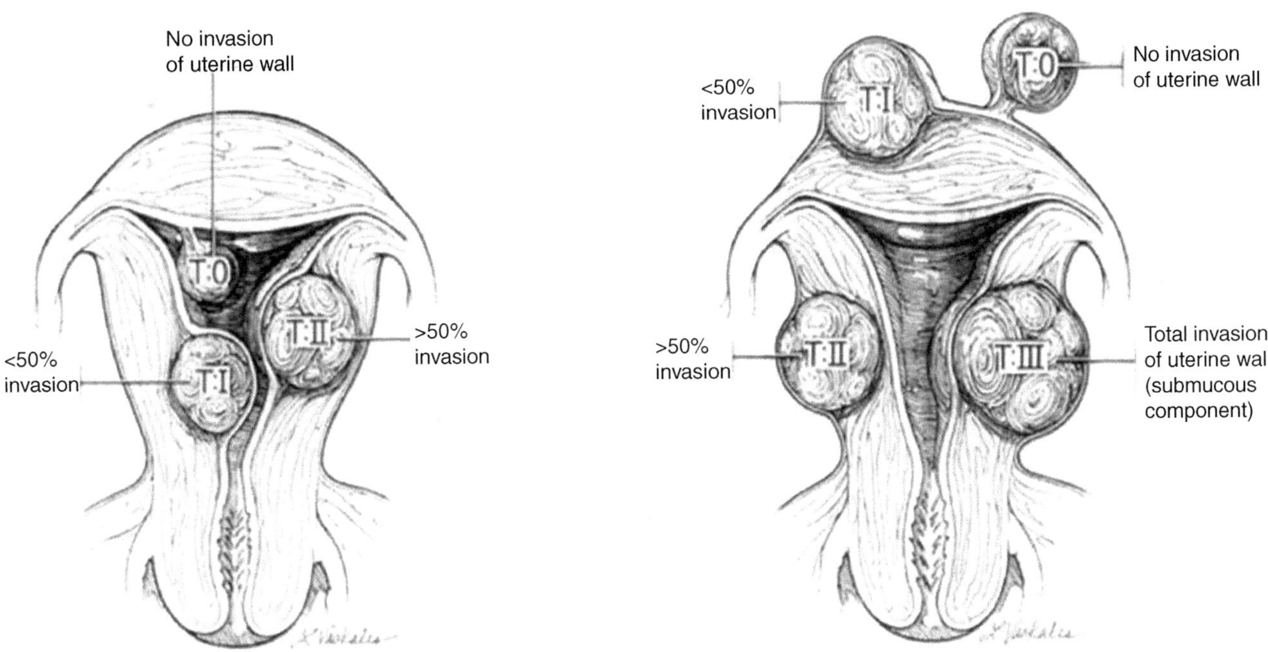

Fig. 31.3 Schematic representation of various invasions of the uterine wall by submucous myomas, on the left. Myomas impinging and penetrating the uterine wall from the periphery of the uterus, on the right (Image taken from: Butram and Reiter [163])

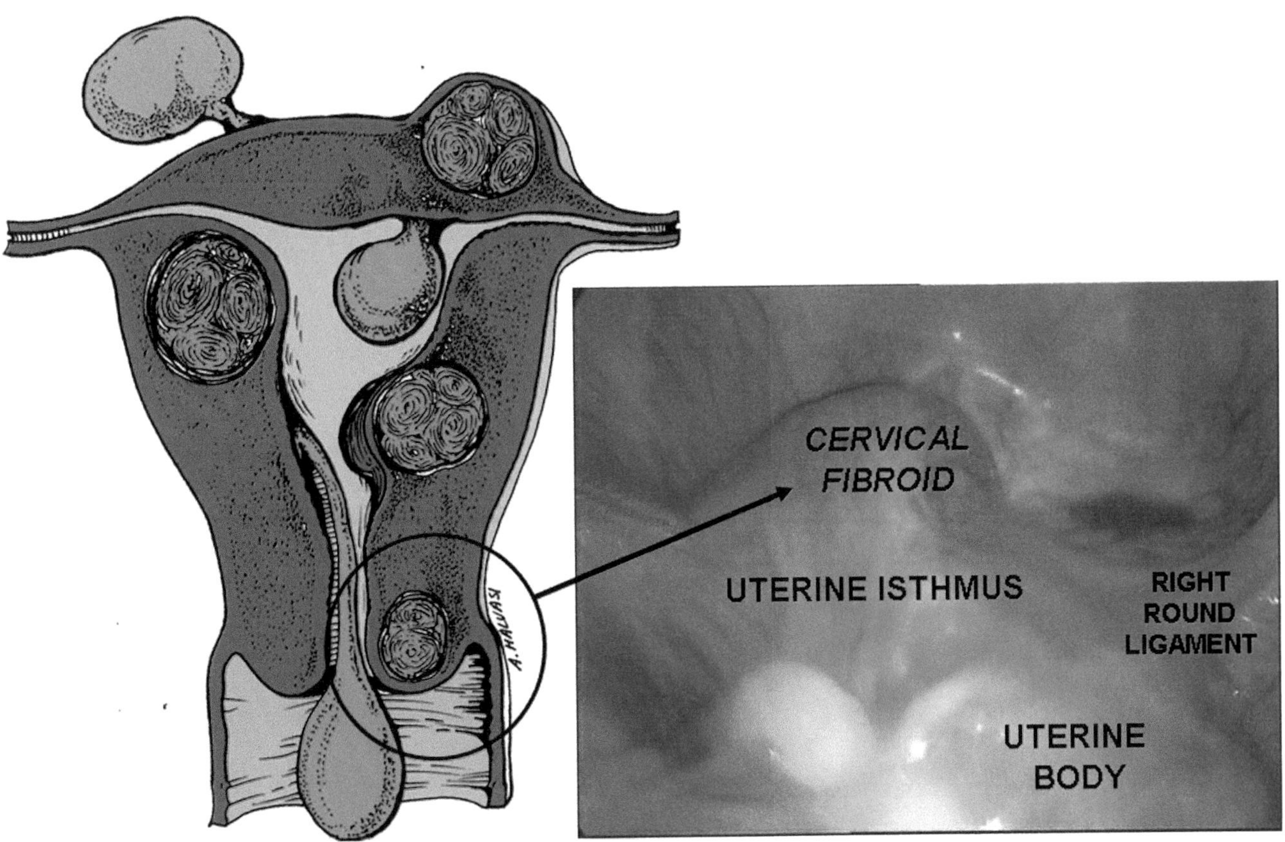

Fig. 31.4 On the left, a schematic representation of the fibroids' location; to the right, the laparoscopic image highlights an anterior cervical uterine myoma, under the uterine isthmus

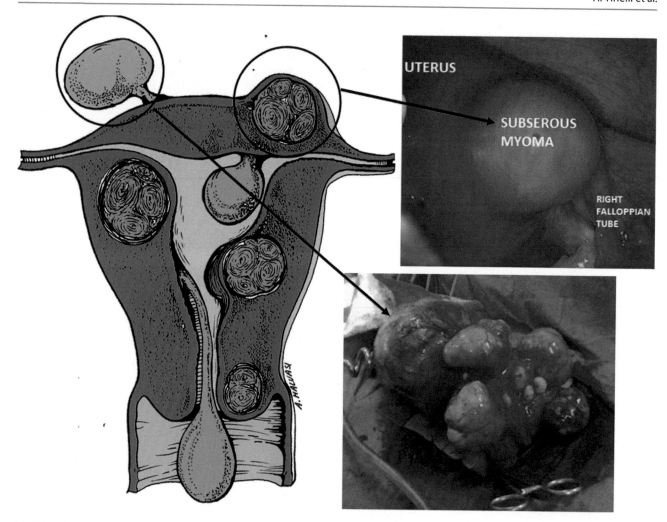

Fig. 31.5 On the left, a representation of fibroids location; on the right, at the top, a laparoscopic image showing a subserosal myoma on uterine body, near right fallopian tube. On the right, below, a laparotomic image showing a myomatosic uterus with several pedunculated fibroids

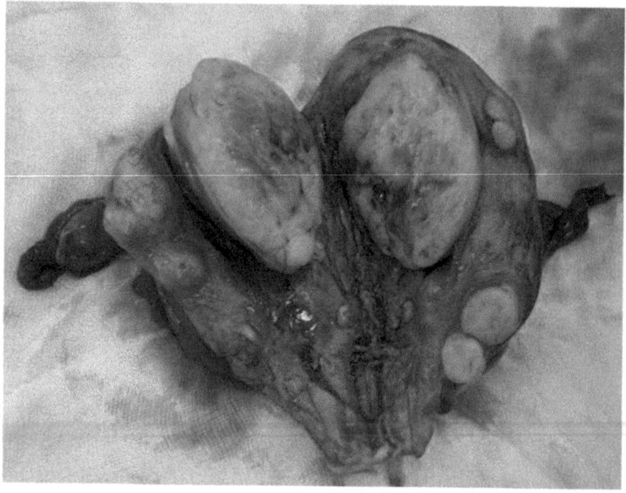

Fig. 31.6 The picture shows a uterus with a large number of myomas, anteriorly dissected from the bottom up to the cervix: fibroids appear well circumscribed, firm, *grey-white* and with a whorled cut surface

Previous epidemiological studies, focusing mostly on symptomatic women, have largely underestimated myoma prevalence [5, 10–12].

Over the past two decades, epidemiological studies have become more accurate, since they investigate a wide range of general population and use advanced non invasive imaging techniques, such as accurate 3D–4D ultrasound screening [1, 10].

Thus, Laughlin et al. [12], demonstrated the prevalence of myomas in 10.7 % of women in the first trimester of pregnancy (Fig. 31.7), which is lower than previously reported.

Some of the data on epidemiologic factors associated with myoma risk are well defined, while the others are not yet fully understood [10].

Documented predispositions in myoma formation and development include: age, race, body mass index (BMI), as well as heritage, reproductive factors, sex hormones, obesity, lifestyle (including diet, caffeine and alcohol consumption, smoking, physical activity and stress), environmental and other pathologies (as hypertension and infection) [1, 10–14].

Fig. 31.7 A traditional transvaginal ultrasonographic image by 2D and Doppler ultrasound probe, showing a posterior subserous myoma and a gestational sac with within the embryo of 6 weeks

Clinical Presentation of the Fibroids

Uterine myomas may be present for years in some women without any symptoms and diagnosed incidentally, during routine gynecological examination or investigation for other illness [15, 16]. In other cases, they are an important cause of morbidity and may result in the need for multiple surgical procedures [16–18].

It is believed that the only 20–50 % of women with uterine fibroids have symptoms. The reasons why some myomas are symptomatic and some not, have not been yet full understood [19], although size, localization and number of fibroids are factors affecting the symptoms [19, 20]. Sometimes women with the fundus uteri reaching the umbilicus do not report any problems, except for the enlargement of the abdomen and the increase in body weight (Fig. 31.8) [19]. It is also unproven that women with multiple fibroids (Fig. 31.9) tend to have more symptoms, compared with those who have only one fibroid [19].

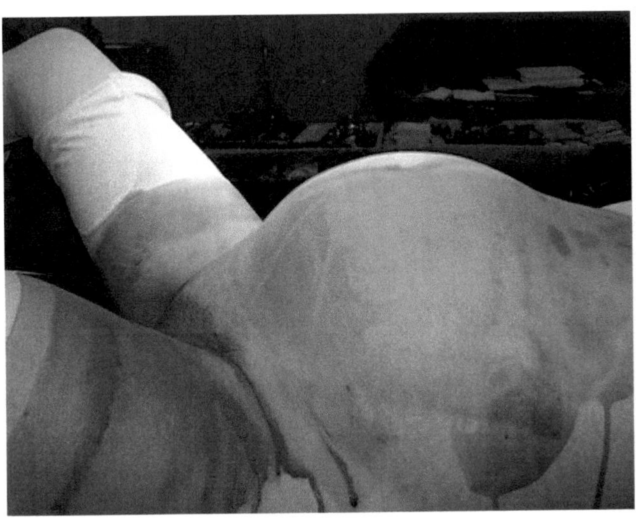

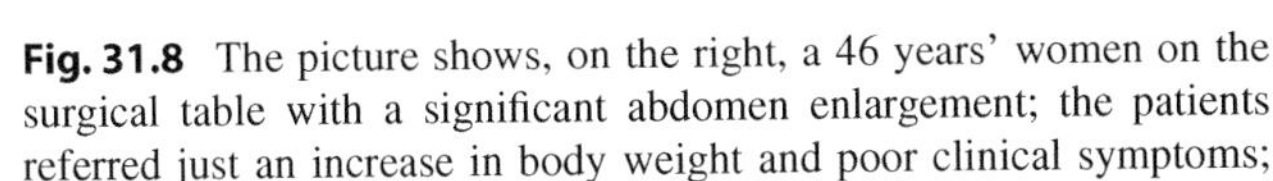

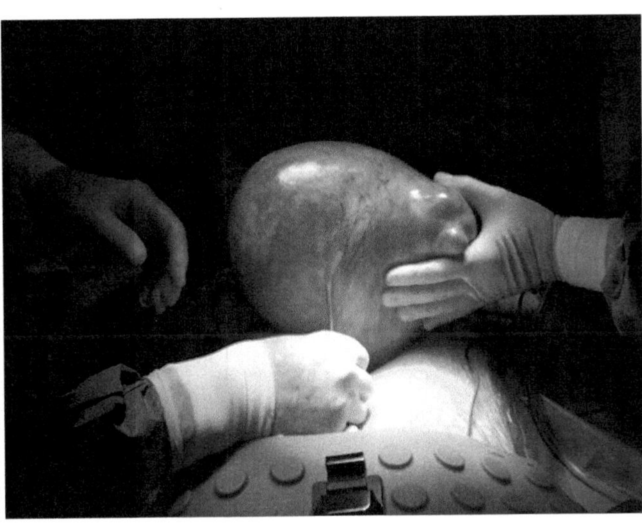

Fig. 31.8 The picture shows, on the right, a 46 years' women on the surgical table with a significant abdomen enlargement; the patients referred just an increase in body weight and poor clinical symptoms; On the right, the laparotomic hysterectomy with a uterus deformed by a huge myoma of 3.5 kg in weight

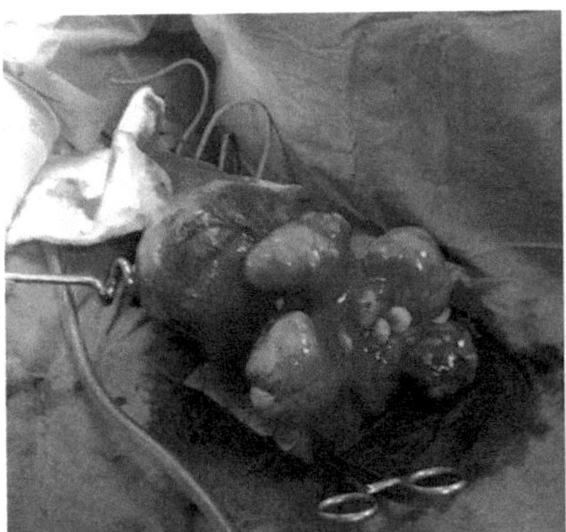

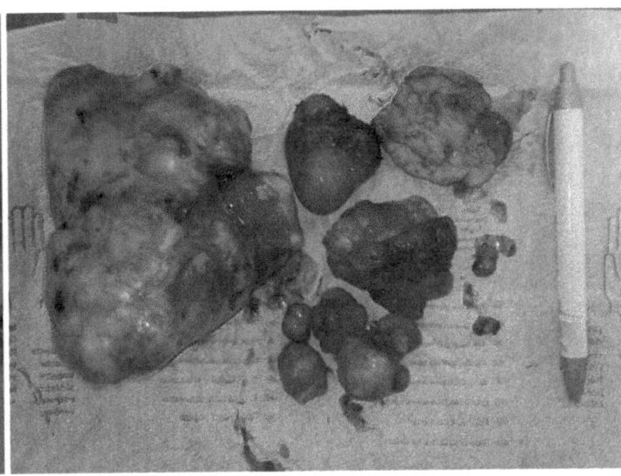

Fig. 31.9 On the left, the picture shows a uterus, deformed by many fibroids, located over the abdomen during a laparotomic myomectomy; on the right, the 11 enucleated myomas

Symptomatic fibroids usually occur in women in their thirties and forties, although they can occur, as well, in other age groups [21, 22]. In 62 % of women affected by uterine fibroids are symptomatic [20].

The most common presenting symptoms of uterine fibroids are: bleeding (menometrorrhagia, metrorrhagia or intermenstrual bleeding), pain, symptoms of compression of adjacent organs, change of the abdomen wall outline and infertility [16, 21, 23].

The Problem of Suspected Fibroid Malignant Alterations

Malignant alteration of uterine fibroids occurs mainly in postmenopausal women and is rarely asymptomatic. The main presenting symptoms of uterine leiomyosarcomas are abnormal vaginal bleeding, pain in the lower abdomen and a pelvic or abdominal mass [40]. In the past, if sudden growth of uterine fibroids is observed, especially after menopause, malignancy should be suspected and these tumors should be surgically removed. Recent evidences indicate that in premenopausal women, "rapid uterine growth" almost never indicates presence of uterine sarcoma [24].

Parker and colleagues examined 1332 women who had undergone a hysterectomy for uterine fibroids as the sole indication for surgery. Only 1 patient out of 371 women operated on for a "'myoma fast-growing" had proved to be a leiomyosarcoma. When the surgeons had judged that the myoma was at "rapid growth", defined as an increase of uterine volume as a womb of 6 weeks of pregnancy in 1 year of observation, none of the 198 patients who had this diagnosis was later shown to a uterine sarcoma at histological examination. Two of these women had instead endometrial stromal sarcoma. A patient of 30 years in the group of patients candidates for hysterectomy showed a normal uterus 22 months before; to gynecological presurgical, had a very large size of the uterus, such as a uterus of 16 weeks. After surgery, histological examination was shown a leiomyosarcoma. None of the 198 patients who had the criteria of "rapidly growing myoma" had a leiomyosarcoma, a mixed mesodermal tumor, or endometrial stromal sarcoma. None of the 17 postmenopausal women admitted for rapid uterine growth proved to be a sarcoma [25].

The uterine leiomyosarcoma (Fig. 31.10) is a very rare condition, has an incidence ranging from 0.5 to 3.3 per 100,000 women per year, with a further incidence of sarcomas in women with myomas at rapid growth of 0.27 % [26].

The transformation of leiomyomas in leiomyosarcoma is very rare [27].

Indisputable scientific data strongly suggest that uterine leiomyosarcomas are solitary lesions and are not commonly found in association with uterine myomas. If there is malignant transformation of uterine leiomyomas, is a rare event. The hypothesis that a uterine leiomyosarcoma derived from a myoma or are the result of malignant transformation of benign leiomyomas is never demonstrated [28].

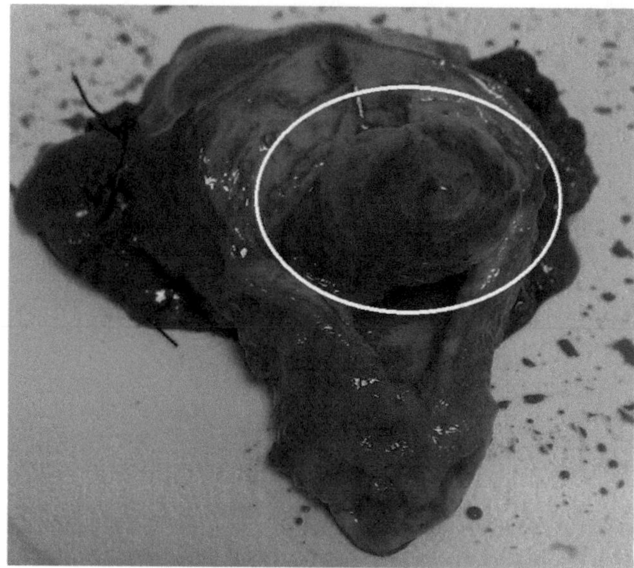

Fig. 31.10 A section uterus by pathologist with, in the white ring, a protruding single leiomyosarcoma of 4 cm, occupying almost the uterine cavity

There is no scientifically validated screening instrument that allow to diagnoses a sarcoma, since the diagnosis of sarcoma is purely histological and sometimes mixed with areas of benign myoma. In fact, to perform a diagnosis of leiomyosarcoma is not easy, even on extemporaneous histological examination. In most medical centers, the frozen section is not the histological technique for the final diagnosis. From one to three slides of a so-called "fibroid" can be routinely assessed when examining the frozen sections. It is more common than you think wrong or missing the diagnosis of uterine leiomyosarcoma in the frozen section [29, 30].

The Histopathology of Myomas

Histologically, the tumor is made up of cells similar to that of the contiguous endometrium (elongated, eosinophilic cytoplasm with central, blunt-ended, pale elongated nucleus, sometimes with clumped chromatin. The cells form whirling fascicles interlaced at right angles. This arrangement clearly distinguishes the leiomyoma (Fig. 31.11) from the surrounding myometrium, which shows a more regular pattern of the muscle fibers (Fig. 31.12). Furthermore, a large number of tumors show a clear border with the myometrium, even forming a valley, exaggerated by fixation artifact, with the

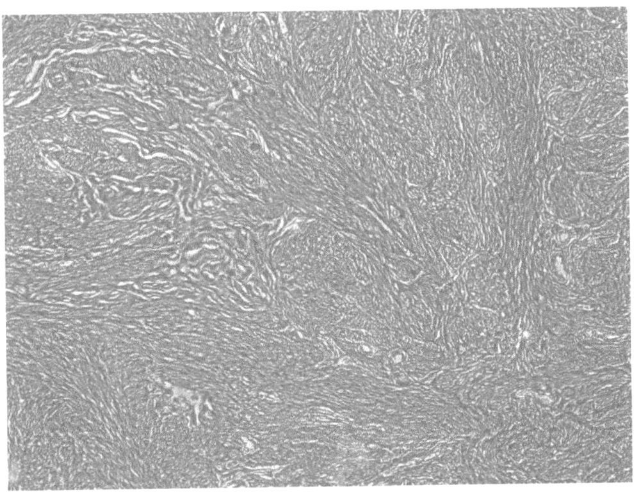

Fig. 31.11 A uterine leiomyoma composed by bundles of spindle cells, similar to those present in the myometrial wall: only the whirling and irregular arrangement of the cellular bundles distinguish the neoplastic proliferation

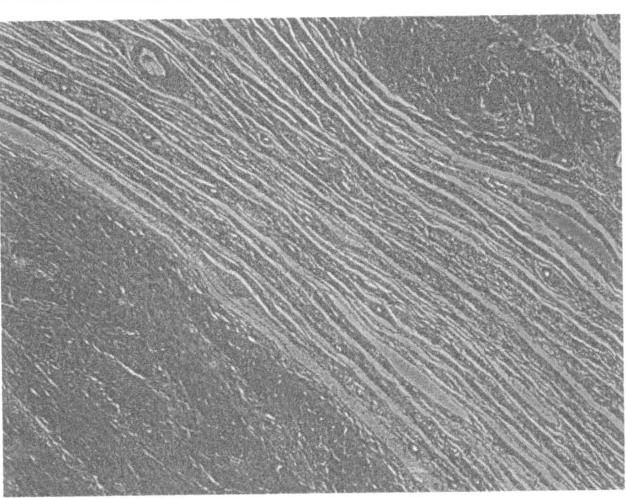

Fig. 31.13 At the center of the image shows a bundle of muscle fibers, collagen tissue and blood vessels are surrounded by extracellular matrix; this is what is known as a myoma pseudocapsule

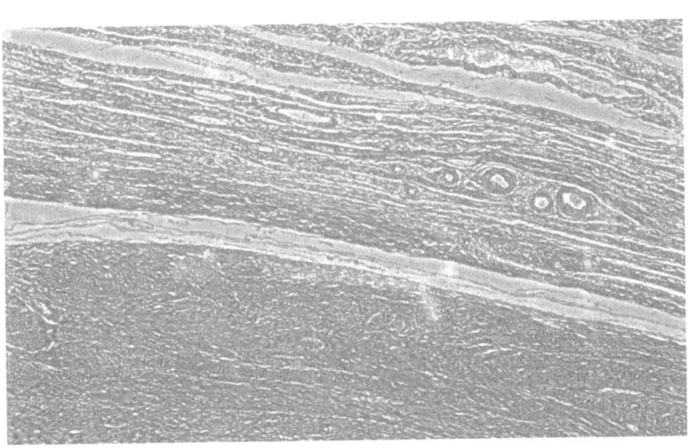

Fig. 31.12 The myometrium (in the *lower part*) surrounding myoma (in the *upper part*) shows a more regular pattern of the muscle fibers

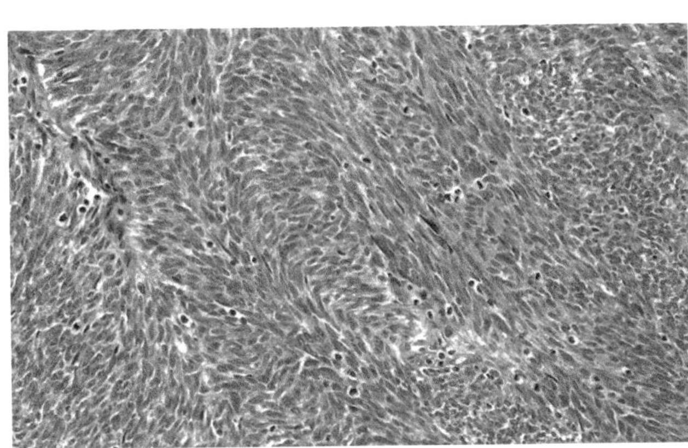

Fig. 31.14 A leiomyosarcoma: other than "tumor cell necrosis", it is detecting the presence of moderate-severe atypia and a mitotic index over 10/10HPF

formation of a ring of compressed myometrial cells, the pseudocapsule. In conservative myomectomy the surgeon exploits this valley to allow an easy excision of the tumor from the uterine wall. This interstitial space is formed from a variable amount of connective tissue (increasing with age and the menopausal state), possible edema and many blood vessels of different caliber, and it is called myoma pseudocapsule (Fig. 31.13).

Leiomyomata variants have differences that can be macroscopic or histological and thereby pose a serious problem of differential diagnosis with leiomyosarcoma.

First of all, there can be "infarct-type" necrosis or hyaline necrosis according to Bell et al. [31], characterized by areas of seemingly coagulative necrosis separated from the rest of the tumor by rings of fibrous or granulation tissue. This type of necrosis must not be confused with "tumor cell necrosis" observed in leiomyosarcoma where the cells are frequently necrotic, there is no separation from the surrounding tumor and often there are clumps of the residue of neoplastic cells surrounding residual vascular structures, commonly known as ghost outlines.

The differential diagnosis with leiomyosarcoma supposes, other than "tumor cell necrosis", the presence of moderate-severe atypia and a mitotic index over 10/10HPF: according to the Bell criteria of Bell [31] the presence of two out of three of these parameters is enough to diagnose leiomyosarcoma (Fig. 31.14). Immunohistochemistry does not bring any further advantages to the differential diagnosis. The borders of the tumor often infiltrate the near myometrium without the presence of the pseudocapsule observed in benign leiomyomata. Clearly malignant tumors express more p16, p21 and p53 immunoreactivity, but this is not helpful in single cases [32].

The expression of Ki 67 is also higher in leiomyosarcomas: in our experience Ki 67 is constantly higher than 40 %,

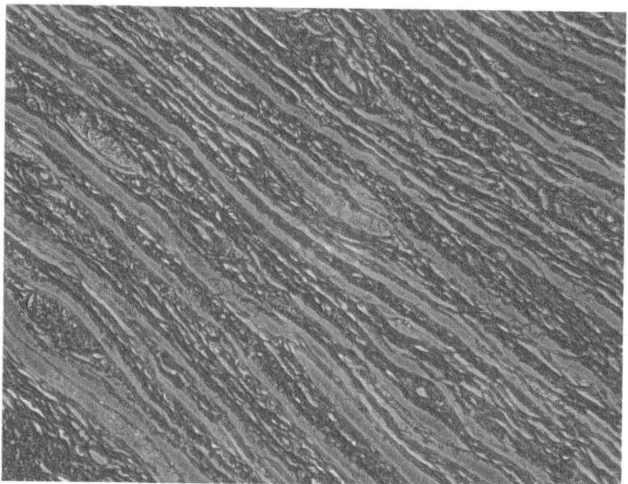

Fig. 31.15 The myometrium surrounding fibroid produce a sort of pseudocapsule, for ischemic phenomena, constituted by a network of: collagen fibers, extracellular matrix, neurofibers and blood vessels, as a separate fibroneurovascular tissue

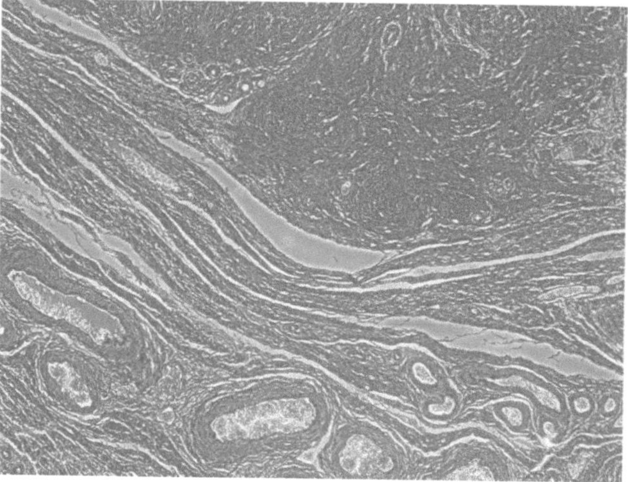

Fig. 31.16 A microscopic section showing the myoma pseudocapsule surface occasionally interrupted by collagen fibers and vessels that anchors the fibroid to myometrium

while in leiomyomata it is always less than 10 %. Necrosis can also be observed beneath the endometrium in tumors that grow into the uterine cavity which ulcerate and bleed, and therefore the necrotic cells are found together with inflammatory infiltrates. Other degenerative changes, more of less common, are: *hyaline transformation* of the stroma, leading to the wide substitution of the tumor, *dystrophic calcification* for a calcium salt deposition in the interstitial stroma (more common in menopausal women), a *hydropic degeneration* that can lead even to the formation of pseudocysts full of clear liquid.

A rarer but important type of change is myxoid degeneration of the fibroid when a gelatinous material is formed and the leiomuscolar cells can appear star-shaped and immersed in a slightly basophile stroma. Here the margins of the tumor must be closely examined as well circumscribed and the mitotic index is an essential point. A myxoid leiomyosarcoma, besides invading the surrounding myometrium, displays evident mitotic figures with only 2 per 10 HPF necessary to presume a malignant behavior. During pregnancy, leiomyomata can undergo necrosis and suffer bleeding (red degeneration), depending on the hormonal situation. Similar degeneration has been seen in hormonal therapy with estroprogestins. GnRH – analogue therapy causes a high degree of cellularity of the tumor which can confuse the pathologist when analyzing the mitotic figures. The increase in cellularity is apparently an effect linked to cell atrophy which reduces the cytoplasm thickness with closer nuclei, often with densely packed chromatin. As we discussed in a previous paper, the arteries we have described alterations of the inner wall agree with the proliferation of muscle cells and distortion or restriction of the lumen [33].

Analyzing leiomyomas composition, they are stiff tumors characterized by an excessive deposition of disordered extracellular matrix (ECM) components, particularly collagen I, III, and IV, proteoglycans, and fibronectin [34]. Matrix metalloproteinases (MMPs) are implicated in leiomyoma remodeling with a higher activity of MMP-2 in leiomyomas than in surrounding myometrium [35], separating by the myoma pseudocapsule.

During its growth, fibroid causes compressive phenomena on the surrounding myometrium, which for ischemic phenomena, seems to produce a sort of pseudocapsule, constituted by a surrounding network of collagen fibers, neurofibers and blood vessels, as a separate fibroneurovascular tissue (Fig. 31.15) [6].

Occasionally the pseudocapsule surface is interrupted by collagen fibers and vessels that anchor the fibroid to myometrium, well represented in microscopic sections (Fig. 31.16). It allows a constitution of a macroscopically clear cleavage plane between fibroid and the pseudocapsule, and between the pseudocapsule and the surrounding myometrium (Fig. 31.17) [36]. The pseudocapsule allows to fibroid only a displacement action (but not destructive) on myometrium, retaining the integrity and contractility of uterine structure [37]. We will discuss the importance of this small structure in the context of the myometrium, for the purpose anatomical, pathophysiological and reproductive systems.

Anatomy of Fibroid Pseudocapsule

Microscopically, the pseudocapsule seems to be as a continuous layer between the fibroid and surrounding myometrium and is made of a thickening of collagen fibers and blood

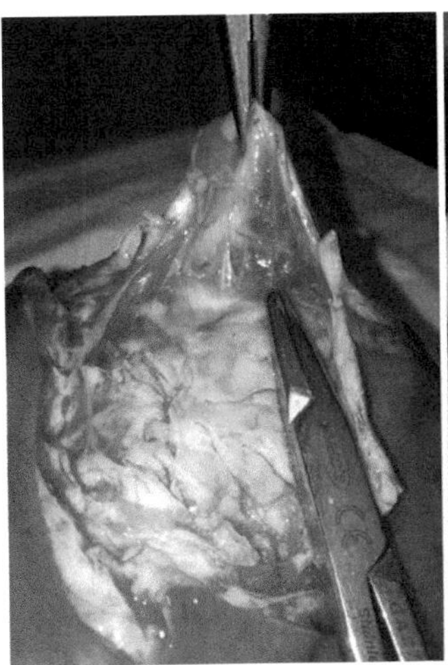
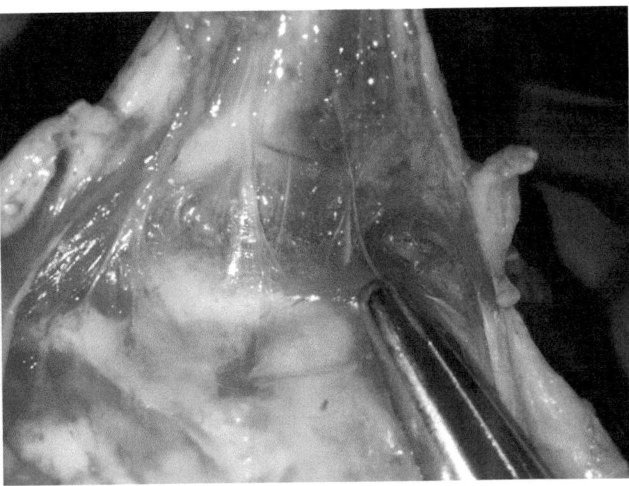

Fig. 31.17 Anatomical section of uterus with intramural myoma detecting myoma pseudocapsule: on the left the clamp shows a clear cleavage plane between fibroid and the pseudocapsule; on the right a surgical image magnification showing the small fibrovascular bridges connecting the pseudocapsule to the fibroid

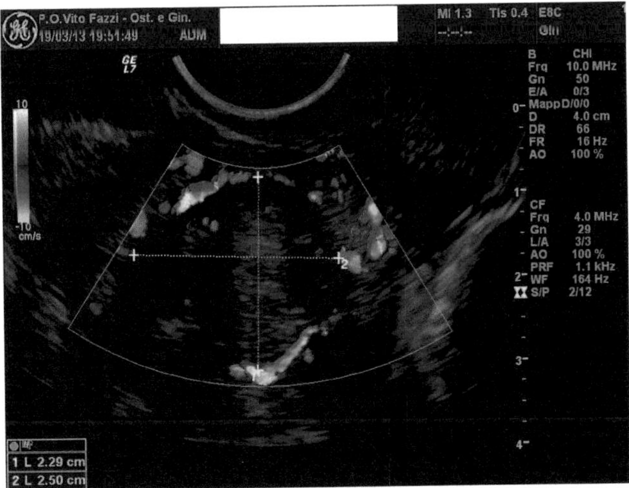

Fig. 31.18 A uterine section by transvaginal ultrasound scan: the pseudocapsule forms a vascular ring around fibroid, sonographically called "ring of fire" by echo-color Doppler, separating myoma from the surrounding myometrium

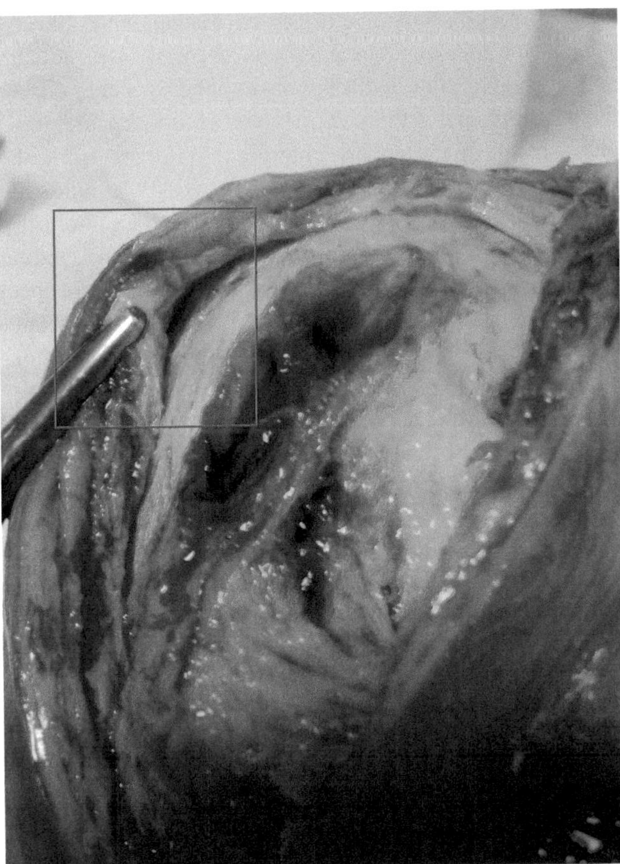

Fig. 31.19 Anatomic section of uterus with intramural myoma showing, in the *red box*, the cleavage plane to identify and to respect during a myomectomy, between fibroid and pseudocapsule

vessels that form a vascular ring, sonographically called "ring of fire" by echo-color Doppler: the pseudocapsule is separated from the surrounding myometrium, sonographically forming a hyperechogenic ring that surrounds and defines myoma (Fig. 31.18) [18]. To help with understanding of the micro-neuroanatomy of the fibroid peripheral area, we should get close with the story of pseudocapsule entity. An anatomical textbook, published at the end of last century, asserted: "*myoma shows a nodular aspect, a round image, well circumscribed, to enucleate even if they miss a pseudocapsule*" [6]. These authors confirmed the existence of the fibroid pseudocapsule and cleavage plane to identify and to respect during a myomectomy (Fig. 31.19) [6]. The first paper that described a fibrovascular system over a fibroid as "a mass of proliferating arteries" was in 1944 [38] and then, Farrer-Brown in 1970 [39] and Awataguchi in 1982 [40] found a fibrovascular plexus around the periphery of the fibroid. Lately, Casey et al. reported significantly higher microvasculature density in the surrounding myometrium in large fibroids; the author discovered that the vascular capsule was a substantial feature of all fibroids, excluding those smaller, and that it reaches the highest density of blood vessels in large tumors [41].

Pathologists examined the relationship between ultrasound and histological findings of the fibroids vascular capsule in the last century, in a series of women using Gn-RH analogues in preoperative treatment before myomectomy [42–44].

Walocha et al. [45] performed a microstructural evaluation of the fibroid pseudocapsule and found that the density of blood vessels increases around myoma. As the fibroid grows, new blood vessels penetrate the tumor from its periphery where "the vascular capsule" network is formed. Some of the vessels in the pseudocapsule connect at the base of the myoma and form a little foot which often bleeds during an extra-capsular myomectomy. These authors analyzed the fibroid vascular system using corrosion casting combined with scanning electron microscopy and affirmed that the pre-existing blood vessels undergo in regression and new vessels invade the tumor from the periphery during the development of myomas. Myoma pseudocapsule originates from small vessels entering the tumor from the periphery, forming a "vascular network" around the myoma, with flattened veins compressed by the tumor [45]. Forssman et al. reported the vascular capsule surrounding myoma of 2 cm of diameter and found that the inner aspect of the capsule contained large vessels that invade the capsule from the periphery [46]. Wei et al. already demonstrated that in large uterine fibroids, the most biologically active zone is the region next to the periphery with a higher level of gene expression, a higher density of blood vessels, a higher proliferative rate, and a lower level of hyaline degeneration [47]. Finally, a preliminary study showed neurotransmitters into the myoma pseudocapsule [48], outline some neuro-biological properties of this structure [49], since the vascular structure has a proper characteristic, similar to cancers [50].

The Ratio of Uterine-Preserving Operative Therapy of Uterus Myomatosus

Uterine fibroid is a multifactorial and still enigmatic pathology. Traditional studies were associated to molecular and genetic investigations, detecting an important role in fibroids' growth and development, with cytogenetic anomalies observed in about 40 % of patients [34, 35]. Starting from the data on myoma and its pseudocapsule mentioned below, we focused our investigations on the morphological and biomolecular properties of myoma pseudocapsule, explaining the ration of uterine-preserving operative therapy.

Uterine Myoma Pseudocapsule Analisysed by Trasmission Electron Microscopy

In such study, we investigated the ultra-structure of myoma pseudocapsule by transmission electron microscopy analysis, to best detail the pseudocapsule structure and its involvement in fibroid growth and removal [51]. In two Universities affiliated Hospitals, ten women with a mean age of 36.7, underwent single laparoscopic intracapsular myomectomy (removing fibroid form its pseudocapsule). The selected patients requested myomectomy for the following associated symptoms: pelvic pain, menorrhagia, and growth of myomatic nodules, verified by ultrasound, with increasing symptoms. Exclusion enrolling criteria for the investigation were: previous uterine surgery (excluding caesarean section), pre-surgical treatment with GnRH-analogues, history of gynecological malignancy and primary sub fertility. Exclusion criteria for preoperative GnRH-analogue treatment was due to reported increased risk of recurrence, a possible delay in the diagnosis of leiomyosarcoma, a risk of massive hemorrhage from degeneration, a greater difficulty in finding the cleavage plane, and a greater extent of hyalinization phenomena [52, 53]. In the study setting, all fibroids were selected through standardized transvaginal ultrasound: all patients had subserous and/or intramural fibroids and transvaginal ultrasound clearly evidenced the fibroid pseudocapsule. The myomas' sizes were between 5 and 8 cm; the 4–9 cm limit was selected by surgeons to avoid longer operation time and pointless uterine trauma for smaller fibroids. To give homogeneity to the intracapsular laparoscopical myomectomy, the authors excluded pedunculated, cervical and intra-ligamentary myomas – because they are extra-myometrium., and suboptimal for authors' purpose. Patients underwent a standardized technique [7, 54] (Fig. 31.20): hysterotomy, pseudocapsule incision, extracting the myoma by stretching and uterine suturing. Samples were taken by scissors from the surface of the pseudocapsule as soon as good hemostasis was reached. Ten myoma pseudocapsule biopsy specimens of approximately 5 mm in depth, which included full thickness of the surrounding myometrium, were collected and processed for transmission electron microscopy (TEM). In semi thin sections the cells are fusiform with a centrally located nucleus. Inflammatory infiltration has not been detected in any section. At the electron microscopy level the cells have the features of the smooth muscle cells. They show nucleus with rounded end, often folded (concertina fashion), notched or with many invaginations. The cytoplasm is packed with thin (about 6 nm thick) filaments; between filaments fusiform dense bodies are interspersed. There are few organelles like mitochondria, glycogen particles and sparse elements of endoplasmic reticulum. Abundant micropinocytotic vesicles

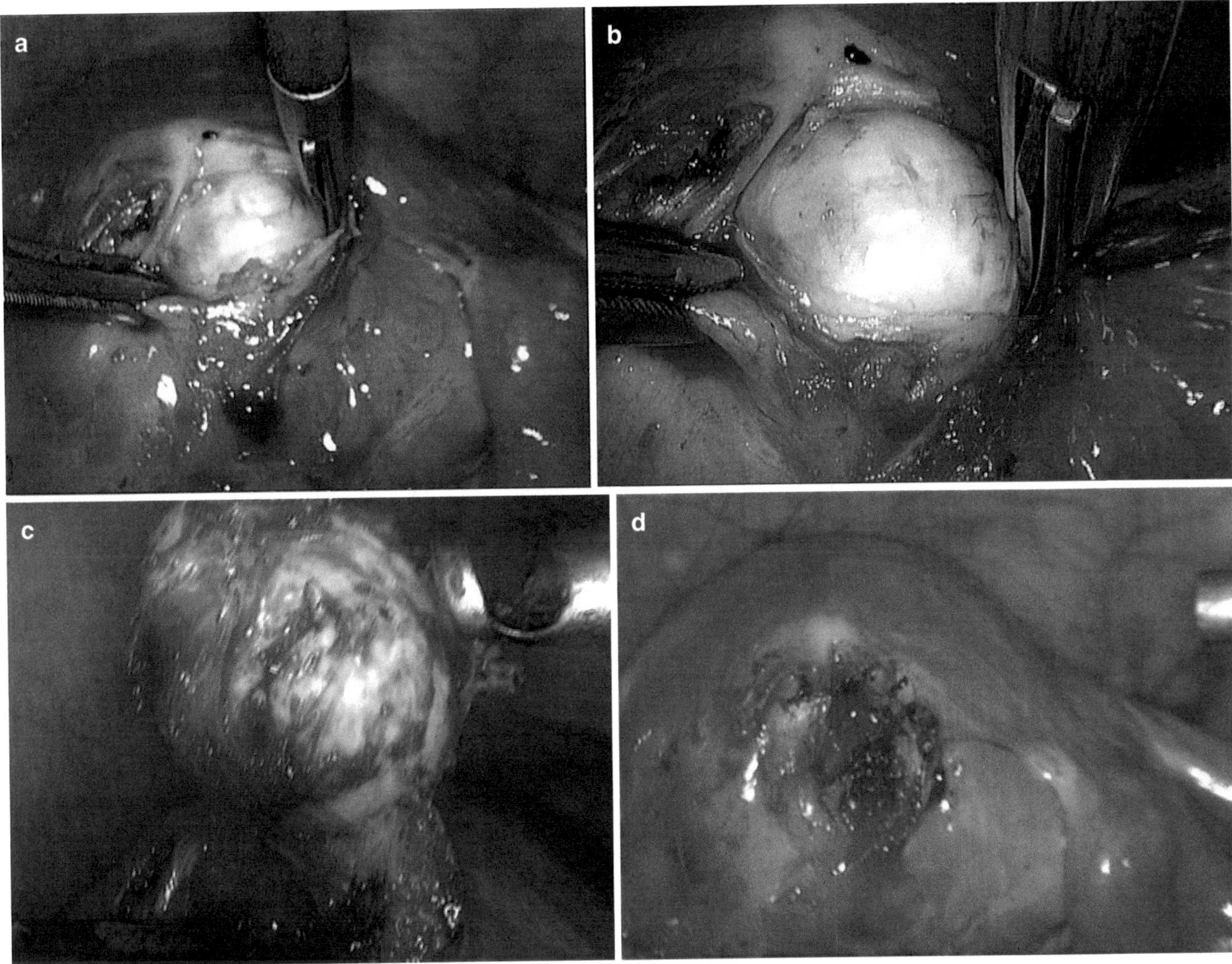

Fig. 31.20 The image shows a laparoscopic intracapsular myomectomy: (**a**) a womb incision over myoma; (**b**) the myoma enucleation by intracapsular technique; (**c**) myoma removal from uterus; (**d**) the minimal uterine bleeding after pseudocapsule sparing

are also present. The cells are surrounded by a thin but distinct basal lamina. The results of this study showed that at the electron microscopy level, the pseudocapsule cells had the features of the smooth muscle cells, as in myometrium. Basing on these findings, myoma pseudocapsule should be a part of myometrium who compresses leiomyoma, being a structure different from leiomyoma. Anatomically, fibroids arise from the uterine myometrium and typically are comprised of fascicles of smooth muscle cells with abundant pink cytoplasm and uniform spindle-shaped nuclei. Fibroids show a monoclonal proliferation of smooth muscle cells with isolated mitoses, minimal atypical nuclei, and an absence of coagulative necrosis and pseudocyst formation. In this investigation, authors investigated the ultra-structure of myoma pseudocapsule by transmission electron microscopy analysis, to best detail the pseudocapsule structure and its involvement in fibroid growth and removal.

Neurotransmitters in Myoma Pseudocapsule

Other investigations [55, 56] showed the presence of neurotrasmitters in myoma pseudocapsule. These studies confirmed the preliminary evidence that pseudocapsules contain neuropeptides together with their related fibers, as a neurovascular bundle, containing a vascular network rich in neurotransmitters like a neurovascular bundle [48, 49].

In the first paper [55], we evaluated the presence of neuropeptide tyrosine (NPY) in pseudocapsule of intramural, corporal, and fundal UMs, as well as in the normal myometrium. In addition, the presence of neurotensin (NT) associated with uterine contraction, and protein gene product 9.5 (PGP 9.5) as marker for uterine innervation, were both evaluated in the same tissues of NPY, in 75 women scheduled for single or multiple myomectomies. The indications for myomectomy were: severe pelvic pain, heavy menorrhagia not responding to conservative treatment, or uncontrolled growth of UMs, as verified by repeated ultrasound. Among the patients, 67 women agreed to sign an informed consent for surgery; pregnancy was ruled out by a β-human chorionic gonadotropin test. All women were Caucasians. The exclusion criteria were: no previous myomectomy or cesarean sections, treatment with gonadotropin-releasing hormone (GnRH) analogs, to avoid eventual influence on results [52, 53] and a history of gynecological tumors. All fibroids were diagnosed using standardized transabdominal and transvaginal ultrasound myoma mapping by expert clinicians. The UMs' location were classified depending on their positions and the ultrasound data were recorded for postsurgical evaluations. Investigated UMs were single or multiple, and were located in the fundus uteri and in the corpus. Pedunculated, subserous, cervico-isthmic, and intraligamentary UMs were excluded. All myomectomies were performed by laparotomy or laparoscopy, depending on their dimensions and the surgeon's preference. The diameters of the UMs were between 4 and −9 cm of diameter. All women were administered a standard prophylactic antibiotic dose of 2 g Cefazolin intravenously. All operations were performed under general anesthesia with endotracheal intubation. All surgical procedures were performed by experienced gynecologists or senior residents who had paramount experience in removing UMs from within the pseudocapsule, as evidence-based data have shown [7, 54]. Once the UM removing and the UM pseudocapsule (PUM) spared on normal myometrium (NM), the surgeons sampled full thickness specimens that included the PUM as well as the surrounding NM from the fundus of the uterus (FU) and the uterine body (UB). These samples were approximately 20 mm in depth, obtained using scissors and were collected in peers, but separately. All samples were sent to the laboratory in a dry-ice container for histological and immunofluorescent analyses. A quantitative analysis of images (QAI) was performed on slides and on microphotographs using a the Quantimet Analyzer (Quantimet 500 Leica Microsystems Imaging Solutions Ltd., Cambridge, UK), equipped with specific software for a detailed evaluation. The densities of NT, NPY, and PGP 9.5 fibers were calculated using a Quantimet Leitz image analyzer that measures the following parameters: (1) detection of NT, NPY, and PGP 9.5 nerve containing fibers counted in 10 fields randomly chosen; (2) the percentage of total area occupied by those fields; (3) the number of observed varicosities; (4) the number of intersections of the nerve fibers; and (5) the total perimeter of NT, NPY, and PGP 9.5 structures in proportion to an average value (100 for each field). Morphometric quantification of the density of each type of nerve fiber was performed on photographs of stained samples using the Quantimet Leica 2000 image analyzer by a single pathologist. The software provided with the analyzer counts and expresses these fluorescent areas in "Conventional Units" or C.U. [48], i.e., as percentages of area occupied by a single type of nerve fiber related to the total observed area. By adding these values (single type of nerve fiber), it is possible to evaluate the sum of the areas occupied by the different types of nerve fibers. The software also calculates the average values and translates them to a single value with a standard deviation, which is reported on the instrument display as the "standard error of the mean (SEM)." Other details about the experimental procedures used for morphometric quantification by the Quantimet Leica are reported in the Anon manual of methods [36]. Statistical analysis of the data was based on the results obtained by the image analyzer software; and the data were averaged to obtain a median value per case. The means ± SEMs were then calculated and reported for each nerve fiber group. Repeated immunofluorescent controls were prepared and the differences were calculated by using Student's *t*-test. A P-value <0.05 was considered statistically significant.

Morphometric quantification of the neurotransmitters was performed on photographs using quantitative image analysis of 67 specimens. Fibers containing neuropeptides were not significantly higher in PUMs than in NM of FUs: 4 ± 0.2 C.U. for NT, 1 ± 0.5 C.U. for NPY, 4 ± 0.3 C.U. for PGP 9.5 in PUMs vs. 3 ± 0.9 C.U. for NT, 2 ± 0.1 C.U. for NPY, 3 ± 0.4 C.U. for PGP 9.5 in NM. Statistical evaluation did not report any significant difference (Table 31.1).

Nerve fibers containing the neurotransmitters increased slightly but not significantly in UBs with respect to FUs; with, 5 ± 0.3 C.U. for NT, 7 ± 0.2 C.U. for NPY, 6 ± 0.5 C.U. for PGP 9.5 in UBs vs. 4 ± 0.9 C.U. for NT, 6 ± 0.8 C.U. for NPY, 5 ± 0.7 C.U. for PGP 9.5 in FUs ($p > 0.05$). Also in such case, statistical evaluation did not report any significant difference among FU and UB neuropeptide concentration (Table 31.2).

Our results showed that NT, NPY, and PGP 9.5 neurofibers are almost equally present in PUF as in NM of a non-pregnant uterus. As all of these neuropeptides are present in the uterine muscle and can affect muscle contractility, uterine peristalsis and muscular healing. A myomectomy respecting the pseudocapsule neurofibers should facilitate smooth muscle scarring and promote restoration of normal uterine peristalsis with a possible positive influence on fertility.

In the second investigation, we compared the quantitative distributions of OXY and ENK in nerve fibers of fibroid pseudocapsules, sampled from uterine fundal, corporal and isthmo-cervical regions. We included 64 women in the study protocol: a well-designed non-randomization controlled trial (Level of evidence: II-1). The following were the inclusion criteria: a large uterus with symptomatic myomas, a myomatous uterus with severe pelvic pain, and menorrhagia, that was not controlled by conservative treatment, or uncontrolled growth of myomas revealed by dynamic ultrasound examinations. The main exclusion criterion was pregnancy,

Table 31.1 Distribution of the neurotensin (NT), the neuropeptide tyrosine (NPY) and the protein gene product 9.5 (PGP 9.5) nerve fibers in uterine fibroid pseudocapsule and in normal myometrium

	Fibroid pseudocapsule	Normal myometrium	*P* value
Neurotensin (NT)	4 ± 0.2 C.U.	3 ± 0.9 C.U.	P > 0.05
	Fibroid pseudocapsule	**Normal myometrium**	**P value**
Neuropeptide Tyrosine (NPY)	1 ± 0.5 C.U.	2 ± 0.1 C.U.	P > 0.05
	Fibroid pseudocapsule	**Normal myometrium**	**P value**
Protein Gene Product 9.5 (PGP 9.5)	4 ± 0.3 C.U.	3 ± 0.4 C.U.	P > 0.05

Table 31.2 Distribution of the neurotensin (NT), the neuropeptide tyrosine (NPY) and the protein gene product 9.5 (PGP 9.5) nerve fibers in uterine fibroid pseudocapsule of uterine body and fundus uteri

	Fibroid pseudocapsule of uterine body	Fibroid pseudocapsule of fundus uteri	P value
Neurotensin (NT)	5 ± 0.3 C.U.	4 ± 0.9 C.U.	P > 0.05
	Fibroid pseudocapsule of uterine body	**Fibroid pseudocapsule of fundus uteri**	**P value**
Neuropeptide Tyrosine (NPY)	7 ± 0.2 C.U.	6 ± 0.8 C.U.	P > 0.05
	Fibroid pseudocapsule of uterine body	**Fibroid pseudocapsule of fundus uteri**	**P value**
Protein Gene Product 9.5 (PGP 9.5)	6 ± 0.5 C.U.	5 ± 0.7 C.U.	P > 0.05

as confirmed by the betaHCG test, performed prior to surgery and women not belonging to the Caucasian group were excluded. Other exclusion criteria included: (1) uterine scarring from previous surgeries (including cesarean section), (2) a treatment history of gonadotropin-releasing hormone (GnRH) analogues, and (3) a history of gynecological tumors. Treatment with GnRH analogues was seen as an exclusion criterion due to their reported association with an increased risk of recurrent myomas, delays in leiomyosarcoma diagnosis, and massive hemorrhages due to difficulties in entering the cleavage plane at a greater extent of hyalinization [52, 53]. Patients with pedunculated, submucous, and intraligamentary fibroids were excluded because of the risk of a distinctly uncommon pseudocapsule that engages the surrounding myometrium following presurgical ultrasound [18] performed by expert clinicians to determine the presence of the ultrasound screen, a white ring surrounding the fibroids, indicated by Doppler sonography as a "ring of fire". The study was designed to include patients of both the single and the multiple fibroid with more than two myomas. Total laparotomic hysterectomies were performed under general anesthesia with endotracheal intubation by experienced gynecologists or senior residents. During surgery, cefazolin (2.0 g) was intravenously administrated as a preventive antibiotic therapy. Following hysterectomy, 3 full-thickness specimens (2 cm wide × 2 cm deep) were acquired from the fundus uteri, corpus, and cervix using a sterile scalpel, referred to Gray's Anatomy Book for the classification of the uterine segments [57].

Separate samples from an identical uterine specimen were collected in peers. The full-thickness specimens contained part of the myoma with its fibroid pseudocapsule and the surrounding myometrium. In patients with multiple myomas, tissues were resected from each site. All tissues were histological examined, prior to analyze them by polyclonal antibodies for the ENK and OXT immunohistochemical assays. Further evaluation of specimens was performed blindly processing samples by their numbers and pathologist was not informed about origin of evaluated samples. The distribution (density) of each type of nerve fiber was performed on digital images of stained samples using a Quantimet Leica 2000 image analyzer (Leica Microsystems Cambridge Ltd., Cambridge, UK) by a single pathologist. The software with the Quantimet Leica 2000 image analyzer enables the counting and expression of fluorescent areas in conventional units (CU) [48], which is the percentage of the area occupied by a single type of nerve fiber relative to the observed area. By adding these values (single nerve fiber types) it is possible to evaluate the sum of the areas occupied by different types of nerve fibers. The software also calculates the average values and translates them into a single value with the standard deviation displayed on the instrument. The density of ENK and OXT fibers was calculated by quantitative analysis using the Quantimet Leica 2000 image analyzer. Results were averaged to obtain a median value per sample and analyzed using one-way analysis of variance (ANOVA) with Bonferroni correction for multiple comparisons of normally distributed data set of 3 groups. Statistical calculations were performed with MedCalc software (version 11.4.1.0). Data are displayed as the mean (m) and standard deviation (SD) overall. Values of $P < 0.01$ were considered statistically significant.

We tested null (Ho) and alternative (Ha) hypotheses for both ENK and OXT positive nerve fibers to distinguish distribution differences of neuropeptides in pseudocapsules depending on localization of fibroids in different uterine regions, i.e., μHo: fundal=corporal=isthmian-cervical region; μHa: fundal≠corporal≠isthmian-cervical region.

Table 31.3 The distribution of neuropeptides enkephalin (ENK) – and oxytocin (OXT) -positive nerve fibers in uterine fibroids pseudocapsules of the uterine fundal, corporal, and isthmian–cervical regions

Parameters	Uterine regions			*Total P*-value
	Fundal	Corporal	Isthmian–cervical	
Number of patients	19 (33.3 %)	18 (31.5 %)	20 (35.2 %)	57 (100.0 %)-
Number of fibroids	22 (33.8 %)	23 (35.4 %)	20 (30.8 %)	65 (100.0 %)
ENK-positive nerve fibers (CU)	0	0	94 ± 0.7	0.01
OXT-positive nerve fibers (CU)	6.3 ± 0.8	15.0 ± 1.4	72.1 ± 5.1	0.01

Sixty-four women were consecutively assessed for eligibility, seven women were excluded and, finally, the study included 57 patients with myomas and hysterectomy. The patients were 36.4 ± 3.6 years old with the body mass index – 23.8 ± 2.5, and the parity index – 1.4 ± 0.3. Analysis of localization of myomas during surgery demonstrated, that in 18 patients myomas were located in restricted uterine regions such as in 5 patients (8.7 %) – in the fundus, in 7 patients (12.2 %) – in the corpus and in 6 patients (10.5 %) – in the isthmian–cervical region, whereas in 39 patients distribution of myomas was expanded with combination of two or all three regions (Table 31.3).

So, in 10 patients (17.5 %) fibroids were found in both fundus and corpus of uteri, in 12 patients (21 %) – in the fundus and isthmian–cervical region, in 13 patients (22.8 %) – in the corpus and isthmian–cervical region and in 4 patients (7 %) – in all 3 regions. Subsequently we obtained samples for ENK and OXT assays in total from 65 fibroid pseudocapsules obtained from 57 removed uteri. Among these, 22 (33.8 %) samples of fibroid pseudocapsules were obtained from fundus, 23 (35.4 %) – from corpus and 20 (30.8 %) – from isthmian-cervix region. Distribution of fibroid pseudocapsule nerve fibers containing ENK and OXT was identified by immunohistochemistry and quantified by morphometric evaluation in relevant number of samples for valid statistical analysis. An absence of ENK-positive nerve fibers was seen in the uterine fundus and corpus fibroid pseudocapsules, whereas ENK values of up to 94 ± 0.7 CU were observed in the nerve fibers in fibroid pseudocapsules obtained from the isthmian–cervical region. OXT-positive fibers were present in fibroid pseudocapsules of all uterine regions. However, density of OXT-positive fibers was comparatively lower in the fundus (6.3 ± 0.8 CU) and at a slightly increased number in the corpus (15.0 ± 1.4 CU), whereas the distribution of OXT-positive fibers was significantly higher in the isthmian–cervical region (72.1 ± 5.1 CU) ($p < 0.01$).

Thus, the uterine cervix, contains a wide amount of immunoreactive nerve fibers filled with a great number of neuropeptides, neurotransmitters play a crucial role in the regulation of woman's sexual and reproductive functions as the central neuronal structure orchestrating the functions of the female tract organs by accepting/activating and passing signals between the central nervous system and all genital tract structures. A high density of ENK and OXT in nerve fibers in the isthmian–cervical region fibroid pseudocapsules highlights the importance of this region for female reproductive and sexual functions, and pregnancy-related complications. The present findings are important to discern the pathophysiology of the female reproductive system and sexual disorders manifesting after surgical procedures in the cervix, including complications during pregnancy and delivery (i.e., miscarriage and cervical dystocia during labor). the uterine cervix, containing a wide amount of immunoreactive nerve fibers filled with a great number of neuropeptides, neurotransmitters play a crucial role in the regulation of woman's sexual and reproductive functions as the central neuronal structure orchestrating the functions of the female tract organs by accepting/activating and passing signals between the central nervous system and all genital tract structures. A high density of ENK and OXT in nerve fibers in the isthmian–cervical region fibroid pseudocapsules highlights the importance of this region for female reproductive and sexual functions, and pregnancy-related complications. The present findings are important to discern the pathophysiology of the female reproductive system and sexual disorders manifesting after surgical procedures in the cervix, including complications during pregnancy and delivery (i.e., miscarriage and cervical dystocia during labor).

Our and literature data confirmed that pseudocapsules contain many neuropeptides and neurotransmitters [48, 49, 55, 56, 58], physiologically active. Moreover, these substances may play a significant role in wound healing and innervation repair [18, 59, 60], and may be essential for reproductive [61–63] and sexual function [64, 65]. Indeed, the lower urinary tract neuropeptide–receptor systems may represent a potential target for therapeutic interventions [66, 67].

The Gentical Analysis of Pseudocapsule

Another of my investigations stated that biochemical growth factors evaluated in the pseudocapsule vessels cause intense angiogenesis in pseudocapsule, probably promoted by the fibroids [68]. The angiogenesis of the myoma pseudocapsule likely leads to the formation of a "protective" vascular capsule responsible for the supply of blood to the growing tumor [69]. However, studies demonstrated a dysregulation of various growth factors and their receptors in uterine myomas [40, 69]. In fact, a research on gene expression analysis in uterine leiomyoma pseudocapsule revealed an angiogenic profile in pseudocapsule [68]. In this investigation we performed, by quantitative real-time RT-PCR method (qRT-PCR), a gene expression analysis of pseudocapsule (PC), matching it with the same analysis in uterine leiomyoma (UL) and uterine myometrium (UM), evaluating the expression levels of IGF-2, used as tumoral marker, and COL4A2, CYR61/CCN1, CTGF/CCN2, VEGF-A and vWF, known to be involved in angiogenic processes. A group of 18 patients underwent laparoscopic myomectomy pseudocapsule sparing. Patients were selected on the basis of their symptoms as pain or pressure, menstrual disorders, large and growing myomas, infertility or reproductive dysfunction. The number, size and location of ULs were assessed for all patients: 11 women had subserous UL (61.1 %) whereas 7 women had intramural UL (38.9 %); ULs were single in 10 patients (55.5 %) and multiple in 8 patients (44.4 %) with the dominant fibroid measured between 3 and 12 cm in diameter. Patients with suspected adenomyosis or adenomyoma were excluded. Pedunculated, small and submucous ULs were also excluded. Preoperative treatment with gonadotropin releasing hormone analogues (GnRHa), known to induce distortion of the UL pseudocapsule [50, 53], has also been considered as an exclusion indication for the purposes of this study. As all women were to be subjected to intracapsular myomectomy, the protocol was primarily explained to the patients and full written consent to operation and protocol was obtained prior surgery. Pre-surgical trans-vaginal (TV) ultrasound (US) was performed to determine the presence of the UL-PC as a white ring surrounding the UL. Laparoscopic myomectomy by intracapsular technique (LIM) was performed as mentioned above [7, 54]. Tissues sampling from the fibroids were taken approximately 20 mm in depth, including full thickness of the UL, UL-PC and the surrounding UM; samples of UL-PC were taken by scissors from its surface, as soon as good hemostasis was reached, while UM tissues were biopsied at 2 cm distance from UL. All samples were orientated as surgeons proceed in case of cervical conization. All samples were collected and stored in saline solution, then sent to the genetic laboratory for successive analysis. To examine the molecular characteristics of PC, the expression levels of CYR61/CCN1, CTGF/CCN2, COL4A2, VEGF-A, vWF, endoglin/CD105 and IGF-2 genes were analyzed in eighteen matched PC, UM and UL specimens. The last gene was chosen because known to be a tumor proliferation marker in UL pathology, the others were selected for their involvement in angiogenesis. mRNA levels were measured by quantitative RT-PCR and corrected against the housekeeping GADPH gene. Normalized data were reported by the medians and interquartile ranges and the degree of variability among the three tissues was statistically determined. The IGF-2 expression varied significantly among the three tissues (p = 0.0011 by Kruskal-Wallis test). In particular, it was significantly higher in UL (0.0165 relative units mean) compared to UM (0.0028 relative units mean; p = 0.033 by Mann-Whitney test) and PC (0.0026 relative units mean; p = 0.032 by Mann-Whitney test). The difference between UM and PC was not significant (p = 0.916 by Mann-Whitney test). Expression levels analysis of endoglin/CD105 revealed a significant difference among the three tissues (p = 0.016 by Kruskal-Wallis test). In particular there was a significant over-expression in PC (0.031 relative units mean) with respect to both UL (0.013 relative units mean, p = 0.020 by Mann-Whitney test) and UM (0.008 relative units mean; p = 0.021 by Mann-Whitney test). The difference between UL and UM was not significant (p = 0.23 by Mann-Whitney test). Both CYR61 and CTGF showed a significant degree of variability among the three tissues in our samples (p =0.044 and p = 0.021 respectively by Kruskal-Wallis test). The down-regulation of CYR61 gene in UL (0.0278 relative units mean) with respect to UM (0.0588 relative units mean) was statistically significant (p = 0.032 by Mann-Whitney test), while difference with respect to PC (0.0479 relative units mean) doesn't reach significance (p = 0.067 by Mann-Whitney test). The difference between UM and PC was no significant as well (p = 0.92 by Mann-Whitney test). The down-regulation of CTGF in UL (0.0049 relative units mean) with respect to UM (0.0121 relative units mean) was significant (p = 0.006 by Mann-Whitney test), while no significant differences were found in the CTGF mRNA level between UL and PC (0.0111 relative units mean; p = 0.090 by Mann-Whitney test) and between PC and UM (p = 0.15 by Mann-Whitney test). Similarly, COL4A2 expression is significantly different across the three tissues (p = 0.018 by Kruskal-Wallis test). Moreover in this case, COL4A2 was expressed at significant higher in UL (2313 relative units mean) than in UM (1157 relative units mean, with p = 0.007 by Mann-Whitney test) while difference with PC (1658 relative units mean) was not significant (p = 0.137 by Mann-Whitney test).

The difference between UM and PC was not significant too (p = 0.154 by Mann-Whitney test).

VEGF-A and vWF mRNA levels showed no significant differences across the three tissues (p = 0.73 and p = 0.24 respectively by Kruskal-Wallis test).

The study' results clearly indicated that the pseudocapsule is a structure anatomically distinguishable from the myometrium and the surrounding fibroid, displaying a significant and specific gene expression profile. The pseudocapsule, as the fibroid, exhibited a significantly reduced expression of the IGF-2 gene, known to be a tumor growth marker, if compared to the fibroid, suggesting that it has a non-fibroid origin and that it has a structural continuity with myometrium. The pseudocapsule also showed a statistical relevant over-expression of the endoglin/CD105 gene, when compared to the myometrium and to the fibroid. Based on these evidences, the over-expression of the endoglin gene, rather than of other angiogenic genes, seemed to indicate the presence of an active angiogenesis correlated with reparative process in the pseudocapsule. All together these data clearly depicted the pseudocapsule as a site of intense angiogenesis linked to the endoglin activation rather than other angiogenic factors such as VEGF-A or vWF. The presence of an active angiogenesis is concordant with the histological studies that describe a parallel array of extremely dense capillaries in the pseudocapsule and in the adjacent myometrium, that are absent in fibroid. This can define the structural and functional features of pseudocapsule that could explain its possible roles in the uterine regenerative process [68].

Although the reported investigations conformed the myometrial origin of pseudocapsule, it has never been established its biological genesis. Thus authors analyzed the nature of this uterine structure by defining the mutational state of Mediator Complex Subunit 12 (MED12) gene, known to be mutated in more that 70 % of fibroids [70], in leiomyoma pseudocapsule by a genetic investigation [71].

MED12 gene encode for a component of the Mediator Complex, which act as a transcription factor involved in general and specific gene regulation. Mutations in MED12 gene could [70] be involved in the overall gene de-regulation commonly observed in fibroids and, as a consequence, in its genesis and evolution [72].

In our prospective, non-randomized, observational study (level of evidence II-2), samples of uterine leiomyomas (ULs) and corresponding uterine myometrium (UM) and PC were collected from 36 females who underwent at laparoscopic myomectomy by the intracapsular technique mentioned above [7, 54]. Patient selection was based upon the following criteria: pain or pressure symptoms, ULs causing infertility or reproductive dysfunction, large and growing UFs, or menstrual disorders. Women taking oral contraceptives, GnRH analogues or other hormonal therapies were not included in this study. Additional exclusion criteria as abnormal uterine bleeding, endometrial hyperplasia, uterine polyps, cervical intraepithelial neoplasia, uterine or cervical cancer, and confirmed or suspected primary adnexal pathology were additionally applied according to the presurgical US examinations, by bidimensional (2D) power Doppler ultrasound (PDU) studies, performed in the first 10 days of menstrual cycle, either with a Logic 7 Pro US system (GE-Kretz, Zipf, Austria), an IU 22 xMATRIX US system (Philips Healthcare, Eindhoven, the Netherlands), or a Voluson 730 US system (GE-Kretz, Zipf, Austria) equipped with a 3.8–5.2 MHz transvaginal transducer. All machines had a standard US setting of Doppler and gray scale, provided by companies. Presurgical vaginal US was performed by 2 well-trained physicians with similar expertise to determine the number, size, and location of any fibroid together with the pseudocapsule, which presents as a white ring surrounding the fibroid and is often colored as a "ring of fire" by Doppler scans. LIM was performed using a standardized method previously described. During the operation, the surgeons sampled specimens for analysis. Tissues sampled from the fibroids were taken to approximately 20 mm in depth, including the full thickness of the UL, the UL-PC interface and the surrounding UM; samples of the PC were obtained using scissors as soon as good hemostasis was achieved, while the UM tissues were biopsied at a distance of 2 cm from the UL. The samples were transported to the laboratory for subsequent analysis.

The patients' ages ranged from 32 to 45 years, with an average of 38.5 years. Twenty females had subserous ULs (55.6 %), 16 females had intramural ULs (44.4 %), 15 had single ULs (41.7 %), and 21 had multiple ULs (58.3 %). Authors investigated MED12 gene mutational state by PCR on genomic DNA followed by direct sequencing from each of the 36 ULs collected and their corresponding PCs. Since up to now most mutations in ULs have been found in intervening sequence (IVS) I and in exon 2 of MED12 gene, we focused our analysis on this portion of the gene. We identified specific already known missense mutation in 12 ULs and different deletions never described before in other 6 ULs (data not shown). We extended the analysis to the corresponding pseudocapsules and we find that none of the pseudocapsules associated to a mutated UL show the corresponding mutation. The same wild type profile was obtained by sequencing of the genomic DNA extracted from randomly selected UMs. To the best of our knowledge, we showed, for the first time, the non tumor origin of the PC, by analyzing the mutational state of the MED12 gene. Mutations in MED12 gene could be involved in the overall gene de-regulation commonly observed in fibroids and, as a consequence, in its genesis and evolution. We confirm the high frequency (18 out of 36) of mutations in MED12 gene among our set of fibroids; then we extend the analysis to the corresponding PCs and we find that each PC show a wild type sequence profile, even when associated to a MED12-mutated UL.

This data clearly indicate the non-tumor origin of the PC and a genomic profile comparable to that of the adjacent healthy myometrium, whose MED12 sequence always results as wild type too. The gene expression profile of PC is well distinguishable from that of the fibroid, as well: in particular it exhibits lower IGF-2 and higher endoglin/CD105 transcript levels when compared to the UL [68]. Since IGF-2 overexpression is known to be a specific leiomyoma marker, this data seem to support the non-tumor origin of PC; by the other side, the high expression level of endoglin gene, involved in neo-angiogenic processes and wound healing [73, 74], could explain the regenerative processes observed at the scar site, after a myomectomy performed by pseudocapsule sparing.

Another genetic investigation [75] involved the analysis of insulin-like growth factor II (IGF-2) and collagen type IV alpha 2 (COL4A2) expression levels in the same set of ULs. To assess whether the MED12 mutational state affects the gene expression profile in UL, we analyzed, using quantitative real-time PCR, the expression of IGF-2 and COL4A2 in our set of ULs. These genes were selected for this investigation because they are known to be up-regulated in UL when compared to matching myometrium. On the basis of the different mutational status, the UL samples were divided into three groups: group A consisted of samples without MED12 mutations, group B consisted of samples exhibiting deletions in the MED12 gene, and group C consisted of samples harboring missense mutations. Firstly, we defined IGF-2 and COL4A2 expression level in UM: we observed that the health tissues always express low level of both genes without any statistical variation depending on the corresponding UL's state ($p = 0.84$ by Kruskal–Wallis test). As a consequence, having ascertained that expression levels in ULs are not influenced by basal levels of expression in the corresponding UMs, we were able to compare the three groups of ULs, directly considering the mRNA relative units of expression of IGF-2 and COL4A2. The analysis of the IGF-2 expression level revealed a significant difference among the groups ($p = 0.0004$ by Kruskal–Wallis test). In particular, the mean relative expression units were significantly higher as assessed by the Mann-Whitney tests in group C (0.017 units mean) compared with group A (0.004 units mean, $p = 0.0004$) and group B (0.003 units mean, $p = 0.002$). The difference between groups A and B was not statistically significant ($p = 0.76$ by the Mann-Whitney test). These data demonstrated a specific correlation between missense mutations in exon 2 of the MED12 gene and IGF-2 overexpression. Conversely, the COL4A2 mRNA levels, although resulted higher in ULs when compared to those expressed by the corresponding UMs, showed no significant differences among the three groups of samples ($p = 0.132$ by Kruskal–Wallis test).

Concluding, the study interestingly revealed that only those with MED12-missense mutations expressed significantly higher levels of the IGF-2 gene. Otherwise, the MED12 gene status does not appear to affect the expression levels of the COL4A2 gene. On the basis of this finding, we suggest that the MED12 status stratified the ULs into two mutually exclusive pathways of leiomyoma genesis with IGF-2 overexpression and the absence of IGF-2 activation. The occurrence of IGF-2 overexpression could be therapeutically targeted in uterine myomas for the non-surgical myoma treatment.

Finally, since pseudocapsule is also genetically different from myoma, all pharmacological and hormonal commonly proposed treatments to prevent the growth of myomas, such as aromatase inhibitor, progestins and anti-progestins, estrogens, Selective Progestin Receptor Modulators (SPRMs), Selective Estrogen Receptor Modulators (SERMs) and GnRH, i.e., should not act on the pseudocapsule as acting on the myoma.

Uterine Myoma Pseudocapsule Analysed by Ultrasound and Histology

Fibroid pseudocapsule sizes, although its biological importance, is often underestimated by surgeons because of difficulties in visualizing the pseudocapsule during laparotomy or laparoscopy so as the pseudocapsule thickness was never morphologically measured in a study. The aim of our study was to measure the myoma pseudocapsule by a feasible and reproducible method, the gynecological ultrasound (US), comparing the thickness with histology according to fibroid location within the uterine wall.

We also hypothesized that pseudocapsule thickness depended on fibroid location within the uterine wall, whether near the endometrial cavity (FEC), intramural (IMF), or subserosal (SSF), and that the pseudocapsule thickness will be equivalent by US and histological measurement. Therefore, we planned to measure in a study [76] the presurgical fibroid pseudocapsule thickness by US and the histological features following hysterectomy in patients undergoing hysterectomy for symptomatic uterine fibroids. Thus, we organized a prospective cohort trial investigating pseudocapsule thickness using US and histology on a total, 90 women with large (from 6 cm in diameter), growing, symptomatic (pain, pressure, or menstrual) fibroids scheduled for hysterectomy. All procedures were conducted in accordance with the guidelines of the Helsinki Declaration on human experimentation. All patients had a heavy menstrual cycle and provided written, informed, and signed consent for the hysterectomy and anonymous use of information concerning fibroid pseudocapsules for research purposes. The following exclusion criteria were applied: abnormal uterine bleeding, endometrial hyperplasia, uterine polyps, cervical intraepithelial neoplasia, uterine or cervical cancer, and confirmed or suspected primary adnexal pathology. The following exclusion criteria were additionally applied according to the presurgical US examinations in order to maintain the homogeneity of fibroid pseudocapsule thickness: adenomyosis or adenomyoma and isthmic-cervical, intraligamentary, or pedunculated fibroids to give analytic homogeneity. Following presurgical US screening, 15 women were excluded and 75 patients were enrolled for further investigation. Bi-dimensional (2D) power Doppler

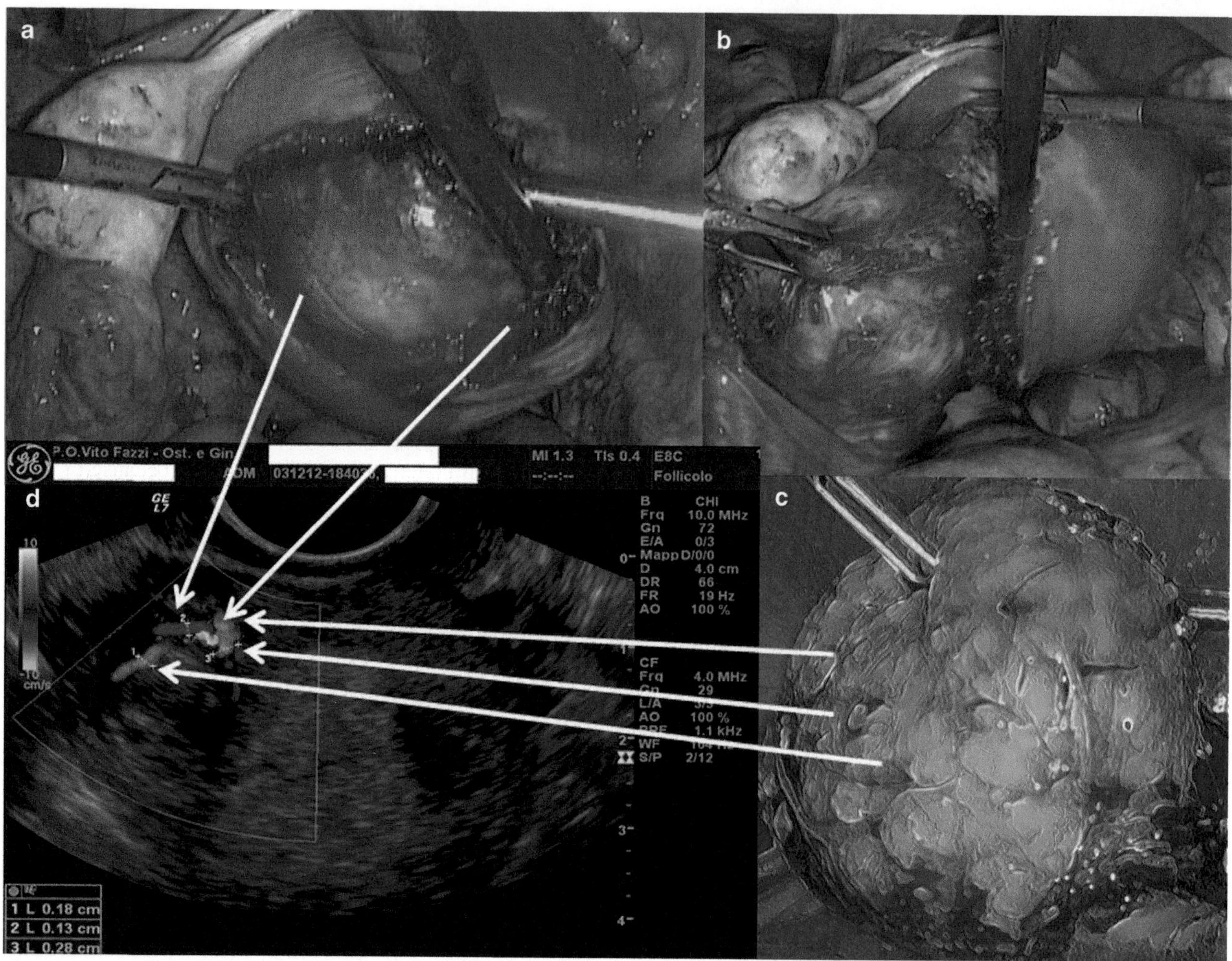

Fig. 31.21 Clockwise, starting from top left: the technique of fibroid enucleation with pseudocapsule sparing (**a–c**). White arrows indicate the pseudocapsule saved during fibroid enucleation, which appears finely covered by a thin fibrovascular matrix (neurovascular bundle). This is joined in the ultrasound image (**d**) to highlight the ring of fire during presurgical evaluation

ultrasound (PDU) studies were conducted in the first ten days of menstrual cycle, either with a Logic 7 Pro US system (GE-Kretz, Zipf, Austria), an IU 22 xMATRIX US system (Philips Healthcare, Eindhoven, The Netherlands), or a Voluson 730 US system (GE-Kretz, Zipf, Austria) equipped with a 3.8–5.2 MHz transvaginal transducer. All machines had a standard US setting of Doppler and gray scale, provided by Companies. Presurgical vaginal US was performed by two well trained physicians with similar expertise to determine the number, size, and location of any fibroid [27], together with the pseudocapsule, which presents as a white ring surrounding the fibroid and is often colored as a "ring of fire" by Doppler scans (Fig. 31.21). The fibroid pseudocapsule thickness was measured by transvaginal 2D-PDU in a clockwise manner in the longitudinal and transversal planes (Fig. 31.22), with 4 measurements: superior–inferior and lateral–lateral; measuring the thickness of two measurements, clinicians added the measurements and split for two, getting the average thickness of the myoma pseudocapsule. The US scanner cursor was placed at the thickest point between the 2 layers on the anterior and posterior pseudocapsule walls, both as regards to the white ring of fire on 2D-PDU. To analyze the fibroid location and pseudocapsule thickness, the uterus was artificially divided in a transverse plane to record each fibroid's location compared to pseudocapsule thickness. In order to strictly standardize the fibroid location in the uterus, we used the leiomyoma subclassification system of Wamsteker et al. (currently used by International Federation of Gynecology and Obstetrics), identifying subserosal fibroids (n° 6 and 5 by Wamsteker classification), intramural fibroids (n° 4), and fibroids near endometrial cavity (n° 3) [18]. All the collected thickness parameters were mapped and recorded. Total hysterectomies were performed either via laparotomy or laparoscopy in the first ten days of menstrual cycle, and the excised uterus was immediately sent to the pathology department

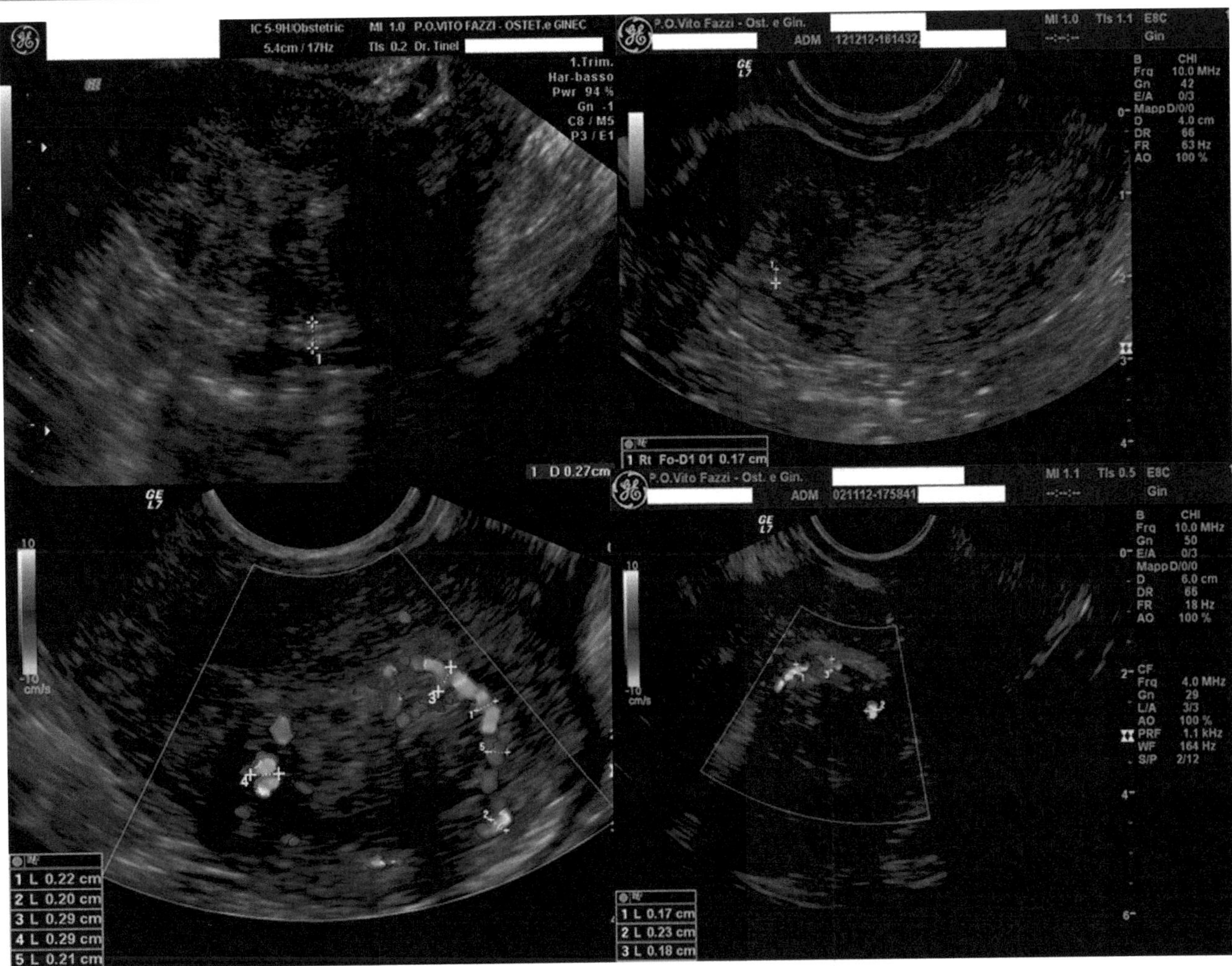

Fig. 31.22 Clockwise, starting from top left: 4 presurgical vaginal ultrasound images demonstrating the presence of the pseudocapsule as a white ring surrounding the fibroid (2 images in the *box above*) or colored as a "ring of fire" by a Doppler scan (in the *box below*)

for macroscopic and histological examination by expert pathologists, already involved in other studies on myoma pseudocapsules. Four fibroid-pseudocapsule–myometrium specimens measuring 2 × 2 cm (superior–inferior and lateral–lateral) were obtained. All specimens were numbered and fixed, before being embedded in paraffin wax for cross-sectional sagittal slices. The sections were obtained at 7-μm intervals and placed on a glass slide for Hematoxylin and Eosin staining. The fibroid-pseudocapsule–myometrium specimen borders were analyzed on each side using conventional light microscopy (10× to 40× magnification) to detail the pseudocapsule thickness.

Pathologists measured the thickness of two measurements, and then they added the measurements and split for two, getting the average thickness of the myoma pseudocapsule for histological evaluation. Artifacts were considered with the correct plane of cleavage of the fibroid from the myometrium. Finally, all US and histological data were matched by an independent researcher for comparison.

All measures are calculated as means ± Standard Deviation (Ultrasound and Histology or U&H). Both variables are normally distributed, because Q-Q plots approximate a diagonal straight line, not showed into the paper. A small difference in the skewness and in the Kurtosis between the two samples (U&H measurements) was observed. Pseudocapsule thicknesses were analyzed by one-way analysis of variance (ANOVA) with Tukey's multiple comparisons and post hoc paired t-test on US and histological measurements. Cut-off levels were defined with receiver operating characteristic (ROC) curves was used to predict sensitivity and specificity. Differences between ultrasonographic and histological pseudocapsule measurements were assessed by Bland Altman method. The nonparametric Kruskal–Wallis test was used to compare US and histological measurements (3 groups of matched measurements). A *p* value of $P < 0.05$ was considered statistically significant. Analyses were conducted with the statistical package for the Social Sciences Version 12.0 (SPSS, Inc., Chicago, IL, USA) and JMP 8 for ANOVA and Kruskal-Wallis. The following hypotheses were tested: H1- Pseudocapsule thickness differs according to fibroid location within the uterine wall sites, i.e., FEC, IMF, and SSF; H2 – Pseudocapsule thickness differs according to the examination technique employed; in this case, either US or histology. All P values are 2 – tailed.

The mean age of the 75 patients was 47 years (range 43–51). Past obstetric history was as follows: 24 %, 41 %, and 35 % had a parity of 1, 2, and ≥3, respectively. Previous delivery was vaginal in 69 % and by cesarean section in 31 %. Past surgical histories included cholecystectomy (12 %), appendectomy (25 %), ovarian cysts (27 %), and surgery for pelvic pain and adhesions (21 %). Multiple past surgeries were recorded for 22 % of the cases. None of the patients reported prior surgical complications. In total, 108 fibroids were sampled, of which 53 were from the uterine body and 55 were from the fundus. The fibroids were subdivided according to their location within the uterine wall into subserosal (n = 57), intramural (n = 33), and near the endometrial cavity (n = 18). There was no significant difference in the mean or median diameter of the fibroid in each location. The first hypothesis (H1) was analyzed by one-way ANOVA, and it was determined that significant differences in pseudocapsule thickness depended on fibroid location within the uterine wall (FEC, IMF, or SSF), independent of measurement technique (P < 0.001). The FEC pseudocapsule walls measured by US were considerably thicker than the IMF (P < 0.001) and SSF (P < 0.001) pseudocapsule walls: 2.64 ± 0.28, 1.70 ± 0.14, and 0.95 ± 0.33 mm, respectively. The thickness measured by histological examination was 2.79 ± 0.25, 1.72 ± 0.21, and 1.03 ± 0.4 mm, respectively. In turn, the IMF pseudocapsule walls were thicker than the SSF pseudocapsule walls (P < 0.001). The results were further analyzed for the second hypothesis (H2), to determine whether US pseudocapsule measurements are comparable with histological measurements. Our measurements revealed a high correlation (correlation coefficient: 0.963) and significance level (P = 0.001) using paired sample t-tests. Only IMF pseudocapsule measurements showed similarity between the histological and US methods (P = 0.625). Conversely, a significant difference was observed between measurements in FEC (P = 0.001) and SSF (P = 0.014) locations. Overall, a difference was observed between US and histological measurements (P = 0.0001) (paired sample t-test). A clear cut-off was observed between FEC pseudocapsule and all other pseudocapsule measurements, i.e., at 2 mm, the difference was significant (P = 0.001). The area under the curve (AUC) was 1 for US measurement and 0.999 for histological measurement. ROC analysis revealed that a cut off value of 2 mm provided almost 100 % sensitivity and specificity for diagnosing a FEC, in this limited sample. Overall Bland Altman limit of agreement analysis revealed that histological measurements tended to be slightly higher than ultrasonographic measurements. However, for 95 % of all cases this difference represented a small range. From a clinical standpoint this difference is unlikely to be significant. The pseudocapsule of fibroids is considerably thicker near the endometrial cavity when compared those of both intramural and subserosal fibroids. Since fibroids closest to the endometrial cavity are the most involved in fertility and infertility and fibroid pseudocapsule is considerably thicker near the endometrial cavity, it is possible to hypothesize an involvement of FP of fibroid near on endometrium, since FP contains many neuropeptides and neurotransmitters that are physiologically active, even if this data may take on a broader meaning in a study on a larger number of patients.

Another investigation [18] evaluated the uterine scar healing after laparoscopic myomectomy, monitored by traditional 2D ultrasound (US) and Doppler velocimetry, in 149 women underwent laparoscopic intracapsular myomectomy (LIM). The indications and surgical techniques were evaluated to consider the benefits and limitations of LIM. The procedures used in the present study were in accordance with guidelines of the Helsinki Declaration on human experimentation. The study protocol was carefully explained to the patients before they entered the study and written consent for operation was obtained. Patient selection was based upon the following criteria: pain or pressure symptoms, UFs causing infertility or reproductive dysfunction, large and growing UFs, or menstrual disorders. Regarding menstrual disorders, the authors used similar criteria established by an international consensus that determined normal limits for menstrual parameters in the mid-reproductive years: excessively frequent menses (each < 25 days), irregular menses (cycle-to-cycle variation greater than 20 days), excessive duration of flow (prolonged 6–8 days) and high volume of monthly blood loss [77]. Presurgical vaginal ultrasound (US) was performed by expert clinician to determine the presence of the pseudocapsule as a white ring surrounding the UF, colored by Doppler as a "ring of fire". The number, size and location of UFs were assessed and patients with suspected adenomyosis or adenomyoma were excluded. All 2D-PDU studies were performed either with a Logic 7 Pro US system (GE-Kretz, Zipf, Austria) or IU 22 xMATRIX US system (Philips Healthcare, Eindhoven, The Netherlands) or with a Voluson 730 US system (GE-Kretz, Zipf, Austria), each equipped with a 3.8–5.2 MHz transvaginal transducer. The uterus and the UF were measured in two planes, sagittal and coronal and all the data were recorded. The Resistance Index (RI) was calculated from the flow velocity waveform of the uterine arteries, at their ascending branch. Magnetic resonance imaging was not used to diagnose fibroids due to expense and time. All UFs were subserous or intramural, single or multiple, and the dominant fibroid measured between 5 and 9 cm in diameter. The study excluded women with UFs that were pedunculated, small (<3 cm in diameter) or submucous. Preoperative evaluation included office hysteroscopy to exclude submucus UFs and other uterine abnormalities. We used the UF classification system of Wamsteker to describe fibroid location, as usually done. Preoperative treatment with GnRH analogues was performed in rare cases, to avoid distortion of the UF pseudocapsule [52, 53, 78]. All patients received prophylactic Cefazolin 2 g I.V prior to laparoscopy and an intrauterine manipulator was used. Laparoscopic myomectomy was performed under general anesthesia by endotracheal intubation with a standardized four port approach: one port for the laparoscope and three lower quadrant ancillary ports (one suprapubic central 10 mm port and two lateral 5 mm ports). The 10 mm central suprapubic port was often changed to 15–20 mm for the introduction of the morcellator at the end of the procedure. Laparoscopic myomectomy by the intracapsular technique was performed without injection of an ischemic solution, as vasopressin, into the myometrium [7]. Its use could mask the musculature vascularization by collapsing vessels, making difficult the selective and gentle pseudocapsule vessel hemostasis during LIM and favouring subsequent intra-myometrial hematomas. Authors used the US to monitor the scar size and the muscular healing following LIM, detailed as following for consistency in the study. The visceral peritoneum was incised in the midline longitudinal plane with monopolar scissors or a crochet needle electrode, quickly proceeding into the myometrium to reach the right plane to detect the fibroid below. Once the pseudocapsule was identified, it was exposed by a Johannes or Manhes clamp or by an irrigator cannula to provide a panoramic laparoscopic view of the pseudocapsule. The pseudocapsule was opened with a longitudinal cut using monopolar scissors or a crochet needle to expose the UF surface. Then the fibroid was secured by a myoma screw or Collins laparoscopic forceps to provide the traction necessary for gentle enucleation, and inserting the irrigator cannula into the space between the UF pseudocapsule and fibroid for assistance. Hemostasis of the small vessels was selectively achieved using a low energy bipolar clamp or by monopolar crochet, to free the base of the UF and the connective bridges from the pseudocapsule, with minimal trauma, minimal blood loss, and pseudocapsule sparing. In cases of deep intramural UFs, chromopertubation was applied via a cervical cannula not only to check tubal patency but also to facilitate the direct recognition of an inadvertently opened uterine cavity. The myometrium was closed in a single (for subserous) or double layer (for intramural) with 1/0 Vicryl (polyglactine; Ethicon, USA), including overlying serosa, with a round CT-1 curved needle, using intra or extracorporeal knots. In sub-serosal myomectomies (types 5 and 6), the edges of the uterine defect were approximated with introflexing U-inverted stitches (myometrium/serosa-serosa/myometrium direction) at 1 cm increments (a baseball-type suture). Interrupted closure or a traditional unidirectional running suture was chosen by the surgeon. Deep intramural UFs (types 2–5 and 3) were closed in two-layers using introflexing baseball-type sutures. If the uterine cavities were accidentally opened during UF enucleation, 2–3 single or continuous sutures were used to close the edge of the uterine cavity. UFs were morcellated with a reusable Rotocut G1 morcellator (Karl Storz GmbH & Co. KG, Germany) or by a Gynecare Morcellex tissue morcellator (Ethicon, Inc., Somerville, NJ, USA). Patients were re-evaluated by transvaginal US on days 1, 7, 30 and 45 after surgery. The myometrial scar pattern was compared to the previous myometrial area occupied by the UF. The scar diameter was measured by placing callipers on the outer edge of the echogenic, heterogeneous, and ill-defined area to determine the healing pattern of the uterine scar after LIM [79–82]. Moreover, authors measured the RI of the uterine arteries at their ascending branch during each US examination. The myometrial area of the scar was calculated as the percentage of the preoperative UF diameter. The parameters were analyzed by an independent statistician using the Student's t-test for paired samples. A significant p-value was considered as $p < 0.05$.

One hundred and thirty-six operated patients completed the study and the follow up. The mean age of our population was 37.2 ± 3.6 years (range 33–40 years), mean BMI was 22.9 ± 2.5 and mean parity was 1.3 ± 0.7. The primary preoperative indications included pelvic pain in 24 %, menorrhagia or metrorrhagia in 23 %, a large growing UF in 13 %, and infertility in 40 %. The size of UFs was 5–6 cm diameter in 35 women (25.7 %), 6–7 cm in 37 (27.2 %), 7–8 cm in 34 (25 %), and 8–9 cm in 30 women (22.1 %). UF were subserosal in 48 women (35.2 %) and intramural in 88 (64.8 %). Of the 136 women, 82 had a single fibroid (60.2 %): 29 subserous (35.3 %) and 53 intramural (64.7 %). Fifty-four had multiple UFs (39.7 %): 19 subserous (35.2 %) and 35 intramural (64.8 %). Of the 48 subserosal fibroids, 29 were type 5 (60.4 %) and 19 were type 6 (39.6 %), with no type 7. Of the 88 intramural UF, 21 were transmural types 2-5 (23.8 %), 38 were type 3 (43.1 %) and 29 were type 4 (33.1 %). Single intracapsular myomectomy was performed for intramural fibroids in 7 women with UF types 2–5 (33.3 %), 16 with type 3 (42.1 %) and 17 with type 4 (58.6 %), and for subserous fibroids in 16 patients with type 5 (55.1 %) and 11 with type 6 (57.8 %). Multiple intracapsular myomectomy was performed for intramural fibroids in 14 women with UF type 2–5 (66.7 %), 22 with type 3 (57.9 %) and 12 with type 4 (41.4 %), and for subserous fibroids in 13 patients with UF type 5 (44.9 %) and 8 with type 6 (42.2 %). Two women (1.4 %) were pre-treated with 3.75 mg leuprolide acetate for 3 months before surgery to shrink the UFs. During surgery, a monopolar crochet needle was used to cut the connective bridges of the pseudocapsule from the surrounding myometrium in 59 women (43.4 %), and bipolar clamp scissors (30 W energy) were used in the remaining 77 (56.6 %). The uterine cavity was entered during myomectomy in 2 women with a single UF (2.4 %) and in 5 with multiple UFs (9.2 %). All laparoscopies were successful without conversion to laparotomy.

On the first and 7th post-operative days, the US pattern of uterine scar area was represented by a highly echogenic area having an-ill defined heterogeneous myometrial texture; from day 30–45 the image shifted to a normal echogenic myometrial texture. There was a progressive reduction of uterine scar. The scar after LIM was 78 % of the previous UF diameter on the first day, 61 % on 7th day, and 19 % on the 30th day, and disappeared (<4 %) on the 45th day. The progressive reduction in size of US pattern of uterine scar area was significant ($p < 0.05$). There was no correlation with the size of the fibroid and the relative reduction in the scar diameter, either on days 1 or 45. There was an increase of the RI value of the ipsilateral uterine arteries from 0.57 of the preoperative day (range 0.45–0.69) to 0.65 on the first post-operative day (range 0.59–0.73). This difference was statistically significant ($p < 0.05$). After 1 week the RI was always elevated to 0.83 (range 0.74–0.92), then the RI decreased to 0.71 (range 0.59–0.83) at the 30th post operative day and to 0.61 (range 0.50–0.72) at the 45th post operative day. All of these comparisons were statistically significant ($p < 0.05$). During the postoperative US evaluations, the authors noted the persistence of small linear hyperechoic points, the stitches of polyglactine that have an absorption time of 50–60 days. No important fluid-filled areas were seen. The authors found a few small anechoic areas < 5 mm at the site of LIM on the first day, and two patients had an anechoic area of 1–2 cm at the myomectomy site (1.5 %), possibly indicating the presence of a hematoma.

Basing on these results, the myometrial area of the scar after LIM can be followed by 2D US and Doppler velocimetry, a non-invasive, safe method to check uterine perfusion, postoperative hematoma and disechogenic, heterogeneous, or an ill-defined scar area, all unfavourable signs for myometrial scarring. Moreover, Doppler transvaginal monitoring, evaluating PI and RI of the uterine arteries at their ascending branch, could identify patients with altered PI and RI parameters, possible markers of impaired wound healing.

The Potential Impact of Pseudocapsule Sparing on Muscular Healing

Uterine muscle is an amazing tissue, specialized to generate force but for that function to be well-served, muscle must be a precisely organized and excitable tissue, in function to pregnancy, labor and delivery. It also shows an impressive ability to adapt to changing functional demands during fetal growth, and provides a major site for energy storage for labor.

Uterine myometrial repair and regeneration that follow surgical injury, as myomectomy, requires that muscle first re-establish homeostasis following the damaging perturbation and then restore the normal structural and functional capacities of the fully differentiated tissue. Restoration of muscle structure and function is a key, early feature in successful repair and regeneration of muscle. However, muscle membrane damage itself can initiate signalling processes that activate muscle regeneration. The synthesis and release of signalling molecules that are activated by muscle fibers subjected to membrane damage can induce the activation and attraction of a diverse population of cells that promote muscle regeneration and growth [83]. Following acute muscle injury, the sequence of muscle injury-repair-regeneration leads to full functional recovery with days to weeks of the initial damage [84].

A vital process in the regeneration of an injured muscle is the vascularization of the injured area. The restoration of vascular supply to the injured area is the first sign of regeneration and a prerequisite for the subsequent morphological and functional recovery of the injured muscle. The new capillaries sprout from the surviving trunks of the blood vessels toward the centre of the injured area to provide the area with an adequate supply of oxygen, subsequently enabling aerobic energy metabolism for the regenerating myofibers [85].

In such regenerative process, there is also the involvement of neuropeptides and neurotransmitters, extremely important in wound healing. In fact, there is evidence that the nervous system and its neurotransmitters, such as Substance P (SP), Vasoactive Intestinal Peptide (VIP), neuropeptide Y (NPY), Oxytocin, Vasopressin (VP), PGP9.5, calcitonin gene-related peptide (CGRP), growth hormone-releasing hormone (GHRH), play a role in mediating inflammation and healing [83, 85–87].

Referring to uterine musculature scar physiology, these peptides sparing enhances a correct healing of a hysterotomy. Most of these neuropeptides have been highlighted in the pseudocapsule, as evidenced [48, 49, 55, 56].

As the neuropeptides are transported to the tissues by the neurovascular network, the myoma pseudocapsule, as neurovascular bundle [49], is therefore a structure rich of neuropeptides. Pseudocapsule vessels were also studied by a preliminary three-dimensional mathematical model [50], who showed an increase vascular tortuosity, disarray, an abnormal branching and the presence of “cul-de-sac” pseudocapsule vessels. All of these features are similar to malignant neoplastic tissue vessels features, present in malignant tumors. It was not possible to clarify if the pseudocapsule vasculature network could be sustained by mechanical and inflammatory effects of myoma on myometrium, or produced by a sort of neoangiogenesis "neoplastic-type", due to the fibroid growth or even to a muscle and tissue healing process, such as a neurovascular preparative reaction of female body to a fibroid expulsion (pedunculated fibroids), necrosis or degeneration, allowing a normal uterine restoration [88].

In human body, difficulties in obtaining serial samples of the hysterotomic scar during myomectomy or cesarean section, are a major barrier to our understanding of the events involved in the post-myomectomy and post-cesarean section remodelling processes of the uterine wound. They can be only monitored by ultrasound or MRI [18].

However, irrespective of the ultimate result, wound healing is a dynamic, interactive process involving neuromediators, angiogenetic factors, neuropeptides, blood cells, extracellular matrix, and parenchymal cells that follows three complex and overlapping phases: inflammation, tissue formation, and tissue remodelling [89].

And the biochemical growth factors evaluated in the pseudocapsule vessels cause intense angiogenesis in pseudocapsule, probably promoted by the fibroids [68].

Anyway, the biological genesis of myoma pseudocapsule sustains the necessity either to better analyze hormonal and pharmacological impacts of drugs on pseudocapsule (based on reducing fibroid growth without compromise pseudocapsule properties), or to remodelling the presurgical uterine fibroid therapy and the post-surgical follow up, in order to preserve uterine functionality, as much as possible.

Translation of Scientific Research on Myoma Pseudocapsule on Medical and Surgical Practice

Since the ultimate goal of scientific research is the application in clinical practice, I tried to translate the studies on the myoma pseudocapsule in surgical practice of reproductive surgery. Fibroids can cause clinical symptoms and myomectomy can significantly improve symptoms and quality of life and, in some clinical situations, improve reproductive outcomes in aged women, who delay childbirth into their 30s and 40s, when the incidence of fibroids is significantly increased. So far, reproductive surgery was supported by a large number of publications that have discussed the benefits of myomectomy. However, very few articles have evaluated, per se, the rationale of the surgical technique, explaining all the steps of the scientific techniques. And this is what I tried to do I explain the rationale for the removal of myomas starting with the preservation of its pseudocapsule, rich of neurotrasmitters and vessels, a neurovascular bundle containing neuropeptides and related fibers surrounding prostate [88].

The idea of a neurovascular bundle surrounding a myoma, inside pseudocapsule, derives from a multidisciplinary discussion among gynecologists and urologists, on analogies of myoma pseudocapsule with the prostate capsule. Based on the purpose of reducing the probability of impotence associated prostate cancer treatment, urologist generally must preserve neurovascular bundles surrounds prostate. Anatomically, the neurovascular bundles are situated on the peripheral to the prostate.

The prostatic neurovascular bundle provide both somatic and autonomic innervations to the continence mechanism. The excision of neurovascular bundle causes more incontinence and impotency than when the neurovascular bundles are preserved [49, 88]. In order to spare the prostatic neurovascular bundles, laparoscopic or robotic assisted prostatectomy are both useful [90], since the magnification facilitates a more gentle dissection with less traction and careful dissection [91].

Although these nerves are microscopic [92], their anatomic location can be evaluated intraoperatively through the use of the capsular vessels as a landmark. An opening in the levator fascia is performed by sharp incision along the anterolateral surface of the prostate starting at the base of the prostate and proceeding toward the apex. This manoeuvre releases the bundle laterally, thus making it easier to make the next step, where the bundle is released posteriorly at the apex. Once the superficial fascia has been released, the site of the neurovascular bundles can be identified by the presence of a thin "groove" on the posterolateral edge of the prostate. The interfascial plane (i.e., between the levator and prostatic fascia) is developed gently using blunt dissection with a fine curved dissector and a gentle diathermocoagulation. Dissection continues in close approximation to the surface of the prostatic fascia in efforts to optimize quantitative cavernous nerve preservation. If bleeding occurs from periprostatic vessels, insufflation pressure can be in the meanwhile increased and pressure applied to the source of bleeding with hemostatic gauze. Hemostasis with high wattage diathermocoagulation or ultrasonic heat energy should be always avoided during dissection near the neurovascular bundles, as these energy sources have been shown to be injurious to cavernous nerve function in the canine model [93].

On the bases of these findings about the importance of the prostatic capsule and the important and physiologic role of nerve-sparing techniques for prostatectomy, and comparing this structure to the fibroid pseudocapsule, the knowledge of peripheral neurovascular bundle of the uterine leiomyoma was challenged and revisited by me and my colleagues (Fig. 31.23).

In fact, literature showed the possibility to perform myomectomy by removing the fibroid from its surrounding structure, the fibroid pseudocapsule [94, 95], I called "intracapsular myomectomy" [7, 79]. It performs by stretching and extracting fibroid directly from the surrounding fibromuscular skeleton, breaking up the fibrous bridges.

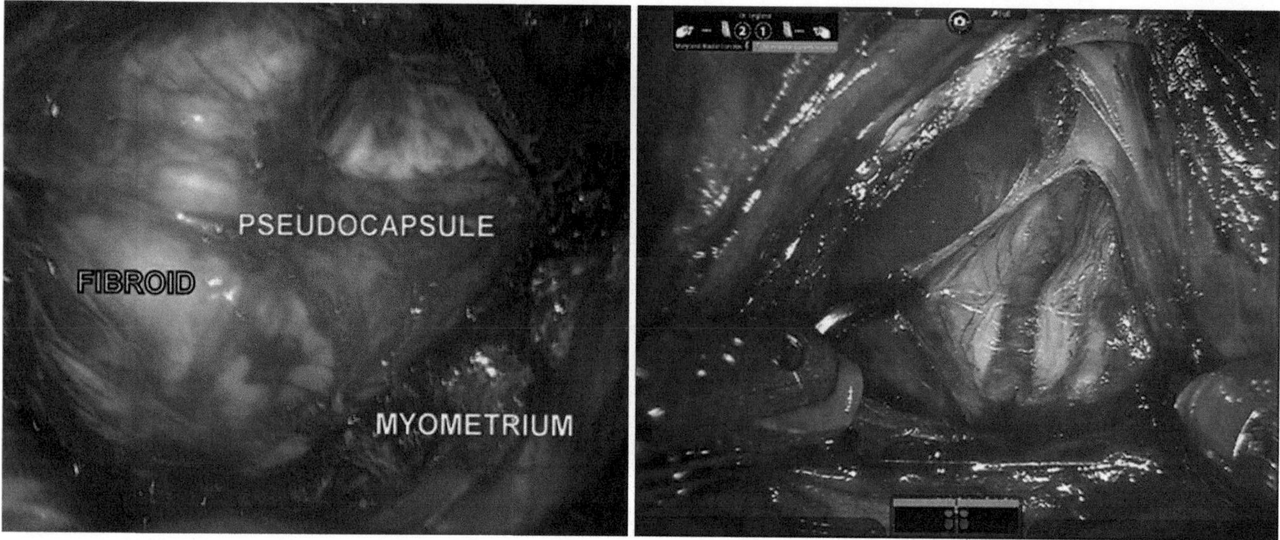

Fig. 31.23 A parallelism between laparoscopic myomectomy sparing pseudocapsule (*on the left*) and radical robotic prostatectomy sparing prostatic vein and neurovascular bundle (*on the right*)

The general myomectomy dogma is that "each surgical fibroid enucleating needs to be gently performed to enhance a correct healing process of the uterine musculature and to facilitate successively the correct uterine musculature anatomical-functional restoring".

So, the main principle of myomectomy is to perform all manipulations as precisely and bloodlessly as possible, and the new surgical technique of intracapsular myomectomy meets this requirement. Nevertheless, the impact of surgical myomectomy differs depending on the technique used [96]. The laparotomic myomectomy is different from the laparoscopic technique, also with same intracapsular method: the laparoscopic access route proved to be the most beneficial. The advantages of the laparoscopic approach are the significantly reduced parameters of both intra- and post-surgical blood loss, decreased bladder pain after Foley removal, the lower number of patients requiring pain relief medication and the shorter hospital stay. In addition, laparoscopic intracapsular myomectomy resulted in slightly improved short-term outcomes in relation to postoperative fever, myometrium scar hematomas, ileus and antibiotic treatment compared to open surgery. Finally, the laparoscopic myomectomy has a favourable impact on blood loss by intracapsular method, aiming to preserve musculature under hysterotomy. The CO2 insufflation can influence blood loss during intracapsular myomectomy, as the increased intraperitoneal pressure can lead to the occlusion of the small blood vessels and capillaries of the pseudocapsule. This effect, combined with less traumatic endoscopic micro-manipulations, could result in beneficial outcomes of surgery. To better clarify these results, I remember that my intracapsular myomectomy was standardized and published [7, 79].

Laparoscopic myomectomies are performed under general anesthesia by endotracheal intubation with a standardized four port approach: one port for the laparoscope and three lower quadrant ancillary ports (one suprapubic central 10 mm port and two lateral 5 mm ports). The 10 mm central suprapubic port is often changed to 15–20 mm for the introduction of the morcellator at the end of the procedure. All patients receive an intrauterine manipulator prior to laparoscopy, to better mobilize uterus. Intracapsular laparoscopic myomectomy of sub mucous and intramural fibroids is generally performed without injection of ischemic solution into the myometrium. The visceral peritoneum is incised in the midline longitudinal plane, by monopolar scissors or crochet needle electrode, proceeding in depth into myometrium to reach the right plane under myometrium, to detect myoma pseudocapsule with the fibroid below.

Once identified the myoma pseudocapsule, it is well exposed by atraumatic clamp or by irrigator cannula, to provide a panoramic laparoscopic view of pseudocapsule of all subserous-intramural leiomyomas. Then surgeon affects the pseudocapsule by a longitudinal cut, performed by monopolar scissors or Hook electrode at low wattage (30 W), to expose the myoma surface. Then fibroid is hooked by a myoma screw or Collins laparoscopic forceps to perform the traction necessary for its gentle enucleating, helping by irrigator cannula to be inserted in the space under myoma pseudocapsule and fibroid. Hemostasis of the small vessels bleeding is selectively achieved by a low wattage bipolar clamp or by Hook electrode or monopolar scissors, always at 30 W, to free the base of the myoma and the connective bridges from the pseudocapsule. In such way, complete minimal traumatic fibroid removal from its pseudocapsule was accomplished with a minimal blood loss and pseudocapsule sparing. In case of pseudo-pedunculated myomas, the pedicle is coagulated by bipolar forceps and cut by laparoscopic scissors or cut after placement of loops or staples, without suturing. In cases of deep intramural myomas, chromopertubation is always applied via a cervical cannula not only to check tubal patency but also to facilitate the direct recognition of an inadvertently opened uterine cavity.

The myometrium closuring is performed by a single (for subserous fibroids) or double layer (for intramurals), including overlying serosa, with a round CT-1 curved needle, using intra or extracorporeal knots. In sub-serosal myomectomies, the edges of the uterine defect were approximated with introflexing U-inverted stitches (myometrium/serosa-serosa/myometrium direction) with intra myometrial knot, at 1 cm increments from the edge of the incision (as a "baseball-type" suture). The closure was by surgeon choice: interrupted closure or traditional unidirectional running suture, stared at the end of one of hysterotomic sides.

Deep intramural fibroids required a two-layer myometrial closure with introflexing sutures, ever by a "baseball-type" suture. If the uterine cavity was accidentally opened during fibroid enucleating, 2–3 deep myometrial single or continuous sutures were applied on the uterine cavity edges. After hysterorrhaphy, fibroids are usually morcellated.

Thus, during myomectomy, as reported by literature [88], the fibroid pseudocapsule neurovascular bundle needs to be always protected, avoiding destructive surgical proceedings such as extensive and high wattage diathermocoagulation (> 30 W) or excessive tissue manipulating or trauma. This method of myomectomy maximally respects the fibroid pseudocapsule neurovascular bundle, rich of neurofibers involved in the correct successive scar healing. The iatrogenic myoma pseudocapsule damage should therefore alter the successive neurotransmitters' function in myometrial repair, with negative effect on uterine healing. Thus, the surgical sequels of an uncorrected myomectomy with pseudocapsule damaging should be: a reduction in neurofibers' presence at hysterotomic site, a deterioration of uterine musculature healing, and a deficit either of myometrial neurotransmission or of muscular impulse and contractility, with final reduced uterine musculature functionality.

The Intracapsular Cesarean Myomectomy

This type of technique to perform a myomectomy sparing pseudocapsule can also be reproduced in another very complex and risky operation: the cesarean myomectomy.

Uterine myomas are observed these days more frequently in pregnancy with an estimated incidence of 2–4 %, because many women are delaying childbearing until their late thirties or the beginning of their forties, the time of greatest risk for myoma growth [97, 98]. Uterine myomas are commonly encountered in women older than 30 years [99] and their growth is directly related to exposure to the circulating estrogens levels. The prevalence of leiomyomas among pregnant women ranges from 0.1 to 3.9 % [99–104]. The effective rate of uterine myomas in pregnancy is unknown; however, they are associated with numerous pregnancy-related maternal and fetal complications like spontaneous abortion, preterm labor, placental abruption, post partum hemorrhage and high rate of cesarean deliveries [99, 105].

Complications in pregnancy, labor and delivery occur almost twice as frequently among women diagnosed with uterine myomas than in those without [99–103]. The literature suggests a high rate of cesarean deliveries in women with myomas up to 39.95 % [106].

Thus, any surgical procedure performed on or around the uterus has the potential of causing severe hemorrhage and, for this reason, uterine myomectomy during cesarean section has consistently been discouraged, in the past years, as a high-risk procedure.

On the contrary, resection of an intramural myoma is inadvisable and contraindicated during cesarean section by some obstetric textbooks [107, 108], due to the risk of profuse uncontrolled bleeding that could lead to hysterectomy.

So, after the development of my well detailed and published technique [7, 18, 79], the intracapsular myomectomy, successfully performed during laparoscopy in non pregnant women with single or multiple fibroids, the authors decided to study their methods of myomas removal during CS, exploring its outcomes (Fig. 31.24).

Thus I prospectively evaluated the surgical outcome of intracapsular myomectomy during CS by a case-control study on 68 patients who underwent intracapsular cesarean myomectomy, compared with a control group of 72 patients with myomatosic pregnant uterus who underwent cesarean section without myomectomy [109].

All operations were ever performed by CS by Stark's method, under regional anesthesia. A routine intracapsular cesarean myomectomy was then done for all anterior fibroids: cervical, body, or fundal, using the same cesarean incision where possible, or utilizing other incisions, when necessary. Each intracapsular cesarean myomectomy was performed after LUS closure. A linear incision was made over the uterine serosa direct to myoma by a scalpel or a monopolar electro-scalpel at low voltage (≤ 30 W), gradually until opening the pseudocapsule, enabling to enter the relatively bloodless plan between the pseudocapsule and its myoma. Once the surface of the myoma was reached and its fibre bridges separated, the myoma was hooked and extracted from its capsule, also by traction and pushing down the capsule using a sharp Metzenbaum scissors. The hemostasis during intracapsular cesarean myomectomy was always reached by gentle low voltage coagulation (≤ 30 W) of pseudocapsule vessels, with minimal blood loss. Generally, 10 I.U. of intravenous oxytocin drip was given as a standard to

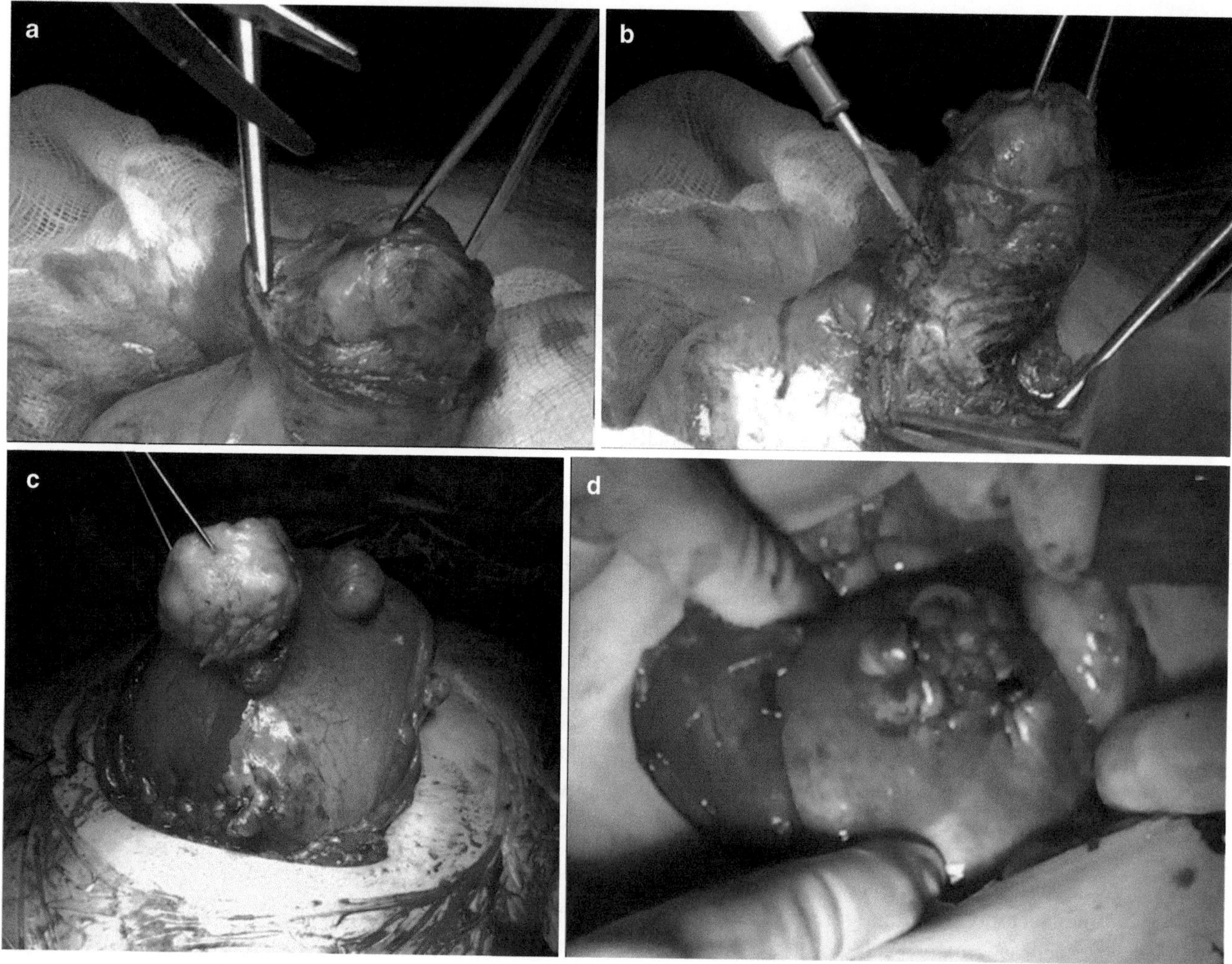

Fig. 31.24 Intracapsular cesarean myomectomy: (**a**) pregnant uterine incision after hysterorrhaphy and myoma pseudocapsule exposure by scissors; (**b**) gentle myoma dissection from myometrium; (**c**) myoma enucleating; (**d**) suture of uterine wall after myoma enucleation

all patients to control bleeding, after enucleating of the fibroid. For myomas located near LUS, we temporarily changed operation' steps: after completion of the CS, an interlocked suture is temporarily placed on the edge of the cesarean uterine incision without closure. Then we performed intracapsular cesarean myomectomies from the edge of the cesarean incision. This also facilitates working from within the uterine cavity or from the outer part of the uterus without significant bleeding from the CS incision. After that, in case of other myomas far from LUS, surgeons made a new incision above the myoma in instances where they were located in a site remote from the CS incision. Suturing of the fibroid base was routinely performed by using two layers of interrupted absorbable sutures (1–0 calibre vicryl) and a baseball-type suture was used for the serosa, using a continuous absorbable suture (2– 0 or 3–0 calibres vicryl), as a third layer. Pelvic irrigation was done with saline solution. Postoperatively, the oxytocin infusion was continued for 12–24 h in parallel with normal saline infusion. Seventy-two control subjects were randomly selected among pregnant women with myomas undergoing CS without myomectomy, at the same Institutions and during the same period, and CS' indications were: breech presentation, more than one previous CS, CS on demand. These women did not receive cesarean myomectomy since they refuse this operations and both myomectomy and control groups were similar in terms of characteristics without any statistical differences.

Most of the removed myomas were subserous or intramural: 48 subserous, 14 intramural and 6 pedunculated. Of these, 12 had multiple sites myomas (17,6 %), but we try to use always the same hysterotomy for neighbours fibroids.

Sites of myomas' removal were: fundal in 37 women (54.4 %), corporal in 22 (32.3 %) and around the lower uterine segment in 9 women (18.7 %), where we temporarily changed operation' steps just in 5 women. The average myoma' size was 8 cm (1.5–20), in 40 women, with 8 myomas measuring 4–6 cm, 14 myomas between 10 and 12 cm and > 13 cm in 6 patients. Differences in blood chemistry and surgical outcome in intracapsular cesarean myomectomy were not statistically significant ($p > 0.05$). Concerning the post-operative course, 5 patients had postpartum fever of 38.8 °C, on average, for two consecutive days after surgery (7.3 %); the blood culture didn't show any bacteria and patients were treated by large spectrum antibiotics. The average duration of hospitalization of intracapsular cesarean myomectomies was 5 days, with six patients requiring more than 5 days of hospital stay (8,8 %); these five patients felt too weak to be discharged, so they preferred to stay in the hospital an extra day.

There was no correlation between complications or duration of hospital stay and patient age, gravidity, parity or indication for CS. None of the patients underwent repeated surgery after intracapsular cesarean myomectomy and no hysterectomy was required after intracapsular cesarean myomectomy. My data show no difference between intracapsular cesarean myomectomy group and control group, in term of pre and post-operative hemoglobin values, mean change in hemoglobin values, incidence of intraoperative hemorrhage, frequency of blood transfusion and of post-operative fever. The only two parameters that affect negatively the group submitted to intracapsular cesarean myomectomy are the duration of operation and the length of hospital stay.

Since obstetricians often confronted with fibroids while performing CS and face the dilemma of how they should be managed, considering the cost-benefit of our study, authors affirmed that intracapsular cesarean myomectomy procedure can be performed with some confidence, without affecting adversely the postoperative course and clinical outcomes.

Hysteroscopic Intracapsular Myomectomy: The Cold Loop Technique

The advent of surgical endoscopy in clinical practice has led to a conservative approach to uterine fibroids, especially for women who want to have children. To date, surgical hysteroscopy is considered an effective and safe treatment for submucous myomas [110]. Hysteroscopic myomectomy is currently the most widely used minimally invasive surgical procedure for the treatment of submucous myomas [111]. Despite its widespread use and ease of implementation, several complications have been reported, some of which are particularly serious [112–115].

Different techniques have been described in the hysteroscopic treatment of submucous myomas, but cold loop myomectomy, ideally performed in a single surgical procedure, seems to be the most effective and safe treatment for G1–G2 myomas [111]. It is an effective method providing greater safety for patients and reducing surgical risks [116].

The technique, conceived by Mazzon and firstly described in 1995 [117], was developed in order to preserve the muscular fibres in the myometrium and ensures the complete removal of the myoma. Indeed, the cold loop technique allows to apply the surgical principles utilized in laparotomic and laparoscopic myomectomy [7, 88, 118] to the hysteroscopic setting.

The importance of pseudocapsule in treating myomas was stressed and a hysteroscopic procedure taking advantage from such anatomic structure was specifically designed. The enucleation of myoma within its pseudocapsule not only ensured a reduced blood loss but it also allowed a complete treatment of the intramural part of myoma. Indeed, since the beginning of hysteroscopy, the intramural extension of myomas represented a challenge for the surgeons, as it influences the possibility to complete the myomectomy in a single-step procedure [111, 119], while increasing the risk for intraoperative complications and repeated surgeries [111, 115, 120]. In case of distention media warning level reached, it is recommended to interrupt the procedure in order to avoid clinical intravasation syndrome, and a second surgery should be scheduled [121].

To ensure a blunt dissection of the fibro-connetival bridges, which anchor the myoma to the pseudocapsule, mechanical loops have been designed (Mazzon's cold loops®, Karl Storz Tuttlingen, Germany). These new instruments allows to avoid the recourse to coagulation or cutting combined with coagulation. In this way the thermal damage of surrounding myometrium and dramatic intraoperative complications, as uterine electrical loop perforation, are theoretically eliminated.

Furthermore, using the cold loop technique, the infiltration of the myoma into the myometrium, which has always been considered a major difficulty in hysteroscopic myomectomy, especially when associated with multiple myomas [111, 120], does not play an important role. Indeed, it makes the intramural extension of the fibroids an intracavitary lesion that is easy to treat.

Before the surgical act, an accurate preoperative diagnostic investigation should be done. A good surgery starts with a good diagnosis. Firstly, to assess the number and size of myomas and the extent of their intramural development, an ultrasonographic evaluation should be carried out in all the patients.

Particular attention must be paid to the measurement of the free myometrial margin (FMM), the thickness of the myometrium between the myoma and the perimetrium, because a reduced FMM is a major risk factor for uterine perforation. In order to avoid such complication, the FMM should be at least 1 cm, nevertheless, even few millimetres of FMM may be considered safe by an expert hysteroscopist. Indeed, it has been shown that this is a dynamic parameter during surgery and tends to progressively grow during the removal of the myoma [122].

However, even in case of uterine perforation, the cold loop allows to avoid the dramatic consequence due to the thermal loop [123–125].

Secondly, a diagnostic hysteroscopy is mandatory for the preoperative evaluation. The knowledge of the number, the position of myomas relatively to the uterine wall, the endometrium thickness, the presence of other intracavitary pathologies and the size of the uterine cavity, may influence the favourable outcome of the hysteroscopic myomectomy. Moreover only with the diagnostic hysteroscopy is possible to really categorize the grading of myoma, according to the classification proposed by Wamsteker [119]. Such classification, officially adopted by the European Society of Gynaecological Endoscopy organizes the myomas based on the intramural development:

- **G0**: completely endocavitary, pedunculated myoma, with no intramural extension;
- **G1**: submucous myoma with less than 50 % intramural extension;
- **G2**: submucous myoma with more than 50 % intramural extension.

Recently, multiple variables and not only the degree of myometrial penetration were considered in the "STEPW classification" proposed by Lasmar et al. [121], to more accurately predict a complete or an incomplete removal of the myoma in one-step procedure before treatment [126].

In addition to the intramural extension, the STEPW classification considered the size, topography, and extension of the base myomas in relation to the uterine wall. The five parameters of STEPW are as follows [121]:

1. Size: the largest diameter found by any of the imaging methods. When the nodule measures ≥2 cm, it is given a score of 0; if it is 2.1–5 cm, it gets a score of 1; and if it measures >5 cm, it gets a score of 2.
2. Topography: defined by the third of the uterine cavity where the fibroid is situated. If it is in the lower third, the score is 0; if in the middle third, the score is 1; and if in the upper third, the score is 2.
3. Extension of the base of the myoma: when the fibroid covers one third or less of the wall, it is given a score of 0; when the base of the nodule occupies between one and two thirds of the wall, the score is 1; and when it affects more than two thirds of the wall, the score is 2.
4. Penetration of the nodule into the myometrium: when the fibroid is completely within the uterine cavity it is given a score of 0; if it has its larger part in the uterine cavity it is given a score of 1; and when it has its larger part in the myometrium it is given a score of 2.
5. Wall: when the fibroid is on the lateral wall, 1 extra point is added regardless of the third that is affected.

In case of a score from 5 to 6, the GnRH analogue (GnRHa) preoperative treatment was suggested by the Authors.

The role of GnRHa before hysteroscopic myomectomy is still controversial in the scientific literature. Concerning the hysteroscopic myomectomy, although some papers reported longer surgical times with GnRHa [127], Muzii in a RCT [128] showed a shorter duration of the procedure. On the contrary, Mavrelos advised against the use of GnRHa before myomectomy as any benefit in such treatment was not identified [53]. A recent meta-analysis [129], including the only 2 available RCT [53, 128], concluded that GnRHa "may improve some outcomes but there is insufficient evidence to support their routine use prior to hysteroscopic resection of submucous fibroids". In order to clarify this issue, randomized controlled trials investigating the efficacy of GnRHa pre-treatment in hysteroscopic myomectomy, especially with cold loop technique, are needed.

Considering the scientific evidence available on the usefulness of the GnRHa therapy before laparoscopic or hysteroscopic myomectomy [129, 130] and based on our experience, we are able to affirm that, waiting for more consistent data, the GnRHa pre-treatment in cold loop myomectomy should be reserved only to the patients with severe anaemia.

At the end of the diagnostic (ultrasonographic and hysteroscopic) evaluation, the surgeon should gain sufficient information about the possibility to perform the procedure in one or two-step.

At the beginning of the cold loop hysteroscopic myomectomy, a dilation of the cervix is carried out.

In the event that dilation proves difficult with this technique, the resectoscope is inserted into the cervical canal to visualize the direction and to complete the dilation.

No drugs should be used for cervical dilation.

Slicing of the Intracavitary Component of the Myoma

The intracavitary component of the myoma is progressively removed up to the surface of the endometrium using the conventional slicing technique (Fig. 31.25). During this phase, an electric loop powered by a 100 W monopolar current in pure cutting mode should be used. When the cleavage plane between the myoma and myometrium is identified, the slicing is stopped.

Enucleation of the Intramural Component of the Myoma

The electric cutting loop is subsequently replaced with a cold loop, which is inserted into the cleavage plane and repeatedly applied along the surface of the myoma (Fig. 31.26). In this way the connective fibers anchoring the myoma to the myometrium are disconnected by blunt dissection (Fig. 31.26). Using the cold loop, the damage of myometrial fibers around the myoma is minimal. The muscle bundles are spared any surgical trauma owing to the thermal damage of electrical cutting.

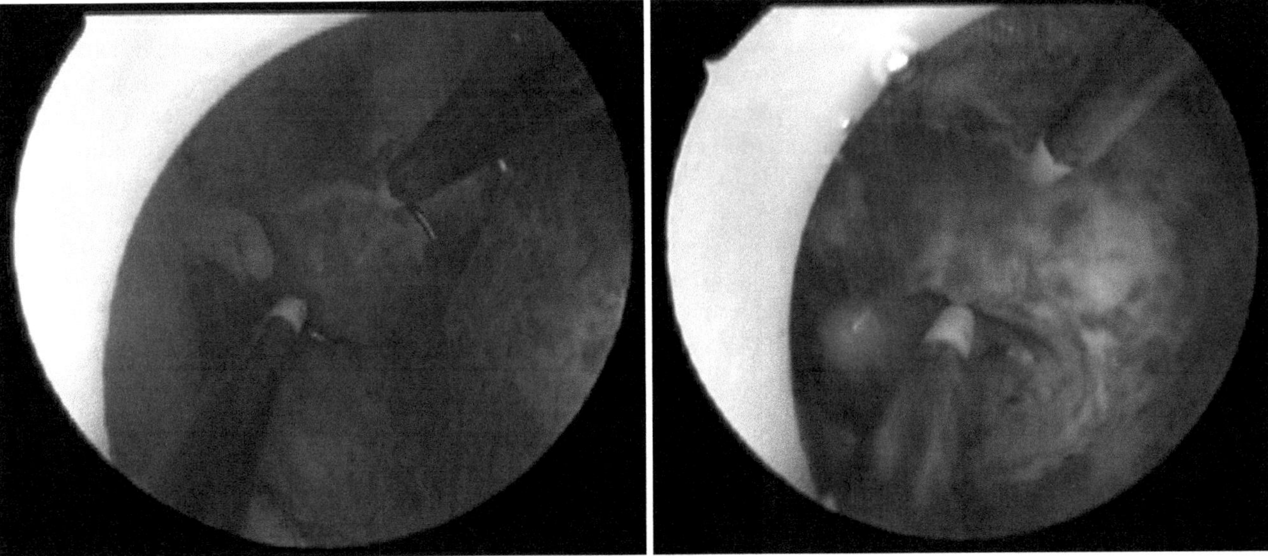

Fig. 31.25 The intracavitary component of the myoma is progressively removed up to the surface of the endometrium using the conventional slicing technique

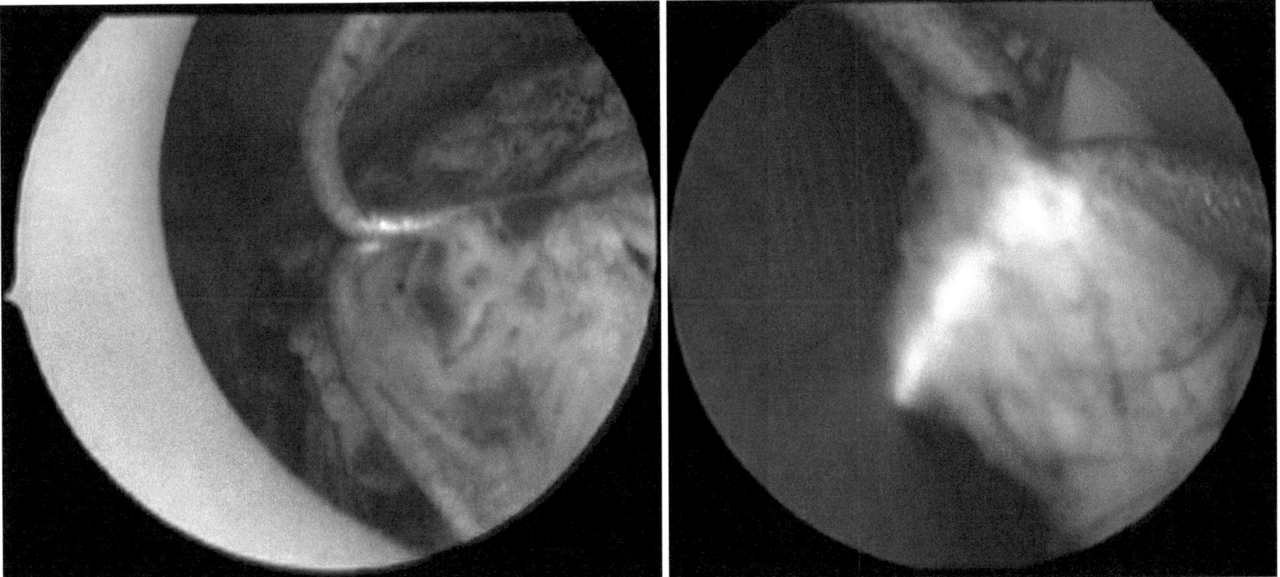

Fig. 31.26 The cold loop is inserted into the cleavage plane and repeatedly applied along the surface of the myoma

Slicing of the Intramural Component of the Myoma

After detachment, the intramural part of the myoma becomes an endocavitary neoformation and is safely removed by slicing as previously described, without damaging the surrounding myometrium (Fig. 31.27). During the slicing phase, the cutting action is always directed from the notch of the myoma towards the uterine cavity and never in the opposite direction: this is done to avoid thermal damage and the risk of accidentally cutting the myometrium around the notch (where the uterine wall is thinnest), or uterine perforation caused by the thermal loop. The electric loop is never used under the endometrial lining.

Control of Uterine Cavity Integrity

The integrity of the cavity and the absence of residual fragments are verified at the end of the procedure, to avoid the risk of inflammation and intracavitary synechiae (Fig. 31.28).

If the surgical procedure is interrupted due to excessive absorption of the distension liquid or other complications, thus the myomas are not totally removed, an additional resectoscopic procedure is scheduled.

The cold loop hysteroscopic myomectomy is usually performed using a 9 mm resectoscope with 0° optical system (HOPKINSII® Karl Storz Tuttlingen, Germany) and glycine 1.5 % for distension of the uterine cavity. For safety reasons, coagulation or blended waveforms are never used: this is also to avoid significant thermal damage deriving from coagulation.

To prevent the risk of clinical intravasation syndrome, the surgeon is constantly informed of the volumetric difference between the inflow and outflow fluid: the surgical procedure must be interrupted when absorption reached 1000 cm^3. The absorption of distending media should be continuously monitored along with the serum sodium level (arterial blood gas analysis). In accordance with the scientific literature [131–133], the critical value limit that we suggest to observe is 125 mEq/l.

Antibiotic prophylaxis should be only administered to patients with specific indications (e.g. cardiac valvulopathies).

According to Hamou who firstly suggested the importance and the usefulness of diagnostic hysteroscopic follow up because of the possibility to directly treat any post-operative adherence [134], 2 months after surgery a diagnostic hysteroscopy should be carried out. Intrauterine adhesions may impair many important reproductive aspects such as menstruation, normal fertility and pregnancy, being able to cause recurrent pregnancy loss, placenta accreta and intrauterine growth restriction. For these reasons, such synechiae have to be considered as a new pathology and not only as a complication or collateral effect correlated to the surgical treatment. According to the American Fertility Society criteria [135], the light synechiae can be easily treated during the endoscopic follow-up using the tip of the hysteroscope.

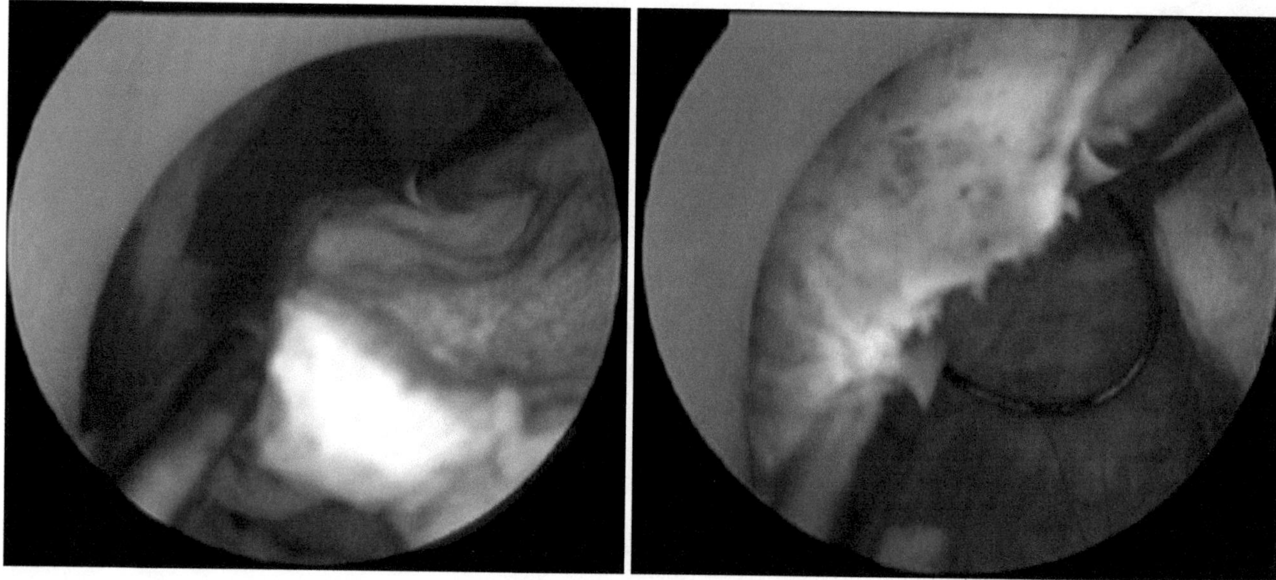

Fig. 31.27 The intramural part of the myoma is now an endocavitary neoformation and is safely removed by slicing, without damaging the surrounding myometrium

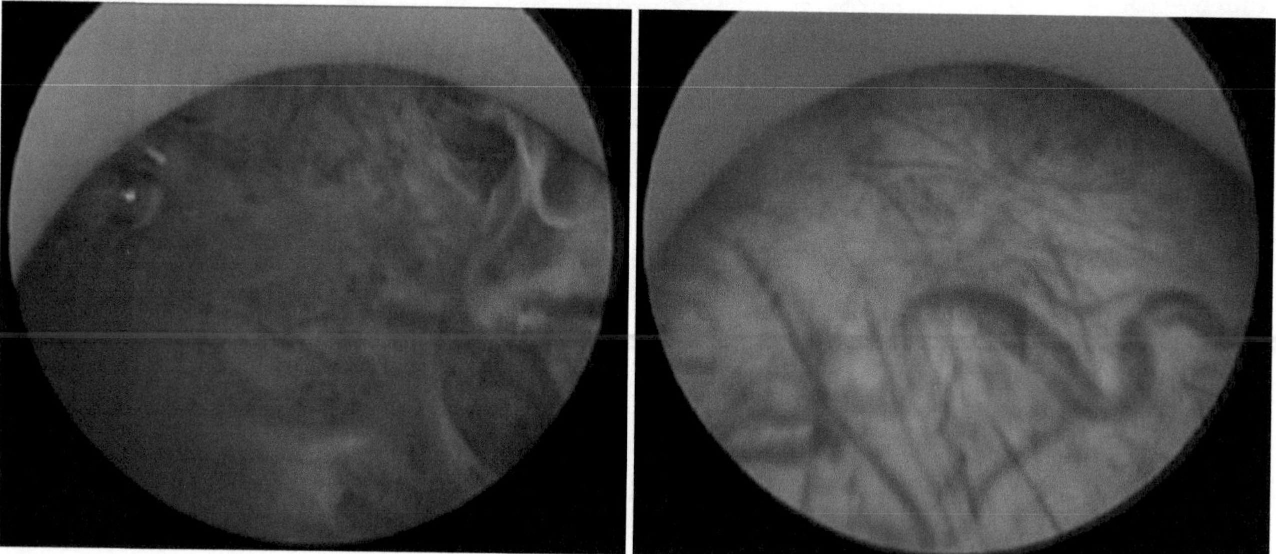

Fig. 31.28 The integrity of the fovea and the absence of sectioned residual fragments are verified at the end of the procedure

Synechiae of the uterine cavity represent the most common post-operative complication following resectoscopic myomectomy [136], and are related to the healing following the removal of myomas or to a possible perforation of the uterine wall [134]. Despite the frequency of this episode, there are few examples available in literature that describe its prevalence [137–140]. Some authors have suggested the use of anti-adherence liquid mixtures, or intrauterine devices aimed at preventing synechiae after resectoscopy [139, 141]. However, other authors have studied the influence of different types of electric energy used during myomectomy and their effect on the formation of adherences [138].

Taskin et al., in a prospective randomised study, reported a rate of synechiae of 31.3 % following resectoscopic myomectomy of a single myoma, reaching a rate of 45.5 % in case of multiple myomas [136]. In 2008 Yang et al. published a study where was reported a rate of 1.5 % in case of the resection of single myoma and a rate of 78 % in case of myomas located one in front of the other. In both groups of patients an IUD after the surgery was placed. The authors remarked the importance of diagnostic hysteroscopy within 2 weeks after the resectoscopic surgical treatment, with the aim to easily treat light intrauterine adherences [140].

In 2014, the results of a retrospective study conducted on a group of 688 patients with one or more G1–G2 myomas showed that the cold loop hysteroscopic myomectomy is a safe and effective procedure capable of ensuring a low prevalence of intrauterine synechiae [116].

The rate of adhesions reported 2 months after resectoscopic myomectomy was approximately 4 %, of which only 0.29 % were represented by fibrous synechiae, even in case of multiple myomas enucleated. The occurrence of synechiae in patients in whom 2 myomas were removed was almost the same as in those with a single myoma treated (4.48 % and 3.22 %, respectively). However, differently from expected, post-surgical synechiae were not found in the group of patients in which more than 2 myomas were removed.

The low rate of adherences can be ascribed to the non-use of electricity in coagulation mode (characterised by a higher thermic damage) and conversely to the use of the cold loop, preventing electric energy, whichever the type (monopolar or bipolar), from getting in contact with the myometrium of the uterine wall and inducing thermic damage which may increase the appearance of synechiae. Moreover, 8 cases of intraoperative complications were reported in in the same series (1.16 %). Furthermore the low rate of complications, such as perforations and the complete absence of damage to the entire layer of the uterine wall caused by thermal loop, might have a positive influence in the low rate of the post-surgical synechiae registered [116]. Moreover, no cases of uterine rupture in subsequent pregnancies were recorded. Several cases have been reported in the literature, some of which with dramatic consequence [142–144]. The possible negative effects on fertility and on pregnancies outcome due to the use of intraoperative monopolar or bipolar coagulation has been already described. The damage of surrounding healthy myometrium is considered as the major risk factor for uterine rupture in pregnancy after laparoscopic myomectomy [143].

In conclusion, it is therefore possible to affirm that the cold loop hysteroscopic myomectomy is a safe and feasible procedure, ensuring the respect of pseudocapsule and of surrounding healthy myometrium. Such technique allows to limit the blood loss during surgery, the damage to healthy myometrium fibers and is associated with a low rate of intraoperative complications. Moreover the rate of adhesions seems to be lower in comparison with the reported literature [18, 116]. These issues are of great importance for fertility patients and the surgeons should pay more attention in pseudocapsule preserving.

Translational Research and Virtual Biomodeling for Personalized Management of Patients with Uterine Myoma: Future Perspectives

Computational simulations of pelvic organs' topographic anatomy is a perspective direction of the translational biomodeling research aimed to design personalized approaches of minimally invasive restorations of women's reproductive health.

Uterine myoma is a common disease with serious consequences for women's well-being by causing such problems as infertility, recurrent miscarriages, dyspareunia, pelvic pain, bowel and bladder dysfunctions, dysmenorrhea, as well as irregular and excessive bleedings are associated with anemia. It is well known that uterine myoma is the most common indication for surgical procedures such as myomectomy and hysterectomy making this condition as an enormous healthcare concern with considerable healthcare expenditures.

From this view it is logical to design a special mathematical tool for preliminary patient-specific structural virtual analysis. It may help to come up with decision on the type of optimal treatment strategy. A mathematical biomodeling would become essential part of patient management. This approach will help to choose conservative or surgical intervention options which will be planned together with patients by demonstrating them virtual events are related with disease and its different treatment options as well as possible risks and beneficial outcomes.

We developed semi-automatic algorithm for constructing personalized virtual 3D anatomical model of uterine myoma which was based on MRI data set of a particular subject as well as on the medical applications of our previous mathematical model-system entitled "Personalized anatomical meshing of human body with applications" [145]. In order to design our semi-automatic technology we have used following algorithms and methods. The medical image segmentation is performed using user-guided active contour segmentation

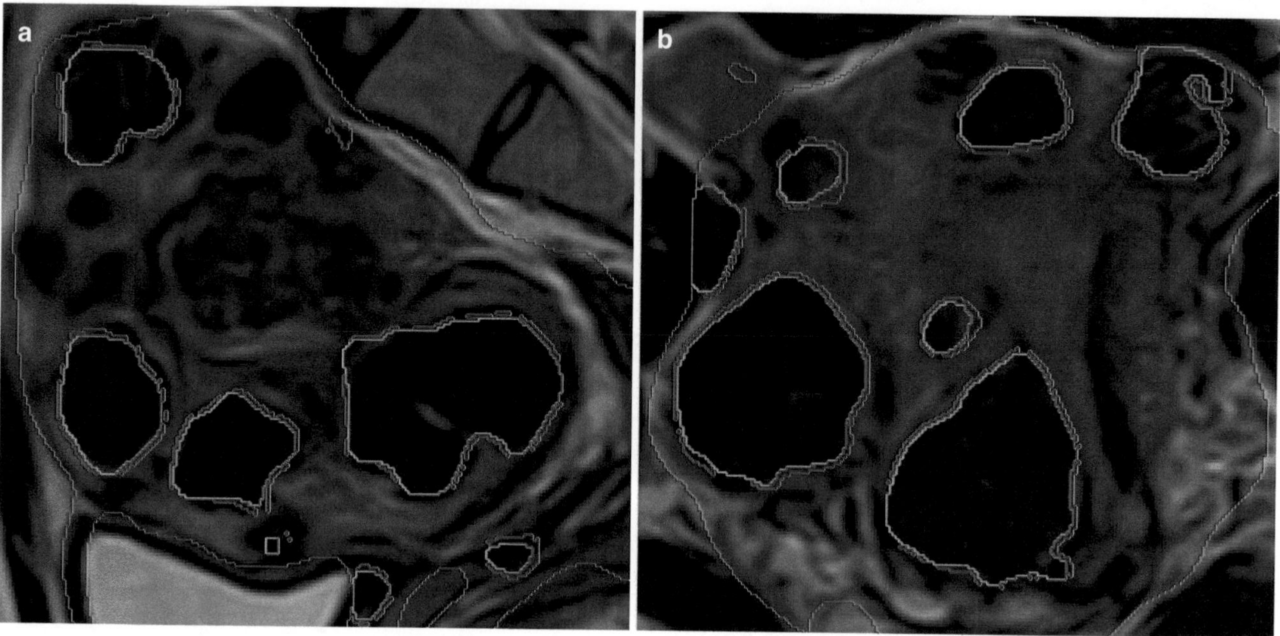

Fig. 31.29 MRI based 2D analysis of myoma pseudocapsule inner and outer boundaries: (**a**) sagittal plane; (**b**) transverse plane

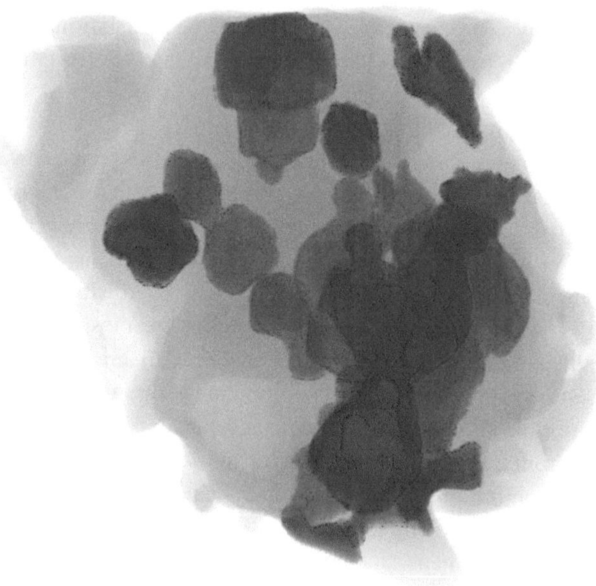

Fig. 31.30 3D reconstruction of multiple large uterine myoma case

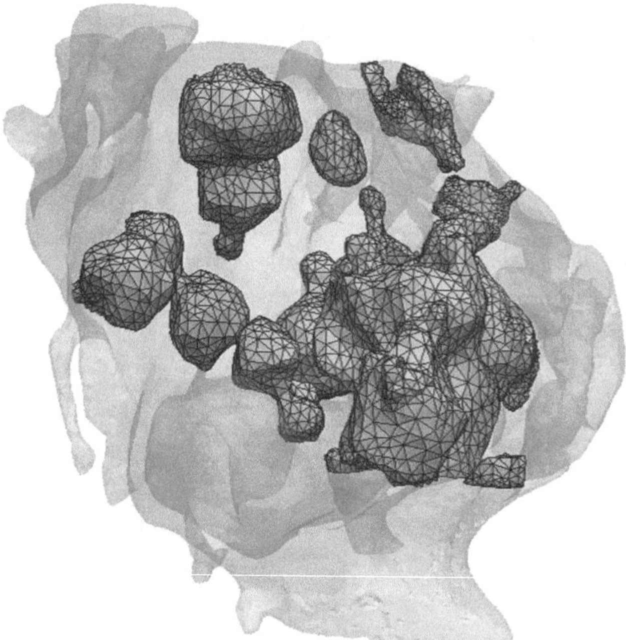

Fig. 31.31 3D computation mesh generated for segmentation results

[146] with supervised random forest classification from ITK-SNAP segmentation software [147]. The inner and outer boundaries of fibroid pseudocapsule can be determined at this stage (Fig. 31.29). Several post-processing algorithms were applied for filling remaining gaps between tissues and final segmented data smoothing. These algorithms are based on Gaussian smoothing, connected-component labelling and mathematical morphology operations: erosion, dilation, opening and closing [148]. As a result, a 3D model of multiple uterine fibroids is produced (Fig. 31.30). This post-processing step is essential for generation of valid mesh, which is suitable for future finite element modelling.

The following algorithms were used for mesh generation: a marching cubes algorithm for surface reconstruction [149]; surface triangulation, smoothing and coarsening techniques [150, 151]; 3D Delaunay triangulation algorithm from the CGAL-Mesh library [152], allowing specific mesh size for each model material; advancing front technique for volume mesh generation [153, 154].

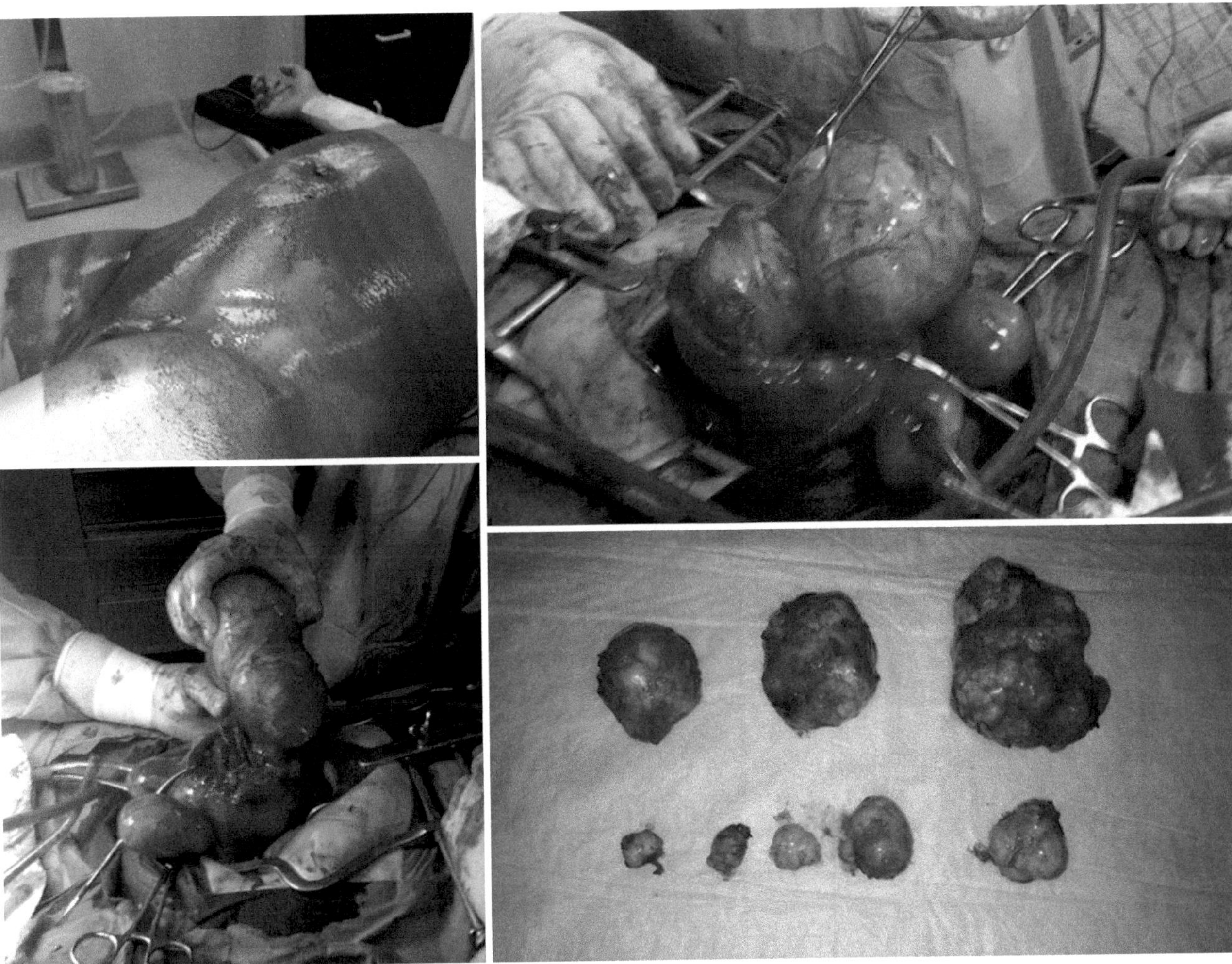

Fig. 31.32 The image shows a 32 years' old patients with multiple fibroids searching pregnancy; the operation was by laparotomic intracapsular multiple myomectomy and uterus reconstruction sparing myoma pseudocapsule

The essential post-processing mesh cosmetics step is applied using Ani3D library [155] in order to increase mesh quality. Preliminary results of our biomodeling cooperation are presented as computational mesh suitable for further computational simulations (A virtual model of multiple fibroids in patient with large uterine myoma) (Fig. 31.31).

In future 3D model will allow us to conduct non invasive virtual topographic anatomical analysis of the individual features of uterine fibroids including number and size of fibroids and their location in the uterine wall (subserosal, intramural, submucosal and pedunculated myomas) as well as in different uterine regions (fundal, corporal and isthmian–cervical) in order to design a personalized management strategy and optimized treatment choice.

Our biomodeling researches will cover wide range of topics are related with uterine topographic anatomy and uterine myoma, such as a mathematical model of fibroid pseudocapsule [156], virtual mechanical soft tissue computational simulations of uterine scar after myomectomy [157] and a virtual 3D model of uterine scar after caesarean section [158], as well as an original concept of angiogenesis initiation and vascular network development during uterine fibroid formation and growth [159].

Conclusions

The morphological and molecular research we conducted on the myoma pseudocapsule produced many interesting scientific results. The fibroid deforms the surrounding myometrium as it grows, giving rise to a dense fibroneurovascular pseudocapsule, rich of neurotrasmitters and growth factors, with a proper angiogenic profile. The discovery of the richness of the fibroneurovascular structure in neurotransmitters and morphological analysis of the pseudocapsule made it possible to translate the results in reproductive surgery and the whole topic of fertility and clinical practice, even for giant fibroids (Fig. 31.32) and during pregnancy (Fig. 31.33). My evidences on the presence of dedicate angiogenesis, neurofibers and neuropeptides in few millimetre structure, the pseudocapsule, suggested to preserve as much as possible such

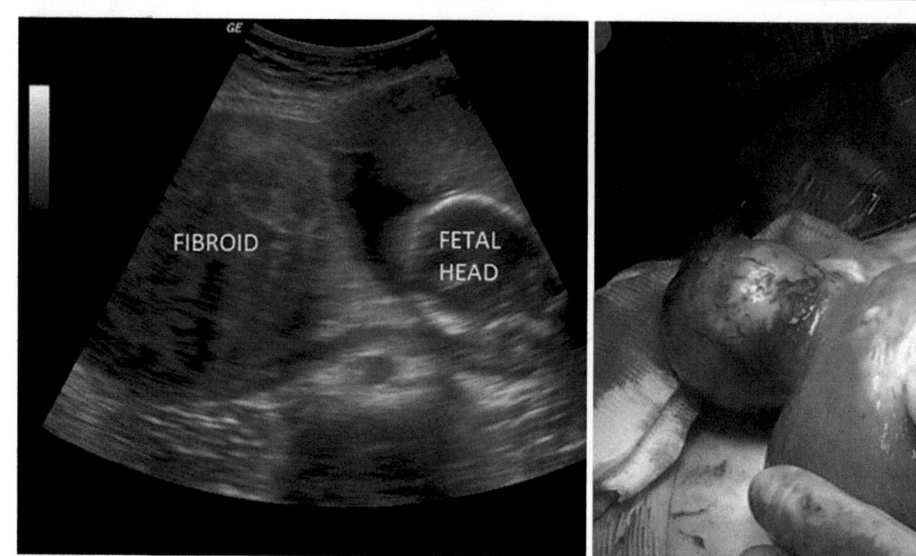

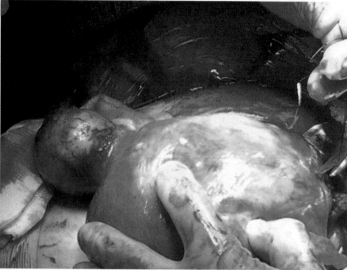

Fig. 31.33 A patient with a subserous fibroid of 4 cm of diameter located near lower uterine segment: on the left, the ultrasonographic image, on the right the image before a cesarean intracapsular myomectomy, after hysterorraphy

structure, during myomectomy. Pseudocapsule sparing during myomectomy should preserve myometrium integrity peripheral to fibroid site, enhancing myometrial healing after myomectomy. Moreover, intracapsular myomectomy, via traditional laparotomy, laparoscopy or hysteroscopy, should favour reproductive outcomes [160] and normal labor and delivery, for less bleeding [13], better neurovascular bundle sparing [88], and post-operative adhesions reduction [37, 116]. So the mix of intracapsular myomectomy and pseudocapsule-sparing by endoscopic "microsurgical" magnification, can be reproduced in all myomectomies, as a safe and feasible minimally invasive technique [7, 18, 54, 116, 161, 162].

Acknowledgement This work was supported by the Russian Science Foundation (grant 14-31-00,024). Some authors are members of the International Translational Medicine and Biomodeling Research Team (http://mathbiomed.crec.mipt.ru).

References

1. Tomasik P, Bomba-Opon D, Krupniewski L, Palczewski P, Wielgos M. Evaluation of uterine myomas during pregnancy using magnetic resonance imaging. Neuro Endocrinol Lett. 2014;35(4):262–4.
2. Downes E, Sikirica V, Gilabert-Estelles J, Bolge SC, Dodd SL, Maroulis C, et al. The burden of uterine fibroids in five European countries. Eur J Obstet Gynecol Reprod Biol. 2010;152(1):96–102.
3. Baskett TF. Hysterectomy: evolution and trends. Best Pract Res Clin Obstet Gynaecol. 2005;19(3):295–305.
4. Fleischer R, Weston GC, Vollenhoven BJ, Rogers PA. Pathophysiology of fibroid disease: angiogenesis and regulation of smooth muscle proliferation. Best Pract Res Obstet Gynaecol. 2008;22(4):603–14.
5. Okolo S. Incidence, aetiology and epidemiology of uterine fibroids. Best Pract Res Obstet Gynaecol. 2008;22(4):571–88.
6. Tinelli A, Malvasi A, Rahimi S, Negro R, Cavallotti C, Vergara D, Vittori G, Mettler L. Myoma pseudocapsule: a distinct endocrino-anatomical entity in gynecological surgery. Gynecol Endocrinol. 2009;25(10):661–7.
7. Tinelli A, Hurst BS, Hudelist G, Tsin DA, Stark M, Mettler L, Guido M, Malvasi A. Laparoscopic myomectomy focusing on the myoma pseudocapsule: technical and outcome reports. Hum Reprod. 2012;27(2):427–35.
8. Evans P, Brunsell S. Uterine fibroid tumors: diagnosis and treatment. Am Fam Physician. 2007;75(10):1503–8.
9. Somigliana E, Vercellini P, Daguati R, Pasin R, De Giorgi O, Crosignani PG. Fibroids and female reproduction: a critical analysis of the evidence. Hum Reprod Update. 2007;13(5):465–76.
10. Wise LA, Laughlin-Tommaso SK. Uterine leiomyomata. In: Goldman MB, Troisi R, Rexrode KM, editors. Women and health. San Diego: Academic; 2013. p. 285–306.
11. Graff-Radford J, Jones DT, Pruthi RK, Flemming KD. A neurological complication of a uterine fibroid. Neurocrit Care. 2013;18(1):93–5.
12. Wise LA, Palmer JR, Harlow BL, Spiegelman D, Stewart EA, Adams-Campbell LL, et al. Reproductive factors, hormonal contraception and risk of uterine leiomyomata in African-American women: a prospective study. Am J Epidemiol. 2004;159(2):113–23.
13. Laughlin SK, Baird DD, Savitz DA, Herring AH, Hartmann KE. Prevalence of uterine leiomyomas in the first trimester of pregnancy. Obstet Gynecol. 2009;113(3):630–5.
14. Wise LA, Ruiz-Narvaez EA, Palmer JR, Cozier YC, Tandon A, Patterson N, et al. African ancestry and genetic risk for uterine leiomyomata. Am J Epidemiol. 2012;176(12):1159–68.
15. Okogbo FO, Ezechi OC, Loto OM, Ezeobi PM. Uterine leiomyomata in South Western Nigeria: a clinical study of presentations and management outcome. Afr Health Sci. 2011;11(2):271–8.
16. Gupta S, Jose J, Mayonda I. Clinical presentation of fibroids. Best Pract Res Clin Obstet Gynaecol. 2008;22(4):615–26.
17. Sparić R, Hudelist G, Berisavac M, Gudović A, Buzadžić S. Hysterectomy throughout history. Acta Chir Iugosl. 2011;58(4):9–14.
18. Tinelli A, Hurst SB, Mettler L, Tsin AD, Pellegrino M, Nicolardi G, Dell'Edera D, Malvasi A. Ultrasound evaluation of uterine healing after laparoscopic intracapsular myomectomy: an observational study. Hum Reprod. 2012;27(9):2664–70.

19. Divakar H. Asymptomatic uterine fibroids. Best Pract Res Clin Obstet Gynaecol. 2008;22(4):643–54.
20. Cramer SF, Patel A. The frequency of uterine leiomyomas. Am J Clin Pathol. 1990;94(4):435–8.
21. Ezeama C, Ikechebelu J, Obiechina NJ, Ezeama N. Clinical presentation of uterine fibroids in Nnewi, Nigeria: a 5-year review. Ann Med Health Sci Res. 2012;2(2):114–8.
22. Stewart EA. Uterine fibroids. Lancet. 2001;357(9252):293–8.
23. Kwon DH, Song JE, Yoon KR, Lee KY. The safety of cesarean myomectomy in women with large myomas. Obstet Gynecol Sci. 2014;57(5):367–72.
24. Barlin JN, Giuntoli 2nd RL. Management of uterine leiomyosarcoma: an update. Exp Rev Obstet Gynecol. 2009;4(5):509–20.
25. Parker WH, Fu YS, Berek JS. Uterine sarcoma in patients operated on for presumed leiomyoma and rapidly growing leiomyoma. Obstet Gynecol. 1994;83(3):414–8.
26. Hyman DM, Grisham RN, Hensley ML. Management of advanced uterine leiomyosarcoma. Curr Opin Oncol. 2014;26(4):422–7.
27. Indraccolo U, Luchetti G, Indraccolo SR. Malignant transformation of uterine leiomyomata. Eur J Gynaecol Oncol. 2008;29(5): 543–4.
28. Mayerhofer K, Obermair A, Windbichler G, Petru E, Kaider A, Hefler L, et al. Leiomyosarcoma of the uterus: a clinicopathologic multicenter study of 71 cases. Gynecol Oncol. 1999;74(2): 196–201.
29. Leibsohn S, d'Ablaing G, Mishell Jr DR, Schalaerth JB. Leiomyosarcoma in a series of hysterectomies performed for presumed uterine leiomyomas. Am J Obstet Gynecol. 1990;162(4): 968–76.
30. Gockley AA, Rauh-Hain JA, Del Carmen MG. Uterine leiomyosarcoma: a review article. Int J Gynecol Cancer. 2014;24(9): 1538–42.
31. Bell SW, Kempson RL, Hendrickson MR. Problematic uterine smooth muscle neoplasms: a clinicopathologic study of 213 cases. Am J Surg Pathol. 1994;18:535–58.
32. Kobayashi H, Uekuri C, Akasaka J, Ito F, Shigemitsu A, Koike N, Shigetomi H. The biology of uterine sarcomas: a review and update. Mol Clin Oncol. 2013;1(4):599–609.
33. Resta L, Sanguedolce F, Orsini G, Laricchia L, Piscitelli D, Fiore MG. Morphometric and histological evaluation of GnRH agonists or progestational agents-treated uterine leiomyomas. Pathologica. 2004;96:35–41.
34. Sozen I, Arici A. Interactions of cytokines, growth factors, and the extracellular matrix in the cellular biology of uterine leiomyomata. Fertil Steril. 2002;78(1):1–12.
35. Bogusiewicz M, Stryjecka-Zimmer M, Postawski K, et al. Activity of matrix metalloproteinase-2 and -9 and contents of their tissue inhibitors in uterine leiomyoma and corresponding myometrium. Gynecol Endocrinol. 2007;23(9):541–6.
36. Tinelli A, Malvasi A, Cavallotti C, Dell'Edera D, Tsin DA, Stark M, Mettler L. The management of fibroids based on immunohistochemical studies of their pseudocapsules. Expert Opin Ther Targets. 2011 Nov;15(11):1241–7.
37. Tinelli A, Malvasi A, Guido M, Tsin DA, Hudelist G, Hurst B, Stark M, Mettler L. Adhesion formation after intracapsular myomectomy with or without adhesion barrier. Fertil Steril. 2011;95(5): 1780–5.
38. Faulkner RL. The blood vessels of the myomatous uteri. Am J Obstet Gynaecol. 1944;47:185–97.
39. Farrer-Brown G, Beilby JOW, Tarbit MH. The vascular patterns in myomatous uteri. J Obstet Gynaecol. 1970;77:967–75.
40. Awataguchi K. Studies on the angioarchitecture of uterine myoma. Nippon Ika Daigaku Zasshi. 1982;49:225–32.
41. Casey R, Rogers PA, Vollenhoven BJ. An immunohystochemical analysis of fibroid vasculature. Hum Reprod. 2000;15(7): 1469–75.
42. Campo S, Garcea N. Laparoscopic myomectomy in premenopausal women with and without preoperative treatment using gonadotrophin-releasing hormone analogues. Hum Reprod. 1999;14:44–8.
43. Lethaby A, Vollenhoven B, Sowter M. Pre-operative Gn-RH analogue therapy before hysterectomy or myomectomy for uterine fibroids. Cochrane Database Syst Rev. 2001;2:CD000547.
44. Pinkerton JV. Pharmacological therapy for abnormal uterine bleeding. Menopause. 2011;18(4):459–67.
45. Walocha JA, Litwin JA, Miodonski A. Vascular system of intramural leiomyomata revealed by corrosion casting and scanning electron microscopy. Hum Reprod. 2003;18:1088–93.
46. Forssman L. Blood flow in myomatous uteri as measured by intra-arterial 133-Xenon. Acta Obstet Gynecol Scand. 1976;55:21–4.
47. Wei JJ, Zhang XM, Chiriboga L, Yee H, Perle MA, Mittal K. Spatial differences in biologic activity of large uterine leiomyomata. Fertil Steril. 2006;85:179–87.
48. Malvasi A, Tinelli A, Cavallotti C, Morroni M, Tsin DA, Nezhat C, et al. Distribution of substance P (SP) and vasoactive intestinal peptide (VIP) in pseudocapsules of uterine fibroids. Peptides. 2011;32:327–32.
49. Mettler L, Tinelli A, Hurst BS, Teigland CM, Sammur W, Dell'Edera D, Negro R, Gustapane S, Malvasi A. Neurovascular bundle in fibroid pseudocapsule and its neuroendocrinologic implications. Expert Rev Endocrinol Metab. 2011;6(5):715–22.
50. Malvasi A, Tinelli A, Rahimi S, D'agnese G, Rotoni C, Dell'Edera D, Tsin DA, Cavallotti C. A three-dimensional morphological reconstruction of uterine leiomyoma pseudocapsule vasculature by the allen-cahn mathematical model. Biomed Pharmacother. 2011;65(5):359–63.
51. Malvasi A, Cavallotti C, Morroni M, Lorenzi T, Dell'Edera D, Nicolardi G, Tinelli A. Uterine fibroid pseudocapsule studied by transmission electron microscopy. Eur J Obstet Gynecol Reprod Biol. 2012;162(2):187–91.
52. De Falco M, Staibano S, Mascolo M, Mignogna C, Improda L, Ciociola F, Carbone IF, Di Lieto A. Leiomyoma pseudocapsule after pre-surgical treatment with gonadotropin releasing hormone agonists: relationship between clinical features and immunohistochemical changes. Eur J Obstet Gynecol Reprod Biol. 2009;144:44–7.
53. Mavrelos D, Ben-Nagi J, Davies A, Lee C, Salim R, Jurkovic D. The value of pre-operative treatment with gnrh analogues in women with submucous fibroids: a double-blind, placebo-controlled randomized trial. Hum Reprod. 2010;25:2264–9.
54. Tinelli A, Malvasi A, Cavallotti C, Hudelist G, Tsin DA, Schollmeyer T, Bojahr B, Mettler L. Single and multiple intracapsular laparoscopic myomectomy. an institutional experience. J Laparoendosc Adv Surg Tech A. 2010;20(8):705–11.
55. Malvasi A, Cavallotti C, Nicolardi G, Pellegrino M, Dell'edera D, Vergara D, et al. NT, NPY and PGP 9.5 presence in myometrium and in fibroid pseudocapsule and their possible impact on muscular physiology. Gynecol Endocrinol. 2013;29:177–81.
56. Malvasi A, Cavallotti C, Nicolardi G, Pellegrino M, Vergara D, Greco M, et al. The opioid neuropeptides in uterine fibroid pseudocapsules: a putative association with cervical integrity in human reproduction. Gynecol Endocrinol. 2013;29:982–8.
57. Gray's Anatomy. The uterus. In: The anatomical basis of clinical practice. 40th ed., ISBN:978-0-443-06684-9. Churchill-Livingstone, Elsevier, USA; 2008. p. 710–4.
58. Sun Y, Zhu L, Huang X, Zhou C, Zhang X. Immunohistochemical localization of nerve fibers in the pseudocapsule of fibroids. Eur J Histochem. 2014;58(2):2249.
59. Delgado AV, McManus AT, Chambers JP. Exogenous administration of Substance P enhances wound healing in a novel skin-injury model. Exp Biol Med (Maywood). 2005;230:271–80.
60. Jiang MH, Chung E, Chi GF, Ahn W, Lim JE, Hong HS, et al. Substance P induces M2-type macrophages after spinal cord injury. Neuroreport. 2012;23:786–92.

61. Collins JJ, Usip S, McCarson KE, Papka RE. Sensory nerves and neuropeptides in uterine cervical ripening. Peptides. 2002;23: 167–83.
62. Tingaker BK, Ekman-Ordeberg G, Facer P, Irestedt L, Anand P. Influence of pregnancy and labor on the occurrence of nerve fibers expressing the capsaicin receptor TRPV1 in human corpus and cervix uteri. Reprod Biol Endocrinol. 2008;6:8.
63. Tingaker BK, Ekman-Ordeberg G, Forsgren S. Presence of sensory nerve corpuscles in the human corpus and cervix uteri during pregnancy and labor as revealed by immunohistochemistry. Reprod Biol Endocrinol. 2006;4:45.
64. Cormio L, Gesualdo L, Maiorano E, Bettocchi C, Palumbo F, Traficante A, et al. Vasoactive intestinal polypeptide (VIP) is not an androgen-dependent neuromediator of penile erection. Int J Impot Res. 2005;17:23–6.
65. Rodríguez R, Pozuelo JM, Martín R, Arriazu R, Santamaria L. Stereological quantification of nerve fibers immunoreactive to PGP 9.5, NPY, and VIP in rat prostate during postnatal development. J Androl. 2005;26:197–204.
66. Arms L, Vizzard MA. Neuropeptides in lower urinary tract function. Handb Exp Pharmacol. 2011;202:395–423.
67. Merrill L, Girard B, Arms L, Guertin P, Vizzard MA. Neuropeptide/Receptor expression and plasticity in micturition pathways. Curr Pharm Des. 2013;19:4411–22.
68. Di Tommaso S, Massari S, Malvasi A, Bozzetti MP, Tinelli A. Gene expression analysis reveals an angiogenic profile in uterine leiomyoma pseudocapsule. Mol Hum Reprod. 2013;19(6):380–7.
69. Stewart EA, Nowak RA. Leiomyoma-related bleeding: a classic hypothesis updated for the molecular era. Hum Reprod Update. 1996;2(4):295–306.
70. Bulun SE. Uterine fibroids. N Engl J Med. 2013;369:1344–55.
71. Di Tommaso S, Massari S, Malvasi A, Vergara D, Maffia M, Greco M, Tinelli A. Selective genetic analysis of myoma pseudocapsule and potential biological impact on uterine fibroid medical therapy. Expert Opin Ther Targets. 2015 Jan;19(1):7–12.
72. Mäkinen N, Mehine M, Tolvanen J, et al. MED12, the mediator complex subunit 12 gene, is mutated at high frequency in uterine leiomyomas. Science. 2011;334:252–5.
73. Dallas NA, Samuel S, Xia L, et al. Endoglin (CD105): a marker of tumor vasculature and potential target for therapy. Clin Cancer Res. 2008;14:1931–7.
74. Valluru M, Brown NJ, Cross SS, et al. Blood vessel characterization in human dermal wound repair and scarring. Br J Dermatol. 2011;165:221–4.
75. Di Tommaso S, Tinelli A, Malvasi A, Massari S. Missense mutations in exon 2 of the MED12 gene are involved in IGF-2 overexpression in uterine leiomyoma. Mol Hum Reprod. 2014;20(10):1009–15.
76. Tinelli A, Mynbaev OA, Mettler L, Hurst BS, Pellegrino M, Nicolardi G, Kosmas I, Malvasi A. A combined ultrasound and histologic approach for analysis of uterine fibroid pseudocapsule thickness. Reprod Sci. 2014;21(9):1177–86.
77. Fraser IS, Critchley HO, Munro MG, Broder M, Writing Group for this Menstrual Agreement Process. A process designed to lead to international agreement on terminologies and definitions used to describe abnormalities of menstrual bleeding. Fertil Steril. 2007;87(3):466–76.
78. Mettler L, Schollmeyer T, Tinelli A, Malvasi A, Alkatout I. Complications of uterine fibroids and their management, surgical management of fibroids, laparoscopy and hysteroscopy versus hysterectomy, haemorrhage, adhesions and complications. Obstet Gynecol Int. 2012;2012:791248.
79. Darwish AM, Nasr AM, El-Nashar DA. Evaluation of postmyomectomy uterine scar. J Clin Ultrasound. 2005;33(4):181–6.
80. Seinera P, Gaglioti P, Volpi E, Cau MA, Todros T. Ultrasound evaluation of uterine wound healing following laparoscopic myomectomy: preliminary results. Hum Reprod. 1999;14(10):2460–3.
81. Beyth Y, Jaffe R, Goldberger S. Uterine remodelling following conservative myomectomy. Ultrasonographic evaluation. Acta Obstet Gynecol Scand. 1992;71(8):632–5.
82. Pun TC, Chau MT, Lam C, Tang G, Leong L. Sonographic evaluation of the myomectomy 'scars'. Acta Obstet Gynecol Scand. 1998;77(2):218–21.
83. Hanna KR, Katz AJ. An update on wound healing and the nervous system. Ann Plast Surg. 2011;67(1):49–52.
84. Tidball JG. Mechanisms of muscle injury, repair, and regeneration. Compr Physiol. 2011;1(4):2029–62.
85. Järvinen TA, Järvinen TL, Kääriäinen M, Kalimo H, Järvinen M. Muscle injuries: biology and treatment. Am J Sports Med. 2005;33(5):745–64.
86. Henderson J, Terenghi G, Ferguson MW. The reinnervation and revascularisation pattern of scarless murine fetal wounds. J Anat. 2011;218(6):660–7.
87. Gouin JP, Carter CS, Pournajafi-Nazarloo H, Glaser R, Malarkey WB, Loving TJ, Stowell J, Kiecolt-Glaser JK. Marital behavior, oxytocin, vasopressin, and wound healing. Psychoneuroendocrinology. 2010;35(7):1082–90.
88. Tinelli A, Malvasi A, Hurst BS, Tsin DA, Davila F, Dominguez G, Dell'Edera D, Cavallotti C, Negro R, Gustapane S, Teigland CM, Mettler L. Surgical management of neurovascular bundle in uterine fibroids pseudocapsule. JSLS. 2012;16:119–29.
89. Vikhareva Osser O, Valentin L. Risk factors for incomplete healing of the uterine incision after caesarean section. BJOG. 2010; 117(9):1119–26.
90. Han M, Kim C, Mozer P, Schäfer F, Badaan S, Vigaru B, Tseng K, Petrisor D, Trock B, Stoianovici D. Tandem-robot assisted laparoscopic radical prostatectomy to improve the neurovascular bundle visualization: a feasibility study. Urology. 2011;77(2): 502–6.
91. Walz J, Burnett AL, Costello AJ, Eastham JA, Graefen M, Guillonneau B, Menon M, Montorsi F, Myers RP, Rocco B, Villers A. A critical analysis of the current knowledge of surgical anatomy related to optimization of cancer control and preservation of continence and erection in candidates for radical prostatectomy. Eur Urol. 2010;57(2):179–92.
92. Lee SE, Hong SK, Han JH, Han BK, Yu JH, Jeong SJ, Byun SS, Lee HJ. Significance of neurovascular bundle formation observed on preoperative magnetic resonance imaging regarding postoperative erectile function after nerve-sparing radical retropubic prostatectomy. Urology. 2007;69(3):510–4.
93. Ong AM, Su LM, Varkarakis I, Inagaki T, Link RE, Bhayani SB, Patriciu A, Crain B, Walsh PC. Nerve sparing radical prostatectomy: effects of hemostatic energy sources on the recovery of cavernous nerve function in a canine model. J Urol. 2004;172 (4 Pt 1):1318–22.
94. Hurst BS. Uterine fibroids. In: Stadtmauer LA, Tur-Kaspa I, editors. Ultrasound imaging in reproductive medicine. New York: Springer; 2014 . p. 117–31.Chapter 10
95. Falcone T, Parker WH. Surgical management of leiomyomas for fertility or uterine preservation. Obstet Gynecol. 2013;121(4): 856–68.
96. Tinelli A, Mettler L, Malvasi A, Hurst B, Catherino W, Mynbaev OA, Guido M, Alkatout I, Schollmeyer T. Impact of surgical approach on blood loss during intracapsular myomectomy. Minim Invasive Ther Allied Technol. 2014;23(2):87–95.
97. Novak ER, Woodruff JD. Myoma and other benign tumours of the uterus, Novaks' gynecologic and obstetric pathology with clinical and endocrine relations. Philadelphia: WB Saunders; 1979. p. 795–801.
98. Ouyang DW. Obstetric complications of fibroids. Obstet Gynecol Clin North Am. 2006;33:153–69.
99. Song D, Zhang W, Chames MC, Guo J. Myomectomy during cesarean delivery. Int J Gynaecol Obstet. 2013;121(3):208–13.

100. Rice JP, Kay HH, Mahony BS. The clinical significance of uterine leiomyomas in pregnancy. Am J Obstet Gynecol. 1989; 160:1212–6.
101. Exacoustos C, Rosati P. Ultrasound diagnosis of uterine myomas and complications in pregnancy. Obstet Gynecol. 1993;82:97–101.
102. Katz VL, Dotters DJ, Droegemueller W. Complications of uterine leiomyomas in pregnancy. Obstet Gynecol. 1989;73:593–6.
103. Incebiyik A, Hilali NG, Camuzcuoglu A, Vural M, Camuzcuoglu H. Myomectomy during caesarean: a retrospective evaluation of 16 cases. Arch Gynecol Obstet. 2014;289(3):569–73.
104. Hasan F, Arumugam K, Sivanesaratnam V. Uterine leiomyomata in pregnancy. Int J Gynaecol Obstet. 1991;34:45–8.
105. Vergani P, Locatelli A, Ghidini A, Andreani M, Sala F, Pezzullo JC. Large uterine leiomyomata and risk of cesarean delivery. Obstet Gynecol. 2007;109:410–4.
106. Coronado GD, Marshall LM, Schwartz SM. Complications in pregnancy, labor, and delivery with uterine leiomyomas: a population-based study. Obstet Gynecol. 2000;95:764–9.
107. Cunningham FG, Leveno KL, Bloom SL, Hauth JC, Gilstrap III LC, Wenstrom KD, editors. Abnormalities of the reproductive tract. In Williams obstetrics. 22st ed. New York: Mcgraw-Hill Medical Publishing Division; 2005.
108. Ludmir J, Stubblefield PG. Surgical procedures in pregnancy. In: Gabbe SG, Niebyl JR, Simpson JL, editors. Gabbe: obstetrics-normal and problem pregnancies. 4th ed. New York: Churchill Livingstone, Inc.; 2002. p. 613.
109. Tinelli A, Malvasi A, Mynbaev OA, Barbera A, Perrone E, Guido M, Kosmas I, Stark M. The surgical outcome of intracapsular cesarean myomectomy. A match control study. J Matern Fetal Neonatal Med. 2014;27(1):66–71.
110. Neuwirth RS, Amin HK. Excision of submucus fibroids with hysteroscopic control. Am J Obstet Gynecol. 1976;126:95–9.
111. Di Spiezio Sardo A, Mazzon I, Bramante S, Bettocchi S, Bifulco G, Guida M, Nappi C. Hysteroscopic myomectomy: a comprehensive review of surgical techniques. Hum Reprod Update. 2008;14:101–19.
112. Jedeikin R, Olsfanger D, Kessler I. Disseminated intravascular coagulopathy and adult respiratory distress syndrome: life-threatening complications of hysteroscopy. Am J Obstet Gynecol. 1990;162:44–5.
113. Sullivan B, Kenney P, Seibel M. Hysteroscopic resection of fibroid with thermal injury to sigmoid. Obstet Gynecol. 1992;80:546–7.
114. Howe RS. Third-trimester uterine rupture following hysteroscopic uterine perforation. Obstet Gynecol. 1993;81:827–9.
115. Murakami T, Tamura M, Ozawa Y, Suzuki H, Terada Y, Okamura K. Safe techniques in surgery for hysteroscopic myomectomy. J Obstet Gynaecol Res. 2005 Jun;31(3):216–23.
116. Mazzon I, Favilli A, Cocco P, Grasso M, Horvath S, Bini V, Di Renzo GC, Gerli S. Does cold loop hysteroscopic myomectomy reduce intrauterine adhesions? A retrospective study. Fertil Steril. 2014;101:294–298.e3.
117. Mazzon I. Nuova tecnica per la miomectomia isteroscopica: enucleazione con ansa fredda. In: Cittadini E, Perino A, Angiolillo M, Minelli L, editors. Testo-Atlante di Chirurgia Endoscopica Ginecologica. Palermo: COFESE; 1995 .chapt XXXIIIb
118. Zhao X, Zeng W, Chen L, Chen L, Du W, Yan X. Laparoscopic myomectomy using "cold" surgical instruments for uterine corpus leiomyoma: a preliminary report. Cell Biochem Biophys. 2014;72:141–6. [Epub ahead of print]
119. Wamsteker K, Emanuel MH, de Kruif JH. Transcervical hysteroscopic resection of submucous fibroids for abnormal uterine bleeding: results regarding the degree of intramural extension. Obstet Gynecol. 1993;82:736–40.
120. Emanuel MH, Wamsteker K, Hart AA, Metz G, Lammes FB. Long-term results of hysteroscopic myomectomy for abnormal uterine bleeding. Obstet Gynecol. 1999;93:743–8.
121. Lasmar RB, Barrozo PR, Dias R, Oliveira MA. Submucous myomas: a new presurgical classification to evaluate the viability of hysteroscopic surgical treatment-preliminary report. J Minim Invasive Gynecol. 2005;12:308–11.
122. Casadio P, Youssef AM, Spagnolo E, Rizzo MA, Talamo MR, De Angelis D, Marra E, Ghi T, Savelli L, Farina A, Pelusi G, Mazzon I. Should the myometrial free margin still be considered a limiting factor for hysteroscopic resection of submucous fibroids? A possible answer to an old question. Fertil Steril. 2011;95:1764–8.e1.
123. Jansen FW, Vredevoogd CB, van Ulzen K, Hermans J, Trimbos JB, Trimbos-Kemper TC. Complications of hysteroscopy: a prospective, multicenter study. Obstet Gynecol. 2000;96:266–70.
124. Hallez JP. Single-stage total hysteroscopic myomectomies: indications, techniques, and results. Fertil Steril. 1995;63:703–8.
125. Aydeniz B, Gruber IV, Schauf B, Kurek R, Meyer A, Wallwiener D. A multicenter survey of complications associated with 21,676 operative hysteroscopies. Eur J Obstet Gynecol Reprod Biol. 2002;104:160–4.
126. Lasmar RB, Xinmei Z, Indman PD, Celeste RK, Di Spiezio Sardo A. Feasibility of a new system of classification of submucous myomas: a multicenter study. Fertil Steril. 2011;95:2073–7.
127. Campo S, Campo V, Gambadauro P. Short-term and long-term results of resectoscopic myomectomy with and without pretreatment with GnRH analogs in premenopausal women. Acta Obstet Gynecol Scand. 2005;84:756–60.
128. Muzii L, Boni T, Bellati F, Marana R, Ruggiero A, Zullo MA, Angioli R, Panici PB. GnRH analogue treatment before hysteroscopic resection of submucous myomas: a prospective, randomized, multicenter study. Fertil Steril. 2010;94:1496–9.
129. Kamath MS, Kalampokas EE, Kalampokas TE. Use of GnRH analogues pre-operatively for hysteroscopic resection of submucous fibroids: a systematic review and meta-analysis. Eur J Obstet Gynecol Reprod Biol. 2014;177:11–8.
130. Fedele L, Vercellini P, Bianchi S, Brioschi D, Dorta M. Treatment with GnRH agonists before myomectomy and the risk of short-term myoma recurrence. Br J Obstet Gynaecol. 1990;97:393–6.
131. Propst AM, Liberman RF, Harlow BL, Ginsburg ES. Complications of hysteroscopic surgery: predicting patients at risk. Obstet Gynecol. 2000;96:517–20.
132. Shveiky D, Rojansky N, Revel A, Benshushan A, Laufer N, Shushan A. Complications of hysteroscopic surgery: "beyond the learning curve". J Minim Invasive Gynecol. 2007;14:218–22.
133. Paschopoulos M, Polyzos NP, Lavasidis LG, Vrekoussis T, Dalkalitsis N, Paraskevaidis E. Safety issues of hysteroscopic surgery. Ann N Y Acad Sci. 2006;1092:229–34.
134. Hamou J. Uterine adhesions. In: Hamou JE, Patrick JT, John JS, editors. Hysteroscopy and microhysteroscopy: text and atlas. New York: Appleton & Lange; 1991. p. 139–50.
135. The American Fertility Society classifications of adnexal adhesions, distal tubal occlusion, tubal occlusion secondary to tubal ligation, tubal pregnancies, müllerian anomalies and intrauterine adhesions. Fertil Steril. 1988;49:944–55.
136. Taskin O, Sadik S, Onoglu A, Gokdeniz R, Erturan E, Burak F, Wheeler JM. Role of endometrial suppression on the frequency of intrauterine adhesions after resectoscopic surgery. J Am Assoc Gynecol Laparosc. 2000;7:351–4.
137. Shokeir TA, Fawzy M, Tatongy M. The nature of intrauterine adhesions following reproductive hysteroscopic surgery as determined by early and late follow-up hysteroscopy: clinical implications. Arch Gynecol Obstet. 2008;277:423–7.
138. Touboul C, Fernandez H, Deffieux X, Berry R, Frydman R, Gervaise A. Uterine synechiae after bipolar hysteroscopic resection of submucosal myomas in patients with infertility. Fertil Steril. 2009;92:1690–3.
139. Guida M, Acunzo G, Di Spiezio Sardo A, Bifulco G, Piccoli R, Pellicano M, Cerrota G, Cirillo D, Nappi C. Effectiveness of

auto-crosslinked hyaluronic acid gel in the prevention of intrauterine adhesions after hysteroscopic surgery: a prospective, randomized, controlled study. Hum Reprod. 2004;19:1461–4.
140. Yang JH, Chen MJ, Wu MY, Chao KH, Ho HN, Yang YS. Office hysteroscopic early lysis of intrauterine adhesion after transcervical resection of multiple apposing submucous myomas. Fertil Steril. 2008;89:1254–9.
141. Metwally M, Watson A, Lilford R, Vandekerckhove P. Fluid and pharmacological agents for adhesion prevention after gynaecological surgery. Cochrane Database Syst Rev. 2006;2:CD001298.
142. Gerli S, Baiocchi G, Favilli A, Di Renzo GC. New treatment option for early spontaneous rupture of a postmyomectomy gravid uterus. Fertil Steril. 2011;96:e97–8.
143. Parker WH, Einarsson J, Istre O, Dubuisson JB. Risk factors for uterine rupture after laparoscopic myomectomy. J Minim Invasive Gynecol. 2010;17:551–4.
144. Pistofidis G, Makrakis E, Balinakos P, Dimitriou E, Bardis N, Anaf V. Report of 7 uterine rupture cases after laparoscopic myomectomy: update of the literature. J Minim Invasive Gynecol. 2012;19:762–7.
145. Vassilevski Y, Danilov A, Ivanov Y, Simakov S, Gamilov T. Personalized anatomical meshing of human body with applications. In book Modeling the heart and the circulatory system. vol 14. Cham, Switzerland: Springer; 2015., p. 221–36.
146. Yushkevich PA, Piven J, Hazlett HC, Smith RG, Ho S, Gee JC, Gerig G. User-guided 3D active contour segmentation of anatomical structures: significantly improved efficiency and reliability. Neuroimage. 2006;31(3):1116–28.
147. ITK-SNAP Medical Image Segmentation Tool. http://itksnap.org/.
148. Convert3D Tool. http://itksnap.org/c3d/.
149. Wu Z, Sullivan JM. Multiple material marching cubes algorithm. Int J Numer Meth Eng. 2003;58:189–207.
150. Taubin G. A signal processing approach to fair surface design. In book Proceedings of the 22nd Annual Conf. on Comp. Graphics and Interactive Techniques, ACM, New York;1995. p. 351–8.
151. Vassilevski YuV, Vershinin AV, Danilov AA, Plenkin AV. Tetrahedral mesh generation in domains defined in CAD systems. In book Matrix methods and technology for solving large problems. Moscow: Institute of Numerical Mathematics, 2005; 21–32, (in Russian).
152. Rineau L, Yvinec M. A generic software design for Delaunay refinement meshing. Comp Geom Theory Appl. 2007;38:100–10.
153. Danilov AA. Unstructured tetrahedral mesh generation technology. Comp Math Math Phys. 2010;50:139–56.
154. Frey P, George PL. Mesh generation: application to finite elements. Paris/Oxford: Hermes Science; 2000.
155. Advanced Numerical Instruments 3D. http://sourceforge.net/projects/ani3d.
156. Danilov AA, Simakov SS, Vassilevski YV, Malvasi A, Ishchenko AI, Kovaleva AM, Mynbaev OA, Tinelli A. A mathematical model of myoma pseudocapsule. The NESA Days 2015. 18–20 September 2015. Berlin, Germany.
157. Danilov AA, Salamatova VYu, Simakov SS, Tinelli A, Malvasi A, Mynbaev OA, Mal'kov PG, Ishchenko AI, Kovaleva AM, Vassilevski YuV. Virtual mechanical soft tissue computational simulations of uterine scar after myomectomy. The NESA Days 2015. 18–20 September 2015. Berlin, Germany.
158. Babenko TI, Danilov AA, Simakov SS, Ryzhkov VV, Kovalev MI, Danilova NV, Mal'kov PG, Mynbaev OA. A virtual 3D model of uterine scar after caesarean section. V International conference on biotechnology and pharmaceutics 'PhystechBIO'. 29–30 April 2015. Moscow Institute of Physics and Technology, Dolgoprudny, Russia.
159. Mynbaev OA, Simakov SS, Danilov AA, Kolobov AV, Mal'kov PG, Polyakov YuV, Kovalev MI, Ishchenko AIL, Tinelli A, Malvasi A, Melerzanov AV, Vassilevski YuV. Angiogenesis initiation and vascular network development during uterine fibroid formation and growth. V International conference on biotechnology and pharmaceutics 'PhystechBIO'. 29–30 April 2015. Moscow Institute of Physics and Technology, Dolgoprudny, Russia.
160. Mazzon I, Favilli A, Grasso M, Morricone D, Di Renzo GC, Gerli S. Is 'cold loop' hysteroscopic myomectomy a better option for reproduction in women with diffuse uterine leiomyomatosis? A case report of successful repeated pregnancies. J Obstet Gynaecol Res. 2014; doi:10.1111/jog.12548. [Epub ahead of print]
161. Camanni M, Bonino L, Delpiano EM, Ferrero B, Migliaretti G, Deltetto F. Hysteroscopic management of large symptomatic submucous uterine myomas. J Minim Invasive Gynecol. 2010;17:59–65.
162. Leone FP, Calabrese S, Marciante C, Cetin I, Ferrazzi E. Feasibility and long-term efficacy of hysteroscopic myomectomy for myomas with intramural development by the use of non-electrical "cold" loops. Gynecol Surg. 2012;9:155–61.
163. Butram VC, Reiter RC. Uterine Leiomyomata: etiology, symptomatology and management. Fertil Steril. 1981;36:433–45.

Laparoscopic Subtotal Hysterectomy (LSH)

32

Bernd Bojahr and Garri Tchartchian

Introduction

Various benign gynecological conditions including dysfunctional uterine bleeding, meno-metrorrhagia due to endometrial hyperplasia, fibroids, diffuse myomatosis, adenomyosis, endometriosis, pressure symptoms related to bowel or bladder function, large uterine fibroids, and treatment of excessive menstrual loss not responding to medical therapy [1–3] are indicative for a laparoscopic hysterectomy. For nonmalignant conditions LSH represents an alternative to total hysterectomy, with a low level of intraoperative and postoperative morbidity [4].

The difference between a subtotal, or supracervical hysterectomy and a total hysterectomy is as follows:

The total hysterectomy removes the entire uterus, including the cervix, whereas in the subtotal or supracervical hysterectomy the excision of the body of the uterus is performed, at or below the level of the isthmus, and conserves the cervix.

Leaving the cervix intact laparoscopically is easier to perform on a technical level, making the Laparoscopic subtotal hysterectomy (LSH) favorable over a total laparoscopic hysterectomy (TLH). With the LSH technique the two pitfalls of TLH, uterine vessel haemorrhage and ureteric injury, can be avoided. The risk of cervical cancer can also be reduced by coring out the entire transformation zone and endocervical canal.

Other advantages can be seen in reports that LSH results in lower levels of sexual, bladder and bowel dysfunction and offers superior protection of the integrity of the pelvic floor compared to total hysterectomy [5–7]. In developed industrial countries there is an increasing uptake rate of LSH [8, 9].

Although laparoscopic surgery is well accepted by gynaecologists worldwide, laparoscopic hysterectomy in Germany is still only performed by a few specialists as it is a highly skilled technique. At the "Klinik für MIC" (a hospital specialized in minimally invasive surgery) in Berlin, Germany, the surgeons are leading experts in laparoscopic subtotal hysterectomy. Between 1998 to December 2014 11,598 LSH procedures were performed there 909 of these extirpated uteri had a weight of more than 500 g and the largest removed uterus had a weight of 4065 g.

This article will describe and illustrate in detail the surgical technique of LSH and will comment on complications, as well as providing some tips and suggestions for implementation.

Surgical Procedure

After bladder catheterism and vaginal disinfection, the patient is placed in a horizontal position, with stretched legs (Fig. 32.1). Positioned on the left side of the patient are the surgeon, the assistant and the surgical nurse, along with instrument tables, facing the monitors and endoscopic tower on the right side of the patient the electronic equipment is set up (Fig. 32.2). No uterus manipulators are needed. A CO_2 pneumoperitoneum to an intra-abdominal pressure of 15 mmHg is established utilizing a Veress needle, placed through an incision in the inferior umbilical fossa. A 5-mm trocar is used for the laparoscopy with 30 ° optics.

Tip When the situs is obscure, and especially in the case of large multimodal myomatous uteri, the excellent image quality provided by the new digital 3-ship camera (STORZ), and the benefits of the 30° telescope can be much appreciated.

The patient is then placed in Trendelenberg position, a maximum (steep) position. Two more 5 mm puncture sites in the lower abdomen are required (Fig. 32.3), the location of which depends on the size of the uterus.

Two additional trocars are introduced left and right lateral to the epigastric vessels in the region of the pubic hair line in cases of a normal sized uterus. The larger the uterus, the further

B. Bojahr (✉) • G. Tchartchian
Klinik für MIC Minimal Invasive Chirurgie, Berlin, Germany

I. Alkatout, L. Mettler (eds.), *Hysterectomy*, DOI 10.1007/978-3-319-22497-8_32

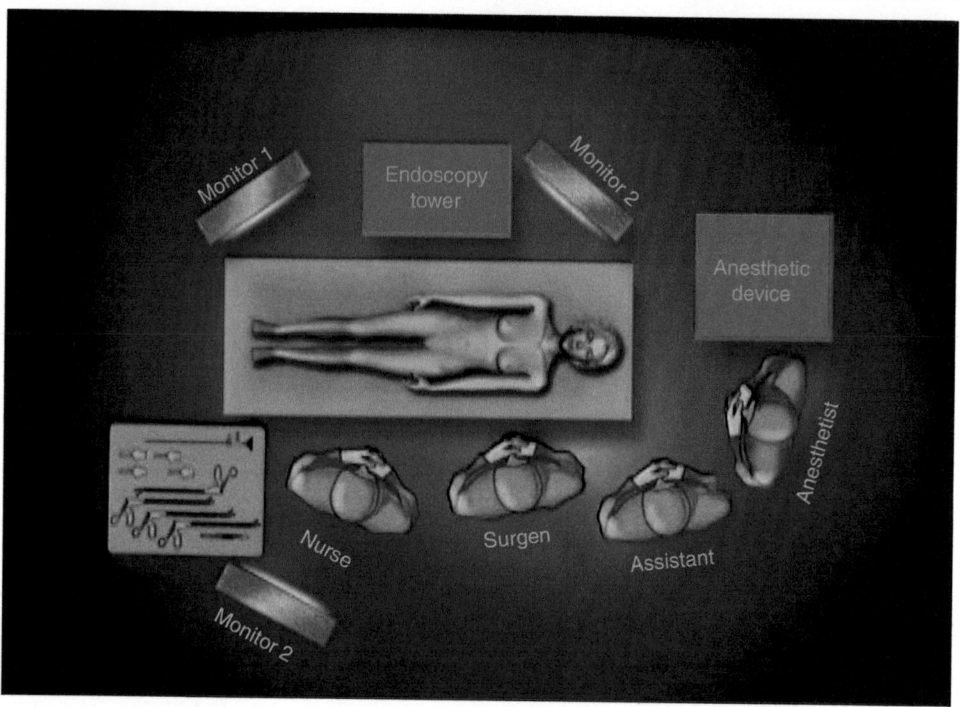

Fig. 32.1 Patient positioning and OR Equipment at MIC Klinik in Berlin

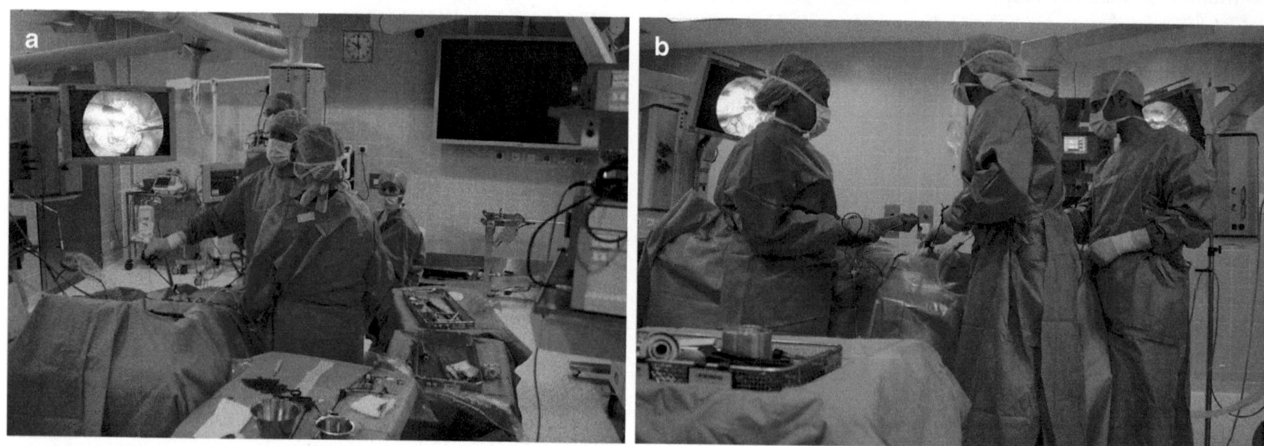

Fig. 32.2 The surgeon, the assistant, the scrub nurse and the instrument table are positioned on the left side of the patient (**a**, **b**)

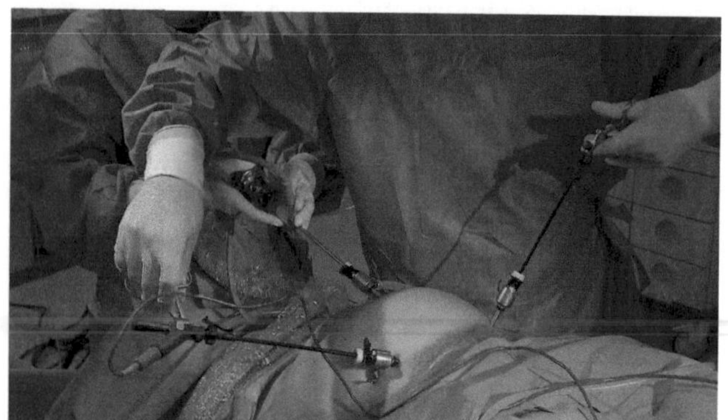

Fig. 32.3 Trocar placement for a LASH (normal sized uterus)

above the symphysis pubis the lateral trocars need to be positioned. In the case of uterus extension as far as the umbilicus, insufflation is performed on the left, below the costal arch with trocar introduction there or in the umbilicus. Correspondingly higher, additional trocars are positioned according to the size of the uterus, to enable the adnexa to be dissected (Fig. 32.4).

Tip With a large myomatous uterus (Fig. 32.5), localization of the two trocars in the lower abdomen depends on the size of the uterus. They are then usually placed two to three centimeters above the pubic hair border. A fourth trocar should be introduced on the left below the costal arch or above the umbilicus to obtain a better overview of the uterus. From there, visualization can be performed with the telescope (Fig. 32.6). The uterus can then be pressed to the right or left using a palpation probe, so as to remove the adnexa laterally. With such large findings, good visualization of the anatomic structures with the 30 ° telescope is essential to avoid unnecessary bleeding.

The only additional re-usable instruments needed for LSH include a bipolar coagulation clamp, Metzenbaum scissors, three various grasping forceps, a needle holder, a unipolar hook, and a suction-irrigation system.

The round ligaments, the fallopian tubes and the ovarian ligaments are coagulated using bipolar forceps for mobilization of the uterus (Fig. 32.7) and subsequently dissected using endoscopic Metzenbaum scissors (Fig. 32.8).

Tip Mobilization of the uterus can also be performed with the ultracision harmonic scalpel. Less frequent instrument changing is required. But also the use of ultracision instruments, monopolar scissors and unipolar loops for the dissection of the corpus uteri has been described [10–12]. Safety,

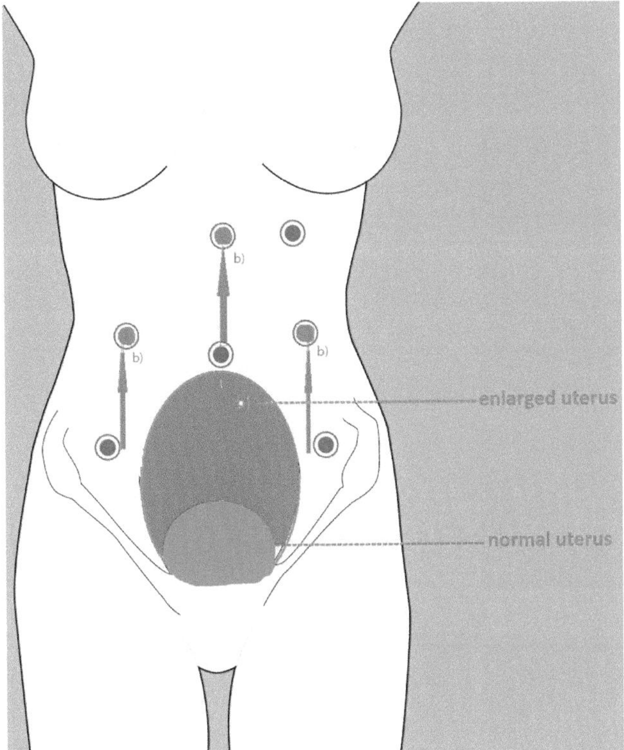

Fig. 32.4 Variations of trocar placement in cases of enlarged uteri

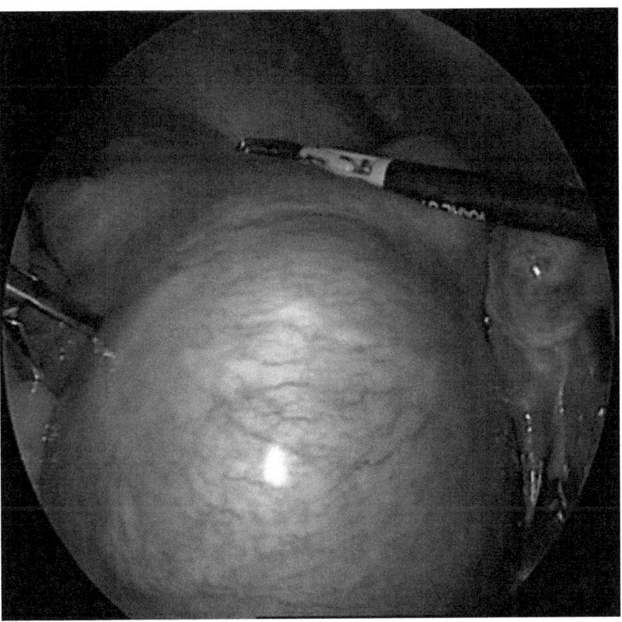

Fig. 32.6 1107 gm Uterus – View from inside

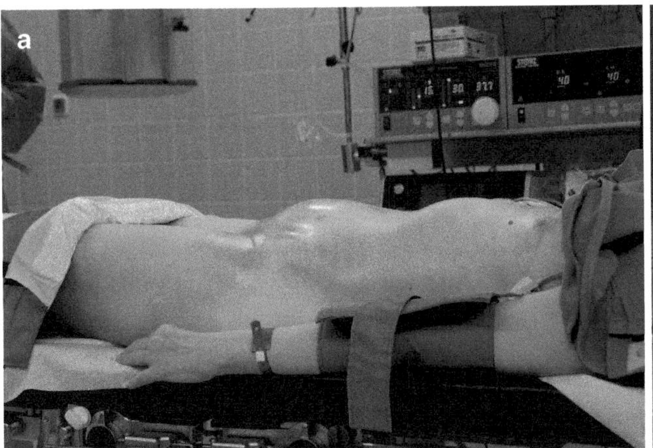

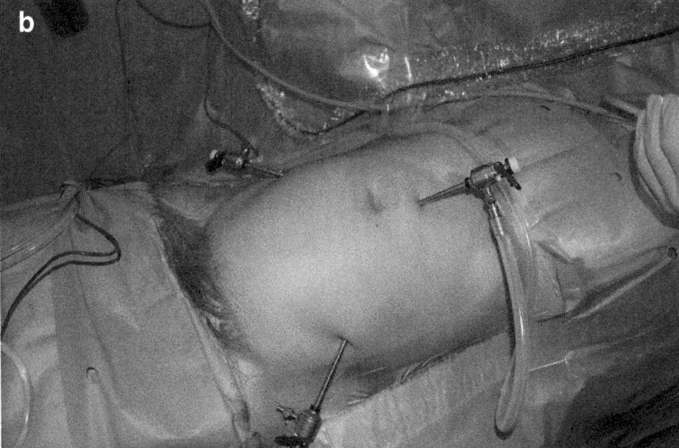

Fig. 32.5 1107 gm Uterus – (**a**) View from outside , (**b**) Trocar placement

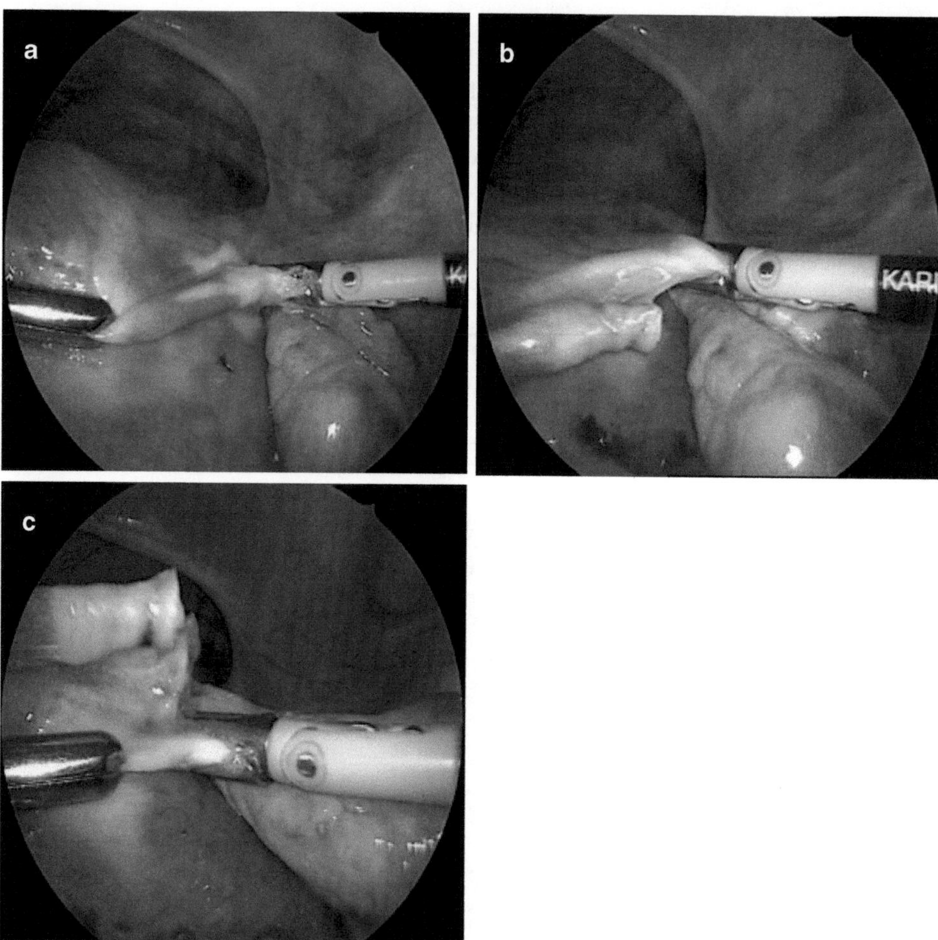

Fig. 32.7 (**a**–**c**) – Bipolar coagulation of the fallopian tube, the round ligament and the ovarian ligament.

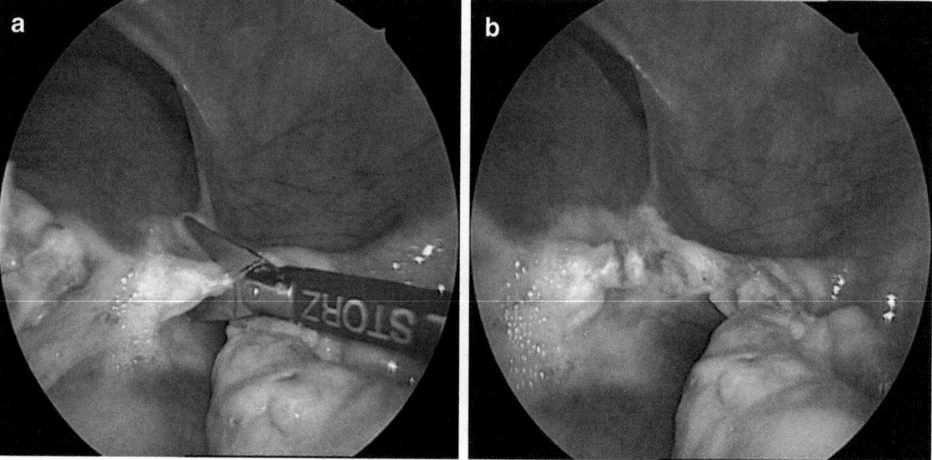

Fig. 32.8 Dissection of the round ligament, fallopian tube and ovarian ligament from the right side with a pair of scissors (**a**) – after the dissection (**b**)

precision of the cut, and shortage of operating time are definite advantages of the unipolar loop arc [10].

Tip In the case of intraligamentous myomas the essential requirements are, on the one hand, sufficient hemostasis and, on the other hand, that dissection is always close up against the myoma. The majority of myomas can be mobilized with a blunt instrument. It is necessary for the ureter to be visualized during and after the removal if the myomas extend as far as the pelvic wall. To ensure that the symptoms complained of before the operation do not persist afterwards if endometriosis foci are present, irrespective of whether they are located in the Douglas, in the area of the round ligaments or in the area of the bladder peritoneum, it is important to also resect these foci completely.

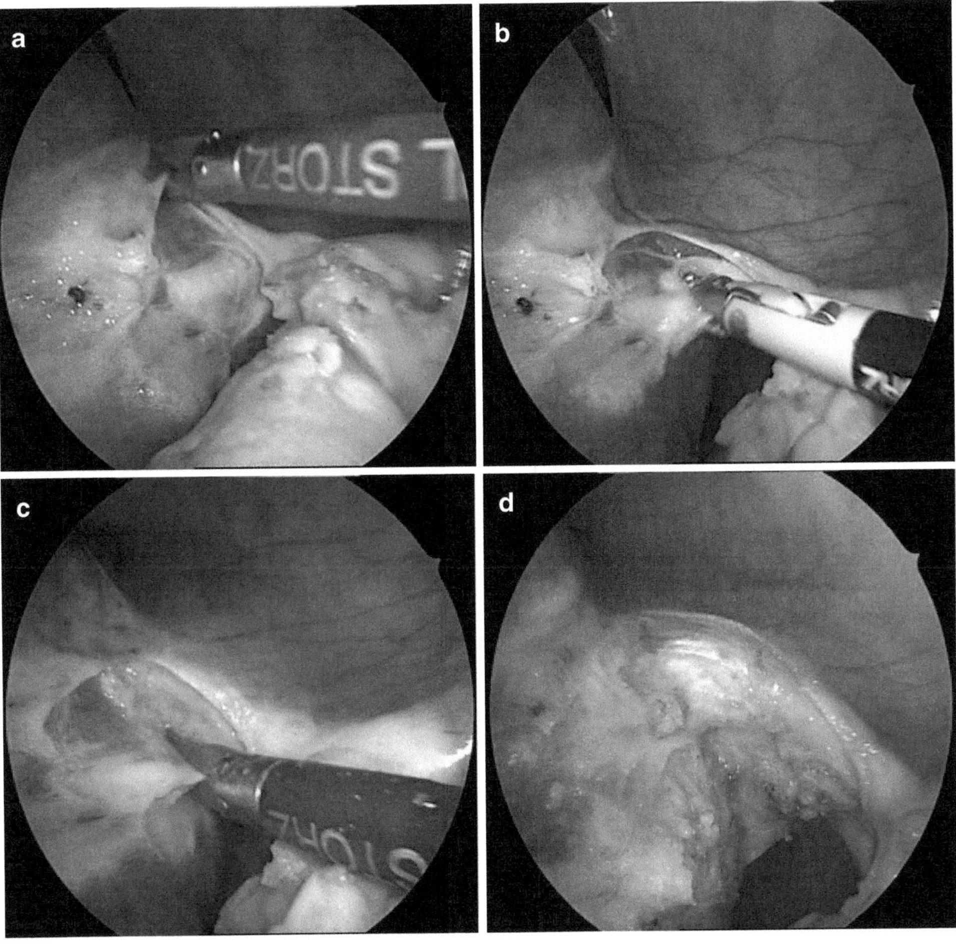

Fig. 32.9 Identification and skeletonization, bipolar coagulation and dissection of uterine vessels on the right side (**a**–**d**)

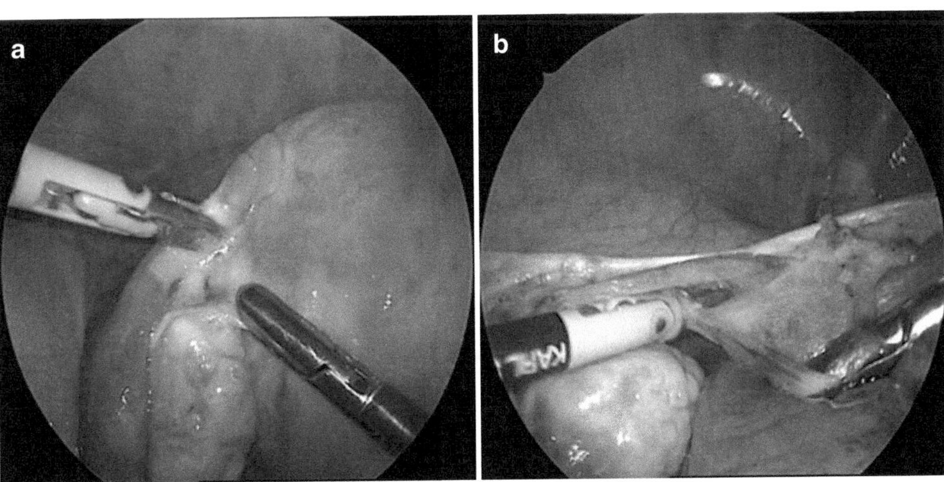

Fig. 32.10 Bipolar coagulation and dissection of round ligament, fallopian tube and ovarian ligament from left side (**a**, **b**)

After identification and skeletonization of the uterine vessels, bleeding is controlled by bipolar coagulation and the vessels dissected using Metzenbaum scissors on the right side (Fig. 32.9).

Grasping forceps are used to pull the uterus to the contralateral side. After separation of the uterus from the ovaries and fallopian tubes and dissection through the round ligaments on the left side (Fig. 32.10) the uterine vessels will be also coagulated and dissected (Fig. 32.11) and a bipolar coagulation zone is placed on the bladder peritoneum for the delineation of the planned direction of incision to open the bladder peritoneum (Fig. 32.12). Once the bladder peritoneum has been separated from the dissected round ligaments using scissors, it can be opened and the bladder pushed slightly caudally. It is not necessary to push away the bladder as it is in total hysterectomy. This is because dissection of the

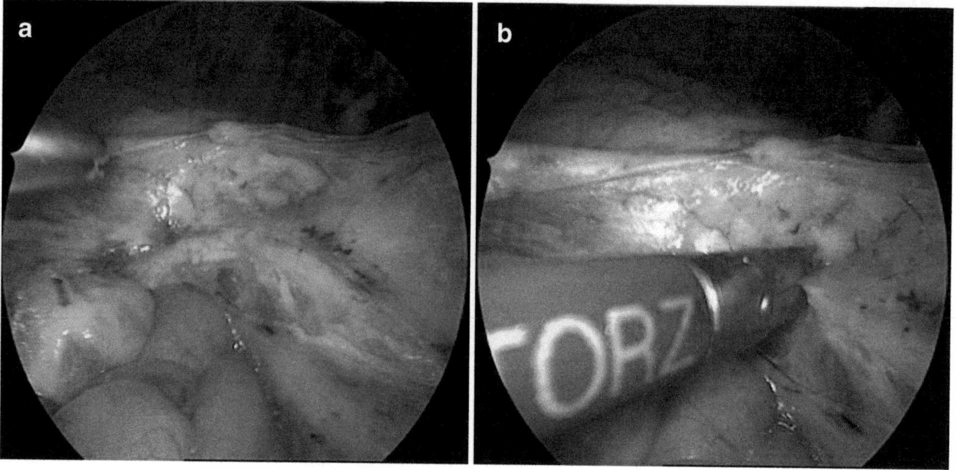

Fig. 32.11 Identification and skeletonization, bipolar coagulation and dissection of uterine vessels on the left side (**a**, **b**)

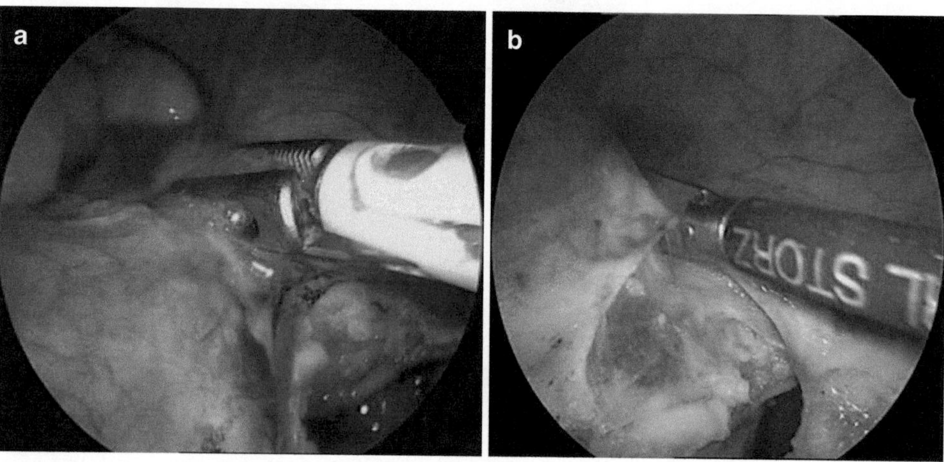

Fig. 32.12 A Coagulation zone is made on the bladder peritoneum (**a**) – Undermining and opening of the bladder peritoneum (**b**)

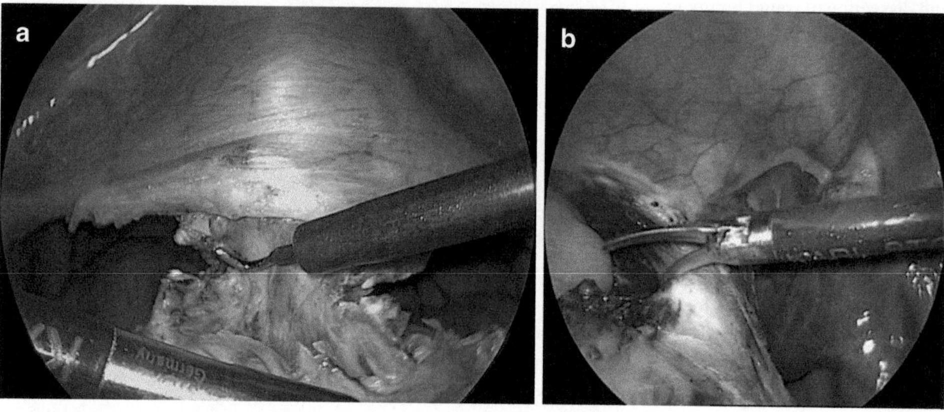

Fig. 32.13 Transection of corpus uteri with unipolar hook (**a**) or with a pair of scissors (**b**)

uterine body with a unipolar hook or with a pair of scissors (Fig. 32.13) is done in the upper third, cranial to where the uterosacral ligaments leave the cervix. If dissection starts from the left side, the uterus is held against the anterior wall using grasping forceps and pulled in cranial direction.

Due to the traction of the uterus to the opposite side (where the dissection is to be performed) space can be created to identify the uterine vessels in the cervical area and the ureter. If coagulation and dissection of the uterine vessels is performed close to the cervix, we do not visualize the ureter. In cases of cervical myomas, even traction of the uterus to the contralateral side is very helpful for visualizing the ureter.

The dissection is done step by step starting from the right using the unipolar hook. In this phase of surgery the surgeon needs clear vision to prevent injuries of adjacent organs; the development of excessive smoke can be prevented by actuating

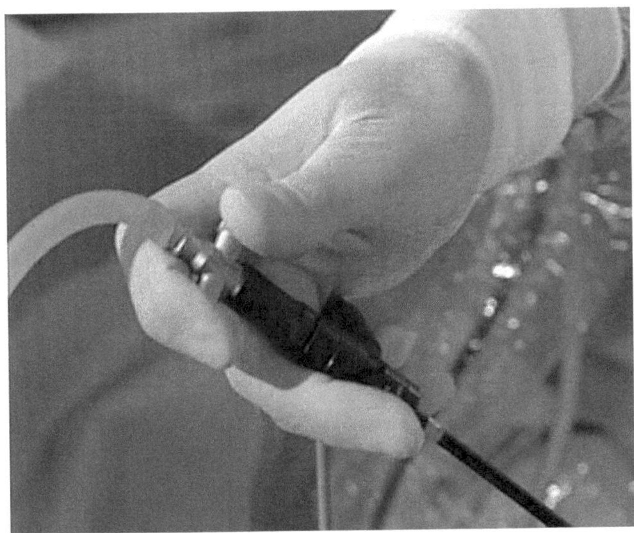

Fig. 32.14 Suction device connected to the unipolar hook

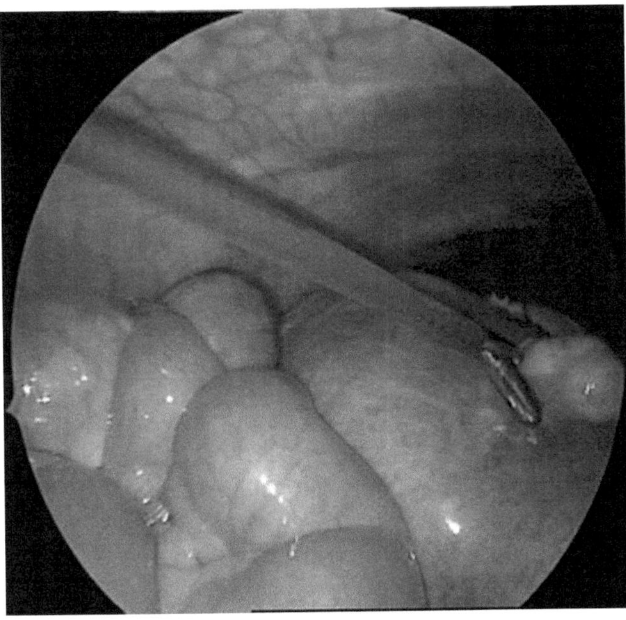

Fig. 32.15 Positionning of the transected corpus in the right-hand mesogastrium

the suction on the hook (Fig. 32.14). The dissected body of the uterus is positioned in the right-hand mesogastrium to enable haemostasis in the wound area (Fig. 32.15), followed by bipolar coagulation of the cervical canal (Fig. 32.16) after efficient haemostasis (Fig. 32.17) in the area of the cervix stump.

Tip The cervix can be held from the left using grasping forceps while searching for the entrance into the cervical canal with the palpation probe or bipolar forceps if identification of the cervical canal is difficult. Coagulation is performed by opening and simultaneously rotating the damp in the cervical canal.

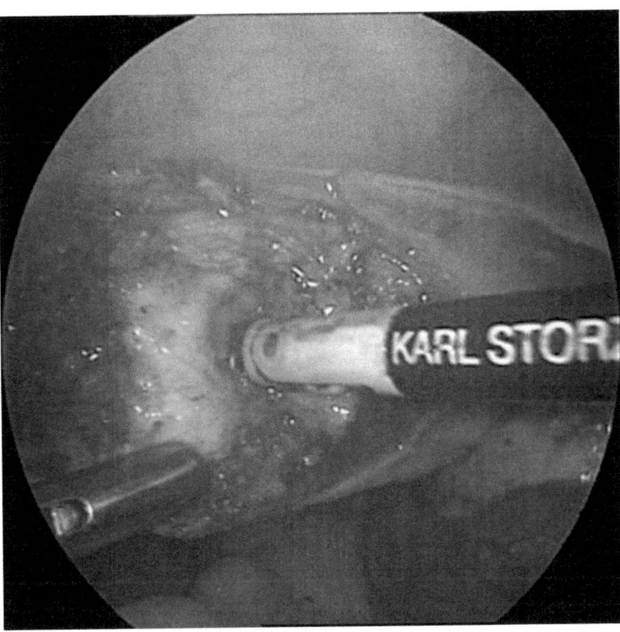

Fig. 32.16 Bipolar coagulation of the cervical canal

A vicryl thread shortened to approximately instrument length is used for peritonealisation of the cervical stump. Under vision, the round needle is introduced through the 5 mm incision (Fig. 32.18). The cervix stump is then covered with peritoneum using a continuous purse-string suture, including both uterosacral ligaments (Fig. 32.19). Following the preparation of a triple knot, the peritoneum is pulled together, with a fourth knot to secure the suture (Fig. 32.20).

The incision is widened to 10–20 mm in the left-hand lower abdomen to remove the uterus. Following injection of a local anaesthetic beneath the wound area of the left-hand incision, an electric morcellator (STORZ® or WISAP®) (Fig. 32.21) is introduced under direct vision. The uterus is then gripped from the left and pulled into the morcellator, which is activated by hand or via foot pedal. It is of utmost importance to keep the sharp rotating blade continuously in vision at the centre of the laparoscopic image to avoid injuries (Fig. 32.22). To remove a large section of tissue in a single piece, it is helpful to assist the process of morcellation with the right-handed grasping forceps so that the blade is always visible on the surface of the uterus (Fig. 32.23). Morcellation is therefore performed around the exterior of the uterus. The uterus is effectively peeled like a potato.

Tip It is particularly important to ensure a good overview during morcellation, and in the case of large uteri a 20 mm morcellator can also be used. This leads to a considerably shorter operation, as the sections of uterus removed in this way are far larger.

Remaining smaller pieces of the uterus or the myoma are retrieved using 10 mm spoon grasping forceps after removal of the uterus (Figs. 32.24 and 32.25).

The operation is completed with lavage and a final checking of the cervical stump (Fig. 32.26). The peritoneum in the area of 15 or 20 mm incisions is closed from the inside using bipolar coagulation. To avoid incision hernias Closure of the fasciae is also necessary. The skin is then closed using single-button sutures. The final position for a normal sized uterus shows 5 mm incisions in the umbilicus and on the right side of the lower abdomen, and a 15 mm incision on the left (Fig. 32.27). If the uterus is noticeably enlarged, an additional 5 mm and a 20 mm incision for the morcellation may become necessary.

Laparoscopic combined hysterectomy (LACH) with "change over technique" – this is a special surgical tech-

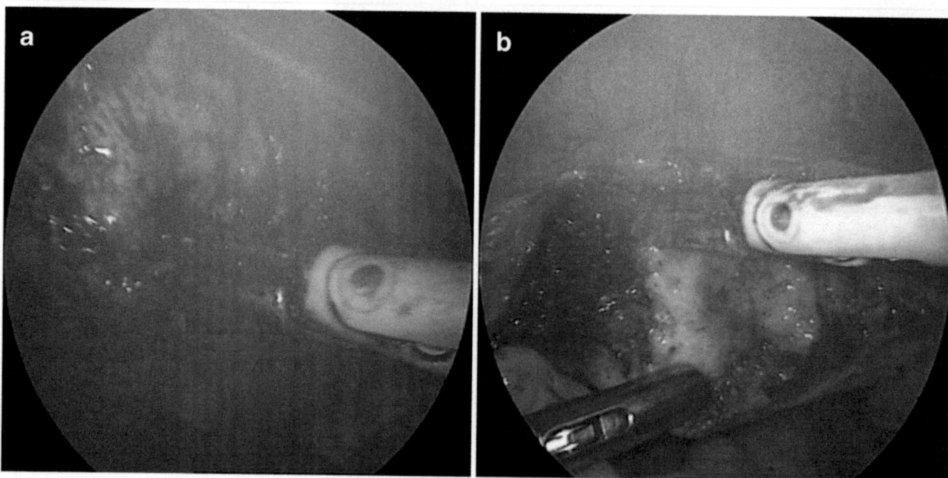

Fig. 32.17 Hemostasis in the area of the cervical stump (**a**, **b**)

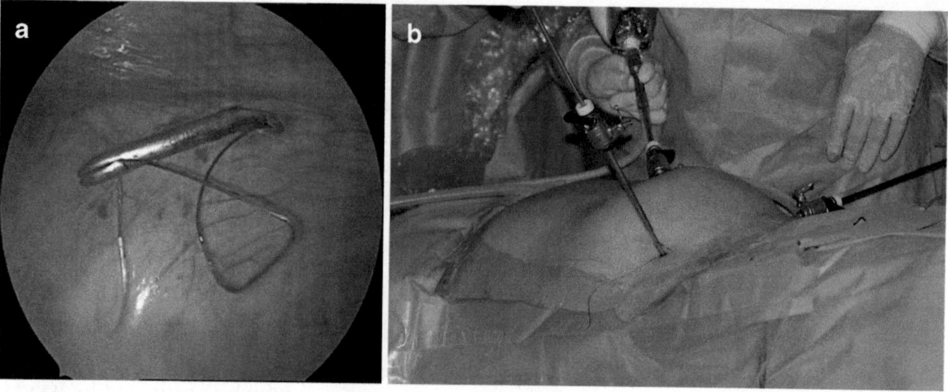

Fig. 32.18 Introduction of a round needle (endoscopic view and view from outside **a**, **b**)

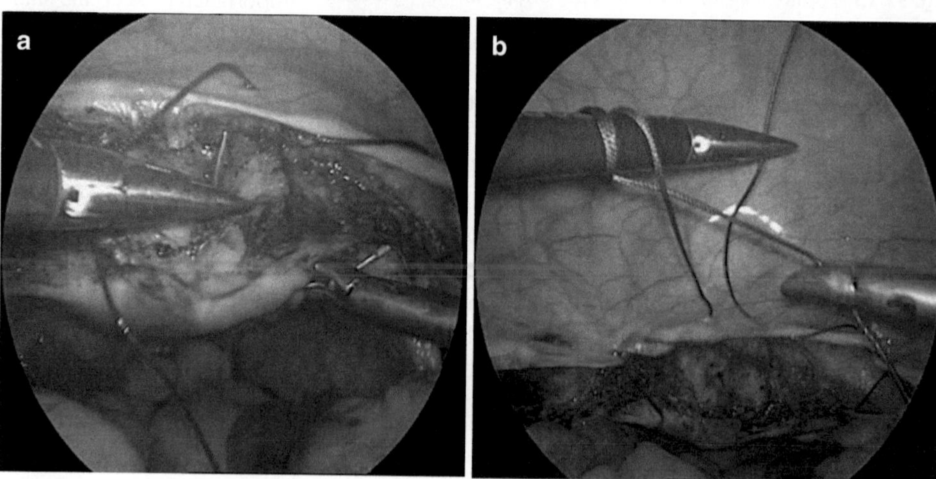

Fig. 32.19 Continuous purse-string suture (**a**, **b**)

nique for the removal of a very large uterus [13, 14]. Here, the uterine corpus is abscised and morcellated laparoscopically. For this, the above mentioned "change over technique" is applied, where the operation-team changes from one side of the patient to the other (Figs. 32.28 and 32.29). The "change over technique" can also be used in LSH given a difficult-case-uterus. The specialty of the "change over technique" lies in the fact that for successful abscission of the uterine corpus in case of very large uterine myomata, the surgeon begins operating on the left side of the uterus, respectively on the left side of the parametrium. After sealing and cutting off the left parametrium and the vascular bundle, the surgeon and the assistant move to the right side of the patient and now operate on the right side of the uterus.

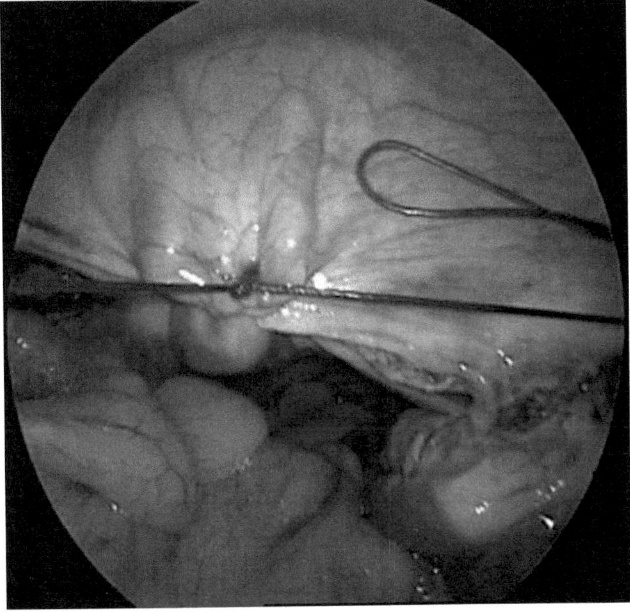

Fig. 32.20 Peritonealization of the cervical stump

Tip Doubtlessly, an umbilical entry of the optical trocar into the epigastrium is possible. However, we always recommend using Palmer's point for the camera trocar on the left side. For the right optical trocar, we use the exact symmetrical counterpoint on the right side. Surgery is always carried out using 5 mm 30 ° optics made by the Karl Storz company. Next, the patient is placed in maximum Trendelenburg position. For the first phase the surgery on the left side we place two more working trocars on the left axillary line of the abdomen, leaving a space of about 8–10 cm between them [14].

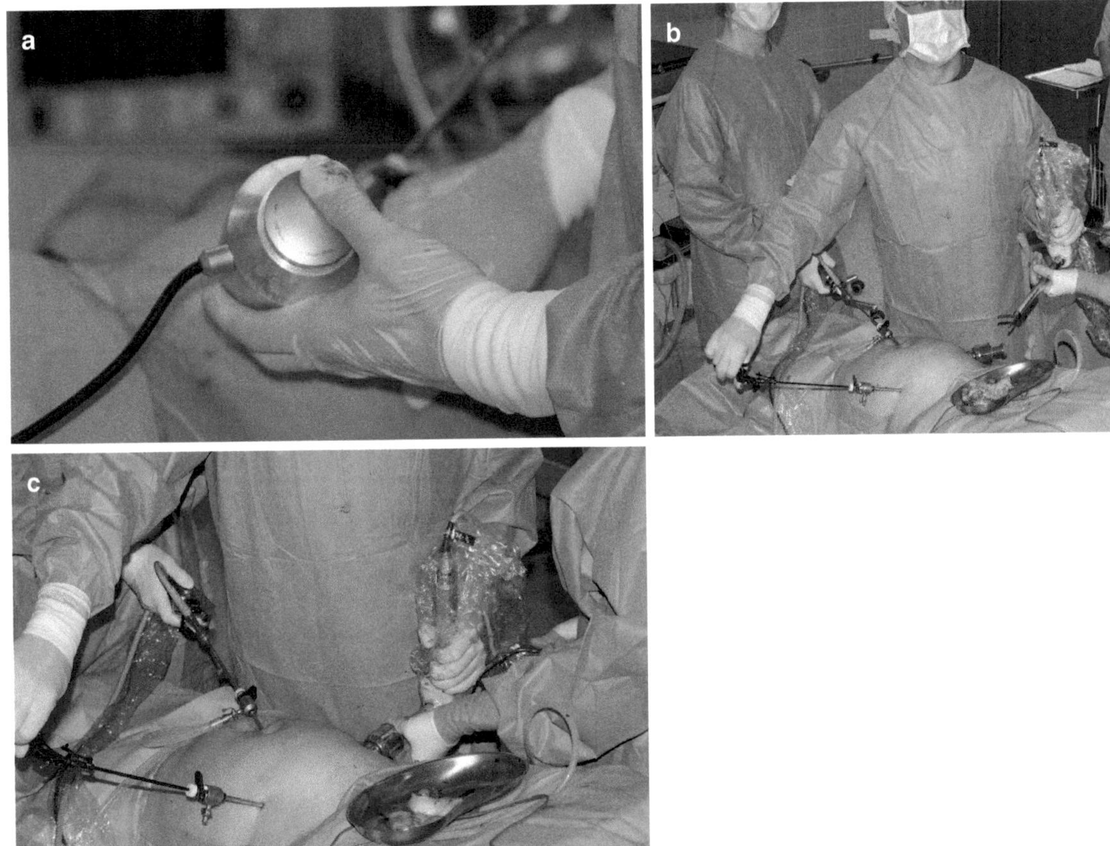

Fig. 32.21 Introduction of a 15 mm Rotocut electric morcellator (Storz) (**a**) or a 20 mm WISAP morcellator (**b, c**)

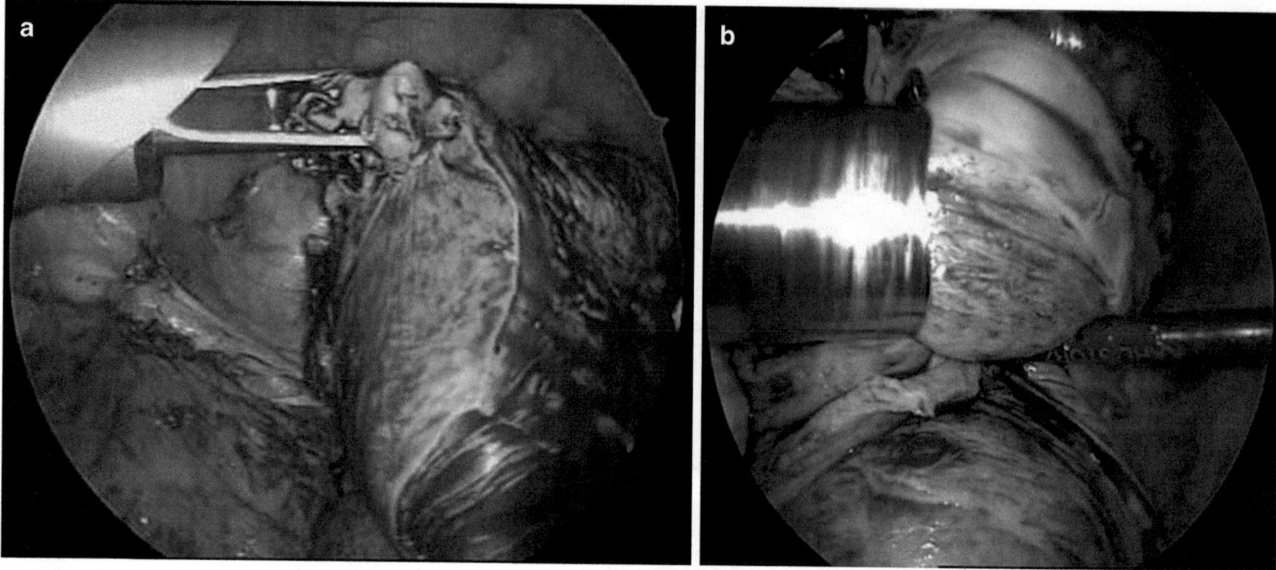

Fig. 32.22 The sharp rotating blade of the morcellator is visible during morcellation (**a** – Rotocut electric morcellator (Storz), **b** – WISAP electric morcellator)

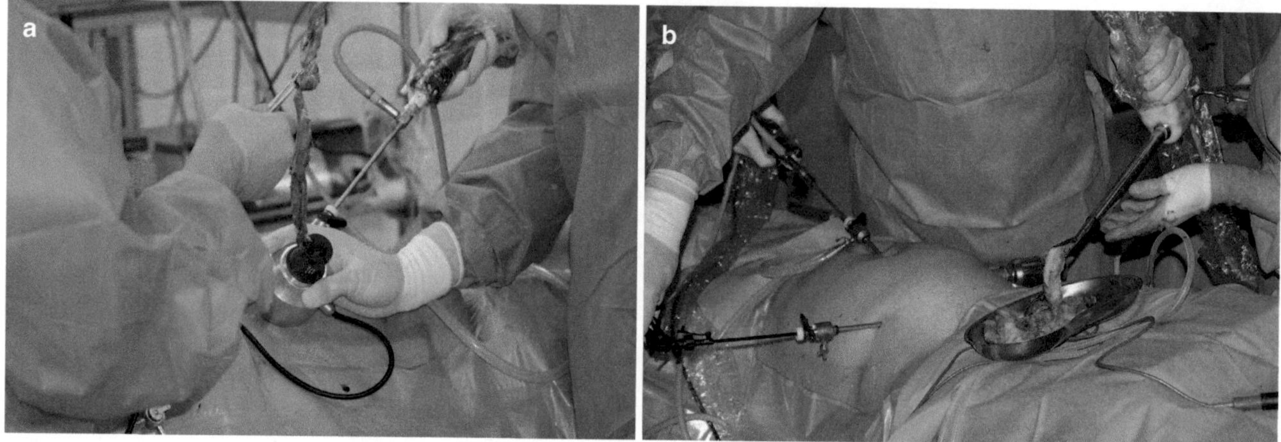

Fig. 32.23 Morcellation - View from outside (**a** – with the Rotocut electric morcellator (Storz), **b** – with the WISAP electric morcellator)

Tip The lower working trocar should be placed at about the height of the uterotubal junction.

After parameterization on the left side is conducted, the second optical trocar is placed in a position symmetrical to the Palmer's point area on the right costal arch under laparoscopic observation for the second phase of the "change over technique". The surgeon and his assistant change their position to the right side of the patient and the operation is resumed from the right. Leaving space of 8–10 cm between them, two further working trocars are placed along the right axillary line.

Complications

Reported complication rates in literature for all different hysterectomy procedures vary tremendously. It appears that complication rates in general are reduced using endoscopic techniques. Complication rates for abdominal hysterectomies are between 13.1 and 48 % [15–17] and for vaginal hysterectomies between 2 and 27.7 % [15, 17–19]. Complication rates for LSH are lower (0–4.35 %) than for TLH (0–18%) [4, 9, 19–23 34].

Compared to vaginal and abdominal hysterectomies, major complications (e.g. haemorrhage, vesicoperitoneal fistula, ureteral injury, rectal perforation or fistula) are more common after laparoscopic hysterectomies, as shown in multicenter studies [24], however the comparison to total laparoscopic hysterectomy shows that LSH has a lower major complication rate [25].

We reported intraoperative and postoperative complication rates of LSH of 0.2 % and 1.2 %, respectively, and a conversion rate of 0.82 % [4], which are similar to the low rates of conversion (0.7 %) and of intraoperative complication (0.1 %) in a second study [26]. Lyons [27] reports low rates

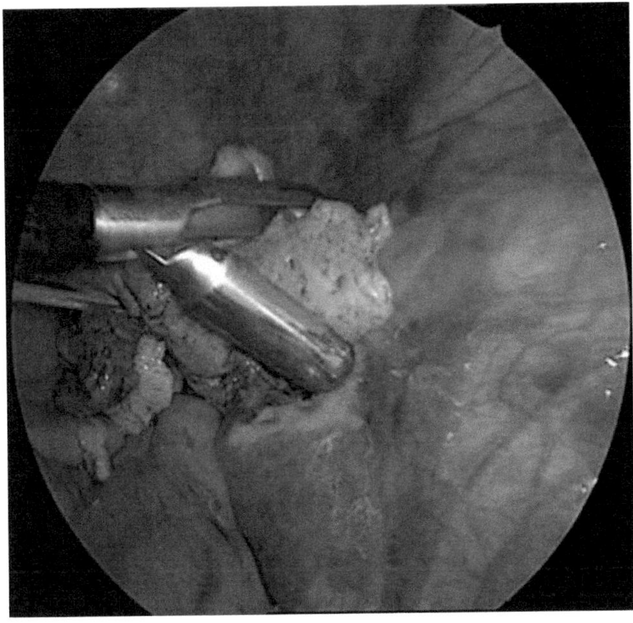

Fig. 32.24 Removal of smaller pieces using a 10 mm spoon grasping forceps

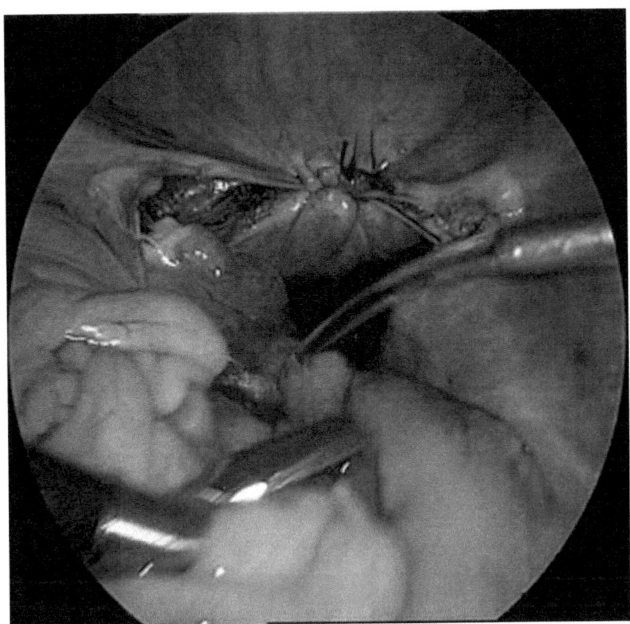

Fig. 32.26 Rinsing of the abdomen

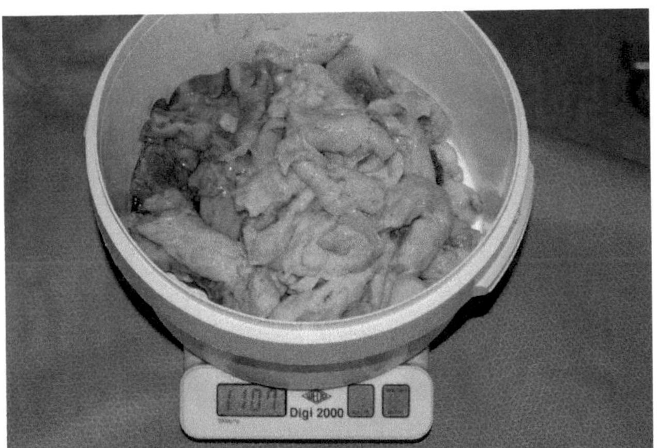

Fig. 32.25 Morcellated pieces of a 1107 g uterus

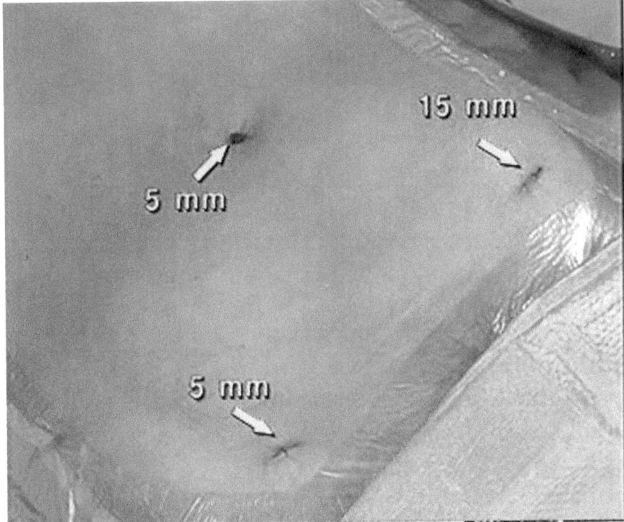

Fig. 32.27 Final abdominal situs

of blood transfusion (0 %), and reoperation (0.001 %), out of 1500 procedures, including patients with severe adhesive disease and severe endometriosis.

The majority of complications associated with a hysterectomy involve injuries to the urinary tract. One multicenter study showed highest complication rates of injury to the urinary tract for TLH (2.26 %) compared to abdominal (0.17 %) and vaginal hysterectomy (0.04 %) [28]. The risk of injury to the ureter or bladder during TLH increases as the bladder is dissected off the vaginal tissue [29]. Because the dissection ends superior to the bladder and ureter during LSH, the risk of direct damage to the ureter and bladder is presumably decreased [28, 30, 31]. Four retrospective studies have reported urinary tract (ureteral) injury rates of less than 1 % out of a total of more than 30,000 laparoscopic hysterectomies [4, 32, 33, 35].

Minor complication rates occurring after LSH are lower (0.25–1.35 %), including bladder incision (0.1–0.25 %), iatrogenic adenomyosis (0–0.56 %) and ileus (0.5 %) [11, 24, 25, 31, 33].

There are several reasons for the conversion of laparoscopic hysterectomies. Uterine size, weight and lack of mobility are clearly limiting factors for laparoscopic surgery, resulting in limited vision available during laparoscopy and higher rates of conversion [26]. Other risk factors are previous gynecological operations [4]. the close proximity of myomas to the cervix or the lateral wall of the pelvis has also made conversion necessary [26], technical difficulties caused

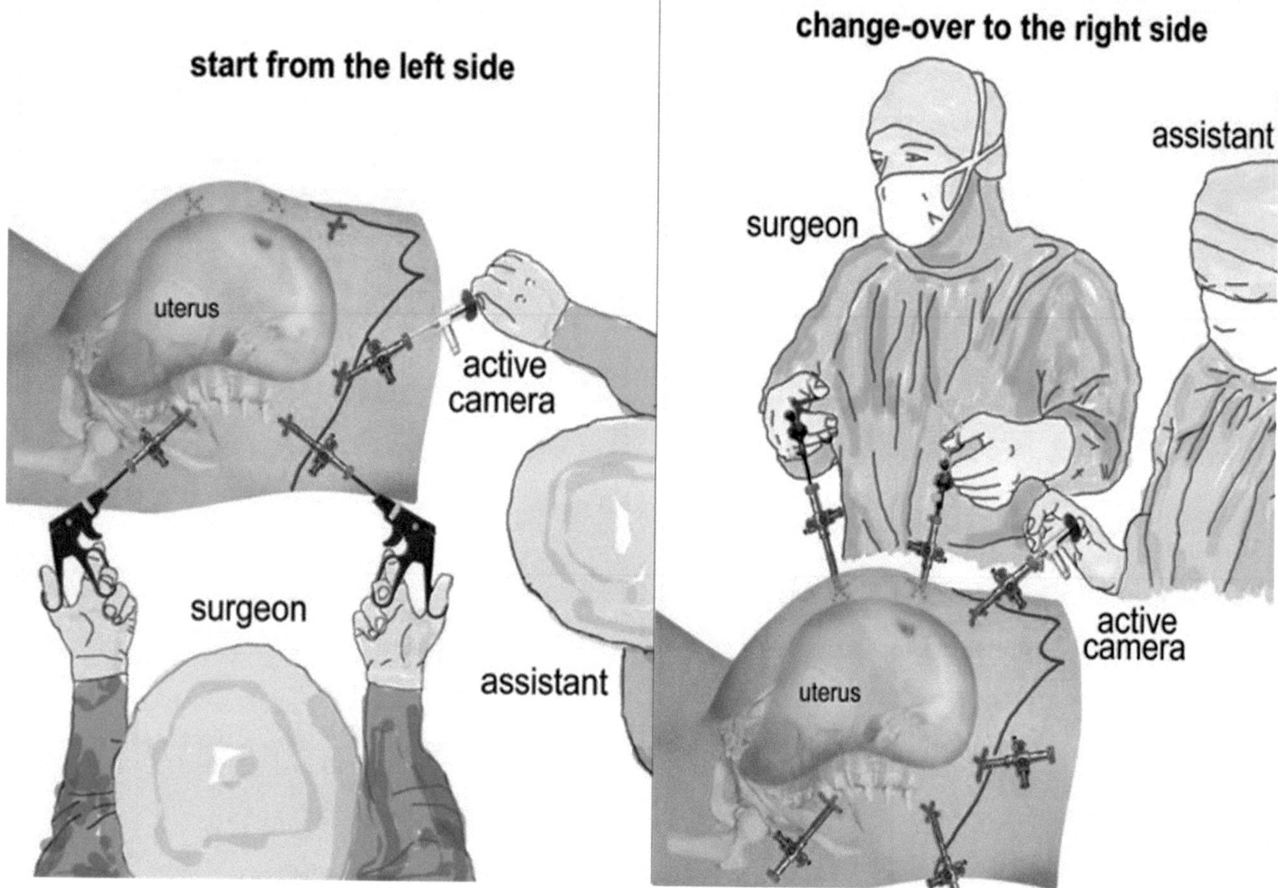

Fig. 32.28 Change Over Technique – Start of parameterization on the left side

Fig. 32.29 Change Over Technique – Operation team changes side. Continuation of parameterization on the right side

by adhesions, difficulty in controlling intraoperative bleeding, or the repair of a complication [33]. Endometriosis is a major challenge to the surgeon [36], and should be completely resected, as further surgery might otherwise become necessary [37].

Further interventions needed due to postoperative complications include postoperative abdominal pain due to adhesions [4]. Other causes of postoperative complications are infections of the cervical stump and of the incision sites [4]. Conservative treatment with antibiotics is indicated.

Remnants of uterine myoma left in the abdominal cavity after morcellation [38] can be rare postoperative complications leading to unclear persisting abdominal pain.

Performed by skilled, experienced surgeons, laparoscopic hysterectomy is a safe procedure resulting in very low rates of complication [35]. Various studies have shown that low complication rates correspond to the level of experience of the surgeons involved, whereas high complication rates observed in other studies are not the result of the technique itself but rather lack of experience. The laparoscopic technique requires a high level of expertise with a learning curve of 30 operations to significantly decrease operating time and complication rates [39].

Conclusion

Minimal morbidity and an equally low complication rate are typically associated with LSH. The majority of complications associated with a hysterectomy are bladder and ureteral lesions and vaginal stump infections. These risks can be reduced significantly as the cervix is conserved, which is reflected in lower surgical morbidity and fewer postoperative complications.

The rate of postoperative complications is lower, hospital stays are shorter, patients recover more quickly and return to normal activity and work after a shorter convalescence compared to abdominal or vaginal hysterectomy. The procedure therefore appears to be beneficial to patients [37, 40–43]. In addition, a comparison to total laparoscopic hysterectomy shows that LSH has a remarkably lower major complication rate [25]. Furthermore, the use of reusable laparoscopic instruments reduces the total cost of the procedure [44].

References

1. Hucke J, DeBruyne F, Wangsatimur BR, Campo RL. Surgical hysteroscopy. Gynäkologie. 1993;26:338–45.
2. Mettler L. Endoskopische Abdominalchirurgie in der Gynäkologie. Stuttgart: Schattauer; 2002.
3. Semm K. Total ablation of uterine mucosa (TUMA) – CURT instead of endometrium ablation. Geburtshilfe Frauenheilkd. 1992;52:773–7.
4. Bojahr B, Raatz D, Schonleber G, Abri C, Ohlinger R. Perioperative complication rate in 1706 patients after a standardized laparoscopic supracervical hysterectomy technique. J Minim Invasive Gynecol. 2006;13:183–9.
5. Kilkku P, Grönroos M, Hirvonen T, Rauramo L. Supravaginal uterine amputation vs. hysterectomy. Effects on libido and orgasm. Acta Obstet Gynecol Scand. 1983;62(2):147–52.
6. Thomas B, Magos A. Subtotal hysterectomy and myomectomy – Vaginally. Best Pract Res Clin Obstet Gynaecol. 2010;25(2):133–52. doi:10.1016/j.bpobgyn.2010.11.003.
7. Vervest HA, de Jonge M K, TM V, JW B, AA H. Micturition symptoms and urinary incontinence after non-radical hysterectomy. Acta Obstet Gynecol Scand. 1988;67(2):141–6.
8. Gimbel H. Total or subtotal hysterectomy for benign uterine disease? A meta-analysis. Acta Obstet Gynecol Scand. 2007;86:133–44.
9. Learman LA, Summit Jr RL, Varner RE, et al. A randomized comparison of total or supracervical hysterectomy: surgical complications and clinical outcomes. Obstet Gynecol. 2003;102:453–62.
10. Pasic R, Abdelmonem A, Levine R. Comparison of cervical detachment using monopolar lap loop ligature and conventional methods in laparoscopic supracervical hysterectomy. JSLS. 2006;10:226–30.
11. Donnez O, Jadoul P, Squifflet J, Donnez J. A series of 3190 laparoscopic hysterectomies for benign disease from 1990 to 2006: evaluation of complications compared with vaginal and abdominal procedures. BJOG. 2009;116:492–500.
12. Giep BN, Giep HN, Hubert HB. Comparison of minimally invasive surgical approaches for hysterectomy at a community hospital: robotic-assisted laparoscopic hysterectomy, laparoscopic-assisted vaginal hysterectomy and laparoscopic supracervical hysterectomy. J Robot Surg. 2010;4(3):167–75.
13. Tchartchian G, Dietzel J, Bojahr B, et al. No more abdominal hysterectomy for myomata using a new minimally-invasice technique. Int J Surg Case Rep. 2010;1(1):7–8.
14. Tchartchian G. Laparoscopic combined hysterectomy using the "Change Over Technique" for very large uterine myomata. In: Schollmeyer T, Mettler L, Rüther D, Alkatout I, editors. Practical manual for laparoscopic and hysteroscopic gynecological surgery. 2nd ed. New Delhi: Jaypee Brothers Medical Publishers; 2013. p. 337–41.
15. Dicker RC, Greenspan JR, Strauss LT, et al. Complications of abdominal and vaginal hysterectomy among women of reproductive age in the United States. The Collaborative Review of Sterilization. Am J Obstet Gynecol. 1982;144(7):841–8.
16. Härkki-Siren P, Sjöberg J. Evaluation and the learning curve of the first one hundred laparoscopic hysterectomies. Acta Obstet Gynecol Scand. 1995;74(8):638–41.
17. Wang PH, Lee WL, Yuan CC, et al. Major complications of operative and diagnostic laparoscopy for gynecologic disease. J Am Assoc Gynecol Laparosc. 2001;8(1):68–73.
18. Daraï E, Soriano D, Kimata P, et al. Vaginal hysterectomy for enlarged uteri, with or without laparoscopic assistance: randomized study. Obstet Gynecol. 2001;97(5 Pt 1):712–6.
19. Sarmini OR, Lefholz K, Froeschke HP. A comparison of laparoscopic supracervical hysterectomy and total abdominal hysterectomy outcomes. J Minim Invasive Gynecol. 2005;12:121–4.
20. Buchele B. Retrospective analysis of 195 laparoscopic supracervical hysterectomies. J Am Assoc Gynecol Laparosc. 2004;11(suppl):S22.
21. Fiaccavento A, Landi S, Barbieri F, et al. Total laparoscopic hysterectomy in cases of very large uteri: a retrospective comparative study. J Minim Invasive Gynecol. 2007;14:559–63.
22. Hoffman CP, Kennedy J, Borschel L, et al. Laparoscopic hysterectomy: the Kaiser Permanente San Diego experience. J Minim Invasive Gynecol. 2005;12:16–24.
23. Johnson N, Barlow D, Lethaby A, et al. Surgical approach to hysterectomy for benign gynaecological disease. Cochrane Database Syst Rev. 2006;19:CD003677.
24. Garry R, Fountain J, Mason S, Hawe J, Napp V, Abbott J, et al. The eVALuate study: two parallel randomized trials, one comparing laparoscopic with abdominal hysterectomy, the other comparing laparoscopic with vaginal hysterectomy. BMJ. 2004;328:1229–36.
25. Cipullo L, De Paoli S, Fasolino L, Fasolino A. Laparoscopic supracervical Hysterectomy Compared to Total Hysterectomy. JSLS. 2009;13:370–5.
26. Bojahr B, Tchartchian G, Ohlinger R. Laparoscopic Supracervical Hysterectomy: a Retrospective Analysis of 1000 Cases. JSLS. 2009;13:129–34.
27. Lyons TL. Laparoscopic supracervical versus total hysterectomy. J Minim Invasive Gynecol. 2007;14:275–7.
28. Härkki-Siren P, Sjöberg J, Tiitinen A. Urinary tract injuries after hysterectomy. Obstet Gynecol. 1998;9:113–8.
29. Jelovsek JE, Chiung C, Chen G, et al. Incidence of lower urinary tract injury at the time of total laparoscopic hysterectomy. JSLS. 2007;11:422–7.
30. Johns A. Supracervical versus total hysterectomy. Clin Obstet Gynecol. 1997;40:903–13.
31. Richards SR, Simpkins S. Laparoscopic supracervical hysterectomy versus laparoscopic-assisted vaginal hysterectomy. J Am Assor Gynecol Laparosc. 1995;2:431–5.
32. Brummer TH, Seppälä TT, Härkki PS. National learning curve for laparoscopic hysterectomy and trends in hysterectomy in Finland 2000–2005. Hum Reprod. 2008;23:840–5.
33. Harmanli OH, Tunitsky E, Esin S. A comparison of short-term outcomes between laparoscopic supracervical and total hysterectomy. Am J Obstet Gynecol. 2009;201:536.e1–7.
34. Karaman Y, Bingol M, Günenc Z. Prevention of complications in laparoscopic hysterectomy: experience with 1120 cases performed by a single surgeon. J Minim Invasive Gynecol. 2007;14:78–84.
35. Donnez O, Donnez J. A series of 400 laparoscopic hysterectomies for benign disease: a single centre, single surgeon prospective study of complications confirming previous retrospective study. BJOG. 2010;117:752–5.
36. Lyons TL, Adolph AJ, Winer WK. Laparoscopic supracervical hysterectomy for the large uterus. J Am Assoc Gynecol Laparosc. 2004;11(2):170–4.
37. Okaro EO, Jones KD, Sutton C. Long term outcome following laparoscopic supracervical hysterectomy. BJOG. 2001;108:1017–20.
38. Hutchins FLJ, Reinoehl EM. Retained myoma after laparoscopic supracervical hysterectomy with morcellation. J Am Assoc Gynecol Laparosc. 1998;5:293–5.
39. Ghomi A, Littman P, Prasad A, Einarsson JI. Assessing the learning curve for laparoscopic supracervical hysterectomy. JSLS. 2007;11(2):190–4.

40. Lyons TL. Laparoscopic supracervical hysterectomy. Obstet Gynecol Clin North Am. 2000;27:441–50.
41. Mettler L, Semm K, Lehmann-Willenbrock L, Shah A, et al. Comparative evaluation of classical intrafascial-supracervical hysterectomy (CISH) with transuterine mucosal resection as performed by pelviscopy and laparotomy – our first 200 cases. Surg Endosc. 1995;33:448–53.
42. Mettler L. Long-term results in the treatment of menorrhagia and hypermenorrhea with a thermal balloon endometrial ablation technique. JSLS. 2002;6:305–9.
43. Reich H, McGlynn F, Sekal L. Total laparoscopic hysterectomy. Gynecol Endosc. 1993;2:59–63.
44. Mettler L, Ahmed-Ebbiary N, Schollmeyer T. Laparoscopic hysterectomy: Challenges and limitations. Minim Invasive Ther Allied Technol. 2005;14(3):145–59.

33 Laparoscopic Supracervical Hysterectomy for Large Uteri

Funlayo Odejinmi and Reeba Oliver

Introduction

Routes of Hysterectomy

The routes of hysterectomy have evolved since ancient times. The first vaginal hysterectomy was performed by Soranus of Ephesus around AD 120 and employment of the vaginal route to remove the uterus continued through the medieval times. The next advance in an alternative route occurred in 1843 when Charles Clay performed the first abdominal hysterectomy in Manchester, England [1]. It was only in 1988 after the advent of modern endoscopic techniques, did the route of hysterectomies evolve again. Harry Reich performed the first laparoscopic hysterectomy in Pennsylvania [1]. Since then, the challenge has always been to push the boundaries of endoscopic surgery to achieve removal of the uterus for all women within the remits of surgical safety.

Once the decision is undertaken that a woman needs a hysterectomy, the route of the hysterectomy is the next debatable issue that is taken into consideration. The decision about the route depends on the patient characteristics, indication for hysterectomy, extrauterine pathology and size of the uterus. Recent reviews comparing routes of hysterectomy suggest that vaginal hysterectomy is the preferred route for hysterectomy for benign conditions and where vaginal hysterectomy is not possible, laparoscopic hysterectomy may avoid the need for an abdominal procedure necessitating a laparotomy [2].

Many perceived barriers to laparoscopic hysterectomy have been identified. The size of the uterus is considered to be a limiting factor to performing most hysterectomies endoscopically. Traditionally the large uterus was exclusively extirpated by the abdominal route, often by a midline incision [3] with the associated risk of infective complications [4].

For the vaginal route, randomised trials have shown that large uteri can be removed vaginallywith no added complications and reduced length of hospital stay [5]. This however requires a higher level of expertise, and even then uterine size has often been cited as a limiting factor and increases the rate of conversion to laparotomy particularly when the vagina is narrow. The use of GnRH analogues to reduce the size of the uterus to allow for vaginal hysterectomy has been advocated [6]. However, the use of GnRH analogues can be associated with unwanted side effects. Thus where vaginal hysterectomy is not possible, and if possible, the laparoscopic approach should be used in order tos avoid abdominal hysterectomy. Randomized trials have shown the benefits of laparoscopic hysterectomy over open abdominal hysterectomy [7].

With the advent of new modern alternatives to the management of menorrhagia such as endometrial ablations and Mirena IUS, most hysterectomies are no longer on "normal sized" uteri. However for the large uterus whatever route is used, uterine size remains a bastion to conquer for the generalist gynaecologist and is often a reason for conversion to abdominal hysterectomy.

Supracervical Hysterectomy

The laparoscopic supracervical hysterectomy (LSH) has become a well-established and proven safe procedure [8] since first described by Semm [9]. It has evolved into an alternative to other forms of hysterectomy, with good short and long term outcomes [10] and patient satisfaction [11]. In some countries up to 40 % of hysterectomies are now performed supracervically [12]. In the absence of the need to remove the cervix for the normal sized uterus it has been shown that the LSH is associated with shorter operating time, less blood loss and less postoperative febrile episodes [13, 14].

F. Odejinmi (✉) • R. Oliver
Department of Obstetrics and Gynaecology, Whipps Cross University Hospital, Barts Health NHS Trust, London, E11 1NR, UK
e-mail: jimi@doctors.org.uk

I. Alkatout, L. Mettler (eds.), *Hysterectomy*, DOI 10.1007/978-3-319-22497-8_33

Although LSH enables the removal of a large uterus laparoscopically with the obvious patient benefits, it has not been without its detractors. There is a perceived risk of developing cervical cancer in the residual cervix necessitating further surgery. But in developed countries where there is cervical screening, the risk of cervical cancer is very low if women do not default from screening programmes. Thus if there is no clinical reason to remove the cervix, LSH with its advantages is an alternative to laparotomy especially in women with high BMI. Again there is the potential risk of leiomyosarcoma. This risk is associated with the morcellation process with the morcellation process. Despite this, current evidence suggests that LSH is a safe and appropriate procedure for the management of benign gynaecological disease. Emphasis should be placed on patient information to aid an informed decision and further diagnostic assessments to allow earlier detection of occult malignancy (see unexpected malignancy).

There are no studies that have looked at long term outcome of women who have had LSH for large uteri. In women with normal uteri, though quality of life in the short term may be better when compared to TLH there is a slightly increased risk of stump haematoma, which can be overcome by careful haemostasis and laparoscopically over-sewing the cervical stump.

In the long term there is an increased risk of spotting. In the series by Tchartchain and colleagues looking at vaginal spotting after LSH they found that vaginal bleeding post procedure can result in a decrease in quality of life. However for myomatous uteri there was no statistical difference in patient satisfaction when compared to women who had LSH for other indications [15]. In the series by Lieng and colleagues 7 % of their cohort went on to have removal of the cervical stump for continued bleeding [16]. The size of the uteri in their cohort was however not specified.

With the advancement of technologies; better laparoscopes, optical systems, endoscopic instruments, vessel sealing technologies and tissue morcellation, it has become possible to push the boundaries of laparoscopic supracervical hysterectomy (LSH). It is now possible not only to perform this procedure in the large uterus but also in the larger patient [17]. Most observational studies demonstrate that LSH for the large uterus is not only feasible but offers a procedure with no added morbidity or complications with good patient satisfaction.

The Large Uterus

There are inconsistencies in literature as what constitutes a large uterus. The uterus was considered large at 280 g but this was the definition used for cut-off for vaginal hysterectomy [18]. With a laparoscope and full visualization of the pelvis a large uterus can be defined as one that extends to or beyond the true pelvis, thus extending above the sacral promontory. In an average sized woman this landmark will extend midway between the pubic symphysis and the umbilicus, equivalent to a 20 week sized fetus or weigh 500 g (Fig. 33.1).

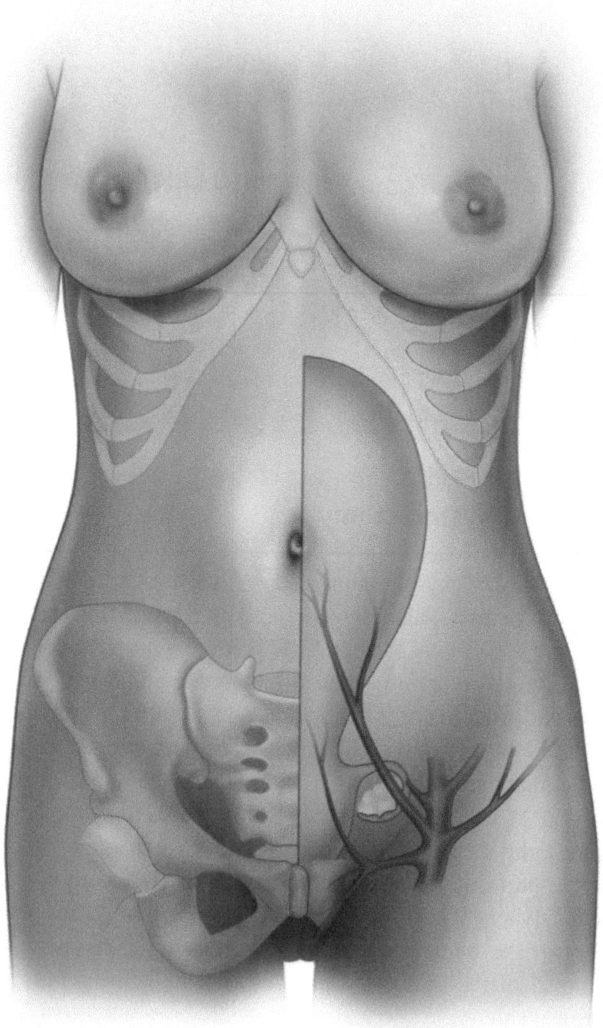

Fig. 33.1 Schematic diagram of a large uterus. Figure 33.1 shows the position of the enlarged uterus in relation to the bony pelvis (Courtesy of Catherine Woodman, BA (Hons))

LSH in Uterus Over 500 g: The Evidence

There have been no randomised studies with outcomes comparing LSH in women with uteri over 500 g with other forms of hysterectomy, thus outcomes can only be extrapolated from observational studies.

In the earliest large series on LSH for large uteri reported by Lyons and colleagues, 67 % of women had uteri larger than 500 g [19]. Alperin and colleagues later published a series of 333 women with uteri larger than 500 g who underwent LSH for large uteri and compared the outcome with 113 women who underwent total laparoscopic hysterectomy (TLH) for uteri larger than 500 g (mean weight 786 g) and found that LSH was associated with a significantly lower operating time than TLH in this group of patients. Additionally, their conversion rate was low and not related to uterine size [3].

In the series by Maclaran et al. where 33 women had a uterine weight of over 600 g, there were no conversions to laparotomy. They found that a combination of elevated BMI and enlarged uterus resulted in 94 % increase in blood loss and 66 % increase in operation duration compared to those with normal weight and uterine size less than 300 g [20]. But in spite of the above, there were no increase in hospital stay or morbidity. Hussain and colleagues in a series of 88 patients undergoing laparoscopic hysterectomy found that with the larger uterus there is significantly more blood loss and longer operating time. Most of the operative time was put down to the added time needed for morcellation. However there was no difference in the length of stay of the patients [17].

In the series of 1584 women by Grosse-Dreiling et al. though there is no data on the sizes of the uteri, the overall conversion rate was 0.88 %. Of the 14 patients that needed conversion to laparotomy, 3 had uteri greater than 850 g and conversions were due to uncontrollable bleeding attributed to uterine size. Uterine size alone contributed to only 20 % of the conversions [21].

In the series of 1000 LSH procedures reported by Bojahr and colleagues of which 68 had uteri weighing 500 g or more, there were 4 conversions in patients with increased uterine weight. The average uterine weight in this group was 976 g, the lightest uterus was 750 g, and the heaviest was 1185 g. The authors note that the conversion to laparotomy was not due to the size alone but the lack of uterine mobility, closeness of myomas to the cervix or the lateral wall of the pelvis [22]. This group again reported on a series of 1952 LSH procedures of which 8.6 % weighed more than 500 g. In this series the overall conversion rate was 0.82 % with 71 % of those conversions due to access related to uterine size [23].

Twijnstra and colleagues reviewing the literature on laparoscopic hysterectomy conversion rates, found that LSH can reduce conversion rates compared to TLH 3 fold, but uteri weighing 500 g or more could increase conversion rates 30 fold [24]. With the large uterus it could be argued that size *per se* is not the limiting factor but rather the shape of the uterus as it is in the TLH procedure [25]. The difficulty in completing the procedure is dependent on the limited pelvic space and the often tortuous and enlarged uterine vessels. Another major factor is the distortion of anatomy caused by uterine fibroids, with conversions to laparotomy being influenced by lower segment or broad ligament fibroids [3]. The mobility of the uterus is also often limited [26]. Access to the cervix and or uterine arteries can be restricted by the presence of fibroids and the approach will depend on the exact location of the fibroids in relation to these structures. Thus irrespective of the definition used, the most important factor in performing a supracervical hysterectomy for the large uterus is access to the uterine vessels and the cervix in order to transect it at the isthmus. Nimaroff and colleagues advised a combined technique of laparoscopic supracervical amputation followed by trachelectomy to enable laparoscopic removal of large uteri weighing more than 450 g [27].

Optimizing the Surgical Outcome

Whatever the route or type of hysterectomy the ideal procedure is one that allows for the procedure to be completed successfully with the least morbidity, fewest complications, allows early recovery and has good patient satisfaction.

Patient Selection

It is thus important that patients are chosen carefully in order to meet these objectives. For the large uterus and in the large patient, recent literature dictates that not only is this a safe procedure and feasible, but it also has good outcomes and satisfaction rates. There have been no studies looking at selection and pre-operative criteria for large uteri for LSH. There have been studies to predict the weight of the uterus using ultrasound or MRI (Fig. 33.2) and comparing this to bimanual examination of the uterus [28]. And though formulae have been developed

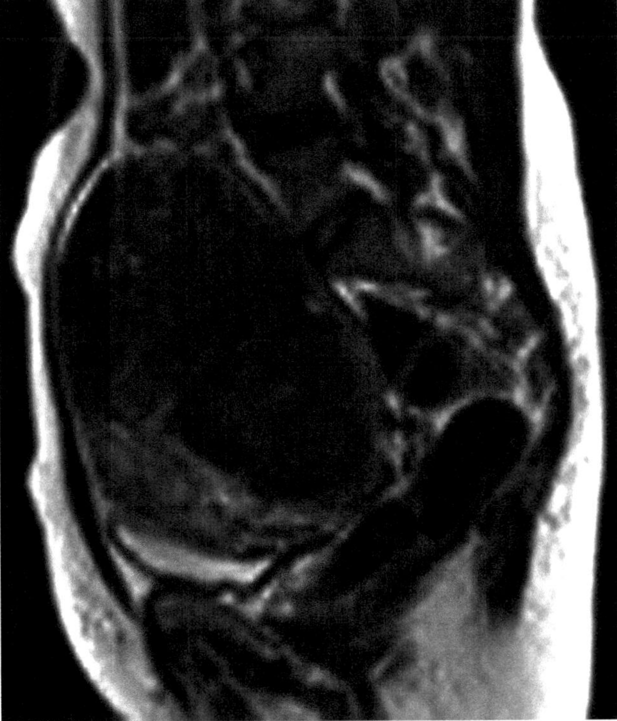

Fig. 33.2 MRI scan of a large fibroid. Figure 33.2 shows a MRI scan of a large fibroid uterus extending out of the true pelvis

to help with the prediction [29], and can be helpful in the evaluation and counseling of the patient as long as there is space to insert the laparoscope beyond the upper margin of the uterus, there is always the possibility of being able to perform the procedure laparoscopically [26].

Counseling the Patient

As with all gynaecological procedures adequate counseling of the patient prior to procedure is necessary. The LSH is associated with reduced hospital stay compared to other forms of hysterectomy and earlier recovery and resumption of intercourse [19]. However, long term sequellae such as spotting and the need for further intervention is increased with subtotal hysterectomy [11].

Though there are no specific studies looking at these issues specifically for large uteri, counseling should also be along the lines of LSH for normal uteri.

There is also the issue of morcellation and the risk of upgrading occult leiomyosarcoma that needs to be discussed with the patients. Clear and written guidelines need to be provided.

Theatre Set Up

The theatre set up is essentially the same as for a standard LSH. It is important that all members of staff are aware of their roles and those responsible for use of modern energy sources are aware of how to trouble-shoot when things go wrong.

As with all forms of laparoscopic surgery that can take over 2 h there is a need to ensure that the patient is warm and adequate anticoagulation measures are taken to prevent thrombosis. The patient will be in the Trendelenberg position for a considerable amount of time and on occasions the angle needed may be quite steep, measures should be used to prevent the patient slipping caudally and to prevent nerve injury.

Patient Habitus

The ideal habitus for a patient for LSH would be one with a "roomy" pelvis that allows visualization of the sides of the uterus and pedicles. There is an increase in obesity in society and this need to be taken into consideration. Performing LSH on the larger patient is not only feasible but safe [17]. Although with the larger patient there is an increased operating time and blood loss [20], this however does not affect the length of hospital stay post operation.

Surgical Technique

The surgical technique of LSH in a large uterus follows that of routine LSH, but with certain modifications to accommodate the distortion in size, shape and lack of access.

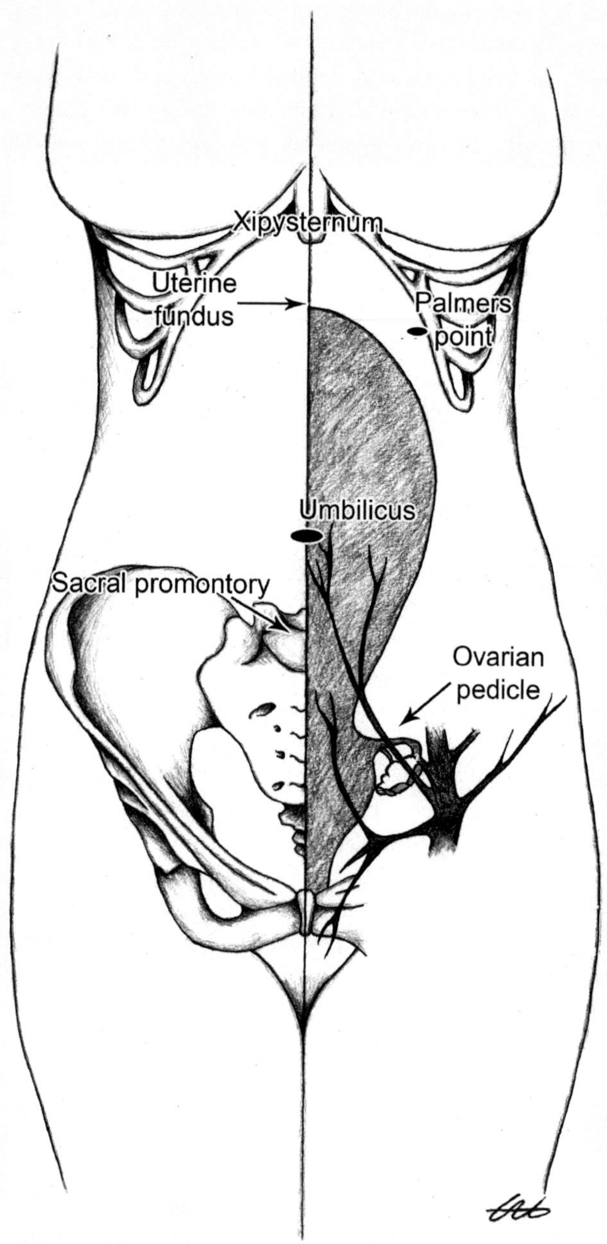

Fig. 33.3 Anterior abdominal landmarks. Figure 33.3 shows the important laparoscopic landmarks of the anterior abdominal wall (Courtesy of Catherine Woodman, BA (Hons))

Land Marks

It is pertinent to be aware of the anatomical landmarks of the whole of the abdominal cavity as the enlarged uterus could rise up to the xiphisternum. Additionally the primary trocar site might have to be varied due to the uterus taking up most of the central abdominal space, and other sites such as the Palmer's point will have to be used (Fig. 33.3). The most important land mark irrespective of the entry point is the ability to visualize both the sides of the uterus below the ovarian pedicles and the neck of the cervix anteriorly and posteriorly.

LSH of a Tall Globular Uterus

The tall globular uterus, as is usually seen with a fundal fibroid, usually does not limit access to the pedicles. The procedure is usually straightforward and follows the routine steps of a LSH (Fig. 33.4).

The procedure begins with placing the ports to allow visualization of the fundus of the uterus as well as the anterior and posterior pouches. This is usually achieved by good manipulation to lift the bulk of the uterus out of the pelvis, and using instruments placed in other available ports for traction and counter traction. It should be remembered that due to the myomas, the uterus may be rotated off its natural axis and therefore every effort should be made to restore this axis as this will allow for exposure of the pedicles.

Because of possible distortion of anatomy which ever pedicle is cephalad, and accessible should be dealt with first followed by the others in descending order until the uterine vessels become visible. Maintenance of strict haemostasis during the preparation and transection of the pedicles is the key to success.

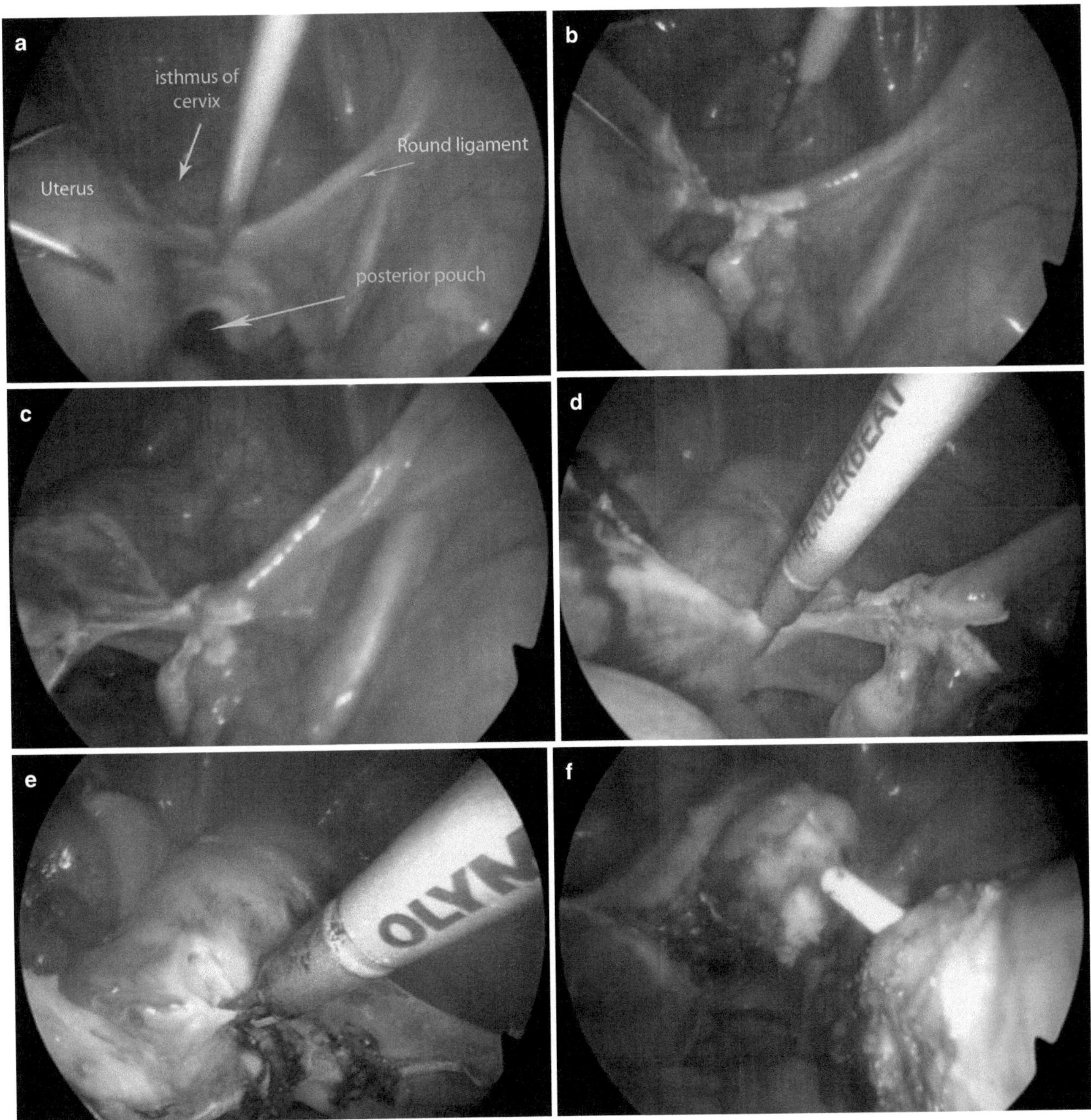

Fig. 33.4 Sequence steps for lash. (**a**) Transection of the broad ligament. (**b**) Transection of the ovarian ligament. (**c**) Skeletisation of the uterine vasculature. (**d**) Transection of the uterine vasculature. (**e**) Transection of the cervix and (**f**) Complete transection of the cervix

Once the adnexal pedicles have been dealt with the bladder flap is then developed to enable the bladder to be dissected and pushed caudally. Care should be taken again if there are uterine fibroids in the lower segment as they may obscure the upper limit of the bladder leading to bladder injury during dissection. The same is true with the presence of adhesions which may be as a result of previous/multiple caesarean sections. Once the bladder flap is developed and the uterine pedicles are exposed the uterine vessels are coagulated and transected either with the use of traditional bipolar instruments and scissors, or with more modern energy sources. It should be remembered that the vessels can be large and multiple thus whilst coagulated it is best not to have the vessels under tension. Where possible the vessels should be approached perpendicular to angle of the uterus as this will prevent shearing during the process of coagulation and transection.

The next step is transection of the cervix as with normal sized uteri. This can be achieved by the use of preformed loops, however it may be difficult to place the loop around and over the fundus of the uterus due to uterine bulk. If this is the case energy sources with a cutting modality can be used to transect the cervix.

Surgical Challenges

Performing a LSH for a large distorted uterus is a very challenging procedure. The technical challenges are specific and can be overcome with the right techniques.

Surgical Challenges for Performing LSH for Large Uteri

The surgical challenges can be summarized as follows:

Distortion due to enlarged uterine size
Distortion due to altered uterine shape
Restricted uterine mobility and limitation of access to structures

Distortion Due to Enlarged Uterine Size

Such a distortion, as it is mostly in the fundus due to fundal fibroids or a uterus enlarged without anatomical distortion as seen in adenomyosis, should afford relatively easy access to the uterine pedicles and to the uterocervical angle for transaction (Fig. 33.5).

Distortion Due to Altered Uterine Shape

Frequently the surgical challenge would be a uterus which is not enlarged in the cranio-caudal axis, but is distorted due to fibroids in the lower segment (Fig. 33.6). Such procedures are technically more challenging and might necessitate myomectomy prior to LSH to facilitate access.

Restricted Uterine Mobility and Limitation of Access

Access to the uterine sides, especially at the utero-cervical junction is paramount as without which the surgery cannot be successfully completed.

Figure 33.7 illustrates the loss of space and limited access which has been restored with good uterine manipulation.

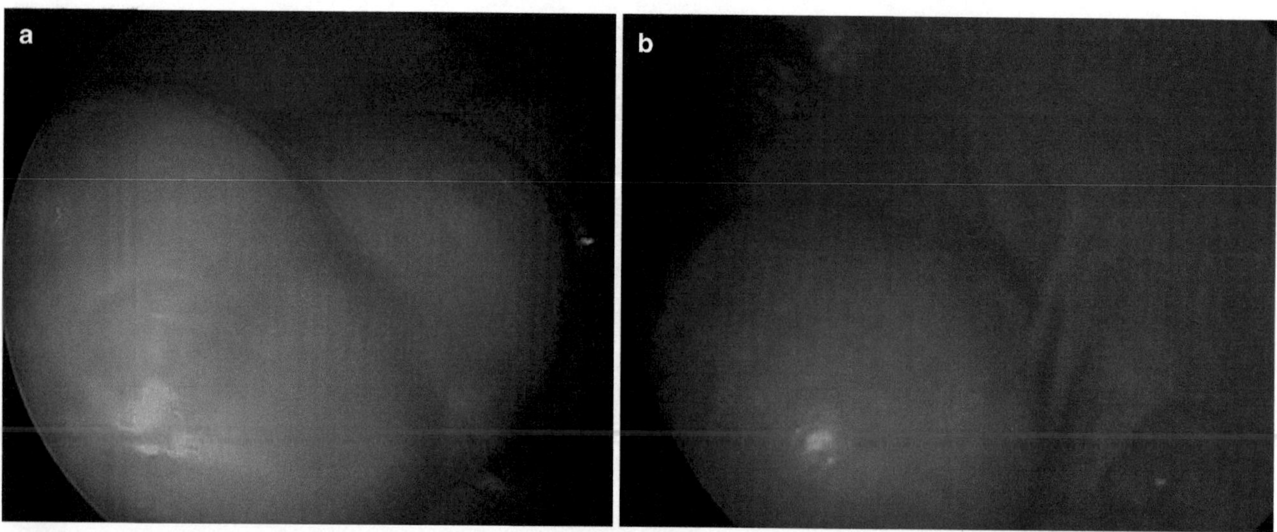

Fig. 33.5 Fundal/non distorted expansion of the uterus. (**a**) Shows uterine enlargement due to adenomyosis and (**b**) shows expansion of the uterine fundus due to fibroids

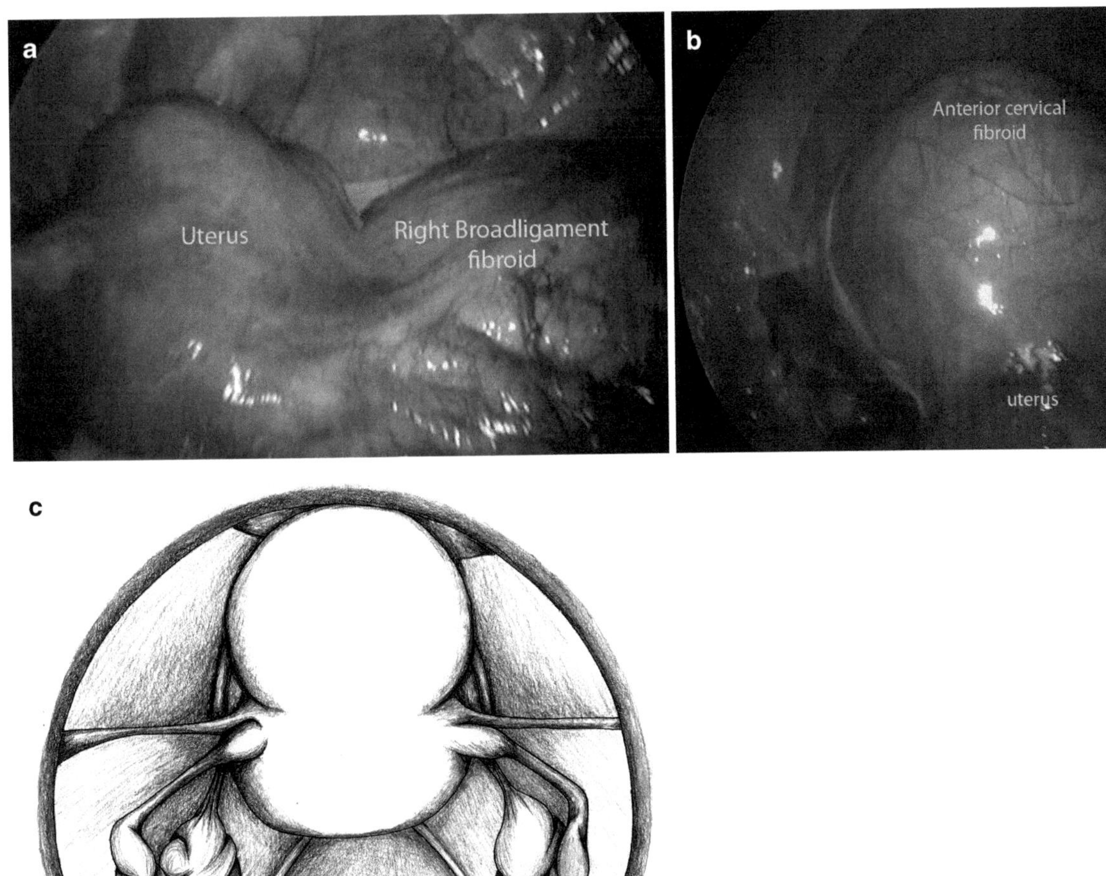

Fig. 33.6 Distortion of the lower segment of the uterus. (**a**) Shows the lower segment of the uterus distorted due to a large broad ligament fibroid and (**b**) shows expansion of the lower segment due to a large cervical fibroid. (**c**) Shows the schematic diagram of the anterior fibroid ((**c**) Courtesy of Catherine Woodman, BA (Hons))

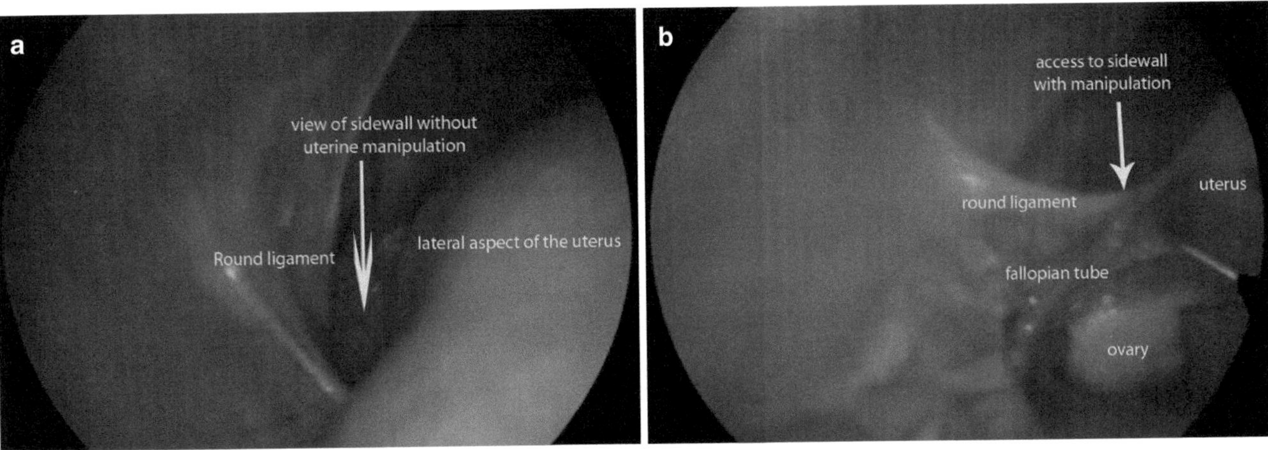

Fig. 33.7 Limited access to side wall structures due to the enlarged uterus. (**a**) Shows the restricted view of the side wall and (**b**) shows the posterior aspect of same uterus with good manipulation

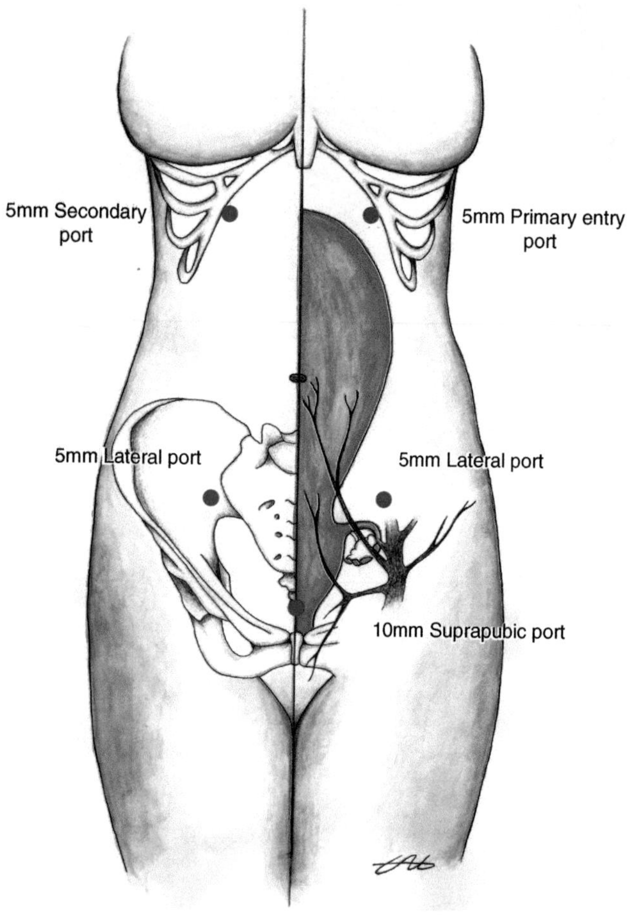

Fig. 33.8 Sites of potential port placements on the anterior abdominal wall. Figure 33.8 shows the possible port sites and the hazards to avoid (Courtesy of Catherine Woodman, BA (Hons))

Overcoming the Surgical Challenges

Most of the limitations for operating laparoscopically on the large uterus can be overcome by good surgical technique, the ability to suture laparoscopically and the use of modern sealing devices.

Port Placement and Utilization and Ergonometrics

In order to perform this procedure it is important to be able to visualize the pelvis (Fig. 33.8). Some surgeons place the entry port above the level of the uterus in the midline [30], this however does not provide complete visualization of both sides of the uterus and runs the risk of injury to the uterus. Shahid and colleagues describe a modified 5-port technique with the first port placed at palmers point and a second 5 mm trocar is placed in the contralateral hypochondrium. Two further ports are inserted in both iliac fossa above the ovarian pedicles. With this technique, though the operating time was longer for uteri greater than 500 g, it did not add to the length of stay of the patients (<500 g = 65 min, >500 g = 103 min, $P = 0.007$) [26].

Others have used 7 trocars with 10 mm tocars above the Bikini line. Though this technique provides adequate access it can have adverse cosmetic results and result in patient dissatisfaction [30, 31]. Some surgeons use a 30 ° laparoscope which provide better visibility into the pelvis [21].

Even when the primary trocar is inserted away from the top of the uterus it is important to remember that surgery is not always limited to that view. On occasion even where visualization of the uterine and ovarian pedicles may seem impossible from the palmers point view rotating to other ports may provide visibility to the pelvic side walls (Fig. 33.9). Thus a handy surgical tip would be to rotate the laparoscope through the different ports to find the best view for execution of the procedure.

Vessel Sealing

Traditionally bipolar technology was used to seal vessels. Currently with the explosion of technology in this area, there is an array of devices including ultrasound devices such as the harmonic scalpel and Ace™ (gynaecare) or Lotus™ (SRA Developments). Though these technologies seal vessels there is a limit to vessel size of about 7 mm and vessels for large uteri often exceed this limit. Hence care needs to be taken to adjust the devices accordingly. There are also "intelligent" sealing devices such as the Thunderbeat™ (Olympus Europa SE & CO) which combine ultrasound and bipolar technology. The Ligasure™ device (Covidien) can also be used with good effect. As these devices seal and cut they have the advantage of decreasing the need to use multiple instruments.

Though these devices can also transect the cervix, once the cervix has been prepared for transection, where available the Laploop™ (Roberts Surgical) or the preformed Linaloop™ (Lina medical) can be used.

Myomectomy Prior to LSH

If there are fibroids obstructing the access to the uterine vessels, then performing a laparoscopic myomectomy may be helpful to aid exposure (Fig. 33.10). It should be remembered that in countries where it is available, the use of Pitressin™ may help with haemostasis. Where it is not other methods of reducing haemostasis during myomectomy may be used [32]. Provided there is adequate space a myomectomy screw may also be used to aid traction and counter traction.

When access to the uterus is limited by the presence of fibroids obstructing vital structures, the decision would be either to perform the laparoscopic supracervical hysterectomy with the fibroids *in situ* or to remove the fibroids to obtain access to the uterine arteries and or the cervix.

Extrapolating from data comparing laparoscopic hysterectomy outcomes with those of myomectomy for the management of uterine fibroids, myomectomy prior to LSH may be associated with increased blood loss [33]. It is thus useful to use techniques to prevent blood loss during myomectomy if this approach is taken. Matsuoka and colleagues describe techniques to perform cervical myomectomy [34]. These techniques can be used to perform cervical myomectomy prior to performing a LSH. Broad ligament fibroids can also be

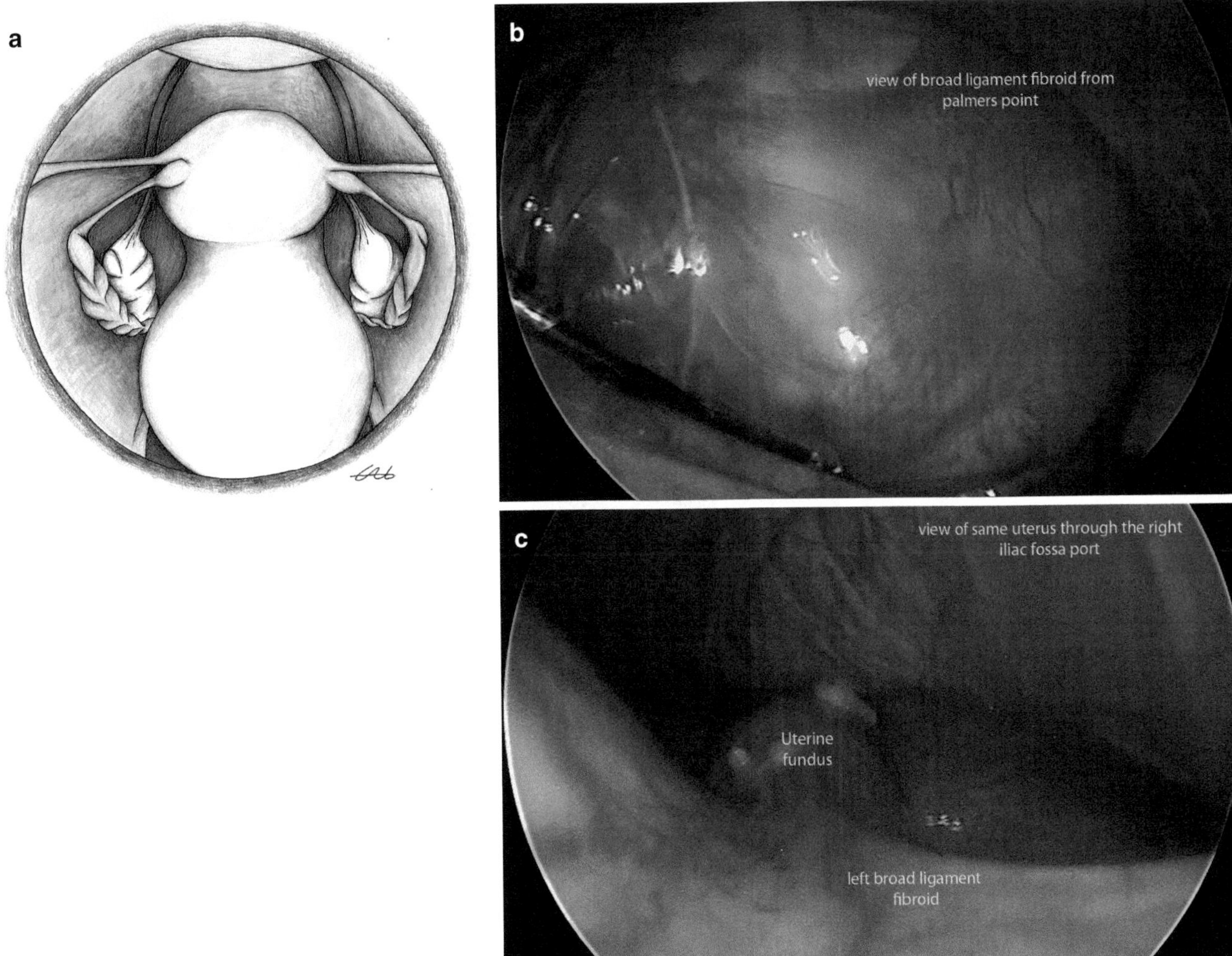

Fig. 33.9 Better identification of anatomy by varying the ports (**a**) shows the schematic diagram of a posterior fundal fibroid. (**b**) Shows view of large uterus from palmers point with fundal 10 cm fibroid and anterior 6 cm fibroid. (**c**) Shows better identification of anatomy with the view from the right lateral port showing the uterus and a broad ligament fibroid ((**a**) Courtesy of Catherine Woodman, BA (Hons))

removed safely with good surgical technique and port placement providing adequate exposure and vision [33, 35, 36].

Retroperitoneal Approach to Hysterectomy

In order to reduce bleeding the retroperitoneal approach to the uterine artery may be used [37]. This allows for the uterine artery to be coagulated and transected at its origin. Roman and colleagues applied this approach to 18 patients undergoing TLH with a mean uterine weight of 540 g [38]. Once the uterus is devascularised, multiple myomectomy may then be performed before the remainder of the procedure is performed. However this is often difficult if there is a broad ligament fibroid obscuring access to the pelvic sidewall (Fig. 33.11). In such cases the broad ligament fibroid will need to be removed before proceeding with the hysterectomy.

Use of Manipulators and Patient Positioning

There are numerous uterine manipulators on the market that facilitate the movement of the uterus. Most have a pivot and do not rely on the habitus of the patient. The important function when performing LSH for the large uterus would be the ability of the manipulator to move the uterus out of the pelvis exposing the posterior and anterior as well as the lateral aspects for the cervix. With low-lying fibroids this aids visualization of the contents of the lesser pelvis (see Fig. 33.7).

Raised Body Mass Index

Though studies have shown that LSH is feasible and safe in patients of high BMI [17], raised BMI has been shown to have adverse outcome on hysterectomy, though not so much for laparoscopic hysterectomy [39]. Paradoxically, it can be easier to perform LSH for the large uterus in larger patients. This is because of the ratio of uterine size to the available space within the patient. There is limited access and visibility when operating on the smaller patient, and this may lead to damage to adjacent organs [20].

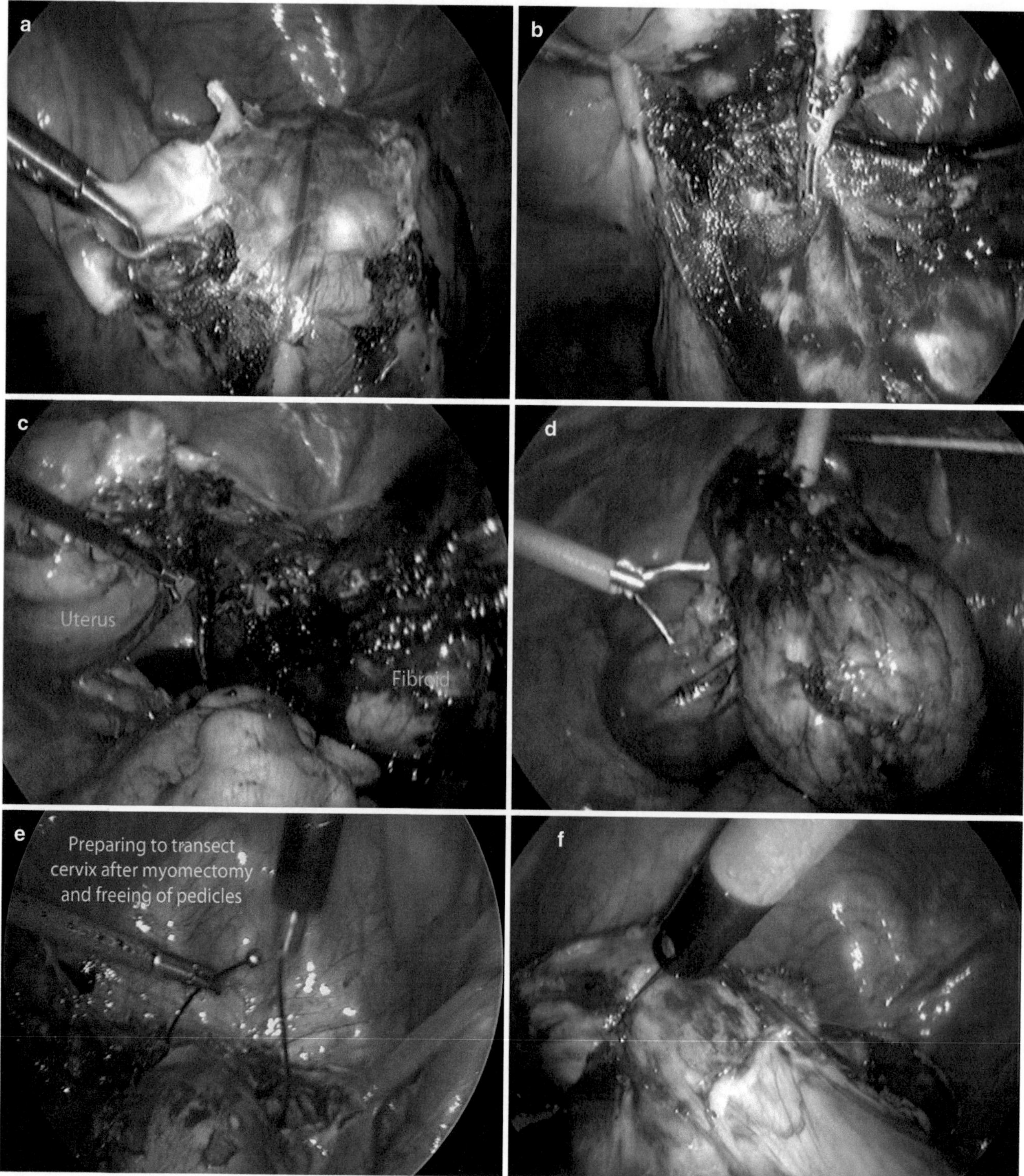

Fig. 33.10 Myomectomy being performed of the fundal 10 cm fibroid and anterior 6 cm fibroid shown in Fig. 33.8, prior to the LSH. (**a**) Reflection of the peritoneum off the anterior cervix, pushing the bladder caudally. (**b**) Use of the harmonic scalpel to separate the fibroid from its attachment to the uterus. (**c**) Demonstration of the fibroid separated from the uterus. (**d**) Fibroid separated from both the uterus and enucleated from the broad ligament. (**e**) Application of the "lap loop" to transect the cervix from the body of the uterus. (**f**) Transecting the cervix

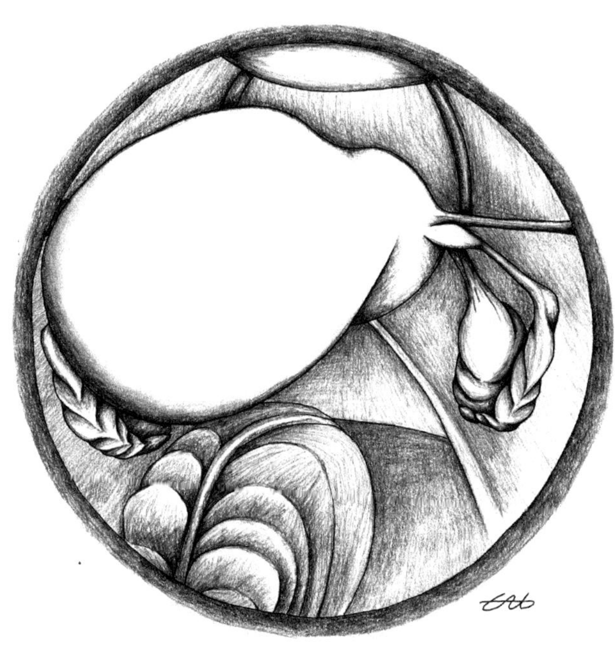

Fig. 33.11 Schematic diagram of a broad ligament fibroid (Courtesy of Catherine Woodman, BA (Hons))

Complications

General Complications

Most studies concur that there is no difference in the complication rate between LSH and TLH. A 16 year study of 3190 laparoscopic hysterectomies by Donnez et al. showed that in experienced hands, laparoscopic hysterectomy is not associated with any increase in major complication rates [40]. Both minor complications (fever >38.5 °C, bladder damage) and major complications (haemorrhage, vesicoperitoneal fistula, ureteral injury, rectal perforation or fistula) have been observed. In the LSH group, the minor complication rate was 0.99 % and the major complication rate 0.37 %. In the TLH group, the minor complication rate was 1.14 % and the major complication rate 0.51 % [40]. Bojahr et al. in their series of 1706 patients found five (0.3 %) intraoperative (three bladder injuries, one ureter injury, and one severe intraoperative bleed) and 20 (1.2 %) postoperative complications [23].

Specific Complications

All the above complications are seen generally in all laparoscopic hysterectomies whether it is done as total hysterectomy or subtotal. There are only a few complications which are specific to the supracervical procedure. Laparoscopic hysterectomy has been associated with higher rates of urinary tract injuries, compared with abdominal hysterectomy (OR 2.61,95 % CI 1.22–5.60) [41, 42, 43]. Later studies performed by Karaman et al. and Bojahr et al. found a lower complication rate (between 0 and 1.4 %) [8, 23].

Bladder Injury

Bladder injury is a complication that can occur in the presence of cervical myoma. It usually occurs as a result of the bladder being stretched over the anterior cervical fibroid [20] a contributory factor in this series was low BMI alluding to poor access. In the series by Grosse-Drieling et al., 2 of the patients had uteri measuring 540 and 595 g and one had a contributory factor of previous surgery [21]. Even though bladder injury appears with cervical myomas, these complications are usually recognized at the time of surgery. The injury can be sutured laparoscopically and have no long-term sequellae. At the end of such procedures even if the complication is unsuspected during the laparoscopy, the catheter bag should be examined before the procedure is completed. If it is found to be inflated this could signify occult bladder injury and further investigations should be carried out to identify the same. The complication of bladder injury at LSH is not unique with large uteri. Donnez and colleagues in a series of 3190 laparoscopic hysterectomies of which 1613 were supracervical had a cystotomy rate of 0.25 % in women with uterine size less than 17 weeks. In this cohort there were also more iatrogenic cystotomies in the total hysterectomy group (0.38 %) [40]. A recent meta-analysis looks at the use for universal cystoscopy at gynaecological surgery to detect urinary tract injury. However though it increases the detection rate intra-operatively it does not decrease the postoperative detection rate [44]. In all the case series reporting on urinary tract injury during LSH for large uteri most injuries were detected intraoperatively. The one reported injury detected postoperatively was managed by catheterisation and allowed to heal spontaneously. For the use of routine cystoscopy to be cost effective it has been estimated that the prevalence of injury would have to be 2 % at laparoscopic hysterectomy [45].

The main recommendation in avoiding bladder injury is being cognisant of limited space particularly in the smaller patient with fibroids in the lower segment, and where patients have had previous surgery. When operating on such patients it is important to look in the catheter bag. If it is inflated with gas, like a balloon it is important to look for the bladder injury and repair the bladder using a 2/0 vicyl suture or equivalent in layers. The patient does not necessarily need to stay in hospital till the catheter is removed. It is our practice to keep the catheter in situ for 7–10 days, the patient is taught how to use a leg bag and discharged home on prophylactic antibiotics. The patient then returns for a cystogram and if the bladder is intact, the catheter is removed and if all is well the patient returns home.

Unexpected Malignancy

Laparoscopic morcellation has enabled the removal of large uteri without necessitating the removal of the cervix. But due to the potential for dissemination of occult uterine cancers the American Association of Gynecologic Laparoscopists (AAGL) stated that, in case of known or suspected uterine malignancy, morcellation is contraindicated [46]. Additionally the Food and Drug Administration (FDA) recently issued a statement discouraging the use of electromechanical morcellation for hysterectomy and myomectomy in most women with uterine myoma [47]. Arkenbout et al. recently assessed the basic "physiology" of the morcellation process and tissue spread and found that LSH and laparoscopic hysterectomy procedures may be at higher risk for tissue scatter than TLH [48].

Bojahret al. analysed data of 10,731 patients who underwent a standardized LSH surgery with electric power morcellation. In total, six sarcomas (0.06 %) and eight endometrial cancers (0.07 %) were documented. This amounts to a very low uterine malignancy rate of 0.13 % [49].

When analysing the risk of malignancy it used to be thought that rapid growth of the uterus is an indication for possibility of malignancy. However, Parker et al. looked at 198 women who had published definition of rapidly growing myoma and none of his cohort on histology were found to have leiomyosarcoma [50]. If there is any suspicion of malignancy the patient should be referred to an oncologist for appropriate investigation and management rather than have a LSH. Pertinent investigations would include LDH estimations and MRI [49]. Thus currently the consensus opinion is not to lose the obvious advantages of a laparoscopic procedure by deferring to an open procedure, but to rely on preoperative diagnosis and clear patient counseling [51].

Conclusion

With the advent of conservative methods of management of normal sized uteri and the evidence skewed towards minimally invasive hysterectomies, it is important that gynaecologists who offer care to women requiring hysterectomy are able to perform LSH for large uteri.

We have outlined the surgical precepts to be followed to achieve a successful outcome. In order to be able to perform the procedure effectively it is imperative to select patients after appropriate pre-operative investigations and consent procedure. It is also imperative for the surgeon to have a good knowledge of anatomy, instruments and modern energy sources and endoscopic skills necessary to achieve a successful outcome.

References

1. Sutton C. Hysterectomy: a historical perspective. Baillieres Clin Obstet Gynaecol. 1997;11(1):1–22.
2. Nieboer TE, Johnson N, Lethaby A, Tavender E, Curr E, Garry R, van Voorst S, Mol BW, Kluivers KB. Surgical approach to hysterectomy for benign gynaecological disease. Cochrane Database Syst Rev. 2009;3:CD003677. doi:10.1002/14651858.CD003677.
3. Alperin M, Kivnick S, Poon KY. Outpatient laparoscopic hysterectomy for large uteri. J Minim Invasive Gynecol. 2012;19(6):689–94. doi:10.1016/j.jmig.2012.06.007.
4. Park SH, Cho HY, Kim HB. Factors determining conversion to laparotomy in patients undergoing total laparoscopic hysterectomy. Gynecol Obstet Invest. 2011;71(3):193–7. doi:10.1159/000317520. Epub 2010 Dec 15.
5. Benassi L, Rossi T, Kaihura CT, Ricci L, Bedocchi L, Galanti B, Vadora E. Abdominal or vaginal hysterectomy for enlarged uteri: a randomized clinical trial. Am J Obstet Gynecol. 2002;187(6): 1561–5.
6. Lethaby A, Vollenhoven B, Sowter M.Pre-operative GnRH analogue therapy before hysterectomy or myomectomy for uterine fibroids Cochrane Database Syst Rev 2001;(2):CD000547.
7. Ferrari MM, Berlanda N, Mezzopane R, Ragusa G, Cavallo M, Pardi G. Identifying the indications for laparoscopically assisted vaginal hysterectomy: a prospective, randomised comparison with abdominal hysterectomy in patients with symptomatic uterine fibroids. BJOG. 2000;107(5):620–5.
8. Karaman Y, Bingol B, Günenç Z. Prevention of complications in laparoscopic hysterectomy: experience with 1120 cases performed by a single surgeon. J Minim Invasive Gynecol. 2007;14(1):78–84.
9. Semm K. Hysterectomy via laparotomy or pelviscopy. A new CASH method without colpotomy. Geburtshilfe Frauenheilkd. 1991;51(12):996–1003.
10. Berner E, Qvigstad E, Myrvold AK, Lieng M. Pain reduction after total laparoscopic hysterectomy and laparoscopic supracervical hysterectomy among women with dysmenorrhoea: a randomised controlled trial. BJOG. 2015;122(8):1102–11. doi:10.1111/1471-0528.13362. Epub 2015 Apr 19.
11. Lieng M, Lømo AB, Qvigstad E. Long-term outcomes following laparoscopic and abdominal supracervical hysterectomies. Obstet Gynecol Int. 2010;2010:989127. doi:10.1155/2010/989127. Epub 2010 Mar 14.
12. Garry R. The place of subtotal/supracervical hysterectomy in current practice. BJOG. 2008;115(13):1597–600. doi:10.1111/j.1471-0528.2008.01956.x.
13. Lyons TL. Laparoscopicsupracervical hysterectomy. A comparison of morbidity and mortality results with laparoscopically assisted vaginal hysterectomy. J Reprod Med. 1993;38(10):763–7.
14. Lethaby A, Mukhopadhyay A, Naik R. Total versus subtotal hysterectomy for benign gynaecologicalconditions. Cochrane Database Syst Rev. 2012;4:CD004993. doi:10.1002/14651858.CD004993. pub3.
15. Tchartchian G, Gardanis K, Bojahr B, de Wilde L. Postoperative patient satisfaction after laparoscopic supracervical hysterectomy. JSLS. 2013;17:107–10.

16. Lieng M, Qvigstad E, Istre O, Langebrekke A, Ballard K. Long-term outcomes following laparoscopicsupracervical hysterectomy. BJOG. 2008;115:1605–10.
17. Hussain M, Odejinmi F. Laparoscopic supracervicalhysterectomy:i mpact of body mass index and uterineweight. Gynecol Surg. 2012;9:351–5. doi:10.1007/s10397-011-0721-5.
18. Darai E, Soriano D, Kimata P, et al. Vaginal hysterectomy for enlarged uteri, with or without laparoscopic assistance: randomised study. Obstet Gynecol. 2001;97:712–6.
19. Lyons TL, Adolph AJ, Winer WK. Laparoscopic supracervical hysterectomy for the large uterus. J Am Assoc Gynecol Laparosc. 2004;11(2):170–4.
20. Maclaran K, Agarwal N, Odejinmi F. Perioperative outcomes in laparoscopic hysterectomy: identifying surgical risk factors. Gynecol Surg. 2015;13:75. doi:10.1007/s10397-015-0914-4.
21. Grosse-Drieling D, Schlutius JC, Altgassen C, Kelling K. ThebenJ. Laparoscopicsupracervical hysterectomy (LSH), a retrospective study of 1,584 cases regarding intra- and perioperative complications. Arch Gynecol Obstet. 2012;285(5):1391–6. doi:10.1007/s00404-011-2170-9. Epub 2011 Dec 16.
22. Bojahr B, Tchartchian G, Ohlinger R. Laparoscopic supracervical hysterectomy: a retrospective analysis of 1000 cases. JSLS. 2009;13(2):129–34.
23. Bojahr B, Raatz D, Schonleber G, Abri C, Ohlinger R. Perioperative complication rate in 1706 patients after a standardized laparoscopic supracervical hysterectomy technique. J Minim Invasive Gynecol. 2006;13:183–9.
24. Twijnstra AR, Blikkendaal MD, van Zwet EW, Jansen FW. Clinical relevance of conversion rate and its evaluation in laparoscopic hysterectomy. J Minim Invasive Gynecol. 2013;20(1):64–72. doi:10.1016/j.jmig.2012.09.006.
25. Leonard F, Chopin N, Borghese B, Fotso A, Foulot H, Coste J, Mignon A, Chapron C. Total laparoscopic hysterectomy: preoperative risk factors for conversion to laparotomy. J Minim Invasive Gynecol. 2005;12(4):312–7.
26. Shahid A, Sankaran S, Odejinmi F. Laparoscopic subtotal hysterectomy for large uteri using modified five port technique. Arch Gynecol Obstet. 2011;283(1):79–81. doi:10.1007/s00404-009-1322-7. Epub 2009 Dec 19.
27. Nimaroff ML, Dimino M, Maloney S. Laparoscopic-assisted vaginal hysterectomy of large myomatous uteri with supracervical amputation followed by trachelectomy. J Am Assoc Gynecol Laparosc. 1996;3(4):585–7.
28. Stoelinga B, Huirne J, Heymans MW, Reekers JA, Ankum WM, Hehenkamp WJ. The estimated volume of the fibroid uterus: a comparison of ultrasound and bimanual examination versus volume at MRI or hysterectomy. Eur J Obstet Gynecol Reprod Biol. 2015;184:89–96. doi:10.1016/j.ejogrb.2014.11.011. Epub 2014 Nov 20.
29. Kung FT, Chang SY. The relationship between ultrasonic volume and actual weight of pathologic uterus. Gynecol Obstet Invest. 1996;42(1):35–8.
30. Lee YS. Benefits of high epigastric port placement for removing the very large uterus. J Am AssocGynecol Laparosc. 2001;8(3):425–8.
31. Wattiez A, Soriano D, Fiaccavento A, Canis M, Botchorishvili R, Pouly J, Mage G, Bruhat MA. Total laparoscopic hysterectomy for very enlarged uteri. J Am Assoc Gynecol Laparosc. 2002;9(2):125–30.
32. Kongnyuy EJ, Wiysonge CS. Interventions to reduce haemorrhage during myomectomy for fibroids. Cochrane Database Syst Rev. 2014;8:CD005355. doi:10.1002/14651858.CD005355.pub5.
33. Odejinmi F, Maclaran K. AgarwalN.Laparoscopic treatment of uterine fibroids: a comparison of peri-operative outcomes in laparoscopic hysterectomy and myomectomy. Arch Gynecol Obstet. 2015;291(3):579–84. doi:10.1007/s00404-014-3434-y. Epub 2014 Sep 13.
34. Matsuoka S, Kikuchi I, Kitade M, Kumakiri J, Kuroda K, Tokita S, Kuroda M, Takeda S. Strategy for laparoscopic cervical myomectomy. J Minim Invasive Gynecol. 2010;17(3):301–5. doi:10.1016/j.jmig.2009.12.020. Epub 2010 Mar 19.
35. Tariq S, Miskry TS, Kindinger LM, Setchell TE. Broad ligament fibroids—a radiological and surgical challenge. Gynecol Surg. 2014;11:19–22.
36. Chandrasekaran D, Agarwal N, Oliver R, Odejinmi F. Evaluation of laparoscopic myomectomy for the management of broad ligament fibroids. Poster presentation. ESGE 2015, ES24-0515. Gynecol Surg. 2015;12(Suppl 1):S1–S494.
37. Gol M, Kizilyar A. EminogluM.Laparoscopic hysterectomy with retroperitoneal uterine artery sealing using LigaSure: Gazi hospital experience. Arch Gynecol Obstet. 2007;276(4):311–4. Epub 2007 Mar 20.
38. Roman H, Zanati J, Friederich L, Resch B, Lena E, Marpeau L. Laparoscopic hysterectomy of large uteri with uterine artery coagulation at its origin. JSLS. 2008;12(1):25–9.
39. Bohlin KS, Ankardal M, Stjerndahl JH, Lindkvist H, Milsom I. Influence of the modifiable life-style factors body mass index and smoking on the outcome of hysterectomy. Acta Obstet Gynecol Scand. 2015;95(1):65–73. doi:10.1111/aogs.12794.
40. Donnez O, Jadoul P, Squifflet J, Donnez J. A series of 3190 laparoscopic hysterectomies for benign disease from 1990 to 2006: evaluation of complications compared with vaginal and abdominal procedures. BJOG. 2009;116:492–500. doi:10.1111/j.1471-0528.2008.01966.x. Epub 2008 Nov 11.
41. Johnson N, Barlow D, Lethaby A, Tavender E, Curr L, Garry R. Methodsof hysterectomy: systematic review and meta-analysis of randomizedcontrolled trials. BMJ. 2005;330:1478.
42. Johnson N, Barlow D, Lethaby A, Tavender E, Curr L, Garry R. Surgicalapproach to hysterectomy for benign gynaecological disease (Review). Cochrane Database Syst Rev. 2006;3:CD003677.
43. Garry R, Fountain J, Mason S, Hawe J, Napp V, Abbott J, et al. TheeVALuate study: two parallel randomized trials, one comparinglaparoscopic with abdominal hysterectomy, the other comparinglaparoscopic with vaginal hysterectomy. BMJ. 2004;328:1229–36.
44. Teeluckdharry B, Gilmour D, Flowerdew G. Urinary tract injury at benign gynecologic surgery and the tole of cystoscopy: a systematic review and meta-analysis. Obstet Gynecol. 2015;126(6):1161–9. doi:10.1097/AOG.0000000000001096.
45. Fischer J. Just Do It!: Routine Cystoscopy Should Be Done at the Time of Gynecologic Surgery. Obstet Gynecol. 2015;126(6):1136–7. - Volume Publish Ahead of Print - doi:10.1097/AOG.0000000000001169.
46. AAGL Advancing Minimally Invasive Gynecology Worldwide. AAGL position statement: route of hysterectomy to treatbenign uterine disease. J Minim Invasive Gynecol. 2011;18(1):1–3.
47. U.S. Food and Drug Administration (2014) Laparoscopic uterinepowermorcellation in hysterectomy and myomectomy: FDA. Safety communication: http://www.fda.gov/MedicalDevices/Safety/AlertsandNotices/ucm393576.htm. Accessed 22 May 2014. DOI 10.1007/s10397-013-0826-0.
48. Arkenbout EA, van den Haak L, Driessen SR, Thurkow AL, Jansen FW. Assessing basic "physiology" of the morcellation process and tissue spread: a time-action analysis. J Minim Invasive Gynecol. 2015;22(2):255–60.
49. Bojahr B, De Wilde RL, Tchartchian G. Malignancy rate of 10,731 uteri morcellated during laparoscopic supracervical hysterectomy (LSH). Arch Gynecol Obstet. 2015;292(3):665–72. doi:10.1007/s00404-015-3696-z. Epub 2015 Mar 28.
50. Parker W, Fu Y, Berek J. Uterine sarcoma in patients operated on for presumed leiomyoma and rapidly growing leiomyoma. Obstet Gynecol. 1994;84(3):414–8.
51. Odejinmi F, Agarwal N, Maclaran K, Oliver R. Should we abandon all conservative treatments for uterine fibroids? The problem with leiomyosarcomas. Womens Health (Lond). 2015;11(2):151–9. doi:10.2217/whe.14.71.

34 Cervical Stump Extirpation

Peter Oppelt

There are both benign and also malignant indications for extirpation of the cervical stump. Techniques of oncological surgery do not form part of this section.

The most frequent indication for cervical stump extirpation is persistent bleeding from the cervical canal, which is reported in the literature as occurring in 0.9–25 % of cases after laparoscopy-assisted supracervical hysterectomy (LASH). Preoperative menorrhagia and endometriosis (adenomyosis tissue in the cervix) appear to be risk factors for persistent bleeding after LASH (Table 34.1) [1–8]. Bipolar coagulation of the cervical stump to ablate any residual endometrial tissue is also regarded differently by various authors [6, 8, 9].

When there is persistent bleeding, only extirpation of the stump may remain as a last resort in some cases. Before such an intervention, however, a recent Pap smear is important in order to exclude cervical cancer.

Two primary surgical options are available:

Vaginal Approach

This is particularly appropriate if the patient has already had a spontaneous vaginal delivery and the cervical stump is sufficiently deep within the vagina.

Laparoscopic Procedure

Laparoscopic cervical stump extirpation is appropriate particularly in nulliparous patients or patients with suspected endometriosis. The length of the cervix should be measured using ultrasound preoperatively. Thanks to the various types of manipulator that are available, it is much easier to perform this operation nowadays. The following surgical steps are carried out using the Hohl uterine manipulator (Storz):

1. A working insert is normally screwed onto the spiral cap. As the cervix has a residual length of around 40 mm, the end of the instrument might break through and possibly injure adherent structures (Fig. 34.1). It is therefore advisable to dispense with the working insert and to rotate the spiral cap (if possible always using the largest one, for better holding) directly into the cervical stump (Fig. 34.2).
2. The best-fitting cover is placed.
3. Laparoscopic inspection of the cervical stump is carried out (Fig. 34.3).

Table 34.1 Contraindications for LASH

Contraindications
Endometriosis recto-vaginal septum
Adenomyosis
Cervical myoma
Dysplasia of the cervix
Malignancy

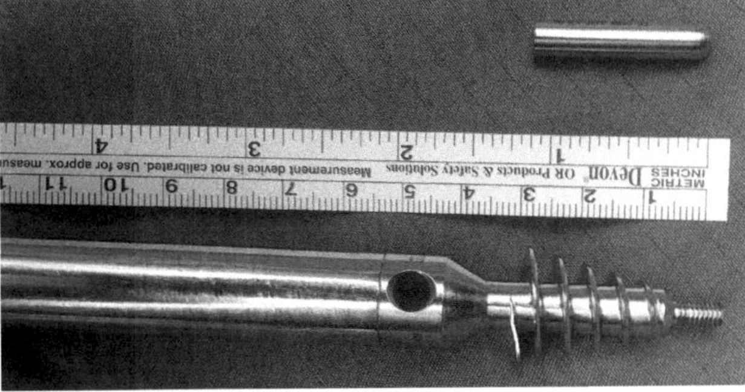

Fig. 34.1 Spiral cab of the "Hohl uterine manipulator2 (don't use the blunt tip on the spiral cab to avoid to break through)

P. Oppelt
Gynecology & Obstetrics, Women's and Children's Hospital Linz, Linz, Austria
e-mail: Peter.Oppelt@kepleruniklinikum.at

I. Alkatout, L. Mettler (eds.), *Hysterectomy*, DOI 10.1007/978-3-319-22497-8_34

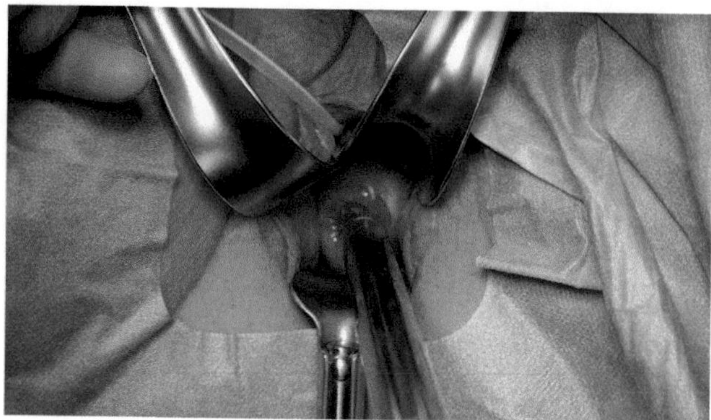

Fig. 34.2 The spiral cab is inserted into the cervical stump

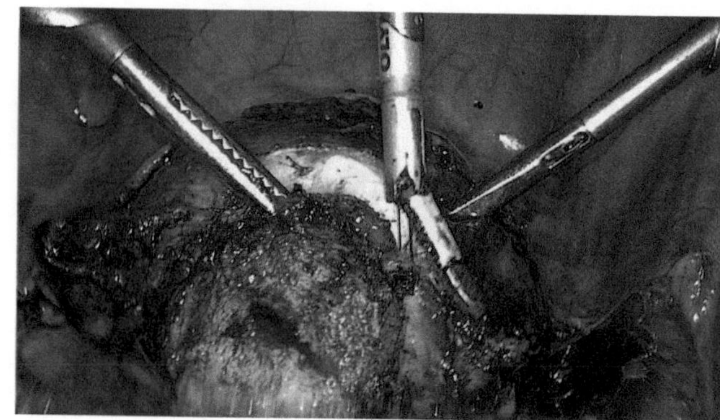

Fig. 34.5 Remove of the cervical stump from the vaginal wall

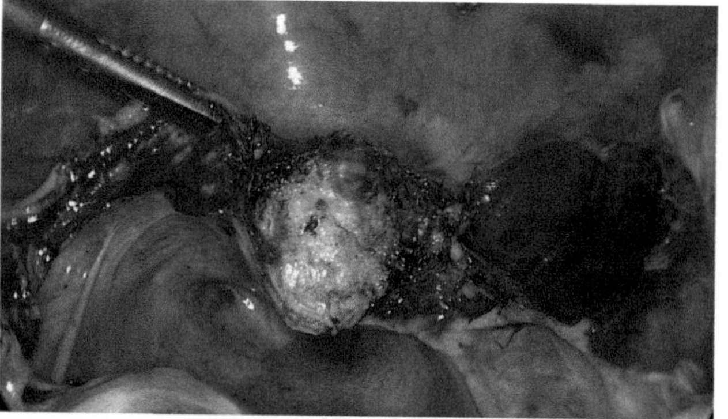

Fig. 34.3 Laparoscopic image of the stump

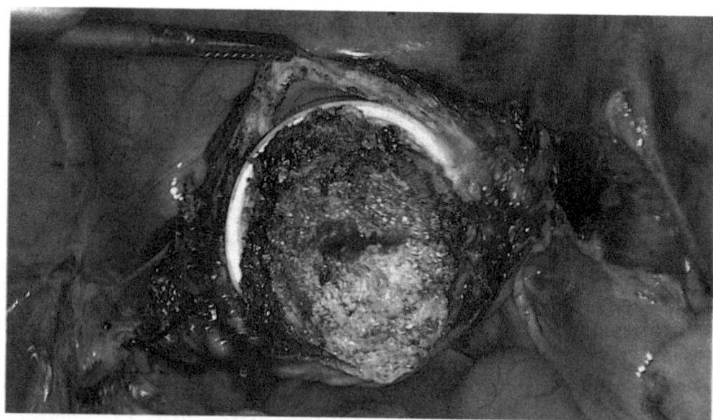

Fig. 34.6 Image of the cap during separation

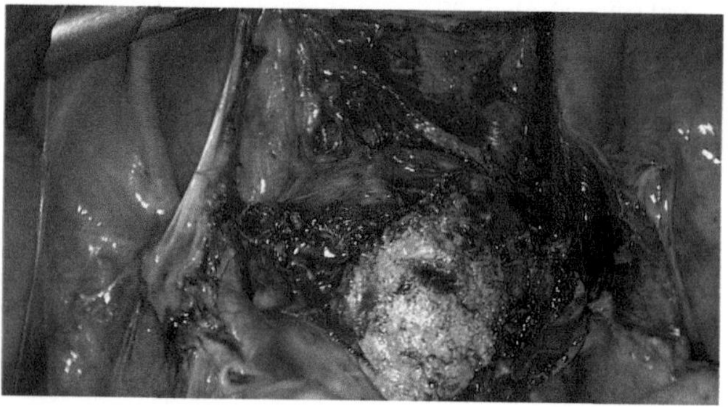

Fig. 34.4 Laparoscopic image of the stump after bladder preparation

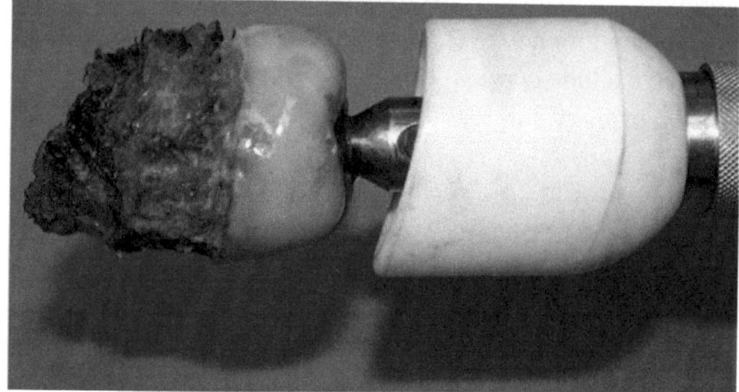

Fig. 34.7 Final operation preparation

4. Tension is applied to the vaginal walls (the manipulator should *always* be inserted straight first of all, and moved to the side under tension; it should never lead directly towards an ovarian fossa. This allows optimal tension to be applied to the vaginal wall, with an optimal distance from the ureters.)
5. An incision is made into the peritoneum and the bladder is pushed away (Fig. 34.4). (In case of an not clear situ, fill up the bladder with 200 ml saline. Push the manipulator straight in. Under this setup, the identification of the structure should be more clearly in an difficult situs).
6. The cervix is released from the parametrial ligaments up to the level of the cap of the uterine manipulator (Fig. 34.5).
7. Since there is no affiliation provided for Peter Oppelt in the chapter opening page, we have taken the affiliation from the Contributor list in the front matter. Please confirm if this is fine. If necessary, coagulation of the cervical part of the uterine artery bilaterally.
8. Separation of the cervical stump at the edge of the manipulator cap with Ultracision / monopolar needle) (Figs. 34.6 and 34.7).
9. Closure of the vagina with endoscopic or transvaginal sutures.

References

1. Morrison JE, Jacobs VR. 437 classic intrafascial supracervical hysterectomies in 8 years. J Am Assoc Gynecol Laparosc. 2001; 8(4):558–67.
2. Kim DH, Bae DH, Hur M, Kim SH. Comparison of classic intrafascial supracervical hysterectomy with total laparoscopic and laparoscopic-assisted vaginal hysterectomy. J Am Assoc Gynecol Laparosc. 1998;5(3):253–60.
3. Gimbel H, Zobbe V, Andersen BM, Filtenborg T, Gluud C, Tabor A. Randomised controlled trial of total compared with subtotal hysterectomy with one-year follow up results. BJOGInt J Obstet Gynaecol. 2003;110(12):1088–98.
4. Van der Stege JG, Van Beek JJ. Problems related to the cervical stump at follow-up in laparoscopic supracervical hysterectomy. JSLSJ Soc Laparoendosc Surg. 1999;3(1):5–7.
5. van Wijngaarden WJ, Filshie GM. Laparoscopic supracervical hysterectomy with Filshie clips. J Am Assoc Gynecol Laparosc. 2001;8(1):137–42.
6. Nouri K, Demmel M, Greilberger U, Fischer E-M, Seemann R, Egarter C, Ott J. Prospective cohort study and meta-analysis of cyclic bleeding after laparoscopic supracervical hysterectomy. Int J Gynecol Obstet. 2013;122(2):124–7.
7. Jenkins TR. Laparoscopic supracervical hysterectomy. Am J Obstet Gynecol. 2004;191(6):1875–84.
8. Ghomi A, Hantes J, Lotze EC. Incidence of cyclical bleeding after laparoscopic supracervical hysterectomy. J Minim Invasive Gynecol. 2005;12(3):201–5.
9. Sasaki KJ, Cholkeri-Singh A, Sulo S, Miller CE. Persistent bleeding after laparoscopic supracervical hysterectomy. JSLSJ Soc Laparoendosc Surg. 2014;18(4):e2014. doi:10.4293/JSLS.2014.002064.

35 Total Laparoscopic Hysterectomy for the Small and Normal-Sized Uterus

Ibrahim Alkatout

Introduction

Hysterectomy is one of the most frequently performed operations in gynecological surgery. International gynecological societies recommend vaginal hysterectomy as the most acceptable technique. However, operative endoscopic methods have gained widespread acceptance in the last two decades, and play a much more important role than the traditional approaches of abdominal and vaginal hysterectomy. With regard to hysterectomies performed for benign disease, the number of abdominal hysterectomies is decreasing, the number of vaginal hysterectomies varies, but laparoscopic and robotic-assisted laparoscopic procedures are on the increase [1]; the trend is visible throughout the world (Fig. 35.1) [2].

The most frequent indications for hysterectomy are uterine leiomyomas (Figs. 35.2, 35.3, 35.4, 35.5, 35.6 and 35.7), adenomyosis (Figs. 35.8, 35.9, 35.10 and 35.11), adenomyoma (Fig. 35.12), diffuse endometriosis (Figs. 35.13, 35.14, 35.15, 35.16, 35.17 and 35.18), uterine prolapse, and therapy-resistant idiopathic bleeding abnormalities. These constitute 60 % and more of the indications for hysterectomy [3]. Alternative therapeutic strategies, such as uterine artery embolization or focused ultrasound therapy have been developed in Germany [4] and other countries [5] over the last ten years. Conservative operative management and the introduction of ulipristalacetate have reduced the number of hysterectomies. Hysterectomy rates depend not only on the indication but also on the age group, family planning, and the centers at which the patients are treated. The indications for hysterectomy in general have now been adapted to the patients' wish to retain their uterus [6, 7]. Hysterectomy is also performed for malignant diseases of the inner genital organs (endometrium or cervix, ovaries and fallopian tube). Endoscopic surgery is only performed for endometrium and cervical cancer. Table 35.1 summarizes the indications for hysterectomy.

Once the decision to perform a hysterectomy has been made, the physician and patient must decide whether the procedure will be performed abdominally, vaginally, or with laparoscopic or robotic assistance [8–10]. Each of these approaches has its advantages and disadvantages, which must be explained to the patient (Fig. 35.19). The surgeon's familiarity with the technique and the economic resources of the hospital are also important considerations (Table 35.2).

The foremost advantage of endoscopic treatment is the fact that the surgeon is able to address other intraabdominal comorbidities simultaneously, such as endometriosis or severe adenomyosis in the adjacent organs (sacrouterine ligaments, cardinal ligament, bladder and/or bowel), as well as adhesions. Although uterine-preserving operative strategies are still controversially discussed and the results are not consistently promising, the only reliable treatment for adenomyosis is total hysterectomy. Since the disease is confined to the uterus, the ovaries can be preserved.

In many cases, conservative medical or conservative surgical treatment signifies undertreatment of the patient, who may then need surgery later on. Subtotal hysterectomy is a compromise that meets the requirements of patients, society and doctors. It is the least invasive approach of hysterectomy. However, the patient must provide her informed consent regarding the disadvantages of the remaining cervix. Only a laparoscopic total hysterectomy (LTH) provides complete protection from renewed fibroids, prevents subsequent carcinoma of the cervix or sarcoma, cell spilling when cutting the corpus and during morcellation, uncontrolled bleeding, and other problems arising from the uterus. The persistence or recurrence of adenomyosis-related symptoms in subtotal hysterectomy continues to be a subject of debate.

I. Alkatout
Gynecology and Obstetrics, Kiel School of Gynaecological Endoscopy, University Hospitals Schleswig-Holstein, Kiel, DE, Germany
e-mail: ibrahim.alkatout@uksh.de; kiel.school@uksh.de

I. Alkatout, L. Mettler (eds.), *Hysterectomy*, DOI 10.1007/978-3-319-22497-8_35

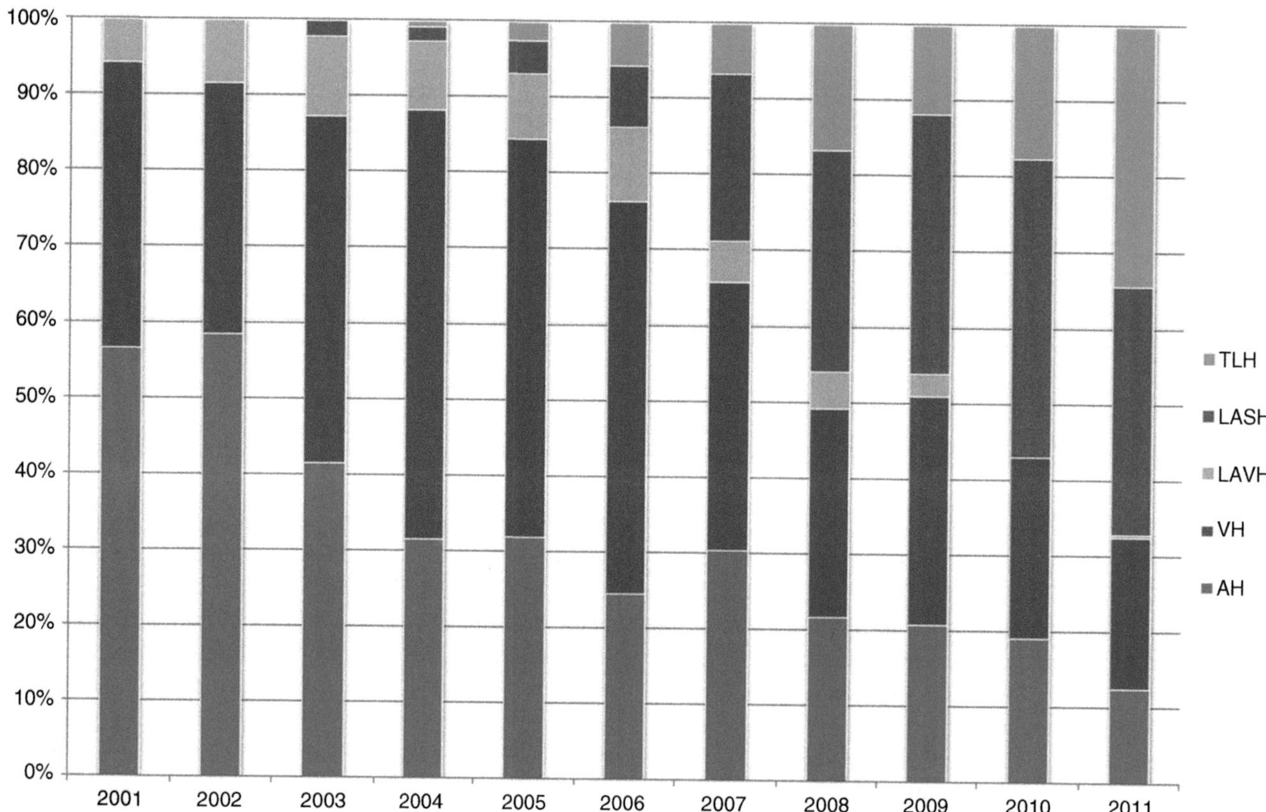

Fig. 35.1 Development of surgical techniques from 2002 to 2010 at the department of obstetrics and gynecology, University of Kiel, Germany. Abbreviations: *AH* abdominal hysterectomy, *LAVH* laparoscopically assisted vaginal hysterectomy, *LSH* laparoscopic supracervical hysterectomy, *TLH* total laparoscopic hysterectomy, *VH* vaginal hysterectomy

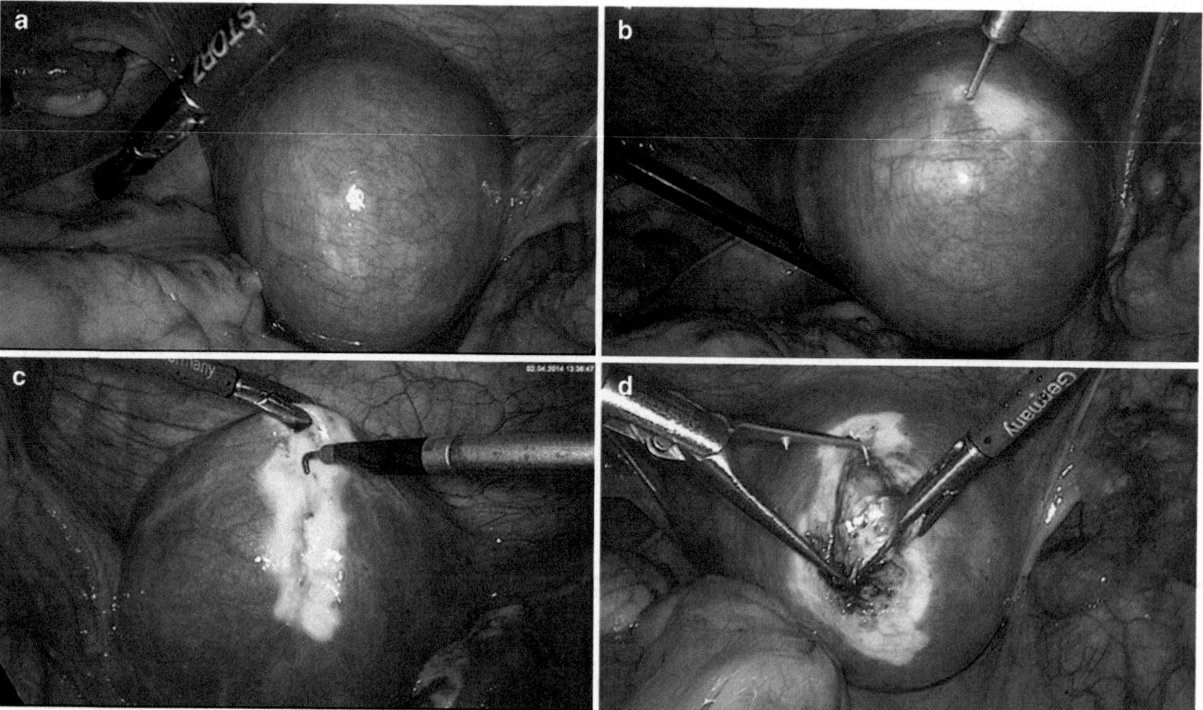

Fig. 35.2 Laparoscopic myoma enucleation. (**a**) Situs of a fundal/anterior wall fibroid. (**b**) Prophylactic hemostasis with 1:100 diluted vasopressin solution (Gylcylpressin) in separate wells between the superficial and healthy tissue of the myometrium, and the capsule/fibroid surface. The purpose of the injection is to separate the pseudocapsule from the fibroid and reduce bleeding. (**c**) Bipolar superficial coagulation of the longitudinal incision strip and opening the uterine wall above the myoma with a monopolar hook or needle until one reaches the myoma. (**d**) Grasping the fibroid and starting the enucleation. The pseudocapsule remains within the uterine wall and is pushed off bluntly

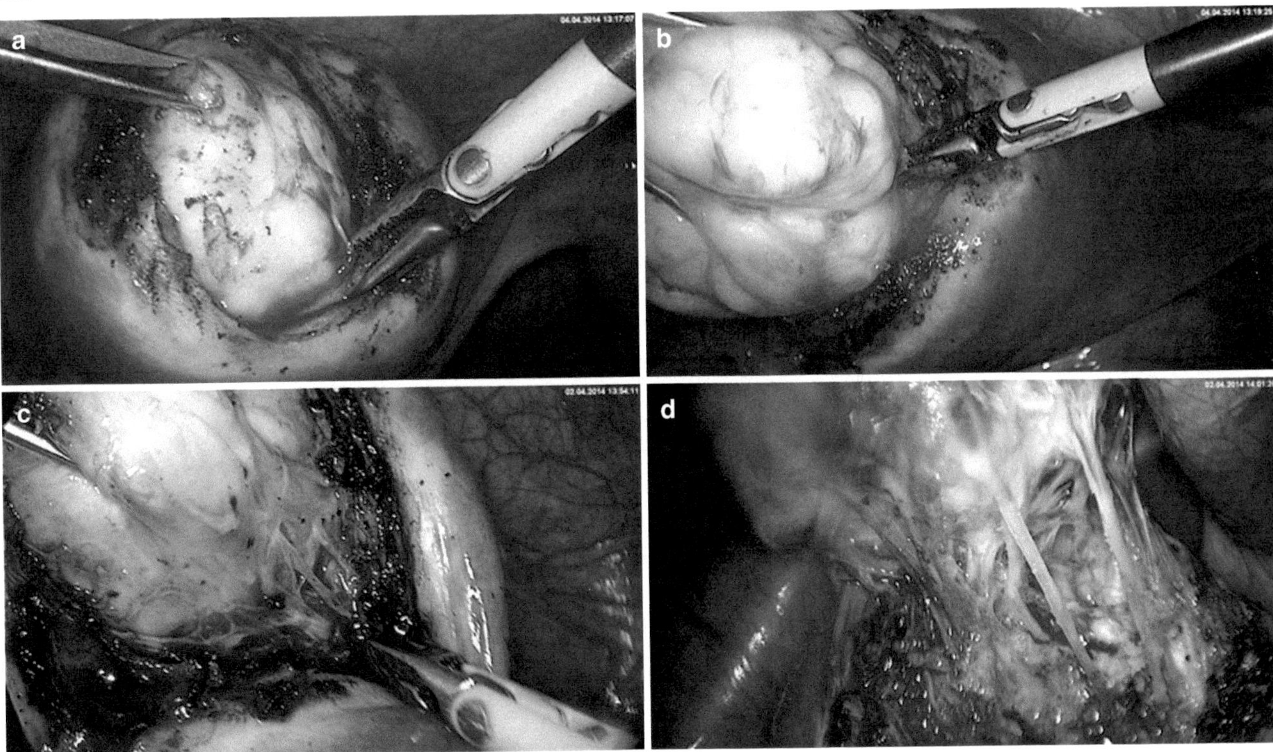

Fig. 35.3 Laparoscopic myoma enucleation. (**a**) Traction of the fibroid with a tenaculum and blunt demarcation from the capsule. (**b**) Focal bipolar coagulation of basic vessels. (**c**) Continuous enucleation of the fibroid under traction and specific coagulation of capsule fibers containing vessels. (**d**) Magnification of the remaining capsule fibers to be coagulated and cut

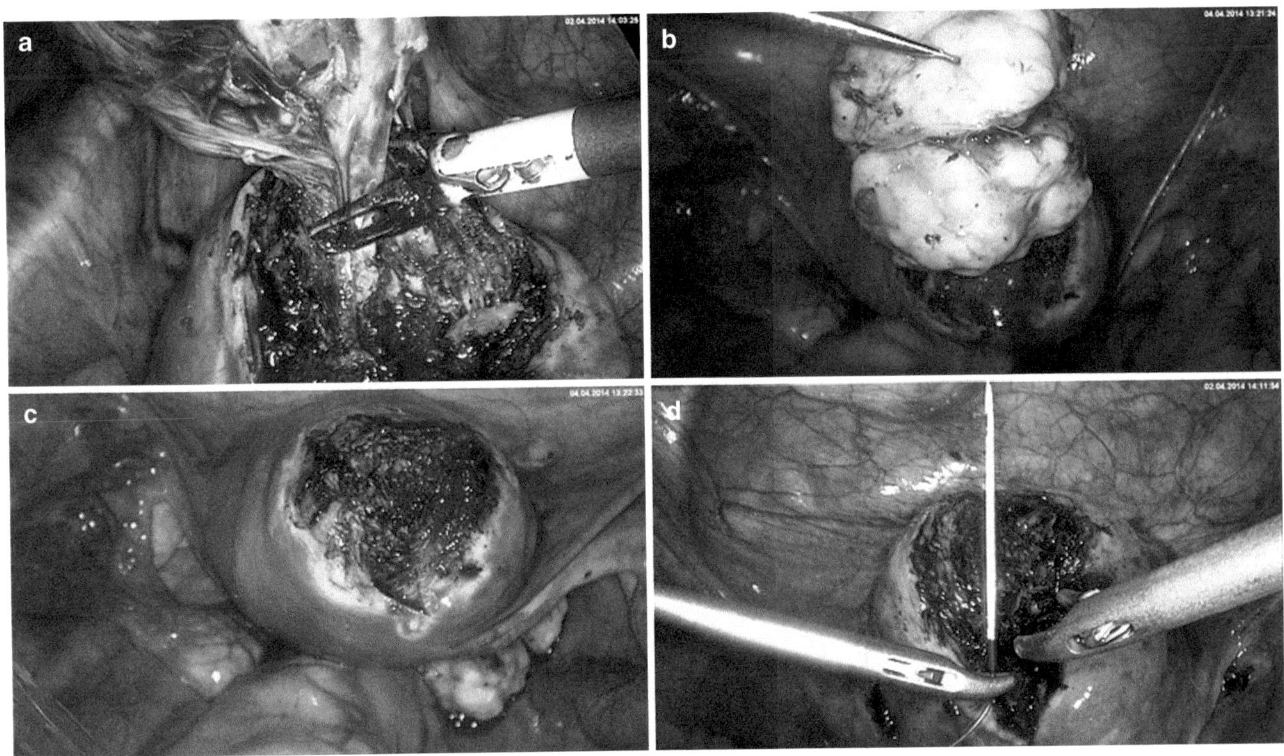

Fig. 35.4 Laparoscopic myoma enucleation. (**a**) Final coagulation of the capsule vessels. (**b**) Double belly fibroid after complete enucleation. (**c**) Minimal coagulation of bleeding vessels under suction and irrigation. (**d**) Approximation of the wound edges with a straight or round sharp needle and a monofilar late-absorbable suture

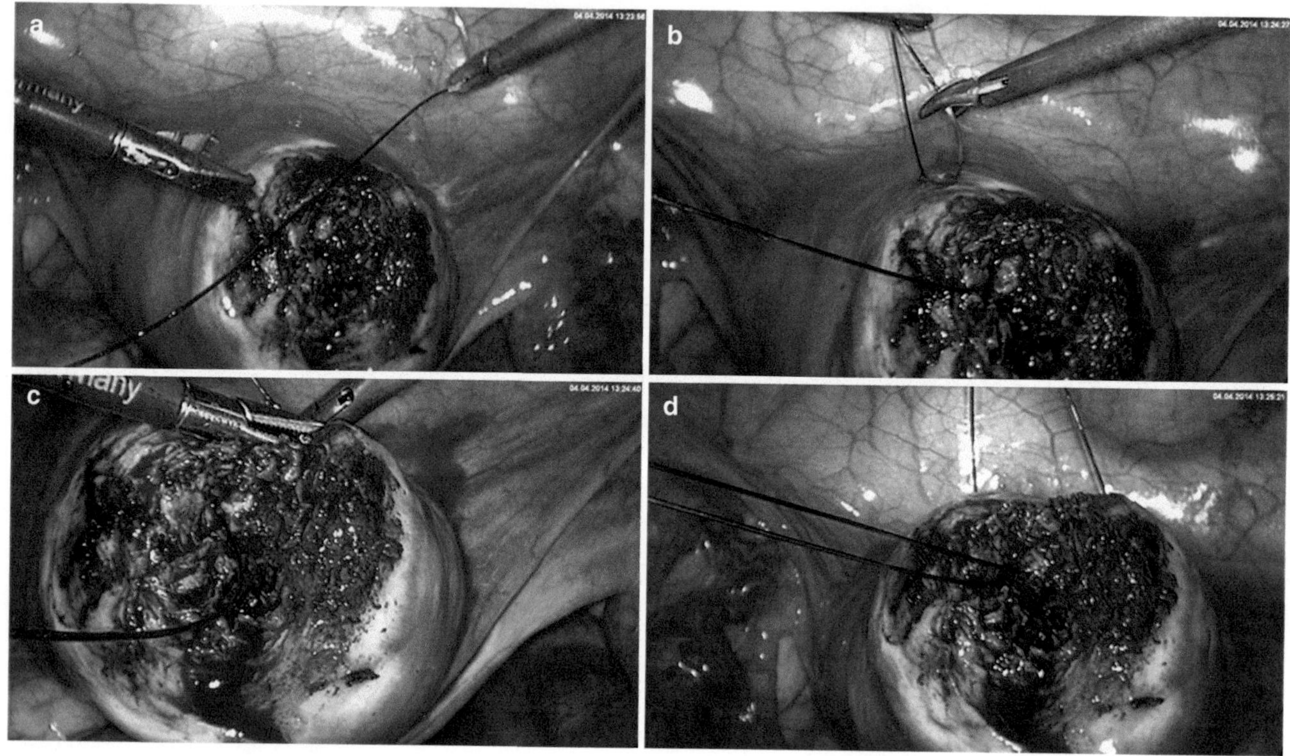

Fig. 35.5 Laparoscopic myoma enucleation. (**a**) Advantages of a circular needle stitch: (**a**) the wound angle is elevated safely and completely when raised with a Manhes forceps, (**b**) deeper layers of the myometrium can be grasped more easily with a circular needle. (**b**) Needle exit and simplified re-grasping with the right needle holder. (**c**) Final stitch to invert the knot. (**d**) Extirpation of the needle, completing the extracorporeal knot, and preparing to push down the extracorporeal knot

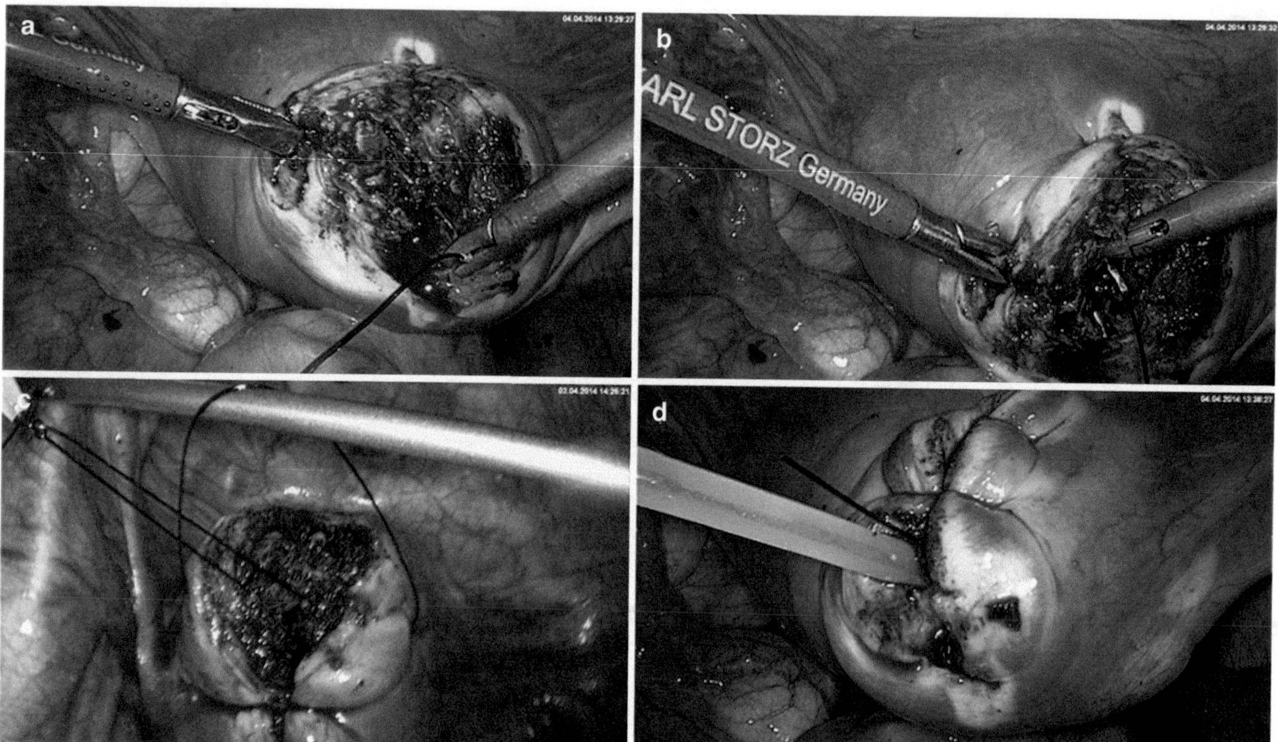

Fig. 35.6 The extracorporeal "von Leffern" knot. (**a**) Pulling out the suture, removing the needle, half hitch. (**b**) Holding the knot with the left hand and reaching over with the right hand. (**c**) Grasping the short end from below and leading it back, exiting before the half hitch. (**d**) Turning back the knot. Holding the straight suture and tightening the knot

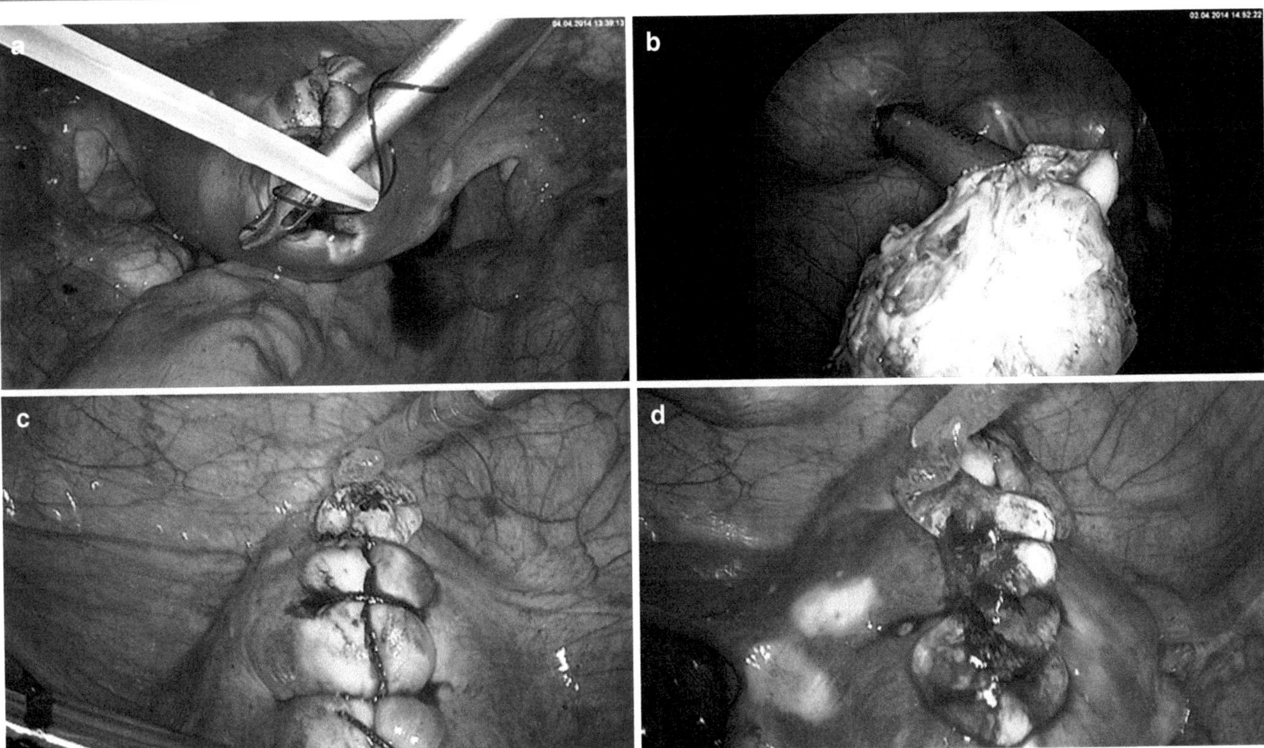

Fig. 35.7 Laparoscopic myoma enucleation. (**a**) Second single suture starting as deep as possible in the uterine wound. (**b**) The needle exits on the left wound margin (immediately adjacent to the Manhes forceps). (**c**) Completing the stitch and preparing the extracorporeal von Leffern knot. The needle holder elevates the thread to avoid tearing the uterine wall when pulling the monofilar thread (PDS). (**d**) Pushing down the extracorporeal knot with a plastic pushrod into the depth of the wound to dump the knot, thus minimizing the size of the external part of the suture

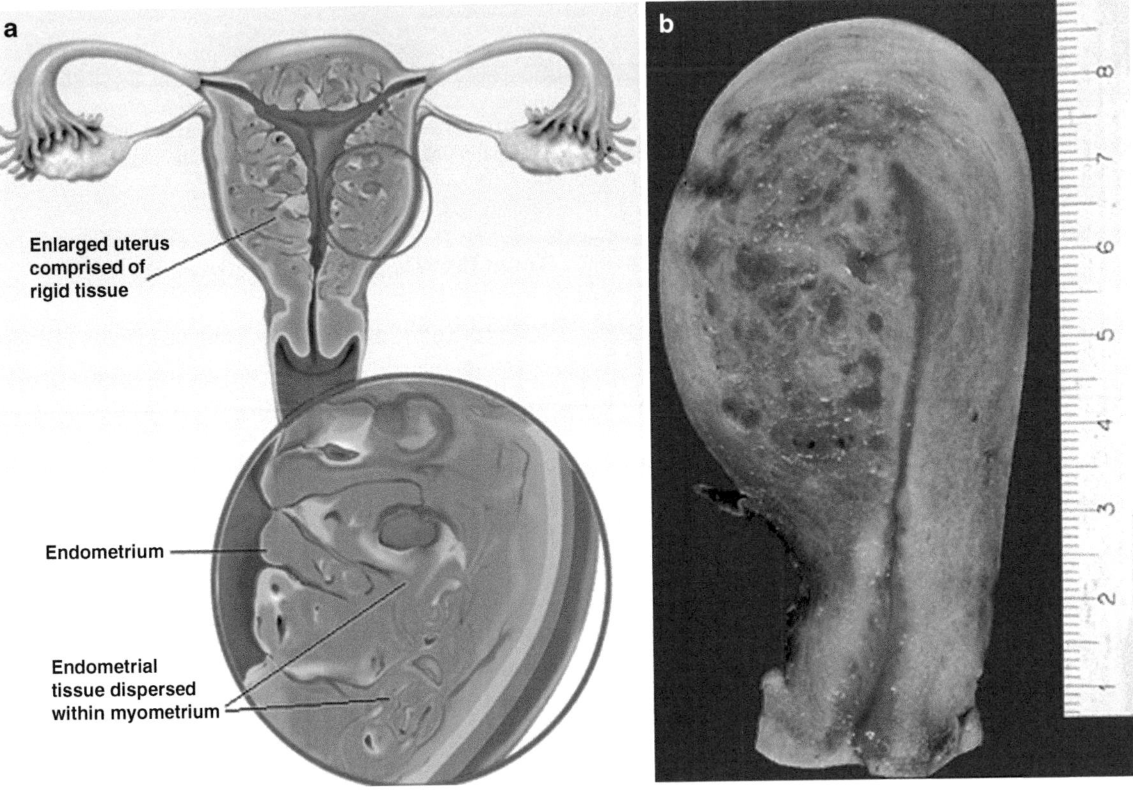

Fig. 35.8 (**a**) Schematic illustration of an enlarged uterus with adenomyosis. Endometriosis glands are dispersed within the myometrium. (**b**) Anatomical specimen in a sagittal cut. The posterior wall is much thicker than the anterior wall, with endometriosis glands spread diffusely in the myometrium wall

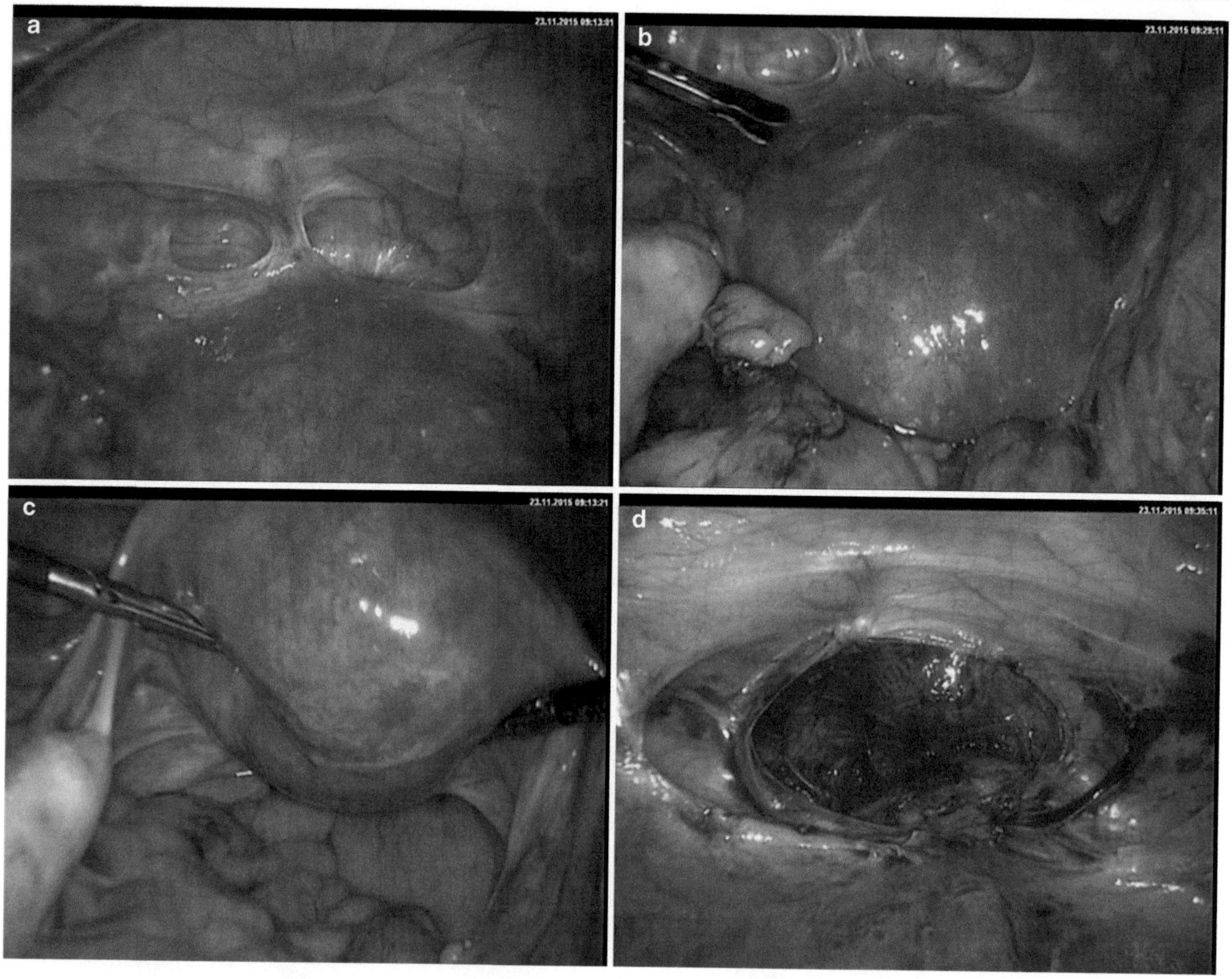

Fig. 35.9 (**a**) Overview of the laparoscopic situs of a patient with severe dysmenorrhea. The uterus is enlarged and soft (**a–c**). The anterior wall is connected to the bladder peritoneum by multiple adhesions. (**d**) After adhesiolysis one has the impression that the adenomyosis has grown through the uterine wall into the adjoining bladder

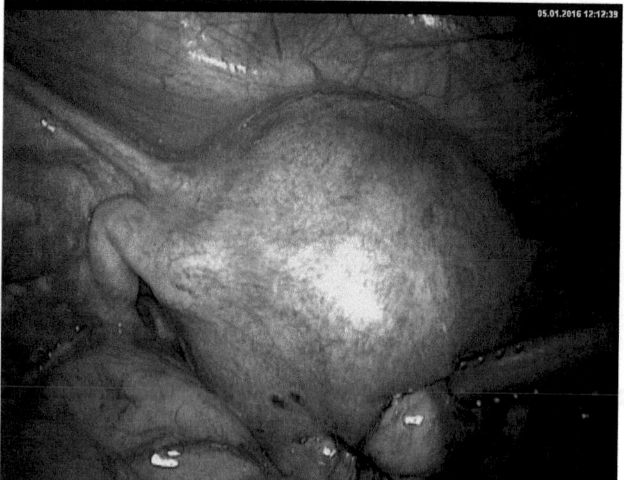

Fig. 35.10 Patient with severe dysmenorrhea and dyspareunia. The injection of blue dye exposes the intramural vessels, which seem to be massively increased. This picture is also typical of adenomyosis of the uterus

Total Versus Subtotal (Supracervical)

Independent of the surgical technique (subtotal or total hysterectomy), endoscopic surgery is a desirable goal. Some women wish to retain their cervix, believing that it may affect their sexual satisfaction after hysterectomy. Removal of the cervix is known to cause excessive neurologic and anatomic disruption, thereby leading to greater surgical and postoperative morbidity, vaginal shortening, subsequent vault prolapse, abnormal cuff granulations, and a propensity for fallopian tube prolapse. These issues were addressed in a systematic review of three randomized trials focused on total versus subtotal hysterectomy for benign gynecological conditions. The conclusions were as follows [11]:

- No difference was noted in rates of incontinence, constipation, or measures of sexual function (sexual satisfaction, dyspareunia).

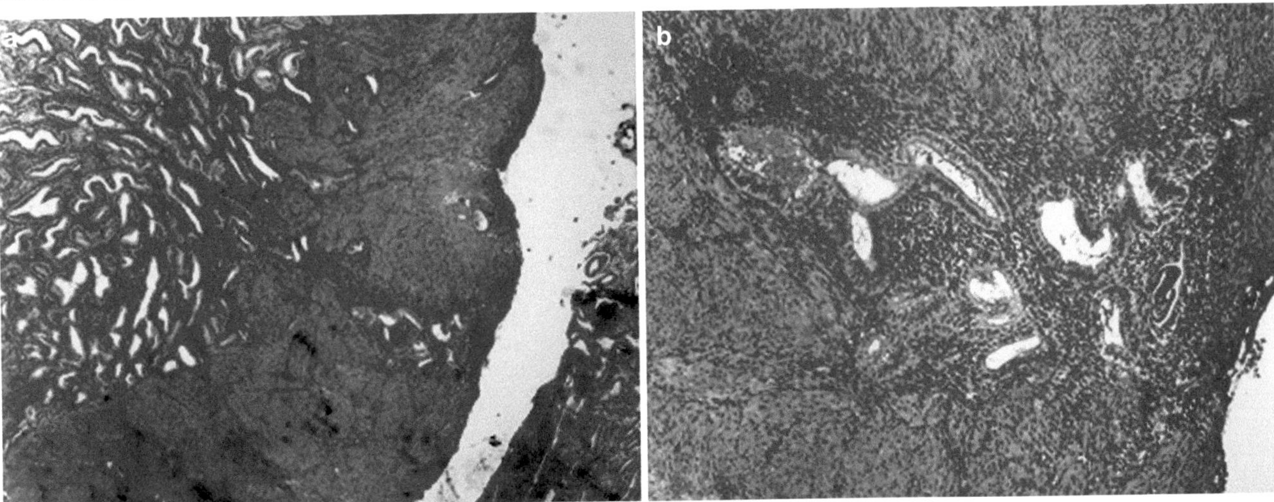

Fig. 35.11 (**a**) Low magnification of a piece of ablated endometrium with the adjoining myometrium tissue in the early secretion phase.(**b**) Islets of endometrium glands in the myometrium stroma with no connection to the uterine cavity. Obviously, the endometrium is fully involved in the endocrine cycle

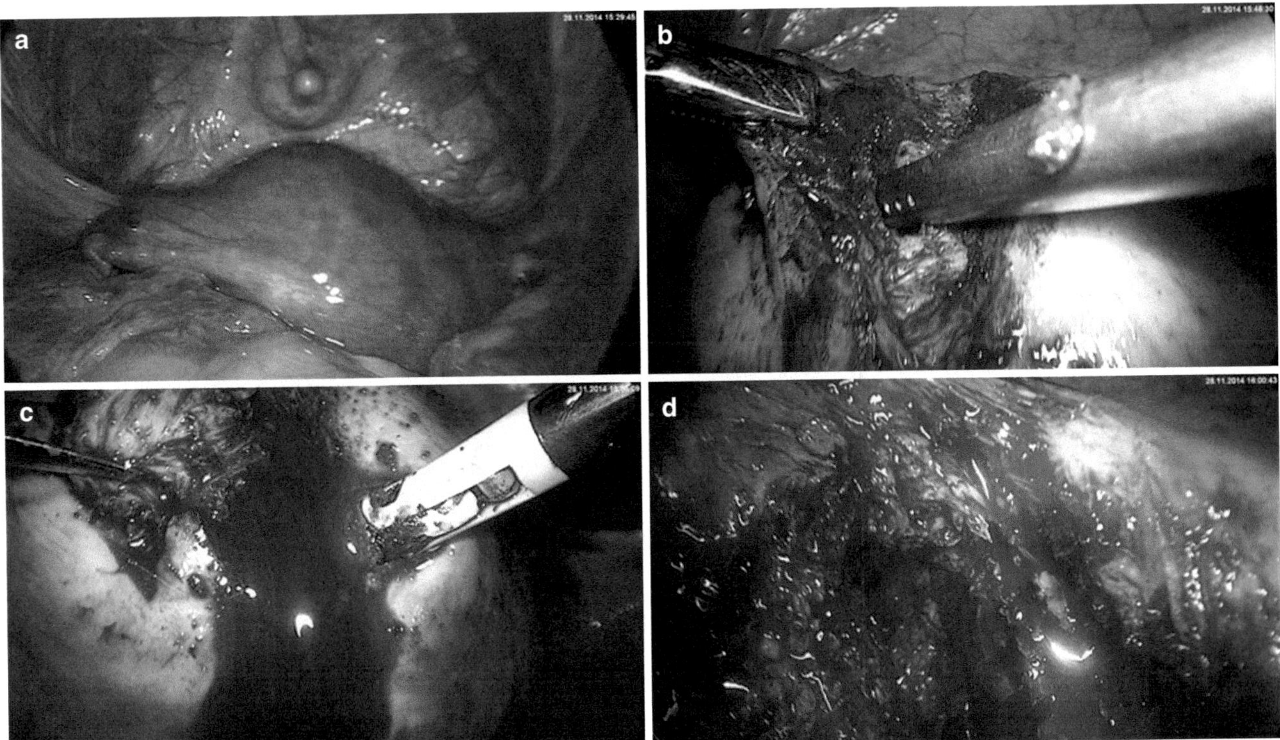

Fig. 35.12 (**a**) Overview of an asymmetrical uterus; endometriosis is suspected at the left tube and a central space-occupying lesion is seen. (**b**) Opening the central intramural lesion, which was suspected to be a fibroid.(**c**) Chocolate-like fluid after entering the adenomyoma. (**d**) On the magnification even the wall layers, including the mid-endometrium tissue can be seen

- The duration of surgery and the quantity of blood loss during surgery were significantly less during subtotal hysterectomy compared with total hysterectomy. However, there was no difference in the likelihood of the patient needing a transfusion.
- Febrile morbidity was less likely and ongoing cyclic vaginal bleeding one year after surgery more likely after subtotal hysterectomy.
- No difference was noted in the rates of other complications, recovery from surgery, or readmission rates.

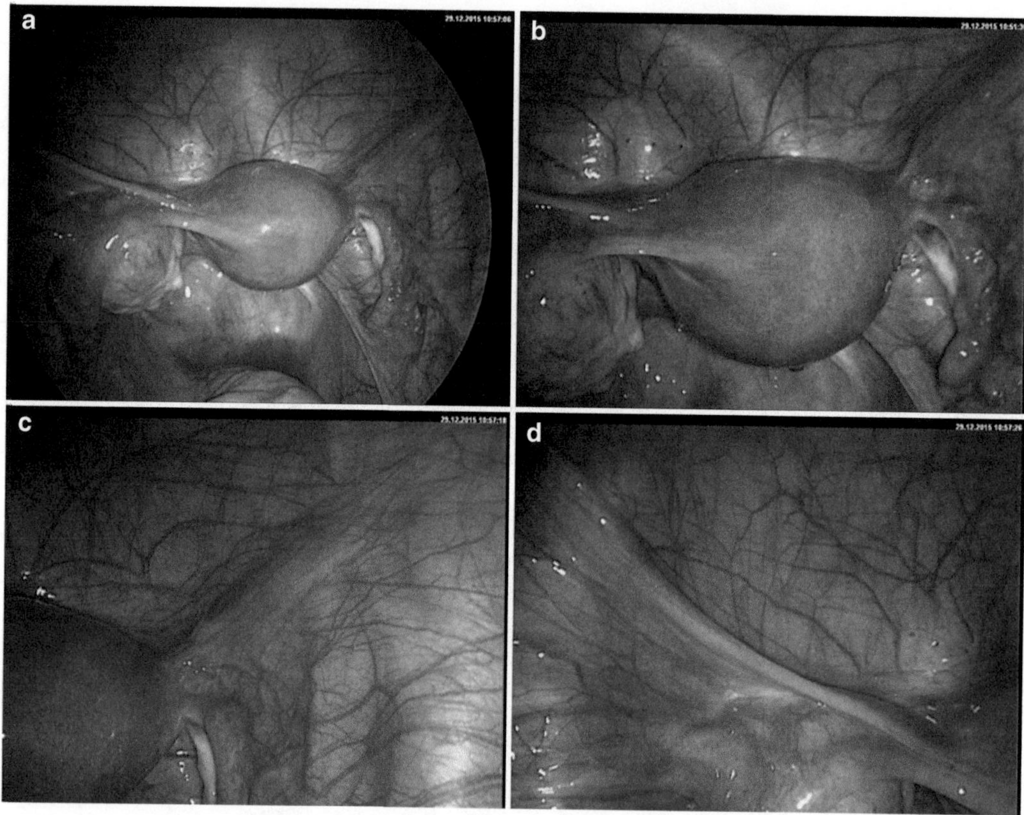

Fig. 35.13 Laparoscopic overview of a patient with dysmenorrhea.(**a**, **b**) An enlarged and irregular uterus with hypervascularization of the serosa. The chronic disease has caused an asymmetry of the round ligaments. (**c**) The right side is much shorter than (**d**) the left side

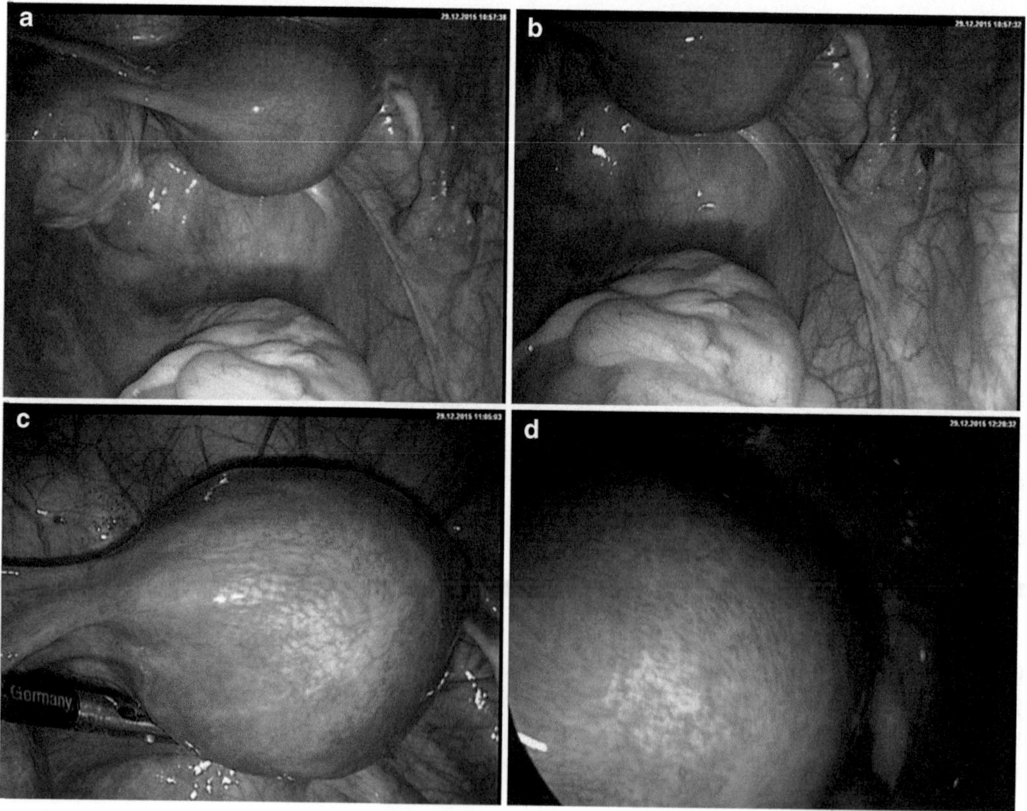

Fig. 35.14 (**a**, **c**) The uterus appears to be less mobile but somehow fixed in the pelvis. (**b**) The peritoneum above the ureter is under tension and can be demarcated from the sacrouterine ligament.(**c**, **d**) The surface of the uterus is hypervascularized; the outflow of the tubes seems to be steep

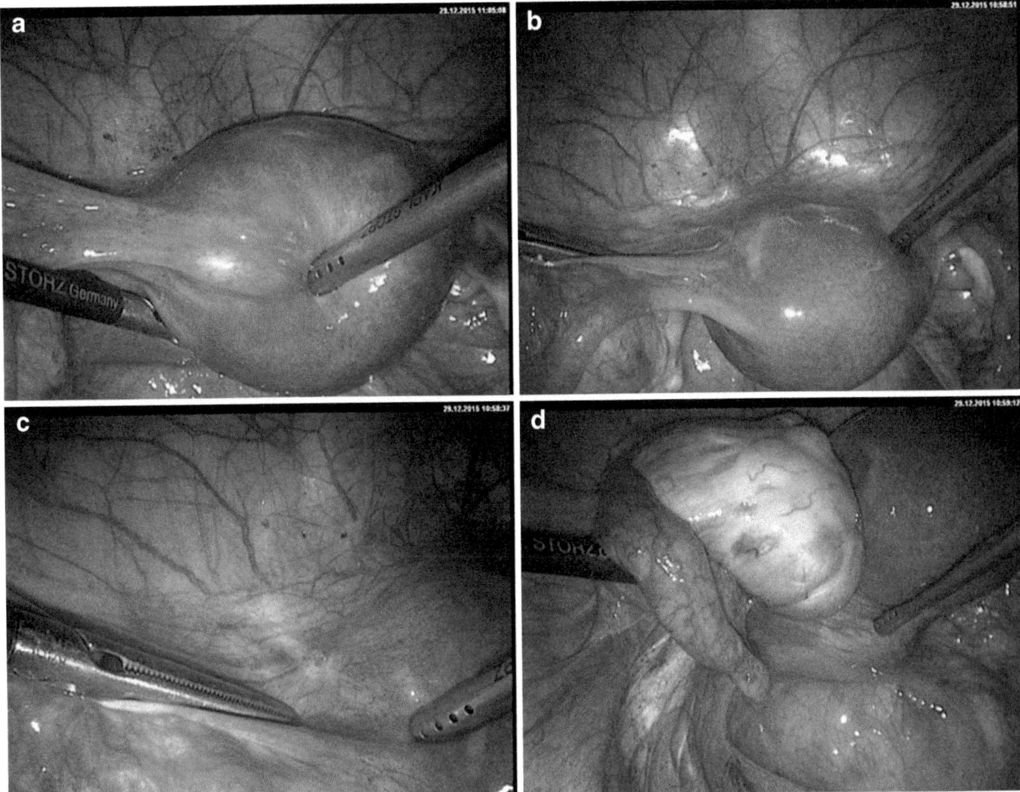

Fig. 35.15 (**a**, **b**) Palpating the uterus with a blunt instrument shows that its consistency is less soft; it is tight but hypervascular.(**c**) Endometriotic nodule on the lower uterine anterior wall.(**d**) Fixed and enlarged cystic left ovary in the ovarian fossa. The ureter can be demarcated behind the peritoneum and is lifted to the fixed area

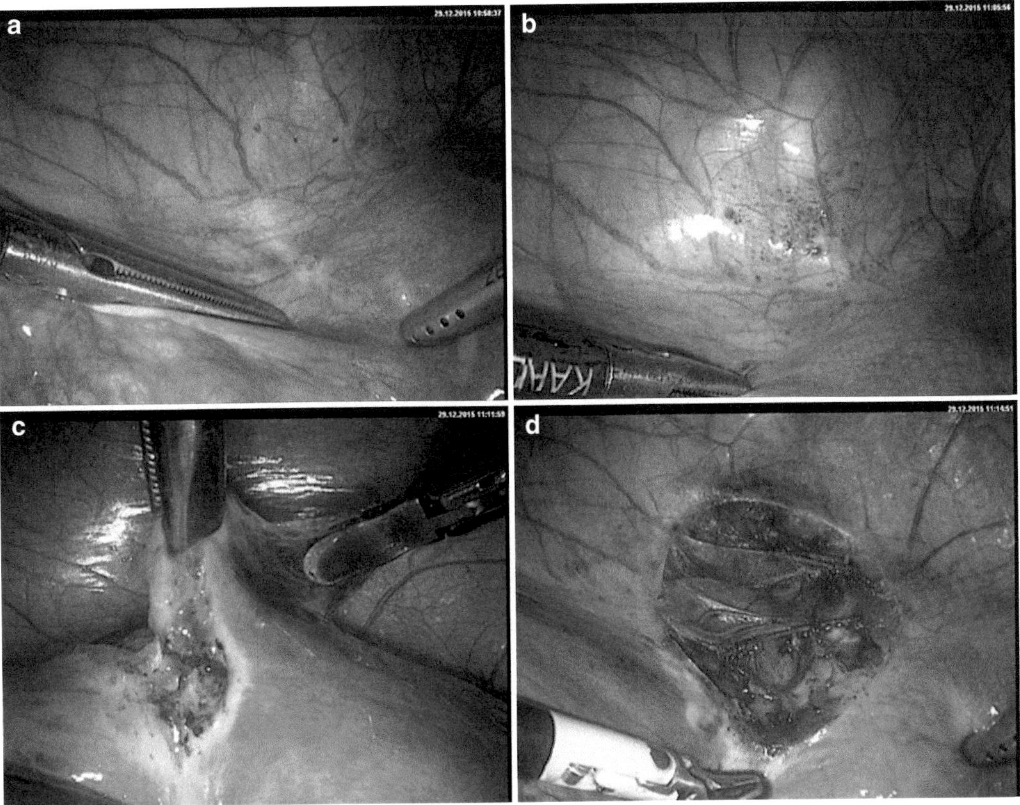

Fig. 35.16 (**a–d**) Excision of the endometriotic nodule of the lower anterior uterine wall.(**b**) Even the adjacent bladder peritoneum appears to be superficially affected because it is hypervascularized and fragile

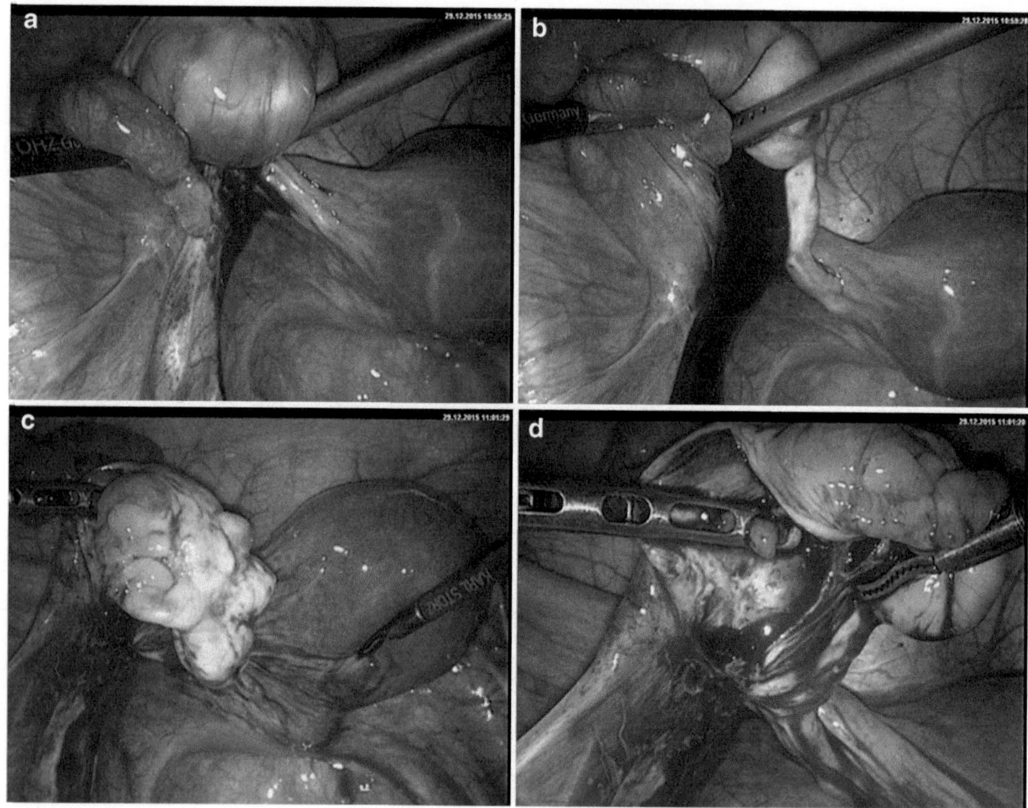

Fig. 35.17 (**a, b**) Lifting the ovary out of the ovarian fossa and releasing it from its peritoneal adhesion leads to opening of the endometrioma. (**c, d**) The depths of the ovarian fossa are affected by disease, as proven by the demarcation of the peritoneal nodule. These nodules are usually connected to the cardinal ligament or the sacrouterine ligament

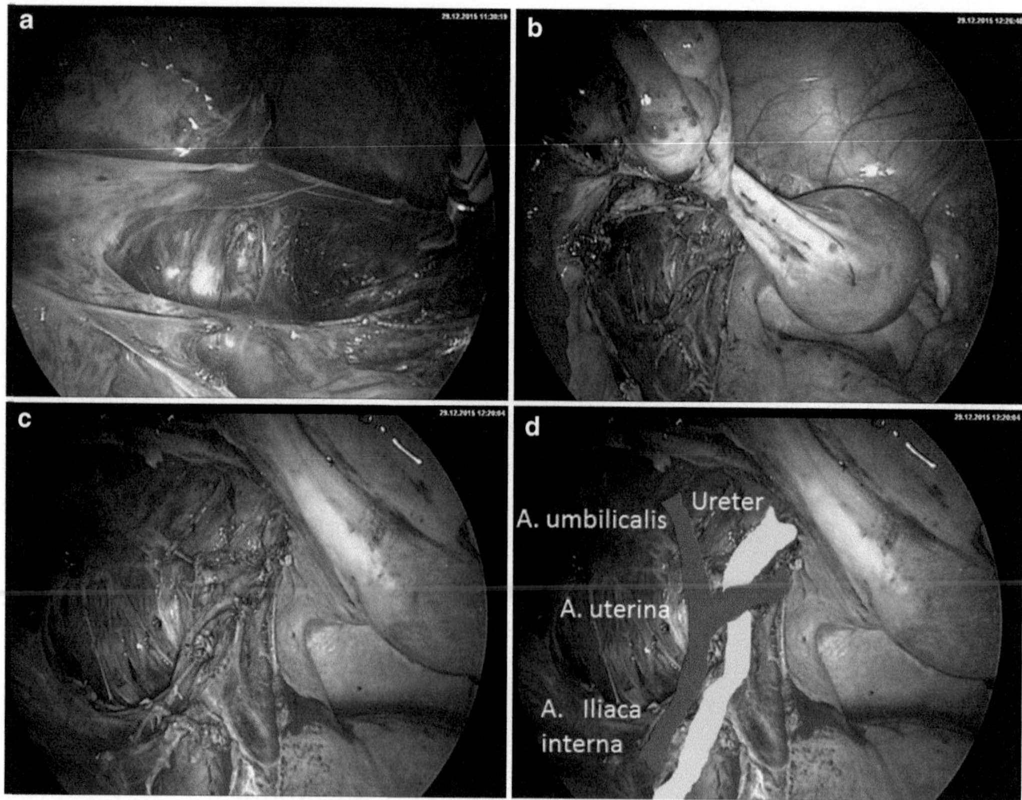

Fig. 35.18 Opening the peritoneal wall for resection of the symptomatic endometriotic nodule. (**a–d**) The ureter and vessels of the pelvic wall can be separated bluntly from the peritoneum and the endometriotic nodule. The ureter or the vessels themselves are very rarely affected. If they are, the condition calls for special surgical treatment

Table 35.1 The five major diagnostic categories that constitute indications for hysterectomy are the following

Uterine leiomyomas
Endometriosis and adenomyosis uteri
Pelvic organ prolapse
Pelvic pain or infection (other than endometriosis): pelvic inflammatory disease, adhesions
Abnormal uterine bleeding of known and unknown origin
Malignant and premalignant disease

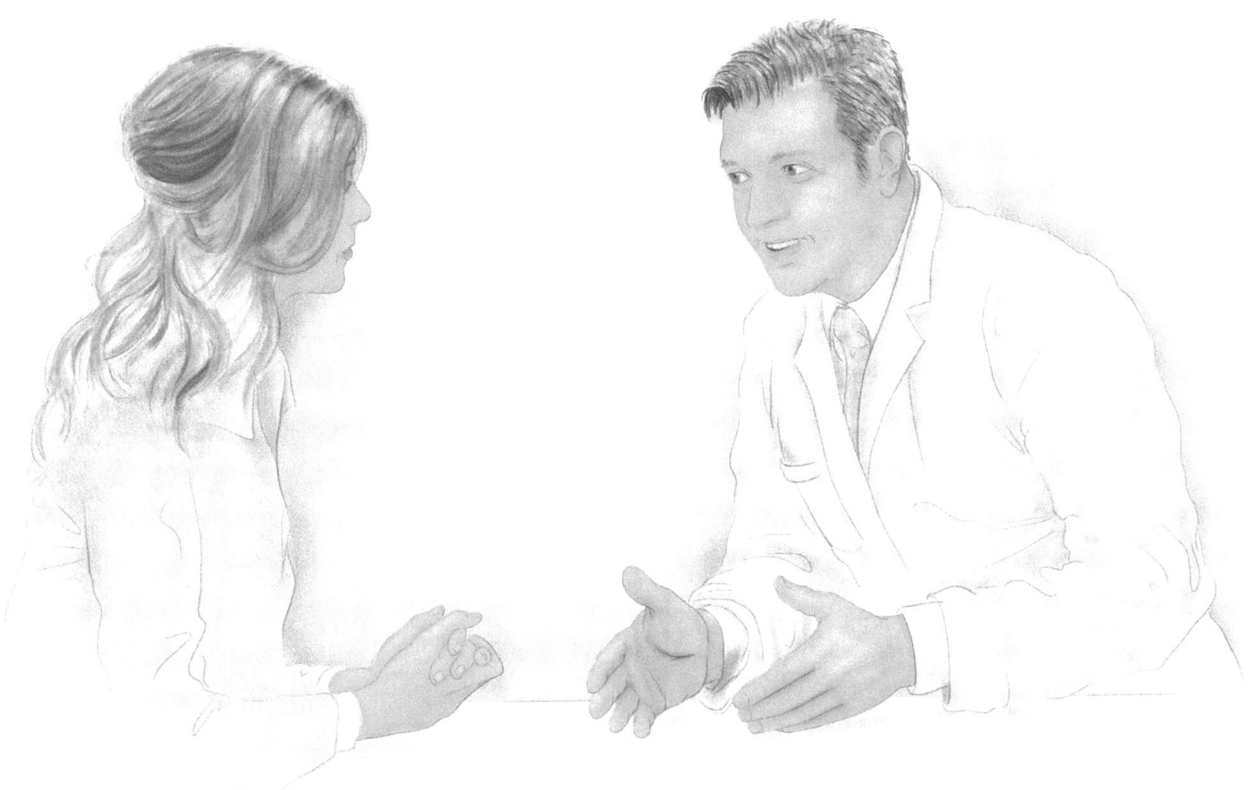

Fig. 35.19 Truly empathetic preoperative counseling must include congruence and respect for the patient

Table 35.2 Vaginal versus abdominal versus laparoscopic hysterectomy. The robotic-assisted laparoscopic hysterectomy is included in the category of laparoscopic hysterectomies

Vaginal hysterectomy compared to abdominal hysterectomy	
Advantages	Shorter hospitalization (mean difference 1 day, 95 % CI 0.7–1.2)
	More rapid return to normal activities (mean difference 9.5 days, 95 % CI 6.4–12.6)
	Fewer infections or fever (OR 0.42, 95 % CI 0.21–0.83)
	Possibility of regional anesthesia
Disadvantages	No simultaneous surgery of comorbidities
	More difficulties in simultaneous adnexal surgery
Laparoscopic hysterectomy compared to abdominal hysterectomy	
Advantages	Less blood loss (mean difference 45.3 ml, 95 % CI 17.9–72.7)
	Shorter hospital stay (mean difference 2 days, 95 % CI 1.9–2.2)
	More rapid return to normal activities (mean difference 13.6 days, 95 % CI 11.8–15.4)
	Fewer wound infections or fever (OR 0.32, 95 % CI 0.12–0.85)
Disadvantages	Longer operating times (mean difference 10.6 min, 95 % CI 7.4–13.8)
	More urinary tract injuries (OR 2.61, 95 % CI 1.22–5.60)
Laparoscopic hysterectomy compared to vaginal hysterectomy	
Advantages	Simultaneous surgery for comorbidities
	Almost independent of the preoperative assessment
Disadvantages	Similar outcomes except longer operating times (mean difference 41.5 min, 95 % CI 33.7–49.4)
	More expensive

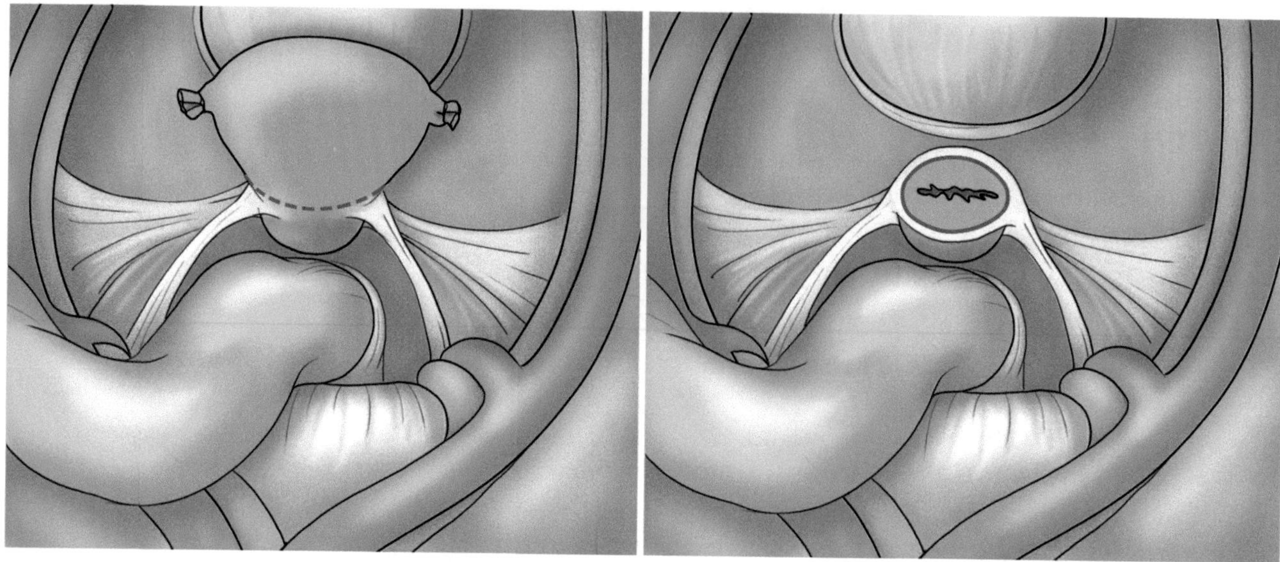

Fig. 35.20 Schematic illustration of subtotal or supracervical hysterectomy with the remaining cervical stump. The sacrouterine ligaments and the cardinal ligament remain untouched. The medial compartment is not opened

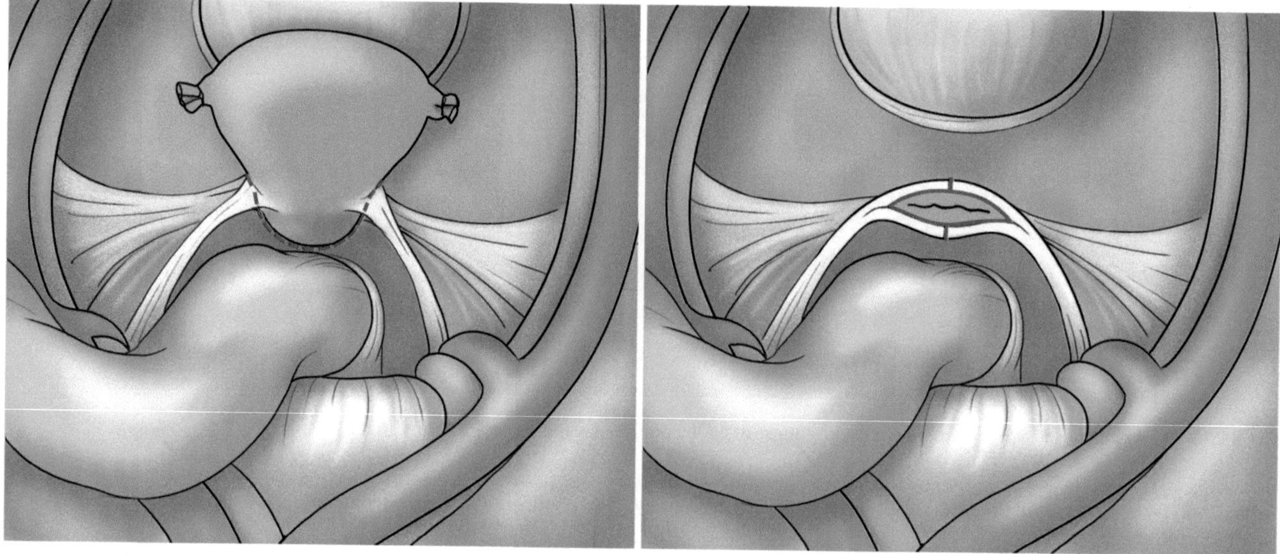

Fig. 35.21 In comparison, in laparoscopic total hysterectomy the middle compartment is opened and the cervix is enucleated out of its bed. In intrafascial hysterectomy the surrounding ligaments remain intact and the vaginal stump is retained

In the short-term, randomized trials have shown that preservation or removal of the cervix does not affect the rate of subsequent pelvic organ prolapse.

The anatomical and therefore functional advantage of the cervix being left in place is that the cardinal and uterosacral ligaments remain in place (Figs. 35.20, 35.21, 35.22, 35.23 and 35.24).

The advantages of supracervical hysterectomy compared to abdominal hysterectomy include shorter operating times and a shorter length of hospital stay when performed laparoscopically. Furthermore, patients who undergo subtotal hysterectomy are able to withstand loads earlier because there is no risk of vaginal cuff dehiscence [12]. Some studies have reported a shorter recovery period following subtotal hysterectomy, but this finding is not supported by data from randomized trials. In a prospective cohort study, supracervical hysterectomy was associated with greater improvement in short term quality of life scores than total hysterectomy, but no difference was registered in postoperative pain or return to activities of daily living [13]. There may also be fewer injuries to the urinary tract because dissection is not performed as close to the cervix or as deep into the pelvis as in total hysterectomy. However, clinical trials designed to demonstrate this clinical observation have not been performed yet.

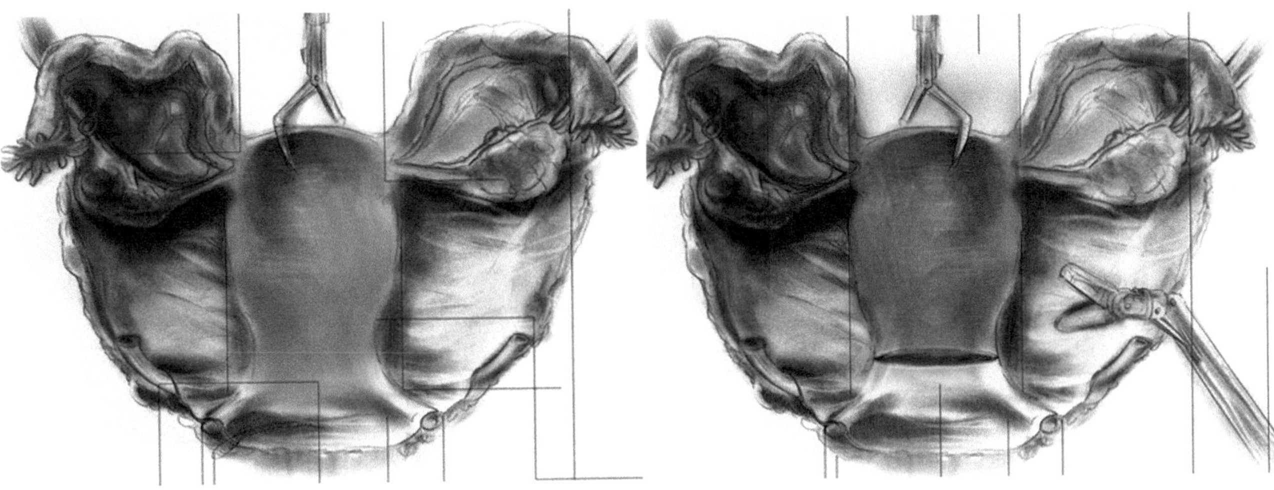

Fig. 35.22 Overview of subtotal and total hysterectomy with reference to the surrounding tissue. The sacrouterine ligaments are omitted in both procedures

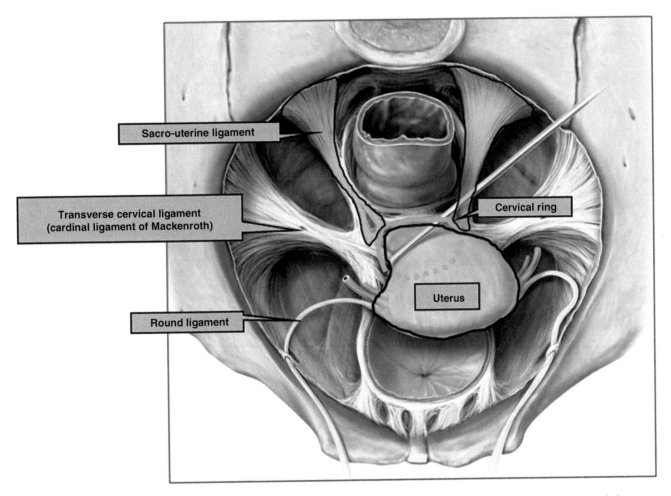

Fig. 35.23 Imaginary transverse plane showing the three compartments and the cervical ring, which is removed in total laparoscopic hysterectomy. The anatomical structure must be reconstructed when closing the vaginal cuff

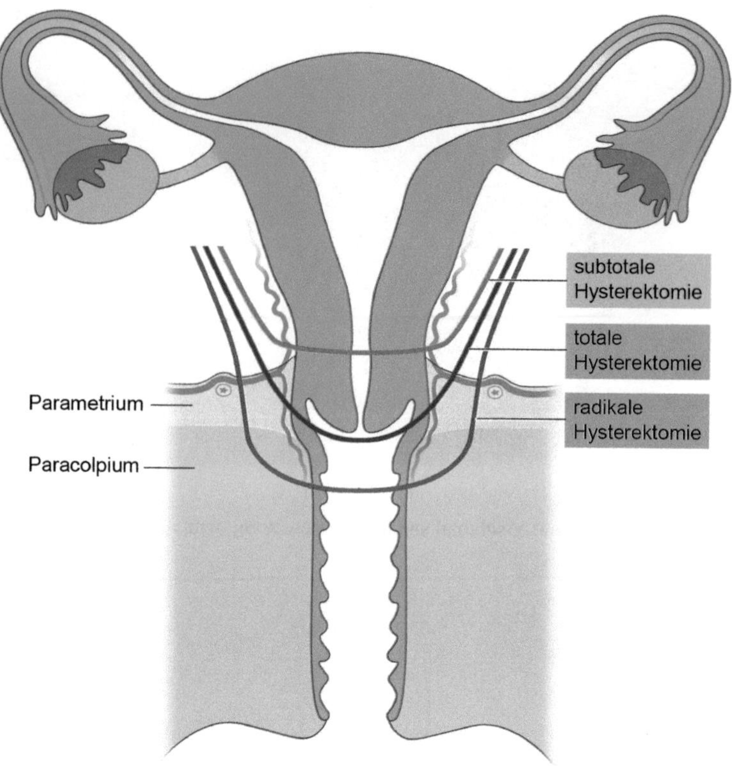

Fig. 35.24 Schematic illustration of the resection line in subtotal, total, and radical laparoscopic hysterectomy. Only the ascending branch of the uterine artery needs to be coagulated and cut with the uterine manipulator in benign cases. When adhering closely to this operative technique, the ureter is located at a safe distance from the coagulation zone (about 2 cm). All radical procedures are associated with a high degree of risk

Other differences include post-hysterectomy body image and health status. Women who underwent subtotal hysterectomy reported a significantly better body image and health-related quality of life than those who underwent total hysterectomy. Both groups reported an improvement in sexual satisfaction [14].

The only absolute contraindication for subtotal hysterectomy is a malignant or premalignant condition of the uterine corpus or cervix.

Extensive endometriosis is a relative contraindication because these women may experience persistent dyspareunia when the cervix is retained. The significance of adenomyosis has been underestimated so far. The uterus is morcellated in the abdomen. If the morcellated uterus is not collected in a bag, adenomyosis may spread into the abdominal cavity. The patient may experience persistent pain in the central segment of the lower abdomen. In laparoscopic supracervical hysterectomy (LSH), the involvement of the cervix or the retrocervical/precervical space is ignored. Very often the sacrouterine ligaments or the lateral cardinal ligaments leading to the ovarian fossa are also affected. In these cases, either the adenomyosis has grown through the uterine wall into the adjacent organs or there is concomitant endometriosis. To rule out all causes of symptoms, it would be advisable to remove all visible endometriosis-associated pathologies. LTH, if performed correctly, is associated with very few additional risks or side effects. Therefore, in cases of adenomyosis of the uterus we explain the situation to the patient in detail and advise LTH [personal statement]. Arguments in favor of LTH include fewer cases of urinary incontinence, less prolapse and cervical stump problems. However, subtotal hysterectomy is performed faster in most cases and seems to be associated with fewer intraoperative and postoperative complications. We lack convincing data concerning the advantages of simultaneous removal of the cervix; the cervix is very rarely involved in the disease [15, 16].

Elective supracervical hysterectomy should be preceded by cervical cytology confirming the absence of cervical intraepithelial neoplasia (PAP smear). Women who have had a supracervical hysterectomy should be screened for cervical cancer according to standard guidelines for their age and risk status. In patients with abnormal uterine bleeding (especially metrorrhagia), endometrial cancer or any type of sarcoma should be ruled out prior to performing a supracervical hysterectomy.

Sometimes the cervix needs to be removed later as a separate procedure. This approach is associated with frequent damage to the bowel and the bladder because the anatomical spaces cannot be exposed clearly and adhesions are common. However, the approach is readily accepted because primary surgery is associated with fewer risks than subsequent procedures. Patients who wish to minimize the likelihood of subsequent surgery may prefer a laparoscopic total hysterectomy (LTH).

Will the Fallopian Tubes and/or Ovaries Be Removed in a Hysterectomy?

Based on the existing data concerning the prevention of ovarian cancer and fallopian tube disorders, we recommend a simultaneous salpingectomy after appropriate counseling.

Notwithstanding the above facts, the number of pelvic floor corrections has increased very markedly throughout the world in recent years. This is a consequence of demographic changes. In 2000, 34.8 million women (12.7 %) in the USA were 65 years or older. By 2030 this number will have risen to 70.3 million (20 %). Similar demographic changes are anticipated in Germany [17]. In 2011, women above the age of 65 years accounted for 20 % of the total population; the percentage will rise to 35 % by 2060. This development will be less striking in other European countries, the United Kingdom, France, the Netherlands and Sweden [17]. The rate of pelvic organ prolapse (POP) repair in women aged 65 years and above is 30–50 % [18];among women older than 80 years it is still 11 % [19].

The reported rates of post-hysterectomy prolapse vary. The cumulative risk has been reported to be 1 % at three years after hysterectomy, and about 15 % fifteen years later. The risk is 5.5-fold higher when hysterectomy is performed for a descensus. Incidence rates of 46 % have been reported elsewhere [19–22]. Apart from the risk of a pre-existing descensus, vaginal deliveries and age are discussed as reasons for the risk doubling with each advancing decade of life [23]. Obviously, the rate of descent also depends on the applied surgical technique and measures for the prevention of descensus [24].

Total laparoscopic hysterectomy involves removal of the uterus and the cervix. The entire procedure is performed laparoscopically. The specimen can usually be removed through the vaginal vault. Laparoscopic-assisted vaginal hysterectomy (LAVH) has been entirely replaced by the endoscopic technique, which has become a standard procedure since the learning curve for laparoscopic suturing is now favorable. Taking into account the advantages of endoscopic surgery (shorter hospital stay, faster recovery, better cosmetic result and fewer infections), the question arises as to whether the risk of post-hysterectomy prolapse after LSH can be reduced by preserving the existing structures of the pelvic floor in the middle compartment or reconstructing them. In cases of pre-existing defects, LTH provides sufficient fixation of the pelvic floor and thus minimizes the risk of a post-hysterectomy prolapse. Mesh implants such as those used for sacrocolpopexy may be employed in both procedures simultaneously.

Our multimodality concept of laparoscopic intrafascial hysterectomy is aimed at the removal of all concomitant pathologies that might also be responsible for the patient's symptomatic condition, and simultaneously reducing the risk of post-hysterectomy prolapse:

1. Removal of all concomitant pathologies, such as adhesions or endometriosis spots, and demarcating the extent of adenomyosis.
2. Intrafascial hysterectomy with preservation of existing ligaments, yet opening the medial compartment when performing total laparoscopic hysterectomy:
   (a) Technique 1: Primary uterine artery clipping/ligation
   (b) Technique 2: Classic intrafascial hysterectomy
3. A technique of stable fixation of the vaginal stump

Development of Laparoscopic Hysterectomy Techniques and Instruments

The popularity of laparoscopic hysterectomy rose gradually after Harry Reich's initial publication of the procedure [25, 26]. A number of approaches evolved, such as laparoscopically assisted vaginal hysterectomy (LAVH), laparoscopic supracervical hysterectomy (LSH), total laparoscopic hysterectomy, and laparoscopic intrafascial hysterectomy (LTH). LTH had a steep learning curve and was initially associated with rather high complication rates [5]. The development of new instruments and consistent training improved the situation. The introduction of the intrauterine manipulator helped to develop the classic intrafascial concept which, today, is the aim of every gynecological surgeon performing total laparoscopic hysterectomy. Hohl used Kurt Semm's procedure of classic intrafascial supracervical hysterectomy (CISH) [27] and developed it further with the use of his manipulator [28]. The majority of the available manipulators are well accepted because they are easy to handle, reusable, and durable. The uterus can be moved in all directions while the elliptical long tip of the manipulator eases out vaginal and paravaginal tissue intraabdominally. The manipulator can be pushed straight towards the field of operation, especially when cutting the uterus off the vagina with the monopolar hook and targeting the tip of the manipulator.

The large majority of manipulators are provided with a ceramic cap that creates a flat surface to work on. Consequently, dissection of the bladder is usually not necessary. It should be noted that the use of the manipulator for bladder dissection is useful and safe even after a cesarean section. The application of the manipulator imitates the classical movements during abdominal hysterectomy; the ureters are kept out of the field of operation. The cap allows intrafascial hysterectomy, which preserves the ligaments and avoids vaginal shortening. The smooth cutting edge is useful for vaginal occlusion (Fig. 35.25).

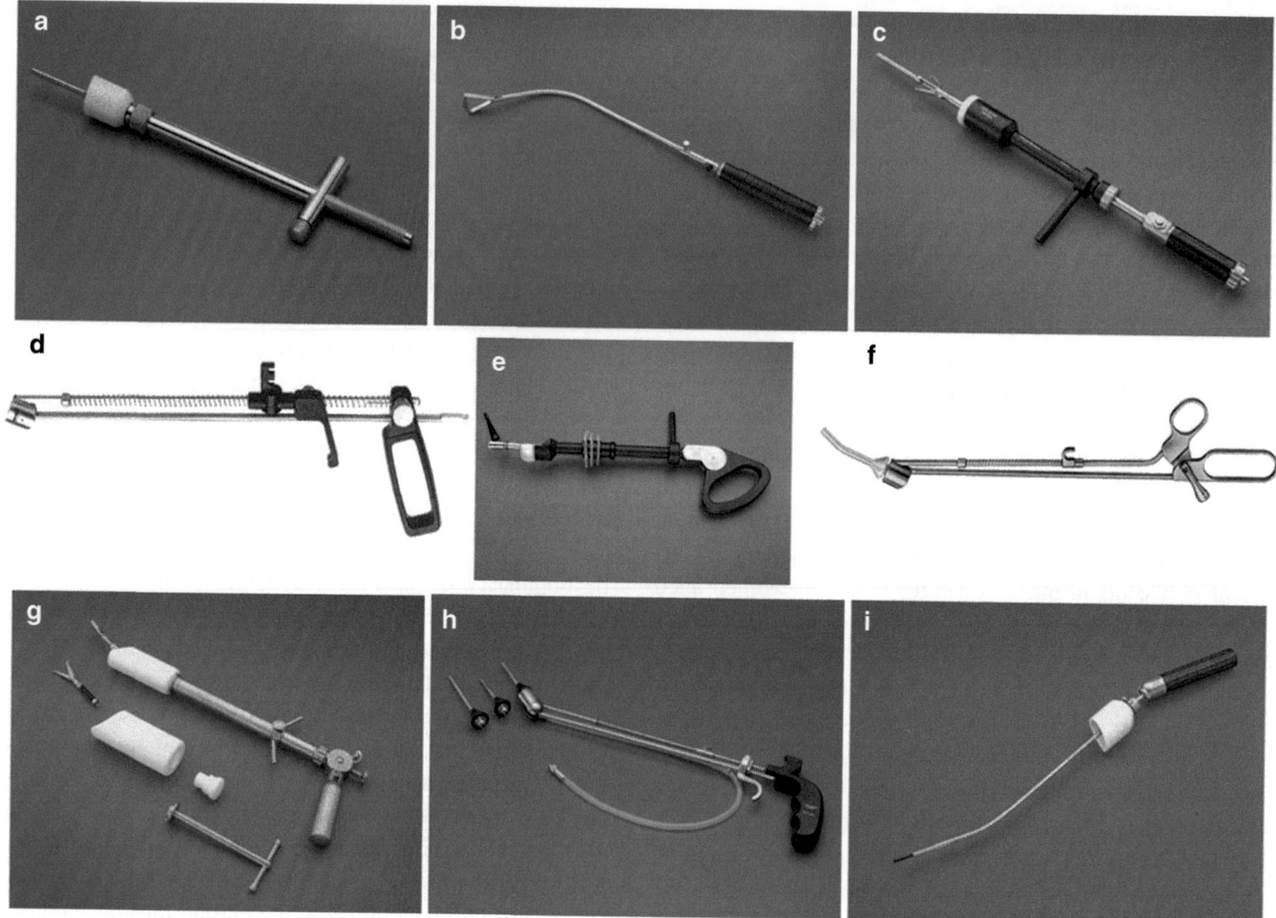

Fig. 35.25 (**a**) Hohl manipulator (Storz). (**b**) Dionisi uterine manipulator (Storz). (**c**) Mangeshikar uterine manipulator (Storz). (**d**) RfQ uterine manipulator. (**e**) Clermont-Ferrand uterine manipulator (Storz). (**f**) Braun uterine manipulator. (**g**) Koninckx uterine manipulator (Storz). (**h**) Tintara uterine manipulator (Storz). (**i**) Donnez uterine manipulator (Storz)

Points to be considered:

- Monopolar electricity can be used on the ceramic cap. Bipolar current causes a larger defect, bearing the risk of subsequent wound healing problems and vaginal cuff dehiscence. The fact that ultrasound is liable to destroy this apparatus must be taken into account when using ultrasound for dissection during hysterectomy.
- Intrafascial hysterectomy involves a much smaller opening to the vagina and preserves the circular ligaments. Large uteruses may need to be morcellated. Extended endometriosis or adenomyosis may involve the circular ligaments, which then have to be removed [28].

The other instruments may be of the disposable or reusable type. Disposable tissue sealing instruments are faster and need not be replaced frequently. However, the instruments are costly and fusion of the layers of tissue results in a less clear overview of the anatomical structures. Bipolar forceps are essential. Extracorporeal sutures (PDS 1.0) are helpful, although intracorporeal sutures (Vicryl) are sufficient for vaginal closure. The monopolar hook facilitates the removal of endometriotic spots and the uterus from the manipulator, but can be replaced by bipolar forceps and scissors. In cases of a large uterus, the tenaculum can be used to lift out the uterus; a morcellator avoids troublesome comminution of the uterus.

Preoperative Considerations and Preparation

When severe endometriosis (Fig. 35.26) is suspected on vaginal examination (Fig. 35.27) and the ultrasound scan is correlated with the patient's medical history, it will be necessary to perform further diagnostic investigations such as MRI, cystoscopy, rectoscopy, or endosonography (Figs. 35.28 and 35.29). Radical interdisciplinary surgery can then be planned and performed (Figs. 35.30, 35.31 and 35.32).

A hysterectomy must always be accompanied by antibiotic protection, such as a second-generation cephalosporin. In cases of suspected bowel involvement, a single

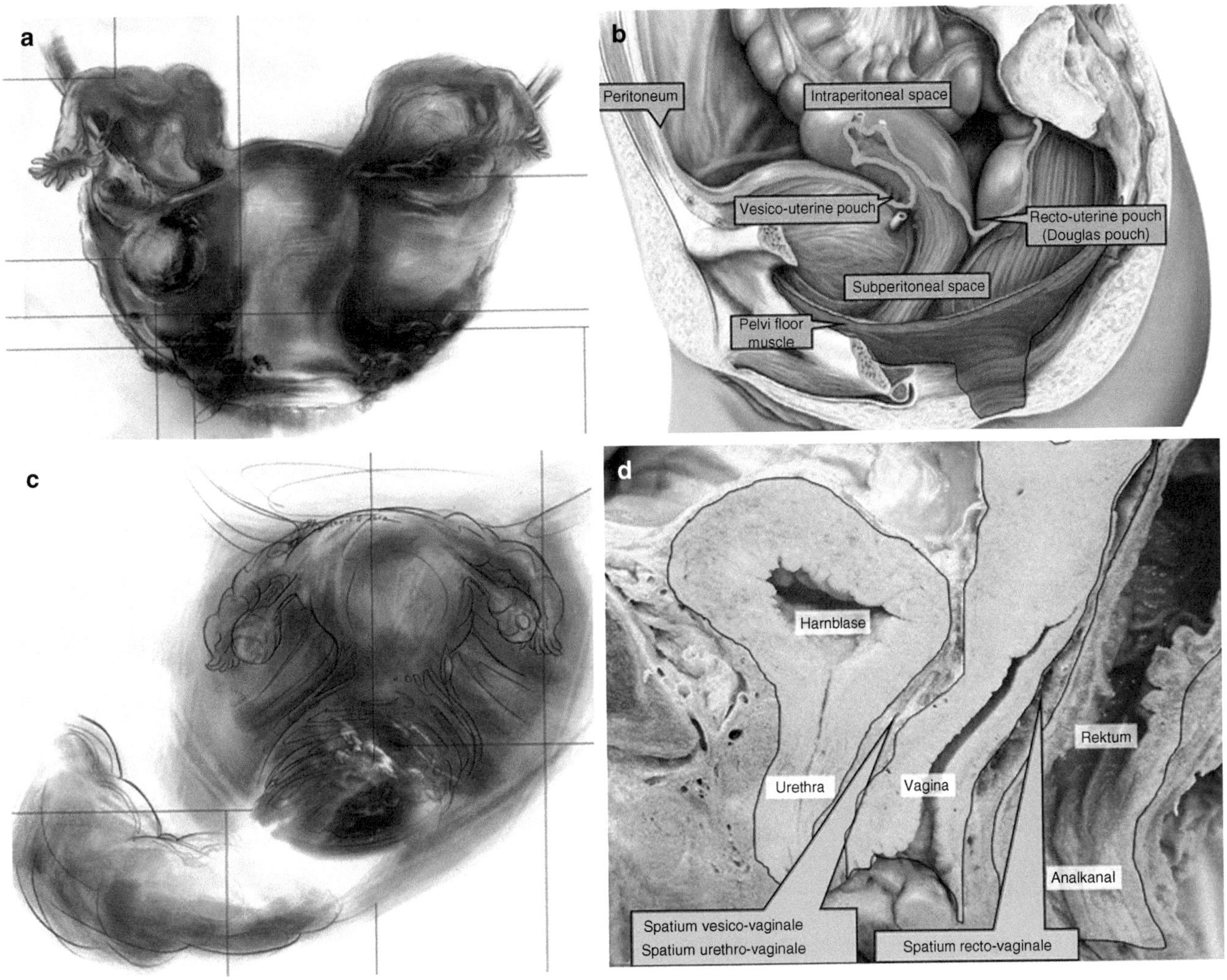

Fig. 35.26 (**a**) Severe endometriosis in relation to anatomical landmarks (**b–d**)

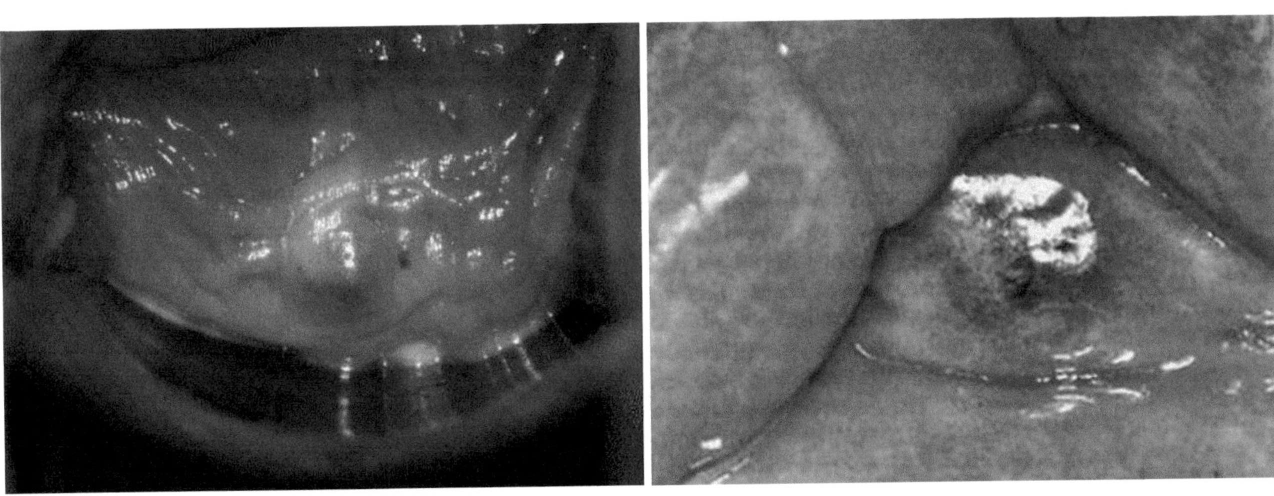

Fig. 35.27 Vaginal photograph of a small endometriotic nodule in the dorsal vaginal wall and another patient with severe deep infiltrating endometriosis involving the vagina

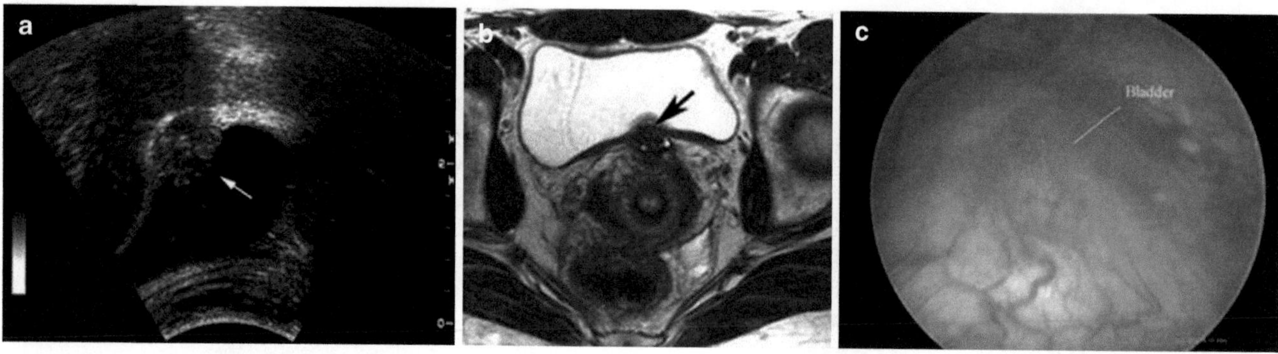

Fig. 35.28 (**a**) Vaginal ultrasound of a solitary nodule between the anterior wall of the uterus and the bladder (vesicovaginal space). (**b**) MRI scan and (**c**) cystoscopy of the same patient

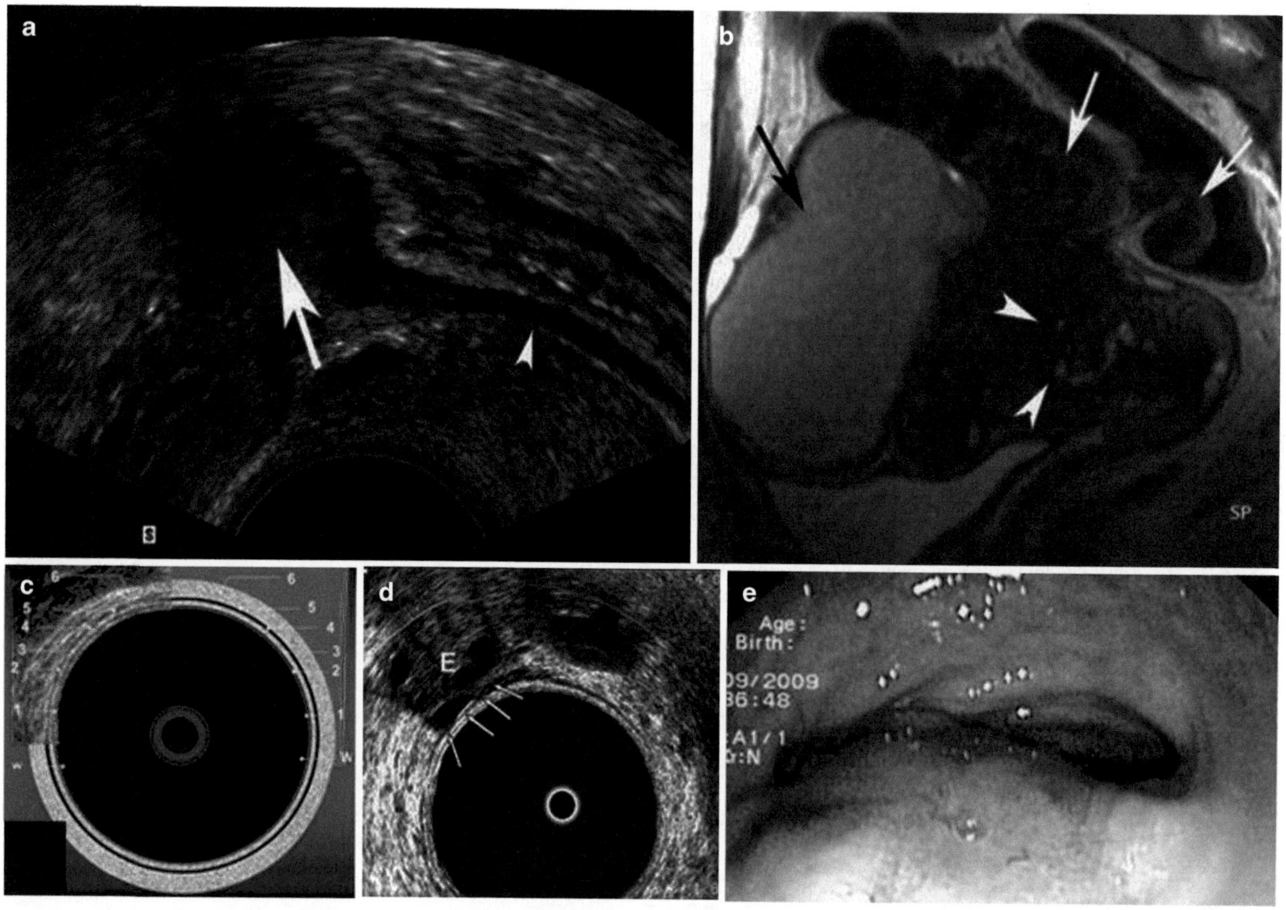

Fig. 35.29 (**a**) Vaginal ultrasound of a solitary nodule between the lower back wall of the uterus/cervix and the rectum (rectovaginal space). (**b**) MRI scan, (**c–d**) endosonography, and (**e**) rectoscopy

shot of metronidazole is also essential. The antibiotic should be applied about 30 min before the start of the operation.

The instruments consist of trocars, a uterine manipulator (for LTH only), needle holders and sutures. Additionally one needs an instrument for coagulation, graspers, scissors, window forceps and a suction irrigation unit. If a robotic set-up is available, the instruments must be adjusted accordingly. A thermofusion device with an integrated knife is optional.

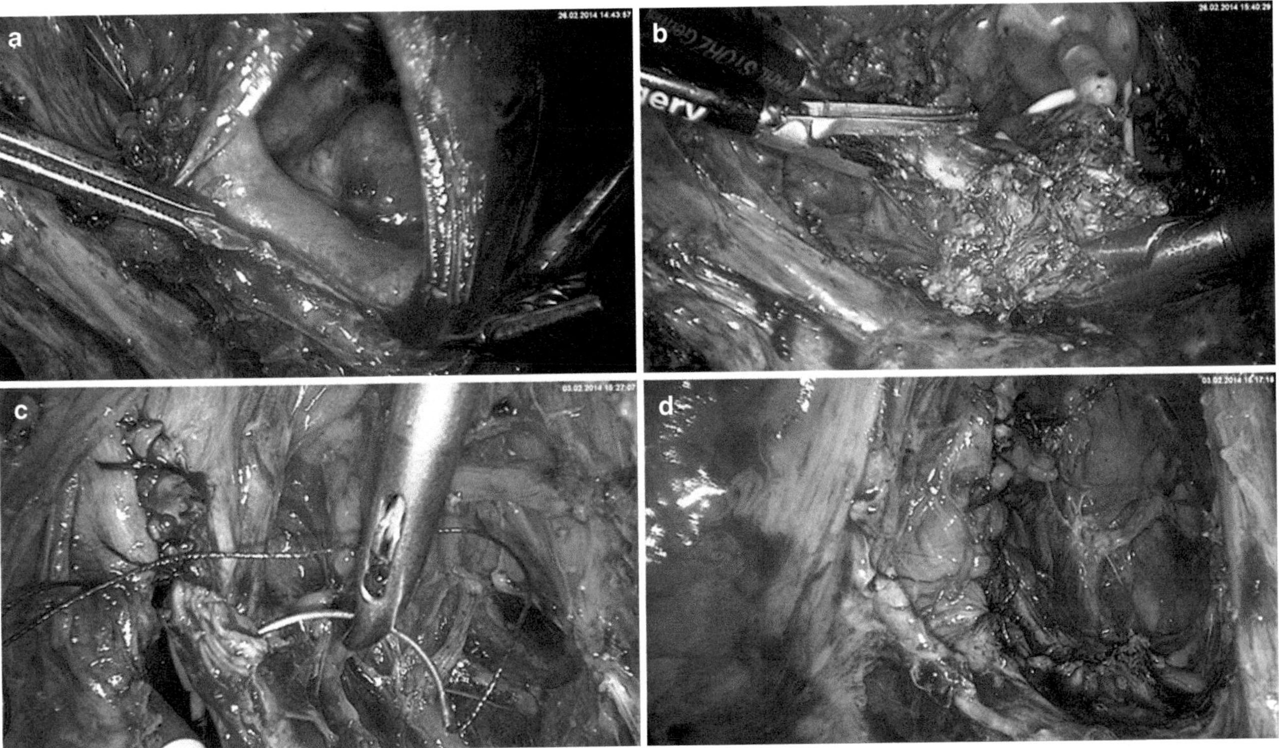

Fig. 35.30 Resection of a solitary nodule in bladder endometriosis. (**a**) The nodule is seen after opening the bladder. Two double J-catheters are placed in both ureters so that (**b**) the nodule can be cut out with an energy device. (**c**, **d**) Closure of the bladder in two layers

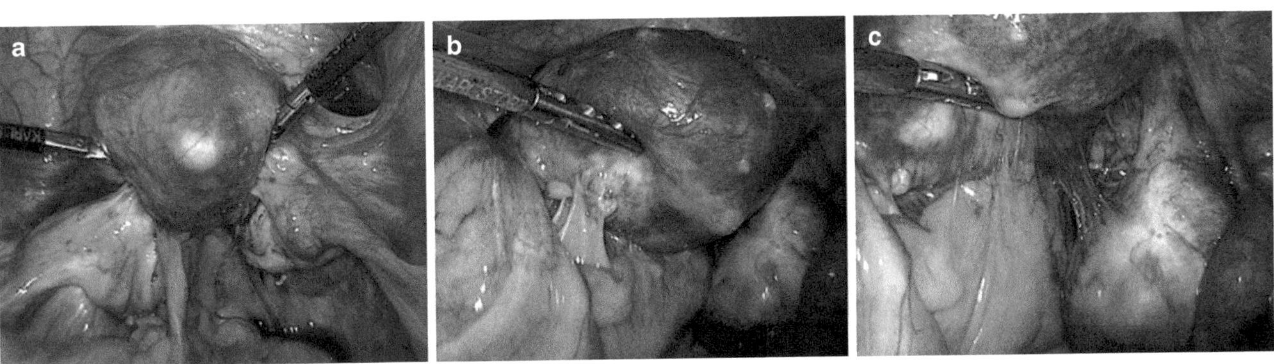

Fig. 35.31 (**a–c**) Overview of severe deep infiltrating endometriosis associated with adenomyosis of the uterus, affecting the lower sigmoid colon/rectum

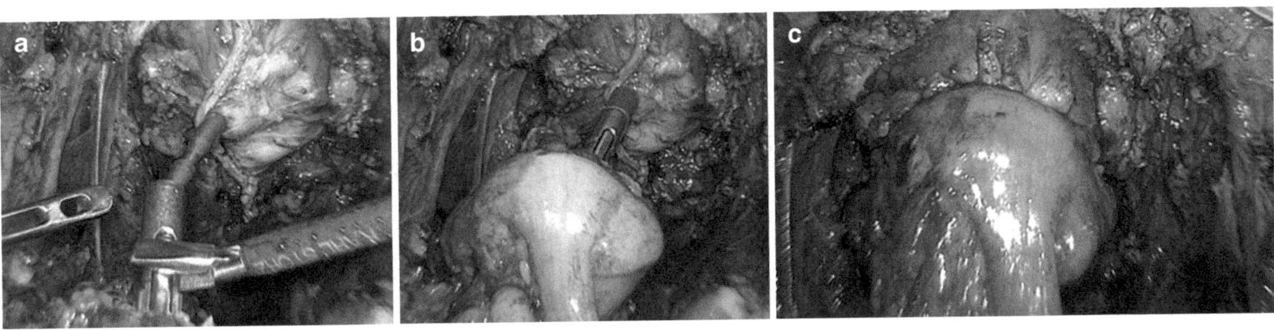

Fig. 35.32 (**a–c**) Endoscopic re-anastomosis can be performed after partial bowel resection

Prerequisites

Obesity or comorbidities, a large uterus or a uterus with multiple myomas is no contra-indication for a laparoscopic procedure. However, in these cases the preoperative assessment and the anesthesia procedure must be discussed with the patient in advance. The trocars may need to be placed higher in the abdominal wall and the surgeon may need more than the usual two ancillary trocars. In cases of a large uterus, the need for morcellation and its risks must be explained to the patient.

Intrafascial Hysterectomy with Preservation of Existing Structures.

Operative Steps of Total Laparoscopic Hysterectomy (LTH)

Step 1

A vaginal examination in anesthesia is performed before using the manipulator. When no further vaginal or rectal pathologies are found, the manipulator is inserted.

Step 2

Port placement

The first step of the operation is placement of the uterine manipulator (Fig. 35.25) [29].

A number of entry techniques are available; direct entry under sight has become very popular in the last few years. Nevertheless, the traditional entry technique described by Kurt Semm and Liselotte Mettler from the University Hospitals Schleswig-Holstein, Kiel, in the 1980s, and still used at the Kiel School of Gynecological Endoscopy is shown here.

Optic Trocar

Veress needle technique and CO_2 gas

To insert the Veress needle, the operating table needs to be in horizontal position. The Trendelenburg tilt is carried out after creating a pneumoperitoneum. The most common site of entry for the Veress needle is the umbilical area. As the wall layers are thinnest at this level, a deep incision will ensure access to the peritoneal cavity. Before incising the skin it would be advisable to palpate the course of the aorta and identify the iliac bifurcation. This will permit inspection and palpation of the abdomen in order to detect any unusual masses (Figs. 35.33, 35.34 and 35.35) [30].

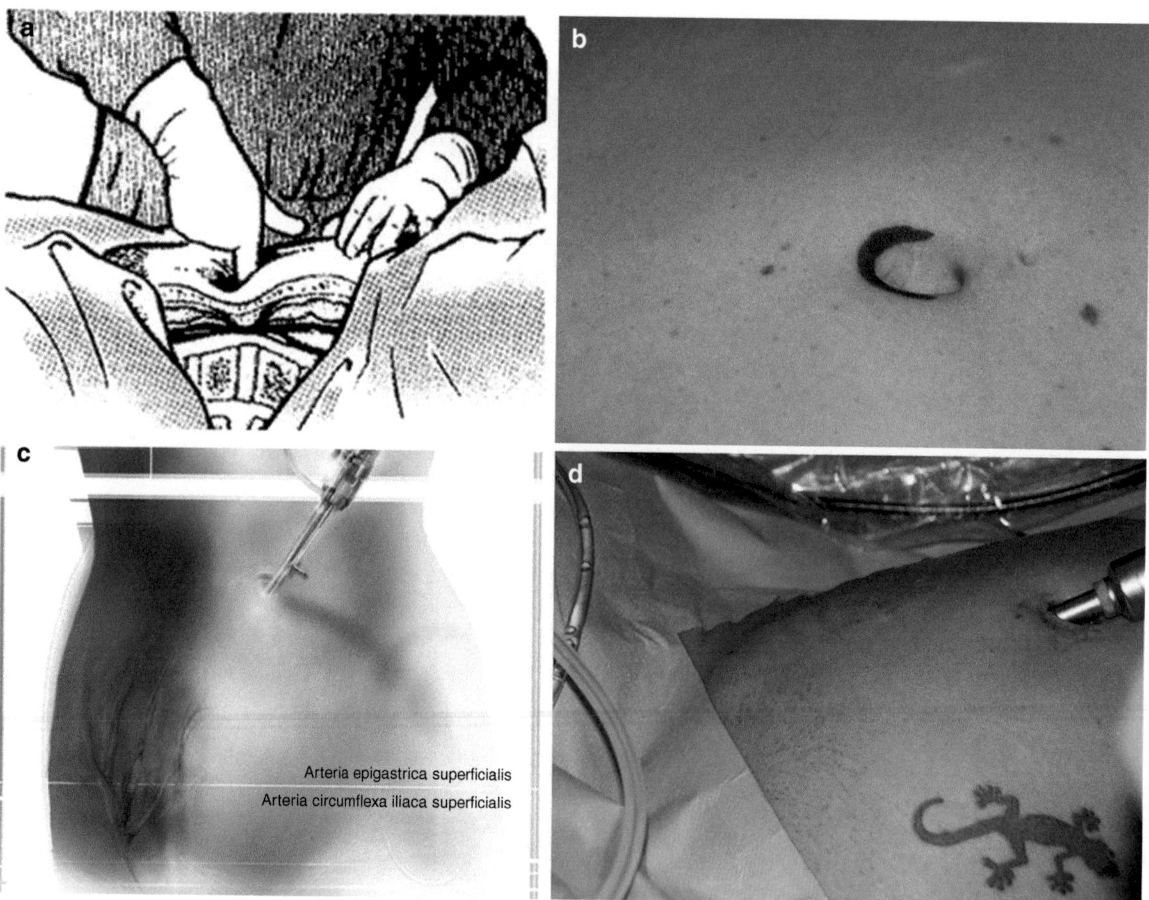

Fig. 35.33 (**a**) Typical point of palpation in the subumbilical region. The fingertip is pointing to the promontory.Subumbilical incision and local palpation reveal the short distance from the skin to the spine (**b–d**). Diaphanoscopy illuminates the region of insertion of the ancillary trocars while demarcating the superficial epigastric artery and the superficial circumflex iliac artery

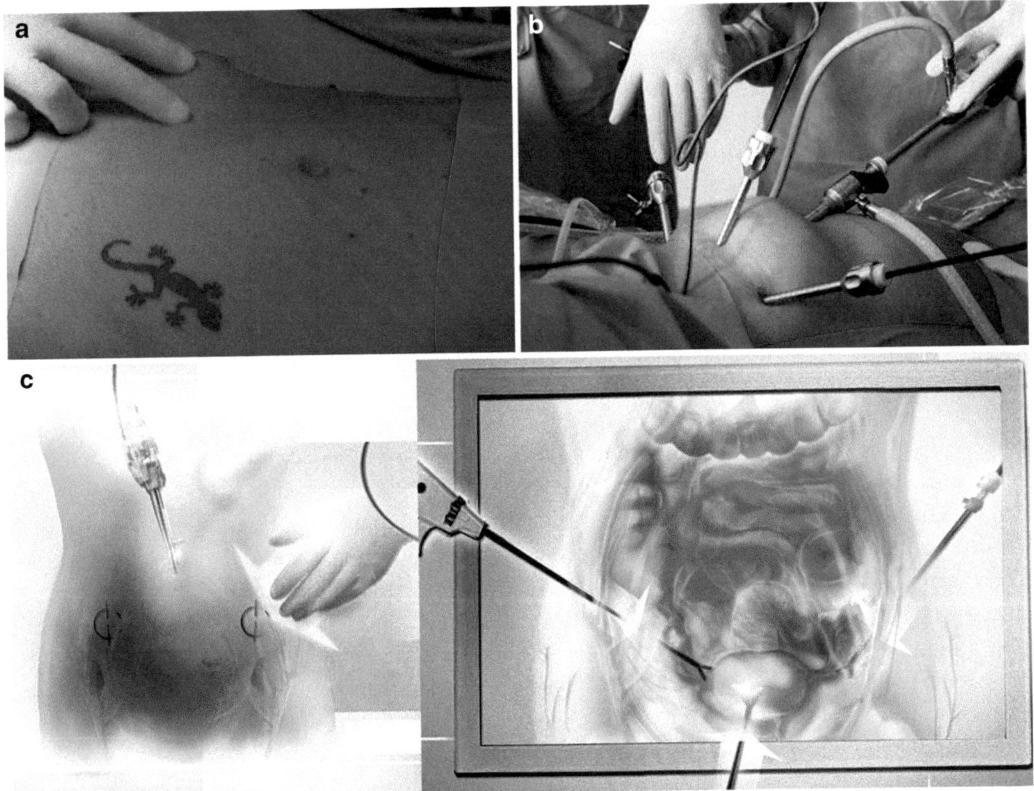

Fig. 35.34 (**a**, **c**) Point of insertion from the outside (two thumbs medial to the anterior superior spine), at a 90 ° angle to the surface, with penetration of all layers of the abdominal wall. Trocar insertion site lateral to the lateral umbilical fold. (**b**, **d**) Overview after insertion of the laparoscope and 3 ancillary trocars

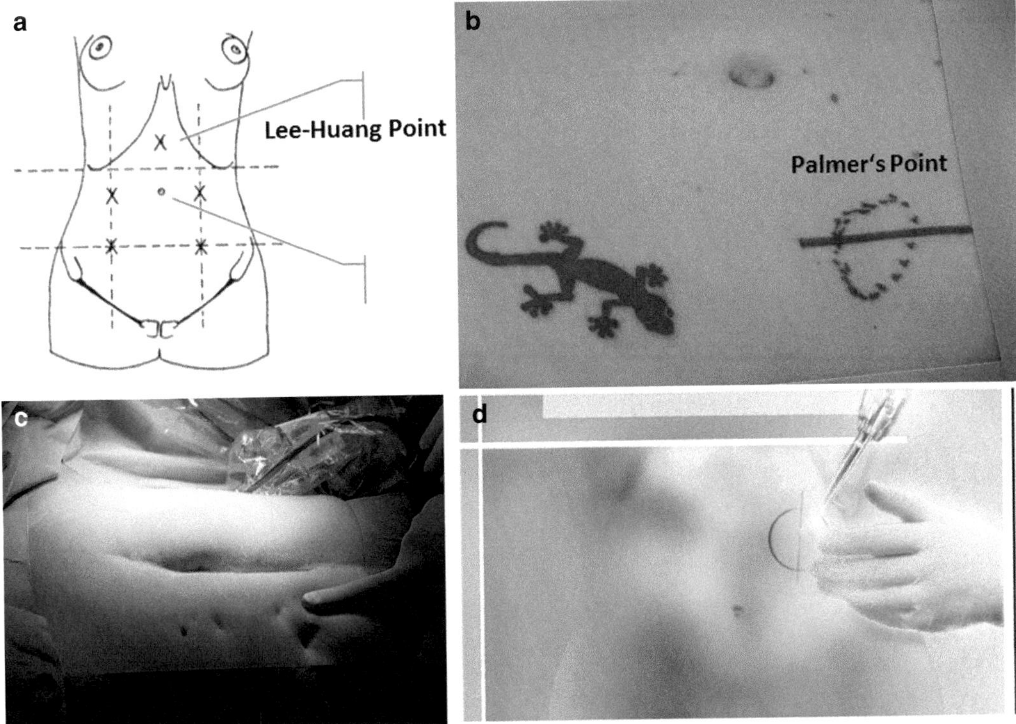

Fig. 35.35 Alternative entry site showing (**a**), in cases of a large uterus, especially at or above the level of the umbilicus, the Lee-Huang point. This point is recommended for video-assisted laparoscopy or in cases of anticipated adhesions in the region of Palmer's point (**c**). (**b**–**d**) Palmer's point is situated in the midclavicular line, about 3 cm below the costal margin

The Veress needle must be tested to ensure that the valve springs, and that gas flow is between 6 and 8 mmHg. In this position the insertion of the primary instrument at a 45° angle toward the uterus involves the least risk of damaging the major vessels coursing downward retroperitoneally. The abdominal wall should be lifted before inserting the instrument. In obese patients the insertion angle is close to 90°, whereas in slim patients the angle is close to 45°. If the first attempt fails, a second attempt is made before selecting an alternative entry site. Before placing the Veress needle, a number of safety checks should be performed in order to minimize the risk of complications:

Usually *two clicks* are heard: the first after perforation of the muscle fascia and the second after perforation of the peritoneum. Proper needle placement is ensured by keeping the Veress needle between the thumb and the index finger. *Aspiration test*: Injection of 5–10 ml of physiological saline solution results in negative aspiration when the Veress needle is correctly placed and yields a blood-tinged aspirate, or one with intestinal contents when the needle is placed in a blood vessel or the intestine. *Hanging drop test and "fluid in flow"*: With the Veress needle placed in the abdominal cavity, lifting the abdominal wall creates negative intraabdominal pressure. A drop of water is then placed on the open end of the Veress needle. If the needle is correctly positioned, the water will move down the shaft.

Any movement of the needle after placement must be avoided as this may convert a small needlepoint injury into a complex and threatening tear. After ensuring that the Veress needle has been positioned correctly, the insufflation is started. Once adequate gas flow and pressure have been achieved, the influx can be raised so that 2–3 l of CO_2 gas can be insufflated per minute until 3–6 l have been insufflated, depending on the patient's size and obesity. After an insufflation volume of about 300 ml, percussion of the liver region will confirm the *loss of liver dullness*, which is a reliable sign of proper positioning of the Veress needle and the creation of a pneumoperitoneum. Abdominal pressure should then be increased to 20–25 mmHg before inserting the primary trocar because this maximizes the distension of the abdominal wall from all underlying structures (Fig. 35.36) [27].

The optic trocar is inserted in two steps. In the first step, a 5-mm optic trocar and the laparoscope are inserted to confirm the pneumoperitoneum and the absence of local adhesions. Dilation to 10 mm is achieved in the second step, either under sight or blindly, thus ensuring optimum visibility during the operation.

Step 1: Entry is performed by a Z *technique*in the following manner: After proceeding forward with the trocar forward to about 1.5 cm, the tip is moved to about 1.5 cm to the right at a 90° angle. The abdominal wall is lifted in the same

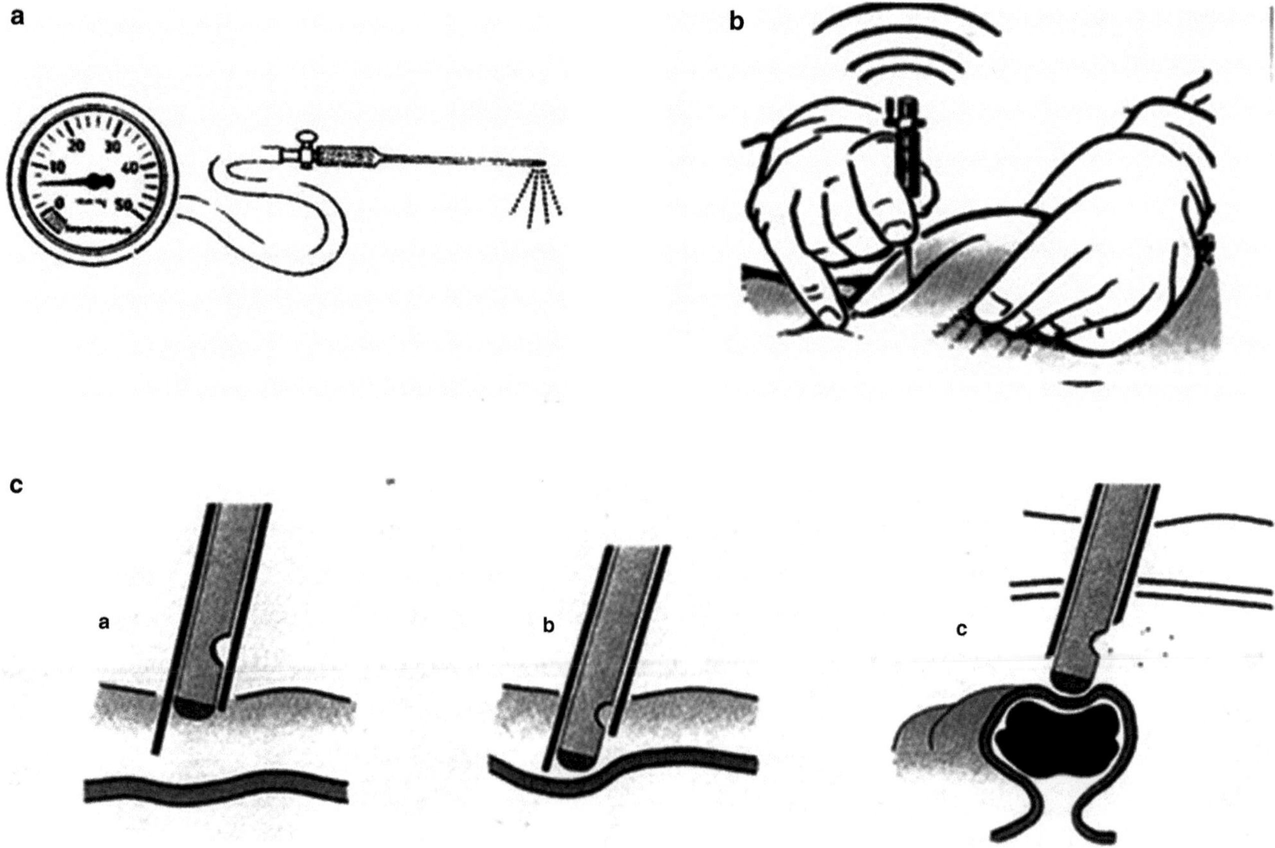

Fig. 35.36 (**a**) Veress needle and its insertion. The pressure going through the needle is measured. (**b**) The safety mechanism avoids damage or injury to the bowel or vessels. By lifting the abdominal wall the distance to the structures below (bowel and vessels) is increased. (**c**) Perforation of the outer skin is performed by the sharp tip of the needle. While running through soft tissue the blunt tip jumps forward by means of a spring mechanism. The same mechanism prevents bowel injury after penetrating the peritoneum

manner as when inserting the Veress needle, and the trocar is screwed with the dominant hand straight into the abdominal wall at a 90° angle, towards the hollow of the sacrum.

Correct placement of the trocar is indicated by a hissing sound when gas escapes through the open valve of the trocar. The obturator is then removed and the trocar is held in place. Before dilating to 10 mm, a 5-mm laparoscope is introduced and rotated through 360° to check visually for any bleeding, intraabdominal abnormality, or adherent bowel loops. If the surgeon suspects adherence of the bowel in the umbilical region, the primary trocar site must be visualized from a secondary port site, such as the lower abdominal wall, with a 5-mm laparoscope.

Step 2: A blunt palpation probe is placed in the 5-mm trocar; the shaft is pulled over the palpation probe and taken out. A 10-mm trocar is then screwed into the abdominal cavity [27].

Subcostal Insufflation Technique (Palmer's Point or Lee Huang Point)

No entry technique is entirely devoid of the risk of gas embolism or injury to vessels, intestines, or the urinary tract. Palmer's point is the safest laparoscopic entry point because it is least likely to be affected by adhesions.

For all patients with a significantly higher risk of adhesion, a history of abdominal surgery including cesarean section, a large fibroid uterus, umbilical hernia, large ovarian cysts, preperitoneal gas insufflation or failed umbilical entry, Palmer described in 1974 an abdominal entry point in the midclavicular line, about 3 cm below the costal margin. Palmer's point can be used for the Veress needle as well as for small trocars. In case adhesions are suspected in the subcostal region on the left side, the Lee Huang point in the midline is a suitable alternative (Fig. 35.35) [27].

Ancillary Trocars

All ancillary trocars must be inserted with an intraabdominal pressure of 15–20 mmHg under direct vision. The inferior epigastric vessels are visualized laparoscopically whereas the superficial vessels can be visualized by diaphanoscopy.

Once the tip of the trocar has pierced the peritoneum, it should be angulated in the direction of the uterine fundus under visual control until the port is placed correctly and the sharp tip can be removed.

Before inserting any ancillary trocars, the patient is moved into the Trendelenburg position. Premature Trendelenburg positioning may increase the risk of retroperitoneal vascular injury because the iliac vessels are located exactly in the axis of a preconceived 45° insertion angle, especially in slim patients with minimal retroperitoneal fat. The number of ancillary trocars is variable; all of them must be inserted under direct vision. If two working trocars are needed, they should be placed in the lower quadrant above the pubic hairline lateral to the deep epigastric vessels from the interior view. From the exterior view the trocars are placed two fingers medial to the anterior superior iliac spine. Two major superficial vessels - the superficial epigastric artery and the superficial circumflex iliac artery - must be avoided. These vessels can be visualized by diaphanoscopy. When a third ancillary trocar is required, the suprapubic midline is the most common site. Diaphanoscopy cannot be relied upon to locate the deep vessels, especially in obese patients (Figs. 35.37 and 35.38).

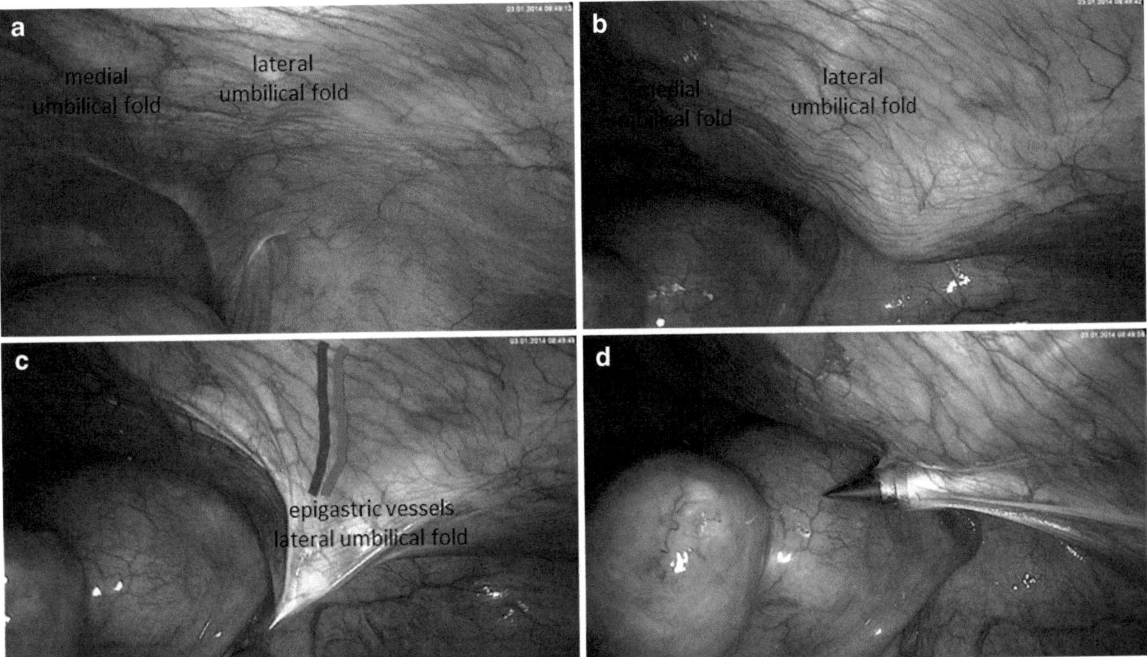

Fig. 35.37 Secondary trocar placement, entry in the right lower abdomen. (**a**) The three different plicae are visualized. (**b**) The palpating finger is showing the area lateral to the lateral umbilical fold. (**c**) Entry of the sharp ancillary trocar lateral to the lateral umbilical fold. (**d**) Once the peritoneum has been penetrated, the trocar points to the fundus of the uterus in order to avoid injury to the major vessels and the bowel

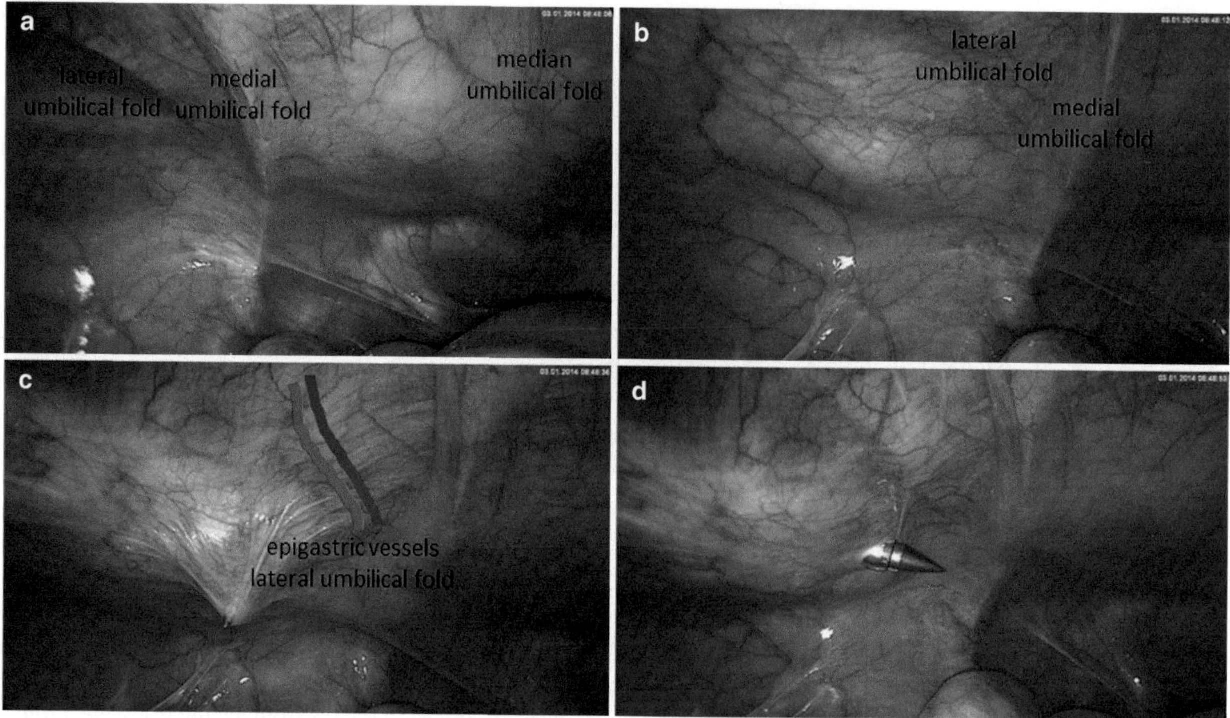

Fig. 35.38 Secondary trocar placement, entry in the left lower abdomen.(**a**) The three plicae are visualized. (**b**) The palpating finger is showing the area lateral to the lateral umbilical fold. (**c**) Entry of the sharp ancillary trocar lateral to the lateral umbilical fold. (**d**) Once the peritoneum has been penetrated, the trocar points to the fundus of the uterus in order to avoid injury to the major vessels and the bowel

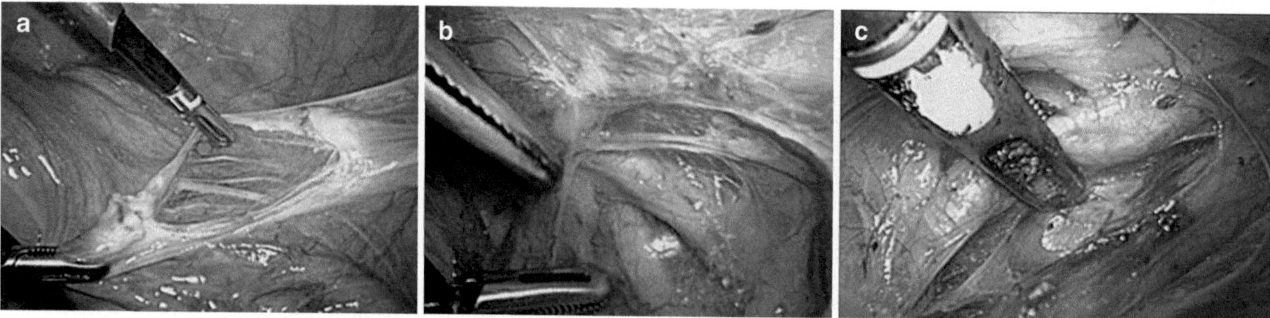

Fig. 35.39 Technique 1: The first step consists of opening the anterior leaf of the broad ligament (**a**). The round ligament is kept intact. The lower crossing of the ureter and the uterine artery are identified (**b**); the uterine artery can be coagulated directly after its point of departure from the internal iliac artery (**c**)

Finger-tapping from the outside can be used to verify correction positioning of the trocar. A small skin incision should be performed before the trocar sleeve is inserted. The trocars must be inserted by the shortest route at a 90° angle to the skin surface so that the risk of injuring structures on the way to the abdominal wall is minimized. When inserting a trocar in the midline, the Foley catheter must be identified in order to avoid accidental bladder perforation [27, 31].

Step 3

Surgical Steps

Resection of endometriosis

The primary sept in hysterectomy is removal of all visible endometriosis spots. These may be superficial and easy to excise (Figs. 35.15 and 35.16), or adherent to more delicate structures and difficult to eliminate (Figs. 35.17 and 35.18).

Laparoscopic Total Hysterectomy (LTH)

In patients being operated on for surgical staging, the surgeon will be able to assess the abdomen, pelvis, obtain pelvic washings, perform salpingo-oophorectomy, lymph node dissection, tissue biopsies and omentectomy in addition to laparoscopic hysterectomy.

(Technique 1: Primary uterine artery ligation)

The next step is to coagulate and separate the round ligament near the pelvic side wall (Fig. 35.39a). The peritoneum is then incised further. The anterior leaf of the broad ligament is opened to the bladder fold and the bladder is pushed downwards. The posterior leaf of the broad ligament is visualized and the ureters are lateralized. The retroperitoneal space is then exposed, the course of the ureters demonstrated, and the site of exit of the uterine artery from the iliac artery visualized (Fig. 35.39b). The crossing point of the uterine artery and the ureter is exposed and the uterine artery coagulated (Fig. 35.39c). The bladder pillar is identified, coagulated, and separated. This is followed by separation of the ovary and the tube from the uterus. If the adnexa – after ensuring a sufficient distance from the ureters – are to be dissected along with the uterus, the infundibulopelvic ligament should be coagulated and the mesosalpinx and mesovarium dissected in the direction of fenestration. The fenestration is a useful point of orientation to safeguard the ureter [32–34] .

(Technique 2: Classic intrafascial hysterectomy):

Surgical Steps

3.1 Inspection of the pelvis, tracing the ureters and planning theoperation (Figs. 35.40 and 35.41)

3.2 Start on the right side. Push the uterus in the opposite direction when separating the adnexa or the ligaments from the pelvic sidewall, with the assistance of the intrauterine manipulator or by traction (Figs. 35.42 and 35.43).

3.3 Division of the infundibulopelvic ligament and round ligament from the pelvic sidewall or, when the adnexa are retained, separation of the adnexa from the uterus (Figs. 35.44, 35.45, 35.46, 35.47 and 35.48).

3.4 Dissection of the broad ligament: The broad ligament is opened and each leaf coagulated separately (Figs. 35.49, 35.50 and 35.51). This is not possible when a sealing and cutting instrument is used, because the two leaves of the broad ligament are sealed together. The direction of exposure is as close to the uterus as possible but as distant as necessary, thus avoiding exposure close to the sidewall and the ureter (Fig. 35.52).

3.5 Separation of the bladder from the uterus by opening the vesicouterine ligament and pushing the bladder downward by about 1–2 cm (Fig. 35.51b and c).

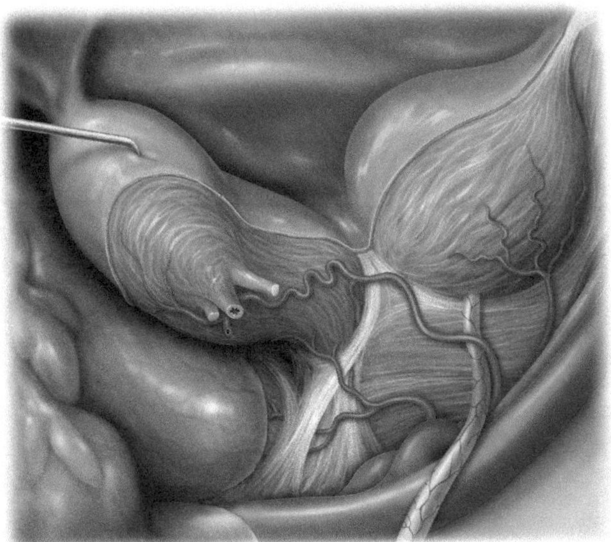

Fig. 35.40 Anatomical illustration showing the relation of the uterine vessel to the ureter in the pelvic wall, compared to its location close to the uterus. The helical course of the ascending branch of the uterine artery can be easily followed. The uterus, bladder and rectum are embedded in a ligament-based pelvic floor

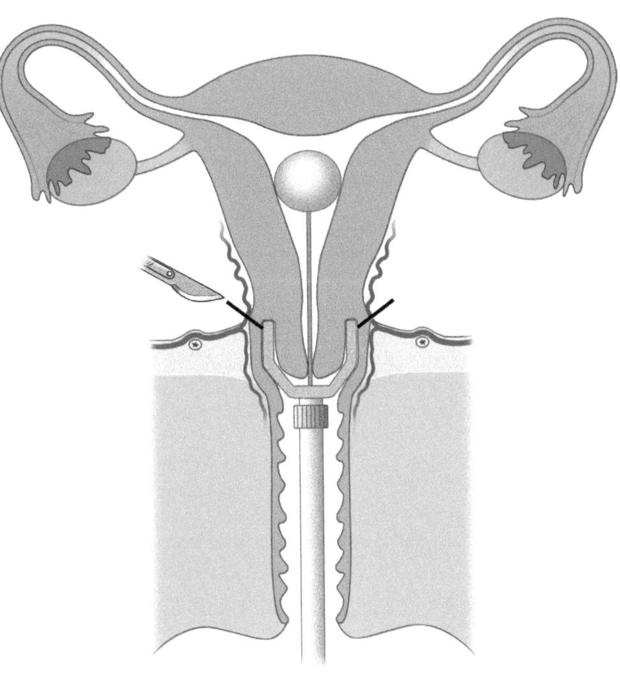

Fig. 35.41 Schematic illustration of the resection line in total laparoscopic hysterectomy. Only the ascending branch of the uterine artery needs to be coagulated and cut on the uterine manipulator. When adhering closely to this operative technique, the ureter is located at a safe distance from the coagulation zone (about 2 cm)

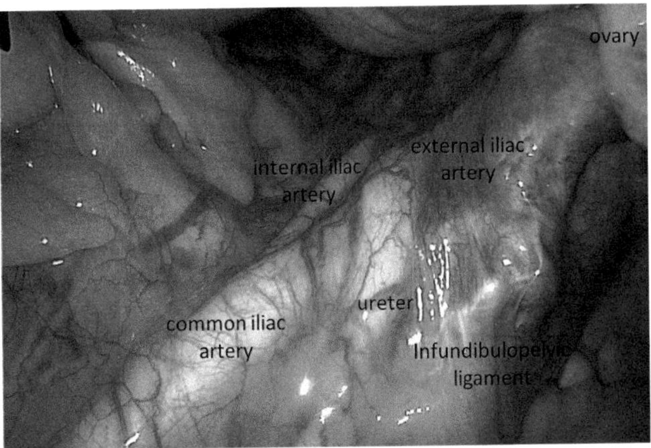

Fig. 35.42 Preliminary inspection of the uterus and the surrounding organs. The lower pelvis as well as the ligaments, vessels and the ureter can be differentiated in relation to the uterus. In slim patients the crossing of the ureter and the common iliac artery can be seen. The infundibulopelvic ligament is identified and held towards the lateral wall in order to obtain a better view of the field of surgery

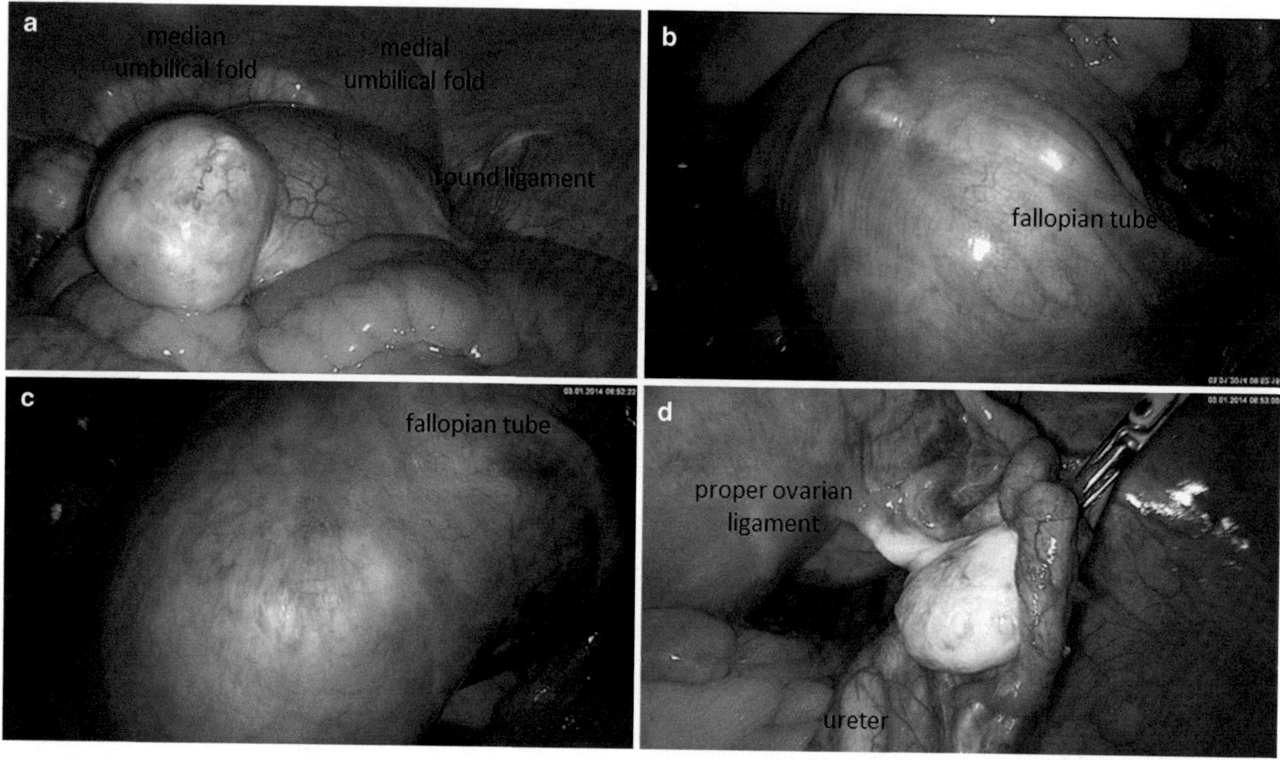

Fig. 35.43 (**a**) Reconstruction of the anatomy of the right pelvic wall. (**b**) Only the fallopian tube is visible at first glance on the right side. (**c**) After mobilization of the uterus a large fibroid on the back wall can be seen. (**d**) The bifurcation of the common iliac artery and the crossing of the ureter are clearly visible. The infundibulopelvic ligament and the ovarian vessels are situated lateral to the ureter. The infundibulopelvic ligament might be fixed to the bowel (especially on the left side) and cause difficulties when exposing the adnexa

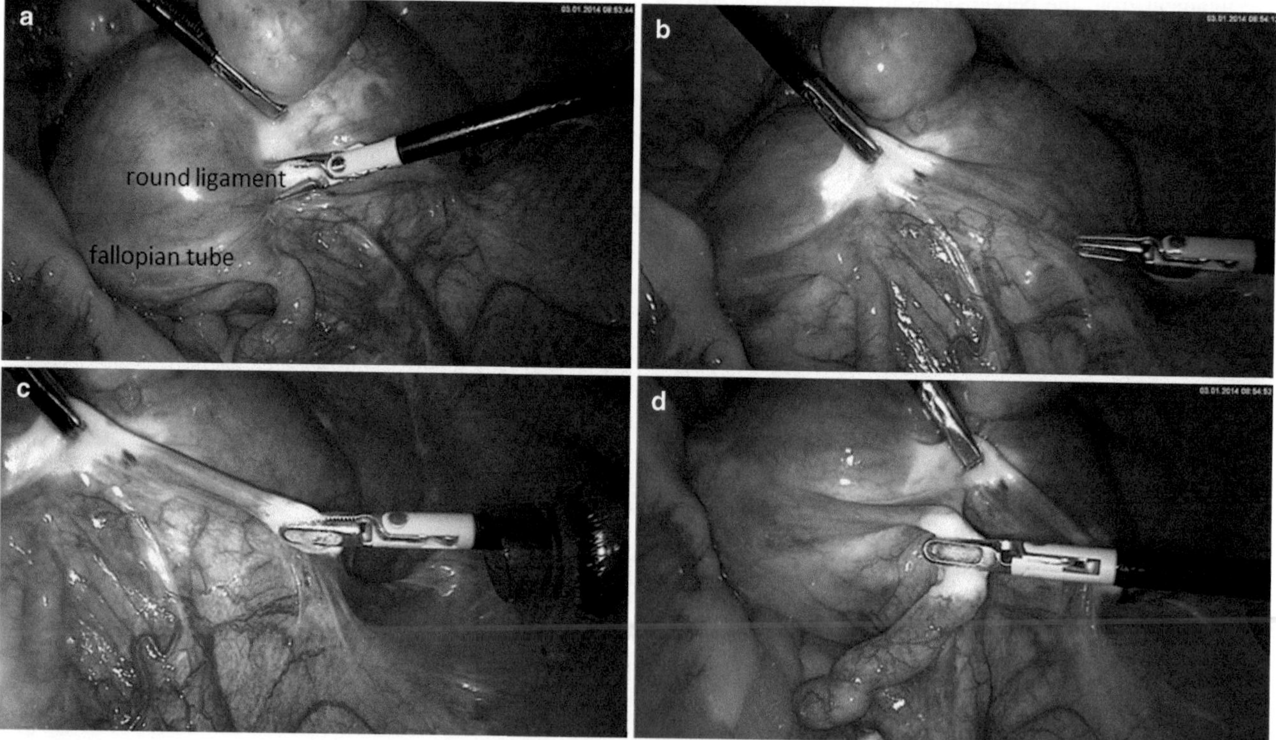

Fig. 35.44 Stepwise bipolar coagulation of the right tube and the right round ligament. (**a–b**) The round ligament is coagulated so that a sharp instrument can be used to pull the tissue without causing bleeding that might impede vision. (**c**) In benign cases the round ligament can be cut close to the uterus, in malignant cases the round ligament is cut very laterally. (**d**) This allows complete inspection of the tube and it can selectively be coagulated and cut

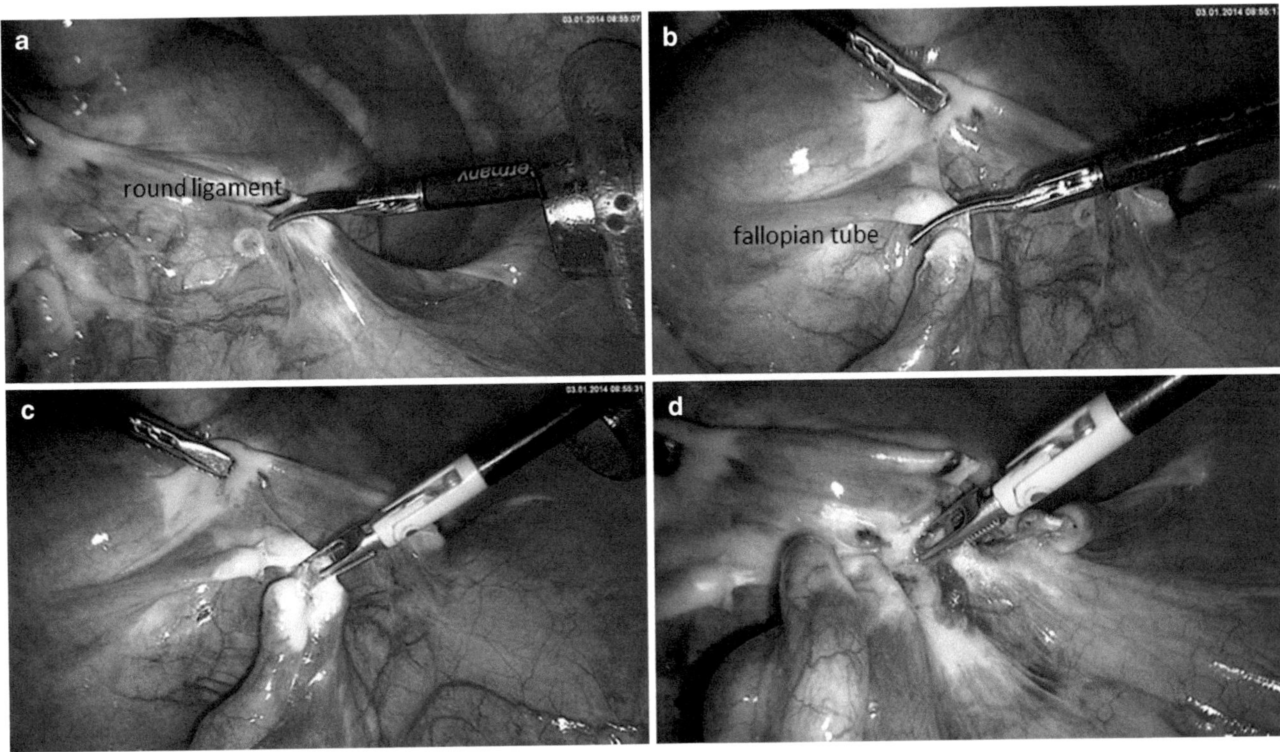

Fig. 35.45 Stepwise dissection of the right tube and the round ligament.(**a**, **b**) The curved scissors are held with the tip away from the uterine wall. (**c**, **d**) After dissecting the fallopian tube, the vessels running underneath must be coagulated before further cutting

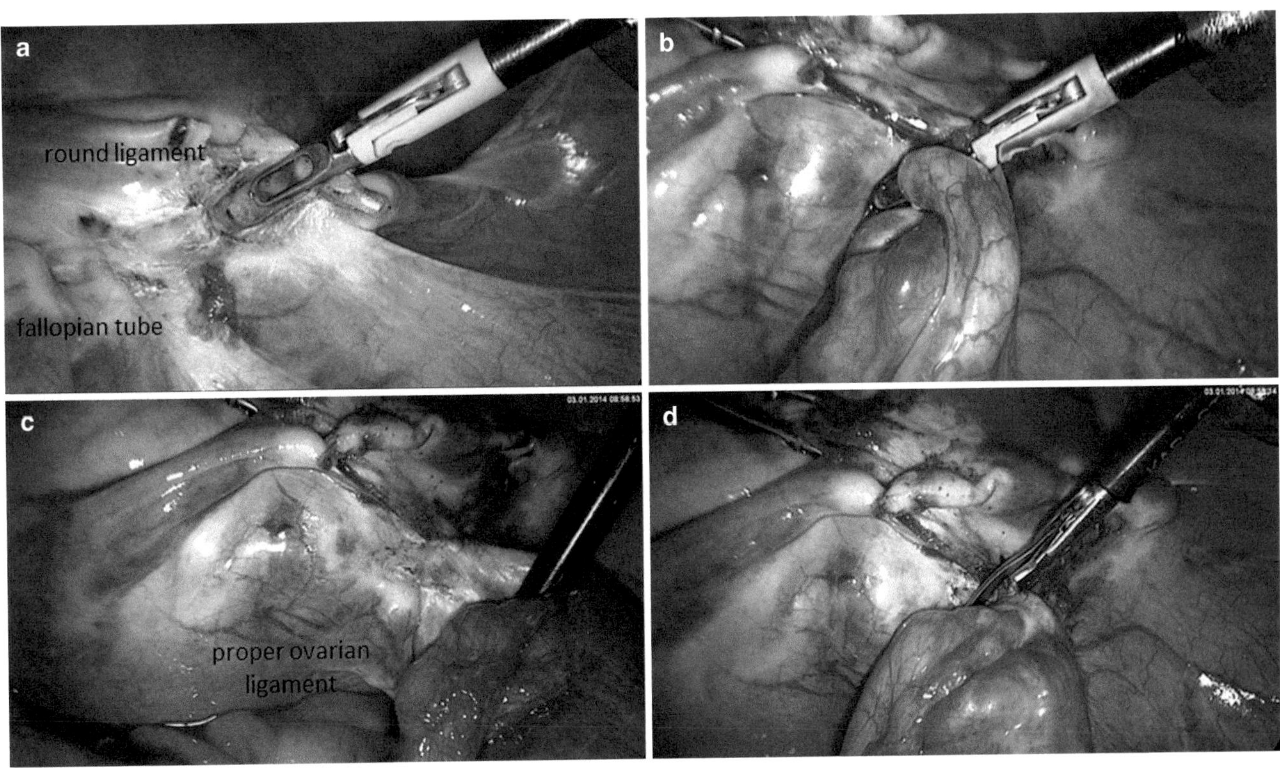

Fig. 35.46 Continuous stepwise dissection and exposure for opening the broad ligament. With traction on tissue, the line of exposure can be easily demarcated (**a**, **c**). Coagulation involves the entire tissue, but the cutting line strictly omits the uterine wall (**b**, **d**). Cutting the tube at this stage provides a better overview for exposure in the following steps. The tube can be removed easily after the hysterectomy

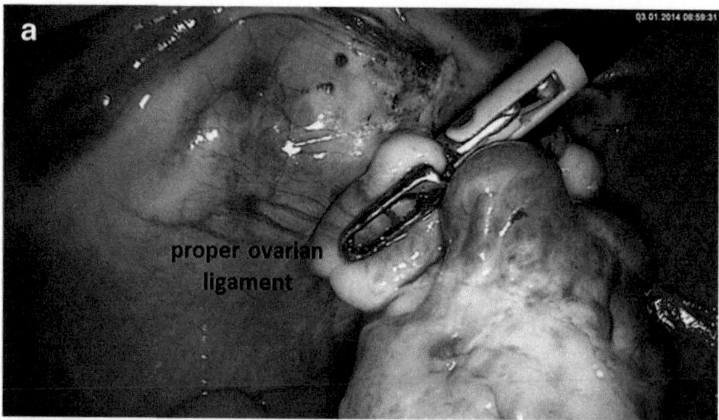

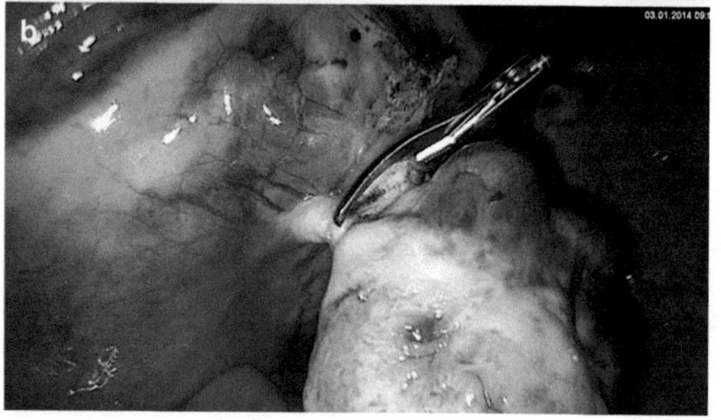

Fig. 35.47 (**a**) Coagulation of the proper ovarian ligament and (**b**) dissection without involving the uterine or the ovarian wall

3.6 Presentation of the ascending branch of the uterine artery and separation of the uterine pedicles (Fig. 35.53).
3.7 Identical stepwise dissection of the left adnexa (Figs. 35.54 and 35.55), opening of the bladder peritoneum and broad ligament (Fig. 35.56), and dissection of the uterine vessels (Figs. 35.57 and 35.58) on the left side. A thorough inspection of the cervix is performed.
3.8 After separation of the bladder from the uterus, the bladder is pushed and dissected down by 2–3 cm to clearly visualize the rim of the cervical cap. In cases of post-cesarean section, a careful, gentle and nearly blunt dissection should be performed (Figs. 35.59, 35.60 and 35.61).
3.9 While lateralizing the ureter by pushing the manipulator upward, the uterine artery and vein with its collaterals are fully coagulated near the cervix and dissected.

The key steps of pushing the bladder down from the anterior vaginal fornix prior to incision and distancing the ureters from the uterine vessels at the cervical/vaginal level can be safely performed by stretching the manipulator firmly cranially, to the contralateral side of the exposure.

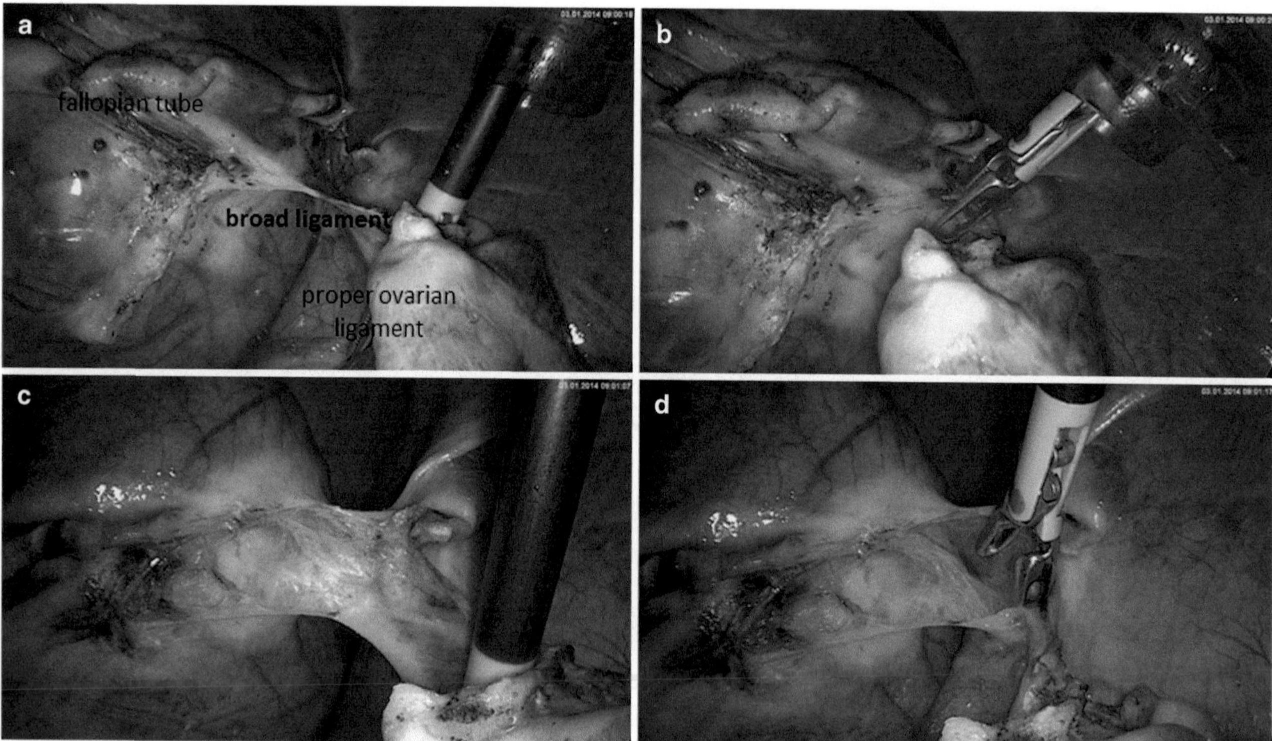

Fig. 35.48 Dissection of the proper ovarian ligament and opening the broad ligament.(**a**) After the proper ovarian ligament has been dissected, the adnexa falls to the lateral aspect. (**b**–**d**) The broad ligament can then be identified and separated into its two leaves

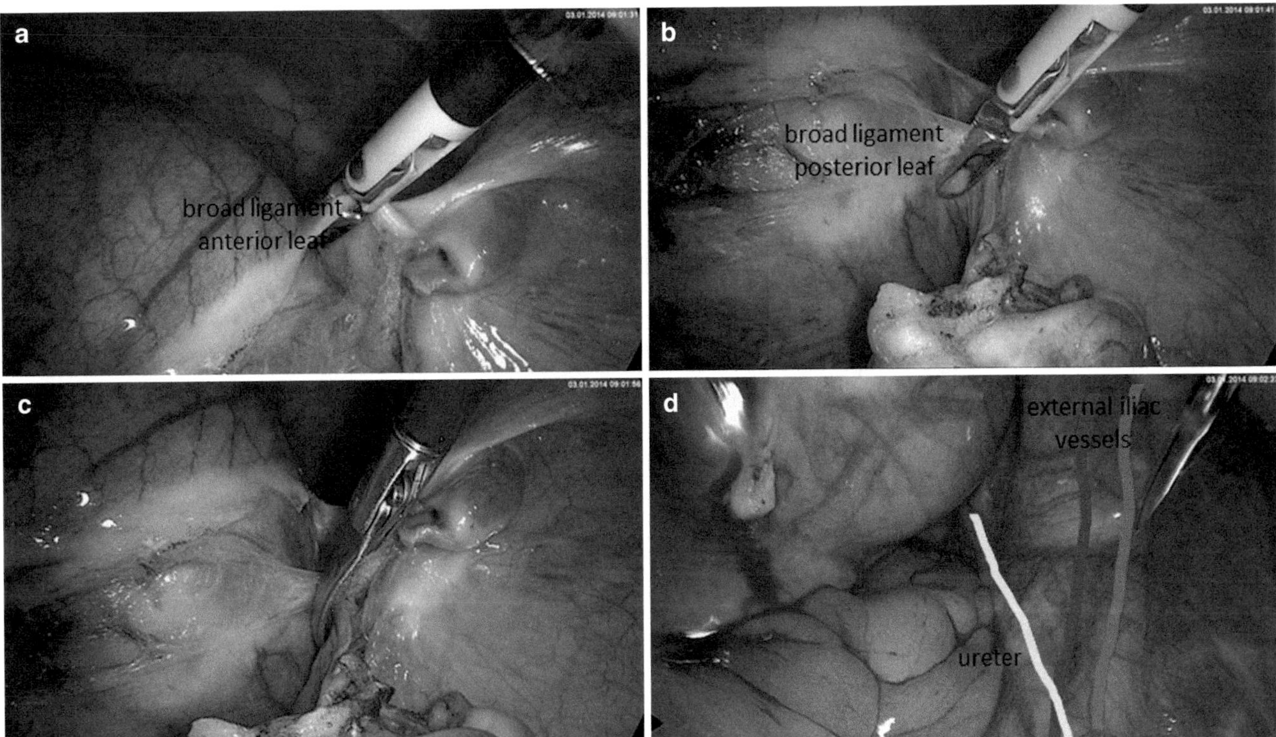

Fig. 35.49 Separation of the anterior and posterior leaf of the broad ligament (**a**–c) in relation to the ureter and the pelvic vessels (**d**).(**a-c**) The broad ligament is coagulated and dissected as close to the uterus as possible without affecting the uterine artery. As the two leaves are separated, the ascending branch of the uterine artery can be visualized easily and omitted. The tip of the scissors is directed strictly away from the uterine wall using the curved blade

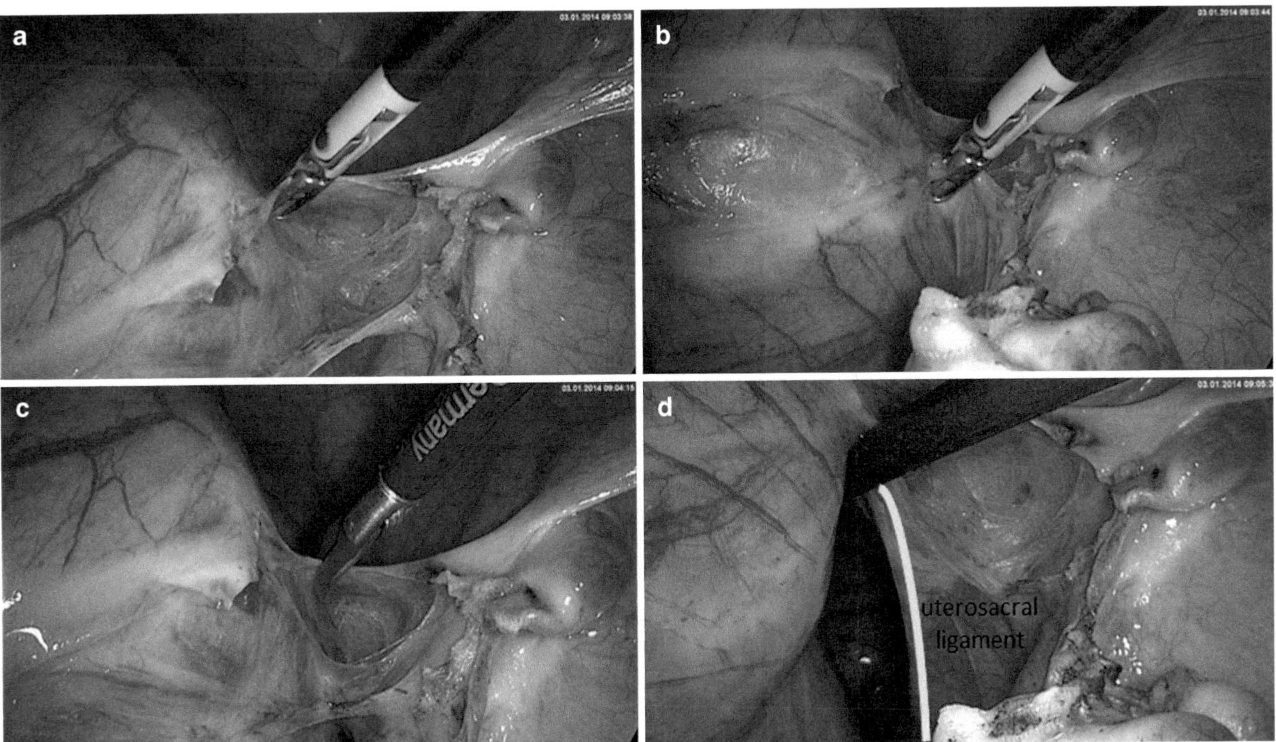

Fig. 35.50 Final separation of the leaves of the broad ligament close to the pelvic floor (**a**–**c**) and the sacrouterine ligament (**d**). The uterus is pushed to the left side; the bladder peritoneum is close by. (**d**) By blunt manipulation the course of the sacrouterine ligament can be visualized; the line of coagulation should omit this part

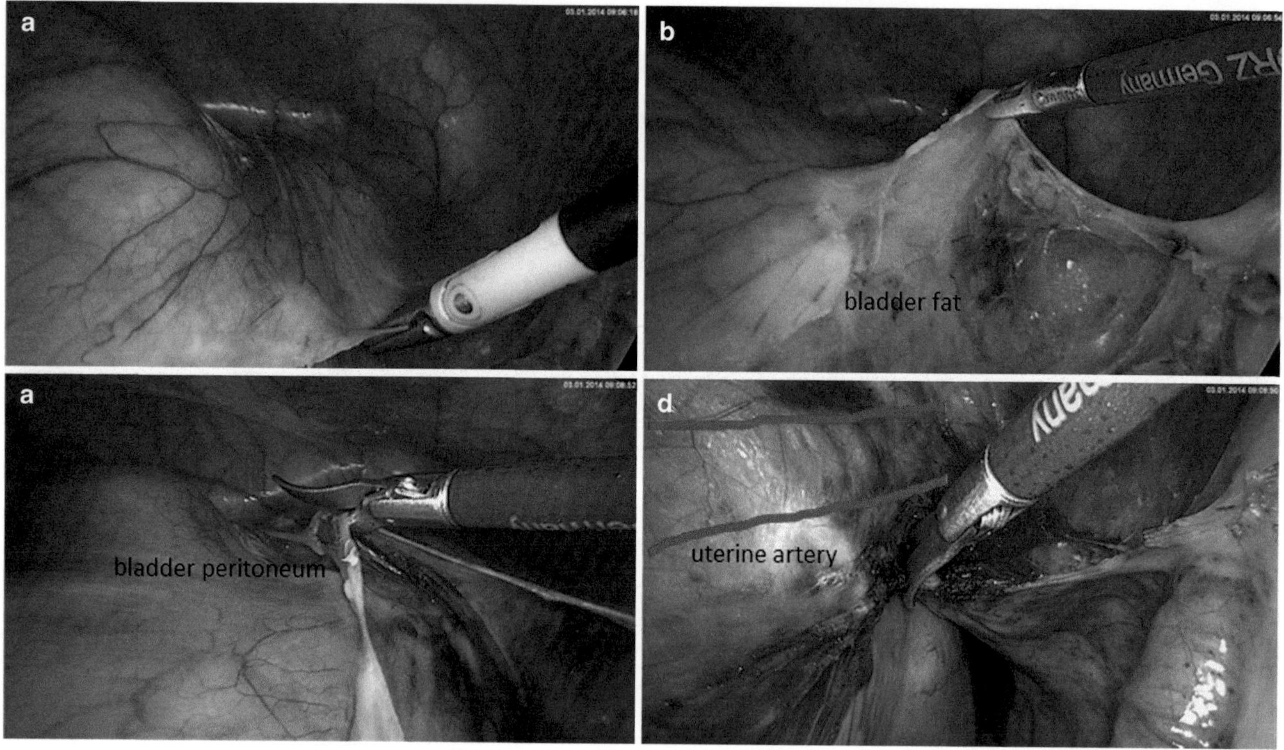

Fig. 35.51 Opening the bladder peritoneum from the right side (**a–c**). The beginning of the bladder peritoneum can be easily demarcated; the cutting line should be neither above this zone nor too far into the caudal aspect. Gas enters the created space and shows the beginning of the bladder pillar. The uterine vessel bundle (**d**) is freed by coagulating and dissecting above and below it. The ureter is at a safe distance lateral to this area of exposure

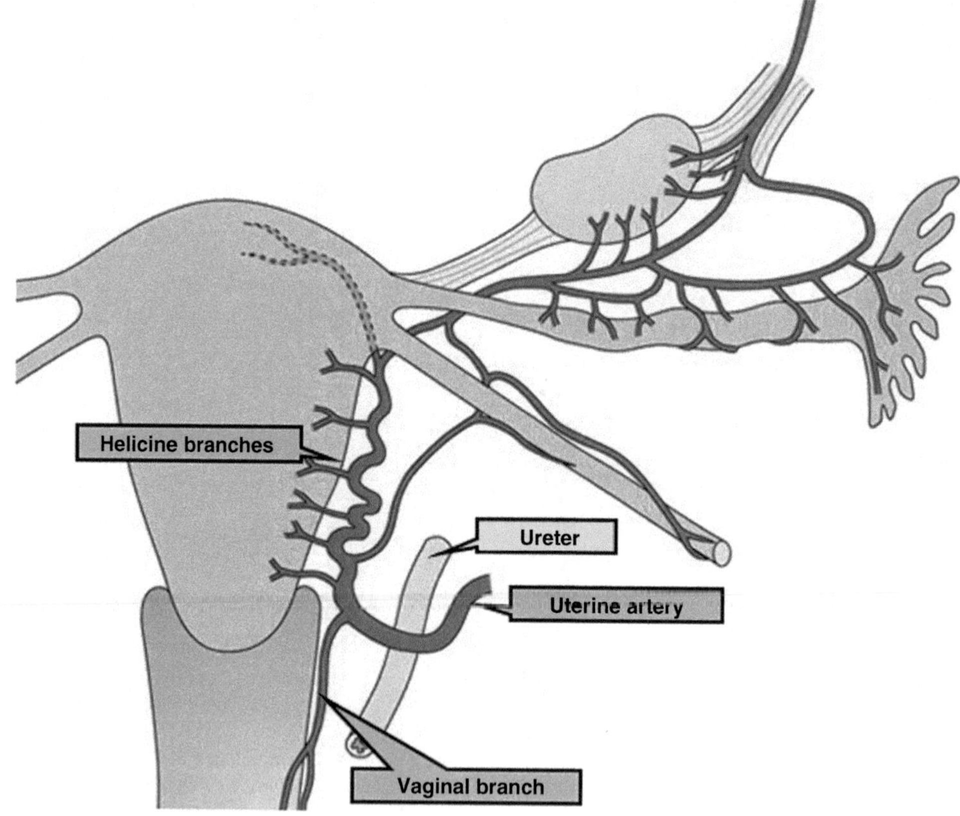

Fig. 35.52 Anatomical schematic illustration showing the spiral structure of the ascending uterine artery. Exposure too close to the uterus may cause arterial bleeding, which can only be stopped after complete coagulation of the uterine artery on the opposite side. The field of surgery would be greatly disturbed by antegrade or retrograde bleeding. The ureter is close to the surgical field only in the lowest part. Pushing the uterus away lateralizes the ureter and moves it to the side

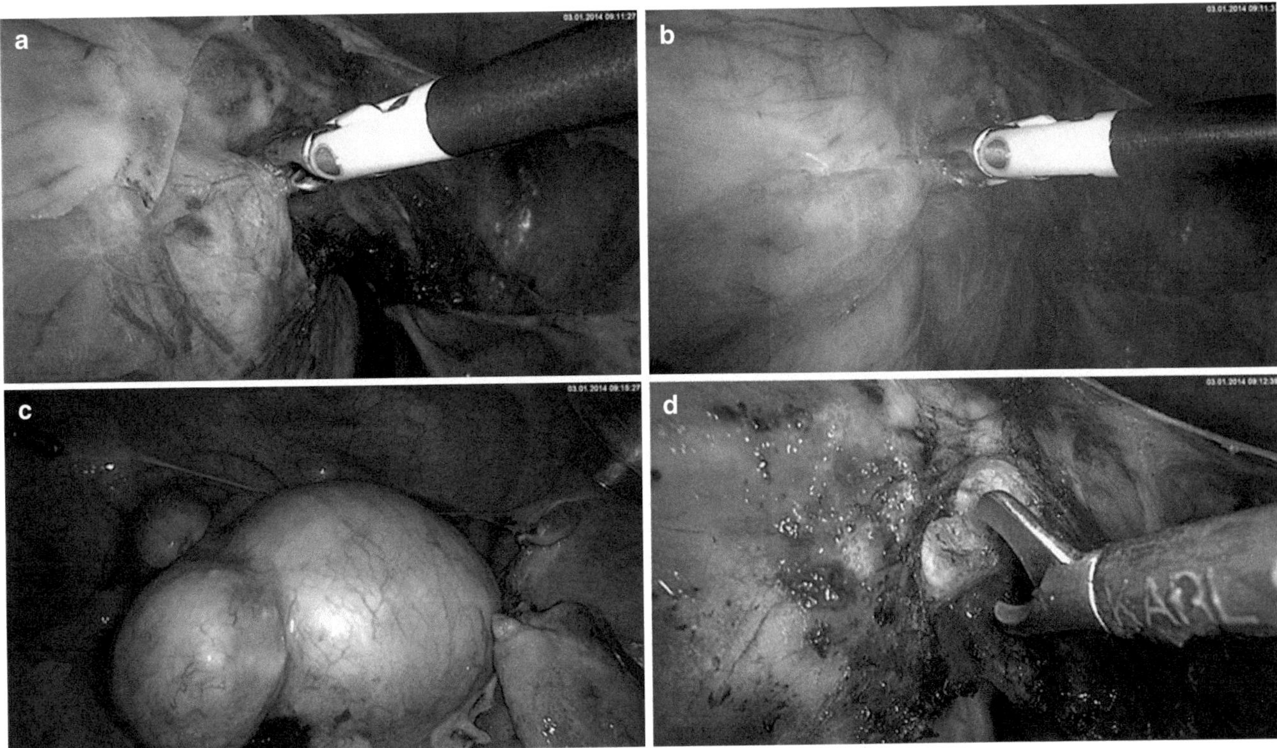

Fig. 35.53 (**a**) Bipolar coagulation and dissection of the uterine vessels. (**b**) The area of coagulation must include the upper part of the artery to avoid retrograde bleeding after dissecting the vessel. (**c**): The color of the uterus changes to whitish/grey. (**d**): A deeper cut can be avoided by using the hook scissors; the uterine artery is dissected in two steps. This allows further coagulation of the tissue lying just behind the artery and avoids cumbersome venous bleeding

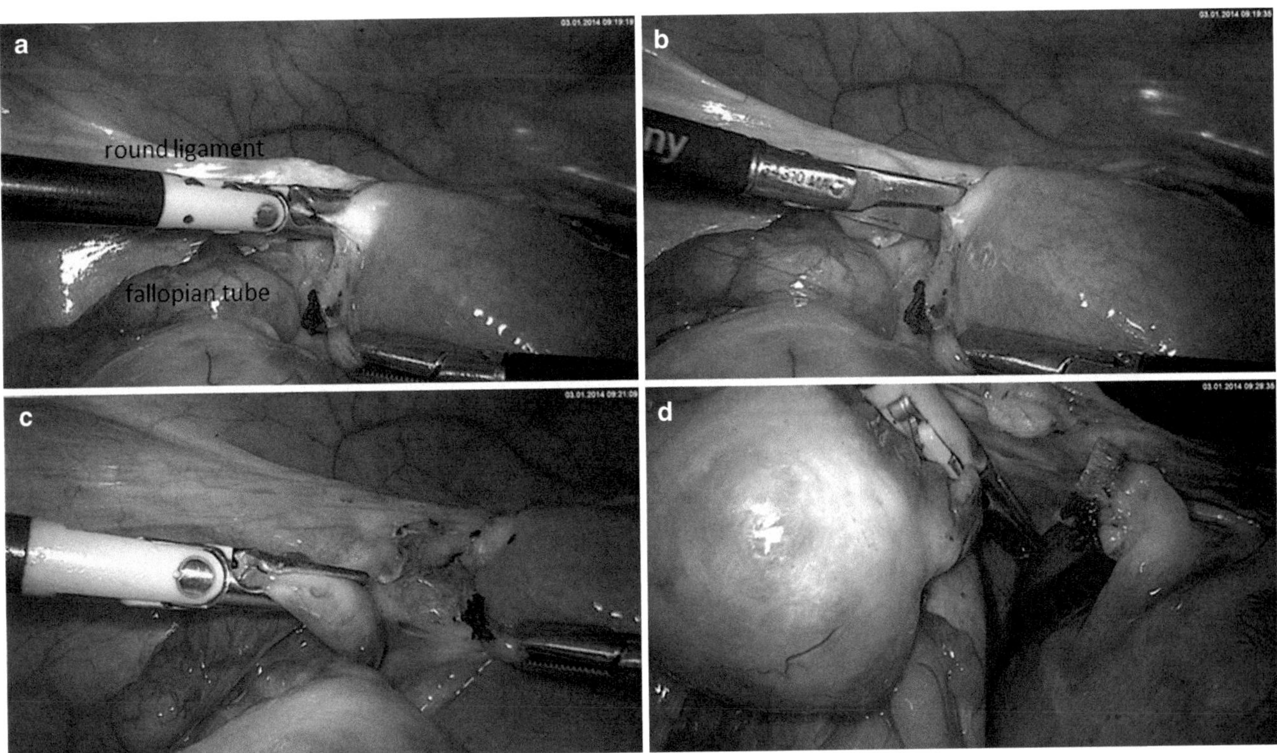

Fig. 35.54 Stepwise coagulation and dissection of the left round ligament and tube (**a**–**c**) and the ovarian ligament (**d**).(**a**, **b**): The curved scissors are held with the tip away from the uterine wall. (**c**, **d**): After dissecting the fallopian tube, the vessels coursing below must be coagulated before further cutting. (**d**): By blunt manipulation the course of the sacrouterine ligament and the uterus can be visualized in patients with lateral myomas. The line of coagulation should omit this part

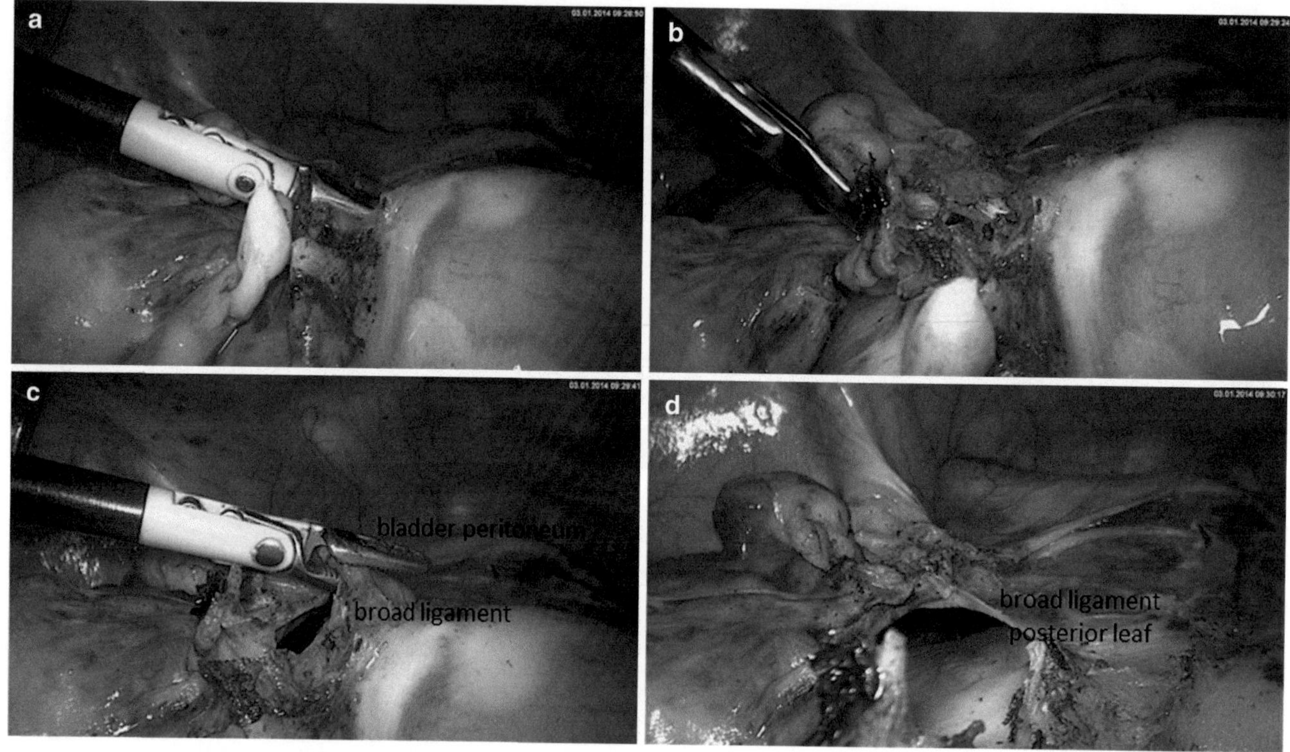

Fig. 35.55 (**a**) Dissection of the bladder peritoneum as well as the anterior and posterior leaf of the broad ligament on the left side. (**b**) Blunt manipulation shows the exact anatomical path of the left adnexa avoiding the wrong surgical route. (**c**) Coagulation is performed as close as possible to the uterus. (**d**) The bladder peritoneum has already been opened from the right side and the posterior leaf of the broad ligament serves as an anatomic landmark for the uterine vessels

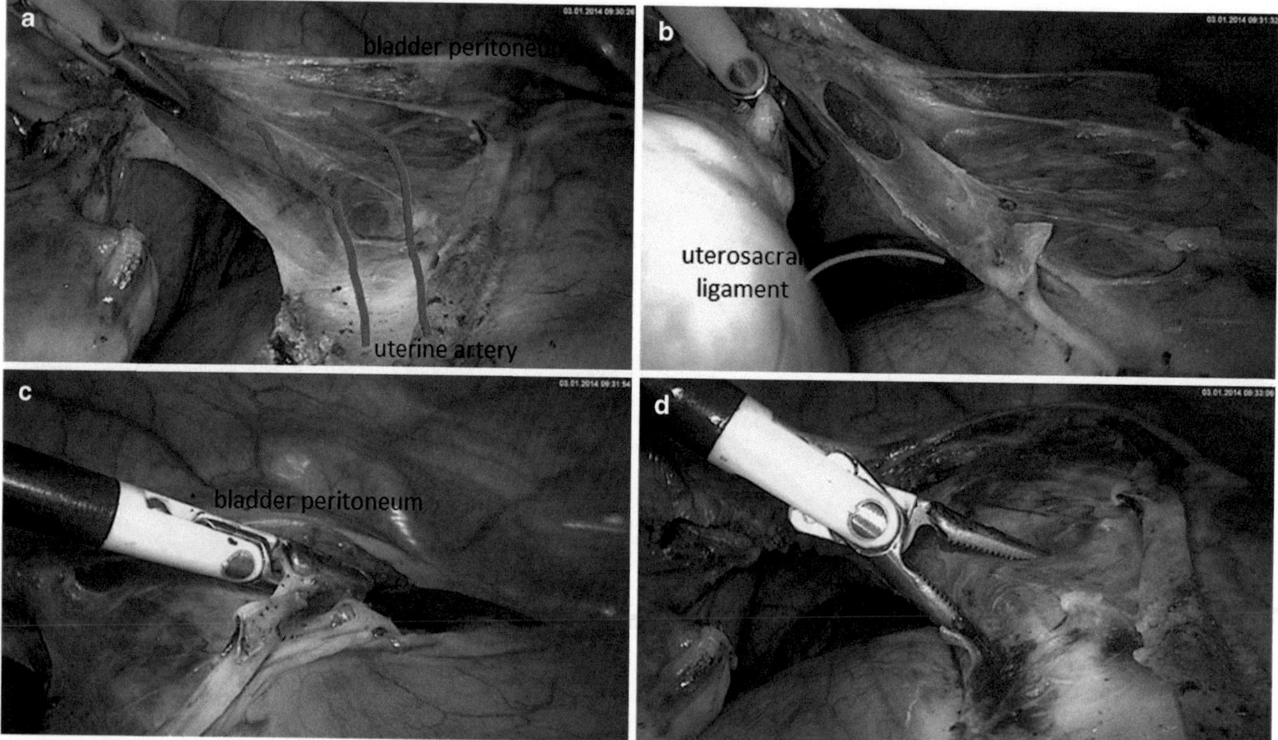

Fig. 35.56 Further opening of the bladder peritoneum and the broad ligament (**a**–**c**), and commencement of coagulation of the left uterine vessels (**d**). The uterine artery functions as an anatomic landmark leading downward (**a**). An intermediate glance at the back of the uterus shows that the cutting edge is above the conjunction of the sacrouterine ligaments

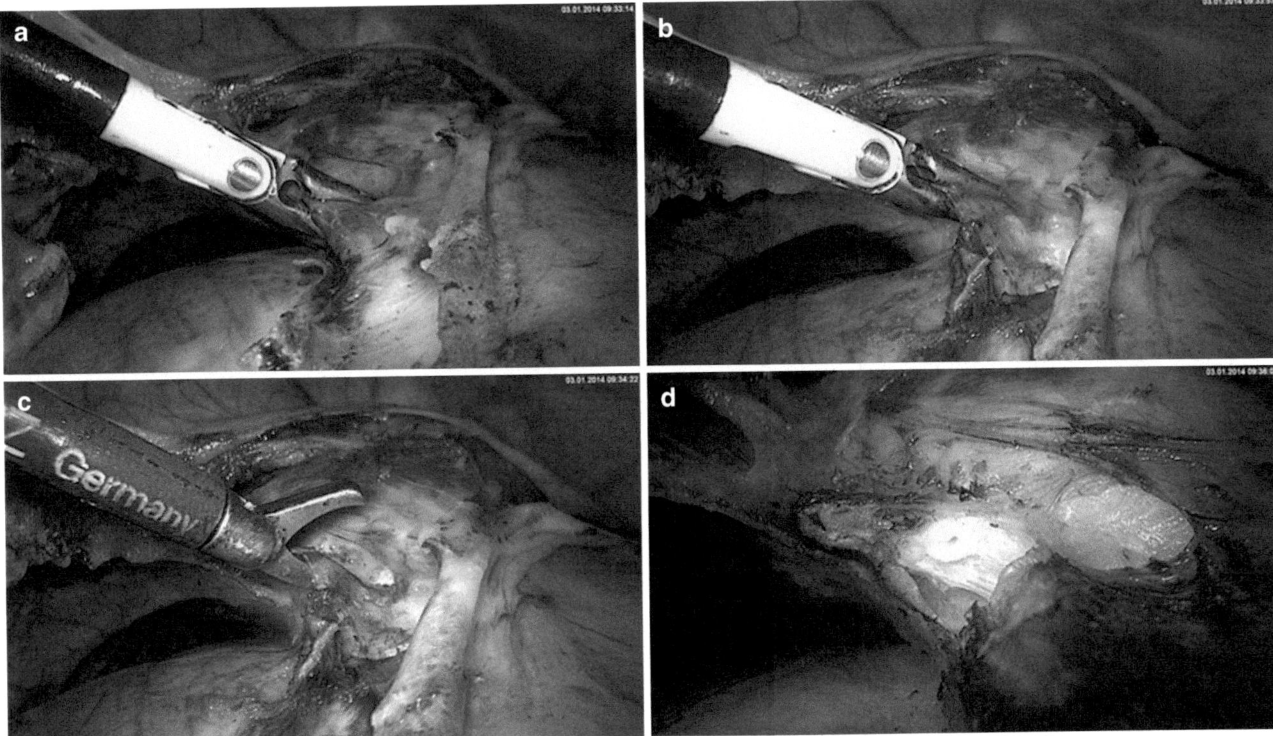

Fig. 35.57 Bipolar coagulation and separation of the uterine vessels on the left side. (**a**) The area of coagulation should include the upper parts of the artery to avoid any retrograde bleeding after dissection of the vessel (**b**). The color of the uterus changes to whitish/grey. (**c**–**d**): A deeper cut can be avoided by using the hook scissors; the uterine artery is dissected in two steps. This allows further coagulation of the tissue lying just behind the artery and avoids cumbersome venous bleeding

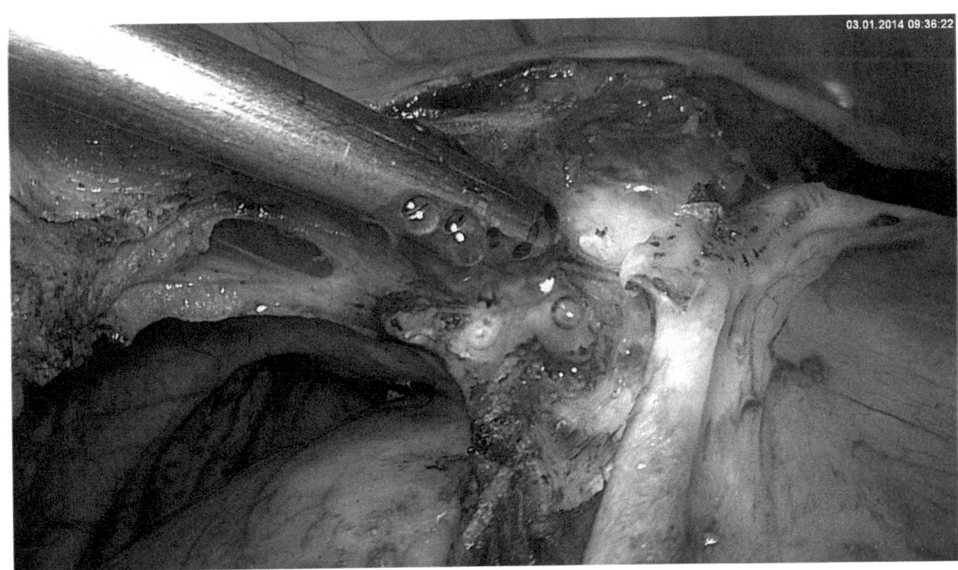

Fig. 35.58 Visualization of the separated left uterine pedicles. A few drops of physiological saline solution render the bipolar coagulation more effective because of better electrolyte flow, especially when the field of operation is very dry

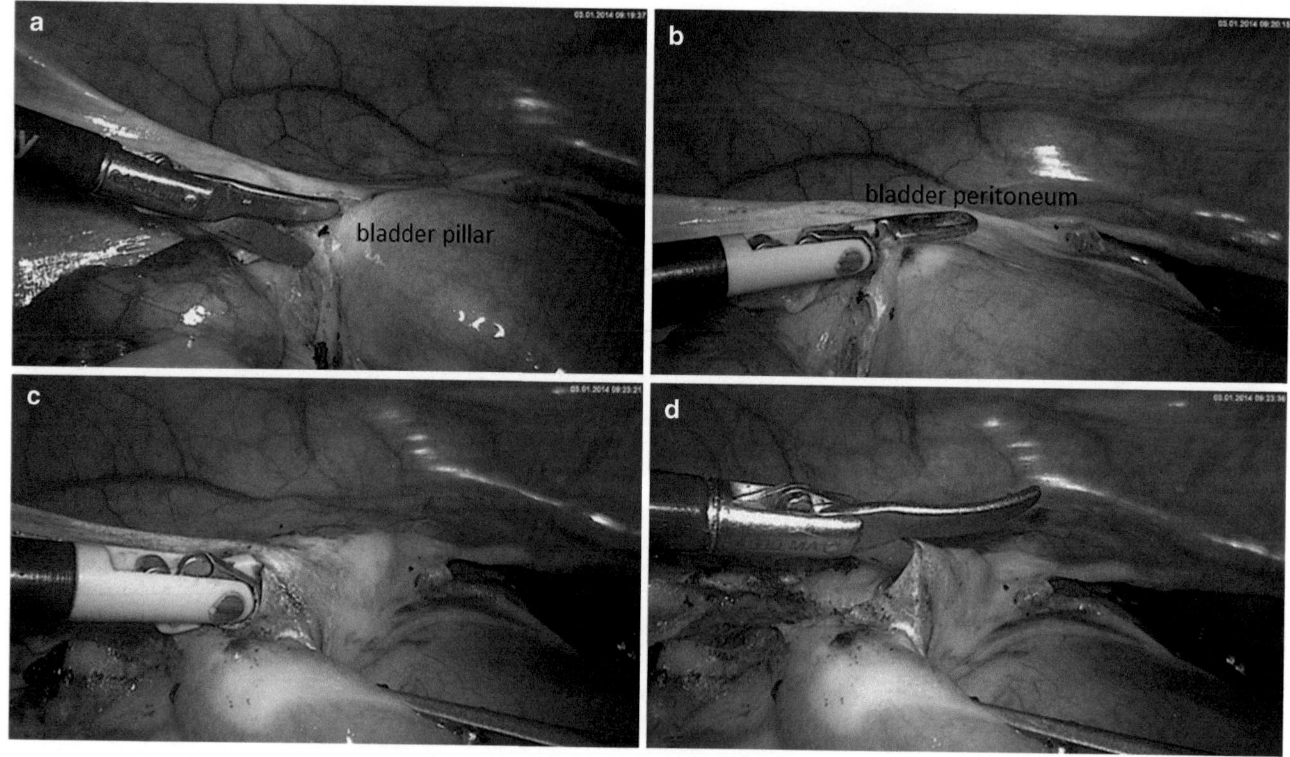

Fig. 35.59 (**a**) Final dissection of the bladder pillar and the bladder peritoneum (**b**) from left to right, (**c**) allowing the CO_2 distension medium to show the way. (**d**) The bladder is pushed safely downward from the field of operation and the peritoneal line of the vesicouterine fold is easily recognized

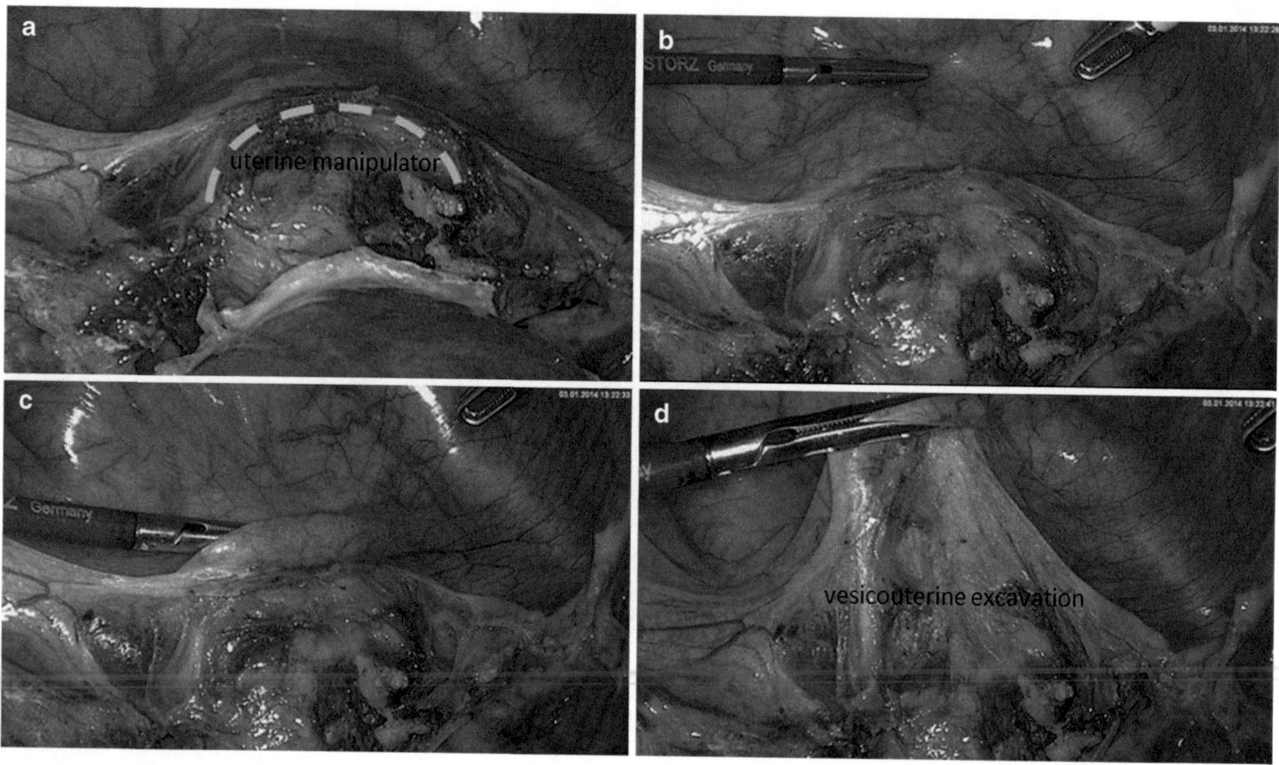

Fig. 35.60 Visualization of the intrauterine manipulator, if inserted (**a**). (**b**, **c**): The bladder cannot be identified immediately in all cases and is safely avoided. The bladder can be localized exactly when a blunt instrument is used to push the suspected bladder towards the cervix from the balloon of the Foley catheter. (**d**) Once the bladder has been identified, it is elevated. Vesicouterine excavation can be used to push the bladder further downward

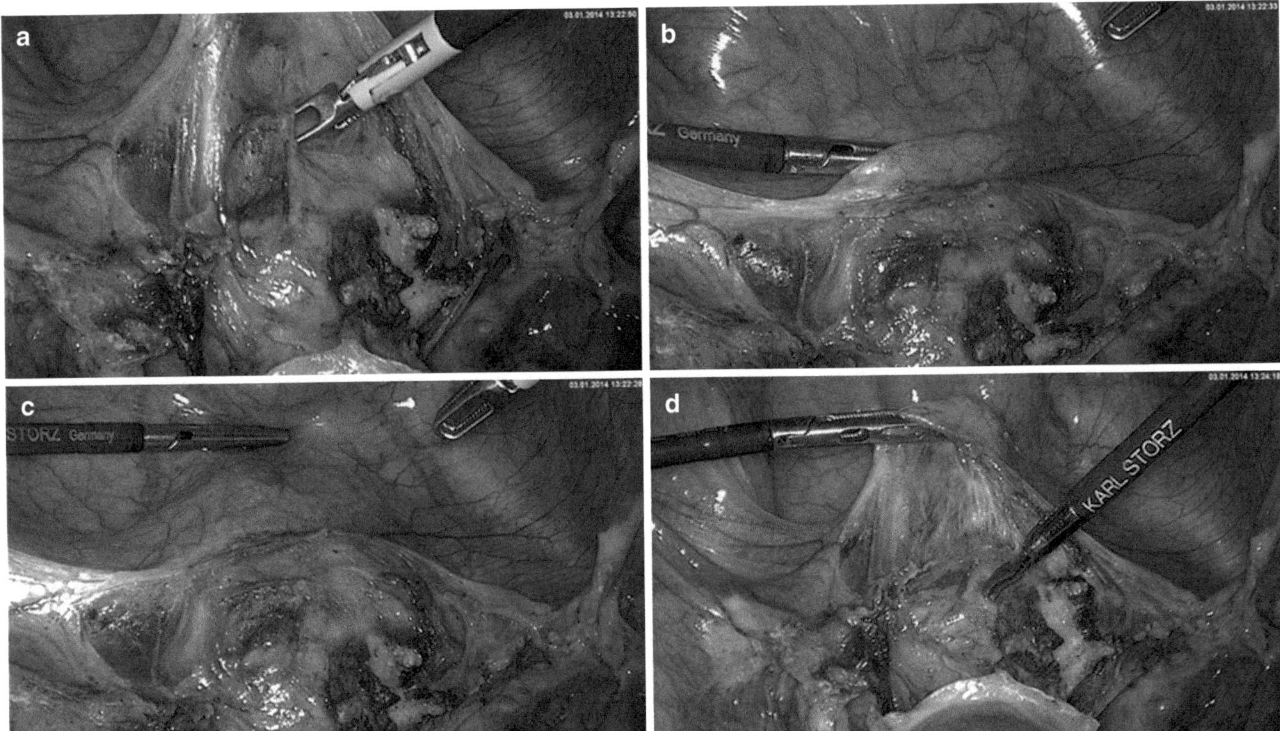

Fig. 35.61 (**a**) Minimal dissection of the bladder peritoneum by about 1 cm for LSH and 2-3cm for LTH, by opening the vesicouterine excavation. (**b**) This is easier when a manipulator is inside the vagina and the cervix is pushed upward. The anatomical landmarks of the bladder are hard to find. Therefore it is easier if the whole organ is pushed upwards and (**c**) back, thereby displaying the anatomical borders. (**d**) The step can also be performed by traction alone. Once the vesicouterine space has been opened, exposure is easily achieved with a blunt instrument while avoiding bleeding

Step 4

4.1 In laparoscopic supracervical hysterectomy, resection of the uterine corpus is performed at this stage of surgery. The steps of exposure are very similar until this point, except for the fact that there is no need for a manipulator and elevation of the uterus is achieved by traction. The corpus of the uterus is cut with a monopolar loop and the cervical channel coagulated to prevent spotting. The cervical channel should be closed because of the risk of ascending infection. Simultaneously, the cervix can be suspended using a strong monofilament suture with extracorporeal knotting (Figs. 35.62 and 35.63).

4.2 Resection of the vagina from the cervix with the monopolar hook by stretching the manipulator firmly cranially. Intrafascial dissection is performed, leaving the sacrouterine ligaments almost completely in place (Figs. 35.64, 35.65 and 35.66).

The uterus is then extracted through the vagina or positioned in the vagina to prevent loss of intraabdominal pressure while still fixed to the manipulator (Fig. 35.67). A large uterus must be morcellated either intraabdominally or transvaginally. In cases of a large benign uterus, visible myomas can be enucleated or the large uterus cut into several smaller pieces which are then extracted through the vagina. As a result, the incision in the lower abdomen need not exceed 5 mm and postoperative pain or the risk of hernia is minimized. Alternatively, a 10–12-mm electromorcellator is used to dissect the material, which is then extracted through the abdominal wall. The cutting edge of the morcellator must always be visible during morcellation. Evidence of the absence of any malignancy must be obtained earlier by appropriate preoperative diagnostic investigation. The patient must be informed in advance about the fact that the uterus, depending on its volume, may need to be morcellated.

Step 5 (Classical Closure)

After removing the uterus, the vaginal cuff and the peritoneum are closed with two Vicryl 0 Z-sutures, or with a running suture with or without separate knotting of the lateral edges. Suturing may be performed intraabdominally or extraabdominally. This simple and economical concept can be adapted to almost all techniques of open surgery.

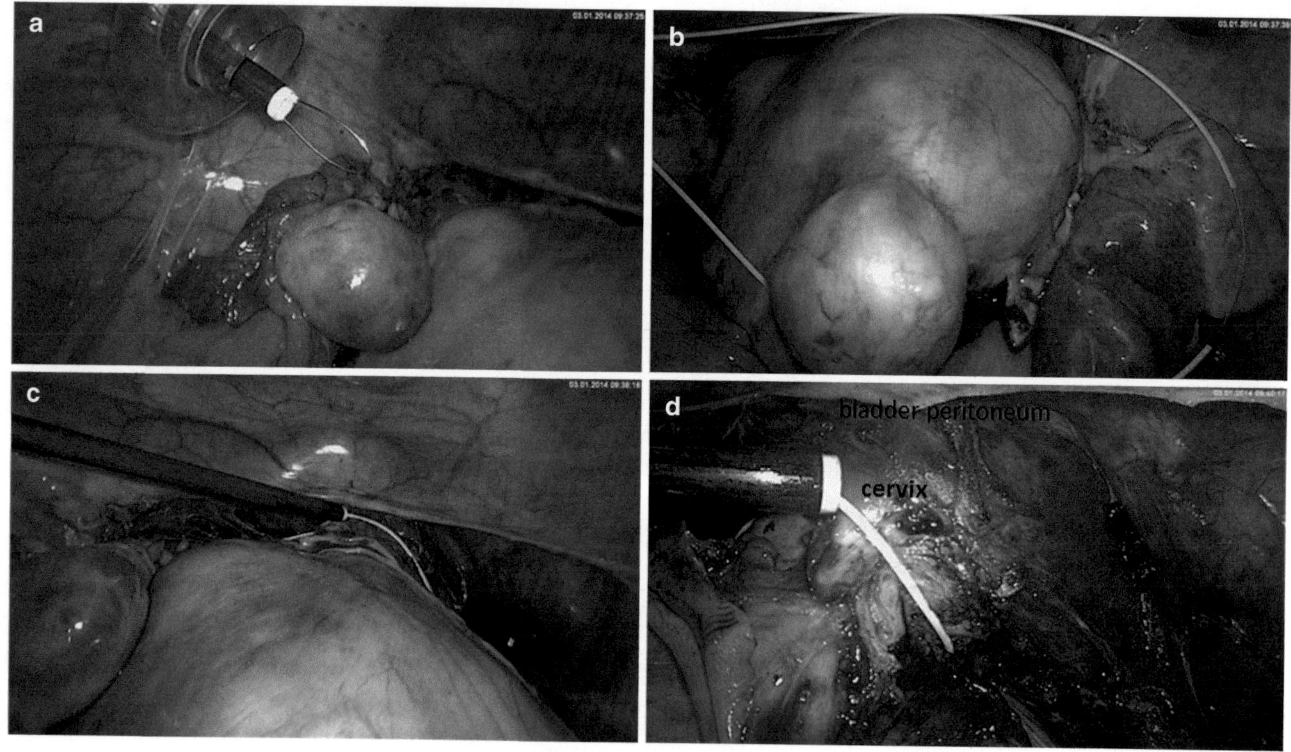

Fig. 35.62 (**a**) Introduction of a monopolar cutting loop for the cervix and (**b**) exact placement prior to activation. (**c**) The whitish uterus is lifted over the loop and (**d**) the loop is tightened gently. Correct placement between the stumps of the uterine artery and above the conjunction of the sacrouterine ligaments is checked

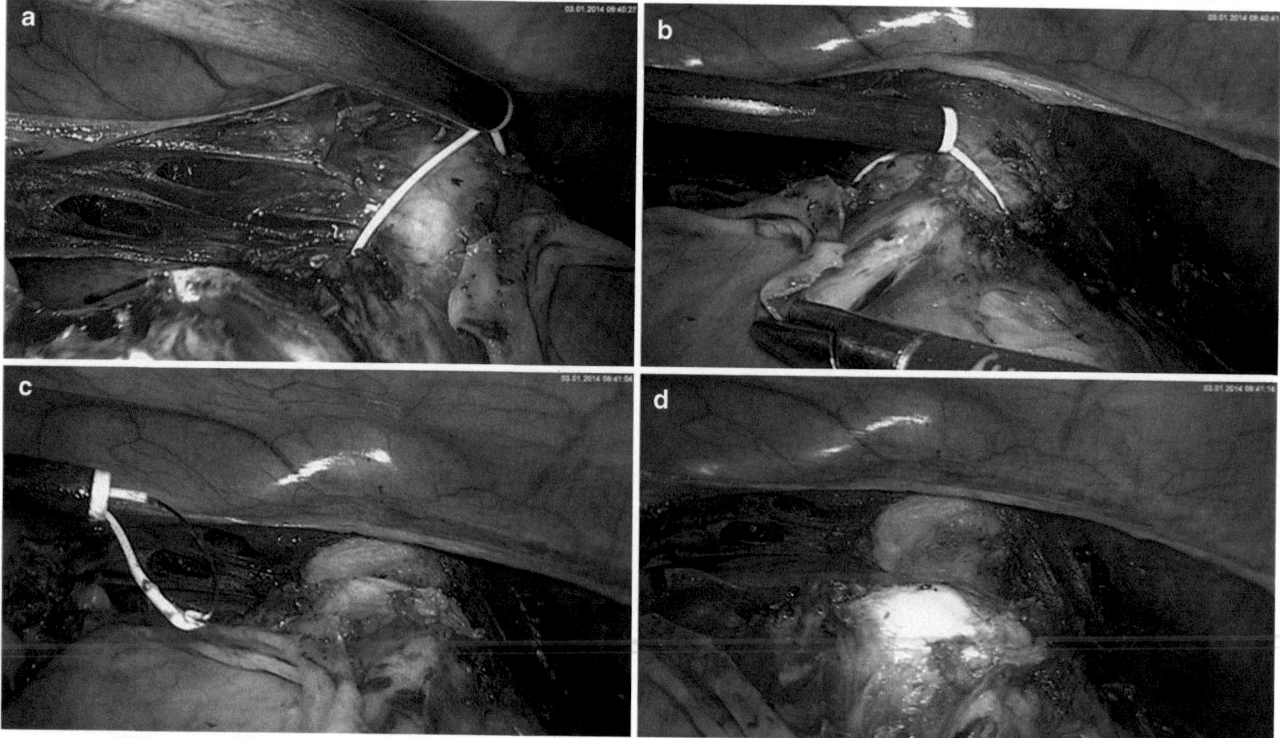

Fig. 35.63 Resection of the uterine corpus from the cervix after placing the cutting loop with the cutting point on the posterior cervix (**a**, **b**). Correct placement between the stumps of the uterine artery and above the conjunction of the sacrouterine ligaments is monitored. Dissection of the cervix and the uterus is performed (**c**, **d**), in this case LSH by monopolar current only in the non-isolated field. When cutting, the uterine corpus is pulled upward to achieve a retrograde conus (**b**, **d**)

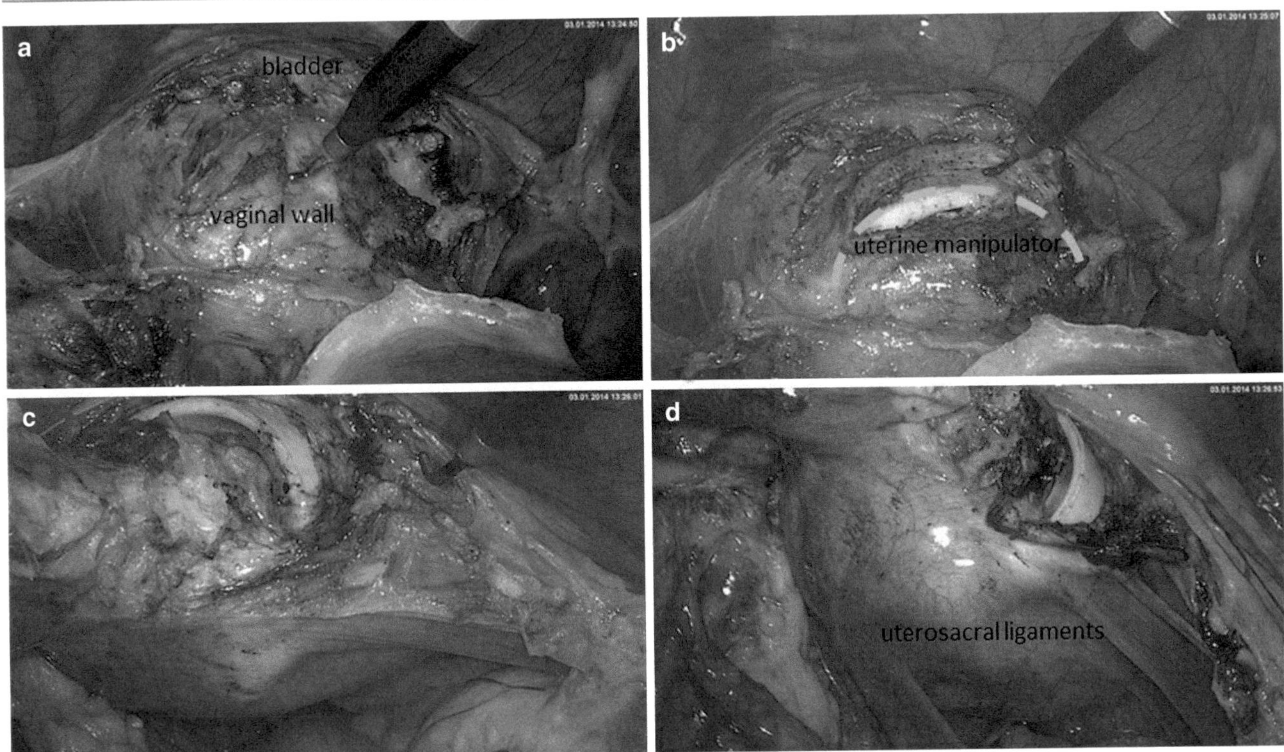

Fig. 35.64 In this case of LTH, the distance between the vagina and the bladder is increased because of exposure of the bladder peritoneum (**a**). The intrauterine manipulator is firmly placed in the abdomen and dissection of the uterus from the vagina is performed in a stepwise manner (**b**–**d**). The conjunction of the sacrouterine ligaments is left in place

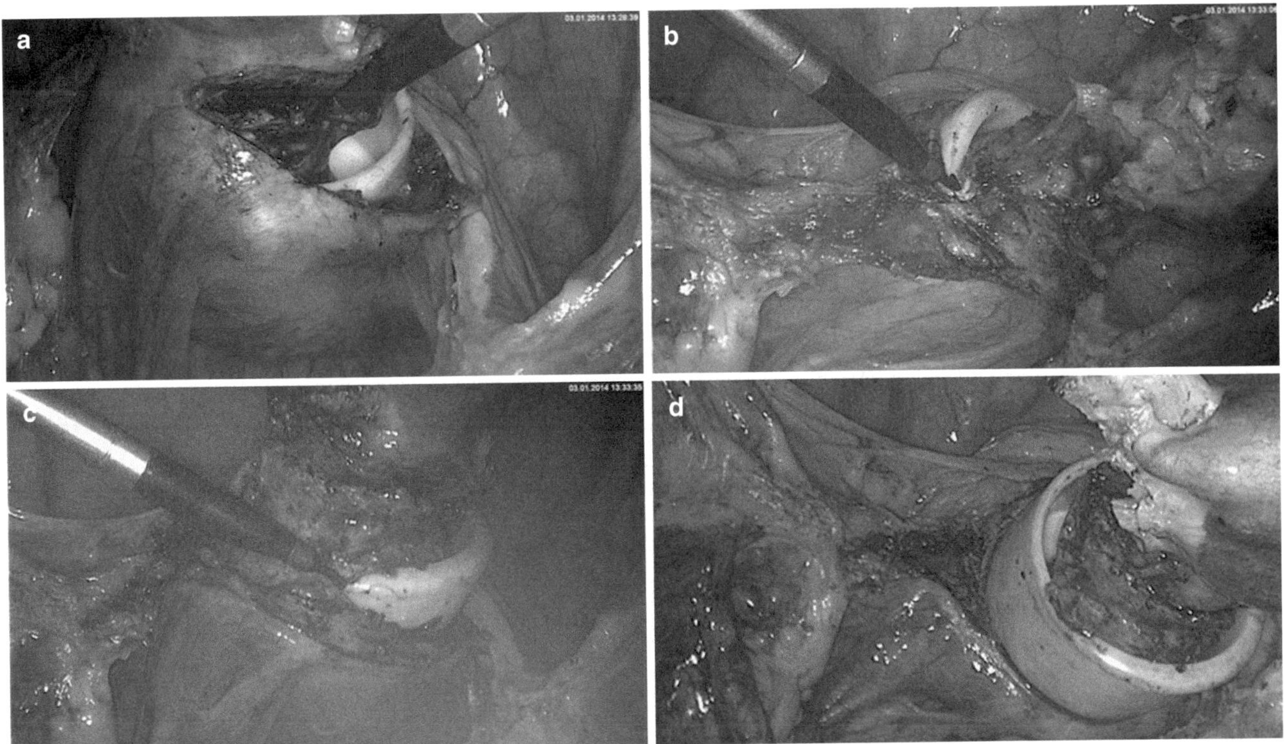

Fig. 35.65 Completion of the dissection of the vagina from the cervix (**a**–**c**) and commencement of retraction of the uterine cervix, still grasped by the manipulator forceps, transvaginally. Excessive lens fogging caused by the monopolar current and the sharpness of the monopolar hook make it necessary to perform precise exposure under full vision. This can be done during simultaneous retraction/manipulation with the use of the 30 ° optic device. (**d**) The surgeon's vision may worsen immediately when CO_2 gas leaks through the colpotomy. Visibility may then become extremely poor and the use of monopolar energy hazardous

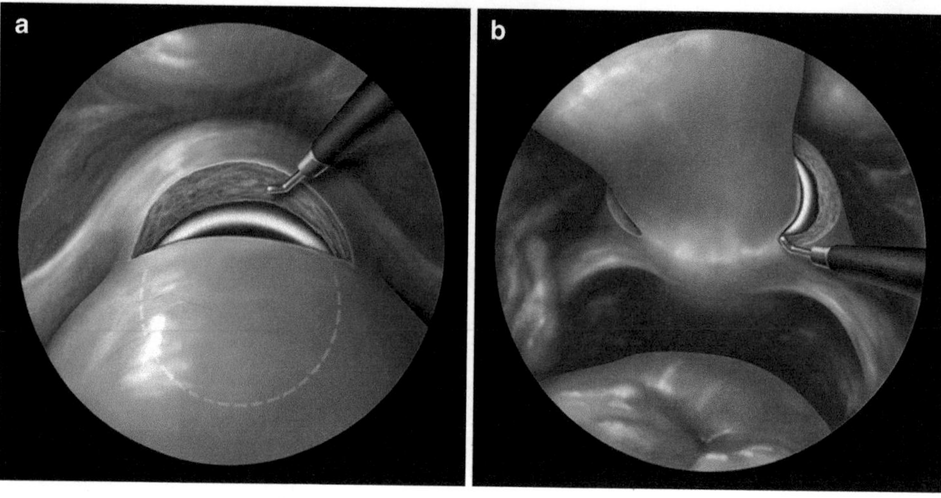

Fig. 35.66 Schematic illustration of uterine dissection. (**a**) Colpotomy is usually started in the anterior part, on the palpable manipulator cap. (**b**) The intrafascial hysterectomy can be completed with the sacrouterine ligaments in view

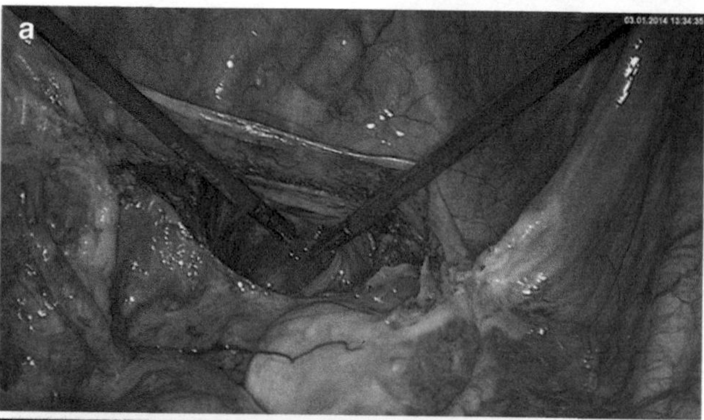

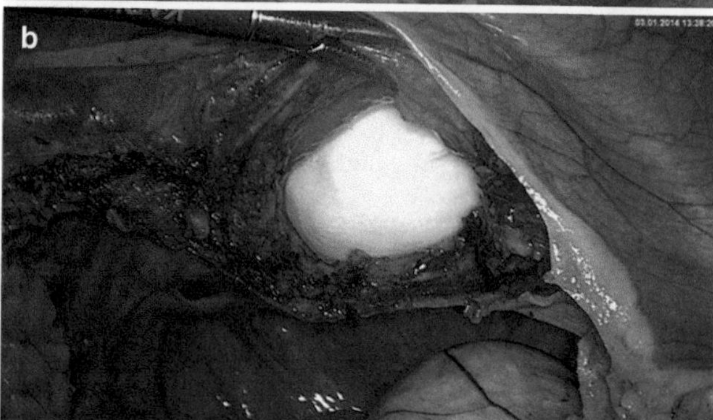

Fig. 35.67 Retraction of uterus through the vagina (**a**).Introduction of a cotton swab-filled glove transvaginally to hinder breakdown of the CO_2 pneumoperitoneum (**b**)

Step 5(Alternative Closure Technique Emphasizing Prolapse Prevention)

A Technique for Stable Fixation of the Vaginal or Cervical Stump

Vaginal closure with Te Linde suturing technique modified by Schollmeyer

Hysterectomy is known to be associated with a high risk of pelvic organ prolapse; the risk is especially high among multiparous women. This may necessitate pelvic organ prolapse surgery. Given the current high life expectancy of women, organ prolapse may pose a problem in later life and also difficulties in surgical repair (thrombosis, embolism, and infection) [35].

The suturing technique of Te Linde, known from abdominal hysterectomy for the closure of the vagina, was modified for laparoscopic use by Bruno van Herendael and further modified by Thoralf Schollmeyer [36, 37].

5.1 Cautious coagulation of the vaginal edge [38] is followed by suturing of the vagina. Coagulation should be performed very carefully to avoid postoperative necrosis of the vaginal stump. Slight residual bleeding is addressed by sutures incorporating the complete vaginal wall. The uterus is either still in the vagina or a glove filled with swabs is placed in the vagina to avoid loss of the pneumoperitoneum. Usually a curved needle and PDS 1–0 is used for single knot suturing, with extracorporeal knots and intracorporeal safety knots. Alternatively, sledneedles or even straight needles can be used for easy handling in and out of the 5-mm trocars.

PDS 1–0 extracorporeal knots are used for the following reasons:

1. The monofilament thread slides easily through the tissue and does not cause additional damage.
2. The monofilament PDS material minimizes the risk of vaginal stump infection.
3. The long half-life of the suture material minimizes the risk of vaginal stump dehiscence [38].
4. Extracorporeal knots provide additional strength.

Optionally, both sacrouterine ligaments may be attached to the posterior vaginal wall to prevent vaginal prolapse (McCall culdoplasty).

5.2 Corner sutures

The peri-cervical ring is pierced by performing a suture in the right vaginal corner, followed by the corresponding vaginal epithelium. The sutures are made at a distance from the urinary bladder to minimize the risk of bladder laceration (Figs. 35.68 and 35.69).

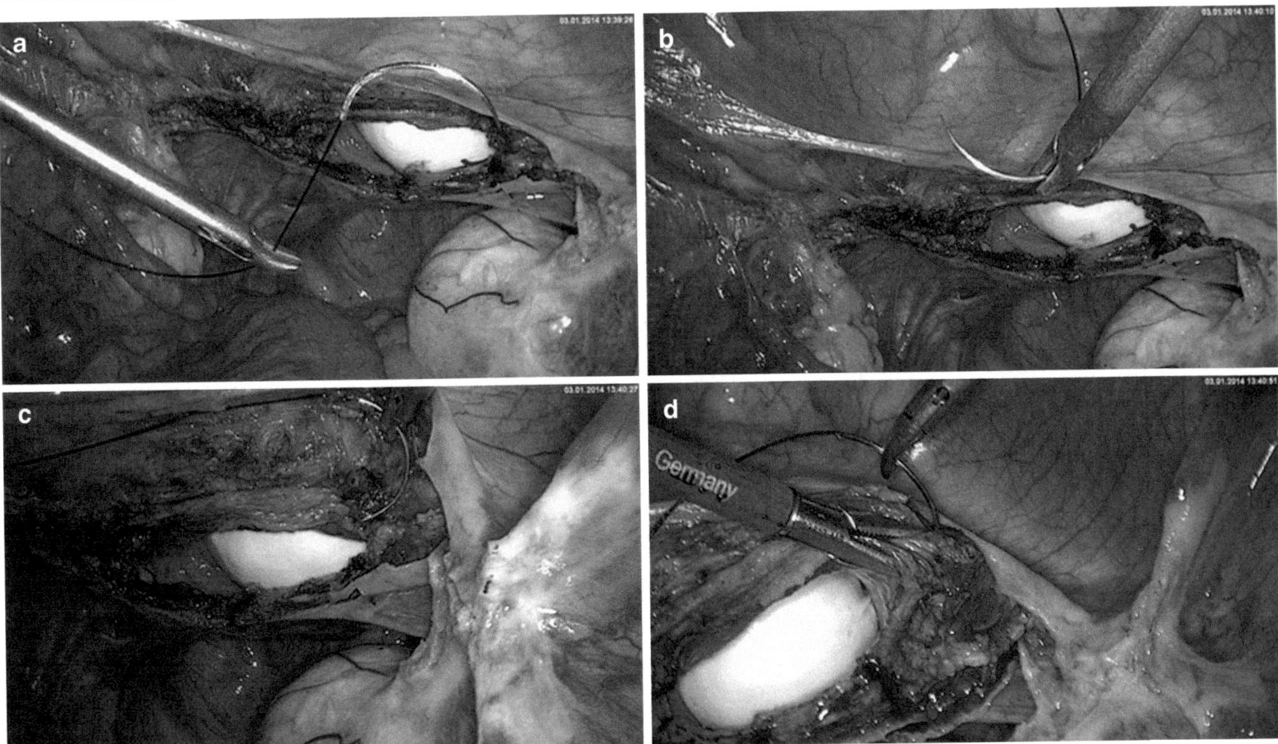

Fig. 35.68 LTH: Right corner suture uniting the anterior and posterior vaginal wall, the posterior peritoneum, and the right sacrouterine ligament. The bladder can be omitted under sight. (**a**) Insertion of the needle and (**b**) positioning of the needle in the needle holder. (**c**) The disadvantages of conventional laparoscopy need to be overcome by surgical quality. (**d**) The forceps must be sharp in order to securely grab the vaginal epithelium. When the suture incorporates the vaginal wall alone and omits the epithelium, there is a high likelihood of postoperative granulomas

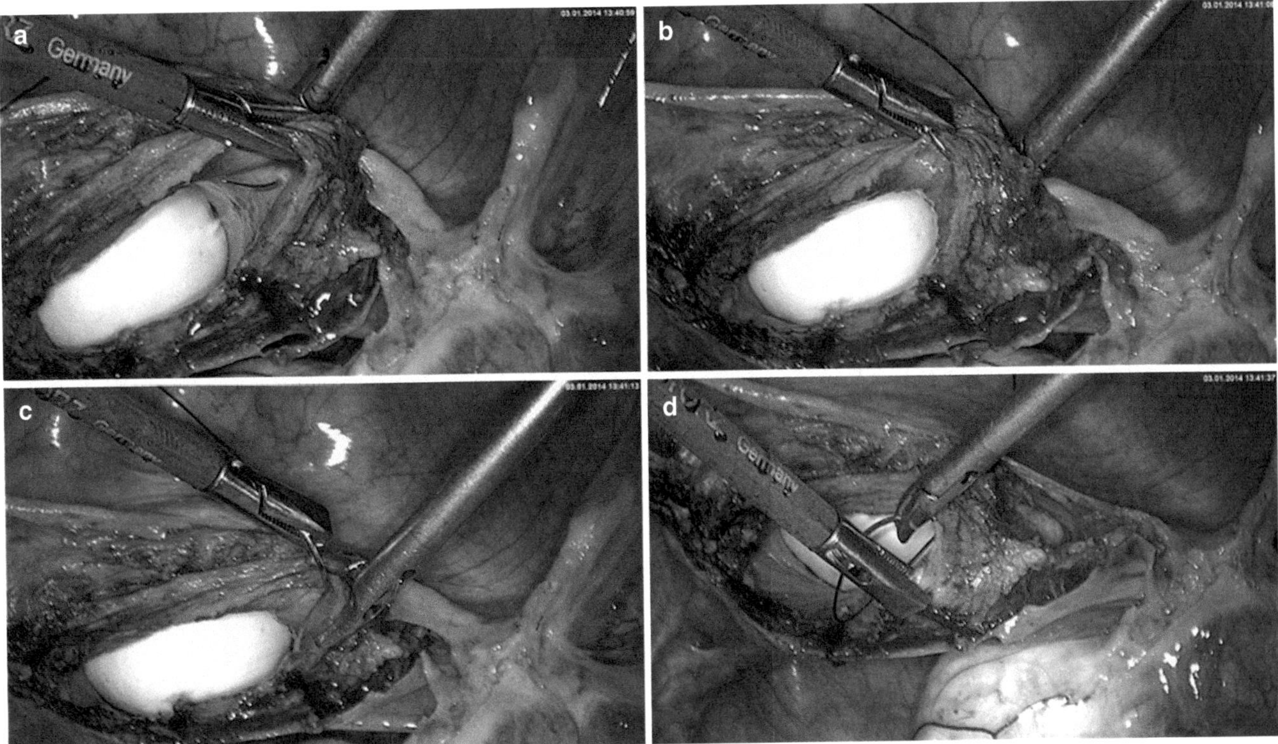

Fig. 35.69 LTH: (**a**) Continuation of the right corner suture. (**b**) The 30° optic device helps to look into the vagina from below when rotating and (**c**) picking up the needle (**d**) from above. The strong paravaginal tissue is grasped in large units

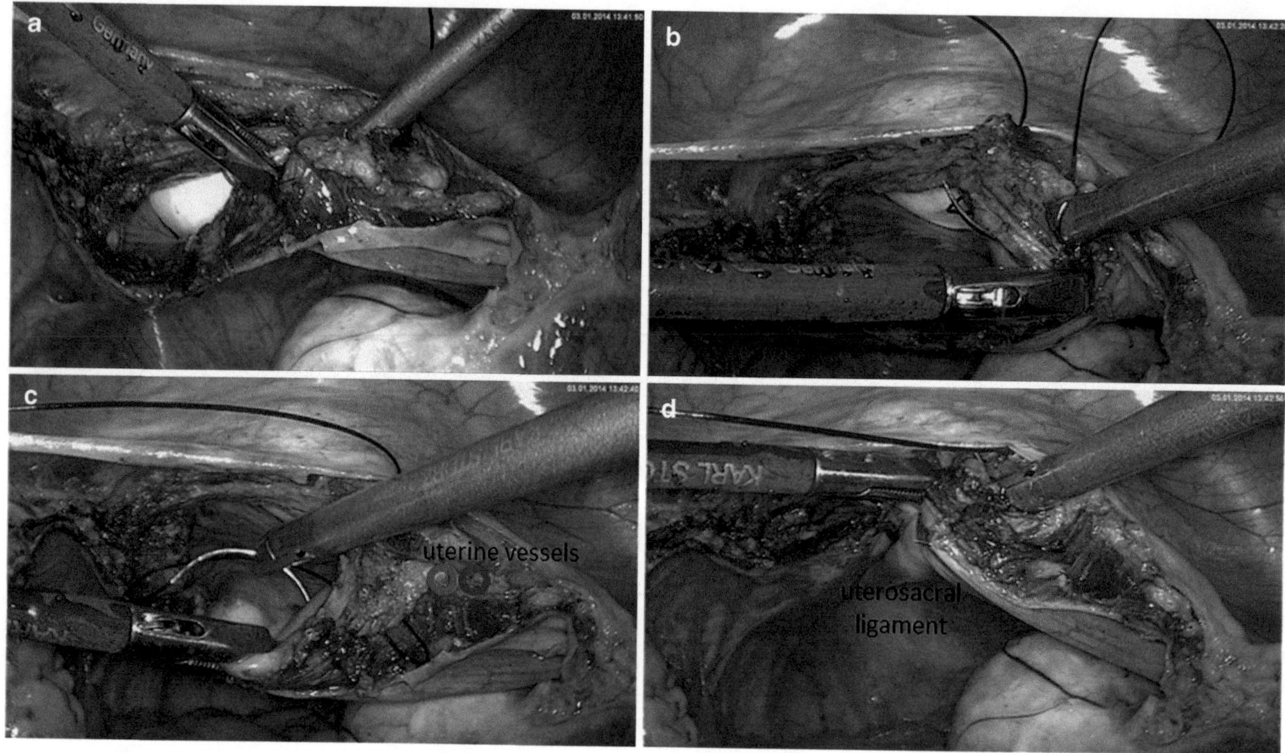

Fig. 35.70 LTH: (**a**) Continuation of the right corner suture while (**b**) leaving out the vessels to the side, (**c**) performing an omega suture (according to Schollmeyer), (**d**) and then grabbing the right sacrouterine ligament. The vessel stumps are omitted and lateralized. When using this type of suture, the vessels are compressed mechanically

5.3 In the second step, the needle is passed through the medial aspect of the cardinal ligament in front of the uterine vessels (Fig. 35.70). The second step involves the structures supporting vaginal wall suspension. Extracorporeal knotting with the placement of a deep and strong monofilament suture allows the surgeon to grasp a large quantity of tissue and smoothly glide through the tissue without causing damage (Figs. 35.71, 35.72 and 35.73).

5.4 Subsequent back-stitching of the vagina is followed by passing the needle through the vaginal epithelium and then, in the third step, through the sacrouterine ligament. The last step may be omitted when the ligament is stitched again once or twice to shorten it. In cases of pre-existing descent, this is absolutely essential.

The needle can now be withdrawn and the suture is completed with an extracorporeal Roeder knot, secured by 2–3 intracorporeal knots (Fig. 35.74). This procedure is repeated on the contralateral side and ensures that all parts of the endopelvic fascia (vesicouterine, cardinal and sacrouterine ligaments) are connected (Figs. 35.75, 35.76 and 35.77).

Step 6

Vaginal Closure

The remaining vaginal opening in the middle can now be closed with two U- or Z-sutures. These ensure both vertical and horizontal compression of the tissue, and minimize the risk of a vaginal stump hematoma. Neither peritonealization nor drainage is necessary (Figs. 35.78 and 35.79). Physiological reperitonealization occurs during the first two weeks after the operation. Any additional peritoneal suturing might cause encapsulation of seroma or hematoma and increase the likelihood of postoperative infection as well as pain. If still inside, the uterus or the swab-filled glove is now taken out of the vagina. Figure 35.80 provides an overview of the procedure.

von Leffern Knot

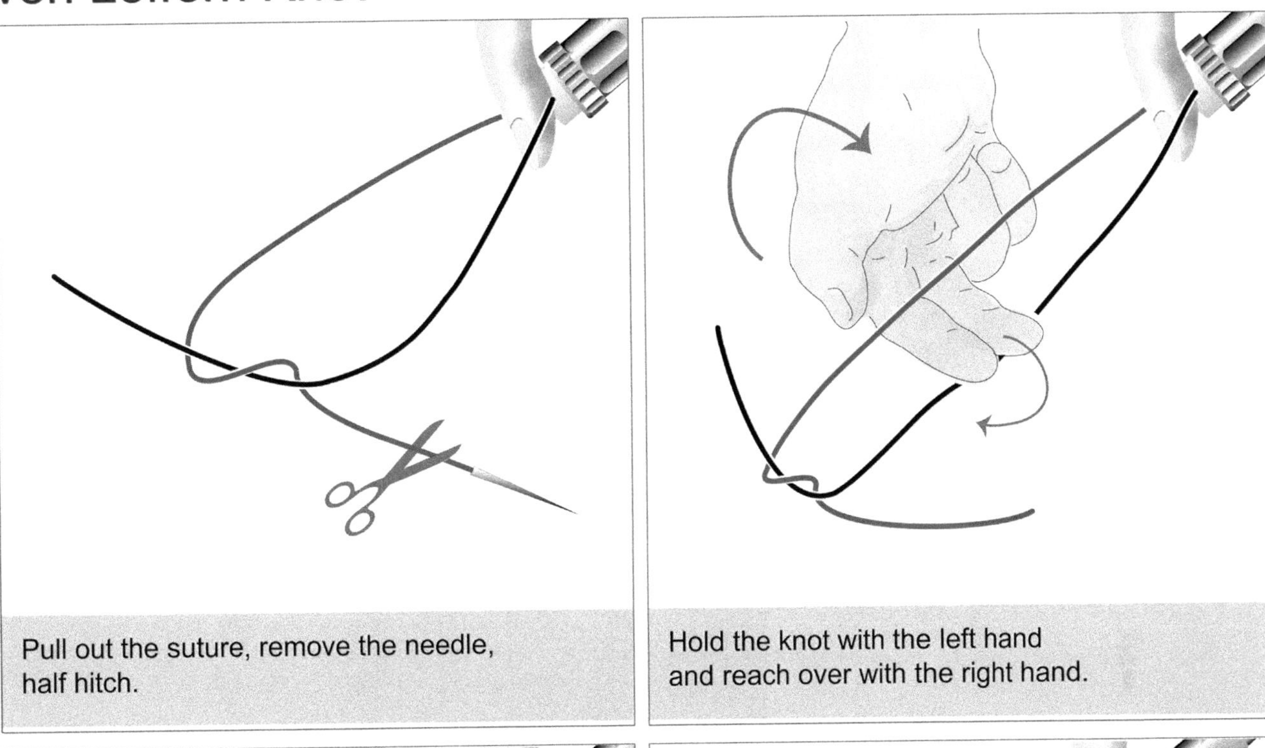

Pull out the suture, remove the needle,
half hitch.
Hold the knot with the left hand
and reach over with the right hand.

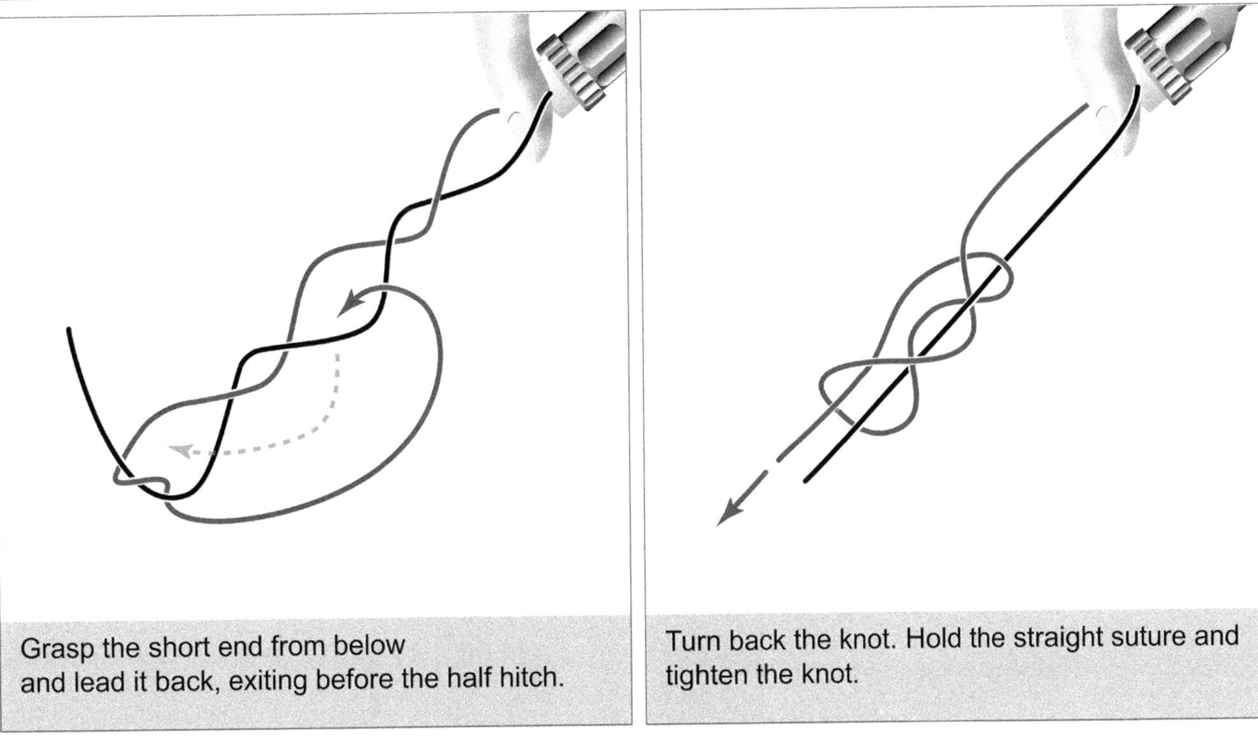

Grasp the short end from below
and lead it back, exiting before the half hitch.
Turn back the knot. Hold the straight suture and
tighten the knot.

Fig. 35.71 LSH: Finalizing the extracorporeal knot of the PDS suture by using the "von Leffern knot"

Roeder Knot

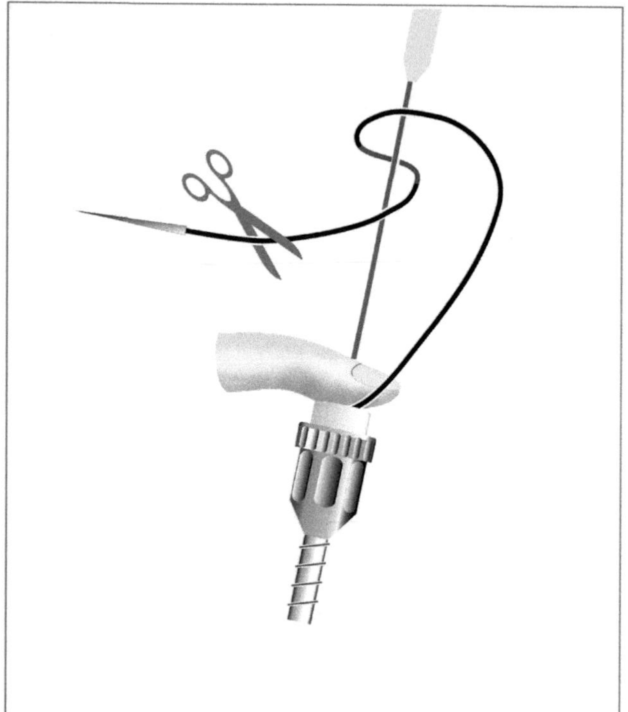

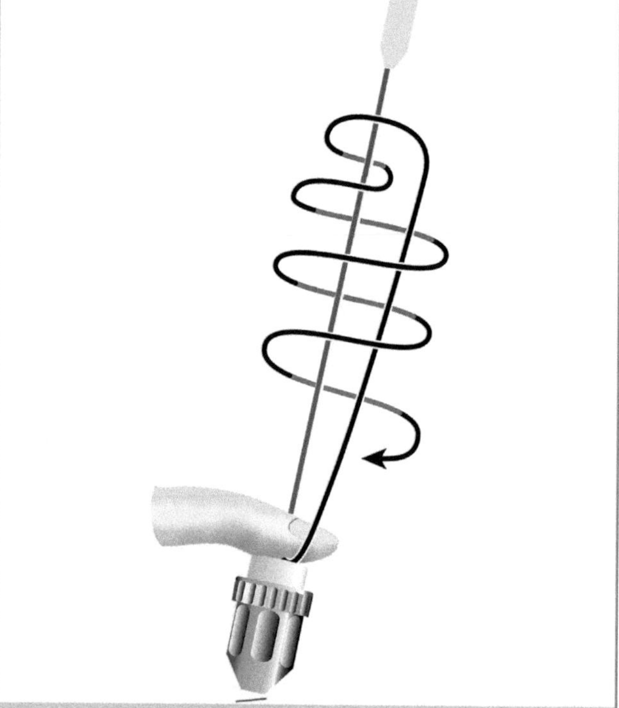

Throw three loops around both strands.
Maintain tension.

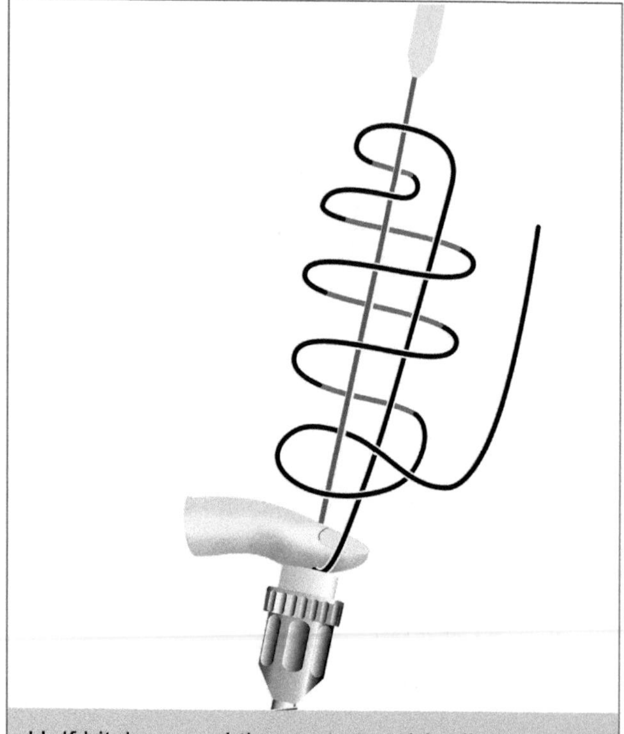

Half hitch around the post strand (red).
Push the knot together.

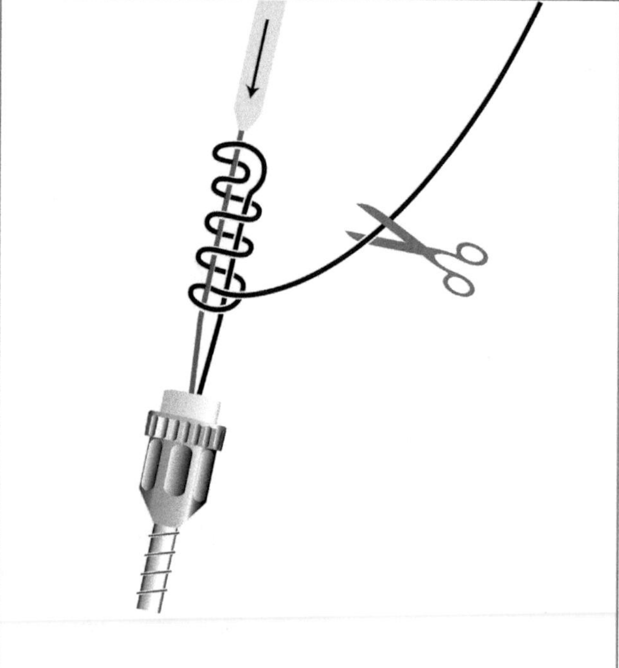

Fig. 35.72 "The Roeder" knot

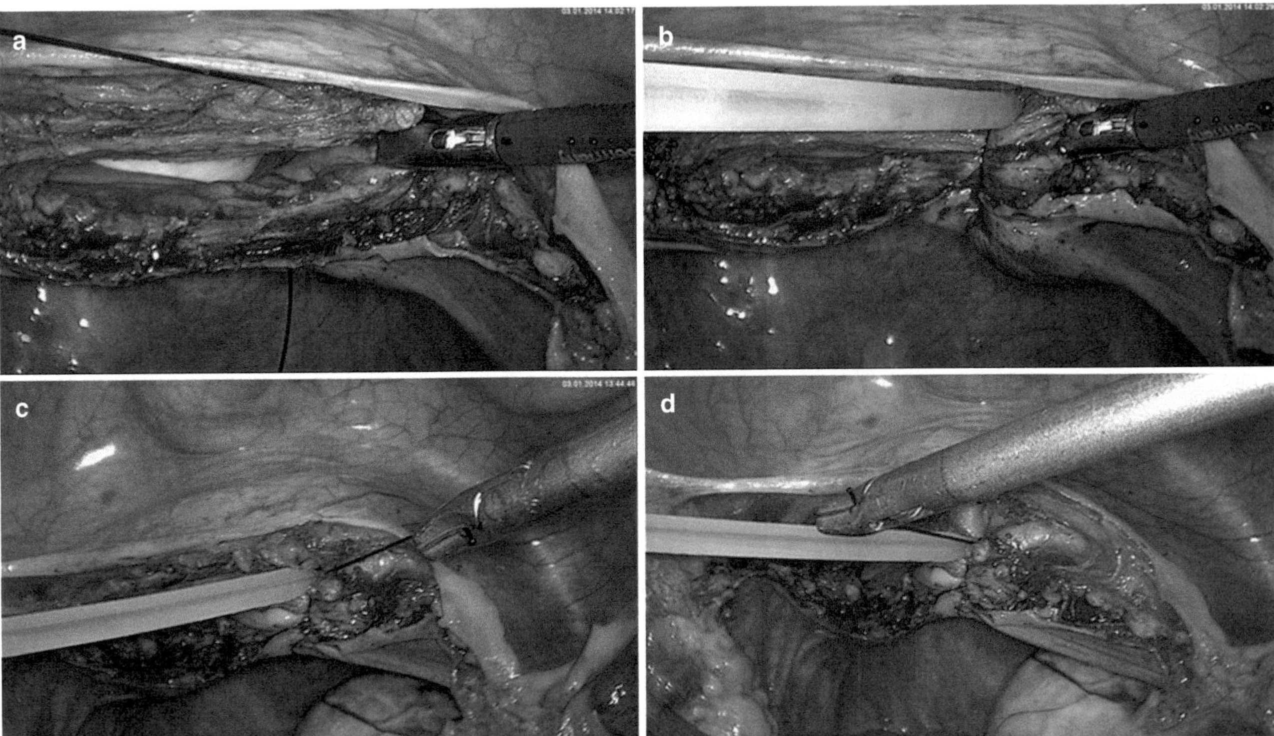

Fig. 35.73 LTH: (**a**) Completion of the extracorporeal "Roeder" or "von Leffern" knot by pushing it down with a plastic pushrod (**b–d**). The edge is pulled into the abdomen to avoid disturbance of intravaginal sensitivity

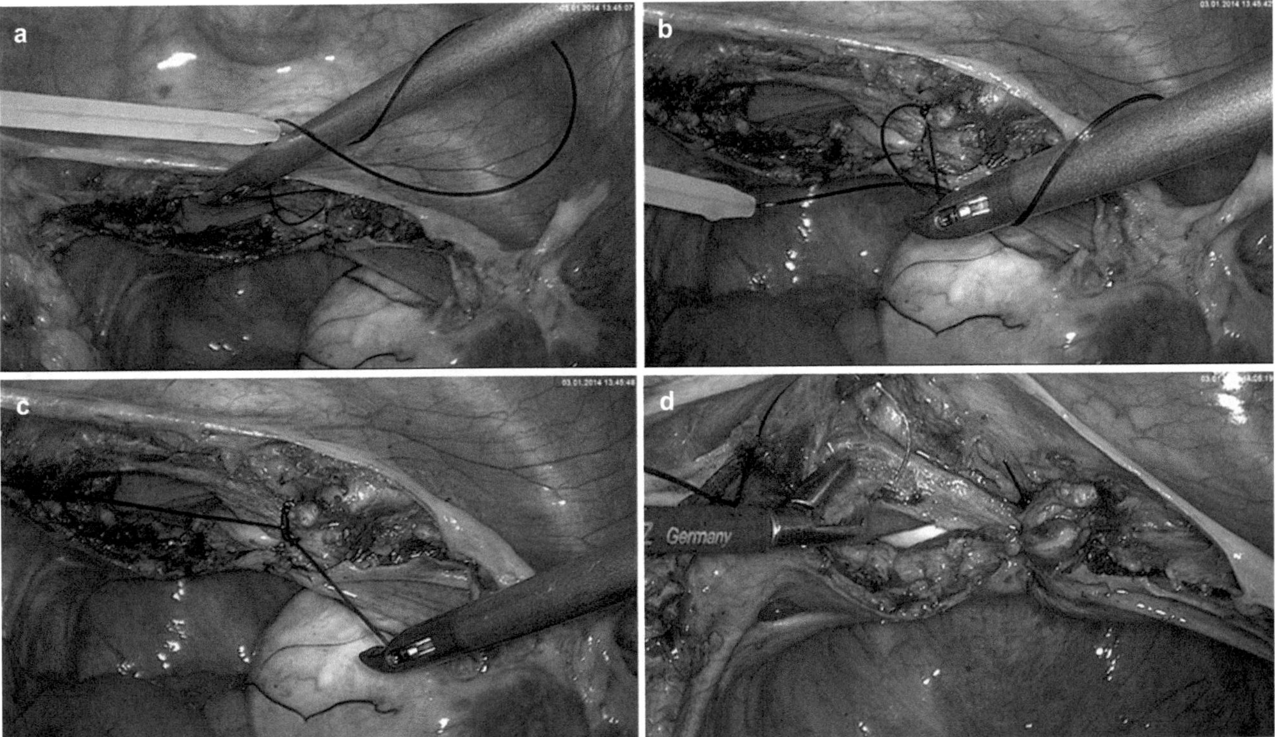

Fig. 35.74 LTH: (**a**) Performance of an intracorporeal safety knot (**b**) by placing the right corner stitch (**c**) and tightening of the threads. Here, it can be clearly visualized that extracorporeal knotting allows the surgeon to push the knot deeper into the tissue than intracorporeal knotting. (**d**) The same knot is performed on the left side, both edges are dry and everted

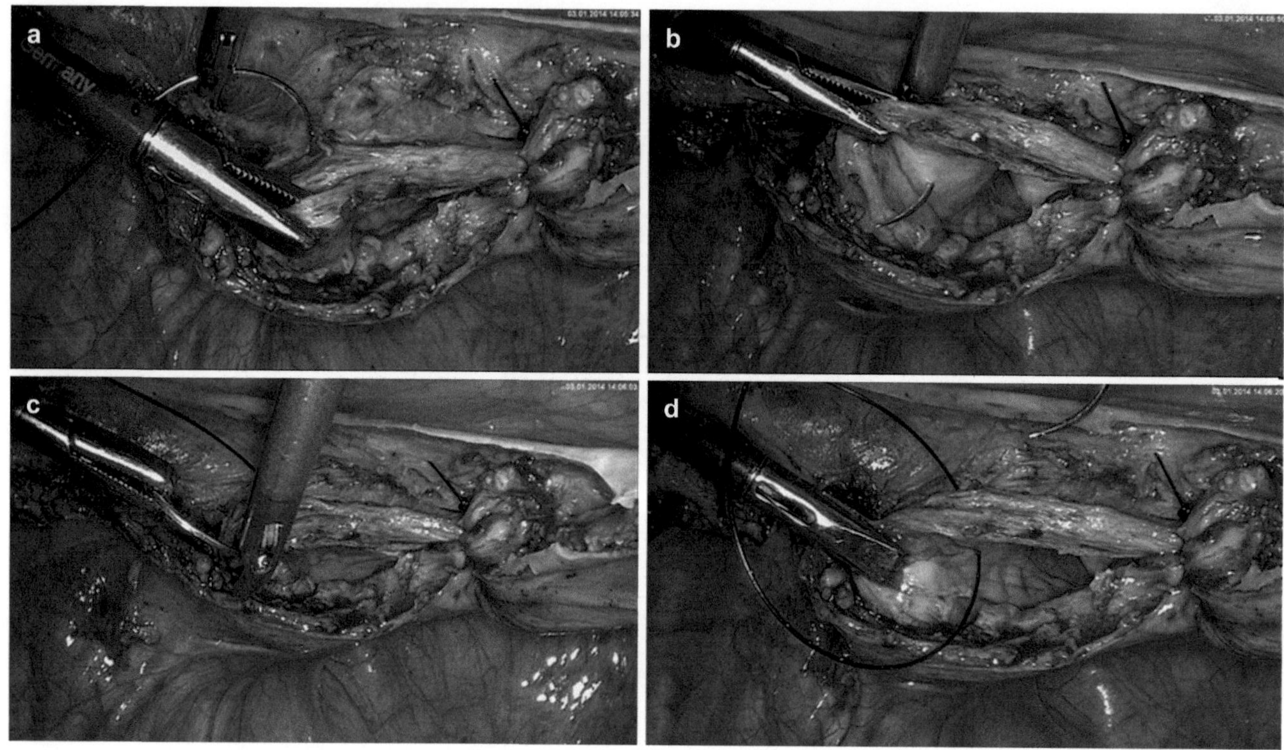

Fig. 35.75 LTH: (**a**) Left corner suture uniting the anterior and posterior vaginal wall, the posterior peritoneum, and the left sacrouterine ligament. The bladder can be omitted under sight. After positioning of the needle, (**b**) paracolpium and epithelium are grabbed and perforated by the needle. (**c**) The grasper of the left hand holds the needle and (**d**) the needle holder only rotates once it has touched the tissue, thereby avoiding tearing of the tissue. The forceps must be sharp in order to securely grasp the vaginal epithelium. When the suture incorporates the vaginal wall alone and omits the epithelium, there will be a high likelihood of postoperative granuloma or bleeding

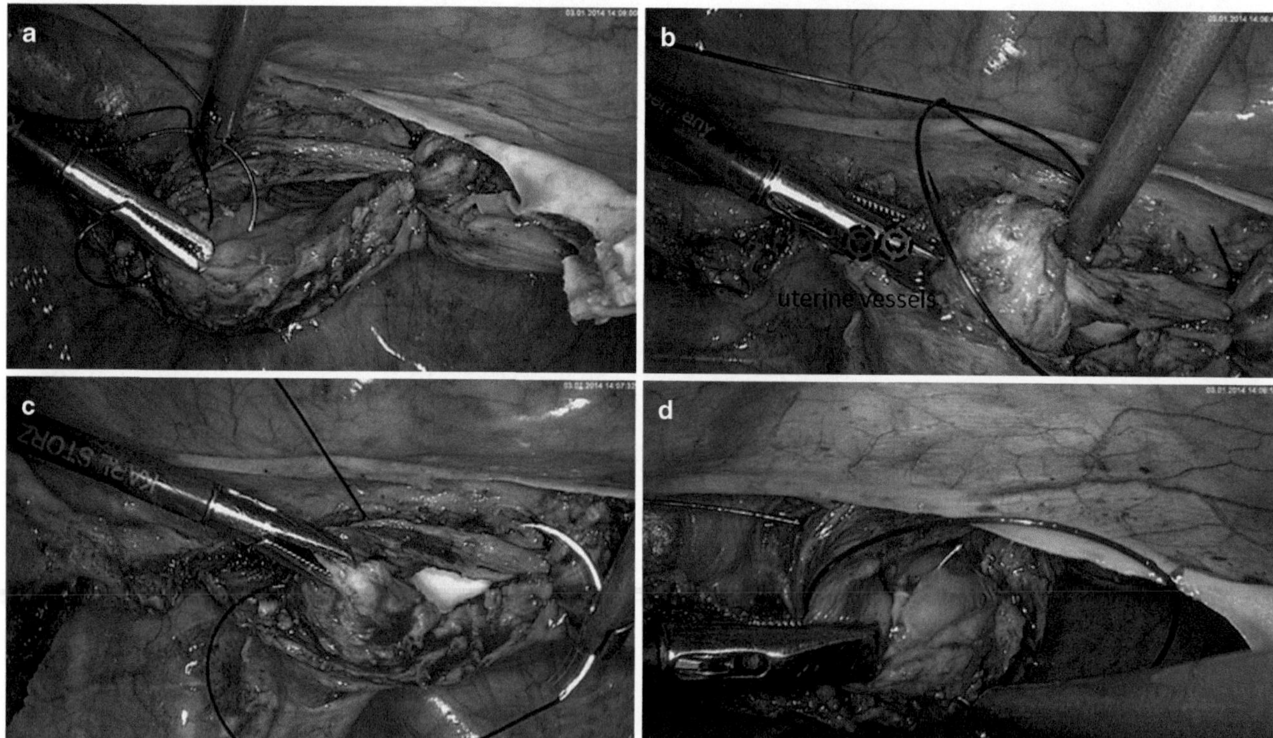

Fig. 35.76 LTH: Continuation of the left corner suture. (**a**) Grabbing and perforation of the dorsal vaginal wall with the needle, (**b**) avoiding the laterally positioned vessels (**c**–**d**) in an omega fashion. When using this type of suture, the vessel stump is omitted and compressed mechanically. Approximately 1 cm of the vaginal wall should be included in the suture

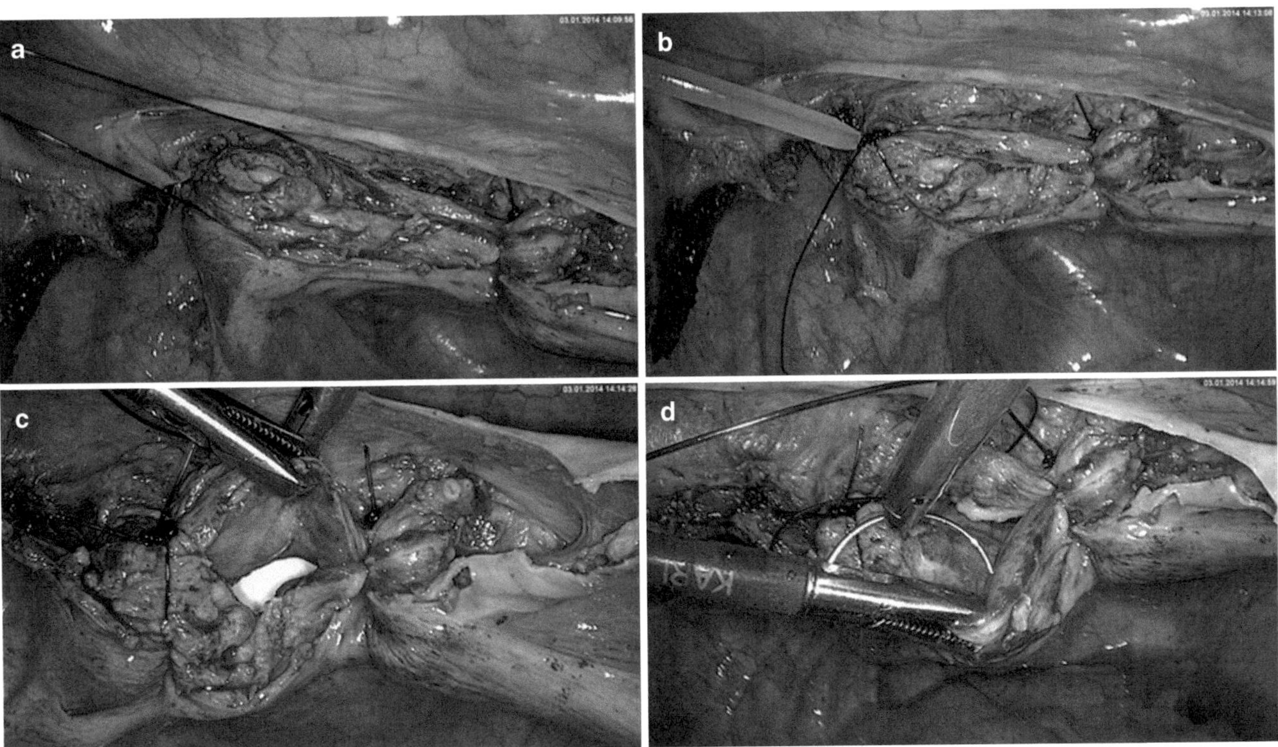

Fig. 35.77 LTH: Completion of the left corner suture.The extracorporeal knot is pushed down by the pushrod (**a–c**). Commencement of a U-stitch or a Z-stitch in the middle (**d**). When the vaginal cuff is not entirely dry, it will be easier to close the edges first. A large part of the bleeding then stops automatically and further coagulation will not be necessary. Severe coagulation on the vaginal wall might increase the risk of vaginal stump infection or dehiscence

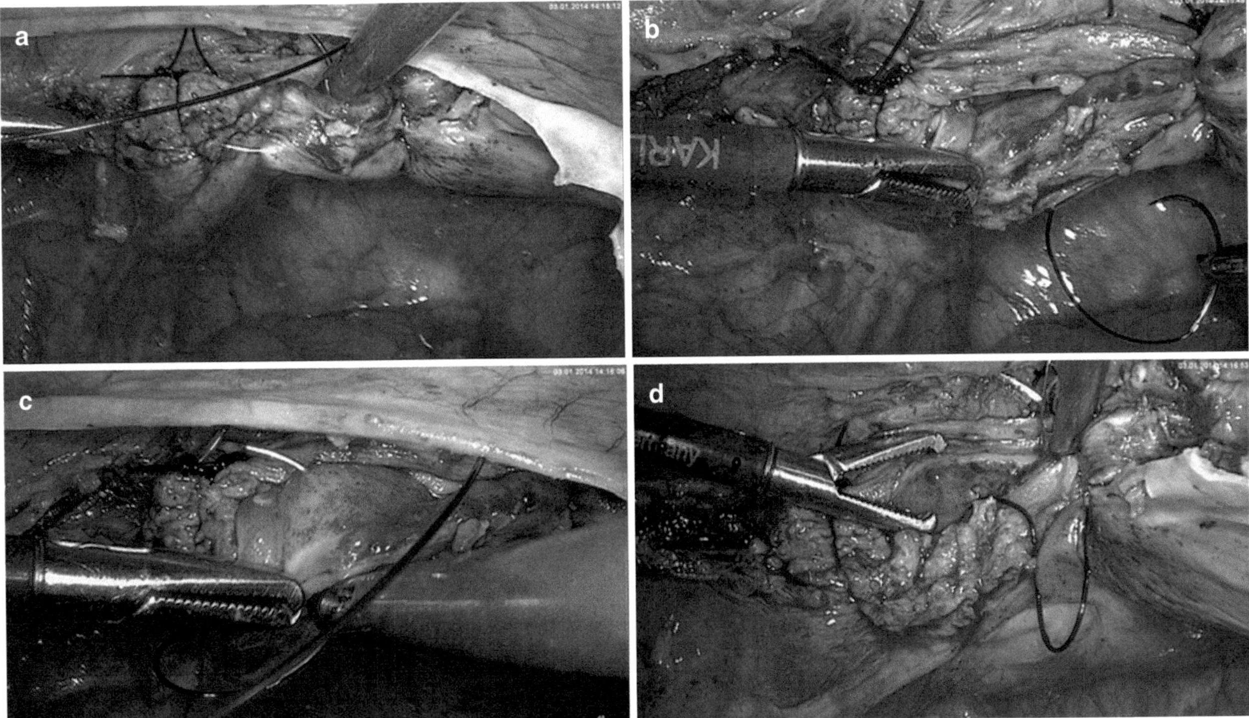

Fig. 35.78 LTH: Final closure of the remaining vaginal opening with (**a**) a U-suture or a Z-suture. (**b**) Grabbing the anterior and posterior wall and (**c**) going straight back. (**d**) The left hand correctly positions the tissue which is to be grabbed, as is necessary in conventional laparoscopy. When using the U-suture, the suture end should reach the bladder to prevent bowel damage

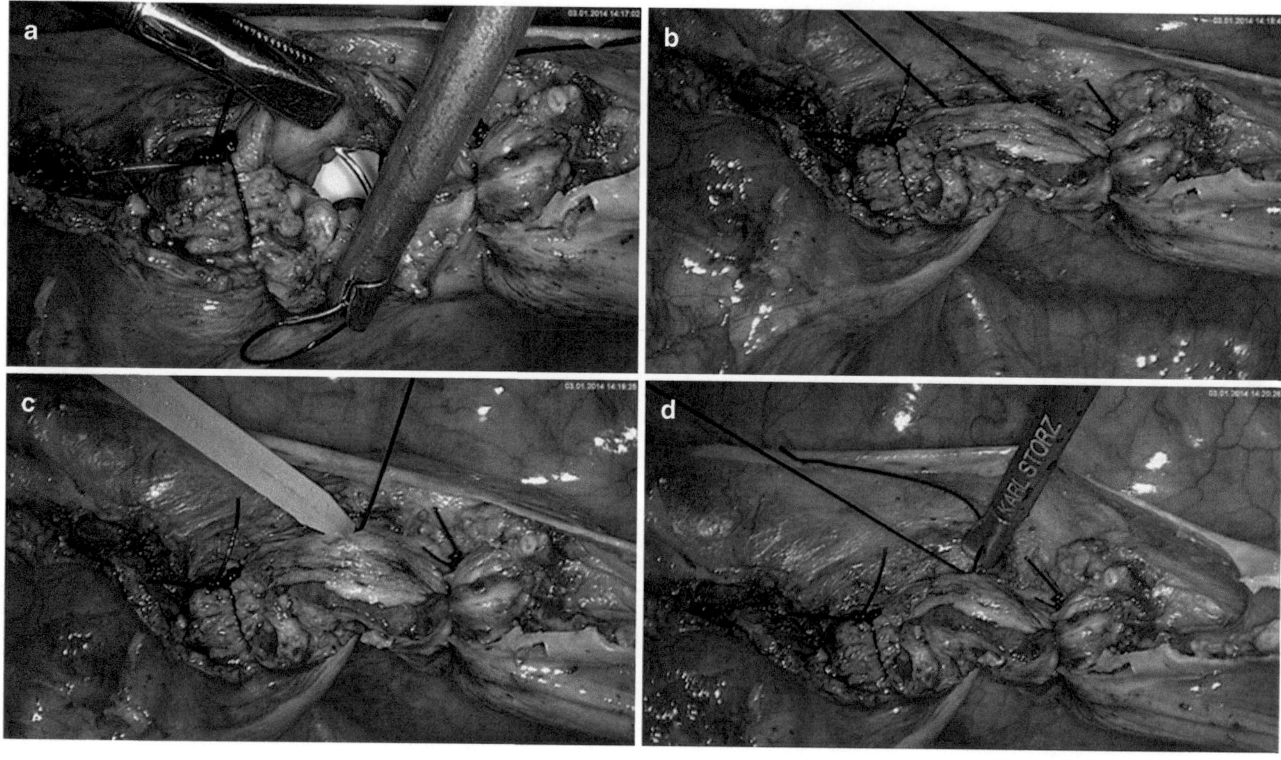

Fig. 35.79 LTH: (**a**) Completion of the central suture with a U-stitch or a Z-stitch. (**b**) Both threads of the U-stitch are pulled out anteriorily and (**c**) after extracorpoeral knotting (**d**) the thread can be shortened. There is no need for extracorporeal suturing because the suture is set ideally and the tissue mass is adequate

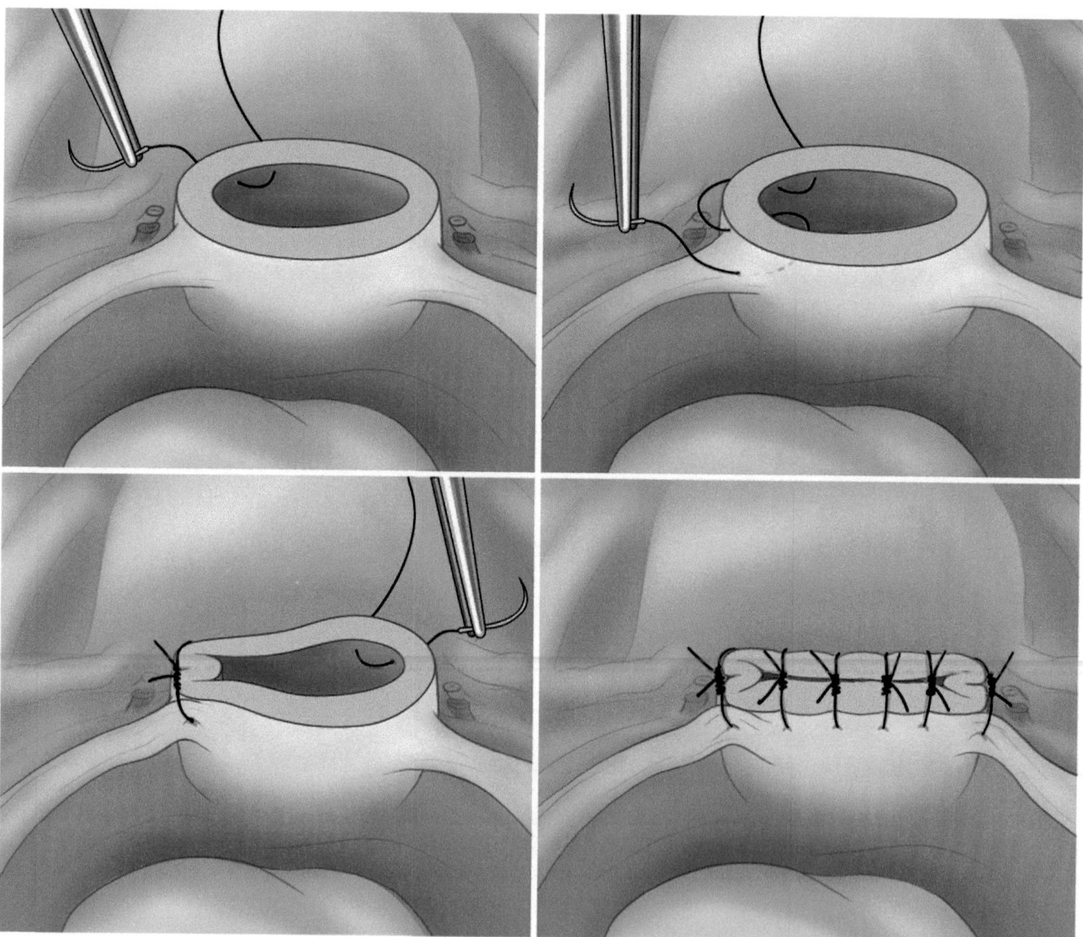

Laparoscopic Subtotal Hysterectomy

In laparoscopic supracervical hysterectomy, resection of the uterine corpus is performed at this stage of surgery. The preceding steps are very similar except for the fact that a manipulator is not needed because the uterus is elevated by traction. The corpus of the uterus is cut with a monopolar loop and the cervical channel is coagulated to prevent spotting. The cervical channel should be closed because of the high risk of ascending infection. Simultaneously, the cervix can be suspended with a strong monofilament suture and extracorporeal knotting. The remaining uterine corpus needs to be morcellated intraabdominally (Figs. 35.81, 35.82, 35.83, 35.84, 35.85 and 35.86).

Figure 35.87 shows the outcome of supracervical and total hysterectomy.

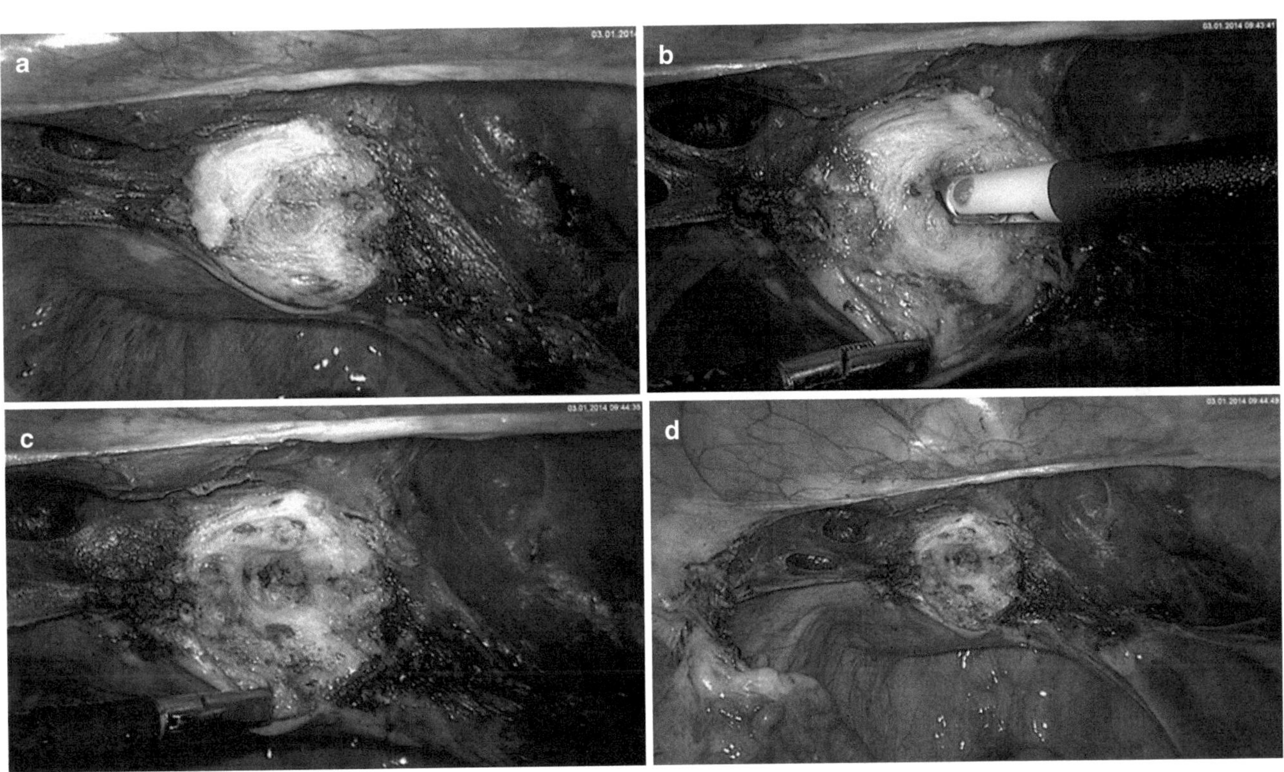

Fig. 35.81 The remaining cervical stump. Especially in cases of bleeding disorders, adenomyosis of the uterus or endometriosis, extended coagulation of the remaining cervical channel should be performed (**a–c**). By pulling the uterus upward when cutting the cervix, resection if performed in the shape of an inverse cone (**d**)

Fig. 35.80 Schematic illustration of vaginal closure after LTH modified by Schollmeyer. A suture is passed through the endopelvic fascia, 1 cm below the cephalad edge of the vaginal epithelium. The needle is pushed from the vaginal lumen through the vaginal wall, passed between the uterine vessels (median part of the broad ligament), and returned through the vaginal lumen. The sacrouterine ligament is identified before the suture is passed through. The needle is pushed from the vaginal lumen through the vaginal wall and the rectovaginal septum, and pierces the sacrouterine ligament. Closure of the vaginal vault with single stiches, U-stiches or Z-stitches. The stitch is drawn through the endopelvic fascia and the vaginal wall, and then out of the vaginal wall and the endopelvic fascia

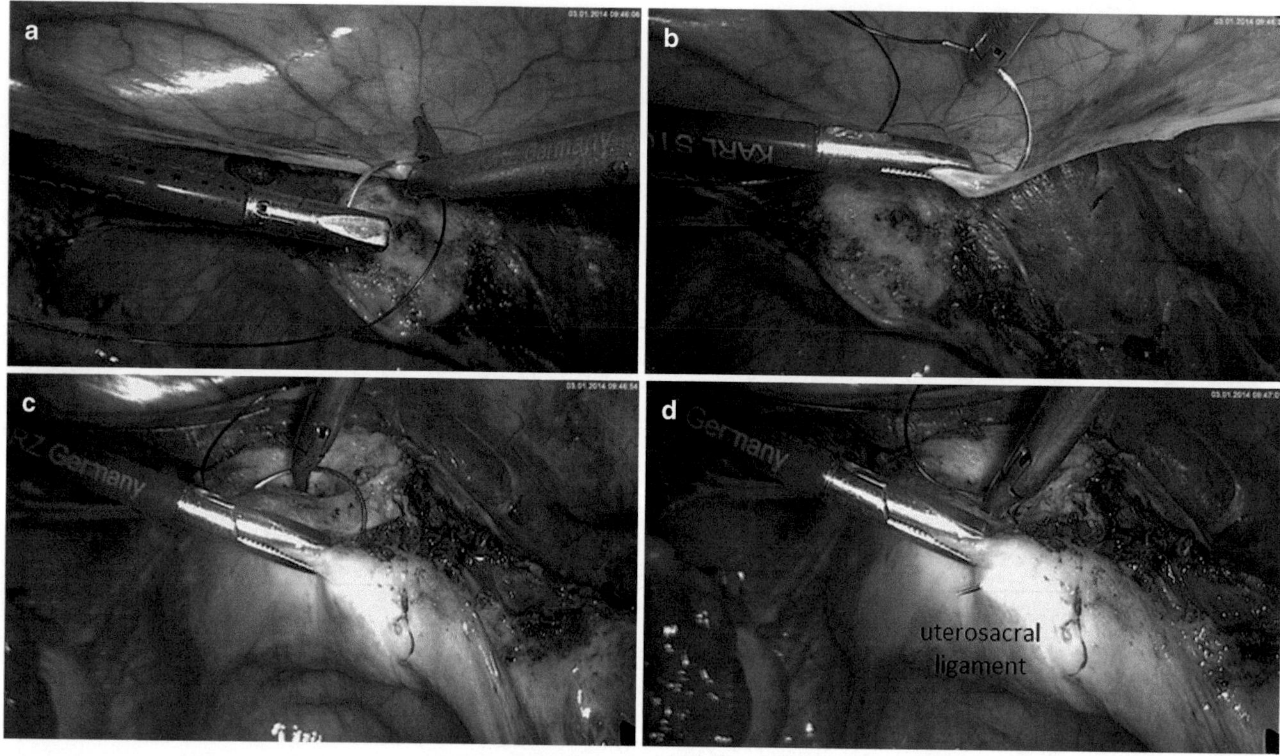

Fig. 35.82 LSH: (**a–d**) As the conjunction of the sacrouterine ligaments has been omitted, the two ligaments are grabbed and included in the suture to achieve cervical suspension (**a**). Connection of the bladder peritoneum to the posterior peritoneum by means of a purse-string suture

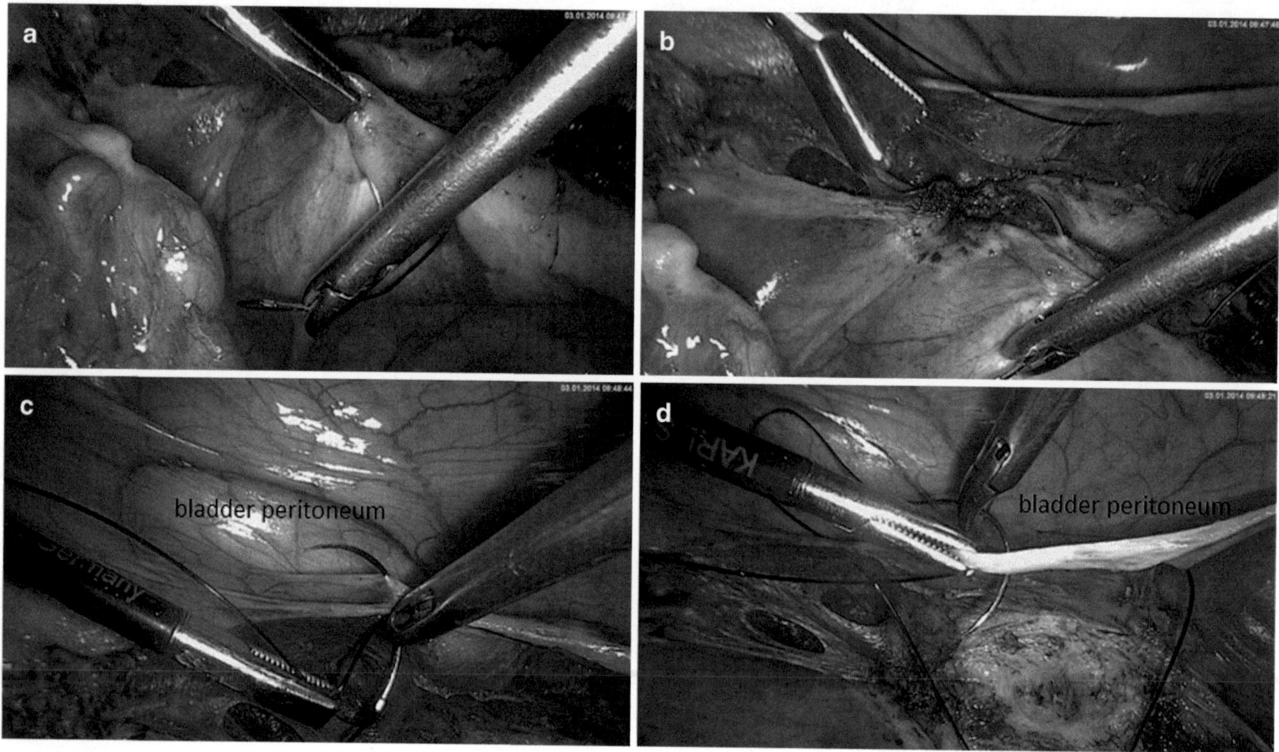

Fig. 35.83 (**a–b**) The sacrouterine ligaments can be identified and included in the closure of the cervical stump.(**c–d**) As the bladder has been slightly exposed during the procedure, there is now enough tissue to functionally close the cervical channel

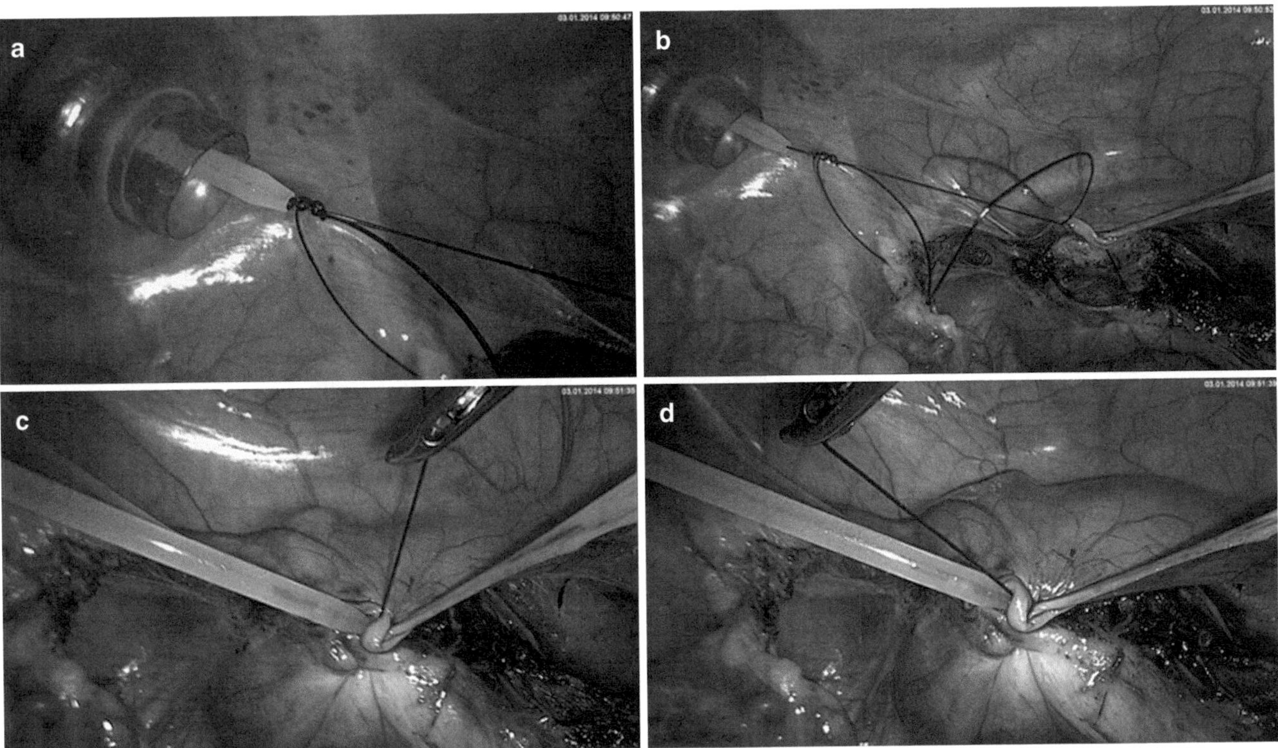

Fig. 35.84 When using the extracorporeal knot, the peritoneum closes the cervical channel functionally and this leads to cervical suspension. (**a**) The extracorporeally performed knot is (**b**) pushed inside. (**c**) Placement on the cervical stump and (**d**) tightening. The omitted sides still permit drainage if necessary

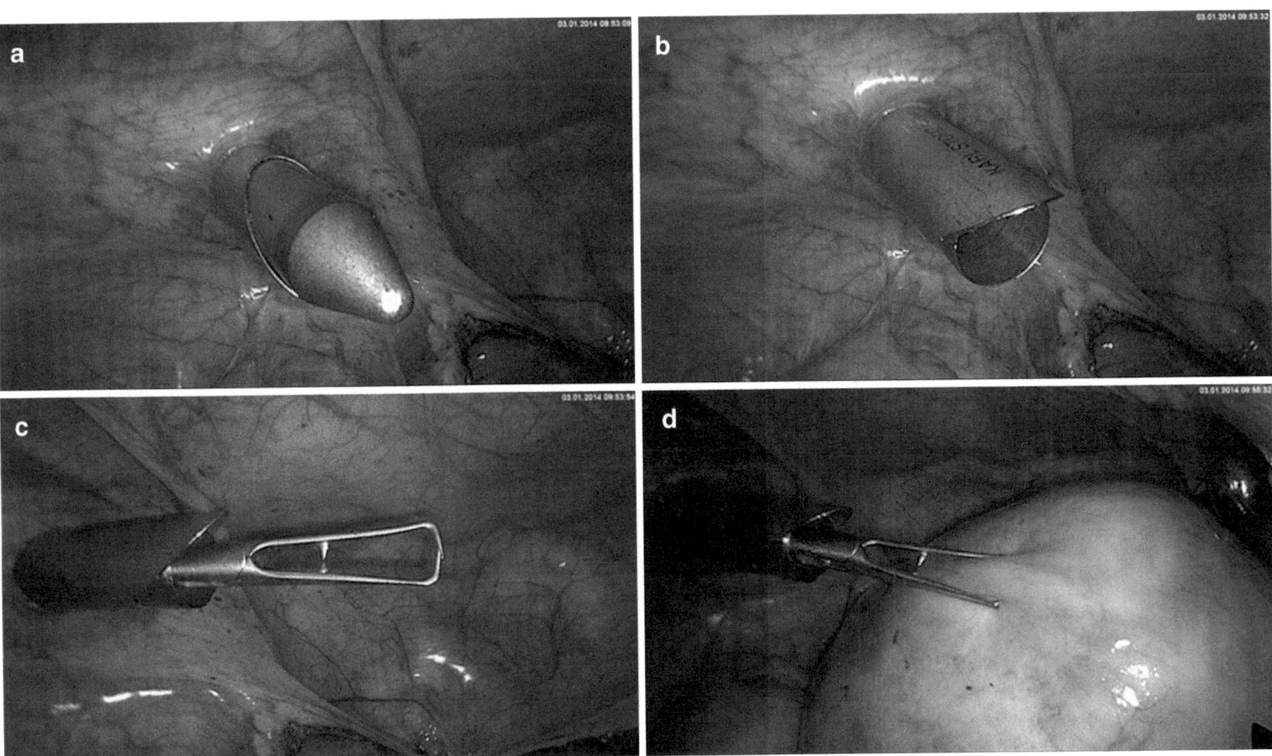

Fig. 35.85 (**a–d**) Introduction of the Roto-Cut morcellator, which is available in diameters of 12 and 15 mm. The knife should be protected by the shield and the tenaculum should be used under direct vision, regardless of the size of the uterus

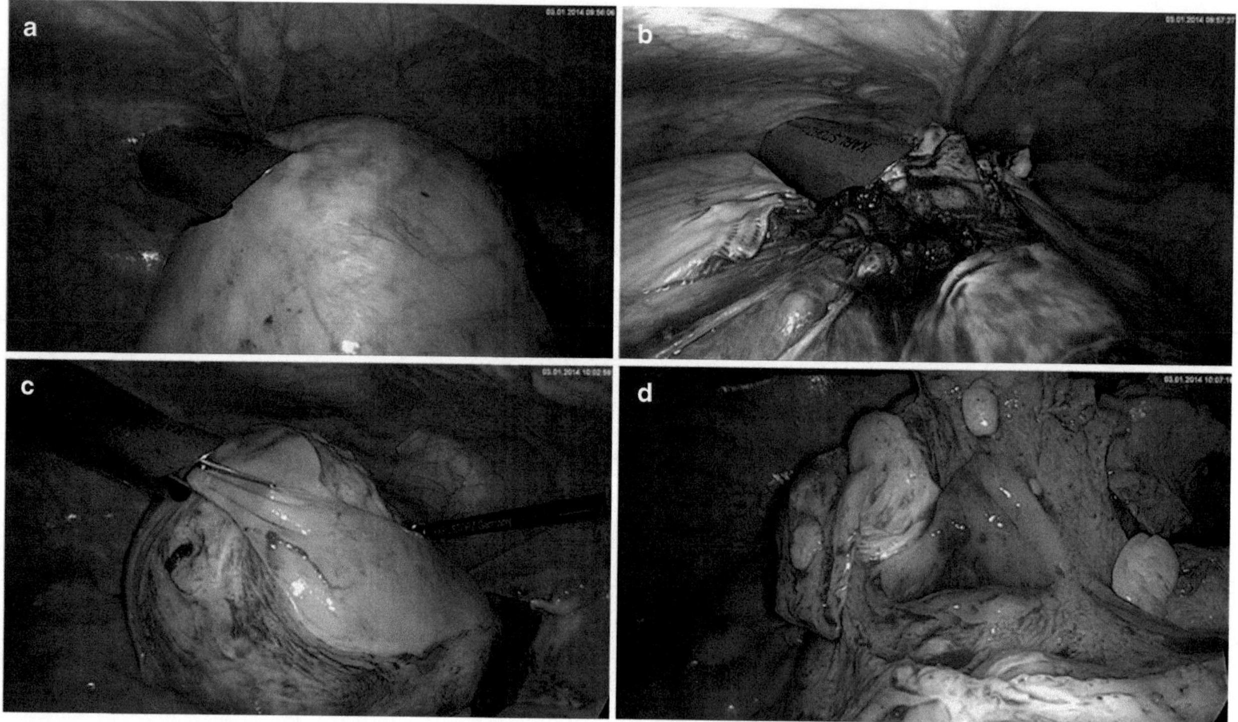

Fig. 35.86 LSH: (**a**) Morcellation of the myomatous uterus (850 g) under (**b**) continuous observation of the rotating cutting edge and (**c**) the protective shield of the morcellator. The protective shield should be directed upward to the abdominal wall in order to avoid cutting the vessels of the abdominal wall. Nevertheless, the lower part, especially the small bowel, must be exposed and kept out of the field of operation. (**d**) The surgeon must be patient and observant in order to avoid cutting into the bowel, which is one of the major complications in the LSH procedure

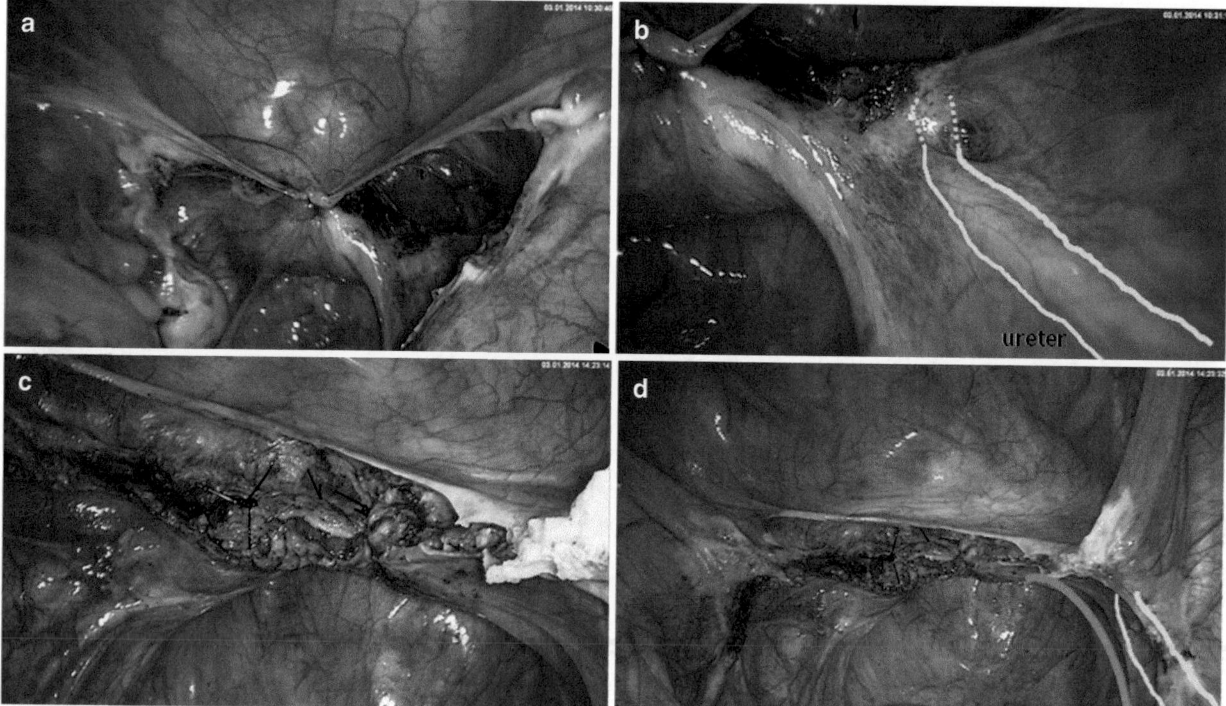

Fig. 35.87 (**a, b**) Final situs after LASH. The cervical channel is covered by peritoneum and both sacrouterine ligaments are under slight tension, thus fixing the middle compartment and the cervical ring. (**c, d**) Final situs after LTH. Closure of vaginal stump has been performed; the sacrouterine ligaments have been elevated by 2 corner sutures. The peritoneum closes the cervical channel, and drainage can be effected on both sides. Both sacrouterine ligaments are under slight tension, thus ensuring colposuspension. Reperitonealization will occur approximately 2 weeks after the operation. The PDS suture allows safe closure and healing of the vaginal cuff because absorption occurs only after about 6 months. The sacrouterine ligaments and the ureter can be clearly identified. Since the anatomy of the ureter has not been affected, opening of the retroperitoneum and its visualization are not necessary

Special Situations

The traditional technique of laparoscopic hysterectomy must be modified in cases of severe adhesions or concomitant deep infiltrating endometriosis. The surgical steps are quite similar to those for oncologic surgery; radical pelvic exposure is essential (Figs. 35.17, 35.18, and 35.40). After adhesiolysis, which may be very extensive in severe endometriosis or adenomyosis, the retroperitoneum is opened (Figs. 35.52, 35.88 and 35.89). The ureter and major vessels are localized, and the crossover of the uterine artery is visualized and exposed (Fig. 35.89). In some cases, clipping of the uterine artery just behind its point of departure from the internal iliac artery (Figs. 35.90, 35.91, 35.92 and 35.93) is useful for the following reasons:

1. More distal preparation and skeletonization of the uterine artery may be difficult or even impossible.
2. Endometriotic scars and nodules are liable to modify the anatomy of the region. This may lead to unexpected bleeding, especially in cases of a larger uterus. Clipping of the initial portion of the uterine artery will minimize intraoperative bleeding.

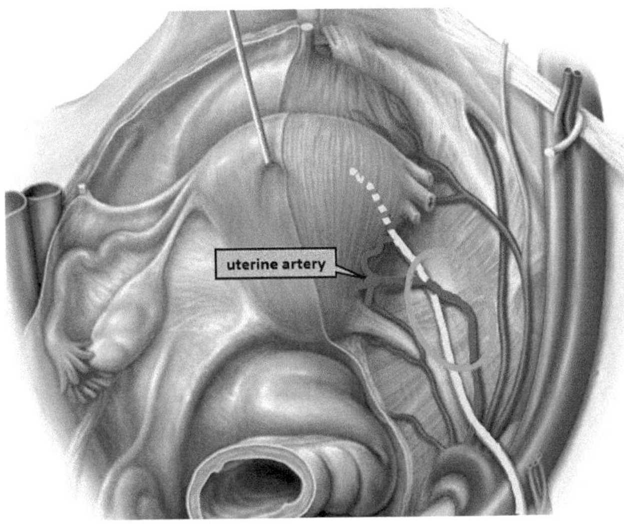

Fig. 35.88 Any uterine pathology may cause major difficulties in exposing the lateral uterine wall and the ascending branch of the uterine artery. Furthermore, all radical hysterectomies include the parametrium and imply a distal resection margin. This might make it necessary to expose the retroperitoneum and localize the departure of the uterine artery from the internal iliac artery

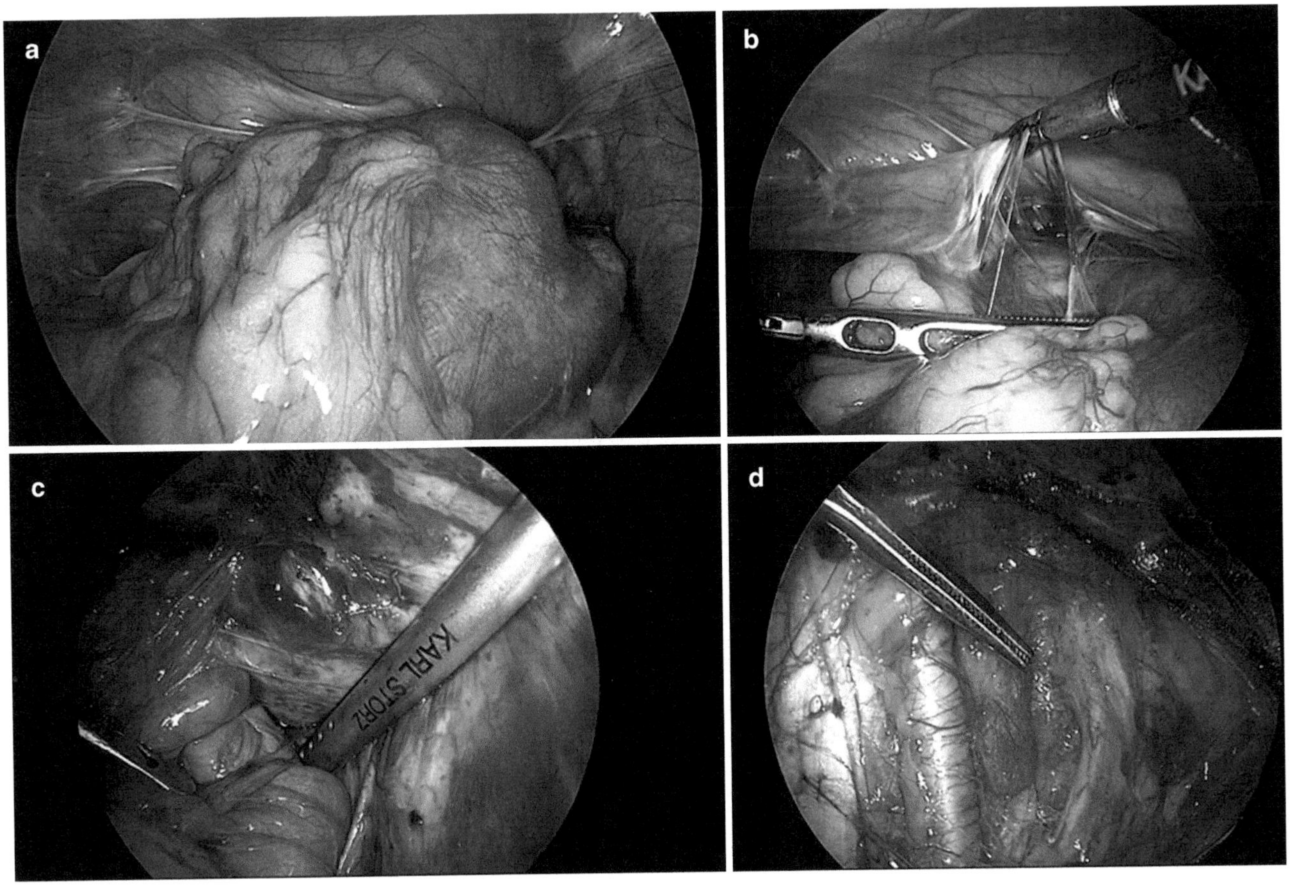

Fig. 35.89 A case of severe adenomyosis of the uterus with subsequent adhesions of the bowel (**a**) and the bladder (**b**) peritoneum. Access to the lateral aspect of the uterus is closed (**c**); retroperitoneal access is necessary (**d**)

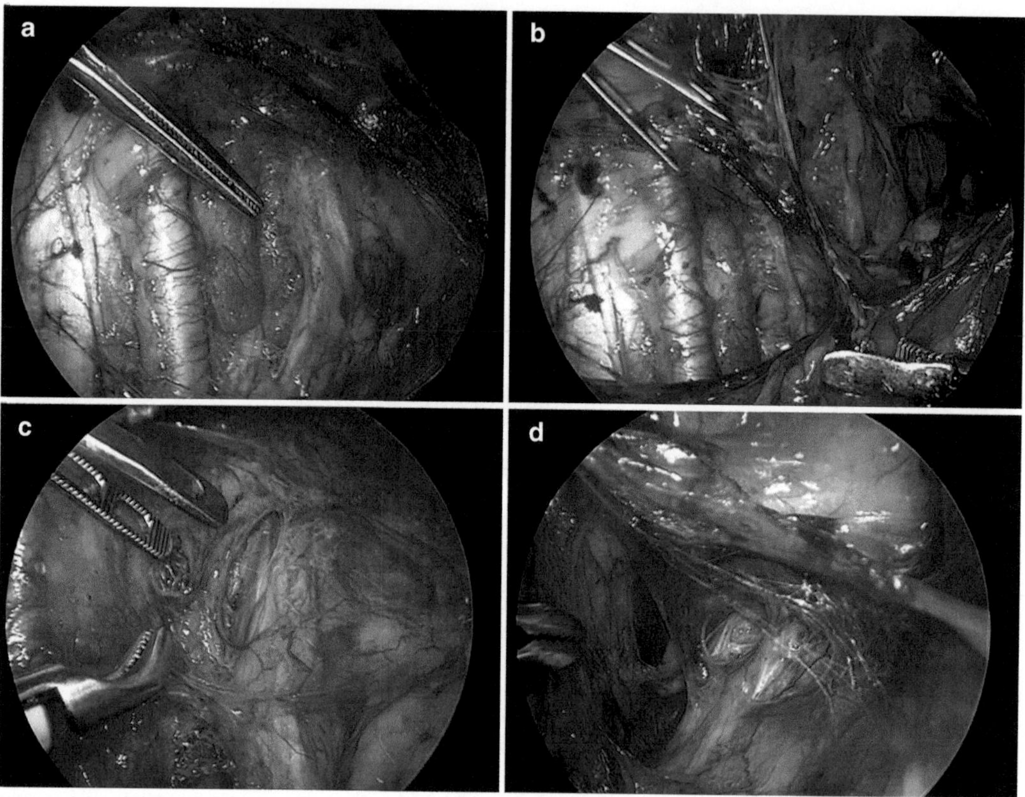

Fig. 35.90 (**a**) After localization of the external iliac artery, the ureter is usually found adherent to the peritoneum. A major lymph node lies in between.(**b**) Opening of the pararectal and (**c**) the paravesical fossa. (**d**) The crossing point of the uterine artery is demarcated, and the ureter is left in its adventitia to avoid skeletonizing and denudation

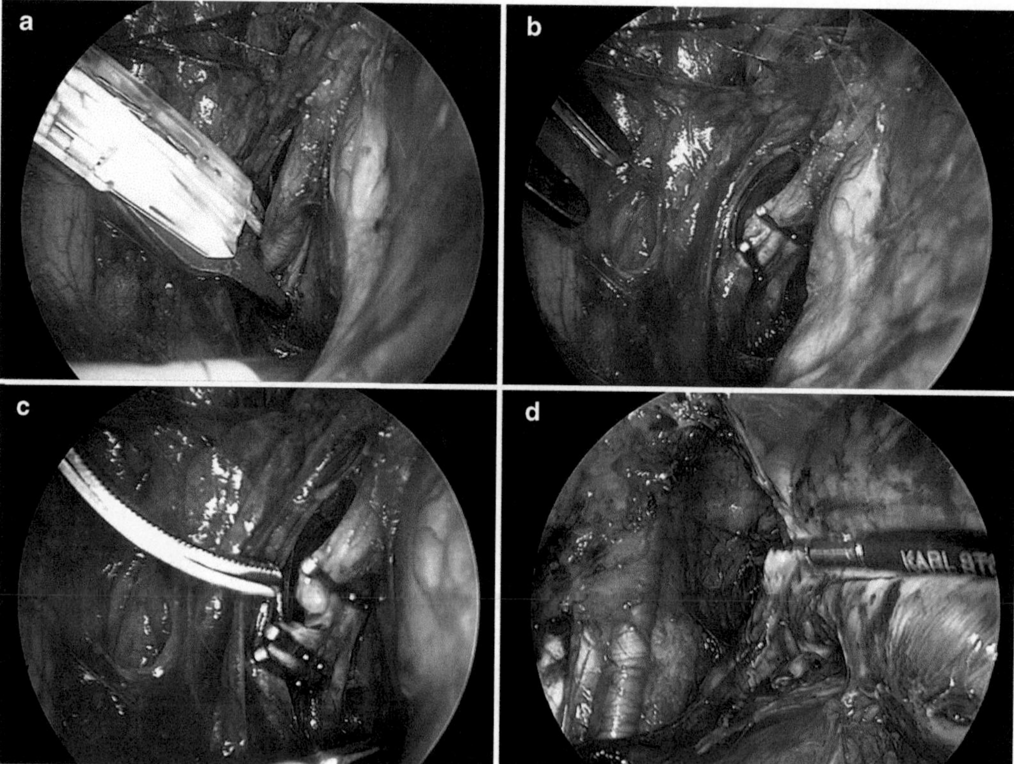

Fig. 35.91 (**a–b**) Clips can be inserted and the artery can be closed and cut (**c**). (**c**) The uterine vein (deep) is seen just beneath the cut artery.(**d**) Overview of the exposed situs. To the right you see the uncolored uterus after closure of both arteries

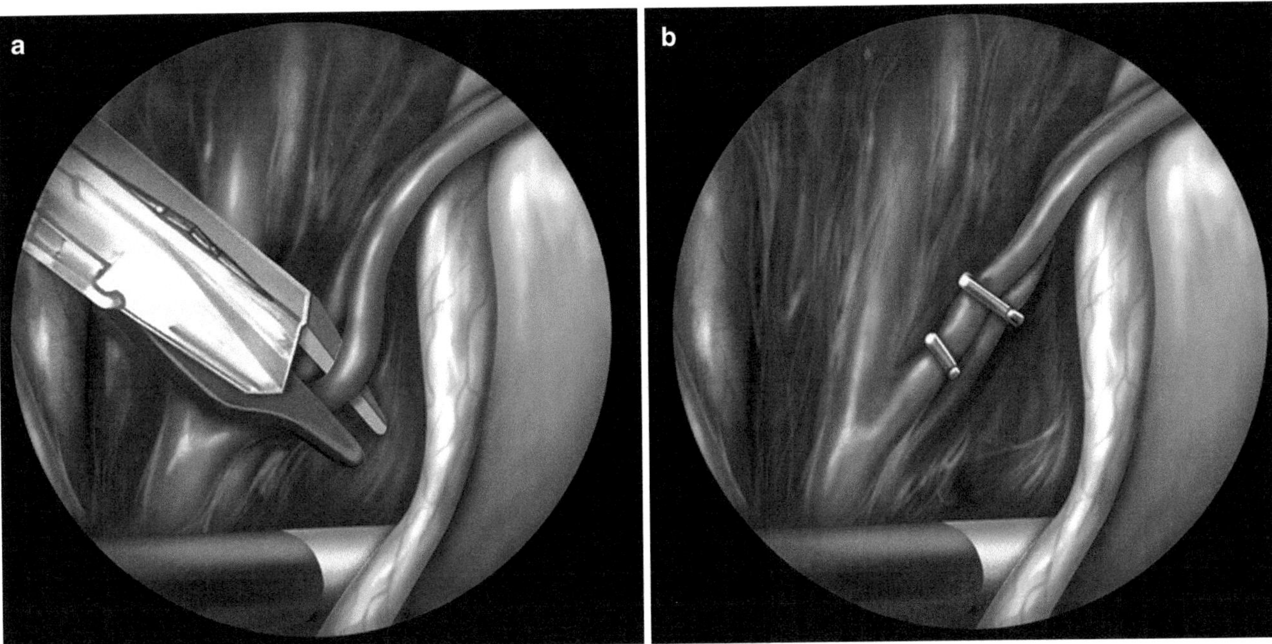

Fig. 35.92 (a–b) Schematic illustration of the retroperitoneal area where the ureter is undercrossing the uterine artery. The uterine vain is usually divided into a superficial part and a deep part. Clips can be set after medializing the ureter

Fig. 35.93 The anatomy of the ureter provides crucial information.(**a**) Vascularization is effected from the upper part: the renal artery, the ovarian artery, and the aorta. In the lower part the ureter is supplied by lateral vessels: the iliac vessels and the uterine artery. Blunt dissection causes minor bleeding at the respective location.(**b**) The histological cross-section shows that vascular supply is located in the adventitia. Therefore, electricity or manipulation causing destruction of the adventitia may lead to secondary fistulas and/or leakage

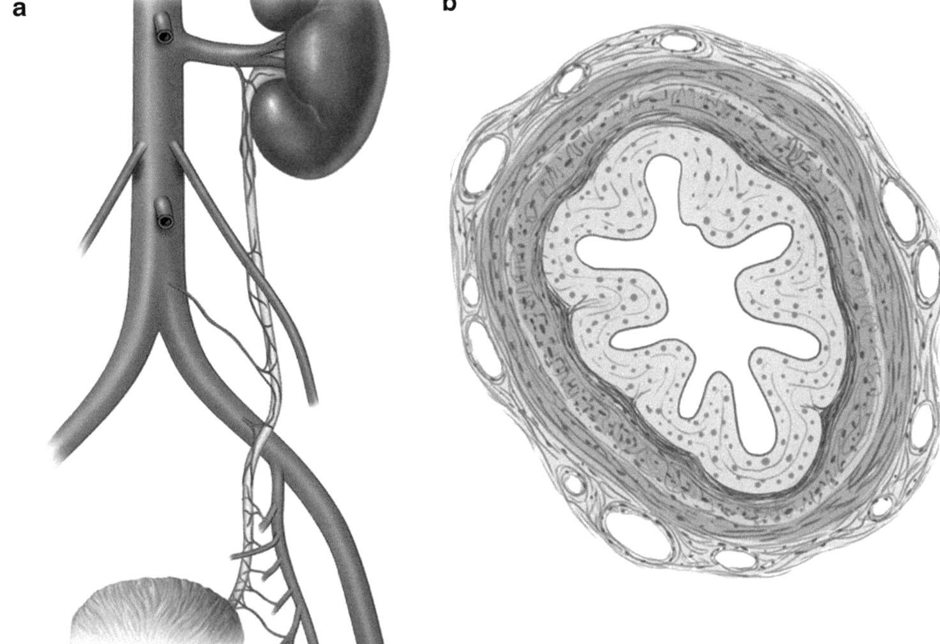

3. The proximity of the uterine artery to the ureter and the thermal spread of bipolar instruments may cause secondary coagulation defects of the ureter, which can be avoided by using vessel clips.

At the end of the procedure the abdominal cavity is irrigated with physiological saline solution and drained. Usually no drains are left in situ (Fig. 35.89).

We established this suture technique because it provides stable fixation of the vaginal end in addition to other safety advantages:

1. As the suture is applied parallel to the urethra, kinking of the ureters is avoided. The thread is led through the medial part of the cardinal ligament, along the anterior-posterior access.

2. Compression of small vessels between the vaginal wall and uterine artery within the cardinal ligament minimizes the risk of bleeding.
3. Despite good suspension there is no relevant displacement of the vaginal access dorsally, which might increase the risk of a cystocele.

Post-hysterectomy Inspection

The pedicles, bladder, ureters and bowel must be inspected under continuous irrigation with Ringer's lactate or Adept (Baxter). Ureter movement is no proof of integrity. In cases of suspected damage to the ureter or kinking of the ureter while closing the vagina, the ureter must be visualized by opening the retroperitoneum and ureterolysis performed until the ureter enters the parametria (Fig. 35.93). Alternatively, methylene blue can be injected. If no dye is seen intraabdominally, severe damage is unlikely. In critical cases the integrity of the ureter can be proven by performing an intravenous pyelogram two to three days after the operation.

Postoperative Management

The urinary catheter is removed; it remains in place only in specific cases. A postoperative cystoscopy is performed in cases of severe endometriosis or adhesions in the upper part of the bladder. Early ambulation a few hours after surgery is good practice. Clear fluids can be ingested 6 h post-surgery, followed by a light diet. Thromboprophylaxis (mechanical and medical) must be used in appropriate cases. The patient can be discharged after 8–12 h. A postoperative ultrasound scan of the renal pelvis should be performed. Ordinary light activities are permitted and the patient may return to work after 4–5 days. Sexual activity, intensive sports and heavy work should be avoided for 6–8 weeks.

Anticipated Problems

Vital symptoms, pain and temperature must be carefully monitored during the first 8 h. A patient who is discharged early must be given a phone number she may call in case of distress or pain. The insertion of a drain is not necessary. Fever, early pain, abdominal distension, delirium, decreased urine output, the shock index and hypotension must be recognized and attended to immediately, as these may be signs of complications.

Summary and Conclusions

In addition to the well-known laparoscopic techniques for myomectomy and hysteroscopic techniques for submucous fibroidectomy, laparoscopic subtotal and total hysterectomy are surgical options for the treatment of multiple fibroids. The surgical procedure is decided upon jointly by the patient and the doctor. The individual steps described in this chapter help the gynecological surgeon to perform a satisfactory operation and eliminate the onerous burden of multiple fibroids in patients who have completed planning their families.

Conclusion

1. The transformation of classic intrafascial hysterectomy into laparoscopic hysterectomy, or even total atraumatic intrafascial laparoscopic hysterectomy (TAIL), is the first step for the prevention of a descensus. The uterine manipulator and the structured procedure have made laparoscopic hysterectomy a much safer option [28].
2. In a comparison of various methods to avoid prolapse during vaginal hysterectomy, McCall culdoplasty proved to be the most effective technique in the short term and after three years [39]. A similar procedure is used for abdominal hysterectomy [40, 41]. The method was modified by Harry Reich and adapted for laparoscopic procedures. One of its disadvantages is the unification of two lateral sutures in the midline, which results in an unphysiological narrowing of the apical pole of the vagina. As transposition of the ureters bears the risk of kinking it would be advisable to use van Herendael's modified suture technique, which avoids this risk [37].

References

1. Kovac SR. Route of hysterectomy: an evidence-based approach. Clin Obstet Gynecol. 2014;57(1):58–71.
2. Schollmeyer T et al. Hysterectomy trends over a 9-year period in an endoscopic teaching center. Int J Gynaecol Obstet. 2014;126(1): 45–9.
3. Lefebvre G et al. SOGC clinical guidelines. Hysterectomy. J Obstet Gynaecol Can. 2002;24(1):37–61. quiz 74–6.
4. Stang A, Merrill RM, Kuss O. Hysterectomy in Germany: a DRG-based nationwide analysis, 2005–2006. Dtsch Arztebl Int. 2011;108(30):508–14.
5. Brummer TH, Seppala TT, Harkki PS. National learning curve for laparoscopic hysterectomy and trends in hysterectomy in Finland 2000–2005. Hum Reprod. 2008;23(4):840–5.
6. Prevention, C.f.D.C.a., Women's reproductive health: hysterectomy fact sheet, D.o.R. Health, Editor. 2009: 1600 Clifton Rd. Atlanta, GA 30333, USA.
7. Hanstede MM et al. Regional and temporal variation in hysterectomy rates and surgical routes for benign diseases in the Netherlands. Acta Obstet Gynecol Scand. 2012;91(2):220–5.
8. Alkatout I et al. Precarious preoperative diagnostics and hints for the laparoscopic excision of uterine adenomatoid tumors: two exemplary cases and literature review. Fertil Steril. 2011;95(3): 1119 e5–8.
9. Alkatout I et al. Principles and safety measures of electrosurgery in laparoscopy. JSLS. 2012;16(1):130–9.
10. Hughes E, et al., Ovulation suppression for endometriosis.Cochrane Database Syst Rev. 2007;(3): p. CD000155.

11. Lethaby A, V Ivanova, NP Johnson. Total versus subtotal hysterectomy for benign gynaecological conditions.Cochrane Database Syst Rev. 2006;(2): p. CD004993.
12. Thakar R et al. Outcomes after total versus subtotal abdominal hysterectomy. N Engl J Med. 2002;347(17):1318–25.
13. Gorlero F et al. Hysterectomy and women satisfaction: total versus subtotal technique. Arch Gynecol Obstet. 2008;278(5):405–10.
14. Roovers JP et al. Hysterectomy and sexual wellbeing: prospective observational study of vaginal hysterectomy, subtotal abdominal hysterectomy, and total abdominal hysterectomy. BMJ. 2003; 327(7418):774–8.
15. Ascher-Walsh CJ et al. Location of adenomyosis in total hysterectomy specimens. J Am Assoc Gynecol Laparosc. 2003;10(3): 360–2.
16. Sarmini OR, Lefholz K, Froeschke HP. A comparison of laparoscopic supracervical hysterectomy and total abdominal hysterectomy outcomes. J Minim Invasive Gynecol. 2005;12(2):121–4.
17. BMI, Demography Report: Report of the German federal government on the demographic situation and future development of the country 2011, German Federal Ministry of the Interior.
18. Nygaard I, Bradley C, Brandt D. Pelvic organ prolapse in older women: prevalence and risk factors. Obstet Gynecol. 2004; 104(3):489–97.
19. Olsen AL et al. Epidemiology of surgically managed pelvic organ prolapse and urinary incontinence. Obstet Gynecol. 1997;89(4): 501–6.
20. Symmonds RE, Pratt JH. Vaginal prolapse following hysterectomy. Am J Obstet Gynecol. 1960:79:899–909.
21. Toozs-Hobson P, Boos K, Cardozo L. Management of vaginal vault prolapse. Br J Obstet Gynaecol. 1998;105(1):13–7.
22. Marchionni M et al. True incidence of vaginal vault prolapse. Thirteen years of experience. J Reprod Med. 1999;44(8):679–84.
23. Swift SE, Pound T, Dias JK. Case-control study of etiologic factors in the development of severe pelvic organ prolapse. Int Urogynecol J Pelvic Floor Dysfunct. 2001;12(3):187–92.
24. Elessawy M et al. The incidence of complications by hysterectomy for benign disease in correlation to an assumed preoperative score. Arch Gynecol Obstet. 2014;292(1):127–33.
25. Reich H. Laparoscopic oophorectomy and salpingo-oophorectomy in the treatment of benign tubo-ovarian disease. Int J Fertil. 1987;32(3):233–6.
26. Mettler L et al. Comparative evaluation of classical intrafascial-supracervical hysterectomy (CISH) with transuterine mucosal resection as performed by pelviscopy and laparotomy–our first 200 cases. Surg Endosc. 1995;9(4):418–23.
27. Semm K. Hysterectomy via laparotomy or pelviscopy. A new CASH method without colpotomy. Geburtshilfe Frauenheilkd. 1991;51(12):996–1003.
28. Hohl MK, Hauser N. Safe total intrafascial laparoscopic (TAIL) hysterectomy: a prospective cohort study. Gynecol Surg. 2010; 7(3):231–9.
29. Schüssler B, Scheidel P, Hohl MK. Hysterektomie update. Frauenheilkunde aktuell. 2008;3:4–12.
30. Veress J. Neues Instrument zur Ausführung von Brust- und Bauchpunktionen und Pneumothoraxbehandlung. Dtsch Med Wochenschr. 1938;64:1480–1.
31. Alkatout I et al. Abdominal anatomy in the context of port placement and trocars. J Turk Ger Gynecol Assoc. 2015;16(4):241–51.
32. Kramer L. Mixed reviews on removing fallopian tubes to prevent ovarian cancer. CMAJ. 2013;185(9):E391–2.
33. Kurman RJ, Shih Ie M. Molecular pathogenesis and extraovarian origin of epithelial ovarian cancer–shifting the paradigm. Hum Pathol. 2011;42(7):918–31.
34. Caceres A, McCarus SD. Fallopian tube prolapse after total laparoscopic hysterectomy. Obstet Gynecol. 2008;112(2 Pt 2):494–5.
35. Altman D et al. Pelvic organ prolapse surgery following hysterectomy on benign indications. Am J Obstet Gynecol. 2008;198(5):572 e1–6.
36. Thompson JD, Warshaw J. Hysterectomy. In: Rock JA, Thompson JD, editors. Te Linde's Operative Gynecology. Philadelphia-New York: Lippincott Raven; 1996. p. 771–854.
37. van Herendael B. Strategies to prevent vaginal vault descent during hysterectomy. In: Mettler L, editor. Manual of new hysterectomy techniques. New Delhi: Jaypee Brothers Medical Publishers (P) Ltd; 2007. p. 82–5.
38. Hur HC et al. Incidence and patient characteristics of vaginal cuff dehiscence after different modes of hysterectomies. J Minim Invasive Gynecol. 2007;14(3):311–7.
39. Cruikshank SH, Kovac SR. Randomized comparison of three surgical methods used at the time of vaginal hysterectomy to prevent posterior enterocele. Am J Obstet Gynecol. 1999;180(4):859–65.
40. Wall LL. A technique for modified McCall culdeplasty at the time of abdominal hysterectomy. J Am Coll Surg. 1994;178(5):507–9.
41. Ostrzenski A. A new, simplified posterior culdoplasty and vaginal vault suspension during abdominal hysterectomy. Int J Gynaecol Obstet. 1995;49(1):25–34.

36 Total Laparoscopic Hysterectomy in Patients with Bulky Uterus

Guenter K. Noé and Michael Anapolski

A big uterus can pose a serious challenge to a gynecologic surgeon in case a total laparoscopic hysterectomy (TLH) is to be performed. Although the basic anatomy of the lesser pelvis does not vary depending on the uterine size, the operative site can present some differences in these patients. Due to the sample size, there is less space in the pelvis and often in the abdominal cavity. This feature restricts the overview and renders more difficult the identification of such anatomical structures as the ureter. If the uterus fills the entire lesser pelvis not only a fast identification and isolation of uterine vessels in the paracervical region is not possible, but also a ligation of the uterine artery leaving the anterior brunch of the hypogastric artery is hardly conceivable. At the same time, the close proximity of the uterus to pelvic walls means a higher risk of an injury to the ureter since its course cannot be easily identified as long as the uterus occludes the field of view. Caused by the uterine size the pedicles of the supplying vessels can often be found in unusual positions (e.g. on the ventral side of the uterus). Due to the larger vessel diameter than in a normal specimen, a bleeding from a uterine artery or vein may result in a serious impairment of the visibility and also lead to a major blood loss. Since the minor branches of the uterine vein can reach the size of a regular normal size uterine vein, they may be mistaken for its major branch. The above mentioned features underline the importance of the correct identification of the supplying vessels prior to their ligation.

Even if the laparoscopic procedure reaches a high level of difficulty, it allows a direct visualization of anatomical structures prior to and during their dissection. This is an important advantage compared to the vaginal approach. Another advantage is the possibility to perform an intrafascial hysterectomy via the laparoscopic route. For hysterectomies scheduled for benign conditions, we prefer this method to conserve as much ligamental and nervous tissue as possible. The intrafascial hysterectomy reduces also the risk of a ureteric injury [1]. This surgical procedure is as a rule possible also in patients with large sized uteri.

The usual preparation sequence of a TLH is a downward dissection that starts in the adnexal region and proceeds towards the uterine vessels. This strategy is not always possible with large uteri since the parauterine and paracervical region may become accessible only after mobilization of the uterus. Such situations require good surgical skills in view of the fact that the usual procedure has to be modified in order to adjust to the situs. We prefer to start with the "easy" side first and proceed to the other side after the uterus gained some mobility. It may be also necessary to switch to the other side before the preparation on the first side is completed. For example, we might dissect the adnexal pedicles on both sides prior to carry on with the dissection on the right side in order to mobilize the uterus and obtain enough space to access the parauterine region. In some cases of bulky uteri, the only accessible region is the anterior aspect of the cervix. Under such circumstances, the dissection should begin here by opening the peritoneal fold. The loose connective tissue in this area can often be pushed away and dissected bluntly towards the lateral aspect of the cervix allowing the access to the uterine vessels. In such cases, the access to the adnexa might be possible only in a retrograde way.

For regular TLH, we usually use an umbilical optic trocar and two working ports – in the left lower abdomen and in the suprasymphysary area. The uterine manipulator is usually handled by the operating nurse. For bulky uteri, we place an additional trocar in the right lower abdomen. The

G.K. Noé (✉)
Department of OB/GYN, University of Witten/Herdecke, Hospital Dormagen, Dormagen, Germany
e-mail: Karl-guenter.noe@kkh-ne.de

M. Anapolski
Obstetrics and Gynaecology, Community Hospital Dormagen, Dr.-Geldmacher-St. 20, Dormagen 41540, Germany
e-mail: michael.anapolski@kkh-ne.de

I. Alkatout, L. Mettler (eds.), *Hysterectomy*, DOI 10.1007/978-3-319-22497-8_36

uterine manipulator can be controlled by an additional person since the operating nurse should avoid any distractions in order to allow a rapid reaction to eventual bleedings. To simplify the preparation and fasten the course of surgery we prefer to use combination instruments, allowing to seal and dissect the tissue without changing the device. Depending on the degree of difficulty, such tools may significantly shorten the time requirement, although the most part of them are designed for a single use and lead hence to higher operative costs.

Although a TLH can be performed in a freehand mode, we prefer the use of a manipulator with a cervical cup. In difficult situations, such as with a bulky uterus, this device helps to increase the distance to bladder and ureter during the dissection process. Different types of manipulators are available on the market with different additional functions and degrees of freedom. We prefer to use manipulators without a uterine spike because it restricts the ability to move the uterus manually within the abdominal cavity.

In a case of a "regular" intrafascial TLH, there is no particular need to expose the ureter in its entire course. With a bulky uterus, the visualization of the ureter prior to and during the dissection is rarely possible, so that it might be reasonable to perform it at least after the uterus removal. If any doubts exist – e.g. in case the dissection was carried out in a close proximity of the ureter – a placement of a ureteric stent should be considered. If a hydronephrosis is known before the surgery, a ureteric stent should be inserted prior to the intervention. To exclude a thermal injury – e.g. a stricture of the ureter – an intravenous pyelogram or a CT-scan can be conducted in the postoperative course. One should bear in mind, that such changes take some time to develop and unsuspicious results might be false negative in case the examination was carried out shortly after the surgery.

Although the closure of the vaginal vault can be performed by a vaginal approach, good endoscopic suturing skills are essential for a TLH since an additional ligation of major uterine vessels might be necessary. We usually perform a continuous endoscopic suturing of the vagina using absorbable material.

As a rule, the uterus can be extracted vaginally after a regular TLH. In case of a bulky uterus, the vaginal route is often not an option to remove the specimen in toto. Under the given conditions, tissue extraction is a serious issue since previously undetected malignancy, premalignant conditions and myoma tissue might be disseminated in the abdominal cavity during power morcellation [2–5]. To address this concern, some authors proposed to carry out a manual vaginal morcellation [6]. Another option is a laparoscopic power morcellation inside an endobag [7–9]. Different devices were developed by the industry recently, but the exact quantification of the risk reduction for spread of uterine sarcoma, endometrial cancer, smooth muscle tumor of uncertain malignant potential (STUMP) and parasitic myoma is not yet available at present.

Technique

A big Uterus is not only defined by weight but also by the volume relatively to the volume of the intra-abdominal space. The problem for the surgeon is primary the lack of space to move and the reduced field of view. Different strategies are suggested as mentioned above.

To obtain a good overview many authors recommend to position the optic trocar 2–4 cm above the umbilicus. According to the position different access-port placements are known (Figs. 36.1, 36.2, and 36.3).

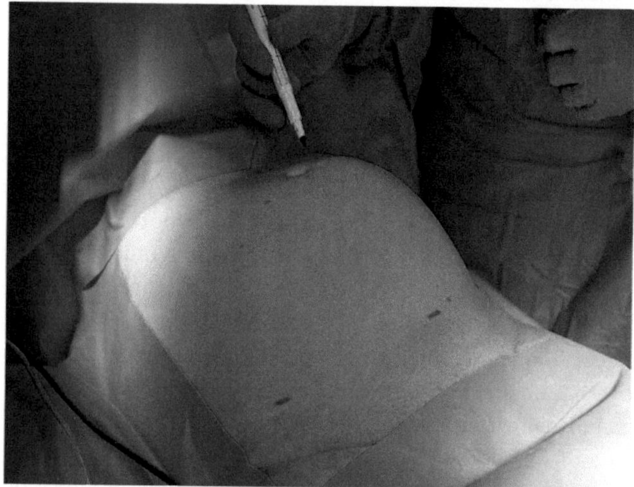

Fig. 36.1 Standard port-position

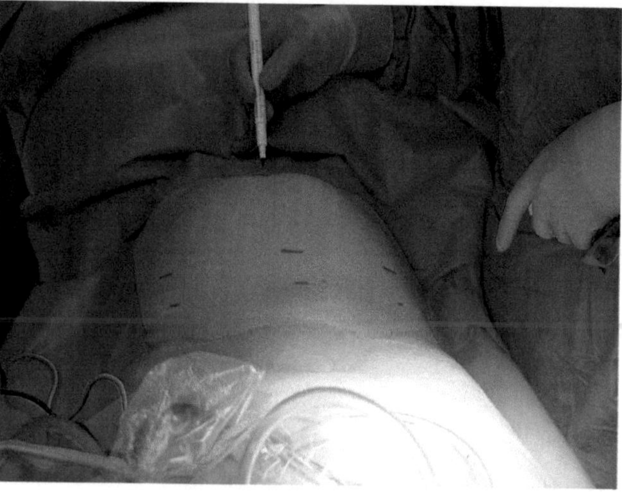

Fig. 36.2 Standard and elevated port-position

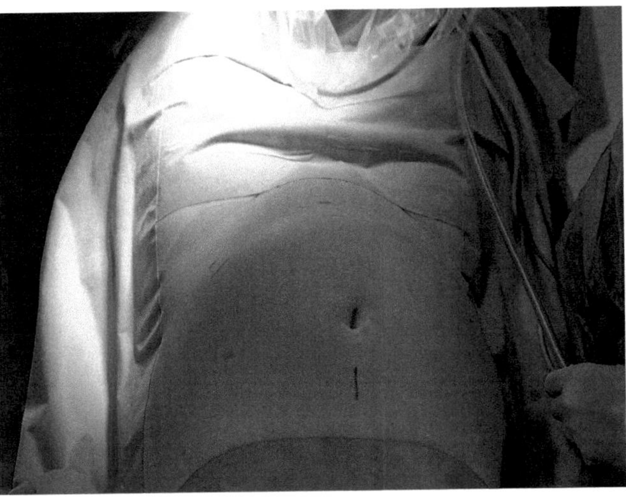

Fig. 36.3 Umbilical and high optic entrance

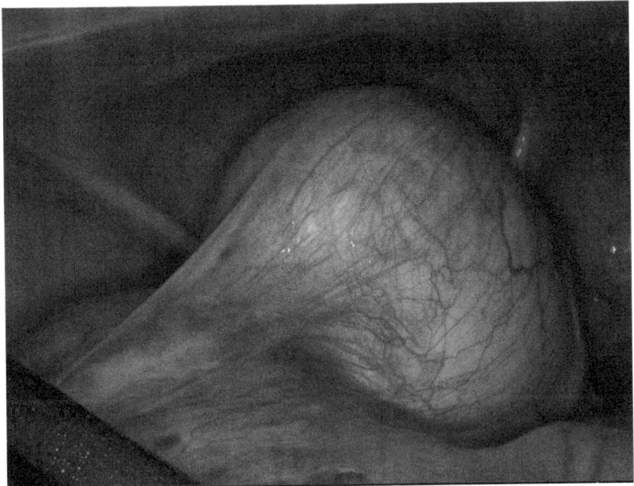

Fig. 36.4 2300 g uterus (all pictures taken on this uterus)

Indeed the higher positioning provides better view and better access to the higher tissue like the adnexa. On the other hand the angel to reach the uterine vessels gets more and more unfavorable the higher the placement of the port is proceeded.

At the end the success or the feasibility of the surgery is related to the access to the blood supply of the uterus. As we describe an approach for uterus 1000 g and more, the access to the uterine origin branch is not possible, the surgeon is forced to get access to the entering branch of the uterine arteries near the cervix from the anterior area. In this region a lot of vessels can be found as well as the ureter is close and the lack of tissue traction can increase the risk of damage.

To have an optimal angle the authors prefer the direct access and place the trocars in a usual setting (Fig. 36.1). One Optic-trocar and three working-port are placed.

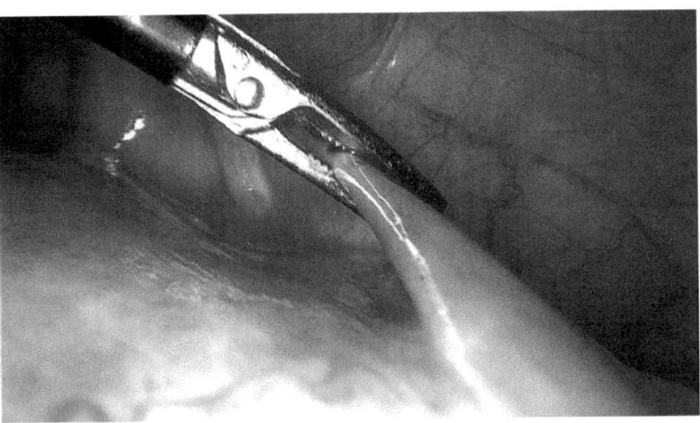

Fig. 36.5 Right round ligament

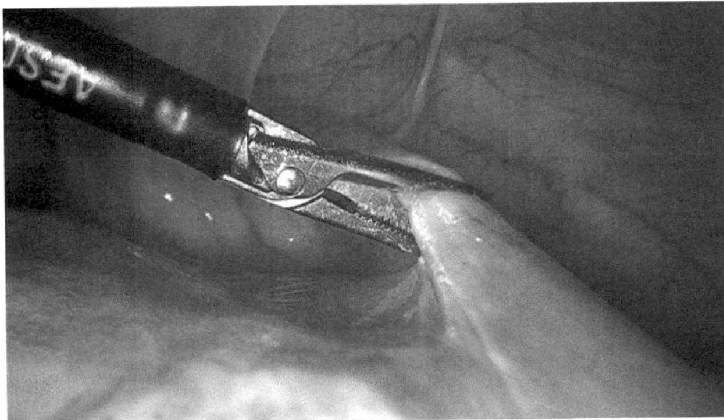

Fig. 36.6 Coagulation and cutting round ligament

Step 1

Visualizing the situation and exposure of the anatomy.

Step 2

Decision:

Is it possible to move the uterus laterally?

Will it be possible to move the uterus cranially after releasing from the round ligaments and the cardinal ligaments?

If these question cannot be answered positively an open procedure should be chosen.

Step 3

Identifying the Round Ligaments and the Peritoneal Border-Line to the Anterior Uterine Wall

The use of a combined instrument (coagulation/sealing/preparation and cutting) is the best advantage in this situation. Unnecessary movements by changing the instruments has to

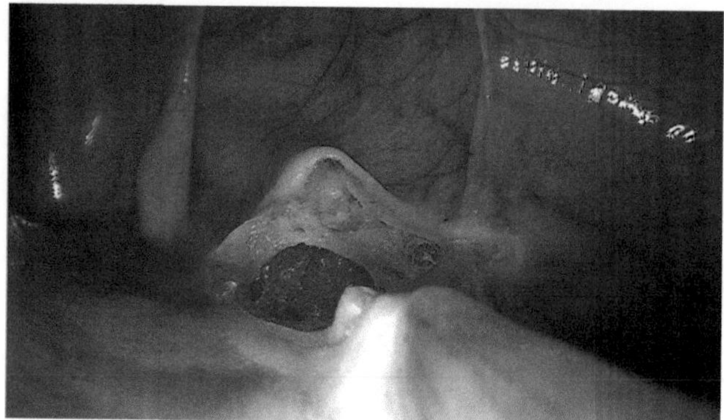

Fig. 36.7 Extension of the ligament

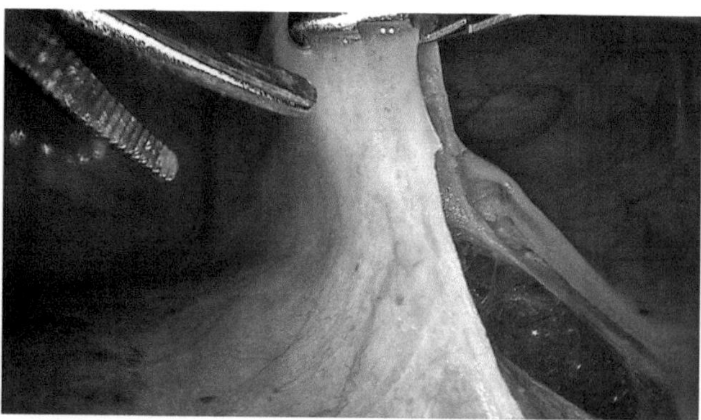

Fig. 36.8 Under traction the CO_2 Gas can stream into the retroperitoneal space

be avoided. It depends on the experience of the surgeon which device is used. We prefer a bipolar combination instrument which provides the possibility to coagulate and cut as well as perpetrate separately.

In a field with poor visibility it is important to do the preparation as dry as possible.

To have the chance to move the uterus we first cut the round ligaments (Figs. 36.4, 36.5, 36.6, and 36.7). The lateral as possible to have a proper access to the retro-peritoneal space is important.

Step 4

Preparation of the peritoneum for identifying the uterine blood supply and get the uterus moved out of the pelvis (Figs. 36.8, 36.9, 36.10, 36.11, 36.12, 36.13, 36.14, and 36.15).

The preparation should be performed in small steps to avoid the rupture of the vein plexus in the lower part of the retro-peritoneal region. We use the gas for the dilution of the spaces and try to prepare as bluntly as possible.

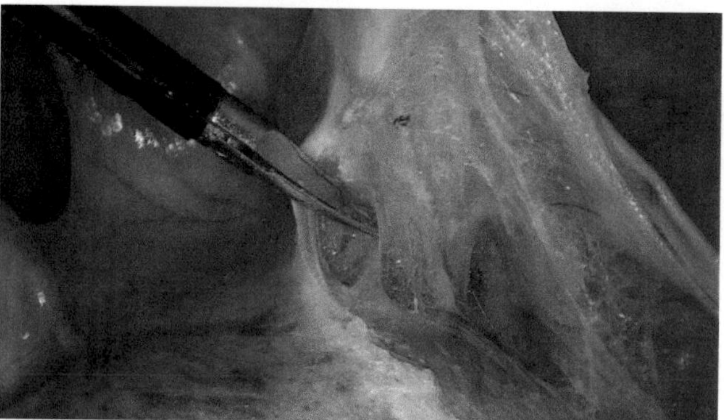

Fig. 36.9 Preparation downwards to the bladder

Step 5

Identifying the Vessel Supply

As the access to the deep branch of the uterine artery is not possible by the bulky uterus, it is necessary to approach the vessels from anterior. To avoid bleedings from the accompanying veins a precise clearing of the margins is useful (Figs. 36.16, 36.17, and 36.18).

A clear and broad sealing of the artery to avoid reverse bleedings from the uterus is important as these bleeding reduce massively the field of view for the rest of the surgery (Fig. 36.19).

Step 6

Approaching the Adnexa (Figs. 36.20, 36.21, 36.22, 36.23, 36.24, and 36.25)

In case of large uterus the access to the adnexa is performed reverse. First the position of the ovary and the tube has to be verified. The protruding masses can make the identification very difficult and the correct direction of the preparation has to be controlled step by step.

The second surgeon can hold the uterus to the contralateral side as far as the tissue allows. Then the first surgeon approaches the tube and the ovarian ligament retroperitoneal.

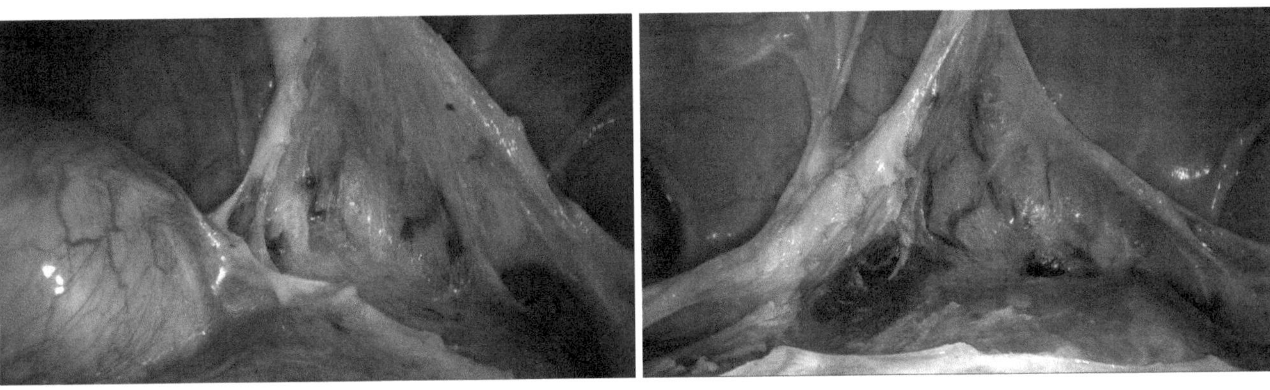

Figs. 36.10 and 36.11 Preparation of the bladder. The identification of the cervix can be difficult as often the cervix is consumed by fibroids

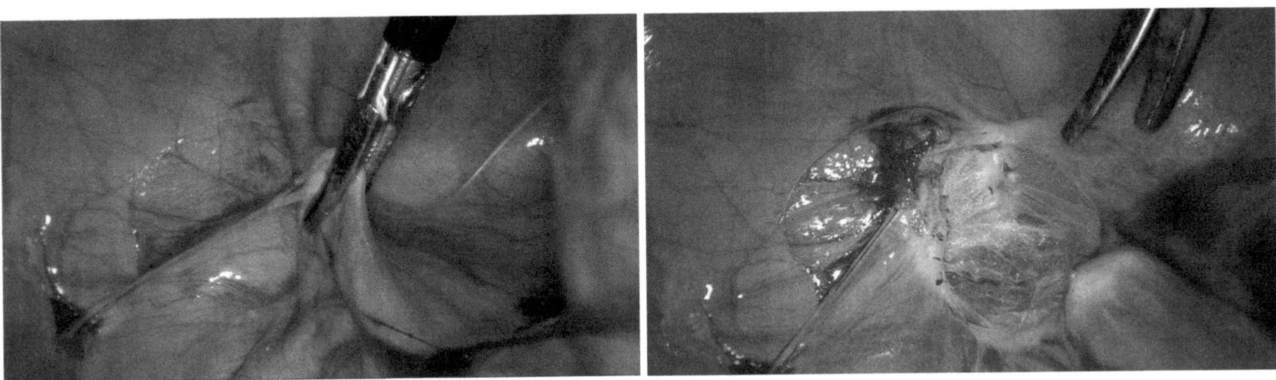

Figs. 36.12 and 36.13 Right round ligament preparation

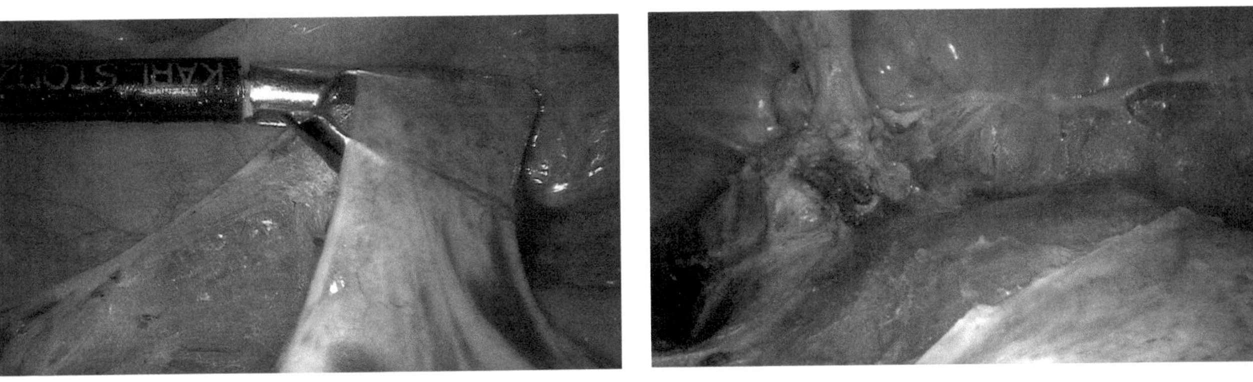

Fig. 36.14 Traction and tunneling the peritoneum to complete the anterior preparation

Fig. 36.15 Exposure bulky, lateral wall

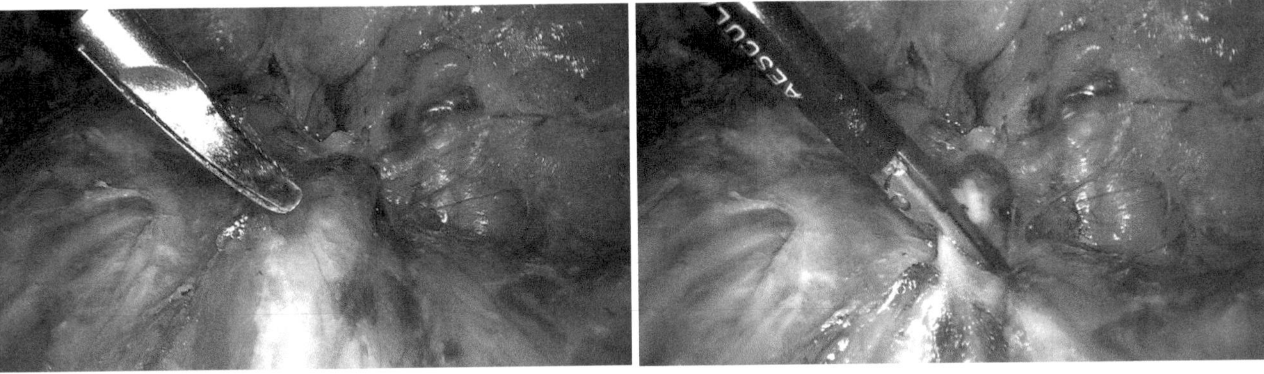

Figs. 36.16 and 36.17 Right uterine artery/exposure and preparation

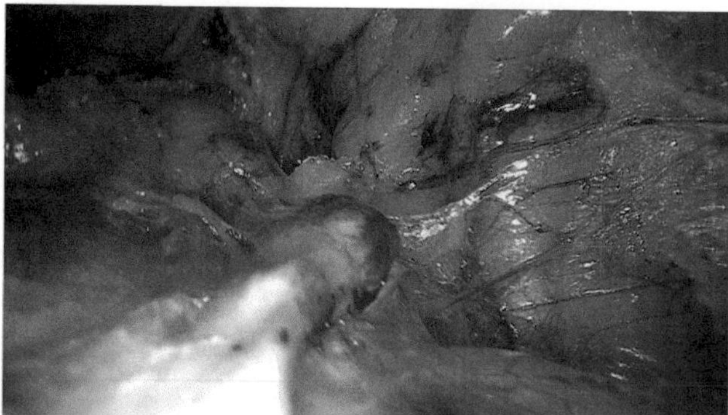

Fig. 36.18 Vain exposure

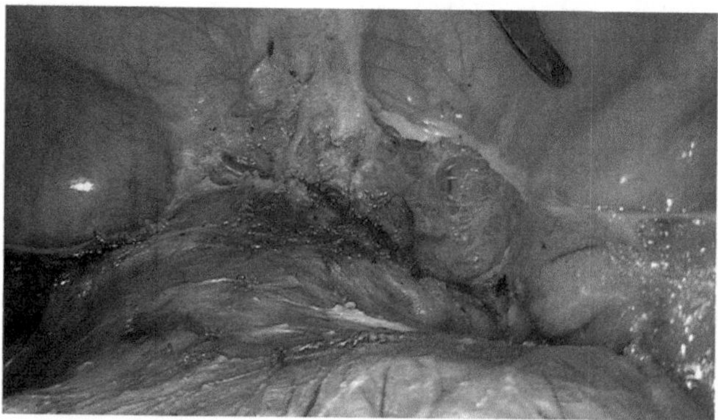

Fig. 36.19 Field after dissecting the artery

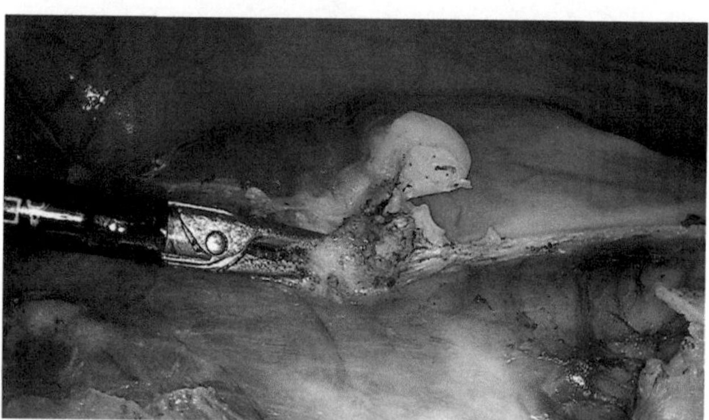

Fig. 36.20 Fallopian tube

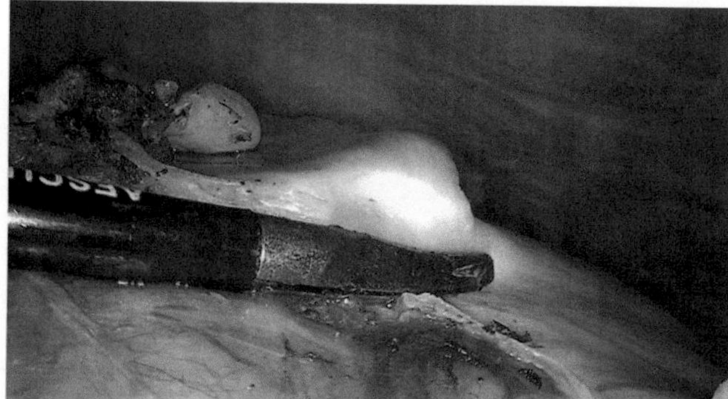

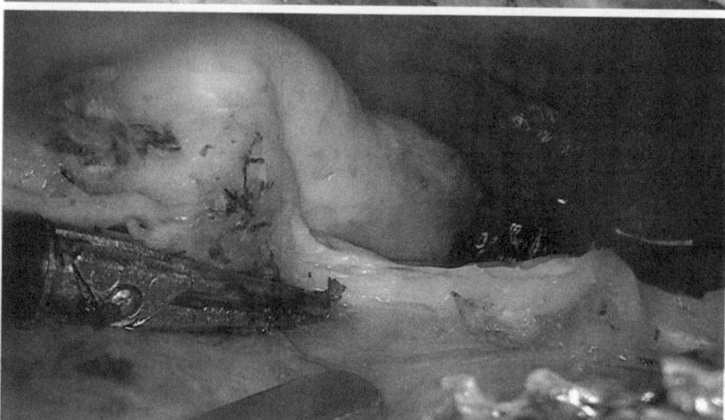

Figs. 36.21 and 36.22 Close preparation to the uterus in small steps

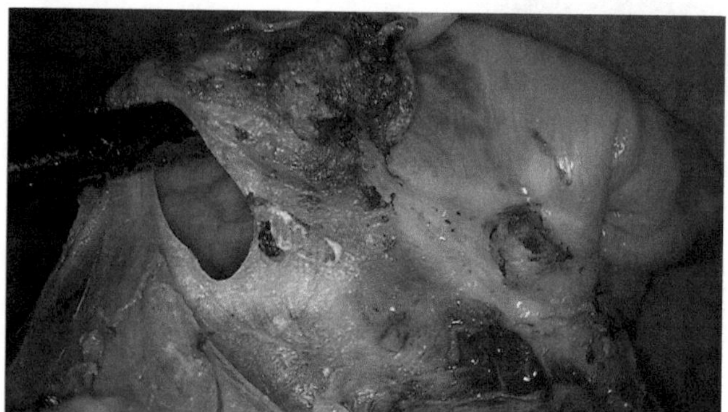

Fig. 36.23 Identification of the proper ovarian ligament

Step 7

Clearing the Margins and Exposure of the Para-Cervical Tissue (Figs. 36.26, 36.27, 36.28, 36.29, and 36.30)

Step 8

Exposure and Preparation of the Cervix (Figs. 37.31 and 37.32)

Upon transitioning of the uterine arteries the uterus can be cut off from the cervix to have an optimal surgical field. This provides the access to the utero-sacral ligaments and they can be spared by an intra-facial dissection. If the pushing up of the uterus is performable optimal, the preparation of the para-cervical tissue is possible and can be done with or without a vaginal adapter.

The TLH or LSH of large uterus is only performable by the use of morcellation. At the moment a uterus larger then 1000 g cannot be morcellated in an enclosed setting. For specimen from 300 to 1000 g we use a bag with three closable access openings to control the morcellation by two hands. It is possible to perform morcellation with only a morcellator in the bag if the tissue is small. It is advantageous to have a helping hand for specimen larger then 300 g controlling the movement of the tissue and provide an optimal view on the rotating knife.

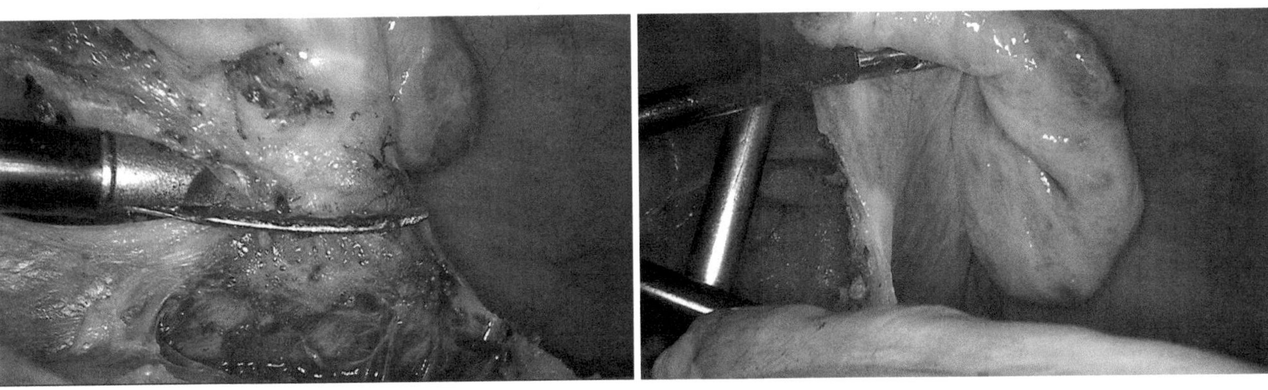

Figs. 36.24 and 36.25 Cutting the proper ligament (*right*)

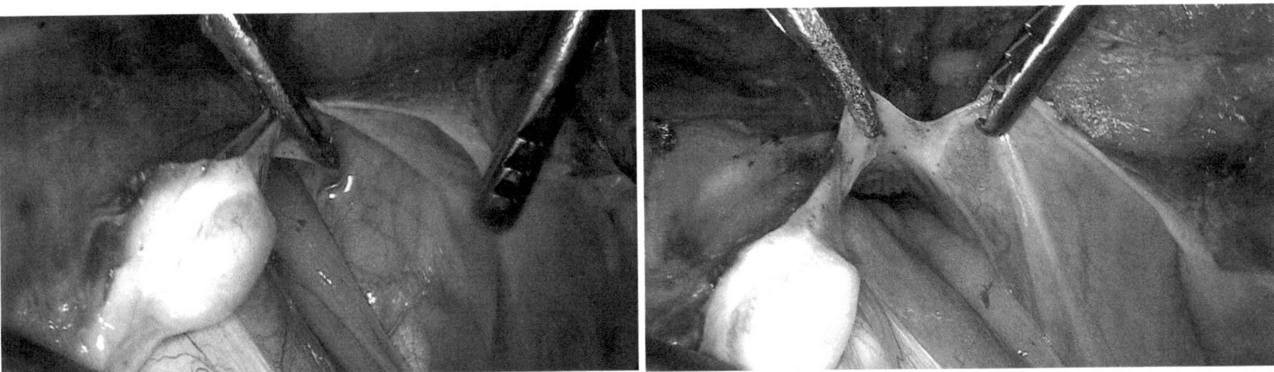

Figs. 36.26 and 36.27 Step by step preparation of the broad ligament

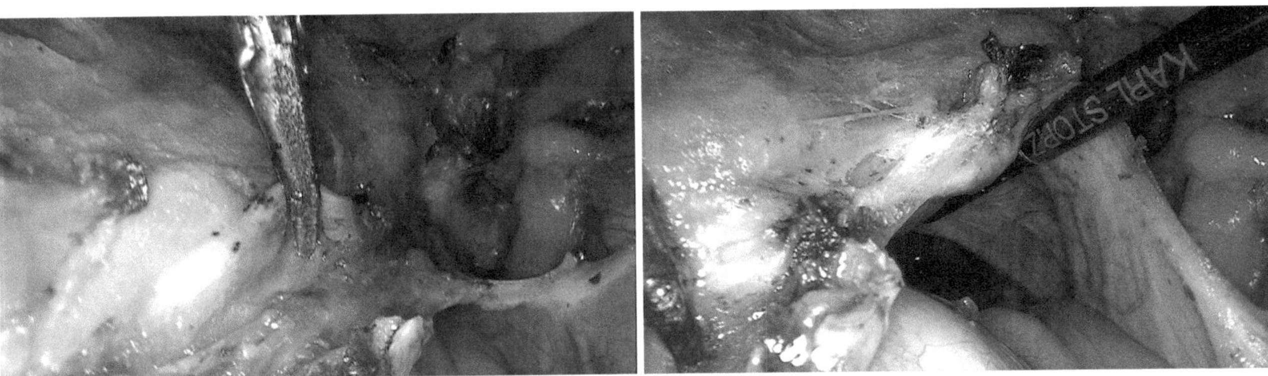

Figs. 36.28 and 36.29 Complete exposure of the right pedicel

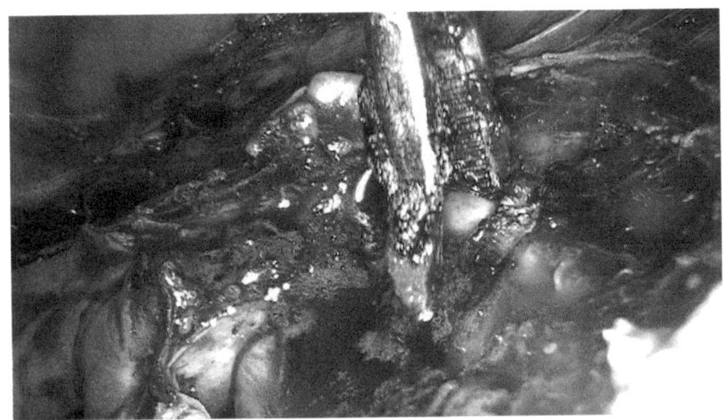

Fig. 36.30 Left uterine artery

As the access openings of the bag are closable we can prevent loosing spillage while extracting the bag after morcellation.

Two liter polyurethane bag with three closable access openings provides a good manageability of large tissue and a proper orientation by the transparency of the polyurethane (Figs. 36.33, 36.34, 36.35, and 36.36).

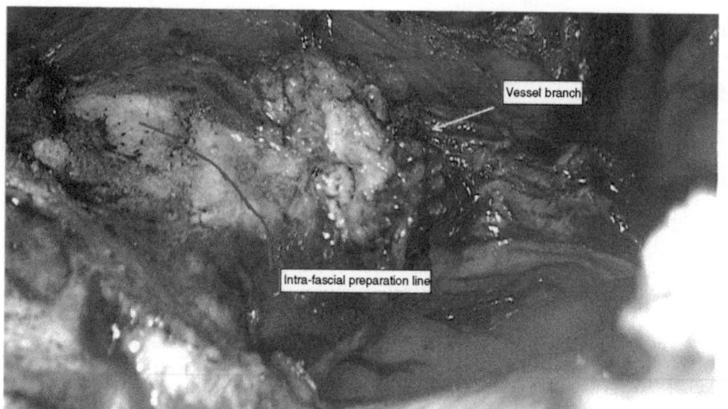

Fig. 37.31 Preparation of the right intra-facial space

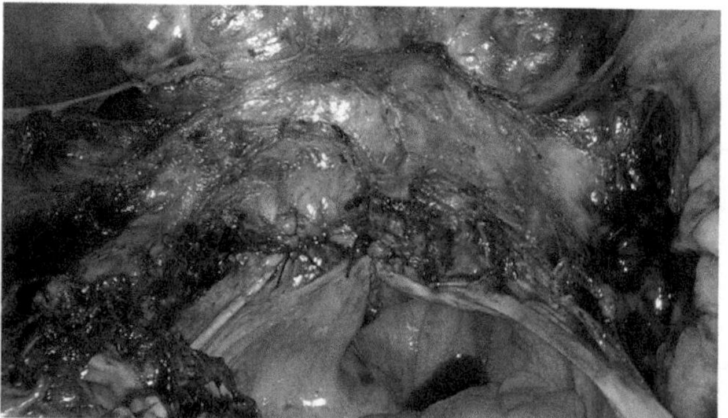

Fig. 37.32 Situs after closing the vagina by a running suture

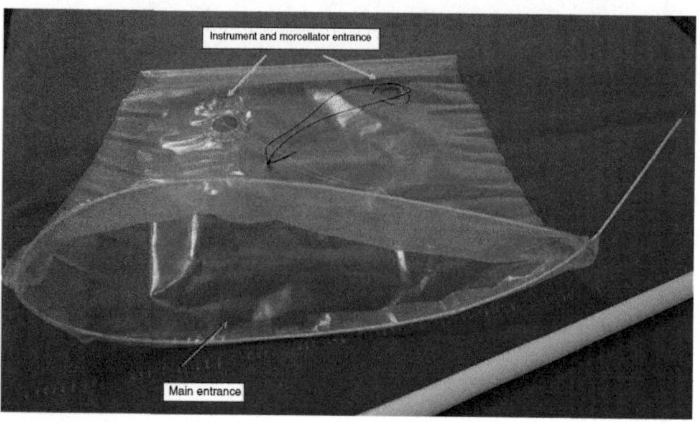

Fig. 36.33 Closable polyurethane bag

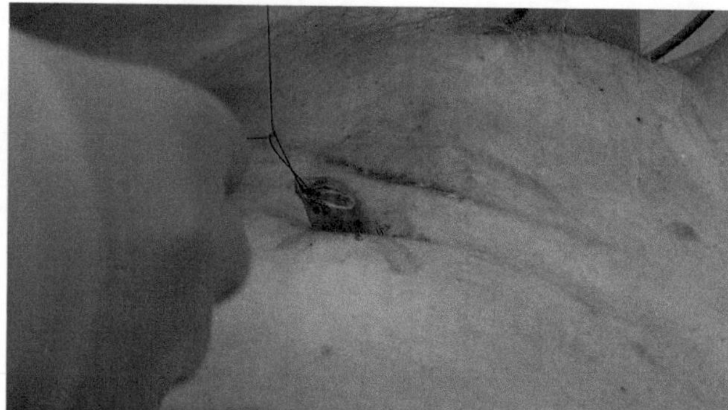

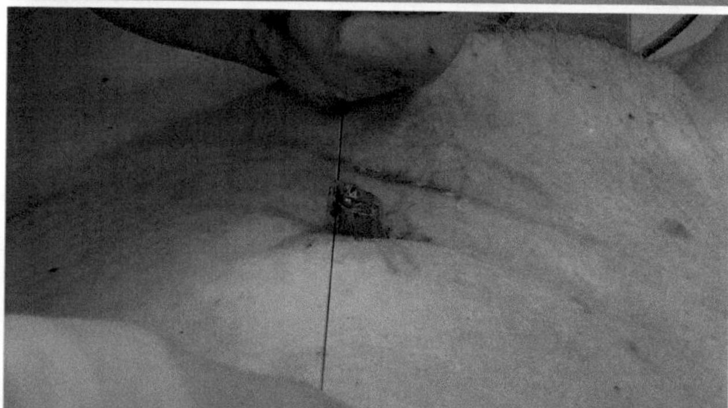

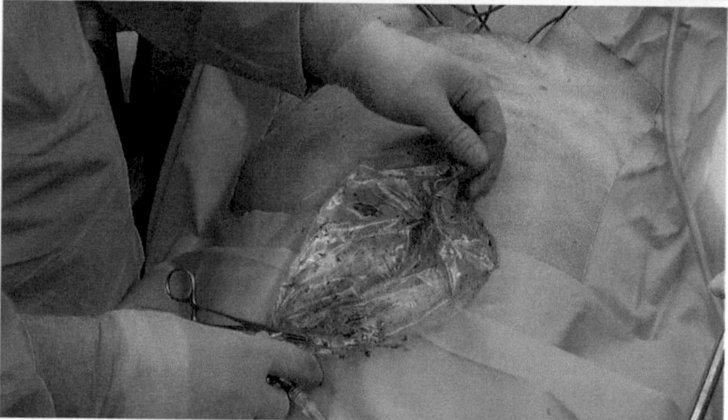

Figs. 36.34, 36.35, and 36.36 Closure of the access port and bag after extraction

References

1. Hohl MK, Hauser N. Safe total intrafascial laparoscopic (TAIL) hysterectomy: a prospective cohort study. Gynecol Surg. 2010;7:231–9.
2. Available at: http://www.fda.gov/MedicalDevices/Safety/AlertsandNotices/ucm393576.htm. Accessed 21 Feb 2015.
3. Brown J. AAGL advancing minimally invasive gynecology worldwide: statement to the FDA on power morcellation. J Minim Invasive Gynecol. 2014;21:970–1.
4. Brown J, Taylor K, Ramirez PT, Sun C, Holman LL, Cone SM, Irwin J, Frumovitz M. Laparoscopic supracervical hysterectomy with morcellation: should it stay or should it go? J Minim Invasive Gynecol. 2015;22:185–92.
5. Nezhat C, Kho K. Iatrogenic myomas: new class of myomas? J Minim Invasive Gynecol. 2010;17:544–50.
6. Montella F, Riboni F, Cosma S, Dealberti D, Prigione S, Pisani C, Rovetta E. A safe method of vaginal longitudinal morcellation of bulky uterus with endometrial cancer in a bag at laparoscopy. Surg Endosc. 2014;28:1949–53.
7. Cholkeri-Singh A, Miller CE. Power morcellation in a specimen bag. J Minim Invasive Gynecol. 2015;22:160.
8. Cohen SL, Einarsson JI, Wang KC, Brown D, Boruta D, Scheib SA, Fader AN, Shibley T. Contained power morcellation within an insufflated isolation bag. Obstet Gynecol. 2014;124:491–7.
9. Harmanli O. Contained power morcellation within an insufflated isolation bag. Obstet Gynecol. 2015;125:229.

Total Laparoscopic Hysterectomy for the Patient with Concomitant Pelvic Organ

37

Shanti I. Mohling, Robert S. Furr, and C.Y. Liu

Pelvic organ prolapse significantly impacts the lives of women throughout the world. Nearly half of women worldwide will suffer from pelvic organ prolapse (POP) in their lifetimes [1]. Prolapse may be devastating as it affects many aspects of daily life including the ability to work, to exercise and to remain continent of urine and stool. It can affect self-esteem and sexual health. While conservative treatment options exist, and should be considered, surgical repair remains a viable option. Indications for surgery include failed conservative management with a pessary or physical therapy, failure or complications of a prior surgery for pelvic prolapse, and patient choice.

Hysterectomy with concomitant repair of pelvic organ prolapse may be performed laparoscopically or robotically, both of which afford excellent visualization of the operative field, thereby resulting in precise repair of pelvic floor defects and improved surgical outcomes. With fewer operative complications and minimal postoperative pain and discomfort, the patient enjoys a shorter recovery period and earlier return to normal activity.

Treatment of Pelvic Organ Prolapse at the Time of Hysterectomy

The primary goal of surgical treatment of POP at the time of hysterectomy is to reconstruct and to restore the integrity of endopelvic fascia. Ultimately, the aim is to restore normal vaginal length, vaginal axis and vaginal support. Because the general principles and detailed surgical techniques of endoscopic hysterectomy for various indications have been described elsewhere in the atlas, this chapter aims to describe the specific techniques of laparoscopic hysterectomy that are unique to the anatomical distortions secondary to POP. This chapter will also be devoted specifically to the concomitant laparoscopic treatment of POP at the time of hysterectomy. Finally, the technique of uterosacral vaginal vault suspension at the time of laparoscopic hysterectomy may also be applicable in the prevention of vaginal vault prolapse.

Anatomic Considerations

Pericervical Ring

The cervix is encircled by thick visceral connective tissue called the pericervical ring. This is the cornerstone of vaginal apical support. The pericervical ring is the convergence of the anterior pubocervical fascia, the posterior rectovaginal septum and the uterosacral ligaments [2]. The pericervical ring constitutes the strongest connective tissue between the ischial spines and is located in the narrowest diameter of the female pelvis. Defects in any of these three components as they converge create varying forms of pelvic prolapse [3]. The location of the ischial spines relative to the structures of the pericervical ring are the most important factors to be considered in reconstructive surgery for pelvic organ prolapse (Fig. 37.1).

Ischial Spine

The ischial spine is a triangular bony eminence projecting from the dorsal border of the ischium. It serves as an attachment point for the sacrospinous ligament, the coccygeus and levator ani muscles, and the pelvic fascia. The space between the ischial spines is the narrowest diameter in the female pelvis and contains the strongest connective tissue.

S.I. Mohling, MD, FACOG (✉)
Fellowship Minimally Invasive Gynecology, Obstetrics and Gynecology, University of Tennessee College of Medicine at Chattanooga, 979 East Third Street, Suite C720, Chattanooga, Hamilton Country, TN, 37403, USA
e-mail: shantimohling@gmail.com

R.S. Furr, MD, FACOG • C.Y. Liu, MD, FACOG
Fellowship Minimally Invasive Gynecology, Obstetrics and Gynecology, University of Tennessee College of Medicine at Chattanooga, 1604 Gunbarrel Road, Chattanooga, Hamilton Country, TN, 37421, USA
e-mail: drfurr@bellsouth.net; Cyliu44@msn.com

I. Alkatout, L. Mettler (eds.), *Hysterectomy*, DOI 10.1007/978-3-319-22497-8_37

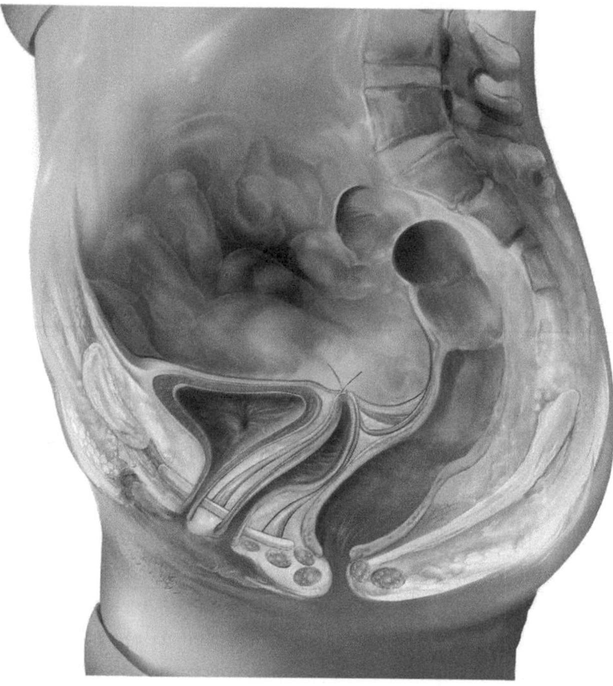

Fig. 37.1 A schematic of reconstructed Pericervical Ring after hysterectomy demonstrating the convergence of pubocervical fascia, the rectovaginal septum and the uterosacral ligament at the level of ischial spine

Pelvic Ureter

During hysterectomy with co-existing POP, one must be keenly aware of the potential for anatomic deviation in the course of the ureter. In the patient without prolapse, the pelvic ureter follows the internal iliac artery, traverses downward from the bifurcation, passes under the uterine artery at the level of the ischial spine, and then turns forward and medially over the anterior lateral vaginal fornix to enter the posterolateral wall of the bladder. At the "knee" of the ureter, the distance between the ureter and the cervix is approximately 1.5–2 cm, however, as the ureter curves forward over the anterior vaginal fornix, this distance can become even smaller, especially with co-existing prolapse.

The surgeon must be vigilant and have a clear idea of the location of the ureter while performing desiccation or ligation of the uterine vessels and while performing the anterior and lateral aspect of colpotomy during hysterectomy. In the setting of utero-vaginal prolapse (especially in the case of chronic uterovaginal prolapse with elongated cervix), anterior enterocele, and cystocele the course of the ureter between the "knee" and the bladder may be displaced, medially or anteriorly. In this area, the ureter can easily be damaged through ligation, thermal injury, transection, or impingement during hysterectomy and during the repair of prolapse.

Uterosacral Ligaments

Many gynecologists hold a traditional concept of the uterosacral ligament believing that it spans from the back of the cervico-vaginal junction curving posteriorly to reach the anterior and lateral aspects of the sacrum. The surgical anatomy of the uterosacral ligament may appear to be readily identified as a dense, strong band of connective tissue medial and posterior to the ischial spine. However, cadaveric and histological studies have generally demonstrated an absence of actual condensed ligamentous structure.

In 2004, Umek and DeLancey used MRI to demonstrate the origin and insertion points of the uterosacral ligament on 61 asymptomatic women. Their study revealed that more than 82 % of uterosacral ligaments actually inserted into the sacrospinous ligament and coccygeus muscle, while only 7 % inserted onto the sacrum [4]. Again, in 2012, DeLancey's group, at the University of Michigan, used dynamic MRI to track the uterosacral ligament on 20 nulliparous women. They found that in 73 % of them, the uterosacral ligaments actually inserted into the sacrospinous ligament and coccygeus muscle. Only 21 % of them had insertions into the presacral fascia. No direct attachment to the sacrum was identified [5]. Therefore, the primary insertion site of the uterosacral ligament is the sacrospinous ligament or coccygeus muscle at the level of the pericervical ring, which holds the cervix and apex of vagina in their normal anatomic position.

Vaginal Tube and Enterocele

Prolapse is the end result of the detachment of endopelvic fascia from its surrounding connective tissue support. Pathophysiologically, prolapse is a condition of herniation – a fascial separation that occurs within the vaginal tube. From a surgical perspective, the vagina is a fibromuscular tube that is completely encapsulated by endopelvic fascia. Anteriorly, this is the pubocervical fascia; posteriorly, the rectovaginal septum, and; superiorly, the uterosacro-cardinal ligament complex. This fibromuscular vaginal tube is lined by vaginal epithelium. Biomechanically, the endopelvic fascia cannot be stretched or attenuated. Thus, it breaks, or separates, under chronic pressure while vaginal epithelium and pelvic peritoneum can be stretched endlessly under pressure.

Fascial separations occurring within the vaginal wall result in pelvic peritoneum having direct contact with vaginal epithelium. Under pressure, both will stretch and protrude, bulging into the vagina forming a hernia sac, or enterocele. Separation between the pubocervical fascia and pericervical ring produces an anterior enterocele. Similarly, a separation in the connective tissue of the rectovaginal septum and pericervical ring presents as a posterior enterocele. Procidentia results from circumferential separation at the pericervical ring together with disintegration of the uterosacral ligament attachments (Table 37.1).

Surgical Considerations

Surgical reconstruction and restoration of the integrity of the pericervical ring will correct a majority of prolapses. In pelvic reconstructive surgery, one must first restore the integrity of the fibromuscular vaginal tube by reattaching the pubocervical fascia to the rectovaginal septum after hysterectomy or by attaching them both to the cervix if the uterus is to be preserved. Next, the apex of the vagina, or the cervix, is suspended to the proximal part of the uterosacral ligaments at the level of the ischial spine. In most cases, this will restore the normal vaginal length and vaginal axis. The latter step can also be accomplished by reattaching the apex of the vagina or the cervix to the sacrospinous ligament, or by performing a sacrocolpopexy with mesh graft. Literature strongly suggests that without proper suspension of the apex of vagina or cervix to the level of the ischial spine, all attempts at prolapse repair will ultimately fail [6].

Because pelvic floor defects are true herniations in pelvic floor fascia, the detached fascia needs to be reconstructed and repairs should be performed using non-absorbable monofilament sutures. In our center, we currently perform laparoscopic uterosacral ligament vault suspension using non-absorbable monofilament suture and laparoscopic or robotic sacrocolpopexy with large pore monofilament polypropylene synthetic mesh. We reserve the use of synthetic mesh for cases of severe prolapse in which the fascia is severely damaged or the patient has had recurrent symptomatic prolapse with failed previous surgical repair.

Following apical suspension, a vaginal examination is performed to ensure that the depth of the vagina has been restored. Frequent intraoperative vaginal examinations, with simultaneous laparoscopic observation, are performed to confirm appropriate correction of anterior and posterior vaginal wall prolapse. In some cases, after the appropriate reconstruction and restoration of the pericervical ring, an anterior or posterior defect will persist. This warrants further reconstruction with either a retropubic paravaginal repair, a midline cystocele repair or vaginal posterior colporrhaphy with perineorrhaphy.

Pre-operative Patient Counseling

If a graft material or non-absorbable synthetic mesh is being considered, the patient must be thoroughly informed and counseled regarding the risks and possible complications associated with the use of these materials. Risks of mesh include erosion into the vagina, dyspareunia, bowel obstruction, infection and pelvic pain. The patient must sign a comprehensive consent prior to surgery.

Additional counseling should include discussion on the possible but rare occurrences of postoperative urinary, bowel and sexual dysfunction. Expected long-term outcomes based on available data should be discussed in detail with the patient. The authors firmly believe that verbalized understanding by the patient of known failure rates, potential complications and potential for *de novo* stress incontinence or urge incontinence can help prevent false expectations and ultimately lead to greater patient satisfaction.

Preoperative Evaluation

A thorough medical history and prolapse history (including urinary, gastrointestinal, and sexual histories) must be carefully taken and recorded in the patient's file prior to surgery. The patient must be examined in both erect and supine position to map out pelvic floor defects in detail. The Pelvic Organ Prolapse Quantification (POP-Q) system is used to quantify, describe, and stage pelvic support. Urinary incontinence must be assessed in the erect and supine positions with and without reduction of prolapse. Assessment of urethral mobility, simple office cystometrics and post void residual are generally adequate for evaluation. A randomized trial, in 2012, demonstrated that for patients with history of uncomplicated, demonstrable stress urinary incontinence, preoperative evaluation in the office alone was not inferior to performing urodynamic testing. This was based on outcomes at one year [7]. In our practice, urodynamic studies are reserved for those with complicated symptoms.

Table 37.1 Fascial separations occurring within the vaginal wall result in pelvic organ prolapse. This table lists traditional nomenclature and pairs it with the precise fascial defect as related to the pericervical ring

Organ prolapse	Anatomical defect
Anterior compartment (anterior enterocele)	Separation of pubocervical fascia from pericervical ring
Posterior compartment (posterior enterocele)	Separation of rectovaginal septum from pericervical ring
Complete procidentia	Separation of the anterior and posterior fascia from the uterosacral ligament attachments and the pericervical ring

Operative Procedures

Patient Positioning

The patient is placed on a non-slip foam pad in the dorsolithotomy position with both legs well supported, as steep Trendelenberg will be maintained throughout most of the procedure. The arms are carefully tucked alongside the body. Attention is taken to ensure that the brachial plexus is not under untoward strain. Padding is placed on all pressure points including the occiput, to prevent neurovascular and ischemic compression injury. The surgeon should have unobstructed access to the perineum and vagina for the use of a vaginal or uterine manipulator, rectal probe and performance of vaginal examination during the surgery. Nasogastric or orogastric tube should be in position prior to subcostal insertion of a Veress needle or trocar to avoid injury to the stomach.

A Foley catheter is always placed at the onset of the surgery.

Placement of Uterine Manipulator

An effective uterine mobilizer capable of uterine anteversion, retroversion and lateral motion is essential. Many options exist for this purpose. A manipulator with a colpotomizing cup is helpful, but not imperative. If the surgeon prefers a non-disposable approach, instruments readily available in any gynecologic procedure tray may be used. In our center, for years we successfully used a simple technique: A single-toothed tenaculum is secured to the anterior lip of the cervix and a uterine sound is placed within the uterus to the fundus. A second tenaculum is placed on the posterior lip of the cervix and subsequently the three instruments are secured tightly together using sterile rubber bands.

Creation of Pneumoperitoneum

Establishing pneumoperitoneum may be one of the most critical steps in the performance of laparoscopic surgery. Many techniques exist with or without the use of a Veress needle, yet no technique has been demonstrated to be superior. In our practice, a Veress needle is usually inserted in the middle of the umbilicus or in the left upper quadrant, a fingerbreadth beneath the costal margin at the mid-clavicular line (Palmer's Point). Saline test or "hanging drop test" confirms ideal placement. Opening pressures for CO_2 gas should be under 10 mmHg, or extraperitoneal placement may have occurred. The patient should be in a flat position during initial placement of the Veress needle. The insufflator pressure may be initially set to 20 mmHg for placement of the trocars, but it should be reduced to 14–15 mmHg for duration of the procedure.

Trocar Placement

Five trocars are inserted after the pneumoperitoneum: a 10 mm umbilical trocar and four 5 mm secondary trocars. A 10 mm laparoscope is used and is inserted through the umbilical trocar sleeve and the patient is placed in steep Trendelenberg position. Two 5 mm trocars are placed lateral to the deep inferior epigastric vessels in the lower abdomen and two 5 mm trocars are placed lateral to the abdominal rectus muscles at or slightly below the umbilical level (Fig. 37.2). The bowels are pushed back to the upper abdomen.

Laparoscopic Hysterectomy and Repair of Concomitant POP

Step 1

Ureteral Identification and Dissection

In the setting of pelvic organ prolapse, the course of the ureter may be distorted. Inspection and exposure of the ureters bilaterally should be accomplished primarily and prior to hysterectomy and any reparative procedures. The transperitoneal approach to ureteral dissection is used in the majority of cases. For those patients who are obese or who have complicated pelvic pathology, a retroperitoneal approach may be necessary.

Transperitoneal Exposure of the Ureters

The ureters on both sides are visualized through the laparoscope (Fig. 37.3). To expose and dissect the ureters, an atraumatic grasper is held open against the peritoneum just above the ureter at the level of the pelvic brim. The peritoneum is incised just below the ureter (Fig. 37.4). A grasper is used to bluntly separate the peritoneum away from the ureter

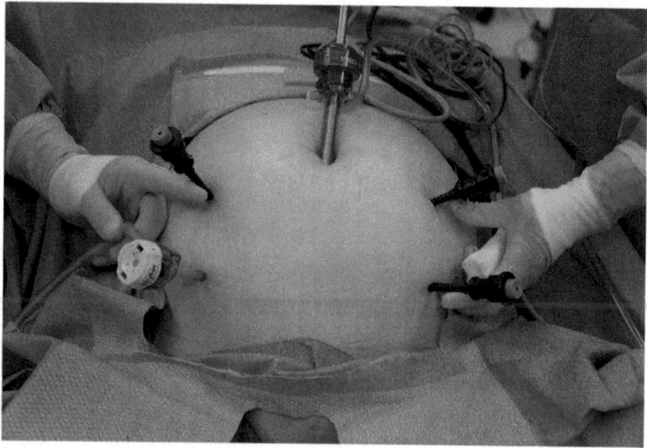

Fig. 37.2 The authors utilize four working 5 mm ports plus a 10 mm umbilical port for the laparoscope

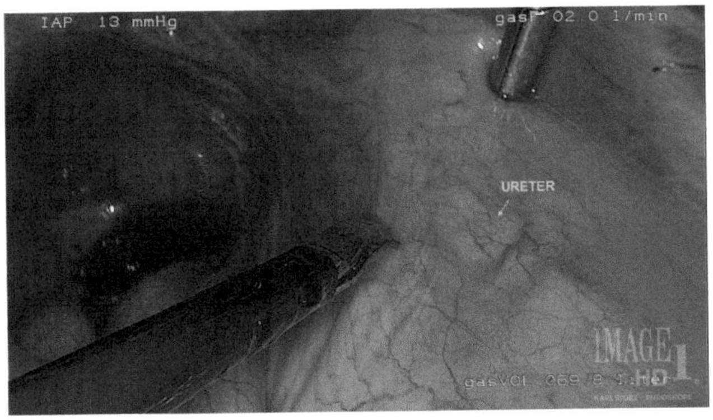

Fig. 37.3 The right ureter is visible coursing beneath the peritoneum. Transperitoneal dissection of the ureter begins by opening the peritoneum just beneath the ureter

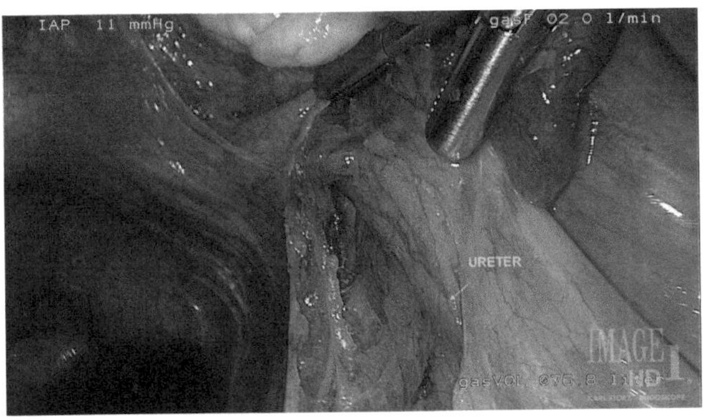

Fig. 37.4 Transperitoneal exposure of the ureter: ureteral exposure is accomplished by opening the peritoneum overlying the ureter. Atraumatic graspers are used to bluntly separate the tissue overlying the ureters and provide counter-traction as the surgeon opens the peritoneum

and a relaxing peritoneal incision is performed. The ureter is exposed to the level where it passes under the uterine artery (Fig. 37.5). This dissection prevents the ureter from becoming tethered, as adjacent tissues are plicated. The procedure is duplicated on the opposite side. It is important to expose the ureters prior to performing the hysterectomy and prolapse support procedures, as visualization of the ureters may become more difficult with retroperitoneal CO_2 gas infiltration, swelling and bleeding.

Retroperitoneal Dissection to Expose the Ureters

Exposure may be accomplished by opening the peritoneum longitudinally between the external iliac artery and the infundibulopelvic ligament (Figs. 37.6 and 37.7). Dissection is carried down posteriorly to the infundibulopelvic ligament to expose the ureter and internal iliac artery (Figs. 37.8, 37.9, and 37.10). Exposure of the ureter should continue until the uterine artery is seen crossing over the ureter (Fig. 37.11). The space between the ureter (medially) and the internal iliac artery (laterally) can be entered posteriorly with ease and is fairly avascular.

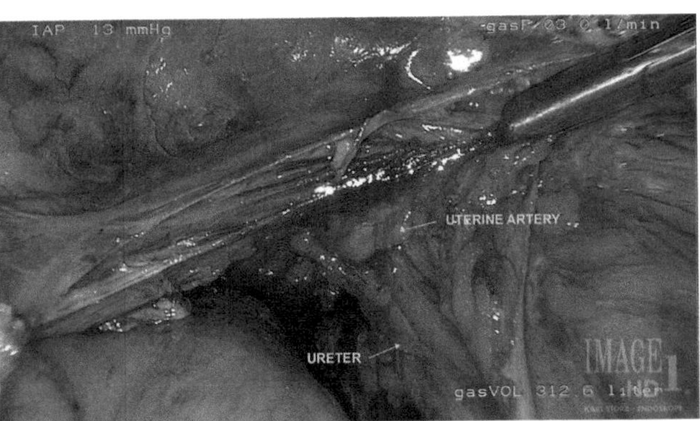

Fig. 37.5 The ureter should be exposed to the level at which it passes beneath the uterine artery. Here the ureter is seen passing just beneath the uterine artery

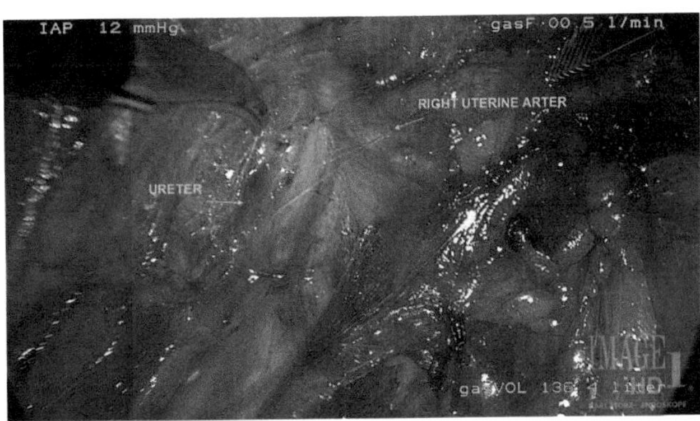

Fig. 37.6 In some patients, habitus or pelvic pathology will dictate the need to expose the ureter by opening the retroperitoneum. This may be accomplished by entering the peritoneum longitudinally, lateral to the infundibulopelvic ligament and medial to the external iliac artery

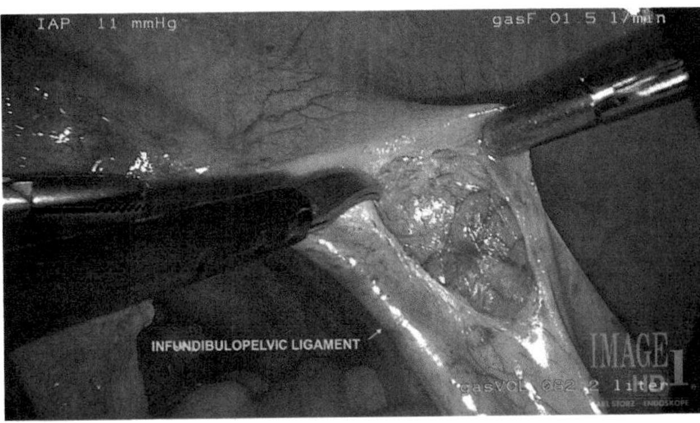

Fig. 37.7 The retroperitoneal space is opened on the right, beginning lateral to the infundibulopelvic ligament

Step 2

Exposure of the Rectovaginal Septum

Regardless of whether the prolapse repair will be performed with mesh or suture, it is crucial to expose and identify the pubocervical fascia and rectovaginal septum before completing the hysterectomy.

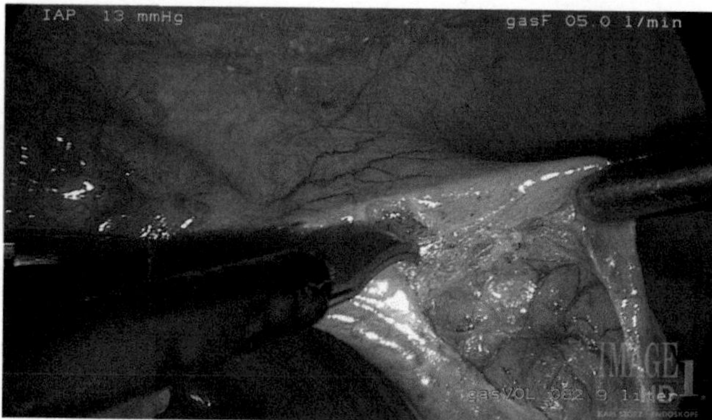

Fig. 37.8 The peritoneal incision is extended caudally

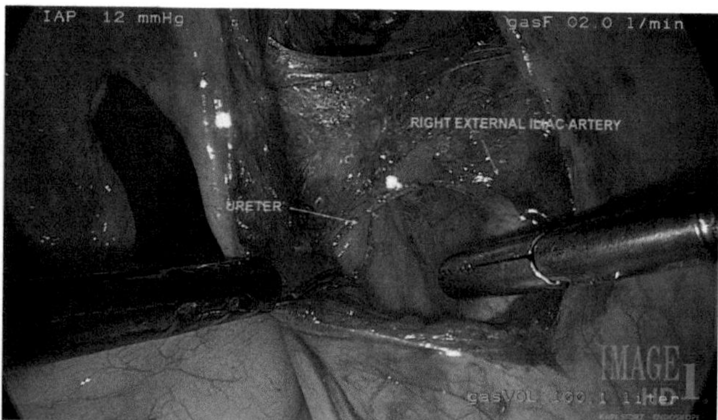

Fig. 37.9 The ureter is identified medial to the external iliac artery

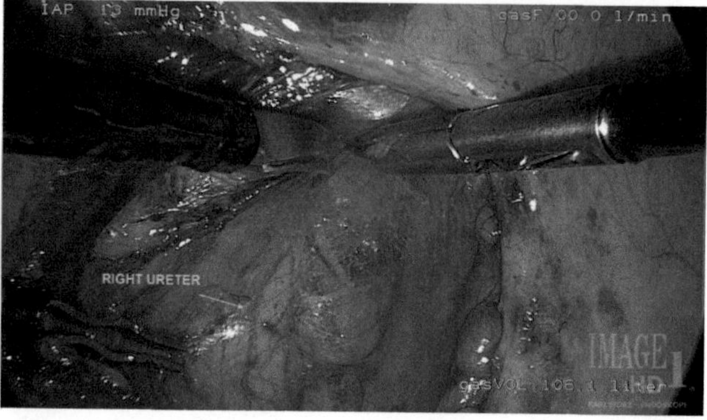

Fig. 37.10 The dissection is continued along the course of the ureter, moving caudally

The assistant, using the uterine manipulator, pushes the uterus anteriorly and superiorly. A rectal probe is helpful in preventing injury of the rectum during the dissection and will facilitate the identification of both the pararectal and rectovaginal spaces. First, the rectal probe is placed and the rectum is deviated toward the patient's left side. A longitudinal incision is made in the peritoneum overlying the right pararectal space, and this is extended caudally toward the rectovaginal space. The rectovaginal space is entered on the right

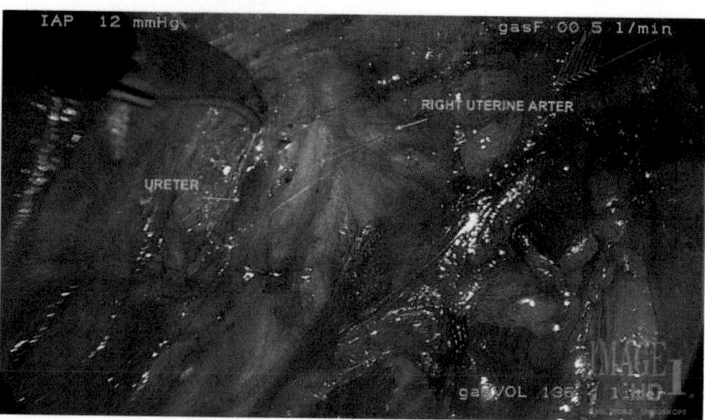

Fig. 37.11 Exposure of the ureter should continue until the uterine artery is seen crossing over the ureter

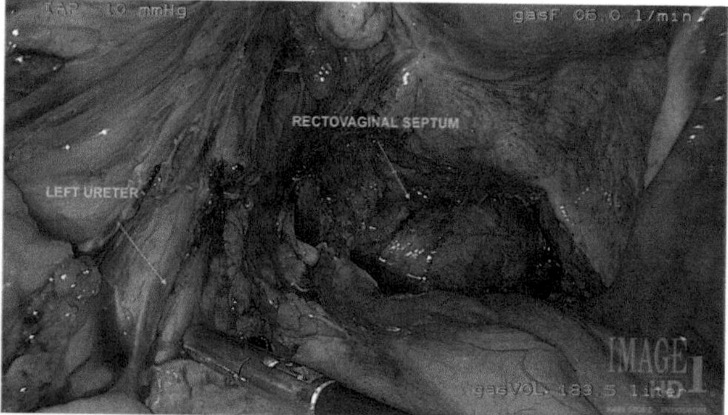

Fig. 37.12 The rectovaginal septum is exposed with simultaneous visualization of the left ureter shown here

side. The same procedure is then performed on the left side with the rectum deviated by the rectal probe to the right during the dissection. The rectal probe can be removed after the rectovaginal space is successfully exposed.

The rectovaginal space is dissected caudally until the rectovaginal septum can be clearly identified (Fig. 37.12). The rectovaginal septum may be confirmed by placing the surgeon's fingers inside the vagina, while simultaneously grasping the rectovaginal septum laparoscopically and forcefully pulling on it. The fingers in the vagina can feel that the entire posterior vaginal wall is being pulled up. In the case of more severe prolapse, the rectovaginal septum will sometimes be found quite low within the space.

Step 3

Exposure of Pubocervical Fascia

To expose the pubocervical fascia, the bladder must be dissected off of the anterior vaginal wall. A transverse incision is made just below the vesicouterine peritoneal fold (Fig. 37.13). To avoid bladder injury during the dissection, after the vesicocervical space is entered, the bladder is grasped with an atraumatic grasping forceps, lifted up and pushed caudally by the

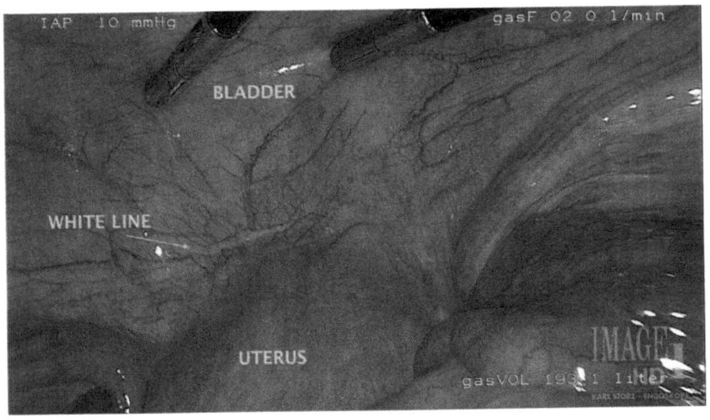

Fig. 37.13 The vesico-uterine peritoneum is seen here with a clearly defined "white line", which lies at the junction between the bladder peritoneum and anterior broad ligament, below which the surgeon will find an ideal plane for creating the bladder flap and exposing the pubocervical fascia

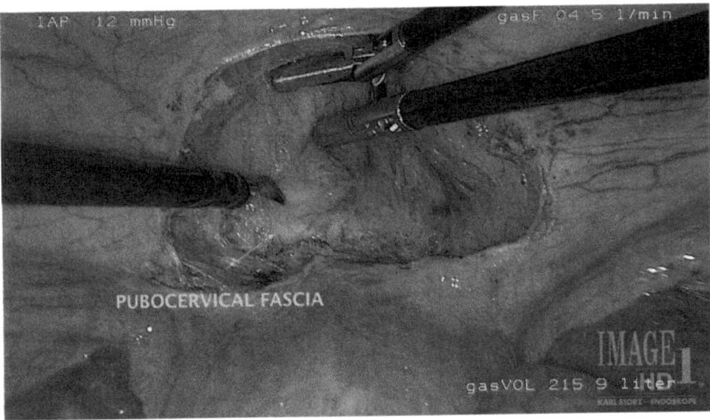

Fig. 37.14 The vesico-uterine peritoneum is entered sharply and dissected to expose the pubocervical fascia

assistant (Fig. 37.14). The vesico-cervical and vesico-vaginal space can then be easily entered and dissected bloodlessly. If excessive bleeding is encountered during the dissection, the possibility of having entered the wrong plane or having caused a bladder injury should be assessed. If it is difficult to distinguish the bladder from the adjacent planes of tissue, the bladder may be backfilled with 200–250 cc of sterile saline to aid in identification of planes. This is done by instilling the bladder with normal saline, through the Foley catheter, and clamping it. The clamp is released once the dissection is completed.

The pubocervical fascia is identified and confirmed by grasping and pulling the fascia laparoscopically while simultaneously placing the surgeon's fingers inside the vagina to appreciate the anterior vaginal wall being pulled upward during laparoscopic traction on the fascia. In the case of a large transverse defect, when the pubocervical fascia has detached from the cervix, it may be found very low in the vagina. This anterior fascia will be incorporated with the rectovaginal septum, in closing the vaginal cuff, to re-establish the integrity of the vaginal tube. When the apex is then attached to the proximal uterosacral ligaments, the pericervical ring is restored.

Step 4

Hysterectomy

Coexisting pelvic organ prolapse presents a unique challenge during hysterectomy, particularly due to the frequent occurrence of an elongated cervix. A study published by DeLancey et al, from 2012, evaluated women with and without prolapse by pelvic MRI. They demonstrated that in 40% of women with prolapse the cervix was elongated [8]. This elongation of the cervix causes displacement and distortion of the course of the ureter. Thus, special care must be taken to visualize the ureter during the ligation and division of the uterine vessels.

Securing the Uterine Vessels

The posterior and anterior leaves of the broad ligament are skeletonized revealing the uterine vessels. The uterine vessels are skeletonized, coagulated and transected being mindful that the ureter passes just lateral and inferior at this point. In lieu of using electrosurgical techniques, we frequently suture ligate the uterine vessels to avoid the potential for thermal injury to the ureter (Fig. 37.15). Following removal of the uterus, often the startling proximity of the ureter to the uterine artery stump may be readily appreciated.

Colpotomy

Most modern uterine manipulators incorporate a colpotomizer cup or ring which simplifies entry into the top of the vagina and enhances ureteral protection by lateralizing these structures. The circumferential colpotomy is performed along the ring or cup (Fig. 37.16), however, in the presence of prolapse, we routinely open the anterior and posterior vaginal fornix first, followed by lateral colpotomy very close to cervix to further reduce the incidence of ureteral injury and to preserve vaginal length. The assistant should maintain cephalad pressure with the manipulator further decreasing the risk of ureteral injury.

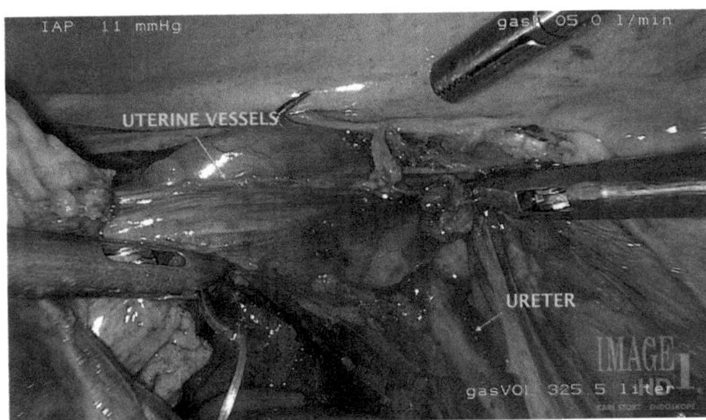

Fig. 37.15 The right uterine vessels have been skeletonized and are suture ligated using extracorporeal knot technique. Note the fully identified and visualized right ureter passing just beneath the uterine artery lateral to the ligation

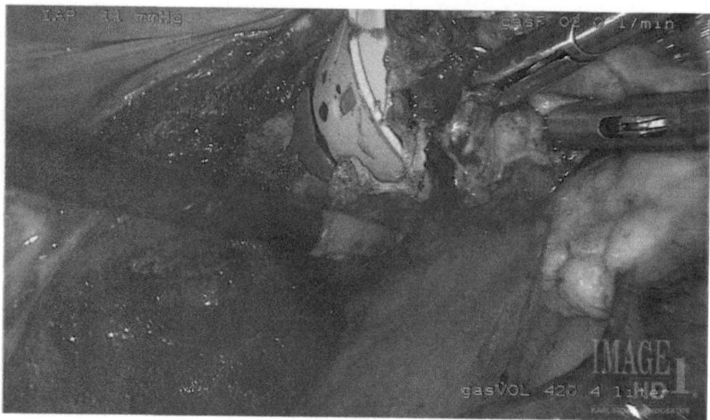

Fig. 37.16 Circumferential colpotomy is performed with the vaginal cuff opened as close to the cervix as possible to preserve vaginal length

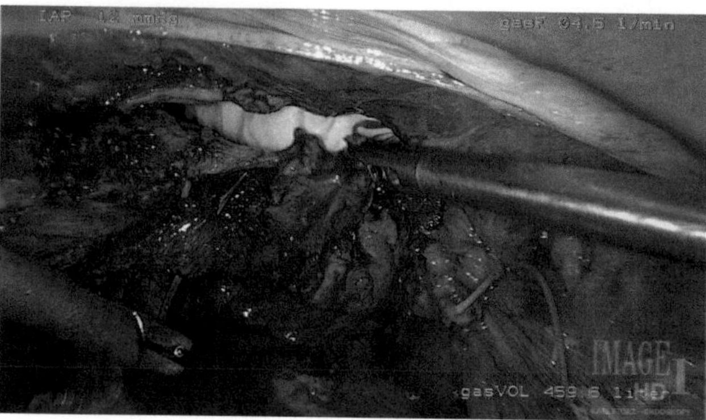

Fig. 37.17 The vaginal cuff is closed using an absorbable monofilament suture. Each bite includes vaginal epithelium and at least 1.5 cm of pubocervical and rectovaginal fascia. Note the presence of a glove in the vagina to maintain pnemoperitoneum

The uterus and adnexa are delivered through the vagina. Rarely, in the case of prolapse, would the uterus be too large to fit through the vagina. Under those exceptions, it will need to be removed using a bag and morcelation or other technique of surgeon preference. Controversy regarding morcelation is outside the scope of this chapter. A vaginal occlusion device is placed in the vagina to maintain pneumoperitoneum throughout the remainder of the procedure or until the cuff is closed.

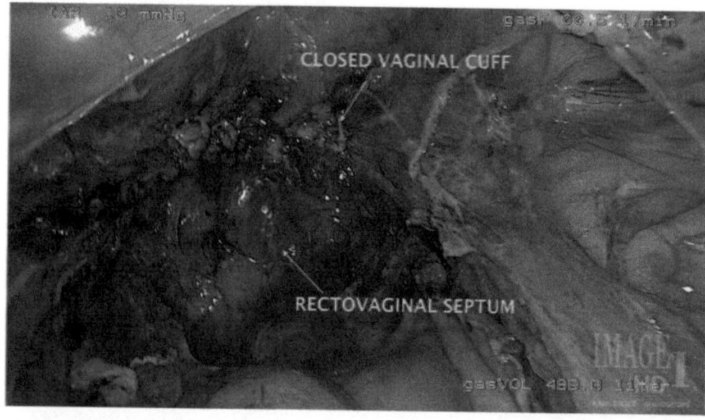

Fig. 37.18 The vaginal cuff is seen fully closed. The right ureter can also be visualized

Step 5

Cuff Closure with Enterocele Repair

For those patients with enterocele, a two-layer closure of the vaginal cuff is performed. The first layer is to close the vaginal epithelium with 3-0 or 2-0 absorbable monofilament sutures followed by a second layer to reapproximate the pubocervical fascia and rectovaginal septum with permanent non-absorbable sutures. Special care must be taken to include adequate fascial tissue in the suture bites.

This step will repair the enterocele and restore the integrity of vaginal fibromuscular tube.

Cuff Closure Without Presence of Enterocele

Closure of the cuff should always re-approximate the rectovaginal septum and the pubocervical fascia. For those patients without enterocele, the vaginal cuff can be closed laparoscopically using a monofilament absorbable suture (Fig. 37.17). Large bites are incorporated that include pubocervical fascia, rectovaginal septum and both anterior and posterior vaginal epithelium (Fig. 37.18). We advocate taking suture bites of at least 1–1.5 cm of tissue for the vaginal cuff closure. Due to the magnifying effect of the laparoscopic view, the surgeon can have a false perception of the amount of tissue included while suturing. Small vaginal cuff suture bites and inadequate hemostasis are the leading causes of postoperative vaginal cuff bleeding and dehiscence.

Step 6

Vaginal Apical Suspension

Uterosacral ligament vaginal vault suspension is performed to re-suspend the apex of the vagina to the level of the ischial spine—the normal anatomical position of the vaginal apex (Fig. 37.19).

To determine the location of the ischial spine, the surgeon places two fingers inside the vagina, palpating the ischial spine, while simultaneously viewing laparoscopically the exact location of the ischial spine from above. A rectal probe can be used to deviate the rectum away from each side of the operative field as the surgeon incorporates the uterosacral ligament complex of tissue at the level of the ischial spine. Using a large-diameter permanent, non-absorbable suture, a deep bite is placed at the point about 1.5–2 cm medial and posterior to the ischial spine (Fig. 37.20). The surgeon should confirm that this stitch truly incorporates the uterosacral ligament by lifting it. It should be a substantial bite that can tolerate significant traction (Fig. 37.21). While elevating the tissue, a second, deeper, bite is taken (Fig. 37.22). This suture is then plicated to the lateral part of the vaginal cuff on the

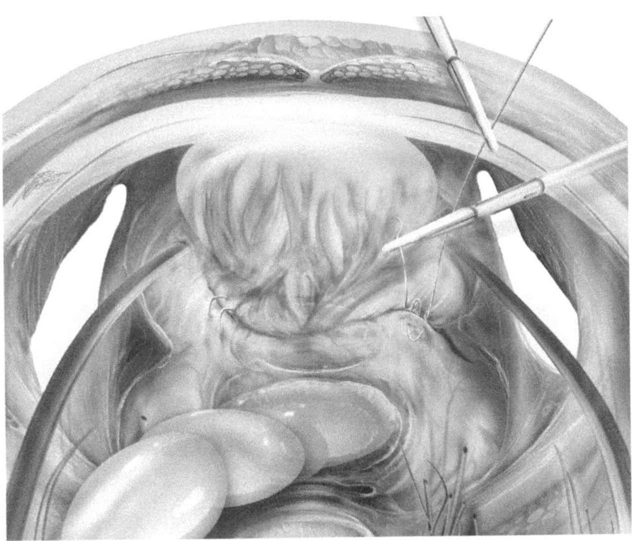

Fig. 37.19 A large permanent suture is used to secure a substantial figure-of-eight bite of tissue at the level of the ischial spine

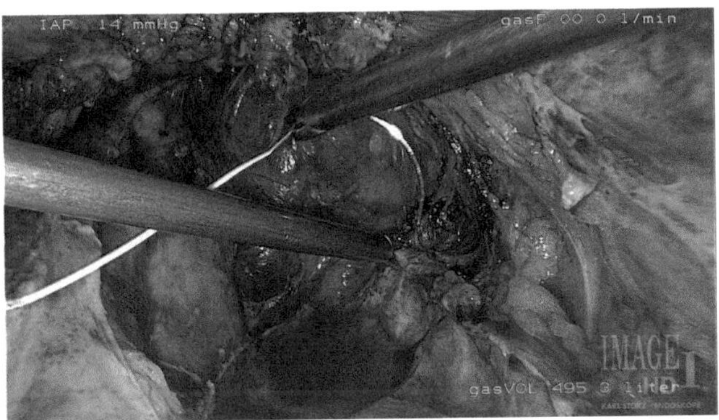

Fig. 37.20 Using two fingers transvaginally, the landmarks of the ischial spines are first identified before placing the first suture. Large suture bites are taken 1.5–2 cm medial and posterior to the ischial spine

ipisilateral side with a sizeable bite of rectovaginal septum and pubocervical fascia (Figs. 37.23, 37.24, and 37.25).

The same procedure is performed bilaterally (Figs. 37.26 and 37.27). Both sutures are tied with extracorporeal knot technique without undue tension (Fig. 37.28). With too much tension there is a higher risk of postoperative pain and discomfort with failure of the suspension.

Care must be taken not to leave any suture gaps. If suture gaps are evident, a second stitch with the same suture material is used to close the gaps (Figs. 37.29, 37.30, and 37.31).

Typically, we use CV-0 Gore-Tex (Gore Medical, Flagstaff, AZ) suture or Number 1 Ethibond (Ethicon) suture for laparoscopic uterosacral ligament vaginal vault suspension, with good result. These sutures should not enter the vaginal canal. Vaginal exposure of those permanent non-absorbable sutures will lead to development of annoying foreign body granulation tissue, vaginal bleeding and possible infection.

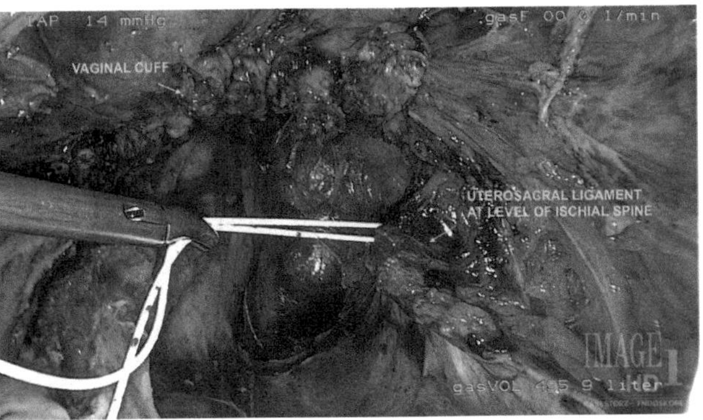

Fig. 37.21 The first bite on the uterosacral ligament at the level of the ischial spines is pulled with enough tension to ensure the strength and depth of tissue is adequate. This elevation will assure an ideal placement of the second bite

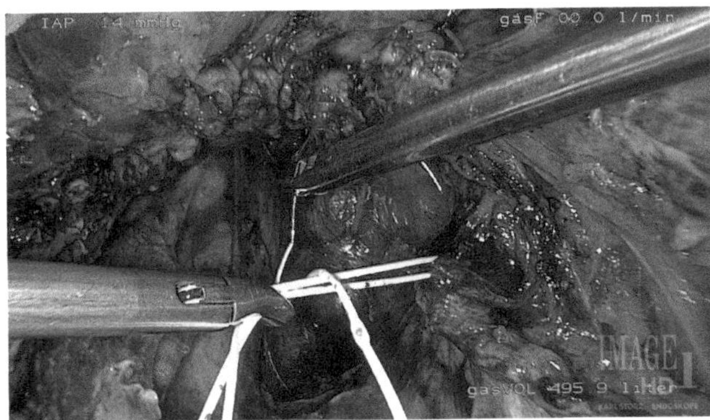

Fig. 37.22 The first suture is lifted and a much larger second bite with the same suture is taken at the same location, that is 1.5–2 cm medial and posterior to the ischial spine

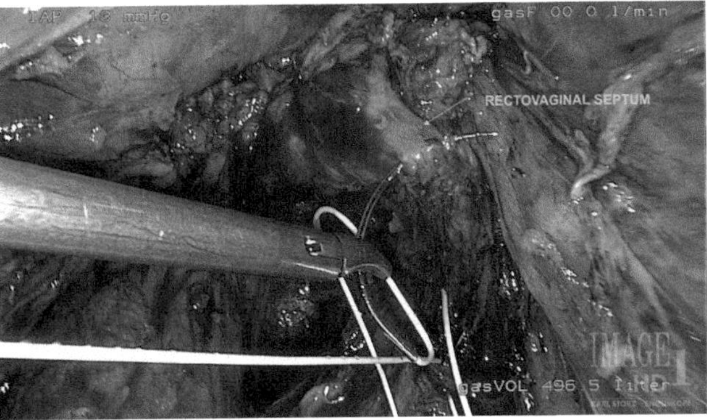

Fig. 37.23 The uterosacral ligament is plicated to the lateral apex of the vagina, incorporating the rectovaginal septum. The uterosacral ligament suture is then continued, plicating it with a large bite of rectovaginal septum close to the closed vaginal cuff. This same suture will continue through the lateral portion of the vaginal cuff, incorporating a large bite of pubocervical fascia just anteriorly above the vaginal cuff

Sacrocolpopexy

The purpose of using mesh in abdominal, robotic or laparoscopic sacrocolpopexy is to replace the failed endopelvic fascia. The risks of mesh are well documented and include

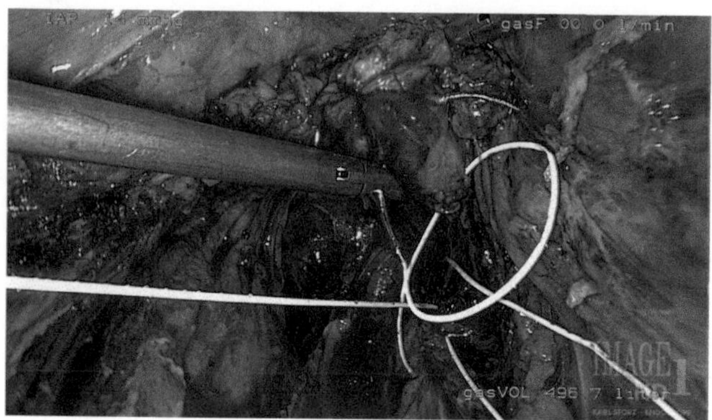

Fig. 37.24 A second bite secures the rectovaginal septum. Occasionally, two bites of rectovaginal septum posteriorly may be taken in cases with more severe prolapse

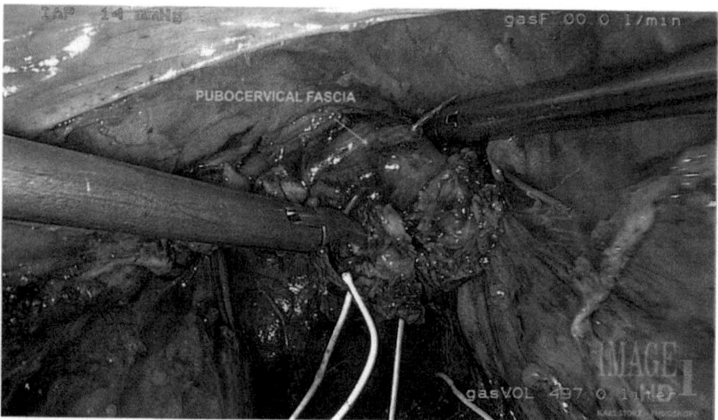

Fig. 37.25 The large bite of pubocervical fascia is incorporated and sutured with the same ipsilateral uterosacral ligament suture

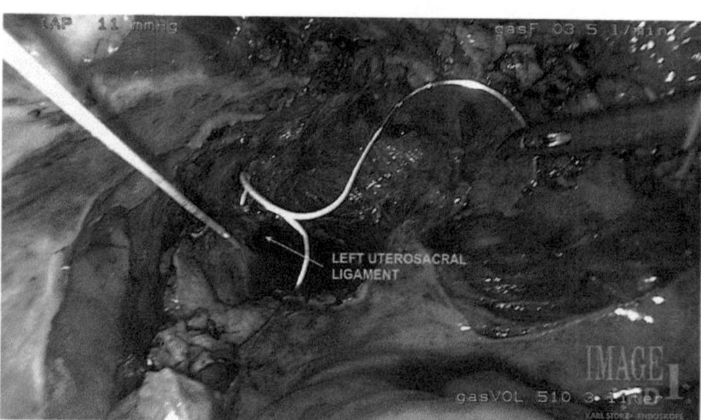

Fig. 37.26 The left uterosacral ligament is secured at the level of the ischial spines

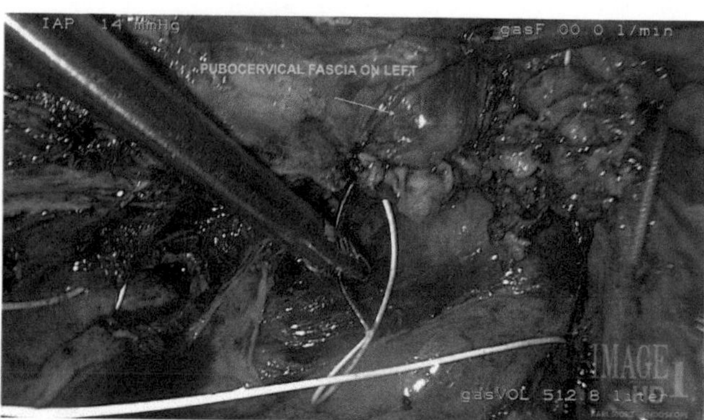

Fig. 37.27 The left uterosacral ligament is plicated to the ipisilateral rectovaginal septum, vaginal apex, and here incorporating the left aspect of the pubocervical fascia

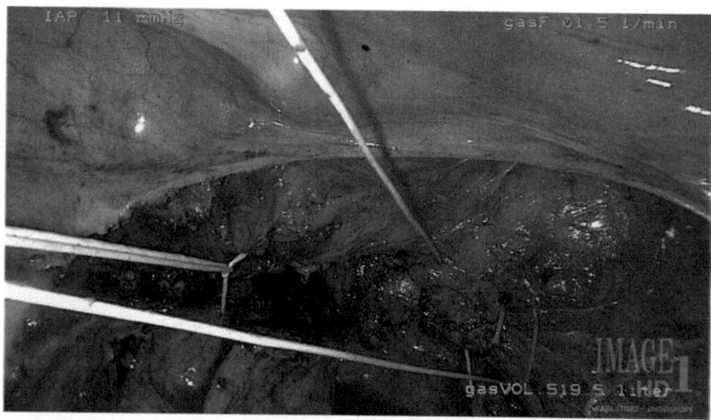

Fig. 37.28 Bilateral uterosacral ligament sutures are seen suspending the apex of the vaginal cuff

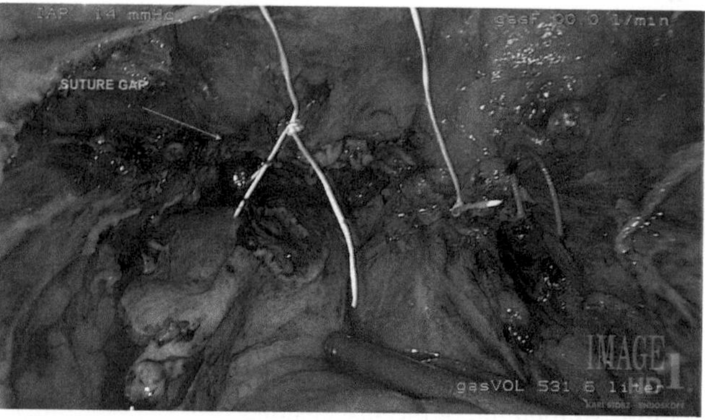

Fig. 37.29 This image demonstrates the gap in the initial suspension stitch on the left. This will be closed using a second suture of the same material. This is shown to illustrate that all suspension sutures are, and must be tied without undue tension

infection, erosion, pain, contraction of the scar and dyspareunia. Multiple studies have demonstrated that some types of mesh are superior to others and it is clear that large pore polypropylene mesh carries the lowest risk of infection, while the ePTFE mesh confers a fourfold increased risk of complications. Concomitant total hysterectomy and smoking increase the risk of mesh complications and are modifiable factors [9].

If a sacrocolpopexy has been planned, a supracervical hysterectomy should be performed, unless contraindicated [9]. Supracervical hysterectomy can easily be accomplished after both uterine vessels are secured and divided. Most menopausal uteri can be placed in a bag and easily removed by slightly extending the fascial incision of the largest laparoscopic or

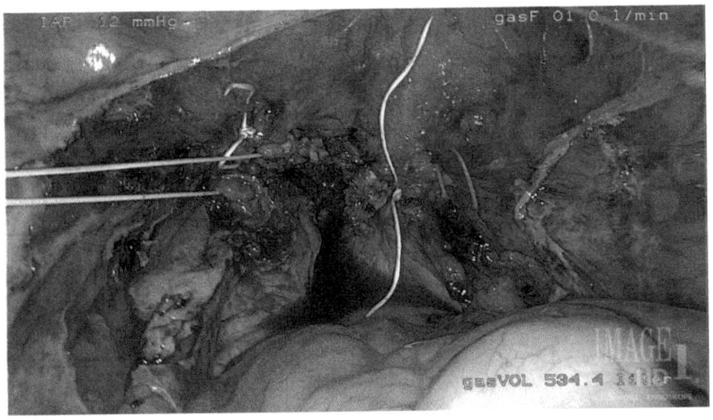

Fig. 37.30 Note how the second suture closes the gap without creating undue tension on the suspension

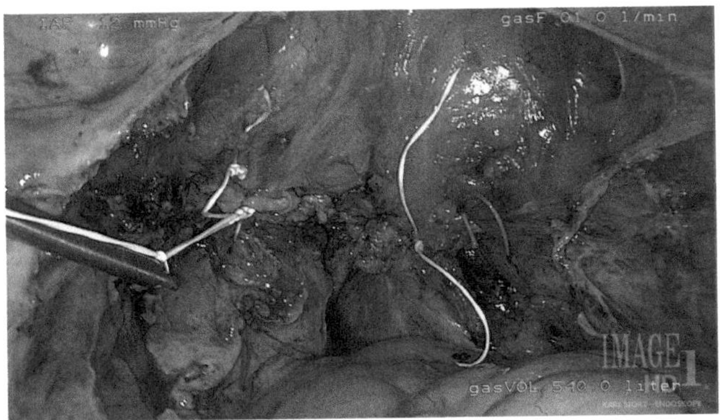

Fig. 37.31 Here we see the completion of the uterosacral ligament suspension and the re-establishment of the pericervical ring

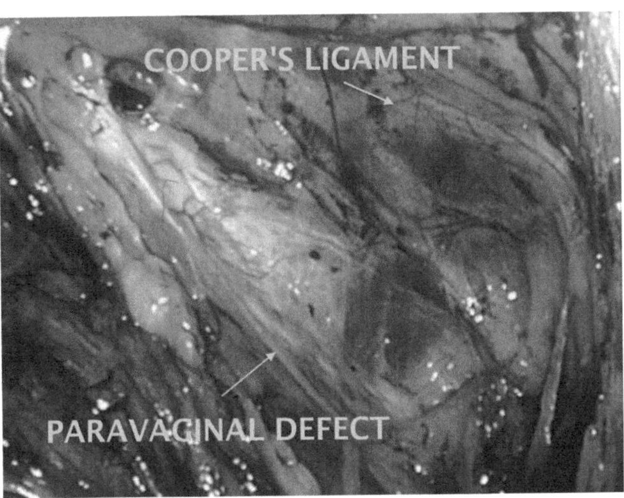

Fig. 37.32 A paravaginal defect can be appreciated in this photo. A paravaginal defect may be responsible for a persistent anterior compartment defect following apical suspension

robotic port. For larger uteri, safe extraction techniques have been described and are beyond the scope of this chapter.

The sigmoid colon is deviated to the patient's left side with the use of a rectal probe. A longitudinal incision is made on the peritoneum overlying the sacral promontory. The incision should be medial to the ureter and common iliac vessels and lateral to the descending sigmoid colon. Careful dissection is carried out along the right side of S-1 and S-2 to expose the anterior longitudinal ligament of the sacrum. Special care must be paid not to injure the middle and lateral sacral vessels in this area. Using a 30° laparoscope will facilitate this dissection. The peritoneal incision is extended caudally to join the longitudinal incision over the right pararectal space, which continues down to the rectovaginal space (see Step 2 above).

If a commercially available Y shaped synthetic mesh is used (Type 1, totally macroporous, Polypropylene mesh), the arms should be trimmed appropriately to fit the exposed fascia. The anterior arm of the mesh is sutured to the previously exposed pubocervical fascia and anterior cervix and the posterior arm of the mesh is sutured to the rectovaginal septum and posterior cervix with 2-0 polypropylene sutures. We typically place one to three rows of three interrupted sutures anteriorly and posteriorly with two on the endopelvic fascia and one on the cervix. An assistant gently pushes the cervix or vaginal vault superiorly, with a vaginal probe until the apex is at the level of the ischial spines. The stem of the Y- mesh is sutured to the anterior longitudinal ligament of the sacrum with two interrupted, non-absorbable sutures. The mesh must be placed snuggly, but without undue tension. Reperitonization with absorbable suture to cover the mesh must also be performed to prevent the rare complication of bowel obstruction secondary to bowel adhesions to the synthetic mesh.

Step 7

Re-evaluation of Pelvic Floor Support

A thorough and systematic vaginal examination must be performed at this time to re-evaluate the pelvic floor support. The apical support and vaginal length, the anterior and posterior vaginal wall support and the status of the perineal body must be carefully evaluated. All of the remaining defects should be corrected.

1. Prolapse of the vaginal apex or cervix.
   (i). The apex of the vagina or cervix must be at the level of the ischial spines.
   (ii). Additional uterosacral ligament suspension sutures should be placed if the apex is not at the level of the ischial spines.
   (iii). In the case of sacrocolpopexy, tighten the mesh to bring the apex of the vagina or cervix up to the level of the ischial spines to restore the normal vaginal length.
2. Persistent anterior vaginal wall defect (Fig. 37.32).

   More than 80% of cystoceles are due to a paravaginal defect and the majority of paravaginal defects will be corrected after the apex of the vagina is restored to its normal position at the level of ischial spine. Therefore, if the anterior wall vaginal defect persists following suspension, one must consider the following three possibilities:

(i). Inadequate or incomplete repair of anterior enterocele.

Re-evaluate the closure of vaginal cuff, to ensure that the pubocervical fascia is well attached to the rectovaginal septum and that the cuff is suspended to the proximal part of the uterosacral ligament at the level of the ischial spine. (Repeat Steps 5 and 6).

(ii). Patient has an extended paravaginal defect.

The retropubic space is entered and dissected laparoscopically, and if paravaginal defect (unilateral or bilateral) is detected, the defect is then repaired by reattaching the pubocervical fascia to the arcus tendineus fascia of pelvis with interrupted stitches using permanent non-absorbable sutures [10].

(iii). Presence of a midline defect: An anterior vaginal colporrhaphy should be performed.

3. Persistent posterior vaginal wall defect.
   (i). Inadequate or incomplete repair of posterior enterocele. Repeat Steps 5 and 6 to evaluate the cuff closure and vault suspension.
   (ii). Rectovaginal septum is detached from the perineal body or the perineal body has been torn or damaged: A vaginal posterior colporrhaphy and perineorrhaphy should be performed.

Step 8

Post Procedure Cystoscopy

Following every laparoscopic hysterectomy and repair of pelvic prolapse, cystoscopy is performed to confirm patency of the ureters and to ascertain no injury to the bladder has occurred. If needed, various agents can be employed to facilitate appreciation of ureteral patency such as indigo carmine, given intravenously at the end of the procedure, or phenazopyridine, given before the case. If bilateral ureteral patency is not observed, then steps must be taken to systematically diagnose the source of the obstruction and resolve the problem. Specific techniques for diagnosing and correcting ureteral injury/obstruction after pelvic reconstructive surgery depend on operator experience and vary by institutional privilege and are thus beyond the scope of this chapter.

Once bilateral ureteral patency is confirmed, a Foley catheter may be left in place until the next post-operative day. A voiding trial may be performed if indicated following removal of the catheter. For patients who fail the voiding trial, the Foley catheter is replaced and they are seen in the office 48 h later for removal of the Foley catheter and a repeat void trial. A suprapubic catheter may alternatively be used.

Conclusion

Coexisting pelvic organ prolapse presents a unique challenge during hysterectomy. Laparoscopic hysterectomy with concomitant surgery for pelvic organ prolapse is effective and minimally invasive. Laparoscopy provides the surgeon with excellent visualization and allows for simultaneous manual examination through the vagina to verify and define the details of repair in a manner not possible through open or robotic procedures.

References

1. Subak LL et al. Cost of pelvic organ prolapse surgery in the United States. Obstet Gynecol. 2001;98(4):646–51.
2. Sprague ML, Furr RS, Rich JS, Liu CY. Treatment of apical prolapse by laparoscopy. In: Bustos-Lopez H, editor. Cirugía Endoscopica en Ginecólogía: Laparoscopia e Histeroscopia. Mexico City: Editorial Médica Panamericana; 2011. p. 177–82.
3. Lin LL, Phelps JY, Liu CY. Laparoscopic vaginal vault suspension using uterosacral ligaments: a review of 133 cases. J Minim Invasive Gynecol. 2005;12:216–20.
4. Umek WH, Morgan DM, Ashton-Miller JA, DeLancey JOL. Quantitative analysis of uterosacral ligament origin and insertion points by magnetic resonance imaging. Obstet Gynecol. 2004; 103(3):447–51.
5. Ramanah R, DeLancey JO, et al. See it in 3D!: researchers examined structural links between the cardinal and uterosacral ligaments. Am J Obstet Gynecol. 2012;207(5):437.e7. doi:10.1016/j.ajog.2012.08.036. Epub 2012 Sep 7.
6. Sprague ML, Furr RS, Liu CY. Laparoscopic surgery for uterine and vaginal vault prolapse. Textbook of gynecological and obstetrical surgery. 2 ed. Ankara: Besevler; 2009.
7. Nager CW, Brubaker L, Litman HJ, et al. A randomized trial of urodynamic testing before stress-incontinence surgery. N Engl J Med. 2012;366:1987.
8. Berger MB, DeLancey JO. Is cervical elongation associated with pelvic organ prolapse? Int Urogynecol J. 2012;23(8):1095–103.
9. Cundiff GW, Varner E, Visco AG, Zyczynski HM, Nager CW, Norton PA, Schaffer J, Brown MB, Brubaker L. Risk factors for mesh/suture erosion following sacral colpopexy. Am J Obstet Gynecol. 2008;199:688.
10. Liu CY. Laparoscopic cystocele repair: paravaginal suspension. In: Liu CY, editor. Laparoscopic hysterectomy and pelvic floor reconstruction. Cambridge: Blackwell; 1996.

Laparoscopic Assisted Vaginal Hysterectomy in Prolapse Situations

38

Hsin-Hong Kuo and Chyi-Long Lee

Introduction

Dr. Harry Reich reported first laparoscopic hysterectomy in 1989, which confirmed the possibility of laparoscopic hysterectomy being employed as a replacement of the vast majority of traditional abdominal hysterectomies.

There are some subdivisions of laparoscopic hysterectomy, which are defined on the basis of the level of laparoscopic operation used to achieve the dissection of the uterus. Total laparoscopic hysterectomy (TLH) involves entire laparoscopic excision of the uterus including laparoscopic closure of the vaginal dome. Laparoscopic assisted vaginal hysterectomy (LAVH) consists of laparoscopic dissection down to the uterine arteries with or without transection of which, and the remainder procedures, including the specimen retrieval, performed through a vaginal approach. For women with prolapse pelvis, the relatively wide vagina route forms a preferable access for vaginal dissection and specimen retrieval. For whom with advanced prolapse uterus, vaginal hysterectomy could be indicated without abdominal wound. The procedures of LAVH are explained steps by steps in the following description. Laparoscopic sacrocolpopexy is an option for the patients with stage two to four uterovaginal prolapses.

H.-H. Kuo (✉)
Gynecologic Endoscopist, Obstetrics and Gynecology, Chang Gung Memorial Hospital, Linko, Taiwan,
No.5, Fuxing St., Guishan Dist., Taoyuan City 33305, Taiwan
e-mail: iamhonghonghong@gmail.com

C.-L. Lee
Chang Gung Memorial Hospital, Keelung Branch,
222 Maijin Road, Anle District, Keelung City 204, Taiwan
e-mail: leechyilong@gmail.com

LAVH Technique- Laparoscopic Dissecting

General anesthesia is required. The patient is placed in the dorsolithotomy Trendelenburg position with both legs protected by elastic bandages. A Foley catheter is inserted for constant urinary drainage. Pelvic examination under anesthesia checks the top of the fundus and makes decision regarding the position of first trocar insertion to have wide surgical view and operating space. A uterine manipulator, generally a setting of Cohen cannula and tenaculum, is placed into the uterus. The axis of the tip of Cohen cannula should be parallel to the axis of uterus to avoid uterine perforating damage while cephalad pushing.

The selection of the size, number and positions of the trocars depend on the circumstanced and surgeon's preferences. But generally speaking, the videolaparoscopy is performed with a midline 10 mm principal trocar introduced through the umbilicus. The ancillary cannulas are placed under laparoscopic visualization: one 5 mm cannula in the right lower quadrant lateral to the inferior epigastric arteries, and one 5 mm cannula in the left lower quadrant. The third 5 mm cannula can be placed in the left or right upper quadrant between the telescope and lateral ports. Once the cannula placement is completed, the patient is placed in a steep Trendelenburg position to allow the bowel out of the pelvis and adhesions are lysed as necessary.

For the case with large uterus, especially at or above the level of the umbilicus, the Lee-Huang point (Fig. 38.1) is recommended for videolaparoscopy.

It locates between the xiphoid process and the umbilicus, which provide a sufficient view of the operative field and adequate space for unimpaired motion of the surgeon's instruments.

The operation begins with the coagulation and dissection of bilateral round ligaments: the anterior leaves of the broad ligaments are opened and incised using unipolar or bipolar electrosurgery to the point of the vesico-uterine pouch (Fig. 38.2a–d). If the tubes and ovaries are to be conserved, the ovarian ligament and the proximal end of tubes are coagulated

I. Alkatout, L. Mettler (eds.), *Hysterectomy*, DOI 10.1007/978-3-319-22497-8_38

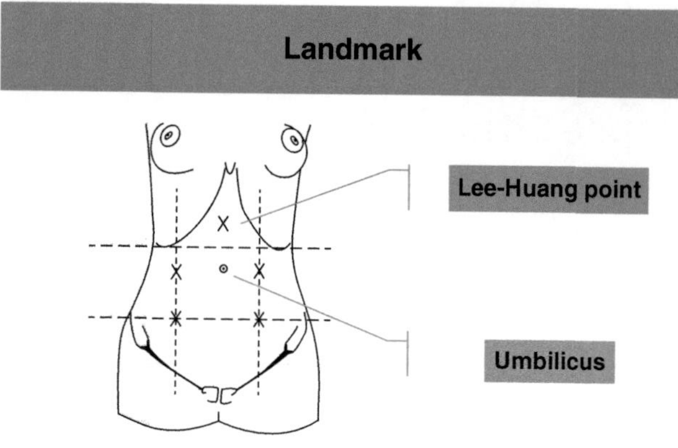

Fig. 38.1 Landmark for Lee-Huang point

and dissected (Fig. 38.3a, b). If the tubes and the ovaries are to be removed with the uterus, the infundibulopelvic (IP) portion of the broad ligament is coagulated and dissected. Before this step, a peritoneal window is created to prevent ureteral damage (Fig. 38.4a–d). The ureter is usually easy to recognize at the level of the pelvic brim, and its peristalsis distinguishes ureter from the pulsating artery. While the IP is elevated gently, the created window is identified in the medial leaf of the broad ligament between the ureter and the IP. The IP is then divided by monopolar and bipolar device. The opening of the medial (or posterior) leaf of the broad ligament can be extended, parallel to the lateral side of the uterus, to the point of origin of the uterosacral ligaments behind the cervix (Fig. 38.5a, b). The ureter should be

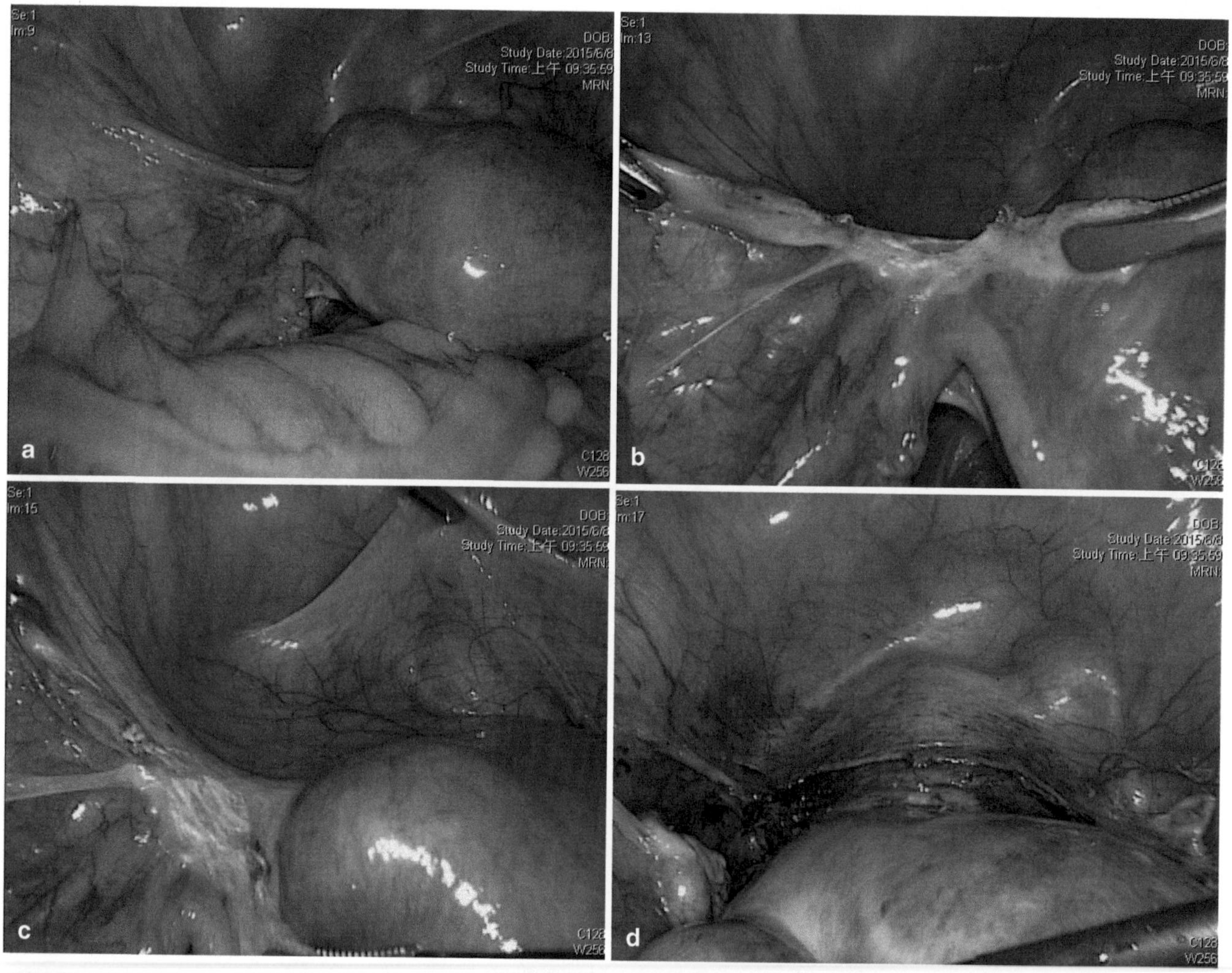

Fig. 38.2 (**a**) Before dissecting the round ligament. (**b**) Dissecting left round ligament with bipolar and unipolary Electrosurgery (**c**) Left round ligament has been dissected. The grasper holds the serosal of bladder. The vesico-uterine pouch locates in the junction between the held serosa and the low uterine corpus. (**d**) The vesico-uterine pouch has been exposed. (**e**) Left leaf of the broad ligament has been exposed. (**f**) A case with history of Cesarean Section. The vesico-uterine pouch is covered by the scarring tissue. (**g**) The dissecting plane is close to the uterus as possible. (**h**) Exposure of bilateral anterior leaves of the broad ligaments and the vesico-uterine pouch. Photos courtesy of Chyi-Long Lee and Kuan-Gen Huang

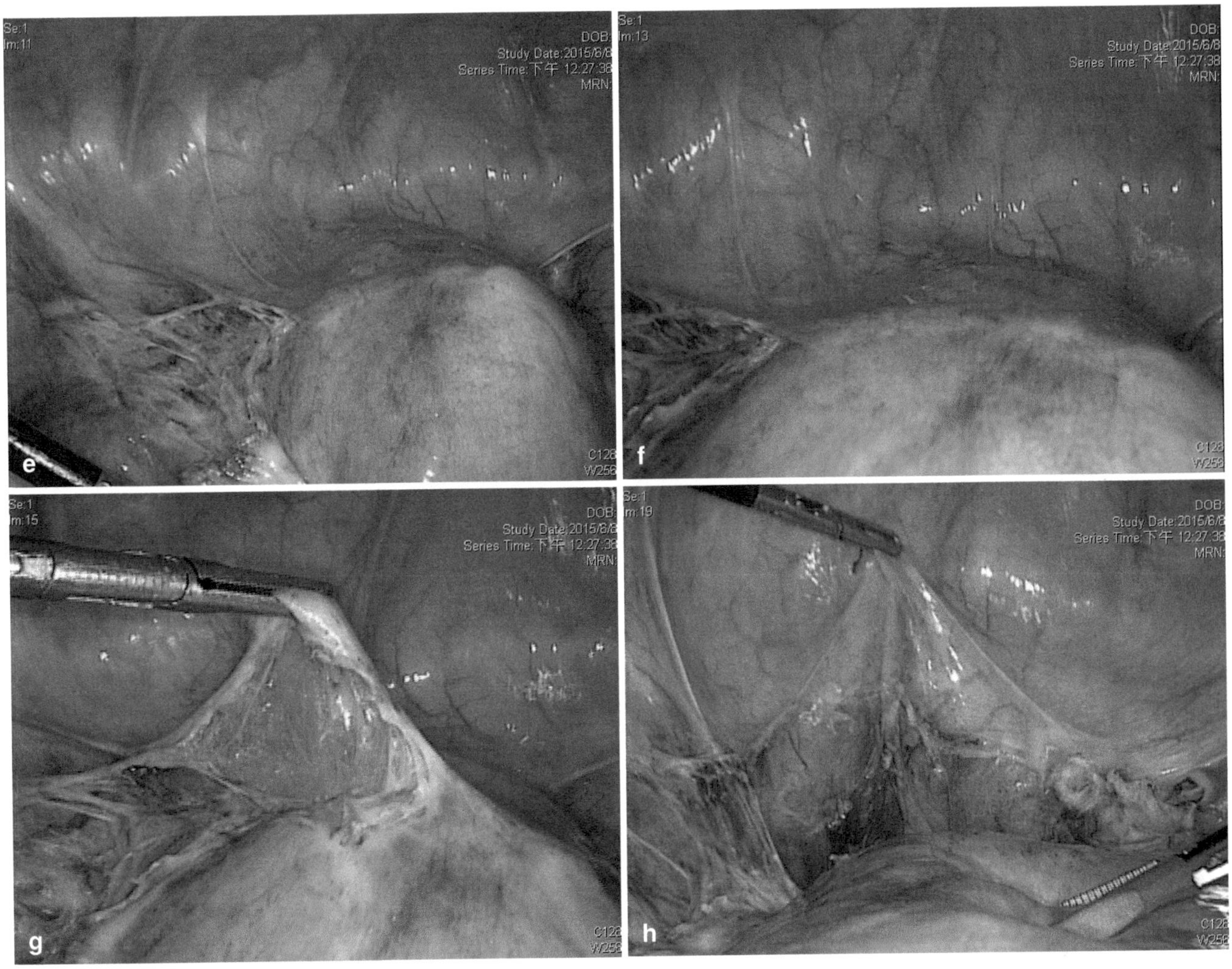

Fig. 38.2 (continued)

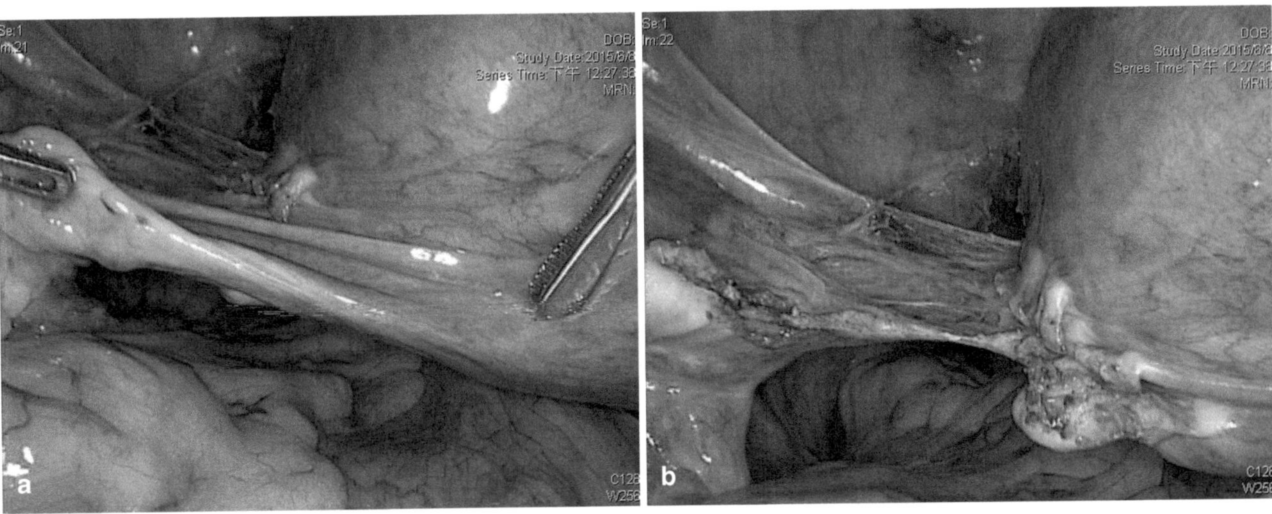

Fig. 38.3 (**a**) Before dissecting left tube and ovarian ligament, (**b**) after dissecting left tube and ovarian ligament. Photos courtesy of Chyi-Long Lee and Kuan-Gen Huang

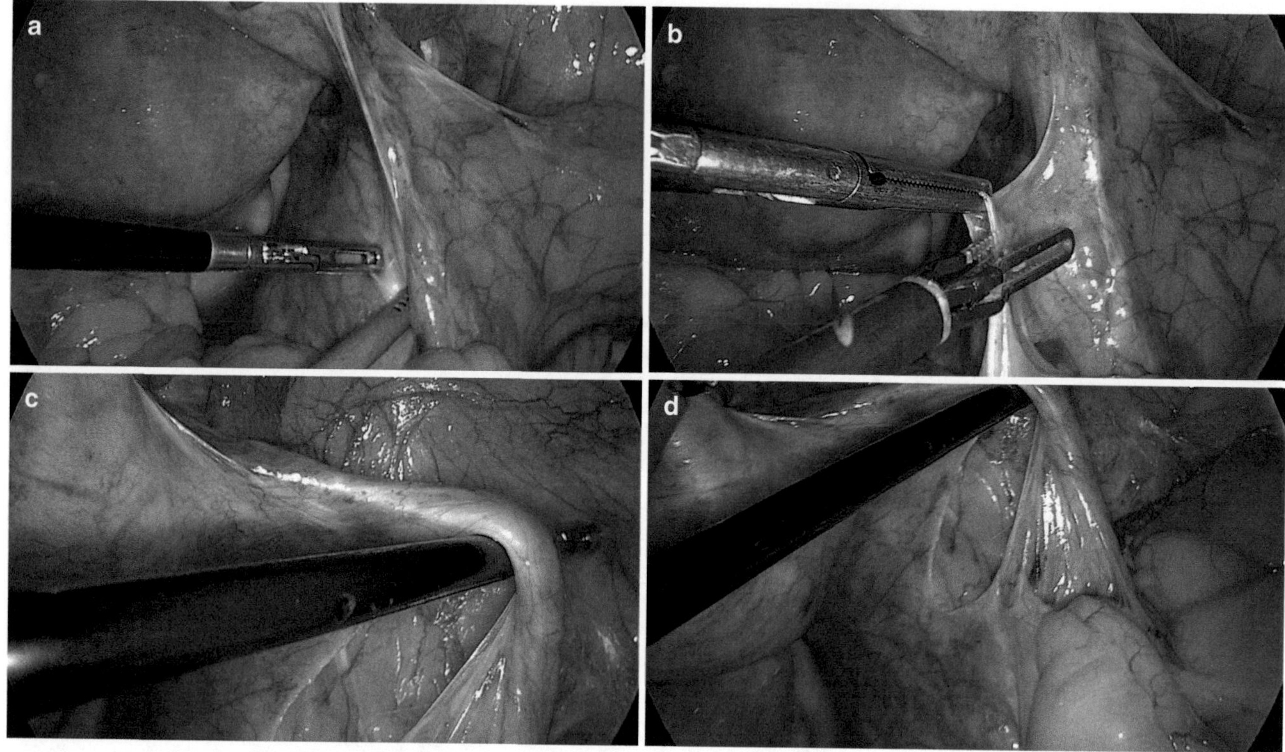

Fig. 38.4 (**a**) The grasper lies between the ureter and the IP (infundibulopelvic) ligament. (**b**) Opening the window between the ureter and the IP ligament. (**c**) The dissecting window for salpingo-oophrectomy. (**d**) The window lies between the ureter and the IP ligament. Photos courtesy of Chyi-Long Lee and Kuan-Gen Huang

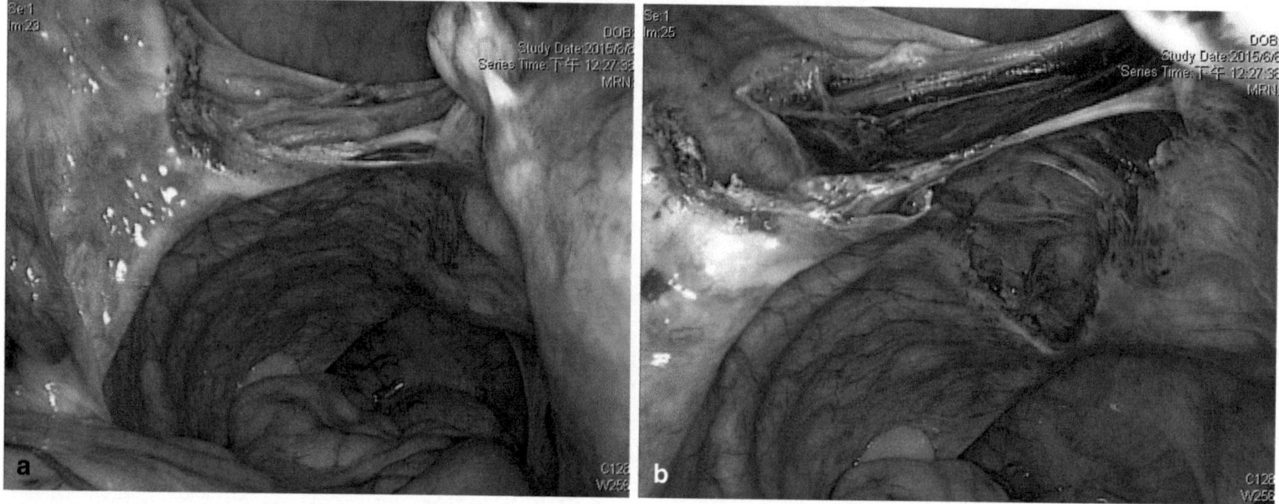

Fig. 38.5 (**a**) The opening of the medial leaf of the broad ligament is seen after the ovarian ligament, tube and round ligament have been dissected. (**b**) The peritoneum is extended, parallel to the lateral side of the uterus, to the point of the uterosacral ligaments

identified medial to the cutting edge of the medial (or posterior) leaf. The same procedure is repeated on another side.

The parametrium is coagulated (or dissected) along the uterus by bipolar and monopolar electrosurgery to the level of the uterine artery near uterine isthmus. Ureteral injury usually happens in this step and some tips should be pointed out. Firstly, the secondary assistant should keep the tension of cephalad by pushing the manipulator to keep the ureter away from the dissecting plane (Fig. 38.6a). Secondary, the principal of the dissecting plane is closely alone with the lateral side of the uterus but its also depends on the level of uterus. The plane near the fundus should be away from the uterus to prevent injury to the ascending branch of the uterine artery (Fig. 38.6b). At the level near uterine isthmus, the plane should just adjacent to the uterus due to the distance between ureter and uterine artery less then 1 cm (Fig. 38.6c, d). The risk of thermal damage of the ureter could be minimized if the safe margin is maximized. Third, some studies reports the incidence of the ureter injuries is prone to occur contralateral to the surgeon side, especially in the case of big uterus. The big uterus leads to difficult manipulating and may prevent the dissecting direction parallel to the lateral side of uterus but toward to the sidewall (Fig. 38.6e, f). In this situation, the surgeon is recommended to shift to the opposite (first assistant) side and the dissecting plane is naturally parallel to the lateral side of uterus (Fig. 38.6g–j).

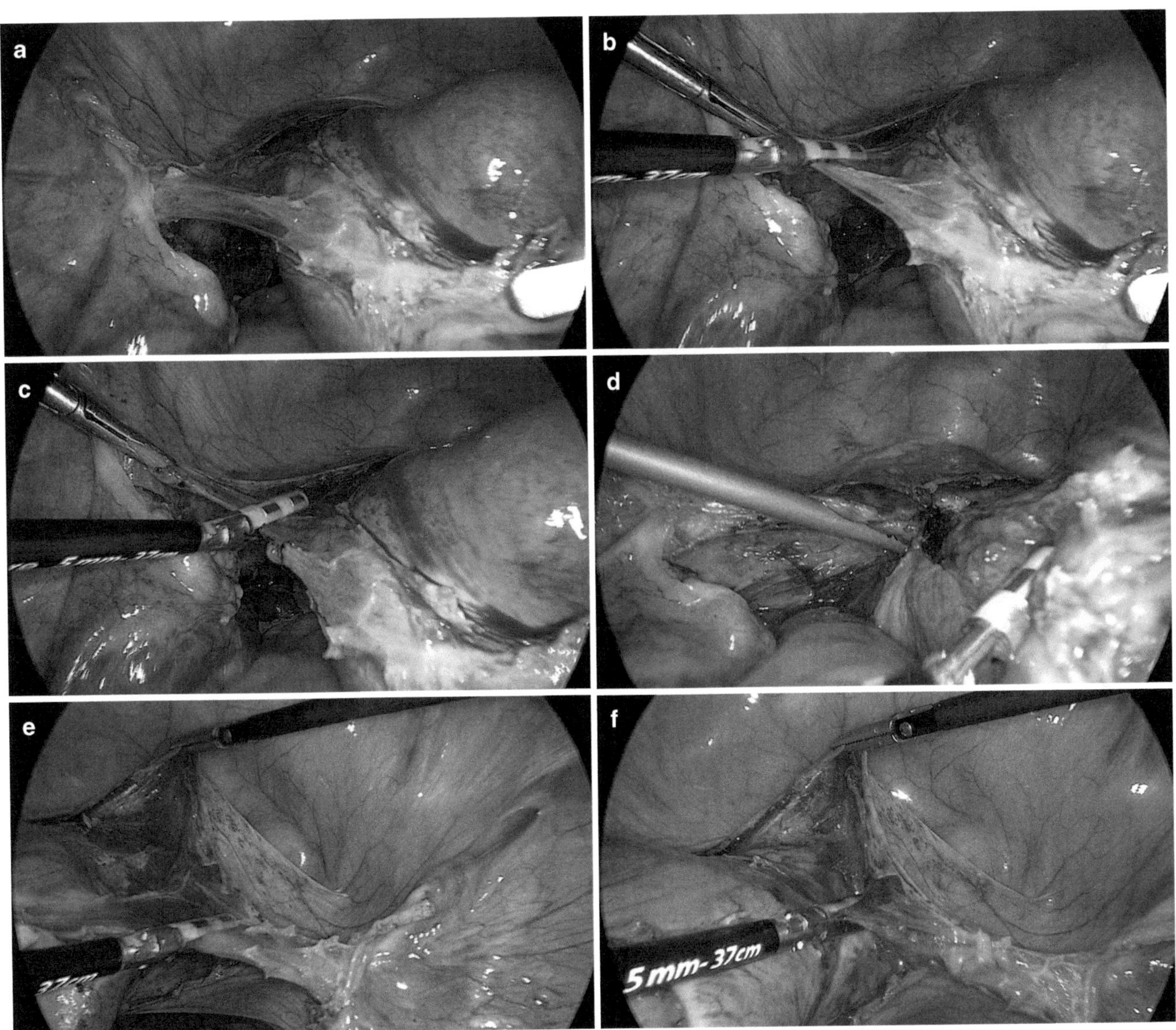

Fig. 38.6 (**a**) The uterus is push cephalad and opposite to the dissecting plane to allow wide operating space and prevent ureteral injury. (**b**) The proximal dissecting plane is away from the uterus. (**c**) During dissecting, the plane is closing to the uterus gradually. (**d**) At the level of isthmus, the dissecting plane should close the uterus. (**e**) In the assistant side, the dissecting plane is toward to the sidewall. (**f**) The surgeon should correct the dissecting plane along with the uterine sidewall. (**g**) Operating in the assistant side, the dissecting plane toward to the uterus, not the pelvic sidewall. (**h**) Through the operating in the assistant side, the uterine artery is dissected with any thermal effect in the pelvic sidewall. (**i**) Before coagulation or dissection of bilateral uterine arteries. A pink uterine corpus. (**j**) The ischemic change of the uterine corpus after the coagulation or dissection of the uterine arteries. Photos courtesy of Chyi-Long Lee and Kuan-Gen Huang

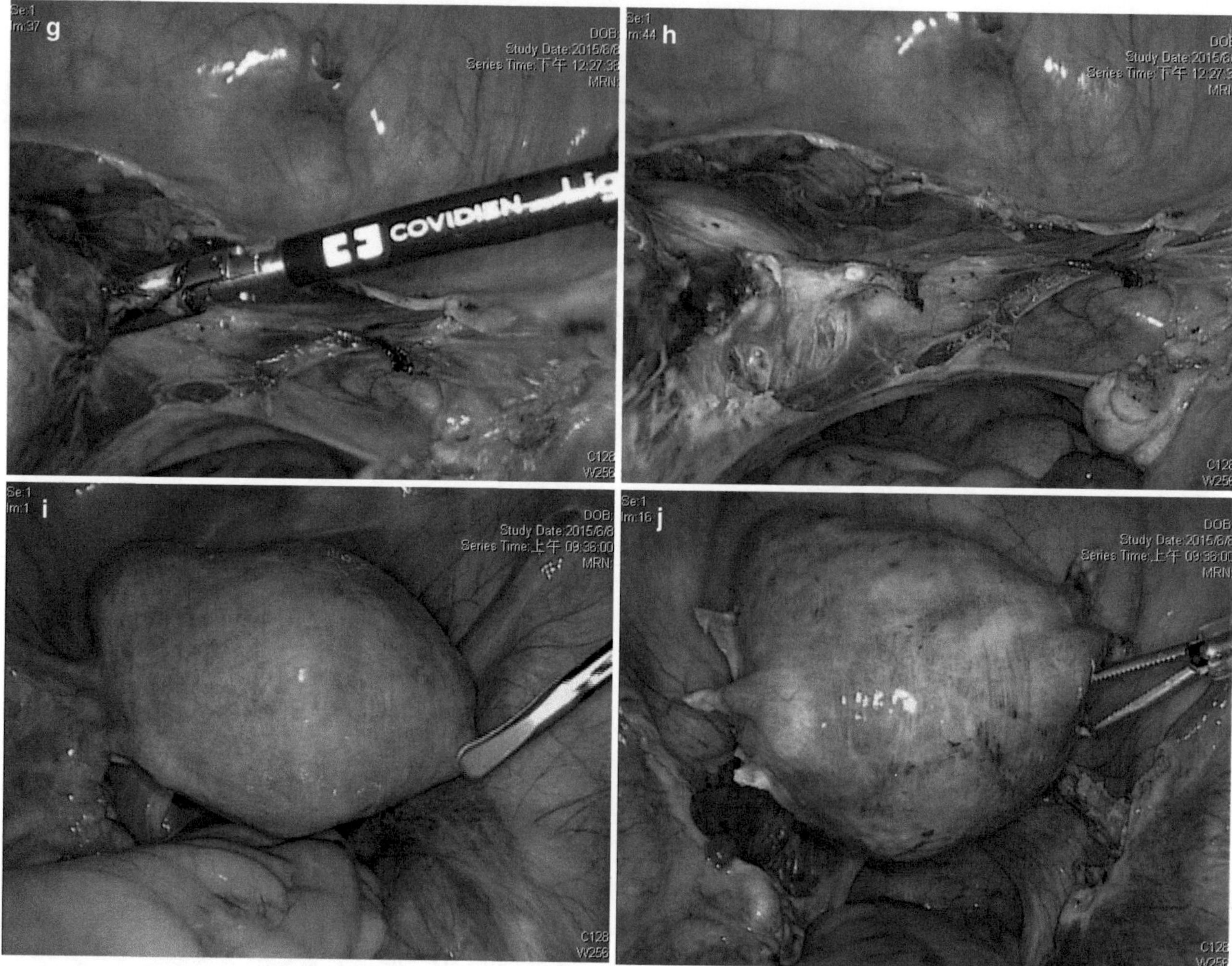

Fig. 38.6 (continued)

The bilateral incision of anterior leaf of the broad ligaments unites in the vesico-uterine pouch. To facilitate dissecting the bladder, a simple method is introduced: the folding gauze clamped by a ring forceps is inserted above the tenaculum (into the anterior fornix) to guide the vesico-uterine pouch and by the gentle pushing of the suction irrigation gear against on the assisted gauzed, separation of the uterus and anterior bladder flap can be easily achieved (Fig. 38.7 a–c). This mechanical procedure is superior to the electro-dissecting to prevent postoperative paralyzing of the bladder. An anterior colpotomy is performed by using monopolar cautery at the level about 1 cm below the cervicovaginal junction. This procedure can be easily evaluated by the exposure of the assisted gauze (Fig. 38.7d). A posterior colpotomy can also be repeated by means of the assisted gauze and unipolar incision method (Fig. 38.7e–g).

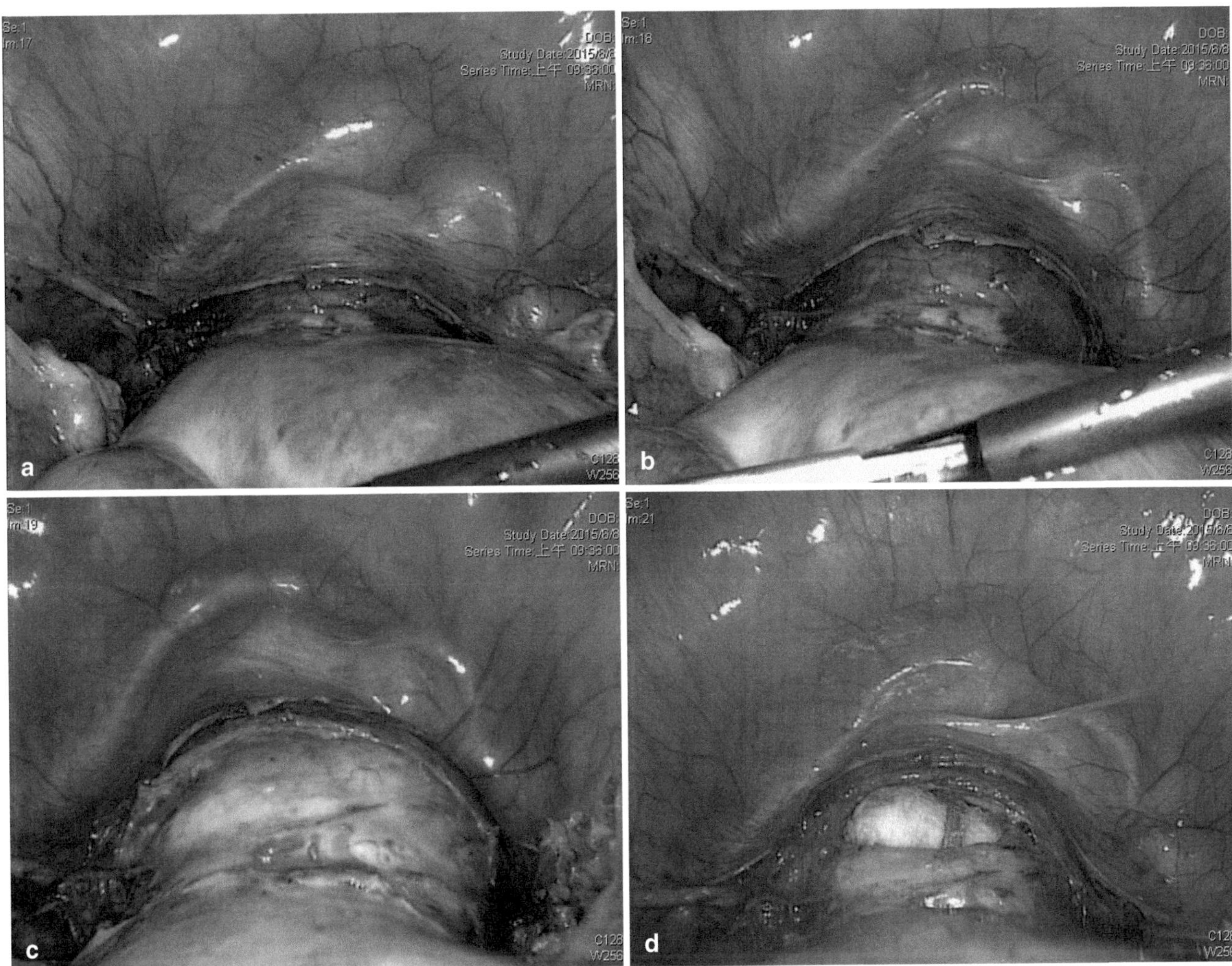

Fig. 38.7 (**a**) Before the assistance of the folding gauze. (**b**) The folding gauze is pushed to the anterior fornix to guide the dissecting of the vesico-uterine pouch. (**c**) The bladder has been dissected away from the vesico-uterine pouch. (**d**) The gauze is exposed. (**e**) Before the assistance of the folding gauze in the posterior fornix. (**f**) The folding gauze is pushed to the posterior fornix. (**g**) The gauze is exposed; the opening of the posterior colpotomy has been finished through abdominal approach. Photos courtesy of Chyi-Long Lee and Kuan-Gen Huang

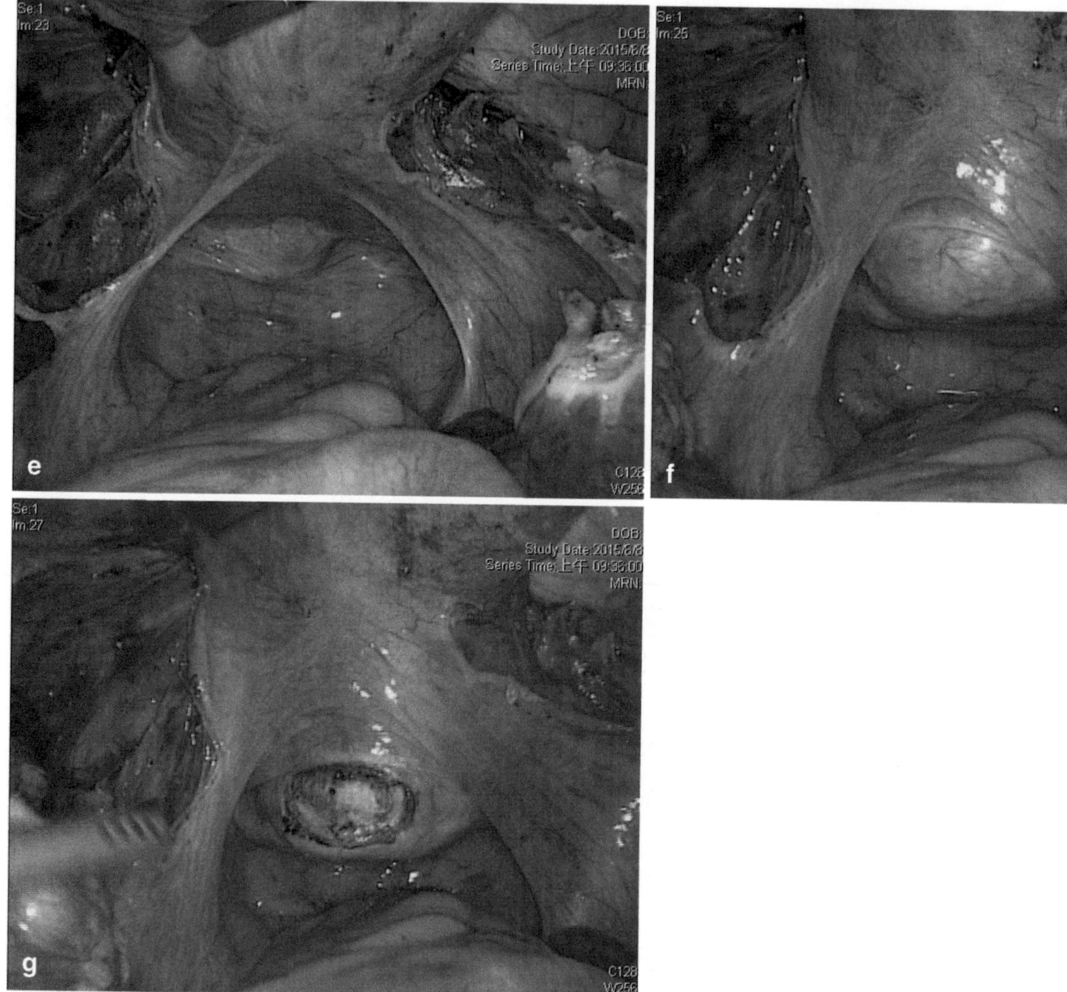

Fig. 38.7 (continued)

LAVH Technique- Vaginal Dissecting

With tractions placed on the uterine cervix by tenaculum, the openings of anterior and posterior colpotomy are extended and the wound retractor maintains the spaces. The bilateral uterosacral ligaments and uterine arteries are clamped by surgical clamp and dissected as the procedures of vaginal hysterectomy (Fig. 38.8a). The detached uterus is removed by manual peeling morcellation (Fig. 38.8b). The vaginal cuff is closed vaginally using a running, non-locking stitch of 2-0 absorbable sutures.

LAVH Technique- Laparoscopic Hemostasis

After the closure of the vaginal cuff, pneumoperitoneum is re-established and the vaginal cuff, bilateral stumps of adnexa and any rough surface are inspected to ensure hemostasis (Fig. 38.9a–h). The peritoneal cavity is irrigated and lavaged until a blood less condition is achieved.

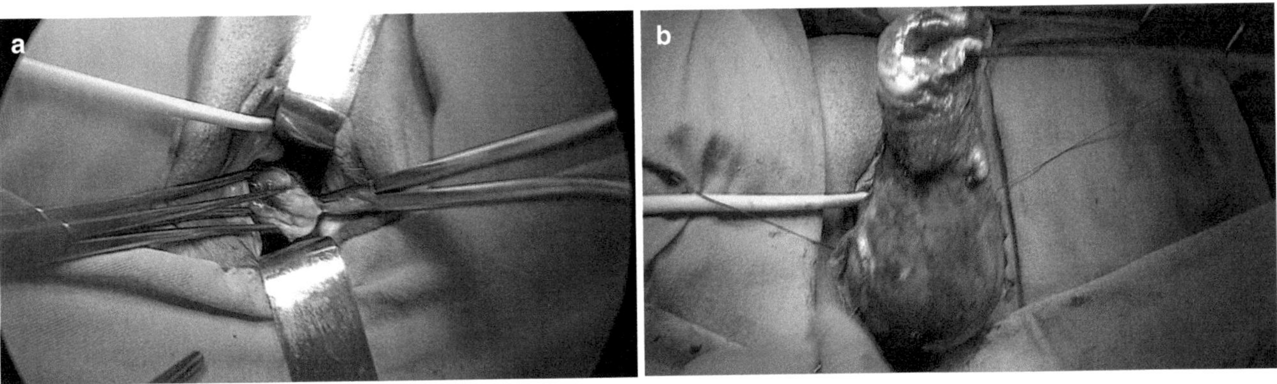

Fig. 38.8 (**a**) The uterosacral ligament is clamped as the procedures of vaginal hysterectomy. (**b**) The specimen is removed through vagina. Photos courtesy of Chyi-Long Lee and Kuan-Gen Huang

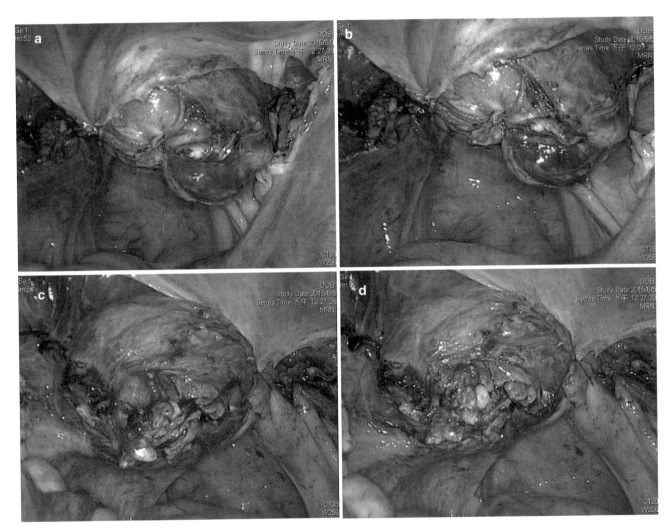

Fig. 38.9 (**a**) Under the assistance of the folding gauze, the right stump of the uterine artery is identified. (**b**) Routine coagulation is made for the distal end of the stump to prevent it bleeding while extubation (increase abdominal pressure). (**c**) Same maneuver (exposure) in the left side. (**d**) Same maneuver (routine coagulation) in the left side. (**e**) Final inspection. (**f**) Well hemostasis of left adnexa. (**g**) Well hemostasis of right adnexa. Photos courtesy of Chyi-Long Lee and Kuan-Gen Huang

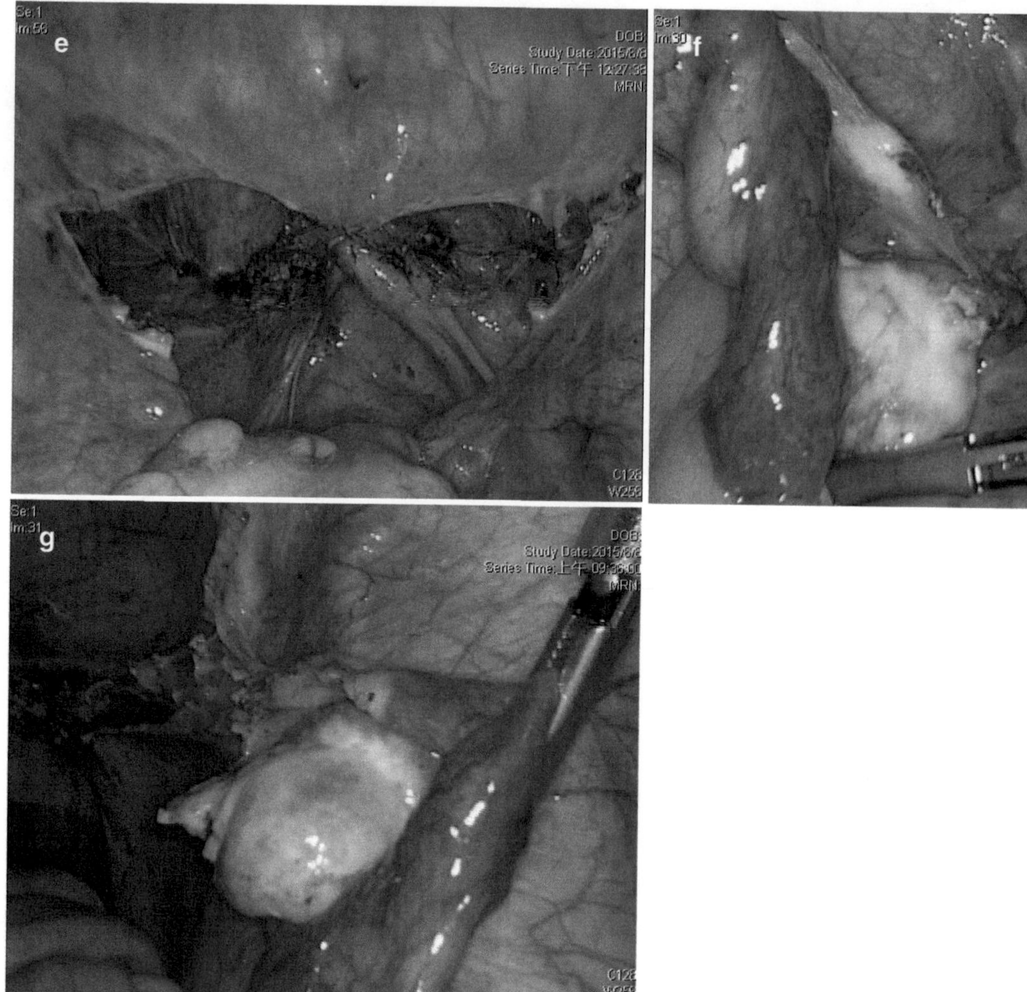

Fig. 38.9 (continued)

Optional Laparoscopic Sacro-colpopexy

The peritoneum superficial to the sacral promontory is incised and an avascular plane in the anterior longitudinal ligament is identified using blunt dissection (Fig. 38.10a, b). This peritoneal window, right of the midline, medial to the right ureter is dissected and continued down to the right uterosacral ligament (Fig. 38.10c, d). The polypropylene mesh is trimmed according to the estimated length between the vaginal vault and the sacral promontory. The distal end is fixed to the vaginal vault exposed by the assistant using the folding gauze (Fig. 38.10e, f). The proximal end of the mesh is interrupted sutured and anchored to the avascular plane in the longitudinal ligament with a total of two non-absorbable sutures (Fig. 38.10g). The exposed peritoneum is approximated with absorbable suture to retroperitoneally cover the mesh (Fig. 38.10h).

LAVH Technique- Routine Cystoscopy

A rigid 70° routine cystoscopy is then performed. Under a direct visualization, the ureteral jets proved the patent of bilateral ureter and the integrity of bladder ruled the penetrating suture materials out (Fig. 38.11a–c).

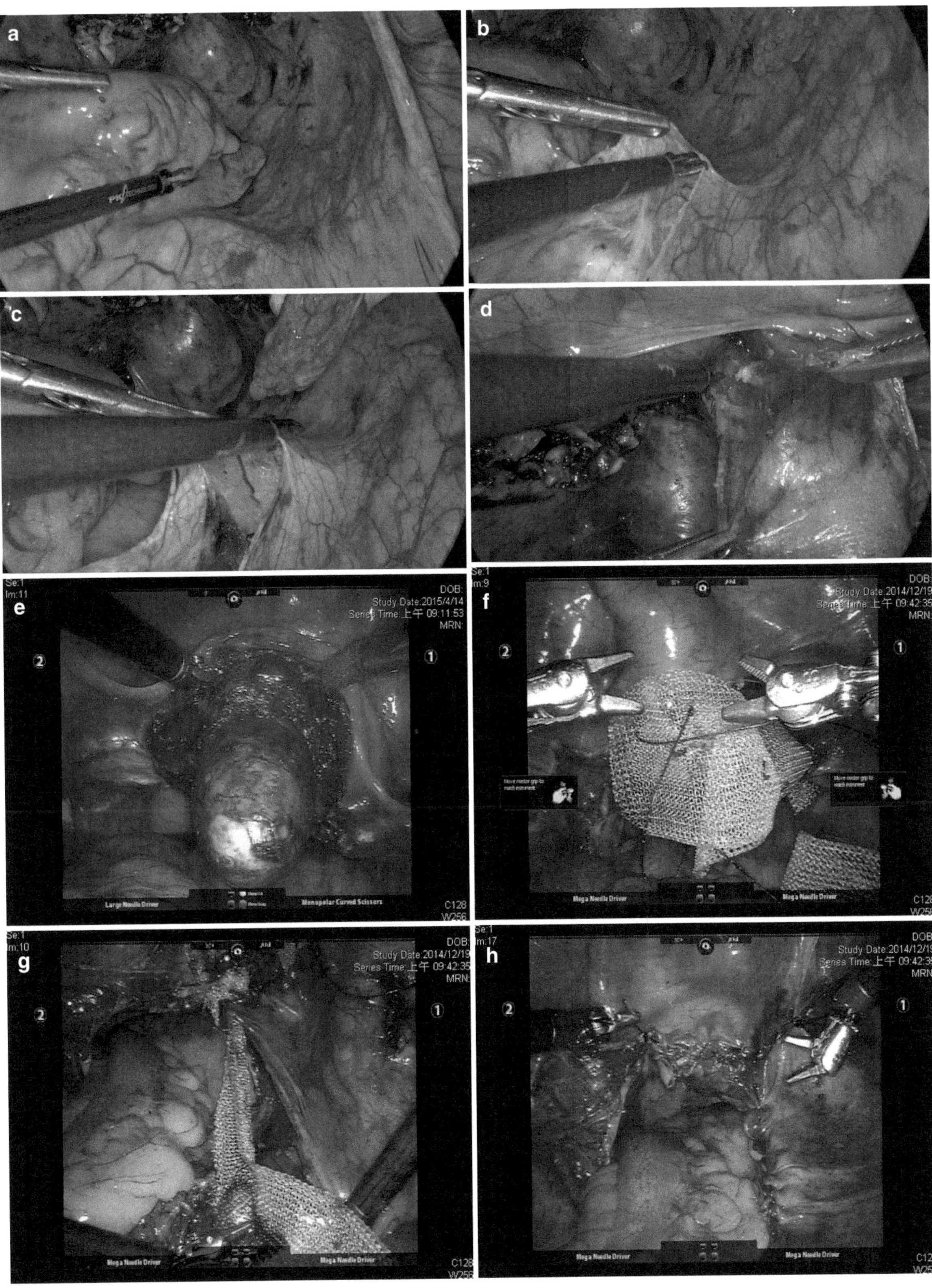

Fig. 38.10 (**a**) The opening of right ureteral orifice. The patent is documented by the urine flow. (**a**) The peritoneum superficial to the sacral promontory. (**b**) The landmark of the bladder dome is air bubble. (**b**) The opening window of the peritoneum superficial to the sacral promontory. The white anterior longitudinal ligament is visualized. (**c**) A papillary lesion is noted in the routine cystoscopy. The biopsy reveals the high grade papillary urothelial carcinoma in the bladder. (**c**) The peritoneal window is extended, right of the midline, medial to the right ureter. (**d**) The peritoneal window is continued to the right uterosacral ligament. (**e**) The vaginal vault exposed by the assistant. (**f**) The distal end of the mesh is fixed to the vaginal vault. (**g**) The proximal end is going to be anchored to the anterior longitudinal ligament. (**h**) A final inspection after approximation of the peritoneum through Robotic camera

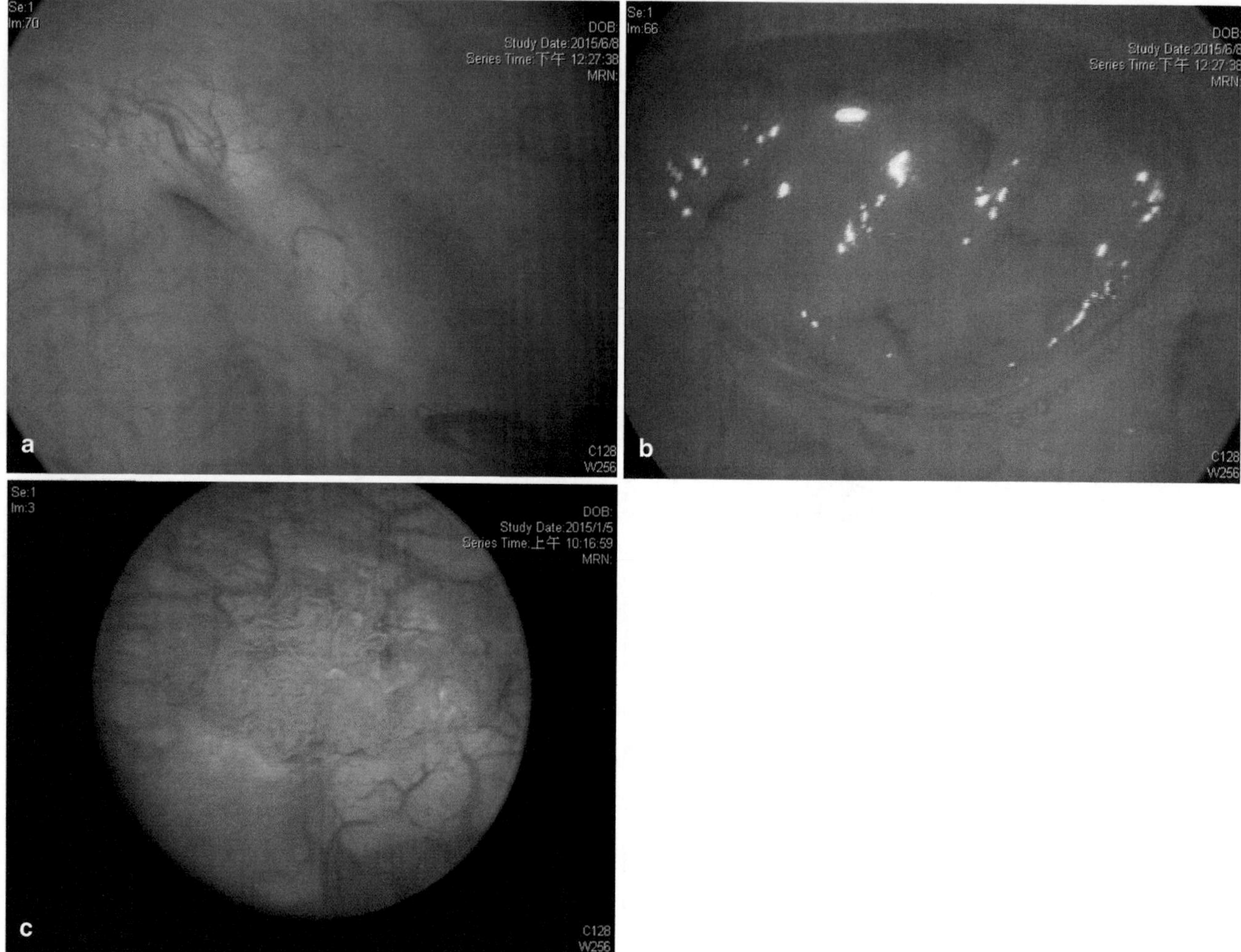

Fig. 38.11 (**a**) The opening of right ureteral orifice. The patent is documented by the urine flow. (**b**) The landmark of the bladder dome is air bubble. (**c**) A papillary lesion is noted in the routine cystoscopy. The biopsy reveals the high grade papillary urothelial carcinoma in the bladder

Radical Hysterectomy and Pelvic Lymphadenectomy (French School)

39

Gabriele Centini, Rodrigo P. Fernandes, Karolina Afors, Rouba Murtada, Marco Fabián Puga, and Arnaud Wattiez

Introduction

The first large series on radical or extended hysterectomy were published in the beginning of the twentieth century by Wertheim [1] in Austria, and later by Okabayashi [2] in Japan and Meigs [3] in the United States.

Since these publications different procedures and classifications have been proposed but none have spread worldwide. The most commonly used classification in the past decade has been the Piver-Smith classification published in 1974 [4].

G. Centini, MD (✉)
Molecular and developmental medicine, Obstetrics and Gynaecology, University of Siena, Ospedale santa Maria alle scotte, Viale Bracci, 16, Siena 53100, Italy
e-mail: Centini.gabriele@gmail.com

R.P. Fernandes, MD
Department of Gynecology Oncology, Instituto do Câncer do Estado de São Paulo – ICESP FM USP, Av. Dr. Arnaldo, 251, São Paulo 01246-000, Brazil
e-mail: ropfernandes@gmail.com

K. Afors, BSc, MBBS, MRCOG
Obstetrics and Gynaecology, King's College Hospital NHS Trust, Denmark Hill, London SE5 9RS, UK
e mail: drkafors@gmail.com

R. Murtada, MD
Department of Gynecology and Obstetrics, Hôpital Jean Verdier, AP-HP, Allee du 14 Juillet, Bondy 93140, France
e-mail: rouba.murtada@gmail.com

M.F. Puga, MD
Departamento de Ginecología, Unidad de Oncología Ginecológica, Instituto Nacional del Cancer- Clínica Alemana de Santiago-Universidad del Desarrollo, Avenida Manquehue Norte 1499, Vitacura, Santiago 765056, Chile
e-mail: marcopugaa@gmail.com

A. Wattiez, MD, PhD
University of Strasbourg, Strasbourg, France

GYN Department, Latifa Hospital, 9115, Oud Metha Road, Al Jadaf, Dubai, UAE
e-mail: arnaud.wattiez@wanadoo.fr

The Piver classification has been criticized on different levels: the description of the five classes was not based on reproducible anatomical landmarks, the boundary between classes was unclear, class I was in fact not a radical hysterectomy and the introduction of a more conservative surgical approach rendered class V excessive in its radicality with regards to the vagina making it obsolete. Moreover, this classification was developed in the United States before the nerve-sparing approach was introduced and adopted into clinical practice and as such is not included in this classification.

For a long time it seemed adequate, however, over time with recent changes in the surgical management of cervical cancer this classification has become outdated. This is largely attributed to the development of endoscopic techniques providing a more detailed knowledge of the anatomy of the parametrium, leading to the development of a new revised classification by Querleu and Morrow in 2008 [5].

The term radical hysterectomy encompassed various techniques based on different anatomical nomenclatures. A common classification was necessary for surgeons to establish a standardised treatment protocol, compare outcomes, as well as for communication and teaching purposes.

Laparoscopy in gynaecological oncology was first introduced in the late 80´s and the well-known benefits of laparoscopy such as early postoperative discharge, pain reduction and faster recovery were already well established for benign surgery [6, 7]. These benefits are particularly relevant for cancer patients, reducing the possibility of thromboembolic events and improving postoperative recovery, allowing patients to begin adjuvant therapy more quickly. In addition, due to the enhanced vision and precision permitted by this technique, laparoscopy progressively demonstrated being not only a safe alternative to laparotomy, but also the preferred route for staging procedures such as lymphadenectomy. After few years of experience, laparoscopy has been extensively adopted for a wide range of gynaecological oncology procedures [8]. Currently extensive data has demonstrated equivocal safety and post-operative outcomes for

I. Alkatout, L. Mettler (eds.), *Hysterectomy*, DOI 10.1007/978-3-319-22497-8_39

laparoscopic oncological procedures, whilst sustaining the benefits of minimally invasive surgery.

There is no doubt that more radical and longer procedures are inevitably associated with complications and morbidities, irrespective of the route used. Of major concern in lymphadenectomy is major bleeding originating in the rich vascular pelvic network. Injury to other surrounding structures such as ureters and nerves although infrequent, can lead to potential complications. In addition, postoperative lymphocele can occur due to the extensive dissection of pelvic lymphatic chains [3, 9].

A comprehensive knowledge of the anatomy, in addition, to a thorough and standardized technique is key in preventing such complications. Pelvic lymphadenectomy (PL) is a stepwise technique where the benefits of laparoscopy can be integrated into surgical practice. However, adequate training is mandatory to master the technique and optimize its use.

In the last few decades efforts have been made to diminish lymphadenectomy complications. Studies have guided surgeons towards a more minimally invasive extraction of lymph nodes: the sentinel node. These nodes can be mapped during laparoscopy by techniques of lymphoscyntigraphy and blue dye test injected in the cervix of the uterus at 3 and 9 o'clock position. Detection of the nodes can be visual or with use of probes depending on the technique used for mapping. Results showed a higher rate of lymphatic drainage to the iliac and obturative nodes [10, 11].

Radical Hysterectomy: A New Classification

All previous classifications were based on a non-standardized anatomical terminology according to the originating school or country. The first step towards a new classification was the standardization of anatomical terms with fixed landmarks in the parametrium clearly defined.

The lateral attachment of the cervix was named "paracervix", incorporating the previously subdivided paracolpium and parametrium, and replacing other terms such as cardinal ligament, Mackenrodt's ligament or parametrium.

The lateral attachments of the bladder and rectum were respectively named lateral ligament of the bladder and rectum. Furthermore, basing itself on anatomical studies, the new classification introduced the two concepts of a nerve-sparing approach to radical hysterectomy, and paracervical lymphadenectomy.

These concepts derived from cadaveric studies demonstrating that the paracervix can be divided into two parts according to types of connective tissue: the medial part, extending from the cervix to the hypogastric artery, is made of dense connective tissue with vessels, nerves, and lymph nodes that should be resected during surgery, whilst the lateral part is node bearing fatty tissue that can be easily isolated from surrounding structures.

This cleavage allows the surgeon to increase the radicality without increasing the morbidity.

Nerve Sparing Approach

The nerve sparing approach was initially developed to reduce the rate of postoperative bladder, bowel and sexual dysfunction caused by damage done to the nerves during a radical hysterectomy procedure and was rapidly demonstrated to be effective.

Surgical experience and cadaveric anatomy studies identified three main surgical steps at high risk of nerve injury during a radical hysterectomy: the resection of the uterosacral ligament, the resection of the paracervix and the resection of the bladder pillars.

The uterosacral ligament, or lateral ligament of the rectum, is in close relation to the hypogastric nerve and the inferior hypogastric plexus making its resection a critical step for potential nerve injuries.

The hypogastric nerve, mainly made of sympathetic fibers, is born from the superior hypogastric plexus at the level of the promontorium, follows an immediately subperitoneal course and joins the inferior hypogastric plexus at the dorsal and lateral part of the pelvis.

In its final third, just before joining the inferior hypogastric plexus, it crosses the ureter while coming from a dorsomedial direction.

At that level and for a few centimeters, the ureter lies close to the lateral ligament of the rectum and is identified and reclined when developing the Okabayshi space (Fig. 39.1).

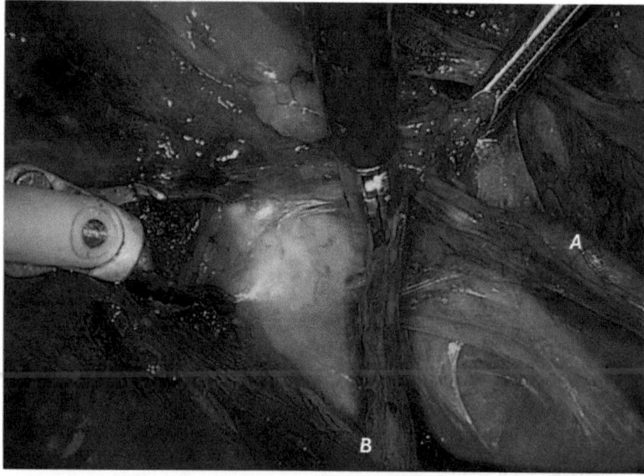

Fig. 39.1 The picture shows the paracervix on the right side after the dissection of the pararectal fossa at the level of the ureteral channel. *A* Uterine artery and paracervix; *B* ureter. *Yellow*: okabayashi space; *Green*: latsko space

The hypogastric nerve and the pelvic splanchnic nerves arising from the sacral roots S2–S4 are brought together to form the inferior hypogastric plexus that lays on the dorsal and lateral part of the pararectal fossa.

This plexus gives branches to the pelvic organs and crosses the paracervix just under the deep uterine vein, which then can be considered a landmark for the sparing of the neural part of the paracervix.

Lastly, a careful dissection needs to be performed when approaching the lateral ligament of the bladder, which is a critical area not only with regards to innervation but also in the proximity of the ureter.

The anatomy of the anterior part of the then called cardinal ligament has been described in details by Fuji as a structure formed by two layers of connective tissue dorsal and ventral to the ureter. According to this description the nerve fibers running to the bladder from the inferior hypogastric plexus pass in the lateral part of this ligament.

In order to spare the lateral part of the lateral ligament of the bladder the fourth space of Yabuki needs to be developed.

Landmarks and Classes

The new classification is based on three fixed and reproducible landmarks: the ureter, the uterine artery and the pelvic sidewall (Fig. 39.2).

These anatomical structures are used to define the four main classes while the deep uterine vein is the landmark used to define two sub-classes, with and without nerve sparing approach.

The four classes are defined according to lateral, anterior, posterior and vaginal extension of the resection as well as in depth of the paracervix. As for the bladder and rectal ligaments the authors considered these structures too short and without clear landmarks and did not define intermediate levels of resection between the cervix and adjacent organs.

Type A is the previously defined extrafascial hysterectomy whereby the paracervix is transsected halfway between the ureter and the cervix and the lateral ligaments of bladder and rectum are resected at the level of the cervix, and less than 1 cm of vagina is removed. This procedure insures the *in toto* removal of the cervix.

Type B is divided into B1 and B2 according to the addition of a paracervical lymphadenectomy. This type of resection was previously known as "modified radical hysterectomy" and its lateral limit is the ureteric tunnel. The ureter is unroofed and at least 1 cm of vagina is resected. The purpose of this procedure is to enlarge the resection of the paracervix while leaving untouched its neural portion, under the deep uterine vein.

Type C is the resection of the uterosacral ligament at the level of the rectum and the vesico-uterine ligament at the level of the bladder. The ureter is mobilized completely and 15–20 mm of vagina starting at the level of the tumor or the cervix is resected.

Performing such an enlarged hysterectomy, the nerve supply to the bladder is threatened and whether it is preserved or not leads to the creation of two sub-classes.

Type C1 is a nerve sparing approach where dissection remains above (ventral to) the deep uterine vein while Type C2 extends resection beyond this landmark and includes the neural portion of the paracervix (Fig. 39.3).

Type D1 is the resection of the entire paracervix, extending to the level of the pelvic sidewall, along with the hypogastric vessels, exposing the roots of the sciatic nerve. Type D2 is D1 with the resection of adjacent fascial or muscular structures

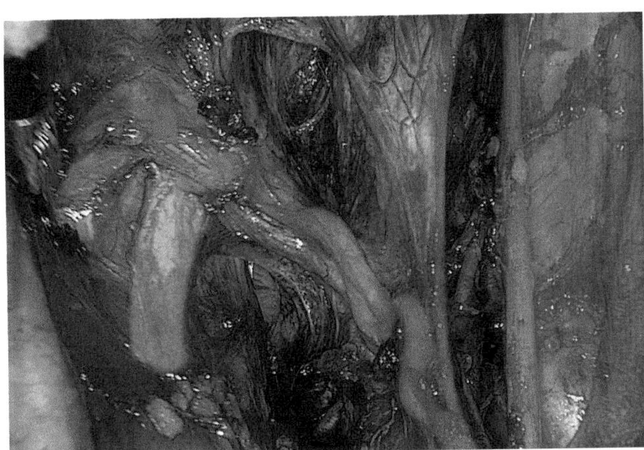

Fig. 39.2 Landmarks in radical hysterectomy. Paracervix after the dissection of the pelvic spaces (*right side*). *Green*: ureter; *Red*: uterine and hypogastric arteries; *Yellow*: pelvic side wall

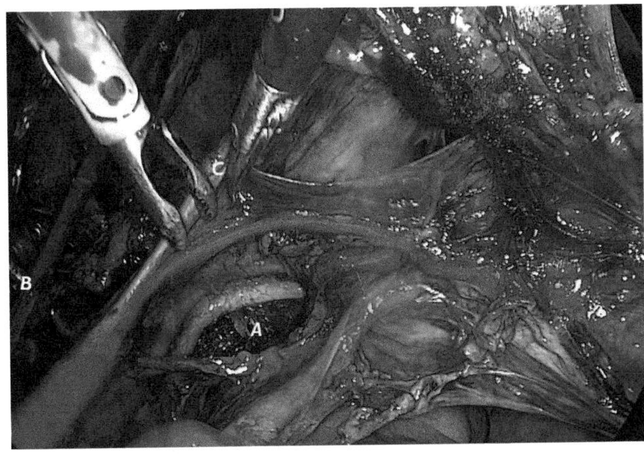

Fig. 39.3 Posterior view of the paracervix on the left side after the dissection. *A* Latsko space; *B* Left obturator nerve; *C* unbilical artery; *Red*: Uterine artery; *Blue*: deep uterine vein; *Yellow*: vaginal artery; *Green*: ureter

The Technique

Radical hysterectomy is one of the most anatomical procedures in gynaecological surgery, as it requires all anatomical spaces of the pelvis to be developed.

In most cases, there is no anatomical distortion and a wide dissection can be performed, guided by reproducible anatomical landmarks.

The procedure begins with the dissection of the lateral spaces of the pelvis in order to identify and isolate the paracervix.

The round ligament is coagulated and sectioned at the level of the umbilical artery and the anterior leaf of the broad ligament is divided. In order to perform this step, an instrument is inserted under the anterior peritoneal leaf until it reaches the uterus and then lifted, exposing the reflection line between peritoneum and uterine serosa. The peritoneum is divided under the point marked with a thin white line between the bladder and the cervix.

The opening reaches caudally the bladder and cranially the psoas muscle exposing the lateral spaces of the pelvis.

The paravesical fossa is divided into its medial and lateral parts using the obliterated umbilical artery as a landmark. The dissection is first carried laterally to the umbilical artery and progresses in a cranio-caudal direction, exposing the obturator area with its homonymous vessels and nerve.

The development of anatomical planes is helped by infiltration of CO_2 into the areolar tissue that fills the spaces, in between the landmarks.

Moving medially between the umbilical artery and the bladder, the medial part of the paravesical fossa is developed, with special care to avoid injury to the superior vesical artery. It arises from the umbilical artery, bringing blood supply to the bladder and is the only artery to cross this space (Fig. 39.4).

The medial part of the paravesical fossa is developed in its dorsal aspect to find the paracervix that marks the limit with the pararectal fossa.

This dissection allows the surgeon to identify the uterine artery and with it the cranial limit of the paracervix.

Following the uterine artery in a ventro-dorsal direction the surgeon enters the Latsko space located laterally to the ureter and dorsally to the paracervix.

A partial ureterolysis is then performed after developing the Okabayashi space, medially to the ureter. During this step, the hypogastric nerve is identified, coursing immediately under the peritoneum and crossing the ureter in its lower third to join the inferior hypogastric plexus (Fig. 39.5).

In thin patients the nerve is easy to identify on the right side as its path is often represented by a peritoneal fold, running from the promontorium through the pararectal fossa, between the ureter and the uterosacral ligament. To the left it is covered by the mesosigmoid.

The dissection then continues into the central spaces, whereby the rectovaginal and vesicovaginal spaces are developed.

To enter the posterior (dorsal) space the assistant grabs the rectum and pulls it in a dorsocranial direction exposing the spaces and the surgeon cuts the peritoneum 1–2 cm under the reflection line of the torus uterinus, below the level of insertion of the uterosacral ligaments.

The procedure continues with the development of the vesicouterine plane. To perform this dissection safely the assistant grabs the bladder and pulls ventrally, removing the bladder from the field, exposing the correct tissue plane (Fig. 39.6).

The right plane is at the level of the pubocervical fascia that is usually visible.

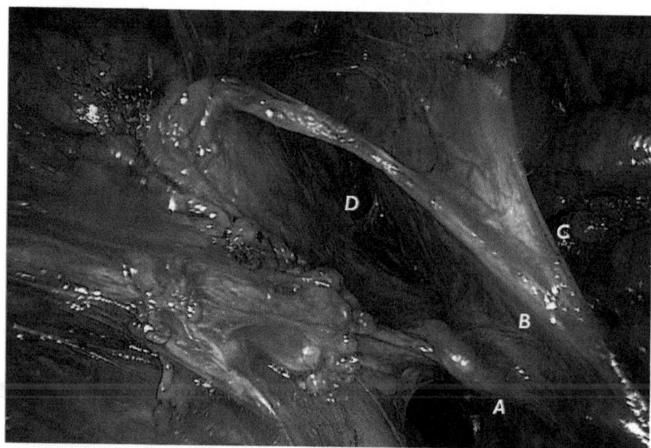

Fig. 39.4 View of the paravesical fossa. *A* Uterine artery; *B* superior vesical artery; *C* umbilical artery; *D* medial part of the paravesical fossa

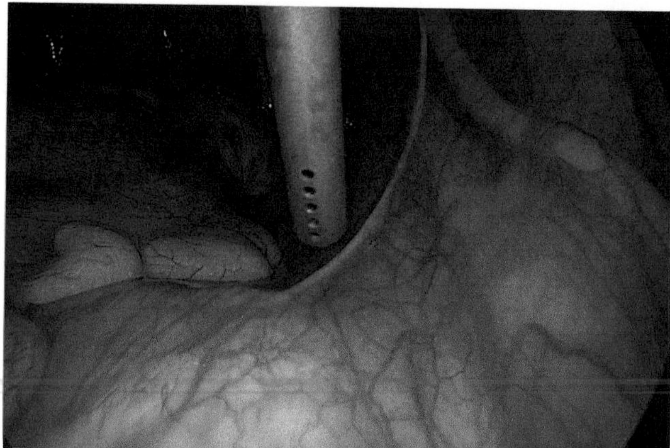

Fig. 39.5 The picture shows the relationship between ureter, iliac vessels and hypogastric nerve. On the right side the ureter cross the external iliac artery and the hypogastric nerve pass under the ureter arising from the promontorium. *Red*: Biforcation of the common iliac artery; *Green*: ureter; *Blue*: hypogastric nerve

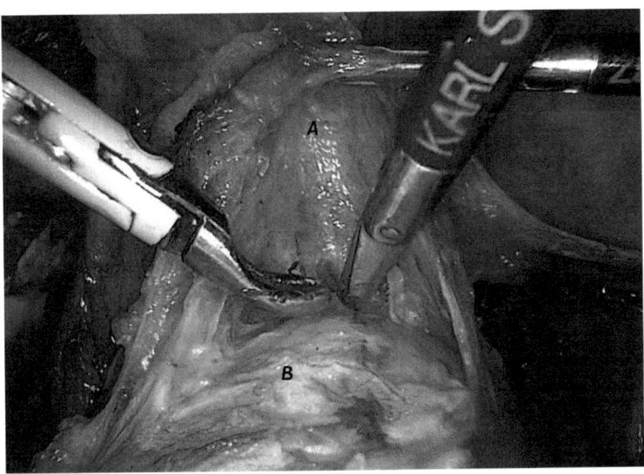

Fig. 39.6 Dissection of the vesicovaginal septum. The assistant lift up the bladder to expose the dissection plane. *A* Bladder; *B* vagina

The development of the vesicouterine space, after the previously developed medial part of the paravesical fossa, isolates the lateral ligament of the bladder.

The dissection of this ligament is one of the most challenging steps of the procedure because of the close proximity of the ureter and the nerve bundles coming from the inferior hypogastric plexus that innervates the bladder.

The anatomy of this lateral ligament of the bladder has recently been found to be more complex than previously thought, with a detailed description reported in Japanese publications in the last decade.

The vesicouterine ligament is in fact made of two different layers, passing over and under the ureter. The superficial layer is made only of connective tissue and small vessels while the deep layer contains the nerve supply to the bladder.

The understanding of the anatomical relationship between the ureter, nerves and the paracervix is crucial to performing a safe procedure (Fig. 39.7).

The ureter crosses the paracervix, coursing in a dorsoventral and craniocaudal direction, passing under the uterine artery and above the deep uterine vein, through the ureteric tunnel. It then turns medially to join the bladder passing between the two layers of the vesicouterine ligament.

To dissect the intraligamentary part of the ureter and at the same time spare the bladder nerve branches, the fourth space of Yabuki is found. This space can be developed dissecting medially to the ureter once passed the superficial layer of the vesicouterine ligament (Fig. 39.8).

Doing so the surgeon can spare the deep layer of the vesicouterine ligament with the branches of the inferior hypogastric plexus arising from the paracervix under the deep uterine vein.

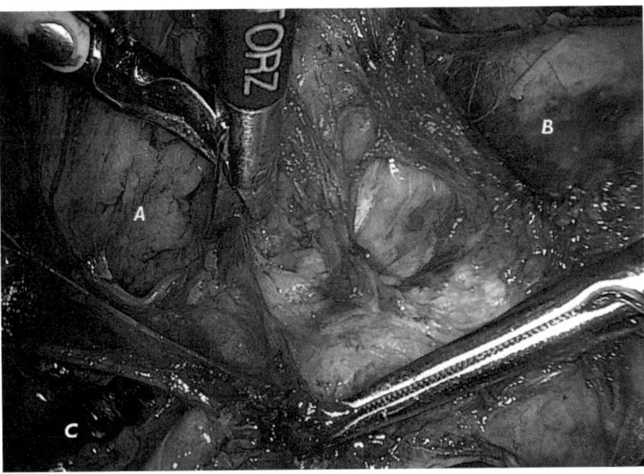

Fig. 39.7 The picture shows the relationship between the superficial layer of the vesicouterin ligament and the ureter (*left side*). This ligament can be divided in i a medial and lateral part. *A* medial part of the paravesical fossa; *B* vesicovaginal plane; *C* pararectal space; *Green*: ureter; *Blue*: superficial layer of the vesicuterine ligament

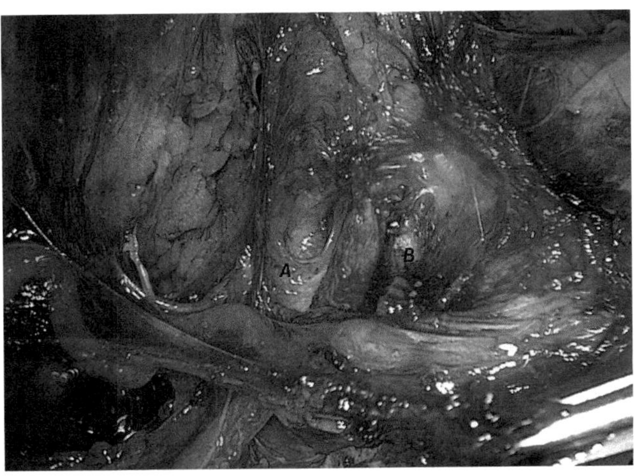

Fig. 39.8 Position of the ureter in the anterior paracervix after the section of the medial part of the ligament. The Yabuky space is located medially to the ureter at the level of the inferior layer of the vesicouterine ligament. *A* Inferior layer of the vesicouterine ligament; *B* yabuky space; *Green*: ureter; *Blue* superficial layer of the vesicouterine ligament; *Red*: uterine artery

Lymphadenectomy

The basic principle consists of identifying the anatomical landmarks by wide dissection of the retroperitoneal space. This is followed by, collection of nodes respecting the anatomical structures. In our technique, the dissection is performed by means of a bipolar forceps and scissors. Nevertheless, other types of energy can be used, notably mechanical energy sources (such as ultrasound) due to the high impedance of the fatty tissue.

Three lymphatic chains are systematically resected during the PL: external iliac, interiliac and obturative. The limits of the pelvic dissection are: Cephalad: iliac vessels bifurcation, lateral: genito femoral nerve. Medial: ureter. Caudal: Circumflex iliac vein.

Adequate exposure is achieved by means of trendelenburg maneuver, uterine manipulator and in some cases organ suspension. The procedure starts with division of the round ligament. The anterior layer of the broad ligament is incised largely in both directions, caudally towards the cervix and cephalad over the psoas muscle. The retroperitoneum is exposed allowing the CO_2 gas to enter the connective tissue facilitating dissection and producing the so-called "bubble effect". The paravesical space (PVS) is then carefully developed using traction and counter traction. Haemostasis should be maintained and is important to reduce contaminating the operative field. The umbilical artery is identified in the middle of the PVS, an important landmark that should be preserved. The connective tissue between the Umbilical artery (UA) and the bladder can then be dissected (Fig. 39.9). Nevertheless, frequently the UA can be left attached to the lateral wall of the bladder and considered as part of the medial limit of the PVS. The pectineal ligament is identified and corresponds to the ventral limit of the space. The dissection is continued deeply until the levator ani muscles are reached. The obturator muscle and fascia with the obturator nerve and vessels run on the lateral aspect of the PVS. Dorsally the dissection continues until the paracervix. Afterwards the pararectal space or Latzko space is developed between the ureter and the internal iliac artery. Once the anatomical landmarks are identified, fatpad resection becomes straightforward.

The lateral aspect of the dissection consists of detaching the nodes from the external iliac vessels. The most lateral aspect of the nodes lies over the genito femoral nerve. By pulling the fatty tissue medially, the nerve can be completely isolated with minimal damage. Continuing with the same medial traction the nodes are separated from the superficial aspect of the external iliac vessels by using selective coagulation. Dissection of the nodes from the external iliac vein is one of the most dangerous steps. In contrast to the artery, traction over the vein leads its walls to collapse making it difficult to identify its limits. Another dangerous step is during anterior dissection of the nodes from the external iliac vein. A branch denominated the *Corona Mortis,* connecting the external vessel to the obturator vein can be frequently found (Fig. 39.10). Variations such as artery to artery and vein to artery shunts have been described. This communication can be sacrificed if needed, but should be performed at a considerable distance from the external iliac vein to avoid injuries of the external iliac vein.

Part of the dissection requires the surgeon to medialize the external iliac vessels, a gesture that should be performed cautiously at all times. The assistant can hold the vessels allowing the surgeon to work close to the lumbosacral fossa. Node dissection at this point should be careful and precise. Branches originating from the external iliac vessels directly into the muscles and foramens of the pelvis can retract and bleed if cut without proper coagulation. After separating the nodes from the external vessels attention should be paid to the deeper limits of the lymph node dissection: the obturator nerve.

The obturator nerve originates on the deepest aspect of the lumbosacral fossa, over the lumbosacral trunk and comprises the lower aspect of the pelvic lymphadenectomy (Fig. 39.11). It leaves the pelvis through the obturator foramen and it is completely surrounded by nodes and fatty tissue demanding greater attention of the surgeon to avoid complete transection. Gentle traction of the nodes is sufficient to isolate them from the nerve.

In cases when surgery is performed together with hysterectomy, the fat pad can be left in place until the end of the surgery and then removed through the vagina. The use of endoscopic bags is highly recommended when removing

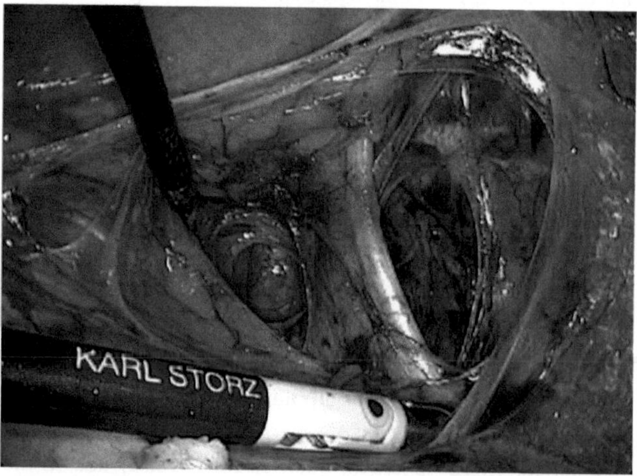

Fig. 39.9 the picture shows the paravesical fossa after the dissection of its both lateral and medial part using the umbilical artery as landmark (*right side*)

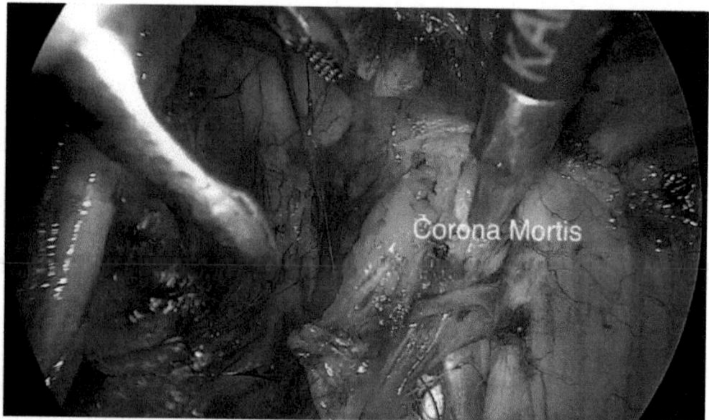

Fig. 39.10 The figure shows the origin of the corona mortis from the external iliac vein (*right side*)

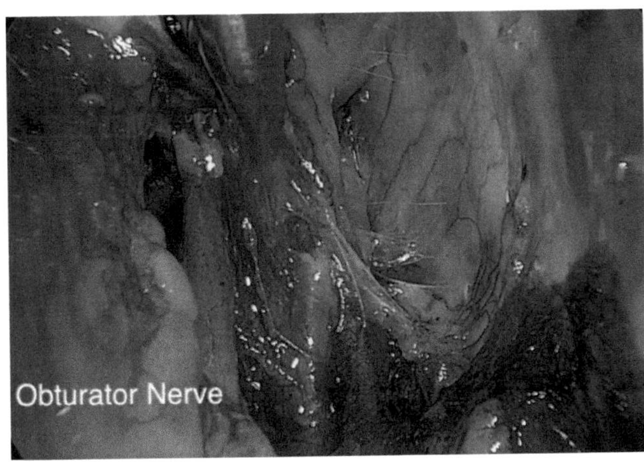

Fig. 39.11 The figure shows the obturator fossa on the right side along with its homonymous nerve artery and vein after the iliac vessels are reclaimed medially

nodes, particularly when they are enlarged or suspicious. In addition, in cases when the vagina is not opened (i.e., traquelectomy and PL, or PL for restaging) the use of bags is mandatory.

Lately surgery has moved towards more minimally invasive procedures and laparoscopy has played a considerable role within this field. Together with the benefits of sentinel node mapping, minimally invasive surgery has further improved outcomes compared to the early introduction of laparoscopy in oncology.

References

1. Wertheim E. The extended abdominal operation for carcinoma uteri (based on 500 operative cases). Am J Obstet Dis Women Child. 1912;66:169–232.
2. Okabayashi H. Radical abdominal hysterectomy for cancer of the cervix uteri. Surg Gynecol Obstet. 1921;33:335–41.
3. Meigs JV. Carcinoma of the cervix – the Wertheim operation. Surg Gynecol Obstet. 1944;78:195–8.
4. Piver MS, Rutledge F, Smith JP. Five classes of extended hysterectomy for women with cervical cancer. Obstet Gynecol. 1974;44:265–72.
5. Querleu D, Morrow CP. Classification of radical hysterectomy. Lancet Oncol. 2008;9(3):297–303.
6. Querleu D, Leblanc E, Castelain B. Laparoscopic pelvic lymphadenectomy in the staging of early carcinoma of the cervix. Am J Obstet Gynecol Elsevier. 1991;164(2):579–81.
7. Nezhat CR, Burrell MO, Nezhat FR, Benigno BB, Welander CE. Laparoscopic radical hysterectomy with paraaortic and pelvic node dissection. YMOB. 1992;166(3):864–5.
8. Köhler C, Klemm P, Schau A, Possover M, Krause N, Tozzi R, et al. Introduction of transperitoneal lymphadenectomy in a gynecologic oncology center: analysis of 650 laparoscopic pelvic and/or paraaortic transperitoneal lymphadenectomies. Gynecol Oncol. 2004;95(1):52–61.
9. Cartron G, Leblanc E, Ferron G, Martel P, Narducci F, Querleu D. Complications des lymphadénectomies cœlioscopiques en oncologie gynécologique : 1102 interventions chez 915 patientes. Gynécol Obstét Fertilité. 2005;33(5):304–14.
10. Abu-Rustum NR, Khoury-Collado F, Gemignani ML. Techniques of sentinel lymph node identification for early-stage cervical and uterine cancer. Gynecol Oncol Elsevier Inc. 2008;111(S):S44–50.
11. Abu-Rustum NR, Khoury-Collado F, Pandit-Taskar N, Soslow RA, Dao F, Sonoda Y, et al. Sentinel lymph node mapping for grade 1 endometrial cancer: Is it the answer to the surgical staging dilemma? Gynecol Oncol Elsevier Inc. 2009;113(2):163–9.

Laparoscopic Radical Hysterectomy with Pelvic Lymphadenectomy (Spanish School)

40

Antonio Gil-Moreno, Sabina Salicrú, Berta Diaz-Feijoo, and Blanca Gil-Ibáñez

Background

In less than two decades, the advent of laparoscopic surgery has definitely contributed to modifying the management of patients with gynecologic cancer. This minimally invasive surgery plays an important role in the basic aspects of gynecologic oncology: diagnosis, staging, and treatment of malignant tumors. All these tasks involve a learning phase for surgeons and a phase of diffusion of these techniques. In cases of cervical and ovarian neoplasms, laparoscopic procedures are technically more difficult and for this reason should be performed by highly specialized teams.

Laparoscopic lymphadenectomy occupies an important place as a diagnostic and staging method in cervical cancer. The first transperitoneal pelvic lymphadenectomies in the management of cervical cancer were originally reported on by Querleu et al. in 1991 [1]. In 1992, Querleu in France and Childers in the United States described transperitoneal para-aortic lymphadenectomy, and in 1995, Dargent showed that extraperitoneal laparoscopy can also be performed at this level [2]. Nowadays, systematic pelvic lymphadenectomy may be substituted by detection and analysis of the sentinel node.

The first laparoscopic hysterectomy for benign diseases was published in 1989 by Reich et al. [3]. Subsequently, laparoscopy was preferentially used in gynecologic oncology to convert radical abdominal hysterectomy into radical vaginal hysterectomy [4–6]. In 1990, Canis et al. [7] and in 1992, Nezhat et al. [8] described for the first time radical hysterectomy performed using the laparoscopic route. During the 90's various clinical series with a limited number of patients showed the possibility of performing radical resections with lymphadenectomy using the laparoscopic approach [9–13]. Different groups have published their experiences showing the feasibility and safety of the procedure and suggesting that prognosis or survival is not adversely affected by the procedure. However, there are few publications on the morbidity and long-term survival of laparoscopic radical hysterectomy.

A. Gil-Moreno, MD (✉) • S. Salicrú, MD • B. Diaz-Feijoo, MD
B. Gil-Ibáñez, MD
Department of Obstetrics and Gynecology, Hospital Universitari Vall d'Hebron Universitat Autònoma de Barcelona, Passeig Vall d'Hebron, 119, 08035 Barcelona, Spain
e-mail: antonioimma@yahoo.es; ssalicru@vhebron.net; bdiaz@vhebron.net; blancalabacin@hotmail.com

Terminology

The term radical hysterectomy implies resection of a vaginal cuff and paracervical tissues besides the uterus. Pelvic lymphadenectomy also constitutes a part of the surgical procedure for early invasive cervical cancer, although it is not included in the current International Federation of Gynecology and Obstetrics (FIGO) staging classification [14]. The operation can be more or less radical according to the tumor size and involvement of paracervical tissue or of the vaginal tissue. Extension to the pelvic wall is performed through the paracervix, usually with involvement of lymph vessels and lymph nodes at this level.

In 1974, Piver et al. [15] pointed out that the term radical hysterectomy involves 'many different operations' and described five classes of extended hysterectomies that have been later summarized or adapted to the two types of radical hysterectomies: proximal, modified or Piver type II hysterectomy (resection of the medial paracervix proximal to the ureters and medial section of uterosacral ligaments) and distal or Piver type III/IV hysterectomy (distal resection of the paracervix at the level of the pelvic wall and removal of the uterosacral ligaments) (see Table 40.1).

In 2008, Querleu and Morrow [16] (Q-M) proposed a new classification of radical hysterectomy based on the lateral extent of resection. Four types of radical hysterectomy (A-D) were described, adding when necessary a few subtypes that look at nerve preservation and paracervical

I. Alkatout, L. Mettler (eds.), *Hysterectomy*, DOI 10.1007/978-3-319-22497-8_40

Table 40.1 Types of radical hysterectomy

Querleu/Morrow type (2008/2011) [16, 17]	EORTC type (Piver 1974) [15]
Type A The fascia of the cervix and lower uterine segment is removed with the uterus	Type I Extrafascial hysterectomy
Type B Removes the cervix, proximal vagina, and parametrial and paracervical tissue The radicality of this operation can be improved by lymph-node dissection of the lateral part of the paracervix. Thus defining two subtypes: B1 and B2, with additional removal of the lateral paracervical lymph nodes.	Type II Modified radical hysterectomy
Type C Requires greater resection of the parametria The issue of nerve preservation is crucial. Two subcategories are defined: **C1 with nerve preservation** Uterosacral ligaments were transected after separation of both hypogastric nerves. The paracervix tissue was transected up to the deep uterine vein. The inferior hypogastric plexus with the splanchnic nerves are identified systematically . Then the bladder branches of the pelvic plexus were identified and preserved in the lateral ligament of the bladder **C2 with a complete parametrial resection** The paracervix is transected completely, including the part caudal to the deep uterine vein	Type III Radical hysterectomy
Type D Differs from type C2 in a feature additional ultraradical procedures, mostly indicated at the time of pelvic exenteration. Excision extends to the pelvic sidewall D1 is resection of the entire paracervix at the pelvic sidewall along with the hypogastric vessels, exposing the roots of the sciatic nerve D2 is D1 plus resection of the entire paracervix with the hypogastric vessels and adjacent fascial or muscular structures	Type IV Radical hysterectomy
	Type V **Pelvic Exanteration**

lymphadenectomy. Lymph node dissection was considered separately and four areas or levels were defined according to corresponding arterial anatomy and radicality of the procedure: level 1, external and internal iliac; level 2, common iliac (including presacral); level 3, aortic infra-mesenteric; and level 4, aortic infrarenal. In addition, it can be adapted to the different types of surgical approaches and is useful for open abdominal, laparoscopic or robotic, and vaginal routes.

More recently, in 2011, Cibula et al. proposed a classification system based on the proposal published by Querleu and Morrow but specifying anatomical landmarks for all types of radical hysterectomy in three dimensions [17].

Types of Radical Hysterectomy (Querleu-Morrow Classification Plus Cibula et al.)

Type A

This type corresponds to the extrafascial hysterectomy, which guarantees full removal of the pericervical tissue up to the attachment of the vaginal fornices. The paracervix is transected medial to the ureter, but lateral to the cervix. The uterosacral and vesicouterine ligaments are not transected at a distance from the uterus. Vaginal resection is generally at a minimum, routinely less than 10 mm, without removal of the vaginal part of the paracervix (paracolpos). The autonomic nerves remain fully preserved.

Type B

This type corresponds to the modified or proximal radical hysterectomy. Partial resection of the uterosacral and vesicouterine ligaments is a standard part. The ureter is only unroofed, dissected from the cervix and displaced laterally, permiting transaction of the paracervix at the level of the ureteral tunel. The nerve supply to the bladder is not treated because the paracervix is not resected caudal to the uterine vein, thereby nerve supply is conserved. At least 10 mm of the vagina from the cervix or tumour is resected.

The radicality of this operation can be improved without increasing postoperative morbidity by lymph-node dissection of the lateral part of the paracervix, thus defining two subtypes: B1 (as described); and B2, with additional removal of the lateral paracervical lymph nodes.

Type C

Type C corresponds to variants of classical radical hysterectomy. This type is transection of the uterosacral ligament at the rectum and vesicouterine ligament at the bladder. The ureter is mobilised completely. 15–20 mm of vagina from the tumour or cervix and the corresponding paracolpos is resected routinely. The Q–M classification system distinguishes between a type C1 procedure, which corresponds to the nerve-sparing modification, and the type C2, which aims for a complete parametrial resection.

In type C1, the uterosacral ligaments were transected after separation of both hypogastric nerves and ureters. The paracervix tissue was transected up to the deep uterine vein. The inferior hypogastric plexus with the splanchnic nerves are identified systematically and preserved (Fig. 40.1). Then the bladder branches of the pelvic plexus were identified and preserved in the lateral ligament of the bladder (Fig. 40.2).

In the C2 type, the paracervix is transected completely, including the part caudal to the deep uterine vein (Fig. 40.3).

Type D

Type D1 is resection of the entire paracervix at the pelvic sidewall along with the hypogastric vessels, exposing the roots of the sciatic nerve. There is total resection of the vessels of the lateral part of the paracervix. Type D2 is D1 plus resection of the entire paracervix with the hypogastric vessels and adjacent fascial or muscular structures. This resection corresponds to the LEER (laterally extended endopelvic resection) procedure.

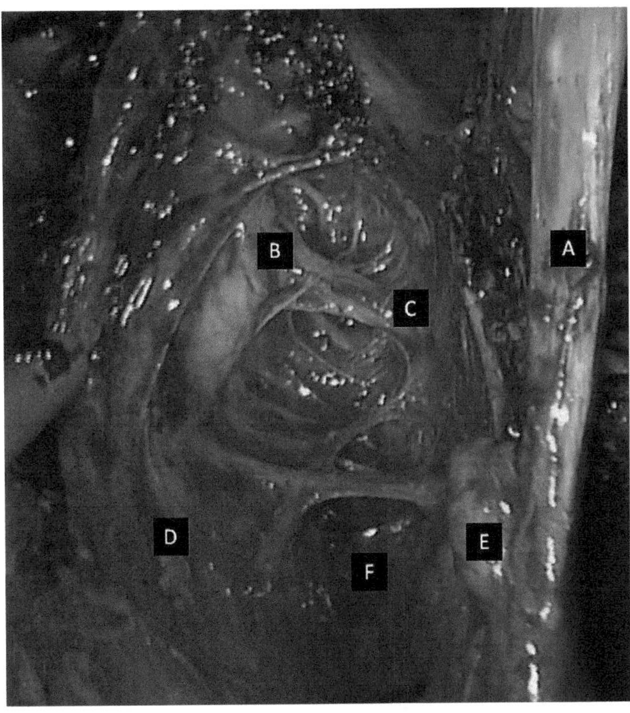

Fig. 40.1 The inferior hypogastric plexus (IHP) has been mobilized laterally from the right uterosacral ligament. The pelvic splanchnic nerves are seen joining the IHP in a perpendicular fashion. *A* Superior vesical artery *B* Inferior hypogastric plexus *C* Pelvic splanchnic nerve *D* Hypogastric nerve *E* Uterine artery *F* Pararectal space

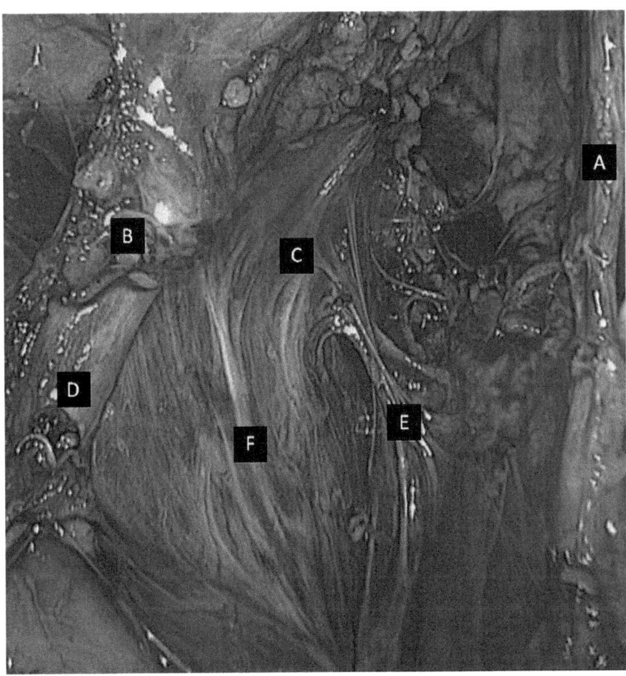

Fig. 40.2 Pelvic autonomic nerves, right side (radical hysterectomy type *C1*). *A* Superior vesical artery *B* Transected uterine artery *C* Inferior hypogastric plexus *D* Ureter *E* Pelvic splanchnic nerve *F* Hypogastric nerve

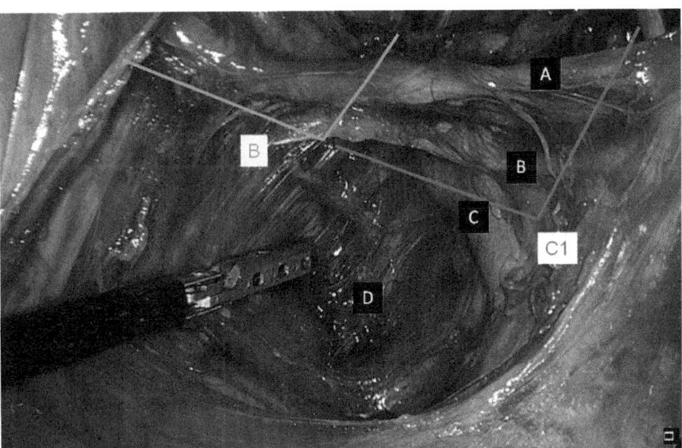

Fig. 40.3 Resection lines on the paracervix for radical hysterectomy type *B* and *C1*. *A* Uterine artery *B* Uterine vein *C* Deep uterine vein *D* Pararectal space

Surgical Procedure Step by Step [18]

Combined general and epidural anesthesia can be used. Patients should undergo bowel preparation and perioperative antibiotics (2 gr of cefazolin intravenously) and low-molecular-weight enoxaparin (40 mg/24 h subcutaneously) should be administered. A uterine manipulator is used. A four-trocar transperitoneal approach is normally used. The laparoscope is introduced through an 11-mm umbilical trocar with a direct-puncture technique (or open technique using a Hasson trocar), and three other trocars are inserted with the patient in the 25–30-degree Trendelenburg position. Two accessory 12 and 5-mm trocars are then placed under direct visualization in the iliac fossas, and one 5-mm accessory trocar is placed at the midline between the umbilicus and the left subcostal margin (Fig. 40.4).

The abdominal cavity is inspected, and the retroperitoneal spaces are opened. The paravesical, pararectal, rectovaginal, and vesicovaginal spaces are developed, thereby delineating the uterosacral ligaments and the parametria (Fig. 40.5).

The pelvic lymph nodes are divided into external iliac, internal iliac or hypogastric, obturator, common iliac and presacral. External iliac nodes are superior and lateral to the external iliac vessels, from the deep iliac circumflex artery to the bifurcation of the common iliac artery. The internal iliac nodes are at the top and side of the internal iliac artery. The obturator nodes are in the obturator fossa below the external iliac vein and above the obturator nerve. Common iliac nodes extend from the bifurcation of the common iliac vessels to the bifurcation of the aorta. Presacral nodes are located below the bifurcation of the aorta and over the left common iliac vein. Lymphs located outside these anatomical areas are usually not involved in the lymphatic spread of uterine malignancies, so their systematic dissection is not justified.

Systematic bilateral pelvic lymphadenectomy is performed with blunt dissection and monopolar/bipolar coagulation from the common iliac artery to the inferior boundary of the circumflex iliac vein. On special occasions we use sealing vessels. Common, internal and external iliac nodes, as well as obturator and presacral lymph nodes, are removed (Fig. 40.6).

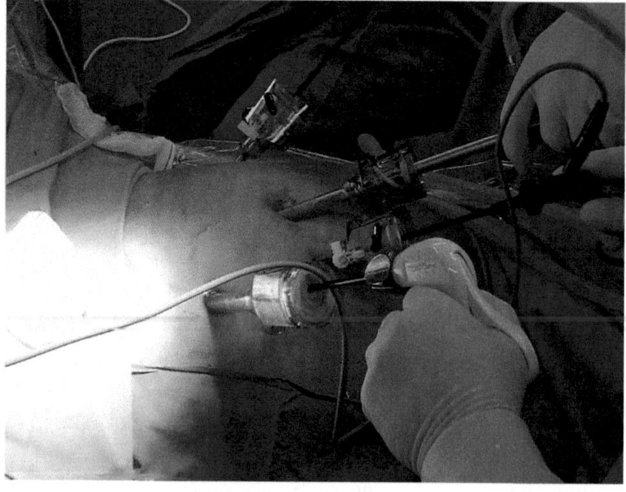

Fig. 40.4 Details of the four-trocar approach

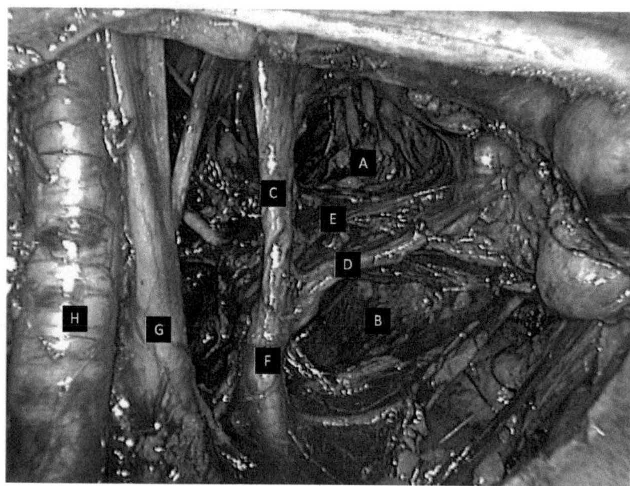

Fig. 40.5 Dissection of the uterine vessels (*left side*). *A* Paravesical space *B* pararectal space *C* superior vesical artery *D* uterine artery *E* uterine vein *F* internal iliac artery *G* external iliac vein *H* external iliac artery

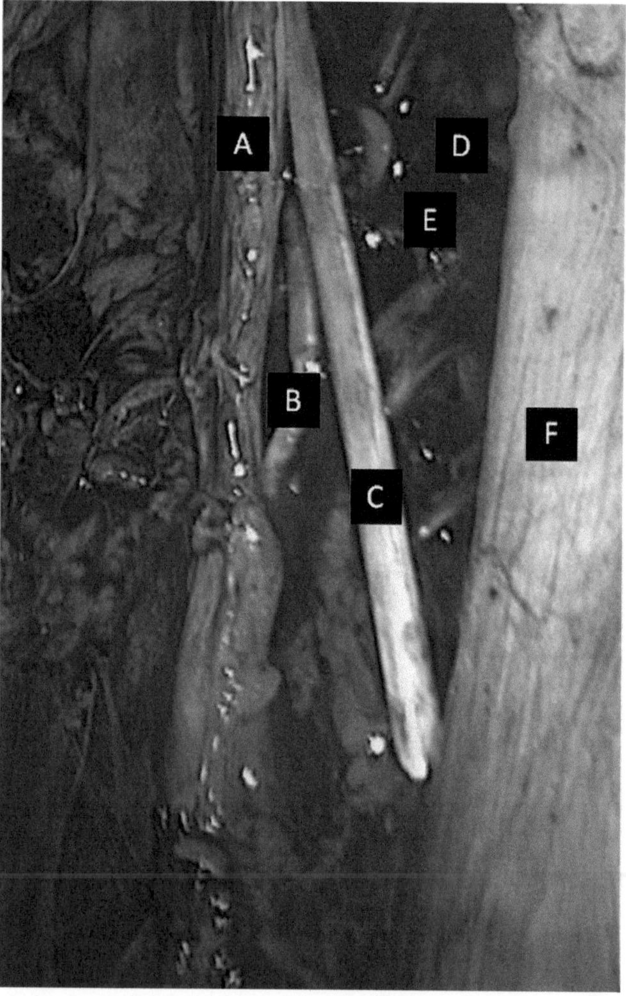

Fig. 40.6 Pelvic lymphadenectomy (*right side*). *A* Superior vesical artery *B* Obturator vein *C* Obturator nerve *D* Intern obturator muscle *E* Obturator fossa *F* External iliac vein

Uterine vessels are identified and cut at their origin from the hypogastric vessels. The uterosacral ligaments are transected after separation of both hypogastric nerves and ureters. The paracervix tissue is transected up to the deep uterine vein (Fig. 40.7).

Dissection of the ureteral tunnel, urinary bladder, and ureteral separation is accomplished with monopolar coagulation using a blunt dissector and with the aid of sealing vessels (Fig. 40.8).

Resection of the proximal paracervical tissues is performed with sealing vessels or monopolar/bipolar coagulation. At the point where the vaginal fornices are encountered bilaterally, the vagina is transected with monopolar coagulation, and the specimen is removed vaginally (Fig. 40.9)

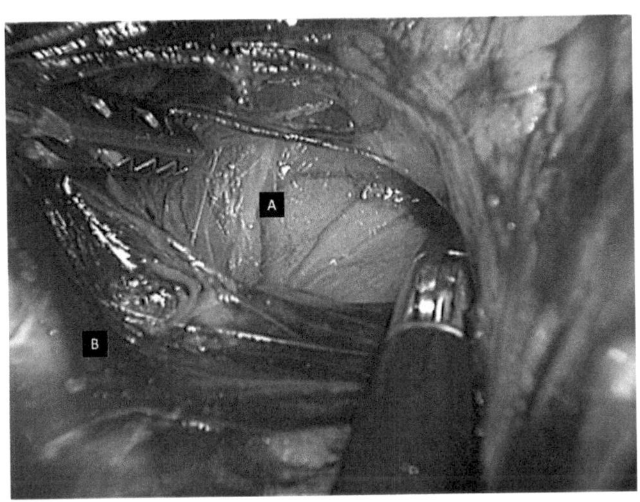

Fig. 40.7 Hypogastric nerves in uterosacral ligament, 2 cm under the ureter. *A* Hypogastric nerve *B* Ureter

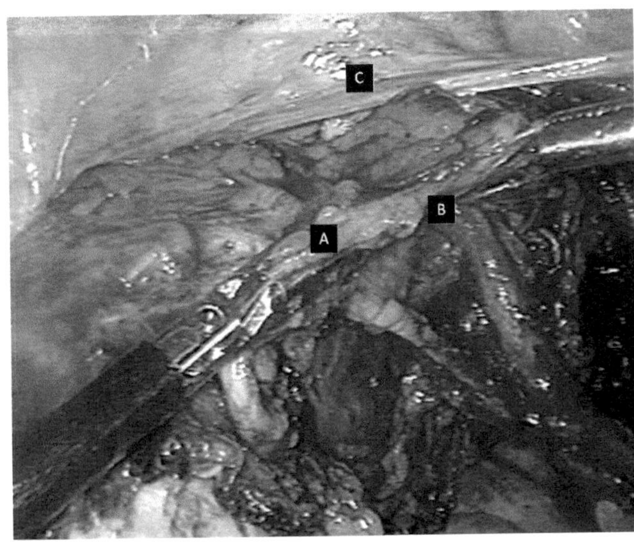

Fig. 40.8 Dissection of the left ureteral tunnel (vesicouterine ligament). *A* Ureter *B* vesicouterine ligament *C* Bladder

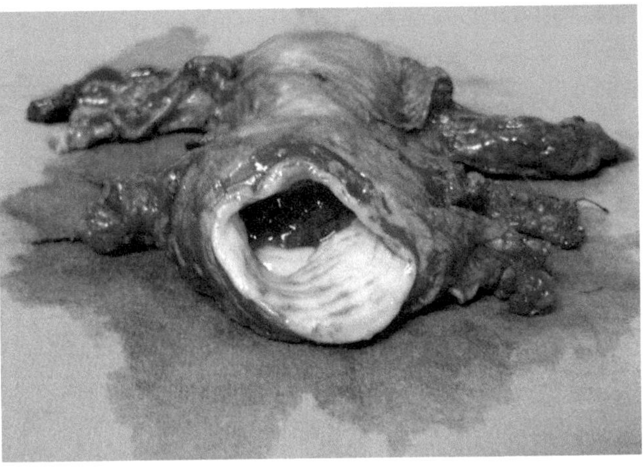

Fig. 40.9 Surgical specimen after total laparoscopic radical hysterectomy (type C1-nerve sparing)

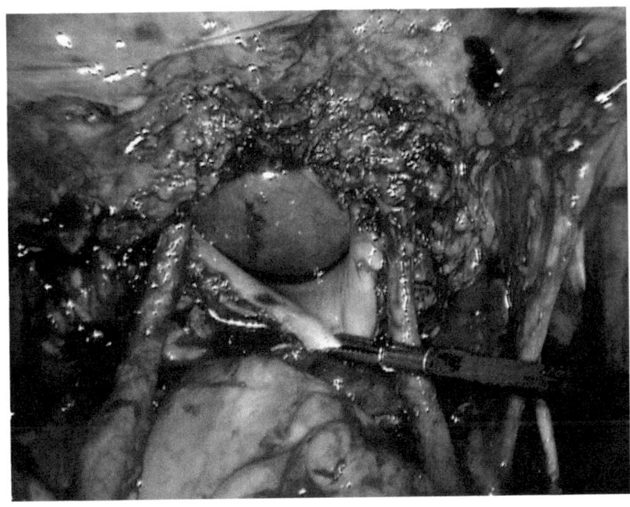

Fig. 40.10 Vaginal cuff before suture through the laparoscopic route

The vaginal cuff is then closed laparoscopically with 2-0 polyglactin continuous sutures. After completing the vaginal procedure, we check for hemostasis and intact ureters, and the peritoneal cavity is thoroughly irrigated and lavaged (Fig. 40.10).

Laparoscopy Radical Hysterectomy Compared with Laparotomy

There have been several studies in the last 10 years in which laparoscopy and laparotomy radical hysterectomy with pelvic lymphadenectomy for the treatment of early invasive Cervical Cancer have been compared.

Duration of Operation

As shown in Tables 40.2 and 40.3, duration of a laparoscopic radical hysterectomy type C operation ranged from 196 min

Table 40.2 Comparative studies of radical hysterectomy by the laparoscopic and the conventional laparotomy route in early invasive cervical cancer

First author, year (References)	Study group	Number patients	FIGO stage	Details	Operative time, min mean	Blood loss, mL, mean	Pelvic nodes mean	Length of stay, days, mean
Lin (2003) [19]	Laparoscopy	10	IA2-IB1 < 2 cm	Type B. Completed vaginally	159	250	16.8	4.1
	Laparotomy	39	IB < 2 cm	Type B	165.7	611.5 *P* < 0.01		8.3 *P* < 0.01
Abu-Rustum (2003) [20]	Laparoscopy	19	IA1-IB1 < 2 cm	Without vaginal surgery	371	301	25.5	4.5
	Laparotomy	195	IA1-IB1		295 *P* < 0.01	639 *P* < 0.01	30.7	9.7 *P* < 0.01
Zakashansky (2007) [21]	Laparoscopy	30	IA1-IIA ≤ 4 cm	Case-control study. Completed vaginally. Advanced laparoscopic training program	318.5	200	31	3.8
	Laparotomy	30	IA1-IIA ≤ 4 cm	NA	242.5 *P* < 0.01	520 *P* < 0.01	21.8 *P* < 0.01	5.6 *P* < 0.01
Li (2007) [22]	Laparoscopy	90	IB1-AII ≤ 5 cm	Type C. Vaginal suture through the vaginal route	263	370	21.3	13.8
	Laparotomy	35	IB1-AII ≤ 5 cm	Type C	217 *P* = 0.001	455	18.8	13.7
Frumovitz (2007) [23, 24]	Laparoscopy	35	IA1-IB1	Type C. Without vaginal surgery	344	319	14	2
	Laparotomy	44	IA1-IB1	Type C	307 *P* = 0.03	548 *P* = 0.009	19 *P* =0.001	5 *P* < 0.001
Díaz-Feijoo (2008) [25]	Laparoscopy	20	IA2-IIA < 4 cm	Sentinel node detection	272	400	19.0	4.9
	Laparotomy	30	IA2-IIA < 4 cm	Sentinel node detection	240 *P* = 0.001	623 *P* = 0.001	21.6	10.7 *P* = 0.001
Malzoni (2009) [26]	Laparoscopy	65	IA1 (n =5, vascular invasion), IA2 (n= 21), Ib1 (n = 39, < 4 cm)	Type II (n = 14), type III (n = 51), paraaortic lymphadenectomy (n = 8)	196	55	23.5	4
	Laparotomy	62	IA1 (n = 3 vascular invasion), IA2 (n=39), Ib1 (n = 39 < 4 cm)	Type II (n = 13), type III (n = 49), paraaortic lymphadenectomy (n = 7)	152 *P* < 0.01	145 *P* < 0.01	25 *P* < 0.01	7 *P* < 0.01
Ditto (2015) [27]	Laparoscopy	60	IA2-IB1 < 2 cm	Type B	215.9	50	25.4	4
	Laparotomy	60	IA2-IB1 < 2 cm	Type B	175 *P* < 0.001	200 *P* < 0.001	34.6 *P* < 0.001	6 *P* < 0.001

in the series of Malzoni [26] to 344 min in the study of Frumovitz [23, 24]. Other groups reporting short operative times are Li et al. [22] and Diaz-Feijoo et al. [25], in which procedures were totally performed using the laparoscopic route.

In a clinical series of 12 patients undergoing laparoscopic radical hysterectomy and lymphadenectomy with intraoperative detection of the sentinel node, Gil-Moreno et al. [28] reported a mean time of 271 min, which is shorter than results published in other series in which the technique of sentinel node detection was not included in the procedure. This study includes patients operated on from March 2001. In the same year, the same group [18], published their experience with laparoscopic radical hysterectomy and pelvis lymphadenectomy in which 27 patients were described (with detection of the sentinel node in 10) and the mean operative time was 285 min. However, patients in this study were included from September 1999, so it can be deduced that the technique of intraoperative sentinel node detection was not

Table 40.3 Comparative studies of radical hysterectomy by the laparoscopic and the conventional laparotomy route in early invasive cervical cancer: complications and follow-up

First author, year (References)	Study group	Complications		Follow-up months
		Intraoperative	Postoperative	
Lin (2003) [19]	Laparoscopy	No	No	11 (1–24)
	Laparotomy	No	No	NA
Abu-Rustum (2003) [20]	Laparoscopy	2 conversions (parametrial bleeding 1, adhesions 1 1 ureteral stent migration replaced at surgery	1 fever of unknown origin 1 transfusion	NA
	Laparotomy	41 transfusions 5 bladder injuries (2.6 %) 5 iliac vein injuries (2.6 %) 1 ureteral lesion (0.5 %)	26 surgical wound infection 25 pelvic/hematoma infections 15 bowel occlusion 13 ileus 4 urinary tract infection 3 bacteremias/sepsis 1 pneumonia 1 *Clostridium difficile* infection 1 deep venous thrombosis 7 lymphedemas	NA
Zakashansky (2007) [21]	Laparoscopy	2 bladder injury	2 *Clostridium difficile* colitis 1 pulmonary thromboembolism 1 deep venous thrombosis 1 ileus 1 bladder dysfunction at 3 weeks	20
	Laparotomy	5 transfusions 1 inferior vena cava injury, small bowel omentum injury	1 thrombosis 1 ileus 1 small bowel occlusion 2 bladder dysfunction at 3 weeks 3 sensory disturbance 2 pyelonephritis	20
Li (2007) [22]	Laparoscopy	2 conversions (iliac vein lesion 1, bladder lesion 1) 4 iliac vein lesions 4 bladder injuries	29 bladder dysfuncton 1 uterocecal fistula 1 vesicovaginal fistula 1 bowel occlusion 4 lymphoceles	26 10 lost to follow-up 13.7 % recurrences 10 % mortality
	Laparotomy	1 iliac vein lesion 2 ureteral lesions	10 urinary retention 1 bowel occlusion 2 lymphocysts 1 dehiscence scar	26 5 lost to follow-up 12 % recurrences 8 % mortality
Frumovitz (2007) [23, 24]	Laparoscopy	11 % transfusions 2 conversions (injury iliac veins 2) 1 lesion inferior epigastric vessels 1 bladder injury	18 % infections 45 % transient bladder dysfunction 3 readmissions (1 fever unknown origin,1 pulmonary embolism, 1 pyelonephritis)	7.2 Recurrence 1
	Laparotomy	15 % transfusions 1 bladder injury	53 % infectious morbidity 31 % transient bladder dysfunction 4 readmissions (fever unknown origin 1, wound celulitis 1, pelvic abscess 1, pulmonary embolism 1)	15.2 Recurrences 2

(continued)

Table 40.3 (continued)

First author, year (References)	Study group	Complications		Follow-up months
		Intraoperative	Postoperative	
Díaz-Feijoo (2008) [25]	Laparoscopy	1 conversion (technical failure) 1 transfusion (5 %) 2 technical failures	Early 0 %, late 20 % 2 urinary incontinence (TVT tape) 3 vaginal suture dehiscence	23.3 100 % survival
	Laparotomy	5 transfusions (16.7 %) 1 disseminated intravascular coagulation (1 death) 1 ureter section	Early 13.3 % 1 urinary tract infection 2 abdominal wall hematomas 1 abdominal wall abscess Late 3.3 % 1 urinary incontinence (TVT tape)	34.6 90 % survival Deaths 3 (recurrent disease 2)
Malzoni (2009) [26]	Laparoscopy	1 bladder injury 2 subcutaneous emphysema	17 bladder dysfunction 1 ureterovaginal fistula 20 lymphorrhea vaginal scar 6 fever episodes	52.5 Vaginal recurrences 5 91 % survival
	Laparotomy	1 bladder injury	19 bladder dysfunction 8 fever episodes 17 lymphorrhea vaginal scar	71.5 Vaginal recurrences 4 93.6 % survival
Ditto (2015) [27]	Laparoscopy	1 bladder injury	1 haemoperitoneum requiring open abdominal surgery 1 uretero-vaginal fistula 2 % urinary retention	31 Recurrences 3 % Death of disease 2 %
	Laparotomy	No	1 lymphocele 1vesico-vaginal fistula 3 % urinary retention	48.7 Recurrences 8 % Death of disease 5 %

initiated until the learning curve of radical hysterectomy with pelvic lymphadenectomy was accomplished.

Regarding the experience of the surgical team and the learning curve for this type of laparoscopic surgery, the study of Pomel et al. [29] provides interesting data. In a group of 50 patients, a mean operative time of 258 min (range 114–540 min, 39 radical hysterectomies type C and 11 type B) was reported. The operative time was not significantly different in patients with and without previous surgery, preoperative brachytherapy or even in relation to body mass index. But the effect of the learning curve was evident. In the first 25 patients, the mean operative time was 290 min, whereas for the last 25 patients, the mean time was 226 min ($P = 0.01$). Moreover, in the last ten patients, the mean operative time decreased to 135 min (range 114–180 min).

In 1995, Sedlacek et al. [30], compared a series of 14 patients undergoing laparoscopic radical hysterectomy type III with lymphadenectomy *vs* the historical group of patients treated in the past 3 years using the laparotomic route, showing a duration of operation of 7 h for the laparoscopy group and 4 h for the laparotomy group, although neither the influence of the surgical experience or the learning curve was considered. Lin [19] published preliminary findings of a prospective and non-randomized study. In the laparoscopic group of ten patients, the mean operative time was 159 min *vs* 165.7 min in the open surgery group (39 patients). It should be noted that the type of hysterectomy was a radical hysterectomy type B and that the procedure was completed by the vaginal route but the surgical time in the two approaches was the same. Abu-Rustum et al. [20] in 2003, carried out a retrospective comparative study of 19 patients undergoing laparoscopic radical hysterectomy with pelvic lymphadenectomy with argon beam coagulation (there were two conversions to open laparotomy, the operative times of which were not included) *vs* a historical cohort of 195 patients who underwent standard laparotomy over an 11-year period. The mean operative time was 296 min in the historical cohort and 371 in the laparoscopy group ($P < 0.01$), but again the learning curve should be taken into account.

Frumovitz and co-workers [23, 24] from the University of Texas M.D. Anderson Cancer Center compared 35 patients operated using the laparoscopic route (two conversions to open laparotomy) with 54 patients undergoing hysterectomy by laparotomy. Surgical times were significantly longer for the laparoscopic group (344 min *vs* 307 min, $P = 0.03$). The authors had two different explanations. Firstly, the learning curve because this was a new technique for the surgical team, and secondly, by the fact that the institution is a teaching center both for gynecologists that want to become specialists in gynecologic oncology and residents that participate in all surgeries. These surgical times are similar to those reported on in the Memorial Sloan-Kettering Cancer Center [20], which is also a university-affiliated hospital. The group of Zakashansky and Nezhat [21] published the results of a case-control study in which 30 laparoscopically-operated patients (the procedure was completed by the vaginal route) were compared with 30 patients operated via laparotomy, emphasizing that the study was performed in a teaching center (with a teaching program for advanced laparoscopic procedures). This is an interesting study because it shows the curve of surgical time by academic year, showing a plateau of 310 min that was not able to be reduced with the experience of the surgeons. When the experience in a teaching program was analyzed, there was an increase in the mean operative time for the laparoscopic procedure *vs* the open route in radical hysterectomies performed by the same alumni. The duration of operation is slightly longer as compared with the same procedure performed by expert surgeons in other series, and approximately coincides with data from other studies of hospitals teaching these procedures [20, 31]. Li et al. [22] compared a group of 90 patients undergoing laparoscopic hysterectomy with suture of the vaginal cuff vaginally with 35 patients operated using the conventional laparotomy approach. The mean surgical time was 263 min *vs* 217 min, respectively ($P = 0.001$). The difference in favor of the laparotomy group was attributed to the learning curve since the duration of operation decreased significantly from 281 min for the first 48 patients to 244 for the last 45 patients ($P = 0.009$).

In 2008, Díaz-Feijoo et al. [25] reported the results of a retrospective non randomized study in which 50 consecutive patients with FIGO stage IA_2, IB_1, and AII disease less than 4 cm underwent radical hysterectomy and lymphadenectomy with intraoperative sentinel lymph node biopsy. The operation was performed entirely by laparoscopy in 20 patients and using the conventional abdominal route in 30. The mean duration of operation was 272.5 min and 240 min. for the laparoscopic and laparotomy groups, respectively ($P = 0.001$).

All studies are consistent with a longer duration of operation for the laparoscopic approach, although the operative time decreases with the surgeon's experience and when the learning curve has been surpassed. However, the laparoscopic technique involves some steps, such as extraction of the lymph nodes using a bag device and insertion of the uter ine manipulator and other laparoscopic instruments which increase the overall operating time.

Intraoperative Blood Loss

A review of the different series published in the literature revealed a mean intraoperative blood loss of 200 mL (see Table 40.2). The learning curve is important to decrease blood loss at the time of surgery. Blood loss in the laparoscopic technique is minimized by a better visualization of the small vessels through magnification of the current optical systems, which allows a careful hemostasis of the operative field [24].

In the first case described by Nezhat et al. [8] in 1992, the estimated blood loss was 30 mL, and in the case reported by Jobling and Wood [32] in 1993, the amount of blood loss was 100 mL. These blood losses were very small bearing in mind the long operating time (420 and 460 min, respectively) and given that procedures were completed by the vaginal route. It is probable that hemostasis was carefully controlled.

When the laparoscopy and the laparotomy routes are compared (Table 40.2), all the studies reported a significantly lower blood loss in the laparoscopic route. Although the significant difference in blood loss (in ml.) may not be clinically important. The clinically important difference is the transfusion rate. Historically, 40–80 % of patients undergoing radical hysterectomy via abdominal laparotomy received blood transfusion.

In the study of Pomel et al. [29] (50 patients) only one patient required blood transfusion in the laparoscopic arm. In the study of Zakashansky et al. [21] published in 2007 (30 patients, procedure completed through the vaginal route), no transfusions were reported. In the study of Malzoni et al. [26], the estimated blood loss was 55 mL and no transfusions were needed. In the study of Díaz-Feijoo et al. [25], the mean blood loss was 623 mL in the laparotomy group and 400 mL in the laparoscopy group ($P = 0.001$). Five patients in the laparotomy group required blood transfusion compared with one patient in the laparoscopy group. In relation to the learning curve, in the largest series of laparoscopic radical hysterectomies lower rates of blood transfusion are generally reported. In the study of Spirtos et al. [33] of 78 patients, the transfusion rate was 1.3 % and in the study of Pomel et al. [29] 2 %.

Pelvic Nodes

The number of pelvic nodes obtained in the different studies published in the literature ranges from 7 to 41. In the largest series, the mean number of nodes removed in the laparoscopic route is around 20 (23.5 in the study of Malzoni et al. [26] with 65 patients, 21.3 in the study of Li et al. [22] with 90 patients and 25.5 in the study of AbuRustum et al. [20] with 197 patients). In other studies, the mean number of lymph nodes obtained is smaller (16.8 in the study of Lin et al. [19] with ten patients) or greater such as 31 in the study of Zakashansky et al. [21] with 30 patients (Table 40.2).

Abu-Rustum et al. [20], reported a mean of 25.5 nodes in the laparoscopic group *vs* 30.7 in the laparotomy group, although significant differences were not found. Malzoni et al. [26] also observed a higher number of nodes obtained in open surgery (25.2) than in laparoscopic surgery (23.5), including a difference in the number of aortic nodes in favor of laparotomy. In the study of Frumovitz et al. [23], a mean of 19 pelvic nodes were obtained during abdominal radical hysterectomy compared with 14 during total laparoscopic radical hysterectomy ($P = 0.001$). However, in the study of Li et al. [22] the mean number of nodes obtained was similar (21.3 laparoscopy *vs* 18.8 laparotomy), whereas Zakashansky et al. [21] showed a significantly higher number in laparoscopic radical hysterectomy than in open abdominal surgery (31 *vs* 21.8, P = 0.01) (Table 40.2).

The decision to perform laparoscopic lymphadenectomy depends on the experience and protocols of each working group. There are, currently, controversial opinions regarding the posibility of comparing the results obtained for each of the different techniques, due to the absence of comparative prospective randomized studies on the effectiveness of each and influence on survival in each type of genital neoplasia.

However, there is not a consensus on the minimal number of nodes which should be removed at the time of a systematic pelvic lymphadenectomy or even if the lymphadenectomy has a therapeutic effect in cervical cancer. With this objective, Suprasert *et al.* [34]retrospectively included 826 patients who were divided into four groups according to the number of nodes removed (with at least 11 pelvic nodes removed). They concluded that the number of removed pelvic nodes was not associated with 5-year disease-free survival nor when stratified by nodal status. These results are opposite to those from the study of Shah et al. [35] who analyzed 5522 women included in the SEER. It concluded that among node-negative women, survival is improved when a greater number of lymph nodes are removed suggesting that the extent of lymphadenectomy in node negative patient influences survival. This could be explained because a greater number of removed nodes could give a better way to detect metastasis or to extract micrometastasis.

Sentinel Lymp Node (SLN)

The sentinel lymph node is defined as the first draining lymph node of an anatomical region, so that a histologically negative sentinel lymph node would predict the absence of tumor metastases in the other non-sentinel lymph nodes. In cervical carcinoma patients, lymph node status is a major prognostic factor and is a decision criterion for adjuvant therapy. In patients with early cervical cancer, pelvic or paraaortic lymph node metastases are detected in only 8 % of women with stage IA2 and in 26 % of women with stage IIA no bulky [36].Thus, many of these patients derive no benefit from pelvic lymphadenectomy. SLN dissections have been associated with decreased short-term and long-term morbidity when compared with complete lymph node dissection such as lymphedema [37]. We should remember that 34.5 % of patients with lymphadenectomy for a gynecological cancer will develop symptomatic linfocysts and 11.4 % a lower-limb lymphedema [38]. Eiriksson and Covens reviewed the reports published on 2333 patients with early cervical cancer and sentinel node dissection. The sensibility was 98.2 % and the predictive negative value was 99.6 %. They suggested that it may be possible that systematic lymphadenectomy can be substituted by detection and analysis of the sentinel node as many groups are making nowadays [39]. The study published by Gil-Moreno et al. in 2005 showed the feasibility of the combination of laparoscopic intraoperative sentinel node mapping and laparoscopic radical surgery in the context of minimally invasive surgery for the management of patients with early cervical cancer [18]. Intraoperative detection of sentinel lymph node status may have significant implications from a clinical management point of view. If the node is positive for tumor metastasis, a radical hysterectomy could be omitted, and adjuvant chemoradiation is commonly given (Fig. 40.11) [40].

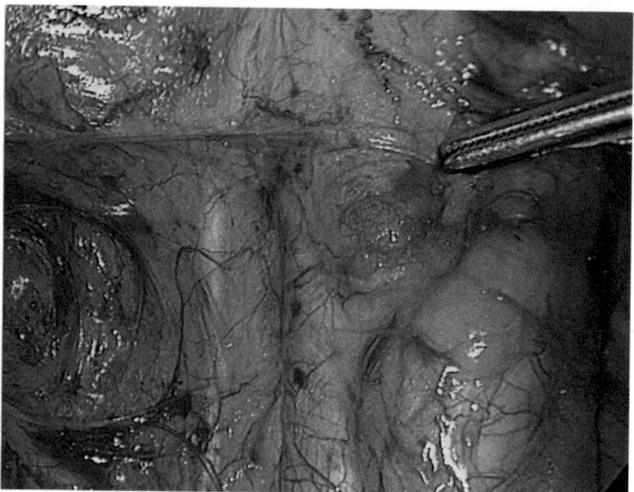

Fig. 40.11 Identification of a blue-positive sentinel lymph node

Intraoperative Complications

Intraoperative complications reported on in the different studies are shown in Table 40.3. Conversion to open surgery has been mostly described in association with vascular injuries [10, 20, 22, 23, 33, 41], bladder injuries [9, 20, 27, 33], pelvic adhesions [9, 20], large uterus [9], or difficulties in maintaining the pneumoperitoneum for technical reasons [18, 25, 33].

Vascular injuries during laparoscopic procedures, including trocar injury at the start of the procedure [23] is one of the most common complications requiring immediate conversion to open surgery and/or blood transfusion, with the external and internal iliac veins [20, 22, 23, 41, 42] and vascular lesions of the abdominal wall being the most frequent. Blood transfusion at the time of surgery or in the immediate postoperative period is also a common complication. Although in the majority of studies higher blood losses are usually reported for conventional laparotomy [20, 21, 23, 25]. A case of secondary hemorrhage requiring relaparoscopy has been also reported [42]. A venotomy of the inferior vena cava during lymph node dissection in the laparotomy group was described by Zakashansky et al. [21].

Intraoperative injuries of the bladder (mostly repaired during the laparoscopic procedure) [23, 27, 29, 31, 33, 41, 42]

and less frequently of the ureters [9, 29, 30, 41, 42] (sometimes documented in the postoperative period) [42] are relatively frequent intraoperative complications. In a review of intraoperative urinary tract lesions in laparoscopic surgery (50 patients) and open surgery (48 patients), no statistically significant differences were observed [43].

Other less frequent intraoperative complications include intestinal damage [41, 42] ,a case of pneumomediastinum immediately following surgery [31], and hypercapnia [41].

In one large serie of laparoscopic radical hysterectomy and lymphadenectomy procedures for invasive cervical carcinoma that included 317 patients, Xu et al. [41] examined complications and analyzed factors associated with conversion to an open surgical procedure. The overall conversion rate was 1.3 % (n = 4). Major and minor intraoperative complications occurred in 4.4 % (n = 14) of the patients. Seven patients had vessel injuries, five of which were repaired or treated laparoscopically. One left external iliac vein required laparotomy, and one patient underwent laparotomy to control bleeding sites. Operative cystotomies occurred in five patients, which were repaired laparoscopically. Two patients underwent laparotomy because of hypercapnia and colon injury. The authors emphasized that these complications were developed in the first 50 laparoscopic procedures, and after those, no intestinal or vascular injuries occurred.

In the majority of studies in which the laparoscopic procedure and open surgery has been compared (see Table 40.3), differences in the rate of intraoperative complications were not found except in the study of Zakashansky et al. [21] regarding the number of patients requiring blood transfusion. Some studies even showed a trend towards a higher number of complications in the laparotomy group [21, 25]. In the laparotomy group in the study of Díaz-Feijoo et al. [25], ureteral injury occurred in one patient and disseminated intravascular coagulation in another. In the laparoscopy group, conversion to open surgery was necessary in one patient.

Postoperative Complications

Postoperative complications are also summarized in Table 40.3. Most relate to infections [12, 20, 21, 23, 28, 29, 33, 42] and bladder dysfunction, as classically reported after radical hysterectomy [12, 18, 21–23, 25, 28, 29, 32, 33, 41, 42]. Voiding difficulties, sometimes requiring intermittent catheterization, may occur between 2 weeks and 6 months postoperatively.

Infectious morbidity is mainly related to urinary tract infection, pelvic abscesses, and abscesses of the vaginal cuff, as well as some cases of fever of unknown origin. Cases of urologic-related sepsis have also been described. Frumovitz et al. [23] showed a higher percentage of postoperative infections in patients undergoing open surgery (53 %) than in those treated laparoscopically (18 %).

Ureterovaginal fistulas and to a lesser extent vesicovaginal fistulas, are also reported on in many studies [12, 22, 29–31, 41, 42, 44]. Surgical repair was necessary in most cases, although some patients have been treated conservatively [44]. In the study of Uccella et al. [43], the rate of postoperative urological complication was similar in laparoscopic and open surgery.

Other uncommon complications include deep venous thrombosis [21, 33, 41], which was reported as the cause of fatal and nonfatal pulmonary thromboembolism [21, 23, 31]. Early mobilization of the patients is highly recommended for the prophylaxis of deep venous thrombosis and pulmonary embolism. However, embolism of the right external iliac artery is a rare postoperative complication of laparoscopic radical hysterectomy [41].

In the study of Díaz-Feijoo et al. [25], 3 months after radical hysterectomy, vagina cuff separation with bowel prolapse after the first sexual intercourse (successfully repaired vaginally)was reported on in three patients in the laparoscopy group. Similar cases have been also described by other authors [29, 31, 44].

Lymphocele is a relatively common complication [22, 31, 33, 41], although most cases are asymptomatic and no treatment is required. Symptomatic lymphocele may be treated by percutaneous puncture, guided by ultrasound or compute tomography. Other complications described in the studies are lymphedema of the lower extremities [12, 41], transient sensory disturbances [29, 41], and colitis caused by *Clostridium difficile* reported both in laparoscopy surgery [21] and in open surgery [20].

Length of Hospital Stay and Costs

Laparoscopic surgery is usually associated with a short hospital stay, ranging between 1 day [31] and 13.8 days [22], although in most studies the mean length of stay varies between 2 and 5 days [8, 13, 18–21, 23–26, 31–33, 44]. (Table 40.2). Studies in which laparoscopy and laparotomy approaches were compared, length of hospitalization was usually shorter for the laparoscopic procedure [11, 19–21, 23, 25, 27] partly, due to early postoperative intestinal motility. In the study of Li et al. [22] there were differences in the bowel recovery time between the open surgery group (2.4 days) and the laparoscopy group (1.96 days) (P = 0.025). Advantages of the laparoscopic procedure include early mobilization and lower pain intensity. On the other hand, Li et al. reported similar lengths of hospital stay for the laparoscopic and open abdominal surgery groups (13.8 *vs* 13.7 days) and argued that patients wanted to be discharged after complete recovery. Moreover, differences in health care delivery systems and culture may account for a large variation in the average hospital stay. Also insurance companies may not be concerned about the duration of hospital stay in cancer patients.

In 1994, Sedlacek et al. [11] estimated the cost of laparoscopic radical hysterectomy as $12,594 in comparison with $12,905 of the open procedure. Reduced costs of laparoscopy were especially associated with a shorter hospital stay.

Outcome and Recurrence

A few cases of port-site metastasis have been reported [42, 44]. Preventive measures include irrigation of port sites with cytotoxic agents, careful tumor manipulation, and use of extraction bags for any suspicious tissue.

Definitive data regarding differences in overall survival, disease-free survival, and recurrence between the laparoscopic approach and conventional open surgery are lacking. Comparative studies of both procedures include small series of patients with relatively short duration of follow-up (Table 40.3). In the study of Li et al. [22], after a mean follow-up of 26 months, the overall mortality in the laparoscopy group was 10 % *vs* 8 % in the laparotomy group, and there was a recurrence rate of 13.7 % and 12 %, respectively. In the study of Frumovitz et al. [23], one recurrence in the laparoscopy group (n = 35) after a mean follow-up of 7.2 months and two recurrences in the laparotomy group (n = 44) after a mean follow-up of 15.2 months was reported. In the series of Díaz-Feijoo et al. [25], the disease-free survival was 100 % in the laparoscopy group after a follow-up of 23.3 months and 86.7 % in the laparotomy group after a mean follow-up of 34.6 months, with an overall survival of 90 %. In the study of Ditto et al. [27] in 2015, the recurrence rate was 3 % in the laparoscopic arm (31 months of follow up) and 8 % in the laparotomy arm (48.7 months of follow up).

Further studies, particularly prospective randomizes studies, with larger study samples and longer follow-up periods are needed to assess the outcome of patients with early-stage cervical cancer undergoing radical hysterectomy with pelvic lymphadenectomy through the laparoscopic approach or conventional open surgery.

Conclusions

In comparison with the conventional abdominal laparotomy, the laparoscopy approach is associated with a lower surgical morbidity in terms of intraoperative blood loss, shorter hospital stay and early resumption of daily activities with an increase in quality of life [25]. Recent advances in laparoscopic instruments simplify training and improve outcomes. Probably magnification yields a better surgical field and shorten operative times by enabling better hemostasis with less tissue damage and easier manipulation. With advances in surgical robotics [45–50], continuation of these trends can be anticipated.

Evidence presented here shows that laparoscopic radical hysterectomy with endoscopic pelvic lymphadenectomy is a safe surgical option in the treatment and staging of early invasive cervical cancer regarding the surgical technique, surgical risk, intraoperative bleeding, perioperative and postoperative complications, and patient's recovery. A decrease in operative time as more procedures are performed and surgeons become more familiar with the procedure may be expected. The laparoscopic technique is more expensive than laparotomy due primarily to laparoscopic instrumentation but the disadvantage of cost is counterbalanced by shorter hospital stay, prompt postoperative recovery, and early resumption of daily activities [11, 30].

In our opinion, minimally invasive surgery (conventional laparoscopy or robotically assisted) should be the standard approach for the surgical treatment of patients with early cervical cancer.

References

1. Querleu D, Leblanc E, Castelain B. Laparoscopic pelvic lymphadenectomy in the staging of early carcinoma of the cervix. Am J Obstet Gynecol. 1991;164:579–81.
2. Leblanc E, Querleu D, Castelain B, et al. Bilan de la cœliochirurgie en oncologie gynécologique en 2000. Bull Cancer. 2000;87:76–85.
3. Reich H, DeCaprio J, McGlynn F. Laparoscopic hysterectomy. J Gynecol Surg. 1989;5:213–6.
4. Dargent D, Mathevet P. Hystérectomie élargie laparoscopico-vaginale. J Gynecol Obstet Biol Reprod (Paris). 1992;21:709–10.
5. Querleu D. Hystérectomies élargies de Schauta-Amreich et Schauta-Stoeckel assistées par cœlioscopie. J Gynecol Obstet Biol Reprod. 1992;20:747–8.
6. Querleu D. Laparoscopically assisted radical vaginal hysterectomy. Gynecol Oncol. 1993;51:248–54.
7. Canis M, Mage G, Wattiez A, JL P, Manhes H, MA B. La chirurgie endoscopique a-t-elle une place dans la chirurgie radicale du cancer du col utérin? J Gynecol Obstet Biol Reprod (Paris). 1990;19:921.
8. Nezhat CR, Burrell MO, Nezhat FR, Benigno BB, Welander CE. Laparoscopic radical hysterectomy with paraaortic and pelvic node dissection. Am J Obstet Gynecol. 1992;166:864–5.
9. Canis M, Mage G, Pouly JL, et al. Laparoscopic radical hysterectomy for cervical cancer. Baillieres Clin Obstet Gynaecol. 1995; 9:675–89.
10. Hsieh YY, Lin WC, Chang CC, Yeh LS, Hsu TY, Tsai HD. Laparoscopic radical hysterectomy with low paraaortic, subaortic and pelvic lymphadenectomy. Results of short-term follow-up. J Reprod Med. 1998;43:528–34.
11. Sedlacek TV, Campion MJ, Hutchins RA, Reich H. Laparoscopic radical hysterectomy: a preliminary report [abstract]. J Am Assoc Gynecol Laparosc. 1994;1(Part 2):s32.
12. Kim DH, Moon JS. Laparoscopic radical hysterectomy with pelvic lymphadenectomy for early, invasive cervical carcinoma. J Am Assoc Gynecol Laparosc. 1998;5:411–7.
13. Spirtos NM, Schlaerth JB, Kimball RE, Leiphart VM, Ballon SC. Laparoscopic radical hysterectomy (type III) with aortic and pelvic lymphadenectomy. Am J Obstet Gynecol. 1996;174: 1763–7.
14. Mutch DG. The new FIGO staging system for cancers of vulva, cervix, endometrium and sarcomas. Gynecol Oncol. 2009;115: 325–8.
15. Piver MS, Rutledge F, Smith JP. Five classes of extended hysterectomy for women with cervical cancer. Obstet Gynecol. 1974;44: 265–72.
16. Querleu D, Morrow CP. Classification of radical hysterectomy. Lancet Oncol. 2008;9:297–303.

17. Cibula D, Abu-Rustum NR, Benedetti-Panici P, Köhler C, Raspagliesi F, Querleu D, Morrow CP. New classification system of radical hysterectomy: emphasis on a three-dimensional anatomic template for parametrial resection. Gynecol Oncol. 2011;122:264–8.
18. Gil-Moreno A, Puig O, Pérez-Benevente MA, et al. Total laparoscopic radical hysterectomy (type II-III) with pelvic lymphadenectomy in early invasive cervical cancer. J Minim Invasive Gynecol. 2005;12:113–20.
19. Lin YS. Preliminary results of laparoscopic modified radical hysterectomy in early invasive cervical cancer. J Am Assoc Gynecol Laparosc. 2003;10:80–4.
20. Abu-Rustum NR, Gemignani ML, Moore K, et al. Total laparoscopic radical hysterectomy with pelvic lymphadenectomy using the argon-beam coagulator: pilot data and comparison to laparotomy. Gynecol Oncol. 2003;91:402–9.
21. Zakashansky K, Chuang L, Gretz H, Nagarsheth NP, Rahaman J, Nezhat FR. A case-controlled study of total laparoscopic radical hysterectomy with pelvic lymphadenectomy versus radical abdominal hysterectomy in a fellowship training program. Int J Gynecol Cancer. 2007;17:1075–82.
22. Li G, Yan X, Shang H, Wang G, Chen L, Han Y. A comparison of laparoscopic radical hysterectomy and pelvis lymphadenectomy and laparotomy in the treatment of Ib-IIa cervical cancer. Gynecol Oncol. 2007;105:176–80.
23. Frumovitz M, dos Reis R, Sun CC, et al. Comparison of total laparoscopic and abdominal radical hysterectomy for patients with early-stage cervical cancer. Obstet Gynecol. 2007;110:96–102.
24. Frumovitz M, Ramirez PT. Total laparoscopic radical hysterectomy: surgical technique and instrumentation. Gynecol Oncol. 2007;104(Suppl):13–6.
25. Díaz-Feijoó B, Gil-Moreno A, Pérez-Benavente A, Morchón S, Martínez-Palones JM, Xercavins J. Sentinel lymph node identification and radical hysterectomy with lymphadenectomy in early stage cervical cancer: laparoscopy versus laparotomy. J Minim Invasive Gynecol. 2008;15:531–7.
26. Malzoni M, Tinelli R, Cosentino F, Fusco A, Malzoni C. Total laparoscopic radical hysterectomy versus abdominal radical hysterectomy with lymphadenectomy in patients with early cervical cancer: our experience. Ann Surg Oncol. 2009;16:1316–23.
27. Ditto A, Martinelli F, Bogani G, Gasparri ML, Di Donato V, Zanaboni F, Lorusso D, Raspagliesi F. Implementation of laparoscopic approach for type B radical hysterectomy: a comparison with open surgical operations. Eur J Surg Oncol. 2015;41:34–9.
28. Gil-Moreno A, Díaz-Feijoo B, Roca I, et al. Total laparoscopic radical hysterectomy with intraoperative sentinel node identification in patients with early invasive cervical cancer. Gynecol Oncol. 2005;96:187–93.
29. Pomel C, Atallah D, Le Bouedec G, et al. Laparoscopic radical hysterectomy for invasive cervical cancer: 8-year experience of a pilot study. Gynecol Oncol. 2003;91:534–9.
30. Sedlacek TV, Campion MJ, Reich H, Sedlacek T. Laparoscopic radical hysterectomy: a feasibility study. Gynecol Oncol. 1995;56:126 (abstract 65).
31. Ramirez PT, Slomovitz BM, Soliman PT, Coleman RL, Levenback C. Total laparoscopic radical hysterectomy and lymphadenectomy: The MD Anderson Cancer Center experience. Gynecol Oncol. 2006;102:252–5.
32. Jobling T, Wood C. Laparoscopic modified radical hysterectomy and lymphadenectomy simulating open operation for stage 1A2 cervical carcinoma. Aust N Z J Obstet Gynaecol. 1993;33:400–3.
33. Spirtos NM, Eisenkop SM, Schlaerth JB, Ballon SC. Laparoscopic radical hysterectomy (type III) with aortic and pelvic lymphadenectomy in patients with stage I cervical cancer: Surgical morbidity and intermediate follow-up. Am J Obstet Gynecol. 2002;187:340–8.
34. Suprasert P, Charoenkwan K, Khunamornpong S. Pelvic node removal and disease-free survival in cervical cancer patients treated with radical hysterectomy and pelvic lymphadenectomy. Int J Gynecol Obstet. 2012;116:43–6.
35. Shah M, Lewin SN, Deutsch I, et al. Therapeutic role of lymphadenectomy for cervical cancer. Cancer. 2011;117:310–7.
36. Benedet JL, Odicino F, Maisonneuve P, Beller U, Creasman WT, Heintz AP, Ngan HY, Sideri M, Pecorelli S. Carcinoma of the cervix uteri. J Epidemiol Biostat. 2001;6:7–43.
37. Robison K, Holman LL, Moore RG. Update on sentinel lymph node evaluation in gynecologic malignancies. Curr Opin Obstet Gynecol. 2011;23(1):8–12.
38. Achouri A, Huchon C, Bats AS, Bensaid C, Nos C, Lécuru F. Complications of lymphadenectomy for gynecologic cancer. Eur J Surg Oncol (EJSO). 2013;39(1):81–6.
39. Eiriksson L, Covens A. Sentinel lymph node mapping in cervical cancer: the future? BJOG Int J Obstet Gynaecol. 2012;119(2): 129–33.
40. Lambaudie E, Collinet P, Narducci F, Sonoda Y, Papageorgiou T, Carpentier P, Leblanc E, Querleu D. Laparoscopic identification of sentinel lymph nodes in early stage cervical cancer: prospective study using a combination of patent blue dye injection and technetium radiocolloid injection. Gynecol Oncol. 2003;89:84–7.
41. Xu H, Chen Y, Li Y, Zhang Q, Wang D, Liang Z. Complications of laparoscopic radical hysterectomy and lymphadenectomy for invasive cervical cancer: experience base on 317 procedures. Surg Endosc. 2007;21:960–4.
42. Puntambekar SP, Palep RJ, Puntambekar SS, et al. Laparoscopic total radical hysterectomy by the Pune technique: our experience of 248 cases. J Minim Invasive Gynecol. 2007;14:682–9.
43. Uccella S, Laterza R, Ciravolo G, et al. A comparison of urinary complications following total laparoscopic radical hysterectomy and laparoscopic pelvic lymphadenectomy to open abdominal surgery. Gynecol Oncol. 2007;107:S147–9.
44. Pellegrino A, Vizza E, Fruscio R, et al. Total laparoscopic radical hysterectomy and pelvic lymphadenectomy in patients with Ib1 stage cervical cancer: analysis of surgical and oncological outcome. EJSO. 2009;35:98–103.
45. Wexner SD, Bergamaschi R, Lacy A, et al. The current status of robotic pelvic surgery: results of a multinational interdisciplinary consensus conference. Surg Endosc. 2009;23:438–43.
46. Sert BM, Abeler VM. Robotic-assisted laparoscopic radical hysterectomy (Piver type III) with pelvic node dissection—case report. Eur J Gynaecol Oncol. 2006;27:531–3.
47. Magrina JF, Zanagnolo VL. Robotic surgery for cervical cancer. Yonsei Med J. 2008;49:879–85.
48. Ramirez PT, Soliman PT, Schmeler KM, dos Reis R, Frumovitz M. Laparoscopic and robotic techniques for radical hysterectomy in patients with early-stage cervical cancer. Gynecol Oncol. 2008;110:S21–4.
49. Nezhat FR, Datta MS, Liu C, Chuang L, Zakashansky K. Robotic radical hysterectomy versus total laparoscopic radical hysterectomy with pelvic lymphadenectomy for treatment of early cervical cancer. JSLS. 2008;12:227–37.
50. Gil-Ibáñez B, Díaz-Feijoo B, Pérez-Benavente A, Puig-Puig O, Franco-Camps S, Centeno C, Xercavins J, Gil-Moreno A. Nerve sparing technique in robotic-assisted radical hysterectomy: results. Int J Med Robot. 2013;9(3):339–44.

Total Laparoscopic Nerve-Sparing Radical Hysterectomy

41

Hiroyuki Kanao and Nobuhiro Takeshima

Introduction

Total laparoscopic radical hysterectomy for cervical carcinoma is currently an accepted surgical procedure not only because of its technical feasibility, but also because of its favorable oncologic outcome [1–6]. However, bladder dysfunction after a laparoscopic radical hysterectomy is likely to decrease the patient's quality of life because of the physical and mental stress that accompany post-operative disorders. The main cause is damage to the pelvic nerve plexus (inferior hypogastric plexus) and its vesical branches during this procedure. These nerve circuits are important for neurogenic bladder control [7–9].

Total laparoscopic nerve-sparing radical hysterectomy has been developed recently for early stage cervical carcinoma using a previously established technical procedure.. The principal features of this technique can be summarized by describing the procedure as one in which the hypogastric nerves, instead of the pelvic nerve plexus and its vesical branches, are preserved at several steps during a classical radical hysterectomy [10, 11]. Consequently, the hypogastric nerves are regarded as the main anatomical landmark of the nerve-sparing radical hysterectomy because they act as the upper limit of the pelvic nerve plexus and the vesical branches.

In this chapter, step-by-step surgical instructions for total laparoscopic nerve-sparing radical hysterectomy are described (with a special focus on the nerve-sparing techniques) and our original research regarding the correlations between the preserved pelvic nerve networks and bladder functions after total laparoscopic nerve sparing radical hysterectomy are introduced.

H. Kanao, MD, PhD (✉)
Department of Gynecologic Oncology, Cancer Institute Hospital, Tokyo, Japan
e-mail: hiroyuki.kanao@vesta.ocn.ne.jp

N. Takeshima
Cancer Institute Hospital, Department of Gynecologic Oncology, Tokyo, Japan

Surgical Procedures

Creation of the Vaginal Cuff

Prior to laparoscopic (LAP) surgery, a vaginal cuff is created (Fig. 41.1). In LAP surgery, an excision of suitable length of the vagina (2 cm from the tumor) is quite difficult due to the loss of tactile sensation; therefore, the creation of a vaginal cuff is essential for an accurate excision of the vagina. Moreover, the creation of a vaginal cuff is also quite useful to prevent the spillage of cancer cells during LAP surgery.

The patient is placed in the lithotomy position. First, 12–15 sutures are placed circumferentially approximately 2 cm from the tumor, and the sutures are pulled to reveal the incision line. Adrenaline at a dilution of 1:1,000,000 is injected into the incision line to reduce bleeding. The vaginal mucosa is then incised circumferentially using electrocautery and the vaginal cuff is doubly closed in a continuous fashion. When the margin of the tumor is difficult to determine, visual inspection with the Schiller test is essential.

Positioning of the Patient and Configuration of the Trocars

The patient is placed in the mild lithotomy position. The legs of the patient are extended slightly and the patent is tilted about 10 ° (Fig. 41.2a). A 12-mm trocar is placed in the umbilicus for a camera port and three 5-mm trocars for forceps are placed as in Fig. 41.2b. A 5-mm extra-long trocar (150 mm length) is placed at the posterior vaginal fornix, and a forceps placed through this port is used as a uterine manipulator. A 1-0 vicryl suture is placed around the uterine body and the uterus is manipulated by a pulling-and-pushing technique of the 1-0 vicryl suture with forceps through the vaginal trocar. In our procedure, a vaginal cuff is created prior to the LAP surgery, thus overcoming the problem of using a uterine manipulator (Fig. 41.2c).

I. Alkatout, L. Mettler (eds.), *Hysterectomy*, DOI 10.1007/978-3-319-22497-8_41

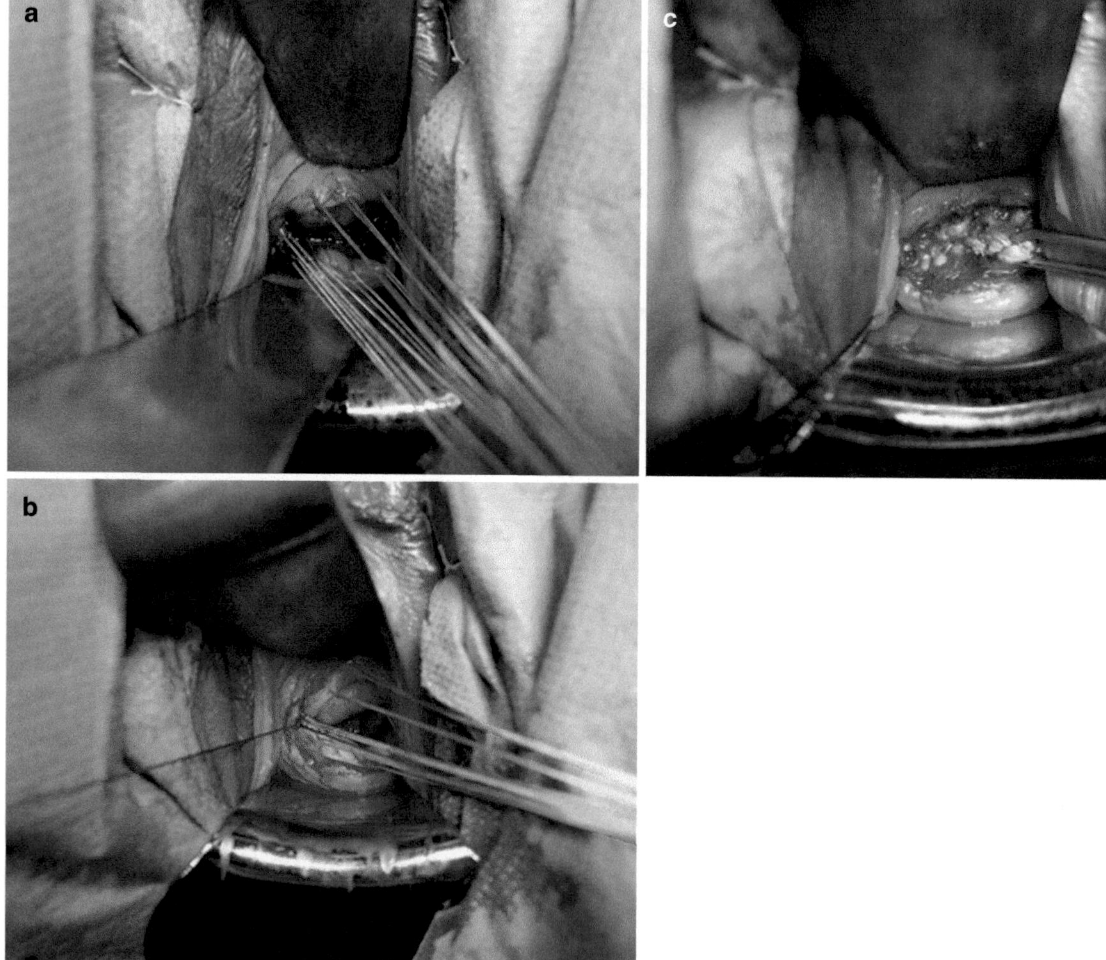

Fig. 41.1 Creation of the vaginal cuff. (**a**) 12–15 sutures are placed circumferentially approximately 2 cm from the tumor. (In this case, Schiller test is performed). (**b**) Incision of vaginal mucosa is made around the sutures and the vaginal cuff closure is started. (**c**) Vaginal cuff closure is completed

Pelvic Lymphadenectomy

Pelvic lymphadenectomy is started by opening the pelvic sidewall triangle, which is the area between the round ligament, the infundibulopelvic ligament, and the external iliac vessels. At first, a wide opening of the pararectal space and paravesical space is developed allowing the exposure of the cardinal ligament between these spaces. These spaces are avascular spaces; therefore, a blunt dissection is sufficient for development. In order to maintain a good surgical view around the paravesical space (and obturator fossa), we suspend an umbilical ligament to the abdominal wall (Fig. 41.3 1).

Next, the space between the psoas muscle and the external iliac vessels is developed widely in order to expose the obturator nerve and vessels (Fig. 41.3 2). The lymphofatty tissue is easily dissected from the obturator nerve and vessels using a blunt dissection technique and the upper end of the lymphofatty tissue (around the common iliac lesion) is clipped and transected (Fig. 41.3 3). The clipping of the cut end of lymph node is particularly important to prevent lymphocele after the surgery. Following the transection of the upper end, the lymphofatty tissue is easily stripped off the external and internal iliac vessels en block (Fig. 41.3 4–6).

For a total laparoscopic nerve-sparing radical hysterectomy, the complete exposure of the pelvic nerve networks (hypogastric nerves, pelvic splanchnic nerves, pelvic nerve plexus, and their vesical branches) is essential; and in order to achieve complete exposure it is very important to perform lymphadenectomy adjacent to the internal iliac region.

After developing a wide pararectal space, the hypogastric nerves can be observed easily along the lateral sides of the mesorectum. The lymph node tissue around the internal iliac region is removed completely; then, the S2–3 roots are identifiable beneath the fascia of the piriformis muscle. Additionally the pelvic splanchnic nerves, which join the pelvic nerve plexus, are visible as visceral branches originating

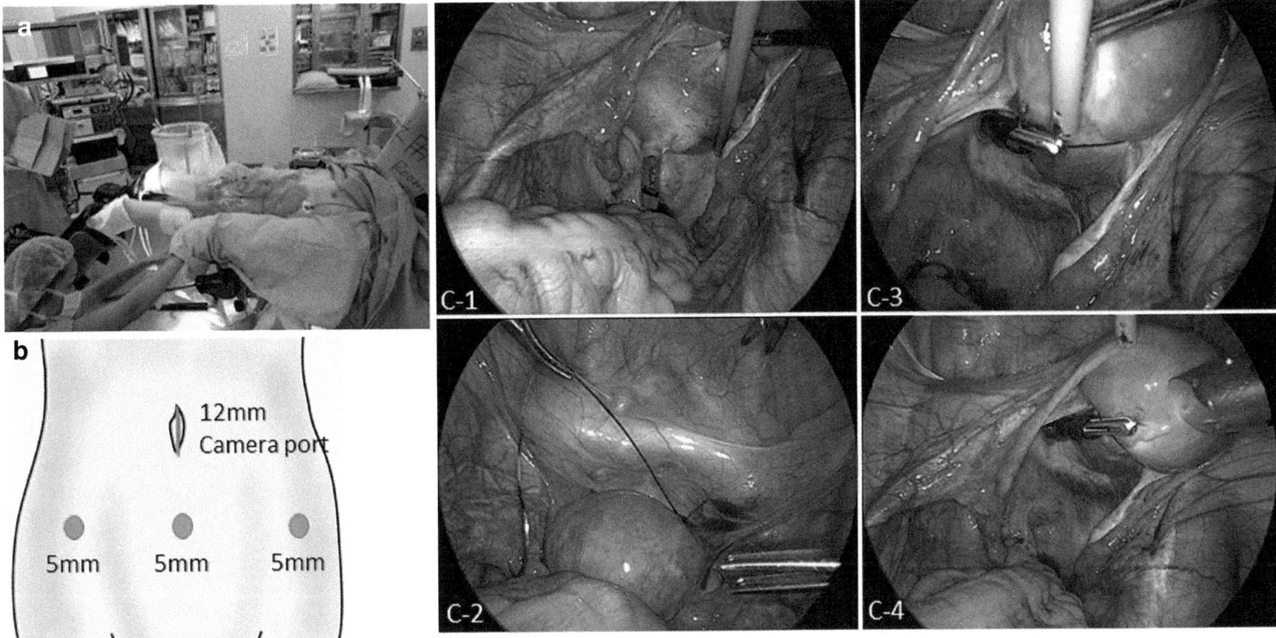

Fig. 41.2 Positioning of the patient and configuration of the trocars. (**a**) patient position, (**b**) trocar position, (**c**) A vaginal additional port. (*C-1*) An extra long trocar is placed at the posterior vaginal fornix. (*C-2*) 1-0 vicryl is placed around the uterine body. (*C-3,4*) This vicryl is grasped by the forceps through this port, and the uterus can be mobilized by this forceps like an uterine manipulator

from the S2–3 roots after the lymph node tissue around the cardinal ligament is meticulously removed (Fig. 41.4). After all lymph nodes are harvested, the nodes are removed with a plastic bag to prevent the scattering of the specimen.

The Transection of Upper Ligaments

The infundibulopelvic ligament or the adnexal ligament (if the patient wants to preserve her ovaries) is desiccated and transected. The round ligament is also desiccated and divided.

The Dissection of the Bladder

The bladder peritoneum is incised using a monopolar knife and the bladder is dissected from the cervix. When the bladder is lifted ventrally enough, an avascular area between the bladder and the cervix can be visualized, and then the dissection of the bladder can easily be performed.

The Transection of the Uterine Artery and the Unroofing of the Ureter

The uterine artery has already been isolated at the pelvic lymphadenectomy step described above; therefore, the transection of the uterine artery is easily performed using a hemoclip. Lifting the end of the uterine artery medially, a branch to the bladder (middle vesical artery) is isolated. After transecting this branch, the uterine artery can be isolated from the ureter completely, and the ureter tunnel can be developed median of the ureter. The bladder pillar is dissected meticulously thus allowing a small vessel to be isolated (cervico-vesical vessels). After transecting these cervico-vesical vessels, the unroofing of the ureter is accomplished.

Steps 4–6 are identical to those of total laparoscopic radical hysterectomy (non nerve-sparing techniques); therefore please refer to the relevant chapter for further details.

The Transection of the Cardinal Ligament

At the pelvic lymphadenectomy step described above, the lymph node of the cardinal ligament is removed; therefore, the vessels and nerves around the cardinal ligament are already isolated at this point. In nerve-sparing procedure described here, only the deep uterine vein is clipped and transected at the pelvic sidewall, and the stump of the deep uterine vein is scraped up to the level of the hypogastric nerves (i.e., the upper end of pelvic nerve networks).

The Transection of the Posterior Layer of the Vesico-Uterine Ligament

This step is essential for the preservation of the vesical branches of the pelvic nerve networks. At the posterior layer of the vesico-uterine ligament, the vesical vessels, nerves, and

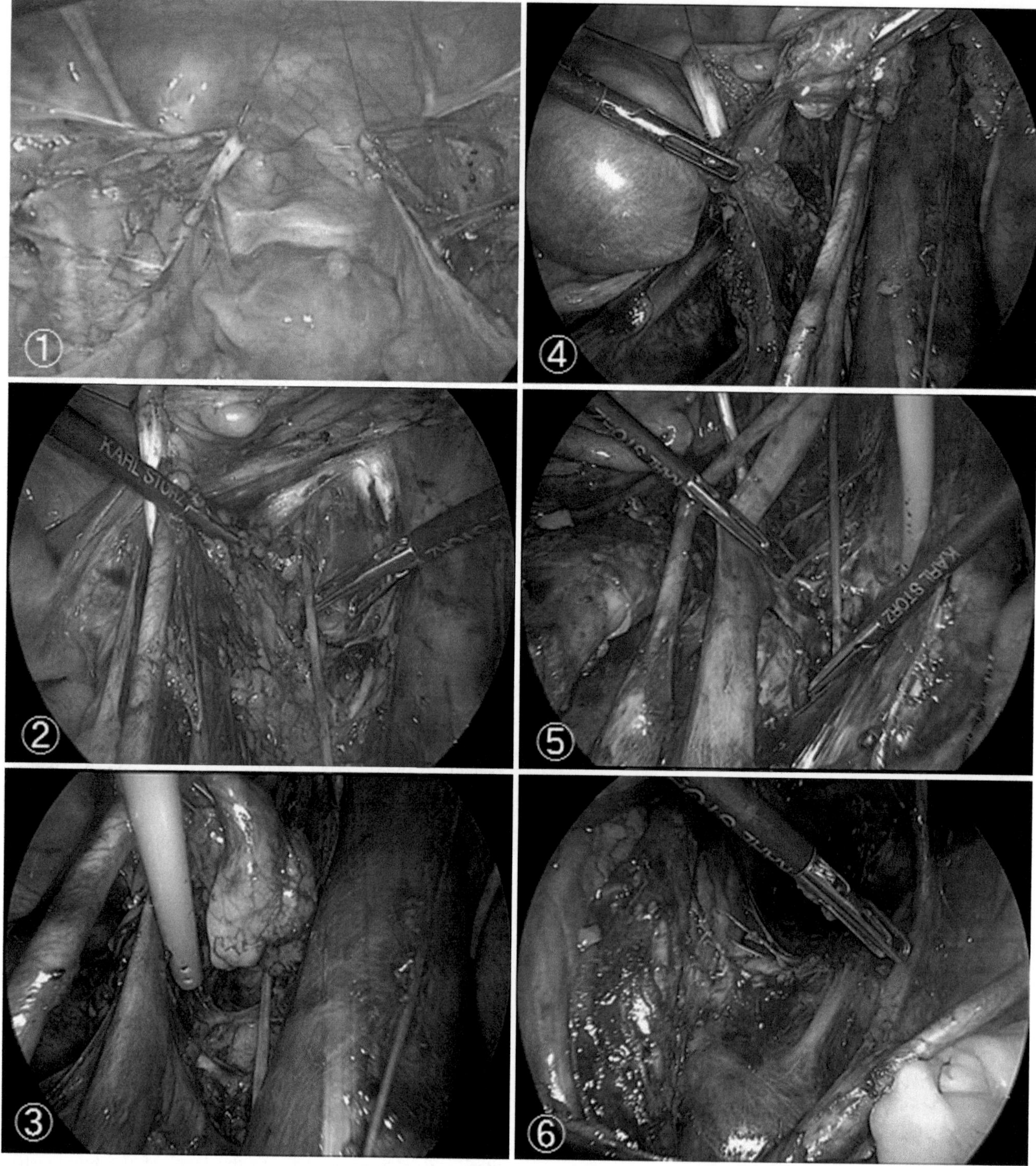

Fig. 41.3 Pelvic lymphadenectomy. (*1*) The umbilical ligament is suspended to the abdominal wall to maintain the good surgical view. (*2*) The space between the psoas muscle and the external iliac vessels is developed widely until the obturator nerve and vessels are exposed. (*3*) The upper end of the lymphofatty tissue(around the common iliac lesion) is clipped and transected. (*4*) Pelvic lymphnode is removed en block. (*5*, *6*) Final view of pelvic lymphadenectomy

adipose tissue are packed by a membrane, therefore a meticulous dissection or "demembranation" is required to expose the two or three vesical veins, which flow into the deep uterine vein; these veins are clipped and transected. The remnant after the transection of these vesical vessels at the posterior layer of the vesico-uterine ligament contains the vesical branches of the pelvic nerve networks. For complete preservation of the function of vesical branches, it is essential to

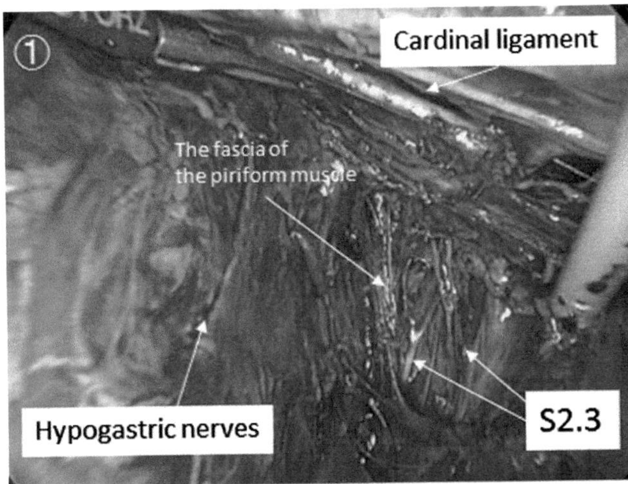

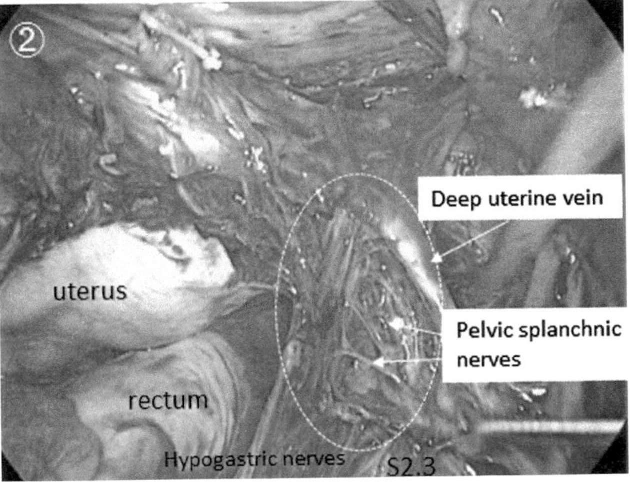

Fig. 41.4 Complete exposure of pelvic nerve networks. (*1*) The lymph node tissue around the internal iliac region is removed completely, then the S2–3 roots are identifiable beneath the fascia of the piriform muscle. (*2*) The complete structure of pelvic nerve plexus is marked by a dotted circle. They are consisted by hypogastric nerves and pelvic splanchnic nerves

prevent thermal injury; therefore, the vesical veins are transected using clips and scissors (Fig. 41.5 1–4).

Transection of the Paracolpium and Sacrouterine Ligament

The Douglas peritoneum is incised and the rectum is dissected until the posterior vaginal wall is exposed. Sometimes, the vaginal wall is opened at this stage because the vaginal cuff has already been created. After dissecting the rectum, the sacrouterine ligament can be exposed. To preserve the pelvic nerve networks, the uterosacral ligament and paracolpium tissue are transected just above the hypogastric nerves.

At this stage, the paracolpium tissue is sutured and ligated to reduce the usage of the energy device and to prevent thermal injury (Fig. 41.5a).

Transection of the Vagina

A vaginal pipe is inserted to extend the vaginal wall. The vaginal cuff has already been created at the first step of this surgery, thus after the transection of rectovaginal ligament, the vaginal wall can easily be transected.

Closure of the Vagina

The specimen is retrieved vaginally. To prevent the scattering of cancer cells, a plastic bag is used for the retrieval of the specimen (Fig. 41.6). The vaginal stump is closed using a 1-0 vicryl interrupted suture. The central part of the peritoneum is closed using a 2-0 vicryl suture, and the lateral part is opened to reduce the occurrence of lymphocyst following the surgery. The drainage tube is placed at the Douglas space.

Figure 41.7 shows the final view of the total laparoscopic nerve-sparing radical hysterectomy for stage Ib2 cervical cancer.

Discussion

Bladder function following conventional total laparoscopic nerve-sparing radical hysterectomy is quite good. However, the degree of radicality of this procedure is insufficient in some cases. Therefore, the applicability of this procedure is expected to be limited to early stage cervical carcinoma [12]. For intermediate-stage or advanced-stage cervical carcinoma, a more radical procedure is necessary. In such cases, nerve-sparing techniques have never been applied. However, in some intermediate-risk cervical carcinoma cases, non-nerve-sparing radical hysterectomy tends to result in overtreatment. We suggest that a different nerve-sparing technique be applied for these cases.

The pelvic nerve plexus appears as a mesh and consists mainly of hypogastric nerves and pelvic splanchnic nerves. The hypogastric nerves are located at the ventral edge and pelvic splanchnic nerves are located at the dorsal edge of the pelvic nerve plexus [13]. Therefore, the pelvic nerve plexus has a somewhat definable anatomical width. In this case, it is possible to apply a different nerve sparing technique, which would likely consist of a more radical procedure than conventional nerve-sparing radical hysterectomy.

To accomplish the innovative nerve sparing technique described here, the complete exposure of the pelvic nerve plexus is necessary. As explained above, the complete exposure of pelvic nerve networks is possible and enables to control the degree of radicality to the point where the uterosacral ligament and paracolpium tissue can be transected. Furthermore, laparoscopic radical hysterectomies can be

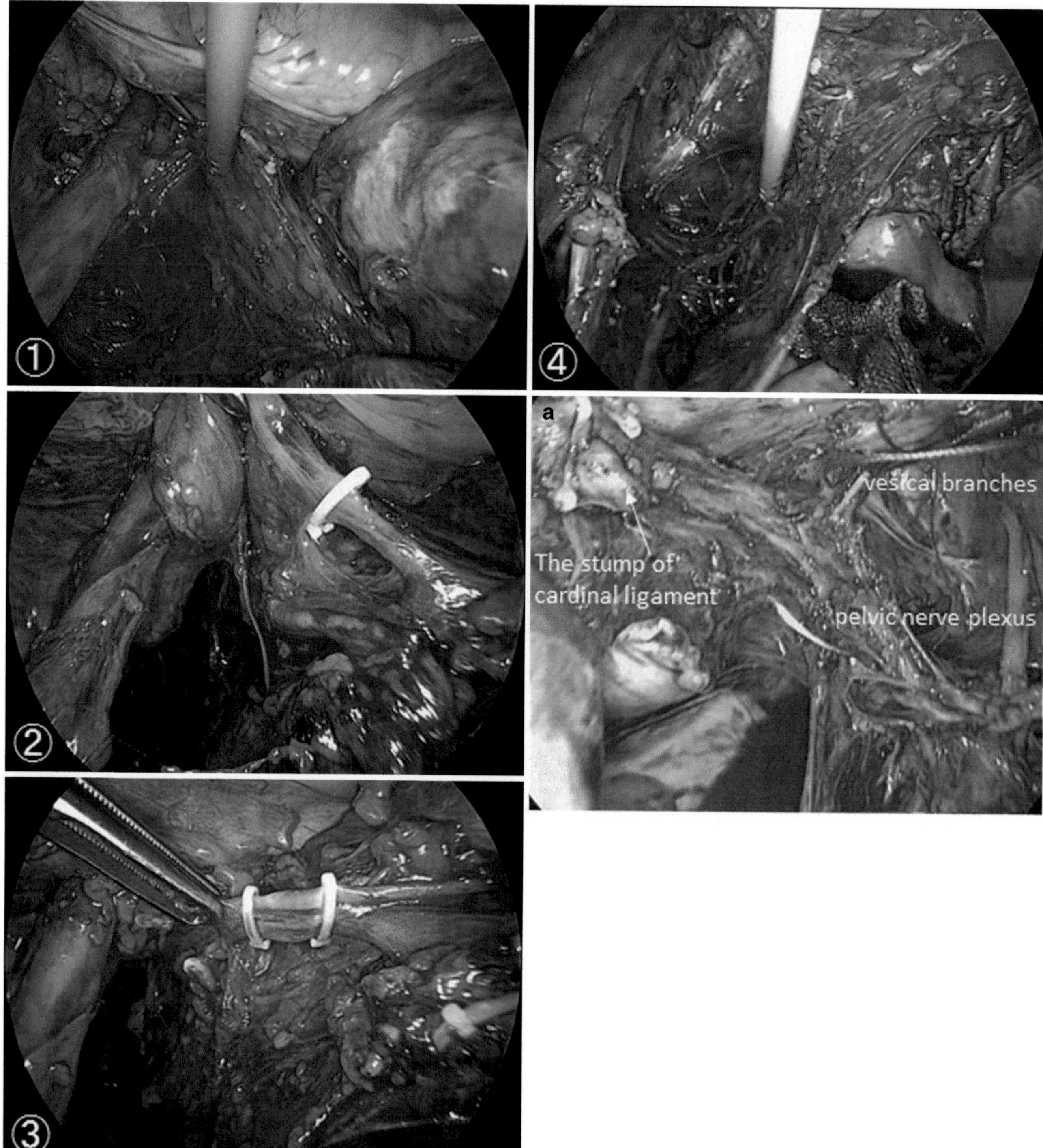

Fig. 41.5 Transection of posterior layer of vesico-uterine ligament and paracolpium tissue. ① The posterior layer of vesico-uterine ligament of left side. Veins, nerves and adipose tissue are packed by a membrane.②③ "Demembranation" expose two or three vesical veins. They are isolated and transected one by one.④ After transection of the posterior layer of vesico-uterine ligament, pelvic nerve networks are exposed. (**a**) To preserved the pelvic nerve networks, the uterosacral ligament and paracolpium tissue are transected just above the hypogastric nerves. At this stage, we suture and ligate the paracolpium tissue to reduce the usage of energy device and to prevent thermal injury

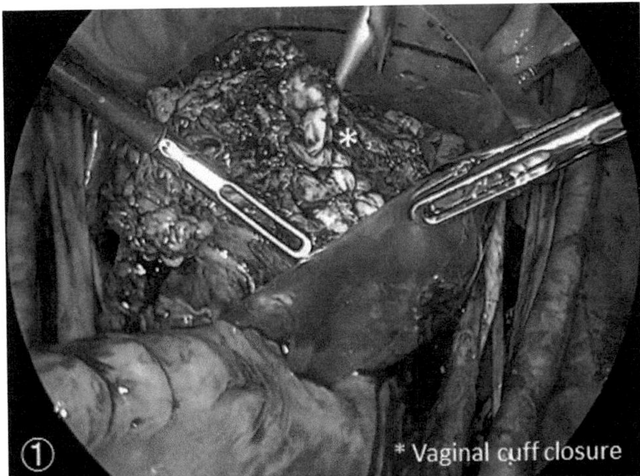

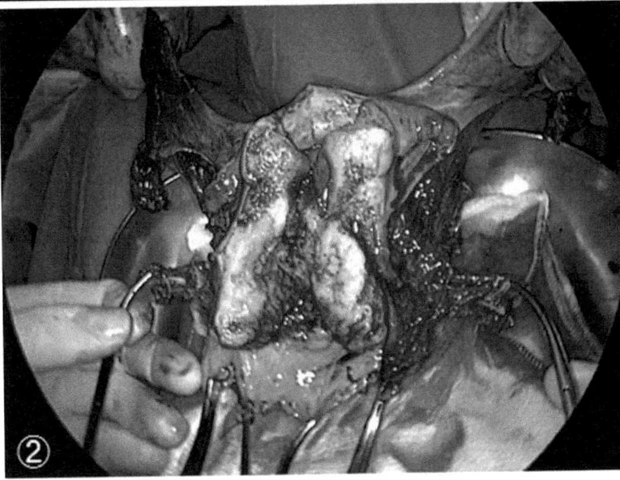

Fig. 41.6 The specimen of total laparoscopic nerve-sparing radical hysterectomy. ① To prevent the scattering of the cancer cells, a plastic bag is used for the retrieval of the specimen. ② This case is stage Ib2 cervical cancer, tumor size is 5 cm, and histological type is SCC. After the retrieval of the specimen, a vaginal cuff is opened to check the surgical margin

categorized into three types depending on the status of the preserved nerve network. The uterosacral ligament and the paracolpium tissue are transected above the hypogastric nerves for the conventional nerve-sparing procedure (group A), between the hypogastric nerves and pelvic splanchnic nerves for the radical nerve-sparing procedure (group B), or below the pelvic splanchnic nerves in the case of nerve-sacrificed radical hysterectomy (group C). We performed 27 cases belonging to group A, 13 cases to group B and 13 cases to group C (Fig. 41.8). Bladder function after these procedures was evaluated using urodynamic studies. Finally, we identified a correlation between the preserved pelvic nerve networks and bladder function after laparoscopic nerve-sparing radical hysterectomy.

Several studies have conducted urodynamic analyses after radical hysterectomy, but no consensus on these procedures has been reached, perhaps because around 80 % of patients with cervical carcinoma already had some degree of bladder dysfunction before the procedure was performed. It is therefore extremely difficult to evaluate the effects of nerve sparing techniques accurately [14]. In this study, we defined our original index (Function Ratio) to control for the scattering of data from urodynamic studies before surgical procedures. Urodynamic studies have many parameters, and among these parameters, the detrusor contraction pressure at maximum flow (PdetQmax) has been chosen to evaluate the motor function of the bladder, and the first desire to void (FDV) to evaluate sensory function, these are defined as:

Function Ratio (FDV) = FDV pre-operative / FDV post-operative.

Function Ratio (PdetQmax) = PdetQmax post-operative / PdetQmax pre-operative.

In fact, the PdetQmax is expected to be proportional to bladder function, and the FDV is expected to be inversely proportional to bladder function. Therefore, the function ratio formulas (FDV, PdetQmax) differ.

Ralph et al. reported that bladder function after radical hysterectomy could improve within 12 months after surgery [15]. Therefore, we analyzed data at 12 months after the operation to ascertain the correlation between the preserved pelvic nerve networks and bladder function after laparoscopic nerve-sparing radical hysterectomy (Fig. 41.9).

Based on the results of this study, it is possible to suggest that the distributions of sensory nerves and motor nerves differ. The sensory nerve is distributed predominantly at the lower (dorsal) half of the pelvic nerve networks. Thus, the sensory functions of group A and B are statistically equivalent, and the sensory function of group C is significantly lower than that of group A or B.

In contrast, the motor nerve is distributed predominantly at the upper (ventral) half of the pelvic nerve networks. Hence, the motor function of group A was significantly more preserved compared to that of either group B or C. The motor functions of groups B and C were damaged to same extent, and thus showed no mutually significant difference. Through this study, we conclude that various types of total laparoscopic nerve-sparing radical hysterectomy are technically feasible, and the sensory and motor functions of the bladder following the operation can be tailored depending on the patient's risk of cervical cancer.

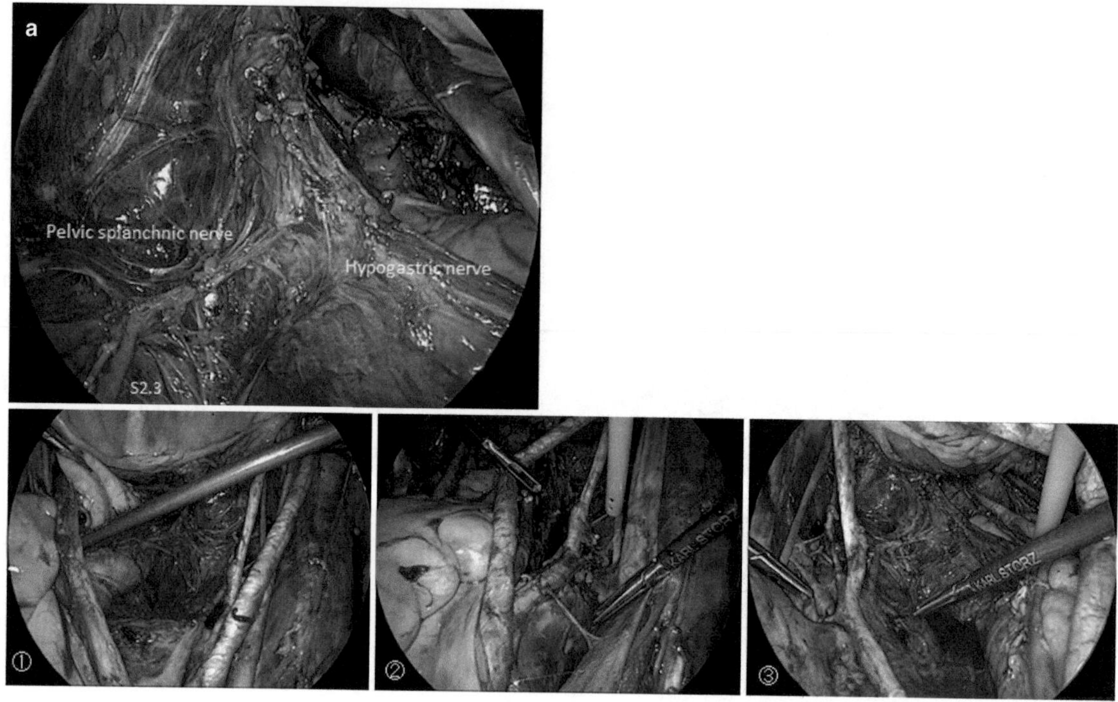

Fig. 41.7 The final view of total laparoscopic nerve-sparing radical hysterectomy for stage Ib2 cervical cancer. (**a**) The status of the preserved nerve networks of left side. ①,② right side ③ left side

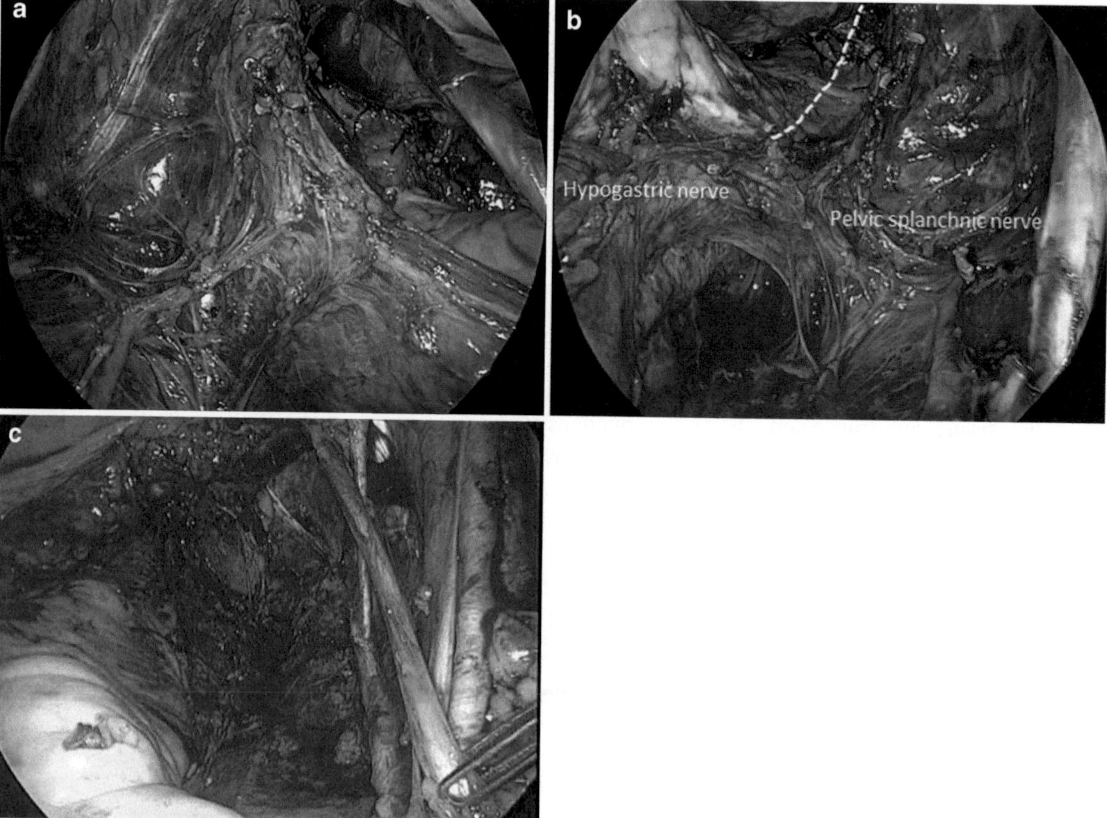

Fig. 41.8 The classification of total laparoscopic nerve-sparing radical hysterectomy. (**a**) Group A. (**b**) Group B (The *dotted line* shows the cutting line of Group A). (**c**) Group C. Patients with mixed pelvic nerve system sparing status (e.g., the right side is categorized into group A, and the left side is categorized into group C) were excluded from this study

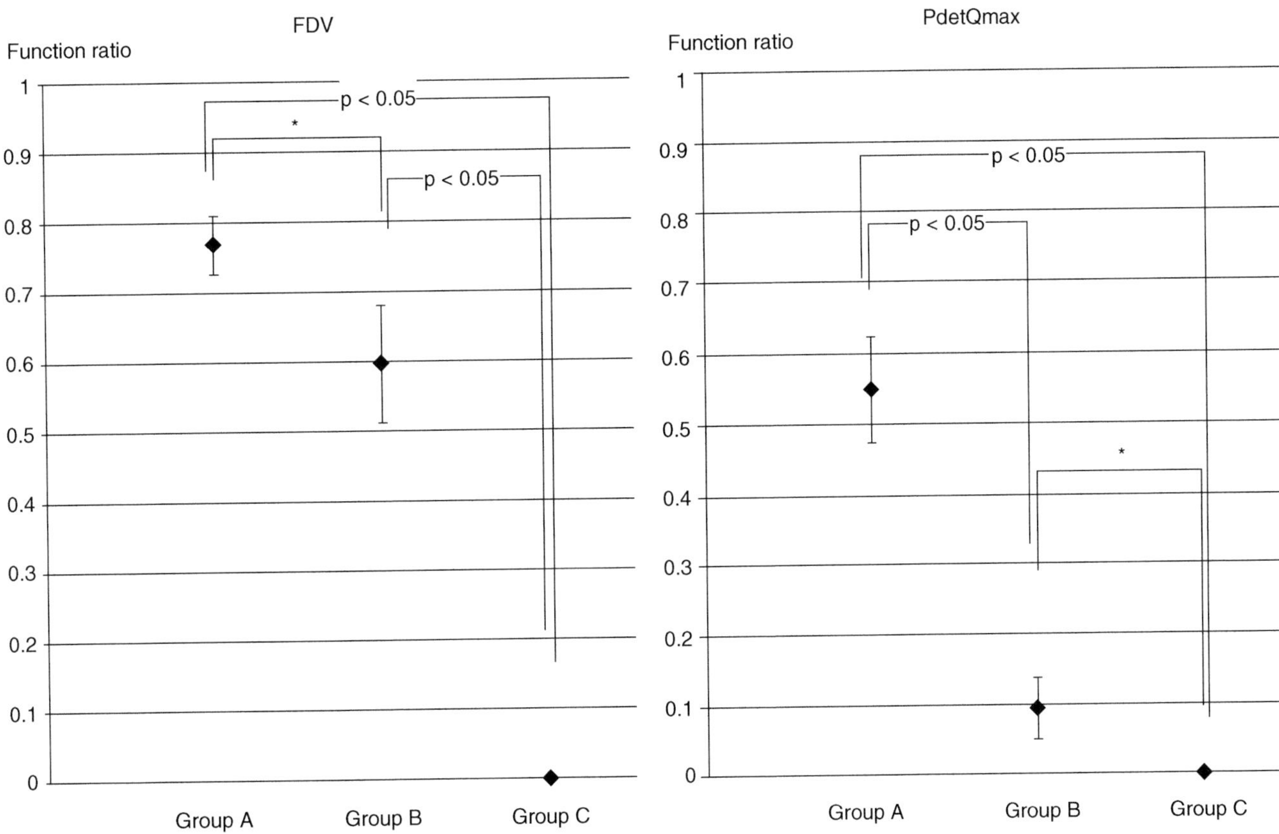

Fig. 41.9 The bladder function of each group at 12 month intervals after the operation

References

1. Malzoni M, Tinelli R, Cosentino F, Fusco A, Malzoni C. Total laparoscopic radical hysterectomy versus abdominal radical hysterectomy with lymphadenectomy in patients with early cervical cancer: our experience. Ann Surg Oncol. 2009;16(5):1316–23.
2. Li G, Yan X, Shang H, Wang G, Chen L, Han Y. A comparison of laparoscopic radical hysterectomy and pelvic lymphadenectomy and laparotomy in the treatment of Ib-IIa cervical cancer. Gynecol Oncol. 2007;105(1):176–80.
3. Taylor SE, McBee Jr WC, Richard SD, Edwards RP. Radical hysterectomy for early stage cervical cancer: laparoscopy versus laparotomy. JSLS. 2011;15(2):213–7.
4. Lee EJ, Kang H, Kim DH. A comparative study of laparoscopic radical hysterectomy with radical abdominal hysterectomy for early-stage cervical cancer: a long-term follow-up study. Eur J Obstet Gynecol Reprod Biol. 2011;156(1):83–6.
5. Sobiczewski P, Bidzinski M, Derlatka P, Panek G, Danska-Bidzinska A, Gmyrek L, et al. Early cervical cancer managed by laparoscopy and conventional surgery: comparison of treatment results. Int J Gynecol Cancer. 2009;19(8):1390–5.
6. Nam JH, Park JY, Kim DY, Kim JH, Kim YM, Kim YT. Laparoscopic versus open radical hysterectomy in early-stage cervical cancer: long-term survival outcomes in a matched cohort study. Ann Oncol. 2012;23(4):903–11.
7. Glahn BE. The neurogenic factor in vesical dysfunction following radical hysterectomy for carcinoma of the cervix. Scand J Urol Nephrol. 1970;4(2):107–16.
8. Seski JC, Diokno AC. Bladder dysfunction after radical abdominal hysterectomy. Am J Obstet Gynecol. 1977;128(6):643–51.
9. Fishman IJ, Shabsigh R, Kaplan AL. Lower urinary tract dysfunction after radical hysterectomy for carcinoma of cervix. Urology. 1986;28(6):462–8.
10. Kavallaris A, Hornemann A, Chalvatzas N, Luedders D, Diedrich K, Bohlmann MK. Laparoscopic nerve-sparing radical hysterectomy: description of the technique and patients' outcome. Gynecol Oncol. 2010;119(2):198–201.
11. Liang Z, Chen Y, Xu H, Li Y, Wang D. Laparoscopic nerve-sparing radical hysterectomy with fascia space dissection technique for cervical cancer: description of technique and outcomes. Gynecol Oncol. 2010;119(2):202–7.
12. Park NY, Chong GO, Hong DG, Cho YL, Park IS, Lee YS. Oncologic results and surgical morbidity of laparoscopic nerve-sparing radical hysterectomy in the treatment of FIGO stage IB cervical cancer: long-term follow-up. Int J Gynecol Cancer. 2011;21(2):355–62.
13. Yamaguchi K, Kobayashi M, Kato T, Akita K. Origins and distribution of nerves to the female urinary bladder: new anatomical findings in the sex differences. Clin Anat. 2011;24(7):880–5.
14. Lin HH, Yu HJ, Sheu BC, Huang SC. Importance of urodynamic study before radical hysterectomy for cervical cancer. Gynecol Oncol. 2001;81(2):270–2.
15. Ralph G, Tamussino K, Lichtenegger W. Urological complications after radical abdominal hysterectomy for cervical cancer. Baillieres Clin Obstet Gynaecol. 1988;2(4):943–52.

Modified Nerve-Sparing Radical-Like Hysterectomy for Deep Infiltrating Endometriosis

42

Stefano Uccella, Jvan Casarin, and Fabio Ghezzi

Introduction

Endometriosis is a common disease characterized by the presence of ectopic endometrial glands and stroma outside the uterine cavity. This heterotopic tissue has the same cyclic estrogen-dependent changes of the eutopic endometrium, according to the various phases of the menstrual cycle.

Endometriosis typically affects young women in their fertile age, being extremely uncommon before menarche and after menopause. The real incidence of this condition is a matter of debate and it is probably underestimated, due to the possible presence of asymptomatic, clinically silent lesions. A large population-based study has shown that this disease affects approximately 11 % of premenopausal women [1]. The average age at diagnosis ranges from 25 to 30 years [2], and it has been estimated that the incidence raises up to 50 % among infertile females [3].

The main symptoms and signs of endometriosis include chronic pelvic pain, dysmenorrhea, dyspareunia, and infertility. The disease can be potentially ubiquitous, but its preferential location is obviously the pelvis. Three different forms of disease have been historically described, according to the site and invasiveness of the implants: peritoneal disease, ovarian endometriomas and deep infiltrating endometriosis (DIE) [4].

In its deeply invasive form, endometriosis grows mainly in the retroperitoneum, and has the potential to infiltrate organs and structures, including the recto-vaginal septum, the lateral parametria (also known as cardinal ligaments or lateral paracervix), the utero-sacral ligaments, the rectosigmoid, the ureters and the bladder. The clinical presentation of DIE is usually characterized by severe chronic pelvic pain, neurologic pain, dyschezia, dysuria, and deep dyspareunia. These symptoms have obvious debilitating consequences on the health and quality of life of reproductive age women.

Complete surgical excision of infiltrative endometriotic lesions by laparoscopy is possible and offers good long-term symptomatic relief, especially in case of failure of pharmacological treatment [5–10].

However, it must be kept in mind that the common locations of DIE are in contiguity with several autonomic nervous structures that exert their control on the function of many pelvic organs. In particular, the pelvic sympathetic and parasympathetic neural pathways (which run through the pelvic ligaments) regulate rectal, bladder, and sexual physiologic activities. Eradication of DIE may therefore disrupt neural fibers, and consequently impair (sometimes definitively) the autonomic control of important vegetative functions.

Rationale for Nerve Sparing

The anatomic proximity of DIE and pelvic autonomic nerves is witnessed by preliminary data from a recent study [11], which show that patients affected by endometriosis involving the recto-vaginal septum and the utero-sacral ligaments have a very high (>90 %) probability of a pre-operative urodynamic diagnosis of detrusor overactivity, even in the absence of bladder symptoms. These results corroborate the observation that pelvic sympathetic and parasympathetic nerves may be encapsulated or at least involved by endometriotic lesions [12]. As a consequence, preservation of neural structures and vegetative functions appears difficult, and may not always be possible at the time of radical surgery for DIE.

However (when neural fibers are not already disrupted pre-operatively), a deep and thorough anatomical knowledge about the routes of the neurogenic control of the pelvis is crucial to try to preserve as much as possible the inervation of the bladder, the rectum and the vagina.

The nerve-sparing approach to hysterectomy for deep infiltrating endometriosis implies the identification and meticulous isolation of the nerves and neural fibers that run

S. Uccella (✉) • J. Casarin • F. Ghezzi
Obstetrics & Gynecology Department, University of Insubria, piazza Biroldi, 1, Varese 21100, Italy
e-mail: stefucc@libero.it; jvancasarin@gmail.com; Fabio.ghezzi@uninsubria.it

I. Alkatout, L. Mettler (eds.), *Hysterectomy*, DOI 10.1007/978-3-319-22497-8_42

in the pelvic ligaments, in order to separate them from the DIE lesions that must be removed [13].

Unfortunately, while the majority of the knowledge on nerve supply to the pelvis relies on anatomical studies on cadavers, the identification of nervous fibers is much more difficult in the operating room.

Autonomic Innervation of the Pelvis [14]

Orthosympathetic Nerves

The efferent orthosympathetic nervous fibers that reach the pelvis take their origin from the inferior thoracic and the superior lumbar (L1-L2) segments of the spine. These descendent branches are accompanied by afferent, ascendant fibers from the same innervated regions and organs.

The first structure contributing to the orthosympathetic innervation of the pelvis, is the inferior mesenteric plexus (IMP). This is a plexyphorm net of sympathetic fibers, covering the aorta from the origin of the inferior mesenteric artery until the promontorium of the sacral bone. At its inferior boundary, the IMP joins with the superior hypogastric plexus (SHP), which is a triangular-shaped net of sympathetic fibers lying in the presacral, retro-rectal space, just in front of the promontorium.

The inferior part of the SHP gives origin to the right and left hypogastric nerves (HN), which first descend laterally to the mesorectum, then they lie in the lateral part of the utero-sacral ligament, following the ureteral course in a dorsal and caudal position. The tissue below the ureter is named "meso-ureter" and should be preserved during dissection, since it contains not only the hypogastric nerves, but also the majority of the parasympathetic neural supply to the pelvis (Fig. 42.1).

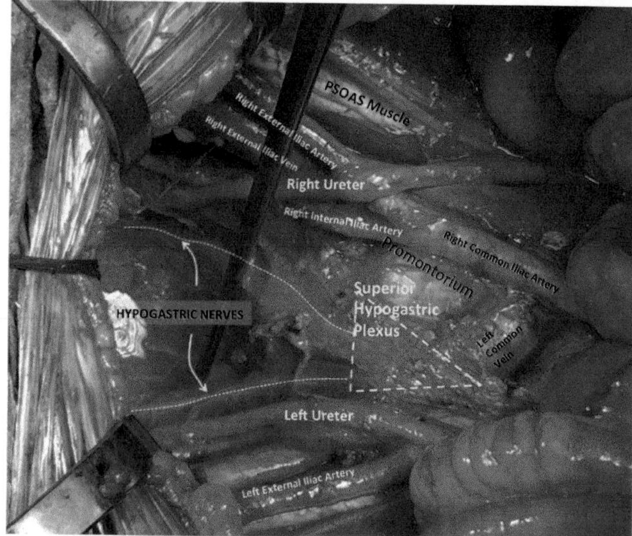

Fig. 42.1 The inferior mesenteric, the superior hypogastric plexus (with its triangular shape) and the two hypogastric nerves running to the pelvis bilaterally

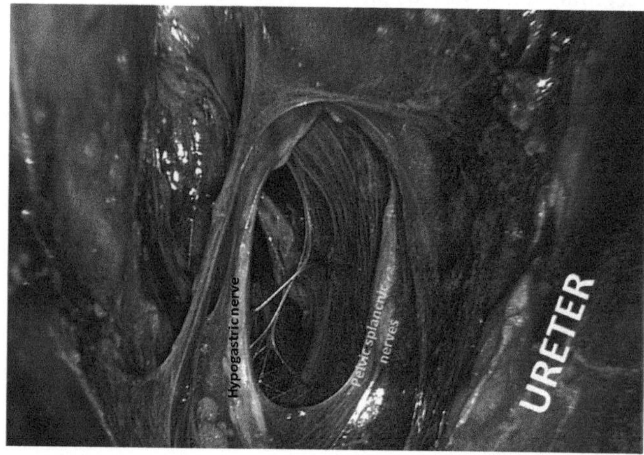

Fig. 42.2 The right inferior hypogastric plexus (also called "pelvic plexus") with its mixed (orthosympathetic and parasympathetic) fibers. The right ureter is lateralized, to expose the hypogastric nerve and the pelvic splancnic nerves, forming the plexus

Parasympathetic Nerves

The parasympathetic innervation of the pelvic viscera, the bladder and urethra, the rectosigmoid and anal canal and the vagina is supplied by the pelvic splancnic nerves (PSN). These tiny neural branches take origin from the anterior rami of the sacral roots between S2 and S4. Lateral to the mesorectum and approximately 3–4 cm laterally and 2–4 cm caudally from the pouch of Douglas, a variable number of parasympathetic PSNs (3–5) pierce the parietal endopelvic fascial sheet covering the ventral aspect of the piriformis muscle. After running in the posterior-lateral aspect of the uterosacral ligaments, below the level of the orthosympathetic routes, the PSNs join the HNs, forming the mixed (orthosympathetic and parasympathetic) inferior hypogastric plexus, also known as pelvic plexus (Fig. 42.2).

Pelvic Plexus, Rectal, Bladder and Vaginal Neural Branches

The pelvic plexus is a pyramid-shaped plexus which is bilaterally located between the posterolateral vaginal fornix and the rectum, ventrally and caudally to the lateral rectal ligaments. This neural network receives ortho- and parasympathetic fibers both descending from the spine and ascending from the pelvic organs. From this anatomical structure, several fine neural branches reach the pelvic organs, mainly following the ligaments and supporting structures of the organs innervated. In particular, neural fibers reach the uterus and the vagina through the parametria and paracolpia; anteriorly, ascending fibers deliver their neural supply to the bladder, running in the vesico-uterine ligaments (bladder branches); posteriorly, the innervation of the recto-sigmoid is delivered by fibers contained in the lateral rectal ligaments (also known as rectal wings).

The deep uterine vein is considered as the limit dividing the vascular part of the parametria (above its level), from their neural portion (below the deep uterine vein), where the pelvic plexus is located. To perform a nerve-sparing procedure that preserves the pelvic plexus, the deep uterine vein is to be identified, and resection should not exceed inferiorly this crucial anatomical landmark.

Pelvic Surgical Spaces for Radical Hysterectomy (Fig. 42.3)

In the pelvis, different anatomical spaces have been described. The knowledge of these regions is of paramount importance to obtain a safe and radical dissection of several oncological and non-oncological diseases in gynecology. In particular, we can recognize two median spaces (the Retzius space in front of the bladder and the presacral retrorectal space behind the rectum), and eight lateral spaces (the median and lateral paravesical and pararectal spaces) bilaterally, for a total of ten different and relatively avascular areas. To perform a radical hysterectomy, the paravesical and pararectal fossae have to be dissected. These virtual spaces must be carefully opened and developed by the surgeon, to make the anatomic landmarks clearer and also to allow a nerve-sparing procedure.

Paravesical Space

The boundaries of the paravesical space are the bladder and the upper part of the vagina, medially, and the obturator internus muscle, the obturator nerve, artery and vein (just beneath the bony arcuate ridge of the ileum), laterally.

This space is created by dissecting, both in dorsal and caudal direction, the loose connective tissue under the peritoneum, laterally to the bladder, until the levator ani muscle is reached. At this level, the external iliac vessels and the obturator nodes made up the lateral wall, while the bladder constitutes the medial landmark.

A useful tip to perform a safe and efficient dissection, is to identify the umbilical obliterated artery, and to develop the tissue laterally to it in a caudal direction. During the development of this space, surgeons have always to look for accessory obturator arteries and veins, which are often present in this area, in order not to damage them during dissection, in particular they have to pay attention to a anastomotic vein between the external iliac vein and the obturator vein, which in surgical jargon is called *corona mortis*.

The longitudinal course of the ureter is the reference for dividing the paravesical space in two different areas, the medial (also known as Yabuki's space) and the lateral paravesical fossa (Fig. 42.4).

Pararectal Space

The pararectal space is a potential space, lateral to the rectum. Dissection of this area usually starts with the development of the retroperitoneum medial to the internal iliac vessels. It is a triangular-shaped space, with an anterior base, represented by

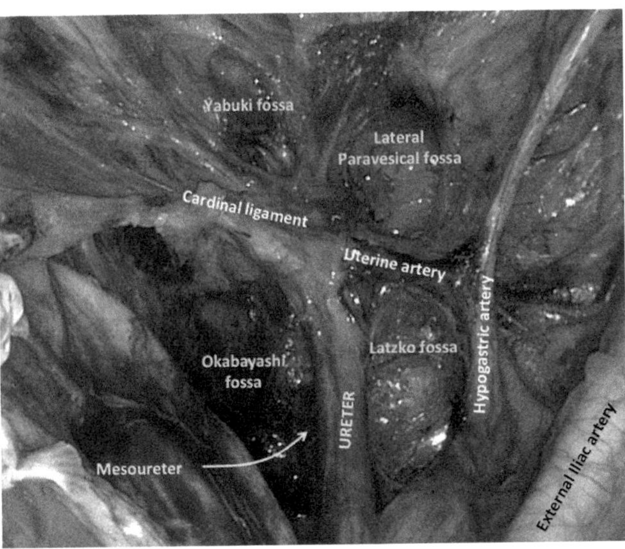

Fig. 42.3 The right paravesical and pararectal spaces, with the course of the ureter and mesoureter, the cardinal ligament and parametrium

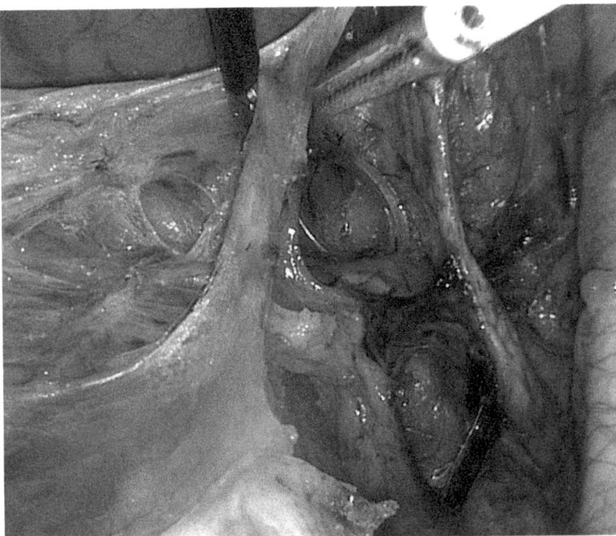

Fig. 42.4 The right lateral and medial paravesical spaces

the cardinal ligament; the medial border is represented by the vagina anteriorly, the peritoneum of the posterior sheet of the broad ligament superiorly, the utero-sacral ligament inferiorly and the rectum posteriorly; the lateral boundary corresponds to the internal iliac artery and vein with their collaterals. The ureter and the mesoureter divide the lateral aspect of the pararectal space (the so-called Latzko's fossa) from its medial aspect (Okabayashi's fossa) (Fig. 42.5).

The identification and development of the paravesical and pararectal spaces with their medial and lateral aspects is the first step to correctly identify the main anatomical structures in the pelvis and to perform a nerve-sparing radical hysterectomy, for both malignancies and endometriosis. Once the ureter with the mesoureter, the internal and external iliac vessels, the cardinal ligament with the uterine artery and veins and the utero-sacral ligament have been identified, the neural fibers of the hypogastric nerves, of the pelvic splancnic nerves and of the pelvic plexus can be localized and possibly spared, if not involved by the disease (Fig. 42.3).

Pre-operative Assessment

Preoperatively, all women should undergo a thorough gynecological examination, including complete medical and surgical history, bimanual visit, pelvic transvaginal and transabdominal ultrasound, to rule out the presence and exact location of the endometriotic lesions, and their relationships with the pelvic organs. In order to evaluate the extent of possible bowel, bladder and ureteral involvement and to better plan the correct surgical approach, pelvic and abdominal MRI with contrast medium may be useful. The administration of colon water distension during MRI is a possible adjunction that allows better visualization of the presence and depth of bowel wall infiltration. Ultrasound scan of the urinary tract may be useful, in order to recognize and quantify the possible presence of hydronephrosis, ureteral dilatation or bladder nodules. Anterograde pyleography is not performed on a routine basis at our department.

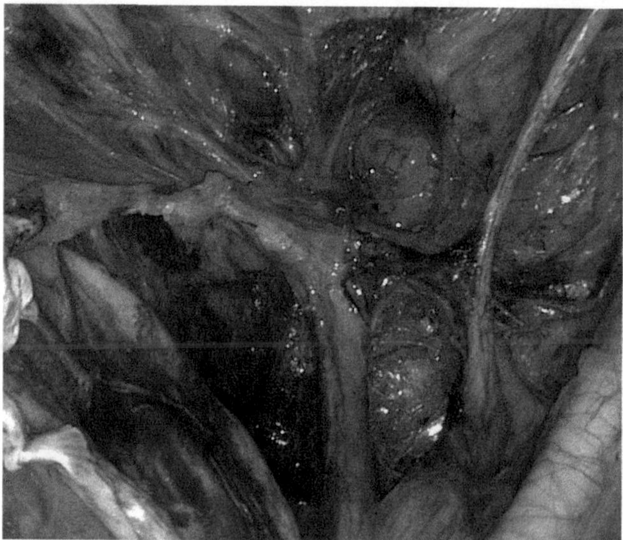

Fig. 42.5 The right lateral and medial pararectal spaces

Women receive one dose of prophylactic antibiotic 1 h before the intervention; antithrombotic prophylaxis is administered with low–molecular-weight heparin (7 days) and compression stockings (until full mobilization). Bowel preparation is not administered on a routine basis, unless bowel resection is planned.

Due to the intrinsic risks of this type of procedures, consisting in difficult recognition and isolation of the anatomical structures, and in the presence of dense adhesions and firm fibrotic nodules that complicate dissection of the surgical planes, pre-operative work-out should include the recognition of the most difficult cases of severe deep infiltrating endometriosis, in order to organize a surgical team of operators with extensive experience in both laparoscopic and open gynecological and intestinal procedures.

Instruments

The list of instruments for laparoscopic modified nerve-sparing radical-like hysterectomy in case of deep endometriosis should include:

- a uterine manipulator (we preferentially use a Rumi uterine manipulator used in conjunction with a Koh cup colpotomizer, [Koh Colpotomizer System; Cooper Surgical, Trimbull, CT]) to allow a safe dissection of the vesico-uterine fold, the delineation of the vaginal fornices and the lateralization of the ureters, obtained by cranial pressure on the instrument.
- Four 5-mm trocars, inserted one through the umbilicus and three suprapubically.
- A 0-degrees laparoscope.
- Scissors.
- Traumatic (Manes forceps) and atraumatic (Matkovic) graspers.
- Bipolar forceps.
- Monopolar hook or spatula.
- A suction-irrigation-system.

The entire procedure may be accomplished with reusable instruments. Only in very particular cases, a disposable combined coagulating/cutting device may be useful.

Surgical Technique

The patient must lie supine in lithotomic position. General endotracheal anesthesia is performed, and during the procedure, Trendelenburg position is maintained, to allow cranial displacement of the bowel loops and optimal exposure of the pelvic organs. The uterine manipulator is positioned vaginally. A Veress needle is inserted in the abdominal cavity and CO_2 is insufflated. After creation of the pneumoperitoneum (10–15 mmHg pressure), a 5-mm trocar is inserted transumbilically for the laparoscope. Under direct visualization, three 5-mm ancillary trocars are positioned suprapubically: one at the level of the midline and two laterally to the epigastric arteries in the left and right lower abdominal quadrants, respectively. The entire abdominal cavity is then inspected.

The third operator, sitting between the legs of the patient, helps the first operator by mobilizing the uterus with the uterine manipulator.

In cases of severe deep infiltrating endometriosis, the pelvis is almost invariably "frozen" by dense adhesions. As a consequence, the procedure starts with meticulous adhesiolysis and adnexal surgery (cystectomy, stripping of endometriomas), if needed. One of the most important rules while performing surgery for DIE is to try to work in healthy tissue, surrounding the disease.

Development of the anatomical spaces is started coagulating and sectioning the round ligament, while the assistant grasps it and pulls it medially to obtain adequate countertraction and exposure. The anterior leaf of the broad ligament is coagulated with bipolar forceps and sectioned, starting from the round ligament up to the vesicouterine fold.

The retroperitoneum is then entered as follows: an incision is made on the peritoneum lateral and parallel to the infundibulopelvic ligamnents and the ureter is identified lateral to the ovarian vessels, when it crosses the iliac bifurcation and enters the pelvis at the level of the pelvic brim.

The lateral pararectal space is dissected medial to the internal iliac artery, and the uterine vessels are identified at their origin from the hypogastric artery and vein. The Okabayashi fossa is then developed by opening the virtual space between the ureter (laterally) and the peritoneum (medially), the cardinal ligament and uterine artery (anteriorly) and the rectum (posteriorly). While moving caudally in the dissection, the medial, fibrous part of the utero-sacral ligament should be separated by its lateral aspect, which contains the neural fibers of the hypogastric nerves and pelvic splancnic nerves. Once the Okabayashi and Latzko fossae have been prepared, the ureter is isolated and the mesoureter is identified and preserved, in order to spare the nervous fibers (hypogastric nerve, pelvic splancnic nerves and pelvic plexus) running in it (Fig. 42.6). If ureteral endometriosis is present, ureterolysis should be accomplished, with the intent of shaving and preserving the ureter whenever possible [5, 7]. Particular attention should be paid during isolation of the ureter to avoid damage to its peri-adventitial vessels, that provide blood supply to this organ, in order to prevent ischemic necrosis and consequent fistulas.

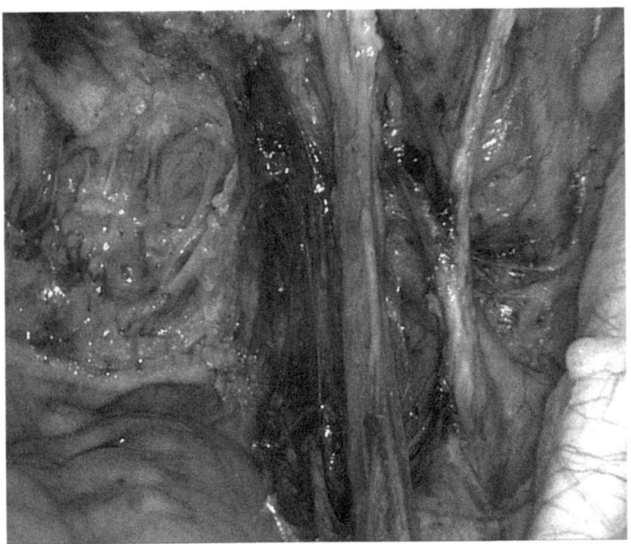

Fig. 42.6 The right ureter and the mesoureter isolated during a modified radical-like hysterectomy for deep endometriosis (the nervous fibers of the hypogastric nerves, pelvic splancnic nerves and pelvic plexus have been identified and spared)

The vesico-vaginal space is dissected and the space of Yabuki is developed only in case of vesical nodules or when the upper part of the anterior vaginal wall has to be removed.

In case of adnexectomy, coagulation and section of the infundibulopelvic ligament is accomplished. If the ovaries have to be preserved, coagulation and section is performed at the level of the tube and utero-ovarian ligament. The posterior leaf of the broad ligament is then opened, down to the level of the uterosacral ligaments.

When the cardinal ligament is involved, partial or total sacrifice of the uterine artery and/or some branches of the internal iliac artery may be necessary before its resection. Resection of the involved cardinal ligament is performed at this time, tailoring the radicality on the basis of the extension of the disease and the anatomical conditions of the patient.

If possible, isolation and preservation of the uterine vessels at the intersection with the ureter is performed. The dissection must never be extended below the level of the deep uterine vein (the border between the vascular portion and the neural portion of the parametrium), in order to spare the hypogastric nerves and the pelvic plexus, unless massive infiltration by the endometriotic process is present below this level.

When a rectovaginal nodule is present, the virtual space between the rectum and the vagina must be opened, starting from the medial pararectal spaces. The decision as to whether bowel resection is necessary, has to be taken on the basis of the percentage of infiltration of the recto-sigmoid wall by the endometriotic lesion. In case of bowel preservation, rectal shaving is accomplished and the nodule is mobilized from the anterior surface of the rectum, leaving it attached to the posterior vaginal wall.

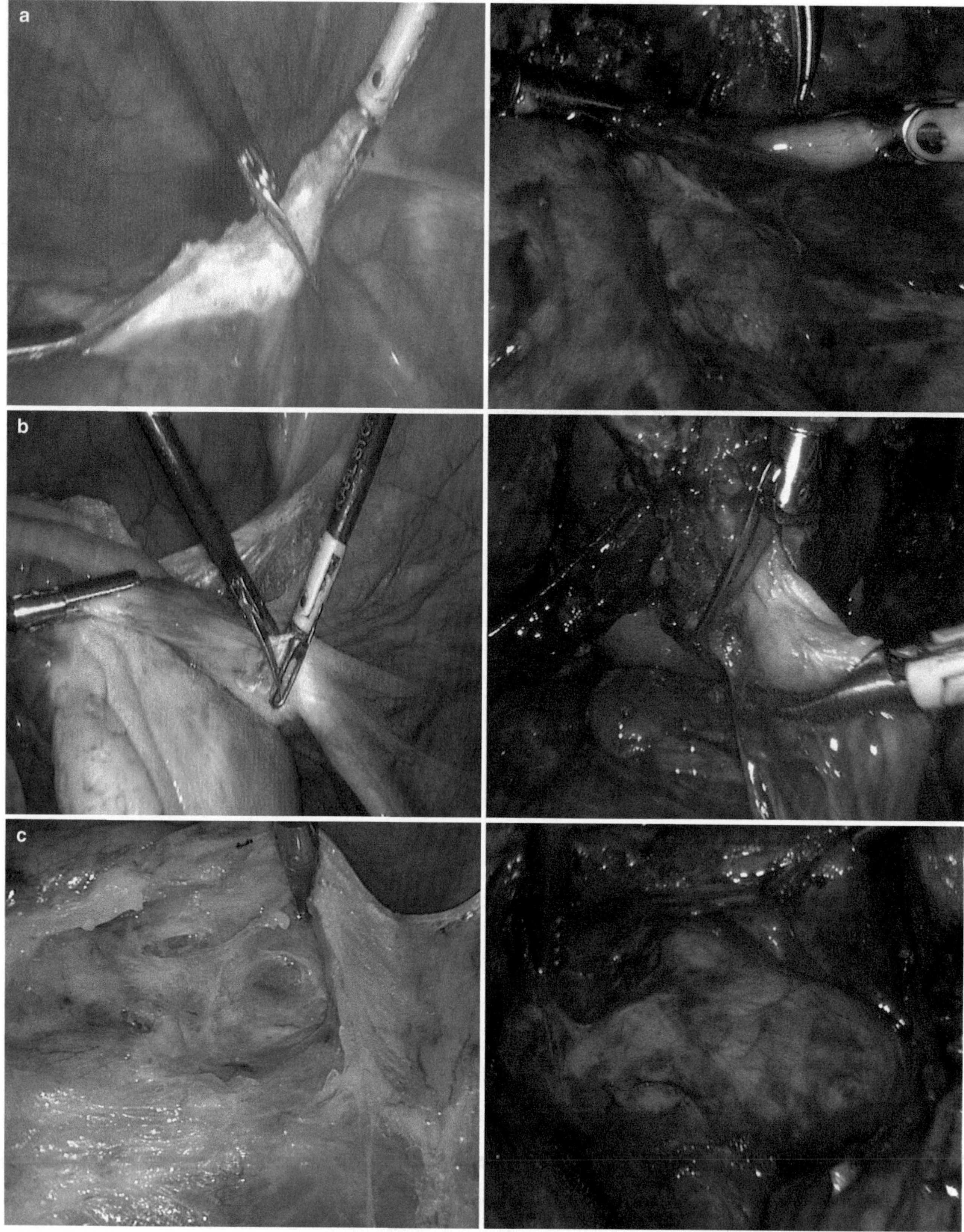

Fig. 42.7 (**a**) Coagulation and section of the round ligament; (**b**) Coagulation and section of the infundibulo-pelvic ligament; (**c**) Development of the vesical flap. Comparison between women without (*left*) and with (*right*) endometriosis. The recognition and dissection of the anatomical structures is more difficult in case of DIE

All the steps described are performed in the same way on both sides.

Once the uterus has been completely detached from its supporting structures, and complete dissection and isolation of the endometriotic process has been accomplished, colpotomy is performed using a monopolar spatula or hook. A colpo-pneumo-occluder inserted through the vagina before the procedure, is useful to prevent loss of pneumoperitoneum during this step of the procedure. Supplementary hemostasis of the vaginal vault with a bipolar forceps could be needed in cases of bleeding during colpotomy.

The extraction is usually performed *en-bloc* through the vagina; in some cases, transvaginal morcellation with cold knife could be necessary.

Once the specimen is extracted, the vaginal vault can be closed by continuous suture either transvaginally or endoscopically [15].

Before trocar extraction, an additional control of the hemostasis should be performed.

Figure 42.7 describes some of the steps of radical hysterectomy, highlighting the differences and the difficulties in the correct recognition of the anatomical structures in patients with vs. without endometriosis.

Post-operative Course

Although the common perception of the operators involved in this type of surgery is that hysterectomy for deep infiltrating endometriosis is associated with a higher likelihood of complications, compared to simple hysterectomy for benign gynecological conditions, the literature is devoid of clear information regarding this specific issue.

Normal post-operative management should include monitoring of the most common post-operative complications. A brief list of specific adverse events possibly related to modified-radical hysterectomy for deep endometriosis include: bladder and ureteral lesions/fistula (usually occurring 7–21 days after surgery), bowel perforation, and urinary, sexual or anal dysfunction, due to failure of nerve-sparing and denervation of the organs involved.

Summary of Key Steps for Modified Nerve-Sparing Approach to Radical Hysterectomy for Deep Infiltrating Endometriosis

- Opening of the retroperitoneum and development of the pararectal and paravesical spaces.
- Isolation of the ureter with preservation of the meso-ureter (in order to spare the hypogastric nerves, the pelvic splancnic nerves and the pelvic plexus).
- Separation of the lateral aspect of the utero-sacral ligament (containing the nervous fibers running to and from the pelvis), from its medial fibrous part, which may be transected, according to the extension of the endometriotic lesion.
- Avoid transection of the cardinal ligament below the level of the deep uterine vein (if possible), in order to preserve the mixed orthosympathetic and parasympathetic pelvic plexus.
- Try to work in healthy tissue surrounding the disease.

References

1. Buck Louis GM, Hediger ML, Peterson CM, Croughan M, Sundaram R, Stanford J, et al. Incidence of endometriosis by study population and diagnostic method: the ENDO study. Fertil Steril. 2011;96:360–5.
2. Giudice LC, Kao LC. Endometriosis. Lancet. 2004;364(9447):1789–99.
3. Dunselman GA, Vermeulen N, Becker C, Calhaz-Jorge C, D'Hooghe T, De Bie B, European Society of Human Reproduction and Embryology, et al. ESHRE guideline: management of women with endometriosis. Hum Reprod. 2014;29:400–12.
4. Nisolle M, Donnez J. Peritoneal endometriosis, ovarian endometriosis, and adenomyotic nodules of the rectovaginal septum are three different entities. Fertil Steril. 1997;68:585–96.
5. Uccella S, Cromi A, Casarin J, Bogani G, Pinelli C, Serati M, Ghezzi F. Laparoscopy for ureteral endometriosis: surgical details, long-term follow-up, and fertility outcomes. Fertil Steril. 2014;102:160–6. e2
6. Ghezzi F, Cromi A, Ciravolo G, Rampinelli F, Braga M, Boni L. A new laparoscopic-transvaginal technique for rectosigmoid resection in patients with endometriosis. Fertil Steril. 2008;90:1964–8.
7. Ghezzi F, Cromi A, Bergamini V, Bolis P. Management of ureteral endometriosis: areas of controversy. Curr Opin Obstet Gynecol. 2007;19:319–24.
8. Redwine DB, Sharpe DR. Laparoscopic segmental resection of the sigmoid colon. J Laparoendosc Surg. 1991;1:217–20.
9. Redwine DB, Wright JT. Laparoscopic treatment of complete obliteration of the cul-de-sac associated with endometriosis: long-term follow-up of en bloc resection. Fertil Steril. 2001;76:358–65.
10. Landi S, Ceccaroni M, Perutelli A, Allodi C, Barbieri F, Fiaccavento A, Ruffo G, McVeigh E, Zanolla L, Minelli L. Laparoscopic nerve-sparing complete excision of deep endometriosis: is it feasible? Hum Reprod. 2006;21:774–81.
11. Serati M, Cattoni E, Braga A, Uccella S, Cromi A, Ghezzi F. Deep endometriosis and bladder and detrusor functions in women without urinary symptoms: a pilot study through an unexplored world. Fertil Steril. 2013;100:1332–6.
12. Anaf V, Simon P, El Nakadi I, Fayt I, Buxant F, Simonart T, et al. Relationship between endometriotic foci and nerves in rectovaginal endometriotic nodules. Hum Reprod. 2000;15:1744–50.
13. Ceccaroni M, Clarizia R, Bruni F, D'Urso E, Gagliardi ML, Roviglione G, Minelli L, Ruffo G. Nerve-sparing laparoscopic

eradication of deep endometriosis with segmental rectal and parametrial resection: the Negrar method. A single-center, prospective, clinical trial. Surg Endosc. 2012;26:2029–45.
14. Ceccaroni M, Fanfani F, Ercoli A, Scambia G. Innervazione viscerale e somatica della pelvi femminile. Testo-Atlante di Anatomia Chirurgica. Roma: CIC Ed. Internazionali; 2006.
15. Uccella S, Ceccaroni M, Cromi A, Malzoni M, Berretta R, De Iaco P, Roviglione G, Bogani G, Minelli L, Ghezzi F. Vaginal cuff dehiscence in a series of 12,398 hysterectomies: effect of different types of colpotomy and vaginal closure. Obstet Gynecol. 2012; 120:516–23.

43 Laparoscopic Total Mesometrial Resection (L-TMMR)

Vito Chiantera, Alessandro Lucidi, and Giuseppe Vizzielli

Oncological Philosophy

Abdominal radical hysterectomy and pelvic lymph node dissection as introduced by Wertheim and Meigs [1–2] first in the beginning of the century is still regarded as "gold standard" in the surgical treatment of the uterine cervix carcinoma, FIGO stages IA2-IB and IIA. The resection of the parametrial and paracervical tissues proposed by the.

conventional radical hysterectomy is based on a "centrifugal diffusion" from the center of the tumor on the direction of the parametrial (dorsal, lateral and ventral) highways.

This imply a classic functional and ligament-focused view of the surgical anatomy.

Local spread of an invasive tumor is currently regarded as an isotropic process of tissue infiltration, irrespective of anatomic boundaries. Malignant solid tumors are thought to permeate locally by invasion of the interstitium or intravasion of lymphatic and venous channels and perineural spread. The conventional oncological surgical practice derived from these concept is a "wide tumor excision" as removal of the malignant tumor with a metrically defined radial margin of macroscopically and microscopically tumor-free tissue. However, despite histopathology confirmed resection within clear margins (R0), local recurrence rate (LRR) in cervical cancer patients still occurs in 10–25 % of the patients [3].

As consequence the clinical results obtained are favorable for small tumor, vascular space negative and free pelvic nodes remaining the necessity of adding adjuvant chemoradiation therapy in patients with histopathology high-risk features.

Those high and intermediate risk patients requiring adjuvant treatment may exceed 50 % in current series with moderate and severe treatment-related morbidity reported for a big percentage of them [4].

V. Chiantera (✉) • A. Lucidi • G. Vizzielli
Department of Oncologic Surgery, Gynecologic Oncology Unit, Campobasso 00168, Italy
e-mail: vito.chiantera@gmail.com; lucidi.alex@gmail.com; giuseppevizzielli@yahoo.it

Hockel theory is based on the concept that local tumor spreads not completely random but follows for a long period of the malignant progression into a permissive compartment morphologically deduced from the embryologic development of the affected organ. Although tumor propagation increase within that compartment during the malignant progression the neoplasm respects the compartment borders for a long period of progression. Only very late adjacent compartments deriving from different embryological origins are invaded and even in these late stages a hierarchy of embryological kinship is maintained.

The logic consequence of this developmental view is a *"Compartment Resection"* as a new principle of radical surgery for local tumor control aiming to a high local tumor control rate without additional post operative radiation.

Höckel et al. first investigated embryonic development of the female reproductive tract with respect to embryological different compartments [5–8] and were able to define three different primordial tissue complexes from cranial to caudal:

- The paramesonephric–mesonephric–Müllerian tubercle complex
- The deep urogenital sinus (UGS) vaginal plate complex
- The superficial UGS-genital folds and tubercle

The pelvic viscera-parietal compartments deduced from the embryonic development define the following pelvic parietal lymph-node basins:

- External iliac
- Paravisceral (i.e.: anterior internal iliac, supraobturator and infraobturator, presciatic)
- Common iliac (including the superior gluteal)
- Presacral (i.e.: posterior internal iliac, aortic, and caval bifurcation)

The high rate of local tumor control following Total Mesometrial Resection (TMMR) without any subsequent

I. Alkatout, L. Mettler (eds.), *Hysterectomy*, DOI 10.1007/978-3-319-22497-8_43

adjuvant radiotherapy in patients with early cervical cancer is impressive [9, 10]. Part of this outcome is achieved with a ultra radical pelvic lymphadenectomy (tLNE), called *"therapeutic lymphadenectomy"*, this differs from the classic staging pelvic LNE where the nodes are removed with the idea to obtain a precise hysto-patological information in order to individualize the adjuvant treatment.

In this version of the pelvic lymphadenectomy the aim of the procedure is to remove every macro or micro metastasis in order to "sterilize" the lateral pelvic surgical field and avoid any necessity of adjuvant treatment. To obtain this a ultra-radical dissection is performed with removing of the external iliac, the superficial obturator and the deep obturator nodes as well as the deep gluteal, pre ischiatic (at the level of the ischial spine), pre sacral (ventrally to the lateral sacral fascia), and internal iliac nodes [10].

Following this theory, the proposed uterovaginal (Müllerian) compartment, identified by bottom-up sectional anatomy as the final differentiation product of the Müllerian structures, as described in previous published data by Höckel et al. [8] are:

(a) The cranial part of the compartment located intraperitoneal that consists of the Fallopian tubes, the mesosalpinx, the uterine corpus with the broad ligament where the latter corresponds to the peritoneal mesometrium
(b) The sub-peritoneal part of the Müllerian compartment (i.e.: the subperitoneal mesometrium) tapers off with bilateral wings made up of dorso-laterally directed supply tissue with the uterine vaginal arteries and veins, lymphatic drainage, and a few lymph nodes (referred to as vascular mesometrium), and dorsally directed suspensory and fatty tissue fused to the anterior and lateral mesorectum continuous with the endopelvic fascia overlying the coccygeus muscles (referred to as ligamentous mesometrium).

Due to the systematic and complete resection of those compartments Hockel achieved impressive results: with a median follow-up of 41 months only three pelvic, two pelvic/distant and five distant recurrences were recorded. A recurrence-free survival of 94 % (95 % CI 91–98) and overall survival of 96 % (93–99) was noticed.

Even more, with the absence of any adjuvant radiation therapy applied to those patients a very low treatment-related morbidity as much as 9 % was reported.

Although it has been questioned whether the confirmation of these findings could change the classification of radical hysterectomy and the indication for adjuvant radiotherapy in early stage cervical cancer [11], various authors have recently described the TMMR as an attractive therapeutic option for the management of this subset of patients [12–15].

The TMMR as a open surgical technique is perfectly standardized and systematic described, Kimmig et al. showed that the principle of compartment based surgery combined with therapeutic lymphadenectomy (tLNE) as described by M. Höckel can systematically be translated to minimally invasive robotic procedures (rTMMR and rtLNE). The method appeared to be feasible and safe. Although the mean follow-up time (18 months) was limited, the number of patients was small and there was some "lack of homogeneity" in the patients' sample composition (six patients at FIGO stage IA and three patients who had prior radiotherapy), it should be noticed that there were no loco-regional tumor recurrence during the observation period.

We have recently reported in a large prospective multicentric experience that compartment based surgery performed as Total Mesometrial Resection combined with therapeutic lymphadenectomy can systematically be translated to laparoscopic procedure (L-TMMR) [16]. Combining the information gained in this two minimal invasive study and despite the limited number of patients or the short follow-up, it should be noticed that altogether only two (2.8 %) early loco-regional tumor recurrences were observed, thus suggesting that LTMMR and R-TMMR techniques may be safe with respect to local tumor control and should be considered at least equivalent to open surgery in term of radicalness.

More in depth, regarding to specific endoscopic surgical procedures, it should be underlined that, exposure of the tumor into the surgical field must strictly be avoided in order to diminishing the risks for a vaginal cuff recurrence and intraperitoneal tumor dissemination.

Regarding the operating time of L-TMMR, it should be noted that it was longer than other series of radical hysterectomy previously published according to the Querleu–Morrow classification [17].

Moreover, especially two steps of the TMMR are particularly demanding if performed laparoscopically: the natural complex eradication of some lymph node stations by laparoscopy (i.e. in the lumbosacral fossa) and the difficulty to obtain the right traction simultaneously both on the uterus, the rectum and the mesometrium in order to complete the dorsal part of the operation. Thus the difference with open surgery in exposing the posterior compartment cannot be neglected. On the other hand, the shorter operating time compared with the historical series by Höckel [5–8] performed by open technique, supports the idea that laparoscopic procedures are time-sparing compared to open technique, especially if performed by a surgical team with a deep experience in the endoscopic approach. Moreover, the two severe postoperative complications reported in the urinary tract and the sole vascular compartment damage are in line with an initial experience on this endoscopic surgical procedure and suggest next future improvements with the increasing of the specific surgical experience. In addition, the low grade post-operative autonomic urinary complications (9.8 %) reported could be justified considering that the L-TMMR technique spares the pelvic nerves that supply the bladder both in the sympathetic and parasympathetic system.

Finally, laparoscopical as well as robotic approach, allowing to finely prepare and completely remove compartment-associated tissue without injuring adjacent structures by respecting the filmy septa at the compartment borders, enables to develop and dissect structures with higher "optical" accuracy than open technique. In our previous experience, laparoscopic elective dissection of the bladder and rectal splanchnic pelvic nerves and consequently, development of a parasympathetic nerve-sparing technique were technically feasible [18]. We believe that this L-TMMR technique is not inferior in terms of *"nerve sparing"* than the previous described laparoscopic approach.

Moreover, compared with the conventional open technique in the L-TMMR patients a notable reduction in global postoperative functional morbidity was demonstrated.

As next step we have compared, with a double-institution case-control study, peri-operative outcomes of R-TMMR and L-TMMR in early stage cervical cancer patients [19]. The few differences registered in this study did not seem clinically relevant, thus making the two procedures comparable, in terms of operative time, estimated blood loss and conversion or complication's rate.

Surgical Procedure

The objective of this chapter is to describe step-by-step the L-TMMR, a modified surgical technique according to the compartment theory based on ontogenetic anatomy proposed by Hockel. The laparoscopic procedure is performed in the modified dorsolithotomy position under endotracheal general anesthesia. A Veress needle is inserted through the umbilicus and the abdomen is insufflated. After pneumoperitoneum and insertion of the laparoscope through an umbilical 10 mm trocar, three suprapubic 5 mm trocars are introduced for ancillary instruments.

Step 1 An initial vaginal step was performed with *"vaginal manchette"* creation in order to encapsulate tumor lesion and reduce tumor spread during uterine manipulation, according to previous published data [20]. To preserve pneumoperitoneum, a wet surgical towel is placed into the vagina caudally to the performed manchette (Fig. 43.1).

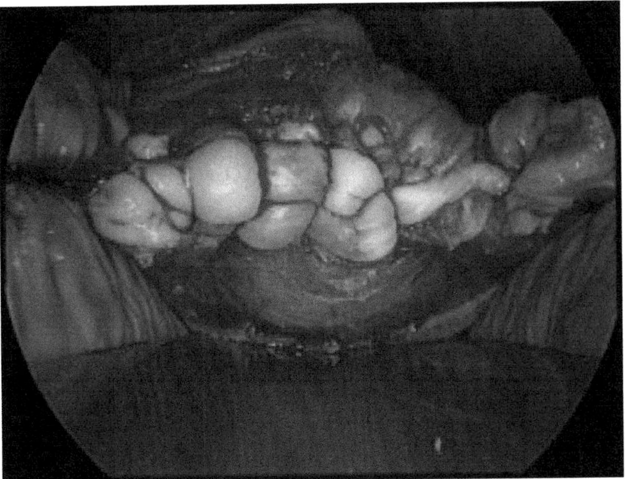

Fig. 43.1 Creation of tumor-adapted vaginal manchette

Tips

The dissection of vescico-vaginal and retto-vaginal septum should be performed without opening of the peritoneum.

Step 2 Exploration of pelvic and abdominal intraperitoneal structures. With the exception of the recto-sigmoid colon, all bowel organs are retracted ventrally and placed in the right upper abdomen. The abdominal retroperitoneum is opened by incising peritoneum at the psoas muscle parallel to the infundibulopelvic ligaments.

Step 3 Exposition of the urogenital mesentery developing anteriorly the paravisceral space with the umbilical artery and the lamina vesicalis dissected from the pelvic wall and tractioned medially

Step 4 Therapeutic systematic pelvic lymphadenectomy [tLNE] according to Höckel is performed and lymph-nodes are examined under frozen section [10]. The parietal nodes of the anterior pelvic compartments (external, internal iliac and obturator) are removed by completely stripping the external and internal iliac artery and vein. The deep pelvic lymph nodes are also removed exposing the proximal sciatic nerves and the lumbar rami of the sacral plexus and removing the paravisceral fat pads up to the sciatic spine (Figs. 43.2 and 43.3). Para-aortic lymph-node dissection is performed in any FIGO stage just in case of pre-operative radiological suspicious or with pelvic positive nodes at frozen section.

Step 5 The infundibulopelvic ligament is coagulated and cut in case of adenocarcinoma histology. In order to obtain more space in the pelvis the uterus–ovarian ligament is cut with separation of the adnexa from the uterus. The adnexa are placed in a bag outside the pelvis and are retained later. Otherwise if conservation of the adnexa were planned, the adnexa are separated form the uterus and dislocated in the upper abdomen at the level of the paracolic spaces on both side. In this case the whole *"peritoneal mesometrium"* (Falloppian tube, mesosalpinx and part of the broad ligament) is accurately dissected and removed separately.

Step 6 The peritoneum is incised again at the level of the right promontorium. The sigmoid colon is mobilized contra-

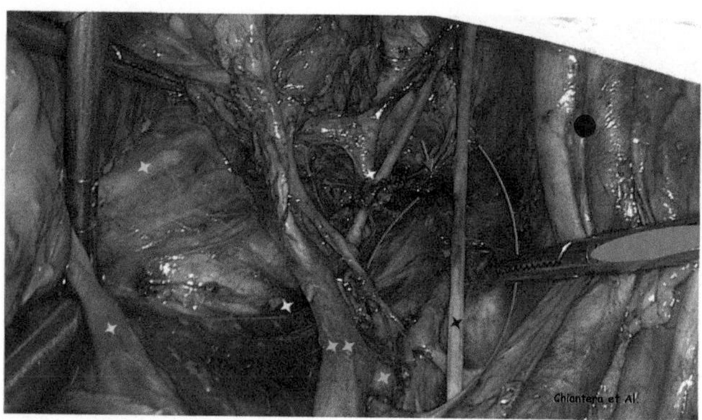

Fig. 43.2 Therapeutic Lymphadenectomy. *Light Green Stars*: right ureter. *Yellow star*: latzko pararectal space. *Double light blue stars*: internal iliac artery. *Single light blue star*: gluteal artery. *White star*: obturator vessels. *Blue star*: right obturator nerve. *Blue circle*: external iliac artery and vein. *Red lines*: borders of the sciatic nerve and sacral plexus. *Red arrow*: sacrospinal ligament

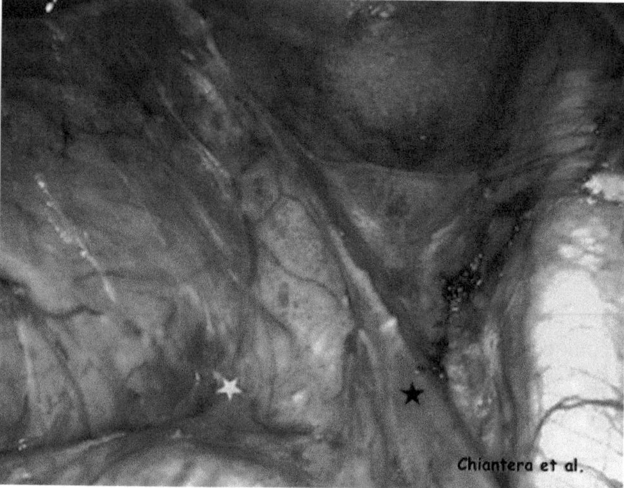

Fig. 43.4 Opening the Parasacral space on the right side and identifying the course of the right hypogastric nerve. *Black star*: right ureter. *Yellow star*: right hypogastric nerve

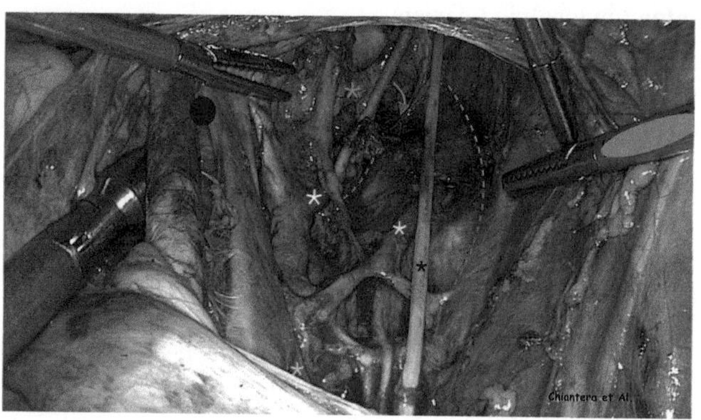

Fig. 43.3 Therapeutic Lymphadenectomy. *Blue circle*: external iliac artery and vein. *White star*: common trunk for the pudendal vein and obturator vessels. *Purple star*: bturator vessels. *Yellow star*: inferior gluteal vein. *Blue stars*: obturator nerve. *Green star*: superior gluteal vein. *Red arrow*: sacrospinal ligament. *Red dotted lines*: borders of the sciatic nerve and sacral plexus

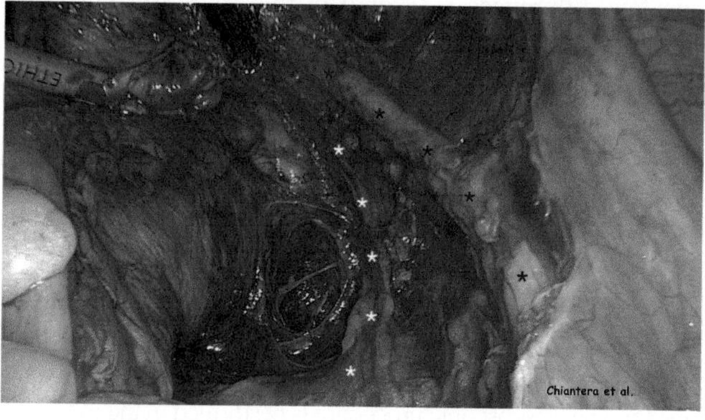

Fig. 43.5 Following the right hypogastric nerve the caudal and dorsal part of the parasacral space is developed up to the lateral border of the dorsal mesometrium.
Black stars: right ureter. *White stars*: right hypogastric nerve

lateral and the hypogastric plexus is identified just caudal the aortic bifurcation. The superior hypogastric plexus is identified at this level and the origin of the two hypogastric nerves is underlined (Fig. 43.4).

Tips

If difficult occurs in the identification of the superior hypogastric plexus the dissection can be further cranially developed up the the level of the aortic bifurcation where the dense tissue of the plexus is easier to identify.

Step 7 Development of the right pre-sacral fossa dorsally the Waldeyer's fascia and ventrally the parietal sacral fascia. Identification and isolation of the right hypogastric nerve adhering medially to the mesorectum (Fig. 43.5).

Step 8 The hypogastric nerve is lateralized in order to completely expose the ligamentous mesometrium. This maneuver is carried out down to the level where the pelvic splanchnic nerves join the right hypogastric nerves to form the right inferior hypogastric plexus.

The proximal inferior hypogastric plexus is mobilized from the lateral surface of the dense subperitoneal connective tissue which encases the rectum enabling the transection of the latter without nerve damage (Figs. 43.6, 43.7, 43.8 and 43.9).

Step 9 A complete uterus anti-version is obtained with the assistant instrument positioned behind the cervix. The Douglas peritoneum is now incised and the recto-vaginal septum is developed up to the level were the previous vaginal dissection was carried. Once the correct traction is obtained and the hypogastric nerves are lateralized, the ligamentum

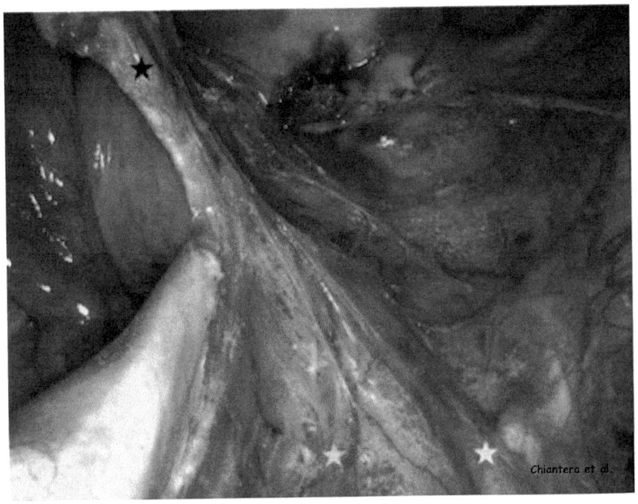

Fig. 43.6 The right hypogastric nerve is lateralized and divided from the posterior mesometrium. Thus the cranial aspect of the dorsal mesometrium is developed. *Black star*: mesometrium. *Yellow star*: right ureter. *Light blue star*: right hypogastric nerve

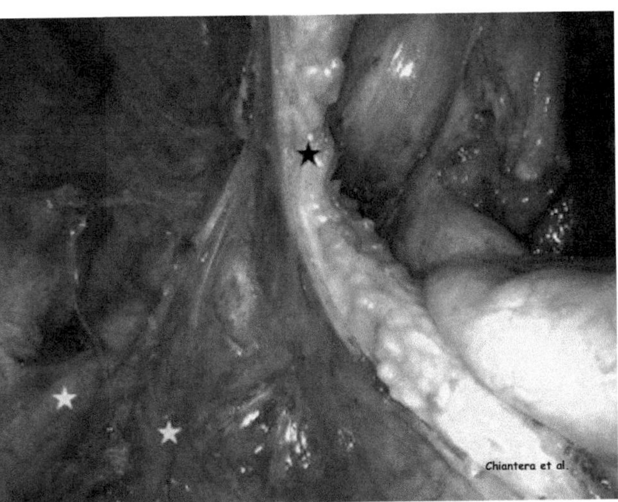

Fig. 43.8 Further lateralization of the left hypogastric nerve from the dorsal mesometrium. *Black star*: mesometrium. *Yellow star*: left ureter. *Light blue star*: left hypogastric nerve

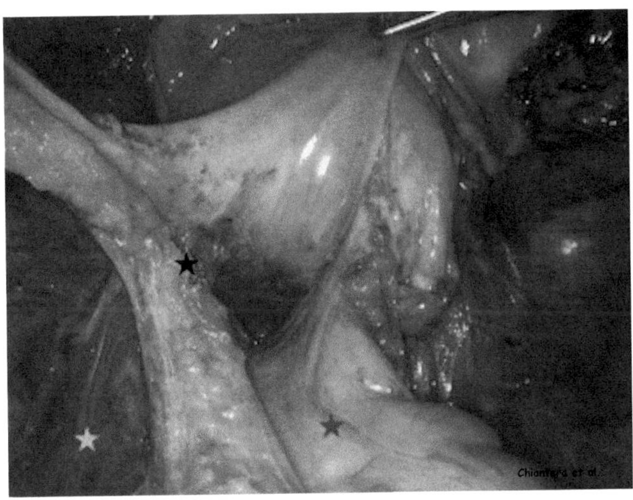

Fig. 43.7 On the left side the same preparation is carried out, the rectovaginal space is cranially dissected at this point. *Black star*: Mesometrium. *Red star*: Rectum. *Light blue star*: right hypogastric nerve

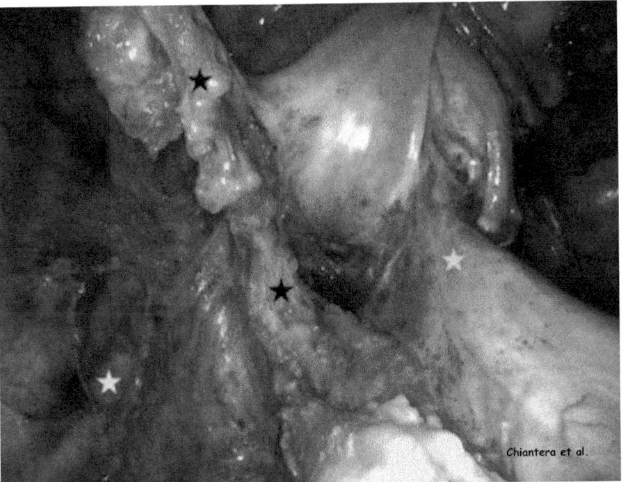

Fig. 43.9 The cranial and caudal part of the dorsal mesometrium is completely divided from the right hypogastric nerve. *Black stars*: cranial and caudal mesometrium. *Yellow star*: left ureter. *Red star*: left hypogastric nerve. *Light blue star*: Rectum

mesometrium. Is transected directly at the level of the anterior surface of the rectum (Fig. 43.10).

Tips

If necessary the rectum is pulled cranial-contralateral and suspended with a suture transfixed into the abdominal wall. Alternatively, the uterus can be suspended ventrally to the abdominal wall with two transfix suture and the assistant can pull the rectum at the level of the promontorium. One of this option is often required in order to obtain the necessary traction thus miming the exposure of the two posterior wings containing the posterior mesometrium as made by laparotomy.

Step 10 The dorsal part of the operation is now concluded (Fig. 43.11), proceeding ventrally the ureter is exposed and its route is completely exhibited until the cross with the uterine vessels (Fig. 43.12).

Step 11 Incision of peritoneum at the level of the vescico-uterine septum with separation of bladder from the anterior cervix and the proximal vagina up to the level of the previous vaginal preparation.

Tips
The vescico uterine septum should be prepared just in his medial aspect in order not to detach the anterior mesometrium from the vescical fascia that has to be keep untouched

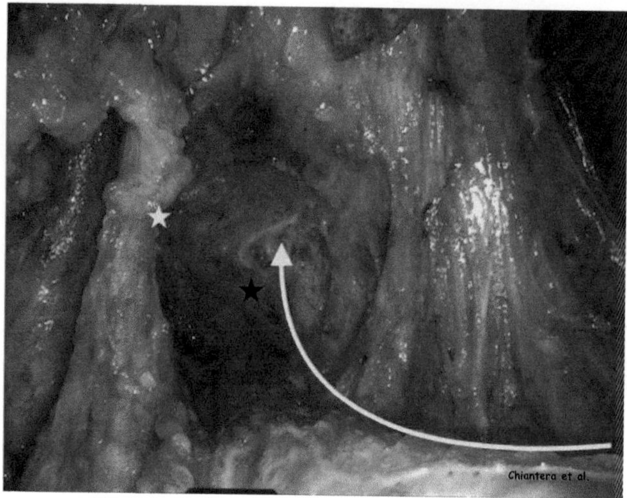

Fig. 43.10 Caudal preparation of the rectovaginal space up to the level of the dorsal vagina, this deep preparation allows a compete explosion of the caudal mesometrium. *Black star*: rectum. *Yellow star*: mesometrium. *Yellow arrow*: line resection of the mesometrium

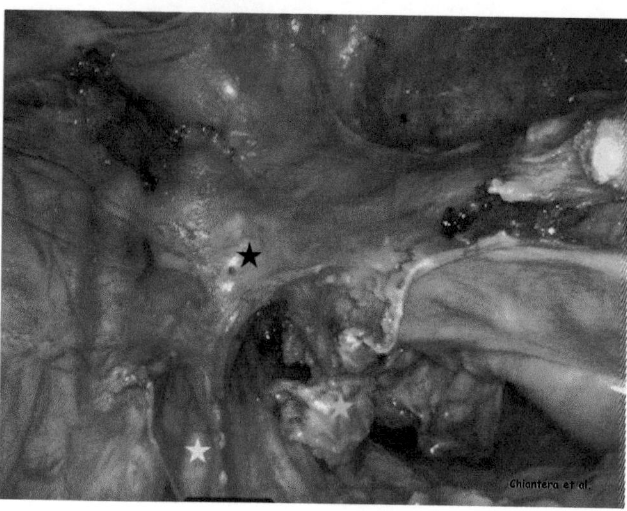

Fig. 43.12 Left vascular mesometrial preparation. *Yellow star*: ureter. *Black star*: vascular mesometrium. *Light blue star*: posterior mesometrium

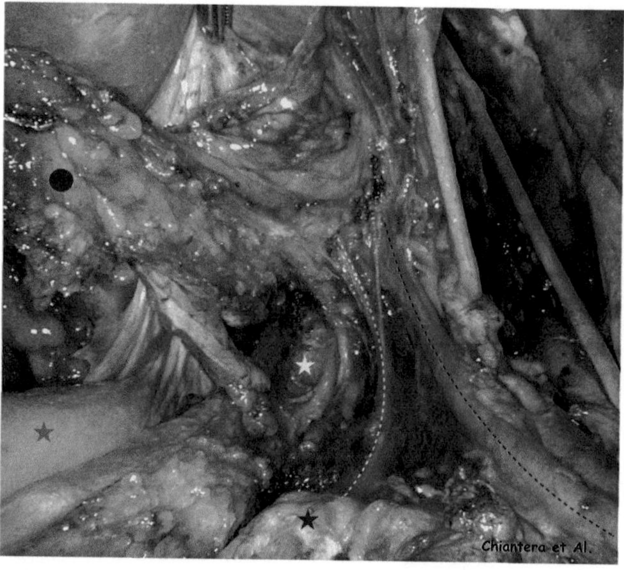

Fig. 43.11 Right side at the end of the dorsal parametrectomy with cranial and caudal mesometrial preparation. Anatomical relations between the ureter, the right nerve and the dorsal mesometrium. *Blue circle*: divided Mesometrium. *Yellow star*: dorsal aspect of the Parasacral space. *Blue star*: sacral promontorium. *Yellow dotted line*: hypogastric nerve and plexus. *Blue dotted line*: right ureter

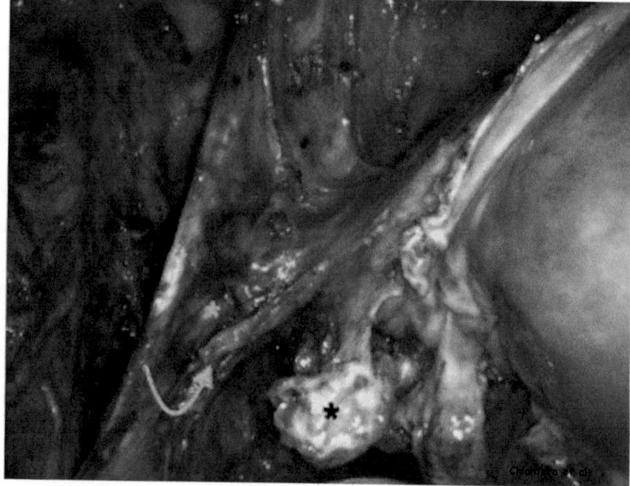

Fig. 43.13 Left vascular mesometrial preparation. *Light blue star*: left ureter. *Light blue arrow*: left vascular mesometrium. *Black star*: posterior mesometrium

until the sharp preparation of the space between the mesometrium and the lateral bladder is completed.

Step 12 The umbilical artery together with the superior bladder mesentery is separated from the anterior mesometrium with sharp dissection in order to isolate the lateral meometrium from the anterior one (Figs. 43.13 and 43.14).

Tips

Differently from the "classic" radical hysterectomy neither the lateral pararectal fossa after Latzko neither the medial one after Okabayashi are developed.

Step 13 The uterine arteries and veins are now coagulated and cut at their origins, this allow the vascular mesometrium to be flipped medially. The lateral mesometrium is mobilized from its origin at the site of the already transected uterine artery and vein(s) towards the uterus beyond the superior surface of the ureter (Figs. 43.15 and 43.16).

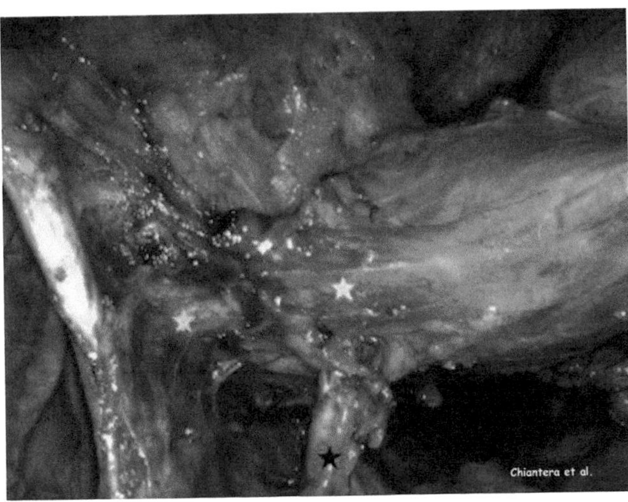

Fig. 43.14 Left vascular mesometrial preparation. *Light blue star*: left uterine artery. *Black arrow*: left ureter. *Yellow star*: ureteral tunnel

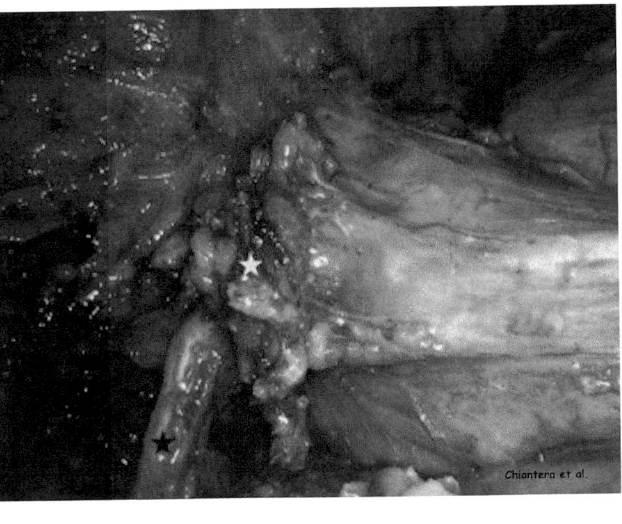

Fig. 43.16 Left vascular mesometrial preparation after the flipping. *Black arrow*: left ureter. *Yellow star*: rolled vascular mesometrium

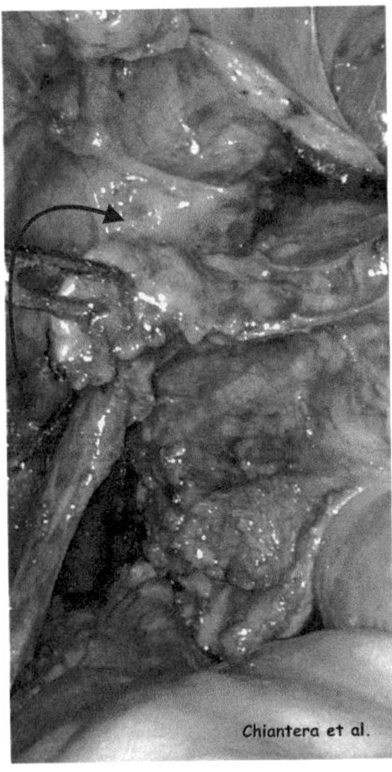

Fig. 43.15 Left vascular mesometrial preparation. Flipping of the vascular mesometrium above the ureter

Tips

The mesoureter has to be divided at the level of the lateral mesometrium in order to permit the medial rotation of the uterine artery and vein above and behind the ureter.

Step 14 The operation proceeds now in the anterior compartment. The vescico-vaginal venous plexus together with the dense subperitoneal connective tissue above the prevescical segment of the ureter is coagulated and divided. After cutting the remaining dorsal attachments the ureter can be completely mobilized laterally together with the dorsal part

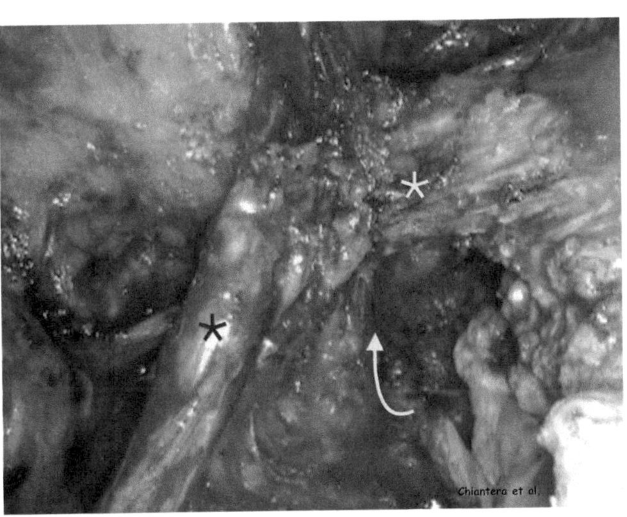

Fig. 43.17 Left vascular mesometrial preparation. Dividing the paravaginal tissue medially to the hypogastric nerve and plexus. *Blue Star: Ureter*, *Yellow Star*: paravaginal tissue, *Yellow arrow*: direction of the hypogastric nerve and plexus

of the dense vescico caginal tissue containing the bladder branch of the pelvic parasympathetic nerve (Fig. 43.17).

Step 15 The paracolpium placed immediately lateral the initial "manchette" is transected connecting the anterior vescico-vaginal space with the posterior retto-vaginal one (Fig. 43.18).

Step 16 The TMMR-specimen is removed through the vagina and the vaginal stump is closed with laparoscopical sutures (Fig. 43.19).

According to Höckel approach no adjuvant radiotherapy should be indicated; although patients with lymph-node

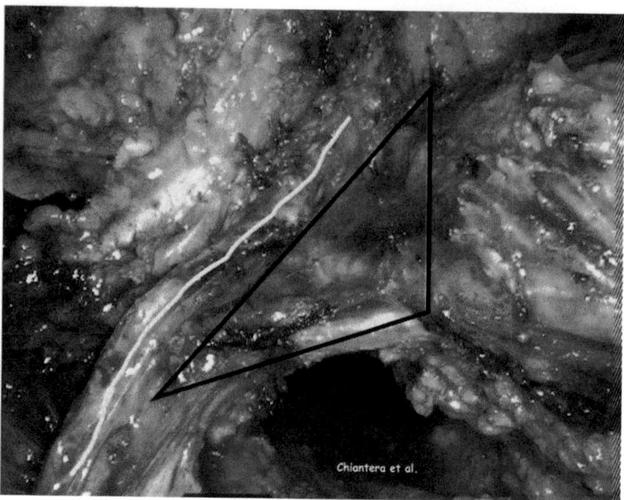

Fig. 43.18 Left vascular mesometrial preparation. Dividing the paravaginal tissue medially to the hypogastric nerve and plexus. *Yellow line*: left ureter. *Black triangle*: left paravaginal tissue

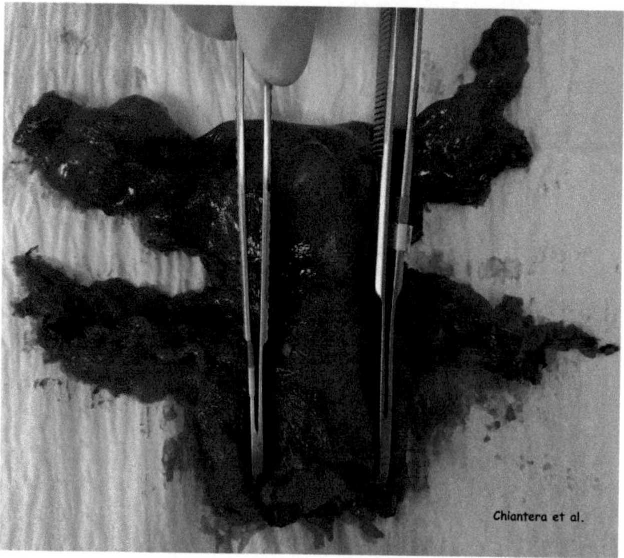

Fig. 43.19 The TMMR surgical specimen with the two of the four "wings"

metastases should be suggested to receive adjuvant chemotherapy with 75 mg/m^2 cisplatin for up to six 3-week cycles, because it had been demonstrated that adjuvant chemotherapy after conventional radical hysterectomy also reduced the incidence of distant metastases in patients with pN1 tumors [21].

Patients should be enrolled in a follow-up program of assessments at 3-month intervals for the first 2 years after surgery, and should be assessed at 6-month intervals thereafter.

It has to be acknowledged that the level of evidence supporting the oncological role of TMMR is still low. The introduction of the ontological surgery in the standard treatment of cervical cancer will probably need more support from the scientific community and further prospective randomized data. However, although the role of TMMR in cervical cancer remains to be definitively established, compelling data from retrospective and prospective series support its role in this clinical setting [11–15]. In conclusion, further larger prospective studies are needed in order to confirm these promising results and to compare this results to the outcome of the classical radical hysterectomy as well as to better define the laparoscopic surgical steps and the subsequent oncological outcome of patients undergoing TMMR compared to a classical open surgical approach.

References

1. Wertheim E. The extended abdominal operation for carcinoma uteri (based on 500 operative cases). Am J Obstet Dis Women Child. 1912;66:169–232.
2. Meigs VJ. Radical hysterectomy with bilateral pelvic lymph node dissections. A report of 100 patients operated on five or more years ago. Am J Obstet Gynecol. 1951;62:854–70.
3. Höckel M, Dornhöfer N. The hydra phenomenon of cancer: why tumors recur locally after microscopically complete resection. Cancer Res. 2005;65:2997–3002.
4. Waggoner SE. Cervical cancer. Lancet. 2003;361:2217–25.
5. Höckel M, Horn LC, Hentschel B, Höckel S, Naumann G. Total mesometrial resection: high resolution nerve-sparing radical hysterectomy based on developmentally defined surgical anatomy. Int J Gynecol Cancer. 2003;13:791–803.
6. Höckel M, Horn LC, Fritsch H. Association between the mesenchymal compartment of uterovaginal organogenesis and local tumour spread in state 1B–2B cervical carcinoma: a prospective study. Lancet Oncol. 2005;6:751–6.
7. Höckel M. Do we need a new classification for radical hysterectomy? Insights in surgical anatomy and local tumor spread from human embryology. Gynecol Oncol. 2007;1:106–12.
8. Höckel M, Horn LC, Manthey N, Braumann UD, Wolf U, Teichmann G, Frauenschläger K, Dornhöfer N, Einenkel J. Resection of the embryologically defined uterovaginal (Müllerian) compartment and pelvic control in patients with cervical cancer: a prospective analysis. Lancet Oncol. 2009;10: 683–92.
9. Höckel M, Kahn T, Einenkel J, Manthey N, Braumann U-D, Hildebrandt G, Leo C, Hentschel B, Vaupel P, Horn L-C. Local spread of cervical cancer revisited: a clinical and pathological pattern analysis. Gynecol Oncol. 2010;117:401–8.
10. Höckel M, Horn L-C, Tetsch E, Einenkel J. Pattern analysis of regional spread and therapeutic lymph node dissection in cervical cancer based on ontogenetic anatomy. Gynecol Oncol. 2012;125: 168–74.
11. Höckel M. Cancer permeates locally within ontogenetic compartments: clinical evidence and implications for cancer surgery. Future Oncol. 2012;8:29–36.
12. Manjunath AP, Girija S. Embryologically based resection of cervical cancers: a new concept of surgical radicality. J Obstet Gynaecol India. 2012;62(1):5–14.
13. Kimmig R. Robotic surgery for cervical cancer. Endoscopic total mesometrial resection and therapeutic lymphadenectomy [Robotic surgery beim Zervixkarzinom. Endoskopische total emesometriale Resektion und therapeutische Lymphonodektomie]. Gynakologe. 2012;45:707–11.

14. Kimmig R, Iannaccone A, Buderath P, Aktas B, Wimberger P, Heubner M. Definition of compartment-based radical surgery in uterine cancer — part I. Therapeutic pelvic and periaortic lymphadenectomy byMichael Höckel translated to robotic surgery (rtLNE). ISRNObstetGynecol.2013;2013:297921.doi:10.1155/2013/297921.
15. Höckel M, Hentschel B, Horn LC. Association between developmental steps in the organogenesis of the uterine cervix and locoregional progression of cervical cancer: a prospective clinicopathological analysis. Lancet Oncol. 2014;15(4):445–56.
16. Chiantera V, Vizzielli G, Lucidi A, Gallotta V, Petrillo M, Legge F, Fagotti A, Sehouli J, Scambia G, Muallem MZ. Laparoscopic radical hysterectomy in cervical cancer as total mesometrial resection (L-TMMR): a multicentric experience. Gynecol Oncol. 2015;139(1):47–51. pii: S0090-8258(15)30071-8
17. Kruijdenberg CB, van den Einden LC, Hendriks JC, Zusterzeel PL, Bekkers RL. Robot-assisted versus total laparoscopic radical hysterectomy in early cervical cancer, a review. Gynecol Oncol. 2011;120(3):334–9.
18. Possover M, Quakernack J, Chiantera V. The LANN technique to reduce postoperative functionalmorbidity in laparoscopic radical pelvic surgery. J Am Coll Surg. 2005;201(6):913–7.
19. Vizzielli G, Lucidi A, Gallotta V, Petrillo M, Dessole M, Fagotti A, Costantini B, Scambia G, Chiantera V. Robotic total mesometrial resection (R-TMMR) *vs.* Laparoscopic total mesometrial resection (L-TMMR) in early cervical cancer: a case-control study. J Minim Invasive Gynecol. 2016;23(5):804–9. In Press
20. Gottschalk E, Lanowska M, Chiantera V, Marnitz S, Schneider A, Brink-Spalink V, Hasenbein K, Koehler C. Vaginal-assisted laparoscopic radical hysterectomy: rationale, technique, results. JSLS. 2011;15(4):451–9.
21. Peters WA, Liu PY, Barrett RJ, et al. Concurrent chemotherapy and pelvic radiation therapy compared with pelvic radiation alone as adjuvant therapy after radical surgery in high-risk early-stage cancer of the cervix. J Clin Oncol. 2000;18:1606–13.

Laparoscopic Radical Hysterectomy for Malignant Indications: Laparoscopic Trachelectomy

44

Vito Chiantera, Alessandro Lucidi, and Marco Petrillo

Cervical cancer is the third most common female cancer and the fourth leading cause of female cancer death worldwide [1]. Approximately 15 % of all cervical cancers are diagnosed in women under the age of 40 years who wish to preserve their fertility [2, 3]. For these reasons, although radical hysterectomy with lymph node dissection represents the standard treatment for early-stage cervical cancer, alternative surgical approaches able to spare reproductive organs have been developed.

In this context, vaginal radical trachelectomy (VRT) with laparoscopic lymphadenectomy represents the gold standard for fertility sparing surgery in early stage cervical cancer patients. This surgical technique was firstly described by Dargent [4] in the 1980s, and to date more than 1000 cases of VRT have been published, with a global pregnancy rate (total number of women who conceived of all who retained fertility) of 24 % [5], and a relapse and death rate of 4.2 % and 2.9 %; respectively [6].

Radical trachelectomy is a surgical procedure in which is removed the cervix with parametria, the upper part of the vagina and pelvic lymph nodes.

Criteria used to select candidates for radical vaginal hysterectomy are:

1. Confirmed invasive cervical cancer: squamous, adenocarcinoma, or adenosquamous
2. FIGO stage IA1 with lymphovascular space involvement, FIGO IA2 L0 or L1 V0 to IB1 L0 or L1 V0
3. Desire to preserve fertility
4. Lesion size < 2 cm
5. No previous history of infertility
6. Limited endocervical involvement at colposcopy (R0 resection possible with surgical margin >5 mm)
7. Estimated length of remaining cervix >1 cm
8. Post-conization adequate resolution of acute inflammation required (usually a 6-week interval between conization and RT)
9. Negative pelvic lymph node status

In this context, although VRT still represents the best surgical approach, only in selected cases laparoscopic radical trachelectomy (LRT) may offer specific advantages.

It has been considered that the age of first pregnancy is progressively increasing; therefore the vast majority of women receiving fertility sparing surgery are nulliparous at the time of surgery.

In these cases, RVT can be technically complex, and the laparoscopic route can be a more reliable strategy. Moreover, LRT represents an alternative to RVT for several gynecologic oncologists who are not proficient in vaginal radical surgery.

In addition, LRT ensures an easier identification of the uterine artery and the hypogastric nerve compared with the vaginal approach, thus allowing a more precious dissection of the parametrium. Therefore, using the laparoscopic route surgeons can better tailor the width of parametrium resection compared with the vaginal approach. In this context, it has to be considered that a novel surgical technique, the total mesometrial resection (TMMR) has been recently proposed as an affective therapeutic strategy in early stage cervical cancer patients [7], with recently published evidences suggesting the feasibility of laparoscopic TMMR [8]. Therefore, LRT may represent an attracting strategy in order to remove mesometrium according with Hockel technique which is not applicable with the vaginal approach.

For these reasons, LRT may be considered in women with tumor dimension > 2 cm receiving fertility sparing surgery which may require a wider parametrial resection. In these

V. Chiantera (✉)
Gynecologic Oncologic Unit, Catholic University of the Sacred Heart, Largo Gemelli, 1, Rome, Italy

Gynecologic Oncologic Unit, Unimol, 86100 Campobasso, Italy
e-mail: vito.chiantera@gmail.com

A. Lucidi • M. Petrillo
Gynecologic Oncologic Unit, Catholic University of the Sacred Heart, Largo Gemelli, 1, Rome, Italy

I. Alkatout, L. Mettler (eds.), *Hysterectomy*, DOI 10.1007/978-3-319-22497-8_44

cases, LRT may be considered only in the context of controlled clinical trials in which a fertility sparing surgical treatment is proposed after neoadjuvant chemotherapy [9]. In this regard, too many case reports and retrospective studies have been presented in literature proposing abdominal trachelectomy as surgical option for patients with tumor dimension >2 cm [10].

In conclusion, we have to point out that for tumor >2 cm LTR may be considered only in the context of controlled clinical trials and at the same time we have to remember that even in patients with tumor dimension <2 cm the real advantage of LRT compared to VRT must be proved necessarily and exclusively through a randomized prospective clinical trial.

In this context, it has to be emphasized that to safely complete LRT is mandatory to perform vaginal manchette to avoid intraperitoneal diffusion of cancer cells during specimen's removal after surgery. We believe that to cure women diagnosed with cervical cancer by fertility-preserving surgery, correct indication and oncologic precautions are more important than the type of approach. During surgical procedures the tumor may be inadvertently manipulated and the tumor cells may have been mobilized [11]. Although it has not yet been demonstrated worsening oncological outcome in cases in which vaginal cuff closure is not performed we consider this procedure essential more so in patients receiving LRT. Indeed, in these cases uterine cervix is exposed in the abdominal cavity to be transected allowing not only a vaginal tumor cell contamination (as for standard radical hysterectomy) but also an intraabdominal tumor spread.

Looking at the literature, a recent review including 485 abdominal radical trachelectomies reported a relapse and death rates of 3.8 % and 2.9 %, respectively [5]; which appears comparable with the results reported for VRT. In particular focusing on the laparoscopic approach, 140 LRT have been described in the literatures (Table 44.1). The operative outcomes are summarized in Table 44.2. The analysis of combined data demonstrates a low average intraoperative complication rate of 0.7 % with an incidence of postoperative complications around 6.4 %. The most common intraoperative complication is represented by the injury of uterine artery occurring during pelvic lymphadenectomy. On the other hand, the most frequent post-operative complications are represented by cervical stenosis, and bladder hypotonia due to the surgical-related damage of the sympathetic and parasympathetic branches of the pelvic autonomic nerve system.

Rates of conversions to laparotomy or secondary surgeries for parametrial bleeding, blood vessel injury, lymphocele, suprapubic, or vulvar hematoma range between 0 %

Table 44.1 Patient characteristics of total laparoscopic radical trachelectomy for early-stage cervical cancer in published studies

Characteristics	Lee et al. [12]	Cibula et al. [13]	Park et al. [14]	Park et al. [15]	Martin et al. [16]	Lu et al. [17]	Ebisawa et al. [18]	Kucukmetin et al. [19]
Number of patient	2	1	4	55	9	25	56	11
Age, years	32	36	29	32	32	29	32	28
Stage, n. patients								
Ia2			1	2	2	10	4	
Ib1	2	1	3	53	7	15	52	11
IIa								
Histologic subtype, n. patients								
Squamous cell carcinoma	2	1	4	42	6	25	42	5
Adenocarcinoma				13	3		12	6
Other							2	

Table 44.2 Operative outcomes after total laparoscopic radical trachelectomy for early-stage cervical cancer in published studies

Characteristics	Lee et al. [12]	Cibula et al. [13]	Park et al. [14]	Park et al. [15]	Martin et al. [16]	Lu et al. [17]	Ebisawa et al. [18]	Kucukmetin et al. [19]
Number of patient	2	1	4	55	9	25	56	11
EBL, ml	650	250	185	NA	NA	120	300	85
Operative Time, min	353	250	250	NA	270	232	349	320
Hospital stay, day	13	6	NA	NA	5.2	3.3	17.5	4
FU, months	11	4	34	NA	28	66	60	9
Intraoperative complication	Injured vessel	No	No	No	No	No	No	NA
Post-operative complications	Bladder hypotonia	No	No	No	No	Voiding dysfunction	Cervical stenosis	NA

and 9 %. Postoperative complications such as dysmenorrhea (24 %), dyspareunia (20 %), menstrual abnormalities (17 %), excessive vaginal discharge (14 %), recurrent candidiasis (14 %), bladder hypotonia (4–16 %), vulvar edema (12 %), lymphocele (3–11 %), chronic pelvic pain (10 %), isthmic stenosis (10 %), amenorrhea (7 %), vulvar hematoma (7 %), suprapubic hematoma (4 %), lymphedema (3 %), urinary tract infection (2 %), and femoro-cutaneous nerve palsy (1 %) are reported.

Focusing on oncologic outcome, the tumour recurrence rate reported with LRT is 2.9 %, which appears superimposable or even lower compared with data reported for VRT (4.2–5.3 %), and abdominal radical trachelectomy (3.8 %) [5, 20]. Furthermore, the risk of recurrence does not seem to be greater after LRT for adenocarcinoma compared with squamous cell carcinoma (2.8 vs. 2.9 %), thus suggesting that tumor histotype does not represent a contraindication to the use of the laparoscopic route.

The obstetric outcomes after LRT for early-stage cervical cancer in the available literature are presented in Table 44.3. Overall, 59 patients attempted to conceive after LRT, and 46 patients successful deliveries were recorded, with a pregnancy rate of 78 % (46/59). Seventeen miscarriages, 14 preterm births and 11 term births have been described. On the other hand, the pregnancy rate in patients attempting to conceive after VRT is 52.8 % [5, 21], thus suggesting that the pregnancy rate after LRT is not lower compared with VRT. Similarly, the pregnancy loss rate is superimposable between vaginal and laparoscopic approach, accounting for 24 % [5, 21]. Unfortunately, regardless of the used surgical strategy, the pregnancy loss rates are significantly higher than that of the general population (12 %) [22]. The preterm birth rate of patients who gave birth after vaginal or abdominal radical trachelectomy is 24.7 %, and 38.7 % respectively. The preterm birth rate after LRT was 24 % in all the published studies, which appears again higher than general population, but superimposable with the vaginal approach [23]. Further investigations are required to establish definitive guideline for preterm birth prevention following radical trachelectomy.

Surgical Procedure

The surgical procedure is similar to that for laparoscopic nerve-sparing radical hysterectomy as described by Querleu [24]. In this chapter we describe our surgical modified technique according to the compartment theory besed on ontogenetic anatomy proposed by Hockel. The laparoscopic procedure is performed in the modified dorsolithotomy position under endotracheal general anesthesia. A Veress needle is inserted through the umbilicus and the abdomen is insufflated. After pneumoperitoneum and insertion of the laparoscope through an umbilical 10 mm trocar, three suprapubic 5 mm trocars are introduced for ancillary instruments.

Step 1 Preserving the integrity of the round ligament, the retroperitoneal space is entered along the lateral pelvic wall, thereby exposing the common iliac, external iliac, internal iliac and umbilical arteries. The pelvic visceroparietal ground plan is exposed by dissecting the areolar fibrous tissue to create a "paravisceral space" down to the pubo- and iliococcygeus muscles and a "presacral space" to the ventral margin of the inferior hypogastric plexus separated by the urogenital mesentery. Laterally to the external iliac vessels the obturator and lumbosacral fossa are developed. We proceed with the identification of the obturator nerves, the lumbosacral trunc, the gluteal vessels and the sciatic nerve. The lymph node dissection include the external and internal iliac nodes and the superficial and deep obturator nodes. We extend the radicality of our lymphadenectomy to the gluteal and pre-ischiatic nodes according to the therapeutic lymphadenectomy described by Hockel (Fig. 44.1) [7]. Lymph nodes are extracted in endoscopic bags through

Table 44.3 Obstetric outcomes after total laparoscopic radical trachelectomy for early-stage cervical cancer in published studies

Characteristics	Lee et al. [12]	Cibula et al. [13]	Park et al. [14]	Park et al. [15]	Martin et al. [16]	Lu et al. [17]	Ebisawa et al. [18]	Kucukmetin et al. [19]
Number of patient	2	1	4	55	9	25	56	11
Attempted to conceive, n. patients	NA	NA	NA	18	4	12	25	NA
Pregnancies, n. patients	NA	NA	NA	14	2	9	21	0
Miscarriages, n. patients	NA	NA	NA	4	0	3	10	0
Preterm birth, n. patients	NA	NA	NA	6	0	1	7	0
Term birth, n. patients	NA	NA	NA	4	1	3	3	0
Ongoing pregnancy, n. patients	NA	NA	NA	0	1	2	1	0

the 10-mm sheath for perioperative histological examination. If the lymph nodes are negative, the procedure is continued.

Tip The pararectal fossa during this step is not developed to avoid uterine artery injury during lymphadenectomy. We proceed with this step later when we have a complete exposition of the pelvic retroperitoneum.

Step 2 A vaginal step is performed with vaginal "manchette" creation (Fig. 44.2a, b) in order to encapsulate tumor lesion and reduce tumor spread during uterine manipulation, according to previous published data [25]. The vescico-vaginal and recto-vaginal septum are opened without peritoneal incision.

Tip A sterile gauze is placed inside the developed septum for a easier identification of the developed space during laparoscopy. A sterile glove with a gauze inside are placed into the vagina to prevent gas loss during laparoscopy.

Step 3 The development of the medial and lateral pararectal space is then performed (Fig. 44.3). The lateral pararectal fossa (Latzko's fossa) is developed until the plan of uterine vein.

Tip Differently from what we have previously reported for radical hysterectomy [26] the parasympathetic nerves plan is not reached and the sacral fascia remains intact along the surface of the sacral root.

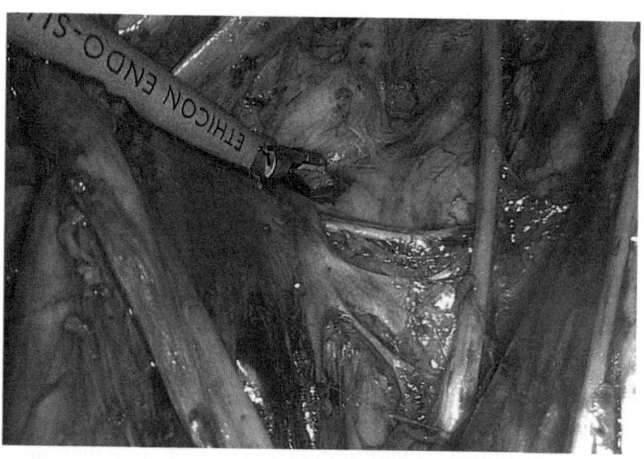

Fig. 44.1 Pelvic side wall after radical lymphadenectomy according to Hockel

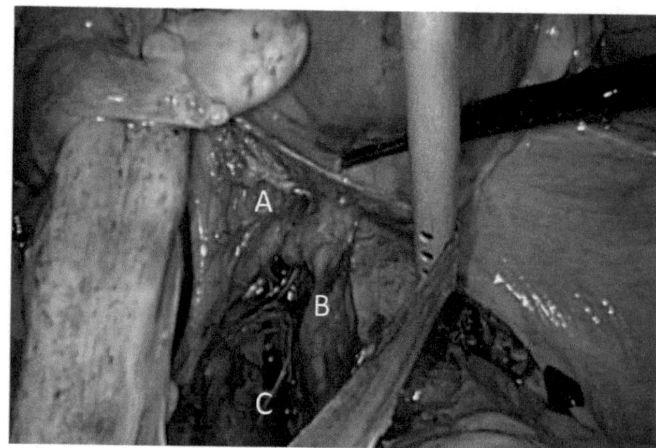

Fig. 44.3 Uterine artery (*A*); Ureter (*B*), Pararectal space (*C*)

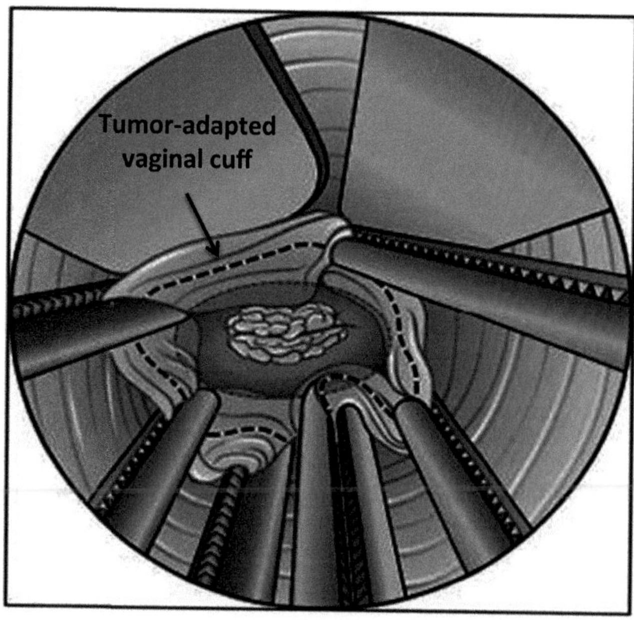

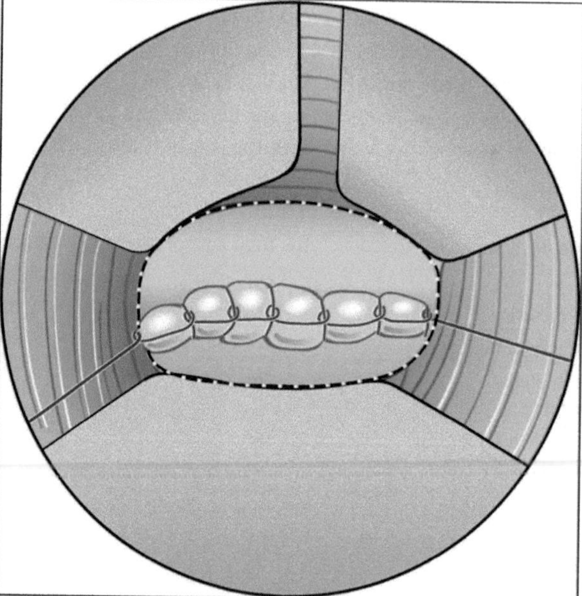

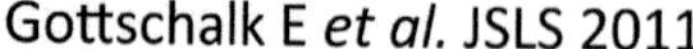

Fig. 44.2 Vaginal manchette

Step 4 The superior hypogastric plexus is isolated at the level of the sacral promontory and the right hypogastric nerve is identified (Fig. 44.4) with the development of the parasacral fossa.

Step 5 A peritoneal incision on the left side is performed at the level of the common iliac artery. The hypogastric plexus and the left hypogastric nerve are identified and the parasacral fossa is developed with reunification on the contralateral space (Fig. 44.5).

Tip At this point the rectum should be cranially pulled. We generally anchored it to the abdominal wall by placing a stitch on the rectal tenia.

Step 6 Hypogastric nerves are bilaterally lateralized and the peritoneum is transected medially to the ureter until the posterior mesometrium (Fig. 44.6) which is then transected at the level of the vaginal manchette (Fig. 44.7).

Tip Before the mesometrial transection Douglas peritoneum should be opened in order to identify the gauze previously positioned during the vaginal step.

Step 7 The pelvic ureter is separated from the broad ligament to the crossing of the uterine artery, and the hypogastric nerve is identified in the space created between the broad ligament and the mesoureter (Fig. 44.8).

Step 8 The uterine vessels and ureters are identified bilaterally (Fig. 44.9). The ascending and descending branches of

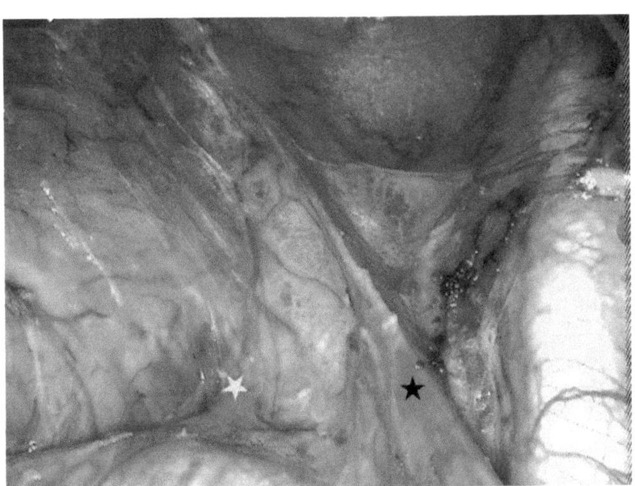

Fig. 44.4 *Black star*: right ureter. *Yellow star*: right hypogastric nerve

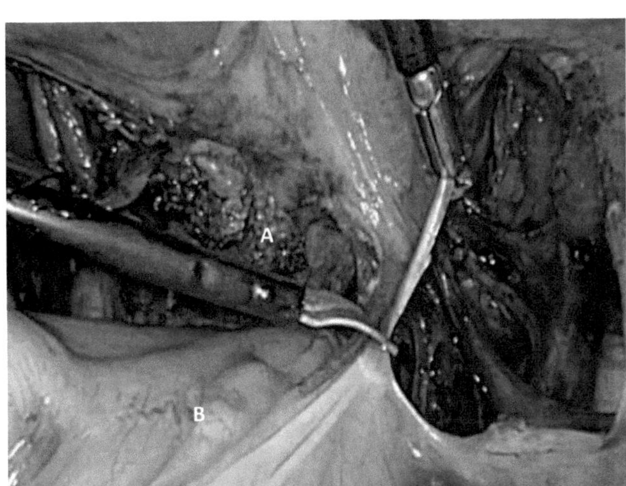

Fig. 44.6 Douglas (*A*); Rectum (*B*)

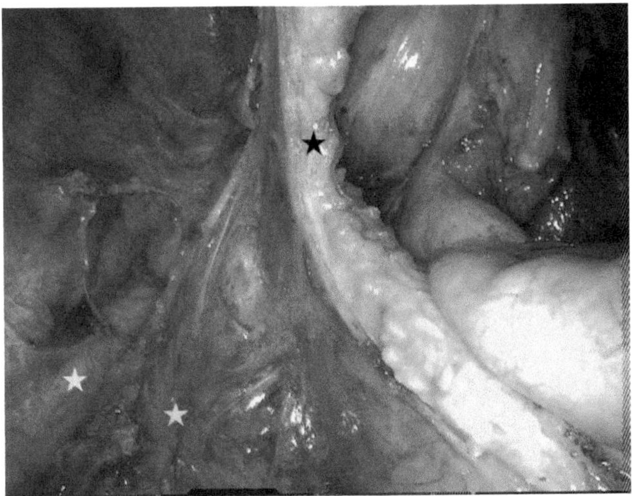

Fig. 44.5 *Black star*: mesometrium. *Yellow star*: left ureter. *Light blue star*: left hypogastric nerve

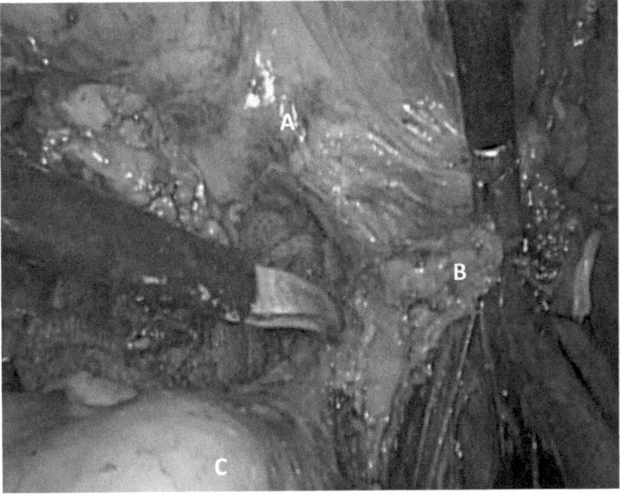

Fig. 44.7 Cervix (*A*); Mesometrium (*B*); Rectum (*C*)

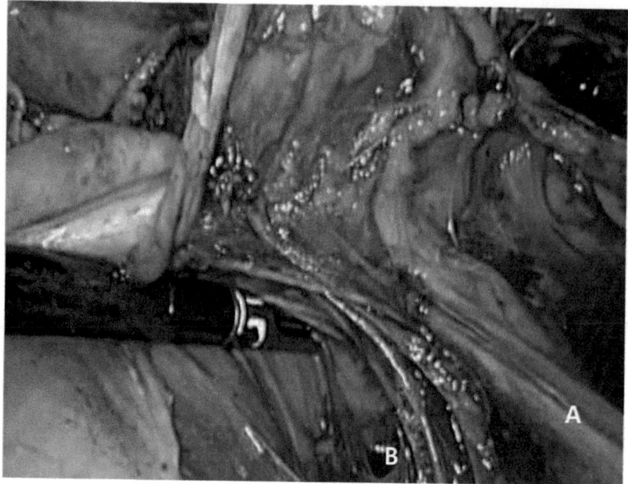

Fig. 44.8 Ureter (*A*); Hypogastric plexus (*B*)

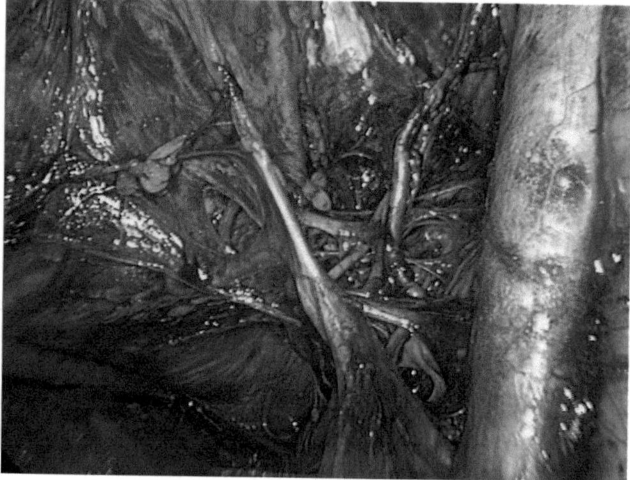

Fig. 44.10 Right lateral parametrium and paravescical space

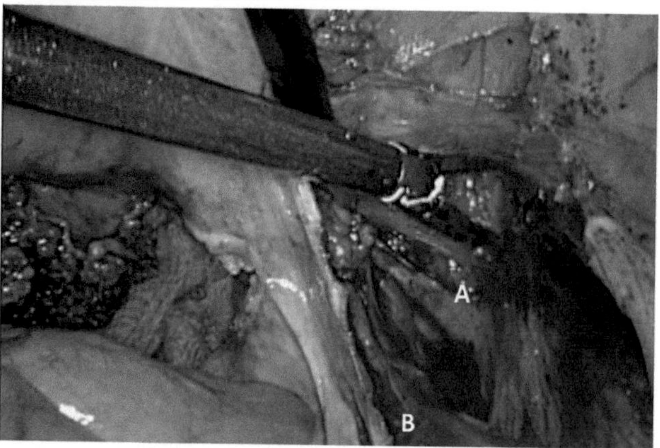

Fig. 44.9 Uterine artery (*A*); Ureter (*B*)

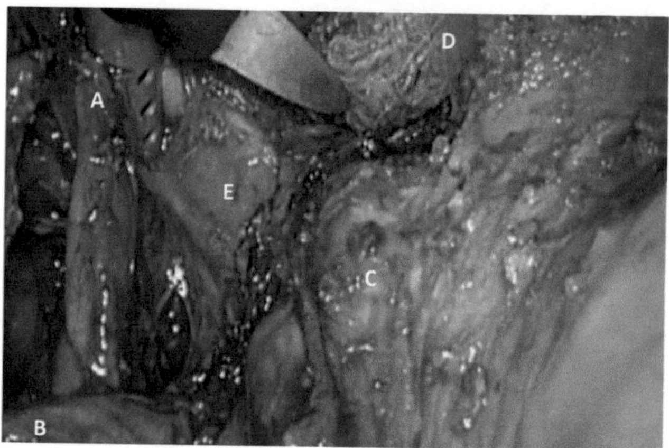

Fig. 44.11 Ureter (*A*); Uterine artery (*B*); Cervix (*C*); Vagina (*D*); Vescico-uterine ligament (*E*)

uterine artery are identified and in our technique uterine artery with both branches is preserved till to final cervical resection from the uterine corpus. The lateral parametrium is resected below (dorsally) the uterine artery (Fig. 44.10). The uterine vein is sectioned at the origin and then the parametrium is rotated below the ureter.

Tip In contrast to our classic radical hysterectomy where the mesouretere remains intact and the parametrium (including uterine artery) is rotated above and medially to the ureter, we prefer to dissect the mesouretere sliding the parametrium (with the uterine artery intact) below ureter.

Step 9 The vescico-vaginal space is opened with the identification of the gauze previously positioned during vaginal step (Fig 44.11).

Tip The two bladder corners are pulled ventrally positioning two stitches through the abdominal wall.

Step 10 The dissection of vescicouterine ligament is performed defining a section plane between the cervix (medially) and the terminal ureter (externally) with the bladder positioned ventraly and the uterine artery dorsally (Fig. 44.11).

Step 11 The uretere is isolated caudally to the uterine artery, surrounded by a rubber strip and anchored to the abdominal wall (Fig. 44.12). In this way we create a kneeling of the uretere caudally to the uterine artery.

Step 12 The infraureteral anterior parametrium, the anterior and lateral paracolpium are transected dorsally to the pulled ureter (Fig. 44.13).

Tip At this point the anterior (vescico-vaginale), lateral and posterior (recto-vaginal) spaces are in communication and the cervix remains pegged to the posterior paracolpium.

Step 13 The remaining paracolpium (Fig. 44.14) is transected caudally to the vaginal manchette.

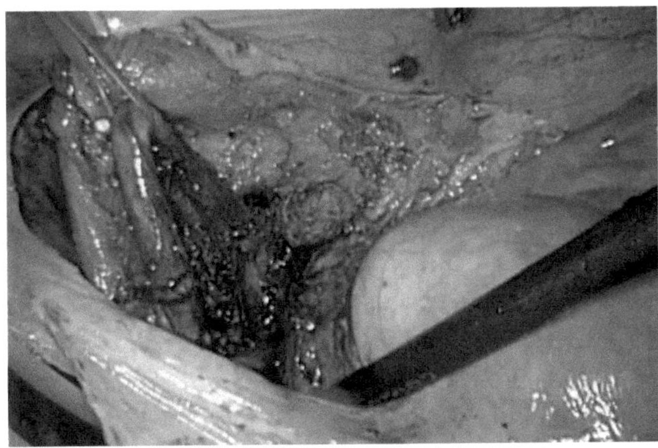

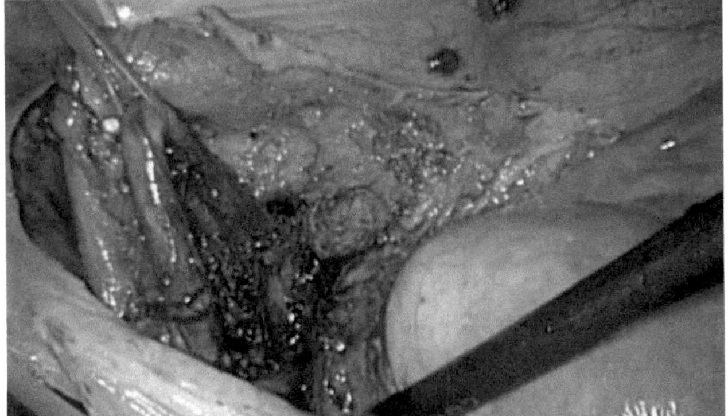

Fig. 44.12 Anchored ureter

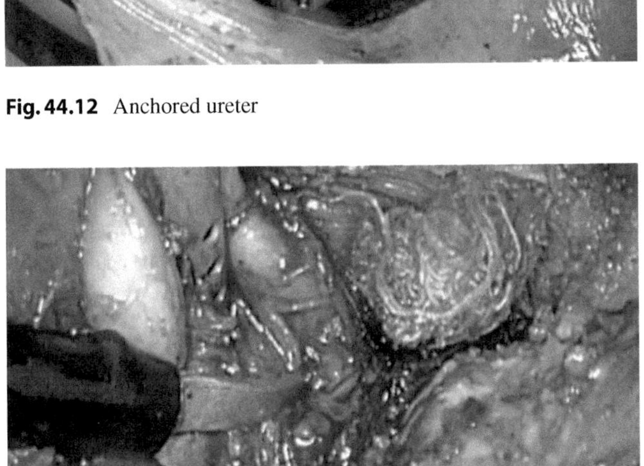

Fig. 44.13 Infraureteral anterior parametrium

Step 14 All these steps are performed bilaterally.

Tip The uterus at this point is held in place by the round ligaments, the uterine arteries and the pelvic infundibula.

Step 15 The vaginal manchette is rotated ventrally in order to expose the isthmus (Fig. 44.15).

Step 11 The descending branch of uterine artery is coagulated, whereas the ascending branch is preserved, then the cervix is then transected approximately few millimetres below the insertion of the uterine artery (Fig. 44.16). The excised cervix is marked and sent for frozen section for the evaluation of surgical margins.

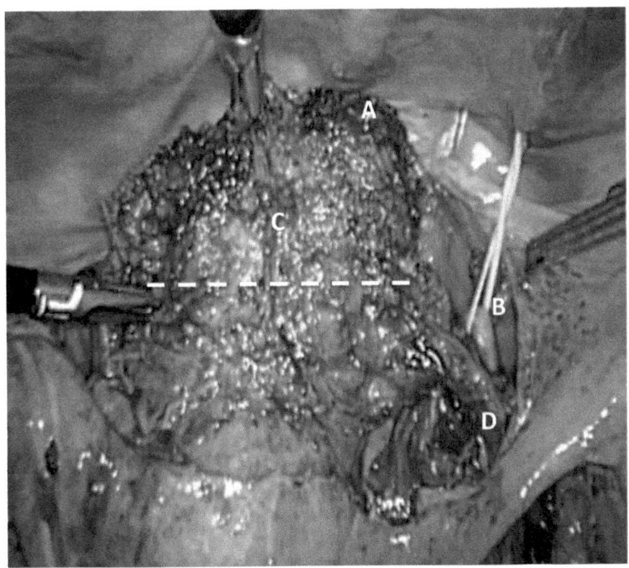

Fig. 44.15 Vaginal manchette (*A*); Ureter (*B*); Cervix (*C*); Uterine artery (*D*)

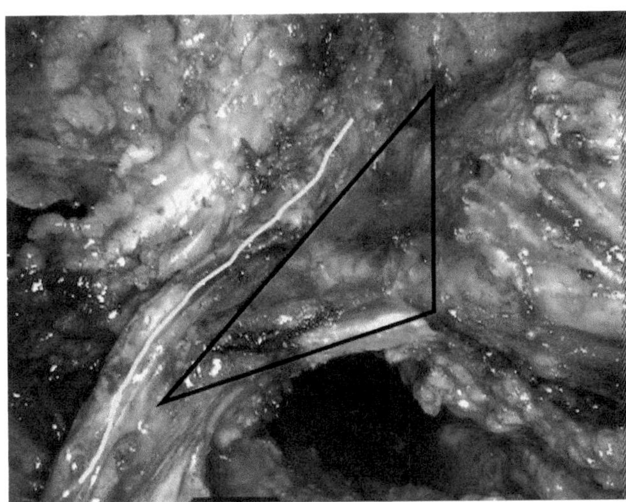

Fig. 44.14 *Yellow line*: left ureter. *Black triangle*: left paracolpium

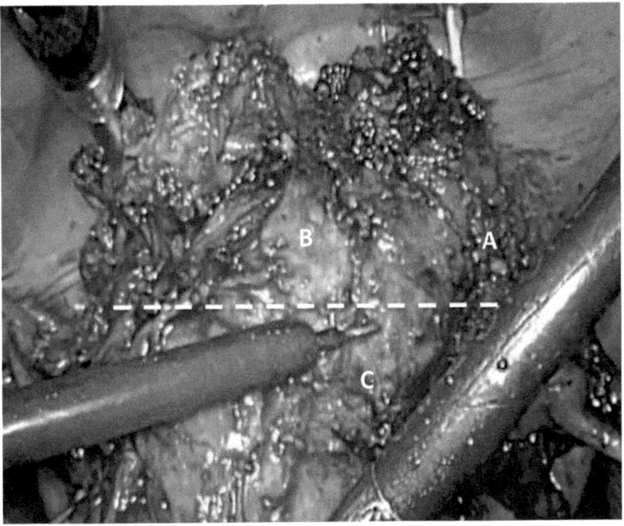

Fig. 44.16 Parametrium (*A*); Cervix (*B*); Isthmus (*C*)

Step 12 Reanastomosis of the uterine corpus and upper vagina is then laparoscopically performed and eight separated stiches are placed (Fig. 44.17).

Step 13 The specimen is sent for extemporaneous histological examination in order to evaluate the the margins of resection (Fig. 44.18).

A Foley catheter is always placed in the isthmus at the end of the surgical procedure.

After LVT, we recommended contraception with oral contraceptives for 6–12 months in patients with squamous cell carcinoma. Patients with adenocarcinomas were recommended non-hormonal contraception. During pregnancy following LVT, we recommended regular visits in short intervals such as in risk pregnancies. Cervical length was assessed on every visit or at least every 2 weeks. In the event of cervical shortening or funnel building, we recommended the Saling procedure between weeks 12 and 14. We recommended examining microbiologic vaginal smears every second week to detect vaginal infection as soon as possible. We advised women to check their vaginal pH twice a week starting in the second trimester. If a patient showed signs of cervical insufficiency, we recommended bed rest and hospitalization. We recommended routinely administering steroid and antibiotic prophylaxis before the 34th week to prevent acute respiratory distress syndrome and premature rupture of membranes (PROM) in patients with cervical insufficiency or suspicious microbiologic smears.

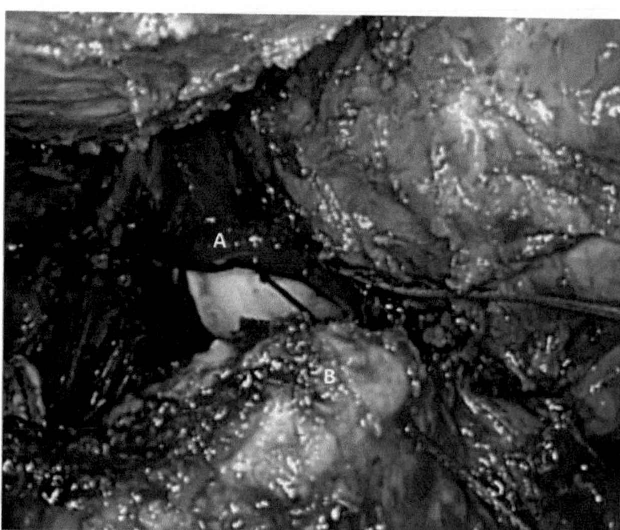

Fig. 44.17 Vagina (*A*); Uterine corpus (*B*)

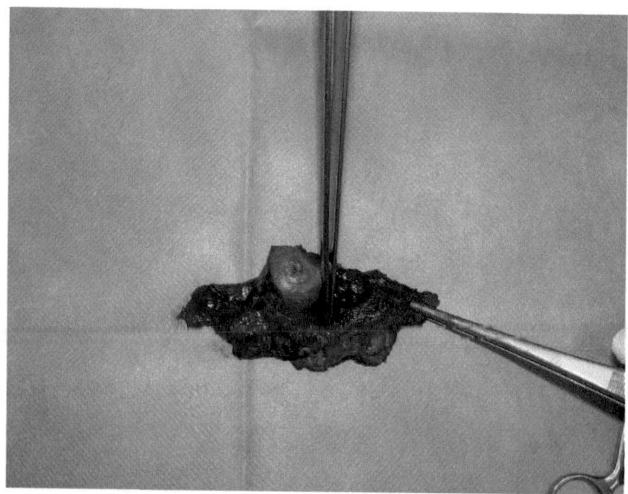

Fig. 44.18 Final surgical specimen

LRT does appear to be a well tolerated treatment for carefully selected patients. The advantages of minimally invasive approaches are visual enhancement, more precise dissection, less blood loss, fewer complications and shorter recovery time. The review of the literature indicates that pregnancy rates are high; however, preterm birth is common. LRT allows a more precious dissection of the parametrium and a wider parametrial resection; however "not always bigger means better". Therefore, VRT remains the gold standard, and LRT should be considered only in the context of clinical trial as an additional surgical approach for selected cases. In tertiary referral centers both surgical techniques must be available to properly tailor surgical management.

References

1. Jemal A, Bray F, Center MM, et al. Global cancer statistics. CA Cancer J Clin. 2011;61:69–90.
2. Rebecca S, Elizabeth W, Otis B, et al. Cancer statistics, 2011: the impact of eliminating socioeconomic and radical disparities on premature cancer death. CA Cancer J Clin. 2011;61:212–36.
3. Covens A, Rosen B, Murphy J, et al. Changes in the demographics and perioperative care of stage IA(2)/IB(1) cervical cancer over the past 16 years. Gynecol Oncol. 2001;81:133–7.
4. Dargent D, Brun L, Roy M. Trachelectomy broaden. An alternative to radical hysterectomy in the treatment of invasive cancers developed on the outer surface of the uterine cervix [in French]. J Obstet Gynecol. 1994;2:292–5.
5. Pareja R, Rendon GJ, Sanz-Lomana CM, Monzon O, Ramirez PT. Surgical, oncological, and obstetrical outcomes after abdominal radical trachelectomy – a systematic literature review. Gynecol Oncol. 2013;131:77–82.
6. Diaz JP, Sonoda Y, Leitao MM, Zivanovic O, Brown CL, Chi DS, et al. Oncologic outcome of fertility-sparing radical trachelectomy versus radical hysterectomy for stage IB1 cervical carcinoma. Gynecol Oncol. 2008;111:255–60.
7. Höckel M, Horn LC, Manthey N, Braumann UD, Wolf U, Teichmann G, Frauenschläger K, Dornhöfer N, Einenkel J. Resection of the embryologically defined uterovaginal (Müllerian) compartment and pelvic control in patients with cervical cancer: a prospective analysis. Lancet Oncol. 2009 Jul;10(7):683–92.
8. Chiantera V, Vizzielli G, Lucidi A, Gallotta V, Petrillo M, Legge F, Fagotti A, Sehouli J, Scambia G, Muallem MZ. Laparoscopic

radical hysterectomy in cervical cancer as total mesometrial resection (L-TMMR): a multicentric experience. Gynecol Oncol. 2015;139(1):47–51. pii: S0090-8258(15)30071-8.
9. Vercellino GF, Piek JM, Schneider A, Köhler C, Mangler M, Speiser D, Chiantera V. Laparoscopic lymph node dissection should be performed before fertility preserving treatment of patients with cervical cancer. Gynecol Oncol. 2012;126(3):325–9.
10. Pareja R, Rendón GJ, Vasquez M, Echeverri L, Sanz-Lomana CM, Ramirez PT. Immediate radical trachelectomy versus neoadjuvant chemotherapy followed by conservative surgery for patients with stage IB1 cervical cancer with tumors 2 cm or larger: a literature review and analysis of oncological and obstetrical outcomes. Gynecol Oncol. 2015;137(3):574–80.
11. Schneider A, Köhler C. Locoregional recurrence after laparoscopic radical trachelectomy: the vaginal cuff must be closed to avoid tumor cell contamination of the peritoneal cavity. Int J Gynecol Cancer. 2015;25(4):550.
12. Lee CL, Huang KG, Wang CJ, et al. Laparoscopic radical trachelectomy for stage Ib1 cervical cancer. J Am Assoc Gynecol Laparosc. 2003;10:11–115.
13. Cibula D, Ungar L, Palfalvi L, et al. Laparoscopic abdominal radical trachelectomy. Gynecol Oncol. 2005;97:707–9.
14. Park NY, Chong GO, Cho YL, et al. Total laparoscopic nerve-sparing radical trachelectomy. J Laparoendosc Adv Surg Tech. 2009;19:53–8.
15. Park JY, Kim DY, Suh DS, et al. Reproductive outcomes after laparoscopic radical trachelectomy for early-stage cervical cancer. J Gynecol Oncol. 2014;25:9–13.
16. Martin A, Torrent A. Laparoscopic nerve-sparing radical trachelectomy: surgical technique and outcome. J Minim Invasive Gynecol. 2010;17:37–41.
17. Lu Q, Zhang Y, Liu C, et al. Total laparoscopic radical trachelectomy in the treatment of early squamous cell cervical cancer: a retrospective study with 8-year follow-up. Gynecol Oncol. 2013;130:275–9.
18. Ebisawa K, Takano M, Fukuda M, et al. Obstetrics outcomes of patients undergoing total laparoscopic radical trachelectomy for early stage cervical cancer. Gynecol Oncol. 2013;131:83–6.
19. Kucukmetin A, Biliatis I, Ratnavelu N, et al. Laparoscopic radical trachelectomy is an alternative to laparotomy with improved peri-operative outcomes in patients with early-stage cervical cancer. Int J Gynecol Cancer. 2014;24:135–40.
20. Martinez A, Poilblanc M, Ferron G, et al. Fertility-preserving, surgical procedures, techniques. Best Pract Res Clin Obstet Gynecol. 2012;26:407–24.
21. Geisler JP, Orr CJ, Manahan KJ. Robotically assisted total laparoscopic radical trachelectomy for fertility sparing in stage IB1 adenosarcoma of the cervix. J Laparoendosc Adv Surg Tech A. 2008;18:727–9.
22. Regan L, Braude PR, Trembath PL. Influence of past reproductive performance on risk of spontaneous abortion. BMJ. 1989;299:541–5.
23. Preterm birth. In: Cunningham FG, Gant NF, Leveno KJ, et al., editors. Williams obstetrics. 21st ed. New York: McGraw-Hill; 2001. p. 689–727.
24. Querleu D. Laparoscopic radical hysterectomy. Am J Obstet Gynecol. 1993;168:1643–5.
25. Gottschalk E, Lanowska M, Chiantera V, Marnitz S, Schneider A, Brink-Spalink V, Hasenbein K, Koehler C. Vaginal-assisted laparoscopic radical hysterectomy: rationale, technique, results. JSLS. 2011;15(4):451–9.
26. Koehler C, Gottschalk E, Chiantera V, Marnitz S, Hasenbein K, Schneider A. From laparoscopic assisted radical vaginal hysterectomy to vaginal assisted laparoscopic radical hysterectomy. BJOG. 2012;119(2):254–62.

Laparoscopic Radical Hysterectomy with Anterior and Posterior Exenteration – Gynecological Perspectives

45

Shailesh P. Puntambekar, Yamini M. Gadkari, Vikrant C. Sharma, Suyash S. Naval, Seema S. Puntambekar, and Natasha U. Singbal

Introduction

Uterine malignancies are a common cause of cancer death amongst women. The incidence has risen in the recent years because of increasing awareness and screening [1, 2]. Radical hysterectomy continues to be the most common surgical approach in treatment of an early stage carcinoma of the cervix and endometrium.

The role of laparoscopy in this setting is to offer all the benefits of a minimally invasive approach, while maintaining equivocal oncological outcomes of an open approach. Since the first radical hysterectomy performed by Clark in 1895 and the Wertheim's technique of radical hysterectomy in 1898 [2], the radical hysterectomy has evolved into a simpler procedure and the surgical approach has evolved over a period of time into a highly specialized and minimally invasive modality. With technological advances we now can perform the radical hysterectomy with minimally invasive techniques like laparoscopy and robotics [3].

Here the author describes his "Pune technique" of laparoscopic radical hysterectomy with operative steps which are standardized. This makes this technique universally acceptable as it is easily duplicable [3].

Advantages of laparoscopic surgery are shorter hospital stay, less postoperative pain, quicker postoperative recovery, cosmetically better, enables the patient to start adjuvant treatment as early as possible. Hence, the acceptance of minimally access surgery in the recent years has increased [2, 3].

S.P. Puntambekar (✉) • Y.M. Gadkari • V.C. Sharma • S.S. Naval
S.S. Puntambekar • N.U. Singbal
Minimal Invasive Surgery, Galaxy Care Laparoscopy Institute Pune, Karve Rd., Pune 411004, India
e-mail: Shase63@gmail.com; yaminingadkari@gmail.com; Vikrant.pgi@gmail.com; navalsuyash@gmail.com; Seemasp4@gmail.com; natashasingbal@gmail.com

Laparoscopic Radical Hysterectomy [2, 3]

Indications

1. Cervical cancer stage IA2 to stage IIA2
2. Endometrial cancer stage II

Preoperative radiation therapy is not a contra-indication for the laparoscopic procedure.

Contraindications

1. Evidence of peritoneal carcinomatosis or distant metastatic disease
2. Evidence of grossly involved lymph nodes

Preoperative

Liquid diet a day prior to the surgery.

Mechanical Bowel Preparation: Polyethylene glycol night before the operative to clear the bowels so as to keep them away from the operative field.

Enema and bowel wash should be avoided as this leads to dilatation of sigmoid colon.

Anaesthesia

Combined regional and general anaesthesia. The regional anaesthesia acts by blocking the sympathetic activity, contracts the small bowel and keeps it away from the operative field.

Patient Position

Patient is placed in modified Lloyd Davis position. A bolster is placed at the level of the anterior superior iliac spine which

I. Alkatout, L. Mettler (eds.), *Hysterectomy*, DOI 10.1007/978-3-319-22497-8_45

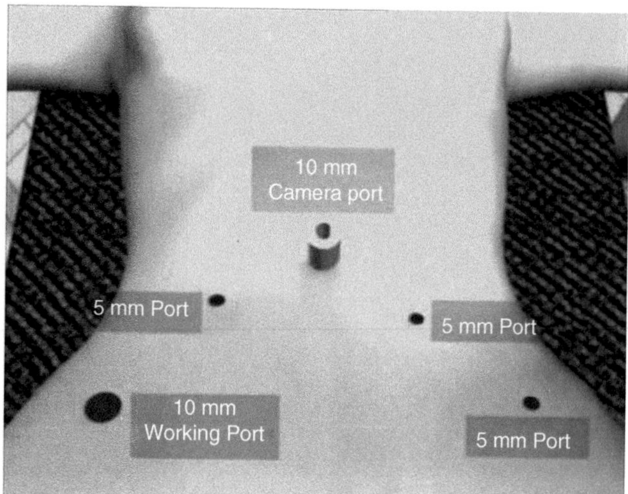

Fig. 45.1 Port positions

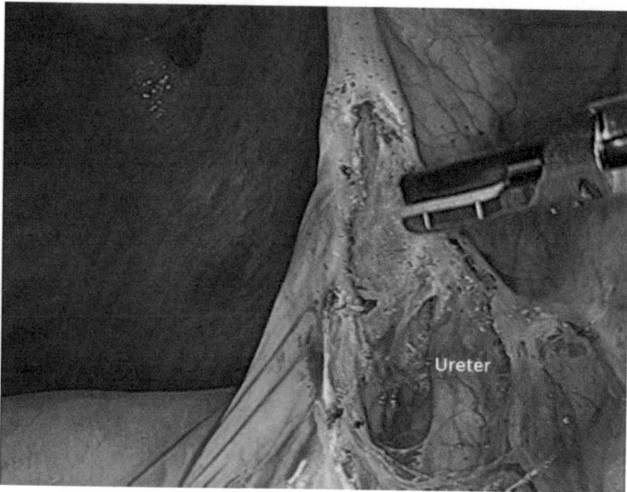

Fig. 45.2 Opening of peritoneum at the level of sacral promontory to expose ureter

causes elevation of the pelvis and results in a drop of the intestines cephalad. A gauze piece is kept in the vagina to prevent the loss of pneumoperitoneum after colpotomy.

Port Positions (Fig. 45.1)

A total of five ports are used.

A 10 mm camera port at the umbilicus.

A 10 mm working port at the Mcburney's point on the right side.

A 5 mm port pararectally (at rectus muscle margin) at the midclavicular line at the level of the umbilicus.

A set of two 5 mm ports are inserted as a mirror image of right side on the left side.

The surgeon stands on the right side, the assistant surgeon on the left side and the camera surgeon also stands on the left side, at the head end.

Procedure

The uterus is manipulated with a myoma screw in cervical malignancy. The myoma screw is introduced from the 5 mm left pararectal port and inserted into the fundus.The uterus is manipulated with a tenaculum in cases of endometrial malignancy.

Step 1: Posterior U- Cut

Uterus is anteverted. The rectum is retracted towards the left side. The right ureter is identified underneath the peritoneum at the level of sacral promontory. The peritoneum is opened medial to infundibulopelvic ligament with the help of harmonic shears to expose the ureter (Fig. 45.2). This cut is extended downwards into the Pouch of Douglas upto the level of uterosacral ligament (Fig. 45.3).The ureter should be on the lateral side and constantly under vision. The same steps are repeated on the left side and both the peritoneal cuts are joined in the Pouch of Douglas forming the posterior U- cut (Fig. 45.4).

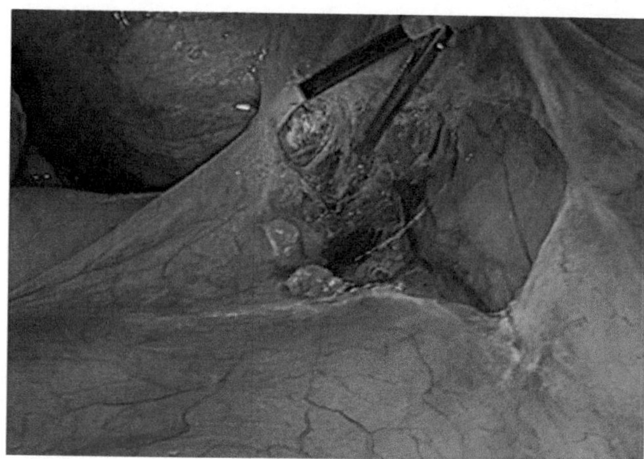

Fig. 45.3 Extending the peritoneal cut towards the Pouch of Douglas

Step 2: Dissection of Rectovaginal Space (Fig. 45.5)

The peritoneum in the Pouch of Douglas is pulled cephalad and the rectum is dissected off the posterior vaginal wall by remaining in between the two layers of Denonvillier's fascia. The plane between the fat and the posterior vaginal wall is dissected keeping in mind the dictum **"the fat belongs to rectum".**

Step 3: Dissection of Pararectal Space

The left ureter is retracted medially, and the posterior leaf of the broad ligament above the ureter is cut. A window is made in the anterior leaf of broad ligament. The ureter is now retracted

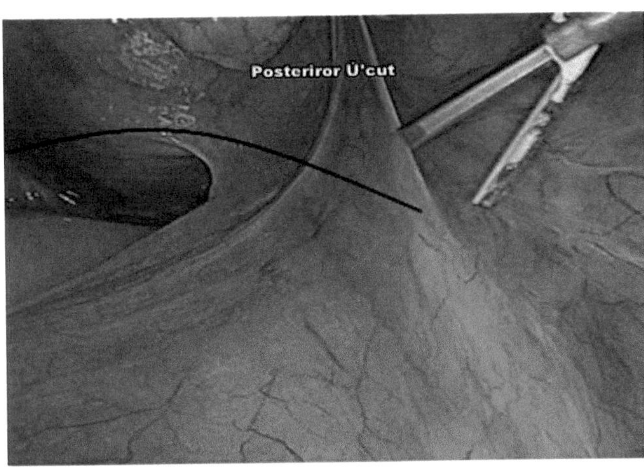

Fig. 45.4 Posterior U-cut

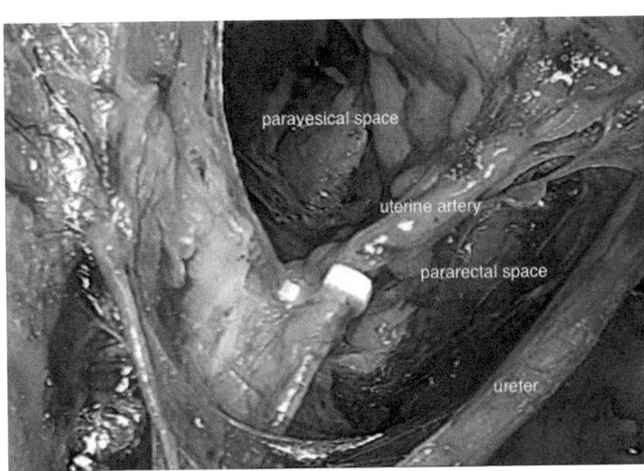

Fig. 45.6 Left pararectal space

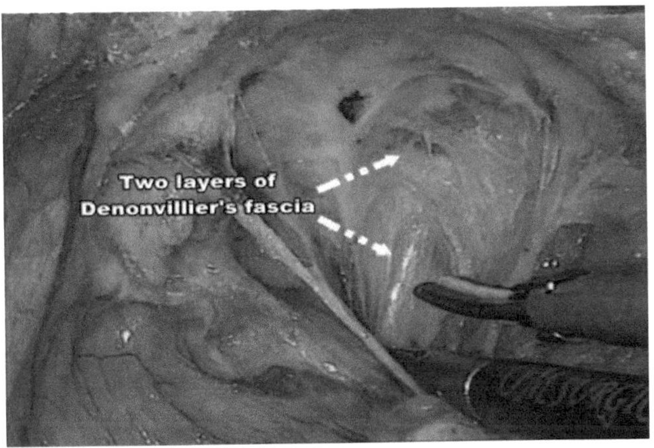

Fig. 45.5 Dissection of rectovaginal space

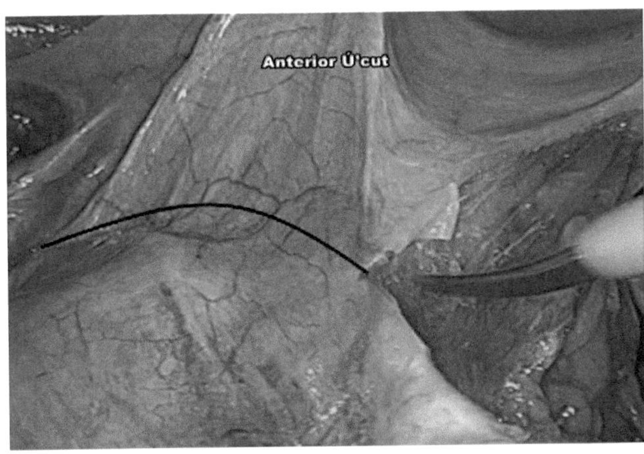

Fig. 45.7 Anterior U-cut

medially and the pararectal space is opened by remaining parallel and lateral to the ureter. The internal iliac artery forms the lateral boundary of this space and is then visualised. The only structure which crosses the pararectal space transversely is the uterine artery (Fig. 45.6). The space anterior to the uterine artery and medial to the obliterated hypogastric artery is dissected. The dissection is continued caudally by remaining parallel to the uterine artery to open the paravesical space upto the levator ani muscle. The uterine vein is seen below the ureter. The ureter always lies in the fork formed by the uterine artery anteriorly and the uterine vein posteriorly. Both the artery and the vein are individually clipped or ligated and then cut. This allows the visualization of the uterosacrals and the mackenrodt's ligament from their origin. The ureter is now retracted upwards and laterally and these ligaments are cut either with the harmonic or ligasure, as laterally as possible. The paracolpos which is continuation with the mackenrodt's ligaments is thus reached. This is divided up to the levator ani muscle. Similar steps are repeated on the right side.

Step 4: Anterior U- Cut

The uterus is retroverted. The peritoneum over the uterovesical fold is cut starting from the round ligament on right side to the left side forming the anterior U- cut (Fig. 45.7).The bladder is dissected off the uterus and cervix by remaining below the fat and above the pubocervicovesical fascia.The dictum used is **"fat belongs to the bladder"**(Fig. 45.8). The peritoneal cut is further extended up to the infundibulopelvic ligaments.

Step 5: Dissection of Ureteric Tunnel (Fig. 45.9)

The uterus is pulled to the left. The right ureter is traced along its entire course towards the bladder. The bladder peritoneum is held and the bladder is retracted upwards by the assistant. The cervicovesical ligaments, also known as the ureteric tunnel, is dissected with the help of Maryland's forceps (Fig. 45.10).There are two veins in the anterior cervicovesical ligament which is clipped and then cut. Similarly the posterior cervicovesical ligament is also clipped and cut. The

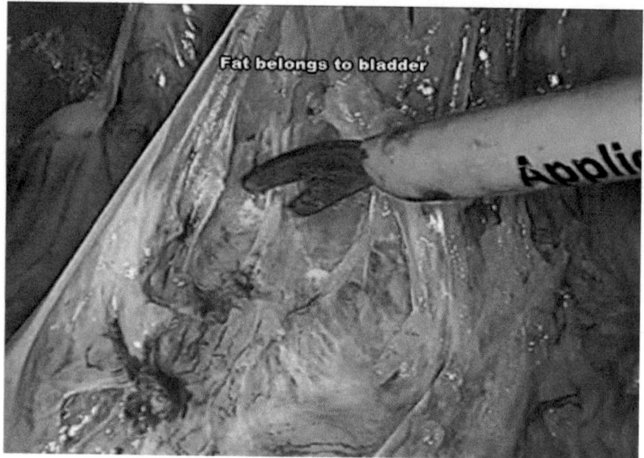

Fig. 45.8 Bladder dissection

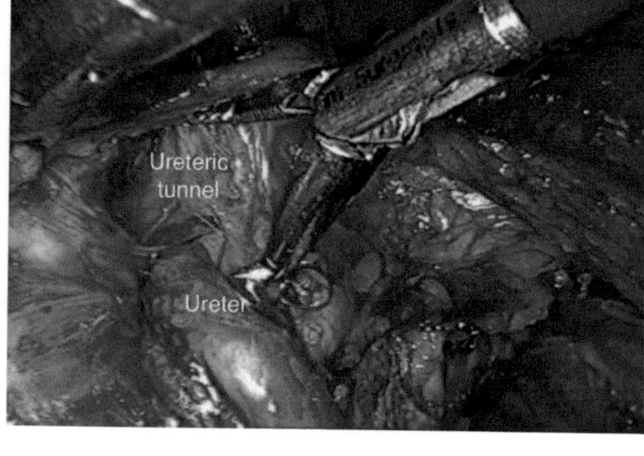

Fig. 45.10 Ureteric tunnel

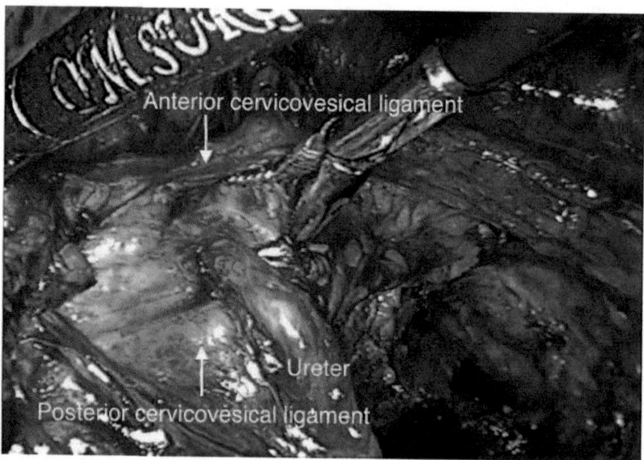

Fig. 45.9 Anterior and posterior cervicovesical ligament

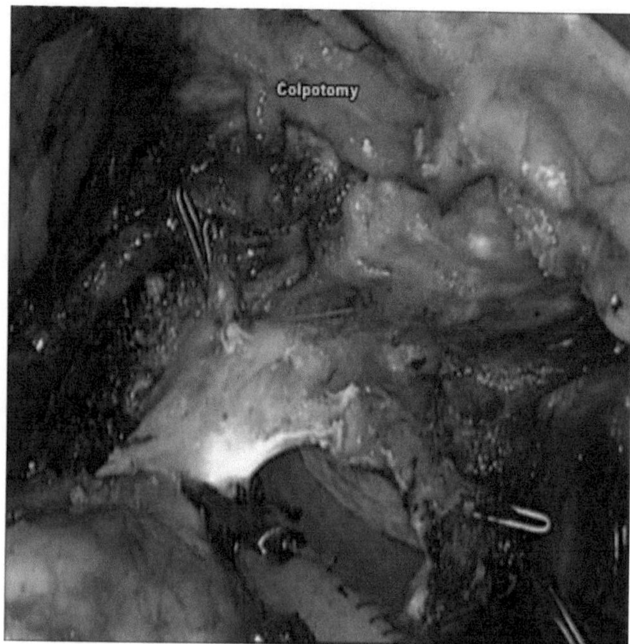

Fig. 45.11 Colpotomy

strands of endopelvic fascia which hold the ureter are cut on the medial side which further lateralises the ureter. The ureter can be seen upto its entry into the bladder. The bladder is pushed further down to achieve a good vaginal cuff, below the growth. The paracolpos is then cut as laterally as possible. These steps ensure that we can obtain maximum amount of paracolpos and the vaginal margin. The same steps are repeated on the left side making the trigonal area visible. Colpotomy is done above this level with the help of harmonic shears (Fig. 45.11). The infundibulopelvic ligaments are then cut and the entire specimen is separated and placed in an endobag.

Step 6: Lymph Node Dissection (Fig. 45.12)

The lymph node dissection is started at the bifurcation of common iliac artery (Fig. 45.13). All the fibrofatty tissue along the external iliac vein and artery is dissected, remaining in a direction parallel to the vessels upto the iliac bone which forms the lateral limit of the dissection. The medial limit is formed by the internal iliac artery and the lower limit is the obturator nerve (Fig. 45.14).Similar dissection is done on the opposite side. The entire nodal tissue obtained is put in the endobag (Fig. 45.15). The endobag is removed vaginally. Haemostatsis is achieved. Vault is closed with continuous locking intracorporeal suturing with vicryl 2–0, which is introduced through the 10 mm working port. Wound is irrigated with normal saline. It is not necessary to use any intra-abdominal drain. The ports are removed under vision and the port sites closed.

The Specimen This technique achieves a Pivers Type III [4]/ Querleu and Morrow [5] Type C Radical Hysterectomy,

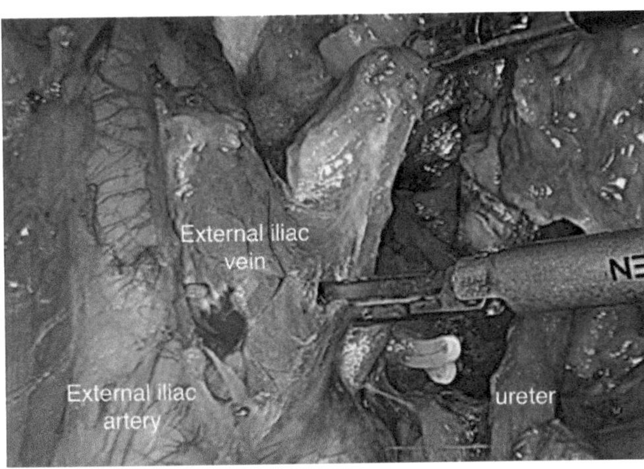

Fig. 45.12 Ilioobturator lymph node dissection

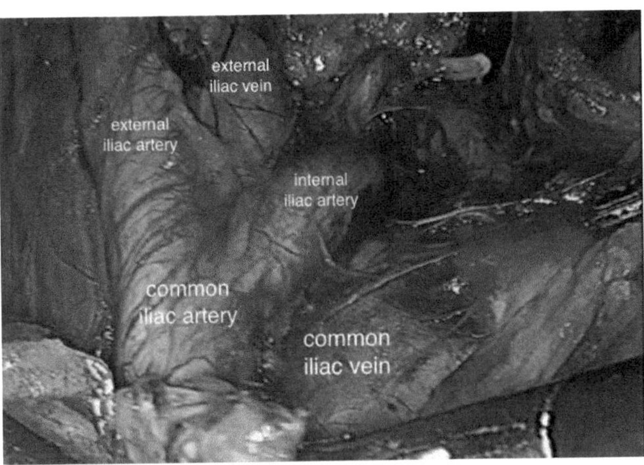

Fig. 45.13 Lymph node dissection of common iliac region

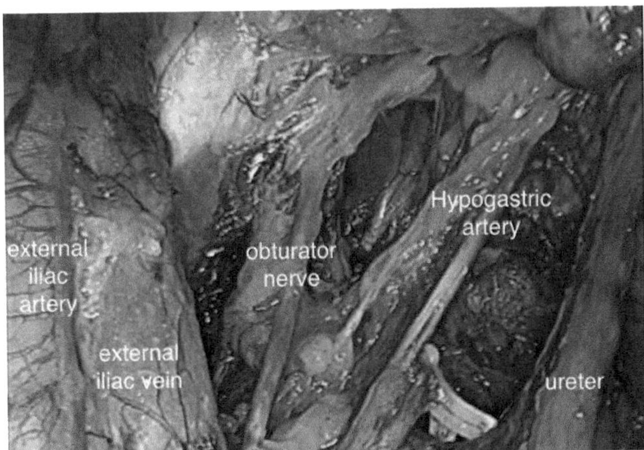

Fig. 45.14 Ilioobturator lymph node dissection

with a paracervical clearance of more than 3 cms, distal vaginal margin of more than 3–3.5 cms, nodal yield of 14–30 nodes.

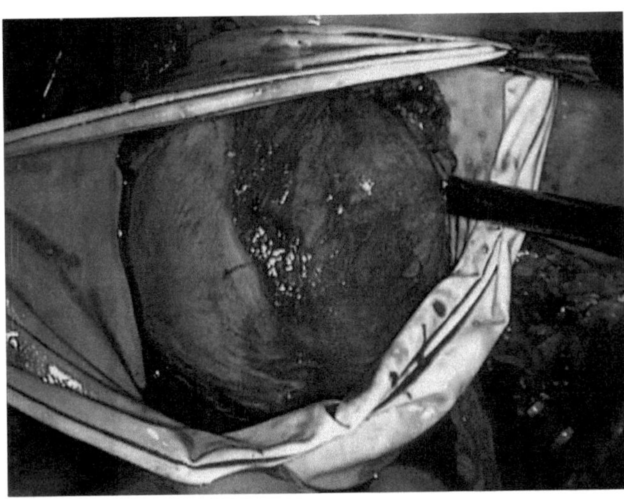

Fig. 45.15 Specimen delivery in endobag

Complications

Haemorrhage
Bladder injury
Ureteric injury
Bowel injury
Fistulas

Laparoscopic Nerve Sparing Radical Hysterectomy [6, 7]

The main disadvantage of laproscopic radical hysterectomy is the bladder dysfunction. This is caused due to autonomic nerve disruption with loss of anatomical bladder neck support and over distension of the bladder. A nerve sparing radical hysterectomy is involves the preservation of superior and inferior hypogastric and the pelvic splanchnic plexus, thus overcoming the complication of bladder dysfunction.

The procedure is the similar as that of laparoscopic radical hysterectomy. The hypogastric plexus lies lateral to the uterosacral ligaments. Thus the dissection at the level of uteroscarals is done carefully. The nerves are identified lateral to the uterosacrals and medial to the ureter.

The branches of the hypogastric nerve going to the uterus are identified in the connective tissue just posterolateral to the vagina and these branches are selectively cut and the nerve plane is lateralized on the posterior side. The bladder branch of the inferior hypogastric plexus is spared by lateralizing the nerve plane and the ureter. The posterior leaf of the vesicouterine ligament contains vesical veins that drain into the deep uterine veins which are individually clipped and cut. The bladder branch that passes just below the inferior vesical vein is also spared. The uterine and cervical branches

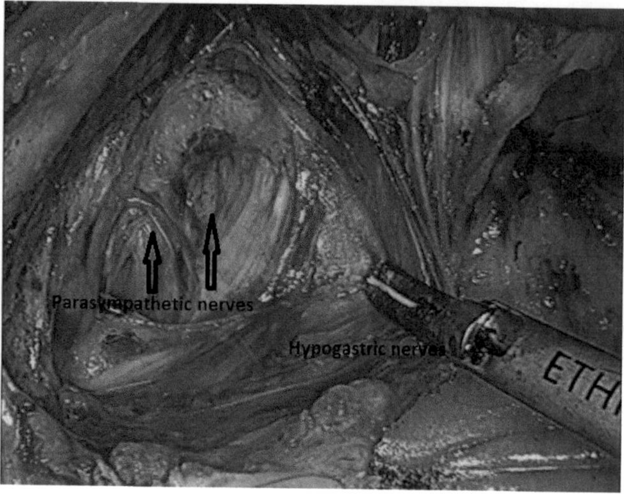

Fig. 45.16 Inferior hypogastric plexus

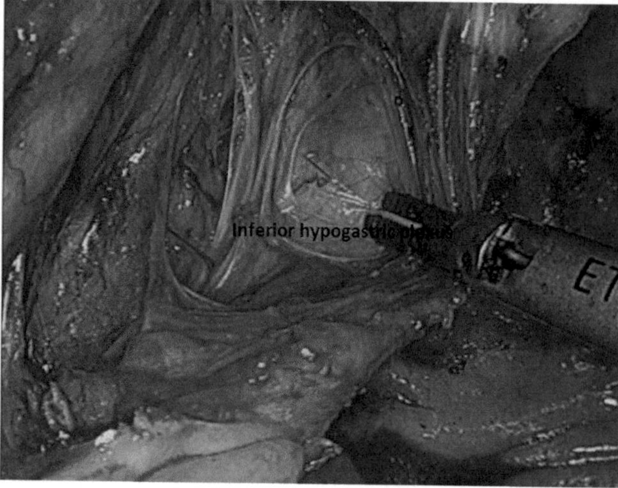

Fig. 45.17 Inferior hypogastric plexus

of the inferior hypogastric plexus in the anterior part are also selectively cut (Figs. 45.16 and 45.17).

The key structure in a nerve sparing radical hysterectomy is the uterine vein. The uterine vein should be cauterised and cut medial to the ureter in order to preserve the nerves.During colpotomy the nerve is lateral to ureter whereas in the initial stages of the dissection the hypogastric nerve and inferior hypogastric plexus were anatomically posteromedial to the ureter. The rest of the procedure is completed in the same way as the laparoscopic radical hysterectomy explained earlier.

Postoperatively the Foley's catheter is removes after 48 h. If urinary retention occurs Foley's catheterization is done again and patient is reassessed every 7 days.

Anterior Exenteration

Currently anterior exenteration is used as one of the modality for treatment of locally advanced cancers of the cervix.The anterior exenteration includes the removal of bladder, lower ureters, perivesical stump, uterus, ovaries and ilioobturator and iliac lymph nodes [8].

The following criteria should be used to decide the operability [9]:

1. Histological documentation of cancer in the palpable mass.
2. Absence of tumour extension to parametrium or pelvic sidewalls.
3. No involvement of the rectum by the growth.
4. Absence of gross pelvic or para aortic lymph node enlargement.
5. No peritoneal implants or bowel involvement.
6. No evidence of distant metastasis.

The absolute contraindications for surgery are:

1. Unilateral or bilateral pedal edema.
2. Sciatica or bone pain.
3. Poor medical condition.

Preoperative Workup

1. Computed tomography of the abdomen and pelvis
2. Chest radiography
3. Liver function tests
4. Cystoscopy

Procedure [10, 11, 12]

Anaesthesia, patient position and port positions are same as laparoscopic radical hysterectomy.

Steps 1 ,2, 3 remain the same as at radical hysterectomy (Fig. 45.18).

Step 4

The anterior dissection is begun by cutting right round ligament and then the anterior leaf of the broad ligament is cut. The peritoneum medial to the obliterated hypogastric artery is cut and the peritoneal cut is extended to the anterior abdominal wall, to separate the bladder from the anterior abdominal wall. Similar steps repeated on the left side.

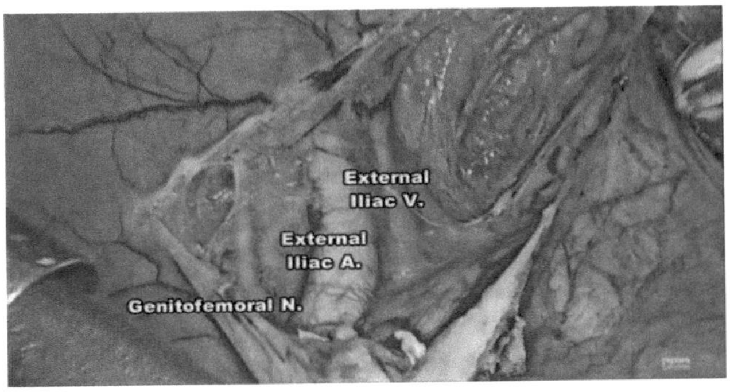

Fig. 45.18 External iliac vessels

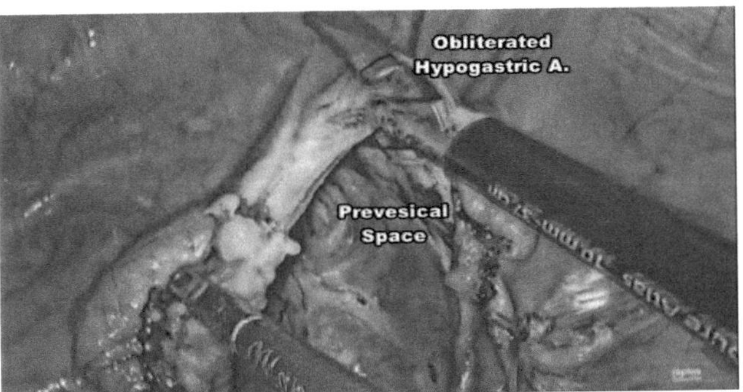

Fig. 45.19 Prevesical space

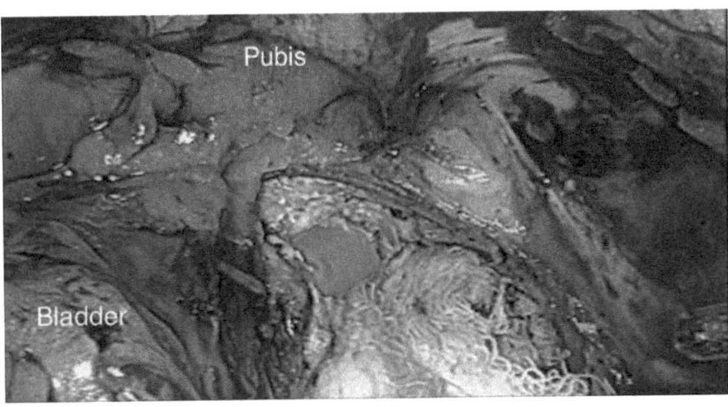

Fig. 45.20 Urethra being cut

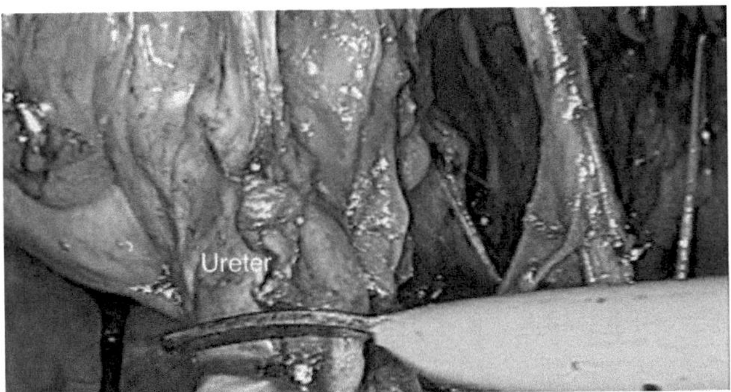

Fig. 45.21 Ureter being clipped and cut

Step 5

The bladder is then brought down from the anterior abdominal wall to enter the retro-pubic space i.e. the Cave of Retzius (Fig. 45.19) The tissue which is anterior and lateral to the urethra and vagina is cut. The urethra is accessed anteriorly (Fig. 45.20). The posterior urethral wall and the anterior vaginal wall are cut. A good length of vagina below the growth is exposed. The aim is to have a distal vaginal cuff of 3 cms.

Step 6

Colpotomy is done. Ilio obturator nodal dissection is done on both the sides and the tissue put in an endobag. Specimen is removed vaginally.

The type of urinary diversion plays an important role in the quality of life.

The various type of urinary diversions which can be done are

- ileal conduit
- ureterosigmoidostomy
- orthotropic illeal neo bladders
- Indiana pouch.

Ureterosigmoidostomy and ileal conduit can be done entirely laparoscopically while Indiana pouch and neo bladder have to be done by opening the abdomen. Here the author describes the ureterosigmoid anastomosis.

Step 7

The right ureter is cut (Fig. 45.21) and transfixed to the sigmoid colon anteriorly over the taenia coli. The end of the suture is held up for better visualization. A cut is made on the ureter which is fashioned into a fish mouth. A cut is also made on the sigmoid, anteriorly overlying the taenia coli (Fig. 45.22). A proximal full thickness stitch is taken, outside-in on colon and is continued inside-out on ureter. Infant feeding tube no. 5 or 6 is inserted in it, to act as a stent across the anastomosis (Fig. 45.23). It is proximally put into the ureter upto the renal pelvis. A note is made of the presence of flowing urine in the tube, to confirm proper placement. It is distally inserted into the opening made in the sigmoid colon. Once the stent is in place, the ureter edges are sutured with a 3:0 vicryl continuous suture. A full thickness continuous suture is taken on one side of the anastomosis, going from proximal to distal. The same suture is taken around and continued from distal to proximal end on the opposite side of the anastomosis. Right edge of ureterosigmoid anastomosis is sutured (Fig. 45.24). The suture is brought around from below the ureter, to be tied to its tail on the left side. A transfixation suture (hypnotic) is taken. The excess tip of ureter is trimmed. The left ureter is brought under the colon and then to the right side.

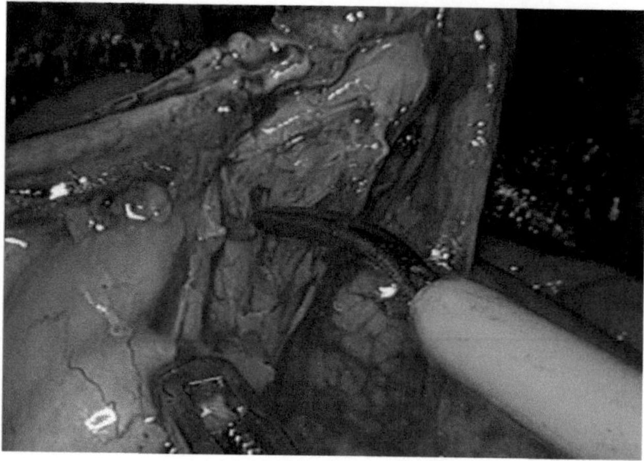

Fig. 45.22 A cut is being made on the sigmoid, anteriorly overlying the taenia coli

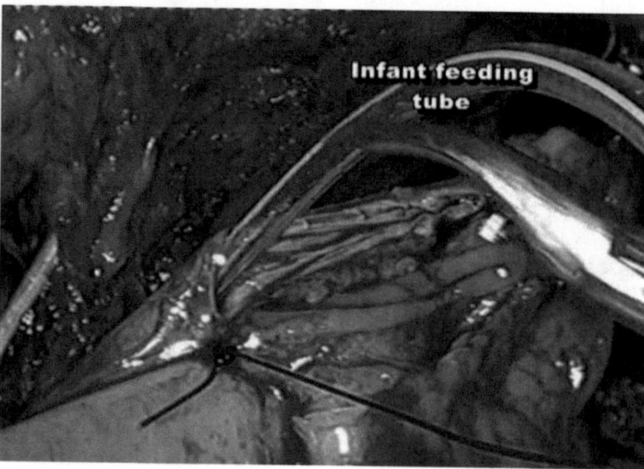

Fig. 45.23 Infant feeding tube no. 5 or 6 is inserted in the ureter to act as a stent across the anastomosis

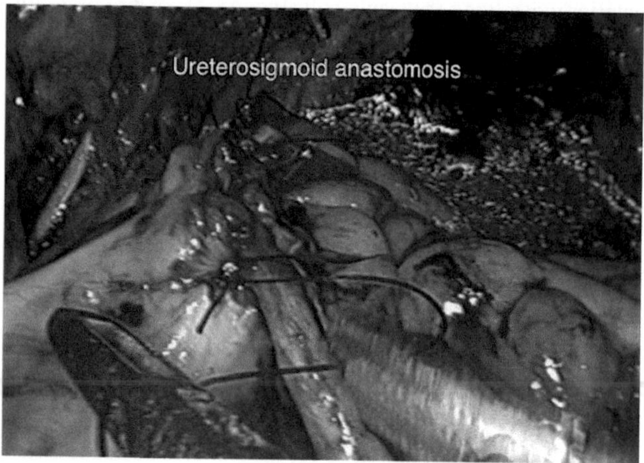

Fig. 45.24 Ureterosigmoid anastomosis

Step 8

The vagina is then sutured with 2:0 vicryl continuous intracorporeal suturing. Haemostasis achieved. An abdominal drain is placed in the pelvis. The ports are then removed under vision and closed.

Posterior Exenteration

Posterior exenteration is one of the treatments described for advanced cancers of the cervix, uterus, ovary, and rectum. Until recently, due to the complexity of the surgery, only the open method was used, however, minimally invasive surgery is now being used as a modality of surgery.

Preoperative Workup

1. Computed tomography of the abdomen and pelvis,
2. Chest radiography,
3. Liver function tests,
4. Cystoscopy
5. Proctoscopy.

All patients are examined under anesthesia before the procedure to confirm the extent of rectal involvement and to assess the feasibility of a stapled colorectal anastomosis.

The need for a temporary colostomy and the possibility of a permanent colostomy is also to be considered and discussed with the patients. The final decision is made at laparoscopy.

Inclusion Criteria

1. Ovarian cancer involving pouch of Douglas
2. Postradiation cervical cancer recurrence localized posteriorly
3. Cervical cancer with rectovaginal fistula
4. Vaginal cancer with rectal involvement

Exclusion Criteria

1. Extrapelvic spread
2. Distant metastasis including para-aortic nodes
3. Involvement of urinary bladder
4. Involvement of ureters
5. Limb edema or sciatic pain
6. Patient medically unfit

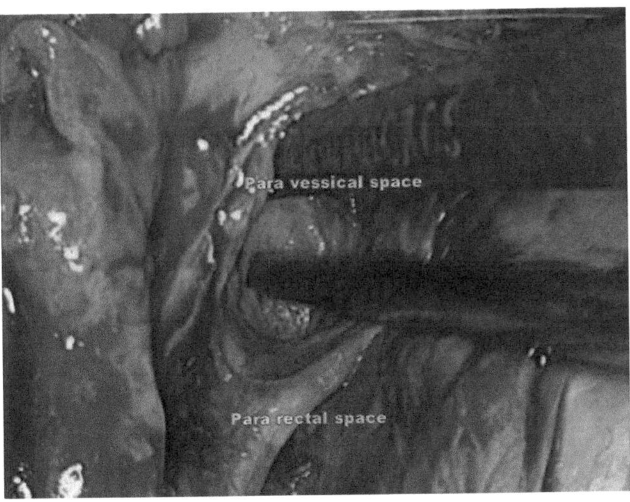

Fig. 45.25 Pararectal and paravesical spaces

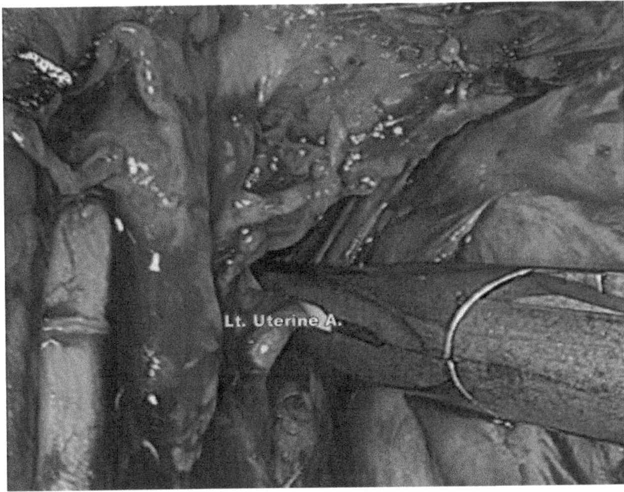

Fig. 45.26 Uterine artery being clipped

Preoperative Bowel Preparation

Routine bowel preparation was with 1 L of oral isosmotic solution (Peglec) taken the night before surgery.

Anaesthesia, patient position, port positions and surgeon position is same as laparoscopic radical hysterectomy.

Procedure [13]

The uterus can be manipulated with the help of a myoma screw or uterine hitch [14].

Step 1

The dissection is begun at the level of sacral promontory after identifying the external iliac vessels and ureters on the left side. A fold of peritoneum is opened and the ureters are lateralised. Infundibulopelvic ligament is skeletonised, clipped and cut.

Step 2

The pararectal spaces on both sides are dissected, remaining parallel and lateral to the ureter. Dissection proceedes anteriorly into the paravesical spaces upto the levator ani, which is used as the distal limit of dissection (Fig. 45.25). The uterine arteries and veins are clipped or ligated (Fig. 45.26). The ureter is further lateralised by dissecting the endopelvic fascia on the medial side. Similar steps are followed on the opposite side.

Step 3

Anterior U cut is made and the urinary bladder is dissected from the uterine cervix(Fig. 45.27).

Involvement of the urinary bladder at this stage would require a total pelvic exenteration.

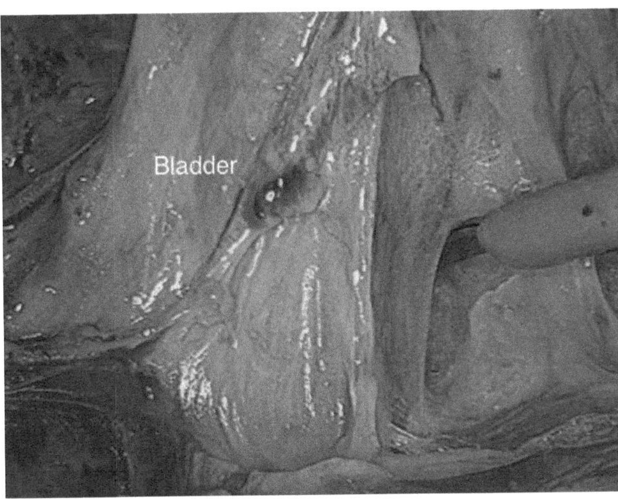

Fig. 45.27 Bladder being dissected using the principle of fat belongs to the bladder

Step 4

The presacral space is dissected between the rectum (Fig. 45.28) and the presacral fascia by following the dictam fat belongs to the rectum (Fig. 45.29). This is an avascular plane, and following this plane distally reveals the levator ani as its inferior limit. The virgin plane is entered between the vaginal wall and the rectum below the level of the Pouch of Douglas. The distal level of rectal involvement is the criterion to decide whether supralevator or infralevator posterior extenteration is to be used.

In supralevator cases rectal continuity be made using endostaping device. In patients with involvement of the sphincter complex, tumor involvement extending very low in the rectum and low malignant rectovaginal fistula require infralevator resection with a permanent colostomy.

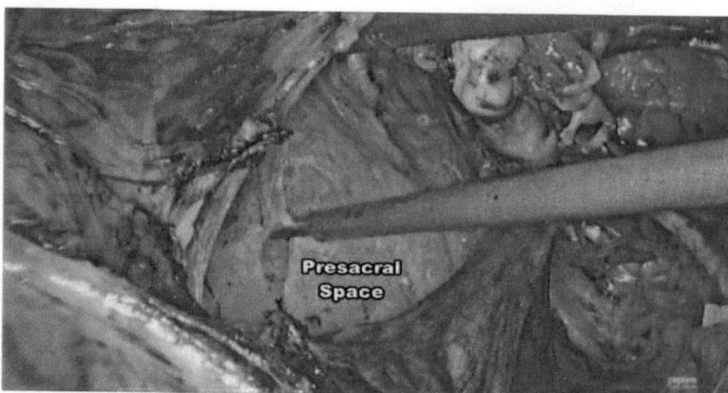

Fig. 45.28 Presacral space

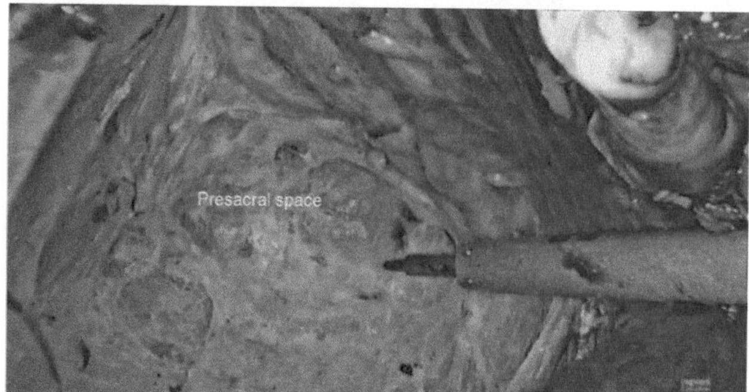

Fig. 45.29 Presacral space opened up using the principle of fat blongs to the rectum

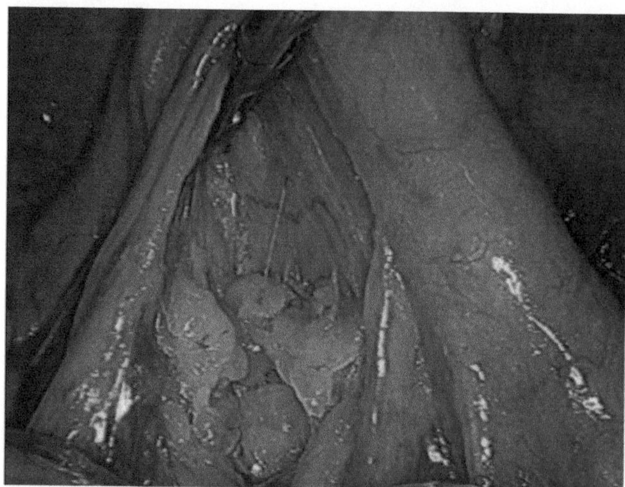

Fig. 45.30 Large bowel being mobilized

Step 5

A low colpotomy is performed.

Step 6

The proximal large bowel is mobilized (Fig. 45.30). The inferior mesenteric artery is clipped and cut at its origin (Fig. 45.31). The rectum distal to the tumor is visualized, which enables transection with the endostapling device (Fig. 45.32).

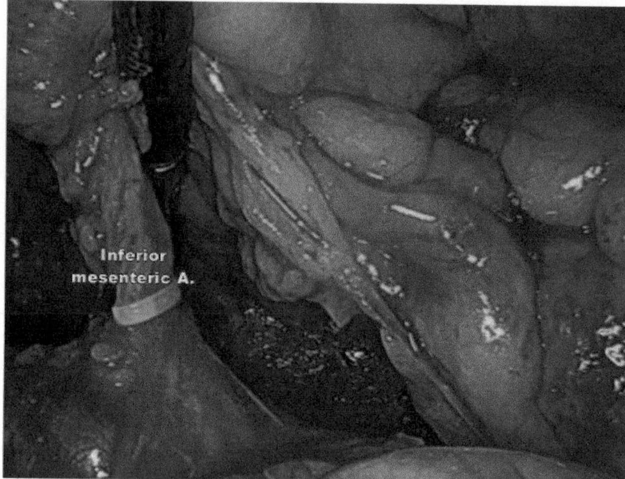

Fig. 45.31 Inferior mesenteric artery being clipped

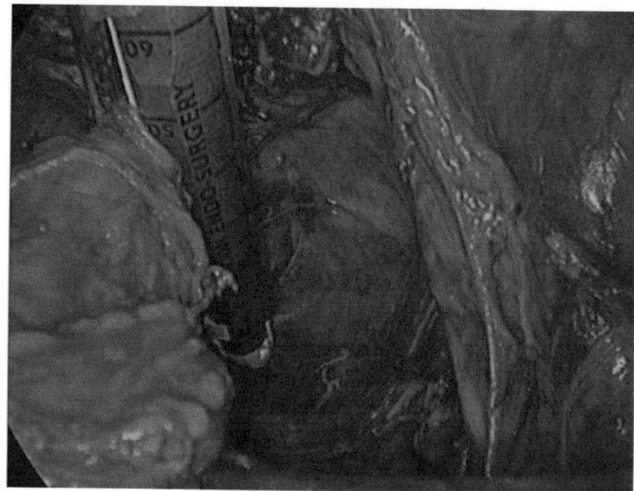

Fig. 45.32 Endostapler

Step 7

Although extraction of the specimen (Fig. 45.33)is possible vaginally, insertion of the anvil of the stapler in the colon is difficult via that route; thus, a suprapubic minilaparotomy of approximately 3 cm is used for specimen extraction. The remainder of the procedure was performed laparoscopically.

Thus, laparotomy is used for specimen extraction, proximal bowel transection and placement of the anvil of the end-to-end anastomotic stapler in the mobilized proximal colon. Circular stapled anastomosis was performed (Fig. 45.34) as well as temporary colostomy. Thus, posterior exenteration involves removal of the rectum, uterus, and vagina, and vulva if necessary.

Step 8

Fibrofatty lymphovascular tissue along the external iliac veins and the obturator nerves is removed (Fig. 45.35). The type of radical hysterectomy performed according to the new classification for radical surgery was type C2.

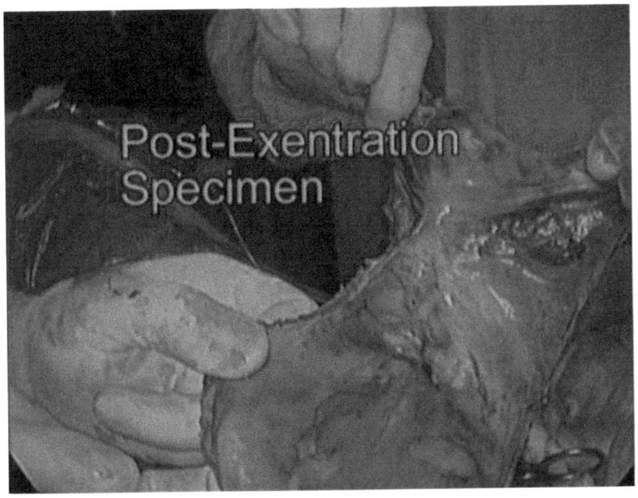

Fig. 45.33 Specimen of posterior exenteration

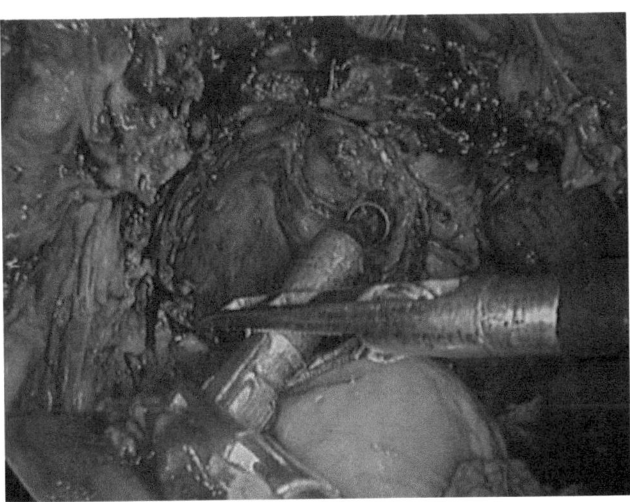

Fig. 45.34 Circular stapler

Complications

- Delayed bladder recovery
- Surgical site infection
- Anastamotic leak
- Prolonged ileus

Successful colostomy reversal is performed after 4–6 weeks in six patients with a temporary colostomy.

References

1. Shanta V, Krishnamurthi S, Gajalakshmi CK, et al. Epidemiology of cancer of cervix: global and national perspective. J Indian med Assoc. 2000;98(2):49–52.

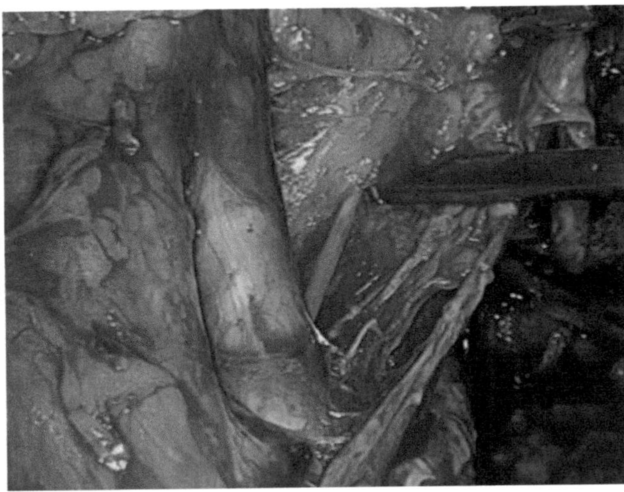

Fig. 45.35 Ilioobturator lymph node dissection

2. Ware RA, van Nagell Jr JR. Radical hysterectomy with pelvic lymphadenectomy: indications, technique, and complications. Obstet Gynaecol Int. 2010;2010 :9. doi:10.1155/2010/587610. Article ID587610
3. Puntambekar S, Palep R, Puntambekar S, Wagh G, Patil A, Rayate N, Agarwal G. Laparoscopic total radical hysterectomy by the Pune technique: our experience of 248 cases. J Minim Invasive Gynecol. 2007;14:682–9.
4. Piver, Ghomi. The twenty-first century role of Piver-Rutledge type III radical hysterectomy and FIGO stage IA, IB1, and IB2 cervical cancer in the era of robotic surgery: a personal perspective. J Gynecol Oncol. 2010;21(4):219–22.
5. Querleu D, CP M. Classification of radical hysterectomy. Lancet Oncol. 2008 Mar;9(3):297–303.
6. Puntambekar SP, Lawande A, Puntambekar S, Joshi S, Kumar S, Kenawadekar R. Nerve-sparing radical hysterectomy made easy by laparoscopy. J Minim Invasive Gynecol. 2014;21(5):732.
7. Puntambekar SP, Patil A, Joshi SN, Rayate NV, Puntambekar SS, Agarwal GA. Preservation of autonomic nerves in laparoscopic total radical hysterectomy. J Laparoendosc Adv Surg Tech A. 2010;20(10):813–9.
8. Brunschwig A. Complete excision of pelvic viscera for advanced carninoma. Cancer. 1948;1:177–83.
9. Brunschwig A. What are the indications and results of pelvic exenteration. JAMA. 1965;194:274.
10. Puntambekar SP, Kudchadkar RJ, Gurjar AM, Sathe RM, Chaudhari YC, Agarwal GA, Rayate NV. Laparoscopic pelvic exenteration for advanced pelvic cancers: a review of 16 cases. Gynecol Oncol. 2006 Sep;102(3):513–6.
11. Jamkar AV, Puntambekar SP, Kumar S, Sharma V, Joshi S, Mitkare S. Laparoscopic anterior exenteration with intracorporeal uretero-sigmoidostomy. J Minim Invasive Gynecol. 2015;22(4):538–9.
12. Martínez A, Filleron T, Vitse L, Querleu D, Mery E, Balague G, et al. Laparoscopic pelvic exenteration for gynaecological malignancy: is there any advantage? Gynecol Oncol. 2011 Mar;120(3):374–9.
13. Puntambekar S, Rajamanickam S, Agarwal G, Joshi S, Rayate N, Deshmukh A. Laparoscopic posterior exenteration in advanced gynecologic malignant disease. J Minim Invasive Gynecol. 2011;18(1):59–63.
14. Puntambekar SP, Patil AM, Rayate NV, Puntambekar SS, Sathe RM, Kulkarni MA. A novel technique of uterine manipulation in laparoscopic pelvic oncosurgical procedures: the uterine hitch technique. Minim Invasive Surg. 2010;2010:836027.

Laparoscopic Radical Hysterectomy (LRH) with Anterior and Posterior Exenteration: Urological Perspectives

46

Jens J. Rassweiler, Ali S. Gözen, Marcel Fiedler, and Jan T. Klein

Introduction

Laparoscopic and robot-assisted radical cystectomy has become an established procedure in the management of muscle-invasive bladder cancer and even accepted in the actual EAU-guidelines [1]. In a recent study coordinated by the EAU-section of uro-technology (ESUT) 18 % of patients were female [2], but the number is increasing due to the higher proportion of smoking women. Even, if there are forms of uterus-sparing of radical cystectomy, the vast majority of women undergo *anterior exenteration* with and without ovarectomy depending on the age of the patient. Based on this, the urologist is familiar with the anatomic details of such an operation regardless whether it is open, laparoscopic or robot-assisted [2, 3]. In gynaecology, the main indications include invasive carcinoma of cervix stage IVA and IVB, respectively advanced endometrial cancer with isolated invasion in the bladder (FIGO IVA) and stage T3 (FIGO III) of vulvar cancer [4–9].

In contrast, *posterior exenteration* is performed very rarely in patients suffering from advanced bladder cancer because the vagina represents an anatomical barrier for tumour infiltration. Such procedures are usually indicated as a salvage procedure (i.e. following radiotherapy of cervix carcinoma; advanced carcinoma of cervix or endometrium with invasion of bladder and rectum (FIGO IVA). Due to the complexity of this operation, it is mainly performed by open surgery in cooperation with a team of abdominal surgeons rather than by means of minimally invasive surgery [10, 11].

Therefore, we want to focus on technical aspects and outcome of *laparoscopic anterior exenteration*, which might be also indicated in advanced stages of cervical and endometrial cancers as well as in rare cases of carcinoma of the vulva respectively other tunours invading the vulva such as melanoma in combination with vulvectomy [6].

Beside the ablative part, the *form of urinary diversion* becomes an important factor with significant impact on the quality of life for the patient, but also regarding complexity and morbidity of the procedure particularly when performed laparoscopically [12–14]. There is an increasing experience with laparoscopic or robot-assisted ileal conduit and neobladders in the literature. Whereas advantages of the ablative part of operation have been demonstrated, it is still controversial about benefits of the complete intra-corporeal technique versus an extracorporeal approach extending the incision required for removal of the specimen [14, 15]. In women, however, the specimen can be extracted via the opening of the vagina [12]. Nevertheless, until now, there is no consensus, which approach offers the best option for the patients.

Indications for Laparoscopic Anterior Exenteration

Since recently, similar oncological outcome could be shown in a large European trial, there are no differ from those of open surgery, including T1–3 stages of bladder cancer. In gynaecology, anterior exenteration is only indicated for advanced stages (FIGO IV) of carcinoma of the cervix uteri, endometrial cancers, as well as vulva carcinoma (FIGO III) respectively as salvage therapy following irradiation and local progression, vesico-bladder fistula [4–9].

Type of Urinary Diversion

The choice of the type of urinary diversion depends on various factors, such as age, compliance, local extension of disease. Basically one has to distinguish between

J.J. Rassweiler (✉) • A.S. Gözen • M. Fiedler • J.T. Klein
Urology, SLK Kliniken Heilbronn,
Am Gesundbrunnen 20-14, Heilbronn 74078, Germany
e-mail: Jens.rassweiler@slk-kliniken.de; asgozen@yahoo.com; marcel.fiedler@gmail.com; JTK171272@gmx.net

I. Alkatout, L. Mettler (eds.), *Hysterectomy*, DOI 10.1007/978-3-319-22497-8_46

Table 46.1 Laparoscopic urinary diversion following anterior exenteration– technical steps and options

Operative step	Options	Comments
Transposition of ureter	Ileal-Conduit	Not for sigmoid-bladder
	Ileal-Neobladder (Studer)	Or ureterosigmoidectomy
		Not for Ileal-Neobladder (Hautmann)
Creation of reservoir	Intracorporeally	Technically difficult
		Stapler for GI-Anastomosis
		V-lock for neo-bladder
	Extracorporeally	Via mid-line incision
		Open technique
Conduit in females	Intracorporeally	Stapler for GI-Anastomosis
		Laparoscopic suture
	Extracorporeally (lap-assisted)	Via mid-line incision
		Open technique
Ureteral anastomosis	Intracorporeally	Sigmoid/Ileal-neobladder
		Sigmoid-pouch
		Ileal conduit
	Extracorporeally	Ileal neobladder (Studer)
		Ileal-pouch
Urethral anatomosis	Intracorporeally	All continent diversions (as first step)
		After re-insufflation (as last step)
	Extracorporeally	With laparoscopic pre-placed stitches

continent and incontinent diversion. The most popular form of incontinent diversion represents the ileal conduit. In selected case with one functioning kidney, ureterocutaneostomy might be an option. Continent urinary diversion includes a modified ureterosigmoidostomy with creation of a reservoir (Mainz-Pouch II), ileal neobladder, and various forms of catherizable pouches attached to the umbilicus (Table 46.1).

Whereas ileal conduit can be performed in almost every patient, ileal (sigmoid) neo-bladder requires some preliminaries: (i) the tumour has not infiltrated the bladder neck, (ii) the patient is able to manage the use of the neo-bladder including possibility to self-catheterize. A pouch can be also performed is almost all situation, however, represents a complex procedure and requires also the ability to self-catheterize [12, 16].

The patient has to be informed about all variation of urinary diversion. For this purpose, we administer an enema of 300 cm^3 of physiologic sodium chloride solution transanally and recod the time, the patient can hold this in the rectum. If the holding time is below 60 min, the patient should not undergo a continent diversion using a sigmoid pouch (ie Mainz-Pouch II). The use of ureterosigmodostomy without pouch has been abandoned. Additionally, we place a urostoma bag filled with 200 cm^3 of normal saline on the right side of the body to check the appropriate position of the stoma of an ileal conduit (Fig. 46.1). Since the rate of hypercontince of a neobladder in women may reach up to 30 %, women should be mentally and physically able to perform self-catheterization.

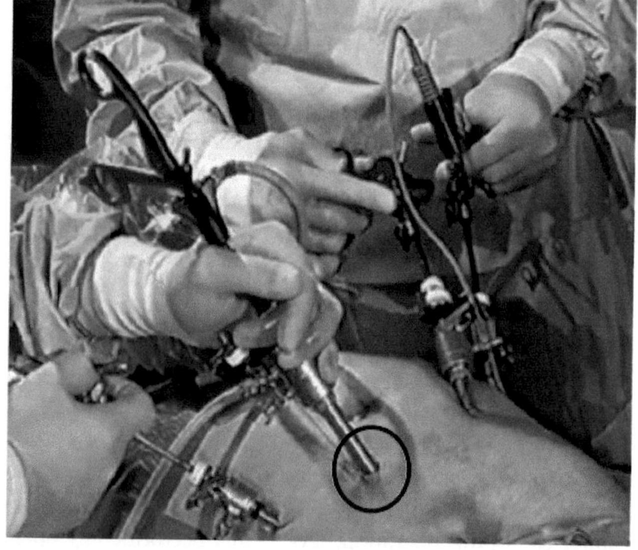

Fig. 46.1 Port placement for laparoscopic anterior exenteration – the right medial trocar entrance is used for the urostoma (*black circle*)

Patient Preparation

Initially, the bowel was prepared by oral self-administration of 2 l of electrolyte lavage solution during two days before the surgical procedure. However, we have changed this to a classical form of bowel preparation by administration of laxatives. It is important to hydrate the patient during the preoperative night (ie. 1500 ml electrolyte solution i.v) to improve renal function during the procedure and minimize the risk of hyperhydration by the anaethesiologist, which has a negative impact on the healing of bowel anatomosis.

Antibiotic prophylaxis with a cephalosporin (2 × 2g) and metronidazole (3x500 mg) is performed from day 1–5 and low molecular weight heparin (4000 units) is administered preoperatively and until the postoperative day 15. Compression stockings are applied as the patient is placed in supine position with the legs apart to allow free access to the vagina. The table is set to a 30 ° Trendelenburg position. An 18F-Foley catheter is inserted to drain the bladder and a nasogastric tube is positioned. As the lower limbs are carefully strapped to the table without compressions, no shoulder pads are necessary.

Technique of Laparoscopic Anterior Exenteration

Equipment

The technique is challenging, requiring state-of-the-art laparoscopic infrastructure and expertise. Using a five- or six-port transperitoneal approach (Fig. 46.1) anterior exenteration in combination with extended pelvic lymph node dissection is performed. Standard laparoscopic surgical equipment with few special instruments is required (Table 46.2). This may include an endoscopic stapler (i.e. Endo-GIA) for control of the pedicles of the bladder and eventually for the intracorporeally performed intestinal anastomosis. The use of an ergonomic chair like ETHOS might be very useful during the procedure (Fig. 46.2).

Table 46.2 Laparoscopic pelvic anterior exenteration–equipment

Standard laparoscopic equipment	
High flow insufflator / Air Seal	1
300 W Xenon light fountain	1
HD-camera (Karl Storz)	1
10 mm 30° laparoscope	1
Trocars	
10–12 mm trocars	2–3
5 mm trocars	3
(reusable trocars preferred)	
Instruments	
Laparoscopic Metzenbaum scissors, 5 mm	1
Laparoscopic bipolar forceps, 5 mm	1
Laparoscopic endo-dissectors, 5 mm	2
Laparoscopic right-angle-dissector, 10 mm	1
Laparoscopic atraumatic prehension forceps	2
Laparoscopic suction irrigation canula	1
Laparoscopy bags (i.e. Storz-Extraction Bag, 800 cm³)	1
Surgical endoscopy 5–10 mm clips appliers	1
Needle-holder (i.e. Duffner, Storz), for both hands	2
Endo-GIA30-stapler (i.e. Covedien)	
Optional	
Harmonic scalpel (i.e. Ultracision, Ethicon), 10 mm device	1
Ligasure® (ie. Covedien) 5–10 mm forceps	1
	1

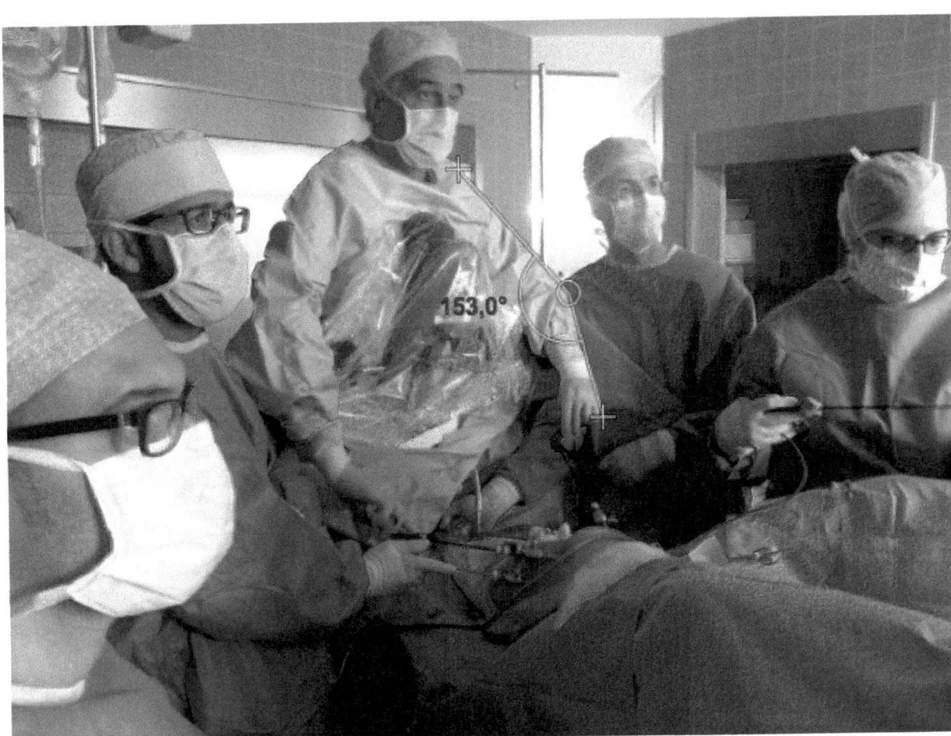

Fig. 46.2 Use of ergonomic chair (ETHOS, United States) with arm rest an chest support during laparoscopic anterior exenteration. The surgeons sits over the head of the patient

Trocar Placement

The patient is in supine position, with the lower limbs slightly (15 °) abducted. A 30 ° flexion is given to the knees, to define accordingly the value of Trendelenburg position. Extension of the hips should be avoided to prevent any backache. In male patients, the technique can be also performed with the legs in a paralell, non-abducted position.

The first 10 or 13 mm trocar is placed 1 cm above the umbilicus, using an open Hasson-technique through a mini-laparotomy. This trocar is reserved for the 30 °-laparoscope. The remaining four ports are placed under endoscopic control after establishment of the pneumoperitoneum (12–15 mmHg, high flow; AirSeal-Insufflator, Dach Medical Group, Freilassing. Germany).

At the « left Mac Burney » point a 12 mm diameter port is used, which can also be used to ease the retrieval of pelvic lymph nodes after dissection. At the true right Mac Burney point, another 12 mm trocar is placed to accept larger instruments (i.e. 10 mm-clip-applicator, right-angle dissector, needle with reducer-sheath, Endoscopic stapler) if necessary. Two 5 mm trocars are placed at the horizontal level of the navel, lateral to the 10/12 mm trocars. Optionally, on the midline, a 5 mm trocar is placed,.

During diagnostic laparoscopy the abdomen and pelvis are inspected focussing on possible peritoneal metastases. If necessary, intestinal adhesions are released by blunt and sharp dissection.

Posterior Dissection

The posterior dissection starts at the level of the recto vaginal space. As described in laparoscopic surgery for prolapse, the posterior vaginal bottom is lifted by the second assistant with a curved metal retractor, exposing immediately the recto- vaginal space to blunt and sharp dissection (Fig. 46.3a). This dissection is extended laterally to the ischio-rectal fossae (Fig. 46.3b).

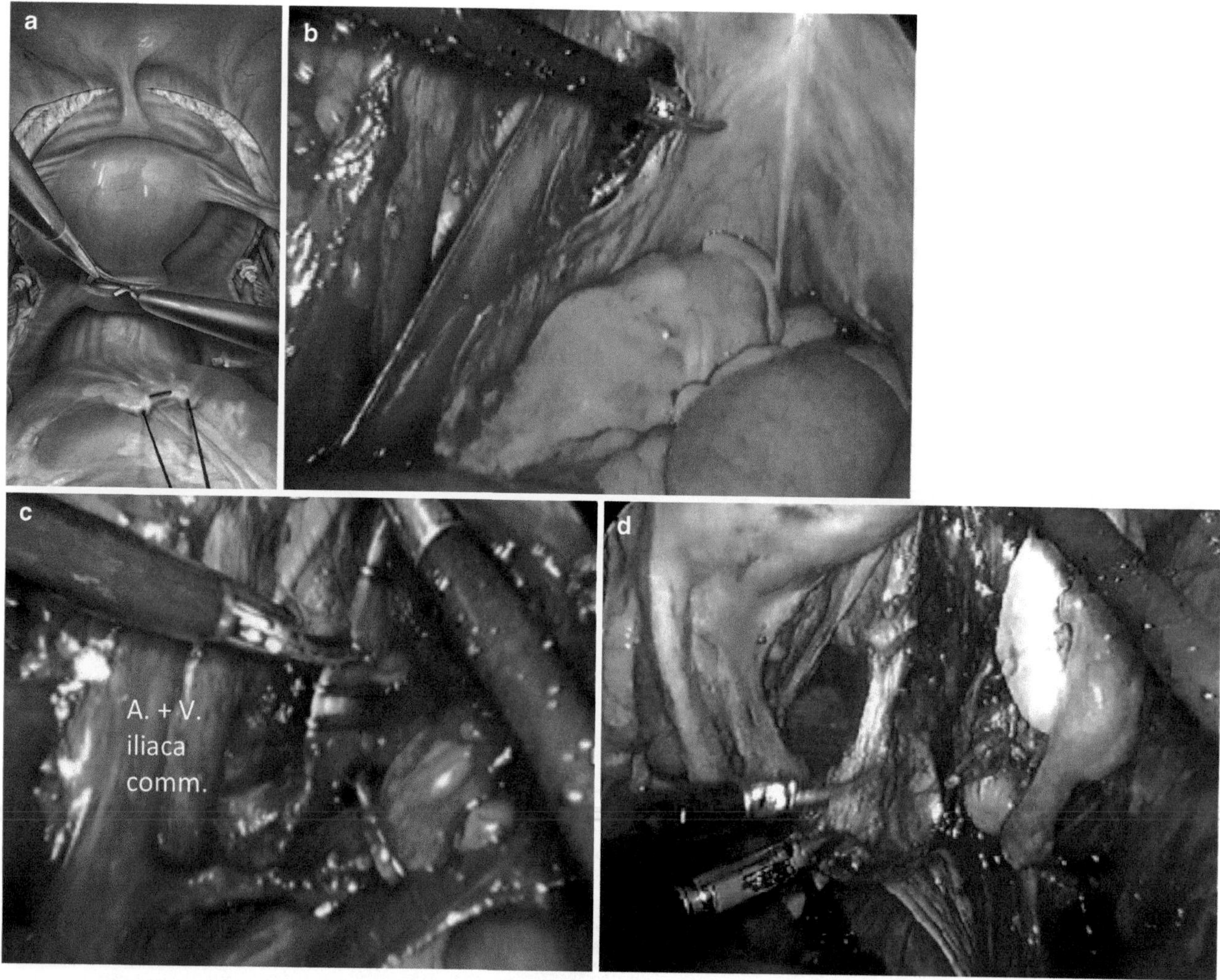

Fig. 46.3 Technical steps of laparoscopic anterior exenteration. (**a**) Posterior approach to the cul de sac, uterus and vagina. Note retraction stich of the sigmoid. (**b**) Incision of the peritoneum cranial to the sigmoid. (**c**) Division of the proximal pedicle (A. vesicalis sup.) on the right side between 10 mm Titanium-clips. (**d**) Transection of adherences between sigmoid and vagina. Both ovaries are included en-bloc in the specimen. Both uterine arteries have been clipped and divided

Table 46.3 Laparoscopic anterior exenteration–technical steps and options

Operative step	Options	Comments
Positioning of Patient	Deflected Supine Lithotomy	For all female patients
Trocar arrangement	Semilunar W-shaped	In case of ileal conduit one port = Urostoma
Transperitoneal access	None	Similar to open surgery
Incision of Douglas Pouch and retrovesical dissection	None	None
Pelvic lymph node dissection	Extended	According to indication
Division of ureters	None	None
Division of ovarian and uterine vessels	Endo-clips	For female patients
Division of umbilical ligaments and pedicles	Endo-GIA Hem-o-lock® Ligasure® Ultracision®	According to surgeon
Suturing of dorsal vein	None	None
Division of urethra	Closed by catheter Closed by clip	According to technique
Incision of anterior vagina	None	None
Entrapment of specimen	Organ-bag intra-abdominally Transrectally	None
Retrieval of specimen	Mini-laparotomy Transvaginal	Periumbilical, mid-line Pararectal Preferable in women

Exposure of Ureter and Iliac Vessels

If pelvic lymph node dissection is done primarily, the peritoneal incision starts at the level of the first peritoneal fold to find and dissect the ureters. The lateral incisions of the parietal peritoneum are extended to the internal inguinal ring. Then, both ligamenta teres are divided and retracted medially to expose the medial aspect of the external iliac vessels. Pelvic lymph node dissection is done on each side, as already described in view of frozen sections. The subsequent dissection and antegrade division of ureters and upper vesical pedicles are then carried out (Fig. 46.3c). In case of an anterior exenteration, removing the bladder and uterus together with the ovaries (Fig. 46.3d), this step includes the division of the ovarian vein (Table 46.3).

Anterior Dissection

Umbilical ligaments and urachus are divided and the prevesical space is opened and bluntly dissected to expose the anterior aspect of the bladder until the bladder neck, urethra and anterior wall of the vagina. Opening of the endopelvic fascia allows the dissection to be continued until the lateral aspects of the urethra, which is dissected completely, secured between clips and transected. A metal retractor might be moved to the anterior vaginal bottom to enable the dissection of the urethro-vaginal space, which is developed in a retrograde way after section of the urethra. Preoperative packing of the vagina can be used for the same purpose.

If an *orthotopic bladder replacement* is planned, a maximal urethral stump is then preserved in view of the anastomosis (Fig. 46.4a–e). According to patient's age and expectations, cystectomy may be carried out with vaginal and uterine preservation [16]. More often, according to the tumour burden and stage, the uterus and part of the vagina may need to be taken with the bladder.

The section of the vaginal anterior wall is carried out with the help of the retractor, giving a flat horizontal shape to vagina ; the gas leak during section of the vagina is prevented by packing the vagina or by the fingers of the assistant. The use of a high-flow insufflator (ie. AirSeal, Dach Medical Group, Freilassing. Germany) is very helpful. Then, the specimen can be extracted transvaginally preferably in an Endobag.

Removal of the Specimen

In advanced cases, even for this manoeuver entrapment of the specimen in an organ-bag is recommended to minimize the risk of tumour cell spillage. Finally, the vagina is repaired and closed with continuous sutures (Fig. 46.5 ; i.e. V-lock, 30 cm, SH-needle).

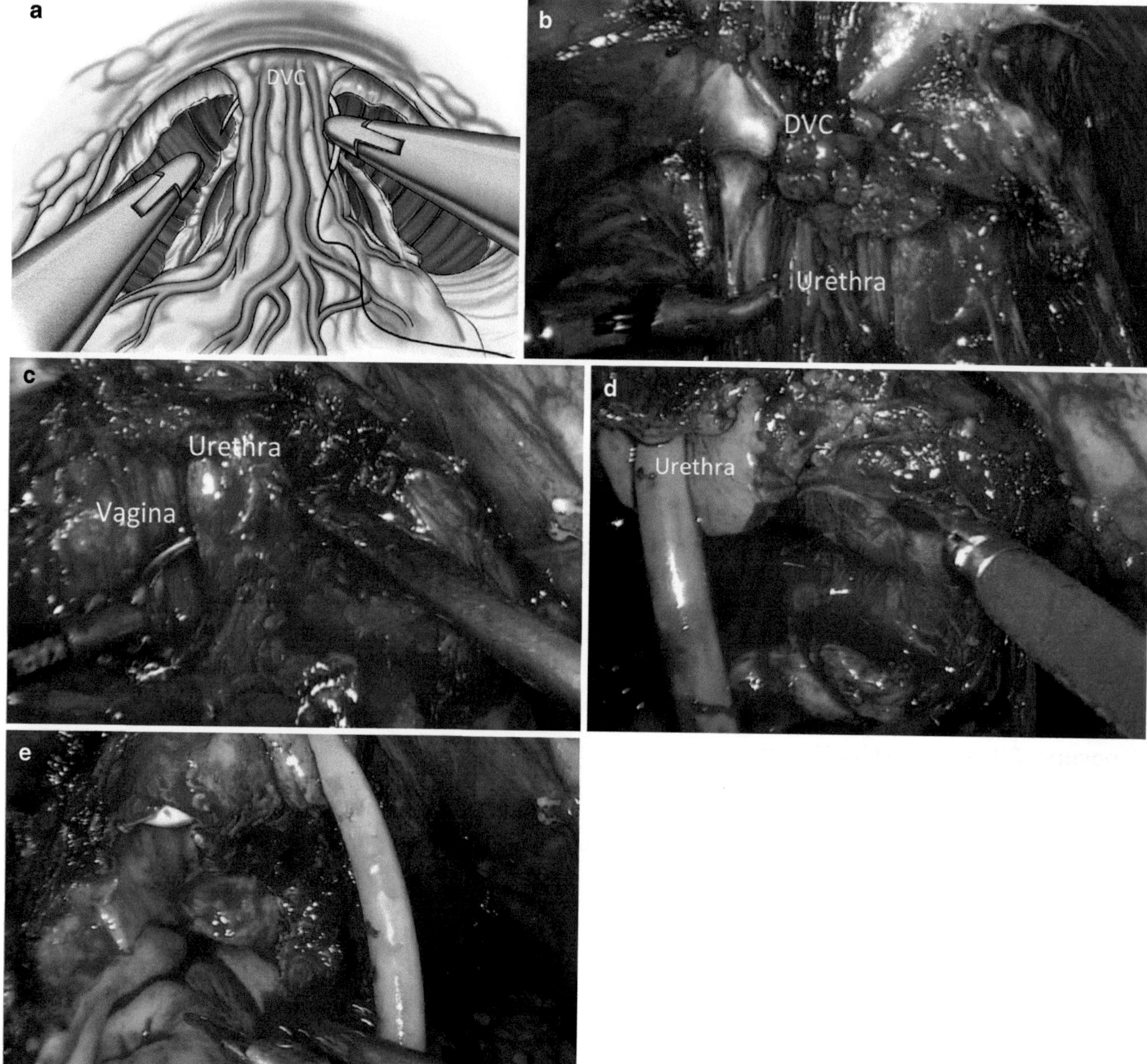

Fig. 46.4 Technical steps of dissection around the urethra during laparoscopic exenteration with formation of an ileal neo-bladder. (**a**) Suturing of the dorsal vein (Santorini's plexus) with an MH-needle (Vicryl, 15 cm or using a barbed suture (V-lock, 30 cm, SH-needle; Ethicon, Conneticut, United States). (**b**) Preservation of pubo-vesical collar and levator fascia lateral to the urethra to improve postoperative continence due to reduced injury to intrapelvic branches of pudendal nerve. (**c**) Posterior dissection of the urethra providing a long urethral stump. (**d**) Transection of the urethra at the level of the bladder neck with indwelling Foley catheter. (**e**) Opening of the vagina preserving a long anterior part. Note the finger of the assistant exposing the urethra and providing sealing of the vagina to minimize loss of carbondioxide

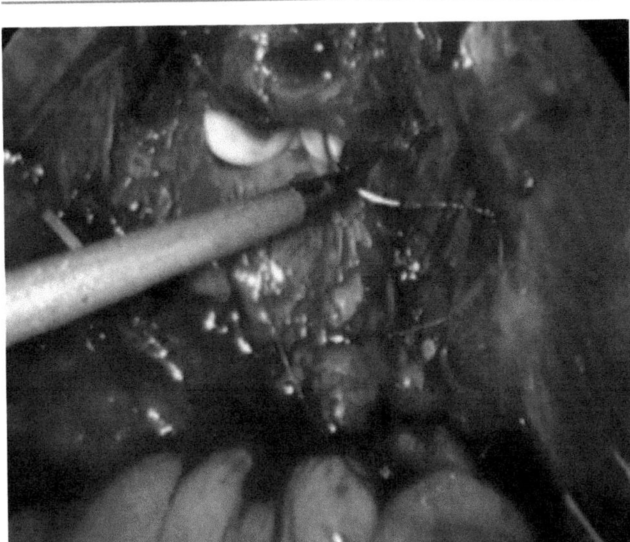

Fig. 46.5 Reconstruction of the vagina over the fingers of the assistant preferably using a barbed suture

Table 46.4 Distribution of urinary diversion in the ESUT-study on laparoscopic cystectomy

Urinary diversion	
Bricker	345 (69 %)
Ureterocutanostomy	10 (2 %)
Mainz II	8 (2 %)
Orthotopic neobladder	128 (25 %)
Continent pouch (Kock, Indiana)	12 (2 %)

Urinary Diversion

Depending on the gender, age of the patient as well as on the specific indication several types and techniques of urinary diversion can be performed (Table 46.4).

Laparoscopic Assisted Ileal Conduit

Completely Intra-Corporeally Construction of Ileal Conduit

In the female patient, following closure of the vagina (Fig. 46.5), the formation of an ileal conduit can be carried out completely laparoscopically. First step represents the transposition of the left ureter (Fig. 46.6a, b). Subsequently a 20-cm ileal segment is isolated by use of an endoscopic stapler (Fig. 46.6c). The ileo-ileal anastomosis is performed with antimesenteric side-to-side stapling and closure of the remaining opening by endoscopic suturing. Then, the distal end of the ileal segment is pulled out via an enlarged trocar incision in the right lower abdomen and sutured to the skin (Fig. 46.6d). Via the so created urostoma, single-J-stents can be introduced, and both ureters are stented and sutured to the ileal conduit in a modified Wallace-type (Fig. 46.6e) technique or individually using interrupted sutures, according to the Bricker's technique (Fig. 46.6d).

Extracorporeal Creation of Ileal Conduit

For most patients, the ileal conduit usually is performed laparoscopically assisted. The extended peri-umbilical mini-laparotomy for retrieval of the specimen is used for the isolation of the 20-cm segment of the distal ileum in an open technique (Fig. 46.7a, b). The ileo-ileal anastomosis is performed by interrupted seromuscular stitches, and the ileum is brought back into the abdominal cavity. Next step represent the uretero-ileal anastomosis using an open technique (Fig. 46.7c). Subsequently, the 10 mm trocar incision in the right lower abdomen is used as ileostoma (Fig. 46.7d): the trocar incision has to be enlarged allowing the pulling of the distal conduit end through the wound, and suture it to the rectus fascia and skin. After placement of two single-J-stents the ileal segment is manipulated back into the abdominal cavity, the periumbilical incision is closed, and the pneumoperitoneum re-established. The separate use of two trocar incisions offers the advantage of a better cosmetic result of the urostoma, and thus minimal problems with the adhesive plates.

Intracorporeal Uretero-Ileal Anastomosis

Alternatively the uretero ileal anastomosis can be performed laparoscopically, the already transposed left ureter is sutured to the right one in a Wallace fashion (i.e. Vicryl 3/0, RB1-needle). Then both ureters are stented by insertion of the single-J-stents, and sutured to the ileal conduit using interrupted or continuous sutures.

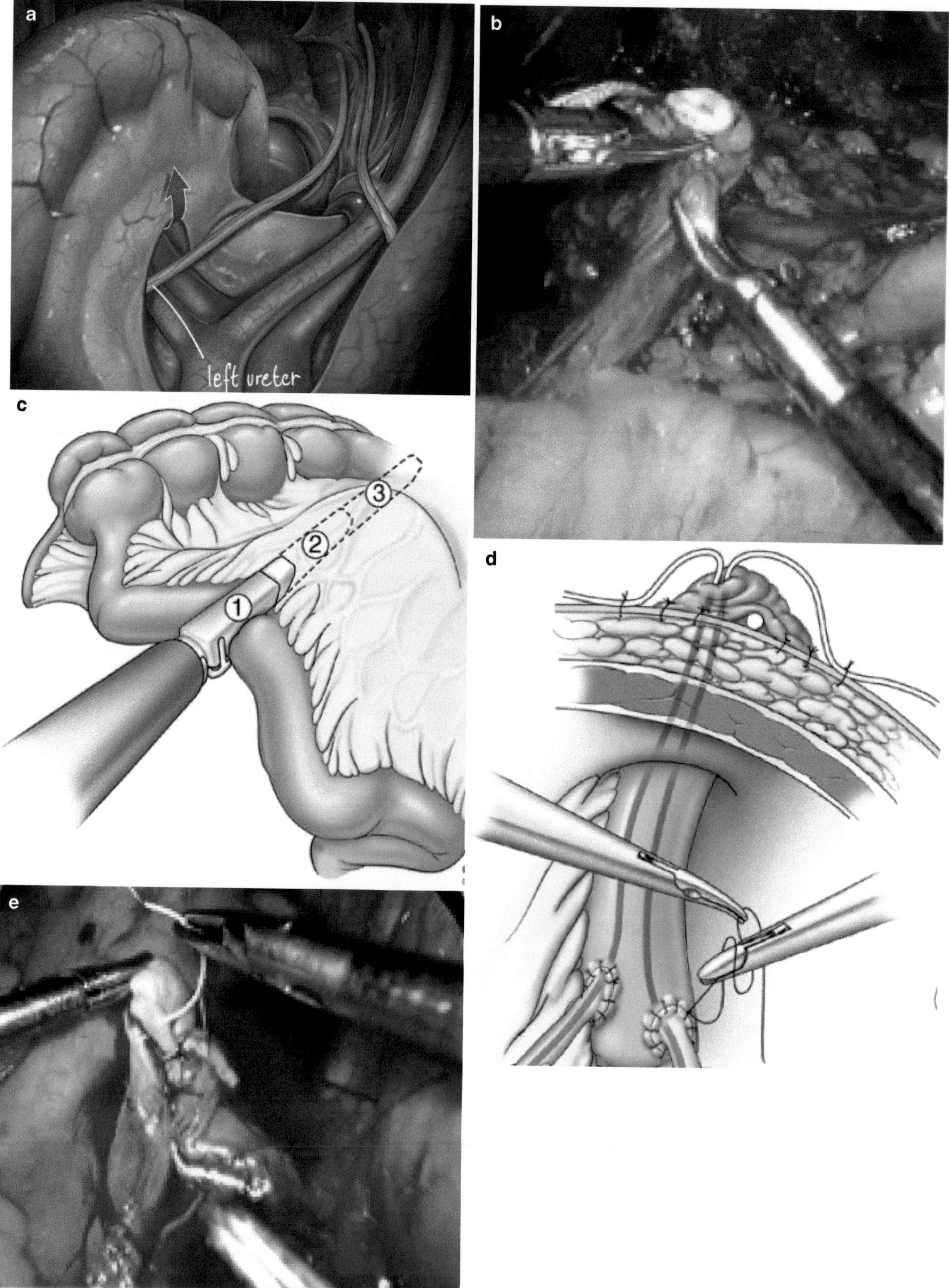

Fig. 46.6 Technical steps of laparoscopic intra-corporeal ileal-conduit. (**a**) Transposition of the left ureter under the meso-sigma, which is facilitated by the previous extended pelvic lymph node dissection (Level I and II). (**b**) Spatulation of the ureter. (**c**) Isolation 20 cm terminal ileum using endoscopic stapler. (**d**) Wallace end-to-side anastomosis of both ureters. (**e**) Fixation of the conduit at the skin; here use of to individual uretero-ileal implantation sites

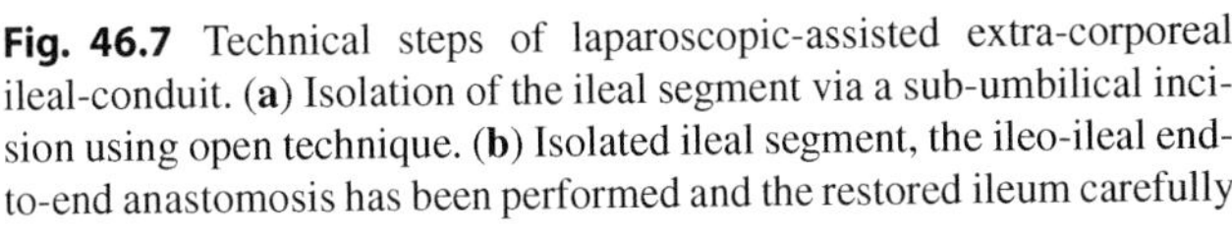

Fig. 46.7 Technical steps of laparoscopic-assisted extra-corporeal ileal-conduit. (**a**) Isolation of the ileal segment via a sub-umbilical incision using open technique. (**b**) Isolated ileal segment, the ileo-ileal end-to-end anastomosis has been performed and the restored ileum carefully replaced intraabdominally. (**c**) Uretero-ileal anastomosis performed in an open technique. (**d**) After accomplishing the urostoma, the abdomen is reinsufflated to check the correct position of conduit and anastomosis

Laparoscopic Assisted Orthotopic Neo-Bladder

This procedure represents the most frequently applied technique of urinary diversion following laparoscopic radical cystectomy, however in the advanced indications in gynaecology they cannot be applied in most cases due to involvement of the bladder neck and urethra.

Extra-abdominal Construction of the Ileal Neobladder

The orthotopic neobladder pouch is created by suturing opened small bowel together to form a new bladder. Like usually, a 55- to 60-cm segment of ileum located 15 cm away from the ileocecal junction is isolated and detubularized, leaving intact a proximal 10-cm isoperistaltic afferent Studer limb segment. As a function of surgeon's skills or preferences, an Hautmann's ileal bladder can be built as well and the bowel prepared accordingly. The continuity of the small bowel is restored outside the body through the incision made for specimen retrieval. Subsequently, a spherical neobladder is constructed extracorporeally. The anterior wall of the reservoir is closed by a running suture (i.e. PDS 3/0 with straight needle; Vicryl 3/0 ; SH-needle) ; the caudal part of this closure is left open in view of the neo-vesico-urethral anastomosis.

Uretero-Ileal-Anastomosis

A termino-terminal uretero-ileal anastomosis is then performed through the same incision, according to Wallace or to Bricker. Ureters are intubated with 8 Fr. smooth catheters

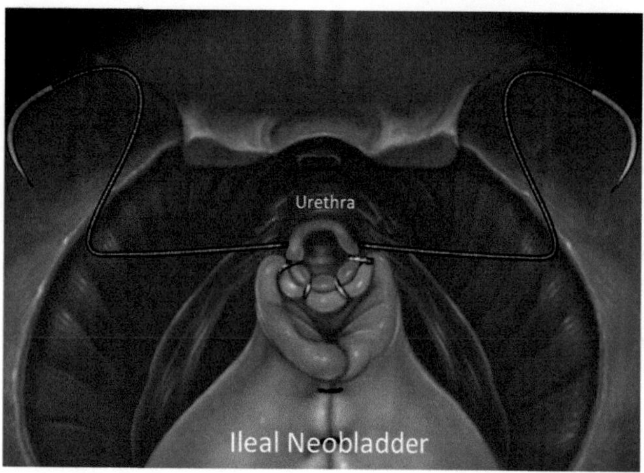

Fig. 46.8 Laparoscopic assisted extracorporeal neo-bladder: urethra-vesical anastomosis using van Veltoven-technique as last step of the procedure

temporarily attached to the posterior wall of the pouch with quickly absorbable sutures (Vicryl rapid ® *2/0)*. Both catheters are exteriorized through the anterior wall of the pouch, and subsequently, will be passed through the abdominal wall.

Urethral Anastomosis

When the pouch is ready, it is placed into the abdomen and the mini-laparotomy is closed classically. The 10 mm trocar is replaced for the telescope in an infraumbilical position and the pneumo-peritoneum re-insufflated.

After appropriate positioning of the ileal neo-bladder in its orthotopic position a « vesico » urethral anastomosis is started between the ileal orifice left open and the urethral stump using a single-knot technique (van Velthoven) minimizing the tension of the tissue (Fig. 46.8). The suture is started at six o'clock on the ileal edge of the suture ; two 6–7 in. of 2/0 PGA monolayer threads knotted together are used ; two hemi-running sutures are then built until twelve o'clock where the only knot tied intracorporeally is done.

When this suture is completed, a Jackson-Pratt drainage is placed into the pelvis ; the tube is exteriorized through a trocar hole in the right fossa. Fascial incisions of 10 mm are closed with interrupted sutures. The skin is closed with surgical staples.

Intra-corporeal Laparoscopic or Robot-Assisted Neo-Bladder

The entire neo-bladder can be also performed laparoscopically as a sigmoid-neobladder [12]. However, most experience exists with the ileal-neobladder replicating the Studer-neobladder. This includes mainly seven steps (Table 46.5). Evidently, this represents a very complicated procedure

Table 46.5 Surgical steps of robot-assisted intra-corporeal laparoscopic orthotopic neo-bladder

Choice of longest ileal segment and urethro-ileal anastomosis
Isolation of 60 cm ileal segment using endoscopic stapler
Ileao-ileal anastomosis using endoscopic stapler
Anti-mesenterial incision of ileal segment preserving the distal end for uretero-ileal anastomosis
Continuous suture of posterior wall of neo-bladder
Closure of anterior wall of neo-bladder
Stenting of both ureters
Uretero-ileal anastomosis

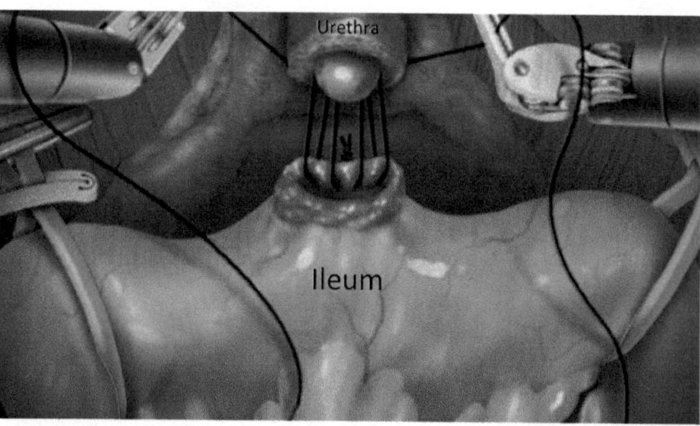

Fig. 46.9 Robot-assisted intracorporeal neo-bladder: anastomosis between urethra and ileal loop ad first step of urinary diversion

even with the assistance of the Da-Vinci-robot [17]. The main advantage represents the fact, that the first step includes urethro-ileal anastomosis (Fig. 46.9) thus minimizing the tension on anastomosis.

Laparoscopic Assisted Sigmoid-Pouch (Mainz-Pouch II)

The Mainz-Pouch II has been used frequently in women, due to the problems of "hypercontinence" with ileal neo-bladders ranging up to 30 % of the patients. However, this technique requires adequate control of the anal sphincter. The procedure can be performed completely laparoscopic or laparoscopic-assisted creating the sigmoid-pouch via a 10 cm- midline incision respectively using a Pfannenstiel incision.

Postoperative Management

In the first night, all patients were monitored on the intensive care unit for vital parameters monitoring and adequate pain management. Parenteral nutrition was continued until complete oral feeding (i.e. day 3–5). The drains are removed

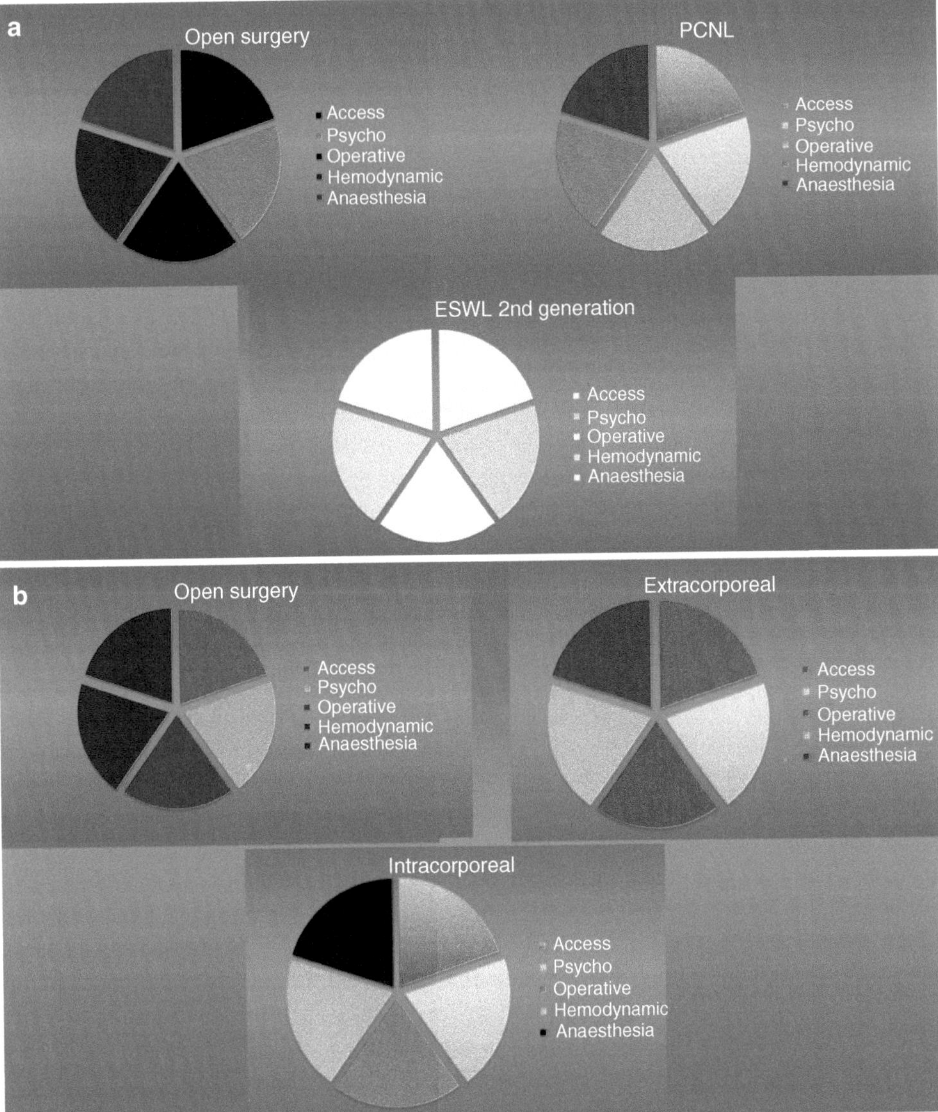

Fig. 46.10 The impact of minimally invasive techniques on the outcome of the procedure (according to Wickham 1991). (**a**) The introduction of percutaneous nephrolithtomy (PCNL) and extracorporeal shock wave lithotripsy (ESWL) significantly improved all five relevant aspects of a surgical procedure (*white* = no problems, *black* = significant problems). (**b**) The introduction of extracorporeal and intracorporeal radical cystectomy with urinary diversion has also reduced some of the five aspects, but on the other hand the associated morbidity might be increased (*white* = no problems, *black* = significant problems)

after reduction of secretion below 50–100 ml. On day 10 and 11, the ureteral stents are removed. Following a cystogram, the urethral catheter of neo-bladders is removed on postoperative day 14–18 (Fig. 46.10), after 48 h of intermittent clamping every 2 h.

Results

Of note, median LN retrieval in the *European Study* was 14 nodes (IQR 9–17). Positive surgical margins (PSM) were detected in 29 specimens (5.8 %): 26/29 PSM were found in patients harboring extravesical disease (11 had pT3, 15 pT4). This underlines, hat laparoscopic technique allows to perform adequate pelvic lymph node dissection.

Minor complications (Clavien I-II) occurred in 39 % (195/503) of patients, with post-operative infections requiring antibiotic therapy being the most frequent (Table 46.6). Major complications instead (Clavien IIIa-IVb) were found in 17 % (85/503) of patients in the early (<30 days) postoperative period. Specifically, 60 patients (12 %) underwent a second surgical operation of which 18 (4 %) due to bowel leak/peritonitis, 8 (2 %) for a urinary leak/fistula, 6 (1 %) for operative management of abdominal wall defects, 5 (1 %) for adhesiolysis due to occlusive syndrome, 3 (0.5 %) for surgical drainage of infected intraabdominal collection and 2 (0.5 %) for post-operative bleeding. Finally six patients (1 %) were re-operated for other causes (including endoarterectomy, ureteral reimplantation, fasciotomy, preputium necrosis), and in 12 patients the cause of re-operation was unknown. Clavien IV complications occurred in five patients (1 %), notably 2 acute respiratory failures (IVa), 1 acute renal failure (IVa), 1 septic multi-organ failure (IVb) and finally 1 patient experiencing both a Clavien IVa (respiratory distress)

Table 46.6 Postoperative complications of European Study on Laparoscopic Cystectomy

Post-op complications	
Clavien I	71 (14 %)
Clavien II	140 (28 %)
Clavien IIIa	29 (6 %)
Clavien IIIb	60 (12 %)
Clavien IVa	4 (1 %)
Hospital stay *(days)*	14 (10–20)
Median (IQR)	18 ± 15

and a Clavien IVb (septic multiorgan failure) complication. The rate of Clavien V complications was estimated at 2 %, with ten patients dying in the early postoperative period principally as a consequence of septic multi-organ failure. Conversion to an open procedure occurred in 12 cases (3.4 %), and depended on different factors ranging from extensive intra-abdominal adhesions to uncontrollable bleeding.

Oncologic Outcomes

There is no doubt, that the prognosis of anterior exenteration for advanced disease (FIGO IV; T4 TCC) is poor. Even in the European Study of laparoscopic cystectomy with D a median follow-up 52 months, 134 recurrences were detected and 118 (23 %) were due to metastatic disease, 14 (3 %) were local and 2 (0.5 %) urethral recurrences. 343 patients are alive and free from disease, 108 died as a consequence of bladder cancer (10 in the early post operative period, 98 due to disease progression), and 52 died of non-cancer specific causes. Actuarial RFS, CSS and OS rates were calculated at 74 %, 82 % and 79 % after 2 years; 66 %, 75 % and 62 % at 5 years; 62 %, 55 % and 38 % at 10 years. Patients with positive surgical margins experienced the worst survival outcomes, with 2- and 5 year OS rates of 31 % and 16 %, respectively. Tumor stage and node involvement were significant predictors of RFS, CSS and OS (all $p < 0.0001$). Notably, no port-site metastases were detected during the entire follow-up of this cohort.

Discussion

Anterior exenteration plays an important role in the management of muscle-invasive bladder cancer in women, representing 18–20 % of patient population [2]. In rare cases of advanced gynaecological tumours stage FIGO IV it may be also indicated [7, 8]. The procedure can be accomplished laparoscopically, but it represents a challenging operation. On the other site, laparoscopy in experienced hands has significantly reduced blood loss of this procedure. Most of the serious complications (Clavien III–IV) are not related to the ablative part, but to the urinary diversion ([7]; Table 46.6).

There is still the debate, whether the urinary diversion should be performed completely intracorporeally or extracorporeally extending the incision required for removal of the specimen. In women, the specimen can be extracted transvaginally. Thus, an additional incision becomes necessary. The main argument against the entire laparoscopic approach represents the technical difficulty of the procedure including bowel anastomosis, uretero-intestinal-anastomosis, stent placement which may be very time-consuming with the hazard of severe postoperative complications (Table 46.6). Even in the hand of the most experienced surgeons the OR-times are very long, which also adds to the associate trauma of the procedure [18].

In case of anterior exenteration for gynaecological indications, usually a neo-bladder is not indicated. This means, that an ileal conduit will be mostly performed. This might be easier, however, we still encountered some complications when doing the procedure intracorporeally, such as a fistula between conduit and ileum at site of intestinal anastomosis. Moreover, it is important to follow all surgical steps established in open surgery to minimize the risk of complications [18]. When using a sigmoid-pouch (Mainz-Pouch) for urinary diversion, we did not perform a sacropexy of the pouch, which resulted in formation of a sigmoidal-vaginal fistula. On the other side, to perform urinary diversion extracorporeally has the advantage of a significantly shorter operating time. Thus, the combination of laparoscopic anterior exenteration with extracorporeal ileal conduit may represent an ideal form of minimally invasive surgery for such extended cases. This can be nicely demonstrated when using the Wickham Wheel ([19]; Fig. 46.10).

In the future, further experience with robot-assisted radical cystectomy and urinary diversion may alleviate to perform the procedure [5, 17, 20]. This could include the use of easier-to construct neo-bladders (i.e. T-pouch, Y-pouch), the use of absorbable staplers and better suturing techniques. Actually, robot-assisted anterior exenteration with intracorporeally urinary diversion is still experimentally.

References

1. Gakis G, Efstathiou J, Lerner SP, et al. ICUD-EAU International Consultation on Bladder Cancer 2012: radical cystectomy and bladder preservation for muscle-invasive urothelial carcinoma of the bladder. Eur Urol. 2013;63:45–57.
2. Albisinni S, Rassweiler J, Abbou CC, Cathelineau X, Chlosta P, Fossion L, Gaboardi F, Rimington P, Salomon L, Sanchez-Salas R, Stolzenburg JU, Teber D, van Velthoven R. Long-term analysis of oncologic outcomes after laparoscopic radical cystectomy in Europe: results from a multi-centric study of EAU-section of Uro-Technology. BJU Int. 2015;115:937–45.

3. Pruthi RS, Wallen EM. Robotic assisted laparoscopic radical cystoprostatectomy: operative and pathological outcomes. J Urol. 2007;178:814–8.
4. FIGO committee on gynecologic oncology. FIGO staging for carcinoma of the vulva, cervix, and corpus uteri. Int J Gynaecol Obstet. 2014;125:97–8.
5. Iavazzo C, ID G. Robotic technology for pelvic exenteration in cases of cervical cancer. Int J Gynaecol Obstet. 2014;125:15–7.
6. Rajaram S, Maheswari A, Srivastava A. Staging for vaginal cancer. Best Pract Res Clin Obstet Gynaecol 2015; ahead of print
7. Martinez A, Fileron T, Vitse L, Querleu D, Mery E, Balague G, Delannes M, Soulie M, Pomel C, Ferron G. Laparoscopic pelvic exenteration for gynaecological malignancy: is there any advantage? Gynecol Oncol. 2011;120:374–9.
8. Mettler L, Meinhold-Heerlein I. The value of laparoscopic surgery to stage gynaecological cancers: present and future. Minerva Ginecol. 2009;61:319–37.
9. Jamkar AV, Puntambekar SP, Kumar S, Sharma V, Joshi S, Mitkare S. Laparoscopic anterior exenteration with intracorporeal urterosigmoidostomy. J Minim Invasive Gynecol. 2015;22:538–9.
10. Odetto D, Saadi J, Saraniti G, Noll F, Salvo G, Perrotta M. Laparoscopic posterior exenteration in cervical cancer: initial experience at Hospital Italiano de Buenos Aires: IGCS-0085 cervical cancer. Int J Gynecol Cancer. 2015;25(Suppl. 1):30–1.
11. Akiyoshi T, Nagasaki T, Ueno M. Laparoscopic total pelvic exenteration for locally recurrent rectal cancer. Ann Surg Oncol. 2015;22(12):3896. epub ahead of print
12. Rassweiler J, Frede T, Teber D, van Velthoven R. Laparoscopicradical cystectomy with and without orthotopic bladder replacement. Minim Invasive Ther Allied Technol. 2005; 14:78–95.
13. Rassweiler J, Godin K, Goezen AS, Kusche D, Chlosta P, Gaboardi F, Abbou CC, van Velthoven R. Radical cystectomy–pro laparoscopy. Urologe A. 2012;51:671–8.
14. Haber GP, Crouzet S, Gill IS. Laparoscopic and robotic assisted radical cystectomy for bladder cancer: a critical analysis. Eur Urol. 2008;54:54–62.
15. Hayn MH, Hellenthal NJ, Seixas-Mikelus SA, et al. Is patient outcome compromised during the initial experience with robot-assisted radical cystectomy? Results of 164 consecutive cases. BJU Int. 2011;108:882–7.
16. Gaboardi F, Simonato A, Galli S, et al. Minimally invasive laparoscopic neobladder. J Urol. 2002;168:1080–3.
17. Collins JW, Wiklund NP. Totally intracorporeal robot-assisted radical cystectomy: optimizing total outcomes. BJU Int. 2014; 114:326–33.
18. De Wilde RL. The danger of time-consuming operative laparoscopies: avoiding severe complications. Geburtshilfe Frauenheilkd. 2012;72:291–2.
19. JE W. Editorial: the concept of minimally invasive therapy. Minim Invasive Ther. 1991;1:1–5.
20. DeBernardo R, Starks D, Barker N, Armstrong A, Kunos C. Robotic surgery in gynecologic oncology. Obstet Gynecol Int. 2011;2011(2011):139867. Epub 2011 Nov 16.

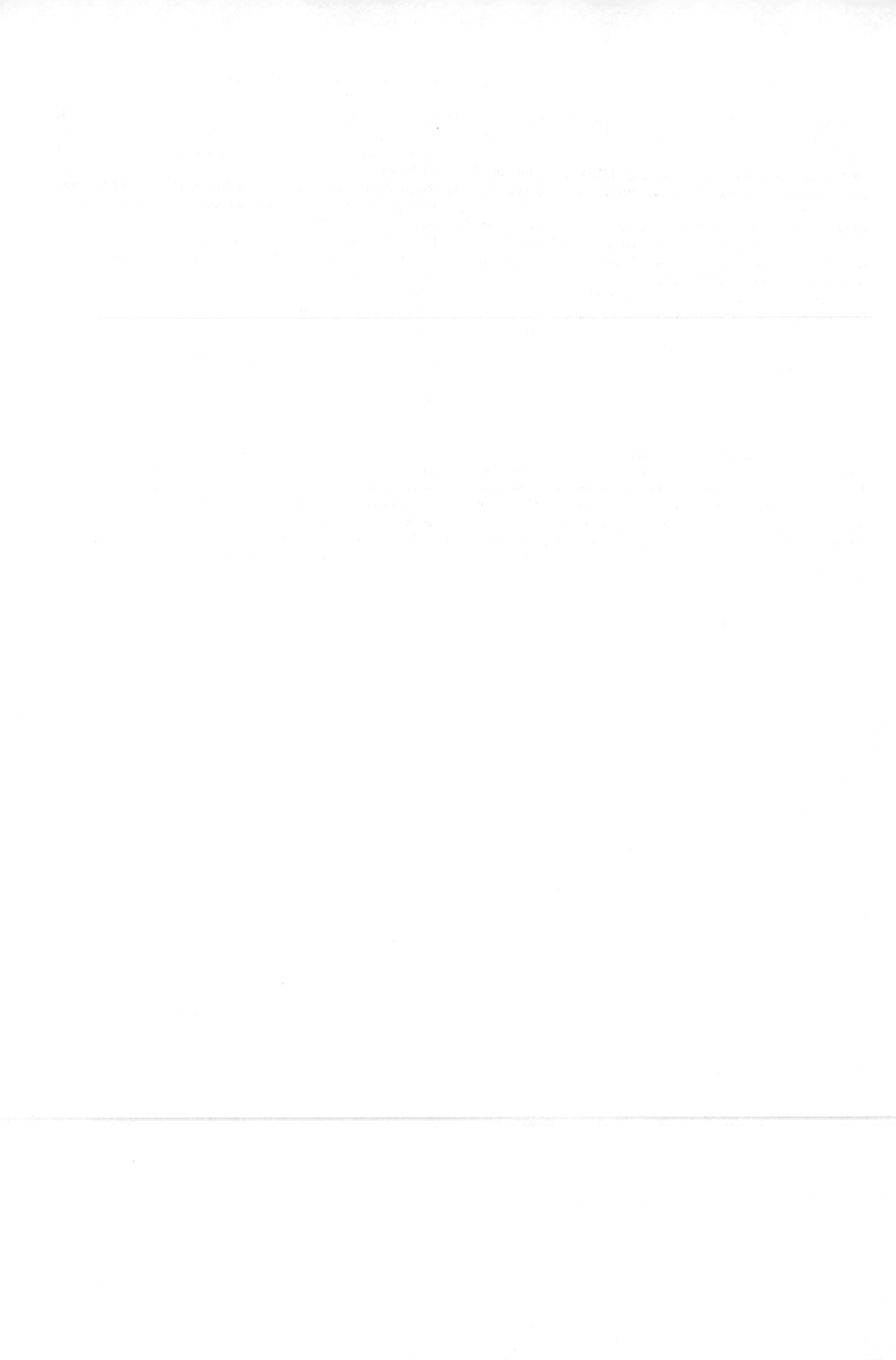

LRH with Anterior and Posterior Exenteration: Surgical Perspectives

47

Gwenael Ferron, Juan J. Torrent, Christophe Pomel, Bernard Malavaud, D. Querleu, and Alejandra Martinez

Introduction

Pelvic exenteration (PE) is the most radical surgery performed in gynecologic oncology. Pelvic exenteration is the only therapeutic approach for the management of pelvic relapse within irradiated fields or in locally advanced tumors resistant to radiochemotherapy.

Over the last decade, the selection criteria have been refined. The surgical technique has substantially evolved, with the development of new haemostatic devices, description of laterally extended endopelvic resection and mainly to the systematization of complex reconstruction techniques of the vagina, perineum, urinary and digestive tract.

Indeed, many reconstructive surgical techniques are available to re-establish pelvic functions lost after an exenterative procedure. Surgical methods have been developed and validated to increase quality of life, enabling assessment of the relevance of reconstructive surgery for patient's well-being. In addition, reconstruction procedures contribute to avoid the empty pelvis syndrome and therefore result in an additional benefit in reducing the pelvic complication rate.

G. Ferron (✉) • B. Malavaud • A. Martinez
Surgical oncology, Institut Claudius Regaud – Institut Universitaire du Cancer, Toulouse 31059, France
e-mail: Ferron.gwenael@iuct-oncopole.fr; Malavaud.bernard@iuct-oncopole.fr; Martinez.alejandra@iuct-oncopole.fr

J.J. Torrent
Gynecology, Hospital Universitari Germans Trias y Pujol, Badalona 08916, Spain
e-mail: Juanjotorrent@yahoo.es

C. Pomel
Surgical Oncology, Jean Perrin Cancer Centre, Clermont-Ferrand 63000, France
e-mail: Christophe.pomel@cjp.fr

D. Querleu
Surgery, Institut Bergonié, Bordeaux 33000, France
e-mail: d.querleu@bordeaux.unicancer.fr

This complex surgery requires highly qualified surgical, anaesthesiology, and paramedical teams. It is associated with a high complication rate and a consequently a long average hospital stay.

The denudated and irradiated pelvis represents the source of complications, such as bowel obstruction and bowel fistula formation. However, the use of non-irradiated colon for urinary diversion decreases fistula rate, and the pelvis filled by a musculocutaneous flap also greatly reduces complications like fistula or abcess. Association of complex reconstruction techniques (myocutaneous flap for vaginal reconstruction associated to a continent colic urinary diversion and digestive's restoration) improves quality of life and also postoperative courses.

Patient Selection for Pelvic Exenteration

An evaluation of the potential oncologic benefit is mandatory before proposing a patient pelvic exenteration, which is a mutilative procedure. Except in rare palliative indications for complex fistulas, only patients with relatively favorable long-term prognosis should be selected. The presence of extrapelvic visceral metastasis, of peritoneal disease, and/or macroscopic aortic lymph nodes metastasis are associated with a poor short-term prognosis and therefore are generally considered as a contraindication.

The objective of the surgery is to achieve free margins. The hypothesis of a residual tumor (R1 or R2) at the end of the surgery must be minimized. The contribution of new imaging techniques such as MRI and PET-CT has improved the preoperative assessment of tumor extent and the detection of distant metastases. Although preoperative imaging is helpful in detecting obvious contra-indications to exenteration, preoperative laparoscopic staging possibly associated with aortic lymph node dissection may be useful to further decrease the rate of abortive surgery.

The type of excision and organ removal must be adapted to the tumor location. The term 'exenteration" encompasses

I. Alkatout, L. Mettler (eds.), *Hysterectomy*, DOI 10.1007/978-3-319-22497-8_47

a variety of surgeries, depending on the involvement of the pelvic organs and the required level of pelvic floor resection. Anterior, posterior, or total exenteration, with or without removal of the pelvic floor and perineum (supralevator, infralevator or extended) are described in the Magrina's classification [1].

Preoperative Preparation of the Patients

The extent of planned surgery determines the information given to the patient. The patient must be informed about potential resections, functional consequences and expected complications, including both body image and sexual function alteration. The available reconstruction techniques, the associated complications and potential benefit must be addressed. Information regarding the day-to-day management of diversion must be provided. Support of a nursing team, stomatologist, dietician and psychologist is mandatory. Placement of stomas must be decided with the patient before the surgery according to her morphotype and clothing habits. In case of continent pouch, urostomy is often placed in the umbilicus.

Even though it is not generally recommended in elective colic surgery, bowel preparation may be useful, particularly in the case of the creation of a continent urinary pouch.

Thorough preoperative assessment of the medical condition of the patient, active anesthesiologic management, including invasive monitoring and peridural analgesia are mandatory. Routine respiratory physiotherapy and early enteral and oral feeding have been found to shorten the postoperative stay.

Patient Selection for Laparoscopic Pelvic Exenteration

Pelvic exenteration as well as reconstruction techniques are feasable by laparoscopy [2]. The contribution of perineal approach to the laparoscopy allows to reduce the mean surgical time as well as to adapt perineal approach to oncologic rules [3].

The use of both new haemostatic tools and automatic suture devices allows to manage in well selected cases this type of surgery with reasonable mean surgical time.

Although the use of this technique is currently undertaken by only a few surgeons, its reproductibility is assured for the ablative phase and also for reconstruction techniques such as Miami continent pouch or ileal loop derivation.

Techniques of vaginal reconstruction are limited in laparoscopic approach with the impossibility to use the current reference rectus abdominis myocutaneous flap.

Indications for lparoscopic approach for PE must be limited to:

- patients with a locally advanced tumor or a small size isolated centro-pelvic relapse.
- non sexually active patients, without the need of "optimal" vaginal reconstruction. For young and sexually active patients, we believe that open surgery with rectus abdomininis flap (or vertical DIEP flap) represents the best option [4].

Gynecologists must keep in mind that such a technically challenging procedure needs to be used with caution, as special laparoscopic and oncologic experience is required.

In this chapter, we report our stepwise surgical procedure of laparoscopic supralevatori anterior (and middle, with complete vaginectomy) pelvic exenteration. In addition, specific steps for rectal resection in case of total PE are described. Lymp nodes dissection are not described here. Indications of pelvic and aortic nodes dissection are depending to results of PET-CT and to the patient medical history. In case of pelvic recurrence, lymphadenectomies have been routenelly previously performed.

Laparoscopic Pelvic Exenteration: A Three Step Procedure

Description of laparoscopic PE can be divided into three different phases [2, 3]:

Step 1: Laparoscopic Ablative Phase

Like in open surgery, anterior (and middle) PE with total vaginectomy represents a multimesovisceral resection including a total mesometrial resection and removal of the ureterovesical compartment. The dissection plans of PE have to be adjusted to the borders of pelvic compartments [5].

The dissection is stopped as soon as laparoscopic dissection is deemed sufficiently complete to later allow en-bloc removal of the specimen via perineal or vaginal approach. Additional steps adapted to each individual case are then performed before the loss of pneumoperitoneum secondary to later removal of the specimen.

Step 2: Laparoscopic Reconstructive Phase with Urinary Diversion Construction (Continent or Not) and Omental J Flap Harvesting

After a complete laparoscopic mobilization of the right colon and both ureters, the urinary diversion is created extracorporeally through a small 5 cm medial minilaparotomy adjacent to the umbilicus or a 5 cm minilaparotomy over the right 10 mm port site.

Step 3: Perineal or Vaginal Approach

The en-bloc specimen is removed through the vagina or after perineal excision adapted to the tumor location.

The vaginal reconstruction is done by using the omental J flap and if needed, additional local flaps.

New haemostatic devices such as vessel sealing combined with ultrasonic and advanced bipolar energy are used to reduce bleeding and instrument changing. Endo-GIA staplers are necessary for bowel section.

Standard laparoscopic instruments are used during this procedure: two non-traumatic graspers, one Leriche dissector, and one needle holder.

Specific instrumentation is required for the continent pouch construction similar to open surgery [6, 7].

Patient Position

The patient is placed in a lithotomy position, with the legs at the same level than the abdomen with complete access to the perineum.

Both arms are placed along the abdomen to facilitate the laparoscopic procedure.

The surgeon operates from the left side and the assistant is on the right. The surgeon can move between both legs to easily access the upper part of the abdomen during omental J flap harvesting and mobilization of the right colon.

Laparoscopic Ports Placement

The umbilicus is used as the port site for the laparoscope. Four operative trocars are placed:

- one 5 mm on each iliac fossa.
- one 10 mm in the placement of preoperative marked stoma site.

Altogether, five trocars are placed. (Fig. 47.1).

Ergonomic placement of trocars is mandatory to access the entire peritoneal cavity, and allows pelvic and supraabdominal procedure with the same ports.

The absence of undefined preoperative intra-abdominal metastatic disease should be confirmed at this time. Since R0 resection is the goal of surgery, and undiagnosed peritoneal or visceral metastases are often unresectable, definitive surgery should be avoided in these cases, except for palliative surgery.

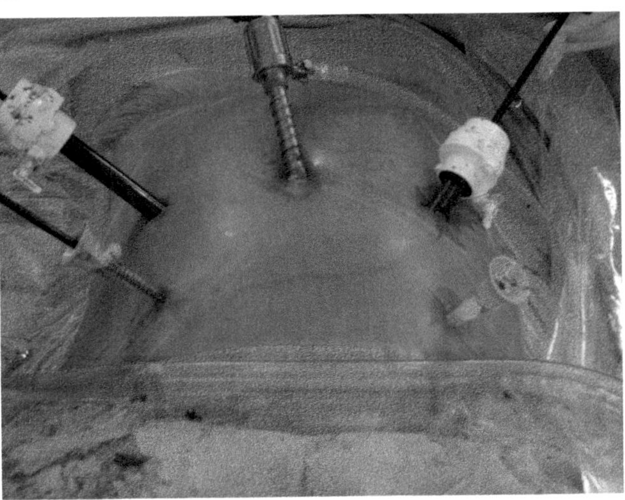

Fig. 47.1 Laparoscopic ports placement

Laparoscopic PE Phase

The abdominal phase is completely performed by laparoscopy.

The patient is placed in Trendelenburg position. Optimal pelvic exposure is required. The small intestine is packed in the upper quadrant after a right paracolic guttier incision.

If necessary, the sigmoid is attached to the left paracolic guttier to empty the posterior pelvis.

Dissection of Retzius and Pelvic Spaces

The anterior visceral peritoneum of the bladder is incised (Fig. 47.2), and the space of Retzius is opened. Both paravesical (Fig. 47.3) and pararectal (Fig. 47.4) spaces are developed.

During this dissection, the ureters still attached to the peritoneum are pouched medially or laterally to widely open the pararectal space.

The pelvic side peritoneum is incised laterally to the rectum.

Ureters Dissection

The infundibulopelvic ligaments are divided. The ureters are obstructed using hemoloks ® then transsected as low as possible in the pelvis (Fig. 47.5).

Of note, the ureters are often located medially in patients who have previously undergone surgery. Preoperative placement of ureteral stents is not required.

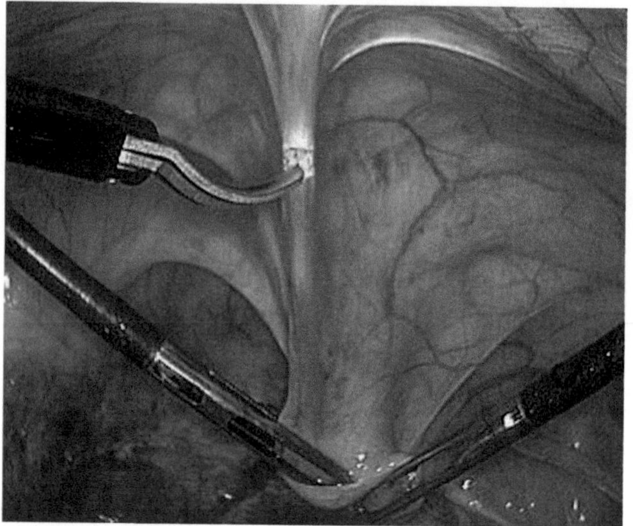

Fig. 47.2 Incision of the anterior visceral peritoneum of the bladder

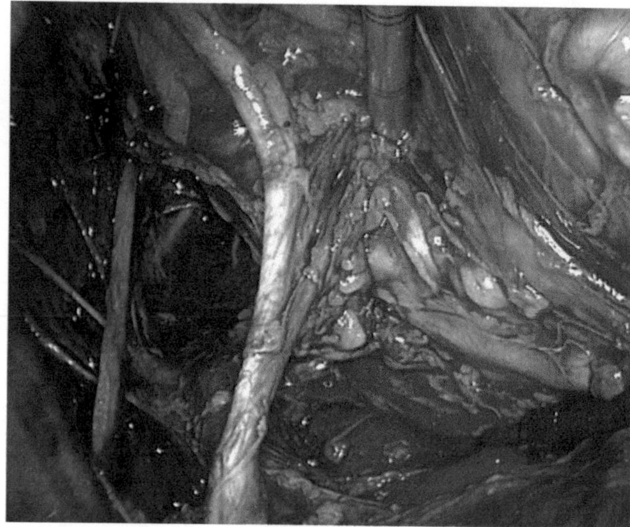

Fig. 47.4 Development of pararectal space

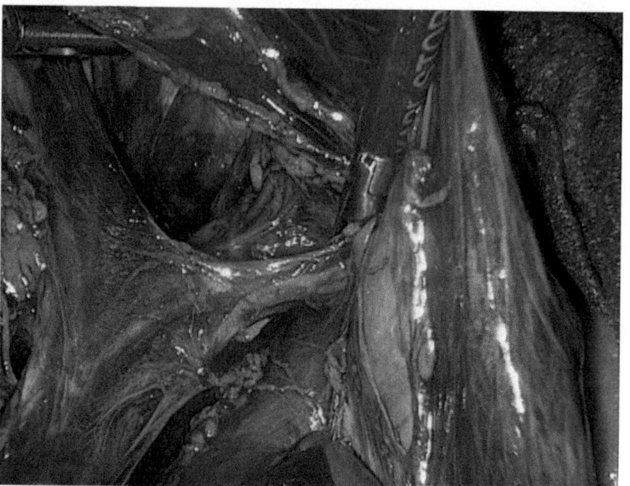

Fig. 47.3 Opening of the Retzius space

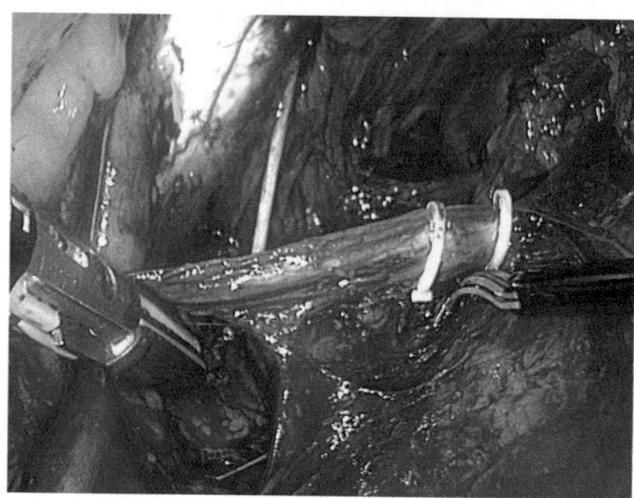

Fig. 47.5 Transsection of the left ureter

Dissection of the Rectovaginal Septa

The peritoneal incision is extended into the Douglas pouch (Fig. 47.6). The anterior aspect of the rectum is separated from the posterior vaginal wall with a blunt dissection (Fig. 47.7).

Coagulation and Section of the Parametrium

The entire specimen is pushed to one side by the assistant. The dissection is started in the pararectal space. The uterine artery and the superior vesical artery are coagulated or clipped (Fig. 47.8). The dissection is carried caudally and medial to the hypogastric pedicle.

The same step is then carried out on the other side.

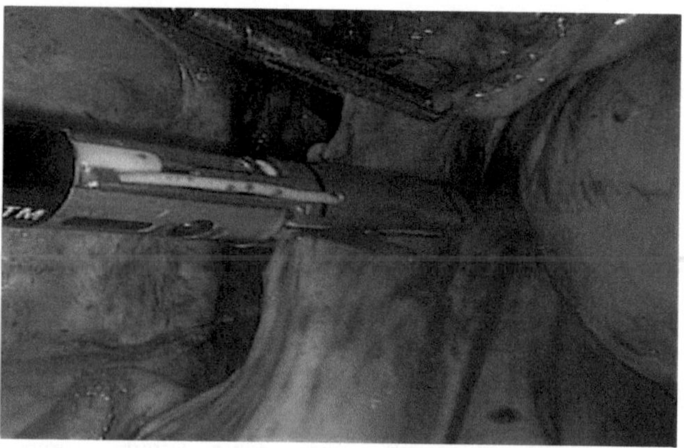

Fig. 47.6 Incision of the peritoneum into the Douglas pouch

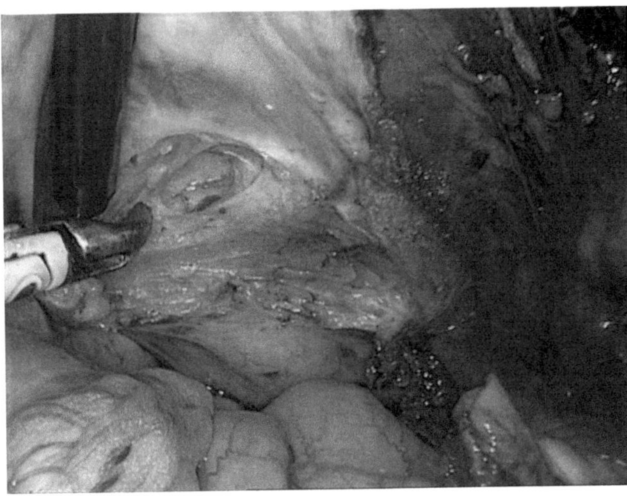

Fig. 47.7 Blunt dissection between the anterior aspect of the rectum and the posterior vaginal wall

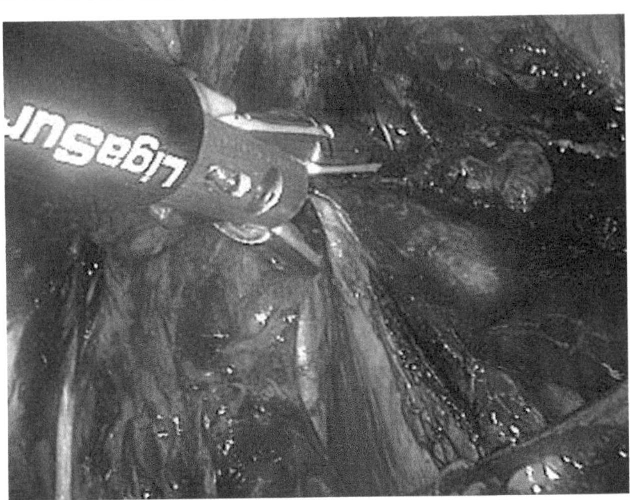

Fig. 47.9 Transsection of the uterosacral ligaments and paracolpos

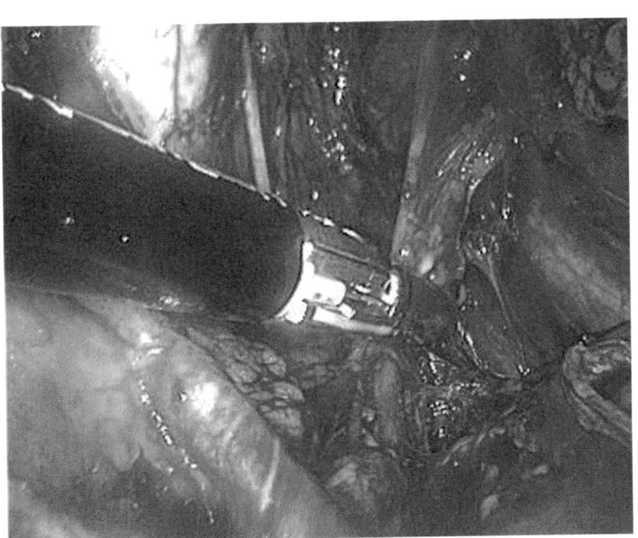

Fig. 47.8 Coagulation of the uterine artery and the superior vesical artery

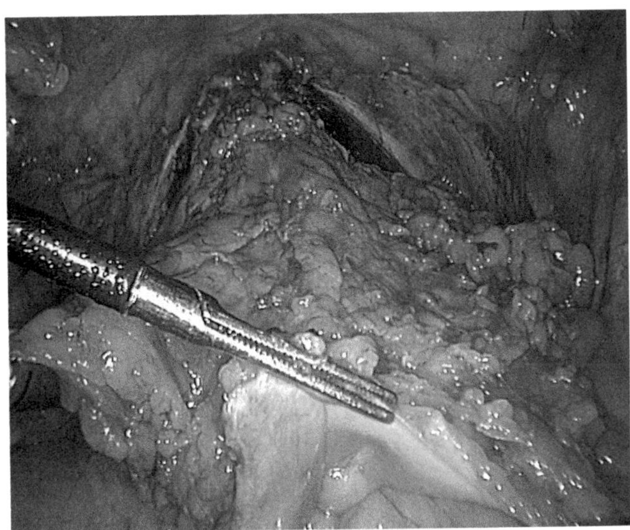

Fig. 47.10 Opening of the endopelvic fascia

Coagulation and Section of Paracervix and Paravaginal Tissue to the Pelvic Floor, and Identifying the Levator Ani

Uterosacral ligaments and paracolpos are transected as laterally as possible according to a complete mesometrial compartmentectomy and removal of the ureterovesical compartment (Fig. 47.9).

The endopelvic fascia is cleaned, and opened in case of infralevator or extended PE (Fig. 47.10).

In Case of Total PE

The rectum is dissected off the sacrum and coccyx by blunt dissection. This is performed by retracting the uterus and distal segment of the rectum anterior and cephalad, inserting an instrument behind the rectum in the presacral space, and freeing the rectum down to the coccyx.

In order to perform a colo-anal or colorectal anastomosis without tension, the left colon including the spleen flexure is widely mobilized.

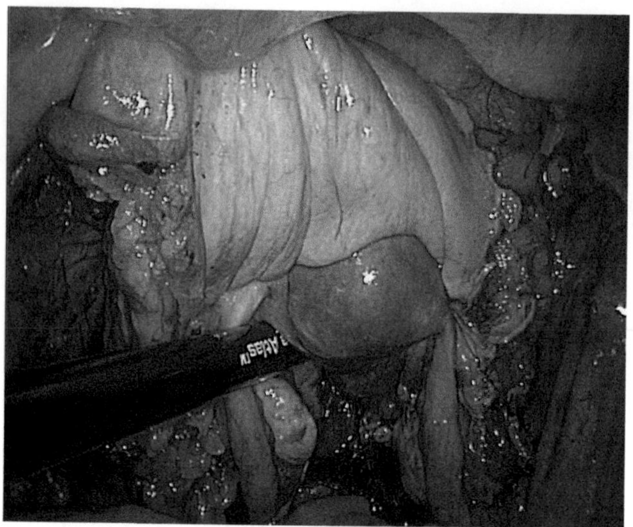

Fig. 47.11 Final laparoscopic view before en-bloc removal via perineal or vaginal approach

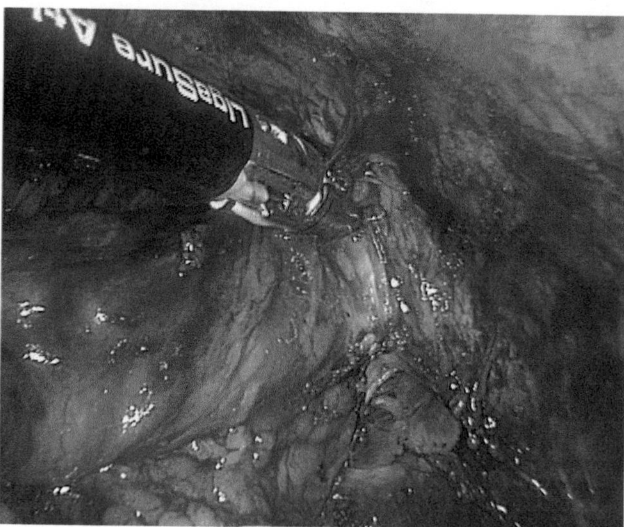

Fig. 47.12 Coagulation of paravesical plexus

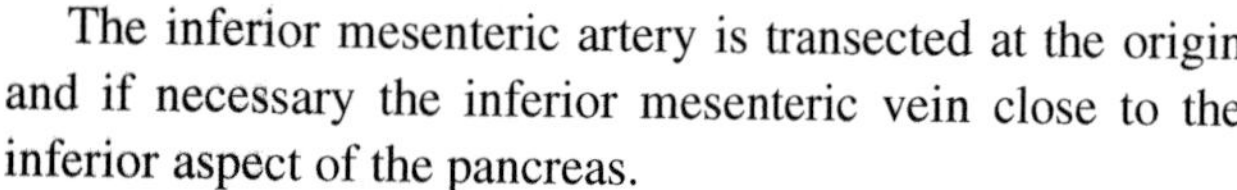

The inferior mesenteric artery is transected at the origin and if necessary the inferior mesenteric vein close to the inferior aspect of the pancreas.

The rectum and the descending colon can be transected by laparoscpy using Endo-GIA staplers or outside after removal of the specimen (see next step).

Later Removal of the Specimen

The dissection is stopped as soon as laparoscopic dissection is deemed sufficiently complete to later allow en-bloc removal of the specimen via perineal or vaginal approach (Fig. 47.11).

By cephalad traction, the urethra can be exposed and transected at this time after coagulation of paravesical plexus (Fig. 47.12).

Additional steps adapted to each individual case are then performed before the loss of pneumoperitoneum, secondary to later removal of the specimen.

In the case of supralevatori PE, some authors have proposed to transect the vagina and remove the entire specimen through the vagina [2, 8]. The vagina is then packed to prevent pneumoperitoneum leakage.

Reconstructive Phase: Urinary Diversion (Bricker Diversion)

Mobilization of Both Ureters

The right ureter is mobilized up to the lower renal pole (Fig. 47.13), whereas for the left, it is dissected above the level of the inferior mesenteric artery and brought across the midline to the right without tension through a window created in the mesentery above the inferior mesenteric artery (Fig. 47.14). This step is facilitated in case of simultaneous aortic lymphadenectomy.

Creation of the Diversion

A 5 cm median incision starting from the umbilical trocar site is performed.

A segment of ileum is mobilized and exteriorized through the incision (Fig. 47.15). A 10 cm ileal segment 15 cm away from the ileocecal junction is isolated to construct the urinary diversion.

Bowel continuity is restored with stapled side-to-side ileo-ileal anastomosis.

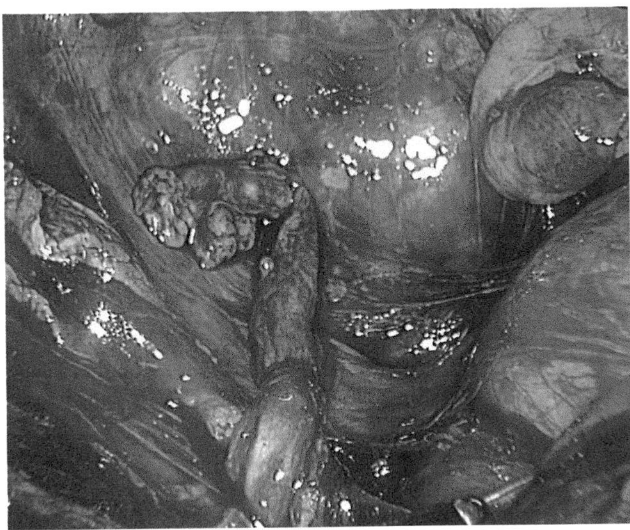

Fig. 47.13 Mobilization of the right ureter

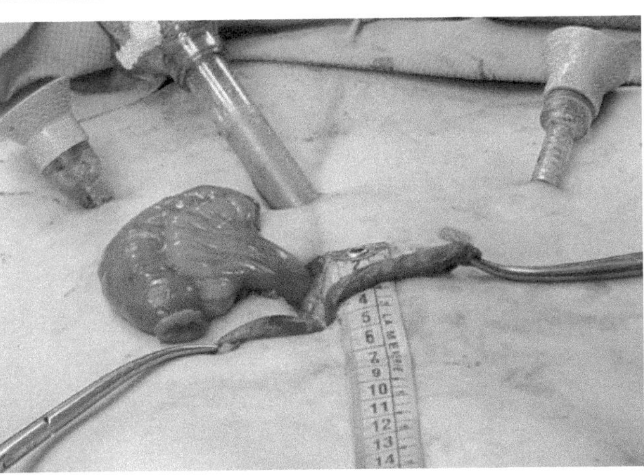

Fig. 47.15 Exteriorization of a segment of the ileum and the both ureters through the ombilical incision before creation of the Bricker diversion

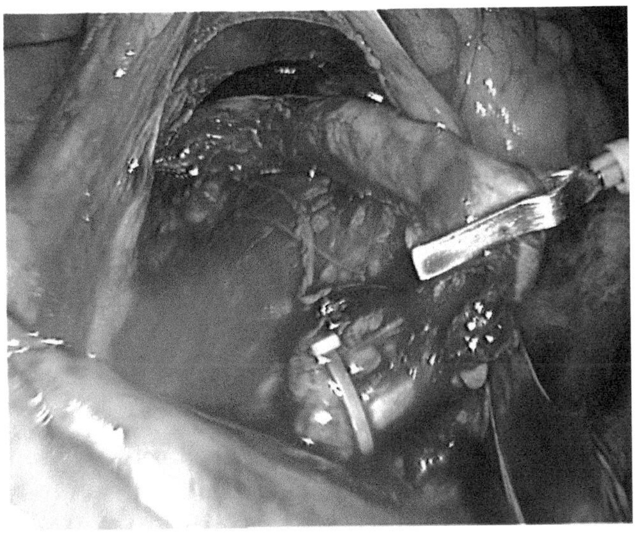

Fig. 47.14 Mobilization of the left ureter after creation of a peritoneal window above the level of the inferior mesenteric artery

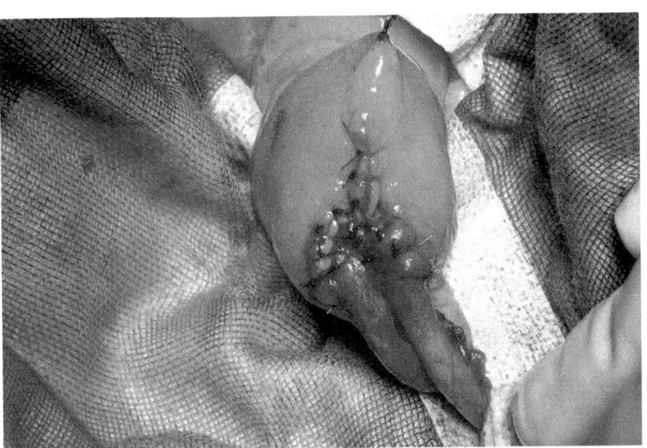

Fig. 47.16 Ileo-ureteral anastomoses in a wallace faction

Ileo-ureteral anastomoses in a Wallace faction are performed extracoporeally (Fig. 47.16). They are bilateral stented (8F Double JJ).

Finally the conduit stoma is fashioned: the end of the ileum is then brought out through a 10 mm port site previously placed in a preoperative marked stoma site.

Reconstructive Phase: Continent Miami Pouch

Right colon Mobilization Up to the Hepatic Flexure and Omental J Flap Harvesting

The patient is then positioned in a 15 ° reversed Trendelenburg with 15 ° left sided rotation to facilitate the mobilization of the ascending and the hepatic flexure of the colon.

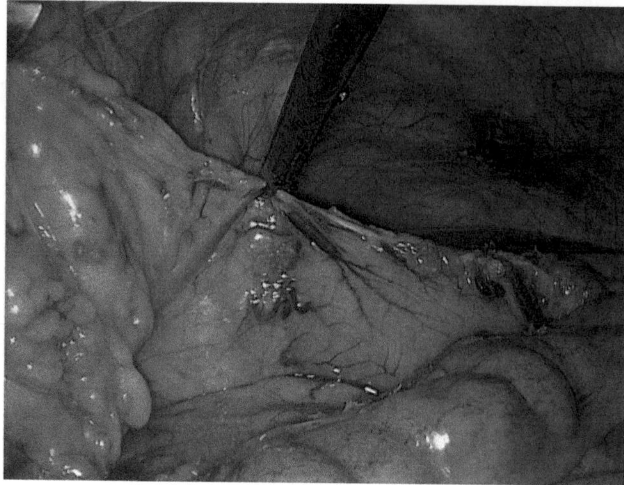

Fig. 47.17 Transection of the omentum off the greater curvature of the stomach

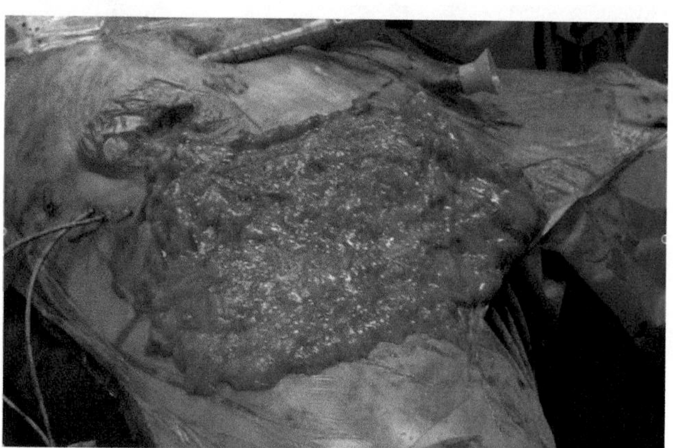

Fig. 47.18 Exteriorization of the omental J flap through the 5-cm iliac incision for neovaginal creation

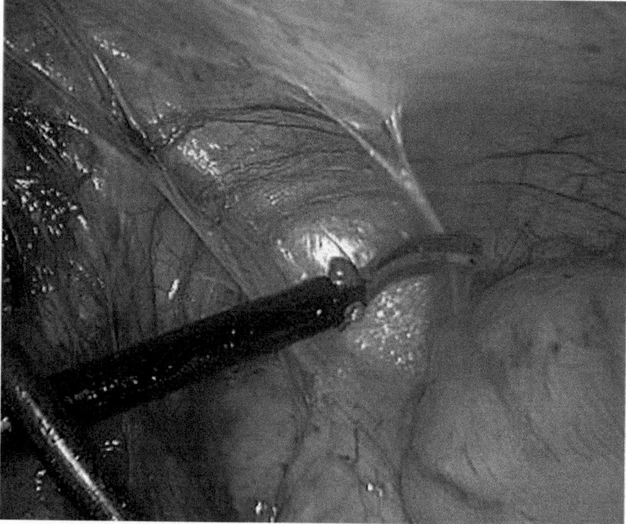

Fig. 47.19 Mobilization of the hepatic flexure

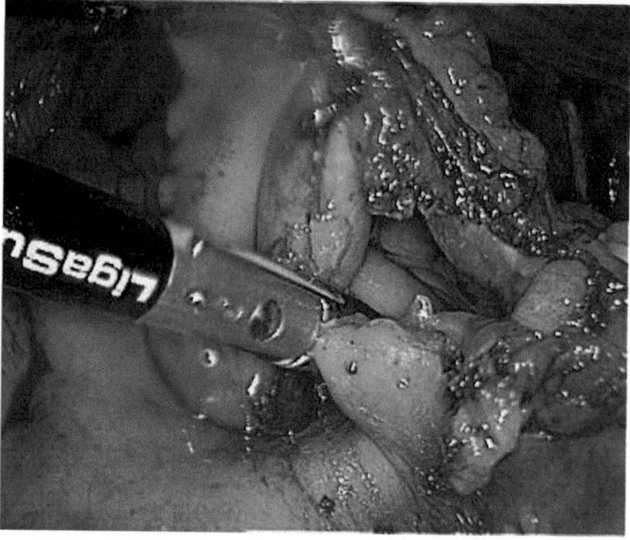

Fig. 47.20 Coagulation of the mesentery

The omentum is liberated from the transverse colon. Omental J flap is harvested at this time, after opening the omental bursa. The omentum is tipped over the anterior aspect of the stomach. The omental J flap is initiated by transecting the omentum off the greater curvature of the stomach (Fig. 47.17). The right gastroepiploic pedicle is skeletonized for the flap vascular supply. The omental J flap is stored at the upper part of the abdomen for the vaginal reconstruction. It will be transferred into the pelvis during the last phase after the removal of the specimen to fill the pelvis and optionally reconstruct the vagina (Fig. 47.18).

Then, the right part of the colon up to and including the hepatic flexure is mobilized (Fig. 47.19). This is to facilitate harvesting of an appropriate length of colon as well as entry into the retroperitoneal space to mobilize the ureters. The colon is transected proximaly to the middle colic artery, thus preserving an important blood supply. Transillumination through the right lower port with a 5 mm endoscope can be useful in identifying this important vessel in obese patients. It is also important to identify the position of the ileocolic artery before dividing the ileal mesentery, because this will be the main blood supply for the pouch. The colon and ileum are skeletonized (Fig. 47.20) and defatted before transection with EndoGIA staplers. 25 cm of colon and 15 cm of the terminal ileum are necessary to create a 250 cc volume pouch.

Mobilization of both ureters:

The right ureter is mobilized up to the lower renal pole, whereas for the left, it is dissected above the level of the

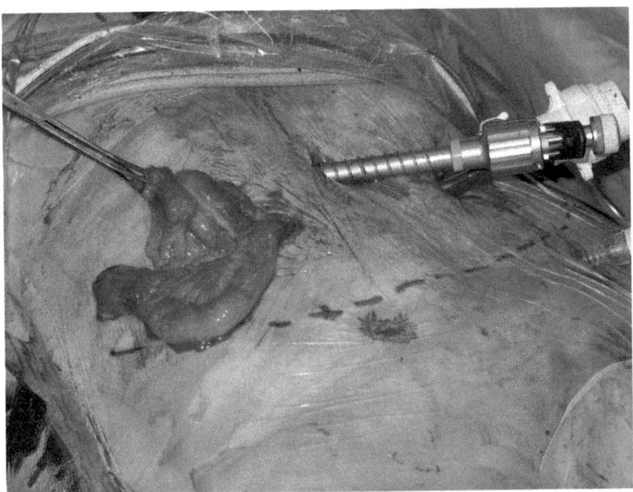

Fig. 47.21 Exteriorization of the ileum and the transverse colon before extracorporeally side-to-side anastomosis

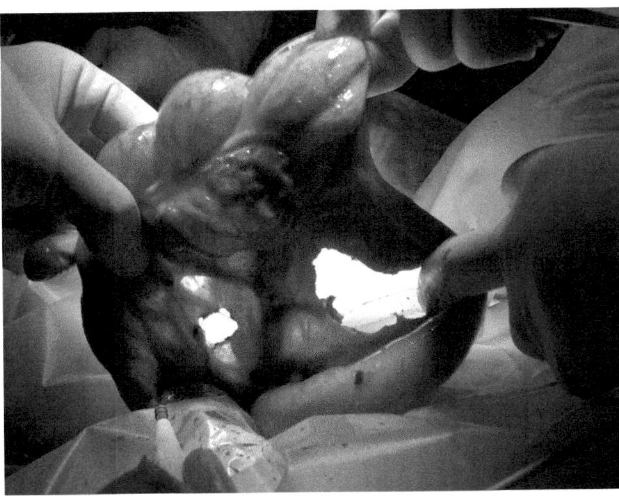

Fig. 47.22 Transillumination of the ileocolic conduit.

inferior mesenteric artery and brought across the midline to the right without tension through a window created in the mesentery above the inferior mesenteric artery. At this point, we prefer to fix the two ureteric ends with sutures near the site for the minilaparotomy to facilitate the exteriorization of the ureters during the next step.

Creation of a 5 cm Lateral Minilaparotomy

Through this, the transected intestinal ends are exteriorized, and a standard ileotransverse anastomosis is performed to restore bowel continuity (Fig. 47.21). We employ a side-to-side technique using two GIA 80 linear staplers.

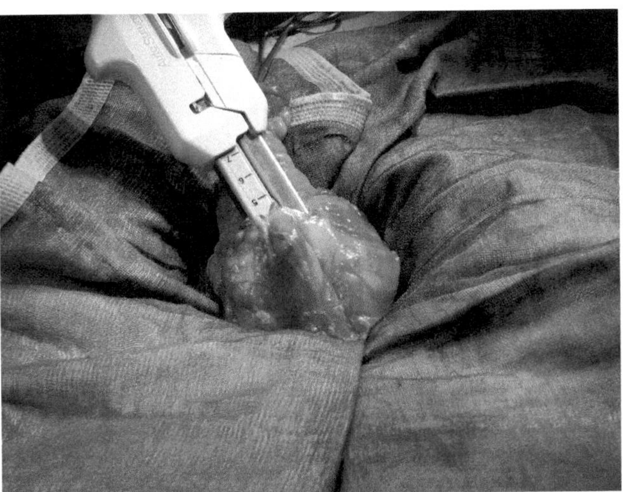

Fig. 47.23 Construction of the reservoir using resorbable staplers

Exteriorization of Ureters and Ileocolic Conduit (Fig. 47.22)

An appendicectomy is performed if it is present.

Creation of the Reservoir

The colon is folded on itself in a « U » configuration, and two sutures are used to maintain the alignment. Two 2 cm colostomies are made at the medial tip of both ends, and detubularization is done with resorbable staples (Poly-GIA) (Fig. 47.23).

The pouch is then unfolded and the detubularization is completed with a second resorbable stapler, thus creating a pouch (Fig. 47.24).

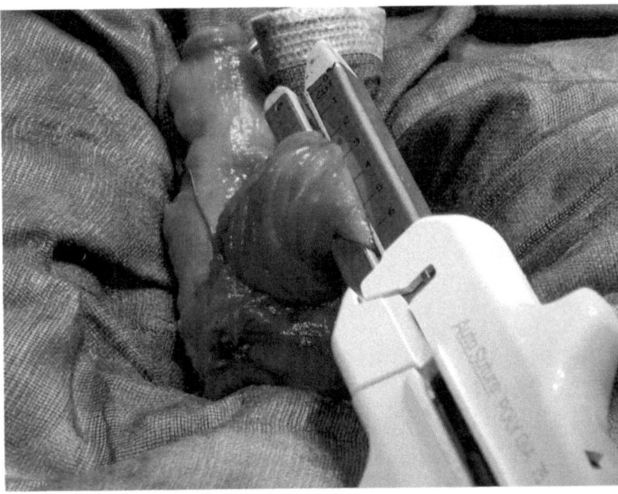

Fig. 47.24 Application of the second resorbable stapler to achieve the detubularization

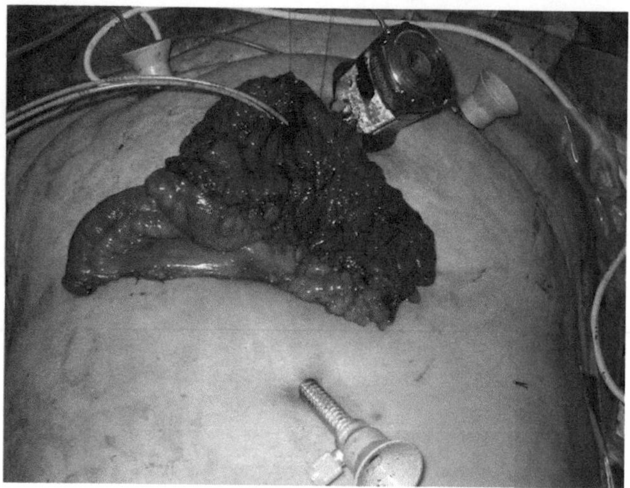

Fig. 47.25 Ureteric anastomosis to continent pouch

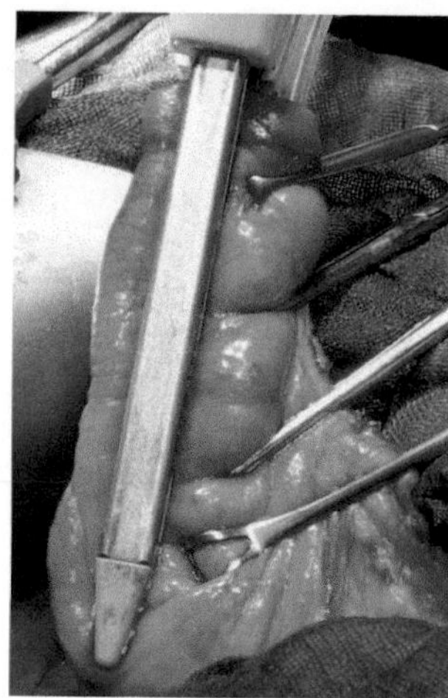

Fig. 47.26 Construction of continent mechanism by tapering of the distal ileal segment

Ureteric Anastomosis to Continent Pouch

Initialy, the ureteric ends were simply spatulated and anastomosed mucosa to mucosa at the base of the pouch with interrupted 4-O PDS sutures (Fig. 47.25).

Currently, in order to provide an efficient antireflux mechanism with a intraluminal valve, the 2 cm end of both ureters are left free into the reservoir and suturred serosa to mucosa at the pouch.

Single J stents (8F) are inserted, and their free ends are tunneled through the right lower abdominal wall to prevent obstruction by irrigation during early postoperative course.

Closure of the Pouch

After the placement of stents, the pouch is closed by a running suture.

Construction of Continent Mechanism: Tapering of the Distal Ileal Segment

A 14F catheter is placed through the ileum, and the ileum is narrowed with a GIA stapler. To obtain an optimal diameter, the 14F catheter is maintained with three or four Babcock forceps on the mesenteric side of the ileum (Fig. 47.26).

Checking the Continence and Integrity of the Pouch

200 mL of blue dye is infused to check for continence and the integrity of the pouch.

Continent Pouch Placement

The pouch is then replaced back into the cavity. The base is sutured to the posterior aspect of the abdominal wall to prevent displacement and torsion of the pouch. The minilaparotomy is then closed, and once the perineal and laparoscopic phases are completed, the ileal conduit is brought through and sutured at the umbilicus.

Specific Post Operative Care

Standard postoperative care includes the use of regular pouch irrigation to prevent mucus accumulation. Permeability of J stents have to be regulary controled and irrigation performed in case of obstruction.

A pouchogram is performed routinely on day 10 to confirm that there is no leakage before removing the J stents and the 14F Foley catheter.

All patients are taught how to self-catheterize with the 14F single-use urinary catheter.

En Bloc Removal of the Specimen Via Perineal or Vaginal Approach Phase

After completion of all required laparoscopic steps, a vaginal approach in type I–II or perineal approach in type III exenterations is used to complete the removal of the specimen.

Vaginal and perineal incision adapted to the extent of disease is followed by dissection with a haemostic device of the attachments of the urethra or vagina to the pelvic wall (Figs. 47.27 and 47.28).

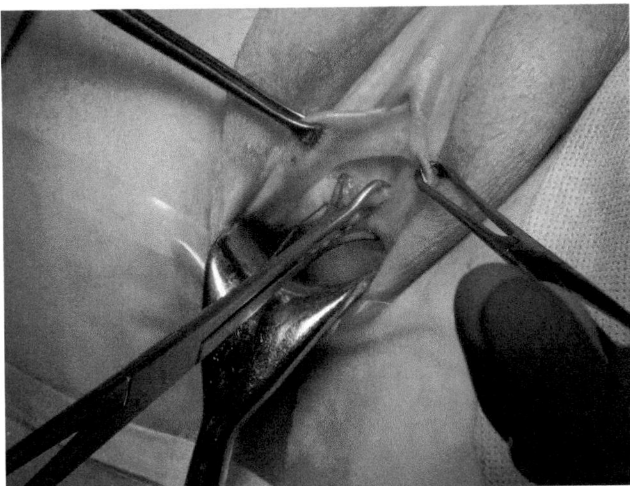

Fig. 47.27 Vaginal and perineal incision adapted to the extent of disease

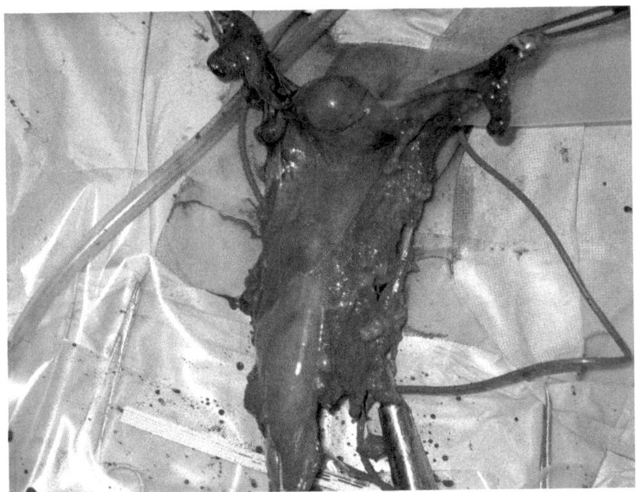

Fig. 47.28 Exteriorization of the anterior and middle PE specimen

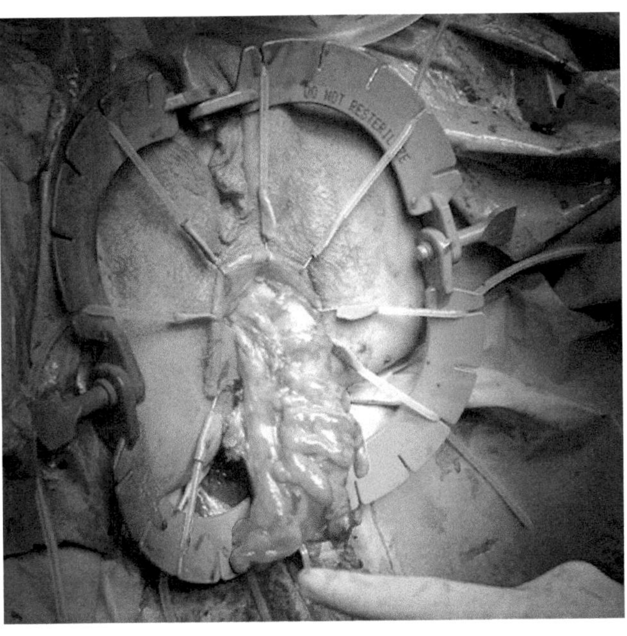

Fig. 47.29 Coloanal anastomosis

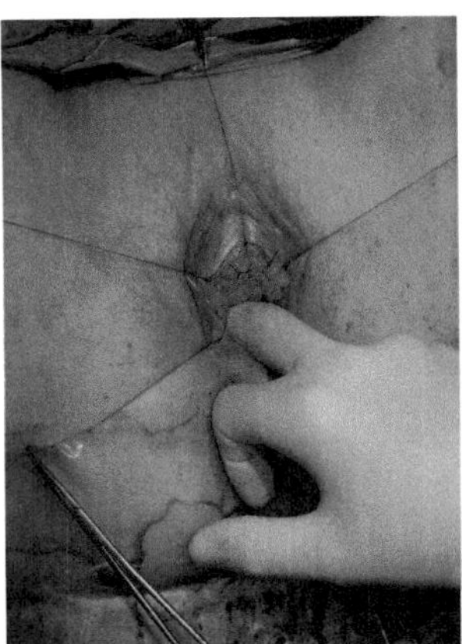

Fig. 47.30 Vaginal reconstruction using an omental J flap

Restoration of Bowel Continuity

The left colon is exteriorized through the anal sphincter to facilitate the colo-anal anastomosis (Fig. 47.29).

If the remain rectum is long, a colorectal anastomosis is performed by laparoscopy using EEA staplers.

A loop ileostomy is performed on left iliac fossa to protect both ileal and colo-anal anastomosis.

Vaginal Reconstruction

The omental J flap, harvested during the previous surgical phase is transferred into the pelvis. It is tubularized and sutured to the introitus or the remaining vagina (Fig. 47.30).

The use of vicryl or biological mesh combined with an omental flap have been described by some authors to reduce the rate of neovaginal prolapse [9].

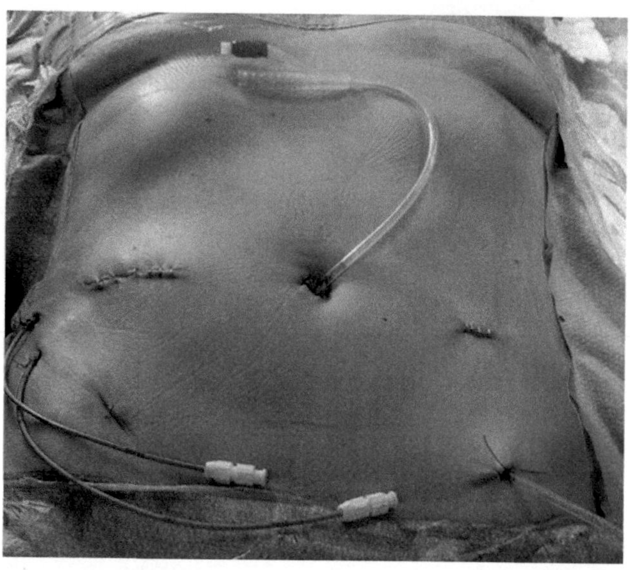

Fig. 47.31 Final view after anterior and middle PE with placement of the urostomy through the umbilicus. Drainage

A vaginal mold is placed and removed each day for irrigation. In our experience, split thickness skin graft is not needed, as spontaneous reepidermization will be completed after several weeks.

An additional local myocutaneous flap can be used if necessary.

Drainage

Abdominal drainage is achieved through the upper umbilical port site and a second one through the vaginal suture (Insert Fig. 47.31).

References

1. Magrina JF. Types of pelvic exenterations: a reappraisal. Gynecol Oncol. 1990;37(3):363–6.
2. Pomel C, Rouzier R, Pocard M, Thoury A, Sideris L, Morice P, Duvillard P, Bourgain JL, Castaigne D. Laparoscopic total pelvic exenteration for cervical cancer relapse. Gynecol Oncol. 2003;91(3):616–8.
3. Ferron G, Querleu D, Martel P, Letourneur B, Soulié M. Laparoscopy-assisted vaginal pelvic exenteration. Gynecol Oncol. 2006;100(3):551–5.
4. Martínez A, Filleron T, Vitse L, Querleu D, Mery E, Balague G, Delannes M, Soulie M, Pomel C, Ferron G. Laparoscopic pelvic exenteration for gynaecological malignancy: is there any advantage? Gynecol Oncol. 2011;120(3):374–9.
5. Höckel M, Dornhöfer N. Pelvic exenteration for gynaecological tumours: achievements and unanswered questions. Lancet Oncol. 2006;7(10):837–47.
6. Penalver MA, Bejany DE, Averette HE, Donato DM, Sevin BU, Suarez G. Continent urinary diversion in gynecologic oncology. Gynecol Oncol. 1989;34(3):274–88.
7. Ferron G, Lim TY, Pomel C, Soulie M, Querleu D. Creation of the miami pouch during laparoscopic-assisted pelvic exenteration: the initial experience. Int J Gynecol Cancer. 2009;19(3):466–70.
8. Puntambekar S, Kudchadkar RJ, Gurjar AM, Sathe RM, Chaudhari YC, Agarwal GA, Rayate NV. Laparoscopic pelvic exenteration for advanced pelvic cancers: a review of 16 cases. Gynecol Oncol. 2006;102(3):513–6.
9. Momoh AO, Kamat AM, Butler CE. Reconstruction of the pelvic floor with human acellular dermal matrix and omental flap following anterior pelvic exenteration. J Plast Reconstr Aesthet Surg. 2010;63(12):2185–7.

Hysterectomy in the Surgical Management of Endometriosis

48

Rouba Murtada, Gabriele Centini, Karolina Afors, and Arnaud Wattiez

Endometriosis is the ectopic presence of endometrial glandular and stromal tissue. It affects 10–20 % of women, and up to 60 % of women suffering from dysmenorrhea [1–4]. As a hormone dependent condition, menopause usually brings an end to its evolution. Infertility and pain are its two major symptoms. The pains most frequently linked to endometriosis are dysmenorrhea, non-menstrual chronic pelvic pain, dyschezia, dysuria and dyspareunia. In certain patients, the severity of symptoms is such that it can cause a significant impact on quality of life, sexual function and psychological physical well-being.

The treatment of endometriosis relies on 2 pillars: hormonal treatment and surgery. In the surgical management of endometriosis, hysterectomy is one of the options. It is generally considered a last resort solution which is to be reserved for severe symptoms, only after failure of other treatments or procedures and after the patient has accomplished her family project.

Few publications are dedicated to the place of hysterectomy in endometriosis. Nevertheless there is evidence to support both the rationale of performing a hysterectomy in endometriosis, and its efficiency in treating painful symptoms.

R. Murtada (✉)
Department of Gynecology and Obstetrics, Hôpital Jean Verdier, AP-HP, Allee du 14 Juillet, Bondy 93140, France
e-mail: rouba.murtada@gmail.com

G. Centini
Molecular and developmental medicine, Obstetrics and Gynaecology, University of Siena, Ospedale santa Maria alle scotte, Viale Bracci, 16, Siena 53100, Italy
e-mail: Centini.gabriele@gmail.com

K. Afors
Obstetrics and Gynaecology, King's College Hospital NHS Trust, Denmark Hill, London SE5 9RS, UK
e-mail: drkafors@gmail.com

A. Wattiez
University of Strasbourg, Strasbourg, France

GYN Department, Latifa Hospital, Dubai, UAE
e-mail: arnaud.wattiez@wanadoo.fr

The Rationale of Hysterectomy for Endometriosis

The Innervation of Eutopic Endometrium

It was demonstrated by Tokushige et al. that patients with endometriosis have a greater density of nervous fibers whithin the eutopic endometrium and myometrium when compared to patients without endometriosis [5].

The same team demonstrated that hormonal treatment significantly decreases the density of nervous fibers within the eutopic endometrium and myometrium, supplying an explanation for their efficacy in treating pelvic pain attributed to endometriosis [6].

Al Jefout et al. went as far as suggesting the immunohistochemical detection of nervous fibers on endometrial biopsy as a diagnostic technique for endometriosis [7]. In a population of 99 women presenting with pelvic pain and/or infertility, they found that this technique had a sensibility and specificity of 83 % and 98 %, and a positive and negative predictive strength of 91 % and 96 %, respectively. Women with endometriosis and pelvic pain had significantly higher density of nervous fibers than women with endometriosis but without pelvic pain (2.3 vs 0.8 /mm2, p = 0.005).

These elements are in favor of a participation of the uterus to nocicetive mechanisms implicated in endometriosis pain.

Nevertheless, Zhang et al. studied the density of nervous fibers in the endometrium of 30 patients with endometriosis, 40 women with adenomyosis, 41 women with uterine fibroids and 47 women with endometriosis and adenomyosis. They demonstrated a greater density in women presenting with pelvic pain as compared to those without painful symptoms, whichever the pathology [8].

Retrograde Menstruation Theory

It is one of the theories concerning the genesis of endometriosis. The persistence of menstrual reflux could contribute

I. Alkatout, L. Mettler (eds.), *Hysterectomy*, DOI 10.1007/978-3-319-22497-8_48

to the maintaining of endometriosis, and its suppression could decrease the genesis of new lesions. Women with endometriosis could have heavier menstrual flux than other women [9, 10]. Also, high levels of prostaglandins have been found in the menstrual flux of women with dysmenorrhea and their recurring outpour into the abdominal cavity could contribute to inflammation and a mechanism of peripheral sensitization [11].

Uterine Dyssynergia

Physiologically, uterine contractions spread from the fundus to the uterine cervix during the menstrual period, which allows the evacuation of uterine debris [12]. These contractions don't occur in women under oral contractives, suggesting a hormonal participation in this phenomenon [13].

These contractions could also occur differently in women with endometriosis, with a hyperkinesia or dyskinesia that could contribute to dysmenorrhea as well as reduce the efficacy of evacuation of the menstrual flux. The pressure of contractions and their frequency were significantly increased in 16 patients with endometriosis in comparison to 14 control patients in a study by Bulletti et al. This inefficacy of uterine contractions resulted in retrograde menstruation, with the previously cited consequences [14].

Adenomyosis Associated to Endometriosis

Adenomyosis, previously called internal endometriosis is the presence of endometriosis within the myometrium. It is a pathology of the fourth and fifth decade and is revealed by menorragia and/or pelvic pain. An association between adenomyosis and endometriosis has been found. It is particularly the case of external adenomyosis, whereby endometriotic lesions principally recto-vaginal nodules, are contiguous to adenomyosis within the myometrium, with a similar histological structure in both lesions [15].

In a radiological study, Kunz et al. found aprevalence in adenomyosis (based on the thickening of the junctional zone) of 79 % in a population of 160 women with endometriosis [16]. Larsen et al. after pathological study of hysterectomy specimens found a prevalence of adenomyosis of 34.6 % in a group of 153 patients with endometriosis, vs 19.4 % in a control group ($p < 0.05$) [17]. Moreover, there was a tendency towards an increase in the prevalence of adenomyosis with the severity of endometriosis: 42,8 % in the ASRM IV group vs 29.4 % in the ASRM I, II and III (NS, $p = 0.10$), as well as in the depth of infiltration of adenomyosis in the myometrium (NS, $p > 0.05$).

The participation of adenomyosis in the persistence of pain after excisional surgery for endometriosis has been studied. Parker et al. studied the thickness of the myometrial junctional zone on MRI, as an indicator for adenomyosis, in 53 patients suffering from pelvic pain [18]. After surgery 40 had histologically proven endometriosis. In these patients, dysmenorrhea and non-menstrual pelvic pain were significantly and three times more likely to persist after surgery when thickness was superior to 11 mm on pre-operative MRI.

Ferrero et al. performed a similar study in women with bowel endometriosis, with or without associated adenomyosis (diagnosis was based on MRI findings) [19]. Dysmenorrhea was significantly improved in patients without adenomyosis or those in whom an excision of focal adenomyosis had been performed, on an 18 months study period. No improvement of dysmenorrhea was obtained when adenomyosis was left untreated. Deep dyspareunia and non menstrual pelvic pain were improved in all groups, as well as specific bowel symptoms.

The presence of adenomyosis could be responsible for an incomplete resolution of painful symptoms in endometriosis after conservative surgery, in particular with the persistence of dysmenorrhea.

The Place of Hysterectomy in Endometriosis

Performing a hysterectomy for a benign condition, all conditions included, generally yields favourable results [20]. Nevertheless, the results of hysterectomy for chronic pelvic pain seem inferior to those obtained in other benign conditions. Indeed, pre-operative pain is a risk factor for post-operative pain in hysterectomy.

In a 2004 study by Hartmann et al. on 1200 patients having undergone a hysterectomy for a benign condition, all indications included, the group of patients presenting with pelvic pain and depression was identified as having a three to five times greater risk of suffering from altered quality of life, dyspareunia and pelvic pain [21]. Nonetheless an improvement was reported in 78–86 % of patients in this sub-group. This observation was again found in a Danish study in 2007 where a questionnaire was sent to 1299 1 year after they had undergone a hysterectomy. It was found that pre-operative pain, as well as pain as an indication for surgery, were risk factors for post-operative pain with respectively odd-ratios of 3.25 and 2.98 [22].

Hysterectomy Is Efficient for Pain Improvement Rather than Pain Resolution

In 1990, Stovall et al. reported the results of hysterectomy by laparotomy for chronic pelvic pain attributed to a uterine cause (leimyomatosis, adenomyosis) one year after surgery

[23]. Pelvic endometriosis cases were excluded. They were surprised to find lower results than expected. 22.2 % of patients had persisting pain, of which 5 % had increased pain. They concluded in the efficacy of hysterectomy for pain improvement, rather than pain resolution. In 1995, Hillis et al. in a serie of 388 patients having undergone a hysterectomy reported similar results with 74 % of pain resolution, 21 % of pain decrease and 5 % of pain increase [24]. A high-risk subgroup, with 40 % of persistent pain, was identified and included patients younger than 30 years, without medical insurance, without an identified pelvic pathology, or with a history of pelvic inflammatory disease.

Hysterectomy Is Efficient in the Treatment of Pain Related to Endometriosis

Endometriosis is one of the causes of chronic pelvic pain. It affects young women, and therefore the surgical management of endometriosis is often focused towards uterine conservation and fertility preservation. Few studies have been dedicated to hysterectomy in endometriosis. Its results are often merged with those of hysterectomy for other indications, and the outcome measures used are heterogeneous throughout literature.

In the study of Hillis et al., the subgroup of patients with histologically proven endometriosis without mention of severity or stage, 81.3 % of patients (n = 13) had no pelvic pain at one year after surgery, 18.7 % had decreased but persistent pelvic pain, and no patient reported increased pain [24]. In a study by Berner et al. on the results of subtotal laparoscopic hysterectomy, all indications included, 37 patients had undergone the procedure for pelvic pain attributed to endometriosis [25]. A significant decrease in pain scores measured on a visual analogic scale was reported at 3 years of surgery, with a mean of 4.01 points. Thirty one percent of patients had residual pain. Nevertheless, the residual pain score was significantly greater than in other pathologies (3.46 vs 0.94, $p < 0.001$).

Despite Imperfect Results, There Is Evidence That Hysterectomy Is Superior to Conservative Surgery in the Treatment of Endometriosis-Related Pain

Hysterectomy in general seems more efficient than conservative procedures. In an observational study of a cohort of 1503 patients reporting a pelvic problem (uterine bleeding, chronic pelvic pain, symptomatic fibroid tumor), Kuppermann et al. studied the impact of hysterectomy, uterine-preserving surgery and non-surgical treatments on health-related quality of life [20]. 13.8 % of patients had undergone a hysterectomy and 9 % a uterine-preserving surgery. An improvement was registered in all parameters of the quality of life questionnaire, in all three categories. Improvement was greater after hysterectomy.

In endometriosis specifically, there is also direct and indirect evidence that hysterectomy is more efficient than conservative surgery for the treatment of pain.

An indirect argument was provided by Weir et al. who studied on a 4 year period the rate of readmission in a population of 7993 patients having undergone surgery for endometriosis [26]. 27 % of patients were readmitted at some point after conservative surgery and 12 % after hysterectomy. Shakiba et al. studied the rate of reoperation in three groups: 107 patients who had uterine preserving surgery, 47 patients who had hysterectomy without oophorectomy and 50 patients who had hysterectomy with oophorectomy [27]. Hysterectomy was performed by laparotomy, laparoscopy or laparoscopically-assisted vaginal way. Patients who had a hysterectomy had a significantly lower rate of reoperation for pelvic pain as compared to the conservative treatment group. At, 2, 5 and 7 years, the percentage of reoperation-free patients was respectively of 79.4, 53.3 and 44.6 % for conservative surgery, 95.7, 86.6 and 77 % for hysterectomy without oophorectomy, 96, 91.7 and 91.7 % for hysterectomy with oophorectomy.

A study by Sinaii et al. compared 802 conservative laparoscopic surgeries for endometriosis to 230 oophorectomies, 209 hysterectomies with ovarian preservation, and 144 hysterectomies without ovarian preservation [28]. 94.6 % of patients had pelvic pain at time of surgery. In the isolated hysterectomy group, 45.9 % of patients considered their procedure to be a complete success for 30.4 % in the conservative surgery group ($p < 0.001$), 37.8 % in the oophorectomy group and 40.3 % in the hysterectomy with oophorectomy group.

Hysterectomy for Endometriosis-Related Pain Should be Part of a Radical Approach

For a long time, hysterectomy with bilateral salpingo-oophorectomy was considered the definitive treatment of endometriosis in that it associates a surgical effect with a hormonal effect due to the removal of the ovaries. Other endometriotic locations were sometimes overlooked, with the idea that the disease would regress after menopause was induced.

There is nevertheless data in favor of the radicality of excision when performing a hysterectomy as the definitive treatment of endometriosis. Fedele et al. compared the results of laparotomic extra-fascial hysterectomy (n = 26) with those of radical hysterectomy comprising a parametrectomy (n = 12) in treating patients presenting with endometriosis and pelvic pain [29]. Pain recurrence occurred in 30 % of patients of the former group and none of the latter. Redwine reported 75 cases of endometriosis occurring after ovarian castration and requiring repeat surgery for excision due to pain recurrence. He concluded that no endometriosis should be left untreated at castration [30].

There Is Conflicting Data on the Importance of Concomittant Bilateral Salpingo-Oophorectomy When Performing a Hysterectomy for Endometriosis

Namnoum et al. compared the results of laparotomic hysterectomy for endometriosis in 29 patients with ovarian preservation and 109 without [31]. They reported a rate of pain recurrence of 62 % in patients of the first group and 10 % in the second, with a reoperation rate of respectively 31 % and 3.7 %. Patients with ovarian preservation had a 6.1 relative risk of painful recurrence and 8.1 of reoperation. In the study of Shakiba et al. the relative risk of reoperation in case of ovarian preservation was of 2,44, although not statistically significant [27]. On the other hand, in the sub-group of patients of ages 30–39 years, BSO did not significantly increase the interval between initial and repeat surgery.

It is also to be taken into consideration that ovarian preservation is preferable in the young patient because of the cardio-vascular risk that comes with early menopause.

For that purpose, bilateral salpingo-oophorectomy is not systematic in our institution when performing a hysterectomy for endometriosis. The adnexae is only considered to be another potential site of involvement, requiring excision only when affected.

Despite Imperfect Results, Hysterectomy for Endometriosis Yields a High Level of Satisfaction

In a personal series of 39 patients having undergone hysterectomy with or without BSO for pain attributed to endometriosis between 2006 and 2012, 30 % responded to being "satisfied" of having had the procedure, and 53 % were "very satisfied", as opposed to "quite satisfied" (7.7 %) and dissatisfied (5.1 %). This came in spite of high rates of significant residual pain, defined by pain described as "important" or "unbearable" in intensity, with nearly 40 % at one year post-operatively and 30 % at 2 years.

Predictors of a high level of satisfaction were patient age, as older patients were more likely to be "very satisfied" and patient request, as patient who had requested the surgery were 50 times more likely to be "very" satisfied.

Predictors of long-term significant residual pain were age and BMI, as a patient was more likely to have pain described as "important" or "unbearable" if she was younger or with a lower BMI.

Age as a predictor is consistent with previously published data whereby age is recurrently stated as being a pejorative factor, whether in conservative surgery for endometriosis, hysterectomy for endometriosis or hysterectomy for pelvic pain in relation to a pathology other than endometriosis. Mac Donald et al. compared the results of hysterectomy for endometriosis related pain in 16 patients of age less than 30 years and 27 patients of age above 40 years [32]. In the two groups, a similar proportion of women considered themselves to be completely treated (80 %). There was no difference with regards to residual dyschezia but dyspareunia persisted in 50 % of patients younger than 30 years versus 17.4 % of patients in the other group ($p = 0.035$). There was no significant difference in the proportion patients regretting having had the procedure. Younger patients had a greater sense of loss.

Far from concluding that hysterectomy for endometriosis should be restricted to women approaching menopause, it does call for a particularly extensive information on the benefits to be expected of the surgery and its imperfect but significant impact on pain. Before performing a surgery marking the end to fertility, the surgeon should be certain that the patient is fully convinced of its usefulness. Performing a hysterectomy at the patient's request was a strong predictor of satisfaction. Therefore, hysterectomy should be suggested with caution to the younger patient, and after a reflection period.

In conclusion, hysterectomy does deserve its attribute of "definitive surgery" in that it is more efficient on chronic pain than conservative surgery, with the lowest reoperation rates. This is true only if hysterectomy is part of a radical approach of the surgical management of endometriosis and is paired with the resection of all associated lesions. The role of concomitant BSO remains to be clarified and its usefulness balanced with its potential morbidity.

Hysterectomy yields a high level of satisfaction from patients, despite an imperfect resolution of pain. Its impact on pain is significant and covers all types of pains associated with endometriosis. Hysterectomy should be suggested to patients older than 40 years as an interim solution before menopause can bring an end to the active phase of the disease. It should be performed with caution in the young patient, even when she no longer wishes to retain fertility. A strong demand coming from the patient is a good indicator of an adherence to the treatment plan and a factor of high level of satisfaction.

Surgical Strategy in Hysterectomy for Endometriosis

Endometriosis is a complex disease which can cause considerable anatomical distortion. It is multicentric and can affect the anterior and posterior compartments of the pelvis as well as the adnexaes and the urinary tract laterally.

In a normal anatomical context, performing a hysterectomy entails the application of a specific surgical approach with reproducible key steps. In case of endometriosis the surgery is a variation on this approach made to include a general strategy. The purpose of this general strategy is three-fold: restore the anatomy, identify landmarks to preserve during dissection (most importantly the ureter) and separate diseased tissue from in sano tissue. Only once these conditions have been fulfilled can the hysterectomy be performed.

The first step is exploratory for a proper assessment of lesions. This starts with a vaginal examination to search for a palpable nodule, and will serve as a benchmark for sequential examination as the nodule is dissected.

A uterine manipulator is placed, and the patient is placed in Trendelenbourg position. Thorough examination of the intra-abdominal cavity is carried. Adhesiolysis is performed, ovaries are liberated from the ovarian fossa and endometriotic cysts are drained. If ovarian preservation is decided their treatment is delayed to the end of the surgery in order to prevent blood spillage from polluting the operative field.

At this point, before undertaking the regular steps of hysterectomy, the ureters should be identified. What is usually achieved through transperitoneal direct visualization isn't possible in the context of severe endometriosis. On the left side it is made possible by removing the physiological attachment of the sigmoid to the left parietal wall. There are four advantages to this step:

1. It allows to mobilize the colon and displace it cranially in order to enhance the working space.
2. It gives direct access to the left adnexae and allows to properly identify the infundibulo-pelvic ligament.
3. The course of the ureter is visualized. This is key in deep endometriosis where it is typically medialized as a result of fibrotic retraction. It is the first structure medial to the infundibulo-pelvic ligament. It can then be lateralized and its distance with the uterus increased during central dissection.
4. It gives access to the left pararectal fossa, an avascular plane which is developed in the case of rectovaginal nodule and/or bowel involvement, or in case of a simple ventral retraction of the rectum with an adhesion to the uterine torus (posterior aspect of the uterus). This space is developed starting at the level of the pelvic brim, or more caudally, laterally to the rectovaginal space, in the absence of anatomic distortion.

During this dissection, special care should be taken in individualizing and preserving the hypogastric nerve which is found immediately underlying the peritoneum.

Once this general strategic sequence has been completed, a specific strategy is adopted depending on the organs affected.

The twin goals of this strategy are: to isolate the uterus from the affected organs in order to perform the hysterectomy, then secondarily remove the residual disease as part of a radical approach. This is the exact opposite of en bloc resection used in oncological cases, and allows a radical but economical approach disregarding the notion of safe margins. Only when the involvement is contiguous to the uterus, such as in the case of a vaginal nodule, can the resection line be displaced in order to include the immediately adjacent disease.

Case 1

The first laparoscopic view (Fig. 48.1) is of a uterus without sign of adenomyosis, but with a retracted left adnexae bearing an endometriotic cyst as well as a hydrosalpynx, adherent to the mesosigmoid. The contralateral adnexae is normal. The first step consists in performing adhesiolysis in order to first liberate the left adnexae from the mesosigmoid through simple cutting action (Fig. 48.2). This reveals fully the endometrioma which is impacted in the ovarian fossa as it is usually the case. The aspiration device is used along with the bipolar to liberate it (Fig. 48.3) and in doing so a spontaneous rupture occurs and the typical chocolate fluid is immediately and progressively aspirated (Fig. 48.4) so as to prevent it from polluting the spaces. For this reason the ovariolysis is always performed with aspirating device in hand. Once the endometrioma has been emptied, a fibrotic retration of the left adnexae is better revealed. At this point, the ureter isn't

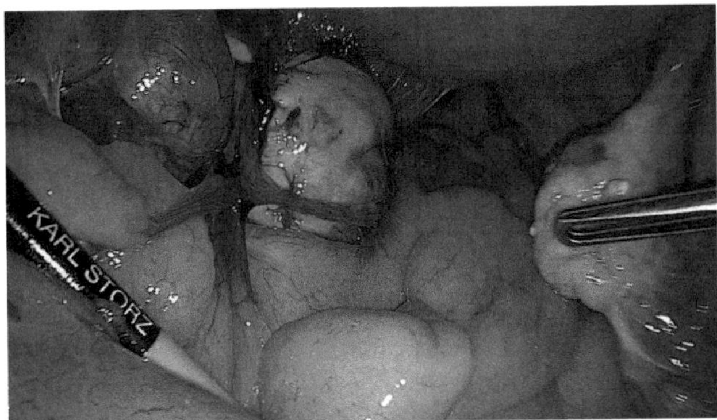

Fig. 48.1 Initial laparoscopic view: endometriosis affects the left lateral compartment

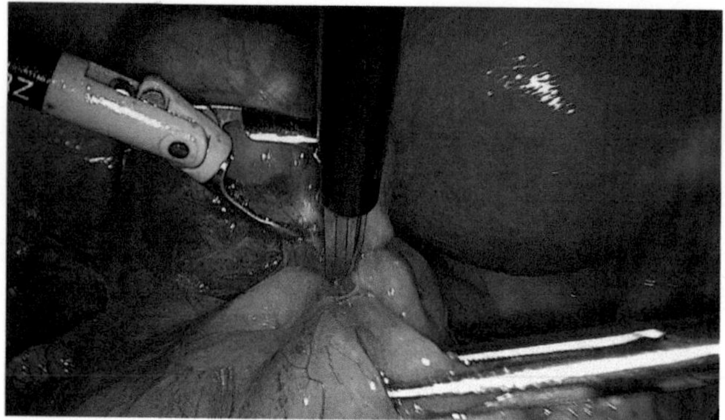

Fig. 48.2 The first step is adhesiolysis: the attachment of the mesosigmoid to the left adnexae is removed

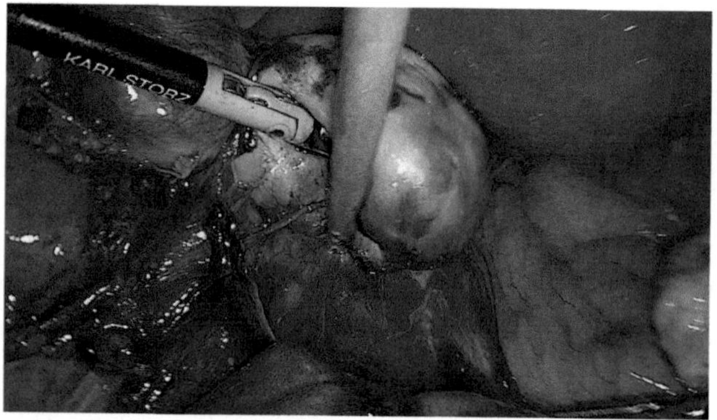

Fig. 48.3 Ovariolysis: the left endometrioma is liberated from the ovarian fossa

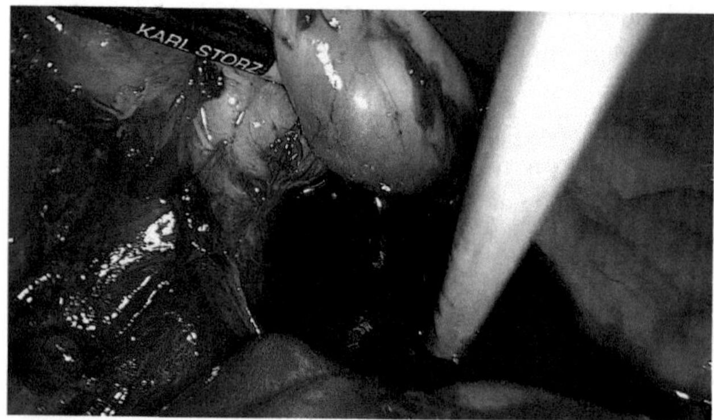

Fig. 48.4 Aspitation of typical chocolate liquid

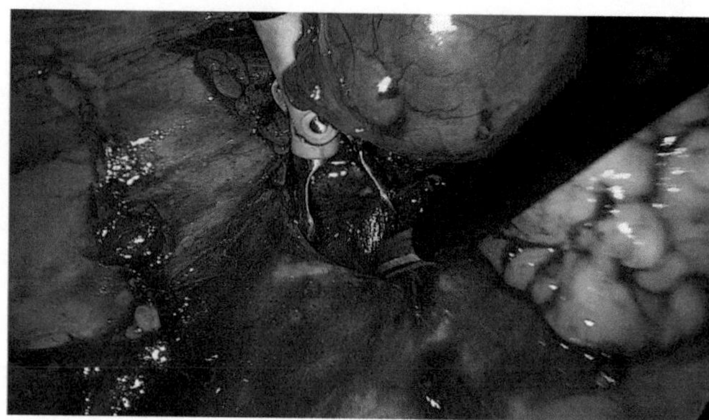

Fig. 48.5 Identify the ureter: the peritoneum is opened at the level of the IP ligament

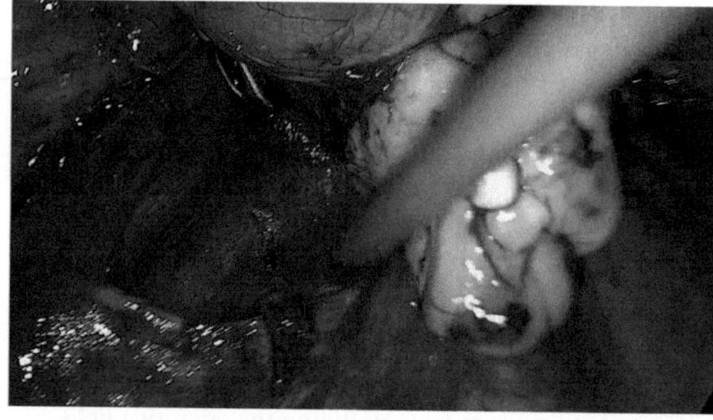

Fig. 48.6 Dividing tissues using divergent forces reveals the ureter, medial to the IP ligament

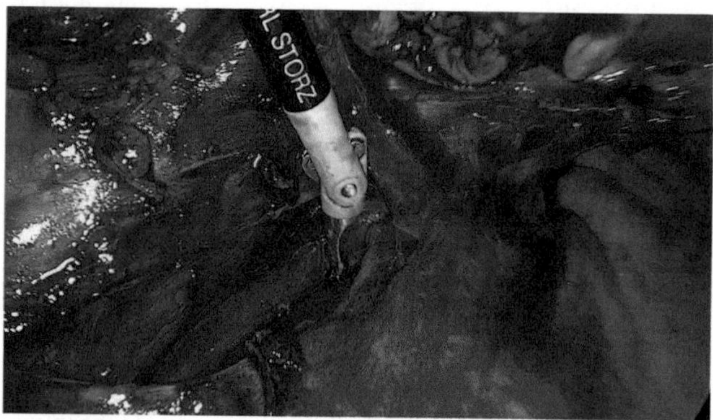

Fig. 48.7 Dissection progresses caudally and left pararectal fossa is entered

identified and it is crucial to individualize it in order to preserve it during further dissection. The peritoneum is opened at the level of infundibulo-pelvic (IP) ligament (Figs. 48.5 and 48.6). Tissues are divided until the ureter becomed apparent, medial to the IP ligament (Fig. 48.7). Dissection is carried caudally and the pararectal fossa is entered (Fig. 48.8). In doing so the ureter is reclined laterally and the bowel is separated from the adnexae. Further ureterolysis is performed to separate it from the IP ligament (Fig. 48.9). Once this preparatory step has been achieved, the hysterectomy can be started as usual with the section-coagulation of the round ligament (Fig. 48.10) and the division of the anterior peritoneum towards the isthmus (Fig. 48.11). Due to the retraction of the adnexae, the IP ligament is not as easily skeletonised as usual, and a further division of the anterior peritoneum is carried

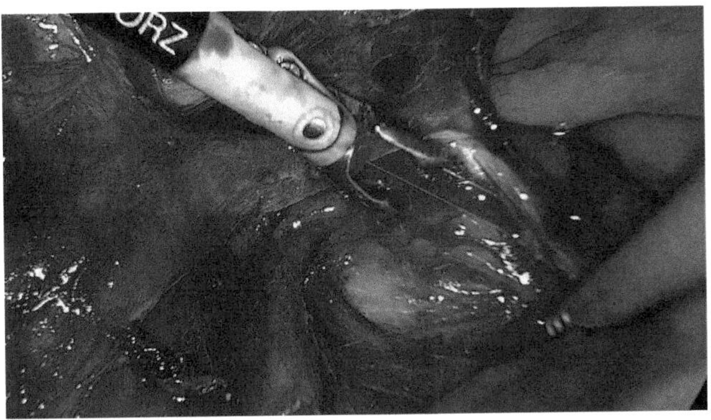

Fig. 48.8 Ureter is reclined laterally, separated from the bowel

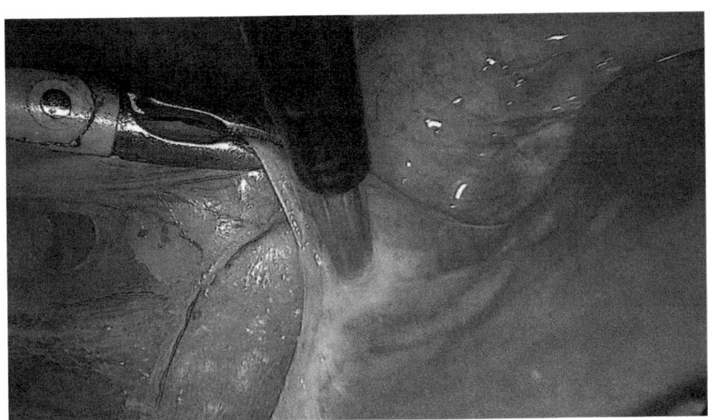

Fig. 48.11 Division of the anterior peritoneum of the broad ligament

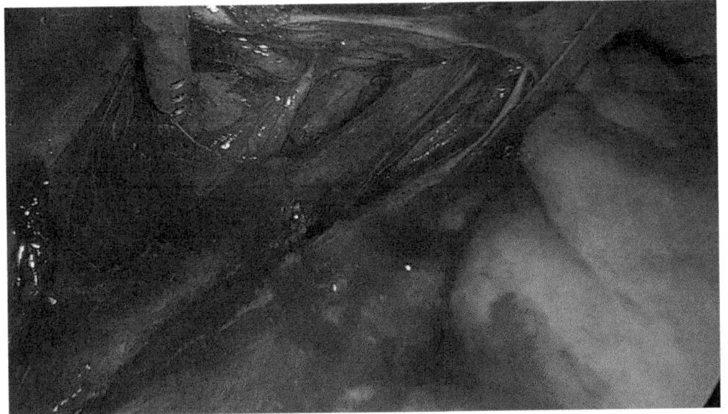

Fig. 48.9 Ureterolysis is pursued in order to separate it from the IP ligament

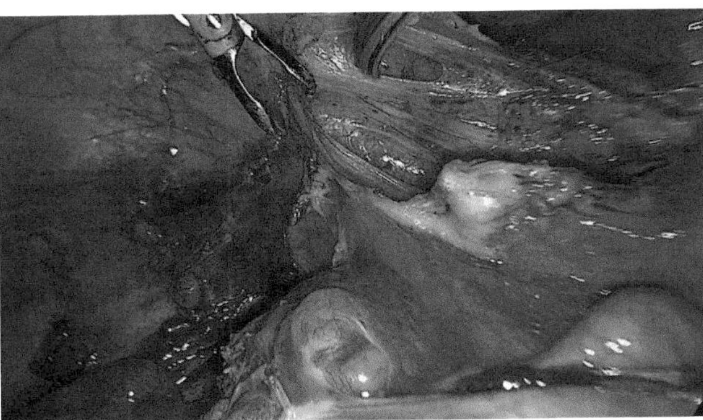

Fig. 48.12 Further division of the anterior fold, cranially, parallel to the IP ligament

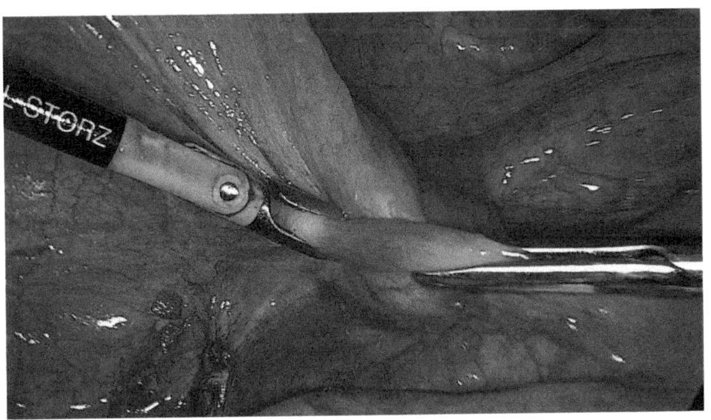

Fig. 48.10 Once the preparatory step has been achieved, the usual steps of hysterectomy can be performed: the round ligament is divided

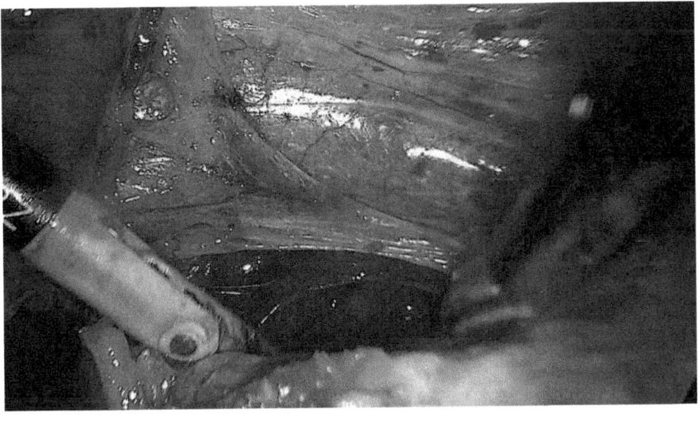

Fig. 48.13 Fenestration of the broad ligament allows to skeletonize the IP ligament

cranially, parallel to the IP ligament in order to better identify it (Fig. 48.12). The posterior peritoneum is fenestrated as usual (Figs. 48.13 and 48.14) and as a further verification measure the bipolar is passed through the opening and to the other side (Fig. 48.15). It then becomes apparent that the ureter is at a safe distance and the section-coagulation of the IP ligament can be performed safely. The rest of the hysterectomy is achieved through the classical steps.

Case 2

In this case, the endometriotic involvement is at the level of the anterior compartment with a retraction of the vesicouterine peritoneum (Fig. 48.16). It is uncertain whether the endometriotic nodule affects the bladder or merely the anterior aspect of the uterus. Two thick lateral folds in the peritoneum are a consequence of the retraction. The dissection is initiated laterally at their level, at a safe distance

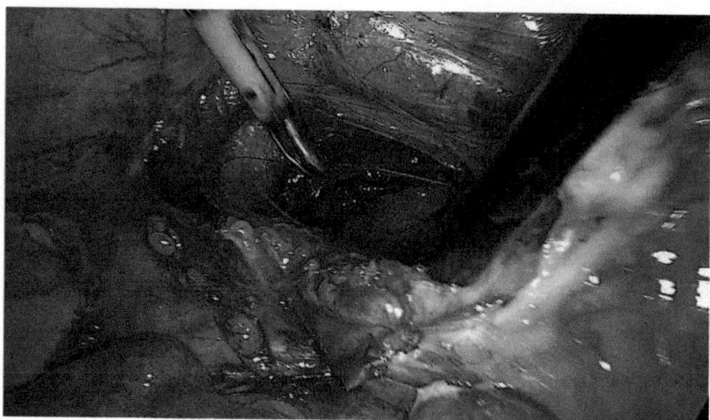

Fig. 48.14 Fenestration is achieved applying divergent forces

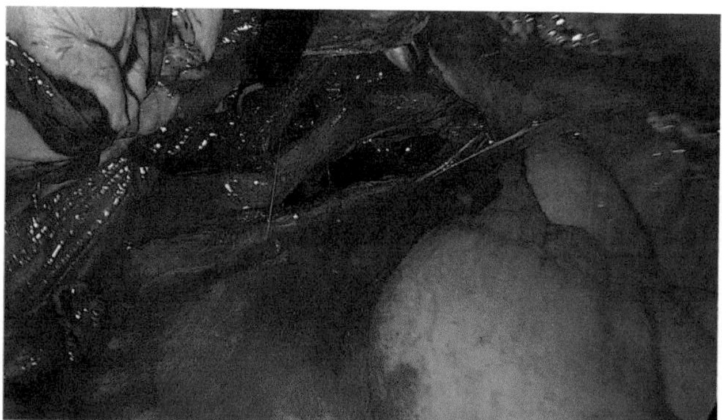

Fig. 48.15 Prior to sectioning the IP ligament, an instrument is passed through the window created in the broad ligament, and seen at a safe distance from the ureter

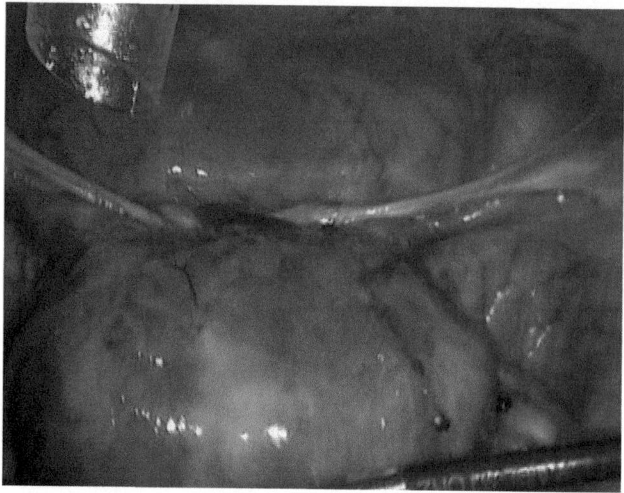

Fig. 48.16 Initial laparoscopic view: endometriotic retraction affecting the anterior compartment

from the bladder (Fig. 48.17). The peritoneum is incised and through pneumodissection, the bubble effect is seen at the level of the paravesical space (Fig. 48.18). The vesico-uterine peritoneum is divided medially (Fig. 48.19),

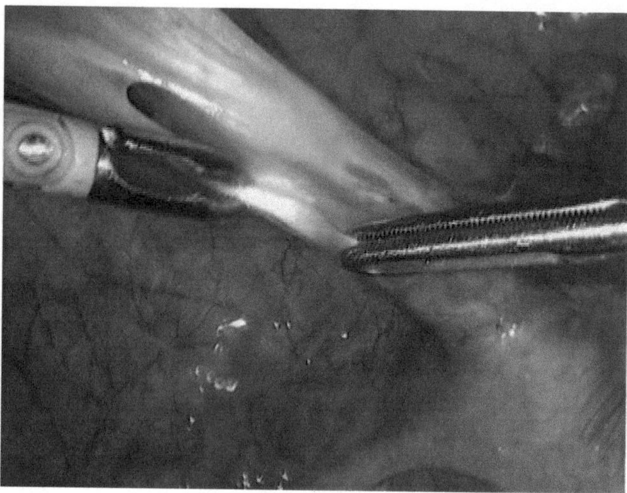

Fig. 48.17 Dissection is initiated laterally in the peritoneal retractile folds, at a safe distance from the bladder

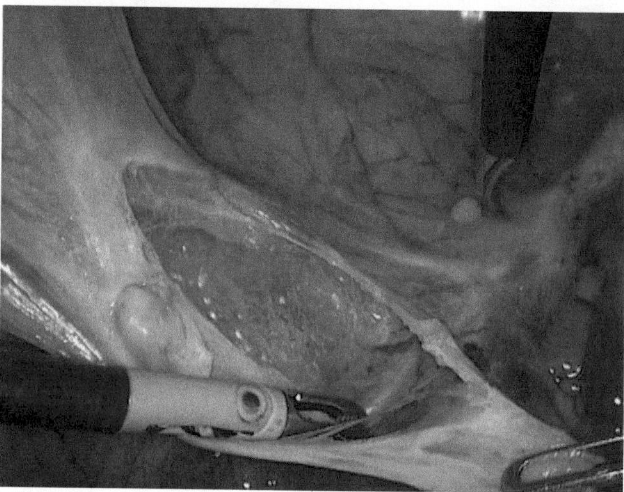

Fig. 48.18 Pneumodissection creating a bubble effect in the left paravesical fossa

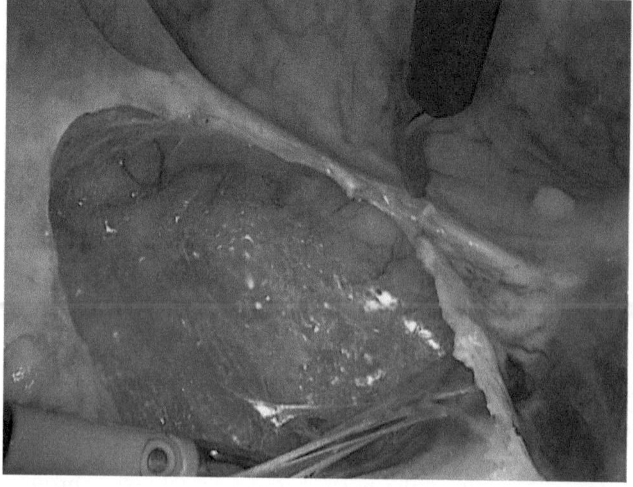

Fig. 48.19 Division of the vesico-uterine peritoneum

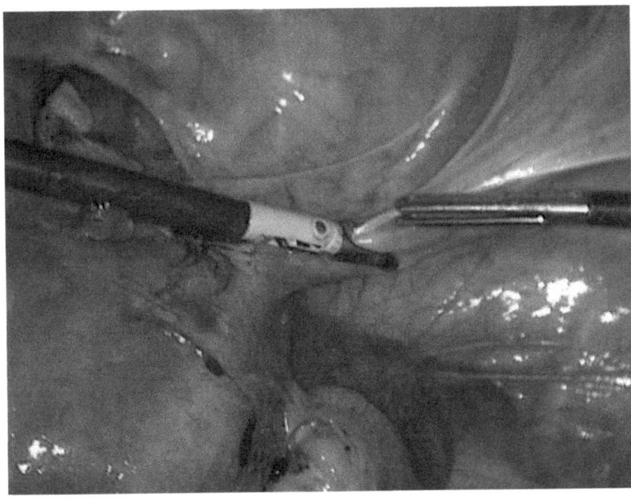

Fig. 48.20 Contralateral dissection

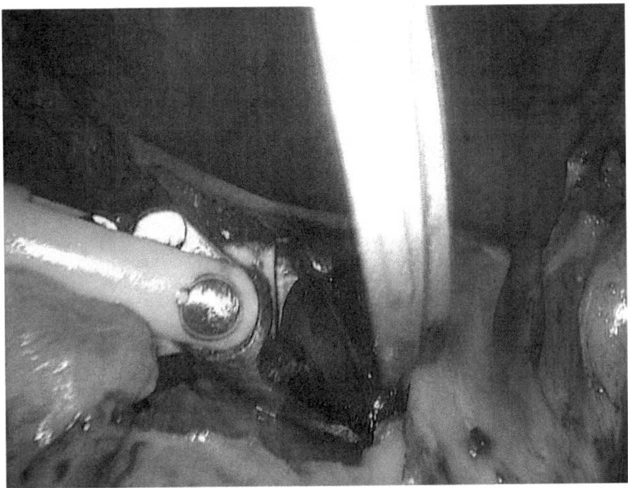

Fig. 48.22 Peritoneum dissected away from the bladder

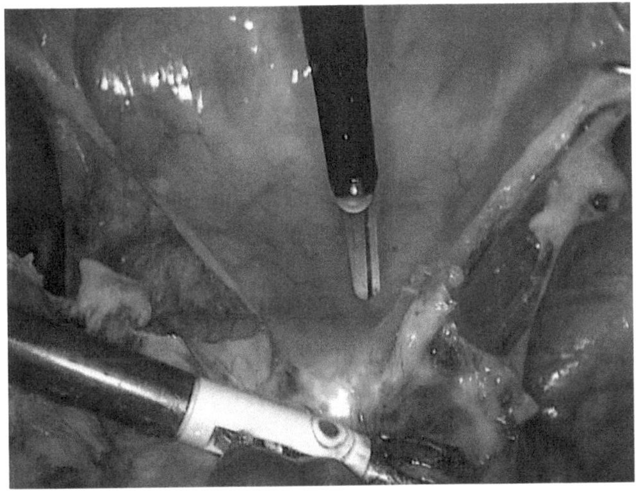

Fig. 48.21 A peritoneal bridge at the level of the bladder lays remnant after bilateral dissection

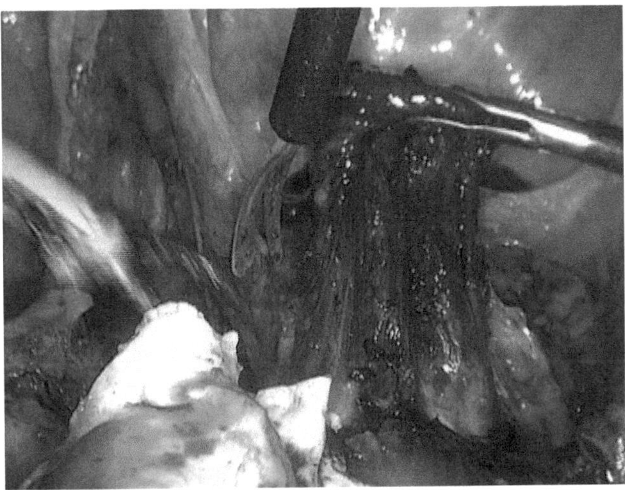

Fig. 48.23 Usual dissection of the vesico-uterine space, the endometriosis affecting the anterior aspect of the uterus, and sparing the bladder

without fully reaching the midline. The dissection is then initiated contra-laterally with the section-coagulation of the right round ligament and safely carried medially (Fig. 48.20). A peritoneal bridge then lays between the two lateral spaces of dissection (Fig. 48.21), close to the bladder. Through divergent movements of the bipolar jaws (Fig. 48.22), the peritoneum is progressively separated from the bladder then divided. It is at that point apparent that the bladder is unaffected. The bladder is seized and the vesico-uterine space is dissected in the usual manner (Fig. 48.23). At the end of the dissection, the endometriotic retraction has been fully separated from the bladder and is entirely on the anterior aspect of the uterus (Fig. 48.24). At that level, the colpotomy will be displaced caudally in order to include the disease. The rest of the hysterectomy can be carried through the usual steps.

In conclusion of these two cases, the usual steps of the hysterectomy apply, but depending on the location of the

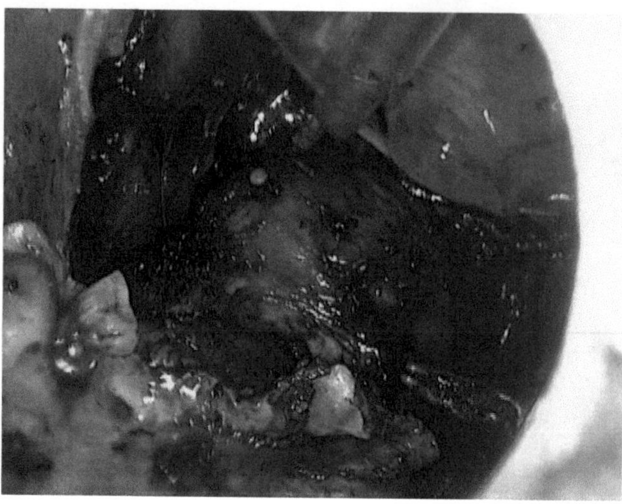

Fig. 48.24 Initiation of colpotomy. The line will be displaced caudally for the hysterectomy to entirely include the endometriotic tissue

endometriosis, a preparatory operative step is necessary. It aims to identify and keep the adjacent organs at a safe distance.

References

1. Eskenazi B, Warner ML. Epidemiology of endometriosis. Obstet Gynecol Clin North Am. 1997;24:235–58.
2. Moen MH, Muus KM. Endometriosis in pregnant and non-pregnant women at tubal sterilisation. Hum Reprod. 1991;6:699–702.
3. Gruppo italiano per lo studio dell'endometriosi. Prevalence and anatomical distribution of endometriosis in women with selected gynaecological conditions: results from a multicentric Italian study. Hum Reprod. 1994;9:1158–62.
4. Waller KG, Lindsay P, Curtis P, Shaw RW. The prevalence of endometriosis in women with infertile partners. Eur J Obstet Gynecol Reprod Biol. 1993;48:135–9.
5. Tokushige N, Markham R, Russell P, Fraser IS. High density of small nerve fibers in the functional layer of the endometrium in women with endometriosis. Hum Reprod. 2006;21:782–7.
6. Tokushige N, Markham R, Russell P, Fraser IS. Effects of hormonal treatment on nerve fibers in endometrium and myometrium in women with endometriosis. Fertil Steril. 2008;90:1589–98.
7. Al-Jefout M, Dezarnaulds G, Cooper M, Tokushige N, Luscombe GM, Markham R, et al. Diagnosis of endometriosis by detection of nerve fibres in an endometrial biopsy: a double blind study. Hum Reprod. 2009;24:3019–24.
8. Zhang X, Lu B, Huang X, Xu H, Zhou C, Lin J. Endometrial nerve fibers in women with endometriosis, adenomyosis, and uterine fibroids. Fertil Steril. 2009;92:1799–801.
9. Cramer DW, Missmer SA. The epidemiology of endometriosis. Ann N Y Acad Sci. 2002;955:11–22.
10. Treloar SA, Martin NG, Heath AC. Longitudinal genetic analysis of menstrual flow, pain, and limitation in a sample of Australian twins. Behav Genet. 1998;28:107–16.
11. Baird DT, Cameron ST, Critchley HO, Drudy TA, Howe A, Jones RL, et al. Prostaglandins and menstruation. Eur J Obstet Gynecol Reprod Biol. 1996;70:15–7.
12. Martinez-Gaudio M, Yoshida T, Bengtsson LP. Propagated and nonpropagated myometrial contractions in normal menstrual cycles. Am J Obstet Gynecol. 1973;115:107–11.
13. Maslow KD, Lyons EA. Effect of prostaglandin and antiprostaglandin on midcycle myometrial contractions. Fertil Steril. 2004;82:511–3.
14. Bulletti C, Rossi S, Albonetti A, Polli VV, De Ziegler D, Massoneau M, et al. Uterine contractility in patients with endometriosis. J Am Assoc Gynecol Laparosc. 1996;3(4 suppl):S5.
15. Koninckx PR, Martin DC. Deep endometriosis a consequense of infiltration or retraction or possible adenomyosis externa. Fertil Steril. 1992;58:924–8.
16. Kunz G, Beil D, Huppert P, Noe M, Kissler S, Leyendecker G. Adenomyosis in endometriosis-prevalence and impact on fertility. Evidence from magnetic resonance imaging. Hum Reprod. 2005;20(8):2309–16.
17. Larsen SB, Lundorf E, Forman A, Dueholm M. Adenomyosis and junctional zone changes in patients with endometriosis. Eur J Obstet Gynecol Reprod Biol. 2011;157(2):206–11.
18. Parker JD, Leondires M, Sinaii N, Premkumar A, Nieman LK, Stratton P. Persistence of dysmenorrhea and nonmenstrual pain after optimal endometriosis surgery may indicate adenomyosis. Fertil Steril. 2006;86:711–5.
19. Ferrero S, Camerini G, Menada MV, Biscaldi E, Ragni N, Remorgida V. Uterine adenomyosis in persistence of dysmenorrhea after surgical excision pelvic endometriosis and colorectal resection. J Reprod Med. 2009;54(6):366–72.
20. Kuppermann M, Learman LA, Schembri M, Gregorich SE, Jackson RA, Jacoby A, et al. Contributions of hysterectomy and uterus-preserving surgery to health-related quality of life. Obstet Gynecol. 2013;122(1):15–25.
21. Hartmann KE, Ma C, Lamvu GM, Langenberg PW, Steege JF, Kjerulff KH. Quality of life and sexual function after hysterectomy in women with preoperative pain and depression. Obstet Gynecol. 2004;104:701–9.
22. Brandsborg B, Nikolajsen L, Hansen CT, Kehlet H, Jensen TS. Risk factors for chronic pain after hysterectomy: a nationwide questionnaire and database study. Anesthesiology. 2007;106(5):1003–12.
23. Stovall TG, Ling FW, Crawford DA. Hysterectomy for chronic pelvic pain of presumed uterine etiology. Obstet Gynecol. 1990;75:676–9.
24. Hillis SD, Marchbanks PA, Peterson HB. The effectiveness of hysterectomy for chronic pelvic pain. Obstet Gynecol. 1995;86:941–5.
25. Berner E, Qvigstad E, Myrvold AK, Lieng M. Pelvic pain and patient satisfaction after laparoscopic supracervical hysterectomy: prospective trial. J Minim Invasive Gynecol. 2014;21(3):406–11.
26. Weir E, Mustard C, Cohen M, Kung R. Endometriosis: what is the risk of hospital admission, readmission, and major surgical intervention? J Minim Invasive Gynecol. 2005;12(6):486–93.
27. Shakiba K, Bena JF, McGill KM, Minger J, Falcone T. Surgical treatment of endometriosis: a 7-year follow-up on the requirement for further surgery (published erratum appears in: Obstet Gynecol. 2008; 112(3):710). Obstet Gynecol. 2008;111(6):1285–92.
28. Sinaii N, Cleary SD, Younes N, Ballweg ML, Stratton P. Treatment utilization for endometriosis symptoms: a cross-sectional survey study of lifetime experience. Fertil Steril. 2007;87(6):1277–86.
29. Fedele L, Bianchi S, Zanconato G, Berlanda N, Borruto F, Frontino G. Tailoring radicality in demolitive surgery for deeply infiltrating endometriosis. Am J Obstet Gynecol. 2005;193(1):114–7.
30. Redwine DB. Endometriosis persisting after castration: clinical characteristics and results of surgical management. Obstet Gynecol. 1994;83:405–13.
31. Namnoum AB, Hickman TN, Goodman SB, Gehlbach DL, Rock JA. Incidence of symptom recurrence after hysterectomy for endometriosis. Fertil Steril. 1995;64(5):898–902.
32. MacDonald SR, Klock SC, Milad MP. Long-term outcome of nonconservative surgery (hysterectomy) for endometriosis-associated pain in women < 30 years old. Am J Obstet Gynecol. 1999;180(6 Pt 1):1360–3.

Laparoscopic Hysterectomy (TLH) in Obese Patients

49

Raffaele Tinelli and Ettore Cicinelli

Introduction

Several studies showed that LPS treatment of obese women with endometrial pathologies offers many advantages compared to the open approach [1–4] primarily considering the less postoperative pain, better visibility of the operative field, and shorter hospital stay as the main benefit [5, 6]; postoperative complications after LPS treatment seems to be reduced or similar [1, 3], likely related to the laparoscopic expertise of the operating surgeons and the patient's co-morbidities.

However, this procedure does not seem to modify the incidence of intra-operative and post-operative complications [3, 7].

It appears from data of several studies that LPS hysterectomy may offer significant advantages over LPT in the comprehensive surgical management of extremely obese women, but it should be performed by advanced laparoscopic gynaecologic surgeons [7].

Surgical Technique of Laparoscopic Hysterectomy

After dilatation with a Hegar dilator (no. 7.5), an uterine manipulator (*Clermont-Ferrand,* Karl Storz, Tuttlingen, Germany) is inserted.

A 11 mm Endopath XCEL® trocar (Ethicon, Johnson & Johnson, USA) that incorporates the zero-degree laparoscope (Karl Storz, Tuttlingen, Germany) was inserted through an umbilical vertical incision, after pneumoperitoneum by Veress needle (Covidien Cares, Minneapolis, MN) has been induced at the level of umbilicus.

Difficulties of entry into the abdomen in obese patients are often associated with the expanded thick fatty layer of the abdominal wall, especially with translocation of the umbilicus which is more caudal to the normal umbilical site and just below the aortic bifurcation.

In our technique, an 11 mm skin incision is created at the superior crease of the umbilical fold, and the underlying subcutaneous adipose tissue is bluntly dissected using the tip of a fine clamp until the umbilical stalk is isolated at the inferior and central part of the incision.

There is a concern that rare but life-threatening complications can occur, including severe bleeding due to damages of major abdominal vessels, as well as other injuries related to bowel and bladder trauma, subcutaneous emphysema and postsurgical infections.

To prevent these complications and risks, the abdominal wall is elevated by upward traction. In obese patients the Veress needle is then inserted nearly perpendicular to the incision and turned toward the pelvis "immediately" after resistance to the needle has been lost.

Three suprapubic ancillary trocars were used: one 5 mm Endopath XCEL® trocar (Ethicon, Johnson & Johnson, USA) trocar was inserted in the midline 3 cm under the umbilicus, and one in each iliac fossa (11 mm on the left side and 5 mm on the right size) laterally to inferior epigastric vessels, respectively.

Before the operative procedure, all the pelvic structures are inspected and the abdomen explored through the laparoscope in a clockwise fashion.

Laparoscopic hysterectomy is performed with the patient in an approximately 30 ° Trendelenburg position to facilitate retroperitoneal exposure by retaining the small intestine in the mid and upper abdomen using gravity and gentle instrumentation. In patients with a prior midline incision, the initial entry into the abdominal cavity was made approximately 2 cm below the left costal margin at the level of the midclavicular line to avoid injury to bowel adherent to the anterior abdominal wall.

R. Tinelli (✉)
Department of OB/GYN, Perrino Hospital, Brindisi 72100, Italy
e-mail: raffaeletinelli@gmail.com

E. Cicinelli
Department of OB/GYN, University Medical School of Bari, Bari, Italy

I. Alkatout, L. Mettler (eds.), *Hysterectomy*, DOI 10.1007/978-3-319-22497-8_49

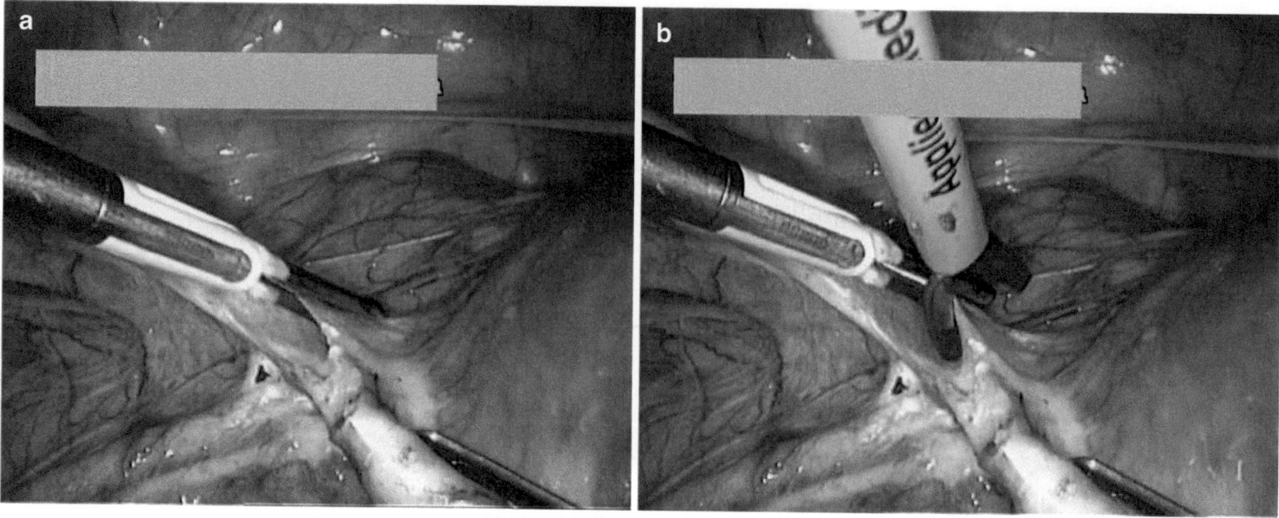

Fig. 49.1 (**a**, **b**) The round ligament is coagulated and transected with endoscopic shears

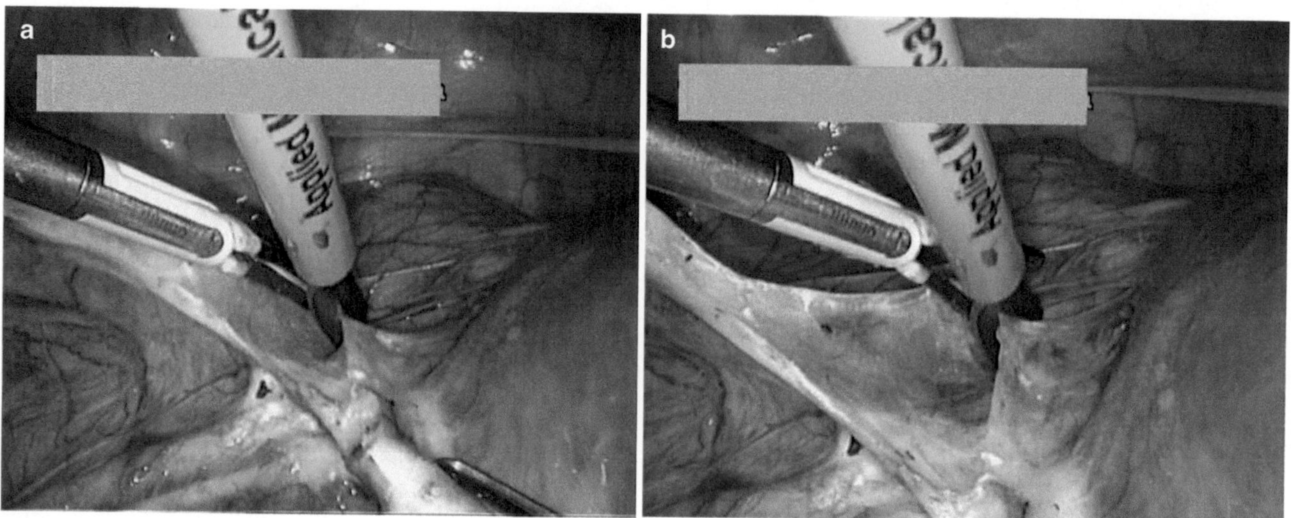

Fig. 49.2 (**a**, **b**) The vesico-uterine fold is grasped and incised

A MiniPort 2 mm single use introducer (MiniPort-Auto-Suture, USSC, Norwalk, CT) and a stopcock for insufflation and desufflation were used to establish the pneumoperitoneum.

The obturator had a spring-loaded, blunt stylet similar in function to a Veress needle. A circular adjustable stopper located on the sleeve of the miniport allowed for adjustment of depth in the cavity. The system was used to establish and maintain the pneumoperitoneum in the abdomen while providing access for a minilaparoscope with a diameter of 1.9 mm and a length of 10 or 12 cm (Karl Storz, Tuttlingen, Germany).

The round ligament is coagulated and transected with endoscopic shears (Fig. 49.1). The vesico-uterine fold is grasped and incised (Fig. 49.2) while the bladder is isolated: after dividing the vesico-uterine fold (Fig. 49.3, the suction-irrigator probe pushes the bladder completely from the upper vagina (Fig. 49.4).

The anterior and posterior peritoneal layers of the broad ligament are opened and the ureter is identified at the pelvic brim, traced into the pelvis and freed from the posterior leaf of the broad ligament. The ovarian ligament is coagulated (Fig. 49.5) with bipolar forceps and transacted with scissors. The uterine vessels are identified allowing an excellent skeletonization of the obliterated artery by preparing the anterior and posterior web. The uterine artery is coagulated and transected.

The vagina is visualized and the vaginal cuff around the cervix is transected with the monopolar needle (Fig. 49.6), incising the vagina circumferentially using the

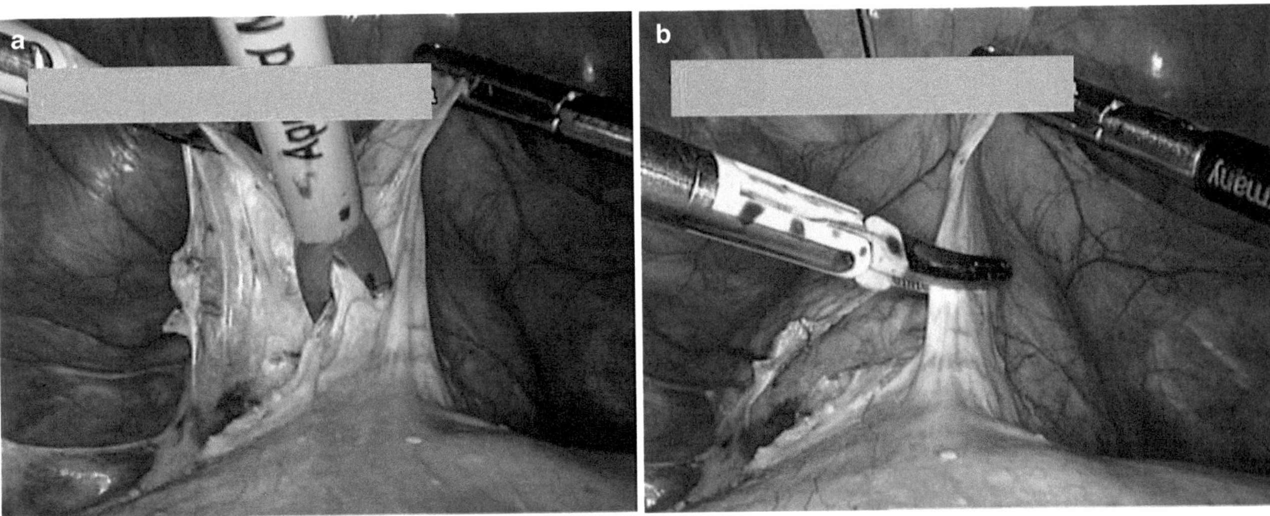

Fig. 49.3 (a, b) The bladder is isolated after dividing the vesico-uterine fold

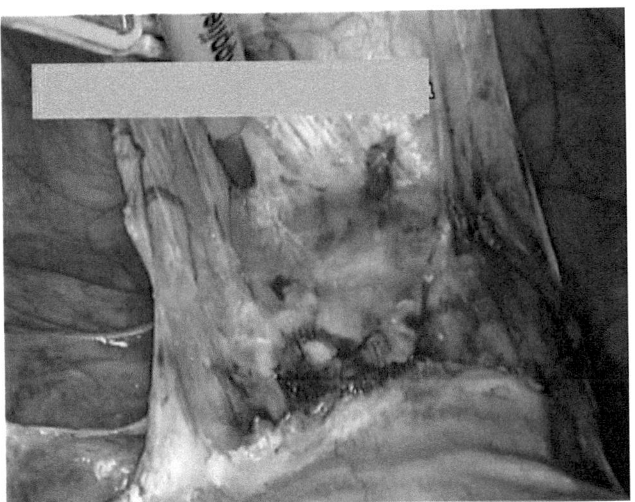

Fig. 49.4 The endoscopic sheras pushes the bladder completely from the upper vagina

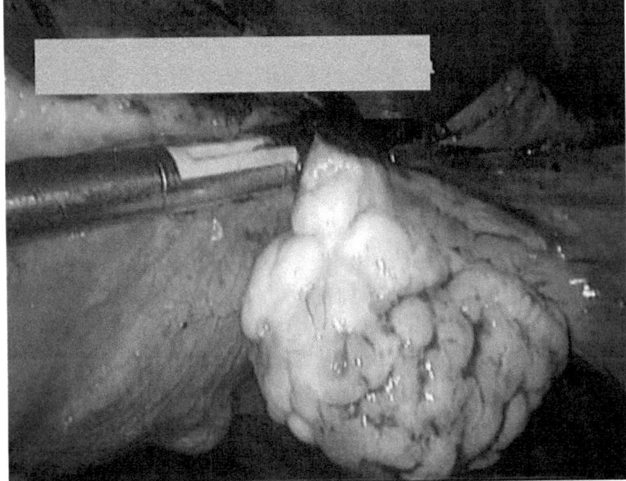

Fig. 49.5 The ovarian ligament is coagulated with bipolar forceps and transacted with scissors

porcelain-valve of the uterine manipulator as a guide; the uterus is removed vaginally. The vaginal vault is closed with continuous 0-polysorb sutures by laparoscopic access and after the laparoscopic control of the haemostasis is performed (Fig. 49.7). The 5- and 10-mm incisions are closed with mattress sutures of 2–0 Rapide Vycril. At the conclusion of the surgical procedure we deflated the abdomen before removing the trocars.

During laparoscopic surgery in obese patients, sufficient intraabdominal workspace is important for the surgeon. Therefore, most surgeons request that their patients be placed in an adequate Trendelenburg position to facilitate retroperitoneal exposure in the case of lymphadenectomy. This leads to retention of the small intestine in the mid and upper abdomen using gravity and gentle instrumentation and reduces bowel injury; however, the effect of an increased workspace is not always sufficient.

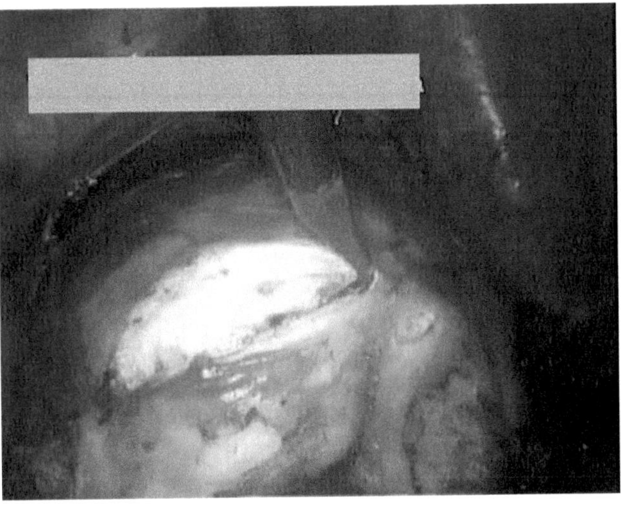

Fig. 49.6 The vagina is visualizated and vaginal cuff around the cervix is transected with monopolar needle

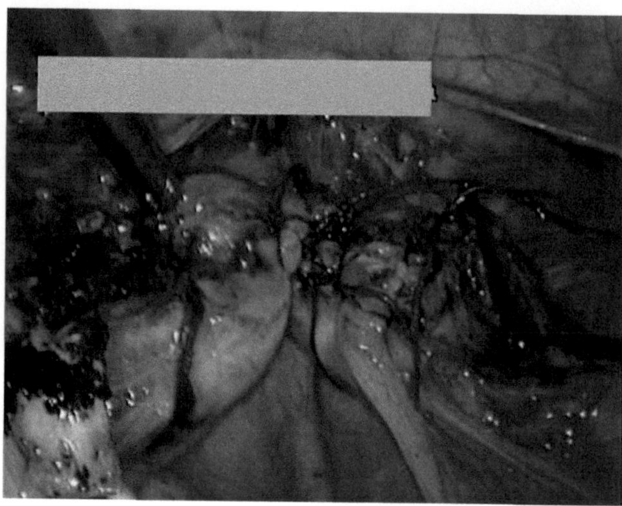

Fig. 49.7 The vaginal vault is closed with continuous 0-polysorb sutures by laparoscopic access and after the laparoscopic control of the hemostasis is performed

Discussion

Obese patients with endometrial cancer patients exhibit a large accumulation and abnormal distribution of abdominal fat; these characteristics seriously affect the exposure of the operative field. In addition, perivascular fat parcels and lipid deposition on vascular walls lead to increased vascular fragility; as a result, slight stretching of blood vessels can easily lead to vascular rupture and bleeding, which severely affect the surgical process and increase surgical difficulty and risk. Furthermore, obesity is frequently associated with many cardiopulmonary and other chronic diseases that decrease operational tolerance.

Many patients with gynaecologic pathologies present with co-morbidity such as obesity, hypertension, and diabetes [8]. Abdominal surgery is therefore exposing patients into increased risk of complications [9].

The role of minimally invasive surgical staging in the management of extremely obese patients with gynaecologic pathologies continues to evolve. Recently, several studies concluded, as others, that the post-operative complications after LPS treatment are reduced or similar [5, 9–12].

Brezina et al. compared the surgical outcomes of 293 obese women undergoing hysterectomy (LPT, vaginal, or LPS). No significant difference was found in obese women between LPS and LPT hysterectomy for operative time and anaesthesia. They concluded that in obese patients for whom vaginal hysterectomy is not possible, LPS hysterectomy should be considered before LPT hysterectomy because the LPS route reduced hospital time and blood loss [13].

Nawfal et al. estimated the impact of body mass index (BMI) on the surgical outcomes of 135 patients undergoing robotic-assisted total LPS hysterectomy for benign indications. They concluded that BMI is not associated with blood loss, duration of surgery, length of stay, or complication rates in patients undergoing robotic-assisted total LPS hysterectomy. Robotic assistance may help surgeons overcome adverse outcomes sometimes found in obese patients [14].

Bardens et al. investigated the influence of the body mass index (BMI) on 200 patients who underwent LPS hysterectomy for benign disease. The group of overweight women had the highest rate of complications and the group of obese women had the lowest. However, the rate of women who required readmission and reoperation was not elevated in the overweight group. They concluded that LPS hysterectomy is a safe and feasible method even in obese and morbidly obese patients. Overweight and obesity increase the time needed to perform LPS hysterectomy but do not seem to relevantly influence the rate of major intra and postoperative complications [15].

Harmanli et al. compared the effect of obesity on perioperative outcomes in women undergoing LPS supracervical hysterectomy (LSH) or LPS total hysterectomy (TLH) for benign conditions in obese (body mass index > or = 30 kg/m^2) and non-obese women. The rates of urinary tract injury, vaginal cuff dehiscence, postoperative fever, and ileus were similar between the groups. Of all seven cuff dehiscences, 5 (71 %) occurred in non-obese women undergoing TLH. They concluded that obesity increased the risk of bleeding requiring transfusion and conversion to laparotomy but did not influence the other perioperative complications. LSH in non-obese women seems to result in best outcomes [16].

In a recent study by Fanfani et al. they analysed perioperative outcomes of Laparo-Endoscopic Single-Site (LESS) hysterectomy in obese and non-obese women in a multicentric retrospective case-control study on 115 women who underwent LESS hysterectomy and were divided into two groups: obese (n = 43, BMI $\geq$ 30 kg/m^2) and non-obese (n = 72, BMI < 30 kg/m^2). No statistical differences regarding perioperative outcomes were observed between the two groups. Conversion to laparotomy occurred in 1 obese (2.3 %) and 3 (4.2 %) non-obese women. Intraoperative complication rate was 11.6 % and 9.6 % in obese and non-obese women, respectively. The early postoperative complication rate was 6.9 % in obese and 4.1 % in non-obese women. This study suggested that obesity (BMI $\geq$ 30) does not preclude successful completion of total LESS hysterectomy [17].

In a recent retrospective study Tinelli et al. compared the safety, complication and recurrence rate after total LPS hysterectomy with lymphadenectomy and LPT hysterectomy with lymphadenectomy for early stage endometrial carcinoma in a series of 75 extremely obese women (BMI > 35).

They performed a multicenter study of all the complications after treatment of 75 consecutive extremely obese patients with clinical stage I endometrial cancer who

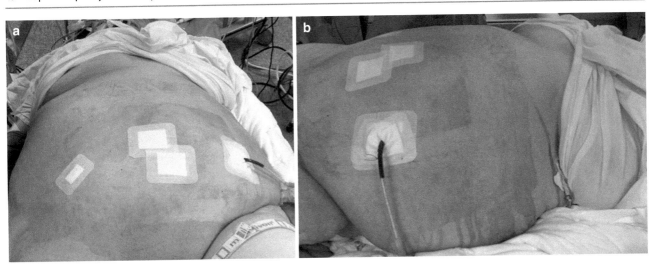

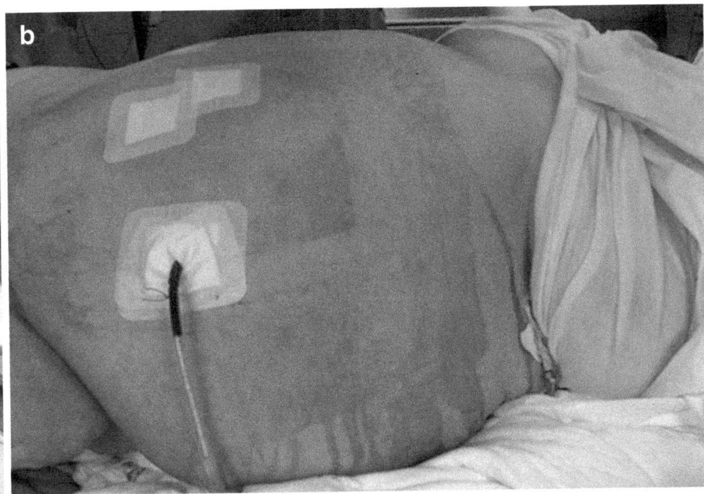

Fig. 49.8 (**a**, **b**) LPS procedures were successfully completed without conversion to LPT and no patient of the two groups required an intraoperative or postoperative blood transfusion

underwent LPS hysterectomy (45 cases) or LPT hysterectomy (30 cases) with pelvic and aortic lymph node dissection.

According to the FIGO staging system, all the patients underwent surgical staging consisting of total hysterectomy, bilateral salpingo-oophorectomy, and in all cases systematic bilateral pelvic lymphadenectomy was performed. In three patients of the LPT group they observed a dehiscence of the abdominal suture with surgical site infection in the first week after surgery that was resutured with interrupted sutured with no sequelae. Postoperative fever was reported in 6 (20 %) patients of the LPT group and in 2 patient of LPS (4.4 %) group.

No case of port-site metastasis, no vascular injury and no wound complications were detected.

In all cases the LPS procedures were successfully completed without conversion to LPT and no patient of the two groups required an intra-operative or postoperative blood transfusion (Fig. 49.8).

One case of bladder injury occurred in the LPS group at the time of utero-vesical fold incision that was laparoscopically sutured.

In this multicentre study, no significant difference in intra-operative complications was observed between groups, whereas postoperative were significantly less common in the LPS than in the LPT group.

We can speculate that LPS hysterectomy in extremely obese women is associated with safety and efficacy outcomes that are similar to those that have been reported for LPT hysterectomy for the treatment of endometrial pathologies [18, 19].

In fact, in almost cases the LPS procedures were successfully completed without conversion to LPT and no patient of the two groups required an intra-operative or postoperative blood transfusion.

Therefore, it appears from data of our studies that LPS hysterectomy may offer significant advantages over LPT in the comprehensive surgical management of extremely obese women, but it should be performed by advanced laparoscopic gynaecologic surgeons.

In fact, a totally LPS hysterectomy is more difficult in the morbidly obese and other patient factors such as associated co-morbidities, adhesive disease, large uteri, fatty mesentery, and inability to tolerate steep Trendelenburg have limited widespread use of this approach in the treatment of uterine pathologies [3–7, 20].

The obese patients with associated co-morbidities had the most to gain from a successfully completed minimally invasive procedure, but also offered the surgeon the greatest challenges to complete the case [21–24].

Moreover, the LPS permits a better exposure of the operative field in association with the advancement of the LPS techniques allowing better dissection of the pelvic spaces; however, it should be outlined that LPS procedures have to be always performed by the same surgical team [4, 7, 12].

Several studies confirm that LPS hysterectomy remains, in expert hands, the procedure better related to the best short-term outcomes in obese women [13–19, 25].

In fact, LPS hysterectomy was associated with a shorter time of post-operative ileus, shorter hospitalization, lower cases of dehiscence of the suture with surgical site infection, reduced cases of postoperative fever, and a reduced time of discharge when compared with LPT fever reducing the costs.

Conclusion

Our data confirm that LPS hysterectomy in extremely obese women improves quality of life in the postoperative period with reduced time of discharge.

The low intra-operative and post-operative complications rate observed in the LPS group highlights the feasibility, safety and efficacy of this surgical approach for the obese patients.

LPS hysterectomy can be considered a safe and effective therapeutic approach for management of e obese women with a better visibility of the operative field, lower postoperative pain, and a significantly lower blood loss, although multicentre randomized trials, long-term follow-up and cost-benefit analyses are required to determine if the use of LPS improves outcomes over standard LPT in obese women and if the advantages of this technique could be extended to a larger proportion of patients.

References

1. Ghezzi F, Cromi A, Bergamini V, Uccella S, Beretta P, Franchi M, Bolis P. Laparoscopic management of endometrial cancer in non-obese and obese women: a consecutive series. J Minim Invasive Gynecol. 2006;13:269–75.
2. Malur S, Possover M, Michels W, Schneider A. Laparoscopic-assisted vaginal versus abdominal surgery in patients with endometrial cancer: a prospective randomized trial. Gynecol Oncol. 2001;80:239–44.
3. Malzoni M, Tinelli R, Cosentino F, Perone C, Rasile M, Iuzzolino D, Malzoni C, Reich H. Total laparoscopic hysterectomy versus abdominal hysterectomy with lymphadenectomy for early-stage endometrial cancer: a prospective randomized study. Gynecol Oncol. 2009;112:126–33.
4. Palomba S, Falbo A, Mocciaro R, Russo T, Zullo F. Laparoscopic treatment for endometrial cancer: a meta-analysis of randomized controlled trials (RCTs). Gynecol Oncol. 2009;112:415–21.
5. Galaal K, Bryant A, Fisher AD, Al-Khaduri M, Kew F, Lopes AD. Laparoscopy versus laparotomy for the management of early stage endometrial cancer. Cochrane Database Syst Rev 2012;(9):CD 006655.
6. Perrone AM, Di Marcoberardino B, Rossi M, Pozzati F, Pellegrini A, Procaccini M, Santini D, De Iaco P. Laparoscopic versus laparotomic approach to endometrial cancer. Eur J Gynaecol Oncol. 2012;33:376–81.
7. Litta P, Merlin F, Saccardi C, Pozzan C, Sacco G, Fracas M, Capobianco G, Dessole S. Role of hysteroscopy with endometrial biopsy to rule out endometrial cancer in postmenopausal women with abnormal uterine bleeding. Maturitas. 2005;50:117–23.
8. Kalogiannidis I, Lambrechts S, Amant F, Neven P, Van Gorp T, Vergote I. Laparoscopy-assisted vaginal hysterectomy compared with abdominal hysterectomy in clinical stage I endometrial cancer: safety, recurrence, and long-term outcome. Am J Obstet Gynecol. 2007;196:248.
9. Litta P, Bartolucci C, Saccardi C, Codroma A, Fabris A, Borgato S, Conte L. Atypical endometrial lesions: hysteroscopic resection as an alternative to hysterectomy. Eur J Gynaecol Oncol. 2013;34:51–3.
10. Mariani A, Webb MJ, Galli L, Podratz KC. Potential therapeutic role of para-aortic lymphadenectomy in node-positive endometrial cancer. Gynecol Oncol. 2000;76:348–56.
11. Lu Q, Liu H, Liu C, Wang S, Li S, Guo S, Lu J, Zhang Z. Comparison of laparoscopy and laparotomy for management of endometrial carcinoma: a prospective randomized study with 11-year experience. J Cancer Res Clin Oncol. 2013;139:1853–9.
12. Walker JL, Piedmonte MR, Spirtos NM, Eisenkop SM, Schlaerth JB, Mannel RS, Spiegel G, Barakat R, Pearl ML, Sharma SK. Laparoscopy compared with laparotomy for comprehensive surgical staging of uterine cancer: Gynecologic Oncology Group Study LAP2. J Clin Oncol. 2009;27:5331–6.
13. Brezina PR, Beste TM, Nelson KH. Does route of hysterectomy affect outcome in obese and nonobese women? JSLS. 2009;13:358–63.
14. Nawfal AK, Orady M, Eisenstein D, Wegienka G. Effect of body mass index on robotic-assisted total laparoscopic hysterectomy. J Minim Invasive Gynecol. 2011;18:328–32.
15. Bardens D, Solomayer E, Baum S, Radosa J, Gräber S, Rody A, Juhasz-Böss I. The impact of the body mass index (BMI) on laparoscopic hysterectomy for benign disease. Arch Gynecol Obstet. 2014;289:803–7.
16. Harmanli O, Esin S, Knee A, Jones K, Ayaz R, Tunitsky E. Effect of obesity on perioperative outcomes of laparoscopic hysterectomy. J Reprod Med. 2013;58:497–503.
17. Fanfani F, Boruta DM, Fader AN, Vizza E, Growdon WB, Kushnir CL, Corrado G, Scambia G, Turco LC, Fagotti A. Feasibility and surgical outcome in obese vs. non-obese patients undergoing Laparo-Endoscopic Single-Site (LESS) hysterectomy: a multicenter case-control study. J Minim Invasive Gynecol. 2014;12:401–10.
18. Barakat RR, Lev G, Hummer AJ, Sonoda Y, Chi DS, Alektiar KM, Abu-Rustum NR. Twelve-year experience in the management of endometrial cancer: a change in surgical and postoperative radiation approaches. Gynecol Oncol. 2007;105:150–6.
19. Seamon LG, Cohn DE, Henretta MS, Kim KH, Carlson MJ, Phillips GS, Fowler JM. Minimally invasive comprehensive surgical staging for endometrial cancer: robotics or laparoscopy? Gynecol Oncol. 2009;113:36–41.
20. Tinelli R, Malzoni M, Cicinelli E, Fiaccavento A, Zaccoletti R, Barbieri F, Tinelli A, Perone C, Cosentino F. Is early stage endometrial cancer safely treated by laparoscopy? Complications of a multicenter study and review of recent literature. Surg Oncol. 2011;20:80–7.
21. Malzoni M, Tinelli R, Cosentino F, Fusco A, Malzoni C. Total laparoscopic radical hysterectomy versus abdominal radical hysterectomy with lymphadenectomy in patients with early cervical cancer: our experience. Ann Surg Oncol. 2009;16:1316–23.
22. Malzoni M, Tinelli R, Cosentino F, Perone C, Vicario V. Feasibility, morbidity, and safety of total laparoscopic radical hysterectomy with lymphadenectomy: our experience. J Minim Invasive Gynecol. 2007;14:584–90.
23. Palomba S, Ghezzi F, Falbo A, Mandato VD, Annunziata G, Lucia E. Laparoscopic versus abdominal approach to endometrial cancer: a 10-year retrospective multicenter analysis. Int J Gynecol Cancer. 2012;22:425–33.
24. Tinelli R, Malzoni M, Cosentino F, Perone C, Fusco A, Cicinelli E, Nezhat F. Robotics versus laparoscopic radical hysterectomy with lymphadenectomy in patients with early cervical cancer: a multicenter study. Ann Surg Oncol. 2011;18:2622–8.
25. Tinelli R, Litta P, Meir Y, Surico D, Leo L, Fusco A, Angioni S, Cicinelli E. Advantages of laparoscopy versus laparotomy in extremely obese women (BMI > 35) with early-stage endometrial cancer: a multicenter study. Anticancer Res. 2014;34:2497–502.

Laparoendoscopic Single-Site (LESS) Hysterectomy

50

Anna Fagotti, Cristiano Rossitto, Francesco Fanfani, and Giovanni Scambia

Introduction

Since its introduction laparoscopic surgery has undergone several advancements. More minimally invasive approaches to further reduce surgical morbidity represent a recent progress in laparoscopy. They consist of a reduction either in port's dimension or in port's number. This last option is called single-site surgery. This approach is performed through a single trans-umbilical multiport device. A multidisciplinary consortium of surgeons, who met at the Cleveland Clinic in July 2008, coined the acronyms of laparoendoscopic single-site surgery (LESS) that included all the techniques performed with a single transumbilical skin incision [1]. Since its first reports [2–5], there has been a considerable surge of interest in LESS as a virtually scarless procedure for a variety of surgical indications in different fields. LESS has been utilized to successfully perform a large number of procedures also in general surgery [6–8]. It was first reported for gynecological procedures in the 1970s for laparoscopic tubal ligations [9]. However, this procedure did not initially gain popularity because of technical challenges. In the last decade, technological advances in flexible optical and coagulation devices allowed performing more advanced procedures, such as total LESS hysterectomy and pelvic/aortic lymphadenectomy. In this period several reports have come out to demonstrate the feasibility and reproducibility of this approach for benign and malignant uterine disease [1, 3, 4, 10, 11].

A. Fagotti (✉) C. Rossitto • G. Scambia
Division of Gynecologic Oncology Policlinico A. Gemelli Foundation, Catholic University Sacred Heart, Rome, Italy
e-mail: annafagotti@libero.it; Cristiano.rossitto@gmail.com; giovanni.scambia@policlinicogemelli.it

F. Fanfani
Department of Medicine and aging science, University G D'Annunzio Chieti, Rome, Italy
e-mail: francesco.fanfani@unich.it

The benefits of single-site surgery seem superior to those reported for standard laparoscopy, including faster recovery, and lower postoperative analgesic requirements and better cosmetic results [12–14].

Or Set-Up and Patient's Positioning

Since single port surgery is a technically complex approach even in case of simple operations, the operating room set up needs to be modified to make the surgeon drive in the most ergonomic position. To this purpose, every single detail should not be overlooked, to avoid difficulties during surgery.

We demonstrated that the OR staff must move around the patient, in an anti clockwise of about half an hour. Accordingly, the first surgeon is positioned at the head of the patient, the first assistant is sitting at her right side, and the second assistant is sitting and moving the uterine manipulator between the patient's legs [10]. The anaesthesiologist and his instrumentation are located between the surgeon and the assistant. The nurse is at the left side of the patients, to easily switch the surgeon's instruments. Finally, two monitors should be positioned at the head and legs of the patient, respectively (Fig. 50.1).

Following the induction of general anaesthesia, the patient is positioned in the dorsal lithotomic position with both legs supported in stirrups with a steep Trendelenburg tilt. In this way, the head of the patient is located at the level of the surgeon's legs. This position allows a number of benefits: (1) small bowel ansae are easily dislocated outside the pelvis; (2) the distance between the working instruments at the umbilicus and surgeon's hands is significantly reduced; (3) the surgeon achieves a very ergonomic position, thanks to the 90 ° angle between the surgeon's arm and forearms.

I. Alkatout, L. Mettler (eds.), *Hysterectomy*, DOI 10.1007/978-3-319-22497-8_50

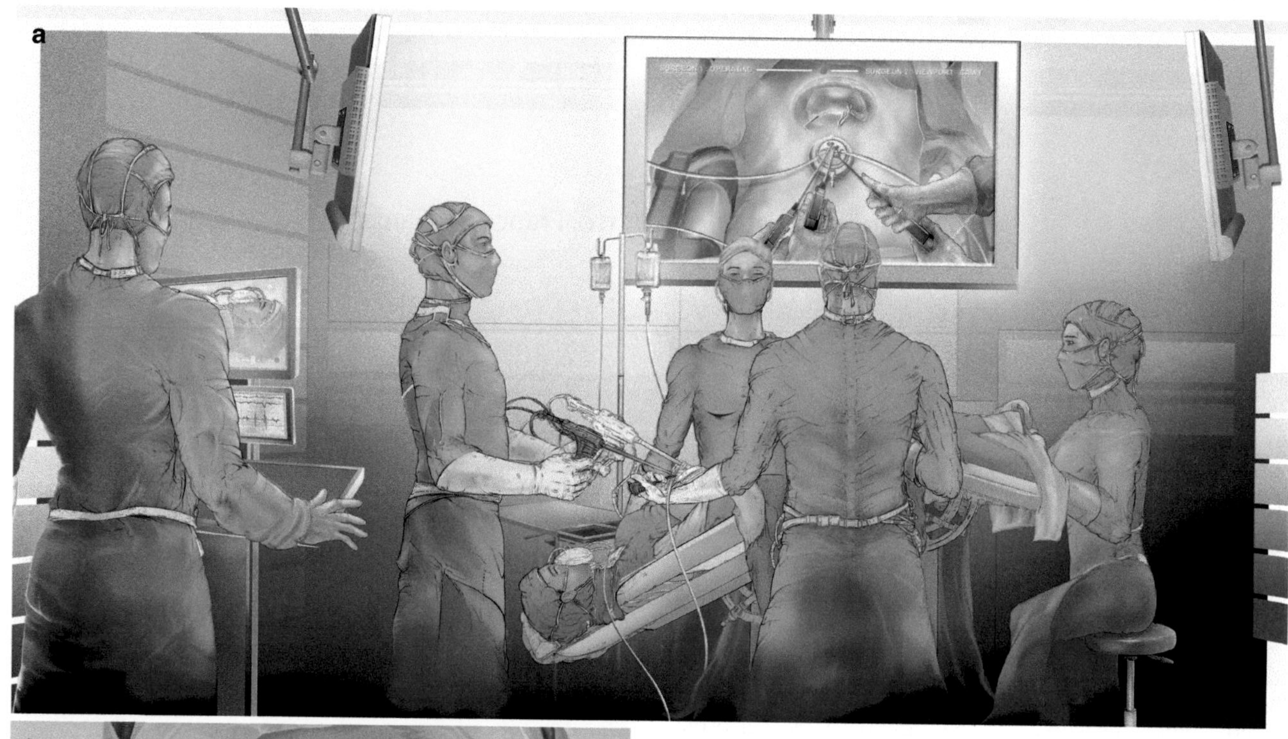

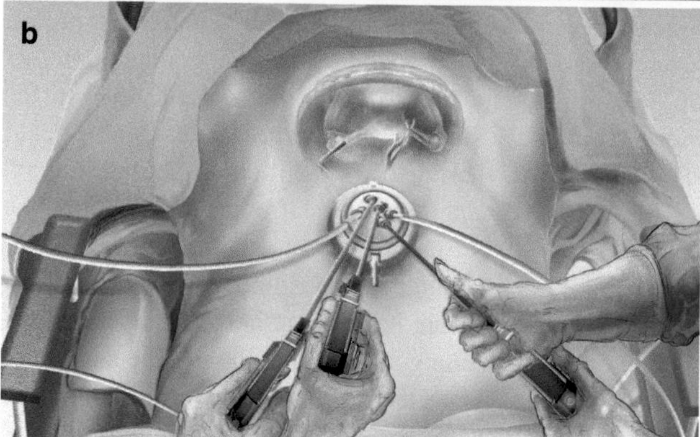

Fig. 50.1 (**a**) OR setting, (**b**) Surgeon's point of view on LESS approach

Instruments

The insertion of the single trocar is obtained by a skin incision within the umbilical scar of about 1.5–2 cm. We suggest performing a larger incision (2.5 cm) in the underlying abdominal fascia in order to avoid any clashing between the instruments and the optic [10]. Single port trocar may have different numbers and sizes of ports for the insertion of the instruments. However, a minimum of three 5 mm ports is required to perform SS hysterectomy.

Dedicated optics to single port surgery allow the best balance between an excellent intra abdominal visualization and no conflict between the camera and the instruments outside the patient. To this purpose, they are usually 5 mm HD telescopes, either with a long and flexible external arm and a 30 ° optic, or with a flexible internal tip and a 0 ° optic.

We strongly suggest using the uterine manipulator to perform single-site hysterectomy. It may partially replace the *third missing hand* with single port surgery, making the indispensable traction on the uterus, and thus resulting much more helpful than in traditional laparoscopy.

Working 5-mm instruments are inserted into the remaining ports, choosing among graspers, bipolar coagulator, cold scissors, suction/irrigation, and a multifunctional device, which grasps, coagulates and transects, simultaneously.

To prevent clashing between instruments and surgeon's hands and to facilitate surgical manoeuvres, the combination of one 33-cm-long instrument with a 43-cm-long straight instrument is suggested. Alternatively, one double bended and one straight instrument could be adopted.

In our opinion, the standard equipment to perform LESS hysterectomy should consist of a 5 mm HD 0 degree optic

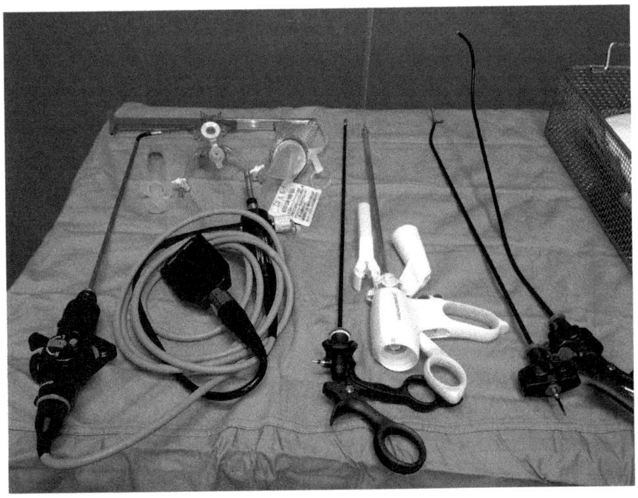

Fig. 50.2 Standard equipment to perform LESS hysterectomy

with flexible tip, a 43 cm long bipolar grasper, a standard multifunctional device, a 43 cm long suction/irrigation, and a uterine manipulator. This set allows the best performances in terms of intra-operative visualization, safe and effective coagulation and cutting, which reflects in a shorter operating time, and lower complication rate (Fig. 50.2).

Surgical Steps and Technique

Surgical steps during LESS hysterectomy should not differ from those described for any abdominal hysterectomy (either laparotomy and traditional laparoscopy). This avoids potential confusion, which may lead to serious intra- and post-operative complications.

Here we present the CUSH (Catholic University of the Sacred Heart) technique for total extrafascial hysterectomy (class A according to Querleu and Morrow) [15].

Coagulation and Section of the Round Ligament

The cutting landmark is the perpendicular projection of the obliterated umbilical artery on the ligament itself (Fig. 50.3). The identification of the correct point allows a safe access to the pelvic retro-peritoneum, through an avascular space, thus avoiding unnecessary bleeding from the small vessels of the broad ligament.

Access to the Pelvic Retro-Peritoneum

Once the round ligament has been sectioned, the wide ligament is opened in a dorso-caudal direction through the surgeon's forceps and CO_2 (Fig. 50.4).

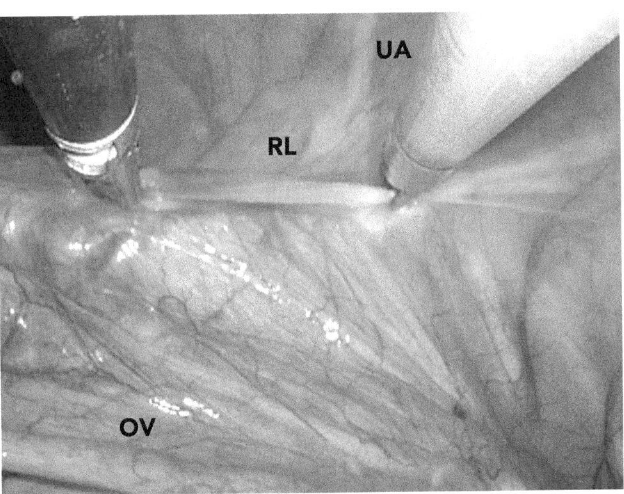

Fig. 50.3 Round ligament (*RL*), coagulated and resected along the vertical projection of the umbilical artery (*UA*). Ovarian vessels (*OV*)

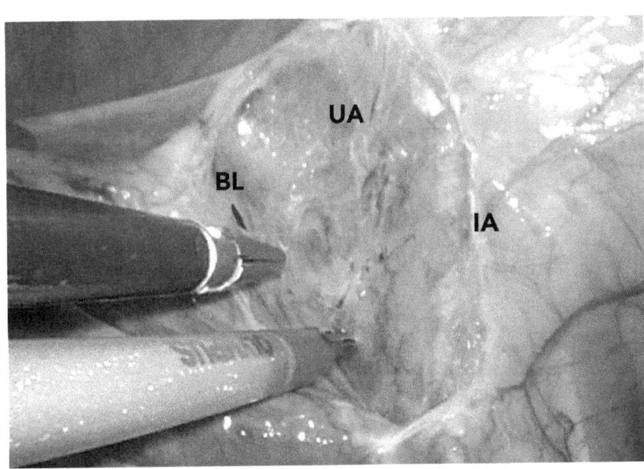

Fig. 50.4 Access to the pelvic retro-peritoneum on the right side. Umbilical artery (*UA*), iliac artery (*IA*), broad ligament (*BL*)

Identification of the Ureter

Through a gentle dissection of the loose connective tissue, the pelvic portion of the ureter is visualized at the posterior layer of the broad ligament. The peristaltic movement of the ureter may be helpful, for its correct identification (Fig. 50.5).

Identification and Closing of the Uterine Artery at Its Origin

In most cases, the uterine artery is the first branch of the obliterated umbilical artery, which is, in turn, a branch of the internal iliac artery. In a small percentage of anatomical variants (about 10 %), it can come directly from the internal iliac or hypogastric iliac artery.

Closing with metal clips the uterine artery at its origin, laterally to the ureter, may serve either as effective haemostats as well as an indirect landmark for the ureter throughout the operation (Fig. 50.6).

Coagulation and Section of the Ovarian Vessels/Utero-Ovarian Ligament

In case of hysterectomy with adnexa removal, we suggest to create a peritoneal window between the ovarian vessels (upper) and the ureter (below) (Fig. 50.7). This procedure moves the ureter further away from the coagulating energy, thus avoiding any ureteral potential injury. The ovarian vessels should be coagulated with extreme caution to avoid any bleeding, in subsequent steps, by alternating between coagulations and cut of small parts of the vessels.

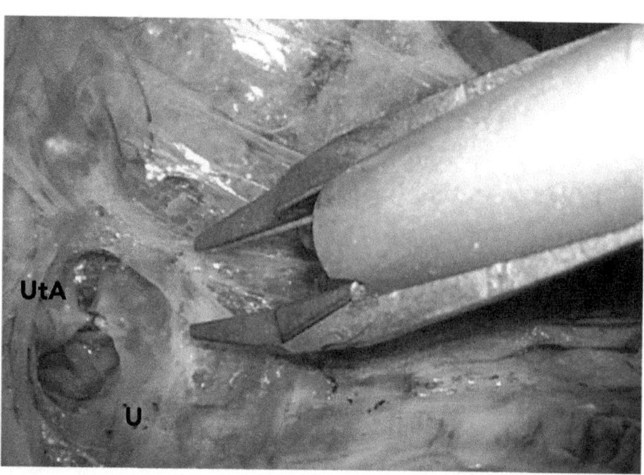

Fig. 50.5 Identification, dissection and closure of the uterine artery (*UtA*) at its origin. The ureter (*U*) passing below the arc drawn by the uterine artery.

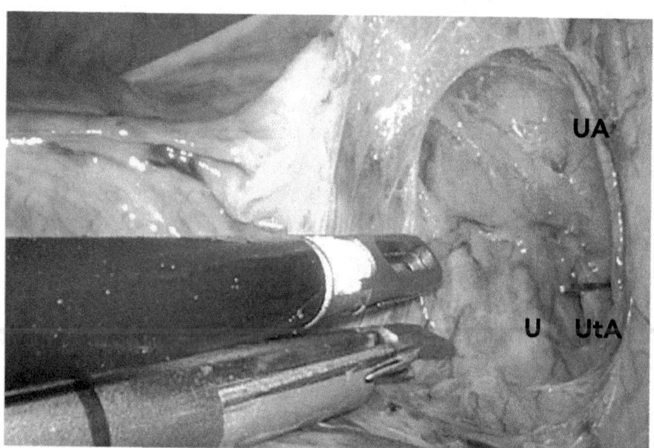

Fig. 50.6 Identification of the retro-peritoneal structures. Uterine artery (*UtA*) closed at the origin with haemostatic clip. Ureter (*U*). Umbilical artery (*UA*)

In case the adnexa will be conserved, the section of the ovarian vessels will be performed proximally to the uterus, at the level of the utero ovarian ligaments. They should be coagulated and cut, leaving 1–2 cm from the uterine body, in order to avoid any bleeding of the cervical branches of the uterine artery.

Section of the Utero-Sacral Ligaments

Detachment and section of the peritoneum covering the utero-sacral ligaments allows colpotomy to be performed more bloodlessly, moves the ureters further away from the energy application and avoids damage to the uterine vessels which remain in the lateral position (Fig. 50.8).

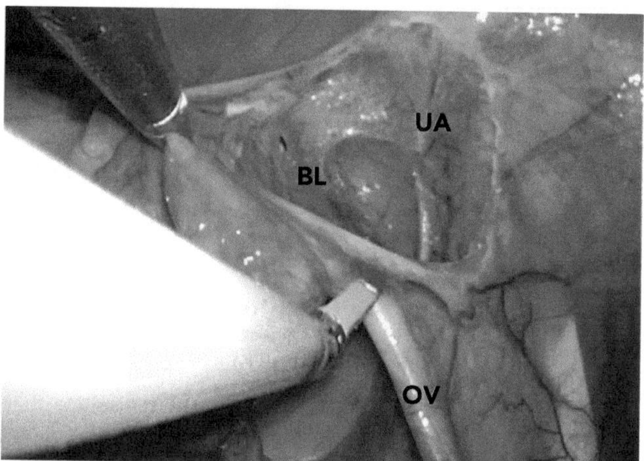

Fig. 50.7 Coagulation and section of the ovarian vessels (*OV*). Umbilical artery (*UA*). Broaf ligament (*BL*)

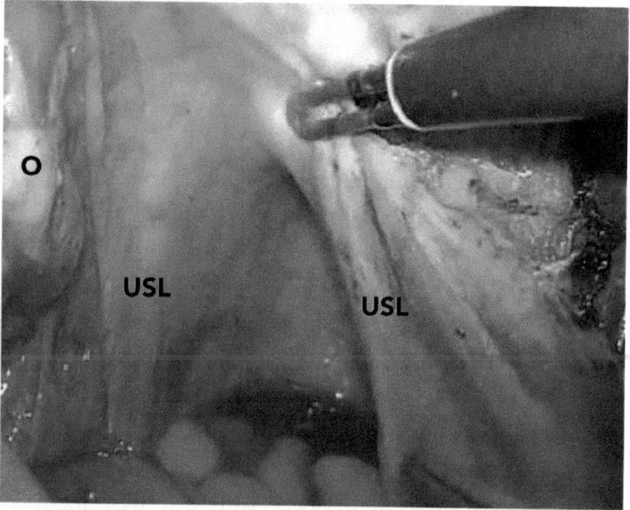

Fig. 50.8 Dissection along the posterior part of the broad ligament, to resect the uterosacral ligaments (*USL*). Ovary (*O*)

Development of the Vesico Uterine and Vesico Vaginal Spaces

Development of the anterior space requires the assistant to apply a strong tension to the uterus in a ventro-medial direction. This tension allows the surgeon to develop the anterior space, between the uterine vessels (dorsal – lateral), the cervix (caudal-medial) and the bladder (anterior). This step must be performed following a latero-medial direction, to avoid any potential risk of damaging the bladder, as in case of previous surgery at this level (i.e. caesarean section). The peritoneal reflection between cervix-vagina and bladder is often very clear. The dissection should be performed 1 cm caudally to this reflection, not to open the cervical fascia. After completing the lateral dissection, both on the right and the left side, the surgeon may grasp the bladder upwards to highlight the peritoneal passage during the central detachment (Fig. 50.9).

Identification, Coagulation and Section of the Uterine Vessels

The coagulation of the uterine vessels in the iuxta-uterine position entails their dissection, so that haemostasis is more precise and safe. After closing the uterine artery at its origin, the vessel coagulation shall be performed progressively since venous reflux bleeding can still occur from the cervical and vaginal branches (Fig. 50.10).

Colpotomy

Colpotomy is a circular incision of the vagina, which is performed closer to the cervix to reduce the vaginal border removal. Colpotomy can be performed with monopolar current (Hook or scissors) or with new multifunctional devices (advanced bipolar or ultrasonic). After closing of the uterine vessels and preparing the anterior and posterior peritoneal planes, this step will be virtually bloodless.

The uterine manipulator valve, introduced into the vagina, will help us to decide on the incision starting point and will guide the operator throughout the colpotomy (Fig. 50.11).

Removal of the Uterus and Closure of the Vaginal Cuff

In the case of histologically proven benign pathologies, the uterus can be removed vaginally, integrally or through cold morcellation. In the case of malignant disease, the uterus must be removed integrally, either through the vaginal approach or by mini-laparotomy (if vaginal removal is impossible). Vaginal suture can occur either laparoscopically or through the vaginal approach. Due to the waste of time, in the single port approach,

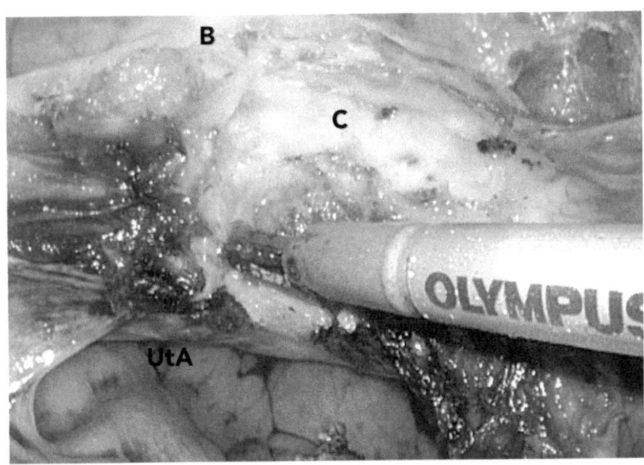

Fig. 50.10 Section and coagulation of the uterine artery (*UtA*), medially to the ureter, at the level of the cervix (*C*). Bladder (*B*)

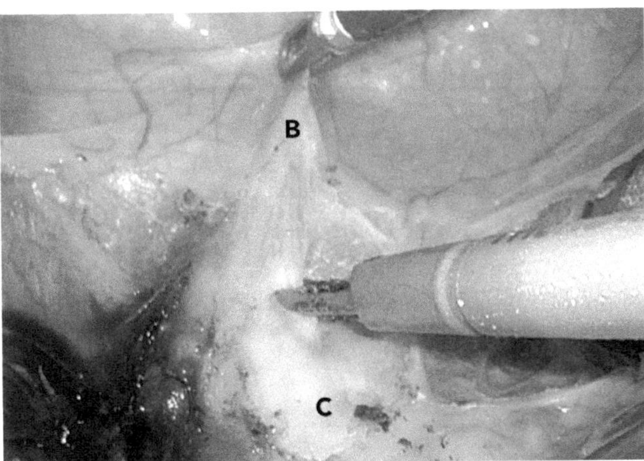

Fig. 50.9 Detachment of vesico-uterine peritoneal reflection. Bladder (*B*), cervix (*C*)

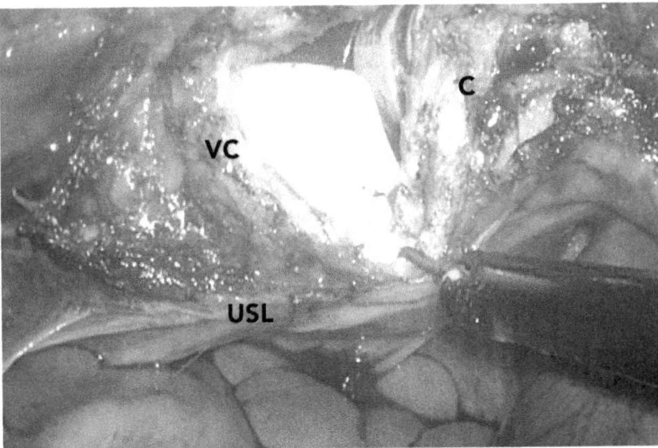

Fig. 50.11 Posterior colpotomy and section of the utero sacral ligament (*USL*). Vaginal cuff, cervix (*C*)

we prefer the vaginal suturing, using a stitch with 1 absorbable wire, first anchoring the vaginal angles and then suturing from right to left with a continuous suture.

Final Control

After suturing the vaginal vault, pneumoperitoneum is re-induced to check haemostats at the trigger points (ovarian pedicles, uterine arteries and utero-sacral ligaments), integrity of the ureter, and the bladder at the idropneumatic test. At the end of the procedure, complete CO2 essufflation should be obtained to avoid patient's pain complain after surgery. The umbilical fascia is closed with a figure-of-eight 0-Vicryl (Fig. 50.12).

Following these simple rules, each surgeon needs about twenty cases to complete his/her learning curve (Fig. 50.13).

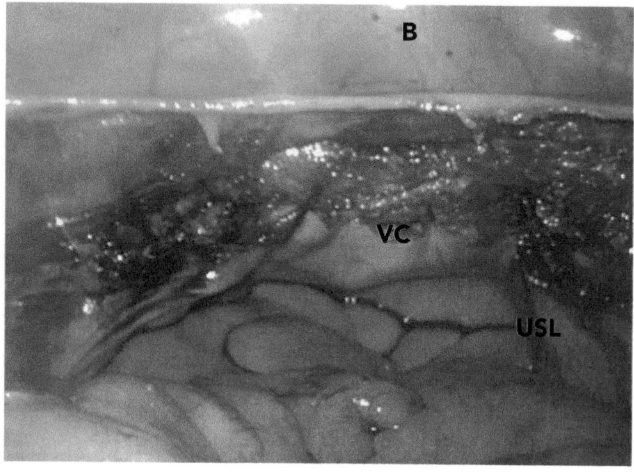

Fig. 50.12 Final imaging after removal of the uterus and vaginal colporrafy. Bladder (*B*), vaginal cuff (*VC*), utero sacral ligament (*USL*)

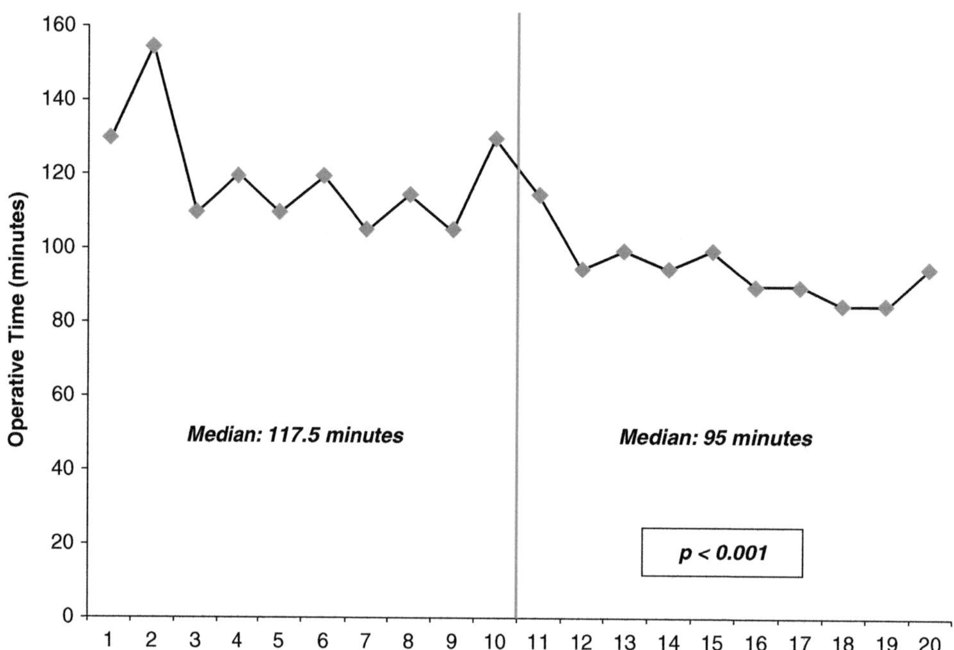

Fig. 50.13 Learning curve for LESS hysterectomy

References

1. Fagotti A, Boruta 2nd DM, Scambia G, et al. First 100 early endometrial cancer cases treated with laparoendoscopic single-site surgery: a multicentric retrospective study. Am J Obstet Gynecol. 2012;206:353.e1–6.
2. Fanfani F, Fagotti A, Gagliardi ML, et al. Minilaparoscopic versus single-port total hysterectomy: a randomized trial. J Minim Invasive Gynecol. 2013;20:192–7.
3. Fader AN, Escobar PF. Laparoendoscopic single-site surgery (LESS) in gynecologic oncology: technique and initial report. Gynecol Oncol. 2009;114:157–61.
4. Yim GW, Jung YW, Paek J, et al. Transumbilical single-port access versus conventional total laparoscopic hysterectomy: surgical outcomes. Am J Obstet Gynecol. 2010;203:26.e1–e6; e1–6.
5. Fanfani F, Fagotti A, Scambia G. Laparoendoscopic single-site surgery for total hysterectomy. Int J Gynaecol Obstet. 2010;109:76–7.
6. Sodergren MH, Aslanyan A, McGregor CG, et al. Pain, well being, body image and cosmesis: a comparison of single-port and four-port laparoscopic cholecystectomy. Minim Invasive Ther Allied Technol. 2014;23(4):223–9.
7. Pini G, Veneziano D, Altieri V, et al. Laparoendoscopic single-site radical nephrectomy for kidney tumor. Surgical technique, cosmetic and postoperative pain control outcomes. Urologia. 2013;80(Suppl 22):16–23.
8. Qiu J, Yuan H, Chen S, et al. Single-port laparoscopic appendectomy versus conventional laparoscopic appendectomy: evidence from randomized controlled trials and non randomized comparative studies. Surg Laparosc Endosc Percutan Tech. 2014;24:12–21.
9. Yoon BS, Park H, Seong SJ, et al. Single-port laparoscopic salpingectomy for the surgical treatment of ectopic pregnancy. J Minim Invasive Gynecol. 2010;17:26–9.
10. Fanfani F, Rossitto C, Gagliardi ML, et al. Total laparoendoscopic single-site surgery (LESS) hysterectomy in low-risk early endometrial cancer: a pilot study. Surg Endosc. 2012;26:41–6.
11. Fanfani F, Fagotti A, Rossitto C, et al. Laparoscopic, minilaparoscopic and single-port hysterectomy: perioperative outcomes. Surg Endosc. 2012;26:3592–6.
12. Li M, Han Y, Feng YC. Single-port laparoscopic hysterectomy versus conventional laparoscopic hysterectomy: a prospective randomized trial. J Int Med Res. 2012;40(2):701–8.
13. Yim GW, Jung YW, Paek J, Lee SH, Kwon HY, Nam EJ, Kim S, Kim JH, Kim YT, Kim SW. Transumbilical single-port access versus conventional total laparoscopic hysterectomy: surgical outcomes. Am J Obstet Gynecol. 2010;203(1):26.e1–6. doi:10.1016/j.ajog.2010.02.026. Epub 2010 Apr 24.
14. Fagotti A, Bottoni C, Vizzielli G, Alletti SG, Scambia G, Marana E, Fanfani F. Postoperative pain after conventional laparoscopy and laparoendoscopic single site surgery (LESS) for benign adnexal disease: a randomized trial. Fertil Steril. 2011;96(1):255–259.e2. doi:10.1016/j.fertnstert.2011.04.006. Epub 2011 May 11.
15. Querleu D, Morrow CP. Classification of radical hysterectomy. Lancet Oncol. 2008;9(3):297–303. doi:10.1016/S1470-2045(08)70074-3.

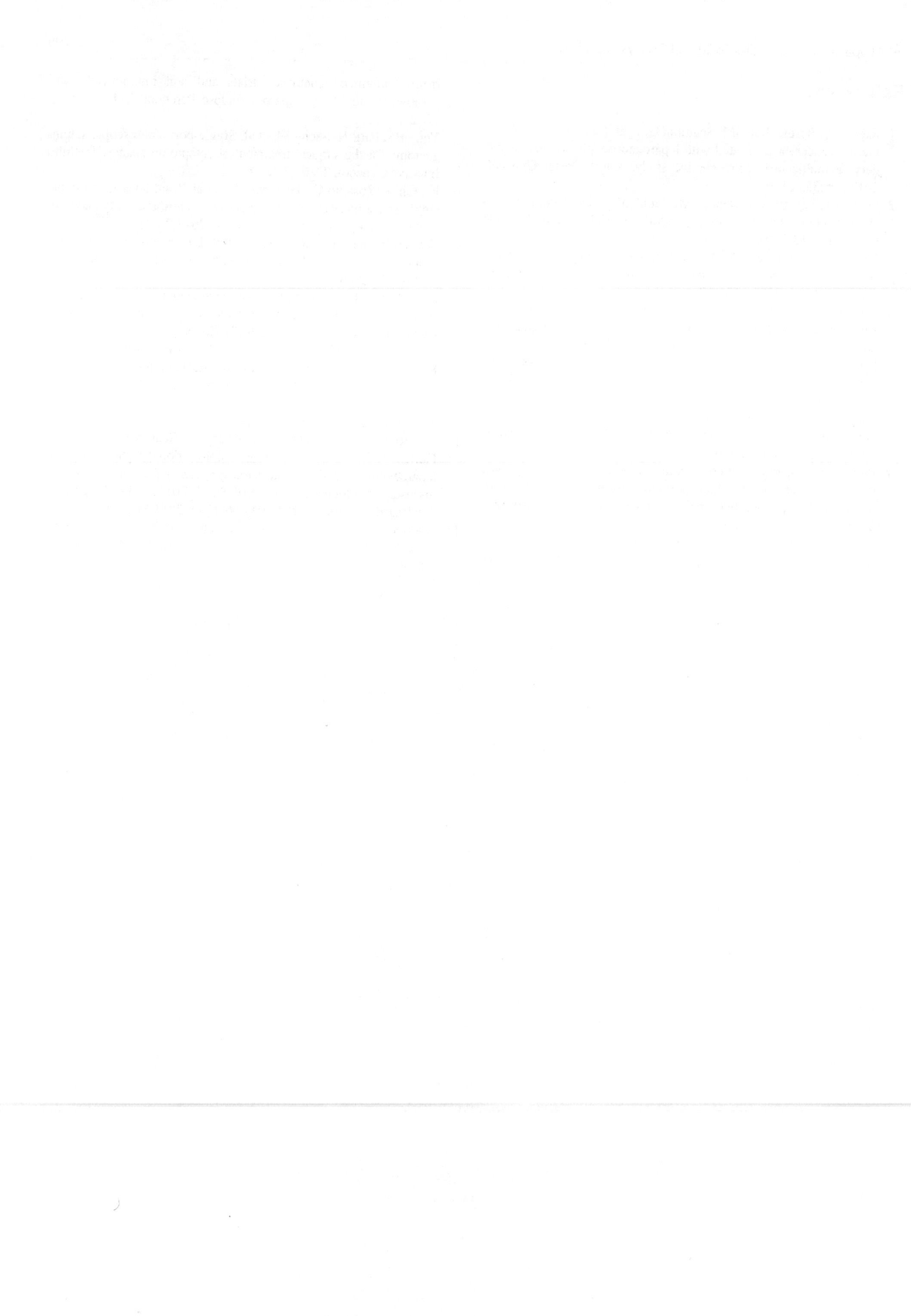

Laparoscopic Pelvic and Paraaortic Lymphonodectomy

51

Bernd Holthaus and Sven Becker

Current Significance of Lymphonodectomy in Gynecologic Oncology

Our current understanding of cancer has its roots in the nineteenth century. At that time the novel techniques of tissue staining – which incidentally have not changed much since – first allowed us to distinguish between normal cells and cancerous growth. The notion that cancer originates within a specific organ, invades locally but ultimately finds its way through the body to metastasize at distant sites remains one of the most fundamental tenements of current oncologic thought.

The question "How does the cancer get from A to B?" logically follows and only two pathways seem obvious: either the bloodstream or the lymphatic drainage system of the body.

It has been and remains exceptionally difficult to systematically detect cancer cells within the bloodstream and reliable technologies have only evolved over the past two decades, spurring a whole scientific industry involved with "Circulating Tumor Cells"and notions of "Liquid Biopsies". At this point, the presence of cancer cells in the bloodstream is documented, a relationship to the prognosis seems established, but the exact significance remains unclear.

The presence of supposedly "migrating" tumor cells within the lymphatic system and particularly within the lymphatic nodes has been documented for much longer. Virchow and his contemporaries were already able to discern these cells using standard hematoxylin-eosin staining.

Linking the presence of micrometastatic cancers cells in lymph nodes to a normally reduced prognosis was yet another milestone in our understanding of cancer.

B. Holthaus (✉)
Department of OB/GYN, Kaukenkaun St. Elisabeth, Damme, Germany

S. Becker
Department of Gynecology and Obstetrics, University Hospital Frankfurt, Kiel, Germany

It is important to stress how much this model or cancer progression, which has been the rock upon which all our treatment concepts have been built, is rooted in the mechanical view of the world that dominated the nineteenth century.

Viewing the cancer as a "runaway" renegade inevitably led to therapeutic concepts of "radical excision" and "removing the bad cells" wherever possible.

If cancerous cells are present in lymphatic nodes and if their presence there leads to a poorer prognosis, surely we can reverse this process by removing the affected lymph nodes.

Because lymphonodectomy is technically challenging and longer operating times only became possible after the introduction of endotracheal intubation after the Second World War, these pathophysiological concepts were not put into action until the 1950s. At this time Joe Vincent Meigs introduced lymph node dissection to the standard oncologic surgery of the day: the radical hysterectomy, originally pioneered by Wertheim, without lymphonodectomy. Hence the now commonly used term for the surgery: "Wertheim-Meigs-Okabayashi".

Lymphonodectomy, by and large, became the standard of all surgical oncologic procedures. Proper "staging" of the tumor became one of the most important advances in standardizing oncologic care, as multimodal treatment approaches depended on stratification to assess the exact treatment.

As a result, no tumor was deemed adequately diagnosed and treated, if the "TNM"-status (tumor, nodal, metastasis) status was not available.

Lost in this great leap forward with regard to overall quality of care was the question at the core of the presence of cancers cells within the lymphatics: Was their presence merely a prognostic marker or would their removal – by removing the "advancing" maximal border of the systemically spreading cancer – improve cure rates?

To this day, there appears to be no definitive answer. In breast cancer, the therapeutic significance of axillary lymph node dissection was unquestioned 20 years ago. Today, as

I. Alkatout, L. Mettler (eds.), *Hysterectomy*, DOI 10.1007/978-3-319-22497-8_51

the molecular markers of the individual disease take the lead in treatment stratification, the removal even of affected lymph nodes has been called into question. Axillary lymph node dissection is now seen as a purely diagnostic procedure without any therapeutic effect.

In gynecologic cancers, the current evaluation of the significance of lymph node dissection is changing, but different approaches are emerging for the different disease entities: endometrial cancer, cervical cancer, ovarian cancer and vulvar cancer.

For the surgeon, deciding who to operate and how to operate, this basic knowledge is decisive as we balance the inherent surgical harm of what we do with the oncologic benefit, a balancing act that – while relying on guidelines and standards – must be made individually for each patient every day.

In endometrial cancer, the available literature – though far from uncontroversial – appears to support a clinical benefit of surgical staging in the form of pelvic and paraaortic lymphonodectomy for all high-risk endometrial cancers, i.e. FIGO IB and above, G3 and non-endometrial cancers irrespective of stage. Statistically, this approach makes sense, as a high proportion of "low-risk" cancers will have negative, non-cancerous lymph nodes.

There is little doubt that removing tumor-free lymph nodes will have no beneficial effect. This argument, however, ignores the fact that statistical probabilities mean little for the individual low-risk patient who is undertreated because she did not have a lymphonodectomy but just happens to be part of the unlucky few.

In fact, it is important to logically stratify the statement: Removing non-affected lymph nodes probably has no survival benefit. Does removal of affected lymph nodes provide a survival benefit, either because the patient will receive additional treatment or because the accessible cancer burden is actually decreased?

When lymph nodes are grossly positive, there is general agreement that they should be removed if possible. This will reduce the residual tumor burden but it might also improve long-term outcome after radiation therapy, as studies have shown that "bulky" lymph nodes larger than 3–4 cm often will not be sufficiently sterilized by radiation. Under these circumstances, laparoscopic – but not laparotomic – lymphonodectomy has the potential to improve the outcome of chemoradiation therapy.

Of course, overall, a reasonable balance between statistical surgical risk and statistical clinical benefit needs to be found. Contrary to chemotherapy or radiation therapy, which can be standardized, the risk of a surgical procedure depends mostly on the two variables "surgeon's skill" and "patient's disposition".

As already mentioned, particularly for cervical cancer, there exists data showing that the removal of grossly affected lymph nodes might confer a survival benefit. While the role of lymphonodectomy for adenocarcinomas such as breast cancer and endometrial cancer has been questioned, squamous lymphatic metastasis appears to be amenable to surgical treatment with curative intention. Furthermore, "oncologic tailoring", i.e. determining the radicality of parametrial resection inevitably depends on histopathologic lymph-node assessment. Because of this, contrary to endometrial cancer, lymphonodectomy remains an integral part of the treatment of all cervical cancers, with the exception of low-risk pT1a1-stages.

In fact, even for non-operable cervical cancer, evaluating lymph nodes, as a means to delineate the limits of the radiation field or to define additional need for systemic chemotherapy, continues to be evaluated.

The role of lymphonodectomy in ovarian cancer is under intense investigation. Laparoscopy does not play a generally accepted role in the staging of early ovarian cancer, where lymphonodectomy is called for under any circumstances. While the existing literature supports the oncologic equivalence of open vs. laparoscopic staging, fear of incompetent use of the difficult laparoscopic techniques has led to a great reluctance to accept the laparoscopic approach within the different national guidelines. Opinions differ along national society recommendations. Overall and globally speaking, laparoscopy is becoming more and more accepted as a staging tool in early ovarian cancer as well as a treatment-stratification tool in advanced ovarian cancer.

For vulva cancer, again a cancer of predominantly squamous histology, the therapeutic effect of adequate treatment of inguinal lymph nodes remains unquestioned – mostly because an inguinal recurrence is basically not treatable and will lead to inevitable death, often after extensive periods of suffering. Laparoscopic pelvic-lymphonodectomy is generally accepted to delineate the limits of subsequent radiation therapy.

Some Remarks About the Access

Laparoscopic pelvic and particularly laparoscopic paraaortic lymphonodectomy remain difficult "high-end" procedures within the spectrum of surgical laparoscopy. As safe laparoscopy relies heavily on patient setup as well as technical and anesthesiologic support, we will now review the key points of patient setup and laparoscopic access.

Adequate Positioning of the Patient

Proper, safe and stable positioning of the patient are key elements of successful laparoscopic surgery.

The patient should be in the regular supine position with adequate dorsal padding. The arms must be "tucked" laterally, i.e. aligned to the body axis (Fig. 51.1a). In very obese patients, this sometimes is not possible, making particularly the pelvic LND much more challenging. Positioning with only one arm tucked to the body is unacceptable as a routine setup. The stability of the patient on the table is less crucial for lymphonodectomy than for hysterectomy, but as the two procedures are often combined and as the same routine positioning should apply to all laparoscopic procedures, the same rules should apply. As the patient needs to be placed in a Trendelenburg position for some time, it is essential to prevent cephalad slide (Fig. 51.1b, c). Consequently, we recommend the use of heavily padded, symmetrically placed shoulder pads (Fig. 51.1d, e). Legs should be in stirrups – the classic position for all gynecologic laparoscopy, allowing easy placement and management of the uterine manipulator. All exposed body parts, such as hands, fingers, elbows etc., need to be safely padded. Particular attention needs to be paid to possible changes of positioning during the surgery, when the patient is completely covered by sterile draping and can no longer been seen directly. Ideally, the patient setup is arranged by the trained scrub-nurse team and reviewed by the surgeon. Usually, the OR nurses are much

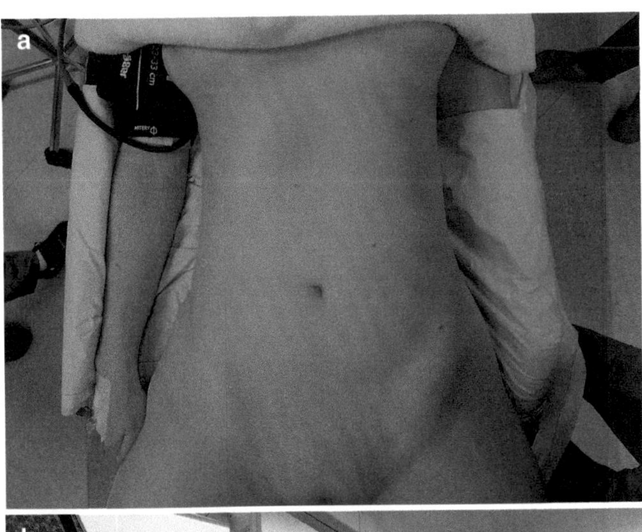

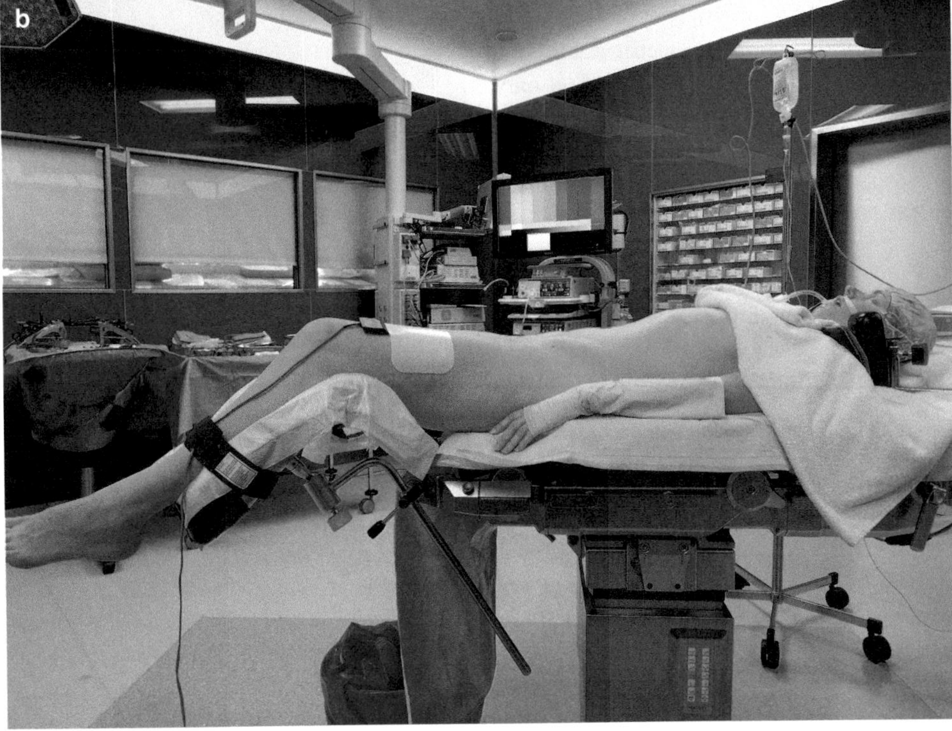

Fig. 51.1 (**a**) Positioning of the patient. Arms always tucked tightly – but well padded – parallel to the thorax. (**b**) Neutral positioning of the OR table. (**c**) "Head-down" >45° i.e. Trendelenburg position during surgery. (**d**) Shoulder padding to prevent positioning injuries. Side view. (**e**) Shoulder padding to prevent positioning injuries. View from *top*

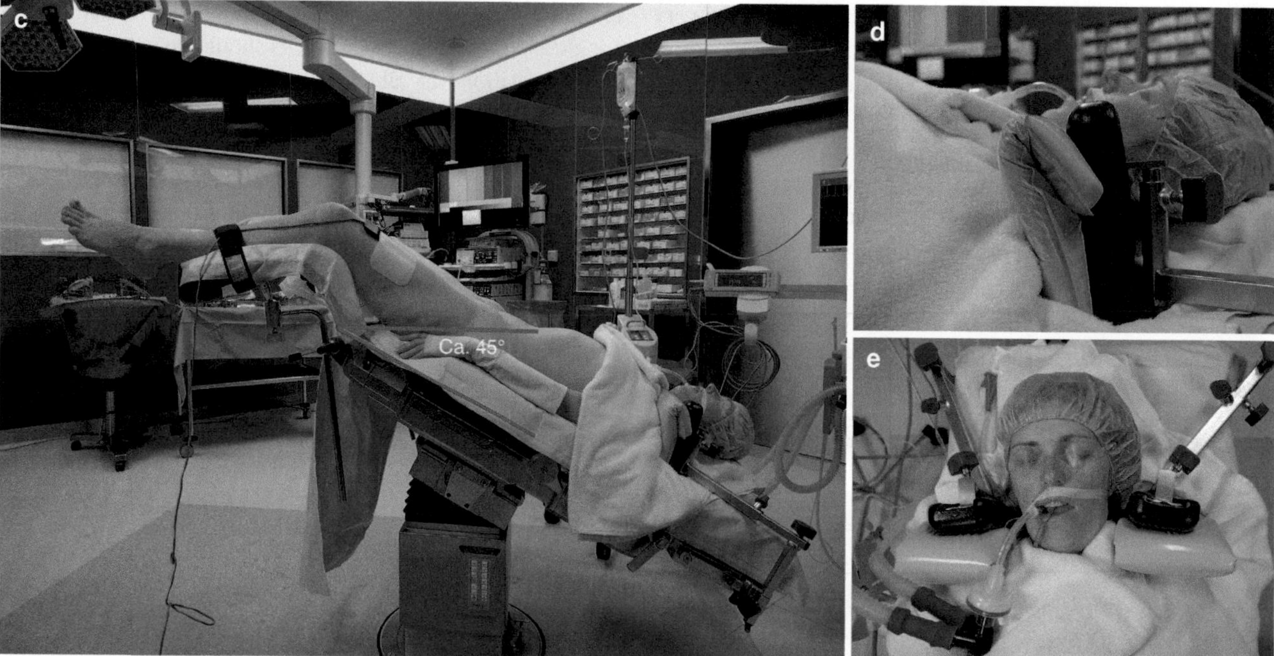

Fig. 51.1 (Continued)

more competent with regard to positioning, but ultimate responsibility rests with the surgeon. Scrubbing the patient for laparoscopy should be no different than for any other patient, but the constant use of electrical energy makes "dry" scrubbing even more important: no amount of scrubbing liquid should run off the patient and moisten dorsal or gluteal parts that could serve as exit points for electrical currents. There are lots of different ways to drape a patient and only the general rules for draping should apply.

Proper Trocar Placement (Figs. 51.2 and 51.3)

As for all advanced laparoscopy, special rules apply to trocar placement. As laparoscopic surgeons are often used to suboptimal situations, they often do not realize the details that make their daily lives more difficult. The central trocar will be placed through the umbilicus after a small vertical incision at the bottom of the umbilical scar. Making this incision too big will lead to inward sliding of the optical trocar, making surgery miserable and more complicated. For all advanced laparoscopic surgery in the pelvis, the lateral trocars should be placed "high and lateral", almost at the level of the umbilicus (but never more than 1–2 cm below that transverse line), and far lateral, but never more medial than 3 cm medial of a sagittal line drawn through the anterior iliac spinal processus. There is less pain for the patient if the placement does not touch the rectal muscle. The working trocar should not be placed in the classic suprasymphysiary position as that inevitably means the surgeon will be working "towards" him or herself. It should be placed midway between the symphysis and the navel, taking care not to go too close to the optical trocar to avoid intraabdominal interference.

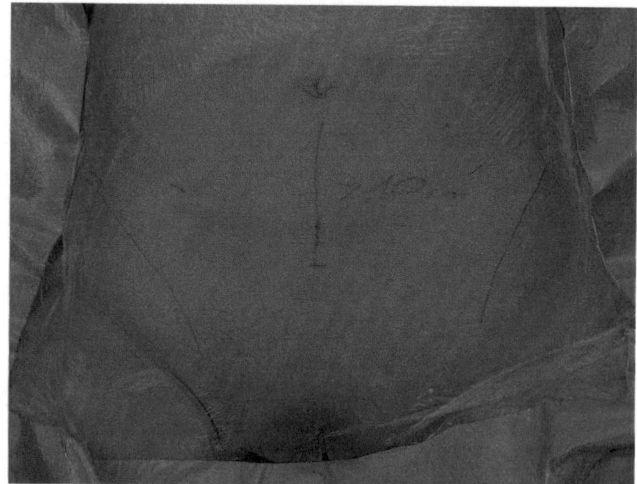

Fig. 51.2 Marking down the trocar positions. The middle, working trocar should be placed sufficiently away from the optical trocar to avoid interference, 10 cm is usually sufficient

All available hands should be used. The first assistant or better the second surgeon should hold the camera and use the right lateral port to hold an atraumatic grasper and assist as the surgery demands. The surgeon should use both hands equally. The left lateral port for traumatic or atraumatic grasping and the medial trocar for cutting, dissection and thermocoagulation. For the surgeon to use the right and left lateral trocars creates unnecessary strain. This will work for cysts, but even then it is awkward although many surgeons used to this approach do not notice this anymore. The use of electrical, harmonic and cutting force, i.e. the use of any potentially dangerous instrument, should be limited to the medial trocar placed between navel and symphysis. Of course, this recommendation needs to be applied reasonably as sometimes (but only rarely) the required angle for cutting will make lateral access better. Generally, however, the medial trocar is the safest access for all potentially dangerous instruments. Only here is the instrument observed in its entirety, irregularity in electrical currents can be immediately realized, and total control is guaranteed.

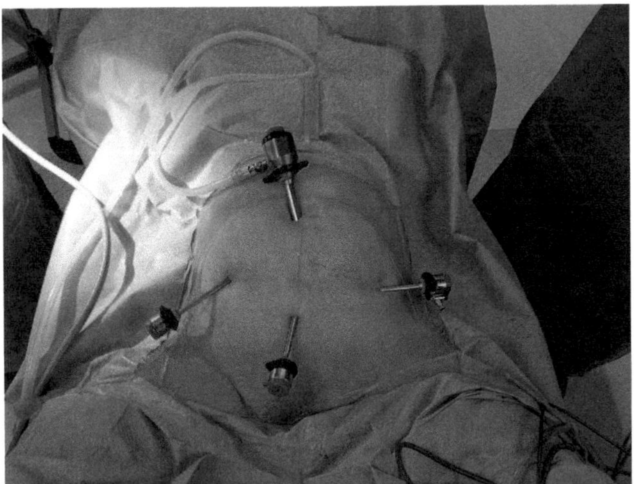

Fig. 51.3 Trocars placed

Very experienced surgeons will be able to use a coagulating grasper through the medial trocar and an electrified scissor through the lateral trocar, but the less experienced surgeon should be wary of such setups.

Having stated how the two authors place their trocars, it should be noted, that trocar placement is ultimately at the surgeon's discretion and will depend also on local traditions and simply on how the individual surgeon was taught. There is no and never will be any scientific evidence as to what is the best placement. An alternative would be the "Indian-Style" placement often seen in the United States, with the two main working trocars placed high and low on the left side of the patient's abdomen.

For removal of the (pelvic) lymph nodes, we recommend placement of a 10 mm trocar in the suprasymphysary position. This trocar will become necessary for placement of the camera during the retrograde approach for the paraaortic lymphonodectomy. An alternative in cases of hysterectomy is to take out the nodes through the opened vagina.

Optimal Positioning of the Surgical Team (Figs. 51.4 and 51.5)

"Optimal" is what works best, and that might very well vary for different surgeons and different teams. However, it is curious to observe how clearly inferior techniques remain long in use, simply because everyone has gotten used to them. Most laparoscopic surgeons were trained in the posi-

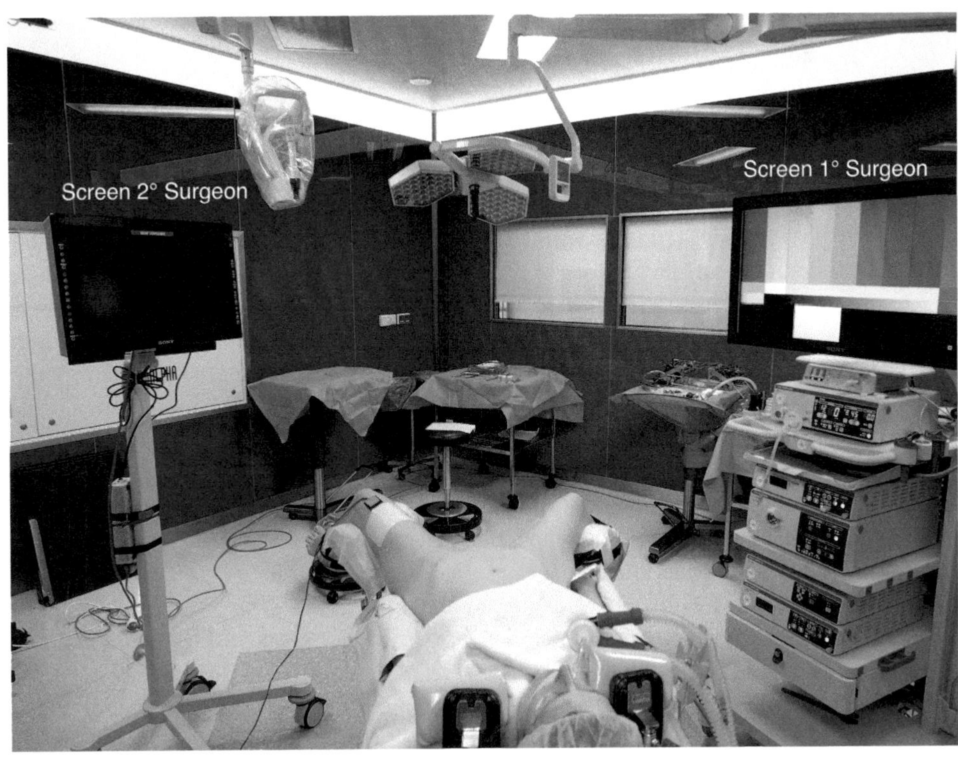

Fig. 51.4 Positioning of the monitors for the first and second surgeon

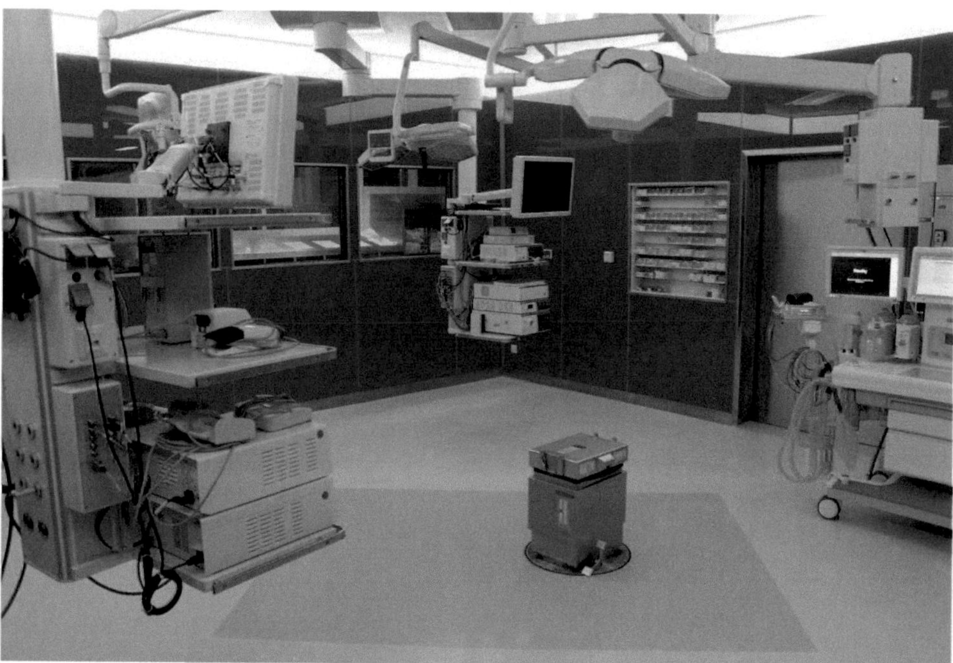

Fig. 51.5 Placement of the generator, insufflator

tion of the first assistant on the right side of the patient and as the responsible surgeon on the left side of the patient.

The second assistant if necessary should sit comfortably between the legs and follow the surgery on an extra monitor placed above the head of the surgeon. If there is a third assistant, ideally, anesthesia will allow for complete draping of the patient and the third assistant will be able to comfortably stand at the head of the patient and hold the camera with both hands. However, this way of draping sadly remains limited to a few centers with highly experienced anesthesia teams as superficially it limits access to the head of the patient although such access really remains immediate at all times by lifting up the drape.

Availability of Necessary Instruments and Video Equipment (Fig. 51.6)

The more complicated the surgery, the better the equipment needs to be. Both pelvic and paraaortic lymphonodectomy can be done using standard equipment: two atraumatic and two traumatic graspers, an Overholt-Clamp for dissection, a clamp for coagulation (curved clamp that can also be used for dissection such as the Kelly-clamp is to be preferred), regular scissors (keeping in mind that monopolar electricity should be used by experienced surgeons only) and suction-irrigation (to be used extremely judiciously and rarely. Particularly irrigation will inevitably make fine dissection more difficult). Any kind of advanced laparoscopy will be easier and speedier for the average laparoscopist if harmonic energy is available, such as Ethicon's Ultracision® or more recently Olympus' Thunderbeat®, the latter combining harmonic and electric energy. With regard to optical instruments, we recommend the routine use of 30° optics, as they allow a better range of vision and a better evaluation, particularly of the field of vision in paraaortic lymphonodectomy, but both surgeries can also be done using zero degree optics. One monitor between the legs and one monitor above the head are the minimum setup required. Ideally, an integrated operating room is available. High resolution camera and video equipment should be available.

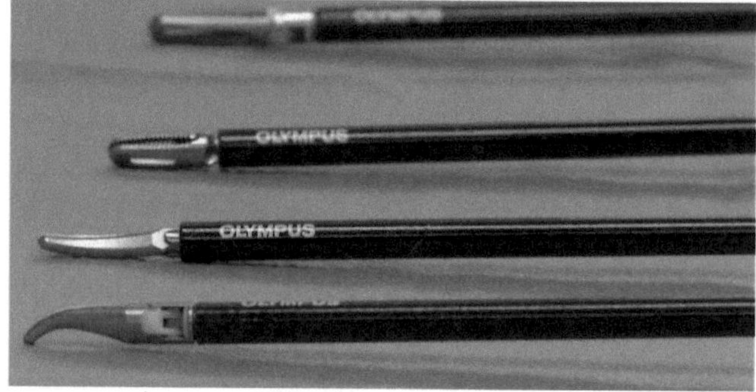

Fig. 51.6 Used laparoscopic instruments for lymphadenectomy

The availability of 3D vision systems will improve overall feasibility particularly of high-end laparoscopic procedures as an increasing body of literature continues to demonstrate.

Optimal Use of Surgical Instruments

Every surgeon will develop a highly individual approach to surgery. However, some principles should be considered: All laparoscopic surgery requires a much higher degree of finesse than abdominal or vaginal surgery. Any kind of bleeding must be avoided during laparoscopy at any time and at all costs as bleeding will disturb the field of vision, obscure the anatomy, require dangerous coagulation, the more so the larger the bleeding. Also, bleeding will make the surgery less beautiful. What does "finesse" mean? The difference between good and bad laparoscopic surgery is the right balance between careful dissection, taking down the tissue sometimes millimeter by millimeter, never cutting were you cannot see, never cutting pedicles that are too thick. It means using the preformed anatomic spaces that can be opened without any sharp dissection at all. It means setting up the vascularized pedicles almost down to the actual artery and vein before sealing the vessels under direct view. It means using the peritoneum as a safe plane of preparation. But it also means doing these things swiftly and decisively to avoid stalling the surgery.

As in all surgery, it means finding the right balance between courage and caution, both based on skill and competence that only time and experience will teach.

Practical little tricks can be important: Try to avoid irrigation, as somehow the crispness of the un-irrigated surgical field will be irrevocably lost after one thorough rinsing. Use suction instead. Train your assistant to focus on proper camera management and sparing interference: "One person only moving" is a simple but important principle. Check the assistant at the uterine manipulator frequently. Uterine manipulation is in essence ureteral distancing and thus protects the single most vulnerable structure in your surgical field.

Technique of Laparoscopic Pelvic Lymphonodectomy

Ultimately, pelvic lymphonodectomy should lead to the representative removal of lymph nodes that reflect the lymphatic drainage of the uterus. This involves the lymphatic axis of the externa iliac vessels as well as the oburatoria fossa, the axis of the internal iliac vessels as well as the common iliac artery. Interestingly, literature looking at patterns of lymphatic spread along these different areas is practically non-existent.

While sentinel lymphonodectomy remains imperfect for endometrial cancer and not yet sufficiently standardized for cervical cancer, the extensive studies surrounding the identification of the pelvic sentinel node all point towards a node of fairly stable location at the bifurcation of common iliac artery to the external and internal iliac artery, towards the appearance of the obturator nerve when accessing the oburatoria fossa medially.

Equally unclear is the desired number of lymph nodes to be removed. Amazing differences exist between the written and unwritten standards of different countries.

We propose a standardized approach. What follows is first an outline of our approach, followed by a detailed explanation of the underlying rationale.

1. Normalization of anatomy – dissection of the ileocoecum cranially and resolution of the sigmoid adhesions in the pelvis
2. Opening of the pelvic sidewall by transecting the round ligament
3. Short extension of the peritoneal incision caudad and medial, towards the bladder
4. Long extension of the peritoneal incision in an arc transversing the external iliac vessels and opening the psoas space
5. Medialization of the infundibulopelvic ligament medially, exposing the ureter as it crosses the pelvic brim
6. Following and dissecting the ureter into the pelvis
7. Separation of the ureter and the internal iliac artery
8. Again moving to the anterior part of our dissection: Isolating the lateral umbilical ligament
9. Opening of the paravesical space
10. Opening of the Fossa obturatoria – Dissection of the obturator nerve
11. Complete lateralization of the axis internal iliac artery – Umbilical Artery/Lateral Umbilical ligament. Finding and dissecting this arterial axis is crucial because it will allow us to do the most important thing gynecologic surgeons do in the pelvic sidewall: Finding where the uterine artery branches off the internal iliac artery.
12. For beginners, managing the arterial axis often appears daunting; however, injuries to big arterial vessels are actually very rare. You really have to directly cut into or puncture these big muscular vessels. Blunt dissection on top of these arteries is easily possible. Of note: There are no significant structures leaving this arterial axis ventrally, laterally or even medially (until the branching of the uterine artery), so it can be used as a safe "preparation" street. In fact, the more vulnerable internal iliac vein lies "protected" behind the artery on both sides and will not be in danger until you have exposed more than half of the arterial circumference
13. Exposing the branching of the uterine artery off the internal iliac artery
14. Opening of the pararectal space
15. Start of the lymphonodectomy at the most distal part of the external iliac artery. Distal limit: Crossing of the circumflex vein. This vein does not need to be coagulated and it has no great significance. Because of the low intravenous pressure, it often appears as a flat, ligamentous structure crossing the artery. To us, it means: "far enough" with regard to the distal end of lymphonodectomy.
16. Avoid disturbing the lateral fatty tissue on the psoas muscle

17. Expose the external iliac artery and remove lymph nodes in a retrograde fashion, using a combination of blunt (80%) and sharp (20%) dissection
18. Try for en-bloc removal
19. At the distal end, expose the internal iliac vein
20. Find the pelvic bone directly "underneath", i.e. medial and dorsal of the internal iliac vein
21. Re-expose the obturator nerve
22. Start removal of the Fossa obturatory lymph nodes
23. Distance the external iliac vessels from the psoas muscle to expose the obturator fossa laterally
24. Use the obturator nerve as a guide to further remove the fossa obturatoria lymph nodes
25. Continue this dissection towards the internal iliac artery lymph nodes
26. Remove the bifurcation node (sentinel node)
27. Cut remaining attachments of the lymph nodes into the fossa obturatoria and to the lateral umbilical ligament
28. Expose branching of the internal iliac vein off the common iliac vein
29. Remove remaining and most proximal external iliac artery lymph nodes into the en-bloc resection tissue
30. Remove lymph nodes using an endobag if at all possible
31. Complete lymphonodectomy by removing the lymph node pads lateral to the common iliac artery (right side).

What follows is a more detailed explanation of the above mentioned step-by-step approach.

Normalization of anatomy – dissection of the ileocoecum cranially and resolution of the sigmoid adhesions in the pelvis (Fig. 51.7a–h)
Ultimately, dissection of the lymph nodes will require sufficient exposure laterally and cranially. If postoperative adhesions pulling the ileocaecum on the right side or the sigmoid colon on the left side towards the pelvis are not removed initially, it will have to be done later, when it tends to be more difficult as the planes are no longer as anatomically pristine.

Particularly the physiologic adhesions of the sigmoid colon towards the left pelvic sidewall are extremely varied. Taking them down requires a certain degree of practice. Opening of the retroperitoneum at this point needs to be avoided. The perfect dissection requires sharp scissors only. Excessive bleeding means the dissection plain is incorrect. Coagulation with electrocautery carries a high risk of thermal bowel injury.

Opening of the pelvic sidewall by transsecting the round ligament (Fig. 51.8a–f)
The classical step. The opening should be performed at the most lateral position. Normally, there are no vessels associated with the round ligament, even though in the English literature, a variable so-called "Sim's artery" is frequently mentioned. Using laparoscopy means the opening of the retroperitoneum allows immediate CO_2 access, leading to distention of this artificial space.

Short extension of the peritoneal incision caudad and medial, towards the bladder (Fig. 51.9a–d)
It is tempting to go further towards the bladder, particularly if a hysterectomy is part of the surgery; however, there is always a danger to run into bleeding or even to injure the bladder.

Long extension of the peritoneal incision in an arc transversing the external iliac vessels and opening the psoas space (Fig. 51.10a–c)
This is the key step at the start of the surgery. Limiting the incision to the peritoneal layer makes this move very safe. The psoas space is one of the "safe" areas. The only danger exists while crossing the external iliac vessels, which theoretically could be injured. Once the psoas space is reached, the incision now bends cranially, going up as far cephalad as possible. At this point, a previous meticulous dissection and removal of the ileocoecum on the right side and the sigmoid colon on the left side becomes crucial. Each further centimeter cephalad helps with the next step: mobilization of the infundibulopelvic ligament medially.

Medialization of the infundibulopelvic ligament medially, exposing the ureter as it crosses the pelvic brim (Fig. 51.11)
This step exposes the ureter. Dissecting the infundibulopelvic ligament always needs to be done with extreme caution. Aside from tearing the ovarian vein (which requires some force…) there are numerous smaller vessels that can tear and cause unnecessary bleeding. This step needs to be done more than once, bluntly, to carefully expose the ureter. This is easier on the right side (no sigmoid).

Following and dissecting the ureter into the pelvis (Fig. 51.12)
This can be either very easy (no previous surgery, no adhesions) or very difficult, when the tissue does not yield easily. Small peritoneal bleeders can be annoying and obscure. Ideally, the ureter is followed caudad easily, leading to the internal iliac artery as it stays close to the pelvic sidewall, while the ureter runs more medial towards the peritoneum of the Douglas space. There are slight differences with regard to the position of the ureter, but they are curiously difficult to describe. On the right side, the ureter sits more "on top" and medial of the internal iliac artery, while on the left side, it runs more laterally to the artery even at the pelvic brim.

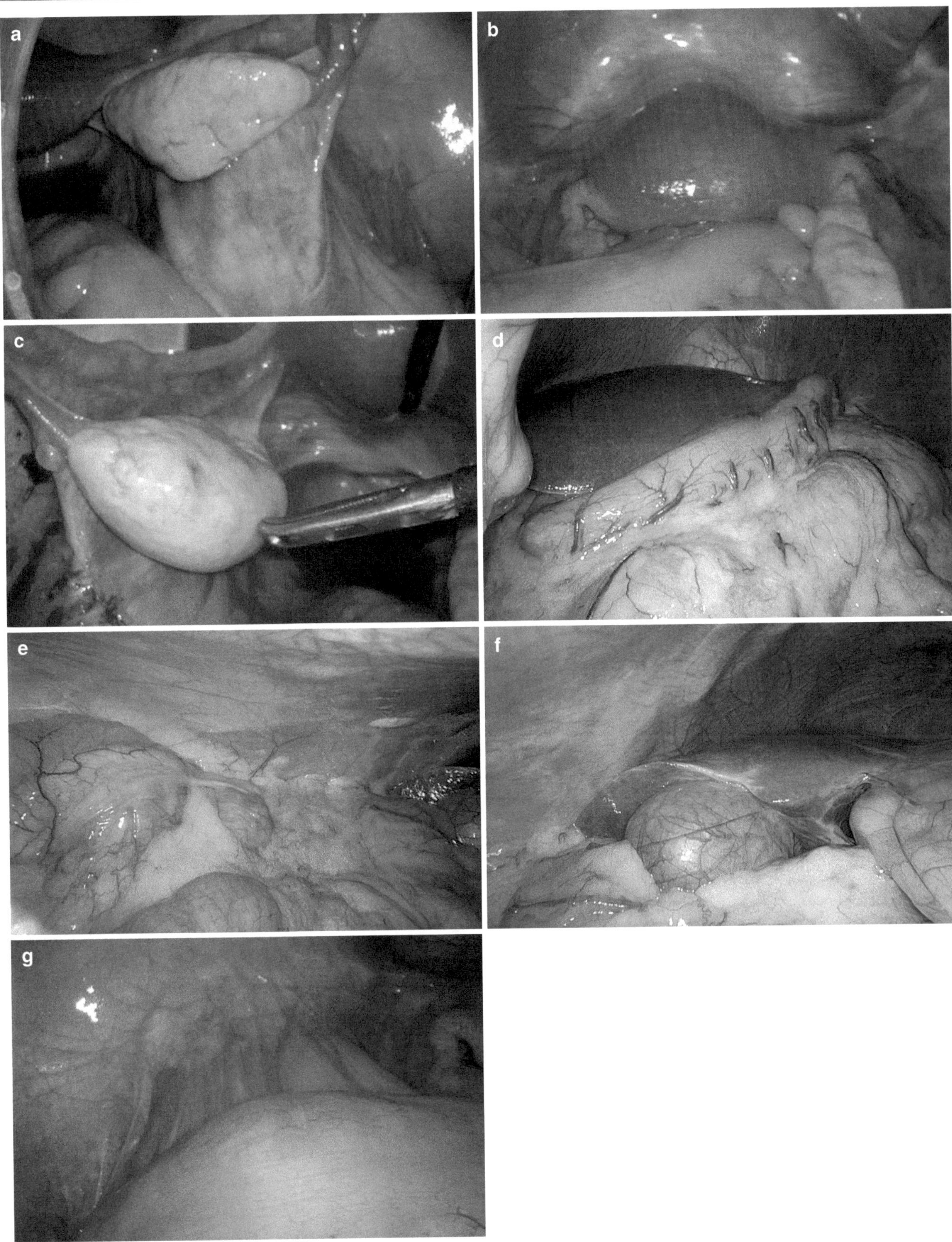

Fig. 51.7 (**a**) Inspection of the pelvis after Trendelenburg positioning. Right adnex. (**b**) Inspection of the pelvis after Trendelenburg positioning. Midline view. Uterus. (**c**) Inspection of the pelvis after Trendelenburg positioning. Left adnex. (**d**) Inspection of the abdominal cavity. Left upper abdomen with liver and stomach. (**e**) Inspection of the abdominal cavity. Right middle abdomen. Coecum. (**f**) Inspection of the abdominal cavity. Right upper abdomen. Liver and gall bladder. (**g**) Inspection of the abdominal cavity. Left middler abdomen. Sigma adhesions to the pelvic side wall

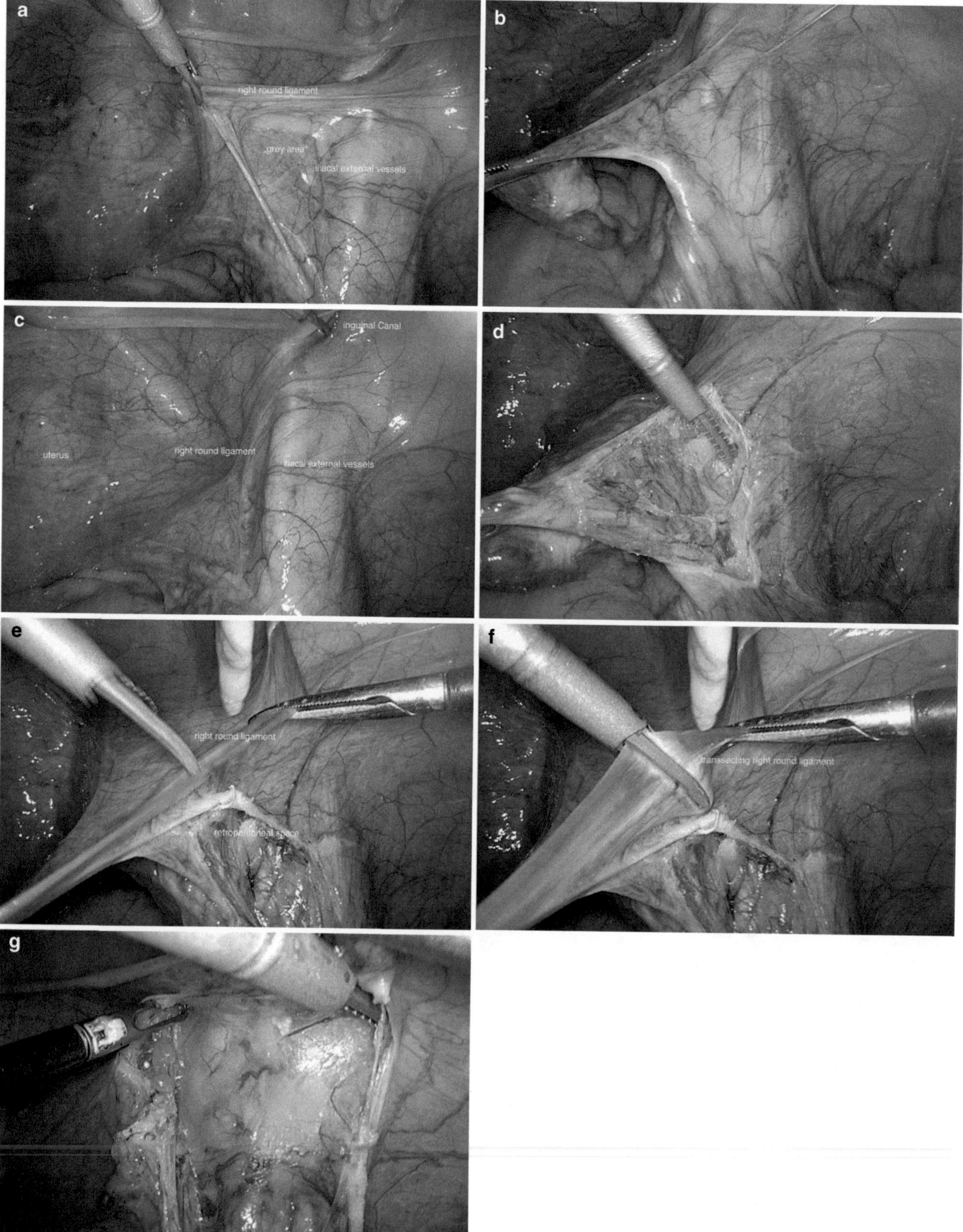

Fig. 51.8 (**a**) Start of the pelvic lymphonodectomy on the right side, exposing the round ligament. (**b**) Identification of the right illiac vessels and psoas muscle. Grasping the right infundibulopelvic ligament. (**c**) Idendification of the right illiac vessels and psoas muscle. (**d**) Incision of the peritoneum above the psoas muscle. (**e**) Tension to the round ligament. (**f**) Transsection of the round ligament. (**g**) Opening of the retroperitoneal space

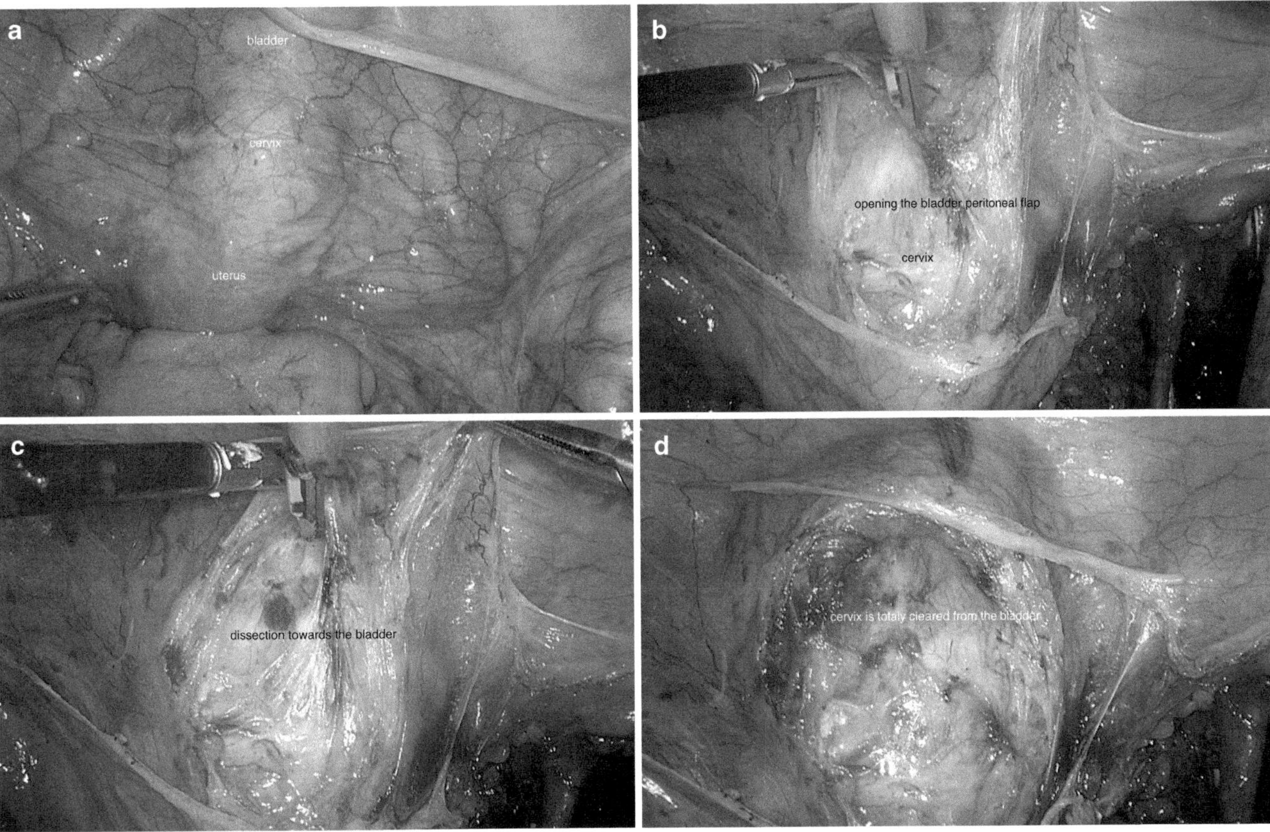

Fig. 51.9 (**a**) Identification of the bladder edge. (**b**) Opening of the bladder peritoneum. (**c**) Downward preparation of the drained bladder. (**d**) Exposing the vesicovaginal fascia

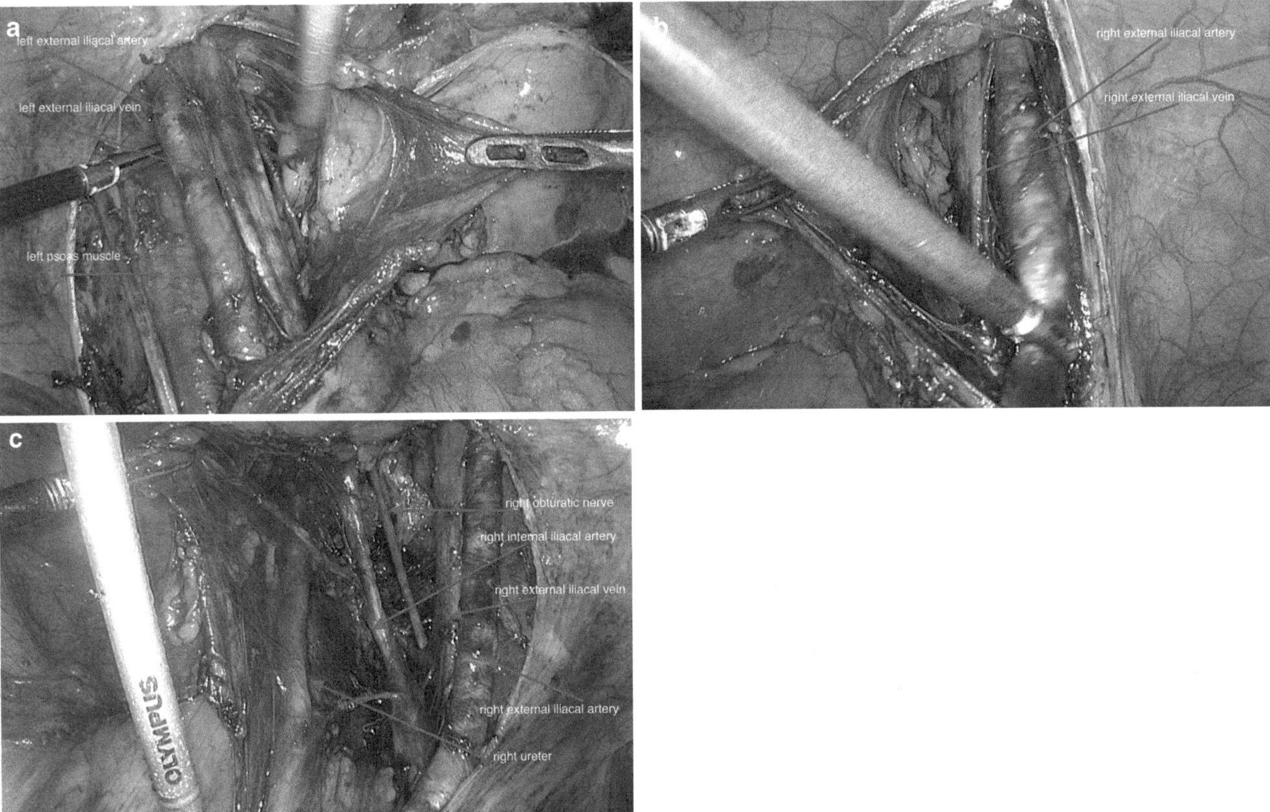

Fig. 51.10 (**a**) Pelvic lymphonodectomy on the left side. Exposition of the external illiac vessels and the psoas muscle. Opening of the obturator fossa. (**b**) Pelvic lymphonodectomy on the right side. Exposition of the external illiac vessels and the psoas muscle. (**c**) Opening of the obturator fossa

If this step is overly difficult, attention can be given to the anterior aspect of the dissection, first.

Separation of the ureter and the internal iliac artery
As already mentioned above, this leads the way to the branching of the uterine artery. At the same time, it prepares access to the pararectal space (opening necessary only when a radical hysterectomy is planned).

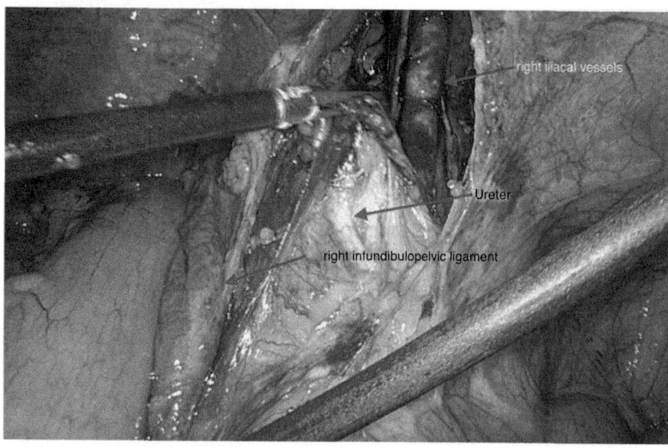

Fig. 51.11 Visualization of the ureter at the level of the right illiac artery bifurcation

Again moving to the anterior part of our dissection: Isolating the lateral umbilical ligament
This step can be performed at any time. Generally, the most important rule of "rules for dissection" is: every operative procedure is different. There is no point in persevering at a particularly difficult part, when other areas can be dealt with more easily. Often, magically, when returning to the difficult area, the anatomy has become kinder and the surgical procedure can move forward, where it was very difficult previously.

No matter how difficult the anatomy or how obese the patient, the lateral umbilical ligament can usually be found on the anterior abdominal wall and followed in a retrograde fashion cephalad, allowing for orientation in the most desperate pelvis.

Opening of the paravesical space (Fig. 51.13)
The paravesical space, immediately medial to the lateral umbilical ligament is the most accessible space of the pelvis. It should be dissected bluntly. The dissection can be carried down almost to the pelvic floor – where unnecessary bleeding awaits, so the last centimeter remains unnecessary and should be avoided. In thin patients, dissecting the paravesical space can sometimes lead to the obturator nerve laterally and the ureter posteriorly.

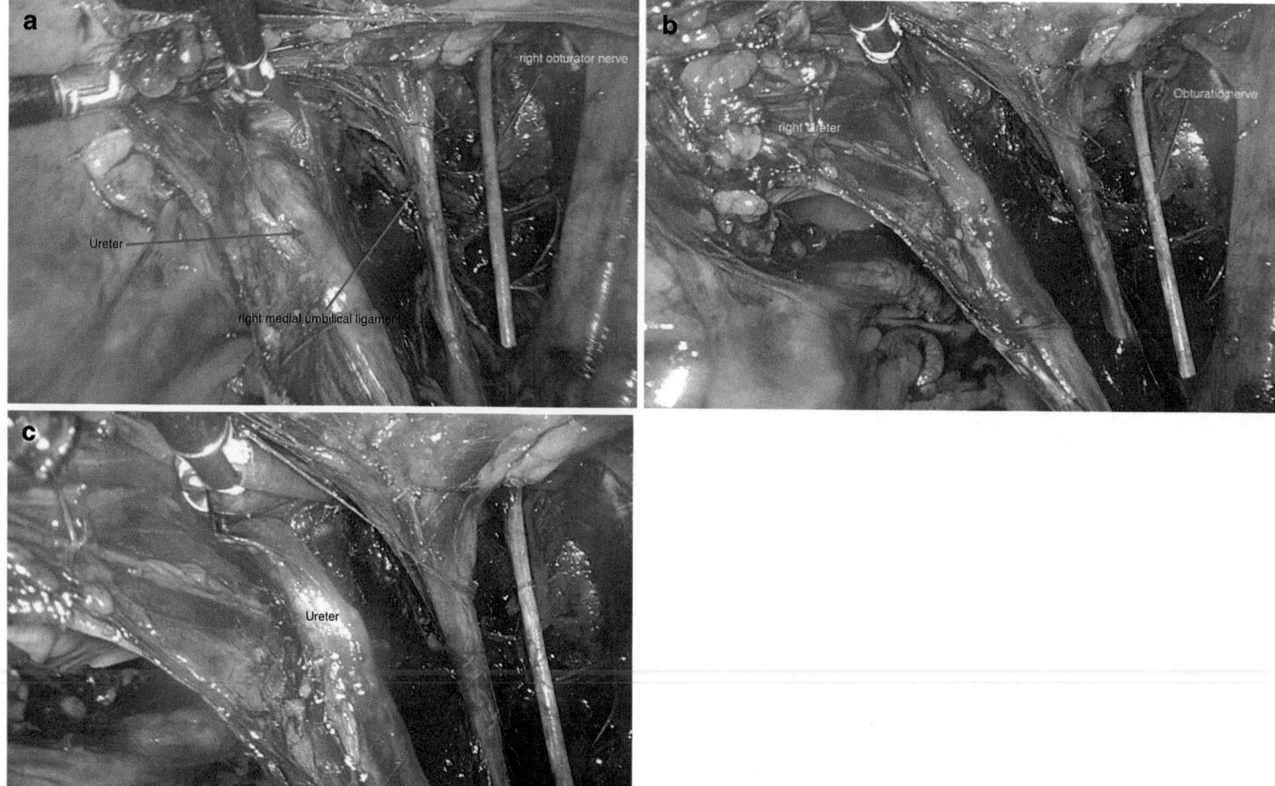

Fig. 51.12 (**a**) Dissection of the right ureter until it is crossed by the uterine artery. (**b**) Visualisation of the right obturator nerve. (**c**) Dissection of the crossing of ureter and uterine atrtery

Opening of the Fossa obturatoria – Dissection of the obturator nerve

Medial of the lateral umbilical ligament (containing the obliterated umbilical artery), the obturator fossa can be accessed. This sometimes requires some sharp dissection as the lateral umbilical ligament can be very lateral, almost attached to the adjacent structures, i.e. the external iliac vein. Because of this, the safe opening of this space should proceed directly lateral of the lateral umbilical ligament, as far away from the pelvic sidewall as possible. The "bottom" of the obturator fossa is the obturator nerve, which needs to be freed from surrounding fatty and lymphatic tissue over some distance to be truly visible during the rest of the surgery. The obturator nerve needs to be frequently checked for its location. It follows the old ureteral rule: "Now you see it, now you don't" and can be easily damaged with electrocautery, thermal energy or by sharp transection. The obturator nerve is the largest nerval structure normally dissected in the pelvis. It is accompanied by the obturator vessels, which rarely need to be coagulated, but can lead to unnecessary and annoying bleeding if not respected. The obturator vein often branches off the *external* iliac vein, in which case coagulation is advised to facilitate lymphonodectomy.

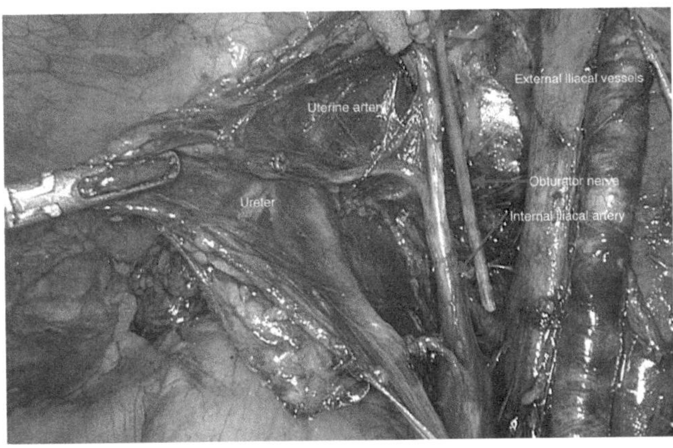

Fig. 51.13 Final view. Preparation and visualization of the crossing of the uterine artery and the ureter

Complete lateralization of the axis internal iliac artery – Umbilical Artery/Lateral Umbilical ligament (Fig. 51.14a)

After a successful approach from caudad and cephalad, this axis often remains attached to the pelvic sidewall. However, other than small peritoneal vessels, there remain no important vessels or other structures so that sharp dissection should carry the most dorsal part of the surgical field down to this vessel axis.

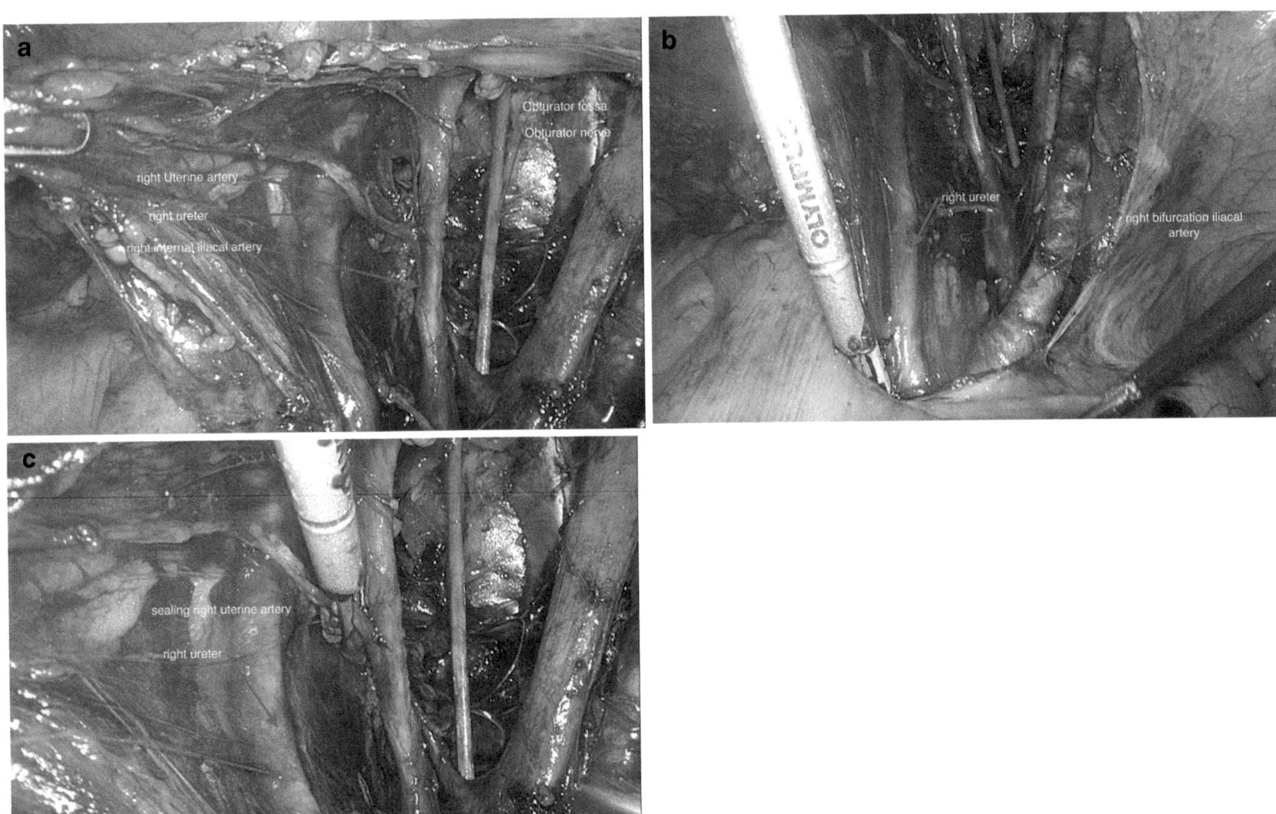

Fig. 51.14 (**a**) Preparation/dissection of the paravesical space. (**b**) Preparation/dissection of the pararectal space. (**c**) Coagulation of the uterine artery at its origin from the internal illiac artery (*right side*)

Exposing the branching of the uterine artery off the internal iliac artery (Fig. 51.14b)
Finding the uterine artery where it branches off (in an almost 90° angle) from the internal iliac artery remains the most critical skill to be mastered by the gynecologic surgeon. It is essential for radical hysterectomy, but extremely helpful in many challenging situations of benign gynecologic surgery. Essentially, it requires a sufficient dissection of the paravesical and the pararectal spaces which are separated by the uterine artery.

Opening the pararectal space (Fig. 51.14c)
Opening the pararectal space is not strictly necessary for pelvic lymphonodectomy, as is the isolation of the uterine artery. It would be necessary as part of the setup for a radical hysterectomy.

Start of the lymphonodectomy at the most distal part of the internal iliac artery (Fig. 51.15a)
Once all the relevant structures have ben delineated and all the spaces opened, lymphonodectomy can safely begin. Grasping of the lymph nodes is usually possible with atraumatic graspers. Lymph nodes tend to bleed, so caution is required. The guiding structure for this first part of the dissection is the external iliac artery.

Distal limit: Crossing of the circumflex vein (Fig. 51.15b)
Care should be take not to go too far into the inguinal canal. Exposing this vein, crossing the external iliac artery is sufficient for the distal limit of dissection.

Avoid disturbing the lateral fatty tissue on the psoas muscle (Fig. 51.16a–e)
Many surgeons believe that the all too easy removal of this lymph node-free fad-pad leads to an increased incidence of lymphoceles/lymph cysts. It certainly does not add to the lymph node count.

Expose the external iliac artery and remove lymph nodes in a retrograde fashion, using a combination of blunt (80 %) and sharp (20 %) dissection
The external iliac artery needs to be exposed and protected. However, it is a sturdy structure and lymph nodes can be "pulled" off the artery in a blunt fashion – as is done in open cases routinely.

Try for en-bloc removal
Particularly on the right side, en-bloc-removal is possible, making later removal from the abdominal cavity easier. However, it is not a goal in itself.

At the distal end, expose the internal iliac vein
After removing the lymph nodes overlying the external iliac artery, the move is medially, down on the very thin and often "empty" (because of the patient's Trendelenburg position) external iliac vein.

The key is to define the "lower" edge of the vein, to make sure that the paper-thin vessel is not accidently injured. The danger is that an injured but "empty" external iliac vein might not immediately bleed.

Find the pelvic bone directly "underneath", i.e. medial and dorsal of the internal iliac vein (Fig. 51.17)
This bony part of the pelvis is a key part of the dissection. It allows safe access to the lateral limits of the obturator space (obturator muscle) and further allows for the safe isolation of the obturator nerve.

Because the obturator lymphatic fat-pad can be easily dissected off the smooth bone, it is also a good starting point for the lymph node resection

Re-expose the obturator nerve
As mentioned above: Again and again, the obturator nerve needs to be visualized. However, this distal part is not the

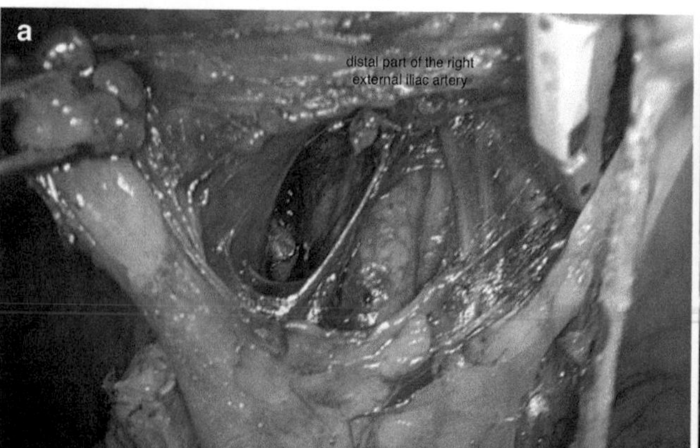

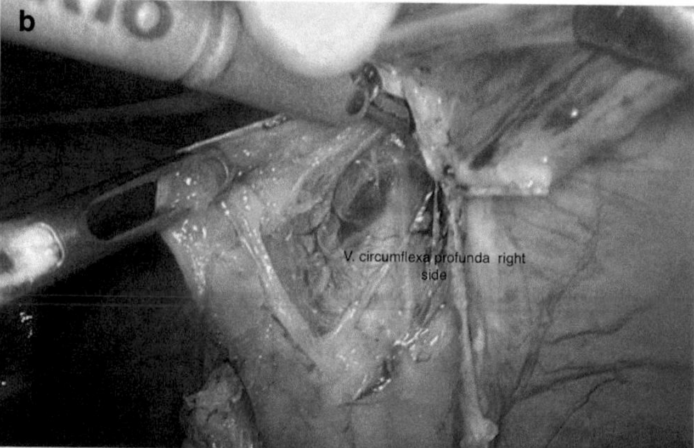

Fig. 51.15 (**a**) Distal limitation of the pelvic lymphonodectomy. Visualization of the distal part of the right external iliac artery. (**b**) Distal limitation of the pelvic lymphonodectomy. Visualization of the V. circumflexa profunda just cranial of the inguinal ligament

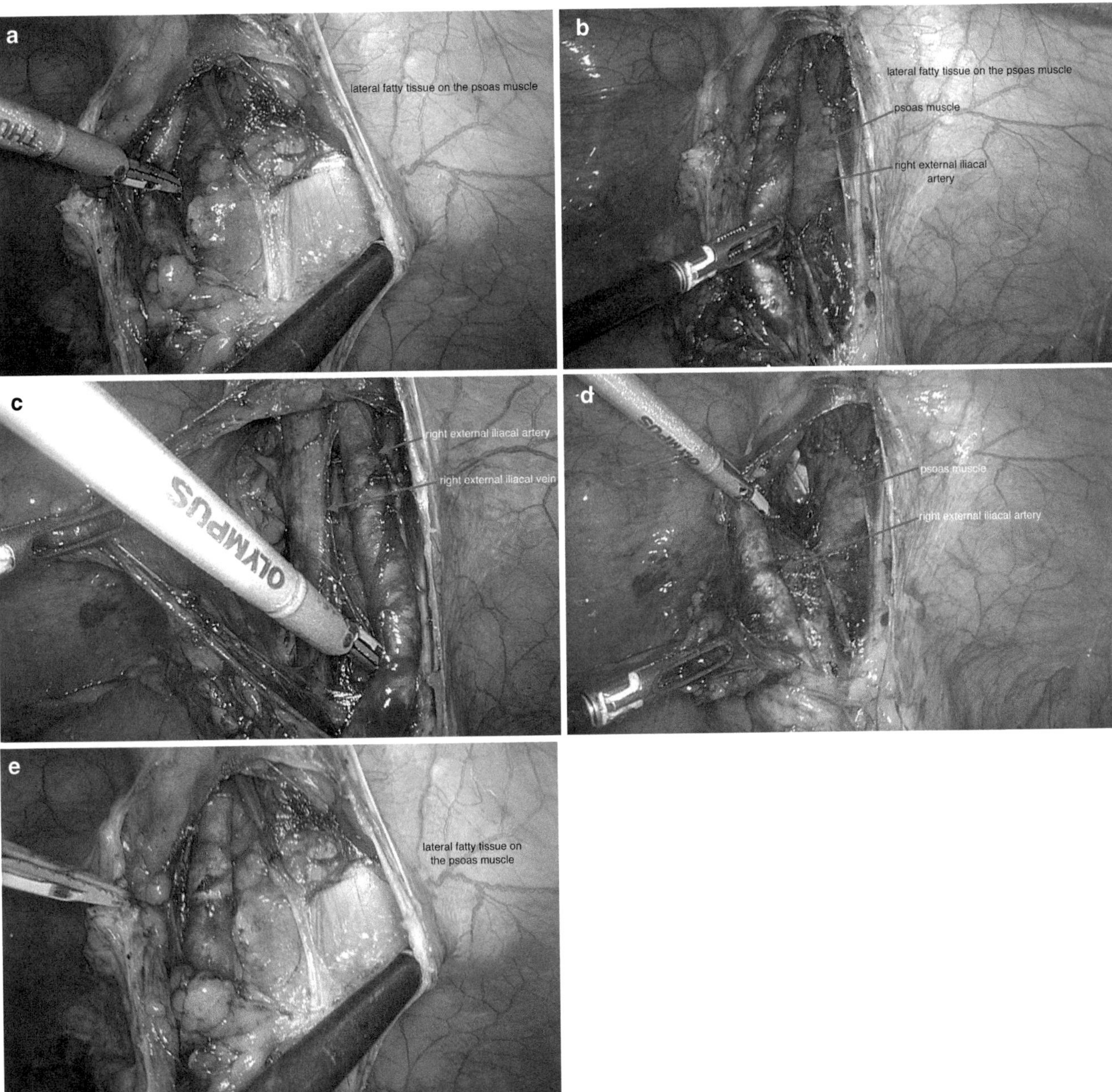

Fig. 51.16 (**a**) The lateral limits of the pelvic lymphonodectomy: psoas muscle and lateral adipose tissue which should not be removed. (**b**) The external illiac vessels are medialized bluntly away from the psoas muscle to allow optimal access to all lymphatic tissue. (**c**) Dissection of the right exteranl artery and vein. (**d**) "Lateral" access to the oburator fossa between psoas muscle and external vessels. (**e**) The lateral border of the lymphonodectomy: psoas muscle

part most likely to be injured. Injuries usually occur right where it appears underneath the external iliac vein into the obturator fossa.

Start removal of the fossa obturatory lymph nodes (Fig. 51.18a–d)
With the external iliac vein safely away and the obturator nerve visualized, lymphonodectomy starts sharply, coagulating and cutting the incoming lymphatic vessels and then removing the lymph node tissue mostly bluntly. Aberrant obturator veins, branching of the external iliac vein need to be watched carefully and usually must be coagulated and transected.

Distance the external iliac vessels from the psoas muscle to expose the obturator fossa laterally
For the laparoscopist, this move does not add much and does not need to be performed at all costs. It allows for slightly better control if bleeding from the obturator muscle perforators occurs. A lot of traditional open surgeons, however, strongly believe that this is an essential part of the pelvic lymphonodectomy,

claiming that the lymph nodes just above the sacral nerves in the area are a common site of recurrence, particularly of cervical cancer, a claim never corroborated by solid evidence nor by the experience of the authors of this chapter.

Also, recent understanding about the lymphatic drainage of the uterus and cervix point to a common sentinel node at a completely different location.

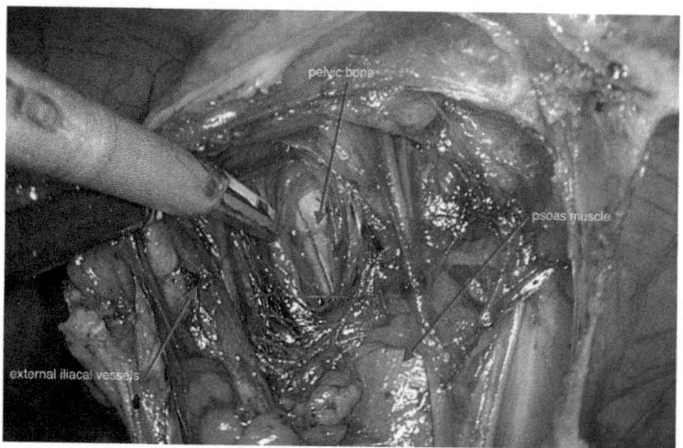

Fig. 51.17 The dorsal limit of the pelvic lymphonodectomy. Vizualisation of the pelvic bones

Still, it is a nice and fairly easy technique to master. Sometime, when all else fails, it might be the only way to find the obturator nerve.

Use the obturator nerve as a guide to further remove the fossa obturatoria lymph nodes
The nerve is a fairly strong structure as far as mechanical force is concerned. Overlying attachments, however, need to be carefully dissected, taking care not to injure the nerve thermally.

Continue this dissection towards the internal iliac artery lymph nodes (Fig. 51.19)
This lymph node, incidentally, is the sentinel node for both endometrial and cervical cancer, making sentinel lymphonodectomy in the area somewhat more tricky than in vulva and breast cancer.

Remove the bifurcation node (sentinel node) (Fig. 51.20a–c)
At this area, the obturator nerve is at its most vulnerable. It is the critical triangle, with strong lymphatic attachments, rich

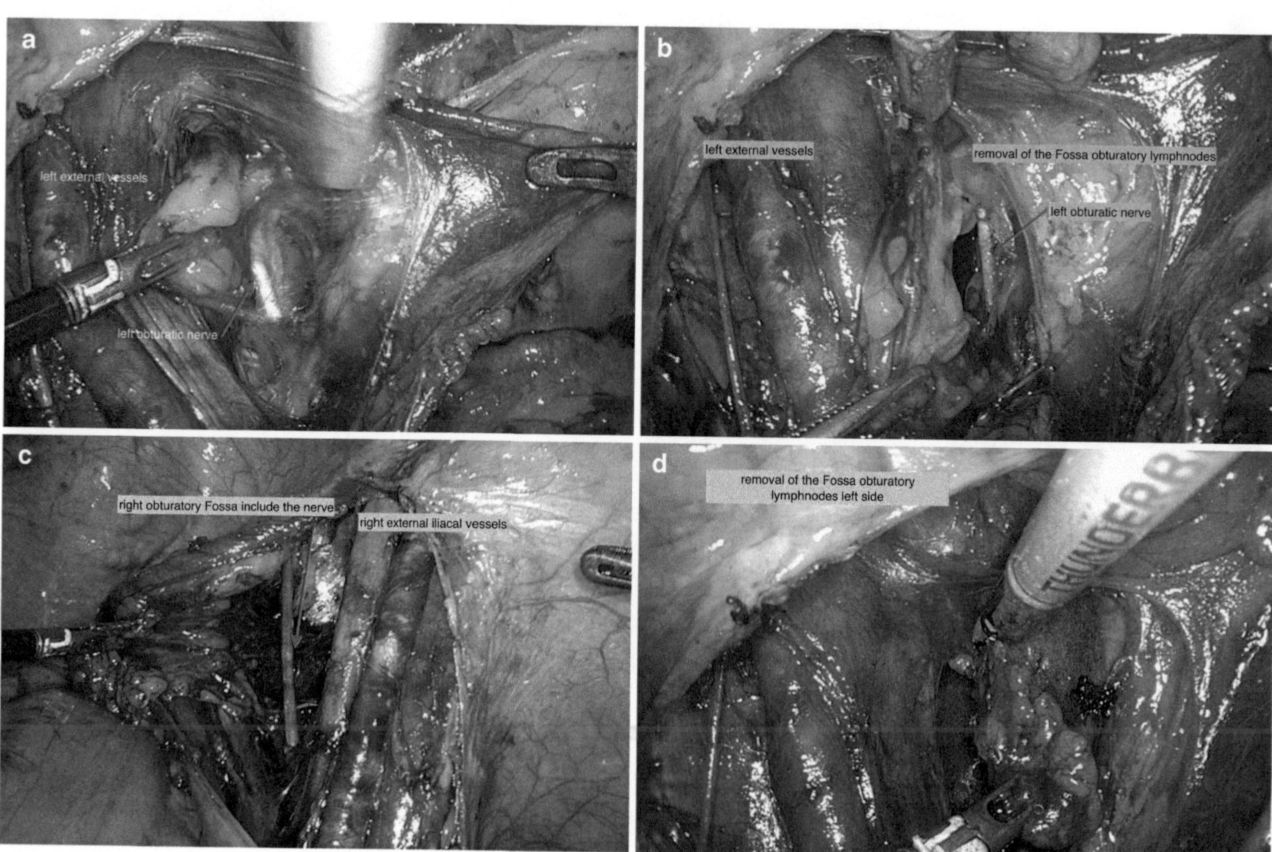

Fig. 51.18 (**a**) Opening of the obturator fossa and identification of the oburator nerve. (**b**) Dissection of the oburator nerve (*left side*). (c) Opening of the obturator fossa and identification of the oburator nerve. Dissection of the oburator nerve (*right side*). (**d**) The "lower" edge of the iliac vein needs to be well exposed before the lymph nodes are removed

microvasculature and numerous dangerous structures underneath or directly lateral (obturator nerve, internal iliac vein).

Cut remaining attachments of the lymph nodes into the fossa obturatoria and to the lateral umbilical ligament
With great caution and care. At this point, tendency is to pull the lymph node package medially, to make these attachments more visible. This, however, dangerously distorts the course of the obturator nerve which must be kept in mind.

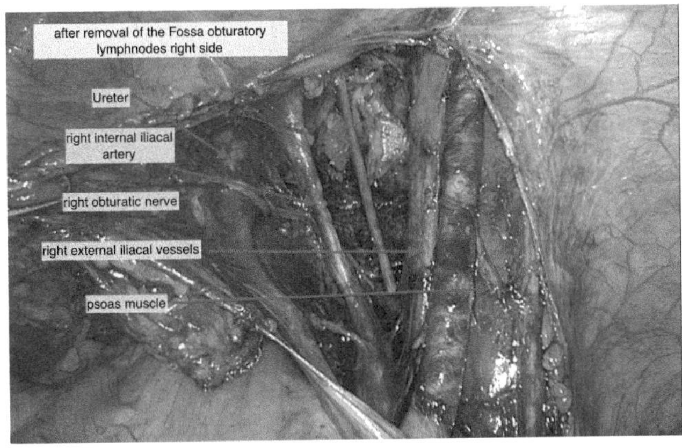

Fig. 51.19 Final view after completed right pelvic lymphonodectomy

Expose branching of the internal iliac vein off the common iliac vein
This is a quality step of the lymph node dissection. If you can actually see this branching, you have certainly done a thorough resection of the most relevant lymph nodes.

Remove remaining and most proximal external iliac artery lymph nodes into the en-bloc resection tissue
Here, the lymphatic chain continuing towards the common iliac artery must be cut at some point.

Remove lymph nodes using an endobag if at all possible (Fig. 51.21)
Other than being aesthetically more satisfying, it also keeps your suprasymphysary 10 mm trocar clean which will be important for the camera positioned there during the paraaortic lymph node dissection.

Complete lymphonodectomy by removing the lymph node pads lateral to the common iliac artery (right side)
Lymph node tissue in this area is usually somewhat flat and patchy. Some bleeding is common.

On the right side, at some point, the posterior limit becomes the inferior vena cava which is not to be injured inadvertently.

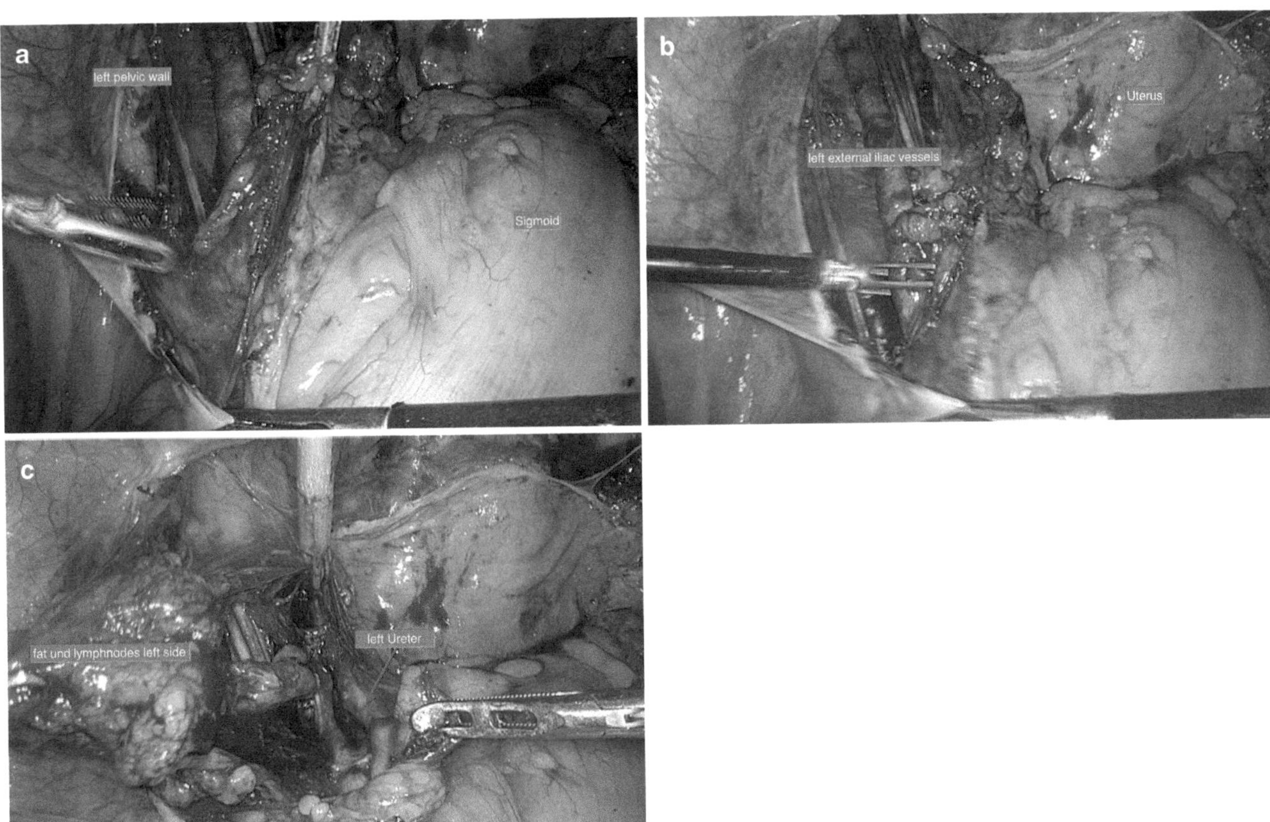

Fig. 51.20 (**a**–**c**) Identification of the left illiac vessels. (**b**) Identification of the ureter. (**c**) Removal of lymph nodes

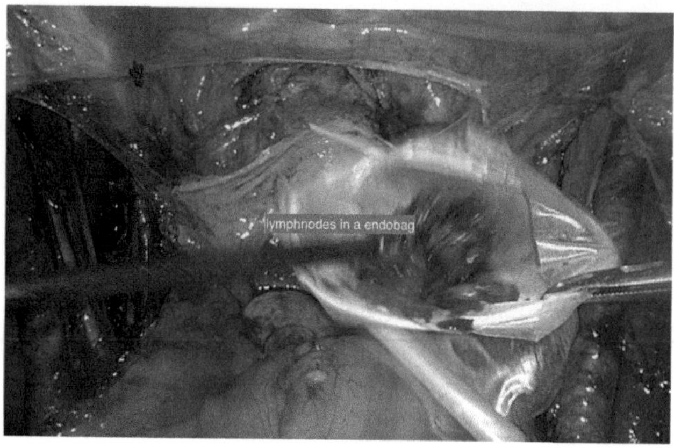

Fig. 51.21 The freed lymphatic tissue is removed separately using endobags

Technique of Laparoscopic Paraaortic Lymphonodectomy

1. Positioning. Retrograde laparoscopy. Camera in the additional suprasymphysary 10 mm port. Second assistant between the legs holding camera only. Surgeon on the patient's right side looking cephalad, First assistant on the patient's left side looking cephalad.
2. Exposing the pelvic brim – starting point is the common right iliac artery.
3. Moving the rectosigmoid to the left side of the abdominal wall and moving the small intestine towards the right side of the abdominal wall. Adjusting Trendelenburg position as needed.
4. Lifting up the peritoneal covering just above the right common iliac artery creates an opening into the retroperitoneal space.
5. Using the arterial trunk, the peritoneal incision is extended upward towards the ligament of Treitz, avoiding all vulnerable structures.
6. In essence, the preparation is about opening the peritoneal tent needed for the surgery.
7. The tent needs to be extended towards the patient's right side, where the ureter needs to be identified separately from the right ovarian vein
8. The right ureter needs to be distanced, exposing the psoas space directly to the right of the vena cava inferior.
9. Delineating the right edge of the vena cava, care must be taken to identify the branching of the ovarian vein – if necessary, the vein needs to be coagulated.
10. Similarly, the crossing of the small right ovarian artery needs to be identified, either to be respected or to be carefully coagulated and transected.
11. After securing the "right side" of the tent, the left side needs to be defined.
12. First, the branching of the interior mesenteric artery needs to be found. It is fairly constant midway between the aortic bifurcation and the crossing of the left renal vein and comes off slightly to the left side of the aorta.
13. Finding the crossing of the left renal vein is challenging. Dissection cannot be sharp: cutting into the lower edge of the left renal vein is a catastrophe that must not happen.
14. About 2 cm towards the left off the aorta, the left ovarian vein starts to descend from the left renal vein. This corner is the most difficult part of the paraaortic lymphonodectomy
15. The tent is now sufficiently defined.
16. Lymphonodectomy can be performed either from cranial to caudal or from caudal to cranial. The decision how to proceed is often situational and depends on the individual anatomy. Distal dissection tends to be more difficult and more dangerous and maybe therefore should be the first step.
17. Preparation on the aorta is unproblematic; dissecting off the vena cava needs to be slow and meticulous. Even pulling on the lymphatic tissue can lead to perforator veins tearing off the vena cave and possible cava bleeders.
18. Cava bleeders need to be closed with pressure immediately. About 90% of them can be stopped by applying sufficient pressure for at least 5 min. What still bleeds after prolonged pressure needs to be sutured with a 4-0 or 5-0 monofilament suture.
19. En-bloc lymphonodectomy down the paracaval and paraaortic spaces is challenging. We recommend a step-by-step approach that takes place in different spaces:
20. Paraaortic area cranial to inferior mesenteric artery (including the difficult angle between the left renal and left ovarian vein).
21. Paraaortic area inferior to the inferior mesenteric artery (careful, the ureter is very close towards the left lateral edge of the preparation and can be easily injured). Visualization of the left ureter remains one of the great challenges. Patient and mostly blunt dissection will eventually allow us to see this important structure. It is deeply imbedded in adipose tissue on the left and does not yield easily to blunt dissection, but sharp dissection is dangerous in this region.
22. Paracaval region, upper half – attention to crossing of the right ovarian artery, branching of the right ovarian vein.
23. Paracaval region, lower half – attention to the perforator veins which are increasing in frequency towards the caudad region.
24. Interaorto-caval region – careful not to injure the lumbar veins going off in a dorsal and downward manner.
25. Paracaval region towards the right side of cava – psoas space. Careful not to injure the right ureter.
26. The key to paraaortic lymphonodectomy is to avoid major bleeding, as it will often require laparotomy.

27. Lymph node tissue is often smaller and can be removed through the umbilical 10 mm trocar.

What follows is a more detailed explanation of the above mentioned step-by-step approach.

Positioning. Retrograde laparoscopy. Camera in the additional suprasymphysary 10 mm port. Second assistant between the legs holding camera only. Surgeon on the patient's right side looking cephalad, First assistant on the patients left side looking cephalad (Fig. 51.22).

These are recommendations only, of course. Each surgeon needs to find out his or her best approach. Some surgeons might want to stand between the legs. However, we strongly encourage our readers to try our approach.

Exposing the pelvic brim – starting point is the common right iliac artery (Fig. 51.23a, b)
This is a test also for the feasibility of this very challenging surgery. If the common right iliac artery cannot be dissected, the surgery might not be possible.

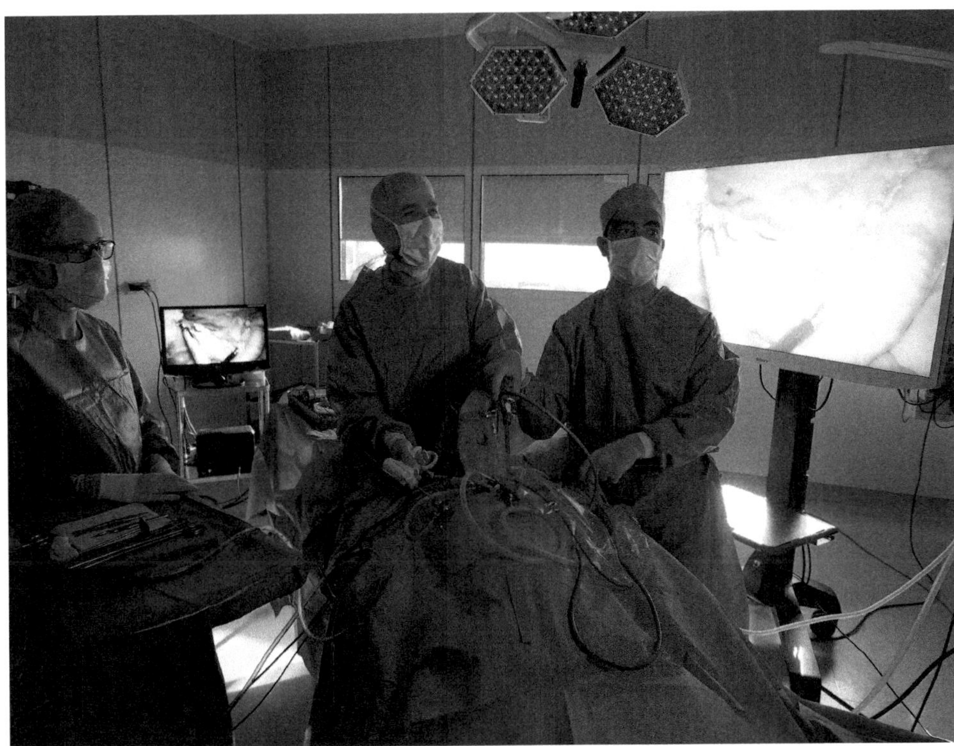

Fig. 51.22 Positioning of the surgeon. Surgeon on the patient's right side looking cephalad, First assistant on the patient's left side looking cephalad

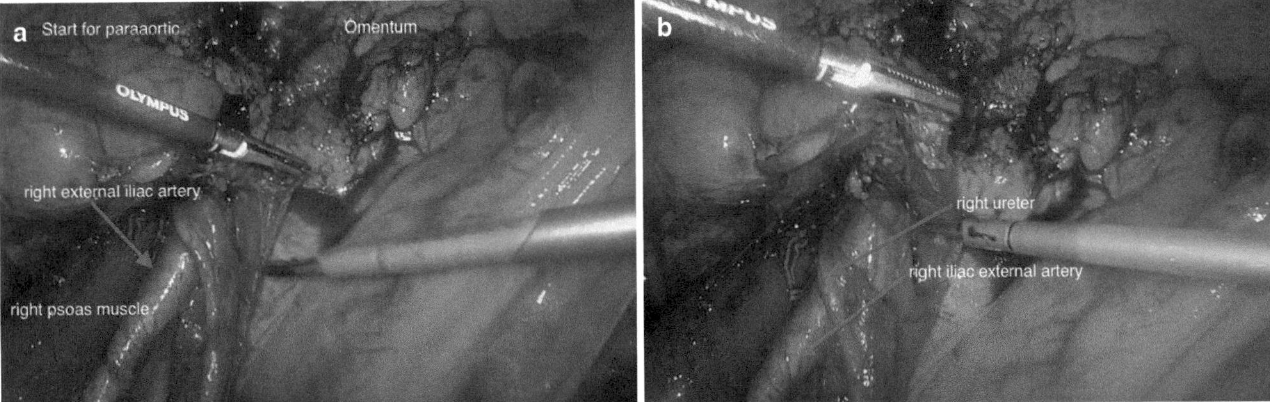

Fig. 51.23 (**a**) The bifurcation of the right common illiac artery is a good starting point for the paraaortic lymphonodectomy. (**b**) Always identify the ureter at this point

Moving the rectosigmoid to the left side of the abdominal wall and moving the small intestine towards the right side of the abdominal wall. Adjusting Trendelenburg position as needed (Fig. 51.24a, b)
At this point, we should discuss the order of the surgery. Oncologically speaking, it is nice to know, if the pelvic lymph nodes are affected. In cervical cancer this might be the reason for performing a paraaortic lymph node dissection. However, given the fact that the paraaortic dissection is the most challenging part of the surgery, with the highest conversion rate (though still very low in the hands of a skilled surgeon), one might consider starting out with this part of the surgery. The advantage is that if the surgeon starts with the paraaortic dissection, the attachments of the sigmoid colon to the left pelvic sidewall have not yet been taken down, helping in the lateralization.

Lifting up the peritoneal covering just above the right common iliac artery creates an opening into the retroperitoneal space
Most laparoscopic oncologic surgery can be done with almost any level of skill on the part of the first assistant. However, paraaortic dissection is different. The presence of at least a minimally skilled assistant is essential.

Using the arterial trunk, the peritoneal incision is extended upward towards the ligament of Treitz, avoiding all vulnerable structures
Again, these first steps are crucial. The oncologic context of the lymphonodectomy needs to be understood. If these first steps are not possible because of bowel obliteration of the field or because of extreme obesity, another, if necessary laparotomic approach must have been discussed with the patient. For this reason, too, the feasibility of the lapararoscopic approach must be established at the beginning of the procedure, just as it needs to be ascertained whether the uterus can be removed vaginally.

In essence, the preparation is about opening the peritoneal tent needed for the surgery (Fig. 51.25a–c)
The laparoscopic paraaortic dissection follows a two-tiered approach: first go upward to create the tent, then go upward to start the lymphonodectomy on the aorta.

The tent needs to be extended towards the patient's right side, where the ureter needs to be identified separately from the right ovarian vein
The difficulties on the right side are always the same: What is the ureter and what is the vein? They look surprisingly similar and waiting for the ureter can be time-consuming. Still, one has to be certain. Sometimes, just extending the dissection on the lateral edge of the vena cava more cranially will solve the problem.

The right ureter needs to be distanced, exposing the psoas space directly to the right of the vena cava inferior (Fig. 51.26a, b)
This space is easily opened and – one more time – the psoas space (this one much more cranial than the first one described during pelvic lymphonodectomy) offers safety.

Delineating the right edge of the vena cava, care must be taken to identify the branching of the ovarian vein – if necessary, the vein needs to be coagulated (Fig. 51.27)
Not coagulating the vein increases the risk of tearing it off, sometimes directly where it comes out of the vena cava, creating a hole that cannot be closed by pressure only.

Similarly, the crossing of the small right ovarian artery needs to be identified, either to be respected or to be carefully coagulated and transected
The ovarian arteries are quite small, but they bleed considerably. Sometimes their coagulation is not even noticed but the lack of coagulation is always apparent on transection. Their identification is not always possible, but they are always there.

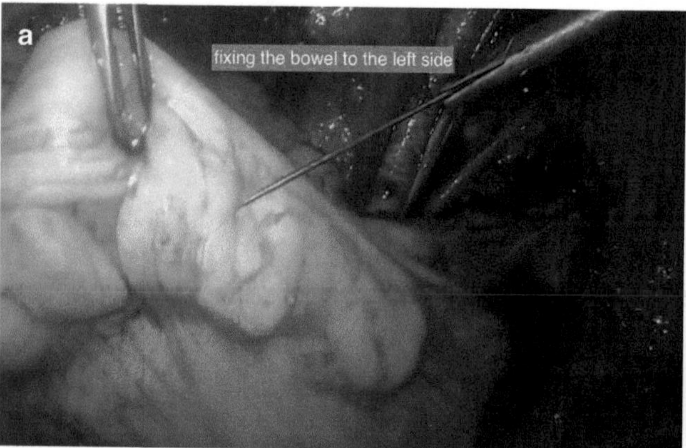

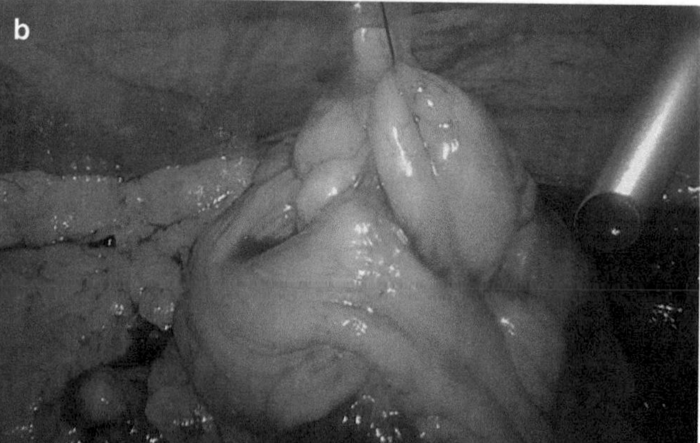

Fig. 51.24 (**a**) To allow optimal access to the aorta, the sigmoid colon is mobilised. (**b**) The sigmoid is fixed towards the left of the patient with a percutan suture

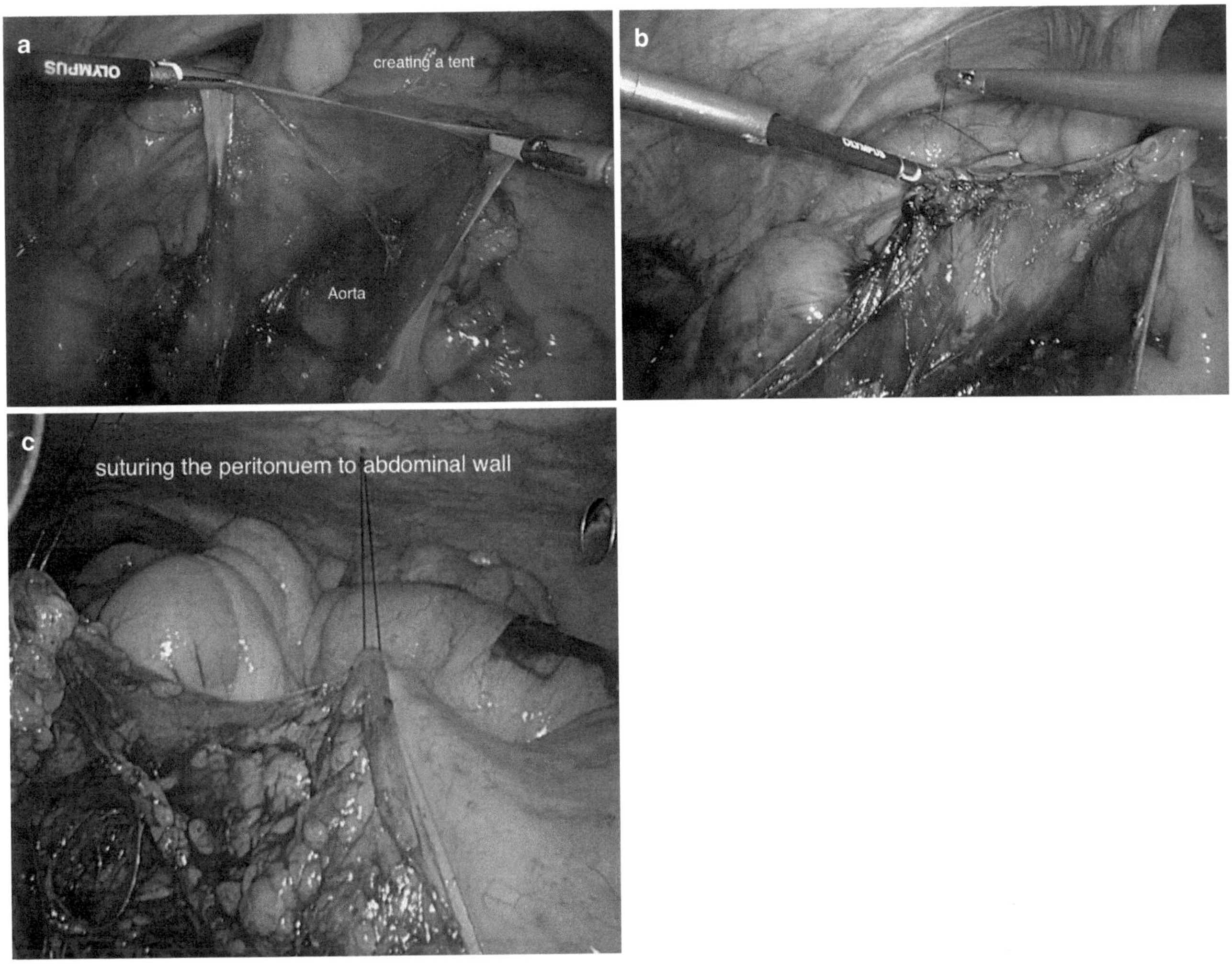

Fig. 51.25 (**a–c**) The peritoneum is opened up to the ligament of Treitz. (**b**) The peritoneum is then fixed towards the abdominal wall with percutaneus sutures. (**c**) The “tent” exposes the surgical field and keeps the small bowel in the upper abdomen

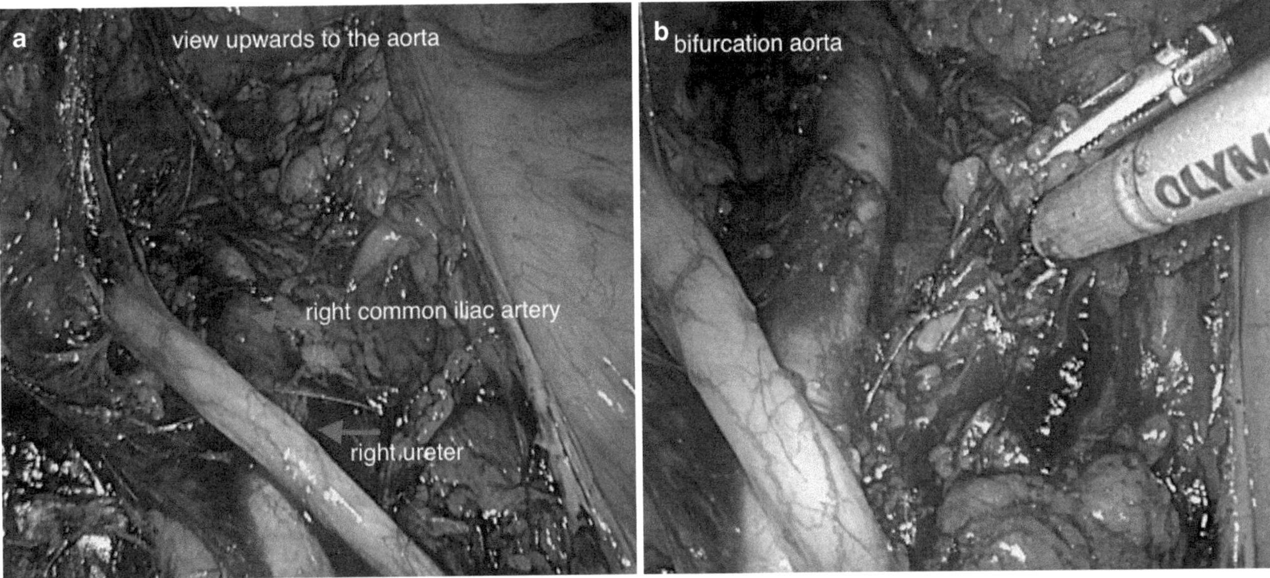

Fig. 51.26 (**a**) Dissection along the right common illiac artery, leading towards the aortic bifurcation. (**b**) The lymphatic tissue below the bifurcation should be removed carefully with the left common illiac vein just below

After securing the "right side" of the tent, the left side needs to be defined (Fig. 51.25c)
On the right side, particularly the right ureter is far more easily visualized than the left ureter.

First, the branching of the interior mesenteric artery needs to be found. It is fairly constant midway between the aortic bifurcation and the crossing of the left renal vein and comes off slightly to the left side of the aorta (Fig. 51.28)
Finding the branching of the inferior mesenteric artery, which serves as a sort of central reference point in the entire field of dissection is the key to all subsequent orientation. With more experience, one realizes that it is relatively constant. Sometimes it can be seen in its lateral trajectory, but ultimately, the branch directly off the aorta needs to be dissected by blunt preparation. We prefer to do this coming from the medial line of aortic preparation.

Finding the crossing of the left renal vein is challenging. Dissection cannot be sharp: cutting into the lower edge of the left renal vein is a catastrophe that must not happen (Fig. 51.29a, b)
The location of the left renal vein is about 4–5 cm cranial of the inferior mesenteric artery. Blunt dissection is essential, can, however, lead to small vessel bleeding which might require coagulation, obscuring the field and making further dissection more difficult. The learning curve of paraaortic laparoscopic lymphonodectomy takes several years, as shown by the group of Achim Schneider, and this is one of the reasons it take time to be comfortable in this region.

About 2 cm towards the left of the aorta, the left ovarian vein starts to descend from the left renal vein. This corner is the most difficult part of the paraaortic lymphonodectomy
Because of the lymphatic drainage of the corpus, these lymph nodes are of particular importance. If they are negative, the paraaortic lymphonodectomy has truly analyzed the complete lymphatic drainage of the uterus.

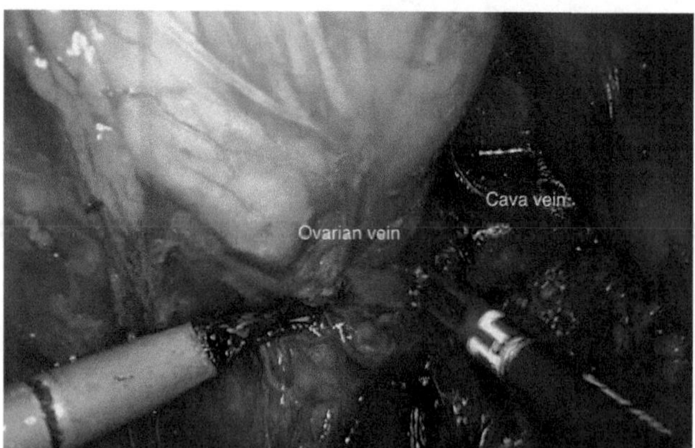

Fig. 51.27 Exposition and dissection of the right ovarian vein

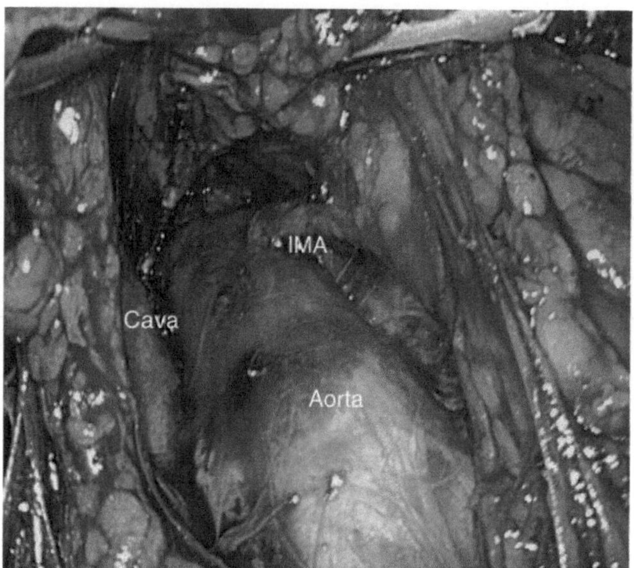

Fig. 51.28 Exposition of the aorta and delineation of the inferior mesenteric artery towards the left and the vena cava toward the right of the patient

The tent is now sufficiently defined
How to best hold the tent open is a matter of debate. We have had good experience with the first assistant opening the tent, as needed, with two blunt instruments. Some surgeons advocate suturing the peritoneal edge to the abdominal wall, others introduces a retractor through an additional trocar in the left upper quadrant.

Lymphonodectomy can be performed either from cranial to caudal or from caudal to cranial
In the end, the order depends on surgeon preference and the actual anatomical situation. Again: The steps of any surgery can be precisely described, but not necessarily their order.

Dissection on the aorta is unproblematic, dissecting off the vena cava needs to be slow and meticulous. Even pulling on the lymphatic tissue can lead to perforator veins tearing off the vena cave and possible cava bleeders (Fig. 51.30a–e)
The aorta is like a well-paved street easily traveled. Blunt dissection is possible. The vena cava tends to be more vulnerable, blunt dissection is to be avoided.

Cava bleeders need to be closed with pressure immediately. About 90 % of them can be stopped by applying sufficient pressure for at least 5 min. What still bleeds after prolonged pressure needs to be sutured with a 4-0 or 5-0 monofilament suture.
Pressure is the most effective hemostatic measure for small cava bleeders. Be careful using clips and sutures too early. Sometimes they make matters only worse.

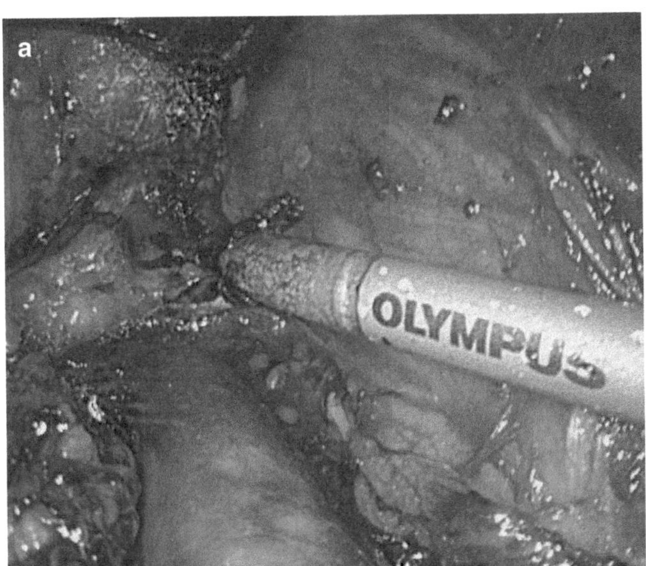

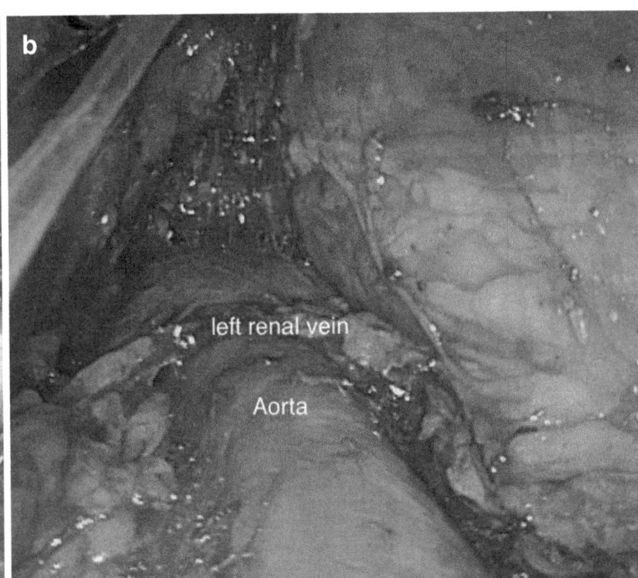

Fig. 51.29 (**a**) Further preparation "upward" i.e. cephalad until the left renal vein crossing the aorta is reached. (**b**) The left renal vein is the upper limit of the gynecologic paraaortic lymphonodectomy

En-bloc lymphonodectomy down the paracaval and paraaortic spaces is challenging. We recommend a step-by-step approach that takes place in different spaces
Lymph nodes should be removed as they become available through the 10 mm trocar at the umbilical position.

Paraaortic area cranial to inferior mesenteric artery (including the difficult angle between the left renal and left ovarian vein) Figs. 51.31 and 51.32a, b)
This is at the same time the most challenging and the most important area of dissection. Even very experienced surgeons continue to find this area very challenging.

Paraaortic area inferior to the inferior mesenteric artery (careful, the ureter is very close to the left lateral edge of the preparation and can be easily injured).
This area – rich in lymph nodes – should be assessed. It is crucial to identify the ureter towards the left lateral side.

Paracaval region, upper half - attention to crossing of the right ovarian artery, branching of the right ovarian vein
Careful dissection includes the identification, coagulation and transection of the above-mentioned structures. Vena cava perforators at this level are rare.

Paracaval region, lower half – attention to the perforator veins which are increasing in frequency towards the caudad region
In the Anglo-American medical community, these perforators are referred to as the "Fellow's veins", indicating that injury is mostly associated with lack of experience, However, here "experience" mostly teaches caution. Blunt dissection will inevitably lead to tearing of these small veins and to holes in the vena cava.

Interaorto-caval region – careful not to injure the lumbar veins going off in a dorsal and downward manner
This is a region rich in lymph nodes, but also rich in big and difficult-to-visualize vessels that are rarely encountered. Careful dissection and reassessment of the oncologic context are important.

Paracaval region towards the right side of cava – psoas space. Careful not to injure the right ureter
This remains one of the most challenging parts. Careful preparation is essential. Respect the trajectory of the inferior mesenteric artery which should remain lateral and cranial of the field. The ureter is difficult to visualize until you have dissected it. Still, it is an important area rich in lymphatic tissue.

The key to paraaortic lymphonodectomy is to avoid major bleeding as it will often require laparotomy
For this step, excellent visualization, using a 30° scope and optimal camera assistance are important. The big dangers are perforator bleeders from the inferior part of the vena cava, the left renal vein, if not exposed carefully, the ovarian veins and the lumbar veins if dissection is performed in a radical manner.

The most common serious source of bleeding will be small holes in the inferior part of the vena cava because of exaggerated pulling on lymphatic tissue, tearing off the small perforator veins. Ninety percent of these bleeders – which are easily diagnosed as venous bleeders because of the dark blue color of the blood – can be stopped by applying at least 5 min of direct pressure on the bleeding site. Patience is the key.

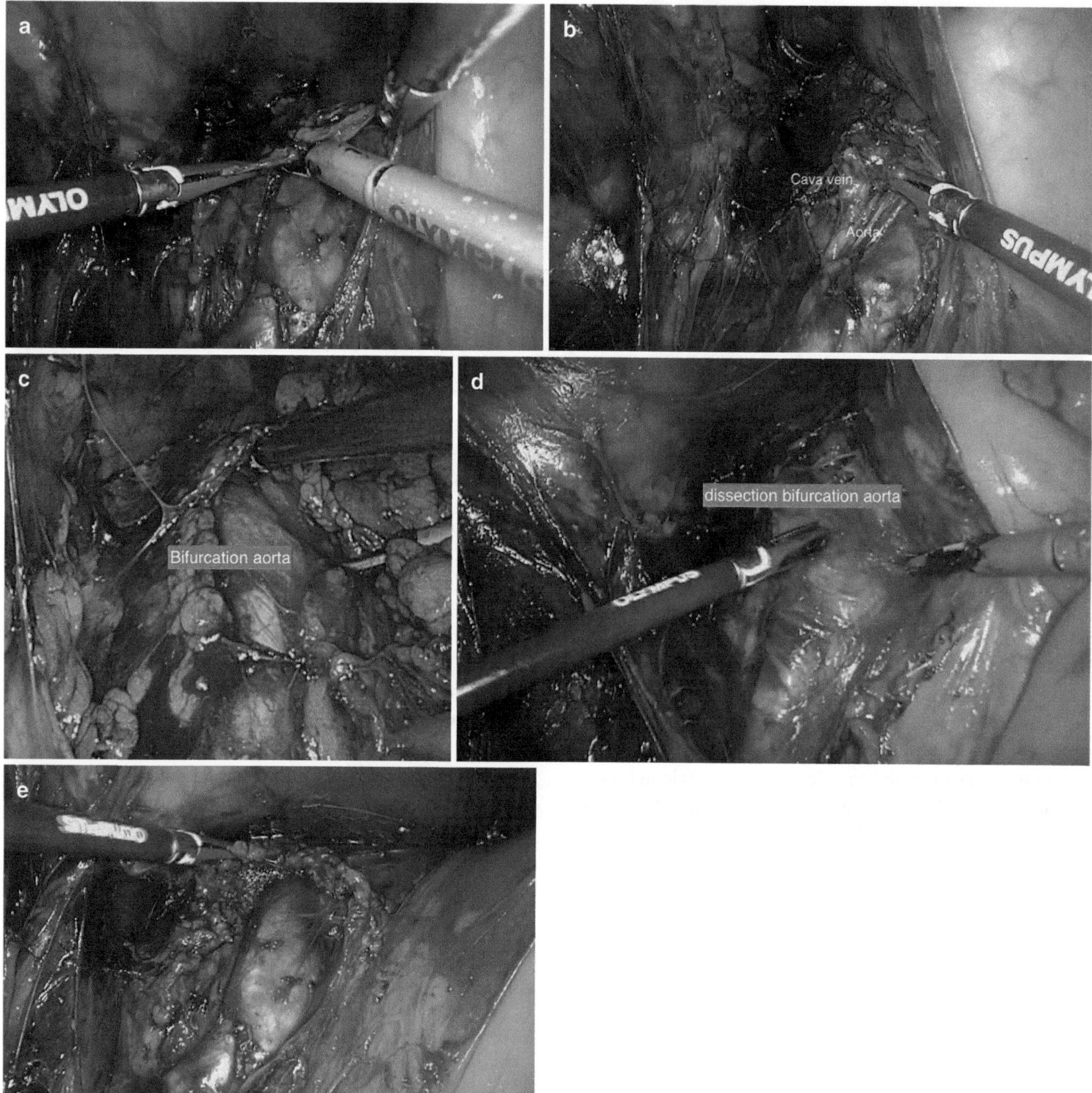

Fig. 51.30 (**a**) The dissection in the aorta is a sharp dissection. (**b**) Sharp dissection on the wall of the aorta. Attention to small perforating vessels. (**c**) First step is to clear the bifurcation of the aorta. (**d**) The use of vessle-sealing devices will facilitate the preparation. (**e**) The surgery follows exactly the course of the aorta

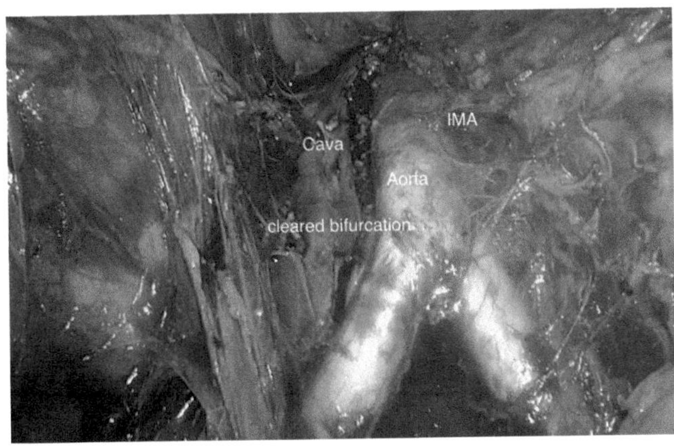

Fig. 51.31 Final view after exposing the aorta and the vena cava inferior

However, if the tear is too large, it needs to be closed with sutures. All venous defects – in fact all vascular defects – need to be closed with monofilament sutures, either 5-0 or 4-0 PDS or, as preferred by some surgeons, permanent sutures. Suturing the vena cava is not only difficult but also dangerous as tearing on the paper-thin venous wall has the potential to catastrophically enlarge the whole, necessitating immediate and urgent laparotomy. It is much better to avoid these bleeders than to control them.

Lymph node tissue is often smaller and can be removed through the 10 mm umbilical trocar

Do not leave small lymph nodes "waiting" in the abdominal cavity. Remove them immediately, lest they should be lost.

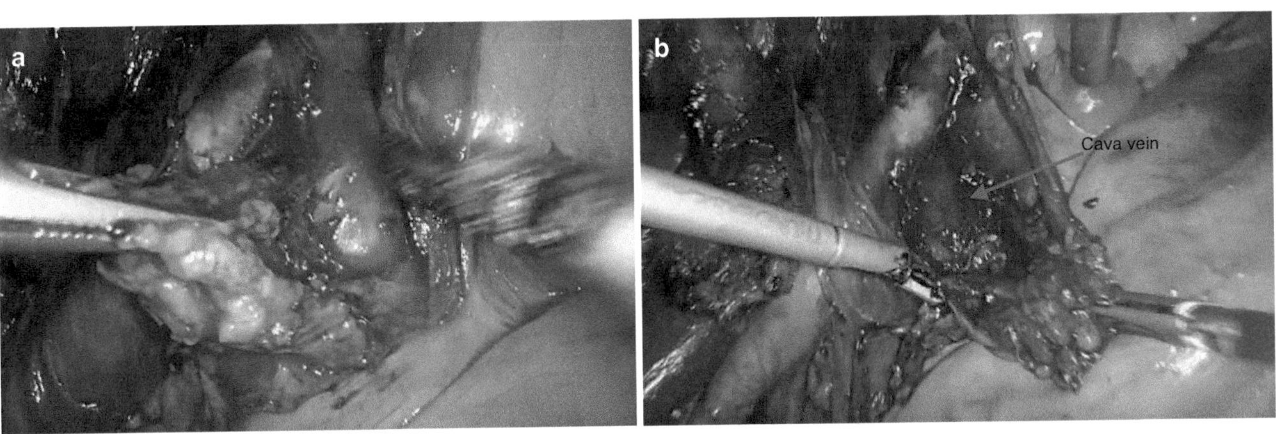

Fig. 51.32 (**a**) Dissesction of lymph nodes downwards the aortic bifurcation. (**b**) Attention! The cava vein is just below the aortic bifurcation

Surgical Techniques of Laparoscopic Omentectomy

52

Jun Ho Lee and Jieun Kim

Introduction

Omentectomy refers to the surgical removal of the omentum. It is usually performed in conditions of malignancies that are likely to transperitoneal metastasis. Omentectomy is a part of standard procedure during surgery for gastrointestinal and genitourinary malignancies like gastric cancer and ovarian cancer. It is a relatively safe procedure once you understand the anatomy and the avascular plane. It is important to be aware of the relationships with adjacent organs that are attached to the omentum to avoid injuries, such as colon, spleen, pancreas, stomach and duodenum. Finding avascular plane by proper traction is the key technique to perform safe omentectomy.

Anatomy and Functions

The greater omentum is a large double layered folds of peritoneum attached from the stomach hanging down to the transverse colon like an apron. It is made up of four layers. The anterior two layers descend from the greater curvature of the stomach and the proximal part of the duodenum, it passes down in front of the small intestines, sometimes as low down as the pelvis. Then they folded on itself and ascend again and attached to the transverse colon. The greater omentum is considered as composition of gastrocolic ligament and gastrosplenic ligament. It is continuous structure but named separately for descriptive purposes. The left border of the greater omentum continuous with the gastrosplenic ligament; and its right border extends as far as the proximal duodenum. Occasionally gastrocolic ligament itself is considered as synonym for "greater omentum" [1].

J.H. Lee, MD, PhD (✉) • J. Kim, MD
Department of Surgery, Samsung Medical Center, Sungkyunkwan University School of Medicine, Irwon-ro 81 Gangnam-gu, Seoul 135-710, South Korea
e-mail: gsjunholee@gmail.com; gskimji@gmail.com

The omentum has been known to play an immunologic role in defending the peritoneal cavity. It is a storage site for lipids, a regulator of peritoneal fluid transit, and a reservoir for immune cells in the peritoneal cavity. It serves as an antibacterial defense, provides hemostasis, reduces intestinal adhesion, and absorbs foreign material from peritoneal cavity. Yet, the omentum remains an understudied organ whose function and role in cancer is not completely understood. Role of omentum in immunology and cancer is still ongoing study [2].

Blood Supply and Lymphatic Drainage

The right and left gastroepiploic vessels provide the blood supply to the greater omentum (Fig. 52.1). The right gastroepiploic artery is a branch of the gastroduodenal artery, which is a branch of the common hepatic artery, which is a branch of the celiac trunk. It runs from right to left along the greater curvature of the stomach except at the pylorus. The left gastroepiploic artery is the largest branch of the splenic artery. It runs from left to right along the greater curvature of the stomach. These arteries lie about a fingerbreadth or more from the greater curvature and anastomose within the two layers of the anterior greater omentum [1, 3].

The right and left gastroepiploic vein run parallel to the same named artery. The right gastroepiploic vein is joined to the anterosuperior pancreaticoduodenal vein then drains into the superior mesenteric vein, and the left gastroepiploic vein drains into the splenic vein. And then, venous blood flow drains to the portal vein and entering the liver cycle.

Generally, the lymphatic drainage of the stomach parallels the vasculature. There are two lymph node groups: those along the left gastroepiploic vessels and those along the right gastroepiploic vessels [3]. Lymph nodes along the left gastroepiploic artey is defined as lymph node station 4sb by Japanese classification of gastric carcinoma [4]. Lymph nodes along the second branch and distal part of the right gastroepiploic artery is defined as lymph node station 4d.

I. Alkatout, L. Mettler (eds.), *Hysterectomy*, DOI 10.1007/978-3-319-22497-8_52

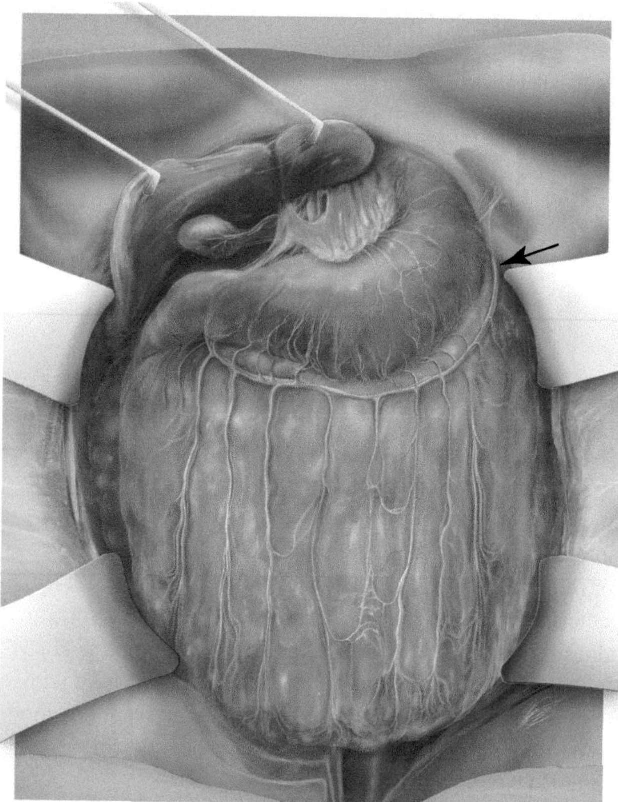

Fig. 52.1 Overview illustration of the omentum and the vessels

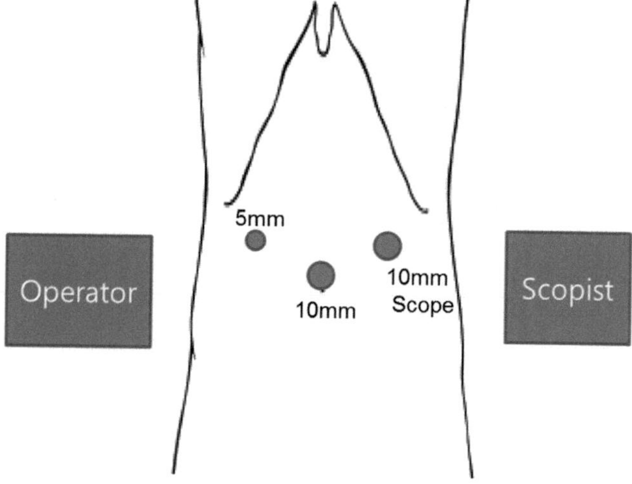

Fig. 52.2 Trocar placement. Five mm port is placed on the patient's right side of abdomen, 10 mm port is placed at the umbilicus, and another 10 mm port is placed at the left side. Five mm port is for the operator's left hand 10 mm port in umbilicus is used for operator's right hand

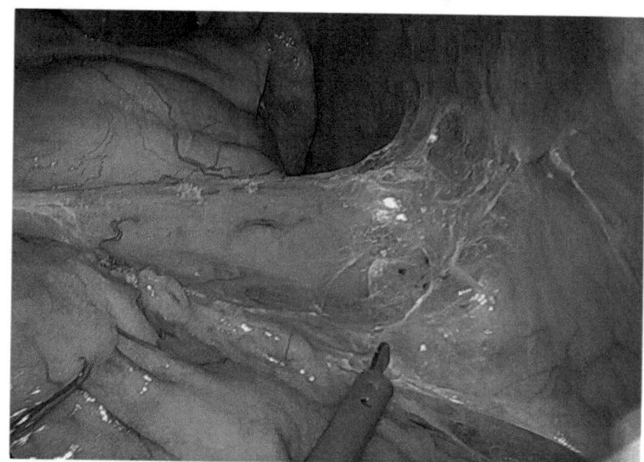

Fig. 52.3 Removing adhesions from the parietal peritoneum

Lymph node stations of 4sb and 4d are regional gastric lymph nodes, which are essential for adequate lymph node dissection during curative resection for gastric cancer [4].

How to Perform Omentectomy

Dissection trough the avascular plane with proper counter traction of the transverse colon can lead to rapid and safe omentectomy during open surgery. In laparoscopic surgery, total omentectomy is time consuming procedure and has potential risk of injury to the adjacent organs. Surgeons not familiar with the upper abdominal anatomy in the laparoscopic view, limited working space, and loss of tactile sense might lead to inappropriate traction and it would make it difficult to find proper dissection plane through overlapped layers of omentum. We would like to introduce some tips to perform omentectomy without an assistant, which could be applied in single incision laparoscopic surgery as well [5].

Total Omentectomy

The patient can be placed in the supine position or lithotomy position, depending on the operator's preference. The operator should stand at either right side of the patient or between the legs of the patient if the patient is in the lithotomy position. After pneumoperitoneum is made and the laparoscopic trocars are in inserted (Fig. 52.2), greater omentum is easy to find in the center of abdominal cavity covering small bowel. Fifteen to twenty degree reverse Trendelenburg position would make a better view to start. Place patient in the left side up position while performing left side omentectomy, begin the procedure by removing all the omental adhesion to the parietal peritoneum. Grasp omentum attached to the parietal peritoneum, and gently pull to the medial side to find avascular white line by operator's left hand (Fig. 52.3). Adhesions can be easily divided with a scissors or electrocautery.

Identify splenocolic ligament by pulling down splenic flexure with operator's left hand (Fig. 52.4). Dividing dense splenocolic ligament could help find dissection plane. Sometimes dividing splenorenal ligament might be neces-

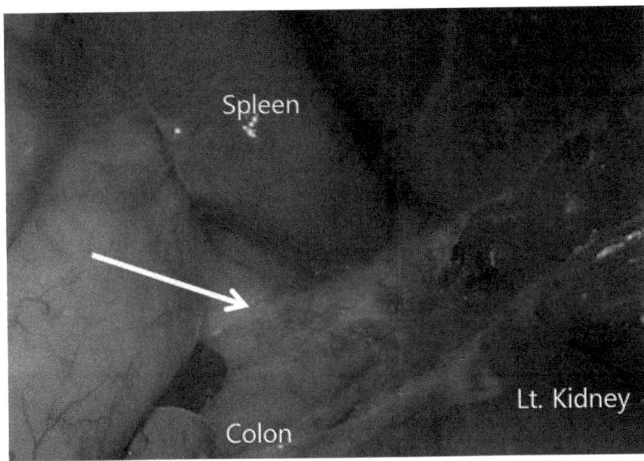

Fig. 52.4 Dividing splenocolic ligament. *Arrow*: splenocolic ligament

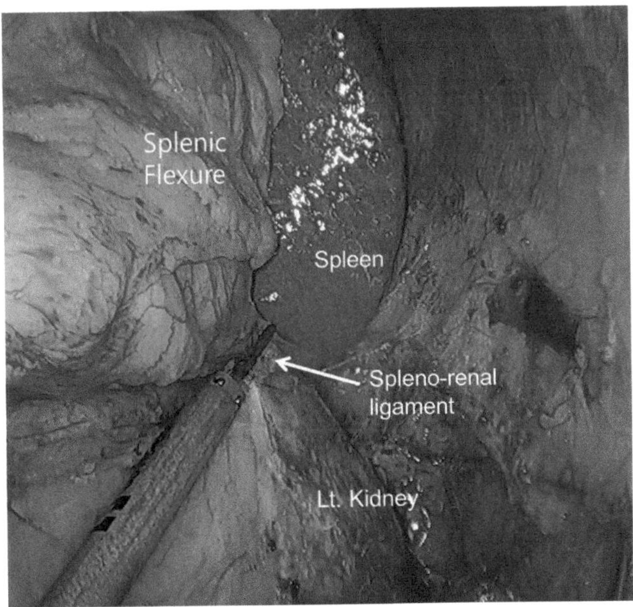

Fig. 52.5 Dividing splenorenal ligament. Left kidney is covered with Gerota's fascia

sary for a better view (Fig. 52.5). Grasp omental tissue 2–3 cm apart from the distal transverse colon with operator's left hand gently lift to the cranial, medial direction. Divide omentum with electrocautrery at the avascular plane just beside transverse colon (Fig. 52.6). Operater's left hand should stay upward direction while operator's right hand should press down transverse colon as if peeling the mesocolon off from the omentum. Continue until tail of the pancreas reveals then follow superior border of the pancreas to the lower pole of the spleen (Fig. 52.7). Occasionally, small vessel branching to inferior pole of the spleen needs to be divided. Careful dissection will identify the root of left gastroepiploic vessels coming up just behind the pancreas tail (Fig. 52.8). The left gastroepiploic vessels are ligated using the hemolock.

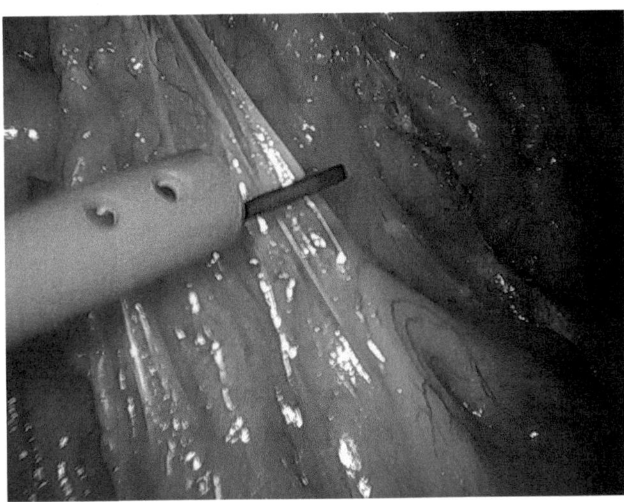

Fig. 52.6 Start dividing omentum with electrocautrery at the avascular plane just beside transverse colon

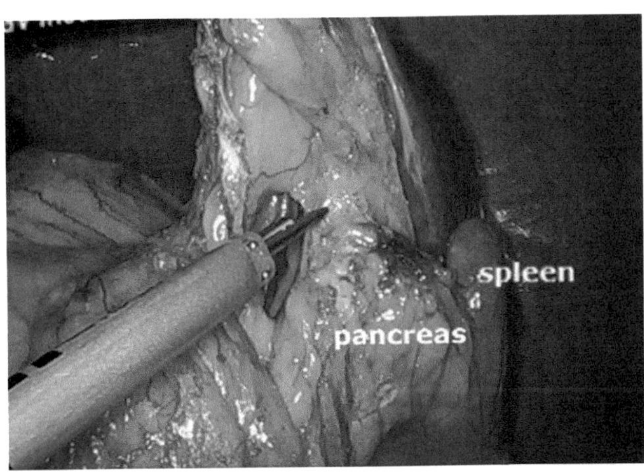

Fig. 52.7 Left side dissection following to the tail of the pancreas

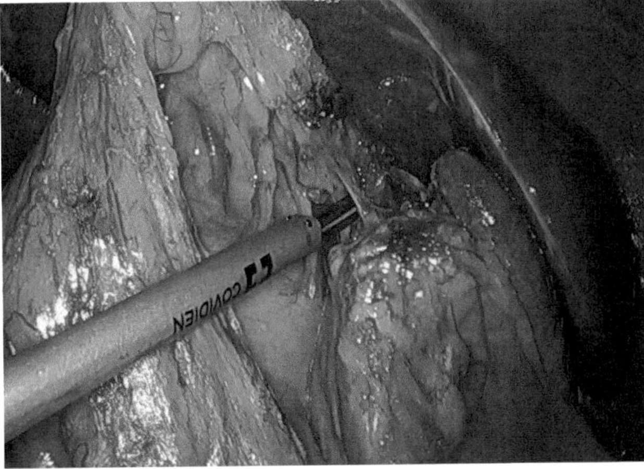

Fig. 52.8 Ligating left gastroepiploic vessels

Continue separating omentum from transverse colon from left to right direction. Keep on upward traction of the ometum with operator's left hand while pressing down transverse colon as previously described (Fig. 52.9). This maneuver will help to minimize injury to the colon. Be careful of the thermal injury of the serosa of the colon by electrocautrery or active blade of ultrasonic shears (Fig. 52.10). If the thermal injury of the serosa is suspected, reinforce suture is needed. Once you divide white line attached to the tenia coli of the transverse colon with an electrocautery, strip off mesocolon from the omentum by gentle push and pull down maneuver with a blunt tip of the monopolar. If you encounter vessels in this layer, mostly it is vessels from mesocolon (Fig. 52.11). Trace the vessels and if it runs horizontal direction, it is vessel from the mesocolon, if the vessel trace up to the vertical direction it is a vessel to the omentum, which you should ligate with the energy device. Gentle press down layer just above the vessel will guide you to the next layer.

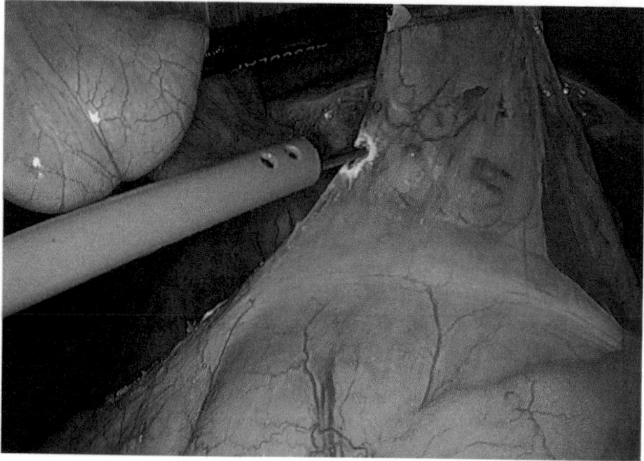

Fig. 52.9 Upward traction of the omentum with operator's left hand while pressing down transverse colon

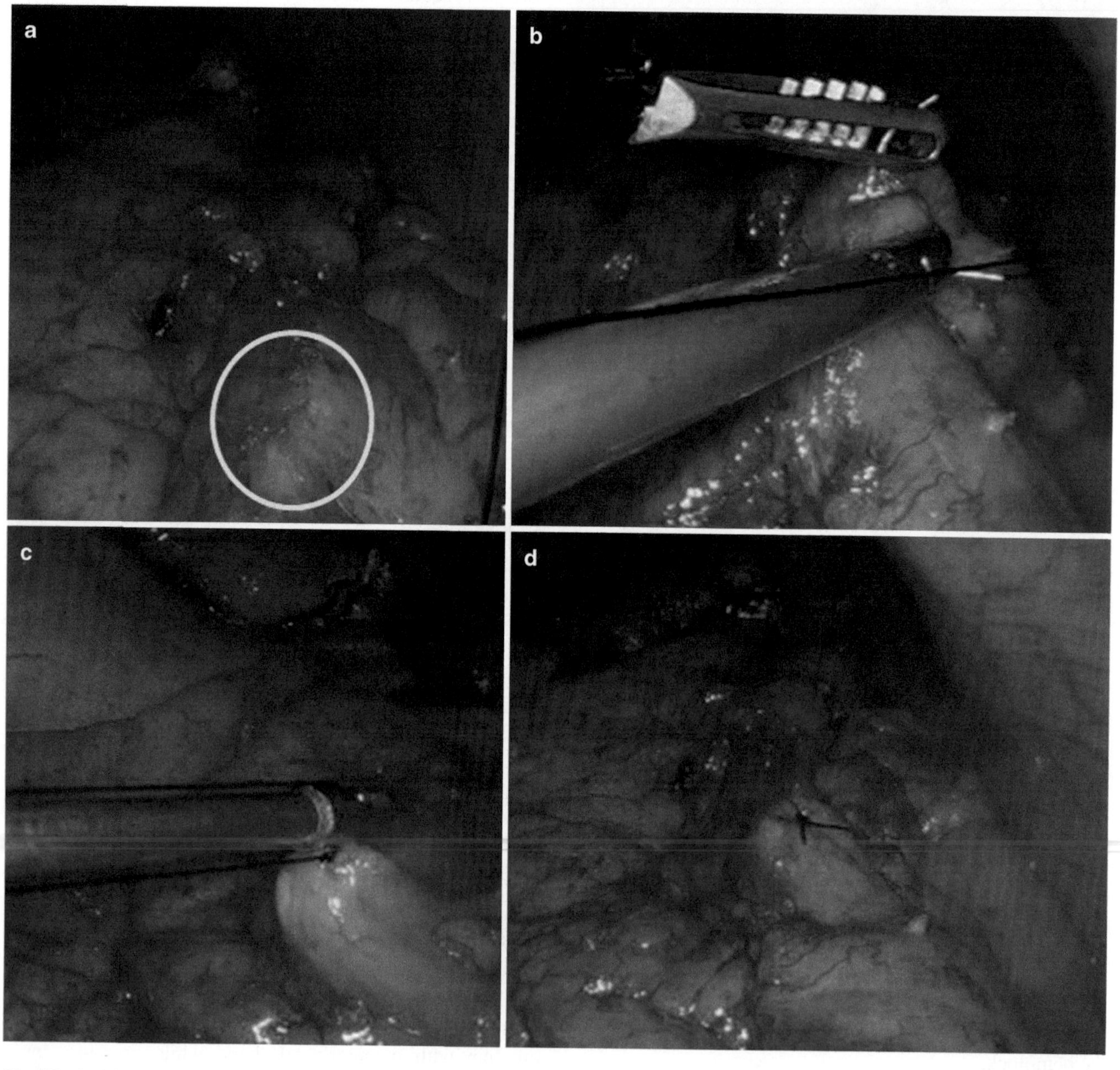

Fig. 52.10 (**a**) *Yellow circle*; Thermal injury to the colon wall. (**b**) Repairing serosa with interrupt suture. (**c**) Making knot with the knot-pusher. (**d**) Final view after serosa repair

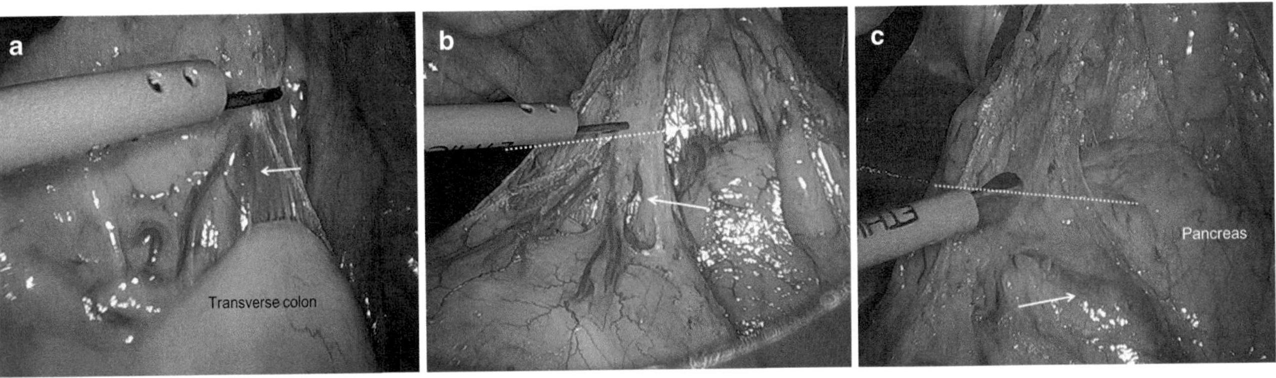

Fig. 52.11 Peeling off mesocolon from the omentum. Be aware of the mesocolic vessels (*arrow*). Dotted line: dissection plane

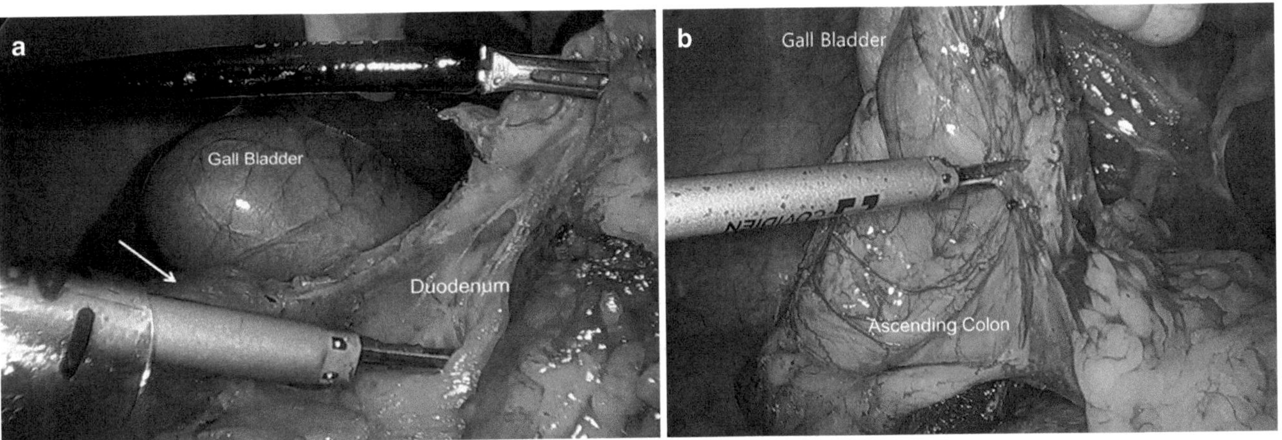

Fig. 52.12 (**a**) Right side omentectomy until the duodenum is seen. *Arrow*: ascending colon. (**b**) Adhesions between the ascending colon and the gall bladder

When you reach right side to the proximal transverse colon, unusual attachment of the omentum may be encounterd. Sometimes colon is folded in hide behind bulky fat tissue in this area. Track down colon until the second portion of the duodenum is seen (Fig. 52.12). Then trace duodenum and trim omentum to the pylorus level.

After separation of the omentum from the transverse colon, flip up the omentum and identify right gastroepiploic vessels arising vertically from the pancreas. Operator's left hand grasp pedicles of the gastroepiploic vessels and stretch to the cranial direction, careful dissection with right hand and ligation of the vessels with the hemolock just above the pancreas (Fig. 52.13). Too much tension before ligating vessels, might cause tearing or injuries to the vessels.

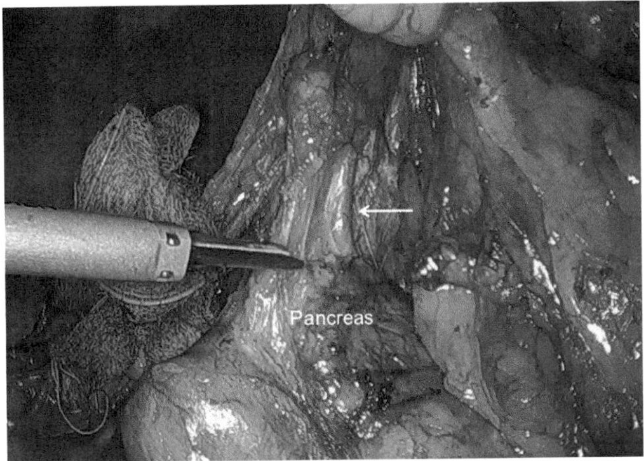

Fig. 52.13 Ligating the right gastroepiploic vessel. *Arrow*: right gastroepiploic artery

Follow ligated gastroepiploic vessels to the greater curvature of the stomach for trimming (Fig. 52.14). Be careful not to injure short gastric vessels inside the gastrosplenic ligament. Once you reach the greater curvature of the stomach, grasp omentum just 2–3 cm apart from the greater curvature with the operator's left hand and trim the greater curvature from left to the right direction with the operator's right hand with the energy device. Hold the omentum upward direction to maintain proper traction, gently pressing down the greater curvature as you divide omentum from the stomach from left to

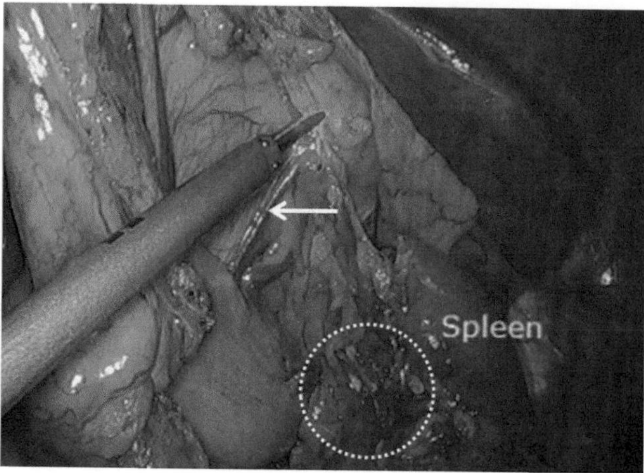

Fig. 52.14 Follow short gastric vessels toward stomach wall for trimming. Arrow: short gastric vessel, *Circle*: ligated left gastroepiploic vessels

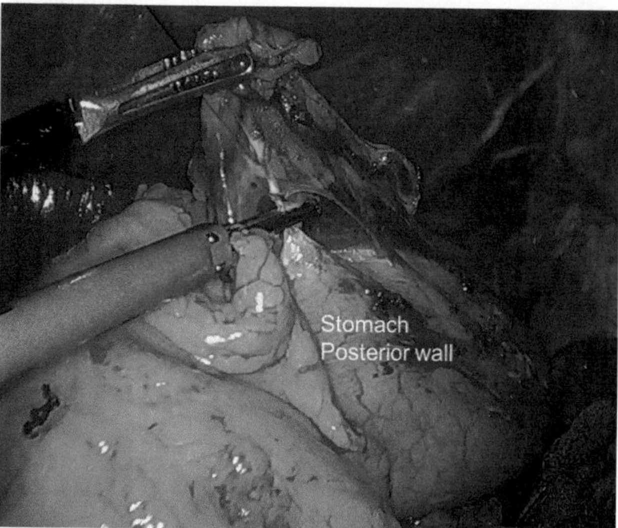

Fig. 52.15 Trimming of the omentum from the stomach

right (Fig. 52.15). This maneuver will show the layers of the dissection plane and minimize the injury of the stomach wall.

Partial Omentectomy

Partial omentectomy is the procedure literally removing only certain part of the omentum. For gastric surgery, partial omentectomy will be removal of the omentum attached to the greater curvature of the stomach including the arcades of the gastroepiploic vessels with the lymph node stations [6, 7]. For gynecologic surgery, terminology of infracolic omentectomy is used [8, 9]. For this case, arcades of the gastroepiploic vessels will be preserved, range of resection would be below gastroepiploic arcades and the rest of the gastrocolic ligament.

Either partial omentectomy or infracolic omentectomy, dissection line should be 4–5 cm apart from the greater curvature of the stomach. The omentum is divided 2–3 cm distance from the gastroepiploic vessels. First, start with making a window at 2–3 cm apart from the arc of the gastroepiploic vessels near lower to mid body of the stomach (Fig. 52.16). Operator's left hand grasp the greater curvature of the stomach and lift upward direction while operator's right hand divide omentum following the gastroepiploic vessels to the left side toward the lower pole of the spleen (Fig. 52.17). When approaching the lower pole of the spleen, it is important to identify the colon to prevent its injury. Make sure colon wall is not in the way of dissecting plane. The left gastroepiploic vessels are ligated as the same method as used for total omentectomy.

The right sided partial omentectomy is mostly same as previously described in the total omentectomy. Follow gastroepiploic vessels to the right side towards proximal duodenum, ligate the right gastroepiploic vessels

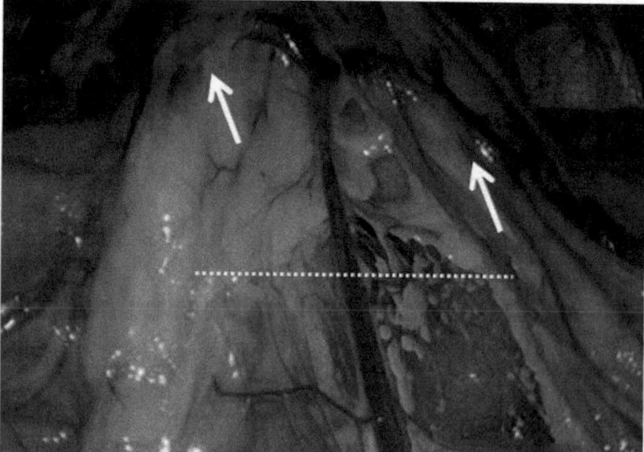

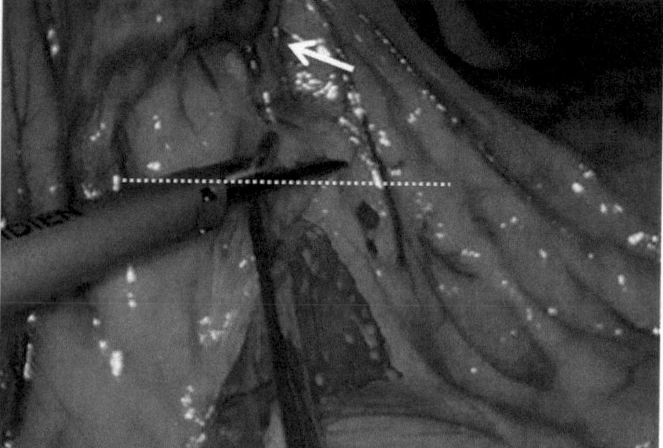

Fig. 52.16 Start partial omentectomy by making a window at 2–3 cm apart from the arc of the gastroepiploic vessels near lower to mid body of the stomach. *Arrow*: gastroepiploic arcade. *Dotted line*: dissection plane

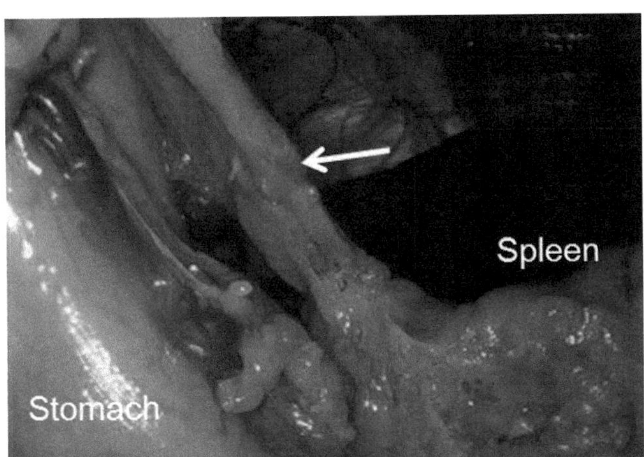

Fig. 52.17 Ligating the left gastroepiploic vessel during the partial omentectomy. *Arrow*: left gastroepiploic vessel

References

1. Moore KL, Agur AMR, Dalley AF. Clinically oriented anatomy. 7 ed. Philadelphia: Lippincott Williams & Wilkins; 2014.
2. Ben Arie A, McNally L, Kapp DS, Teng NN. The omentum and omentectomy in epithelial ovarian cancer: a reappraisal. Part I – omental function and history of omentectomy. Gynecol Oncol. 2013;131(3):780–3. doi:10.1016/j.ygyno.2013.09.014.
3. Lee JH, Kim CY, Kodera Y, Fujiwara M. Dissection of the greater omentum and left gastroepiploic vessels. In: Kitano S, Yang HK, editors. Laparoscopic gastrectomy for cancer. Japan: Springer; 2012. p. 65–74.
4. Japanese Gastric Cancer A. Japanese classification of gastric carcinoma: 3rd English edition. Gastric Cancer Off J Int Gastric Cancer Assoc Jpn Gastric Cancer Assoc. 2011;14(2):101–12. doi:10.1007/s10120-011-0041-5.
5. Kim SM, Lee SH, Ha MH, Seo JE, Kim JE, Choi MG, et al. Techniques of the single-port totally laparoscopic distal gastrectomy. Ann Surg Oncol. 2015;22 Suppl 3:S341. doi:10.1245/s10434-015-4839-y.
6. Kim DJ, Lee JH, Kim W. A comparison of total versus partial omentectomy for advanced gastric cancer in laparoscopic gastrectomy. World J Surg Oncol. 2014;12:64. doi:10.1186/1477-7819-12-64.
7. Kim SM, Lee JH, Lee SH, Ha MH, Seo JE, Kim JE, et al. Techniques of reduced PRT Laparoscopy-Assisted Distal Gastrectomy (Duet LADG). Ann Surg Oncol. 2014;22(3):793. doi:10.1245/s10434-014-4087-6.
8. Nezhat FR, Pejovic T, Finger TN, Khalil SS. Role of minimally invasive surgery in ovarian cancer. J Minim Invasive Gynecol. 2013;20(6):754–65. doi:10.1016/j.jmig.2013.04.027.
9. Arie AB, McNally L, Kapp DS, Teng NN. The omentum and omentectomy in epithelial ovarian cancer: a reappraisal: part II – the role of omentectomy in the staging and treatment of apparent early stage epithelial ovarian cancer. Gynecol Oncol. 2013;131(3):784–90. doi:10.1016/j.ygyno.2013.09.013.

Final Steps and Postoperative Considerations

53

Monika Martina Wölfler

Final Steps After Hysterectomy Via Laparoscopy

Upon finalizing the hysterectomy by removing the uterus transvaginally and closure of the culdotomy or removing the uterine corpus via morcellation in case of a subtotal hysterectomy, extensive lavage of the peritoneal cavity to remove debris and clots and inspection of the entire operating field are essential. Meticulous inspection of the culdotomy, the adnexal region or site of salpingoophrectomy, all peritoneal edges, blood vessels and vascular pedicles for bleeders and good hemostasis after irrigation and suction of fluids reduce the risk of postoperative hemorrhage.To identify small bleeders it might be helpful to temporarily reduce the intraperitoneal pressure. Bipolar electrocauterisation under direct vision is standard for steady hemostasis. Additionally, hemostatic agents, tissue sealants and compression suture clips can be used, however, good evidence is scarce [1].

Irrespective of the dimension of the operative procedure, be it a standard laparoscopic hysterectomy in an outpatient setting or major surgery for deep infiltrating endometriosis or a radical hysterectomy including lymphonodectomy, at the end of the procedure it is important to visualize normal ureteral peristalsis and document whether the urine is clear in the urinary catheter. Normal ureteral peristalsis is certainly not a proof for the absence of for instance thermic ureteral lesion, however, forensically it is substantial to at least address the macroscopic integrity of the ureter intraoperatively.

After major surgery the application of an intraperitoneal drain might be requested although there is no scientific evidence to favor the use of drains at all. Furthermore, data from randomized trials underline that routine use of drains does increase the risk of wound infection. In case drains are inserted they should be removed as soon as possible [2].

When finishing the laparoscopy, the removal of the accessory trocars should be carried out carefully and under direct vision. Small bleeders can mostly be controlled with pressure or electrocauterisation,otherwise a full thickness suture should be placed. For 12 mm accessory trocars and the laparoscope trocar fascial closure is required to prevent herniation. After removing the laparoscope, extensive deflation of carbon dioxide prior to removing the trocar avoids postoperative discomfort caused by residual gas [3].

For the closure of all cutaneous incisions intracutaneous absorbable monofilament sutures will guarantee for optimal aesthetic outcome. All wounds need to be covered with sterile dressings. Alternatively, for the small incisions tape strips and dressings or a skin adhesive dressing can be used.

Postoperative Considerations

The perioperative management was subject to major changes in recent decades, hence checklists for the prevention of complications and for the improvement of patients´ safety are nowadays standard in most clinics and are explicitly recommended by several gynecologic and surgical societies (see also Fig. 53.1 displaying the checklist used at our clinic as an example).Data from abdomino surgical studies underline the superiority of the "fast-track surgery" concept and enhanced postoperative recovery programs compared to traditional concepts in perioperative management [2, 4]. Data from these studies refer to major abdominal surgery and patients with mostly advanced morbidity. Since the majority of gynecologic patients scheduled for hysterectomy are American Society of Anesthesiologists category 1 or 2 (ASA1 healthy or ASA2 mild systemic disease) they might benefit even more from the "fast-track surgery" concept. For the postoperative management in particular several issues need to be addressed.

M.M. Wölfler
Obstetrics and Gynecology, Medical University of Graz, Auenbrugger Platz 14, Graz 8036, Austria
e-mail: Monika.woelfler@medunigraz.at

I. Alkatout, L. Mettler (eds.), *Hysterectomy*, DOI 10.1007/978-3-319-22497-8_53

Preoperative Checklist

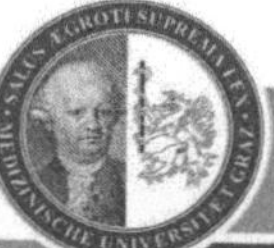

Department of Gynecology and Obstetrics — Medical University of Graz

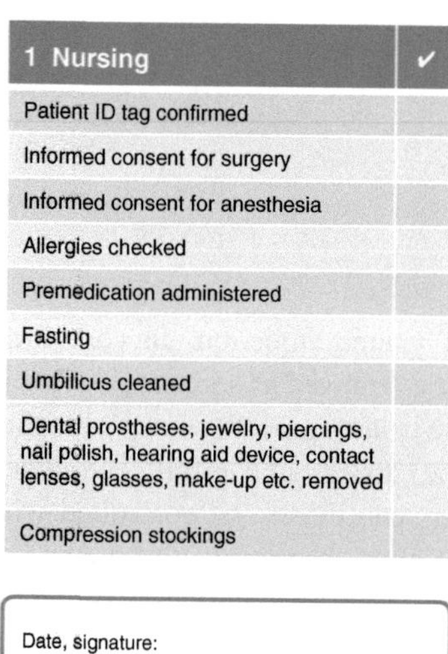

1 Nursing	✔
Patient ID tag confirmed	
Informed consent for surgery	
Informed consent for anesthesia	
Allergies checked	
Premedication administered	
Fasting	
Umbilicus cleaned	
Dental prostheses, jewelry, piercings, nail polish, hearing aid device, contact lenses, glasses, make-up etc. removed	
Compression stockings	

Date, signature:

2 Gyn. Surgeon	✔
Surgical listing confirmed	
Site of surgery checked	
Previous abdominal surgery and relevant diagnoses checked	
Informed consent for surgery	
Anesthesic protocol checked	
Allergies checked	
Surgical consultants informed	
Diagnostic imaging reviewed	
Biobank consent	

Date, signature:

3 Anesthesiologist	✔
Cleared for anesthesia	
Informed consent for anesthesia	
Labs reviewed	
Allergies checked	
Blood products	
Anesthesia modality	
Postoperative requirements	

Date, signature:

Patient ID

Intraoperative Checklist

Modified according to the WHO recommendations

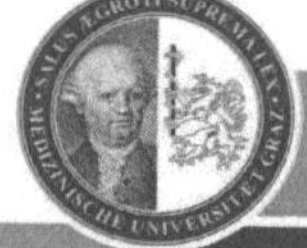

Department of Gynecology and Obstetrics — Medical University of Graz

1 Sign in	✔
Nursing	
Patient ID confirmed	
Preoperative checklist reviewed	
Allergies checked	
Special hygiene issues checked	
Patient positioning	
Equipment for operation checked	
Metal implants	
Anesthesiologist	
Patient ID confirmed	
Difficult airway/aspiration risk	
Anesthesia equipement checked	
Anesthesia modality checked	
Blood products available	

2 Team Time Out (prior to operation)	✔
Patient ID confirmed	
All team members introduced themselves by name and role	
Surgical procedure confirmed	
Imaging studies available	
Site of operation identified	
Positioning of patient checked	
Allergies known	
Antibiotic prophylaxis within the last 60 minutes	
Questions	

OP-date	
OP-room	
Signature surgeon	

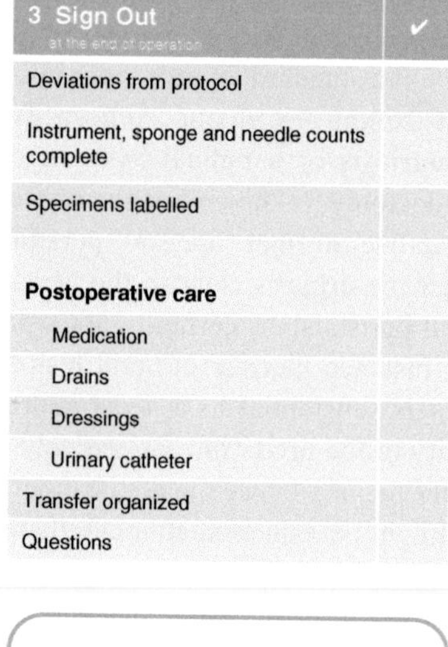

3 Sign Out (at the end of operation)	✔
Deviations from protocol	
Instrument, sponge and needle counts complete	
Specimens labelled	
Postoperative care	
Medication	
Drains	
Dressings	
Urinary catheter	
Transfer organized	
Questions	

Patient ID

Fig. 53.1 Preoperative checklist(Courtesy of the Department of Gynecology and Obstetrics, Medical University of Graz. Adapted English version 2015)

Discharge Checklist

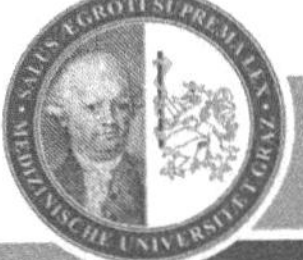

Department of Gynecology and Obstetrics — Medical University of Graz

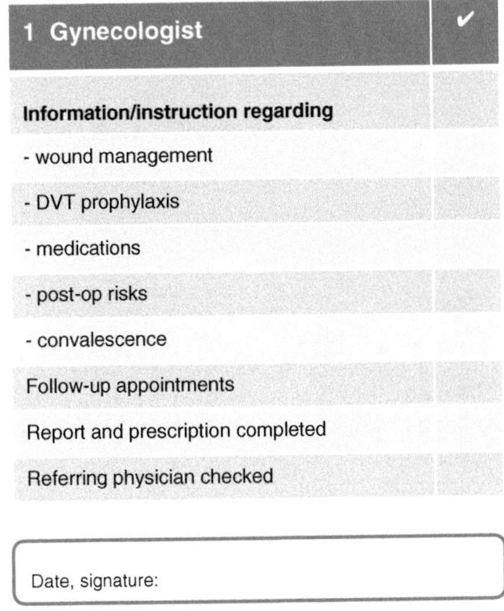

1 Gynecologist	✔
Information/instruction regarding	
- wound management	
- DVT prophylaxis	
- medications	
- post-op risks	
- convalescence	
Follow-up appointments	
Report and prescription completed	
Referring physician checked	

Date, signature:

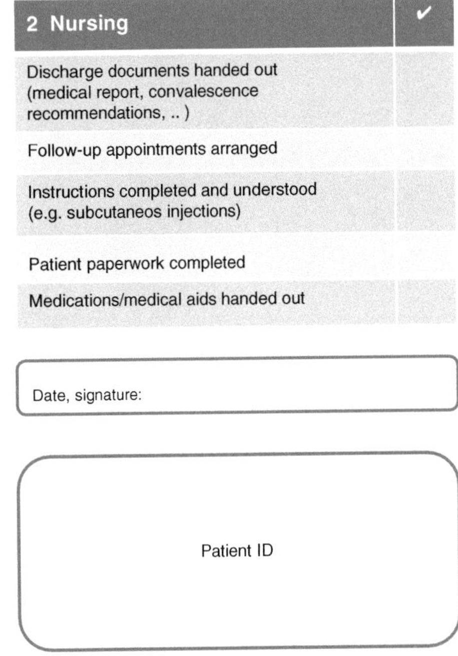

2 Nursing	✔
Discharge documents handed out (medical report, convalescence recommendations, ..)	
Follow-up appointments arranged	
Instructions completed and understood (e.g. subcutaneos injections)	
Patient paperwork completed	
Medications/medical aids handed out	

Date, signature:

Patient ID

Fig. 53.1 (continued)

Analgesia

Effective analgesia that allows early mobilization is a fundamental prerequisite for improved postoperative recovery. Especially in case of extensive surgery epidural analgesia followed by multimodal non-opioid analgesia is the most effective evidence-based method [2]. Epidural analgesia, however, is not indicated in the vast majority of laparoscopic hysterectomies and can be replaced by opioid-sparing multimodal analgesia, including oral paracetamol, non-steroidal anti-inflammatory drugs, gabapentanoids and local anesthetics [5]. For vaginal hysterectomy recent data have shown that preemptive local analgesia prior to hysterectomy is associated with significantly lower pain scores and a reduction in narcotic use postoperatively [6, 7]. Patients undergoing laparoscopic hysterectomy might benefit from paracervical analgesia as well. Additionally, there is substantial evidence that transversus abdominis plane (TAP) blocks (see also Fig. 53.2) and local anesthetic infiltration of trocar insertion sites in several laparoscopic procedures result in reduced pain scores and analgesic requirement [8–10]. TAP block in laparoscopic hysterectomy in particular was associated with lower use of opioids in the postoperative phase [11]. A recent study on extended assisted ventilation with an open umbilical trocar valve after laparoscopic hysterectomy showed that this is an effective and safe method to reduce postoperative pain levels, in particular abdominal and shoulder pain [3].

For efficient postoperative pain treatment it is crucial that clinical standards of care provide anticipatory pain management and that the use of opioids is evited.

Postoperative Nausea and Vomiting (PONV)

Besides postoperative use of opioids, non-smoking status and history of PONV or motion sickness, female gender per se is a risk factor for PONV according to the Apfel risk score [12]. This risk score and an individual risk based multimodal PONV prophylaxis is advocated by evidence-based guidelines as standards of care. Tailored anesthesia and pain management in particular avoiding too liberal dosing of anesthetics and opioid analgesics is essential in order to reduce the risk for PONV [13].

Thus multi-modal opioid sparing analgesia and a risk-based prophylaxis should be provided to every patient

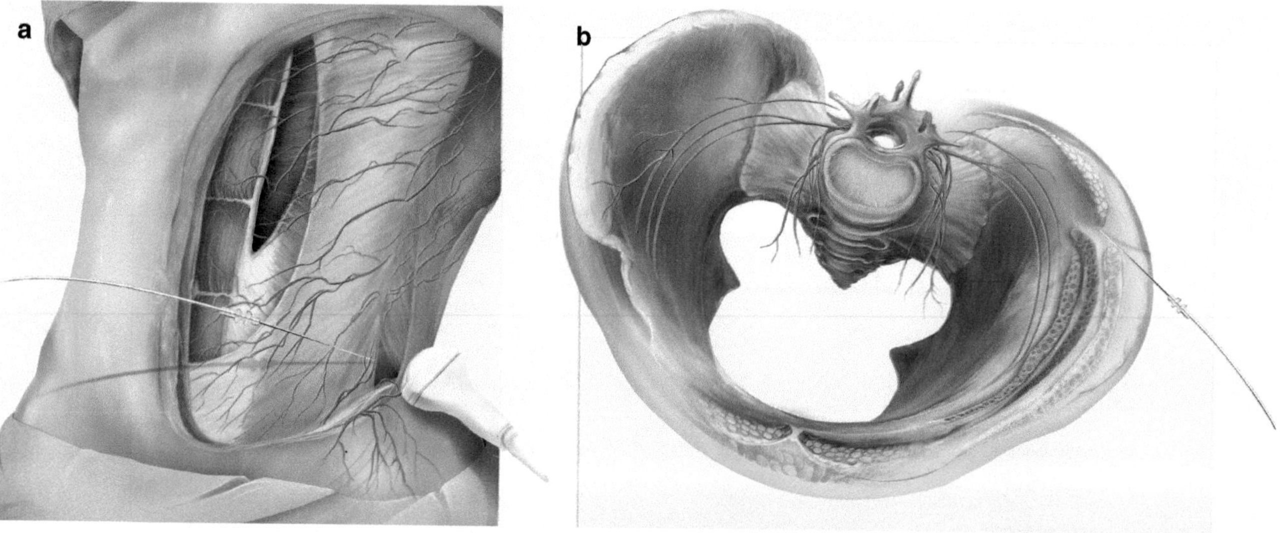

Fig. 53.2 The anatomical background for performing the transversus abdominis plane (TAP) block. The original technique described by Rafi et al. in 2001 [14] was a "blind" TAP block injecting a local anesthetic through the triangle of Petit on the lateral abdominal wall, whereas currently the ultrasound guided insertion of the needle is performed in an anterior to posterior manner to the plane of the rectus abdominis muscle [15]. Therefore, the ultrasound probe is placed diagonally over the lateral abdominal wall at the level of the mid axillary line (**a**). The extent of analgesia which can be achieved by TAP block is from the umbilical to the suprapubic region (block of the innervation of the anterior abdominal wall by the tenth thoracic intercostal nerve to first lumbar nerve) (**b**)

undergoing laparoscopic hysterectomy in order to minimize the occurrence of PONV.

Urinary Catheter, Drains and Tamponades

A recent meta-analysis of randomized controlled trials on immediate and delayed removal of urinary catheters following uncomplicated hysterectomy suggests that delayed catheter removal increases the incidence of postoperative bacteriuria and symptomatic urinary tract infection but reduces the risk of re-catheterization [16]. For laparoscopic radical hysterectomy and extensive resection of deep infiltrating endometriosis of the pelvis no such evidence is available albeit the removal of the urinary catheter upon mobilization is advisable. Functional bladder dysfunctions are common following nerve-sparing radical hysterectomy. Systematic bladder training, however, does not influence the rate of urinary retention or readmissions for bladder catheterization and is therefore not indicated [17].

There is no scientific evidence to favor the use of drains and tamponades. Several randomized trials addressing intraperitoneal drainage have shown that routine use of drains does increase the risk of wound infection, causes discomfort and postoperative pain and should therefore never be used routinely. In case drains are inserted they should be removed as soon as possible [2].

According to data from a recent Cochrane Database systematic review, patients with gynecological malignancies undergoing pelvic lymphadenectomy do not benefit form the placement of retroperitoneal tube drains to preventlymphocyst formation. When the pelvic peritoneum is left open, tube drain placement is associated with an even higher risk of short and long-term symptomatic lymphocyst formation [18].

Antibiotic Prophylaxis

There is no evidence for antibiotic prophylaxis in the postoperative phase. Antibiotic medication should only be initiated upon specific indication.

Venous Thromboembolic Event Prophylaxis

The rate of venous thromboembolic events (VTEs) including deep venous thrombosis and pulmonary embolism among women undergoing gynecologic surgery is high, particularly for women with a gynecologic malignancy. Current guidelines recommend VTE prophylaxis in the immediate postoperative period for patients undergoing open surgery. However, the VTE prophylaxis recommendations for women undergoing minimally invasive gynecologic surgery are not as well established. The risk of VTEs in patients undergoing minimally invasive surgery of intermediate complexity such as laparoscopic hysterectomy appears to be low based on retrospective analyses [19]. To date, there are no established guidelines that specifically provide a standard of care for patients undergoing minimally invasive gynecologic surgery for benign or malignant disease [20].

Pelvic surgery in general increases the risk of VTEs. The expositional risk after laparoscopic hysterectomy is considered to be intermediate and the dispositional risk of any patient is individual and needs to be addressed separately. Besides mechanical compression by graduated compression stockings the use of low molecular weight heparins (LMWH) is the standard postoperative pharmacologic prophylactic strategy based on multiple high-quality randomized trials [21–24].There is insufficient evidence to recommend graduated compression stockings alone in intermediate and high-risk surgical patients. According to a very recent evidence-based review the duration of prophylaxis should be extended to 28–35 days for patients undergoing abdominal/pelvic cancer surgery and higher doses of LMWH should be considered in obese patients [24]. In all studies the importance of early mobilization is emphasized.

Mobilization

Mobilization of patients at an early stage after surgery reduces postoperative complications and improves recovery and is one of the vital issues in the "fast-track surgery" concept [2]. For standard laparoscopic hysterectomy this can be within a few hours after surgery and even after extensive operative procedures mobilization on the day of surgery should be aspired.

Nutrition

In the past few years the dominating dogma of fasting periods after vaginal or laparoscopic hysterectomies was abandoned in favor of early food intake [25]. Even after major abdominal gynecologic surgery for either benign or malignant conditions early postoperative intake of fluids and food appeared to be safe without increased gastrointestinal morbidities or other postoperative complications according to a systematic Cochrane Database review. The benefits of this early postoperative feeding approach include faster recovery of bowel function, lower rates of infectious complications, shorter hospital stay, and higher satisfaction scores [26].

Daily Care, Monitoring and Diagnostics

The provision of a detailed nursing-care programme for each postoperative day is mandatory, and details about the care programme and the expected duration of hospital stay should be provided to patients (and relatives) upon indication for surgery and detailed planning of the surgical procedure for as well in-patients and out-patients [2, 4]. Intensive care observation is rarely necessary after laparoscopic hysterectomy and may be due to the patient's individual risk factors. Most clinics have standards for postoperative monitoring including recordings of pain, digestion, urination, vaginal bleeding and discomfort, daily ward rounds and if indicated physical examination. Any further diagnostic evaluation or examination should be symptom-driven and not be performed routinely. For instance, there is substantive evidence that routine hemoglobin level testing has little clinical benefit following elective laparoscopic hysterectomy and should be reserved for patients who develop signs or symptoms suggestive of acute anemia [27].

Very recent data suggest that e-health interventions providing personalized pre- and postoperative instructions on the resumption of daily activities, and tools to improve self-empowerment and to identify recovery problems result in a faster return to work, a higher quality of life and less pain during postoperative recovery after inter alia hysterectomy for benign conditions [28]. Thus, besides efficient nursing-care it is effective to inform patients in detail about the process of convalescence, instruct them and empower their responsibility.

Discharge and Recommendations to the Patient

After an uneventful postoperative recovery a general physical examination and conversation with the patient about the laparoscopic procedure, subsequent medical checkups, and instructions for the phase of convalescence are recommended and should be documented. There is no evidence to conduct a gynecologic examination or sonography prior to discharge without specific indication. It is important to make sure that the patient is mobile, urinating freely, has regular digestion and adequate pain control, and does not have excessive vaginal bleeding. Most clinics have checklists for the management of discharge and provide brochures with convalescence recommendations on daily activities (avoid heavy lifting, no sexual intercourse, no bath tub and swimming for up to 6 weeks, etc.). There is no scientific evidence to sustain these concrete recommendations, however. A Dutch interdisciplinary team defined convalescence recommendations rooted in expert-based knowledge for gynecological surgery. For laparoscopic hysterectomy his expert panel recommends the resumption of light, moderate and heavy activities after 1, 2 and 4 weeks respectively. These recommendations reflect an average functional recovery time for a healthy woman, but certainly the specialist in charge will take the presence of co-morbidities or potential complications into account for individual recommendations to a patient [29] (see also Table 53.1).

Table 53.1 Multidisciplinary convalescence recommendations

	Examples	Considered medically possible from (days/weeks after day of surgery)				
		Lapsc– Adn	LSH	TLH	VH	AH
Light activities	Lifting or carrying 5 kg	2 dy	1 wk	1 wk	2 wk	2 wk
	2 h sustained sitting					
	30 min sustained standing and walking					
Moderate activities	Lifting or carrying 10 kg	1 wk	2 wk	2 wk	3 wk	3–4 wk
	Pushing or pulling 15 kg					
	Riding a bicycle					
	Vacuum cleaning					
Heavy activities	Lifting or carrying 15 kg	2 wk	3 wk	3 wk	4 wk	6 wk
	Standing and walking during entire working day					
Resumption of (average) job	+/– 8 h a day	2 wk	3 wk	3–4 wk	4 wk	6 wk
	+/– 40 h a week					

Source: VonkNoordegraaf et al. [29]
Abbreviations: *Lapsc Adn* laparoscopic adnexal surgery, *LSH* laparoscopic supracervical Hysterectomy, *TLH/LAVH* total laparoscopic hysterectomy/laparoscopic assisted vaginal Hysterectomy, *VH* vaginal hysterectomy, *AH* abdominal hysterectomy
Time schedule: *dy* day (s), *wk* week (s)

Ambulatory Care Setting

Recent data suggest that ambulant care appears to be safe and does not have higher rates of complications or readmissions even in advanced laparoscopic surgery such as laparoscopic hysterectomy [30–32].

In an ambulatory care setting, the patient is monitored for discomfort in the recovery room for a few hours postoperatively. The evaluation of vital signs every 30 min should provide sufficient safety. Preemptive analgesia, early mobilization and fluid and food intake at an early stage are recommended. The minimal duration of surveillance after general anesthesia is 2 and 4 h after application of opioids, respectively. After a final checkup by the anesthesiologist and gynecologic surgeon the patient can be discharged. Information about convalescence and practical instructions for daily activities should be provided to the patient prior to surgery and handing out brochures providing this information upon discharge are beneficial.

References

1. KlinglerCH, RemziM, MarbergerM, JanetschekGHaemostasis in laparoscopy. EurUrol.2006;50:948–56; discussion 956–47.
2. Kehlet H, Dahl JB. Anaesthesia, surgery, and challenges in postoperative recovery. Lancet. 2003;362:1921–8.
3. Radosa JC, Radosa MP, Mavrova R, Rody A, Juhasz-Boss I, Bardens D, Brun K, Solomayer EF, Baum S. Five minutes of extended assisted ventilation with an open umbilical trocar valve significantly reduces postoperative abdominal and shoulder pain in patients undergoing laparoscopic hysterectomy. EurJObstetGynecolReprod Biol. 2013;171:122–7.
4. Kehlet H. Fast-track colorectal surgery. Lancet. 2008;371:791–3.
5. White PF, Kehlet H, Neal JM, Schricker T, Carr DB, Carli F. The role of the anesthesiologist in fast-track surgery: from multimodal analgesia to perioperative medical care. AnesthAnalg. 2007;104:1380–96. table of contents
6. Long JB, Eiland RJ, Hentz JG, Mergens PA, Magtibay PM, Kho RM, Magrina JF, Cornella JL. Randomized trial of preemptive local analgesia in vaginal surgery. IntUrogynecolJ Pelvic Floor Dysfunc. 2009;20:5–10.
7. O'Neal MG, Beste T, Shackelford DP. Utility of preemptive local analgesia in vaginal hysterectomy. AmJ Obstet Gynecol. 2003;189:1539–41; discussion 1541–32.
8. Keir A, Rhodes L, Kayal A, Khan OA. Does a transversus abdominis plane (tap) local anaesthetic block improve pain control in patients undergoing laparoscopic cholecystectomy? A best evidence topic. Int J Surg. 2013;11:792–4.
9. Siddiqui MR, Sajid MS, Uncles DR, Cheek L, Baig MK. A meta-analysis on the clinical effectiveness of transversus abdominis plane block. JClinAnesth. 2011;23:7–14.
10. CharltonS, CynaAM, MiddletonP, GriffithsJDPerioperative transversus abdominis plane (tap) blocks for analgesia after abdominal surgery. Cochrane Database SystRev.2010;(12):CD007705.
11. Pather S, Loadsman JA, Gopalan PD, Rao A, Philp S, Carter J. The role of transversus abdominis plane blocks in women undergoing total laparoscopic hysterectomy: a retrospective review. AustN ZJ ObstetGynaecol. 2011;51:544–7.
12. Apfel CC, Laara E, Koivuranta M, Greim CA, Roewer N. A simplified risk score for predicting postoperative nausea and vomiting: conclusions from cross-validations between two centers. Anesthesiol. 1999;91:693–700.

13. Obrink E, Jildenstal P, Oddby E, Jakobsson JG. Post-operative nausea and vomiting: update on predicting the probability and ways to minimize its occurrence, with focus on ambulatory surgery. Int J Surg. 2015;15C:100–6.
14. Rafi AN.Abdominal field block: A new approach via the lumber triangle. Aneasthesia. 2001;56:1024–1026.
15. Hebbard P, Fujiwara y, Shibata y, Royse C: Ultrasound-guided transversus abdominis plane (TAP) block.Aneasthesia and intensive care. 2007;35:616–617.
16. Zhang P, Hu WL, Cheng B, Cheng L, Xiong XK, Zeng YJ. A systematic review and meta-analysis comparing immediate and delayed catheter removal following uncomplicated hysterectomy. IntUrogynecol J. 2015;26(5):665–74.
17. Fanfani F, Costantini B, Mascilini F, Vizzielli G, Gallotta V, Vigliotta M, Piccione E, Scambia G, Fagotti A. Early postoperative bladder training in patients submitted to radical hysterectomy: is it still necessary? A randomized trial. ArchGynecolObstet. 2015;291(4):883–8.
18. CharoenkwanK, KietpeerakoolC: Retroperitoneal drainage versus no drainage after pelvic lymphadenectomy for the prevention of lymphocyst formation in patients with gynaecological malignancies. Cochrane Database SystRev.2014;(6):CD007387.
19. Nick AM, Schmeler KM, Frumovitz MM, Soliman PT, Spannuth WA, Burzawa JK, Coleman RL, Wei C, dos Reis R, Ramirez PT. Risk of thromboembolic disease in patients undergoing laparoscopic gynecologic surgery. ObstetGynecol. 2010;116:956–61.
20. Ramirez PT, Nick AM, Frumovitz M, Schmeler KM. Venous thromboembolic events in minimally invasive gynecologic surgery. JMiniInvasive Gynecol. 2013;20:766–9.
21. Eppsteiner RW, Shin JJ, Johnson J, van Dam RM. Mechanical compression versus subcutaneous heparin therapy in postoperative and posttrauma patients: a systematic review and meta-analysis. World J Surg. 2010;34:10–9.
22. Falck-Ytter Y, Francis CW, Johanson NA, Curley C, Dahl OE, Schulman S, Ortel TL, Pauker SG, Colwell Jr CW. Prevention of vte in orthopedic surgery patients: antithrombotic therapy and prevention of thrombosis, 9th ed: American college of chest physicians evidence-based clinical practice guidelines. Chest. 2012;141: e278S–325S.
23. SachdevaA, DaltonM, AmaragiriSV, LeesT.Elastic compression stockings for prevention of deep vein thrombosis. Cochrane Database SystRev.2010;(7):CD001484.
24. Bell BR, Bastien PE, Douketis JD. Prevention of venous thromboembolism in the enhanced recovery after surgery (eras) setting: an evidence-based review. CanJAnaesth J Canadien d'anesthesie. 2015;62:194–202.
25. Reif P, Drobnitsch T, Aigmuller T, Laky R, Ulrich D, Haas J, Bader A, Tamussino K. The decreasing length of hospital stay following vaginal hysterectomy: 2011–2012 vs. 1996–1997 vs. 1995–1996. Geburtshilfe und Frauenheilkunde. 2014;74:449–53.
26. CharoenkwanK, MatovinovicE: Early versus delayed oral fluids and food for reducing complications after major abdominal gynaecologic surgery. Cochrane Database SystRev.2014;(12):CD004508.
27. Chamsy DJ, Louie MY, Lum DA, Phelps AL, Mansuria SM. Clinical utility of postoperative hemoglobin level testing following total laparoscopic hysterectomy. AmJ ObstetGynecol. 2014;211:224 e221–7.
28. Vonk Noordegraaf A, Anema JR, van Mechelen W, Knol DL, van Baal WM, van Kesteren PJ, Brolmann HA, Huirne JA. A personalised ehealth programme reduces the duration until return to work after gynaecological surgery: results of a multicentre randomised trial. BJOG: IntJ ObstetGynaecol. 2014;121:1127–35. discussion 1136
29. Vonk Noordegraaf A, Huirne JA, Brolmann HA, van Mechelen W, Anema JR. Multidisciplinary convalescence recommendations after gynaecological surgery: a modified delphi method among experts. BJOG Int J ObstetGynaecol. 2011;118:1557–67.
30. Nezhat C, Main J, Paka C, Soliemannjad R, Parsa MA. Advanced gynecologic laparoscopy in a fast-track ambulatory surgery center. JSLS J SocLaparoendosc SurgSocLaparoendosc Surg. 2014;18: e2014.00291.
31. de Lapasse C, Rabischong B, Bolandard F, Canis M, Botchorischvili R, Jardon K, Mage G. Total laparoscopic hysterectomy and early discharge: satisfaction and feasibility study. JMiniInvasive Gynecol. 2008;15:20–5.
32. Lassen PD, Moeller-Larsen H. P DEN: same-day discharge after laparoscopic hysterectomy. Acta Obstet Gynecol Scand. 2012; 91:1339–41.

Extraperitoneal Hysterectomy-Total Pelvic Peritonectomy Combined with the Segmental Resection of the Rectosigmoid

54

Massaki Andou

The Extraperitoneal Hysterectomy

Theoretically, total removal of the pelvic peritoneum is the most beneficial tactic for disease restricted to the pelvis. With the total removal of the pelvic peritoneum in mind, we developed our laparoscopic extraperitoneal hysterectomy. The goals for this surgery are the complete eradication of tumor cells for stage II ovarian cancer and this surgery is also implemented as optimal cytoreductive surgery for selected stage III patients who have massive residual pelvic disease after previous surgery or neoadjuvant chemotherapy, where upper abdominal tumors have been completely controlled.

Ovarian cancer has the possibility to be extensive disease, with a traditionally invasive approach to treatment. Because ovarian cancer requires the most invasive surgery in gynecology, making this surgery patient friendly is a necessary theme. The feasibility and efficacy of laparoscopic staging and cytoreductive surgery in ovarian cancer is demonstrated in our series. Laparoscopic surgery for ovarian cancer is traditionally regarded as a contraindication. However, the standard laparotomy is a very invasive procedure which is sometimes difficult to perform with very poor performance status patients, and also potentially causes the delay of the main therapy; chemotherapy. In contrast, laparoscopic optimal cytoreduction allows quick recovery from surgery meaning a quick return to primary treatment. It also has the advantage of decreasing bowel morbidity, which also frequently causes delays in administration of chemotherapy.

M. Andou, MD, PhD
Obstetrics and Gynecology, Kurashiki Medical Center, 250 Bakuro-cho, Kurashiki, Okayama 710-8522, Japan
e-mail: ichi-195@mvc.biglobe.ne.jp

Procedure

Four ports are used in this surgery- a 12 mm port in the umbilicus, another 12 mm port is placed in 4 cm median and 4 cms above the right iliac crest. One 5 mm port is placed at the same position on the opposite side. Another 5 mm port is placed directly between these two ports. The patient is placed in the lithotomy position with a slight Trendelenberg tilt. Standard laparoscopic instruments are used for most of the procedure. We also used a linear stapler and circular stapler for bowel reconstruction.

The extraperitoneal hysterectomy begins with a peritoneal incision starting from the pelvic sidewall triangle at the level of the pelvic brim (Fig. 54.1). The incision is extended anteriorly, curving along the upper edge of the public bone and finally arriving at the same point on the left side of the pelvis. The next step is the dissection of the bladder peritoneum from the bladder wall. The bladder peritoneum is dissected until the uterine cervix appears. The bladder is then dissected off from the cervix. After mobilization of the peritoneum of the bladder and pelvic

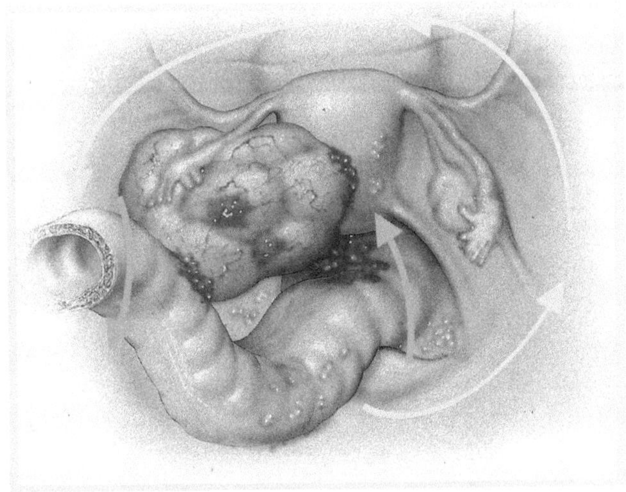

Fig. 54.1 Incision line of the pelvic peritoneum

I. Alkatout, L. Mettler (eds.), *Hysterectomy*, DOI 10.1007/978-3-319-22497-8_54

sidewall, the extraperitoneal transection of the parametria is started (Fig. 54.2).

After the ureter is detached from the posterior layer of the broad ligament, the ureter is dissected down until the entrance of the ureteral tunnel is reached. Then, the cardinal ligament is bipolar desiccated and transected (Fig. 54.3). The vagina is exposed and transected.

The second stage of this procedure is the removal of the rectosigmoid. As the peritoneum of this portion cannot be detached from the organ, the procedure requires the segmental resection of this segment. The rectosigmoid is mobilized starting from the dissection of the presacral space. This dissection continues until the pelvic diaphragm is reached. The mesosigmoid is divided using a harmonic scalpel. After full mobilization of the mesosigmoid, the upper portion of the segment is transected using a linear stapler (Fig. 54.4) and the caudal portion of this segment is also transected. After all of these procedures have been completed, the uterine body along with the rectosigmoid are put into a protection bag to stop the spilling of tumor cells in the abdominal cavity, and removed through the vagina (Fig. 54.5). Finally, the rectum is anastomosed to the sigma using a circular stapler (Fig. 54.6).

All cases underwent a hysterectomy, bilateral salpingo-oophorectomy, retroperitoneal lymph node dissection, sampling of ascitic fluid, multiple peritoneal biopsy, appendectomy and omentectomy. Some selected cases underwent cytoreductive procedures including elimination of peritoneal dissemination using an argon beam coagulator, removal of the pancreas tail and spleen because of metastatic tumors to the splenic hilus, resection of the total pelvic peritoneum including extraperitoneal hysterectomy, segmental resection of the rectosigmoid due to dissemination to the pelvic peritoneum and/or bowel wall

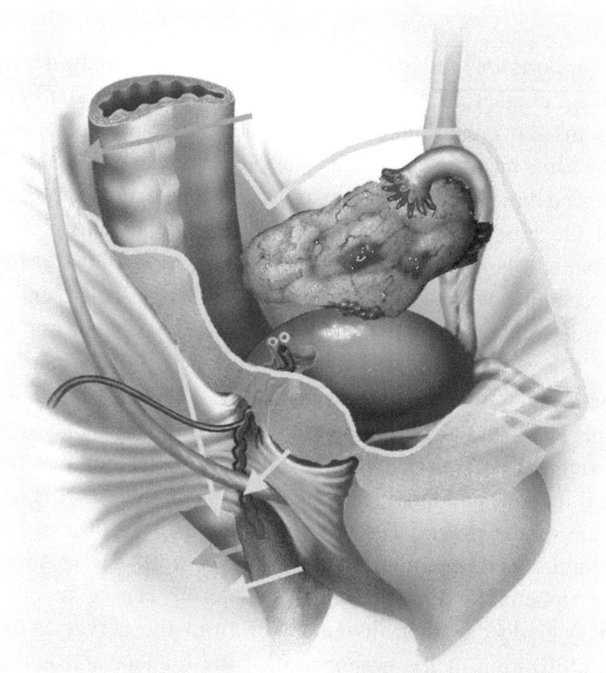

Fig. 54.2 Extraperitoneal resection of the parametria

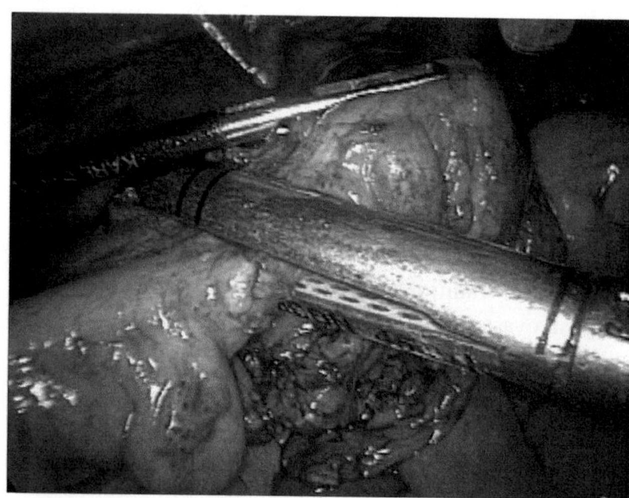

Fig. 54.4 Transection of the rectosigmoid

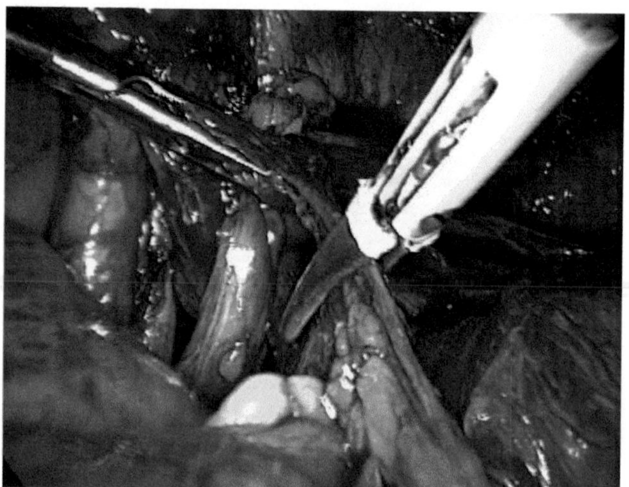

Fig. 54.3 Transection of the left cardinal lig

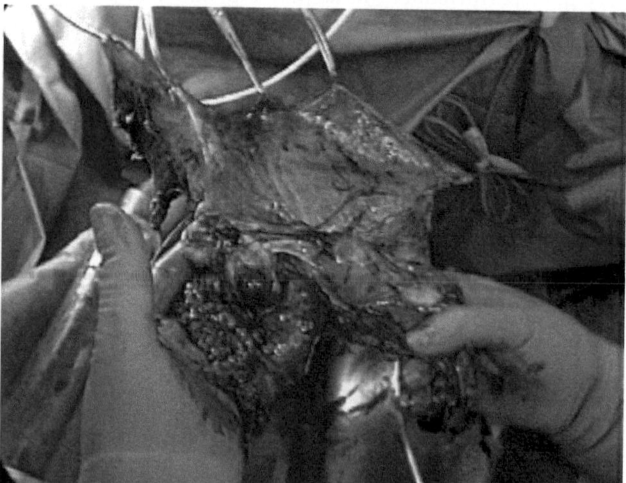

Fig. 54.5 Retrieved specimen

invasion (Fig. 54.7). Although the indications for this surgery are not broad, it is efficacious and safe for patients who require extensive pelvic resection or cytoreduction. Through this procedure, it has become possible to achieve complete tumor eradication if the tumor is located in the pelvis.

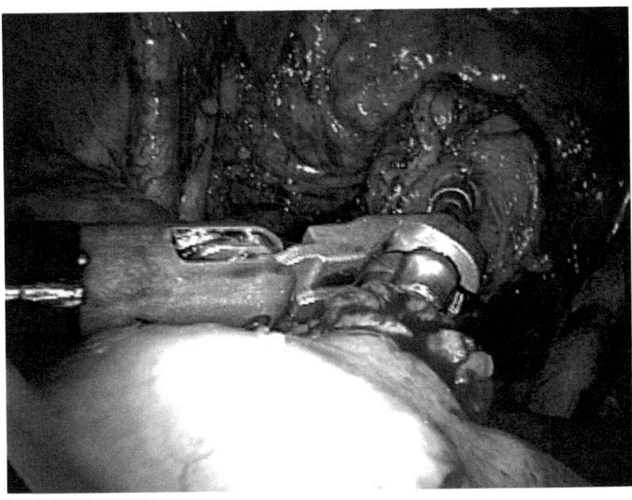

Fig. 54.6 Anastomosis of the rectosigmoid

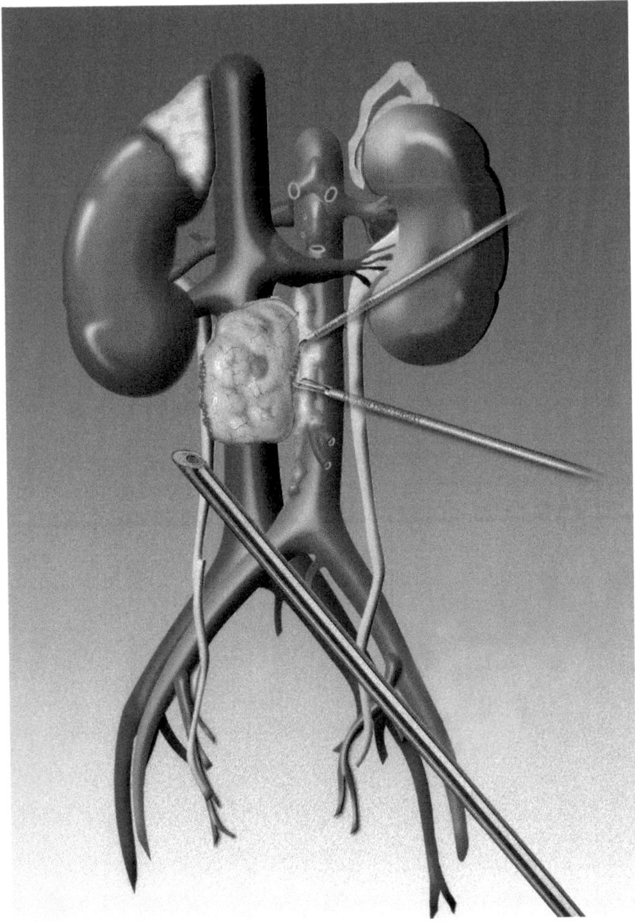

Fig. 54.7 Illustration showing the metastatic lymph node fixed to the inferior vena cava in debulking lymphadenectomy

Additional Cytoreductive Procedures

Because of the aggressive nature of ovarian cancer, many cases suffer from extensive tumor distribution or dissemination. For these cases it is necessary to find ways to manage the broad extension of the disease while considering the quality of life of the patient. We have introduced some additional procedures for laparoscopic cytoreductive surgery for advanced ovarian cancer such as a debulking lymphadenectomy, diaphragma stripping, omentectomy, and segmental resection of the small bowel or the rectosigmoid.

In the case of the debulking lymphadenectomy we use the paraortic dissection followed by the transperitoneal approach in the pelvis (Fig. 54.8). We use very fine bipolar forceps to grasp the base of the adhered metastatic lymph node and then simultaneously coagulate the connected area and slice off the lymph node in a sweeping motion (Fig. 54.9). The resected lymph nodes are retrieved from the port site after being placed in a retrieval bag to prevent the spillage of tumor cells.

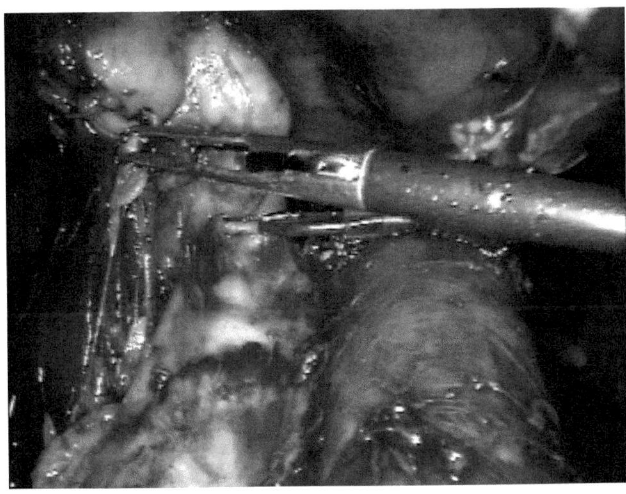

Fig. 54.8 Dissection of metastatic lymphnodes using bipolar forceps

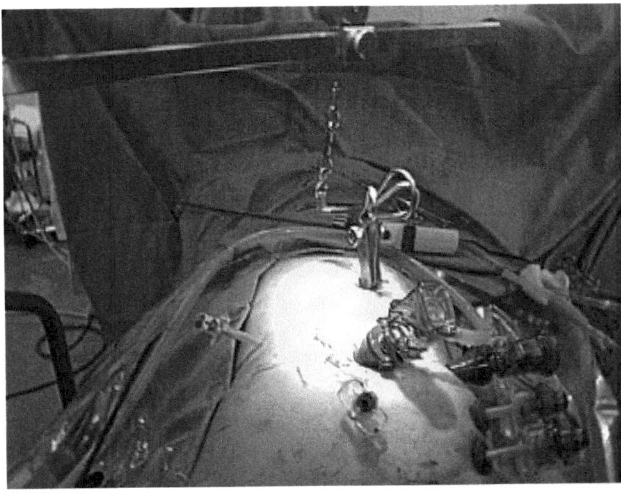

Fig. 54.9 Gasless technique for diaphragma-stripping

As for diaphragma stripping we use gasless laparoscopy at the very end of the entire procedure (Fig. 54.10). The reason for this is to prevent barotraumas like pneumothorax. We infiltrate diluted pitressin between the diaphragma fascia and the diaphragma muscle to create space (Fig. 54.11). Then we use a harmonic scalpel to remove the fascia layer. We do not use electrocautery to avoid the contraction of the diaphragma (Fig. 54.12a–d).

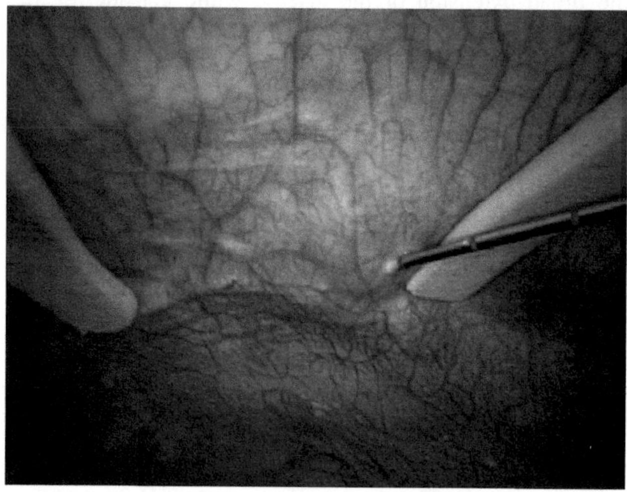

Fig. 54.10 Infiltration of diluted pitressin as aquadissection (diaphragma -stripping)

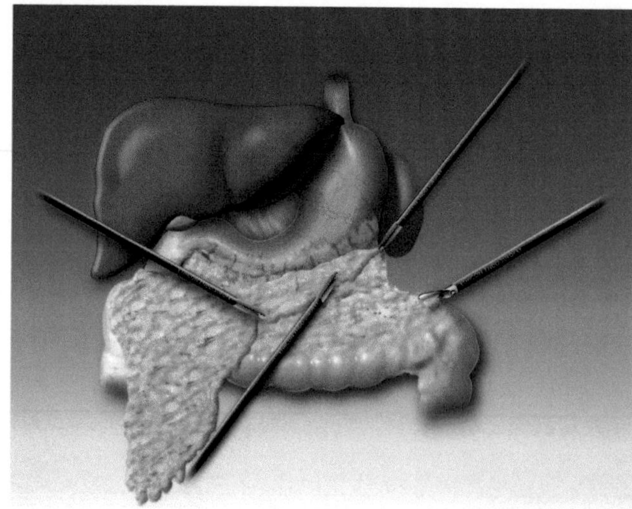

Fig. 54.12 Infragastric omentectomy- the omentum is removed below the gastroepiploic artery

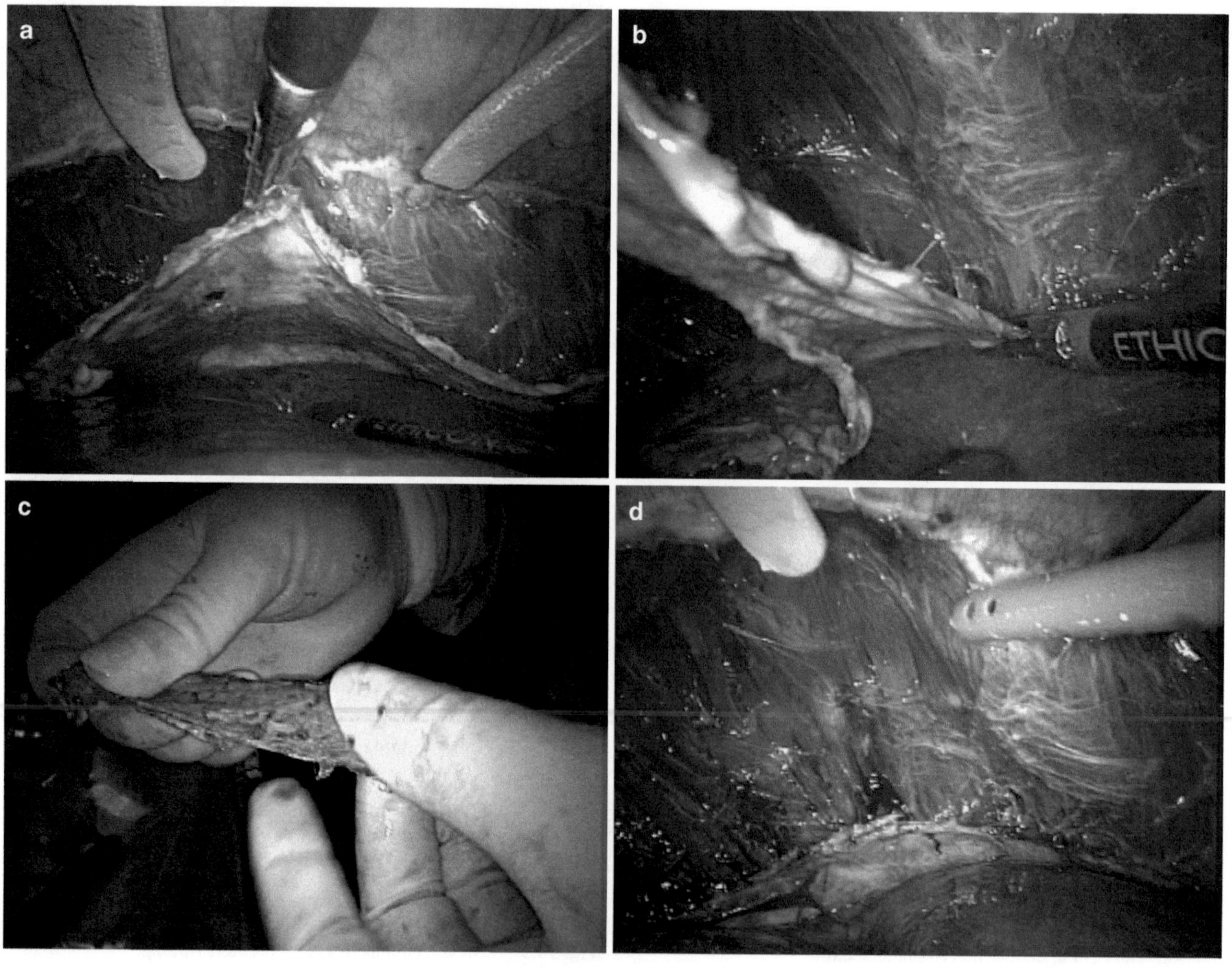

Fig. 54.11 (**a**) Dissection using harmonic scalpel (diaphragma-stripping). (**b**) Removal of dissected diaphragma (diaphragma-stripping). (**c**) Retrieved specimen after diaphragma-stripping. (**d**) Status after diaphragma-stripping

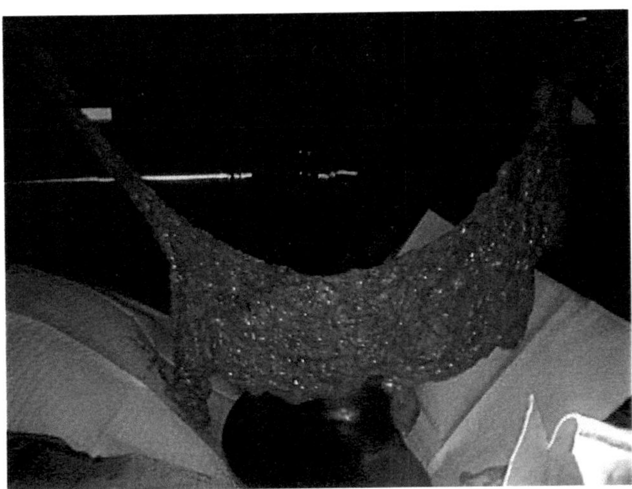

Fig. 54.13 Specimen after omentectomy

The omentectomy we perform is an infragastric omentectomy. The goal of this procedure is to remove as much of the tumor as possible. Initially, we cut the omentum from the transverse colon (Fig. 54.13) and dissect until the upper boundary, just under the gastroepiploic artery, with a harmonic scalpel (Fig. 54.14).

For resection of the bowel, we employ reconstructive techniques. Segmental resection of the bowel requires stapling, using both a linear and circular stapler. For the small bowel, functional end-to-end anastomosis using four linear staples produces the best result (Figs. 54.15 1–14, 54.16, 54.17, and 54.18). After transection of the segment of the small bowel using two 45 mm linear staples, anastomosis of the residual bowel stumps can proceed. The antimesenteric sidewall of both bowel stumps is approximated using a 3-0 stay suture. Each fork of a linear stapler is inserted into each of the orifices of the oral and anal stumps of the small bowel. Firing of the linear stapler results in side-to-side anastomosis. The open cut end of connected bowel stumps is stapled and closed using a 60 mm linear stapler.

For cases with extensive peritoneal implants, we eliminate peritoneal dissemination using an argon beam coagulator (Fig. 54.19). Some cases underwent resection of the pancreas tail and spleen because of metastatic tumors to the splenic hilus. We used a linear stapler to transect the pancreas tail. As a result of performing these additional procedures, we can offer optimal cytoreduction tailored to individual patients.

Results

From June 2000 to date, 21 patients have undergone pelvic peritonectomy with or with out rectal resection combined standard procedure. For some patients, the procedure had to be divided into two operative sessions due to the extensive nature of their disease. All patients underwent a hysterectomy and bilateral adnexectomy and retroperitoneal lymphadenectomy and omentectomy. Some patients also required an appendectomy. Six patients with one stage IIc, (clear cell carcinoma), five IIIc (serous papillary adenocarcinoma) and one IV (papillary adenocarcinoma) underwent he standard procedure plus a pelvic peritonectomy with LAR. Fourteen cases underwent the standard procedure plus a pelvic peritonectomy without LAR. These cases ranged from stage Ia to stage IV, diagnosed with granulose cell carcinoma, clear cell carcinoma, serous papillary adenocarcinoma, papillary adenocarcinoma and mucinous adenocarcinoma.

The average observation period is 87 months (range 16 months to 168 months). Of the patients who underwent rectal resection, two patients are alive with disease, five patients are alive with no evidence of disease. Of the 14 patients who did not undergo rectal resection seven patients are alive with no evidence of disease. Six of these patients have died from disease and we have no data on one patient. No major complications requiring reoperation occurred during the surgical procedures and the post-operative courses of all patients was uneventful and recovery was very quick.

Discussion

Although we cannot draw any definite conclusions for survival advantage in this retrospective analysis as we only have a limited number of cases over a relatively short period, the quality of life of patients who underwent this minimally invasive surgery is obviously better. There are some problems with this minimally invasive approach such as, the occurrence of port site metastasis and the difficulty in mastering the necessary surgical skills. Evaluating the treatment methods for patients with malignancy is difficult when considering the small number of patients with advanced ovarian cancer. We believe that the limit of traditional therapy may have already been reached. In order to achieve a new stage in management and to increase the quality of life of patients, it is necessary to break traditional patterns and attempt a new approach. This was our motivation in applying this technique to ovarian cancer cases.

Laparoscopic surgery, with its minimally invasive advantages, is vital for achieving a more patent friendly approach, even when dealing with diseases like advanced ovarian cancer. Through the kind of extensive debulking techniques described here, optimal cytoreduction can be achieved completely laparoscopically. Laparoscopy allows the possibility of expanding the radicality of surgery to match the needs of patients with advanced and recurrent gynecologic malignancy, without increasing the invasiveness of the surgery itself. Additionally, by also applying reconstructive techniques, it is possible to ensure full resection of all questionable tissue, a necessity for cases with malignant disease. Minimally invasive surgery benefits those who must undergo the most radical procedures and laparoscopy provides the necessary platform for reaching a new stage in malignancy management.

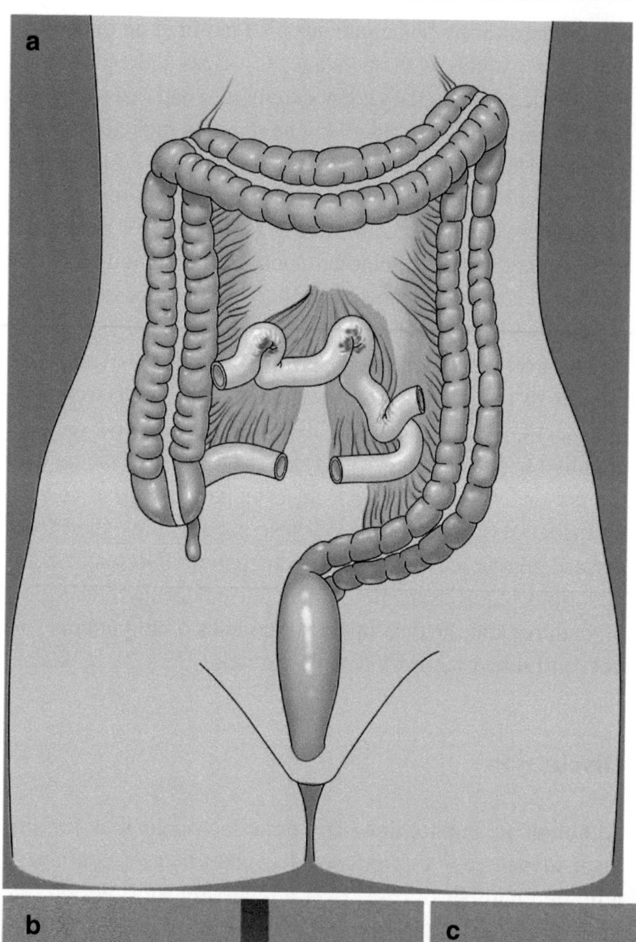

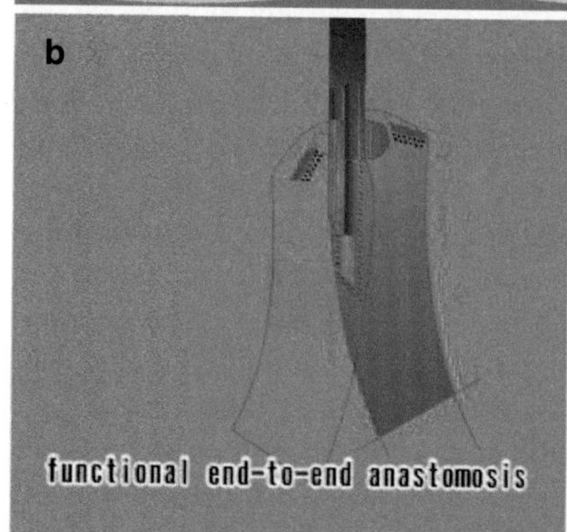

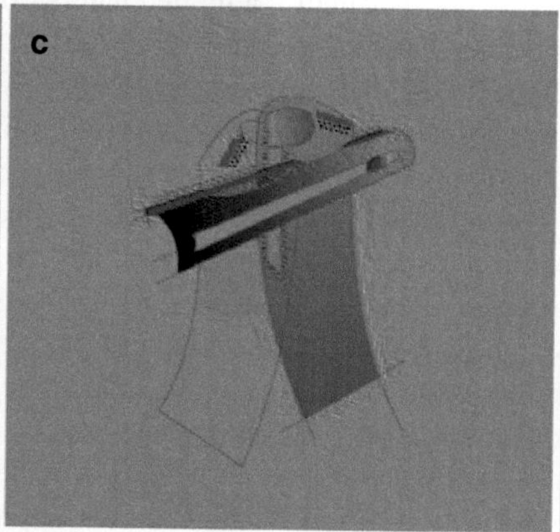

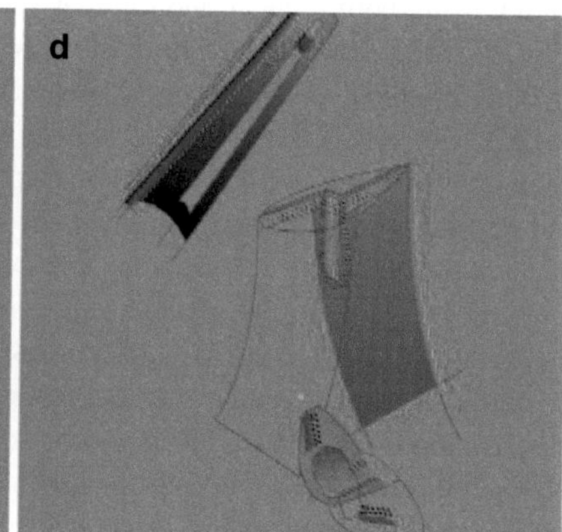

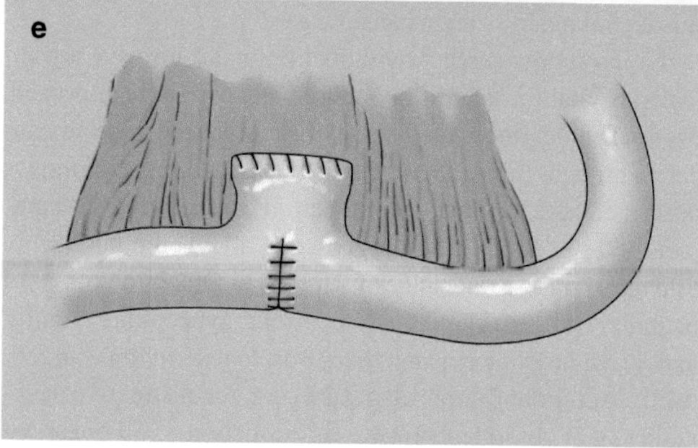

Fig. 54.14 (**a**) Dissemination to the small bowel- the resected segment of the small bowel is infiltrated by ovarian cancer metastasis. (**b**) Functional end-to-end anastomosis. This technique is required when large tracts of the small bowel need to be resected due to extensive invasion or numerous smaller invasion sites that cannot be resected individually. (**c**) Connection of the two bowel loops. (**d**) Creation of a new flow. (**e**) Status after functional end-to-end anastomosis

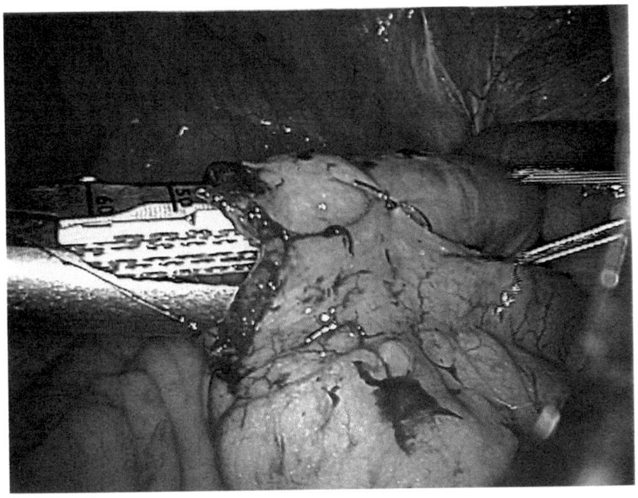

Fig. 54.15 The antimesenteric sidewall of both bowel stumps are approximated and stapled (side to side fixation)

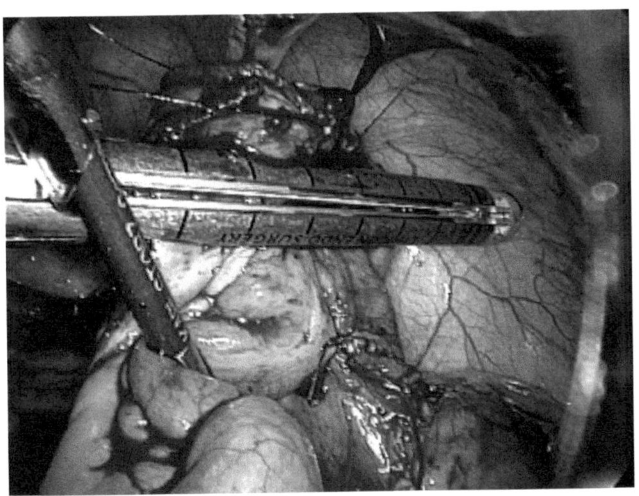

Fig. 54.16 Closure of the open cut end of the connected bowel stumps using a 60 mm linear stapler

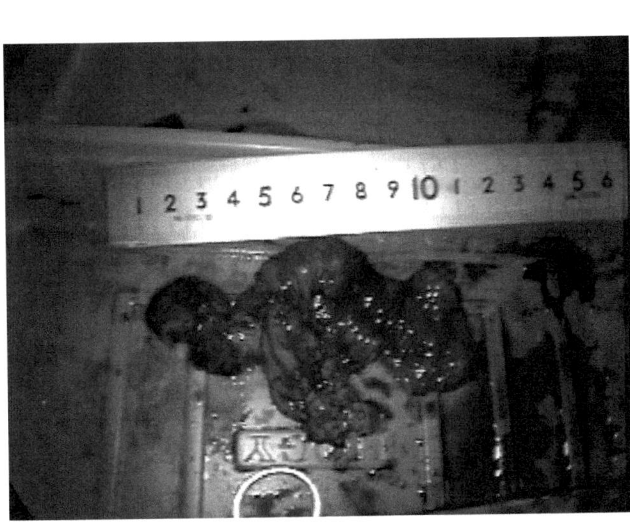

Fig. 54.17 Specimen after small bowel resection

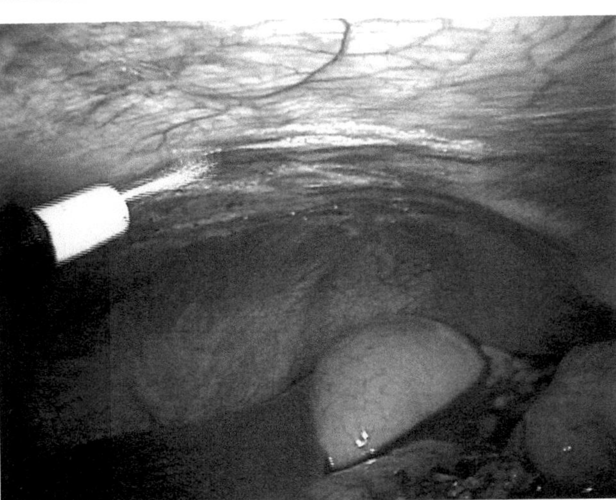

Fig. 54.18 Elimination of peritoneal dissemination using an argon beam coagulator

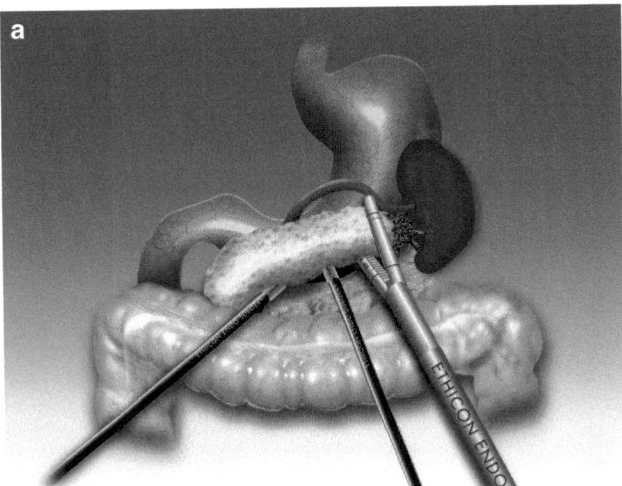

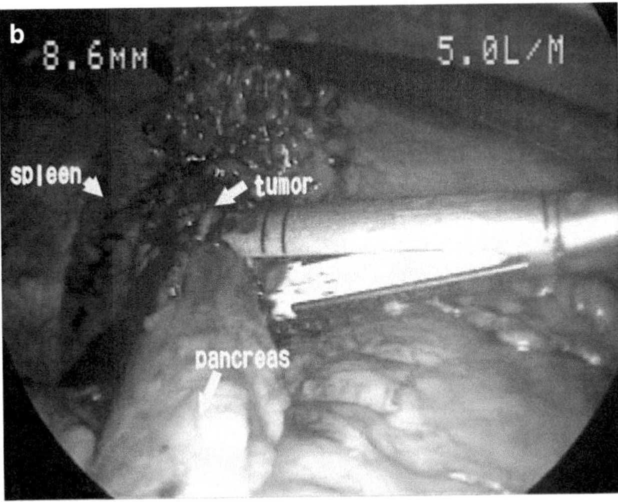

Fig. 54.19 (**a**) Removal of the pancreas tail and spleen because of metastatic tumors to the splenic hilus. (**b**) removal of the pancreas tail and spleen because of metastatic tumors to the splenic hilus

Part IX

Robotic-Assisted Laparoscopic Hysterectomy and Extended Procedures for Benign and Malignant Indications

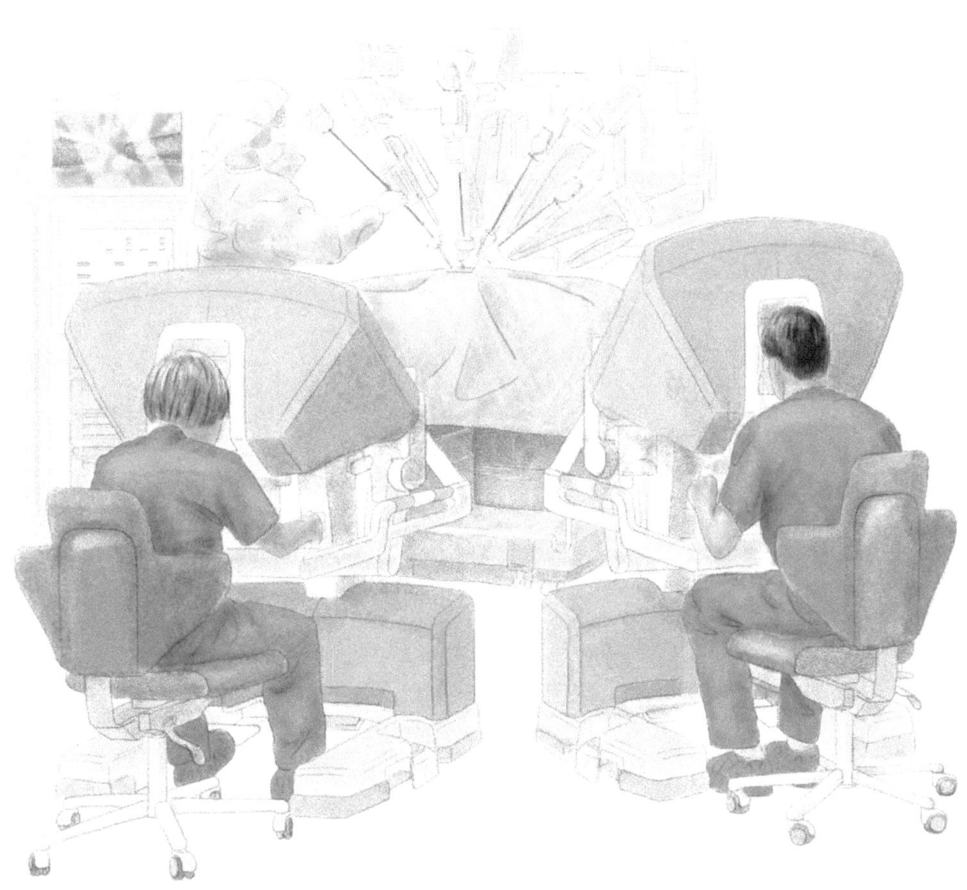

55 Indications and Contraindications to Robotic-Assisted Hysterectomy

Melissa H. Lippitt, Edward J. Tanner III, and Amanda Nickles Fader

Introduction

Hysterectomy is one of the most common surgical procedures performed during a woman's lifetime. In 1998, there were approximately 540,000 hysterectomies performed in the U.S. This decreased to 430,000 by 2010 [1], due to introduction of more conservative approaches to management of uterine fibroids and abnormal uterine bleeding, the most common indications to hysterectomy. While the overall number of hysterectomies performed in the U.S. and Europe has declined substantially over the past decade, the use of minimally invasive techniques (MIS), including laparoscopic and robot-assisted approaches, has increased. Level I studies have shown the benefit of minimally invasive surgery compared with laparotomy, including improved perioperative outcomes, shorter hospital stays, improved quality of life and faster return to daily functions [2]. With regards to minimally invasive hysterectomy techniques, the first elective hysterectomy utilizing a vaginal approach was performed in Germany in 1801. Almost 200 years later, the first total laparoscopic hysterectomy was performed in 1988 [3], which was followed in 1999 with the first published case of robot-assisted gynecologic surgery [4]. After several iterations were developed by different U.S. companies, in 2005, the da Vinci Surgical System® (Intuitive Surgical, Sunnyvale, CA), was approved by the Food and Drug Administration for use in gynecologic surgery (Figs. 55.1 and 55.2).

Currently, robotic-assisted surgery is performed for both benign and oncologic gynecologic indications (Table 55.1) [5]. Gynecologists may perform a wide variety of robotic-assisted procedures, including hysterectomy, myomectomy, excision of endometriosis, tubal re-anastomosis to restore fertility, sacrocolpopexy, adnexal cyst removal, repair of vesicovaginal fistulas and staging of cervical and endometrial cancers [6–12]. The potential benefits of robotic surgery over conventional laparoscopy include improved depth perception with three dimensional stereoscopic vision, wristed instruments for improved dexterity, tremor canceling software to improve surgical precision, improved range of motion, optimization of ergonomics and autonomy, decreased learning curves and potentially decreased incisional pain [2, 13] (Table 55.2). The limitations of robotic surgery include the lack of haptic feedback, bulky platform, and increased cost compared with laparoscopic platforms and instrumentation.

M.H. Lippitt • E.J. Tanner III • A.N. Fader (✉)
Kelly Gynecologic Oncology Service, Department of Gynecology and Obstetrics, Johns Hopkins Medicine, Baltimore, Maryland, USA
e-mail: mweinro1@jhmi.edu; Etanner4@jhmi.edu; Afader1@jhmi.edu

Indications

Benign Indications

Robotic surgery for benign gynecologic disease is on the rise since the approval of the da Vinci Surgical System® in 2005. A recent study by Wright et al. examined the rate of hysterectomy for benign gynecologic disorders at 441 U.S. hospitals. During 2007 to 2010, robotically assisted hysterectomy rates increased from 0.5 % in 2007 to 9.5 % of all hysterectomies, while laparoscopic hysterectomy rates increased from 24.3 to 30.5 % [14]. Additionally, the authors found that the abdominal hysterectomy rates decreased among hospitals where robotic-assisted hysterectomy was both performed *and* not performed. A contemporary Cochrane review in 2014 concluded, "We are uncertain as to whether robotic assisted surgery (RAS) or conventional laparoscopic surgery (CLS) has lower intraoperative and postoperative complication rates because of the imprecision of the effect and inconsistency among studies when they are used for hysterectomy

I. Alkatout, L. Mettler (eds.), *Hysterectomy*, DOI 10.1007/978-3-319-22497-8_55

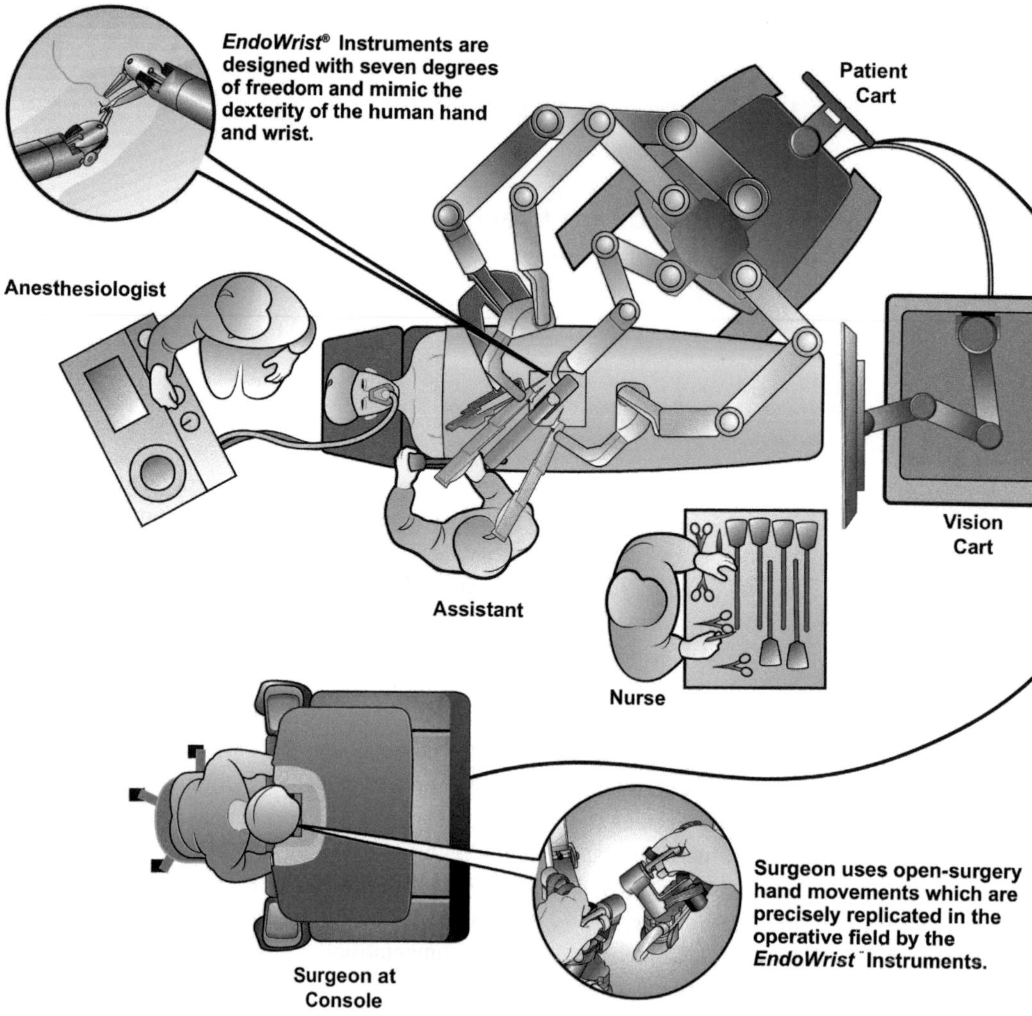

EndoWrist® Instruments are designed with seven degrees of freedom and mimic the dexterity of the human hand and wrist.

Patient Cart

Anesthesiologist

Vision Cart

Assistant

Nurse

Surgeon uses open-surgery hand movements which are precisely replicated in the operative field by the *EndoWrist*™ Instruments.

Surgeon at Console

Fig. 55.1 da Vinci Si operating room schematic (©2016 Intuitive Surgical, Inc Used with permission)

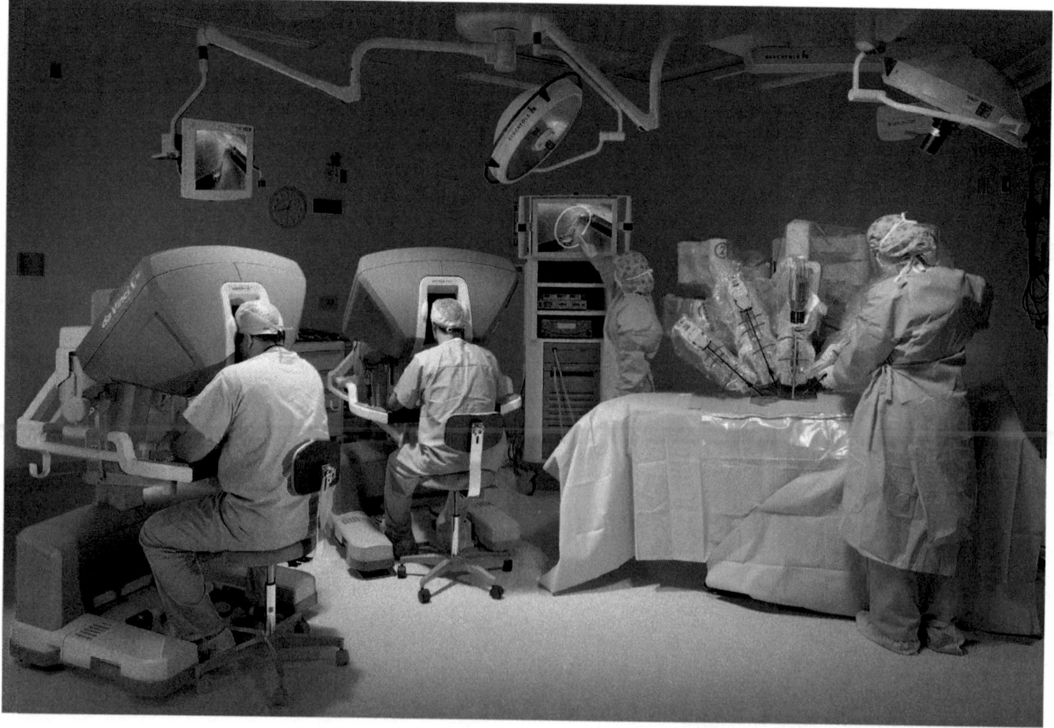

Fig. 55.2 da Vinci Si operating room (©2016 Intuitive Surgical, Inc Used with permission)

Table 55.1 Indications for robotic-assisted hysterectomy

Benign indications	Large uteri
	Leiomyomas
	Endometriosis
	Severe adhesive disease
	Cervical dysplasia
	Benign adnexal mass or cysts
	Sacrocolpopexy
	Morbid obesity
Malignant indications	Endometrial cancer
	Cervical cancer
	Early ovarian cancer
	Risk reducing surgery for women with familial cancer syndromes

Table 55.2 Benefits and limitations of robotic surgery compared to conventional laparoscopy

Benefits	Limitations
Improved depth perception with three dimensional stereoscopic vision	Lack of haptic feedback
Wristed instruments for improved dexterity	Possible increased operative time
Tremor canceling software to improve surgical precision	Lack of direct access to the patient
Improved range of motion	Cost
Optimization of ergonomics and autonomy	
Decreased learning curves	
Decreased incision pain	

and sacrocolpopexy. Moderate-quality evidence suggests that these procedures take longer with RAS but may be associated with a shorter hospital stay following hysterectomy. Ongoing trials are likely to have an important impact on evidence related to the use of RAS in gynecology [15]." Currently, robotic surgery is used to treat a variety of benign gynecological diseases including large uteri, uterine leiomyomas, endometriosis, severe adhesive disease, cervical dysplasia, benign adnexal masses or cysts, management of pelvic organ prolapse and sacrocolpopexy.

Large Uteri and Leiomyomas

Payne et al. reported the feasibility of robotically assisted hysterectomy in women with large uteri in five community practices. The largest uteri removed in this study weighed 3020 g. The study showed that women with large uteri (uterine weights greater than 250 g) may successfully undergo robotically- assisted hysterectomy with low morbidity, low blood loss, and minimal risk of conversion to laparotomy [16]. A subsequent retrospective review compared outcomes of mini-laparotomy versus robot-assisted laparoscopy for uteri weighing at least 500 g. Unadjusted mean blood loss, rate of hemorrhage, and rate of blood transfusion were all higher with mini-laparotomy than with robot-assisted surgery, while the median postoperative stay was significantly shorter with robotic surgery [17]. Additionally, given the wristed instrumentation of the robotic platform, suturing and knot tying in the repair of myomectomy defects may be technically less challenging to perform with robotic-assistance than with conventional laparoscopy.

Endometriosis and/or Severe Adhesive Disease

In the hands of experienced surgeons, robot-assisted laparoscopic hysterectomy may facilitate hysterectomy for patients with endometriosis and/or severe adhesive disease who may otherwise not have been offered a minimally invasive approach. Advincula et al. published a feasibility study in 2005 and reported on the success of robot-assisted laparoscopic hysterectomy in patients with a scarred or obliterated anterior cul-de-sac [18]. More recently, a retrospective cohort study compared robotic versus laparoscopic approach of hysterectomy in patients with severe pelvic adhesions [19]. Robotic surgery was associated with a shortened operation time and reduced blood loss in patients with severe adhesions compared with laparoscopy. They also reported a lower post-operative pain score in the robotic group as compared to the laparoscopic group.

Pelvic Organ Prolapse – Sacrocolpopexy

The gold standard procedure for the surgical treatment of severe pelvic organ prolapse is open abdominal sacrocolpopexy. An alternative approach to laparotomy includes laparoscopic sacrocolpopexy and more recently robot-assisted laparoscopic sacrocolpopexy. A recent systematic review of conventional laparoscopic sacrocolpopexy versus robot-assisted laparoscopic sacrocolpopexy reported the clinic outcomes (estimated blood loss, intraoperative and postoperative complications) of prolapse surgery are similar, but robotic surgery is less efficient in terms of cost and time [20]. Laparoscopic sacrocolpopexy is technically more challenging because it requires the surgical skills to perform suturing with knot tying and the ability to accurately determine the correct planes for safe dissection of the vesicovaginal and rectovaginal spaces [21]. Robotic technology overcomes some of these limitations, allowing a surgeon who may be uncomfortable with laparoscopy to still be able to offer a minimally invasive approach.

Obese Patients

Obesity represents one of the most common causes of death in the Western hemisphere [22]. The robotic technique can optimize the surgical approach and recovery of obese patients with equally, if not better outcomes, compared to open and/or laparoscopic techniques. Advantages of the robotic approach include minimal blood loss, low conversion to open rates, no need for drain use and quicker recovery period [23]. Robotic assisted hysterectomy is feasible in patients with all classes of obesity, including super obesity. A patient with a BMI of 98 successfully underwent a robotic-assisted hysterectomy [24].

Malignant Indications

In 2012, the Society for Gynecologic Oncology released their consensus statement on the use of robotic-assisted surgery in gynecologic oncology, stating "Robotic-assisted surgery has had a significant impact on the minimally invasive surgical approach to patients with gynecologic malignancies in the United States [25]." Currently, the robotics platform is used in the treatment of endometrial cancer, cervical cancer, and less commonly for ovarian cancer and resection of recurrent, oligometastatic disease.

Endometrial Cancer

Endometrial cancer is the most common gynecologic cancer in the United States and it has the most common use of the robotic platform [25]. Minimally invasive surgery approach is the accepted standard of care for endometrial cancer surgical staging. Eight randomized controlled trials, including the U.S. Gynecologic Oncology Group LAP2 study in 2009 demonstrated an improvement in surgical outcomes for patients undergoing laparoscopy for endometrial cancer staging when compared with those operated on by laparotomy [26–28]. While more data is needed to compare robotic surgery directly to laparoscopy, the adoption of the robotic platform has led to an increase in the total number of patients who were offered minimally invasive surgery [27, 29, 30].

In 2011 Paley et al. published a large, prospective, nonrandomized study of 377 consecutive robotic surgical staging procedures for endometrial cancer compared with 121 staging procedures performed by laparotomy for the same indication. Overall, serious complications, such as wound dehiscence, bleeding, and urologic injury were found to be three times more likely in the laparotomy group. However, this study did not include a laparoscopy arm for direct comparison. Gaia et al. [28] published a systematic review of 1591 patients, from eight studies, undergoing robotic-assisted surgeries compared with traditional laparoscopic or laparotomy techniques for the treatment of endometrial cancer. The study found that the estimated blood loss was reduced in robotic hysterectomy compared with laparotomy ($P < 0.005$) and laparoscopy ($P=0.001$), length of stay was shorter for both robotic and laparoscopic cases compared with laparotomy ($P < 0.01$) and operative time for robotic hysterectomy was similar to laparoscopic cases but was greater than laparotomy ($P <0.005$). Conversion to laparotomy was more than double in the laparoscopy group (4.6 % vs. 9.9 %), but this was not statistically significant ($P = 0.06$). The mean number of lymph nodes and perioperative complication rates, which included gastrointestinal injury, urologic injury, and vaginal cuff dehiscence, were the same in the three study arms.

Sentinel lymph node mapping for endometrial cancer at that time of hysterectomy and staging results in reliable mapping of relevant lymph nodes that drain the uterus (Fig. 55.3). Advantages of SLN mapping including reduction of lymphedema and intraoperative complications and improved detection of positive lymph nodes with ultrastaging techniques. Sinno et al. published a study in 2014 comparing colorimetric versus flurometric sentinel lymph node mapping during robotic surgery for endometrial cancer, suggesting that fluorescence imaging with indocyanine green may be superior to colorimetric imaging with isosulfan blue in women undergoing sentinel node mapping for endometrial cancer. Currently, the robotic platform remains the most feasible method for performing accurate sentinel lymph node mapping [31–33].

Cervical Cancer

The standard of care for a patient with early cervical cancer (FIGO stage IA2 – IIA) is a radical hysterectomy, with 5-year overall survival rates of 62–90 % [34]. The intricacies of radical hysterectomy, which include a sophisticated

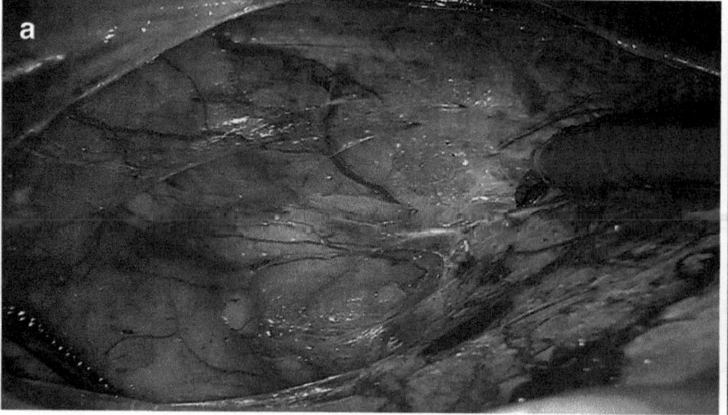

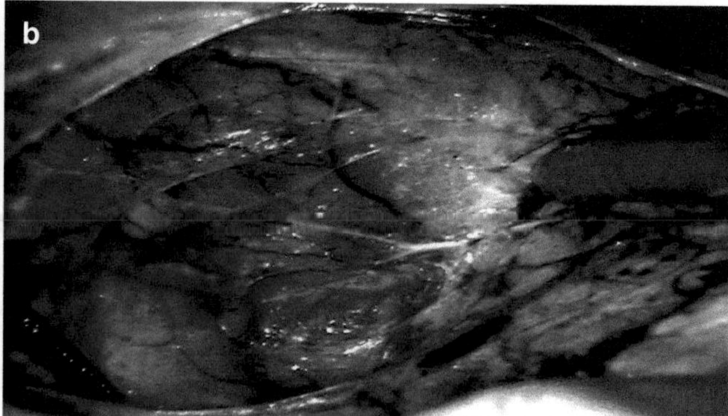

Fig. 55.3 Sentinel node mapping with indocyanine green: (**a**) without fluorescence, (**b**) addition of firefly fluorescence

dissection of the parametria, unroofing of the ureter from the ureteric canal within the cardinal ligament, and an en block resection of the uterus, cervix, parametria, and uterosacral ligaments, make it an ideal procedure to perform on the robotic platform, especially as only a small number of surgeons adopted the laparoscopic technique for this complex procedure [2]. Multiple studies have assessed the feasibility and safety of robotic-assisted radical hysterectomy (RRH) [35–38]. Boggess et al. [35] showed RRRH versus radical abdominal hysterectomy (RAH) to be associated with reduced operating room time, estimated blood loss, and length of surgery as compared to radical abdominal hysterectomy; Magrina et al. [38] showed improved outcomes for RRH vs total laparoscopic radical hysterectomy and RAH; Cantrell et al. [36] showed similar progression free survival and overall survival compared to RAH. One study, Soliman et al. [13] showed overall decreased intravenous opioid administration compared with the total laparoscopic radical hysterctomy (TLRH).

The robotic platform is also quite useful for radical trachelectomy in select patients with early-stage cervical cancer desiring fertility preservation [39]. Radical trachelectomy is a complex procedure, and the superior optics and wristed hand motions offered by the robotic platform compared with conventional laparoscopy are particularly attractive in this setting [2].

Ovarian Cancer

Comprehensive surgical staging in ovarian cancer requires exploration of the entire peritoneal cavity, from the diaphragm to the pelvic floor. The new fourth generation system allows multi-quadrant surgery without needing to undock and rotate patients. More research is needed to determine whether initial ovarian cancer debulking surgery will become a common use of robotic-assisted surgery in the future. Data suggests that robotic surgery is feasible for early stage ovarian cancer staging and select patients with recurrent ovarian cancer, in the absence of carcinomatosis, may be candidates for secondary surgical cytoreduction via a robotic approach [40, 41].

Contraindications

The only absolute contraindication to robotic hysterectomy is an anesthetic contraindication to pneumoperitoneum. Relative contraindications would include need for laparotomy to control bleeding, advanced malignancy and poor visualization or exposure, which may occur in a patient who has undergone multiple abdominal surgeries and has extensive adhesive disease. Additionally, in order to ensure a safe working environment, it is essential for the surgeon, bedside assistant and scrub technicians to be well versed and comfortable using the robotic surgical platform.

Additional Considerations

Single Site Robotic Assisted Hysterectomy

Laparoendoscopic single-site surgery may offer advantages versus conventional laparoscopy, including fewer operative complications related to trocar insertion, a cosmetically more pleasing incision, and a larger surface area for specimen retrieval in the post-power morcellator era [42, 43]. One of the first robotic assisted laparoendoscopic single-site surgeries was described by Escboar et al. in 2009, in which a hysterectomy was performed for a BRCA mutation carrier [44]. In this initial case report, a GelPort along with standard robotic trocars and standard robotic instruments were used. Today, Intuitive Surgical has developed a single-site apparatus that can be used with the Si da Vinci Surgical System. It utilizes novel robotic instruments with curved instrument cannulae and semi-rigid instruments, thereby optimizing the single site robotic-assisted hysterectomy (Fig. 55.4). Scheib et al. [45] presented one of the first series of robotic laparoendoscopic single-site surgery in 40 patients for the treatment of various gynecological conditions. A case report in 2015 reported the feasibility of sentinel lymph node biopsy and hysterectomy utilizing the single incision robotic surgery platform [46]. Further studies are needed to better define the ideal benign and malignant gynecological conditions for this new technology.

Cost Considerations

A controversy with robotic surgery remains the high cost associated with performance of the procedure. Proponents of robotic surgery have suggested that the technology can be made more cost-effective, especially as the learning curve improves and shorter operating times are optimized [2]. A large portion of the cost includes the initial purchase cost of

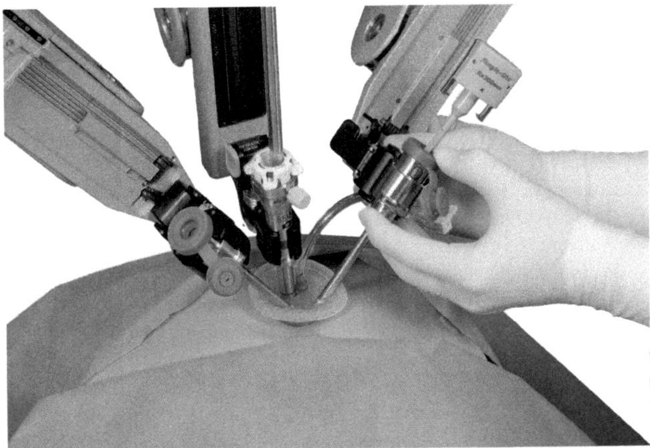

Fig. 55.4 da Vinci single-siteTM instrumentation for the da Vinci Si system (©2016 Intuitive Surgical, Inc Used with permission)

the robot as well as routine maintenance. In 2014, Wright et al. [47] performed an economic analysis to examine the influence of procedure volume, variation in hospital accounting methodology and use of various analytic methodologies on cost of robotically assisted hysterectomy for benign gynecologic disease and endometrial cancer. The authors concluded that the cost of robotic gynecologic surgery decreases with increasing procedure volume. However, in all of their scenarios, robotically assisted hysterectomy remained substantially higher in cost than laparoscopic hysterectomy. For surgeons who performed more than 50 procedures, robotic hysterectomy for benign indications cost $924 more than laparoscopic hysterectomy, and was $688 more for endometrial cancer. Compared to laparotomy, minimally invasive surgery has additional economic benefits including decreased complication rates leading to societal and indirect economic benefits of an earlier return to work [48]. While robotic surgery may remain more costly than laparoscopic surgery, the introduction of robotic surgery has led to an overall decline in the rate of open abdominal hysterectomy [14], and thereby decreasing the overall societal cost of hysterectomies. We expect to see the costs of robotic surgery continue to decrease as other technologies are introduced to the marketplace.

Conclusion

Minimally invasive surgery, including vaginal, laparoscopic and robotic approaches, should be the standard of care for hysterectomy when feasible. Many studies support the feasibility of robotic surgery for benign and malignant gynecologic indications. As robotic surgery continues to gain more popularity, we expect to see more studies exploring the benefits of the robot for benign and malignant gynecologic indications. Ideally, we will see a future with continued increases in the rates of minimally invasive surgery and therefore improved patient outcome.

References

1. Wright JD, Herzog TJ, Tsui J, Ananth CV, Lewin SN, Lu Y-S, et al. Nationwide trends in the performance of inpatient hysterectomy in the United States. Obstet Gynecol. 2013;122(2 Pt 1):233–41.
2. Sinno AK, Fader AN. Robotic-assisted surgery in gynecologic oncology. Fertil Steril Elsevier. 2014;102(4):922–32.
3. Sutton C. Past, present, and future of hysterectomy. J Minim Invasive Gynecol Elsevier Ltd. 2010;17(4):421–35.
4. Falcone T, Goldberg J, Garcia-Ruiz A, Margossian H, Stevens L. Full robotic assistance for laparoscopic tubal anastomosis: a case report. J Laparoendosc Adv Surg Tech A [Internet]. 1999;9(1):107–13. Available from: http://www.ncbi.nlm.nih.gov/entrez/query.fcgi?cmd=Retrieve&db=PubMed&dopt=Citation&list_uids=10194702
5. Escobar P, Falcone T. Atlas of single-port, laparoscopic, and robotic surgery. New York: Springer; 2014.
6. Lenihan JP, Kovanda C, Seshadri-Kreaden U. What is the learning curve for robotic assisted gynecologic surgery? J Minim Invasive Gynecol. 2008;15:589–94.
7. Nezhat C, Saberi NS, Shahmohamady B, Nezhat F. Robotic-assisted laparoscopy in gynecological surgery. JSLS. 2006;10(3):317–20.
8. Cela V, Freschi L, Simi G, Tana R, Russo N, Artini PG, et al. Fertility and endocrine outcome after robot-assisted laparoscopic myomectomy (RALM). Gynecol Endocrinol. 2012;3590(January): 1–4.
9. Göçmen A, Şanlıkan F, Uçar MG. Comparison of robotic-assisted laparoscopic myomectomy outcomes with laparoscopic myomectomy. Arch Gynecol Obstet. 2013;287(1):91–6.
10. Caillet M, Vandromme J, Rozenberg S, Paesmans M, Germay O, Degueldre M. Robotically assisted laparoscopic microsurgical tubal reanastomosis: a retrospective study. Fertil Steril. 2010;94(5):1844–7.
11. Hemal AK, Kolla SB, Wadhwa P. Robotic reconstruction for recurrent supratrigonal vesicovaginal fistulas. J Urol. 2008;180(3):981–5.
12. Melamud O, Eichel L, Turbow B, Shanberg A. Laparoscopic vesicovaginal fistula repair with robotic reconstruction. Urology. 2005;65(1):163–6.
13. Soliman PT, Langley G, Munsell MF, Vaniya HA, Frumovitz M, Ramirez PT. Analgesic and antiemetic requirements after minimally invasive surgery for early cervical cancer: a comparison between laparoscopy and robotic surgery. Ann Surg Oncol. 2013; 20(4):1355–9.
14. Wright JD, Ananth CV, Lewin SN, Burke WM, Lu Y-S, Neugut AI, et al. Robotically assisted vs laparoscopic hysterectomy among women with benign gynecologic disease. JAMA. 2013;309(7):689–98.
15. Liu H, Lawrie TA, Lu D, Song H, Wang L, Shi G Robot-assisted surgery in gynaecology. Cochrane Database Syst Rev. 2014;(12): CD011422.
16. Payne TN, Dauterive FR, Pitter MC, Giep HN, Giep BN, Grogg TW, et al. Robotically assisted hysterectomy in patients with large uteri: outcomes in five community practices. Obstet Gynecol. 2010;115(3):535–42.
17. Smorgick N, Dalton VK, Patzkowsky KE, Hoffman MR, Advincula AP, As-Sanie S. Comparison of 2 minimally invasive routes for hysterectomy of large uteri. Int J Gynecol Obstet. 2013;122(2):128–31.
18. Advincula AP, Reynolds RK. The use of robot-assisted laparoscopic hysterectomy in the patient with a scarred or obliterated anterior cul-de-sac. JSLS. 2005;9(3):287–91.
19. Chiu L-H, Chen C-H, Tu P-C, Chang C-W, Yen Y-K. Comparison of robotic surgery and laparoscopy to perform total hysterectomy with pelvic adhesions or large uterus. J Minim Access Surg [Internet]. 2015;11(1):87. Available from: http://www.journalofmas.com/text.asp?2015/11/1/87/147718
20. Pan K, Zhang Y, Wang Y, Wang Y, Xu H. A systematic review and meta-analysis of conventional laparoscopic sacrocolpopexy versus robot-assisted laparoscopic sacrocolpopexy. Int J Gynecol Obstet. 2016;132:284–91.
21. Clifton MM, Pizarro-Berdichevsky J, HB G. Robotic female pelvic floor reconstruction: a review. Urology. 2016;91:33–40.
22. Fontaine K, Redden D, Wang C, Westfall A, Allison D. Years of life lost due to obesity. JAMA. 2003;289(2):187–93.
23. Iavazzo C, Gkegkes ID. Robotic assisted hysterectomy in obese patients: a systematic review. Arch Gynecol Obstet [Internet]. 2016;293(6):1169–83. Available from: http://www.ncbi.nlm.nih.gov/pubmed/26861466
24. Stone P, Burnett A, Burton B, Roman J. Overcoming extreme obesity with robotic surgery. Int J Med Robot Comput Assist Surg. 2010;6(4):382–5.
25. Ramirez PT, Adams S, Boggess JF, Burke WM, Frumovitz MM, Gardner GJ, et al. Robotic-assisted surgery in gynecologic oncology: a society of gynecologic oncology consensus statement developed by the society of gynecologic oncology's clinical practice robotics rask force. Gynecol Oncol. 2012;124:180–4.
26. Walker JL, Piedmonte MR, Spirtos NM, Eisenkop SM, Schlaerth JB, Mannel RS, et al. Laparoscopy compared with laparotomy for

comprehensive surgical staging of uterine cancer: gynecologic oncology group study LAP2. J Clin Oncol. 2009;27(32):5331–6.

27. Paley PJ, Veljovich DS, Shah CA, Everett EN, Bondurant AE, Drescher CW, et al. Surgical outcomes in gynecologic oncology in the era of robotics: analysis of first 1000 cases. Am J Obstet Gynecol Elsevier Inc. 2011;204(6):551.e1–9.
28. Gaia G, Holloway RW, Santoro L, Ahmad S, Di Silverio E, Spinillo A. Robotic-assisted hysterectomy for endometrial cancer compared with traditional laparoscopic and laparotomy approaches: a systematic review. Obstet Gynecol. 2010;116(6):1422–31.
29. Holloway RW, Ahmad S, DeNardis SA, Peterson LB, Sultana N, Bigsby GE, et al. Robotic-assisted laparoscopic hysterectomy and lymphadenectomy for endometrial cancer: analysis of surgical performance. Gynecol Oncol. Elsevier Inc. 2009;115(3):447–52.
30. Hoekstra A V., Morgan JM, Lurain JR, Buttin BM, Singh DK, Schink JC, et al. Robotic surgery in gynecologic oncology: impact on fellowship training. Gynecol Oncol. Elsevier Inc. 2009;114(2):168–72.
31. Abu-Rustum NR, Khoury-Collado F, Pandit-Taskar N, Soslow RA, Dao F, Sonoda Y, et al. Sentinel lymph node mapping for grade 1 endometrial cancer: is it the answer to the surgical staging dilemma? Gynecol Oncol. Elsevier Inc. 2009;113(2):163–9.
32. Tanner EJ, Sinno AK, Stone RL, Levinson KL, Long KC, Fader AN Factors associated with successful bilateral sentinel lymph node mapping in endometrial cancer. Gynecol Oncol. Elsevier Inc. 2015;138(3):542–7.
33. Cormier B, Rozenholc AT, Gotlieb W, Plante M, Giede C Sentinel lymph node procedure in endometrial cancer: a systematic review and proposal for standardization of future research. Gynecol Oncol. Elsevier Inc. 2015;138(2):478–85.
34. Landoni F, Maneo A, Colombo A, Placa F, Milani R, Perego P, et al. Randomised study of radical surgery versus radiotherapy for stage Ib-IIa cervical cancer. Lancet. 1997;350(9077):535–40.
35. Boggess JF, Gehrig PA, Cantrell L, Shafer A, Ridgway M, EN S, et al. A case-control study of robot-assisted type III radical hysterectomy with pelvic lymph node dissection compared with open radical hysterectomy. Am J Obstet Gynecol. 2008;199(4):357.e1–7.
36. Cantrell LA, Mendivil A, Gehrig PA, Boggess JF. Survival outcomes for women undergoing type III robotic radical hysterectomy for cervical cancer: a 3-year experience. Gynecol Oncol. Elsevier Inc. 2010;117(2):260–5.
37. Estape R, Lambrou N, Diaz R, Estape E, Dunkin N, Rivera A. A case matched analysis of robotic radical hysterectomy with lymphadenectomy compared with laparoscopy and laparotomy. Gynecol Oncol. 2009;113:357–61.
38. Magrina JF, Kho RM, Weaver AL, Montero RP, Magtibay PM. Robotic radical hysterectomy: comparison with laparoscopy and laparotomy. Gynecol Oncol. 2008;109(1):86–91.
39. Ramirez PT, Schmeler KM, Malpica A, Soliman PT. Safety and feasibility of robotic radical trachelectomy in patients with early-stage cervical cancer. Gynecol Oncol [Internet]. Elsevier Inc. 2010;116(3):512–5. Available from: http://dx.doi.org/10.1016/j.ygyno.2009.10.063
40. Minig L, Padilla Iserte P, Zorrero C, Zanagnolo V. Robotic surgery in women with ovarian cancer: surgical technique and evidence of clinical outcomes. J Minim Invasive Gynecol [Internet]. Elsevier Inc. 2016; 23(3):309–16. Available from: http://dx.doi.org/10.1016/j.jmig.2015.10.014
41. Escobar PF, Levinson KL, Magrina J, Martino MA, Barakat RR, Fader AN, et al. Feasibility and perioperative outcomes of robotic-assisted surgery in the management of recurrent ovarian cancer: a multi-institutional study. Gynecol Oncol [Internet]. Elsevier Inc. 2014;134(2):253–6. Available from: http://www.ncbi.nlm.nih.gov/pubmed/24844594.
42. Fagotti A, Bottoni C, Vizzielli G, Alletti SG, Scambia G, Marana E, et al. Postoperative pain after conventional laparoscopy and laparoendoscopic single site surgery (LESS) for benign adnexal disease: a randomized trial. Fertil Steril [Internet]. Elsevier Ltd. 2011;96(1):255–9.e2. Available from: http://dx.doi.org/10.1016/j.fertnstert.2011.04.006.
43. Song T, Park J-Y, Kim T-J, Lee Y-Y, Choi CH, Lee J-W, et al. A prospective comparative study of cosmetic satisfaction for three different surgical approaches. Eur J Obstet Gynecol Reprod Biol [Internet]. Elsevier Ireland Ltd. 2015;190(January 2011):48–51. Available from: http://www.ncbi.nlm.nih.gov/pubmed/25978858.
44. Escobar PF, Fader AN, Paraiso MF, Kaouk JH, Falcone T Robotic-assisted laparoendoscopic single-site surgery in gynecology: initial report and technique. J Minim Invasive Gynecol Elsevier Ltd. 2009;16(5):589–91.
45. Scheib SA, Fader AN. Gynecologic robotic laparoendoscopic single-site surgery: prospective analysis of feasibility, safety, and technique. Am J Obstet Gynecol [Internet]. Elsevier Inc; 2015;212(2):179.e1–179.e8. Available from: http://dx.doi.org/10.1016/j.ajog.2014.07.057.
46. Sinno AK, Fader AN, Tanner EJ. Single site robotic sentinel lymph node biopsy and hysterectomy in endometrial cancer. Gynecol Oncol [Internet]. Elsevier Inc. 2015;137(1):190. Available from: http://dx.doi.org/10.1016/j.ygyno.2014.12.033.
47. Wright JD, Ananth CV, Tergas AI, Herzog TJ, Burke WM, Lewin SN, et al. An economic analysis of robotically assisted hysterectomy. Obstet Gynecol. 2014;123(5):1038–48.
48. Advancing Minimally Invasive Gynecology Worldwide A. AAGL position statement: robotic-assisted laparoscopic surgery in benign gynecology AAGL advancing minimally invasive gynecology worldwide. J Minim Invasive Gynecol. 2013;20:2–9.

56 Preparation of Robotic-Assisted Laparoscopic Hysterectomy

Martin Heubner

Planning robotic hysterectomy, special conditions and requirements have to be taken into account. The positioning of the patient is a crucial aspect regarding safety as steep Trendelenburg position, which is associated with special risks, is mandatory. The set-up of the robotic device, including draping and positioning of the patient cart again are issues concerning the technical functionality of the robotic system. Even more than other operative techniques, robotic surgery has to be regarded a team task in which communication and interaction between surgeons, nurses and anesthesiologists is mandatory to achieve good results.

History of the Patient

Noteworthy aspects of history taking involve precedent surgical procedures and preexisting comorbidities. It is important to recognize that patient positioning in robotic surgery is substantial for good results and is –in contrast to classic laparoscopy- not alterable during the operation.

Previous operations, especially abdominal operations should be recognized in order to estimate the extent and the location of adhesions, which is especially important considering the placement of the camera trocar. Open laparoscopy might be an option if extensive adhesions are suspected in the mid-abdomen. Heart, lung and cerebral diseases might be important considering the ability of steep Trendelenburg positioning of the patient.

Especially patients with obesity can benefit from the use of robotic surgery as it might avoid laparotomy with subsequent complications and intraoperative problems. There is no upper limit with respect to the patients' BMI. However, the prospects of anaesthesiological ventilation can be impaired to high ventilation pressure, especially in Trendelenburg position of the patient [1]. A useful indicator is whether the patient is able to sleep in a flat position without heightening of the upper part of the body. Special instrument, especially extra-long trocars should be held available for obese patients.

Important preexisting illnesses comprise heart diseases, especially higher grade heart valve failures or pulmonary hypertension, pulmonary illnesses such as chronic obstructive lung disease and vessel problems such as cerebral aneurysms. Orthopedic musculoskeletal problems are also important to recognize. All these and further yet unmentioned aspects may result in impaired options of patient positioning and require conference with the anaesthesiological team. Allergies are of importance as perioperative antibiotics are usually applied during surgery.

Informed Consent of the Patient

The preoperative information of the patient should cover all common complications and risks of other techniques of hysterectomy. Still, some special aspects should be considered. Steep Trendelenburg position requires special handling and can result in special complications such as ventilation problems, extremely rare ophthalmologic problems (corneal abrasion, ischemic optic neuropathy, visual loss) and postoperative orthopedic problems (e.g. shoulder problems or distension of the brachial plexus if shoulder pads are used). It is noteworthy that some authors report a higher rate of vaginal cuff dehiscence after robotic surgery; hence, this should be mentioned. As the size of the trocars regularly exceeds 7 mm, port-site hernias are also of importance.

Operative Set-Up

Patient positioning has to be carried out with great caution. Trendelenburg position of at least 30° is mandatory to assure adequate access to the pelvis. To prevent the patient from

M. Heubner
Department of Gynecology and Obstetrics, Kantonsspital Baden, Baden, Switzerland
e-mail: Martin.Heubner@ksb.ch

I. Alkatout, L. Mettler (eds.), *Hysterectomy*, DOI 10.1007/978-3-319-22497-8_56

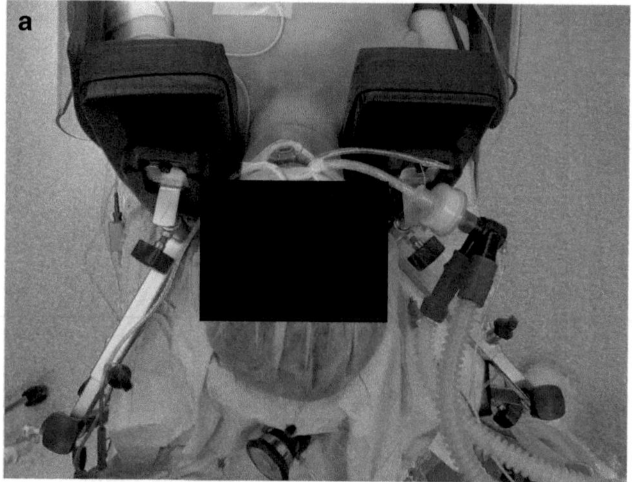

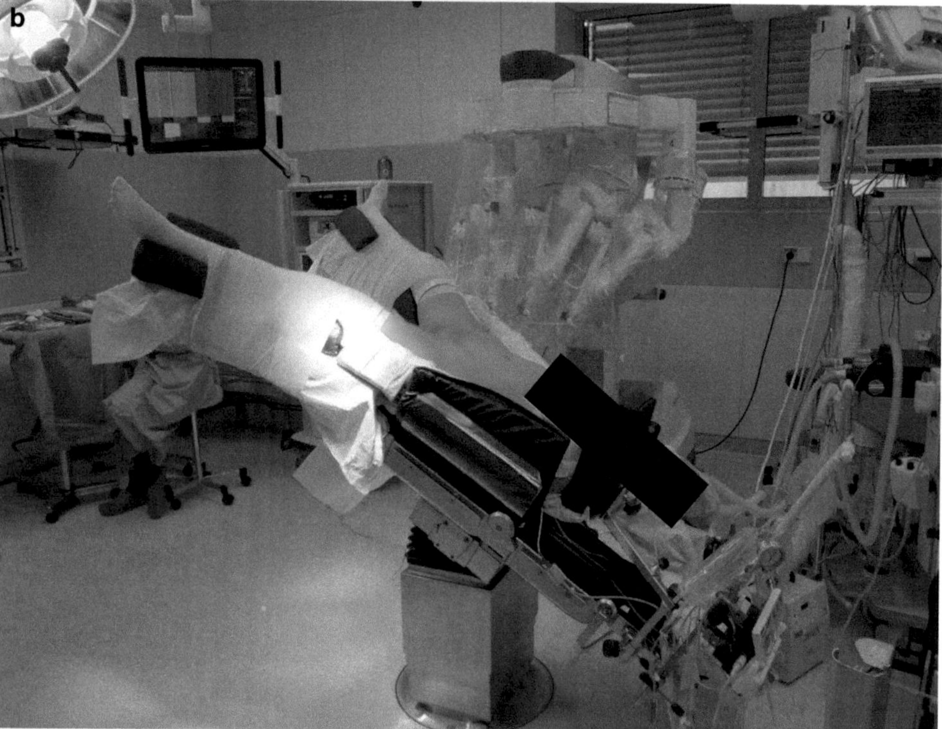

Fig. 56.1 Shoulder pads can be used to provide the patient from sliding (**a**), allowing steep Trendelenburg position (**b**)

sliding off the operating table, different technical options are available. Fixated shoulder pads, vacuum mattresses or boot-type leg holders are devices which might be useful, the preference is certainly individual (Fig. 56.1). The resulting forces acting upon the respective body parts in Trendelenburg position must not be underestimated. Positioning should be controlled before disinfection and during the operation and is a team task demanding involvement of surgeons, anesthesiologists and nurses. A skilled and experienced team is the major key to avoid complications and docking problems.

Docking should be carried out according to the manufacturers' instructions. The technique differs between different types of robotic systems. However, it is important to recognize that a professional docking is one of the most important aspects for a successful operation. Mistakes in the docking procedure occur frequently in the introduction phase of a robotic system and can grossly impair handling of the instruments during surgery. The position of the arms has to be considered not only in the start position but also extrapolated to future potential movements which again depend on the planned operating field. In this regard, it has to be ensured that moving robotic arms will not impair the patient, members of the OR-team or OR-equipment. This aspect appears self-evident. However, a surgeon beginning with robotic surgery technique faces a completely new situation: not being physically present at the operating table with no haptic or optical feedback apart from the direct operating field inside the abdomen. Thus, the permanent critical surveillance by assistants and immediate feedback to the console surgeon is crucial.

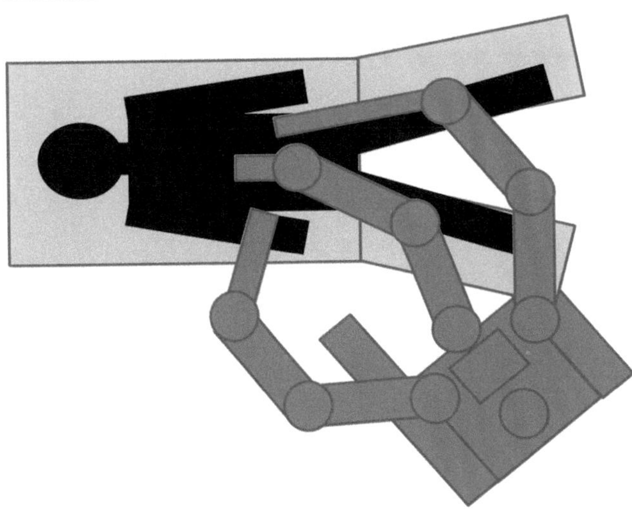

Fig. 56.2 Schematic sketch of side docking approaching over the right hip of the patient

There are different ways of approaching the patient with the patient cart. Placing the patient cart between the patients' legs usually makes the docking procedure easy as the resulting symmetrical geometry gives maximum space between the robotic arms. However, the prospects of vaginal manipulation are impaired by this method. **Side docking** in a 30° angle, usually approaching from caudally over the right hip of the patient, is a feasible method allowing access for vaginal manipulation and docking of the robotic arms without interference (this applies to the da Vinci® Si system or lower; see Fig. 56.2).

The type of docking also depends on the model of robotic device that is used. It is recommended that representatives of the accordant company and/or skilled physicians with experience on the respective device attend the first operations to give advice.

General Aspects: Introduction of Robotic Surgery as a Team Task

Introducing robotic surgery, it is certainly beneficial if the whole OR team including surgeons and anesthesiologists attend the first attempts of patient positioning, disinfection, draping and docking, as perspectives may differ within the team. E.g., potential movement dysfunctions of the robotic arms caused by wrong draping may be better foreseen by the surgeon while potential impairments of sterility aspects are often better estimated by the OR nurses. Patient positioning again has to offer good access to the surgical field for the surgeon and access to the patient for the anesthesiologist and has to ensure the patients' safety. In general, experience shows that it is helpful if the whole team is familiar with all aspects of the setup. This allows quick development of know-how and efficacy and helps to avoid demotivation throughout the whole staff.

Disinfection and draping should be carried out according to the standards of the surgical unit. It should be kept in mind that a switch to open surgery might become necessary and this should therefore be considered. Draping of the robot-arms and their handling under aspects of sterility is a complicated procedure requiring training and experience. It is important to consider the necessary free moving space of the robotic arm, tension should strictly be avoided. Wrong draping can result in functional errors of the robotic arms. The OR team should undergo several training sessions before conducting the first operation on a patient.

Although emergency transition to open surgery is very rare, draping should be conducted in a manner also allowing open access to the abdomen without necessity of additional draping/undraping or disinfection.

The perioperative application of a single-shot antibiotic prophylaxis should be carried out 30 min before surgery. A combination of ampicillin/sulbactam is feasible. Alternatively, e.g. in case of allergy to penicillin and its derivates, clindamycin can be administered. A prolonged treatment with antibiotics beyond the time of surgery cannot be recommended.

Reference

1. Wysham WZ, Kim KH, Roberts JM, Sullivan SA, Campbell SB, Roque DR, Moore DT, Gehrig PA, Boggess JF, Soper JT, Huh WK. Obesity and perioperative pulmonary complications in robotic gynecologic surgery. Am J Obstet Gynecol. 2015;213(1):33.e1–7. doi:10.1016/j.ajog.2015.01.033. Epub 2015 Jan 28.

Instruments, Apparatuses and Uterine Manipulators for Hysterectomy with Special Focus on Robotic-Assisted Laparoscopic Hysterectomy

57

Mona E. Orady

Introduction

Hysterectomy is the surgical removal of the uterus. It may also involve removal of the cervix, ovaries, fallopian tubes and other surrounding structures [1]. Hysterectomy is the most common procedure performed for gynecological disorders. Overall hysterectomy rates vary from 1.2 to 4.8 per 1000 [2]. Removal of the uterus renders the patient unable to bear children (as does removal of the ovaries and fallopian tubes) and has surgical risks as well as long-term effects, hence surgery is only recommended when other treatment options are not available or have failed. It is expected that the frequency of hysterectomies for non-malignant indications will decrease as there are good alternatives in many cases [3]. However, hysterectomy will remain as the definitive treatment of uterine pathology. Uterine myomas are the most frequent indication for abdominal hysterectomy, accounting for 40 % of all hysterectomies, with other indications including endometriosis (12.8 %), malignancy (12.6 %), abnormal uterine bleeding (9.5 %), pelvic inflammatory disease (3.7 %) and uterine prolapse (3.0 %). Utero-vaginal prolapse is the indication for 44 % of all vaginal hysterectomies. In recent years, non – descent vaginal hysterectomy (NDVH) is being tried for most benign conditions and uteri of up to 12 weeks gestational size or more can be safely removed intact vaginally [2]. However, large leiomyomas, severe pelvic inflammatory disease, malignancy (invasive cervical cancer, endometrial carcinoma, ovarian and fallopian tube cancer, and gestational trophoblastic tumors) and most suspicious adnexal masses are still often approached via laparotomy [2].

The introduction and rapid advancement of laparoscopy has allowed for the development of alternative minimally invasive approaches to hysterectomy thus avoiding the morbidity associated with an abdominal hysterectomy when the vaginal approach is not feasible [4, 5]. Initially utilized in laparoscopic assisted vaginal hysterectomy, the laparoscope allowed the treatment of adnexal pathology or endometriosis and assistance in the release of the uterine structures and bladder flap from above, facilitating the vaginal approach in more complex cases. As tools and techniques advanced, a greater proportion of the hysterectomy procedure was undertaken using the laparoscopic approach leading to the first total laparoscopic hysterectomy successfully completed via laparoscopy in 1989 [4].

Following this, the development of tools that facilitated dissection, vessel sealing and suturing were developed in order to simplify and improve the procedure. The advantages of the minimally invasive approach for the patient included reduced pain, hospital stay, blood loss, and a much shorter recovery as compared to abdominal hysterectomy [5, 6]. This led to the desire to utilize this approach even in complex hysterectomy procedures, obese patients, and cancer surgeries. This motivated surgeons and the industry as whole to push the limits of the surgery, and to develop and explore other laparoscopic approaches such as single port surgery, mini-laparoscopy, natural orifice surgical procedures (NOTES) and combinations of the above, to see if the procedure could be accomplished with even less scarring, pain, and time required for recovery [7].

The most advanced and expensive tool used to date for the performance of minimally invasive hysterectomy procedure is the daVinci™ surgical robot (Fig. 57.1). After receiving FDA approval for use in gynecology in 2005, the frequency of daVinci robotic assisted total laparoscopic hysterectomy has exponentially increased [8, 9]. It offers all the benefits of the laparoscopic approach, but affords the surgeon improved vision utilizing a three dimensional magnified high definition camera and scope as well as superior control over articulating instruments with 7° of freedom. These features enable the surgeon to accomplish more difficult procedures by making it easier to work in areas deep within the pelvis or work around large fibroids which would otherwise restrict the

M.E. Orady, MD, FACOG
Gynecologic Surgeon, Director of Robotic Surgery Services, Department of Surgery, St. Francis Memorial Hospital, Dignity Health Medical Foundation, San Francisco, California, USA
e-mail: oradymd@gmail.com

I. Alkatout, L. Mettler (eds.), *Hysterectomy*, DOI 10.1007/978-3-319-22497-8_57

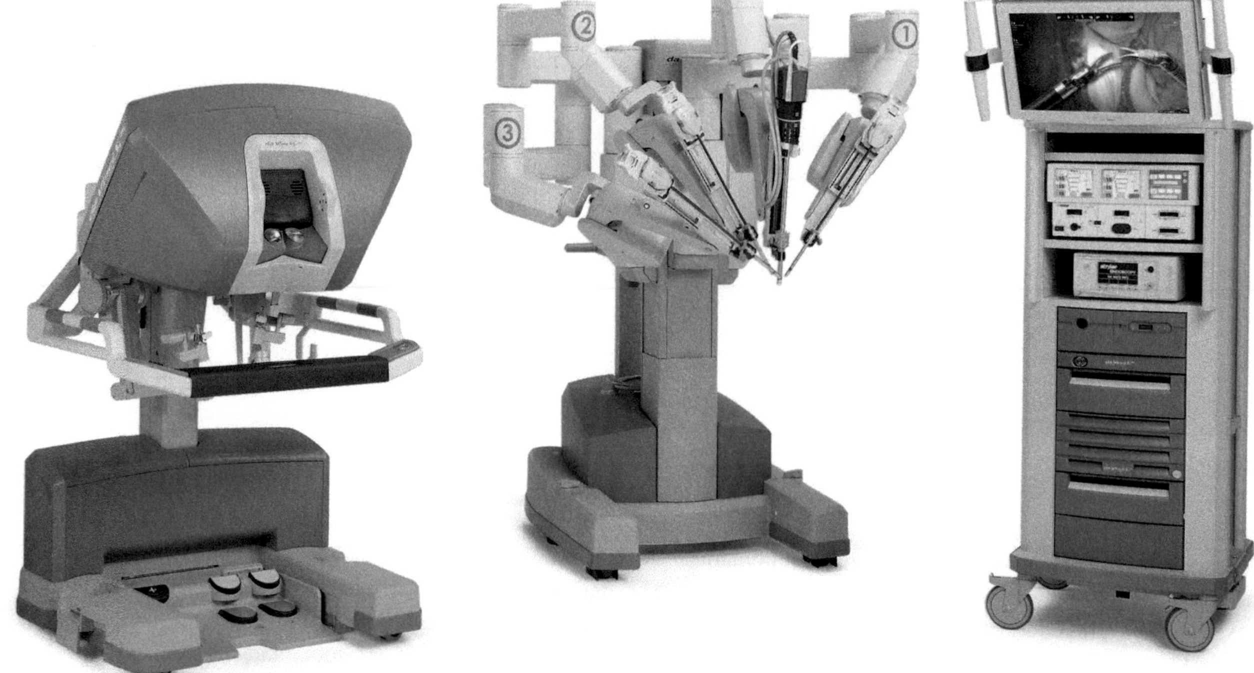

Fig. 57.1 The DaVinci surgical system TM is comprised of three components. The Vision Tower, Robotic Patient-side cart and the Surgeon Control Console. The tower contains light and energy sources as well as the vision monitor. The robot consists of the arms which attach to the robotic trochar cannulas, the robotic instruments, and the robotic camera, which pass through the robotic trocars, providing surgeon with direct intuitive control of the instruments, camera, and energy from the surgeon console. Some systems come with two consoles (Dual Console) which allow the surgeon to train a resident, fellow, or colleague giving the instructing surgeon the ability to take over control at any time, telestrate, or direct the learning real time during a case

Table 57.1 Comparison between traditional laparoscopy and robotic assisted laproscopy

	Traditional laparoscopy	Robotic assisted laparoscopy
Number of ports	3–5 ports	Tends to average one more than laparoscopy
Size of ports	Three 5 mm and one 10 mm on average	Three to Four 8 mm and one 5–12 mm on Average
Vision	2-D vision although some 3-D Scopes are becoming available	3-D HD 10 X vision Autofocus and Auto white balance available on newer models
Control of instruments	Camera and opposing instruments controlled by assistant but instruments easily interchangeable between ports	Camera and Opposing instruments controlled by surgeon but assistance must do all instrument exchanges and troubleshooting
Precision of movement	Straight instruments with fulcrum effect	Wristed instruments with 7° of movement
Ability to scale movements	Direct control	Console allows surgeon to allow scaling to 1:1, 3:1, or 5:1 ratio of hand movement to instrument movement to allow for fine motor control
Energy devices available	All ultrasonic and Advanced energy devices compatible with instrument ports	Only traditional monopolar and bipolar devices, as well as a single vessel sealing device and a PK dissector utilizing PK energy are available. Harmonic device lacks wristing
Tremor	Amplified by fulcrum effect	Filtered by console programming

movement and reach of conventional laparoscopic instruments [10, 11]. Table 57.1 provides a comparison of robotic assisted versus conventional laparoscopy for hysterectomy. This chapter will review the different tools that are utilized in hysterectomy procedures and the optimal tool selection methods appropriate for each individual procedure method.

Instruments for Access and Exposure

The most important aspects of surgery are access and exposure. Without access to and exposure of the relevant anatomy, the procedure cannot be performed. The three main approaches to hysterectomy require different vantage points of access in order to achieve the appropriate exposure. More often than not, the perceived inability to achieve the required access and exposure of the anatomy in question via one approach is what leads a surgeon to selecting one modality over another.

Abdominal Hysterectomy

For abdominal hysterectomy, access is achieved directly through the abdominal wall, either through a transverse or vertical incision. The transverse Pfanennstiel incision is the most common in benign procedures while the midline vertical incision is more favored in oncologic procedures (Fig. 57.2). Vertical Incisions can be extended to accommodate larger or more complex pathology or allow access to para-aortic lymph nodes by extending it above the umbilicus. In turn, using a Maylard or Churney incision allows for increased exposure through a transverse incision, which is often preferred due to decreased pain, risk of hernia, and improved cosmesis [12].

Once the incision is made, the choice of retractor will aid in attaining the appropriate exposure. The most commonly used retractor in benign abdominal hysterectomy is the Balfour retractor which comes with wrenched side blades, an attachable bladder blade and an optional upper blade. For more complicated or larger pathology, the Bookwalter retractor allows attachment of multiple retractor blades of multiple sizes and configurations to a metal ring which is placed floating above the incision attached to a metal arm fastened to the operating table. More recently, disposable plastic double ring wound retractors such as the Alexis wound retractor can be useful in thicker abdominal walls providing retraction of skin, subcutaneous fat, muscle, fascia and peritoneum within a plastic sheath, thus providing maximal retraction and exposure with an even distribution of pressure. This can be useful for performance of a hysterectomy in obese patients, in whom obtaining exposure is often challenging [12] (Fig. 57.3).

Vaginal Hysterectomy

Vaginal exposure for vaginal hysterectomy yields its own challenges. Generally, the best candidates for vaginal hysterectomy are multiparous patients with some degree of uterine descensus and adequate room in the vagina to obtain exposure of the cervix. Most gynecologists will use vaginal sidewall retractors as well as a long posterior retractor in order to obtain exposure and protect the rectum such as a weighted Steiner retractor with a long lip that will reach the posterior vaginal cuff to retract it inferiorly. Anteriorly, either a long bladed Deaver or Right angle retractor can be used to protect and retract the bladder superiorly. Briesky or Jackson vaginal retractors can also be used to retract laterally as needed. The labia may be retracted using a suture or a Lonestar retractor

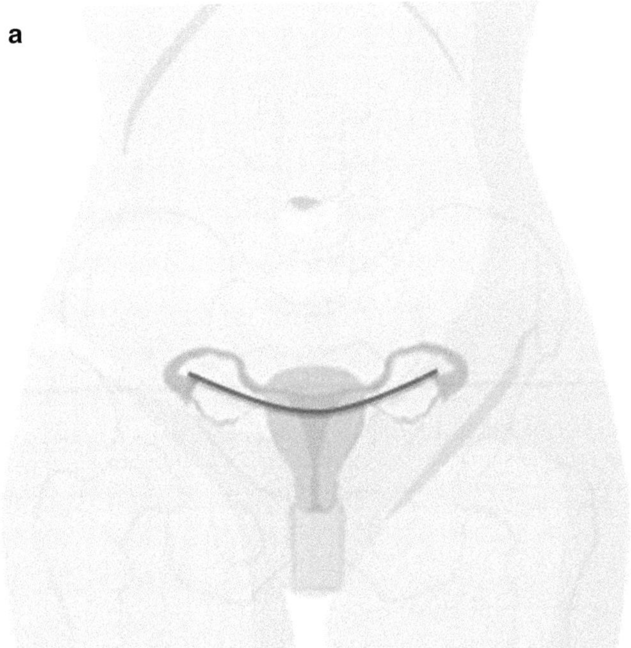

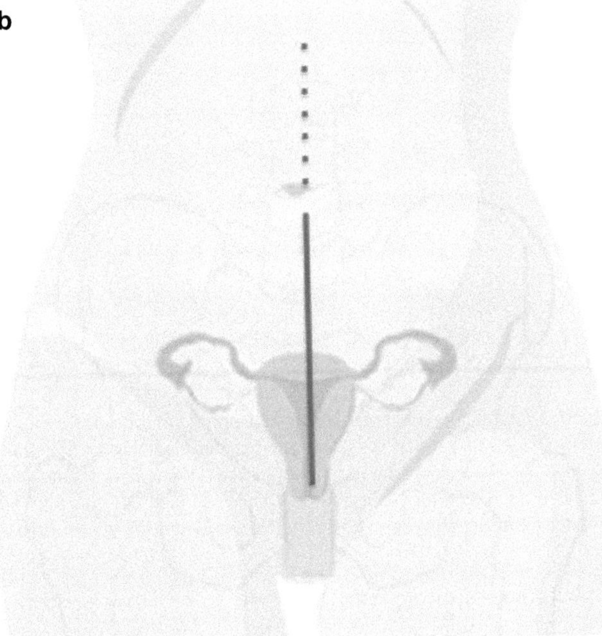

Fig. 57.2 Abdominal hysterectomy incisions: (**a**) Transverse Incision includes the options of a Pfanennstiel incision, Maylard Incision, or Cherney Incisions, depending on whether rectus muscles are separated, cut, or detached from insertion on the pubis. (**b**) Vertical incisions can remain below umbilicus or be extended above as needed and thus provide the opportunity to extend the incision in order to increase visualization, and are thus the most versatile. However, they cause more pain, worse cosmesis, and a greater risk for hernia than transverse incisions

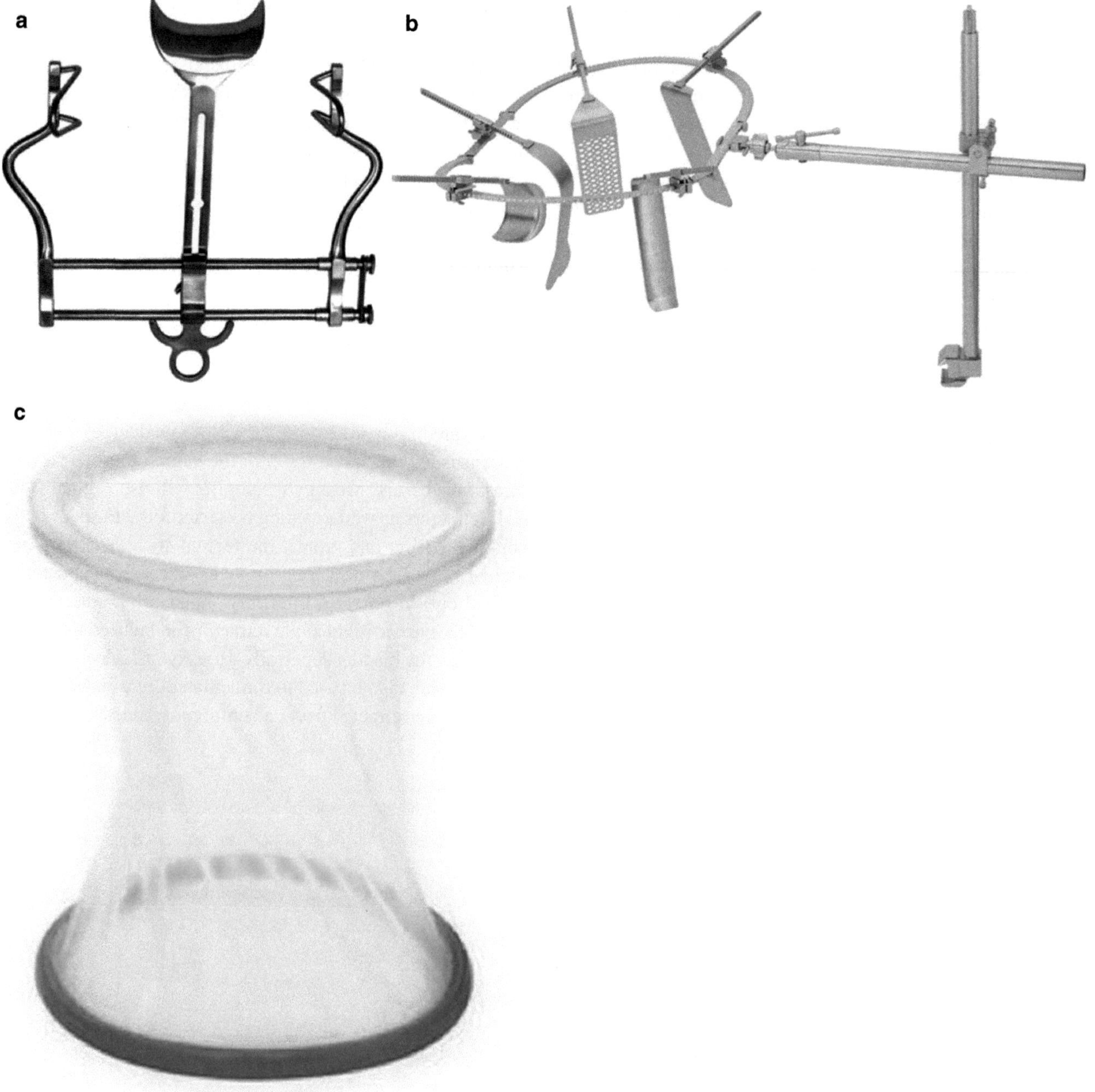

Fig. 57.3 Retractors for abdominal hysterectomy. (**a**) Balfour Retractor provides side wall retraction as well as a bladder blade for retraction of the bladder. (**b**) Bookwalter Retractor is the most versatile and can retract in all directions with many options for blades. It can thus be adjusted to the anatomy more easily. (**c**) Alexis Wound Retractor is useful for thick abdominal walls when limited visualization is needed or if an incision is meant to be kept small as in a mini-laparotomy. It provides 360° of retraction in all directions but is disposable and thus is just for single use

which consists of a plastic ring with hooks that grasp the labial folds or vaginal muciosa in order to obtain retraction at the introitus. A Bookwalter type of retractor (Bookwalter® Magrina II Retractor System) has also been developed for use in vaginal hysterectomy and is very useful to obtain stable, controlled retraction for efficient performance of a vaginal hysterectomy [13] (Fig. 57.4).

Laparoscopic Hysterectomy

For all the laparoscopic approaches to hysterectomy, including single port, mini-laparoscopy and robotic assisted laparoscopy, retraction is provided by insufflation of the peritoneal cavity, which creates space to work within the abdominal cavity without directly opening the abdominal wall. The Trendelenburg position then provides gravity

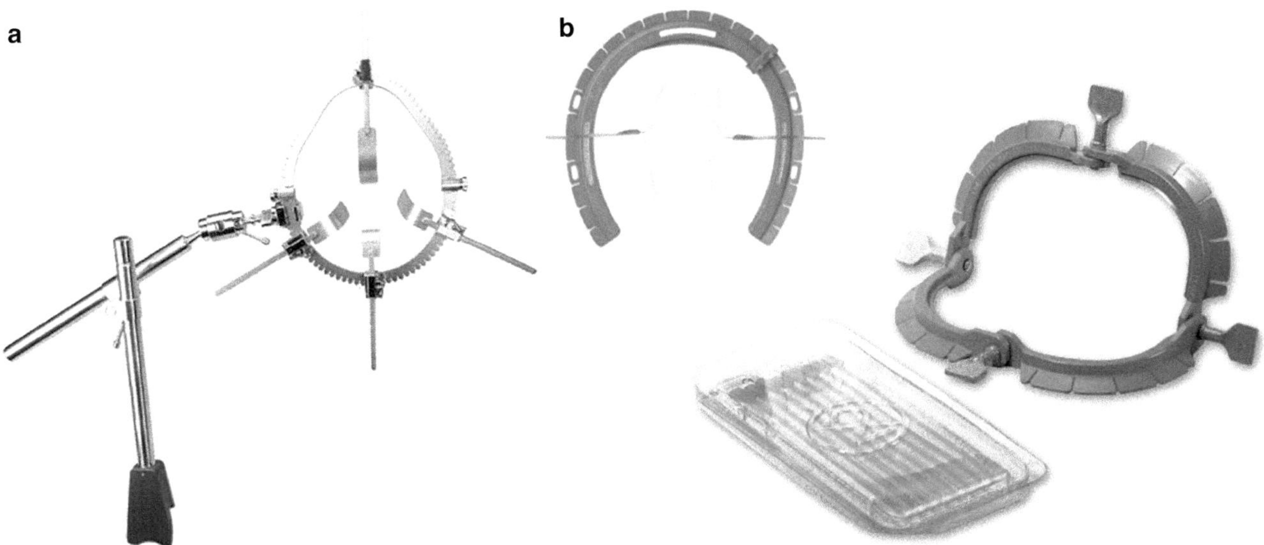

Fig. 57.4 Retractors for vaginal hysterectomy. (**a**) Bookwalter Magrina II Retractor System is similar to the abdominal bookwalter retractor but was developed specifically for vaginal hysterectomy providing adjustable blades in order to maximize visualization into the vagina. (**b**) Lonestar Vulvar Retractor is useful to enhance visualization during vaginal hysterectomy by using adjustable minimally traumatic hooks to retract away labia allowing easier access to the vagina

assisted retraction of the bowel while the uterine manipulator elevates the uterus allowing visualization and access to the uterus and surrounding structures for the performance of the hysterectomy. Passages through the abdominal wall then allow a camera to obtain visualization and instruments to be placed through the abdominal wall in order to perform the surgical procedure. Thus, the key is obtaining access to the intraperitoneal space, then placement of trochars through the abdominal wall, followed by utilizing an appropriate camera to provide visualization and an appropriate vaginal manipulator to provide manipulation and exposure of the vascular pedicles for the performance of the hysterectomy procedure [14].

None of the laparoscopic methods of hysterectomy differ on these two points but only differ on the size, number and location of the passages through the abdominal wall and the specific instruments used through these passages in order to perform the procedure. Thus, the advantages of each relate to the instruments used for the procedure since ultimately the end result of a hysterectomy is accomplished in a similar manner of isolating and sealing ovarian and uterine pedicles, transecting the uterus, removal of the specimen, and then closing the vaginal cuff if needed. All methods share the benefit of minimally access surgery for the patient including small scars and a fast recovery. The advantage of the robotic instrument relates to its precision, enhanced vision, and greater control, which allows more complex or difficult hysterectomies to be accomplished in a safe and efficient manner. Thus, patients who are morbidly obese, have extensive adhesions resulting from multiple prior surgeries or endometriosis, or have very large or obstructing fibroids may benefit from the surgeon choosing this instrument. For relatively straightforward hysterectomies in which the best cosmetic result is desired, either the vaginal, or mini-laparoscopic approach should be considered. If patients desire only a single incision then either single port laparoscopy or single port robotic assisted laparoscopic approach may be considered. Standard laparoscopy however remains the most utilized approach as all the other approaches are modifications of this approach and are highly dependent on the availability of specific instruments that facilitate the other approaches.

Initial Entry Techniques

Three forms of access or initial entry exist in Laparoscopy. Open (Hassan) technique, Veress Needle technique, and Direct entry. In the Open technique a disposable or re-usable trochar is placed directly into the peritoneal cavity after a small incision is made using retractors and a scalpel. The incision is then carried through the fascia and peritoneum. The Hassan cannula is then secured using sutures placed at the angles of the fascia and tied to the Hassan cannula. This technique can be useful if there is suspicion for severe adhesions or risk of adherence of bowel to the anterior abdominal wall. This method of entry is the method utilized in single port laparoscopy only a larger 1.5–3 cm incision is often needed. After this various single port access devices such as the Covidien SILSTM Port or the GELPORT by Applied Medical, and the Triport or Quadraport by Advanced Surgical Concepts are placed into the umbilical incision providing channels through which the instruments and the camera can then be introduced into the peritoneal cavity. Another option is to group small low profile laparoscopic trochars in a single incision made at the umbilicus [7] (Fig. 57.5).

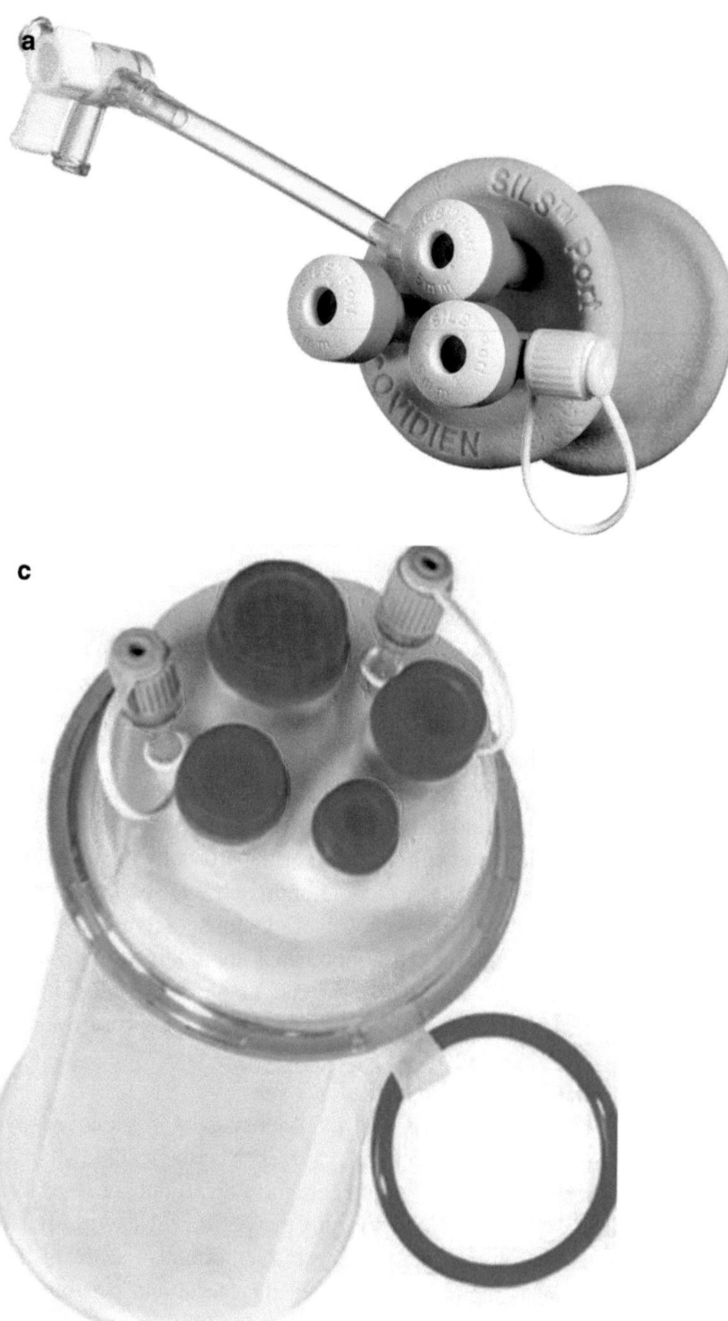

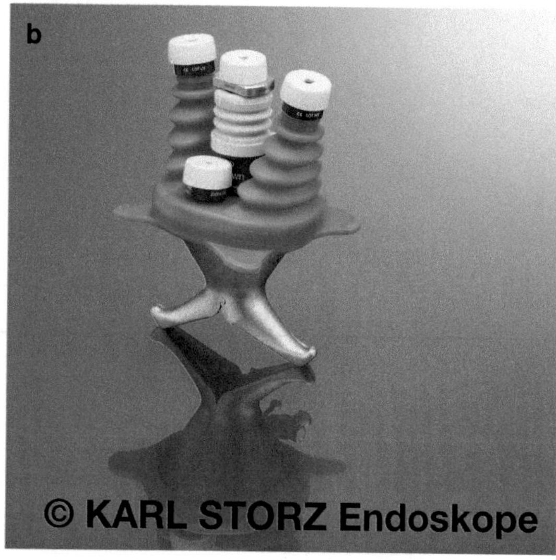

Fig. 57.5 Port options for single port or single incision Hysterectomy. (**a**) Covidien SILS Port has instrument ports built in with an insufflation access point laterally and an additional vent available for smoke evacuation. (**b**) Storz Single port system also has three active port as well as an insufflation port. Its advantage is that it is re-usable and similar to the Covidian port does not require additional trochar because instruments can be passed directly through the ports (©2015 Photo Courtesy of KARL STORZ Endoscopy-America, Inc.) (**c**) ASC Triport and quadraport by advanced surgical concepts is another disposable multi-instrument access port for single incision laparoscopic surgery requiring a 2.5 cm incision that allows up to four instruments to be used simultaneously. (**d**) The GelPOINT Advanced Access Platform by Applied Medical allows low profile ports to be placed through a gel port seal which thus gives greater versatility for port placement but may thus sometimes requires a slightly larger incision for access. However, he integral Alexis wound protector/retractor offers atraumatic retraction and protection for specimen removal

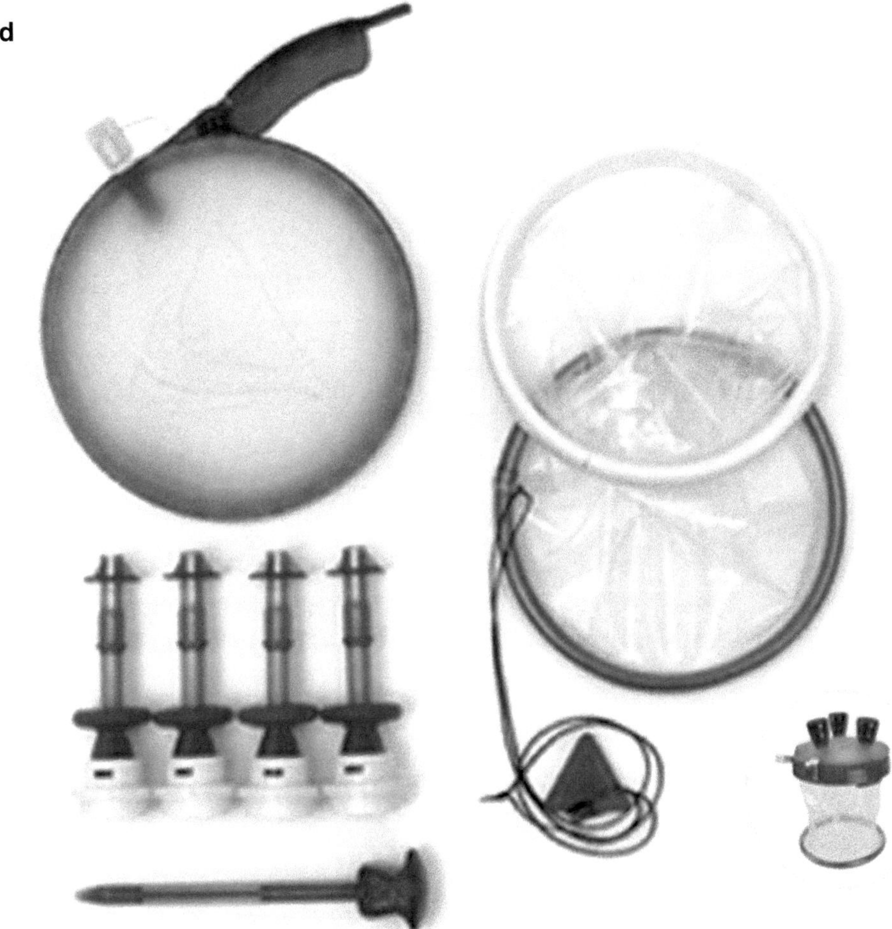

Fig. 57.5 (continued)

For robotic single port surgery access is obtained in the same manner as for laparoscopic single port surgery, but currently a special port and cannulas are used that then attach to the robotic instrument (Fig. 57.6). Prior to these cannulas and ports being developed specifically for this platform surgeons would use the straight robotic cannulas placed through a GELPORT access port placed at the umbilicus. The 8 mm robotic camera and 8 mm robotic instruments would then be introduced through the approximately 2.5–3 cm umbilical entry point, occasionally with a hybrid 5 mm assistant port. This allowed the surgeon to have some wristed movements but there were still some issues with instrument clashing and difficulty in triangulation around relevant anatomy. The subsequently released single port robotic platform reduced the size of the umbilical incision down to 1.5–2 cm with a port similar to the SILS port and reduced the diameter of the cannulas down to 5 mm and added a curved shape in order to improve triangulation. However, reducing the diameter of the instruments and allowing them to bend to follow the curve of the cannula removed the wristing feature from the instruments and thus greatly decreased the range of motion of the instruments as compared to the straight 8 mm robotic instruments. Recently a needle driver with 4° of movement has been developed in order to allow some increased range of motion to facilitate suturing.

In the Veress technique a disposable or re-usable Veress needle (Fig. 57.7) is introduced into the peritoneal cavity via the umbilicus or left upper quadrant at Palmer's point in order to obtain insufflation of the peritoneal cavity with CO_2 gas prior to the introduction of initial cannula and trochar. The purpose of insufflation is to tense the abdominal wall and create a distance between it and the bowel and blood vessels with the intention of making an introduction of the blind trochar easier and safer. However, there is no concrete evidence that this technique reduces initial entry tochar injury. Initial trochar may then consist of a re-usable trochar with a sharp tip versus various configurations of re-usable trochars with bladed, blunt, or spreading tips. The advantage of spreading tips which are designed to spread rather than cut the muscle and fascia fibers is to reduce trauma to these fibers and reduce the size of the remaining defect once the cannula is removed. This may reduce pain at the trochar site and risk of hernia

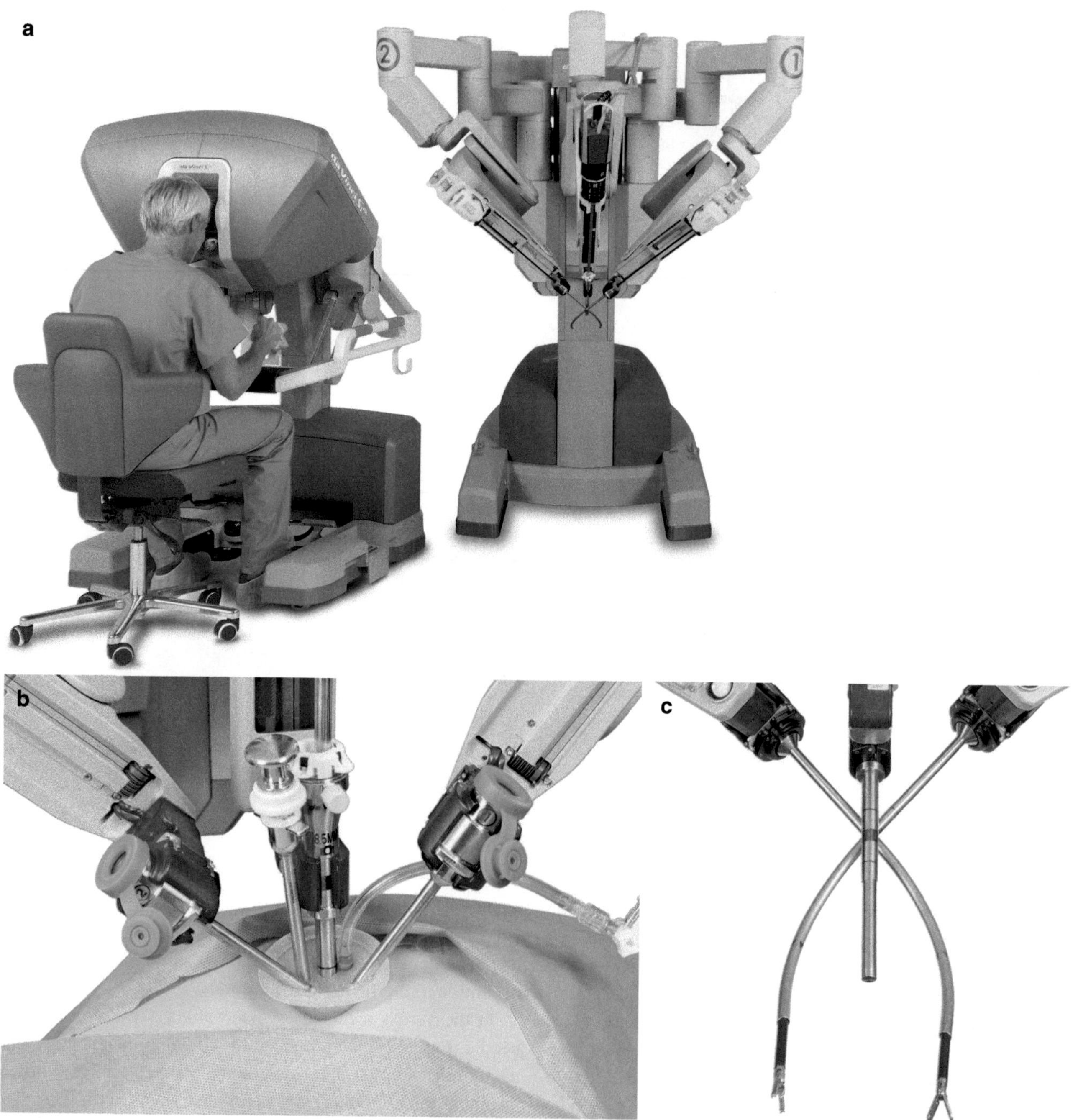

Fig. 57.6 Single port platform for DaVinci Robot. (**a**) The Si and Xi daVinci Systems have the possibility of use with a single port platform, which consists of a five-lumen SILS access port through which instruments and camera pass and cross. Remote center technology minimizes cannula collisions, arm interferences and port-site movement while the daVinci System software corrects for the crossing in order to intuitively coordinate the surgeon's hands with the instruments movements. (**b**) The five lumen port is placed through a 1.5–2 cm incision and provides access for two 5 mm curved instrument cannula, through which two semi-rigid 5 mm instruments pass, as well as the regular 8.5 mm 3D endoscope as well as a 5/10 mm accessory assistant port and the insufflation adaptor. (**c**) The curved architecture of the instrument cannulas allow the semi-rigid instruments to curve in order to optimize triangulation while minimizing external collision and crowding of instruments

formation. Some of the disposable trochars available include the possibility of visual entry via a camera channel within the trochar which allows the surgeon to visualize the layers of the abdominal wall as they are penetrated. The Versastep system includes a Veress needle with a sheath surrounding it, which may then be dilated using a blunt trochar allowing a completely blunt entry into the peritoneal cavity after access is secured with the needle at the site of needle placement. The only re-usable spreading visual entry trochar is the Ternamian trochar with a screw like blunt entry through the abdominal

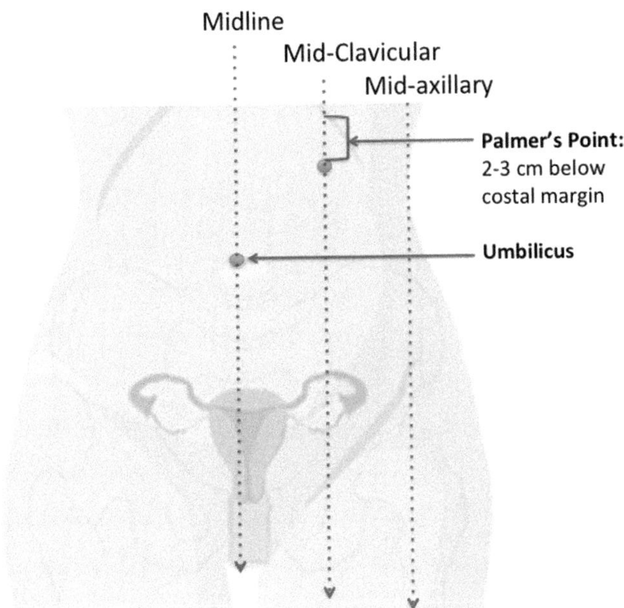

Fig. 57.7 Veress needle and points of entry. Palmer's point is 2–3 cm below left costal margin in Mid-clavicular line may be utilized if adhesions are suspected at umbilicus from prior surgeries. Contraindications to utilizing Palmer's point include right upper quadrant surgery such as prior gastrectomy or splenectomy

wall which allows the layers to be visualized as the trochar is screwed through them thus spreading the fibers [15].

The final method of entry into the peritoneal cavity is direct entry through the umbilicus without prior insufflation. In this method the abdominal wall is elevated via superior traction with the surgeons non-dominant hand or towel clip and the initial trochar is introduced directly into the peritoneal cavity either using a visual entry blunt-tipped or non-visual entry sharp disposable or re-usable trochar. Access is then confirmed via introduction of the camera, followed by insufflation through the port. In all methods, once access with initial trochar is obtained remaining trochars may then be introduced under direct visualization.

In robotic surgery, since the camera port can often be above the umbilicus, especially in the case of the large fibroid uterus extending above the level of the umbilicus, this needs to be taken into account when deciding on entry technique. Thus, open entry or the Hassan technique may not be optimal as it is more difficult to use the open technique above the umbilicus. Few surgeons are comfortable with direct entry above the umbilicus, and thus when a supra-umbilical camera port is desired most surgeon's will insufflate using a Veress needle, then either place the camera port first and then introduce remaining ports under direct vision. The author's preferred method is to place a 5 mm left upper quadrant visual entry port after insufflation and then use this port to survey the pelvis and decide on locations of both the robotic camera port and robotic re-usable ports dependent on the pathology. This is preferred as by optimizing camera and robotic ports according to pathology in difficult cases, one can obtain maximal vision and range of motion and prevent clashing of instrument arms or restriction of movement. As in other single-port procedures, single port robotic assisted procedures utilize open entry at the umbilicus and this location cannot be varied for the pathology, which is one of the limitations of single port surgery in general.

In mini-laparoscopy, small mini-laparoscopy ports measuring less than 3 mm in diameter are introduced laterally or in the suprapubic location after the initial camera port is placed at the umbilicus. Some mini-laparoscopy instruments measuring 2.5 mm in diameter do not require cannulas and are introduced directly through the skin into the peritoneal cavity. Generally, the initial port will consist of a 5 or 10 mm camera port placed at the umbilicus and mini-instruments are used laterally unless the small 3 mm mini-scope is available in which case this mini-scope is placed at the initial entry point.

As outlined above, the choice of type of entry and trochar type and tip is extremely surgeon specific. However, all surgeons should understand the different types of trochars that exist including advantages and disadvantages of each when selecting their preferred method of entry, torchar type and placement location [15]. After a preferred method is chosen, the surgeon should utilize this method as much as possible and only vary as needed for the case, as repetition prevents injury and several studies have shown that the highest rates of entry related complications occur immediately after changing a trochar type or entry method used by the surgeon. Figures 57.8 and 57.9 highlight the differences in access ports as well as port locations for the various approaches.

Visualization

Camera and scope technology are continuously evolving leading to the development of smaller, more maneuverable visualization tools that provide significantly improved vision while performing surgical procedures. Currently, laparoscopic scopes are available in the 10, 5, and 3 mm sizes (Fig. 57.9) and the 10 and 5 mm laparoscopes are available in either the 0 or 30° fields of view. The 30° increases the field of view in order to look around, above, or underneath structures and is most useful when operating deep in the pelvis with deep endometriosis or when performing hysterectomy for a very large uterus. The 3 mm camera by Storz is most useful in the performance of mini-laparoscopic hysterectomy, or for initial survey from the left upper quadrant in complex cases in which entry at palmer's point is preferred. Camera's with a flexible tip are (Fig. 57.9) available through Olympus are most useful for single port hysterectomy as they allow the camera tip to bend in order to obtain a better view for triangulation so that a surgeon's hand do not clash with the camera. It is also useful for NOTES procedures in which a Natural Orifice is used for introduction of the scope. Since one of the main advantages of robotic surgery includes the 3D HD

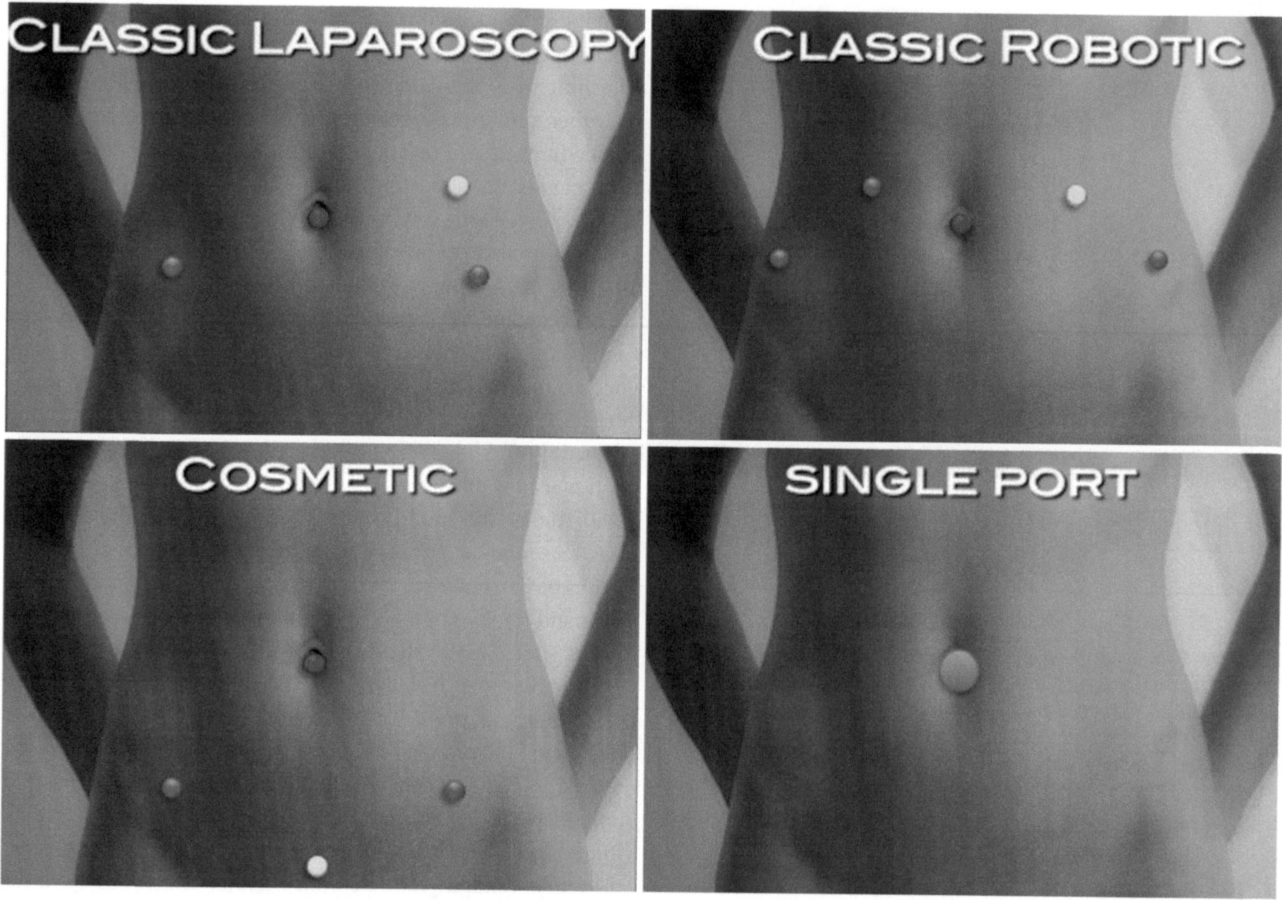

Fig. 57.8 Port placement in laparoscopic, robotic, single port, and mini-laparoscopy procedures. In Classic Laparoscopic hysterectomy four 5–10 mm ports are place as shown, although the accessory port (*yellow*) may vary in placement to opposite side or to the suprapubic area depending on surgeon preference. In classic robotic surgery port placement is usually in an M configuration or slight arc varied according to the pathology. Laparoscopic or robotic procedures can be made more cosmetic by lowering lateral ports or placing them more ultra laterally. However, the wristed instruments of the robotic platform make these more cosmetic port locations much easier to use with the wristed instruments of the robotic platform. Single port or single incision procedures always utilize the umbilicus. The incision incision is usually larger than laparoscopic ports measuring 2–3 cm and thus has a higher rate of herniation and wound complications. The advantage of mini-laparoscopy is that ports are only 2–3 mm and thus do not need closure and produce very minimal scars and have little to no risk of hernia formation

magnified vision for the surgeon, some companies such as Olympus have released a 3D laparoscopic scope and camera in order to provide a similar view for the laparoscopic surgeon. However, it does not duplicate the magnification and the complete immersion in the three dimensional environment provided by the surgeon console in robotic procedures.

Exposure and Uterine Manipulation

Uterine manipulators with a colpotomizer are a very important part of any of the laparoscopic approaches to hysterectomy, whether traditional laparoscopy, mini-laparoscopy, or robotic assisted laparoscopy. The uterine manipulator fulfills many functions (Table 57.2). However, the main purpose of the uterine manipulator is exposure. It assists in the elevation and movement of the uterus upwards and out of the pelvis to help provide exposure to the uterine vasculature and bladder flap while increasing the distance away from the ureters in order to avoid direct or indirect injury. This increases the safety of a laparoscopic hysterectomy. In addition, the colpotomy ring, cup, or blade can be used to push the ureters more laterally, and the uterine artery superiorly, while delineating the junction between the cervix and the vaginal fornices tenting them upwards. Tenting the vaginal fornices upwards will provide the necessary exposure aiding in the dissection of the bladder flap and cervicovaginal fasica as well as delineating the site for colpotomy incision at the apex of the vagina such that the incision will not shorten the vagina significants. This also provides the tissue tension required to swiftly make the colpotomy incision with minimal energy in order to avoid tissue necrosis and complications such as cuff cellulitis or dehiscence [16].

Many different uterine manipulators exist including some that are disposable, reusable, or have both re-usable and disposable components (Figs. 57.10 and 57.11). Some have straight handles and others are arched or curved. Arched manipulators allow the user to follow the arc of the sacrum

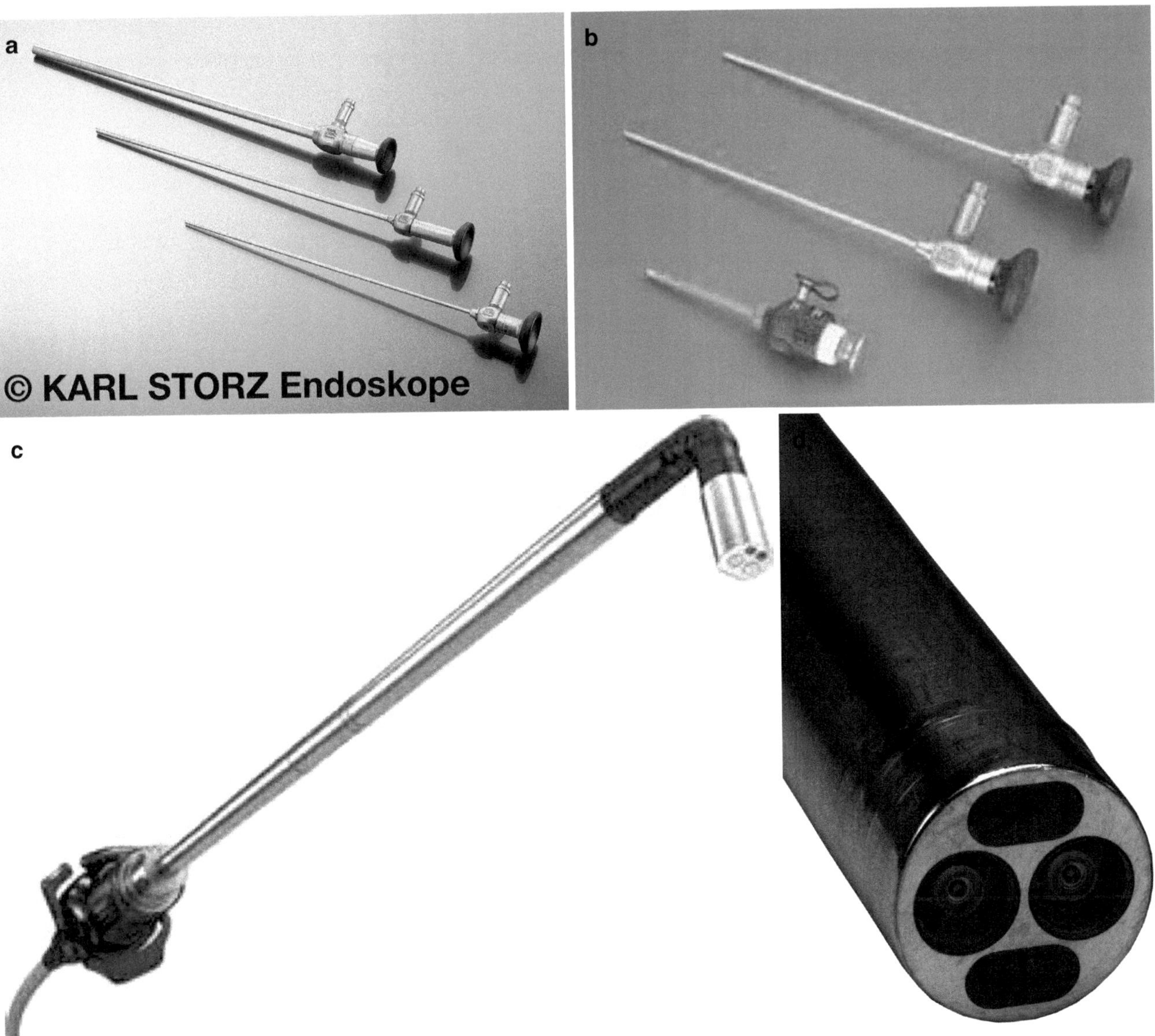

Fig. 57.9 Various cameras and scopes utilized in laparoscopic, robotic, single port, and mini-laparoscopy procedures. (**a**) Traditional laparoscopic Ports come in either 5 or 10 mm scopes providing a 0 or 30° scope angle. Bariatric 30° scopes assist with larger pathology or in single port procedures in order to move the camera away from other instruments to prevent clashing. ©2015 Photo Courtesy of KARL STORZ Endoscopy-America, Inc. (**b**) Mini-laparoscopy scopes are also now available measuring a mere 3.5 mm diameter, which is very useful in simpler or diagnostic procedures in which minimization of the port site may be desired. (**c**) Olympus has developed an articulating 5 mm scope as well as an articulating 5 mm 3-D scope designed for optimal visualization for singe port or notes procedures. (**d**) The scope providing the best visualization for precise intricate surgery is the scope and camera designed for the DaVinci Robotic instrument. This scope provides extremely detailed High definition vision utilizing both a right eye and a left eye in order to give the surgeon a 10X magnified 3D view inside the patient at the surgeon console. The camera is controlled by the surgeon from the surgeon console providing optimal control. With the newest Xi system the camera also has newer features of auto focus, auto white balance, and instant switch from 30° up to 30° down view. The camera can also now be placed at any position and be controlled by any of the robotic arms which greatly facilitates multi-quadrant surgery

and thus manipulate in a more anatomical fashion allowing for maximal elevation of the uterus out of the pelvis and away from the ureters. Straight manipulators, may be assisted by (articulation) in order to antevert or retrovert the uterus for exposure. Metal manipulators are sturdier and thus are less likely to bend or break with a larger uterus or severely deformed or deviated pathology such as in patients with large lower segment fibroids or severe endometriosis. [17].

In the United States the two most commonly used uterine manipulators for laparoscopic hysterectomy are V-care, which is entirely disposable, and Cooper Surgical's uterine manipulators including the Rumi, Rumi arch, Rumi II, and Advincula arch manipulators which work with a Koh ring and disposable tips. Recently the Koh ring has been incorporated into a back-loading disposable piece which also incorporated the vaginal occluder balloon. One of the advantages of the Rumi and Arch

Table 57.2 Functions of the uterine manipulator

Functions of the uterine manipulator [11, 13]
Mobilizes the uterus including anteversion, retroversion, lateral and elevation movements
Clearly identifies and distends the vaginal fornices to enable a circular incision of the vaginal apex
Elevates and defines the cervico-vaginal junction to enable a safer dissection of the vesico-uterine fold and fascia
Enables the elevation of the uterus upwards in the abdomen, in order to obtain a good visualization of the uterine artery and its elevation above the ureter
Maintains pneumoperitoneum during colpotomy
Raises the uterus and brings it closer to the laparoscopic surgical instruments, facilitating the procedure
Manipulates the uterus, thus stretching and presenting the side being operated upon
Increases the distance between the uterus and the bladder, the ureters, and the rectum, thus reducing the chance of injury
Can be used pull the uterus out vaginally after its complete detachment
Facilitates the identification of the uterovesical peritoneum, the cul-de-sac, and the vaginal cuff just below the cervical attachment

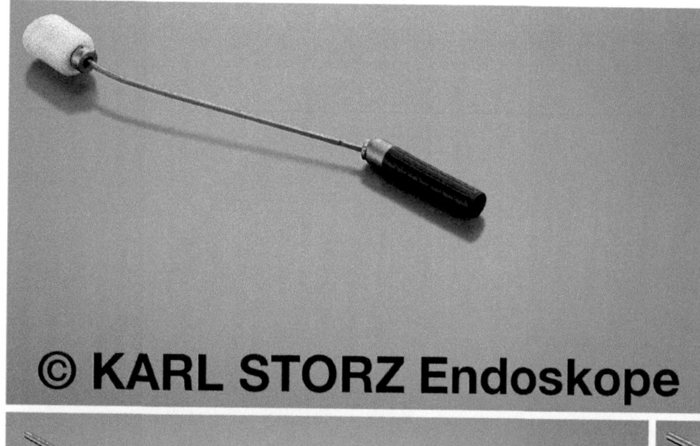

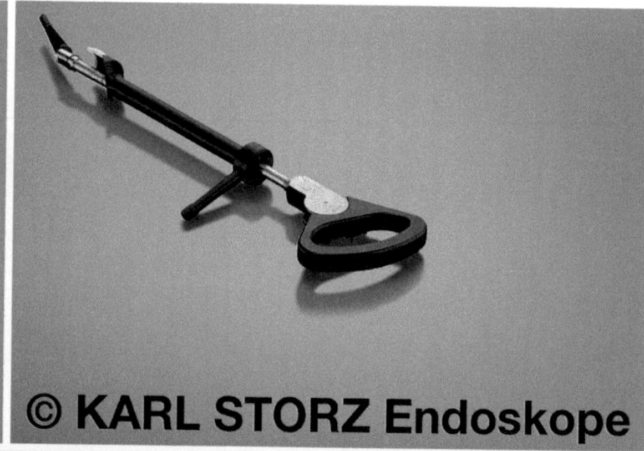

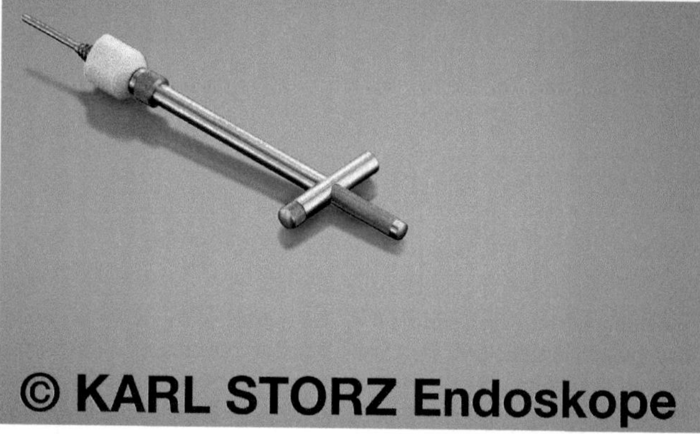

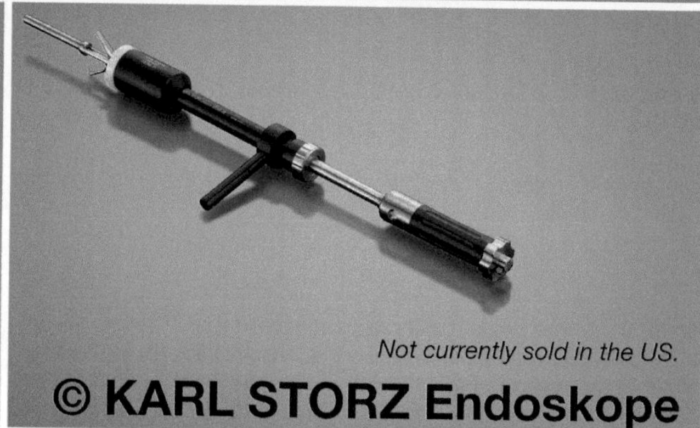

Fig. 57.10 Examples of re-usable uterine manipulators. Many different re-usable uterine manipulators that consist of a manipulator portion and a colpotomizer system exist. Some examples include the Donnez, Clermont-Ferrand, Hohl and Mangeshikar uterine manipulators sold by Storz. Some of the features of these manipulators are reviewed in Table 57.4 (©2015 Photo Courtesy of KARL STORZ Endoscopy-America, Inc)

manipulators is that they are attachable to Copper Surgical's Uterine Positioning System (UPS) (Fig. 57.12). This device attaches to the operating room bed and holds the manipulator firmly in position using a hydraulic system which allows the manipulator to be moved in any direction and then holds the position without drifting. This precludes the need for a vaginal assistant to constantly hold and push up on the manipulator and affords the surgeon several advantages, especially in more complicated, difficult, or long cases. First, the surgeon can personally position the uterus as desired at any time, knowing that the position will not change. Second, it provides stability such that there is no drifting downwards as occurs when the assistant fatigues which often places the ureter at risk. Third by stabilizing and securing the anatomy, the surgeon can focus on dissection of the important anatomical structures without the position changing as the surgeon is working near or around the uterus [18].

Many other disposable manipulators exist including ones with a lighted ring in order to aid colpotomy. However, in Europe and other areas of the world re-usable manipulators predominate in an attempt to limit disposable instruments utilized in surgical procedures. Many re-usable manipulators

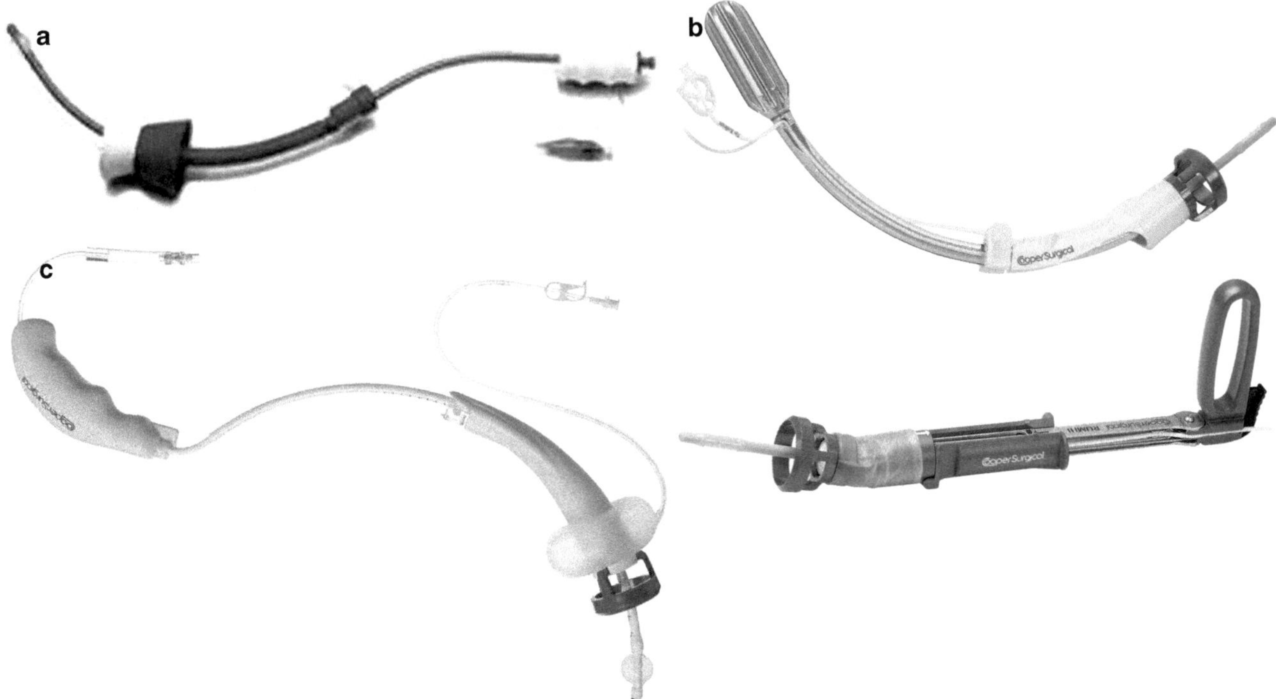

Fig. 57.11 Examples of disposable or partially disposable uterine manipulators. (**a**) V-Care uterine manipulator is fully disposable and has three cup sizes. It is shaped as an S shape for easier manipulation. (**b**) Copper surgical utilizes the Koh colpotomizer ring which is fenestrated and more cup shaped and thus provides clearer delineation of the colptomy site and lateralizes the ureter away from the uterine artery. The colpotomizer and occluder balloon section is disposable and comes in various sizes, as do the balloon tips which secure the uterus to the manipulator. Two manipulator bodies exist. One is a curved metal arc (Advincula Arch) which takes the curve of the vagina and is most useful for larger pathology. The other is the Rumi II system which allows anteversion and retroversion of the uterus via the handle. (**c**) Recently Cooper surgical has released a completely disposable version of the Advincula Arch which has the same advantaged of the KOH colpotomy ring and vaginal occluder balloon built in but has more of the S-shaped curve giving it easier handling for the user and less need for assembly. However, for larger pathology it may not be as sturdy as the metal arch

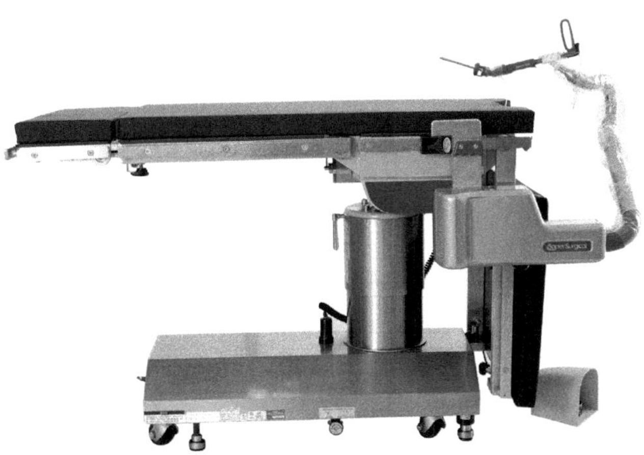

Fig. 57.12 Uterine positioning system. The uterine positioning system produced by Cooper surgical is compatible with either the Advincula arch or Rumi uterine manipulators. It is a device which attaches to the operating room table and holds the uterine manipulator with a hydraulic arm which remains fixed in place until the surgeon changes the position using a foot-pedal to release the hold. This allows the surgeon to position the uterine manipulator and uterus into any position and fixes it in place so that it does not drift or move. This thus takes the place of a vaginal assistant and allows the surgeon precise control of the uterus which greatly assists in difficult laparoscopic or robotic hysterectomy procedures

Table 57.3 Factors to consider in choosing a uterine manipulator

Factor for consideration	Ideal quality
Cost	Re-usable preferred
Ease of assembly	Minimal number of parts
Material	Metal or indestructible material
Range of motion	Pivoting head or arched shape
Placement into uterus	Easy placement with minimal cervical dilation required
Fixation into uterus	Method of fixation into uterus
Adjustability	Variable tip lengths and cup sizes to adjust for size of the uterus and cervix
Delineation of vaginal fornices	Circular cup or ring preferred over rotating valve
Vaginal occlusion	Method of occlusion to prevent loss of pneumoperitoneum

are present on the market. All share similar components of a method of fixation to the uterus, a cervical cup for delineation of fornices, and a method of vaginal occlusion. Most are straight rather than curved and several have the capability of anteversion and retroversion of the uterus. Table 57.3 lists some factors that should be taken into consideration when evaluating a uterine manipulator while Table 57.4 provides a comparison of some of the uterine manipulators available.

Table 57.4 Comparison of uterine manipulators

Manipulator	Re-usable	Number of parts	Pivoting head	Shape	Variable tip lengths	Method of fixation in uterus	Number fornix delineator sizes	Method of delineation of fornix
V-care	No	1	No	S-Shape	Yes	Balloon	4	Ridged cone
Rumi II	Partial	3	Yes	Straight	Yes	Balloon	4	Fenestrated cup
Advincula Arch	Partial	3	No	Arched	Yes	Balloon	4	Fenestrated cup
Donnez	Yes	3	No	Slight Curve	No	None	3	Cap
Clermont-Ferrand	Yes	6	Yes	Straight		Screw	3	Rod
Konninckx	Yes	4	Yes	Straight	No	Intrauterine clamp	1	Rotating cap
Hohl	Yes	4	No	Straight	Yes	Screw	3	Curved cap
Mangeshikar	Yes	6	No	Straight	Yes	Forceps	5	Cap
Minneli	Yes	4	No	Straight		Screw	3	Rotating valve

Ultimately cost and a surgeon's preferences determine which manipulator is used during a case [17].

Instruments for Dissection and Hemostasis

In general terms, a Hysterectomy has three components:

1. Isolation, sealing, and ligation of either the utero-ovarian or infundibulopelvic ligament depending on desire for ovarian preservation
2. Isolation, sealing, and ligation of uterine vasculature
3. Colpotomy or uterine amputation dependent on desire to preserve the cervix, followed by assurance of hemostasis and closure of openings including the vaginal cuff if needed.

All three components require dissection of the two vascular bundles, the bladder flap, and cervical vaginal fascia and transection with hemostasis of the two vascular bundles at the uterine isthmus and the adnexa [19].

Abdominal Hysterectomy

The standard instruments for surgeons are a clamp, scissors, and suture for ligation, and forceps and a needle driver for suturing. Thus, in abdominal hysterectomy, the clamp traditionally used is the Heaney clamp. However, the Seppelin clamp is more frequently used in oncologic procedures as the Z-configuration of clamp minimizes tissue slippage and need for a pedicle so that the cut can be made directly on the clamp with scissors or a scalpel. The neeldle driver tends to be a long handled but heavy needle driver in order to drive bites of suture through thicker ligaments such as the cardinal or uterosacral ligaments, and then used later for closure of the vaginal cuff which also consists of thick tissue and fascia. A monopolor current via bovie, is often used for dissection, cutting, and hemostasis while vasclular bundles are ligated generally using suture unless hand-held advanced bipolar instruments are used as an alternative. Vaginal hysterectomy is similarly performed but in the reverse order with dissection performed again with a scalpel, scissors, and bovie, while division of vascular pedicles is performed using a curved Heaney clamp to clamp, curved mayo scissors to cut, and a Heaney needle driver to suture the pedicles and for vaginal cuff closure.

Vaginal Hysterectomy

Since the advent of Laparoscopic surgery, many devices for dissection, hemostasis, and advanced vessel sealing have been developed and are even now slowly being incorporated into abdominal and vaginal procedures secondary to ease of use and speed of control of vascular pedicles. The main goal of energy devices is to seal vessels and attain hemostasis with or without cutting of the pedicle. Since exposure is usually adequate in abdominal surgery, there is little need to avoid the traditional clamp, cut, and tie rhythm. Thus, in abdominal hysterectomy, using these devices may add expense and save an insignificant amount of time. However, for difficult vaginal hysterectomies and in the vagina in general, where exposure is limited, a vessel sealing device can ease the procedure as it is often difficult to suture and tie pedicles in the tight vaginal space. Therefore, utilization of either a re-usable or disposable energy vessel sealing and cutting device may be advantageous. All are shaped similar to the curved Heaney clamp and thus may be applied in a similar manner to seal and divide the uterosacral or cardinal ligaments, followed by the uterine artery and broad ligaments, then either the infundibulopelvic or utero-ovarian ligaments in order to remove or preserve the ovaries. Re-usable devices include

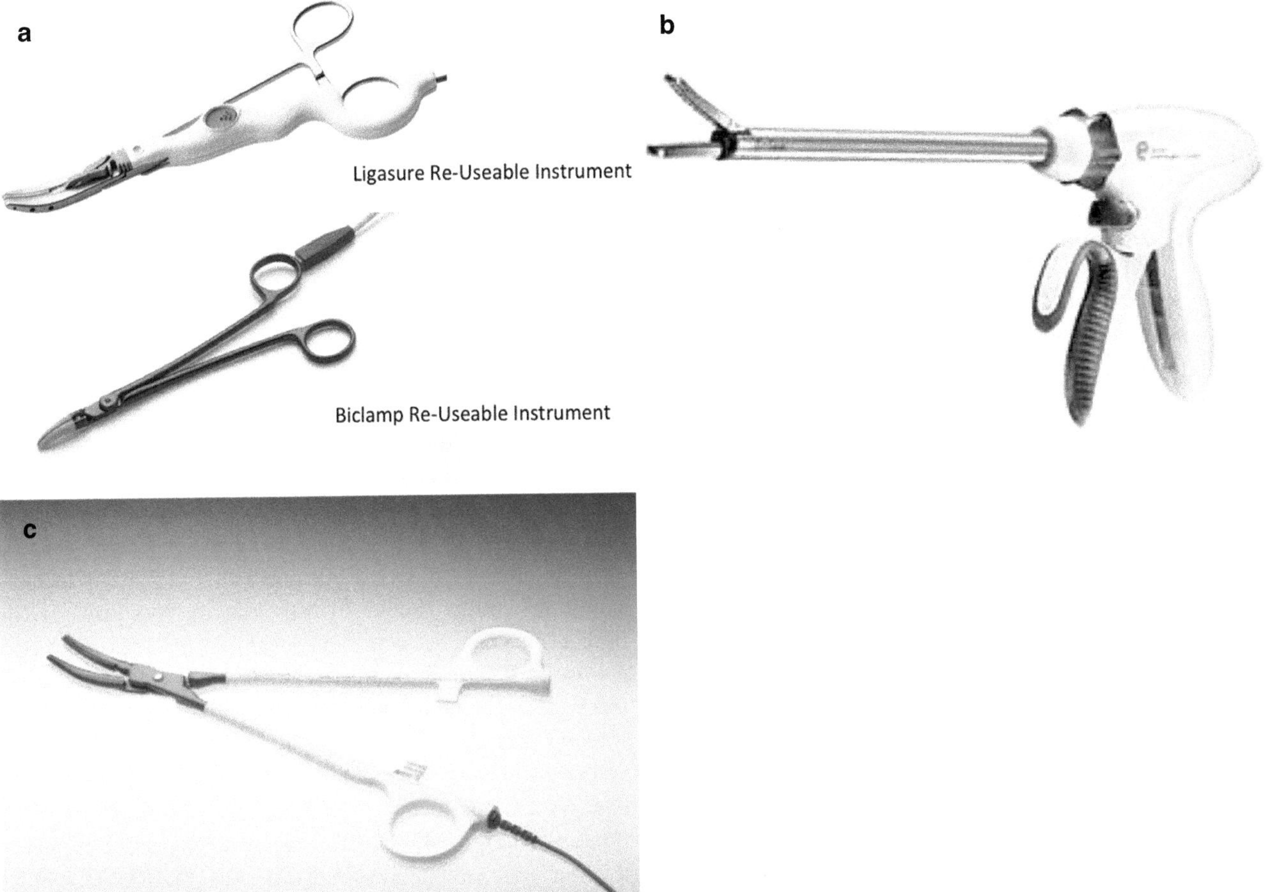

Fig. 57.13 Energy devices for vaginal hysterectomy. Bipolar instruments can be useful for expediting vaginal hysterectomy, used to seal vessels instead of suturing. (**a**) Re-usable instruments like the Ligasure or Biclamp are the most economic but only seal without seal and cut features. (**b**) Disposable instruments exist with the Enseal allowing sealing and cutting to occur simultaneously. (**c**) One of the first disposable instruments which was also used for vessel sealing in vaginal hysterectomy was the PKS Seal open forceps

the Biclamp or re-usable Ligasure devices, both of which have advance bipolar energy with Ligasure also utilizing additional pressure for vessel sealing. Disposable devices include the Gyrus SEAL, ENSEAL, and the Disposable Ligasure (Fig. 57.13). The Gyrus was the original advanced bipolar device using PK energy, followed by Ligasure and then the ENSEAL. Both Ligasure and Enseal utilize pressure, heat, and advanced bipolar energy to seal and cut the vessels. As the blade in Enseal applies pressure as it cuts, the pressure is more evenly distributed rather than decreasing near the tip as in Ligasure. However, Ligasure, like the Gyrus SEAL allows the surgeon to seal without cutting, thus providing the surgeon with more control [20]. Hysterectomy by using them to seal vascular pedicles instead of suture ligation. Re-usable instruments like the Ligasure or the Biclamp are overall the most economical but only seal without seal and cut features. The disposable Enseal allows sealing and cutting to occur simultaneously but this can be a disadvantage if the seal is not complete and does cost more per case. The PK seal open forceps was one of the first disposable instruments used for vessel sealing in vaginal hysterectomy but did not have the same cut feature as the PK used in laparoscopy. Thus, when choosing a device the advantages and disadvantages of each must be considered.

Laparoscopic Hysterectomy

Advanced Laparoscopic Surgeries such as total laparoscopic or supracervical hysterectomy have really been revolutionized by the advanced energy vessel sealing devices that have been developed for laparoscopy. The original energy utilized in Laparoscopy was monopolar energy, which is most useful for cutting (rather than sealing) such as in the use of monopolar scissors. Bipolar energy allowed passage of energy between the two blades of a grasper or forceps such as a Maryland and thus became utilized for coagulation of vessels in hysterectomy procedures. However, inadequate sealing of vessels secondary to charring and desiccation of tissue surrounding the vessel which did not allow adequate passage of energy into the center of the vessel. This often resulted in inadequate sealing of the vessel and either immediate or delayed bleeding. In addition, other problems included lateral thermal spread to surrounding tissue, and sticking of the vessels and tissue to the clamp used to apply the energy with surface charring of the tissue. Thus, their use was limited especially when desiring to seal larger vessels. For this reason, early developers of the total laparoscopic hysterectomy procedure such as Harry Reich, would often suture uterine vessels rather than trying to seal them with energy [21]. Modern laparoscopic vessel sealing devices were later developed and have greatly facilitated the performance of laparoscopic hysterectomies. These devices may be categorized into advanced bipolar or ultrasonic energy devices or a combination of the two. All devices effectively seal vessels up to 7 mm in diameter and some have built in tissue transection capabilities. A comparison of these devices is provided in Table 57.5.

The first advanced bipolar energy system was the plasmakinetic pulsed bipolar system named the PK Gyrus (Olympus). It had an impedance dependent feedback-controlled method of delivery pulsed bipolar energy to the tissue causing vapor pulse coagulation induced sealing of vessels upto 7 mm in diameter. The intermittent and automatically adjusted pulses of bipolar energy produced by the plasma kinetic generator cause minimal lateral thermal spread and prevented sticking of tissue to the plasma kinetic forceps blades after coagulation. The Gyrus then offered a sharp blade for cutting the sealed pedicle with a hand control. The PK energy type could also be used with a dissecting forcep, spatula, needle-point, and hook in order to avoid the need for mono-polar energy during a case.

Other advanced bipolar devices include Ligasure, Bicision, and EnSeal. Advanced bipolar devices possess active feedback control over the power output, adjusting the energy according to the measured impedance of the tissue between the blades. Heat production is kept below 100 °C and the energy is pulsed to allow cooling [22]. However, there is no simultaneous tissue division and a cutting blade or mechanism is required for division or transection of the sealed vessel or tissue. Ultrasonic devices such as the ACE harmonic scalpel combine both the sealing and cutting steps into a single process and thus may increase dissection speed. However, the literature had reported that ultrasonic devices can create temperatures of up to 200 °C which can potentially put adjacent tissue at risk to lateral damage [21]. This concern has been partially addressed by adding a Teflon coating in newer ACE Harmonic devices which may decrease the peak temperature of the device.

Although many comparative studies have been performed, neither type of device has been proven superior. In general terms however, advanced bipolar devices ultimately produce less heat than ultrasonic devices. Both advanced bipolar and ultrasonic devices efficiently seal vessels ($\leq$7 and $\leq$5-mm diameter, respectively), and most also have built-in tissue transection capabilities. Bipolar devices are said to seal slightly larger vessels but do not seal and cut simultaneously or as efficiently as ultrasonic energy. Ultrasonic energy is best known for efficient dissection reflected by its ability to use the device in a cutting mode, and low lateral thermal spread to adjacent tissue. However, the device itself reaches higher temperatures and remains at this high temperature for an extended period resulting in initial concern of a higher rate of thermal injury to the ureter or bowel during hysterectomy procedures [23]. All Ultrasonic energy devices are disposable, as are most advanced bipolar energy devices, and thus add to the cost of the procedure. A reusable Biclamp using and Erbe generator is available and is frequently used in Europe for laparoscopic as well as vaginal hysterectomy as it is available in both a Maryland dissector and standard bipolar Forceps tips for use in laparoscopic hysterectomy. For vaginal hysterectomy it had a heavy ridged curved clamp similar to the Haney Clamp.

Only one device combines both bipolar and ultrasonic energy in order to try to combine the advantages of both types of energy [24]. The Thunderbeat (Olympus, Japan) is the first device to integrate both ultrasonically generated frictional heat energy and advanced bipolar energy in one instrument. This multifunctional device can interchangeably deliver the energies via two separate control buttons allowing the surgeon to favor advanced bipolar energy for sealing larger vessels and surface coagulation, while ultrasonic energy is preferred for quick cutting and sealing. The jaw is designed in a thin dissector design facilitating tissue dissection and increasing the multifunctional uses of the instrument.

Two publications involving animal models using this newer device compared the Thunderbeat with other commercially available energy devices in the market, namely, Harmonic Ace (Ethicon Endo-Surgery, USA), LigaSure (Covidien, USA), and EnSeal (Ethicon Endo-Surgery, USA) in the porcine model [24]. Compared with the other three devices, the Thunderbeat showed faster dissection speed, similar bursting pressure, and similarly acceptable thermal spread. The device was proven to be safe in cutting, coagulating, and tissue dissection. In another experiment led by Seehofer et al. [25] the Thunderbeat was compared to the Harmonic Ace and LigaSure in a pig model. Temperature profile, seal failures, maximum burst pressure, and cutting speed were measured. In this study, the Thunderbeat was faster than Harmonic Ace in terms of dissection while equaled the sealing efficacy of the LigaSure with a similar heat production.

Table 57.5 Comparison of advanced bipolar devices used in laparoscopy

Device	Energy type	Description	Positive features	Negative features
PK Gyrus (Olympus)	Plasma kinetic technology (Advanced bipolar)	Delivers a high current and very low voltage to the tissue. A series of rapid pulses allows a cooling phase decreasing lateral thermal spread	Holds onto the tissue being desiccated without slipping or sticking	Disposable
			A blade can be manually deployed through the forceps to transect tissue	Jaws can be traumatic
			Facilitates Dissection	Unreliable on vessels >7 mm
		The vessel is sealed by denaturing the protein within the vessel walls, forming a coagulum which occludes the lumen	Both a 5 and 10-mm version is available	Consistency somewhat dependent on user
			A Gyrus spatula is also available and can be used as both a cutting and coagulating instrument	
Ligasure (Covidien)	Advanced bipolar energy with pressure	Delivers high current, low voltage along with pressure from the jaws to tissue	Fast seal using combination of advanced bipolar energy and pressure	Disposable
			Compresses surrounding tissues to seal with the vessel	Hinders dissection secondary to bulky jaws and sealing of surrounding tissue
		The system monitors the energy expended while denaturing the collagen and elastin within the vessels walls. During the cooling phase of the cycle, cross-linking re-occurs creating a new seal	Both a 5 and 10 mm version is available	Unreliable on vessels >7 mm
				Pressure decreases near tip of the jaw
				Consistency less dependent on user
Enseal (Ethicon)	Advanced bipolar energy with pressure	Uses a bipolar electrode to concentrate energy on tissue within the plastic jaws of the instrument	Sealing using combination of advanced bipolar energy and pressure	Disposable
		Temperature sensitive matrix (nanopolar thermostats) within the jaws controls the energy delivered to the electrode-tissue interface	Easier to dissect with than Ligasure secondary to slim Jaws	Cutting may occur prior to adequate sealing as sealing is still occurring during cutting phase
			Has an articulating version which facilitates single port procedures and improves angles for vessel sealing	Unreliable on vessels >7 mm
		Pulsing of energy according to temperature allows cooling		Proper use requires a certain level of surgical skill thus is surgeon dependent
				Less efficient than some other devices
BiClamp (Erbe)	Advanced bipolar	A bipolar electrosurgical current produced by the ERBE VIO system ,with an optimally adjusted waveform, voltage and current density is applied and the tissue is coagulated and sealed	Tissue structures can be coagulated over larger areas and surgeon has greater control over width of area coagulated that seal and cut devices	Is a seal only device, therefore requires a separate instrument (usually laparoscopic scissors) for cutting once the vessel is sealed. This may decrease efficiency of the procedure
		The particular features of the ERBE BiClamp create a parchment-like coagulation seam during bipolar coagulation, thus sealing the vessel	Highly economical as the ERBE BiClamp is reusable	
			Auto stop and plug and play feature is user-friendly and adjusts automatically for different procedures	

(continued)

Table 57.5 (continued)

Device	Energy type	Description	Positive features	Negative features
Harmonic ACE (Ethicon)		High frequency ultrasonic transducer with active titanium blade vibrates at 55,000 cycles per second	Fast seal and cut	High external temperature
		Mechanical energy causes a breakdown of protein creating a coagulum. Vessel and tissue sealing is dependent on the power setting as well as the pressure exerted and the tissue tension	Low lateral thermal spread	Vessel sealing ideal <5 mm
			5 mm instrument	Poor reliability on vessels ≤7 mm
			Good for efficient dissection	
		A straight and curved blade is available	Lower working temperature causes less charring and sticking	Consistency is highly dependent on the user
			Variability of energy delivered can be adjusted by the surgeon ,depending on the need and tissue being transected	
			The active bade can also be used as a cutting knife useful for colpotomy	
Thunderbeat (Olympus)	Ultrasonic and advanced bipolar energy	Integrates both ultrasonically generated frictional heat energy and advanced bipolar energy in one instrument as a multifunctional device	Multifunctional device can interchangeably deliver the different energies	Disposable
			Allows the surgeon to simultaneously seal and cut vessels up to 7 mm in size with minimal thermal spread	Unreliable for vessels above 7 mm
			The jaw is designed to provide precise, controlled dissection and continuous bipolar support with grasping allowing for efficient dissection and hemostasis	Ease of use required practice and training of the surgeon

Specialized Laparoscopic Hysterectomy

For single port laparoscopic procedures, if an advanced energy device is desired for vessel ligation the surgeon must either try to present the vessels and tissue to the vessel sealer that they normally use for laparascopic hysterectomy or choose an articulating vessel sealing device. To date the only vessel sealer that is available with the ability to bend or articulate is the Enseal system by Covidien. The articulation of the instrument facilitates triangulation in single-port procedures.

In mini-laparoscopy, one of the main limitations to the performance of hysterectomy was the lack of bipolar energy devices. Thus, a 5 mm port was often utilized in a hybrid laparoscopic technique in either a "single port" or traditional laparoscopic orientation in order to seal the vascular pedicles. Storz has now released 3.5 mm ROBI Bipolar Graspers and Scissors providing energy application through a mini-laparoscopic port (Fig. 57.14). Other 2 or 2.5 mm instruments do not provide energy and thus mainly function as graspers, scissors, or dissectors but not as vessel sealers. As the energy devices advance in mini-laparoscopy instruments, it is likely that the performance of hysterectomies using "mini" ports will increase.

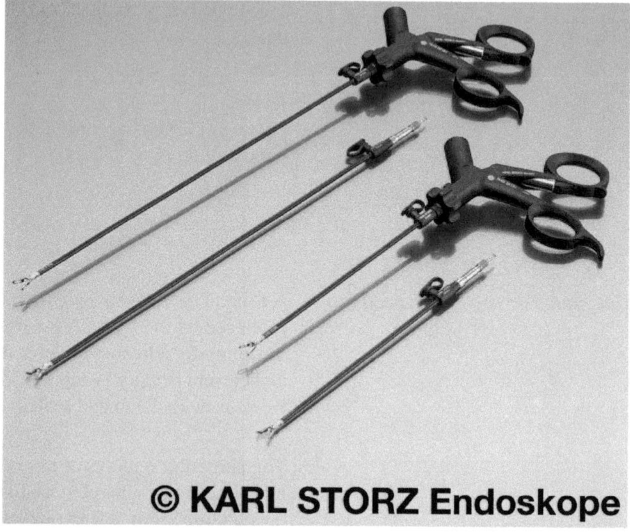

Fig. 57.14 ROBI bipolar graspers and scissors for mini-laparoscopy procedures. 3.5 mm instruments that allow bipolar energy application have been developed by KARL STORZ. These include graspers, dissectors and scissors. The ROBI bipolar grasper can be used to seal infundibulopelvic ligaments as well as uterine vasculature in laparoscopic hysterectomy procedures (©2015 Photo Courtesy of KARL STORZ Endoscopy-America, Inc)

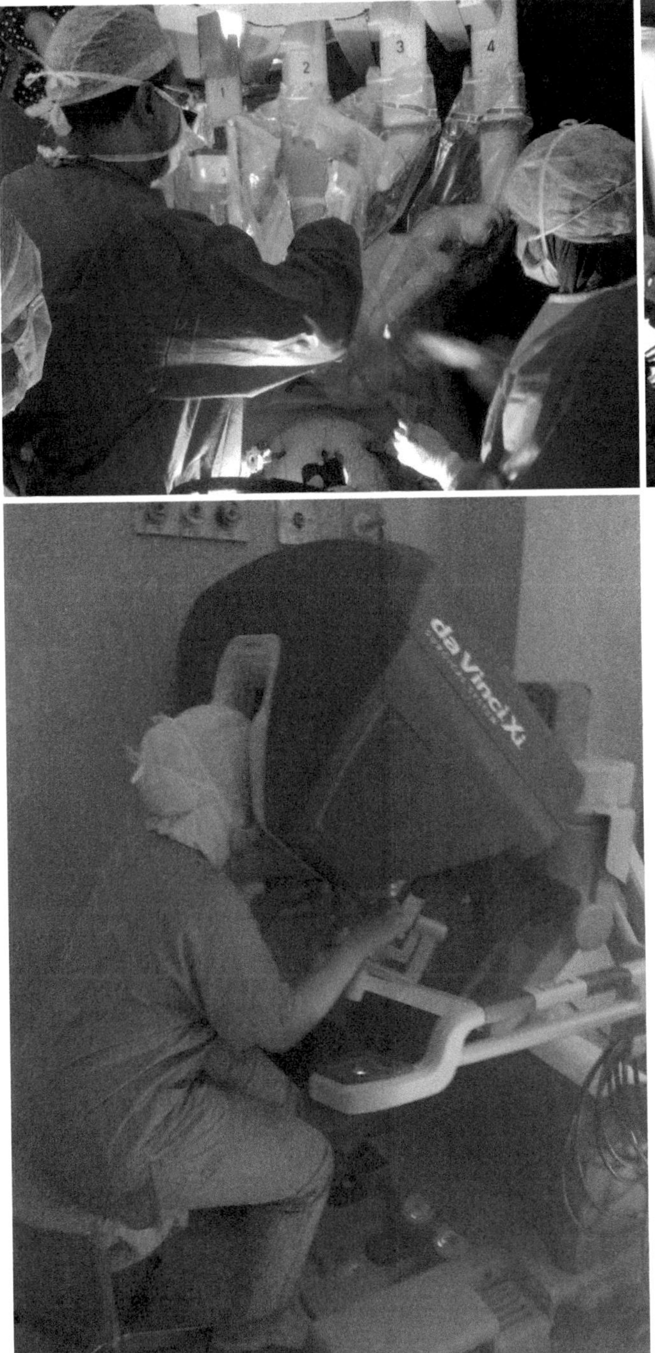

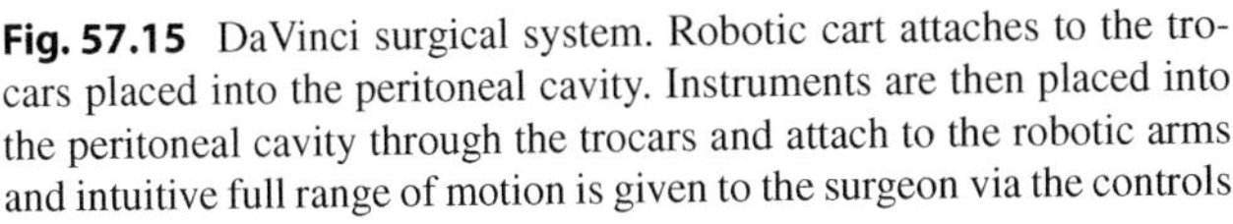

Fig. 57.15 DaVinci surgical system. Robotic cart attaches to the trocars placed into the peritoneal cavity. Instruments are then placed into the peritoneal cavity through the trocars and attach to the robotic arms and intuitive full range of motion is given to the surgeon via the controls at the Surgeon Console. Assistants stand at the bedside and help with instrument exchanges, camera management and retraction. The surgeon controls the robotic instruments, energy, and camera from the surgeon console

The daVinci robotic surgical system (Fig. 57.15) is one of the most expensive and advanced tools available for the performance of hysterectomy, greatly extending the ability of a surgeon to push the limits of laparoscopy. However, one of the criticisms of the system is its extensive reliance on traditional bipolar and monopolar energy thus requiring the surgeon to understand the proper use of this type of energy and its effect on tissues in order to reduce risk of injury resulting from thermal spread. The disadvantages of traditional bipolar energy can be overcome using the concepts of adequate tissue dissection down to the vessel wall, made easier by the superior vision and articulating precisely

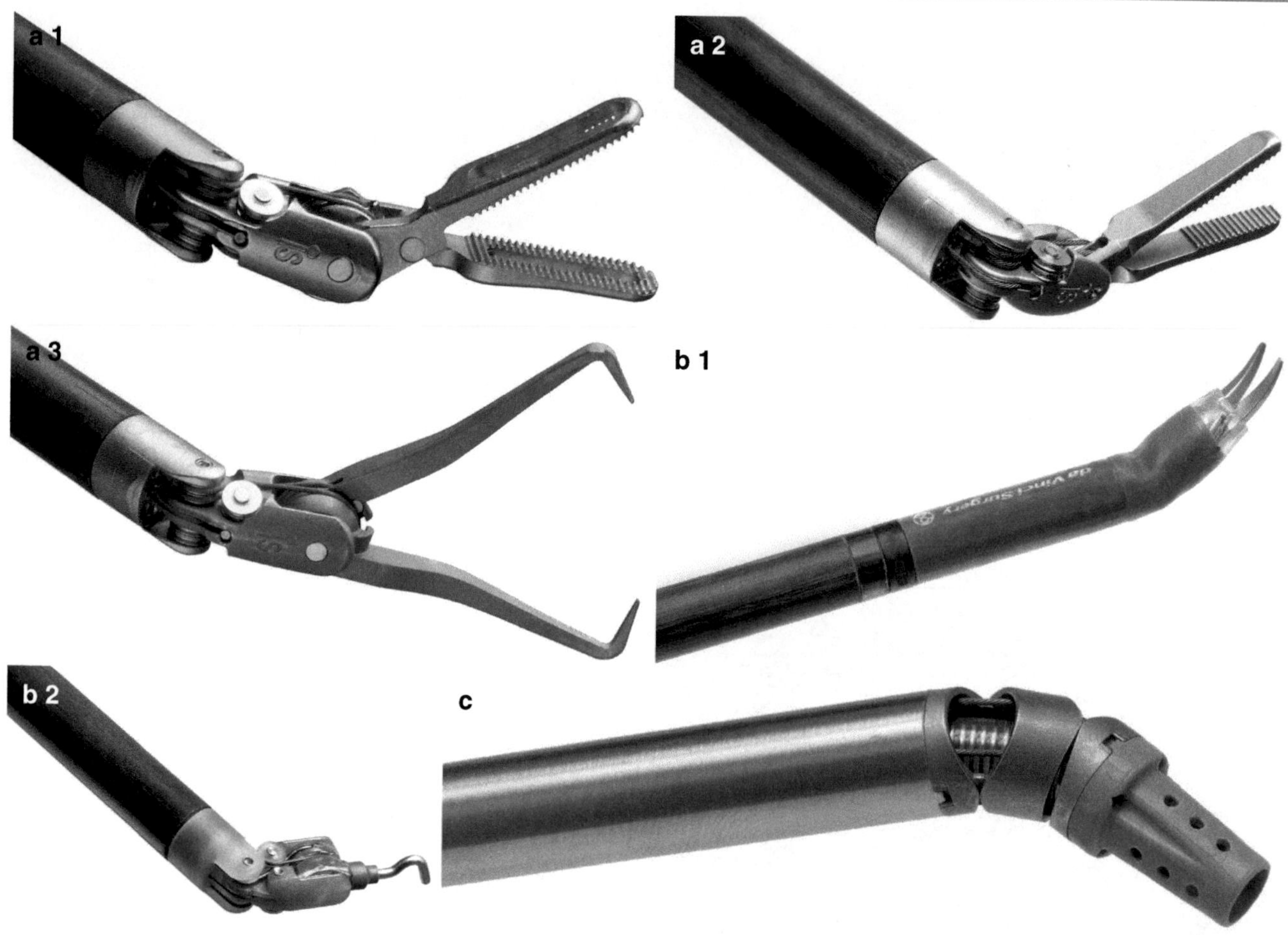

Fig. 57.16 Typical instruments used in DaVinci Hysterectomy. (**a**) Grasping instruments include the prograsp, long-tipped forceps, and robotic tenaculum. (**b**) Cutting devices include the mono-polar scissors, mono-polar hook, and mono-polar spatula. (**c**) Other useful instruments include the clip applier and suction irrigation device. The only other instruments required are some kind of bipolar vessel sealing or coagulation instruments reviewed in Fig. 57.17

controlled instruments. Bipolar energy can then be applied, applied directly to the vessel with intermittent manually pulsed application allowing heat and charring to dissipate so that the energy transmits further into the vessel. This thus mimics the pulsed bipolar energy of advanced devices but without the ability to adjust power for tissue impedance. Similarly, using appropriate tension and counter-tension techniques and principles of utilizing a larger surface area for coagulation and smaller surface area with a swift movement with tissue on tension for cutting using the mono-polar scissors reduces tissue damage and thermal spread (Fig. 57.16). These swift movements and precision in energy application is greatly facilitated by the wristed instruments that mimic the surgeons' hands exactly to a set scale (1:1, 1:3, 1:5 depending on the setting). Therefore, in experienced hands the energy can be used safely and effectively since the surgeon has much greater control over the movements and the precision of the dissection and energy application as compared to traditional laparoscopy. Thus, if the energy is utilized precisely and selectively only when needed, a safe and efficient dissection and hemostatic control of pedicles can be acheived with the added possibility of decreasing blood loss over laparoscopy.

As far as advanced bipolar energy use with the daVinci robotic surgical system, the S and Si Systems are compatible with a PK gyrus generator utilizing the PK dissector instrument for vessel sealing (Fig. 57.17). This instrument has the advantages of advanced bipolar energy and is optimally shaped for both dissection and vessel sealing, although it does not function well as a grasper and thus does not have the multi-purpose advantages of the fenestrated bipolar or bipolar Maryland instrument which utilize traditional bipolar energy. Thus, when choosing the instrument the surgeon must compromise one of two functions and compare that to the preference for type of energy. The PK dissector is slim and long and is optimal for careful dissection around vessels or in retroperitoneal space but does not grasp peritoneum or tissue well. However, its vessel sealing ability is superior secondary to the pulsed PK advanced energy. Thus, surgeons who utilize this instrument have a style of surgery focused on dissection and selective vessel sealing and use the blades of the PK dissector much like a Kelley instrument in abdominal

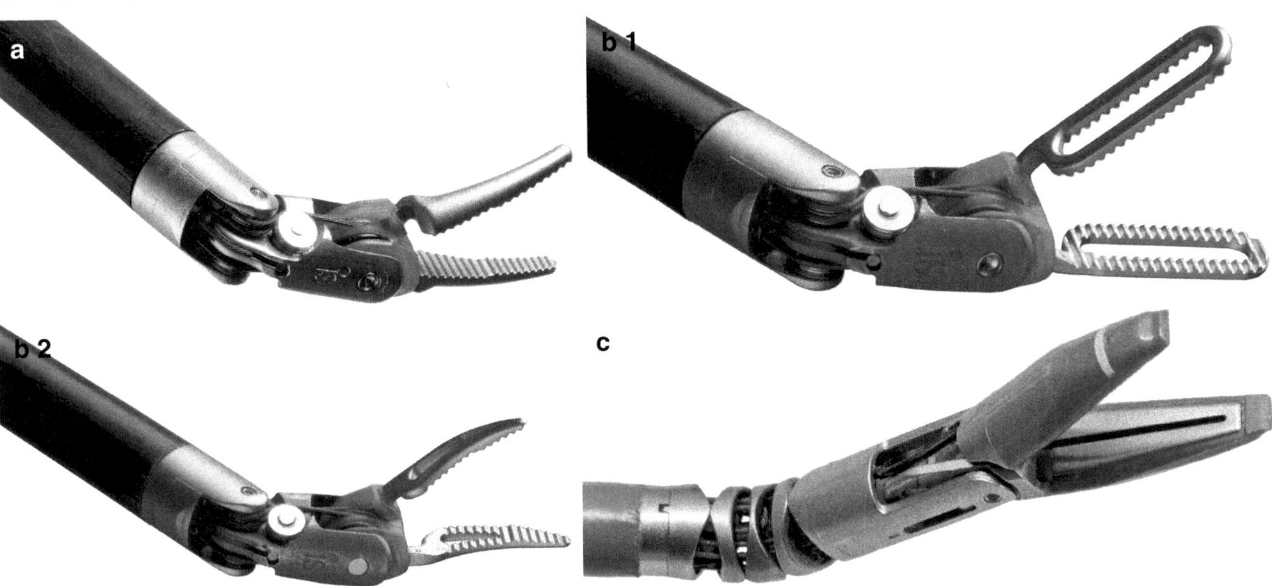

Fig. 57.17 Bipolar Instruments for use with DaVinci surgical System. (**a**) The PK dissector allows application of advanced bipolar energy for optimal vessel sealing. Its thin jawline also allows dissection of anatomy down to the vessel wall. (**b**) The fenestrated bipolar and bipolar Maryland apply traditional bipolar energy and thus require manual pulsing of the jaws in order to allow tissue to cool between pulses thus reducing sticking and charring and increasing efficiency during vessel sealing. (**c**) The newest instrument is a vessel sealer employing Ligasure-like technology to seal and cut vessels efficiently and rapidly. However the instrument is not multifunctional and thus functions poorly as a grasper or a dissector

surgery, utilizing the monopolar energy to cut tissue that is elevated between the blades. (Figure) Surgeons, who utilize the fenestrated bipolar or bipolar Maryland, tend to use more blunt dissection and traction of tissue and peritoneum to open spaces and will need to apply more energy in order to accomplish similar vessel sealing. Thus, the style of the surgeon also determines the instrument chosen for the task.

A newer vessel sealing and cutting instrument (Fig. 57.17) has also been released for the Si and Xi systems which has a similar seal and cut technology as the Ligasure device but its thickness and bulk make it function poorly as a dissector or a grasper. As such, it may not provide much advantage over the PK dissector for hysterectomies [26, 27]. Surgeons, that utilize this instrument prefer the combined sealing and cutting as compared to the seal and then cut seal and then cut with scissors or monopolar hook stating that this may save time by the combined sealing and cutting of pedicles. This is especially useful for colectomy, or other general surgery procedures. In hysterectomy, if a surgeon wishes to mimic the laparoscopic approach of sealing and cutting utero-ovarian or infundibulopelvic ligaments then sealing and cutting the broad ligament along the uterus until the uterine artery is reached then this instrument may accomplish this effectively. However, authors caution that if the broad ligament is not opened, allowing the ureter to fall ever further inferiorly or laterally, that this may decrease the distance between the ureter and vascular pedicles. This is especially important in cases of distorted anatomy such as in patients with a large fibroid uterus or severe endometriosis. In addition, as this instrument functions poorly as a dissector, the vascular pedicles may not be skeletonized as effectively potentially compromising vessel sealing especially if the vessel size is large such as in patients with large fibroids. It is thus extremely important that surgeons understand the instruments and energy that they are utilizing and watch different surgery styles using these instruments before selecting the method that will achieve both safety and efficiency in their hands.

Instruments for Tissue Extraction

Once a hysterectomy is performed the tissue needs to be removed from the abdominal cavity. In abdominal or vaginal hysterectomies, the pathology is removed via the incision used to obtain access, either abdominally or vaginally. When the laparoscopic approach is undertaken, removal of the specimen is dependent on the type of hysterectomy performed. If a total laparoscopic hysterectomy is performed, then extraction may occur vaginally through the colpotomy incision. Even if the uterus is enlarged, by placing vaginal retractors similar to those utilized in vaginal hysterectomy and using either long single, double, or triple toothed graspers on the uterus, the uterus can be extracted using wedge or strip cutting of the specimen until it is completely removed. If containment of the tissue is a concern, the specimen may be placed into a laparoscopic bag first then by pulling the opening of the bag out through the vagina and placing the retractors within the bag, morcellation can be performed via the vaginal route in a contained fashion (Fig. 57.18).

If the specimen is too large to pull into the vagina, a small 2–4 cm suprapubic or umbilical incision can be made, placing a small Alexis wound retractor into the wound, grasping the tissue with towel clips or triple toothed graspers and similarly cutting the specimen in a systematic fashion in order to remove it. Again, if containment is desired, the specimen may be placed within a bag first then by pulling the bag up through the incision and placing the alexis retractor within, then morecellation can be performed in a contained environment. Newer bags with the retraction ring already built in have also been released and may be utilized for the same purpose (Fig. 57.19).

For supra-cervical hysterectomy, the cervix is spared and there is no colpotomy incsion. Therefore, the only options for extraction of the uterus with or without the adnexa are mini-lap morcellation or mechanical morcellation. Again consideration should be made for containment of the specimen if required. Mechanical morcellators are devices introduced into the peritoneum through a trochar site which is extended to 15–20 mm with a revolving blade that cuts the specimen into strips for extraction as a grasper pulls the tissue towards to blade pulling the strip out through the morcellator channel. Most mechanical morcellators are disposable and utilize a sharp blade for cutting. Although an energy based morcellator was available from Gyrus, lack of efficiency and excessive smoke production were limiting factors. The rotacut morcellator from Stortz is a re-usable mechanical morcellator in which only the blade is disposable. It is relatively strong and efficient but does require some assembly and does not have a retractable safety guard similar to disposable morcellators. There are several completely disposable morcellators available on the market that vary in their features but are limited by cost and durability. Table 57.6 compares the available morcellators. The Gynecare Morcellex was one of the

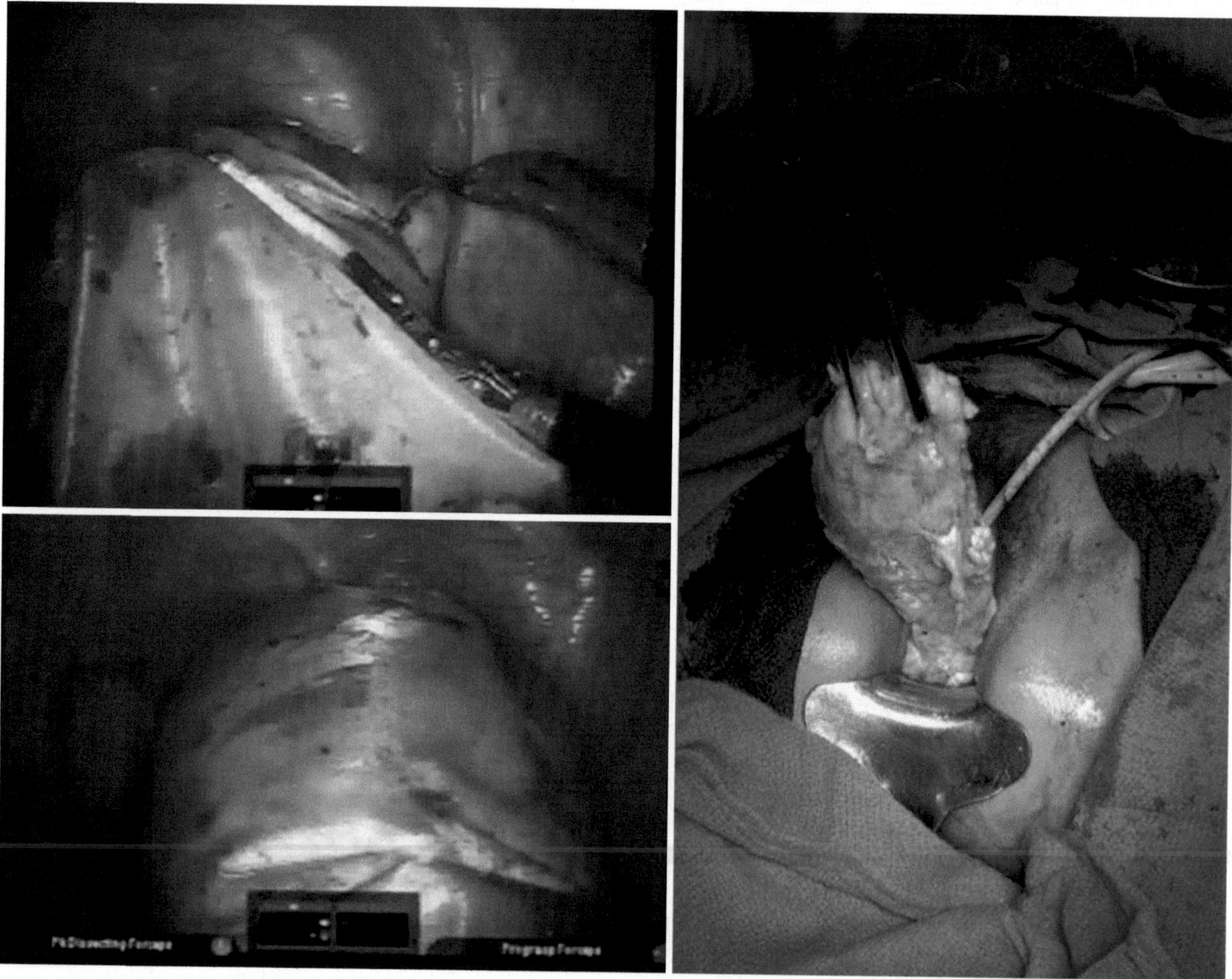

Fig. 57.18 Uterine specimen removed vaginally after placement within a specimen bag and hand scalpel morcellation within the bag. The bag is introduced through the vagina after the colpotomy is completed. The uterus can then be placed within the bag and the bag pulled out through the vagina. Vaginal retractors can then be placed and the uterus can be wedge resected or morcellated with the assistance of a scalpel until it is completely removed

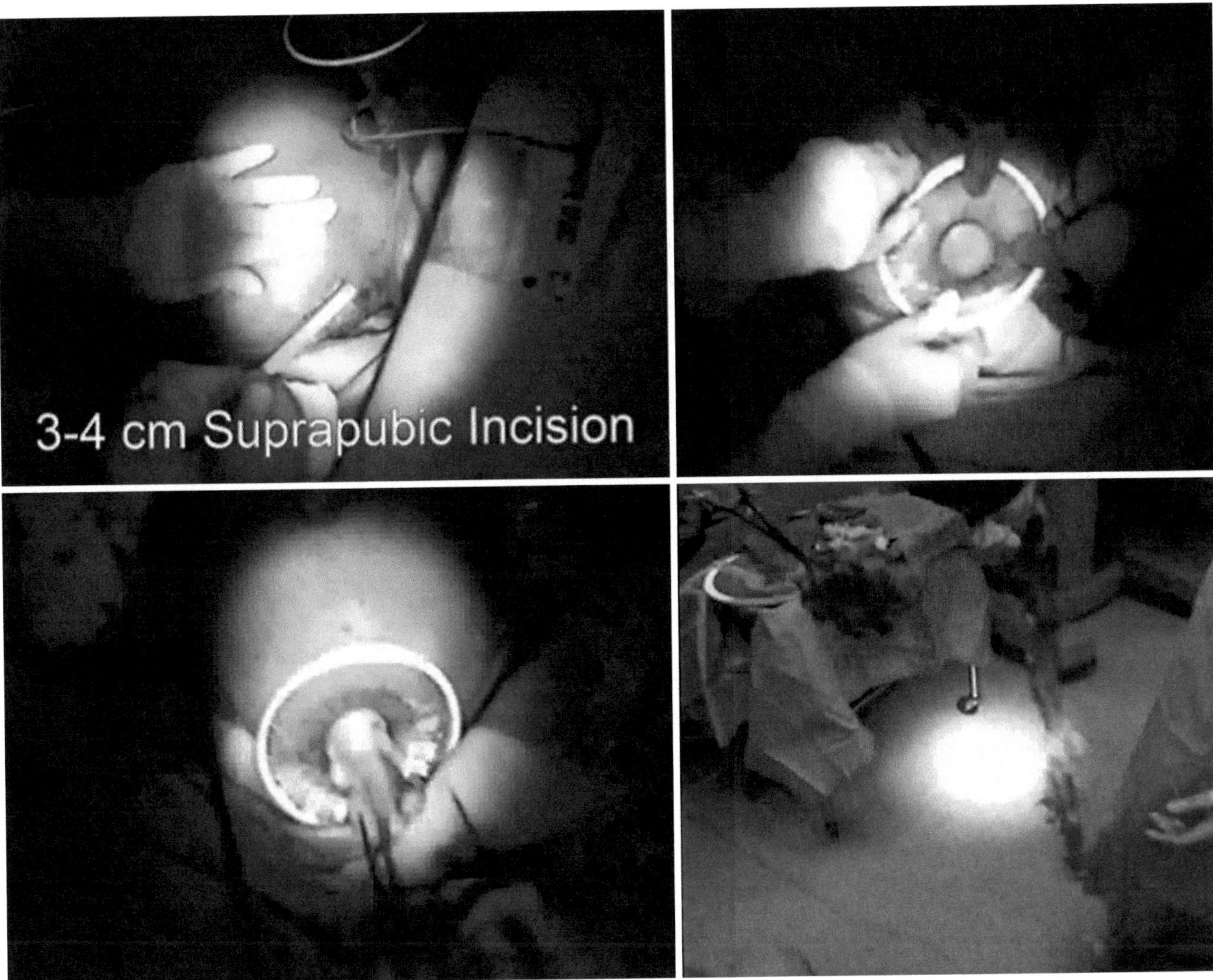

Fig. 57.19 Minilap Morcellation. Specimen is placed within a bag and pulled out through a suprapubic or umbilical incision measuring 2–3 cm. Wound protector/retractor is placed within the bag and scalpel is used to extract specimen using hand morcellation techniques

Table 57.6 Comparison of mechanical morcellators

Morcellator	Disposable	Cordless	Safety guard	Detachable from port	Sizes available	Criticisms
STORZ Rotocut Morcellator	No Disposable Blade	No	Yes Cannula without safety also available for coring	No	15 mm	Bulky and heavy in size Assembly required
LiNA Xcise	Yes	Yes Battery operated	Yes	No	15 mm	Battery life is a limitation Hand control is only option
Blue Endo MOREsolution Tissue Morcellator	Yes	No	Yes	Yes Allows for extraction of tissue that may get stuck in the port	15 mm 20 mm Allows choice to increase size for larger specimen	As does disassemble some practice needed to keep morcellator from detaching from port
Gynecare Morcellex Tissue Morcellator	Yes	No	Yes First to be developed	No	15	Inefficient blade Tissue fragmentation appears to be excessive
The PKS Plasma Sword Bipolar Morcellator	Yes	No	No	No	15 mm	Extremely inefficient compared to bladed systems Excessive smoke production Thermal injury is a concern

first disposable morcellators on the market and included the safety guard to protect the blade when not in use. It initially did lack some durability and when the blade dulled it tended to shred tissue leading the surgeon to have to use a second morcellator to complete the case. The Lina morcellator is completely cordless and functions off a battery pack. The Blue endo morcellator comes in both 15 and 20 mm sizes, allowing surgeons to extract larger pathology more easily. In addition, it detaches from its port so that if tissue gets caught within the channel it can be pulled out. Both of these also have a safety guard in their design. The use of morcellators in hysterectomy has been declining since the FDA warning was released in 2013 and many registries and studies are taking place to evaluate possible use of morcellation within containment systems to prevent spread of tissue within the peritoneal cavity during morcellation [28].

Instruments for Vaginal Cuff Closure

Closure of the vaginal cuff in both the Abdominal and Vaginal hysterectomy approaches is relatively simple as compared to Laparoscopic approaches. Although there were a few now abandoned attempts at staple devices used initially in an attempt to expedite abdominal hysterectomy, most surgeons close the vagina using either continuous or interrupted sutures incorporating the cardinal and uterosacral ligaments into the angles in order to provide support. Only a toothed forceps and long handled heavy needle driver are required. Similarly, in Vaginal hysterectomy a heavy Haney needle driver can make suturing the cuff at the apex of the vagina simpler. Again uterosacral ligaments are usually incorporated into the cuff closure in order to provide support and help prevent prolapse of the apex at a later time.

Although, with practice and persistence, laparoscopic suturing can be performed relatively efficiently utilizing either intracorporeal or extracorporeal knot tying utilizing a knot pusher, it is this area in which some devices have been developed in order to assist in vaginal cuff closure or laparoscopic suturing in general. These can be especially useful in single port hysterectomy procedures in which the lack of triangulation makes vaginal cuff suturing extremely challenging. Therefore, some surgeons may choose to either close the vaginal cuff using a vaginal approach or utilize a device to assist with suturing or knot placement. Two categories of such devices exist. The first are devices that assists in passing the needle through tissue and may also expedite knot tying, and another are devices that assists with knot tying by utilizing pre-loaded Roeder knots that are placed after the needle is passed through the tissue using standard laparoscopic suturing techniques. Although some of these devices are re-usable, all require purchasing of suture with needles specifically designed for each particular device and thus the cost of this suture should be accounted for in addition to the cost of the device.

Two examples of devices that assist with knot tying are the Pare Surgical Inc. Quik-Stitch re-usable knot tying device and the Ethicon Endo-Surgery Suture assistant. Quik-Stitch is re-usable, while Endo-surgery Suture assistant can only be reloaded 5 times. Both are 5 mm in diameter and function in a similar manner allowing the surgeon to pass the suture into the peritoneal cavity with a grasper at the end of the device, then after passing the needle through the tissue utilizing standard laparoscopic needle drivers the device is used to place and synch the knot in place.

There are several devices that assist with passing the suture through the cuff, as well as knot tying, by toggling a needle back and forth between tips of the grasping end of the device. Endo evolution Endo360° Reusable Stainless Steel Suturing Device is a 10 mm re-usable device with a curved tip and needle that may be used for vaginal cuff closure purposes as well as other applications. The suture with needle is specifically made for this device and thus must be purchased separately. Covidien has also developed a 10 mm single use device. Covidien Endo Stitch™ single use suturing device uses a straight needle that passes from one jaw to the next after grasping the tissue through which the needle needs to be passed. A similar articulating device, the SILS™ Stitch articulating suturing device performs a similar function but is designed specifically for single port surgery. Again, suture with needles need to be purchased separately. In addition to the expense, the disadvantages of these devices is that it is difficult to compensate for different tissue thickness or to adjust the size of the bites taken as well as with traditional suturing and thus there may be concern for inadeqate closure if not used properly.

Development of a needle driver with a small diameter for mini-laparoscopy that is strong enough to drive a needle through thick vaginal tissue did take some time and surgeon's performing hysterectomy by mini-laparoscopy often resorted to suturing vaginally, as did the surgeons' performing single port hysterectomy. Storz did develop an adequate needle driver which is re-enforced by a low-friction cannula that prevents the needle driver from bending when passing needles through tougher tissue. This now can allow surgeons to utilize a 3.0 mm port site in order to close the vaginal cuff. Both the trochar/cannula set and the needle driver are re-usable stainless steel instruments and thus are cost efficient.

For Hysterectomy, the robotic instrument has simplified vaginal cuff closure by greatly simplifying suturing and knot tying because of the ergonomic intuitive movements of robotic instrument arms completely mimicking open surgical technique allowing suturing in any angle. Although the single port platform still includes instruments that are not wristed, this will also soon change and will simplify single

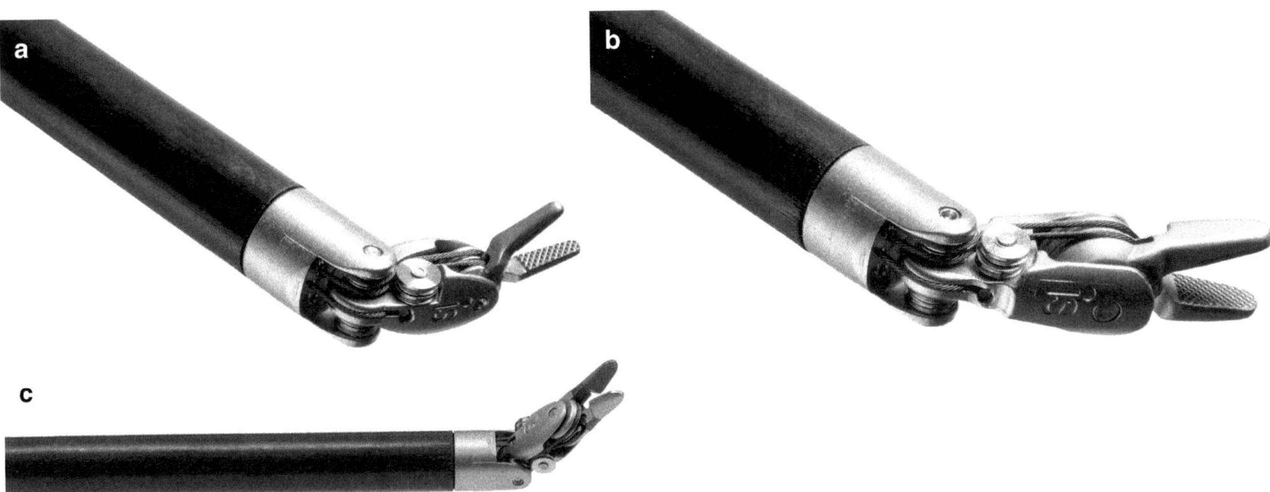

Fig. 57.20 DaVinci Suturing Instruments. For robotic hysterectomy there are two sizes of needle drivers that are available for use in vaginal cuff closure. The large needle driver (**a**) however is not as heavy or as sturdy as the mega needle driver (**b**) which is easier to use on thick vaginal tissue. Both also come as a suture-cut needle driver (**c**) which has a suture scissor in the shank thus allowing the surgeon to save time cutting suture. Initially 5 mm single port robotic needle drivers were not wristed and thus gave the surgeon more difficulty in suturing the cuff, but recently a wristed 5 mm single port needle driver was released greatly simplifying vaginal cuff suturing with the single-port platform

port robotic hysterectomy as well. Options for instrumentation for grasping the vaginal cuff include the Pro-grasp (often used for retraction with fourth arm during the case), the toothed cobra grasper, the long-tipped forcep, or the bipolar instrument utilized during the case such as the bipolar Marylyn or fenestrated bipolar instrument. As each robotic instrument utilized during the case costs money, most surgeons will try to use one of the instruments used earlier during the case for elevation and manipulation of the vaginal cuff rather than choosing a specific instrument solely for this purpose. For optimal suturing however, a needle driver should be used for driving the needle and trying to drive the needle with one of these other instruments may be cumbersome and cost time. In general, the heaviest option for needle driver should be chosen as the vaginal cuff tends to be relatively tuff tissue as compared to bowel or bladder for which a smaller (Large) needle drive is often used. One may choose either the option which incorporates scissors into the needle driver (Mega-Suture cut) or the needle driver on its own (Mega) needle driver and utilize their assistant for cutting the suture [26] (Fig. 57.20).

Conclusion

A well-informed surgeon should study and know the uses and limitation of the instruments available before selecting the appropriate instrument for the procedure and task at hand. Hysterectomies are one of the most commonly gynecologic procedures performed in women. The ultimate goal of a surgeon is to perform the procedure efficiently and safely while causing the least amount of trauma to the tissue and patient. Technology and devices is now allowing these procedures to be performed in most women utilizing minimally invasive surgical techniques, minimizing the need for laparotomy. Whether the vaginal, laparoscopic, mini-laparoscopic, single port, or robotic approach is undertaken, both patient selection and the choice of the appropriate instruments will determine the overall success of the procedure.

References

1. Duhan N, Al-Hendy A. Techniques of hysterectomy, hysterectomy (Ed.). 2012. ISBN: 978–953–51-0434-6.
2. Wu JM, Wechter ME, Geller EJ, Nguyen TV, Visco AG. Hysterectomy rates in the United States. Obstet Gynecol. 2003;110:1091–54.
3. Bahamondes L, Bahamondes MV, Monteiro I. Levonorgestrel-releasing intrauterine system: uses and controversies. Expert Rev Med Devices. 2008;5:437–45.
4. Reich H, Roberts L. Laparoscopic hysterectomy in current gynaecological practice. Rev Gynaecol Pract. 2003;3:32–40.
5. Einarsson JI, Suzuki Y. Total laparoscopic hysterectomy: 10 steps toward a successful procedure. Rev Obstet Gynecol. 2009;2:57–64.
6. Johnson N, Barlow D, Lethaby A, Tavender E, Curr L, Garry R. Methods of hysterectomy: systematic review and meta-analysis of randomised controlled trials. BMJ. 2005;330:1478–86.
7. Uppal S, Frumovitz M, Escobar P, Ramirez PT. Laparo-endoscopic single-site surgery in gynecology—a review of the literature and available technology. J Minim Invasive Gynecol. 2011;18:12–23.
8. Reynolds RK, Advincula AP. Robot-assisted laparoscopic hysterectomy: technique and initial experience. Am J Surg. 2006;191: 555–60.
9. Beste TM, Nelson KH, Daucher JA. Total laparoscopic hysterectomy utilizing a robotic surgical system. J Soc Laparoendosc Surg. 2005;9:13–5.
10. Orady M, Hrynewych A, Nawfal AK, Wegienka G. Comparison of robotic-assisted laparoscopic hysterectomy to other minimally invasive approaches. J Soc Laparoendosc Surg. 2012;16:542–8.

11. Orady ME, Aslanova R, Paraiso MFR. Hysterectomy for benign indications. Minerva Ginecol. 2014;66(1):13–21.
12. Stone HH, Hoefling SJ, Strom PR, et al. Abdominal incisions: transverse vs vertical placement and continuous vs interrupted closure. South Med J. 1983;76:1106–8.
13. Wong WSF, Lee TCE. Hybrid approach for difficult vaginal hysterectomy. Vaginal Hysterectomy. 2nd edn., Jaypee Brothers Medical Publishers Pvt Ltd. 2014:180–186.
14. Vilos GA, Ternamian A, Dempster J, Laberge PY. Laparoscopic entry: A review of techniques, technologies, and complications. SOGC. 2007;193:433–47.
15. Vilos GA, Ternamian A, Dempster J, Laberge PY. Laparoscopic entry: a review of techniques, technologies, and complications. J Obstet Gynaecol Can. 2007;29(5):433–65.
16. Van den Haak L, Alleblas C, Nieboer TE, Rhemrev JP, Jansen FW. Efficacy and safety of uterine manipulators in laparoscopic surgery. A review. Arch Gynecol Obstet. 2015;292(5):1003–11. doi:10.1007/s00404-015-3727-9.
17. Ornella Sizzi. Overcoming technical limits to laparoscopic hysterectomy. Ob Gyn. 2006. http://www.obgyn.net/.
18. Swan K, Kim J, Advincula AP. Advanced uterine manipulation technologies. Surg Technol Int. 2010;20:215–20.
19. Brill AI, Stamos MJ. Perpendicular blood vessel sealing in surgical practice. 2012;1:13.
20. Campbell PA, Cresswell AB, Frank TG, Cuschieri A. Real-time thermography during energized vessel sealing and dissection. Surg Endosc Other Interventio Tech. 2003;17:1640–5.
21. Emam TA, Cuschieri A. How safe is high-power ultrasonic dissection? Ann Surg. 2003;237:186–91.
22. H. Z. Lin, Y. W. Ng, A. Agarwal, Y. F. Fong. Application of a new integrated bipolar and ultrasonic energy device in laparoscopic hysterectomies. ISRN Minimally Invasive Surg. 2013;2013:Article ID 453581.
23. Seehofer D, Mogl M, Boas-Knoop S, et al. Safety and efficacy of new integrated bipolar and ultrasonic scissors compared to conventional laparoscopic 5-mm sealing and cutting instruments. Surg Endosc. 2012;26:2541–9.
24. Milsom J, Trencheva K, Monette S, et al. Evaluation of the safety, efficacy, and versatility of a new surgical energy device (THUNDERBEAT) in comparison with Harmonic ACE, LigaSure V, and EnSeal devices in a porcine model. J Laparoendosc Adv Surg Tech A. 2012;22:378–86.
25. Seehofer D, Mogel M, Boas-Knoop S, Under J, Schirmeir A, Chopra S, Eurich D. Safety and efficacy of new integrated bipolar and ultrasonic scissors compared to conventional laparoscopic 5-mm sealing instruments. Surg Endosc. 2012;26(9):2541–9. doi:10.1007/s00464-012-2229-0. Epub 2012 Mar 24
26. Payne TN. Advancements in robotic hysterectomy, ACS Surgery News, 2013.
27. Hoste G, Van Trappen P. Robotic hysterectomy using the vessel sealer for myomatous uteri: technique and clinical outcome. Eur J Obstet Gynecol Reprod Biol. 2015;194:241–4. doi:10.1016/j.ejogrb.2015.09.030.
28. Barron K, Richard T, Robinson PS, Lamvu G. Association of the U.S Food and Drug Administration Morcellation warning with rates of minimally invasive hysterectomy and myomectomy. Obstet Gynecol. 2015;126(6):1174–80.

58 Diagnostic Laparoscopy via the Da Vinci Robot in General and Site Recognition

Agnieszka Oleszczuk-Cosse

Introduction

The robot assisted surgery is an innovative technique to perform laparoscopic procedures that is still evolving and is open for new operative possibilities. Robotic precision in tumor excision, easier intracorporal suturing and favorable ergonomics for the surgeon make the da Vinci robot particularly suitable for performing complex laparoscopic microinvasive surgical operations [1]. However, diagnostic laparoscopic procedure needs to be performed before every operation with the Da Vinci robot. Ongoing efforts to improve the morbidity and cosmesis have led to minimization of size and number of ports required for laparoscopic surgery. Single port laparoscopy or Laparo-Endoscopic Single Site surgery (LESS) represent the latest innovation in minimally invasive surgery. The advantages of the LESS via Da Vinci robot, with the use of only one port for a 3D camera and intuitive instruments together with the option to perform a tissue biopsy and a variety of therapeutic interventions through only one incision could be used also specifically for a diagnostic laparoscopy in a future.

The robotic surgery provides also the possibility of: performing an intraoperative ultrasound as well as through a Firefly™ Imaging System blood or lymph vessel or bile duct flow, now used in gynecologic oncology for real-time lymphangiography.

Thanks to better ergonomics of minimal invasive procedure, 3D stable visualization of enlarged operations field, and improvement of dexterity, as well as a use of a second console for assisted learning and also the intraoperative possibility of drawing lines on the screen showing the actual surgical site, the robot assisted surgery is the most effective way to teach and to learn pelvic anatomy and new surgical techniques due to a better site recognition. Through the extensive knowledge of the anatomy, the identification and the appropriate exposure of the surgical region with a safeguard of relevant structures like: ureter and depending on the operation also uterine artery and/ or pelvic nerves, almost every operation via the Da Vinci robot has a potential to be performed near to bloodless.

Dr. med. A. Oleszczuk-Cosse
Department of Gynecology, Charité University Hospital Berlin, Charitéplatz 1, Berlin, Germany
e-mail: a.cosse@charite.de

Diagnostic Laparoscopy via the Da Vinci Robot in General

Diagnostic laparoscopy via the Da Vinci robot is a minimally invasive method for identification of all relevant abdominal and pelvic structures and for the diagnosis of intra-abdominal diseases by direct inspection of intra-abdominal and intrapelvic organs with a possibility for a tissue biopsy, a culture acquisition, and a variety of therapeutic interventions.

Indication

The diagnostic laparoscopy is performed before every minimal-invasive operative procedure via the Da Vinci robot (Table 58.1). However, some surgeons preceding the previously planned robotic operation still prefer to perform the diagnostic laparoscopy by a gold standard method through a conventional laparoscopy [2].

The diagnostic laparoscopy via Da Vinci robot as a staging procedure of early cervical and endometrial cancer is useful for making a definitive clinical diagnosis whenever there is a diagnostic dilemma even after routine diagnostic workup. By enabling accurate staging, diagnostic laparoscopy permits patient selection for curative resection or a neoadjuvant chemotherapy while avoiding nontherapeutic laparotomy, which is associated with a delay in initiation of chemotherapy.

However, for other indications like: identifying the cause of infertility, acute or nonspecific abdominal pain, suspected intra-abdominal injuries or anatomical pathologies is the

I. Alkatout, L. Mettler (eds.), *Hysterectomy*, DOI 10.1007/978-3-319-22497-8_58

Table 58.1 Indications for a diagnostic laparoscopy via the Da Vinci robot and via the conventional standard method with advantages and disadvantages of the Da Vinci robot in comparison to the conventional laparoscopy

Indications for a diagnostic laparoscopy	Via the Da Vinci robot	Via the conventional laparoscopy	Advantages of the da Vinci over the conventional laparoscopy	Limitations of the da Vinci in the shadow of the conventional laparoscopy
Laparoscopic operative probedure	Before every robotic operative probedure	Before every (robotic or conventional) laparoscopic operative probedure	Ergonomics Intuitive instruments 3D	Higher costs of the system An absence of a tactile feedback Additional time for docking Additional learning curve
Cervical or endometrial cancer	Before planned lymphadenectomy by an early cervical or endometrial cancer	Just to examine the abdomen and pelvis with or without planned lymphadenectomy		
Infertility	Only before a specific operative procedure	Just to examine the abdomen and pelvis with or without planned operative proceure		
Abdominal pain	Only characteristic pain before a specific operation for example on an endometiose	Acute and non-specific with or without planned operative proceure		
Suspected abdominal injuries	Only before a specific operation	With or without planned operative proceure		
Anatomical pathologies	Only before a specific operation	With or without planned operative proceure		

standard conventional laparoscopy the procedure of choice and the use of Da Vinci robot is until now still suboptimal. Although the robotic surgery is very advantageous through better ergonomics and intuitive instruments, for a short basic procedure as a diagnostic laparoscopy those advantages are not able to overwhelm still existing limitations of the robotics like much higher costs of the system maintenance and disposables per case as well as the absence of tactile feedback.

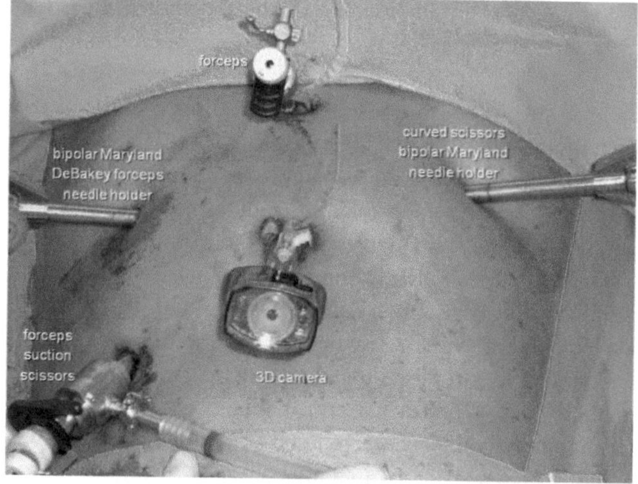

Fig. 58.1 Possible placement of trocars for a diagnostic and an operative laparoscopy via Da Vinci robot with an example of the instruments used in those trocars. A long 12-mm trocar at the umbilicus: is for 3-dimensional robotic camera; two 8-mm trocars are placed in the left and right lower quadrants are for: bipolar Maryland, DeBakey forceps, needle holder; and curved scissors, bipolar Maryland, needle holder, respectively; a left upper quadrant accessory entrance for: forceps, suction, scissors, or a special trocar a 3-mm microlaparoscope

Procedure

Before the start of every robotic case, a patient is placed in low dorsal lithotomy position with arms padded and tucked at the sides of the patient after general anesthesia is administered. The bladder is drained with an indwelling urinary catheter, and if needed: a uterine manipulator, and alternatively an intrauterine catheter for chromopertubation is placed to assess tubal patency intraoperatively. Typically four trocars are used after pneumoperitoneum is obtained. A long 12-mm trocar is placed usually at the umbilicus or above it (depending on the size of the pelvic pathology or art of the planned operative surgery). This trocar serves the 3-dimensional robotic camera. Previously, it is possible to place an entry with a 3-mm micro-laparoscope in a left upper quadrant to help guide all other operative trocarplacements in patients with enlarged pelvic pathology or who may are at risk for intra-abdominal adhesions. Further, two 8-mm trocars are placed in the left and right lower quadrants, respectively. A fourth trocar as an accessory port can be placed between the camera port and the right lower quadrant port or also in the left upper quadrant. This trocar is typically 12 to 15 mm to enable an introduction of other laparoscopic instruments for suction-irrigation, traction and countertraction or a possibility for introduction of a suture or probe for microbiologic examination. Additionally one 5-mm trocar above the symphysis can be placed for traction/ countertraction as needed.

Once all trocars are in place (Fig. 58.1), the patient can be placed in steep Trendelenburg position and the surgical cart with three robotic arms can be brought between the patient's legs and docked. Then, each trocar can be attached to the assigned robotic arm with the exception of the accessory port(s) that are manipulated by the bedside surgical assistant(s). The robotic arms are docked to the assigned trocars: right and left operating robotic arms directly to the right and left lower quadrant trocars, respectively, whereas the robotic camera arm to either umbilical or supraumbilical trocar. Then the diagnostic laparoscopy can be performed while adhering to the basic principles of conventional diagnostic laparoscopic technique. A systematic examination of the abdominal and pelvic sites as well entire abdominal and pelvic viscera, including the peritoneum, omentum, liver, uterus, fallopian tubes, ovaries and bladder is performed to identify any pathology and its extension.

After the diagnostic procedure and depending on the diagnosed, abdominal and pelvic status, the planned operative procedure via Da Vinci robot can begin. If there is, however, an evidence of widespread or peritoneal-based disease, or for example bladder, rectum or depending on the operation lymph node metastasis diagnosed, or when there is a direct extension of the pathology to surrounding structures that preclude its respectability, the diagnostic laparoscopy procedure via Da Vinci robot may need to be terminated after taking confirmatory biopsy specimens.

To end the procedure, an adequate hemostasis and correct instrument and gauze and sponge counts is ensured. Ports are removed under direct visualization to prove that there is no visceral herniation or bleeding. A decompression of the abdominal cavity by expelling the pneumoperitoneum to reduce postoperative shoulder pain is performed. All port sites greater than 5–10 mm should be closed with an absorbable suture and skin is closed with either continuous or interrupted subcuticular sutures.

Possible complications typical for laparoscopy are the same for conventional as well as via Da Vinci robot and include fatal gas embolism, problems due to hypercarbia, postoperative crepitus, and pneumothorax, as well as procedure-specific complications for the diagnostic laparoscopy such as uterus, bladder, bowel, nerves and/or vessels injury.

Further Possibilities through Innovations

Ongoing advancements in surgical instruments, optics, and ports have allowed the development of new options for intraoperative procedures with the Da Vinci robot.

Single Port Surgery

LESS is surgical term used to describe various techniques that aim at performing laparoscopic surgery through a single, small skin incision concealed within the umbilicus. Single port techniques may help to reduce postoperative pain, promote earlier return to daily activities, and improve cosmesis and patient satisfaction. There is also a potential reduction in other complications associated with multiple incisions, such as port-site hernias and hemorrhage [3]. Recently published outcome data demonstrate feasibility, safety and reproducibility for LESS in gynecology in general but comparative data and prospective trials are required to determine the clinical impact of LESS in treatment under gynecologic conditions [4]. The Da Vinci robotic system with articulating instruments can also be integrated with LESS for many gynecologic surgical procedures. However, we are still far from the ideal robotic platform. Significant improvements are needed before this technique might reach widespread adoption beyond selected centers [5].

Advantages of the single-port robotic surgery over conventional multi-port laparoscopy include better cosmesis from a hidden umbilical scar, a possible decrease in morbidity that can result from visceral and vascular injury during trocar placement, a decrease in post-operative wound infections, hernia formation, an elimination of multiple trocar site closures, 3D visualization, and improvement of dexterity. Escobar et al. found, using robotic-assisted LESS for bilateral salpingo-oophorectomy and total hysterectomy, that the Da Vinci robotic LESS attempts to further enhance cosmetic benefits and reduce morbidity of minimally invasive surgery in gynecology, and the use of LESS improved patient recovery time and cosmesis [6].

Significant advances have been achieved in the field of robotic LESS since the first reported clinical series in 2009. The ideal robotic platform should have a low external profile, the possibility of being deployed through a single access site, and the possibility of restoring intra-abdominal triangulation while maintaining the maximum degree of freedom for precise maneuvers and strength for reliable traction [5]. A very promising new robotic development in form of instruments created for a combined use with one single port is da Vinci Sp Single Port Robotic Surgical System (Intuitive Surgical ®) that consists of three articulating endoscopic instruments and an articulating endoscopic camera inserted through a single robotic port (Fig. 58.2). The patient side cart uses the same basic cart as the da Vinci Surgical System, but the configuration of the surgical arms and manipulators are changed to manipulate the unique EndoWrist Sp instruments and a 3D high definition camera through a single port: a 25 mm cannula. This device is already available and approved by FDA up until now for special urologic procedures only. The robotic intuitive instruments available to be used by the system include flexible endoscopes, blunt and sharp endoscopic dissectors, scissors, forceps, needle holders, endoscopic retractors, electrocautery and accessories for manipulation of tissue, including grasping, cutting, blunt and sharp dissection, approximation, ligation, electrocautery and suturing. The instruments have also two more degrees of freedom than the da Vinci Single-Site instruments previously

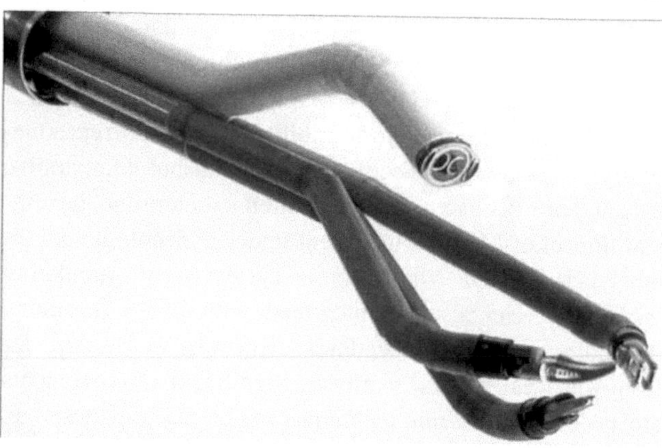

Fig. 58.2 Da Vinci Sp Single Port Robotic Surgical System (Intuitive Surgical ®) that consists of three articulating endoscopic instruments and an articulating endoscopic camera inserted through a single robotic port

available allowing substantially more control for the surgeon. This da Vinci Sp Single Port Robotic System could further overwhelm the limitations of robotics and be very advantageous for cosmesis especially by performing as basic as a diagnostic procedure.

Laparoscopic Ultrasound

For a diagnostic purpose, to evaluate organs that are not amenable to inspection during an operative laparoscopic procedure via Da Vinci robot, also a laparoscopic ultrasound is possible to be performed by using a unique specialized ultrasound transducer for robotic-assisted surgery (BK Medical ProART™ 8826 Robotic "Drop-in" Transducer, Intuitive Surgical®) that fits through a standard robotic trocar.

Ultrasound during diagnostic laparoscopy via the Da Vinci robot, already used during urologic procedures, could be very useful especially proceeding oncologic procedures for example to see intraoperative high resolution real-time borders of a tumor on the same screen as an robotic operative field.

Fluorescent Robotic Lymphangiography

The ability to view intraoperative blood or lymph vessel, or bile duct flow provides a Firefly™ Fluorescence Imaging System, now used in gynecologic oncology for robotic real-time lymphangiography. The Firefly™ Imaging System is build inside the Da Vinci 3D camera and forms the Da Vinci Fluorescence Imaging Vision System for the Da Vinci Surgical System. During a sentinel lymphadenectomy operation for cervical or endometrial cancer, when indicated, this specifically built camera enables the performance of diagnostic real-time fluorescent lymphangiography, called also near-infrared (NIR) fluorescent robotic lymphangiography [7, 8].

Before the diagnostic lymphangiographic procedure an indocyanine green (ICG) fluorescent glowing dye is injected into the cervix. The ICG naturally binds to albumin that flows in lymph vessels. The da Vinci® Fluorescence Imaging Vision System is a special Da Vinci camera with excitatory light source for laser (Firefly™) built inside the scope. The Firefly Imaging System is intended to be used along with the usual white light as usual during an operation and, when indicated, the light source for laser (Firefly) can be activated and intraoperative real-time lymphangiography can be performed. For that, while operating, a surgeon turns on the Firefly through the console, then from the Firefly source in the scope the 803 nm wave length laser illuminates the surgical scene, the ICG dye is excited and glows green signal, showing the path of vessels to the Da Vinci camera and this into the vision cart. That enables surgeons to see the in real-time the green lymph vessels as the tissue without lymph flow appears gray. This provides the ability to view a real-time imaging of lymphatic tissue during lymphadenectomy.

Near-infrared (NIR) fluorescence imaging with intracervical ICG injection using the robotic platform has a high bilateral sentinel lymph node detection rate and appears more favorable than using blue dye alone and/or other modalities [8].

Site Recognition via the Da Vinci Robot

By operating via the Da Vinci robot it is important to recognize not only the surgical site where the 3-D camera is directed but also the structures that are in that region before and during a performed dissection.

Transperitoneal Site: Before any Dissection

During the diagnostic laparoscopy via the robot Da Vinci many additional key vascular structures can be identified transperitoneally before any dissection:

- The internal iliac artery runs parallel and just posterior to the ureter.
- The external iliac artery is several centimeters anterior to it on the psoas muscle.
- The external and internal iliac arteries can be followed superiorly to find the bifurcation of the common iliac arteries at the pelvic brim overlying the sacroiliac joint. This is an ideal place to identify the ureter transversing the point of bifurcation as it enters the pelvis.
- The right common iliac artery can be followed superiorly to the bifurcation of the aorta, above the presacral space at approximately the fourth lumbar vertebra.
- The left common iliac artery is difficult to identify because of the overlying mesentery of the sigmoid colon.

– The left common iliac vein is located just medial and inferior to the left common iliac artery in the presacral space. It may also cover the entire space between the both common iliac arteries [11].

Retroperitoneal Site: During Abdominal Dissection

The recognition of structures in an abdominal site and a presacral region are important for procedures like paraaortic lymphadenectomy or ovarian transposition. The structures, important to recognize for paraaortic lymphadenectomies are from right to left: the psoas muscle; ovarian vessels; the right ureter that runs medial at this point to the psoas muscle and lateral to the inferior vena cava (Fig. 58.3); vena cava that runs to the right lateral of the aorta; aorta and both common iliac arteries. Below the bifurcation of the aorta superficially in a presacral region is the superior hypogastric nerve plexus and the presacral nodes, and beneath them, the left common iliac vein crossing from the left to the right. On the left side of the aorta are further: the inferior mesenteric artery, the sigmoid colon, and its mesentery. Deeper medially, there are the lumbar veins and artery; laterally is the left ureter (Fig. 58.4) and on the far left is the psoas muscle.

Retroperitoneal Site: During Pelvic Dissection

The pelvic site is the main operating field in the gynecology. Therefore, through the knowledge of the anatomy and the identification of the three vascular pelvic regions: the pelvic brim, the pelvic sidewall and the base of the broad ligament, position of the ureter, as well as of the eight avascular spaces and through exposure and safeguard of the relevant anatomy, the operation via the Da Vinci robot can be performed near to bloodless. Therefore it is crucial to identify the structures and where is the ureter running within those regions.

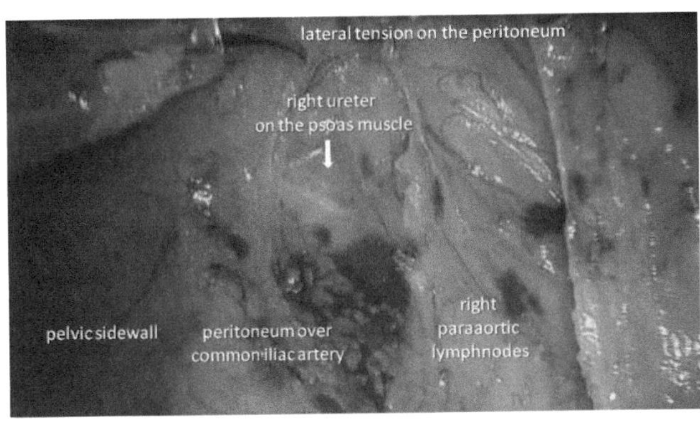

Fig. 58.3 Before the right paraaortic lymphadenectomy: identification of the right ureter. The right ureter runs medial to the psoas muscle

Vascular Regions

At the **pelvic brim** region we find vertically peritoneum, underneath that ovarian vessels in the infundibulopelvic ligament and medially is the ureter crossing over the bifurcation of the common iliac to internal and external artery (Fig. 58.5), underneath that is common iliac vein, further underneath is obturator nerve: exiting the psoas muscle medially to pass over the pelvic brim to the pelvic sidewall; and underneath that is the sacroiliac joint. The pudental nerve and the ureter comes into the pelvic brim in a vertical fashion, and then rotates in 90° to enter the pelvic sidewall.

In the **pelvic sidewall** region there are three surgical layers. The first pelvic sidewall layer is the ureter layer, where the ureter is enveloped in its own visceral sheet of visceral connective tissue [10]. There, an ureterolysis is performed posteriorly to the base of the broad ligament (Fig. 58.6). It leads inferiorly further to the pararectal space. The second pelvic sidewall layer is a vascular layer, which is also a safe zone for coagualtion and cutting that consists of the internal iliac vessels and their branches (Figs. 58.6 and 58.7). And last but not least, the third pelvic sidewall layer is a parietal

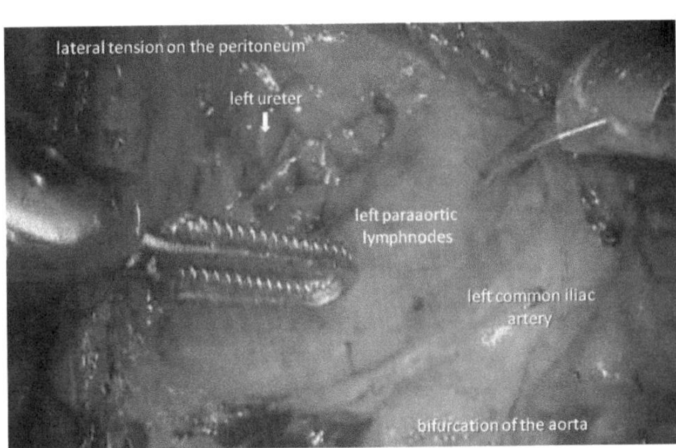

Fig. 58.4 Before the left paraaortic lymphadenectomy: identification of the left ureter. On the left side of the aorta laterally is the left ureter

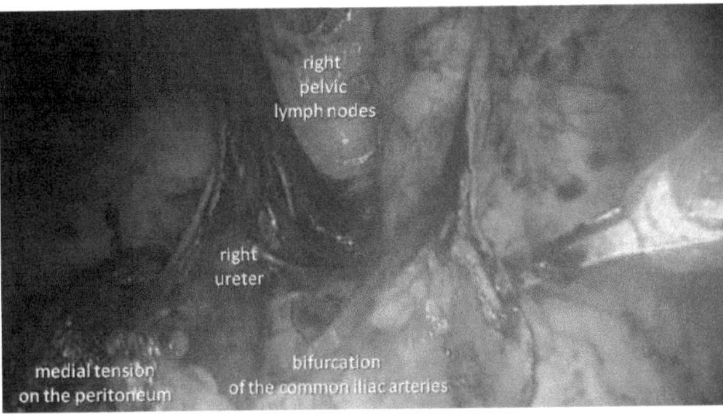

Fig. 58.5 Before the right pelvic lymphadenectomy identification of the right ureter in a peritoneal flap. At the pelvic brim region medially is the ureter crossing over the bifurcation of the common iliac to internal and external artery

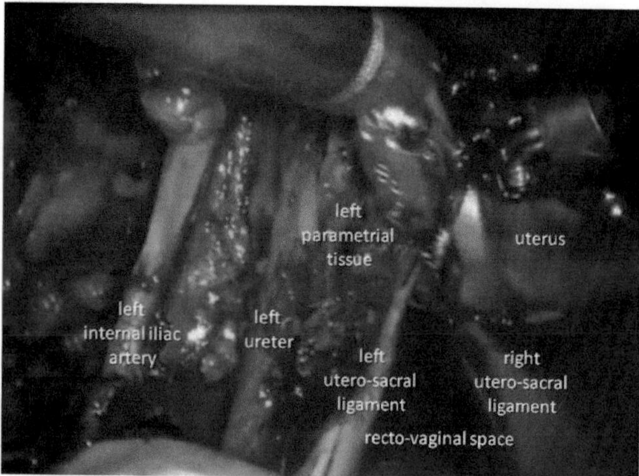

Fig. 58.6 After the ureterolysis and the dissection of uterine artery just before the arametrectomy on the left side by performing robotic radical hysterectomy. The rectovaginal space was previously entered vaginally. In the first pelvic sidewall layer is the ureter layer, where the ureter is enveloped in its own visceral sheet of visceral connective tissue. There is performed ureterolysis posteriorly to the base of the broad ligament

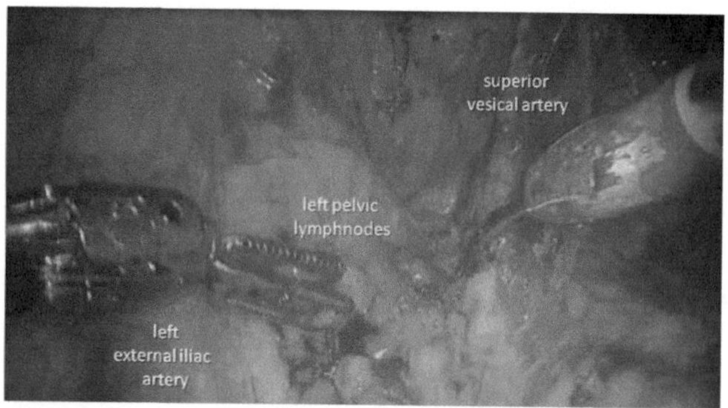

Fig. 58.7 Before the left pelvic lymphadenectomy: identification of the left superior vesical artery. The second pelvic sidewall layer is a vascular layer, which a safe zone that consists of the internal iliac vessels and their branches (here superior vesical artery)

layer that consists of the external iliac vessels on the medial board of the psoas muscle and obturator vessels and nerve on the anterior portion of the obturator internal muscle (Fig. 58.8). The base of the pelvic sidewall is a base of the broad ligament.

By every laparoscopic hysterectomy technique also performed by the robot Da Vinci the broad ligament is dissected. Anteriorly to the dissected ligament the bladder flap is developed in a vesico-vaginal space, posteriorly to the dissected ligament the posterior peritoneum of the uterus is dissected toward the base of the uterosacral ligaments where the uterosacral ligaments meet the cervix (Fig. 58.9). With the push-press dissection technique the uterine artery is identified and skeletonized laterally from there. Then the uterine artery is followed to find the ureter in the base of the broad ligament.

The **base of the broad ligament** region is a place to find where the ureter passes underneath the internal iliac artery (Fig. 58.10), 1–2 cm medial to the cervix but 2–3 cm medial

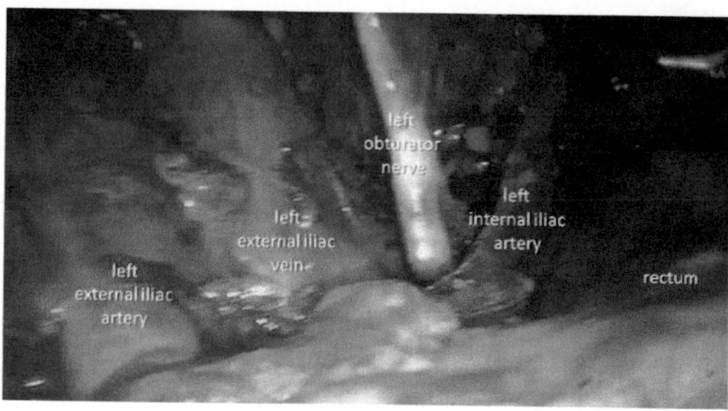

Fig. 58.8 Situs after the left pelvic lymphadenectomy. The third pelvic sidewall layer is a parietal layer that consists of the external iliac vessels and obturator nerve

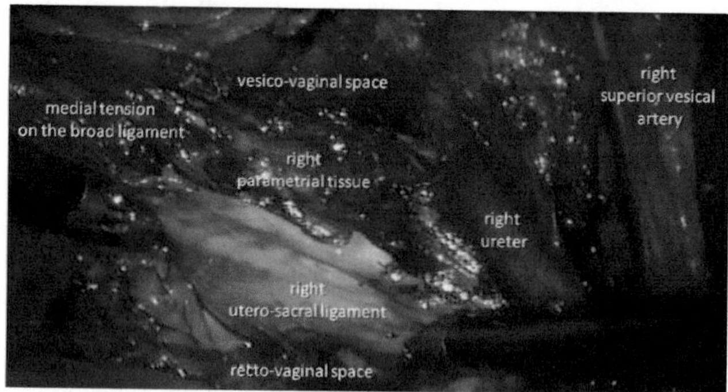

Fig. 58.9 After the ureterolysis, during the right parametrectomy by performing the robotic radical hysterectomy on the right side. The avascular vesico-vaginal and recto-vaginal spaces were previously entered vaginally. The dissection of the base of the broad ligament: anteriorly to the parametrial tissue is a vesico-vaginal space, posteriorly is the utero-sacral ligament. Here the rectovaginal space was previously entered vaginally

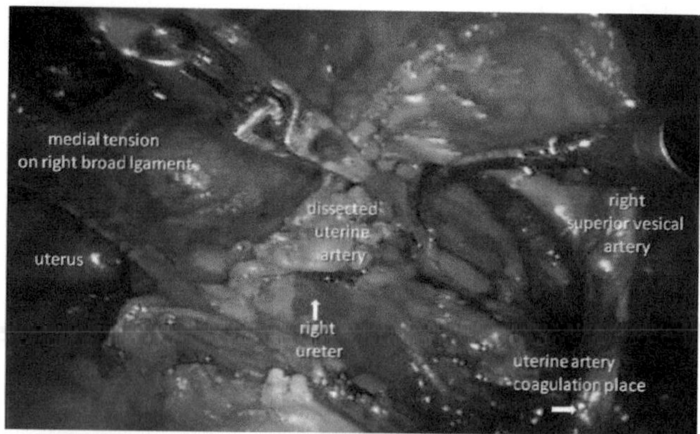

Fig. 58.10 After a dissection of the right uterine artery running over the right ureter, during robotic radical hysterectomy procedure. The ureter passes underneath the internal iliac artery at the base of the broad ligament region

and superior to the ischial spine. It is also the base of the cardinal ligament. The dissection allowed at the base of the broad ligament region is without cutting, only tenting, traction and counter-traction, push-press technique.

The further dissection anteriorly and inferiorly from the base of the broad ligament leads to the paravesical space which is simply also a paravaginal space and then more anterior and medial dissection leads into retropubic space of Retzius. The dissection posteriorly and inferiorly from the base of the broad ligament leads to the pararectal space.

Avascular Spaces

Three pairs of ligaments: uterosacral ligament (rectal pillars), cardinal ligament and vesicouterine ligament (bladder pillars) divide the pelvis into six potential avascular spaces with some vascular boarders: presacral, pararectal space, rectovaginal space, vesicovaginal space, paravesical/ paravaginal/ obturator space, prevesical (retropubic) space of Retzius [12].

The **presacral (retro-rectal or perlumbal) space**: is boarded laterally on the right side with the right ureter, on the left side with the left common iliac artery. It begins at the bifurcation of the aorta into the common iliac which boarder this space and lead into the pelvic brim. At the base of the mesosigma just inferior to the aortic bifurcation, the superior hypogastric plexus can be identified.

The **pararectal space**: is triangular, with the base of the cardinal ligament representing the anterior boarder. The medial boarder is the ureter and the rectal pillars (uterosacral ligament) with the rectum and the hypogastric nerve adhering medially to the mesorectum (Fig. 58.11) and the lateral border is the internal iliac artery and the iliococcygeus fascia and muscles. The hypogastric nerve is a continuation of the superior hypogastric plexus on either side. Inferiorly the hypogastric nerve, where the pelvic splanchnic nerves and the sacral splanchnic nerves join, form the inferior hypogastric plexus on the lateral surface of the uterosacral ligament (Fig. 58.12). On the floor is levator ani muscle and it leads to ischial spine and sacrospinous ligaments. The pararectal space is crossed by the vesical and rectal nerve plexuses. This space can be easily developed by bluntly dissecting

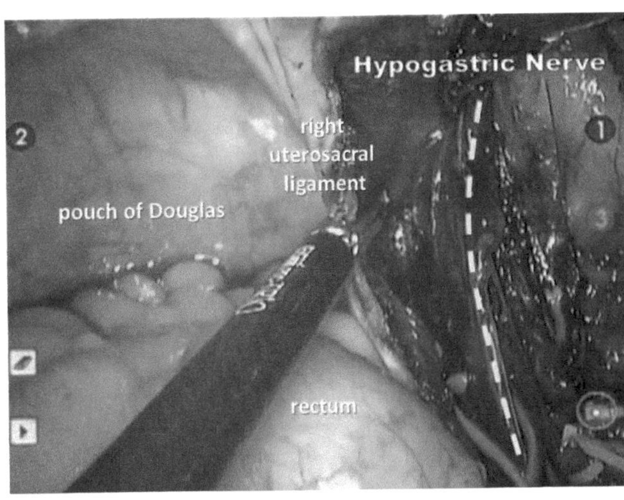

Fig. 58.11 Right pararectal space is triangular, the medial boarder is the right ureter and the right rectal pillars (uterosacral ligament) with the rectum and the right hypogastric nerve (right pelvic nerve) adhering medially to the mesorectum, to the lateral side of the right uterosacral ligament (rectal pillars). The right hypogastric nerve will be isolated till the cut end of the uterine vein and will be preserved by the devision of the right uterosacral ligament during nerve-sparing hysterectomy (Photo from educational video by Maggioni [9])

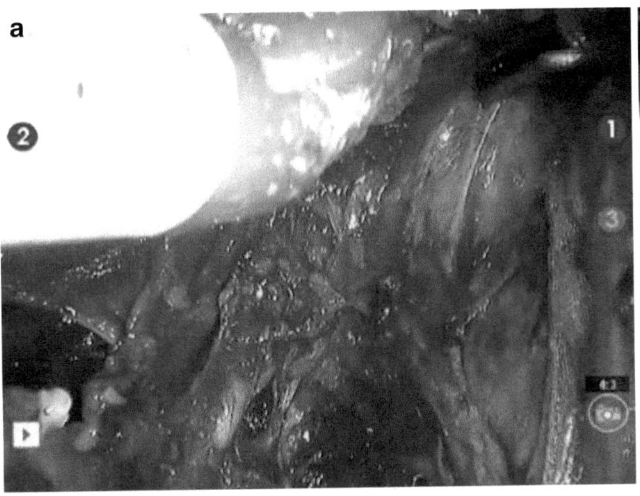

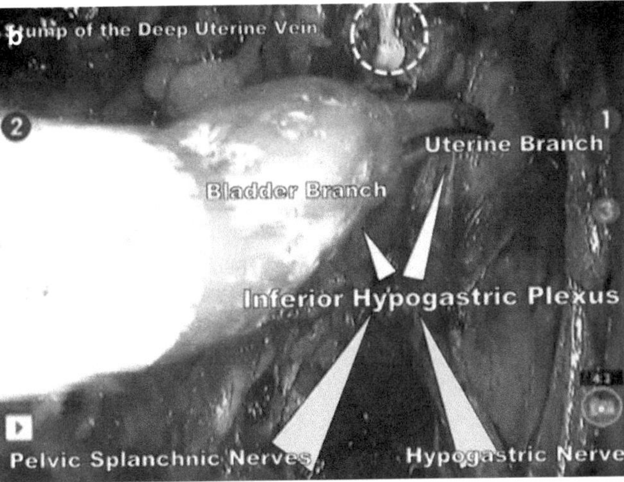

Fig. 58.12 Inferior hypogastric plexus (pelvic plexus) on the lateral surface of the uterosacral ligament. It is formed as a junction of splanchnic nerves and hypogastric nerve and has the bladder and the uterine branch. Only the uterine branch of the inferior hypogastric plexus is resected by the nerve-sparing radical hysterectomy. Left pararectal space after isolation and transsection of: the uterine artery, the superficial uterine vein and the deep uterine vein. The stump of the deep uterine vein is elevated up the level of hypogastric nerve (Photos from educational video by Maggioni [9])

posteriorly to the origin of the uterine artery and lateral to the ureter.

The **rectovaginal space**: is a safe avascular space, what is used for repair of the posterior vaginal wall defects or rectocel. It is framed by: superiorly with cul-de-sac peritoneum and utero-sacral ligaments; laterally: with iliococcygeus muscles; posteriorly: with rectum and its visceral fascial capsule with rectal fat; anteriorly: with vagina and its visceral fascial capsule; inferiorly: with perineum. It builds rectovaginal fascia/ septum. It is necessary to perform initially the ureterolysis on the both sides and then the dissection of the uterosacral ligaments to get to and dissect safely this rectovaginal space. To enter the space of the rectovaginal septum a transverse incision is made over the posterior cervix superiorly between the two uterosacral ligaments, also known as the medial-rectal-pillars. Then, the rectum is dissected inferiorly until the uterosacral ligaments are identified and transsected, thereafter, the rectovaginal space may be entered.

The **vesicovaginal space**: is a potential space between the bladder and the vagina (Fig. 58.13). Therefore, it has to be developed to mobilize the bladder of the lower uterine segment and the upper third of the vagina. Its lateral boarder is: the bladder pillars with ureters on the both sides. It is covered by the anterior peritoneal reflection and must be dissected for the completion of the hysterectomy to develop the bladder flap as a crucial part of that operation (Fig. 58.14). The dissection in this space is important to be performed medially and centrally, away from the bladder pillars in which are vascular vessels as well as the ureter. Once the dissection is done from both sides the bladder can be dissected of the cervix with cold scissors using push-(from below to the bladder)-cut-spread technique.

The **paravesical and paravaginal, and obturator space**: is anterior and inferior to the base of the broad ligament. Its boarders are: medial: the bladder and anterior vagina; lateral: obturator internus fascia with obturator nerve and vessels; floor: fascia endopelvina and the "white line": the arcus tendineus of the pelvis; posterior: internal iliac vessels and ischial spine; anterior: back of pubic bone. During dissection in the obturator space: in a straight line underneath the place where the obturator nerve enters the obturator foramen is the ischial spine with the pudental nerve behind the sacrospinal ligament. The obturator space and paravesical space are particularly important in pelvic lymphadenectomy, paravaginal space in nerve-sparing radical hysterectomy (Figs. 58.7 and 58.15).

The **prevesical (retropubic) space of Retzius** is the retropubic continuation of the paravesical space. It is located between the posterior part of the pubic bone and Cooper's ligament, which is its anterior boundary. Posteriorly is the anterior part of the bladder, lateral: the internal obturator

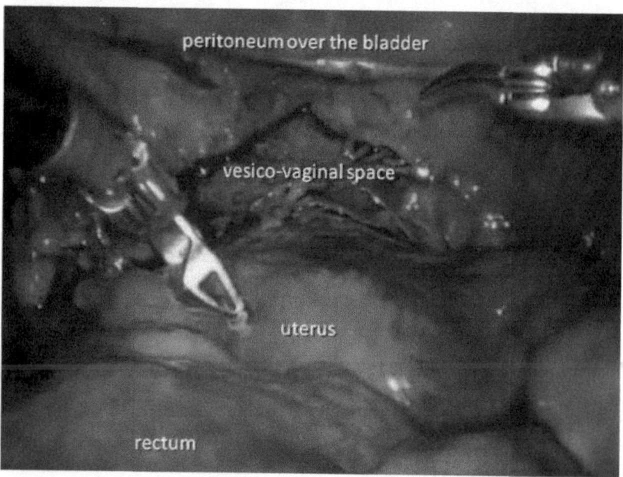

Fig. 58.13 After opening of the vesico-vaginal space before the robotic radical hysterectomy. The vesicovaginal space is a potential space between the bladder and the vagina

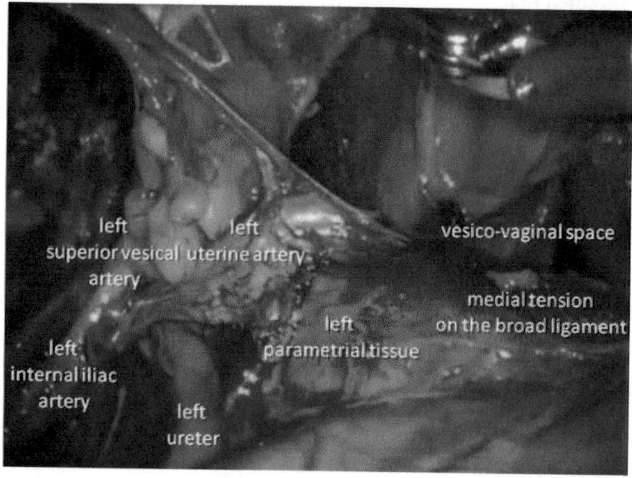

Fig. 58.14 After the ureterolysis, before the robotic radical hysterectomy on the left side. In the vesicovaginal space: the bladder flap was developed

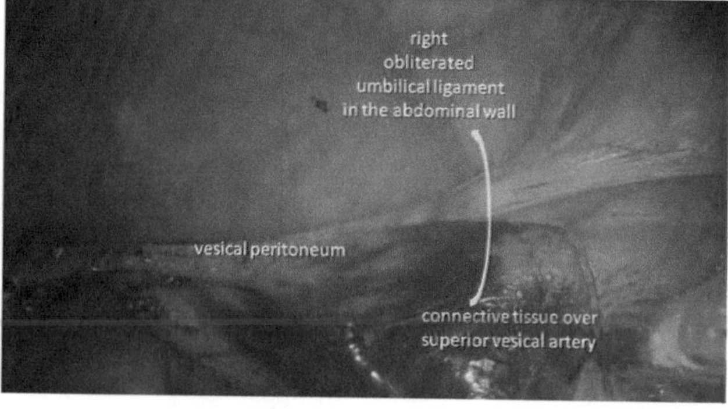

Fig. 58.15 An opening of the right paravesical space. By pulling up and down on the obliterated umbilical ligament the superior vesical artery can be easily identified and medial to that the paravesical space opened. After identification of the superior vesical artery and following it cranially the first medial branch of it is the begin of the uterine artery

muscle and it is continued posteriorly with the vesicovaginal space. The floor is the pubocervical (paravaginal) fascia, inserted into the tendinous arch in the internal obturator fascia. During the Retzius space development with blunt and sharp dissection of fibrofatty tissue a special care needs to be taken to avoid periurethral neurovascular injury.

Laparoscopic Identification of the Ureter, the Uterine Artery

For every gynecologic laparoscopic procedure via the Da Vinci robot, the previous anatomic surgical knowledge and the key gynecologic structures, especially where of the **ureter** is running in the abdominal and pelvic regions is essential for its intraoperative identification and to guarantee a safe gynecologic procedure. The lumbar ureter lies on the psoas muscle medial to the ovarian vessels (Fig. 58.3). It enters the pelvic cavity just superficial to the bifurcation of the common iliac artery and just deep to the ovarian vessels, which lie in the infundibulopelvic ligament at the pelvic brim. It lies in the anterior medial leaf of the broad ligament as it winds toward the bladder and can be recognized by its characteristic peristaltic motion. The ureter then passes just lateral to the uterosacral ligament, approximately 2 cm medial to the ischial spine through the upper part of the cardinal ligament at the base of the broad ligament. Here it lies just beneath the uterine artery, approximately 1.5–2 cm lateral to the side of the cervix. The ureter forms a "knee" turn under the uterine vessels and at from this point travels medially and anteriorly to pass on the anterolateral fornix of the vagina to enter the bladder at the junction of the upper and middle third of the vagina [11]. Therefore, special attention must be given after the hysterectomy by closing the vaginal cuff, where at the lateral angle of the vagina, as well as anterior and anterio-lateral in the upper third of the vagina is the ureter.

Before every operative procedure with the Da Vinci robot, in which the **uterine artery** needs to be ligated, in order to guarantee a hemostasis and a safe procedure, even before identification of the uterine artery, previously performed ureterolysis via the Da Vinci robot is of great importance. For the ureterolysis, the ureter can be found on the pelvic sidewall medial to the infundibulopelvic ligament as it crosses the external iliac. The peritoneum superior to the ureter is gently grasped and entered. The ureter is in the medial tenting sheet to the infundibulopelvic ligament. The peritoneal incision is extended: by tenting of the further peritoneum and cutting with millimeter by millimeter progression only of what can be seen or determined. The medial traction is placed on the medial edge of the peritoneal incision of the first pelvic sidewall layer to open retroperitoneal space, and the dissection is continued in a fat-nonfat interface (fat belongs to the rectum, the dissection is performed superior to the fat) until the ureter is identified medially in the opened space that further inferiorly leads to the pararectal space. There are two main structures after opening the peritoneum of the pelvic sidewall, that go down in the pelvis: first medial, that peristalses, that is the ureter; and the second lateral, that pulsates, that is the internal artery (Fig. 58.16) that branches medially to the uterine artery (Fig. 58.17). With further medial traction of the peritoneum, the ureterolysis is performed with push-spread-push-spread, traction-countertraction as well as millimeter snaps and millimeter wipes dissection technique continued to the level of the cardinal ligament.

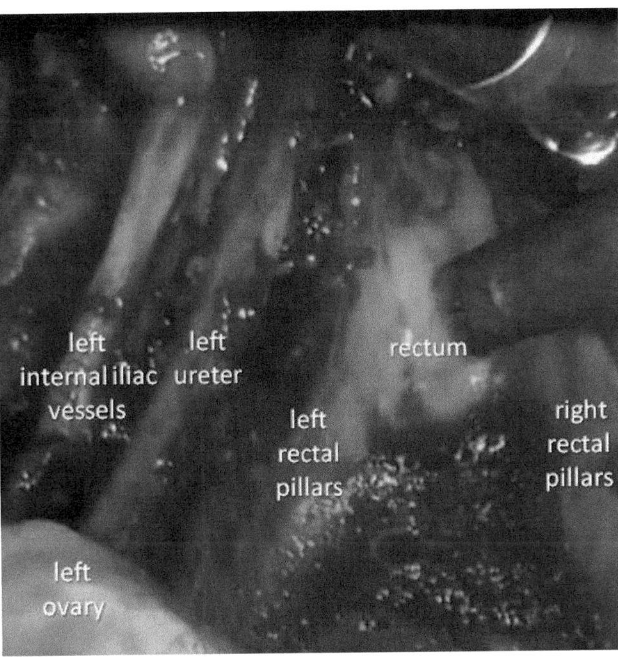

Fig. 58.16 Situs after a robotic radical hysterectomy without salpingectomy. There are two main structures that go from the pelvic sidewall down into the pelvis: first medial, that peristalses, that is the ureter; and the second lateral, that pulsates, that is the internal artery

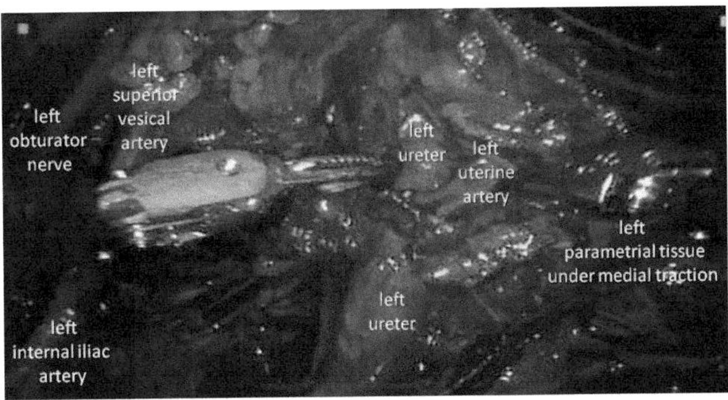

Fig. 58.17 After a pelvic lymphadenectomy and ureterolysis but before radical hysterectomy on the left side. The internal artery branches medially into the uterine artery that crosses from above the ureter in order to run into the uterus

In order to find the uterine artery, first, identification of the obliterated umbilical ligament can be helpful as a continuation of the superior vesical artery on the anterior abdominal wall (Fig. 58.15). Moving this ligament provokes a movement of the superior vesical artery, that lead straight further to the internal iliac artery (named also the hypogastric artery) coming from the bifurcation of the common iliac artery. The medial branch of the internal iliac artery is always the uterine artery (Fig. 58.14). Medial to the branching of the uterine artery from the internal iliac artery is the ureter, as the uterine artery crosses the ureter on its top aiming to the uterus. The ligation of the uterine artery is performed as lateral from the ureter as possible (at the uterus by total hysterectomy or at the internal iliac artery by radical hysterectomy procedure).

Laparoscopic Identification of the Hypogastric (Pelvic) Nerve, Splanchnic Nerves and Inferior Hypogastric (Pelvic) Plexus

Especially the Da Vinci robot with 3D stable and enlarged site view enable the surgeons to recognize the parts of the autonomic nerve system in the pelvis in order to preserve them during oncologic procedures and perform nerve-sparing operations. Those autonomic nerves that could be damaged during oncologic operations are: lumbar splanchnic nerves during periaortic lymph node dissection; superior hypogastric plexus during presacral lymph node dissection; hypogastric nerve during resection of the uterosacral ligaments (rectal pillars); proximal inferior hypogastric plexus during a division of the uterosacral ligaments and cardinal (transverse cervical) ligaments; and distal inferior hypogastric plexus during transection of the vesicouterine (pubocervical) ligaments.

The **hypogastric nerve (pelvic nerve)** can be identified in the pararectal space through an opening of the pararectal space between the internal iliac artery and the ureter, posteriorly to the uterine artery. There the hypogastric nerve runs parallel and approximately 2 cm inferior to the ureter (Fig. 58.18). The hypogastric nerve can be also found in the para\rectal space as adhering fibers to the lateral side of the uterosacral ligament (rectal pillars) (Fig. 58.11). The hypogastric nerve will be isolated until the cut end of the uterine vein to be preserved during the division of the uterosacral ligament by the nerve-sparing radical hysterectomy [9].

The hypogastric nerve inferiorly in a site where the pelvic splanchnic nerves and the sacral splanchnic nerves join, form **the inferior hypogastric (pelvic) plexus** with two branches (bladder and uterine branches) on the lateral surface of the uterosacral ligament (Fig. 58.12). In order to identify the hypogastric (pelvic) plexus: the ureter is separated from the posterior leaf of the VUL (vesico-uterine ligament) up to the loose tissue of the entrance of paravaginal space. The ureter is than shifted laterally. Then one can see: the posterior leaf of the left vesicouterine ligament that consists of left vesical veins that are draining into the deep uterine vein in the posterior layer of the vesicouterine ligament (VUL) (Fig. 58.19). The transsection of the vessical veins expose the bladder branch of the inferior hypogastric plexus (pelvic plexus) that runs posteriorly to the posterior part of the VUL. The exposure of the bladder branch (Fig. 58.12) is needed for its preservation during the nerve-sparing hysterectomy as only the anterior layer of the VUL is resected, where the uterine branch of the pelvic plexus runs.

In order to identify the **pelvic splanchnic nerves** the following structures need to be recognized: the uterine artery that is running just superior and parallel to the superficial uterine vein. Just inferior and parallel to the superficial uterine vein is the deep uterine vein (all those vessels are isolated and transected by the nerve-sparing radical hysterectomy) (Fig. 58.18). Just inferior and parallel to the deep uterine vein there are the pelvic splanchnic nerves localized. The pelvic splanchnic nerves are laterally to the hypogastric nerve that is running inferiorly to the ureter. If we follow the fibers of the hypogastric nerve further anteriorly, we can observe that they run just below the deep uterine vein (Fig. 58.18c).

Through a better site recognition, 3D stable view as well as magnification of the surgery area with better ergonomics, with the Da Vinci robot it is possible not only to learn and to teach the laparoscopic surgical anatomy but also to perform advanced laparoscopic operations that have been performed almost only by an abdominal approach before.

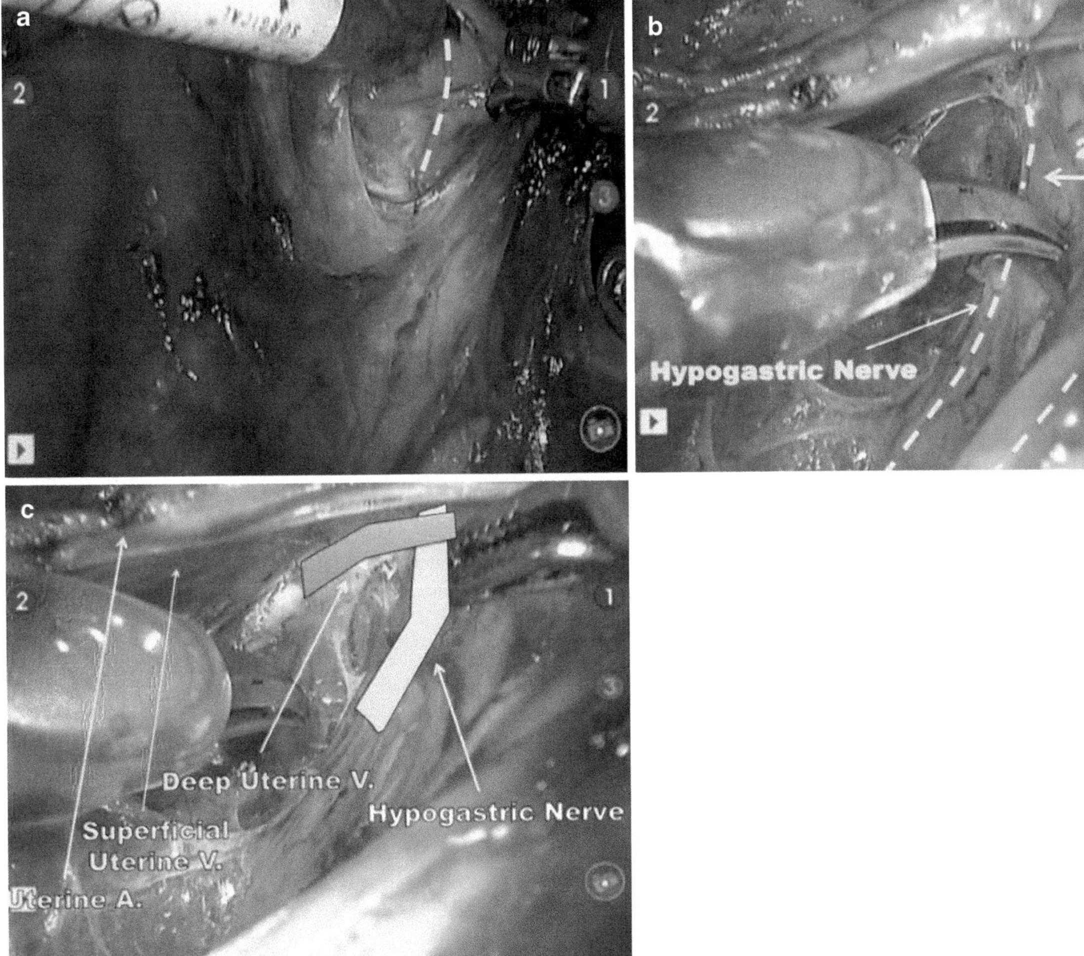

Fig. 58.18 Left pararectal space. The hypogastric nerve (pelvic nerve) can be identified in the pararectal space through an opening of the pararectal space between the internal iliac artery and the ureter, posteriorly to the uterine artery. There the hypogastric nerve runs parallel and approximately 2 cm inferior to the ureter. (**a**). An opening of the left pararectal space (between the left internal iliac artery and the left ureter, posteriorly to the left uterine artery) looking for the left hypogastric nerve (marked *yellow* here). (**b**). In the opened left pararectal space: the left hypogastric nerve is approximately 2 cm inferior to the left ureter. (**c**). The uterine artery is running just superior and parallel to the superficial uterine vein. Just inferior and parallel to the superficial uterine vein is the deep uterine vein (all will be isolated and transsected by the nerve-sparing radical hysterectomy) and just inferior and parallel to the deep uterine vein there are the pelvic splanchnic nerves localized. The pelvic splanchnic nerves are lateral to the hypogastric nerve, that is running inferior the ureter. If we follow the fibers of the left hypogastric nerve further anteriorly, we can observe that they run just below the left deep uterine vein (Photos from educational video by Maggioni [9])

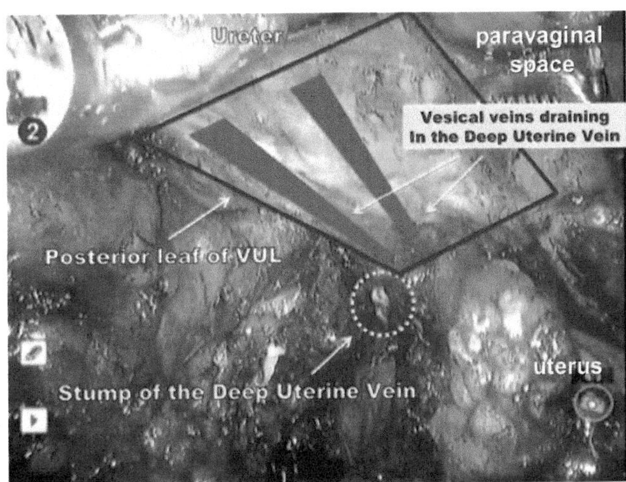

Fig. 58.19 Left vesicouterine ligament. The posterior leaf of the left vesicouterine ligament that consists of left vesical veins that are draining into the deep uterine vein in the posterior layer of the vesicouterine ligament (VUL) (Photo from educational video by Maggioni [9])

References

1. Mettler L, Schollmeyer T, Boggess J, Magrina JF, Oleszczuk A. Robotic assistance in gynecological oncology. Curr Opin Oncol. 2008;20(5):581–9.
2. Oleszczuk A, Kohler C, Paulick J, Schneider A, Lanowska M. Vaginal robot-assisted radical hysterectomy (VRARH) after laparoscopic staging: feasibility and operative results. Int J Med Robot. 2009;5(1):38–44.
3. Bedaiwy MA, Franjoine SE, Ali MK. Laparoendoscopic single-site (LESS) surgery in gynecology: Current status and future directions. Middle East Fertil Soc J. 2013;18(1):1–8.
4. Fader AN, Cohen S, Escobar PF, Gunderson C. Laparoendoscopic single-site surgery in gynecology. Curr Opin Obstet Gynecol. 2010;22(4):331–8.
5. Autorino R, Kaouk JH, Stolzenburg JU, Gill IS, Mottrie A, Tewari A, et al. Current status and future directions of robotic single-site surgery: a systematic review. Eur Urol. 2013;63(2):266–80.
6. Escobar PF, Fader AN, Paraiso MF, Kaouk JH, Falcone T. Robotic-assisted laparoendoscopic single-site surgery in gynecology: initial report and technique. J Minim Invasive Gynecol. 2009;16(5):589–91.
7. Rossi EC, Jackson A, Ivanova A, Boggess JF. Detection of sentinel nodes for endometrial cancer with robotic assisted fluorescence imaging: cervical versus hysteroscopic injection. Int J Gynecol Cancer. 2013;23(9):1704–11.
8. Jewell EL, Huang JJ, Abu-Rustum NR, Gardner GJ, Brown CL, Sonoda Y, et al. Detection of sentinel lymph nodes in minimally invasive surgery using indocyanine green and near-infrared fluorescence imaging for uterine and cervical malignancies. Gynecol Oncol. 2014;133(2):274–7.
9. Maggioni, A. Robot-assisted laparoscopic nerve sparing Okabayashi's radical hysterectomy according to Shingo Fujii's Technique [educational video]. European Institute of Oncology Milan, Italy; 2010.
10. Rogers RM. Pelvic anatomy seen through the laparoscope. In: Pasic RP, Levine RL, editors. A practical manual of laparoscopy: a clinical cookbook. Lancashire: Parthenon Publishing Group; 2002. p. 7–17.
11. Yadav J, Datta MS, Nezhat C, Nezhat C, Nezhat F. Intraperitoneal and retroperitoneal anatomy. In: Nezhat C, Nezhat F, Nezhat C, editors. Netzhat's operative gynecologic laparoscopy and hysteroscopy. 3rd ed. Cambridge: Cambridge University Press; 2008. p. 70–82.
12. Barbosa C, Wattiez A, Mencaglia L. Gynecologic laparoscopic surgical anatomy. In: Mencaglia L, Minelli L, Wattiez A, editors. Manual of gnecological laparoscopic surgery. 2nd ed. Tuttlingen: Endo-Press; 2007. p. 57–71.

General Aspects and Their Handling: Adhesions

59

Alexander Di Liberto and Kubilay Ertan

Introduction

Peritoneal adhesions, this means mainly non congenital, abnormous fibrous connections between tissues, that are normally anatomically not conjoined, are an ubiquitous problem in abdominal surgery that could appear after every surgical intervention of each kind, including robot-assisted interventions and in this context robot-assisted hysterectomies, but with different likelihood.

Prior surgical interventions respectively post-inflammatory alterations in the upper abdomen (state after cholecystectomy, after pancreatitis and also after extensive surgical interventions via laparotomy) are mostly not relevant for the predominant proportion of laparoscopic interventions in the lesser pelvis respectively concerning the laparoscopic access points, but can cause problems and challenges just as the trocar positions would be shift to a more cranial localization, this means above the umbilicus (for example for the access to the paraaortic lymph node regions or to perform hysterectomy procedures in big uteri), especially in robot-assisted interventions, where generously a cranial shifting of the trocars have to be performed.

Basical problem is the preoperative estimation of the extent of adhesions, just after surgical interventions in the lower abdomen and lesser pelvis at the colon and small intestine or localised adhesions in the lesser abdomen and pelvis (e.g. after pelveoperitonitis due to adnexitis or severe endometriosis, but also after cesarean sections were unexpected large-area and firm adhesions between the anterior uterine wall and the abdominal wall can be found). In the state after peritonitis in particular generalised peritonitis respectively four-quadrant peritonitis extensive peritoneal adhesions have to be anticipated, so that the laparoscopic respectively robot-assisted methods of entrance to the peritoneal cavity have to be adapted correspondingly. The most commonly consequences of intraperitoneal adhesions are chronic pain syndroms in the lower abdomen, small intestine obstruction up to ileus, for the gynaecological patient cohort primary or secondary sterility and dyspareunia as well as the formation of pseudocysts in the lesser pelvis (with the partially difficult differential diagnosis to genuine cystic lesions and, for this reason, hindered decision-making for or against surgical clarification), and relating to subsequent operative interventions in the peritoneal cavity a higher risk of organ injury, especially bowel lesion (serosal defects, enterotomy, primary detected or unnoticed during surgery), major blood loss, and a increased rate of conversions to laparotomy (Table 59.1).

Adhesion-related complaints themselves frequently result in re-operations (the SCAR3 trial demonstrated an incidence of 10 % concerning adhesion-related hospital stays within 5 years postoperatively [1]) and are, in a great extent, both very questionable regarding the primary surgical outcome (i.e. elimination of the complaints), and concerning the long-term course, because the likelihood of recurrence of adhesion formation in identical or other localizations is very high, in spite of application of substances and materials for adhesion prophylaxis.

This leads to a significant long-term impairment of the quality of life on the one hand and a considerable charging of costs in the healthcare systems on the other hand.

Robot-assisted laparoscopic interventions are affected at least in an equal measure related to the complex of problems concerning peritoneal adhesions, both regarding preexisting adhesion (of any origin), and the induction of de novo adhesions, the last one perhaps in a higher degree, because just complex operative interventions are performed robot-assisted (notably complex hysterectomies, oncological therapy, surgical interventions in higher-degree endometriosis, complex myomectomies, etc.).

A. Di Liberto (✉) • K. Ertan
Department of Gynaecology and Obstetrics,
Leverkusen Municipal Hospital, Leverkusen 51375, Germany
e-mail: diliberto@klinikum-lev.de

I. Alkatout, L. Mettler (eds.), *Hysterectomy*, DOI 10.1007/978-3-319-22497-8_59

Table 59.1 Medical and surgical consequences of peritoneal adhesions

General medical and surgical aspects	Gynaecological aspects
Chronic pain syndroms (localised or generalised in the abdomen)	Primary/secondary sterility; increased rate of ectopic pregnancies
Small intestine obstruction up to ileus	Dyspareunia
Subsequent operative interventions (with higher risk of organ lesions, major blood loss and laparotomy)	Formation of pseudocysts in the lesser pelvis (diagnostic dilemma)
Socio-economic consequences	Increased complexity of gynaecological operations

Particularly in oncological interventions in cervical and endometrial cancer, which are exceedingly eligible for the robot-assisted technique, large-area accesses to the retroperitoneum have to be established, by what substantial peritoneal traumata occur.

In comparison to traditional laparoscopy the robot-assisted interventions are characterized by the utilization of a higher number of trocars and a larger trocar diameter leading primary to a greater surgical trauma in the area of the peritoneal entrances, but no data or reports are available on this topic, especially in comparison to traditional laparoscopy.

Surgical Principles of Prevention of Adhesions and of Adhesiolysis

In general, for robot-assisted laparoscopic interventions in gynecology the same surgical principles are valid for prevention of adhesions and of adhesiolysis.

For prevention of adhesiolysis, finally representing the most effective potential to avoid respectively to reduce adhesion-associated morbidity, the principles of "good surgical technique" are valid; this are beside the general awareness which pathophysiological mechanisms constitute for formation of adhesions the minimisation of direct and indirect surgical trauma at the parietal peritoneum and other serosal surfaces, provided that these are not related to the therapeutical target area. Therefore, this means gentle handling of tissues and organs, the reduction of HF surgical-caused heat effect at the peritoneum and other surfaces (i.e. sparing coagulation), the avoidance of ischemic change, this means especially the diminuation of bleeding not only by coagulation but by accurate and anatomical dissection and by conservation of smaller vessels, the avoidance of desiccation, which is particularly relevant in laparoscopic interventions concerning the capnoperitoneum, the reduction of application of external material and foreign bodies, the shortening of operation time, and, if necessary, the application of materials of adhesions prevention (see Chap. 6).

The basic principles of correct adhesiolysis are the careful and accurate dissection of adhesions, as possible without additional injury and trauma of the peritoneum and serosal surfaces, the economic use of electrocoagulation with concurrent avoidance of bleedings. Finally, the extent of adhesiolysis also depends on the mode of intervention and the dimensions of the required surgical field, and, eventually apparent complaints concerning adhesions.

Adhesions which do not impair the access to the surgical area or the surgical target area, and which do not cause anamnestic and/or clinical complaints, and are not a potential future menace, for example provoking intestinal/small bowel obstruction, should better be left and not to be touched.

However, even if they seem not to present a direct obstacle to the surgical activity, adhesions can constitute a risk factor for sticking with laparoscopic instruments and therefore causing delayed noticed bleedings or unnoticed blunt tissue trauma up to higher grade organ injury and complications.

For the traditional laparoscopy, which is characterized in comparison to open abdominal surgery by reduced formation of postoperative adhesions, there exist additional problems concerning the complex of problems of the capnoperitoneum, generally the gas pressure leading to microtrauma at the hole peritoneum, and the consecutive desiccation of the peritoneal surface – all of these constitue risk factors for the formation of adhesions, at least contribute to adhesions. However, these risk factors can be influenced by various methods and techniques: Adding of O_2 to the carbonic dioxide, limitation of gas pressure to a minimum limit (with the disadvantage of a potential diminished visualisation or an increase of bleeding in the surgical area), and a continuous humidification of the peritoneal cavity via the insufflation system or by an intermittend irrigation.

Robot-assisted laparoscopic operations allow a decreased gas pressure or a minimum of pressure of some mmHg because the abdominal wall is stretched tent-like by the anchorage of the trocars at the patient side cart, thus imitating a "gasless" laparoscopic intervention. In addition, the robotic technique provides the potential to perform adhesiolysis more precisely (better visualisation [higher image resolution and particularly spatial view], and the higher flexibility and dexteritiy of the robotic instruments and for this reason a pinpoint adhesiolysis, selective and punctual coagulation of small vessels in adhesion threads, respectively the avoidance of bleeding by increased visualisation. Robot-assisted adhesiolysis is carried out in close analogy to traditional laparoscopy by grasping the adhesion with a smooth grasping forces (e.g. of eligible EndoWrist™

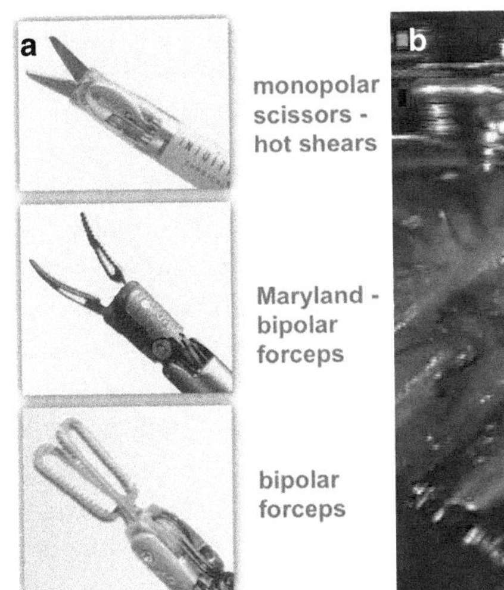

Fig. 59.1 (**a**) Eligible EndoWrist instruments for robot-assisted adhesiolysis (Source: Intuitive Surgical, Sunnyvale, California, with permission). (**b**) Arrangement of instruments in robot-assisted adhesiolysis (above: Grasping Forceps, bottom left: Maryland Bipolar Forceps; bottom right: Monopolar Curved Scissors, "Hot Shears")

instruments: Maryland Forceps or Bipolar Forceps, Fig. 59.1a), slight to moderate tension of the adhesion for delineation of the borders to normal peritoneum or other neighbouring organs (uterus, adnexa, bowel), as required selective and punctial coagulation of vessels in the adhesion and cutting the adhesion with monopolar scissors (e.g. of eligible EndoWrist™ instrument: Monopolar Curved scissors, Hot Shears, Fig. 59.1a), as necessary careful shifting and pushing of adjacent tissue structures respectively neighbouring organs under minimisation of bleedings, tissue trauma and especially serosal defects. Figure 59.1b shows a typical arrangement of instruments in robot-assisted adhesiolysis.

However, possible disadvantages of robot-assisted interventions are the generally higher number of inserted trocars leading to a larger peritoneal wound area (reduction of the peritoneal trauma by availability and application of a robot-assisted single port technique, which is already in use, but to date it is limited concerning complex minimal invasive procedures; for the future a flexible robotic single port technique is under way, which might overcome the current limitations of single port techniques), the absence of haptic and tactile feedback endangering a gentle handling of peritoneal and serosal surfaces, the increased view can compensate the latter only partially. There are no comparative and descriptive studies on this topic up to now.

Risk Factors for Adhesions/Planning of Operations in Expected Adhesions

Essentially, risk factors for existing peritoneal adhesions result from the patient's history, i.e. the indicated and presumed previous operations; the presumed previous operations are commonly only apparent by existing scarring at the abdominal wall because the patients oftenly do not remember operations which have been long ago, especially elderly patients.

Besides the medical history of an operation respectively the existence of an operation scar the antecedent of inflammatory disease (concerning the gynaecological sector these are adnexitis, resp. Pelveoperitonitis or simply chronic lower abdominal pain), and the history of endometriosis are relevant. Particularly in chronic inflammatory diseases of the bowel (Crohn's disease, ulcerative colitis) the presence of peritoneal adhesions with different extent must be anticipated.

This applies similarly both for robot-assisted and traditional laparoscopic interventions, and especially for hysterectomies.

Within the scope of the planning and preparation of operations the patient has to be informed about possible accesses to the peritoneal cavity (trocar placement), their situative variability (modification of the number of the trocars and their position), the higher risk of a conversion to laparotomy (including the information of and discussion about the particular incision line: Pfannenstiel incision versus longitudinal incision) and of an intraoperative neighbouring organ injury, particularly an enterotomy respectively an increased postoperative complication rate.

In addition, the constitution of the surgical team, if necessary the stand-by of a visceral surgeon has to be considered; furthermore, a longer operation time has to be taken into account (both concerning the medical resilience of the patient and the allocation of a sufficient logistic prearrangement [positioning, the patient warming, anaesthesiologic monitoring]). Finally, the essential items about this have to be documented in the informed consent.

In this connection there are no fundamental differences between robot-assisted laparascopic interventions and traditional laparoscopic operations, whereupon, in most cases, the primary more complex intervention would be accommodated.

Laparoscopic and Robot-Assisted Accesses in Presence of Adhesions

For robot-assisted intervention there are only a few differences concerning the accesses to the abdominal cavity compared to traditional laparoscopic procedures. Due to the major importance of the distance of the camera to the top of the uterus in robot-assisted operations (reduced flexibility of the daVinci™ camera, respectively the restrictation of fast camera movements), i.e. always a sufficient distance has to be given, this corresponds to a hand, in these interventions the trocar positions are in most cases more cranial as compared to traditional laparoscopic trocar positions (Fig. 59.2a–c). Just in operations of big uteri the camera trocar has frequently be placed above the umbilicus, so that especially in existing adhesions in the lower abdomen and in the pelvis the trocar positioning is primary outside of the hazardous zone. Insofar the Palmer's point can be utilized as access way as well as in traditional laparoscopy and later for replacement of the Veres needle with a daVinci™ working trocar. Here, plenty of surgeons apply previously of placing the daVinci™ camera a traditional endoscope to get a picture of the situation inside of the abdominal cavity. Likewise, an open sky technique can be applied in robot-assisted interventions; in this technique the abdominal cavity is opened under visual control both in the area of the lower umbilicus and supraumbilical, similarly to traditional laparoscopic open accesses, the so-called open sky access, whereas special open sky trocars for robotic-assisted surgery are not available.

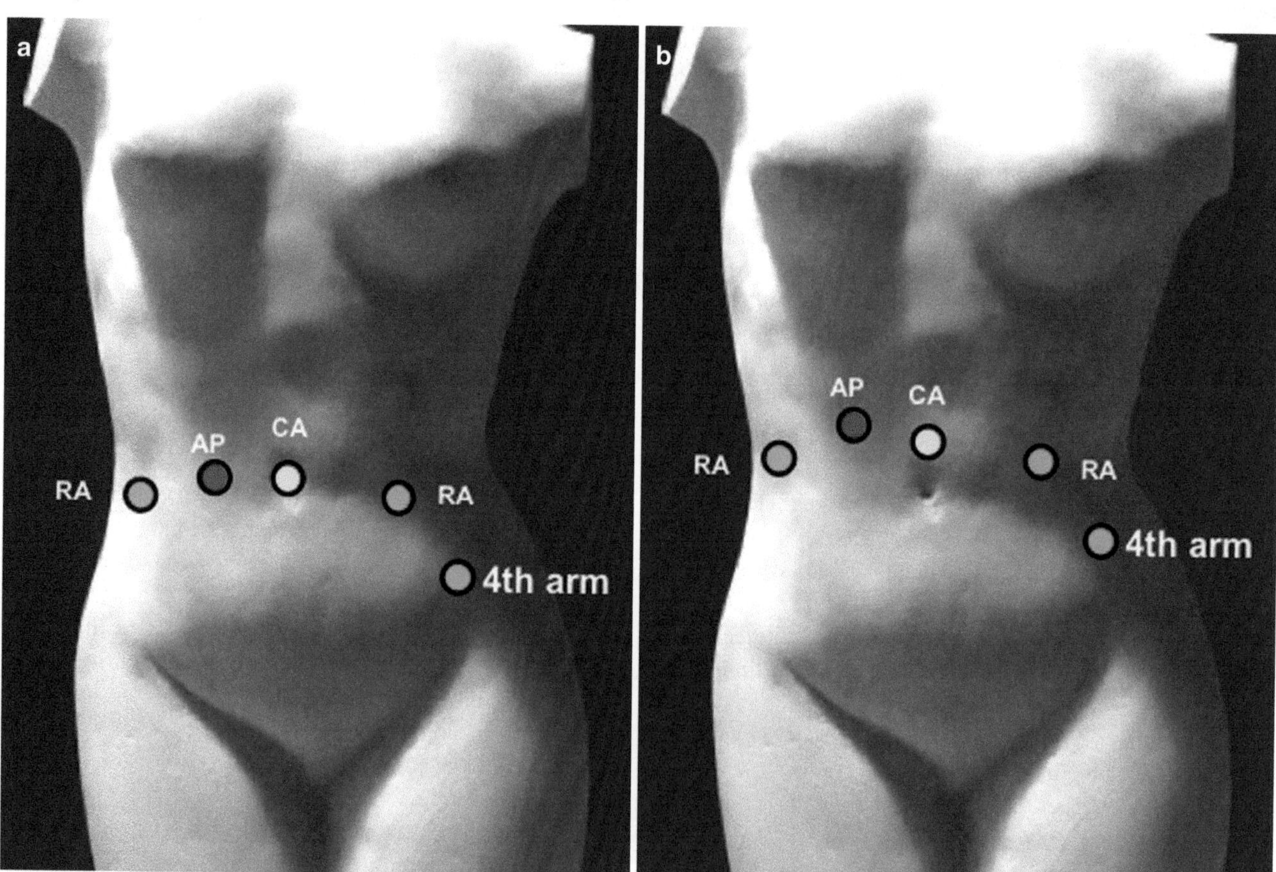

Fig. 59.2 (**a**) Suggestion for umbilical placement and arrangement of the camera and robotic trocars in case of adhesions in the lesser pelvis. (**b**) Suggestion for supraumbilical placement and arrangement of the camera and robotic trocars in case of adhesions in the lower abdomen and lesser pelvis and/or enlarged uterus. (**c**) Suggestion for subcostal placement and arrangement of camera and robotic trocars in case of upper abdominal adhesions and/or huge uterus

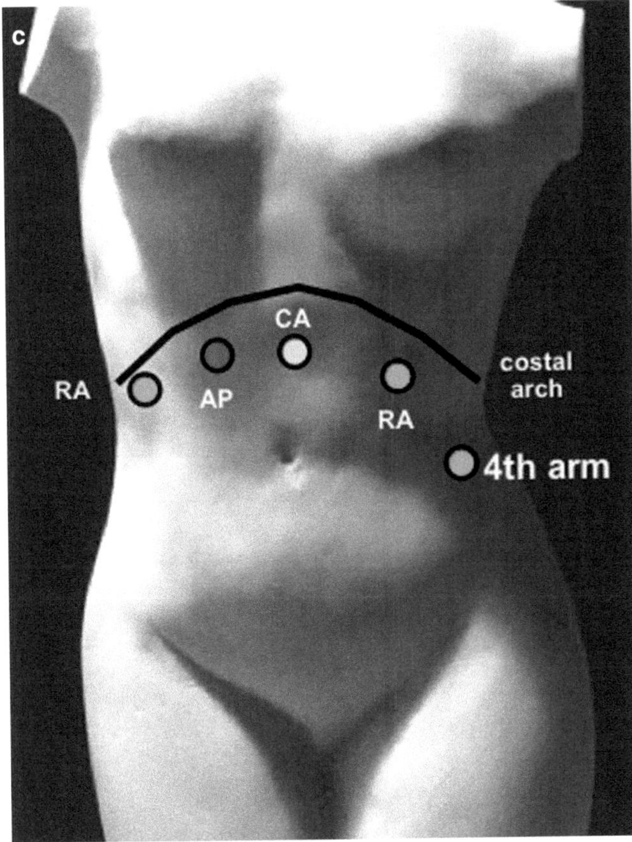

Fig. 59.2 (Continued)

Traditional Laparoscopic/Robot-Assisted Management of Adhesions (Before and After Docking of the Patient Side Cart)

In the case of existence of adhesions in the area of the trocar accesses the required flexibility of the robotic arms is limited in robot-assisted surgery. In this connection a traditional laparoscopic adhesiolysis is required until enough space, i.e. a sufficient surgical field for a sufficient mobility of the robotic arms is achieved in the proper surgical field in order to place all the needed daVinci™ trocars in the middle and lower abdomen.

Not till then, the patient side cart can be placed, the robotic arms can be docked and the operation can be continued from the surgeon's console.

In the event of adhesions in the lower abdomen and in the lesser pelvis adhesiolysis can be continued with the daVinci™ system after establishment of a sufficient surgical visual field, docking maneuver and taking over of the operation at the console.

Here, adhesiolysis can be performed much easier than in traditional laparoscopy due to the three-dimensional view, the superiority of instrument flexibility, and the higher number of freedom degrees of the EndoWrist™ instruments; for example, combined with the fixed camera position and the magnification of the daVinci™ optical system vessels can better be visualized in adhesional threads and can accurately be coagulated, and, thus, bleedings can be reduced at the best and thermal effects can be limited to a minimum.

In case of a required mobilisation of the intestinum for a better accessibility to the lesser pelvis (i.e. pelvic and para-aortic lymh node dissection) an adequate adhesiolysis has to be performed via traditional laparoscopy in the middle abdomen prior to the docking of the patient side cart so that the small intestine and the colon can be shifted to the middle and upper abdomen sufficiently by Trendelenburg positioning.

After docking of the patient side cart and installation of the camera the visual field is limited to the upper regions of the abdomen; this constitutes a relevant confinement of the robotic technique (the daVinci™ camera cannot pivoting more than 90° cranially; this limitation is largely eliminated in the daVinci™ 4th generation device, the daVinci™ Xi).

Application of Techniques for Prophylaxis of Adhesions.

All techniques of adhesion prevention and prophylaxis (e.g. oxidised regenerated cellulose [Interceed™], expanded polytetrafluoroethylene [Gore-Tex™], sodium hyaluronate and carboxymethylcellulose [Seprafilm™], icodextrin 4 % [Adept™], dextrane 32 %, carboxymethylcellulose and polyethylene oxide [Oxiplex™], polyethylene gylcol gels [Spraygel™], hyaluronic acid based gel [Hyalobarrier™], ferric hyaluronate gel 0.5 % [Intergel™], and others) are applicable in robot-assisted interventions as well as in traditional laparoscopic operations, at which the application of the particular medium and technique will be done after termination of the console phase and after undocking of the patient side cart at the end of the operation.

Available Data About Postoperative Adhesions After Robot-Assisted Operations

Regarding the influence of robot-assisted laparoscopic operations on the postoperative formation of adhesions there are no clinical or experimental trials from the gynecological sector available demonstrating a reduction or increase of adhesions on the one hand, and analyzing the performance of adhesiolysis in terms of effectivity and complication rate on the other hand, both in comparison to traditional laparoscopy and to open abdominal surgery.

There is only one experimental trial existing, from the urological sector [2], in which advantages of robot-assisted operations compared to open abdominal operations have been demonstrated in robot-assisted laparoscopic ileocystoplasty (RALI) on the basis of a porcine model.

The fact, that there is a higher amount of inserted trocars in robot-assisted surgery (at least 1 more trocar compared to traditional laparoscopy), the larger incisions as well as the presumably stronger traction and shear forces at the abdominal wall by a quasi suspension of the abdominal wall at the patient side cart, and consequently a more intense trauma to the peritoneum, and the bias of a so-called negative selection, i.e. a case selection, which is primarily more complex due to the robotic case selection profile (both concerning anatomical alterations and surgical pretreatments) let at least suppose that the advantages of the more precise adhesiolysis and the operation technique of robotic surgery are revoked hereby.

Conclusions

Existing adhesions in the context of robot-assisted operations and especially robot-assisted laparoscopic hysterectomies are treated according to the basic principles as well as traditional laparoscopic operations. The establishment of an adequate field of action is carried out for the robot-assisted technique with the daVinci™ system with means of traditional laparoscopy. Adhesiolysis in the lesser pelvis can be performed effective and precise with the daVinci™ technique related to their advantages (3D view, flexibility and dexterity of the EndoWrist™ instruments, tremor free surgery, amount of magnification of the daVinci™ endoscope) (Fig. 59.3a–h).

To which extent de novo adhesions are fewer respectively the effectiveness of adhesiolysis in robot-assisted surgery is superior to traditional laparoscopic operations has to be investigated in further research.

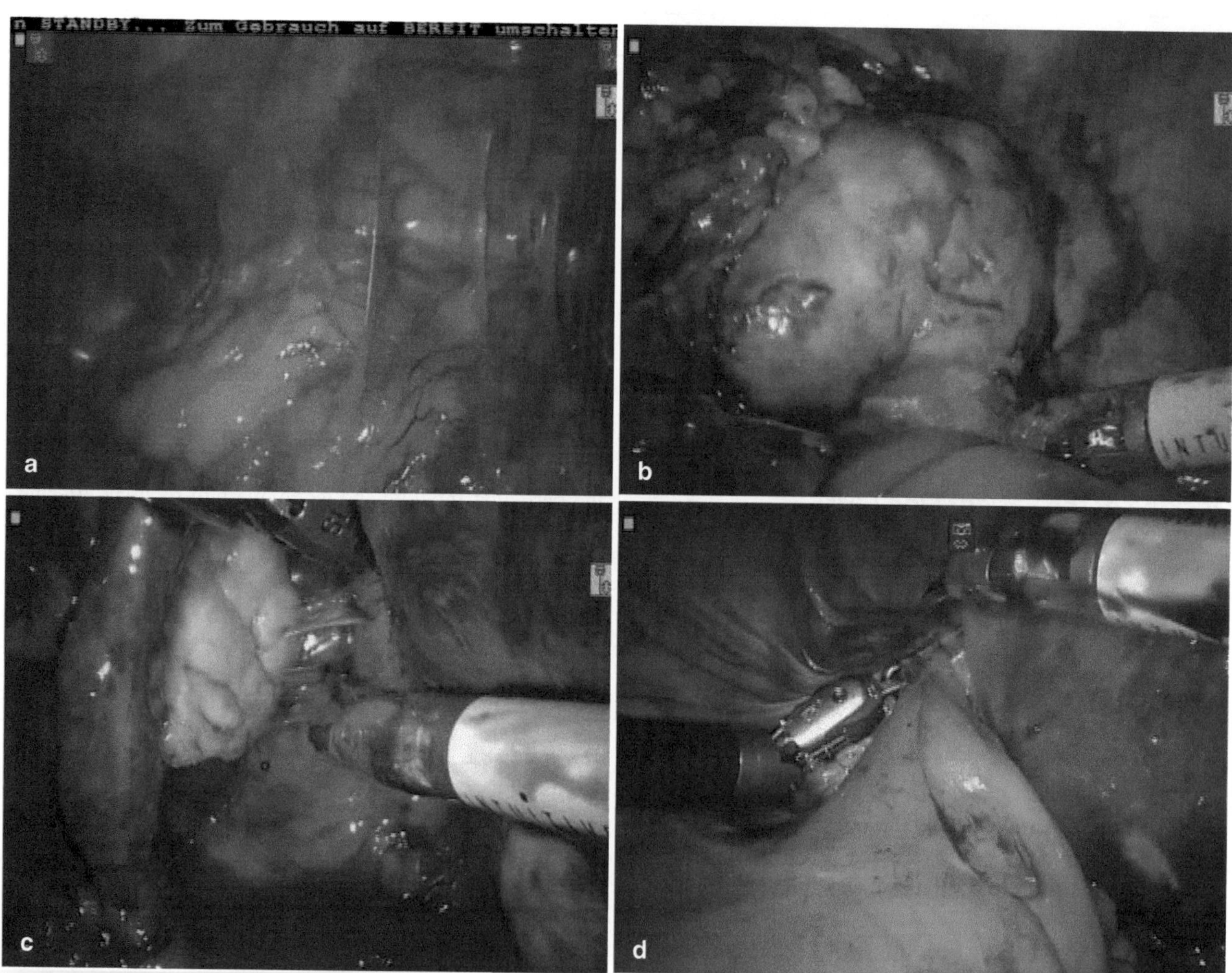

Fig. 59.3 (**a**) Robot-assisted hysterectomy due to uterus myomatosus and myoma necrosis with consecutive pelveoperitonitis; initial view into the lesser pelvis; recent adhesions. (**b**) Robot-assisted hysterectomy due to uterus myomatosus and myoma necrosis with consecutive pelveoperitonitis; after exposing of a necrotic myoma; recent adhesions. (**c**) Robot-assisted hysterectomy due to uterus myomatosus and myoma necrosis with consecutive pelveoperitonitis; adhesiolysis of the adnexa in concomitant adnexal inflammation, recent adhesions. (**d**) Robot-assisted hysterectomy with concomitant endometriosis; endometriotic adhesion between colon sigmoideum, left adnexa and left round ligament. (**e**) Robot-assisted hysterectomy with concomitant endometriosis, adhesiolysis of the right adnexa. (**f**) Robot-assisted hysterectomy with concomitant endometriosis with obliteration of the rectovaginal excavation (pouch of Douglas); sharp and blunt adhesiolysis. (**g**) Robot-assisted hysterectomy with accidental finding of concomitant endometriosis; initial aspect. (**h**) Robot-assisted hysterectomy with accidental finding of concomitant endometriosis; adhesiolysis of the right adnexa with involved colon and small intestine

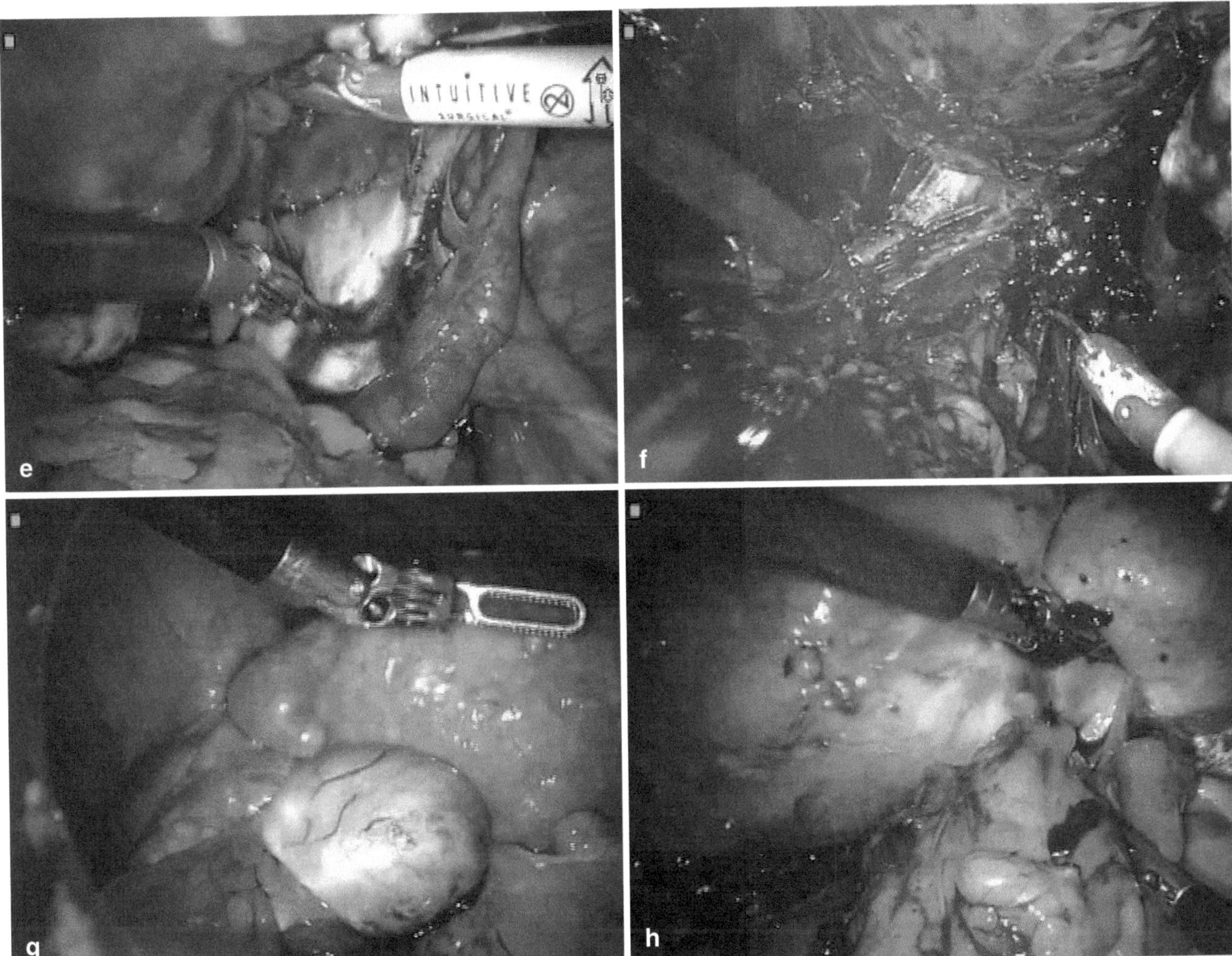

Fig. 59.3 (Continued)

References

1. Parker MC, Wilson MS, Menzies D, Sunderland G, Clark DN, Knight AD, Crowe AM. The Scar-3 study: 5-year adhesion-related readmission risk following lower abdominal surgical procedures. Colorectal Dis. 2005;7(6):551–8.
2. Razmaria AA, Marchetti PE, Prasad SM, Shalhav AL, Gundeti MS. Does robot-assisted laparoscopic ileocystoplasty (RALI) reduce peritoneal adhesions compared with open surgery? BJU Int. 2014;113:468–75.

Suggested Reading

Ahmad G, Mackie FL, Iles DA, O'Flynn H, Dias S, Metwally M, Watson A. Fluid and pharmacological agents for adhesion prevention after gynaecological surgery. Cochrane Database Syst Rev 2014; 9(7). Art No.: CD001298. doi: 10.1002/ 14651858. CD001298.pub4.

Al-Jabri S, Tulandi T. Management and prevention of pelvic adhesions. Semin Reprod Med. 2011;29:130–7.

Anderson SA, Beierle EA, Chen MK. Role of laparoscopy in the prevention and in the treatment of adhesions. Semin Pediatr Surg. 2014;23:353–6.

Arung W, Meurisse M, Detry O. Pathophysiology and prevention of postoperative peritoneal adhesions. World J Gastroenterol. 2011;17(41):4545–53.

Audebert A, Darai E, Bénifla JL, Yzbeck C, Déchaud H, Wattiez A, Crowe A, Pouly JL. Postoperative abdominal adhesions and their prevention in gynaecological surgery: What should you know? Gynecol Obstet Fertil. 2012;40:365–70.

Awonuga AO, Saed GM, Diamond MP. Laparoscopy in Gynecologic Surgery: Adhesion development, prevention, and use of adjunctive therapies. Clin Obstet Gynecol. 2009;52:412–22.

Blackburn SC, Stanton MP. Anatomy and physiology of the peritoneum. Semin Pediatr Surg. 2014;23:326–30.

Brokelman WJA, Lensvelt M, Borel Rinkes IHM, Klinkenbijl JHG, Reijnen M. Peritoneal changes due to laparoscopic surgery. Surg Endosc. 2011;25:1–9.

Chiu LH, Chen CH, Tu PC, Chang CW, Yen YK, Liu WM. Comparison of robotic surgery and laparoscopy to perform total hysterectomy with pelvic adhesions or large uterus. J Minim Access Surg. 2015;11(1):87–93.

Diamond MP, Wexner SD, Di Zereg GS, Korell M, Zmora O, Van Goor H, Kamar M. Adhesions prevention and reduction: current status and futur recommendations of a multinational interdisciplinary consensus conference. Surg Innov. 2010;17(3):183–8.

Hackethal A, Sick C, Szalay G, Puntambekar S, Joseph K, Langde S, Oehmke F, Tinneberg HR, Muenstedt K. Intra-abdominal adhesion formation: does surgical approach matter? Questionnaire survey of South Asian surgeons and literature review. J Obstet Gynaecol Res. 2011;37(10):1382–90.

Hindocha A, Beere L, Dias S, Watson A, Ahmad G. Adhesion prevention agents for gynaecological surgery: an overview of Cochrane reviews. Cochrane Database of Syst Rev 2015; (1). Art No:CD011254.doi:10.1002/14651858.CD011254.pub2.

Molinas CR, Binda MM, Manavella GD, Koninckx PR. Adhesion formation after laparoscopic surgery: what do we know about the role of the peritoneal environment? Obstet Gynecol. 2010;2(3):149–60.

Ott DE. Laparoscopy and adhesion formation, adhesions and laparoscopy. Semin Reprod Med. 2008;26(4):322–30.

Ten Broek R, Kok-Krant N, Bakkum EA, Bleicrodt RP, Van Goor H. Different surgical techniques to reduce post-operative adhesion formation: a systematic review and meta-analysis. Hum Reprod Update. 2013;19(1):12–25.

Vettoretto N, Carrara A, Corradi A (Associazione die Chirurghi Ospedalieri Italiani – ACOI) et al Laparoscopic adhesiolysis: consensus conference guidelines. Colorectal Dis 2012; 14: e208–e215

Wallwiener M, Koninckx PR, Hackethal A, Brölman H, Lundorff P, Mara M, Wattiez A, De Wilde RL. A Eurpean survey on awarness of post-surgical adhesions among gynaecological surgeons. Gynecol Surg. 2014;11:105–12.

General Aspects and Their Handling: Comorbidities

60

Celine Lönnerfors and Jan Persson

Medical and Surgical Comorbidities

In medicine, the term "comorbid" entails medical condition(s) existing simultaneously, but independently, with another condition.

Medical conditions known to increase the risk of surgery include bleeding disorders, diabetes mellitus, heart disease, obesity, liver disease, infectious disease, chronic respiratory disease, obstructive sleep apnoea, substance abuse and immunological disorders [1, 2], (Table 60.1).

In addition, the presence of extensive intraabdominal adhesions, advanced endometriosis and obesity are conditions associated with an increased surgical risk.

An understanding of the potential morbidity associated with surgery and different surgical approaches, as well as the impact of comorbidity, is important to offer the patient optimal treatment. For women with malignant disease, a higher surgical risk is acceptable than for women with benign disease and for women with significant comorbidities a thorough preoperative evaluation including patient information, optimizing patient status, and a comprehensive consideration of alternative, less invasive treatment options are key.

Minimally invasive hysterectomy is associated with less postoperative pain and a lower rate of morbidity, shorter hospital stay and convalescence [3–6]. An effort put into preserving the clinical benefits of laparoscopic surgery and facilitating the performance of more advanced surgery has led to the development of robotic surgery. The uptake of robot-assisted surgery was rapid. In 2008, only 3 years after the introduction, one in five hysterectomies for benign disease in the United States were performed robotically [7]. Three randomized, controlled trials comparing laparoscopic to robotic hysterectomy for benign disease have been published where the studies by Paraiso et al. and Sarlos et al. found a similar clinical outcome but an increased cost for robotics [8, 9]. In contrast, the randomized trial from our clinic showed that robotic hysterectomy for benign disease could be economically feasible if performed as excess capacity at a high volume center [10]. A recent Cochrane review on surgical approach to hysterectomy for benign disease concluded that when a vaginal hysterectomy is unfeasible, a laparoscopic hysterectomy is preferable to an abdominal approach. In addition, although the present evidence does not suggest that robotic hysterectomy is of benefit in this population, further evaluation is needed. The study further concluded that the benefits and hazards associated with different approaches is dependent on surgical expertise and that the approach to hysterectomy should be decided by the woman in discussion with her surgeon [11].

Patients with both substantial medical and surgical comorbidities are patients in whom surgery is particularly hazardous and where a minimally invasive approach might be particularly beneficial. Leonard et al. demonstrated that BMI, uterine size, leiomyoma size, and previous abdomino-pelvic surgery are all independent risk factors for intraoperative conversions from laparoscopy to laparotomy and Bonilla et al. showed that a large uterus increased the risk of a longer hospital stay, morbidity, and blood loss [12, 13]. These characteristics thereby provide a measure of the complexity and potential difficulty of a surgery and as such these high-risk surgeries have traditionally been performed by laparotomy [14]. Robotic surgery was introduced to overcome some of the limitations of traditional laparoscopy and to expand the patient population being offered minimal invasive surgery.

Robotic surgery is laparoscopic surgery utilizing an advanced tool. However, contrary to laparoscopic surgery, the requirement of a steep Trendelenburg position, large machinery impeding direct access to the patient, and an increased number of advanced, time consuming procedures all present additional management challenges for the surgical team [15], (Table 60.2).

C. Lönnerfors (✉) • J. Persson
Department of Obstetrics and Gynecology, Skåne University Hospital, Lund 22185, Sweden
e-mail: celine.lonnrfors@med.lu.se; jan.persson@med.lu.se

I. Alkatout, L. Mettler (eds.), *Hysterectomy*, DOI 10.1007/978-3-319-22497-8_60

Table 60.1 Medical conditions that increase the risk of surgery [1, 2]

Condition	Type and reason for increased risk
Bleeding or clotting disorder	Increased risk of bleeding or developing blood clots during and after surgery
Cardiovascular disease	Increased demands on the myocardium to maintain cardiac output due to surgical stress Increased susceptibility to surgical factors such as blood loss and volume shifts Enhanced myocardial oxygen demand caused by increased heart rate and blood pressure as a result of surgical stress
Chronic respiratory disease	Reduced ability to compensate for any alteration in the acid-base balance Increased risk of hypoventilation due to depressed respiratory function during anesthesia Changes in ventilation impair the diaphragm resulting in reduced volumes and lung capacities Increased risk of postoperative pulmonary complications due to risk of exacerbation of bronchial inflammation and increased risk of bronchospasm and postoperative pneumonia
Diabetes mellitus	Increased risk of infection and impaired wound healing due to altered glucose metabolism and associated impaired tissue perfusion Increased risk of lower limb ischemia and pressure sores Disruption and worsening of diabetes control Increased risk of postoperative acute myocardial infarction
Immunological disorders	Increased risk of impaired wound healing and infection
Chronic kidney disease	Impaired tubular excretory function of the kidney cause elevation in levels of creatinine and blood urea nitrogen Impaired synthetic function leads to a decrease in the production of erythropoietin (resulting in anemia) and active vitamin D-3 (causing hypocalcemia, secondary hyperparathyroidism, and hyperphosphatemia), accumulation of acid, potassium, sodium and water excretion (causing acidosis, hyperkalemia, hypertension, and edema), and platelet dysfunction (promotes bleeding) Drugs usually eliminated by the kidney including anesthetic drugs can accumulate to toxic levels Renal insufficiency is a risk factor for cardical complications in surgical patients
Liver disease	Decreased synthesis of plasma-binding proteins Impaired drug metabolism and elimination Impaired hormonal response to surgical stress Increases the risk of morbidity (bleeding, impaired wound healing, renal dysfunction, hepatic failure, infection) and mortality in the postoperative period
Nutritional status	Malnutrition further exacerbates the catabolic state induced by surgical stress Increased risk of postoperative infection and impaired wound healing for both obese and underweight women Obesity increases risk of having other comorbidities

Table 60.2 Anesthesiological challenges specific to robotic surgery [11]

Patient positioning	Steep Trendelenburg	Compromised hemodynamics and oxygenation. Restricted intraoperative airway access Increased risk of postoperative respiratory stress, nerve injury, occult blood loss, corneal abrasion
Pneumoperitoneum		Increased peak inspiratory and plateau airway pressures and end-tidal CO_2 tension while decrease in lung compliance and vital capacity leading to ventilation-perfusion mismatch, atelectasis, subcutaneous emphysema and gas embolism
Restricted access		Might impact patient care in emergency situations

Communication and teamwork are vital to create a safe, effective and efficient environment to minimize complications and optimize the perioperative period for the patient. Proper training and experience with the procedure in low-risk patients is important prior to undertaking surgery in high-risk patients.

To perform robotic gynecologic surgery optimal exposure of the pelvis is necessary and this is possible through a steep Trendelenburg position [16]. Without proper exposure, the procedure is prolonged and there is an increased risk of intra-operative complications [17]. The dorsal lithotomy position can have significant physiological consequences. Most susceptible to the head-down extreme position are the cardiac, respiratory, and central nervous systems and patients with underlying disease might be especially vulnerable [18]. The cranial movement of the diaphragm by pneumoperitoneum and abdominal contents, can decrease pulmonary compliance and functional residual capacity, cause pulmonary edema, and exacerbate ventilation/perfusion mismatch, which can be particularly perilous in the morbidly obese or in patients with underlying chronic lung disease [19–21] The establishment of pneumoperitoneum can result in increased postoperative complications in patients with underlying lung disease. Patients with chronic obstructive pulmonary disease are less efficient in eliminating excessive CO_2, which can lead to postoperative respiratory hypercarbia and acidosis [22, 23]. In addition, the development of subcutaneous emphysema contributes significantly to the total amount of CO_2 absorbed [15]. Obese women have less efficient ventilation during pneumoperitoneum and are at higher risk of coronary artery disease, pulmonary dysfunction, and diabetes [24, 25]. The combination of the steep Trendelenburg position with pneumoperitoneum influences cardiopulmonary physiology; increased left ventricular filling pressure and systemic vascular resistance and decreased cardiac output [26–28]. Prolonged surgery places the patient's cardiorespiratory capacity under pressure for longer [29].

The president of the American Congress of Obstetricians and Gynecologists released the following statement in 2013: *Patients should be advised that robotic hysterectomy for benign disease is best used for unusual and complex clinical conditions in which improved outcomes over standard minimally invasive approaches have been demonstrated* [30]. No randomized studies on the optimal hysterectomy approach for women with significant medical or surgical comorbidities or for complex cases such as severe adhesions, extensive endometriosis or difficult anatomical conditions are available, i.e. cases where robotic surgery has been suggested to be most beneficial.

Retrospective and prospective studies on the impact of surgical comorbidities are available and several studies have indicated robotic surgery to be feasible and safe in women with complex benign disease. Boggess et al. found robotic hysterectomy in 152 consecutive cases with complex benign disease (obese patients, patients with one or more prior pelvic or abdominal surgeries, patients with moderate to severe endometriosis or leiomyomas, and patients with large uteri) to be associated with short hospital stay, minimal blood loss and no conversion to laparotomy. They concluded that robotics allows for a safe and efficient surgery in patients with complex pathology [14]. Several study groups have reported on the feasibility of complex endometriosis surgery using robotics and several studies have indicated that robotic surgery is feasible and safe in women with other complex benign disorders such as large uteri, pelvic fistula or in case of previous intraabdominal surgery [18, 24, 31–42]. In addition, several publications indicate that robotic surgery is utilized to an increased extent in women with comorbidities [24, 33, 34, 43, 44]. Patzkowsky et al. compared the perioperative outcome of 288 robotic and 257 laparoscopic hysterectomies for benign disease and found that even though more complex cases were being performed robotically the surgical outcome was similar in both groups [45]. This selection case bias where more difficult cases are chosen for a robotic approach, is increasingly evident at our clinic where the referrals specifically indicating a wish for robotic surgery has increased substantially.

The impact of obesity has been most extensively studied, particularly in women undergoing hysterectomy for endometrial cancer. Obese patients are more likely to have additional comorbidities that may increase the risk of surgical and anesthetic morbidity and mortality when compared with women of normal weight [46–48].

Due to the increasing prevalence of obesity, it is important to develop surgical techniques to manage these patients appropriately. Three large randomized controlled trials found laparoscopic surgery to be a valid alternative to laparotomy for surgical treatment of endometrial cancer [5, 49–51]. The complexity of advanced traditional laparoscopic procedures in obese women has hindered a general adoption of laparoscopic surgery for this group of patients.

For morbidly obese patients (BMI ≥ 40 kg/m^2) laparoscopic surgery is particularly challenging but also more advantageous compared to open surgery [52–54]. A recent study evaluating the impact of obesity on the outcomes of surgical treatment of endometrial cancer by either laparoscopy or laparotomy found laparoscopy to be associated with a better clinical outcome [55]. However, the conversion rate increased and the lymph node yield decreased in women with BMI exceeding 40, the latter was true even for women operated by laparotomy. In the Lap2 study, the overall conversion rate was 25.8 %, although for women with BMI ≥ 40, the rate was 56 % [5]. Wound related complications are the most common complications for obese women undergoing laparotomy. Decreasing the rate of laparotomy while retaining an acceptable oncological outcome is highly important in obese women.

Extreme obesity has traditionally been considered a relative contraindication to laparoscopic surgery; thicker panniculus reducing the range of instrument motion, the effect of steep Trendelenburg position on the respiratory system and the redundancy of bowel interfering with optimal exposure of the pelvis [56].

Robotic surgery for gynecological disease has been found to be feasible in obese women [44, 57–62]. Concerns about whether or not robotic surgery is safe in obese patients has been raised, particularly due to the need for a very steep Trendelenburg position during the procedure. Several recent publications have concluded that robotic surgery is safe in this group of patients. Wysham et al. found a low incidence of pulmonary complications and overall complications in 1032 obese women following robotic surgery for gynecological disease and Corrado et al. reported a perioperative complication rate of 10 % and no conversions to laparotomy in their study on 70 morbidly obese patients [60, 63]. A large cohort study by Zakhari et al. showed that although women undergoing robotic surgery were more likely to have a much higher burden of comorbidities as well as significantly more often being obese or morbidly obese, a greater rate of lymph node dissection, a decreased length of hospital stay as well as comparable postoperative morbidity and mortality was seen when compared to laparoscopy [44]. This trend towards a higher utilization of robotics in higher BMI categories has also been demonstrated in urology [64].

The intraoperative management of extensive intraabdominal adhesions is a surgical challenge. Adhesiolysis is associated with a prolonged operative time and an increased risk of intraoperative and postoperative complications, especially inadvertent bowel injury [65–67]. Unlike other postoperative complications, the consequences of adhesion formation comprise a lifelong risk of various clinical entities [65, 68–72]. The presence of adhesions increases the risk of small bowel obstruction, the need for emergency surgery with adhesiolysis as well as decreased pregnancy rates, increased need for fertility treatments, and chronic abdominal pain [65, 66, 72–77].

Data about the incidence of adhesions differ considerably, although most studies report an incidence of between 20 and 93 % [78–82]. These significant variations may be explained by diverse procedures and entry techniques as well as by varying underlying disease [83]. Pediatric and lower gastrointestinal surgery is associated with a majority of adhesion-related problems whereas the rate is lower following urological and gynecological procedures [77]. The presence of adhesions is more probable in patients with a history of laparotomy or extended surgery. Laparoscopy reduces, but does not prevent, the occurrence of adhesion-related complications [79, 84].

For laparoscopic and robotic surgery, the presence of adhesions in the umbilical area must be considered as the insertion of a trocar can lead to bowel injury. In their study on 814 patients, Audebert and Gomel found the rate of umbilical adhesions to be 0.68 % of patients with no previous abdominal surgery, 1.6 % following laparoscopic surgery, 19.8 % following a previous horizontal suprapubic incision, and 51.7 % after a midline incision [85]. In addition, the study demonstrated that the presence of severe adhesions involving the bowel was low in women with no previous surgery, after laparoscopic surgery or after a horizontal incision (0.42–6.87 %), but 31.46 % in women with a previous midline incision [85]. Sepilian et al. found the incidence of umbilical adhesions and bowel adhesions to be 21.2 and 2.6 % in patients with a history of laparoscopy through an umbilical incision [86]. Consequently, in patients with a history of laparoscopy or laparotomy, an alternative access to the abdominal cavity such as the Palmer's point should be considered to minimize the risk of inadvertent organ perforation during trocar entry. The occurrence of adhesions at the Palmer's point after previous operations is unlikely because most abdominopelvic operations are conducted farther from this anatomical region [83]. Since 2012, direct access at Palmers point using the 12 mm semi blunt assistant trocar has been the preferred method for gaining access to the abdominal cavity for robotic procedures at our clinic. During the last 3 years performing approximately 900 procedures, one complication (bleeding from mesenteric vessels in a women with low BMI) has occurred following direct entry at Palmers point. The overall complication rate during port placement at our institution is low (0.3 %) and known or suspected adhesions are considered an indication rather than a contraindication for robotic surgery [87].

Lysis of adhesions is associated with a prolonged operative time and an increased risk of intraoperative and postoperative complications [65, 66, 77]. Adhesions precluding acceptable exposure are, in addition to unanticipated carcinomatosis, the most commonly stated reasons for conversion to laparotomy in robotic surgery.

The conversion rate during robotic hysterectomy for benign disease is low. Most studies report rates of less than 1 % [8–10] and even in women with complex benign disease the rates are in the range of 0–1.7 %. [14, 45]. For robotic hysterectomy for malignant disease most report rates <4 %, although in a recent publication by Jones et al. the rate was 8.7 % [62, 87–91]. The latter publication evaluated the risk factors for conversions from robotic surgery to laparotomy in 459 patients and found bowel injury, increasing BMI and non-White race but not prior surgery, medical comorbidities or malignant disease to be associated with conversion to open surgery [91]. The Lap2 study, a randomized study comparing staging for endometrial cancer by laparoscopy and laparotomy found increasing BMI, age and metastatic disease to be associated with an increased risk of conversion [5].

The conversion rate in the first 1000 robotic procedures performed at our institution for malignant or benign disease was 3.7 %; 41 % of the conversions were due to intraabdominal adhesions and 3 % due to an intraoperative complication [87]. Overall, 36 % of the women had at least one previous laparotomy and 24 % had intraabdominal adhesions necessitating adhesiolysis. An intraoperative complication occurred in 3.3 %. A urinary injury (ureter or bladder) occurred in 1.7 %, a bowel injury in 0.8 %, a vessel injury in 0.6 % and a neural injury in 0.2 % of the patients. Sixty-five per cent of patients with an intraoperative complication had major intraabdominal adhesions. The conversion rate and the rate of intraoperative complications in patients with adhesions was 5.8 % and 5.4 % respectively [86].

In a later study on our first 949 hysterectomies for malignant and benign disease, the overall conversion rate was 2.4 %; 46 % was due to intraabdominal adhesions. In 70 % of the conversions, the decision was made prior to docking the robot and the conversion rate among women in whom the robot was docked was 0.8 %. The conversion rate in the 240 women undergoing hysterectomy for benign disease was 0.4 % [87]. In 2013/2014, one (1.2 %) conversion and no intraoperative complications occurred during a hysterectomy for benign disease even though 66 % had at least one complicating factor (ASA ≥3, severe endometriosis, > one previous midline incision, BMI >40 kg/m^{2,} uterine size >200 g). The conversion was due to extensive intraabdominal adhesions in a woman with several previous midline incisions.

The presence of adhesions is associated with a somewhat higher risk of conversion and intraoperative complications. The latter can, in a majority of cases, be managed robotically and adhesions should not dissuade from performing a robotic procedure if other factors favor this approach.

Dry-lab studies have shown that the robot is more advantageous compared to traditional laparoscopy when the procedure becomes technically more challenging regardless of the level of the surgeons experience [92]. Even though no randomized controlled trials comparing laparoscopy and robotics for patients with significant comorbidities within this patient group are available, several studies indicate that even with an experienced and skilled surgeon, obese patients, patients with prior abdominal surgeries, or patients requiring lengthy and high-risk surgeries are likely to benefit from robotic surgery. In addition to a thorough preoperative evaluation, intraoperative monitoring, teamwork, good communication and a heightened awareness of the possible problems that might arise are important to achieve a successful surgery and an uncomplicated postoperative period. Training, experience and refinement of practice has, at our institution lead to a decrease in the overall rate of intraoperative-, postoperative-, and ≥ grade 3 complications according to the Clavien-Dindo scale by 46 %, 44 % and 76 % respectively. This decrease has occurred over a seven-year period and illustrates that the effort and time needed to implement a successful robotic program should not be underestimated.

Robotic surgery for benign disease has been suggested to be beneficial primarily in complex cases or in high-risk patients. The development a standardized, reproducible method of hysterectomy for all benign cases called **safe, simple hysterectomy** is in our opinion key to minimize the risk of complications for all patients. This method mimics surgery for malignant disease where the pelvic sidewalls are opened and the ureters identified, dissected and visualized during the entire surgery and the vascular pedicels are skeletonized and secured. Proper training and experience with this method in non-complex cases is important prior to undertaking the more challenging procedures. In high-risk surgeries aberrant anatomy due to endometriosis or adhesions, decreased visibility due to obesity, enlarged uteri or suboptimal pneumoperiotoneum or Trendeleburg's positioning due to anaesthesiological issues are challenges that must be overcome to successfully complete the case. The predictability of this method for the console surgeon, the bedside assistant and the operating room nurse optimizes the chances of the surgery being uneventful. This allows for swift damage control when necessary, and thereby decreases the risk of intraoperative complications, intraoperative bleeding, and conversion to laparotomy as well as the risk of reoperation, which is particularly important for this high-risk population.

Safe, Simple Hhysterectomy: Surgical Technique

All models of the da Vinci robots can be used. Ports should be placed as for standard pelvic surgery. Central docking or side docking at surgeon's discretion for the Si robot whereas the Xi robot is usually docked 90 ° from the side. Suitable robot instruments are: monopolar scissors, a bipolar forceps, and a prograsp. The latter can, in most cases, be used for closing the vaginal cuff. For the assistant, a 10–12 mm trocar is used for suction/irrigation, insertion of sponges, clips, and needles.

For identification of the vaginal fornices, a vaginal tube is placed at onset of surgery.

Initial entry into the abdomen is usually achieved through direct entry at Palmers point in the upper left quadrant with the assistant trocar or with Verress needle or open entry at the midline. A midline entry is avoided in case of previous extensive intraabdominal surgery.

Triangulation and tensioning of the tissue is created using the fourth arm with the infindibulopelvic (IP) ligament, the round ligament and the pelvic sidewall as the parameters (Fig. 60.1) and the peritoneum is opened approximately 1 cm lateral to the IP ligament (Figs. 60.2 and 60.3). The areolar, avascular space is identified and, when possible, dissection is performed in this space to minimize bleeding. The ureter is identified (Fig. 60.4), the pararectal space is developed (Figs. 60.5 and 60.6) and the uterine artery is identified (Fig. 60.7), skeletonized (Fig. 60.8) and sealed with a hemostatic clip

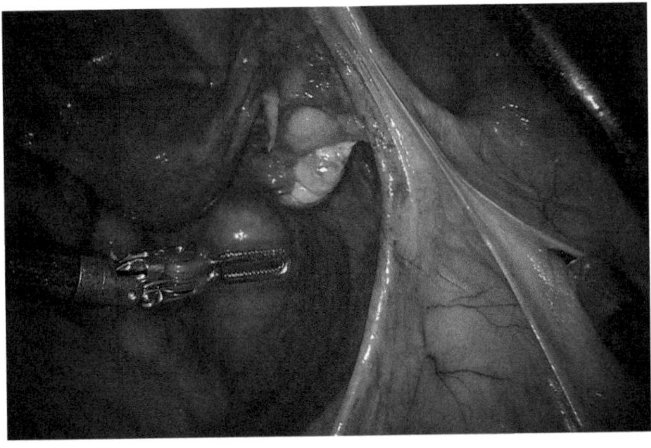

Fig. 60.1 Triangulation of the peritoneum to gain access to the pelvic sidewall

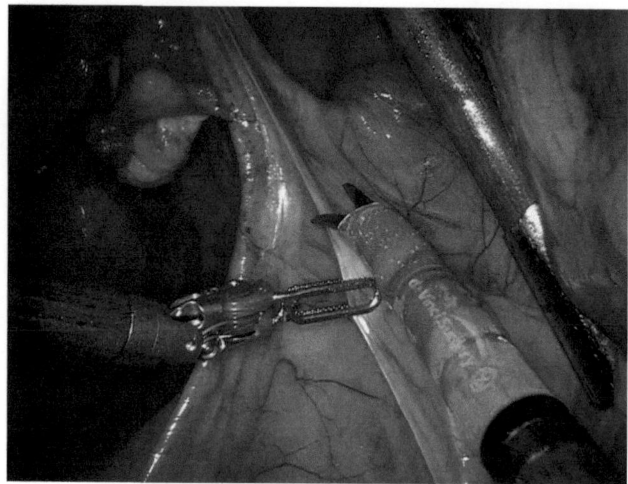

Fig. 60.2 Opening of the peritoneum approximately 1 cm lateral to the IP ligament

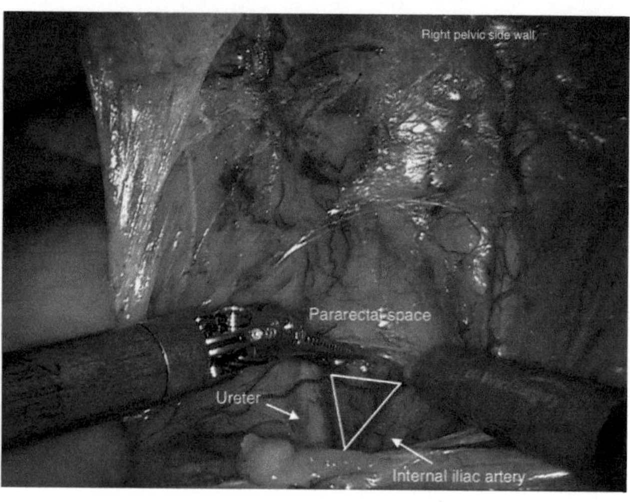

Fig. 60.5 Identifying and developing the pararectal space

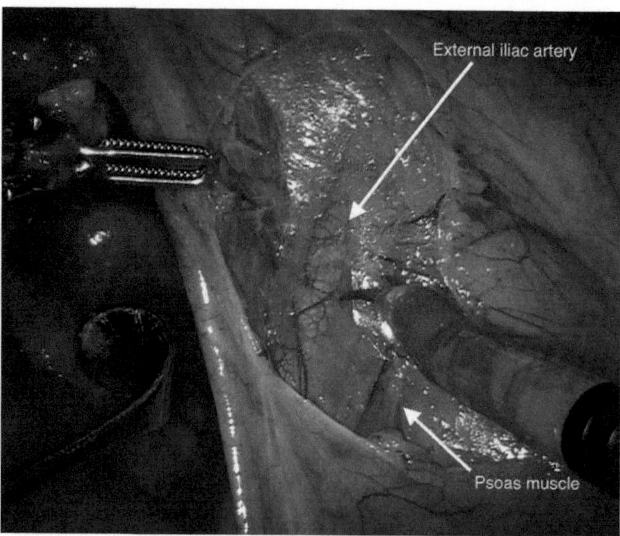

Fig. 60.3 Visualizing the anatomy of the pelvic sidewall including the psoas muscle and the external iliac artery

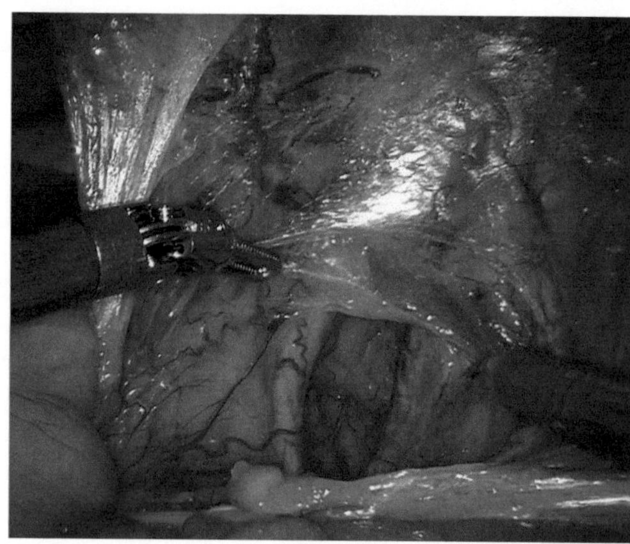

Fig. 60.6 Further atraumatic development of the pararectal space

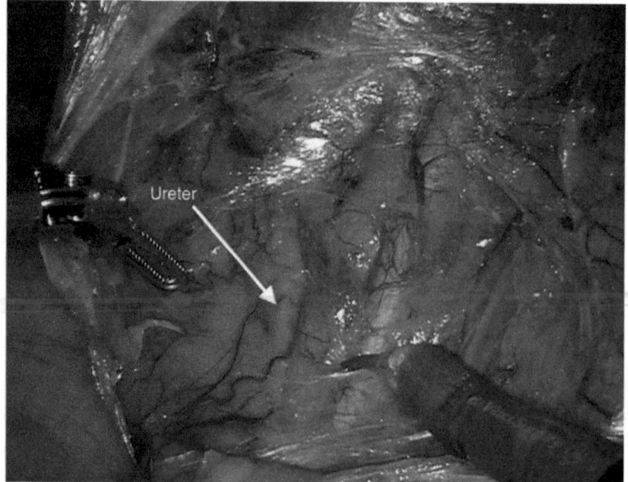

Fig. 60.4 Identifying the ureter

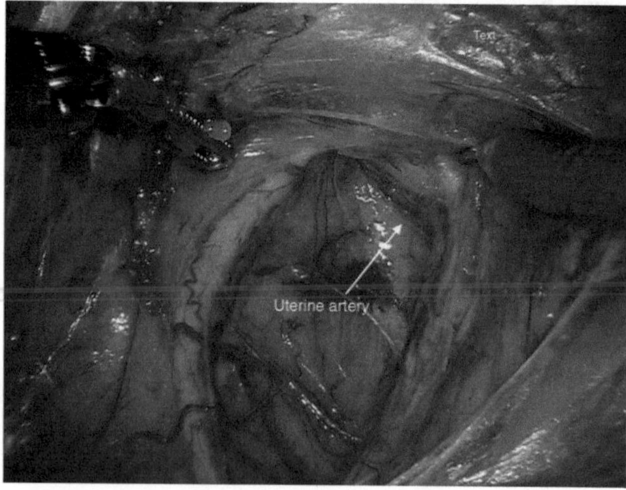

Fig. 60.7 Identifying the uterine artery

(Figs. 60.9 and 60.10). The ureters are dissected off the posterior peritoneum, carefully lateralized to maintain blood supply (Fig. 60.11). The previous steps are performed on the contralateral side. In case of ovarian preservation, the fallopian tubes are removed (Fig. 60.12). The medial broad ligament is opened (Figs. 60.13 and 60.14), the IP ligament is skeletonized, and in case of a bilateral salpingoophorectomy, a hemostatic clip is placed (Figs. 60.15 and 60.16). When preserving the ovaries careful coagulation of the ovarian ligament including the parametrial veins is performed (Fig. 60.17). The Okabayashis space is developed (Figs. 60.18 and 60.19) and the rectovaginal space is opened (Figs. 60.20, 60.21 and 60.22). The round ligaments are divided, (Figs. 60.23 and 60.24) the anterior peritoneum opened (Figs. 60.25 and 60.26), the vesicouterine peritoneal fold is identified and, using the vaginal tube as a guide, the bladder is mobilized off the lower uterine segment (Figs. 60.27 and 60.28). The vaginal tube facilitates identification of the vaginal fornices as well as moving the ureters laterally. Desiccate and divide the uterine vessels at the level of the lower isthmus

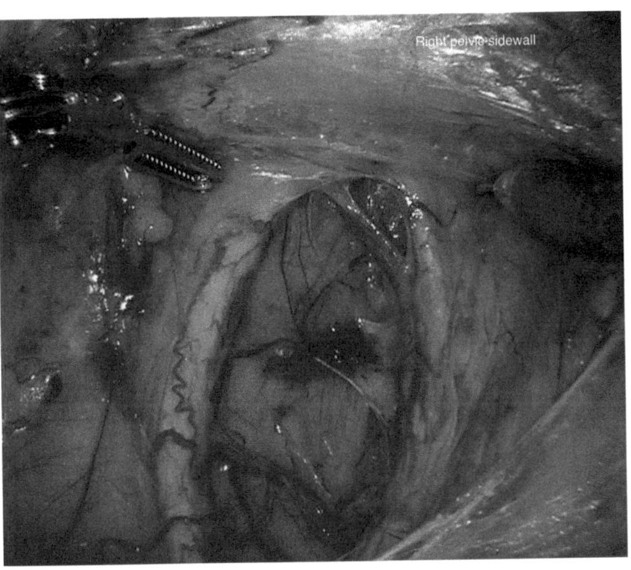

Fig. 60.8 Skeletonizing the uterine artery

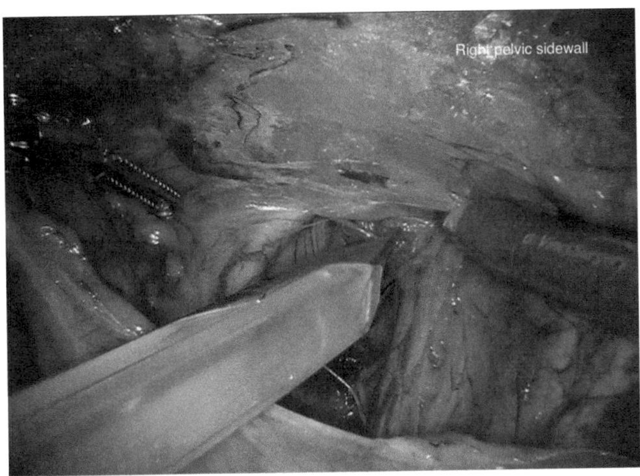

Fig. 60.9 Placing a hemostatic clip on the uterine artery at its origin

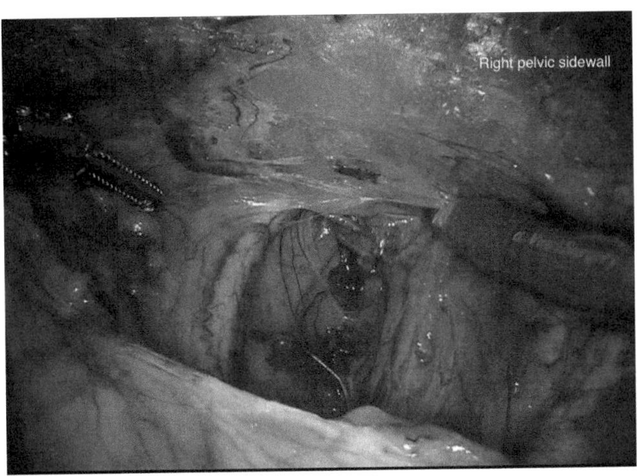

Fig. 60.10 Clips on the uterine artery at the pelvic sidewall

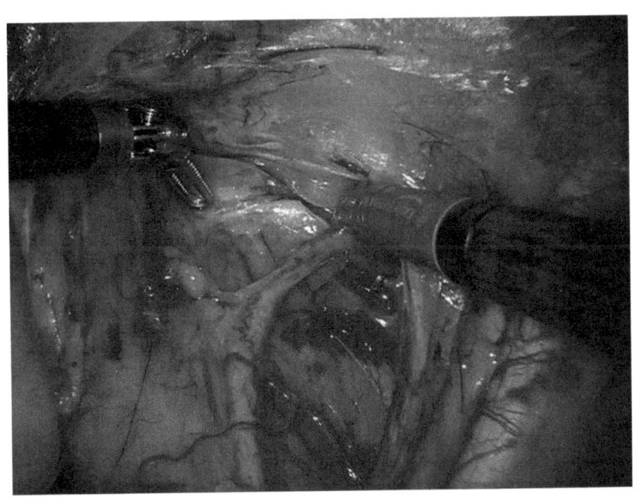

Fig. 60.11 Lateralizing the ureter

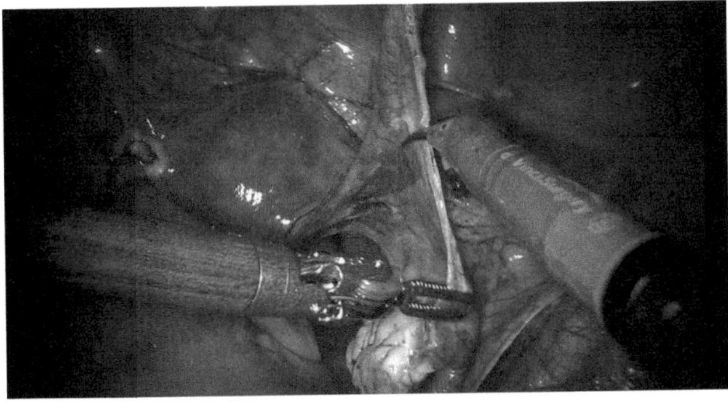

Fig. 60.12 Dissection of the fallopian tube in case of ovarian preservation

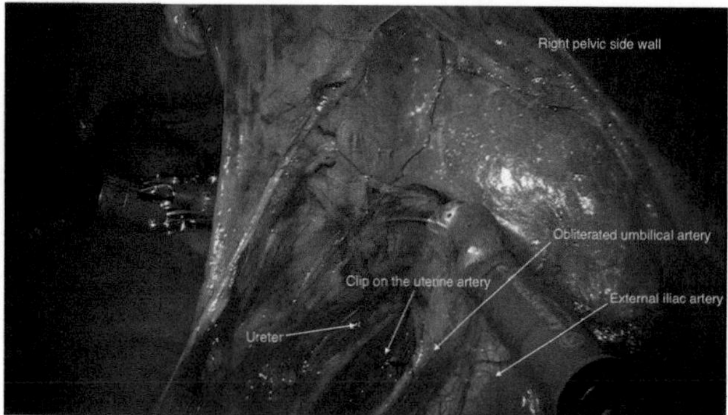

Fig. 60.13 Opening of the broad ligament

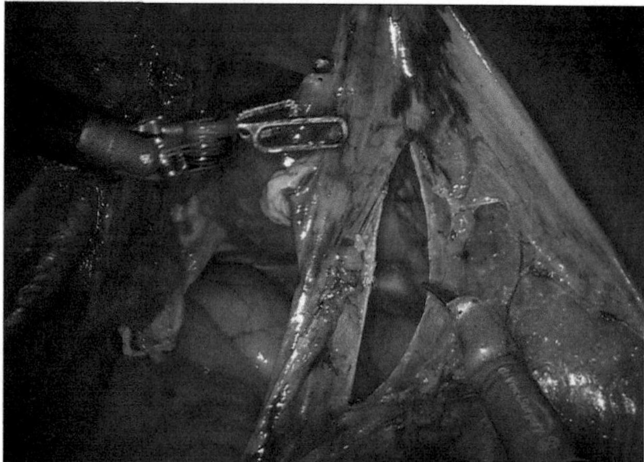

Fig. 60.14 Skeletonizing the ovarian ligament

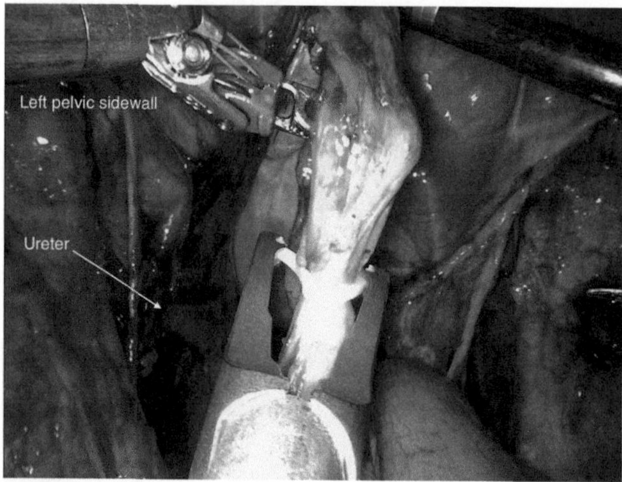

Fig. 60.15 Placing a hemostatic clip on the ovarian ligament when performing a salpingoophorectomy

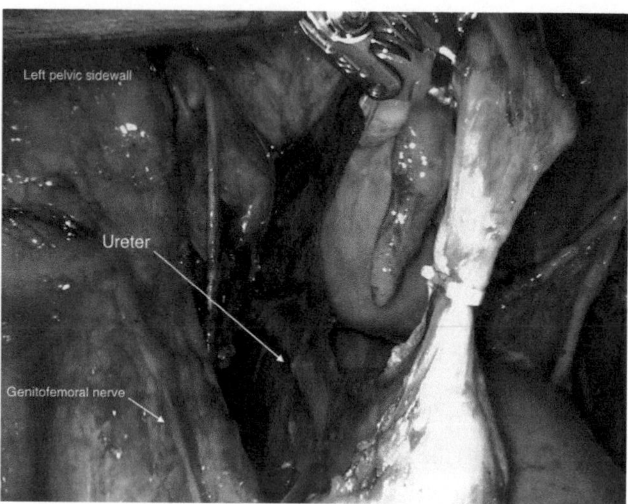

Fig. 60.16 Hemostatic clip on the ovarian ligament

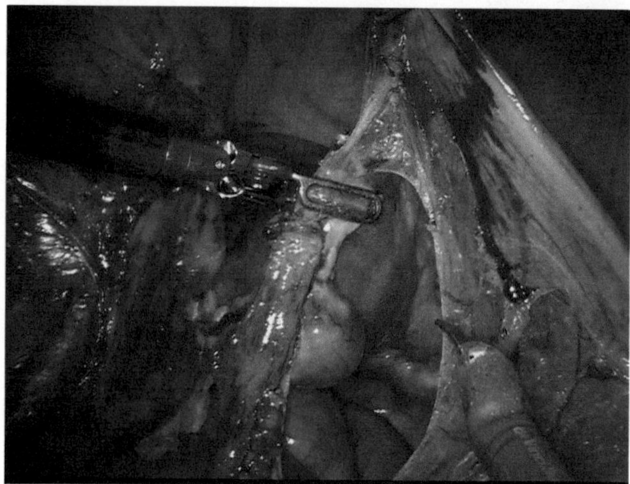

Fig. 60.17 Coagulation of the ovarian ligament

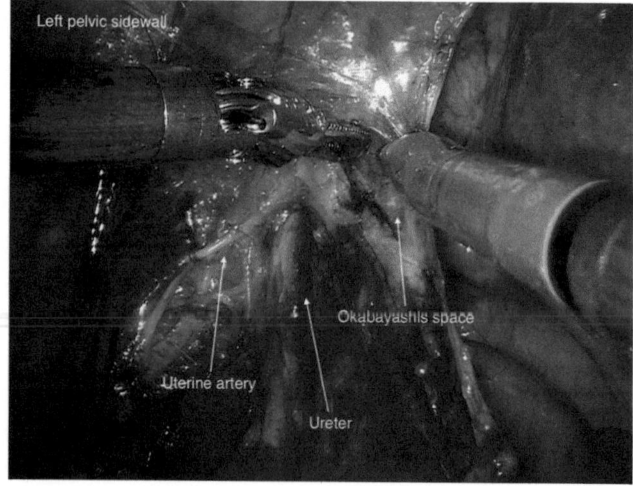

Fig. 60.18 Development of Okabayashis space

(Figs. 60.29 and 60.30) and thereafter dissect medially to the uterine vessels down to the vaginal tube to minimize the risk of ureteral injury to provide a vascular pedicle that can be

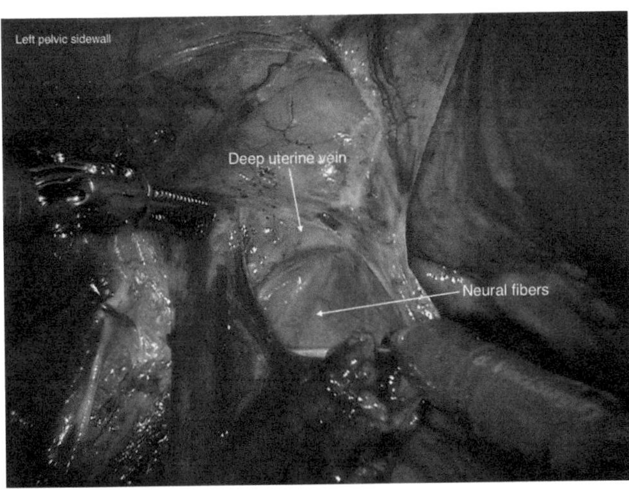

Fig. 60.19 Further development of Okabayashis space

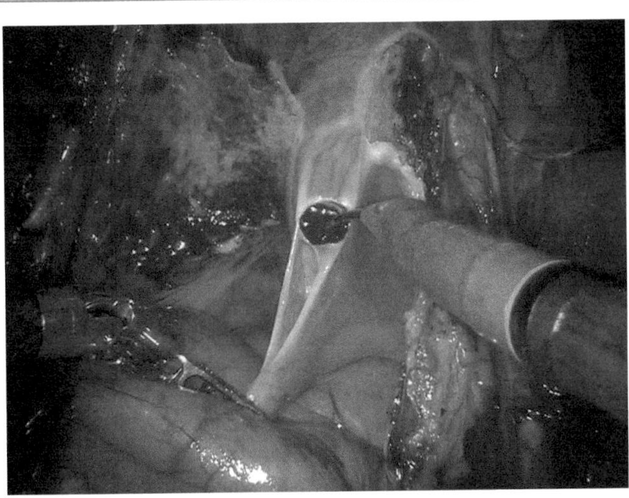

Fig. 60.22 Opening of the peritoneum in the rectovaginal space

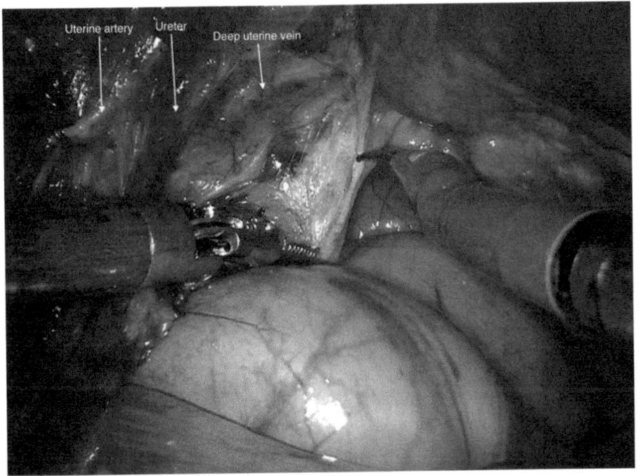

Fig. 60.20 Opening the rectovaginal space

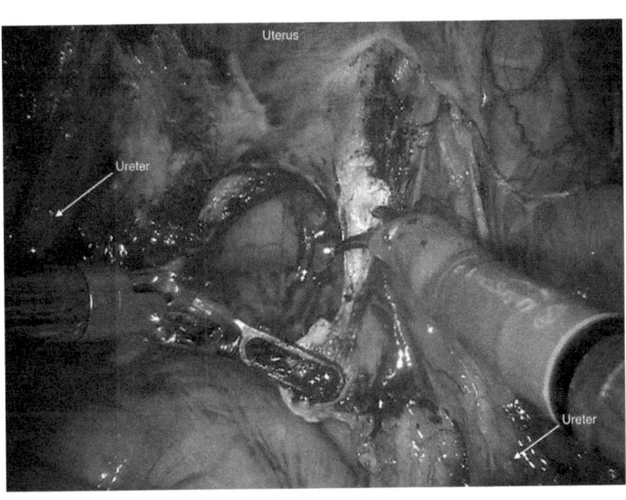

Fig. 60.23 Tissue tension during dissection helps to identify the correct plane

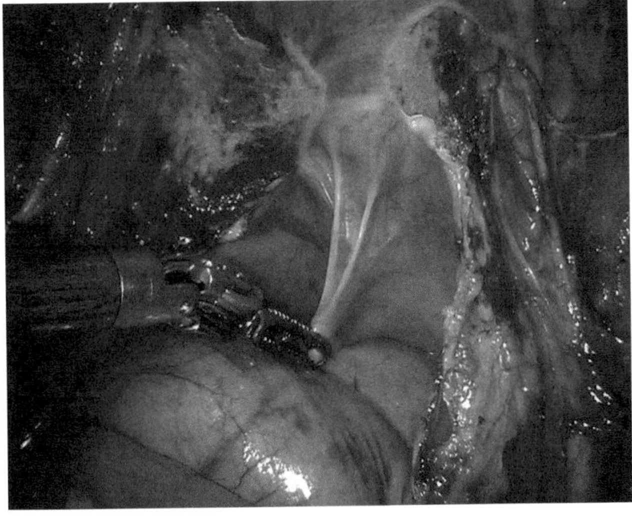

Fig. 60.21 Identifying the correct plane to dissect in the rectovaginal space

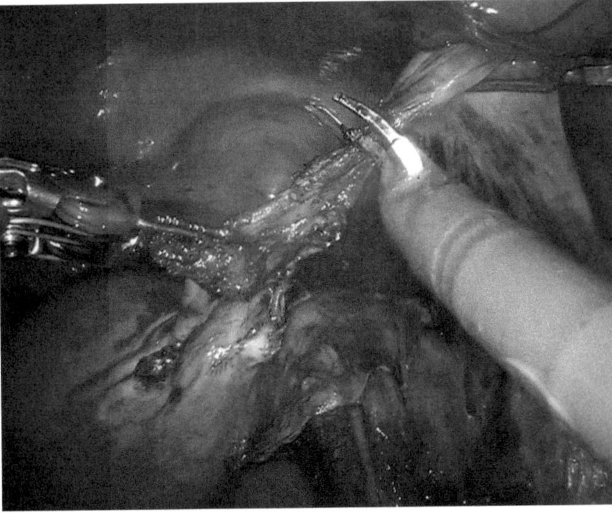

Fig. 60.24 Coagulation and division of the round ligament

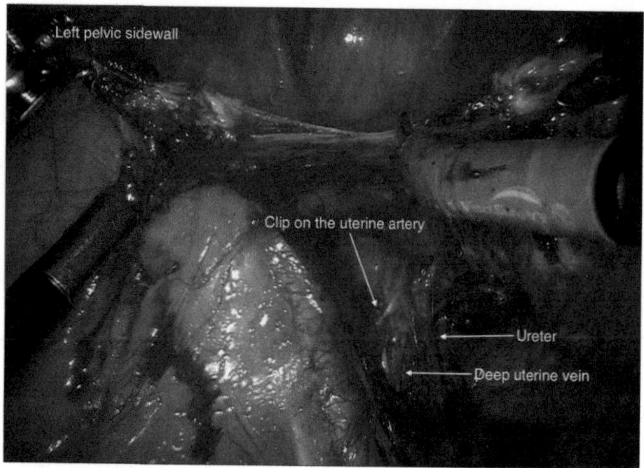

Fig. 60.25 Division of the anterior peritoneum utilizing tissue tension with visualization of the ureter and uterine artery

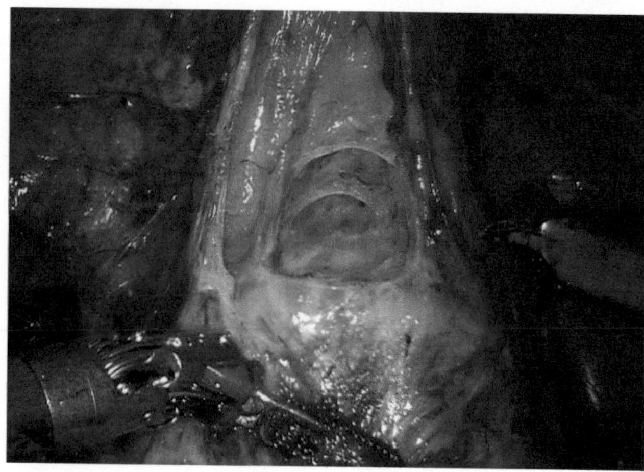

Fig. 60.28 Further mobilization of the bladder

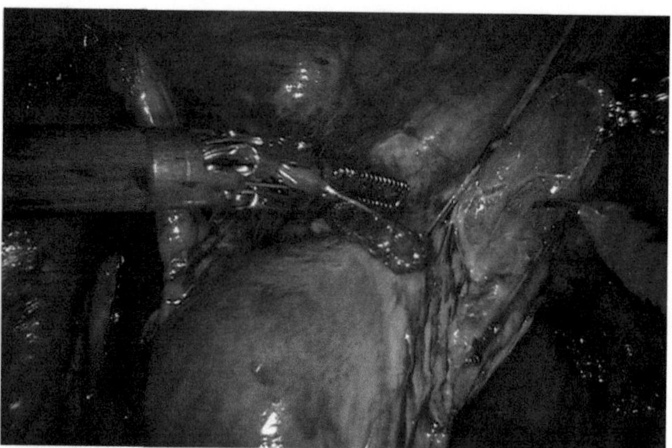

Fig. 60.26 Further division of the anterior peritoneum

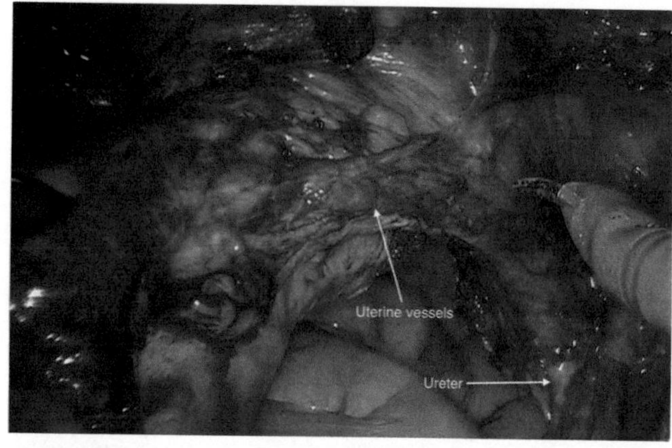

Fig. 60.29 Skeletonized uterine vessels

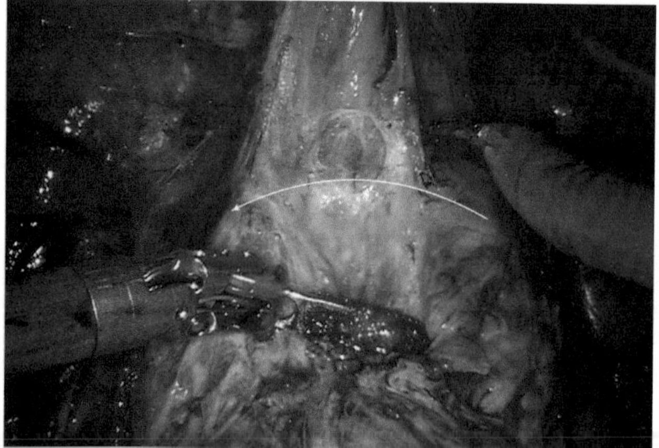

Fig. 60.27 Mobilizing the bladder using the edge of the vaginal tube as a guide to identify the correct plane

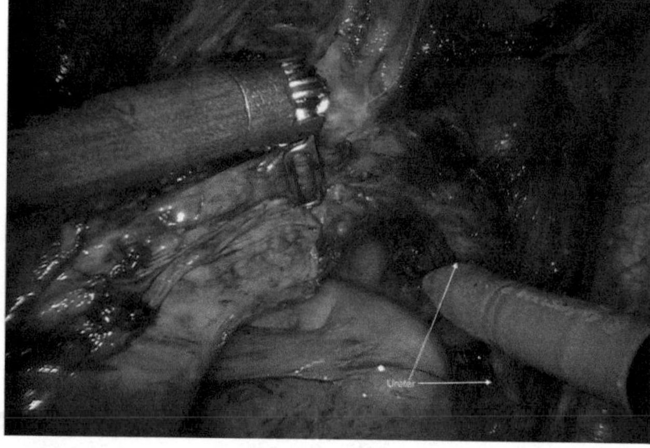

Fig. 60.30 Coagulation of uterine vessels

safely desiccated further in the event of bleeding (Fig. 60.31). To optimize cuff closure and healing, dissecting and mobilization of 7–10 mm of the vagina is desirable (Fig. 60.32).

The colpotomy is performed using the tip of the monopolar scissors in cutting mode (Figs. 60.33, 60.34 and 60.35). Vaginal cuff closure is performed (Figs. 60.36 and 60.37).

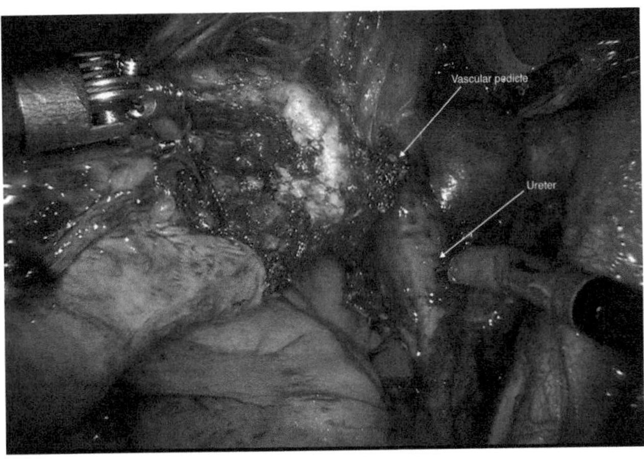

Fig. 60.31 The uterine vessels have been divided and further dissection is performed medially to the vascular pedicle

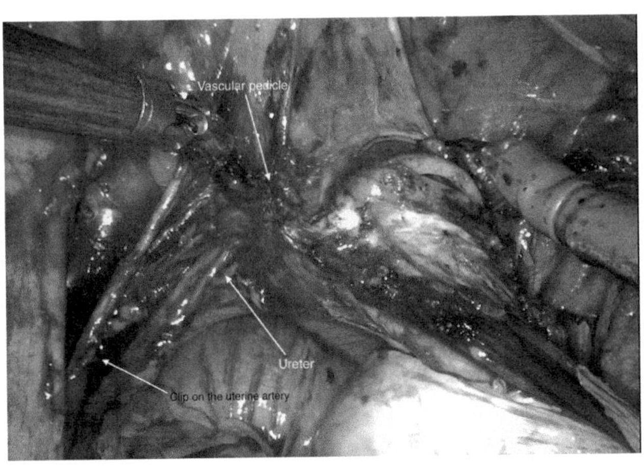

Fig. 60.34 The colpotomy is performed at a safe distance from the ureters

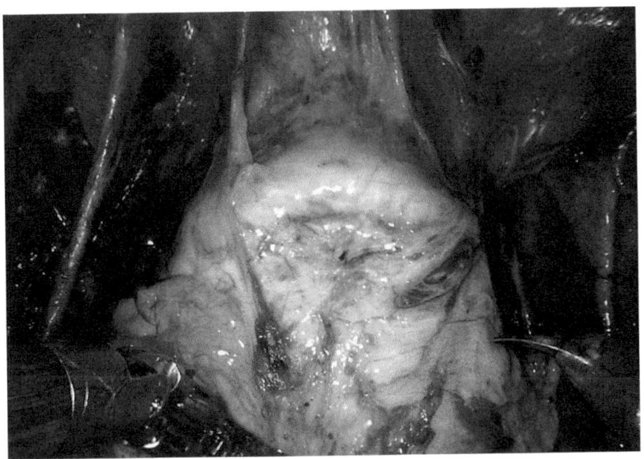

Fig. 60.32 Preparation of the vaginal cuff

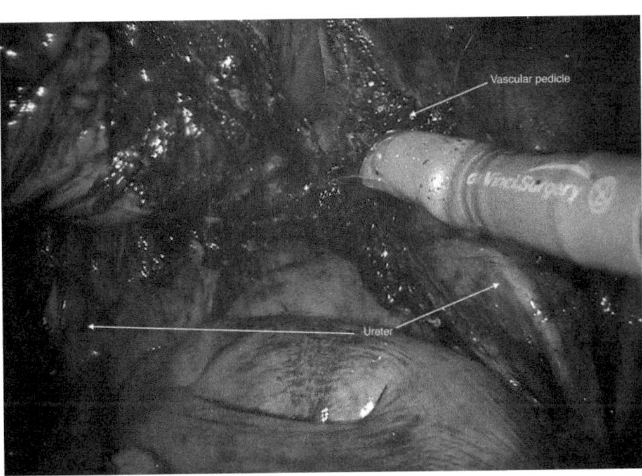

Fig. 60.35 Colpotomy on the lateral/posterior part of the vagina

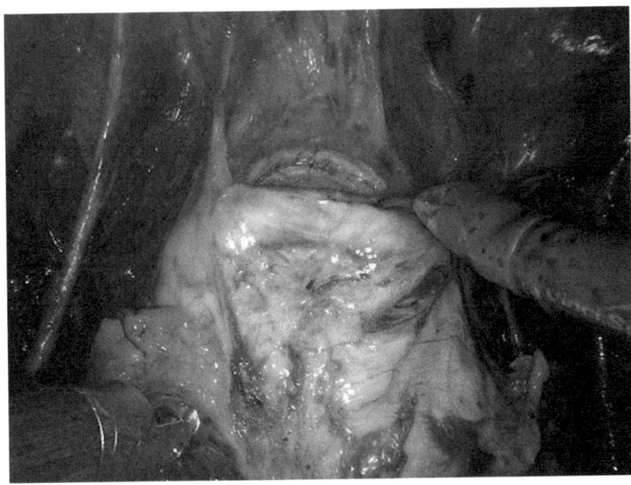

Fig. 60.33 Colpotomy using monopolar cutting current

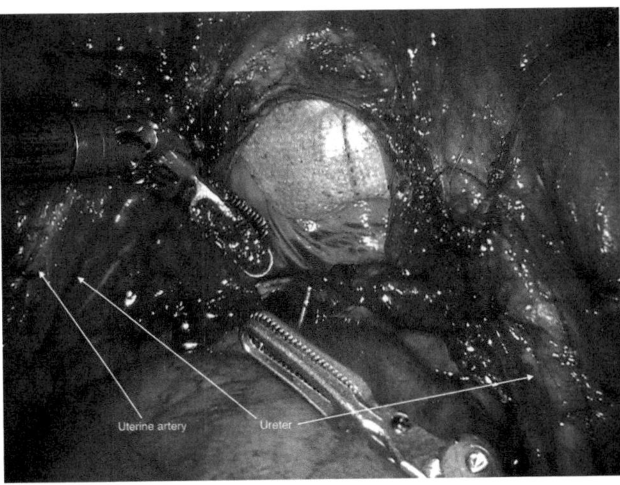

Fig. 60.36 Suturing the vaginal vault

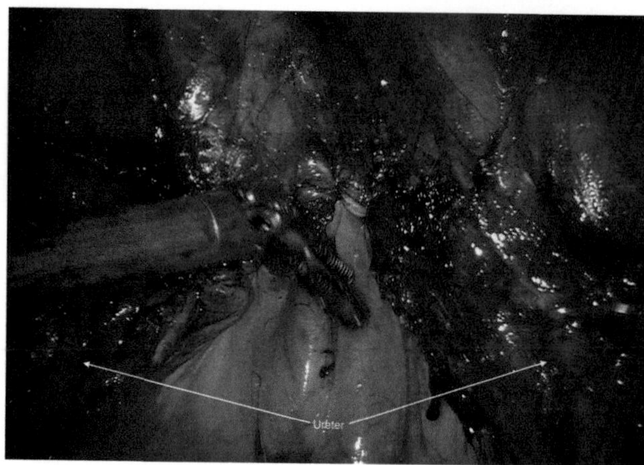

Fig. 60.37 Completed cuff closure

Key Points

- Identify patients with significant comorbidities
- Proper indications for surgery
- Adequate patient information, informed consent
- Optimize the patient prior to surgery
- Be aware of the increased risks of performing surgery in patients with comorbidities
- Training and experience in non complex cases before undertaking complex cases
- Use a standardized, reproducible, safe surgical approach
- Be prepared for all possible medical or surgical complications during surgery
- Teamwork and communication

References

1. Potter PA, Perry AG, Ross-Kerr JC, et al. Canadian fundamentals of nursing. 5th ed. Toronto: Elselvier; 2014.
2. Hoffman B, McGowan T. Chapter 18: Surgery in the patient with kidney disease. In: Merli GJ, Weitz HH, editors. Medical management of the surgical patient. 3rd ed. Philadelphia: Saunders Elsevier; 2008. p. 605–33.
3. Nieboer TE, Johnson N, Lethaby A, et al. Surgical approach to hysterectomy for benign gynaecological disease. Cochrane Database Syst Rev. 2009;8(3):CD003677.
4. Jacoby VL, Autry A, Jacobson G, et al. Nationwide use of laparoscopic hysterectomy compared with abdominal and vaginal approaches. Obstet Gynecol. 2009;114(5):1041–8.
5. Walker JL, Piedmonte MR, Spirtos NM, et al. Laparoscopy compared with laparotomy for comprehensive surgical staging of uterine cancer: Gynecologic Oncology Group Study LAP2. J Clin Oncol. 2009;27(32):5331–6. Epub 2009 Oct 5.
6. Galaal K, Bryant A, Fisher AD, et al. Laparoscopy versus laparotomy for the management of early stage endometrial cancer (Review). Cochrane Database Syst Rev. 2012;(9):CD006655. doi: 10.1002/14651858.CD006655.pub2.
7. Wright JD, Ananth CV, Lewin SN, et al. Robotically assisted vs laparoscopic hysterectomy among women with benign gynecologic disease. JAMA. 2013;309(7):689–98. Epub 2010 May 14.
8. Paraiso MF, Ridgeway B, Park AJ, et al. A randomized trial comparing conventional and robotically assisted total laparoscopic hysterectomy. Am J Obstet Gynecol. 2013;208: 368.e1–7.
9. Sarlos D, Kots L, Stevanovic N, Schaer G. Robotic compared with conventional laparoscopic hysterectomy: a randomized controlled trial. Obstet Gynecol. 2012;120:604–11.
10. Lönnerfors C, Reynisson P, Persson J. A randomized trial comparing vaginal and laparoscopic hysterectomy vs robot-assisted hysterectomy. J Minim Invasive Gynecol. 2015;22(1):78–86. Epub 2014 Jul 19.
11. Aarts JW, Nieboer TE, Johnson N, et al. Surgical approach to hysterectomy for benign gynaecological disease. Cochrane Database Syst Rev. 2015;8:CD003677. doi:10.1002/14651858.CD003677.pub5.
12. Leonard F, Chopin N, Borghese B, et al. Total laparoscopic hysterectomy: preoperative risk factors for conversion to laparotomy. J Minim Invasive Gynecol. 2005;12:312–7.
13. Bonilla DJ, Mains L, Whitaker R, et al. Uterine weight as a predictor of morbidity after a benign abdominal and total laparoscopic hysterectomy. J Reprod Med. 2007;52:490–8.
14. Boggess JF, Gehrig PA, Cantrell L, et al. Perioperative outcomes of robotically assisted hysterectomy for benign cases with complex pathology. Obstet Gynecol. 2009;14(3):585–93.
15. Kaye AD, Vadivelu N, Ahuja N, et al. Anestetic considerations in robotic-assisted gynecologic surgery. Ochsner J. 2013;13(4):517–24. Review.
16. Klauschie J, Wechter ME, Jacob K, et al. Use of anti-skid material and patient-positioning to prevent patient shifting during robotic assisted gynecologic procedures. J Minim Invasive Gynecol. 2010;17(4):504–7.
17. Ramanathan R, Carey RI, Lopez-Pujals A, Leveillee RJ. Patient positioning and trocar placement for robotic urologic procedures. In: Patel VR, editor. Robotic urologic surgery. 2nd ed. London: Springer; 2012. p. 107–20.
18. Sener A, Chew BH, Duvdevani M, et al. Combined transurethral and laparoscopic partial cystectomy and robot-assisted bladder repair for the treatment of bladder endometrioma. J Minim Invasive Gynecol. 2006;13(3):245–8.
19. Kalmar AF, Foubert L, Hendrickx JF, et al. Influence of steep Trendelenburg position and CO(2) pneumoperitoneum on cardiovascular, cerebrovascular, and respiratory homeostasis during robotic prostatectomy. Br J Anaesth. 2010;104(4):433–9. Epub 2010 Feb 18.
20. Hirvonen EA, Nuutinen LS, Kauko M. Hemodynamic changes due to Trendelenburg positioning and pneumoperitoneum during laparoscopic hysterectomy. Acta Anaesthesiol Scand. 1995;39(7): 949–55.
21. Choi SJ, Gwak MS, Ko JS, et al. The effects of the exaggerated lithotomy position for radical perineal prostatectomy on respiratory mechanics. Anaesthesia. 2006;61(5):439–43.
22. Carry PY, Gallet D, Francois Y, et al. Respiratory mechanics during laparoscopic cholecystectomy: the effects of the abdominal wall lift. Anesth Analg. 1998;87(6):1393–7.
23. Koivusalo AM, Lindgren L. Respiratory mechanics during laparoscopic cholecystectomy. Anesth Analg. 1999;89(3):800.
24. Lowery WJ, Leath 3rd CA, Robinson RD. Robotic surgery applications in the management of gynecologic malignancies. J Surg Oncol. 2012;105(5):481–7.
25. Sprung J, Whalley DG, Falcone T, et al. The impact of morbid obesity, pneumoperitoneum,and posture on respiratory system mechanics and oxygenation during laparoscopy. Anesth Analg. 2002;94(5):1345–50.

26. Barnett JC, Hurd WW, Rogers Jr RM, et al. Laparoscopic positioning and nerve injuries. J Minim Invasive Gynecol. 2007;14(5):664–72.
27. Lestar M, Gunnarsson L, Lagerstrand L, et al. Hemodynamic perturbations during robot-assisted laparoscopic radical prostatectomy in 458 Trendelenburg position. Anesth Analg. 2011;113(5):1069–75. Epub 2011 Jan 13.
28. Joris JL, Noirot DP, Legrand MJ, et al. Hemodynamic changes during laparoscopic cholecystectomy. Anesth Analg. 1993;76(5):1067–71.
29. Bird VG, Winfield HN. Laparoscopy in urology: physiologic considerations. In: Fallon B, editor. Hospital physician urology board review. Wayne: Turner White Communications, Inc.; 2002.
30. Choosing the route of hysterectomy for benign disease. ACOG Committee Opinion 444. Obstet Gynecol. 2009;114:1156–8.
31. Cadiére GB, Himpens J, Germay O, et al. Feasibility of robotic laparoscopic surgery: 146 cases. World J Surg. 2001;25(11):1467–77.
32. Nezhat C, Saberi NS, Shahmohamady B, Nezhat F. Robotic assisted laparoscopy in gynecologic surgery. JSLS. 2006;10(3):317–20.
33. Liu H, Lawrie TA, Lu D, et al. Robot-assisted surgery in gynaecology. Cochrane Database Syst Rev. 2014;10:12.
34. Weinberg L, Rao S, Escobar PF. Robotic surgery in gynecology: an updated systematic review. Obstet Gynecol Int. 2011;2011:852061. Epub 2011 Nov 28.
35. Swan K, Advincula AP. Advances in urogynaecological robotic surgery. BJU Int. 2011;108(6 Pt 2):1024–7.
36. Advincula AP, Xu X, Goudeau S, Ransom SB. Robotic-assisted, laparoscopic, and abdominal myomectomy: a comparison of surgical outcomes. Obstetrics & Gynecology. 2011;117(2, part 1):265–56.
37. Giep BN, Giep HN, Hubert HB. Comparison of minimally invasive surgical approaches for hysterectomy at a community hospital: robotic-assisted laparoscopic hysterectomy, laparoscopic-assisted vaginal hysterectomy and laparoscopic supracervical hysterectomy. J Robot Surg. 2010;4(3):167–75.
38. Silasi DA, Gallo T, Silasi M, et al. Robotic versus abdominal hysterectomy for very large uteri. JSLS. 2013;17(3):400–6.
39. Payne TN, Dauterive FR, Pitter MC, et al. Robotically assisted hysterectomy in patients with large uteri: outcomes in five community practices. Obstet Gynecol. 2010;115(3):535–42.
40. Liu C, Peresic D, Samadi D, Nezhat F. Robotic-assisted laparoscopic partial bladder resection for the treatment of infiltrating endometriosis. J Minim Invasive Gynecol. 2008;15(6):745–8.
41. Chammas Jr MF, Kim FJ, Barbarino A, et al. Asymptomatic rectal and bladder endometriosis: a case for robotic-assisted surgery. Can J Urol. 2008;15(3):4097–100.
42. Barakat EE, Bedaiwy MA, Zimberg S, et al. Robotic-assisted, laparoscopic, and abdominal myomectomy: a comparison of surgical outcomes. Obstet Gynecol. 2011;117:256–65.
43. Magrina JF, Espada M, Munoz R, et al. Robotic adnexectomy compared with laparoscopy for adnexal mass. Obstet Gynecol. 2009;114(3):581–4.
44. Zakhari A, Czuzoj-Schulman N, Spence AR, et al. Laparoscopic and robot-assisted hysterectomy for uterine cancer: a comparison of costs and complications. Am J Obstet Gynecol. 2015;213(5):665.e1–7. Epub 2015 Jul 15.
45. Patzkowsky KE, As-Sanie S, Smorgick N, et al. Perioperative outcomes of robotic versus laparoscopic hysterectomy for benign disease. JSLS. 2013;17:100–6.
46. Bamgbade OA, Rutter TW, Nafiu OO, Dorje P. Postoperative complications in obese and nonobese patients. World J Surg. 2007;31(3):556–60.
47. National Institute for Health and Care Excellence. Obesity: identification, assessment and management of overweight and obesity in children, young people and adults. London: NICE; 2014. p. 64.
48. Adams JP, Murphy PG. Obesity in anaesthesia and intensive care. Br J Anaesth. 2000;85(1):91–108.
49. Mourits MJ, Bijen CB, Arts HJ, et al. Safety of laparoscopy versus laparotomy in early-stage endometrial cancer: a randomised trial. Lancet Oncol. 2010;11(8):763–71.
50. Janda M, Gebski V, Brand A, et al. Quality of life after total laparoscopic hysterectomy versus total abdominal hysterectomy for stage I endometrial cancer (LACE): a randomised trial. Lancet Oncol. 2010;11(8):772–80. Epub 2010 Jul 16.
51. Zullo F, Falbo A. Palomba. Safety of laparoscopy vs laparotomy in the surgical staging of endometrial cancer: a systematic review and metaanalysis of randomized controlled trials. Am J Obstet Gynecol. 2012;207(2):94–100. Epub 2012 Jan 13. Review.
52. Pitkin RM. Abdominal hysterectomy in obese women. Surg Gynecol Obstet. 1976;142(4):532–6.
53. O´Gorman T, MacDonald N, Mould T, et al. Total laparoscopic hysterectomy in morbidly obese women with endometrial cancer. Anaesthetic and surgical complications. Eur J Gynaecol Oncol. 2009;30:171–3.
54. Eltabbakh GH, Shamonki MI, Moody JM, Garafano LL. Hysterectomy for obese women with endometrial cancer: laparoscopy or laparotomy? Gynecol Oncol. 2000;78(3 Pt 1):329–35.
55. Uccella S, Bonzini M, Palomba S, et al. Impact of obesity on surgical treatment for endometrial cancer: a multicenter study comparing laparoscopy vs open surgery with propensity-matched analysis. J Minim Invasive Gynecol. 2016;23(1):53–61. E pub 2015 Aug 14.
56. Palomba S, Nelaj E, Zullo F. Visceral fat amount as predictive factor for early laparotomic conversion in obese patients with endometrial cancer. Gynecol Oncol. 2006 Jul;102(1):128–9.
57. Seamon LG, Cohn DE, Henretta MS, et al. Minimally invasive comprehensive surgical staging for endometrial cancer: robotics or laparoscopy? Gynecol Oncol. 2009;113(1):36–41.
58. Tang KY, Gardiner SK, Gould C, et al. Robotic surgical staging for obese patients with endometrial cancer. Am J Obstet Gynecol. 2012;206(6):513.e1–6. Epub 2012 Jan 12.
59. Backes FJ, Brudie LA, Farrell MR, et al. Short- and long-term morbidity and outcomes after robotic surgery for comprehensive endometrial cancer staging. Gynecol Oncol. 2012;125(3):546–51.
60. Wysham WZ, Kim KH, Roberts JM, et al. Obesity and perioperative pulmonary complications in robotic gynecologic surgery. Am J Obstet Gynecol. 2015;213(1):33.e1–7. Epub 2015 Jan 28.
61. Gallo T, Kashani S, Patel DA, et al. Robotic-assisted laparoscopic hysterectomy: outcomes in obese and morbidly obese patients. JSLS. 2012;16(3):421–7.
62. Geppert B, Lönnerfors C, Persson J. Robot assisted laparoscopic hysterectomy in obese and morbidly obese women: surgical technique and comparison with open surgery. Acta Obstet et Gynecol Scand. 2011;90:1211–7.
63. Corrado G, Chiantera V, Fanfani F, et al. Robotic hysterectomy in severely obese patients with endometrial cancer: a multicenter study. J Minim Invasive Gynecol. 2015;23(1):94–100. pii: S1553-4650(15)01510-1. doi: 10.1016/j.jmig.2015.08.887. [Epub ahead of print].
64. Sundi D, Reese AC, Mettee LZ, et al. Laparoscopic and robotic radical prostatectomy outcomes in obese and extremely obese men. Urology. 2013;82(3):600–5.
65. Ten Broek RP, Strik C, Issa Y, et al. Adhesiolysis-related morbidity in abdominal surgery. Ann Surg. 2013;258:98–106.
66. Van Der Krabben AA, Dijkstra FR, Nieuwenhuijzen M, et al. Morbidity and mortality of inadvertent enterotomy during adhesiotomy. Br J Surg. 2000;87:467–71.
67. LeBlanc KA, Melvin JE, Corder JM. Enterotomy and mortality rates of laparoscopic incisional and ventral hernia repair: a review of the literature. JSLS. 2007;11:408–14.
68. Van Goor H. Consequences and complications of peritoneal adhesions. Colorectal Dis. 2007;9(suppl 2):25–34.

69. Taylor GW, Jayne DG, Brown SR, et al. Adhesions and incisional hernias following laparoscopic versus open surgery for colorectal cancer in the CLASICC trial. Br J Surg. 2010;97:70–8.
70. Nieuwenhuijzen M, Reijnen MMPJ, Kuijpers JHC, van Goor H. Small bowel obstruction after total or subtotal colectomy: a 10-year retrospective review. Br J Surg. 1998;85:1242–5.
71. Ellis H, Moran BJ, Thompson JN, et al. Adhesion-related hospital readmissions after abdominal and pelvic surgery: a retrospective cohort study. Lancet. 1999;353:1476–80.
72. Ording Olsen K, Juul S, Berndtsson I, et al. Ulcerative colitis: female fecundity before diagnosis, during disease, and after surgery compared with a population sample. Gastroenterology. 2002; 122:15–9.
73. Parikh JA, Ko CY, Maggard MA, Zingmond DS. What is the rate of small bowel obstruction after colectomy? Am Surg. 2008;74: 1001–5.
74. Ng SS, Leung KL, Lee JF, et al. Long-term morbidity and oncologic outcomes of laparoscopic-assisted anterior resection for upper rectal cancer: ten-year results of a prospective, randomized trial. Dis Colon Rectum. 2009;52:558–66.
75. Leung TT, Dixon E, Gill M, et al. Bowel obstruction following appendectomy: what is the true incidence? Ann Surg. 2009;250:51–3.
76. Ahmad G, Duffy JM, Farquhar C, et al. Barrieragents for adhesion prevention after gynaecological surgery. Cochrane Database Syst Rev. 2008;2:CD000475.
77. Ten Broeck RPG, Issa Y, van Santbrink EJP, et al. Burden of adhesions in abdominal and pelvic surgery: systematic review and met-analysis. BMJ. 2013;347:f5588.
78. Dubuisson J, Botchorishvili R, Perrette S, et al. Incidence of intraabdominal adhesions in a continuous series of 1000 laparoscopic procedures. Am J Obstet Gynecol. 2010;203:111e1e3.
79. Tinelli A, Malvasi A, Guido M, et al. Adhesion formation after intracapsular myomectomy with or without adhesion barrier. Fertil Steril. 2011;95:1780e5.
80. Trew G, Pistofidis G, Pados G, et al. Gynaecological endoscopic evaluation of 4 % icodextrin solution: a European, multicentre, double-blind, randomized study of the efficacy and safety in the reduction of de novo adhesions after laparoscopic gynaecological surgery. Hum Reprod Update. 2011;26:2015e27.
81. Brill AI, Nezaht F, Nezhat CH, et al. The incidence of adhesions after prior laparotomy: a laparoscopic appraisal. Obstet Gynecol. 1995;85:269e72.
82. Menzies D, Ellis H. Intestinal obstruction from adhesions-how big is the problem? Ann R Coll Surg Engl. 1990;72:60e3.
83. Herrmann A, De Wilde RL. Adhesions are the major cause of complications in operative gynecology. Best Pract Res Clin Obst Gynaecolo. 2015;35:71–83. pii: S1521-6934(15)00193-5. doi: 10.1016/j.bpobgyn.2015.10.010. Epub ahead of print.
84. Ten Broek RP, Kok-Krant N, Bakkum EA, et al. Different surgical techniques to reduce post-operative adhesion formation: a systematic review and meta-analysis. Hum Reprod Update. 2013;19:12–25.
85. Audebert AJ, Gomel V. Role of microlaparoscopy in the diagnosis of peritoneal and visceral adhesions and in the prevention of bowel injury associated with blind trocar insertion. Fertil Steril. 2000;73(3):631–5.
86. Sepilian V, Ku L, Wong H, et al. Prevalence of infraumbilical adhesions in women with previous laparoscopy. JSLS. 2007;11:41–4.
87. Lönnerfors C, Persson J. Implementation and applications of robotic surgery within gynecologic oncology and gynecology; analysis of the first thousand cases. Ceska Gynekol. 2013;78(1):12–9.
88. Lönnerfors C, Reynisson P, Geppert B, Persson J. The effect of increased experience on complications in robotic hysterectomy for malignant and benign gynecological disease. J Robot Surg. 2015;9(4):321–30.
89. Paley PJ, Veljovich DS, Shah CA, et al. Surgical outcomes in gynecologic oncology in the era of robotics: analysis of first 1000 cases. Am J Obstet Gynecol. 2011;204:551.e1–9.
90. Reynisson P, Persson J. Hospital costs for robot-assisted laparoscopic radical hysterectomy and pelvic lymphadenectomy. Gynecol Oncol. 2013;130:95–9.
91. Jones N, Fleming ND, Nick AM, et al. Conversion from robotic surgery to laparotomy: a case-control study evaluating risk factors for conversion. Gynecol Oncol. 2014;134(2):238–42.
92. Kaul S, Shah NL, Menon M. Learning curve using robotic surgery. Curr Urol Rep. 2006;7(2):125–9.

61 General Aspects and Their Handling: General Surgery Conditions and Techniques for Robotic Hysterectomy

Jan-Hendrik Egberts

During the last 30 years, minimal invasive surgery has revolutionized many general and especially oncological surgical techniques. After a controversial debate about the safety and efficacy of this new surgical approach, it is now widely accepted. For colorectal cancer, several prospective and multicenter studies have demonstrated the potential advantages of minimal invasive techniques [1, 2]. However, even today the rate of minimal invasive resections for colorectal cancer is still limited due to technical limitations, the long learning curve and other reasons.

The application of robotic assistance in minimal invasive surgery has been a logical development over the last years. Today, robotic assisted surgery is gaining acceptance in all surgical fields, such as thoracic surgery, upper GI surgery, HPB surgery and transplantation surgery, with encouraging results [3].

Especially in anatomical regions like the pelvic or the thorax with limited access, the advantages are obvious. The first use in colorectal surgery was for a segmental colonic resection for a benign disease in 2002 [4] and for a low anterior rectal resection in 2006 [5]. In 2012 a prospective multicenter study was initiated, investigating the safety and efficacy of robotic-assisted vs. laparoscopic low anterior rectum resection (ROLARR-study) [6]. The recruitment was recently completed.

Besides the technical improvements in surgery, another milestone in rectal cancer surgery was the description of the "holy plane" by Heald [7]. Based on the embryology of the rectum with the development of the complex anatomy of the pelvic floor, the distribution of lymphatic nodes and vessels and nerval structures becomes more systematic. The surgeon should follow the embryological fasciae (i.e. perirectal fascia and the pelvic fascia which is called the "holy plane") in order to achieve the best optimal oncological specimen by preserving the autonomic pelvic nerves that comprise the superior hypogastric plexus, the right and left hypogastric nerves and the right and left inferior hypogastric plexuses. The precise preparation in this plane, developing the whole rectum with perirectal tissue, is called "total mesorectal excision (TME)" [8].

Knowledge of embryology might be of special interest for the oncological resection of other compartments in the pelvic region, such as urological and gynecological cancers. Especially in tumors infiltrating the rectum, for example ovarian cancers or in cases of deep endometriosis, the gynecological surgeon might be in a position to dissect this tissue.

In the following section, the set-up and technique for a low anterior resection, as an example of a pelvic surgical procedure, is described.

Setup

Patient Positioning

Due to the current limitation in the movement of the patient table, the patient positioning gains even more importance before the docking maneuver since the procedure sometimes requires an extreme positioning of the patient. Also, several surgical procedures require a dual docking, in which the robot arms are disconnected and re-docked after the re-positioning of the patient. Future developments will synchronize the robot arms with the table in order to move the patient during the robot procedure similar to the conventional laparoscopic technique.

For procedures in the pelvic region, such as low anterior resections, the patient is placed supine in a modified lithotomy position. The legs are abducted with flexed knees and the arms alongside the body. It is important to standardize the set-up for different procedures in order to maximize the safety and efficacy.

J.-H. Egberts
Department of Visceral-, Thoracic, Transplantation-, and Pediatric Surgery, University Hospitals Schleswig-Holstein, Campus Kiel, Kiel 24105, Germany
e-mail: jan-hendrik.egberts@uksh.de

I. Alkatout, L. Mettler (eds.), *Hysterectomy*, DOI 10.1007/978-3-319-22497-8_61

OR Set-Up

A 12 mmHg pneumoperitoneum is achieved by a mini-laparotomy and the ports are introduced as follows:

- Two 12 mm conventional laparoscopic trocars (camera and assistant trocar)
- Three 8 mm robotic trocars

Once the camera trocar is inserted, an assessment of the entire abdomen is performed and the trocars are placed at their optimal sites.

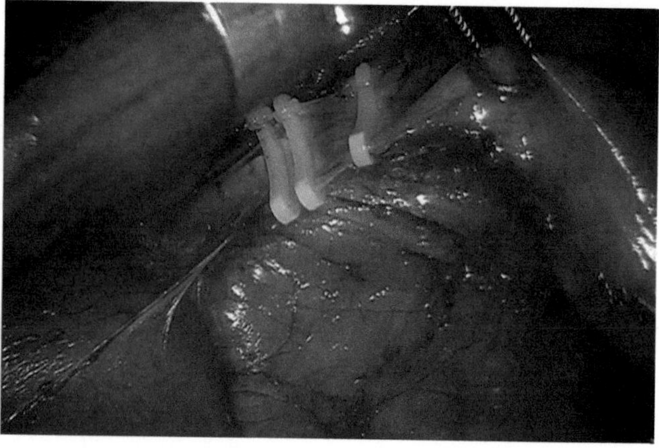

Fig. 61.2 Inferior mesenteric vein after central ligation close to the duodenum (left lower corner)

Elements of the Procedure

The major elements of a low anterior resection (LAR) for rectal cancer are:

- central ligation of the inferior mesenteric artery (IMA) and inferior mesenteric vein (IMV)
- mobilization of the left colon/ splenic flexure
- rectal resection with total mesenteric excision (TME)
- specimen removal and anastomosis

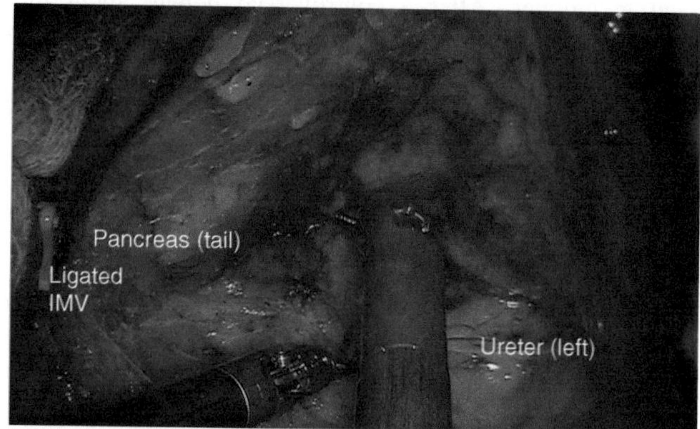

Fig. 61.3 Medial to lateral view after left flexure mobilization

The operation for LAR starts with a visual inspection of the abdomen (especially the liver for metastases) and a central ligation of the IMA and IMV. A so-called "medial to lateral approach" begins with the incision of the peritoneum after lifting the sigmoid colon and upper rectum. The incision starts at the level of sacral promontory. The superior rectal artery will be seen and followed to its origin of the IMA after identification of the left colonic artery and sigmoidal artery. These structures should be free of other tissue in order to avoid an injury of the ureter. The ligation of the artery can be taken by the surgeon's preferred method as shown in Fig. 61.1.

The dissection in this plane will be continued in the layer of the anteriorly localized IMV and colonic mesentery and the posteriorly localized retroperitoneum (Fig. 61.2). In this layer the retroperitoneal structures, such as the pancreas, ureter and vessels, can be detected and saved by blunt dissection. The surgeon dissects the tissue laterally to the left colonic flexure and cranially the pancreas tail (Fig. 61.3). During this dissection the IMV is ligated near the ligament of Treitz. The final mobilization of the left colon and splenic flexure is then performed from a lateral approach.

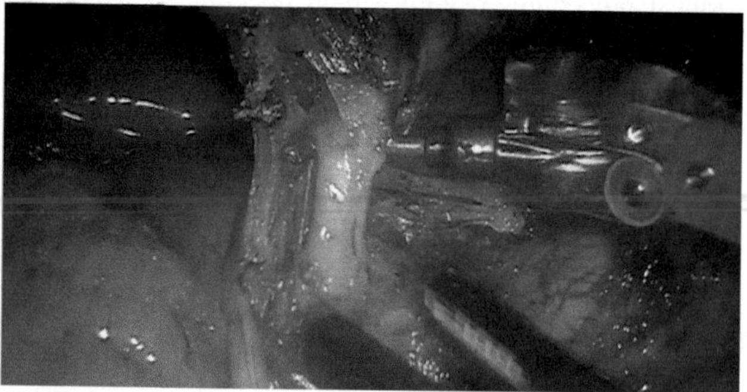

Fig. 61.1 Inferior mesenteric artery prior to central ligation

The removal of the rectum and mesorectum (total mesorectal excision –TME) is carried out according to Heald's principles [7]. By staying in the avascular plane between the endopelvic visceral fascia and the endopelvic parietal fascia, an avascular space is developed. In this plane the hypogastric nerve plexus becomes visible and can be preserved. Also, the sacral venous plexus, located deep in the parietal layer, will be untouched. During this preparation it is essential to use the robot arms to provide upward traction and counter traction by cautious and frequent repositioning in order to avoid damage to the TME specimen. The dissection in this plane is completed posteriorly to the level of the pelvic floor. The lateral stalks are then dis-

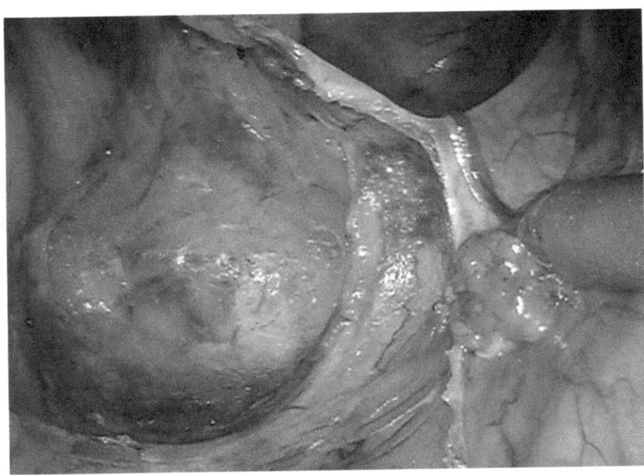

Fig. 61.4 View in the pelvic after dorsal mobilization of the rectum

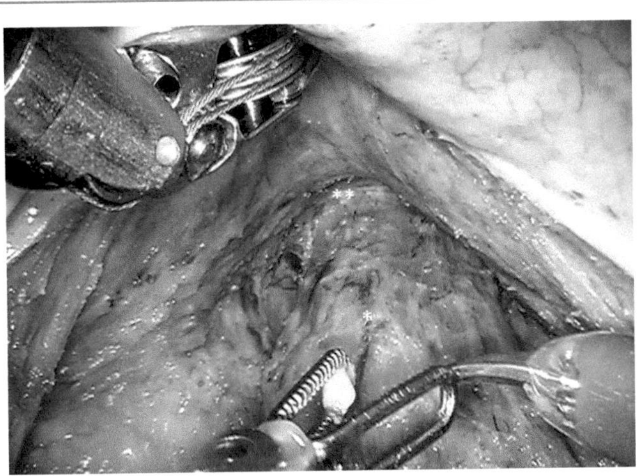

Fig. 61.6 View in the pelvic after complete ventral mobilization of the rectum

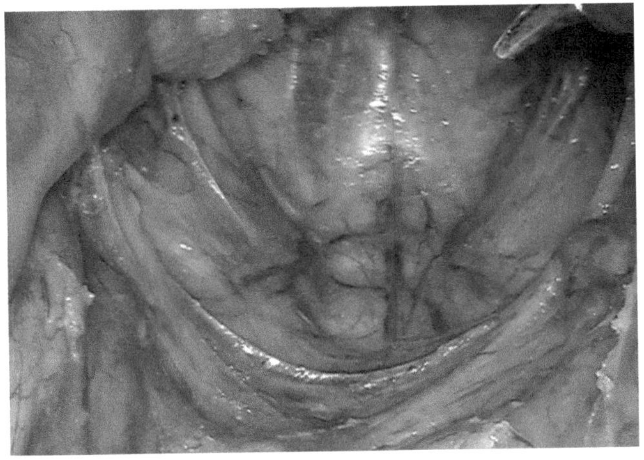

Fig. 61.5 View in the pelvic after complete dorsal mobilization of the rectum

sected. Here the vagina or the seminal vesicals and prostate are dissected free and protected (Figs. 61.4, 61.5 and 61.6). The autonomic nerves are localized laterally on the pelvic wall and should be protected during these dissecting steps.

The dissection is continued until the pelvic floor is reached (bare rectum area) and finally divided with a stapler device. The removal of the specimen is now possible and performed by an incision.

The anastomosis and reconstruction is usually performed by a circular stapler device with a side-to-end anastomosis. If adequate colonic length is present, a colonic J pouch is performed.

Up until now, the anastomosis and reconstruction is performed in a standard laparoscopic approach since no robotic instruments are available so far.

Conclusions

The robotic approach for surgery for rectal cancers appears promising. It creates new opportunities and allows a perfect view and mobility in the limited area of the pelvic region.

In general and thoracic surgery, the number of robotic-assisted procedures is increasing. There is a wide range of indications for procedures that can be performed with robotic assistance, extending the limitations of the minimal invasive approach.

References

1. Dalibon N, Moutafis M, Fischler M. Laparoscopically assisted versus open colectomy for colon cancer. N Engl J Med. 2004; 351(9):933–4. author reply -4
2. Jayne DG, Thorpe HC, Copeland J, Quirke P, Brown JM, Guillou PJ. Five-year follow-up of the Medical Research Council CLASICC trial of laparoscopically assisted versus open surgery for colorectal cancer. Br J Surg. 2010;97(11):1638–45.
3. Spinoglio G, editor. Robotic surgery: current applications and new trends (updates in surgery). Milan: Springer; 2014. p. 238.
4. Weber PA, Merola S, Wasielewski A, Ballantyne GH. Telerobotic-assisted laparoscopic right and sigmoid colectomies for benign disease. Dis Colon Rectum. 2002;45(12):1689–94. discussion 95–6.
5. Diana M, Marescaux J. Robotic surgery. Br J Surg. 2015;102(2):e15–28.
6. Collinson FJ, Jayne DG, Pigazzi A, Tsang C, Barrie JM, Edlin R, Garbett C, Guillou P, Holloway I, Howard H, Marshall H, McCabe C, Pavitt S, Quirke P, Rivers CS, Brown JM. An international, multicentre, prospective, randomised, controlled, unblinded, parallel-group trial of robotic-assisted versus standard laparoscopic surgery for the curative treatment of rectal cancer. Int J Colorectal Dis. 2012;27(2):233–41.
7. Heald RJ. The 'Holy Plane' of rectal surgery. J R Soc Med. 1988;81(9):503–8.
8. Weaver KL, Grimm Jr LM, Fleshman JW. Changing the way we manage rectal cancer-standardizing TME from open to robotic (including laparoscopic). Clin Colon Rectal Surg. 2015;28(1):28–37.

Robotic Assisted Supracervical Hysterectomy

62

Noam Smorgick

Introduction

Supracervical (subtotal) hysterectomy refers to the removal of the uterine corpus with preservation of the uterine cervix. This subtype of hysterectomy is technically simpler compared with total hysterectomy because it does not require an extensive dissection of the cardinal ligaments and the vesico-uterine fold, nor suturing of the vaginal cuff. Thus, with the advent of laparoscopic and robotic hysterectomy, the rates of supracervical hysterectomy from all hysterectomies increased considerably. More recently, robotic assisted supracervical hysterectomy combined with sacral colpopexy has been found to be an excellent treatment for apical (level I) prolapse, further increasing the use of this procedure. Nevertheless, because supracervical hysterectomy requires some type of morcellation for specimen extraction, recent concerns regarding dissemination of leiomyosarcoma during power morcellation may limit the use of this procedure. Similar to total hysterectomy, the debate regarding the benefits and challenges of the robotic platform for supracervical hysterectomy continues. This debates centers on the relative advantage of converting an open hysterectomy to a minimally invasive hysterectomy by using the robotic platform when taking into account its higher cost.

Indications for Robotic Supracervical Hysterectomy

The main indications for this procedure are:

1. Hysterectomy for benign indication in women without cervical pathology. Robotic supracervical hysterectomy is an acceptable alternative to total hysterectomy in women requiring removal of the uterus for benign indications such as uterine fibroids, abnormal uterine bleeding and pelvic pain. As for total hysterectomy, the robotic platform may enable performing a minimally invasive hysterectomy in women with high surgical complexity (such as large fibroids or extensive pelvic adhesive disease from prior abdominal surgeries or pelvic inflammatory disease) who may not have been candidates for laparoscopic hysterectomy. Of note, supracervical hysterectomy is contraindicated in cases of cervical dysplasia for obvious reasons. Supracervical hysterectomy is less recommended for women with advanced endometriosis and pelvic pain because of higher rates of persistent postoperative pelvic pain [1].
2. Removal of the uterine corpus combined with sacral colpopexy in cases of pelvic organ prolapse. Sacral colpopexy for repair of level I pelvic floor defect (i.e., apical prolapse) is considered an excellent treatment for this pathology, and has been found to be superior to vaginal repair in a recent Cochrane review [2]. This procedure is often combined with total or supracervical hysterectomy. Sacral-colpopexy requires extensive suturing for placement of the mesh on the cervix and the anterior and posterior vaginal walls, which may be simplified with the use of the robotic platform. Moreover, supracervical rather than total hysterectomy has the advantage of lower risk of mesh erosion [3].
3. Patient desire and request. Some women may elect to preserve the cervix when it is unrelated to the uterine pathology (i.e., in case of uterine corpus leiomyoma) because of personal preference. The surgeon should provide appropriate counseling regarding advantages and disadvantages of supracervical hysterectomy (see below) in order to allow for patient's informed decision and consent.

N. Smorgick
Obstetrics and Gynecology, Assaf Harofe Medical Center, Zeriffin, Beer Yaakov 70300, Israel
e-mail: Noam_yossi@yahoo.com

I. Alkatout, L. Mettler (eds.), *Hysterectomy*, DOI 10.1007/978-3-319-22497-8_62

Advantages of Robotic Assisted Supracervical Hysterectomy

To date, no studies have directly compared robotic assisted total and supracervical hysterectomy. However, related trials have been performed comparing abdominal total and supracervical hysterectomy. Most of these studies have not found a significant difference between the two surgeries in long term outcomes. A highly quoted 2002 randomized controlled trial by Thakar et al. found similar outcomes regarding bladder, bowel, and sexual function at 12 months [4]. In addition, the rate of pelvic organ prolapse was similar between the two groups. Nevertheless, short term outcomes such as postoperative hospital length of stay and rates of postoperative fever and wound hematoma were lower in the supracervical hysterectomy group [4]. On longer follow up of 14 years using a mailed questionnaire, no differences were found in rates of urinary incontinence, pelvic organ prolapse, pelvic pain, sexual function and quality of life [5].

Despite similar long term outcomes when compared to total hysterectomy, supracervical hysterectomy remains popular because it is considered technically "simpler" compared with total hysterectomy. Supracervical hysterectomy requires less dissection of the cardinal ligaments and the vesicouterine fold (i.e., bladder flap), and more importantly does not require suturing for closure of the vaginal cuff. This advantage is very important for the laparoscopic approach, since laparoscopic suturing is a relatively advanced surgical skill. Furthermore, the main surgical complication associated with vaginal cuff closure, vaginal cuff dehiscence, which is more common in laparoscopic and robotic assisted hysterectomy compared with abdominal and vaginal hysterectomy, is practically non-existent in supracervical robotic and laparoscopic hysterectomy [6]. Accordingly, supracervical hysterectomy constitutes up to 80 % of laparoscopic hysterectomies in Germany [7], as well as a large share of robotic assisted hysterectomies.

Disadvantages of Subtotal Hysterectomy

The risk of cervical cancer in the remaining cervix has been considered a disadvantage of subtotal hysterectomy. However, recent high quality studies have concluded this risk to be less than 0.1 % when appropriate pre-operative patient selection is performed [8]. Cyclic vaginal bleeding caused by remnants of endometrial tissue in the cervical stump occurs in up to 15 % of women [9].

Tissue extraction remains the main disadvantage of subtotal hysterectomy. In the absence of vaginal vault opening, the only means of extraction of the uterine corpus are power morcellation (using commercially available morcellators) or "cold knife" hand morcellation through incisions in the abdominal wall or the pouch of Douglas. As discussed below, recent concerns regarding the dissemination of malignant fibroids by use of power morcellation are currently a major limitation of this technique.

Morcellation

Until recently, the usual method for specimen extraction in supracervical hysterectomy was the use of laparoscopic power morcellators through a 12–15 mm port. The unquestionable disadvantage of this method is intraperitoneal spread of uterine and fibroid fragments. It was assumed that those fragments may cause dissemination of malignant fibroids (leiomyosarcoma) or stromal sarcoma, but these events were considered extremely rare, in the range of 1/1000 [10]. However, following claims that dissemination of leiomyosarcoma may be more common than previously thought, the US Food and Drug Administration (FDA) issued a statement in 2014 warning against the use of power morcellators in the majority of women undergoing hysterectomy [11].

Setting aside the FDA warning and its impact on medical practice, the actual rate of inadvertent leiomyosarcoma morcellation in a patient undergoing supracervical hysterectomy for fibroids presumed benign is debatable. The FDA concluded that the risk of unsuspected uterine sarcomas and leiomyosarcomas in patients undergoing hysterectomy for presumed benign fibroids is 1 in 352 and 1 in 458, respectively. However, this report was based on retrospective studies originating from referral centers with high risk patients with possible selection bias [11]. Furthermore, due to the lack of high quality studies, the impact of unsuspected sarcoma dissemination by power morcellation on the patient's ultimate survival is also unknown. More recent studies have attempted to investigate the risk of a sarcoma being inadvertently morcellated. A large Norwegian study which included 4791 women undergoing various gynecologic procedures concluded that the incidence of leiomyosarcoma among women suspected of having benign fibroids was 0.5 % (1 in 183 women), while the risk of unintended morcellation of a leiomyosarcoma was much lower, 0.02 % (1 in 4791 women) [12].

In view of the medical and medico-legal issues that are currently associated with the use of power morcellators [13], other methods for specimen removal which may be used for supracervical hysterectomy have been suggested. These include cold knife hand morcellation through the abdominal wall (after the specimen is placed in a retrieval bag) and contained power morcellation, i.e. power morcellation of the specimen within a closed bag. The former technique is straightforward to perform, but may require an extension of the port incision (especially when the specimen removed is large) and longer operative time. The latter technique is more cumbersome, and has mostly been described in vitro [14]. However, future development of contained power morcellating devices may once again make this technique both safe and easy to use.

Prophylactic Removal of the Adnexa or Fallopian Tubes

Removal of the adnexa or the fallopian tubes may be performed in conjunction with supracervical hysterectomy for benign conditions. Removal of the fallopian tubes with ovarian preservation carries minimal surgical risks and presumably low risk of premature ovarian failure, but may provide some protection from ovarian carcinoma in the future [15]. Furthermore, prophylactic bilateral salpingectomy prevents the benign post-hysterectomy complication of hydrosalpings (which may appear on ultrasound as ovarian cysts and may lead to unnecessary future surgery) [16]. Thus, we favor prophylactic salpingectomy in all patients undergoing hysterectomy.

The decision to perform prophylactic oophorectomy is more complex and depends on the patient's age, menopausal status, and their personal or familial history of breast and ovarian cancer. Prophylactic oophorectomy in pre-menopausal women would cause early surgical menopause, associated with increased risks for coronary artery disease, osteoporosis, and possibly dementia [17–19]. These risks may be partially overset by replacement estrogen therapy. On the other hand, the overall risk of ovarian cancer in those women without family history of breast/ovarian cancer whose ovaries were preserved during benign hysterectomy is low, ranging from 0.03 to 1.96 % [17]. Thus, the risks and benefits of this procedure should be considered and appropriate patient's consultation should be provided. The current recommendations of the American College of Obstetrics and Gynecology [20] and the Society of Gynecologic Oncologists [21] are to favor ovarian preservation in pre-menopausal women with average risk for ovarian cancer. The recommendations for ovarian preservation versus removal in menopausal women with average risk for ovarian cancer are inconclusive due to lack of sufficient studies. In women with higher risk for ovarian cancer due to family history or BRCA1/BRCA2 mutation, the risk-reducing bilateral oophorectomy is recommended in pre-menopausal women when childbearing is complete, factoring in the age at onset of cancer in affected family members.

The Step-by-Step Use of the Robotic Platform for Subtotal Hysterectomy

Patient's Positioning and Preparation

As for laparoscopic and robotic total hysterectomy, patient's positioning and operating room organization is of the utmost importance for the successful completion of this surgery. Following general anesthesia and endotracheal intubation, the patient is placed in a dorsal lithotomy position, with the buttocks slightly protruding outside the operating table. The arms are padded and tucked to the patient's sides. The legs are placed in stirrups, preferably padded "boot" stirrups which allow placing most of the patients' weight on their heels as well as easy upward and downward movement of the legs during surgery, if required (Fig. 62.1). Use of pneumatic compression device is recommended. Robotic hysterectomy, especially when combined with sacral-colpopexy, requires positioning in steep Trendelenburg position, often for several hours. As a result, patients' positioning on the operating table must be secure in order to avoid cephalad slippage during the surgery. This may be accomplished by using shoulder braces, vacuum positioning systems, or specially designed mattresses such as the "egg-crate" mattress. A grounding electrode is placed on the patient's thigh.

Following patient's positioning, the vagina and the abdomen are prepped and draped. A Foley catheter is routinely placed. A uterine manipulator, although not always deemed necessary for removal of a small uterus, is often very helpful for performing subtotal hysterectomy. Uterine manipulators containing a cervical ring, which helps delineate the vaginal margins when performing the colpotomy incision during total hysterectomy, are also useful for subtotal hysterectomy by elevating the uterine vessels further away from the ureters and possibly decreasing the risk of thermal injury during the coagulation of these vessels. These manipulators are manufactured in reusable and non-reusable forms. The choice of specific uterine manipulator is usually guided by surgeon's preference. Our own preference is to use easy to handle manipulators containing colpotomy rings such as the VCare (Conmed, Utica, New York, USA) or the RUMI (Cooper Surgical, Trumbull, Connecticut, USA) (Fig. 62.2).

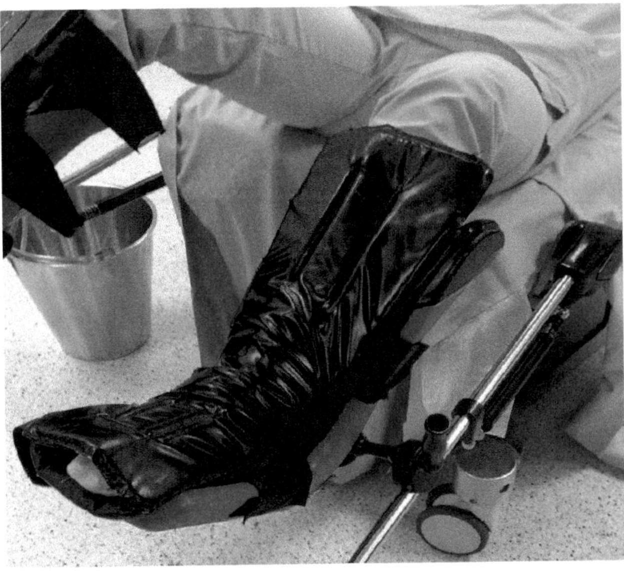

Fig. 62.1 "Boot" stirrups allowing for comfortable positioning of patients in a lithotomy position during long surgeries, as well as easy movement of the legs from low to high lithotomy position

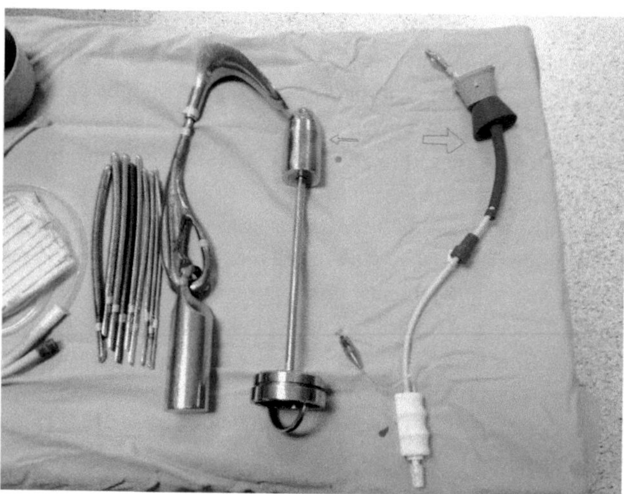

Fig. 62.2 Operative vaginal table prepared for robotic supracervical hysterectomy and sacral colpopexy. A plastic uterine manipulator containing a cervical ring (in this figure, the VCare) and an end-to-end anastomosis sizer are shown

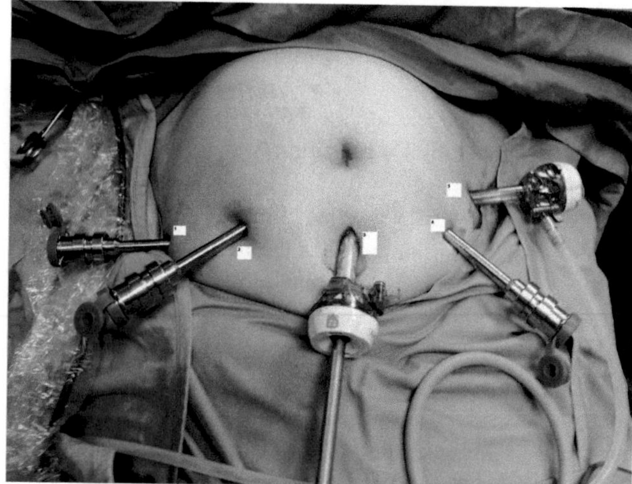

Fig. 62.3 Port configuration for robotic supracervical hysterectomy and sacral colpopexy. The camera port is located about 3 cm above the umbilicus. One robotic port is placed on the right side and two other robotic ports are placed on the left side. The bed-side assistant port is placed on the right side

Setup of the Robotic Platform

The basic setup includes the surgeon operating from the robotic console and controlling the robotic camera and 2 or 3 robotic arms, a bedside assistant using a laparoscopic port and standing on the right or left side of the patient (according to the port configuration – see below), and a second assistant sitting between the patient's legs and handling the uterine manipulator. The scrubbed surgical technician is often positioned in front of the first surgical assistant, on the other side of the patient. This positioning allows for easy reach to each of the robotic arms, required for instrument replacement and troubleshooting. A "vaginal" table is placed within arm's reach of the second surgical assistant. On this table are placed surgical instruments required for the insertion of the uterine manipulator (i.e., speculum, uterine sound and cervical dilators) and other vaginal instruments which may be required for sacral-colpopexy (i.e., sizers and spatula retractors). It is extremely important to place monitors in the room to allow for comfortable viewing of the surgery by the two surgical assistants and the surgical technicians. The robot may be docked in a direct line over the lower part of the patient's body, or on the left side or right side of the patient (i.e., side docking). The side docking technique allows for more comfortable seating for the second surgical assistant, which often translates into easier manipulation of the uterine manipulator.

Initiation of Pneumoperitoneum

According to surgeon's preference, pneumoperitoneum may be initiated with the closed technique (using a Veress needle), the open technique (i.e., the Hasson method) or the direct entry technique. The latter was recently modified with the introduction of optical trocars, which allow "under vision" direct entry.

Port Configuration for Robotic Subtotal Hysterectomy

Similar to other types of robotic hysterectomy, the usual port configuration for robotic subtotal hysterectomy will include -

1. *The robotic camera port (either 8 or 12 mm)*: this port should be placed at least a handbreadth (i.e., 10 cm) above the uterine fundus. For normal size uteri to mildly enlarged uteri (up to ~12 gestational weeks size), the typical placement is the umbilicus. For enlarged uteri, this port is moved cephalad. In cases of combined subtotal hysterectomy and sacral-colpopexy, although most often a normal sized uterus is removed, it is helpful to place the camera port a few centimeters above the umbilicus to allow for optimal visualization of the sacral promontory area (Fig. 62.3).
2. *Two lateral ports for robotic instruments*: the typical placement is a right sided 8 mm port for the monopolar shears and a left sided 8 mm port for the bipolar forceps (or similar electrosurgical instruments such as the Plasma Kinetic forceps). These two ports may be used later on to introduce needle drivers, in case a suture is placed on the cervical stump or on the vaginal walls for sacral-colpopexy.
3. *A third robotic arm*: this arm may be placed when an additional grasping instrument is required, most often in

cases of large uteri, peritoneal adhesive disease, or when a concomitant sacral-colpopexy is performed. The robotic instruments often used for these purposes are the pro-grasp or the tenaculum. The third robotic arm is usually placed between the camera port and the lateral robotic port, either on the right side or on the left side. When a concomitant sacral-colpopexy is performed, it is convenient to place the third robotic arm of the left side to allow for retraction of the sigmoid colon and easier exposure of the sacral promontory area. When the procedure includes only the subtotal hysterectomy without sacral-colpopexy, it is more convenient to place the third robotic arm on the right side of the patient in order to allow the surgeon a control of robotic grasping instruments on both side of the pelvis.

4. *Laparoscopic port for bedside surgical assistant*: this port is usually placed on the opposite side of the third robotic arm. In cases only two robotic arms are used, this port is usually placed on the left side of the patient. This port is used for introduction of laparoscopic graspers, suction irrigator and sutures as required. The size of the port can range from 5 mm (in case only graspers and suction/irrigation are used) to 12 mm (in case multiple sutures are used, i.e. in a sacral-colpopexy procedure).

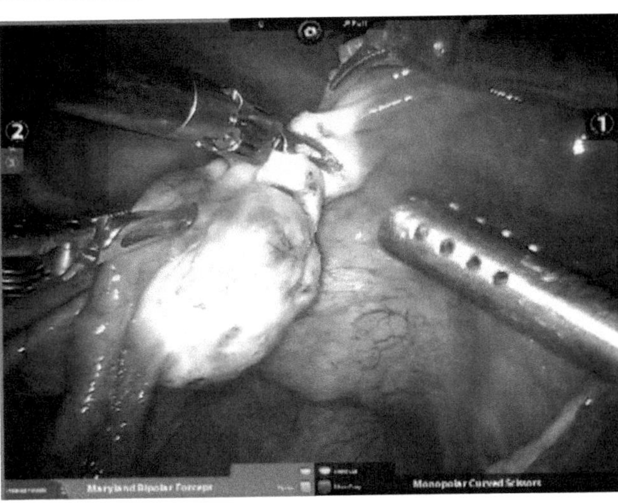

Fig. 62.4 Coagulation of the utero-ovarian ligaments

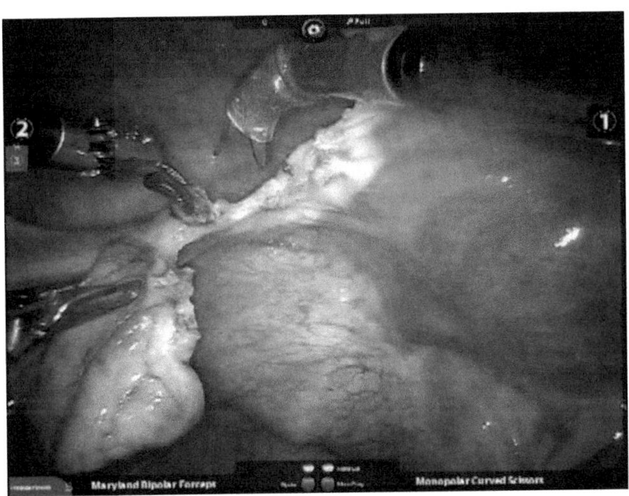

Fig. 62.5 Division of the round ligament

Surgical Steps for Robotic Assisted Supracervical Hysterectomy

The surgical steps are similar to laparoscopic and open supracervical hysterectomy. The pelvis and the abdomen are surveyed, and any adhesions which may hinder the hysterectomy steps are taken down with sharp or blunt dissection. The course of the ureters from the pelvic brim downward is identified. When a concomitant sacro-colpopexy is planned, the sacral promontorium is identified. In cases of a large fibroid uterus, the uterus is moved with the manipulator and the robotic/laparoscopic instruments in order to evaluate the access of the vascular pedicles and the visibility of the colpotomy ring.

1. *Separation of the adnexa from the uterus*: The hysterectomy itself may begin with coagulation and division of the utero-ovarian ligaments and the fallopian tubes, even in those cases when removal of the adnexa is planned (Fig. 62.4). This step allows a good visualization of the posterior leaf of the broad ligament and the posterior side of the uterus. The adnexa may be removed later on separately when indicated.
2. *Division of the round ligament and anterior leaf of the broad ligament*: The round ligaments are coagulated and divided, and the incision is carried anteriorly to the vesico-uterine pouch (Fig. 62.5). The upper margin of the colpotomy ring may serve as a guide to the location of this incision, with the manipulator pushed cephalad.
3. *Dissection of the vesico-uterine pouch (i.e., the bladder flap)*: The vesico-uterine pouch is developed by using blunt and sharp dissection of the areolar tissue separating the urinary bladder from the cervix and the upper part of the vagina (Fig. 62.6). In most cases, this is easily accomplished with a downward pressure using the blunt side of the monopolar shears while the bladder is held with a grasping instrument to provide counter-traction, combined with the cephalad traction by the manipulator. In women with prior cesarean section or endometriosis, this step of the surgery is often more complicated because of dense adhesions. In those cases, the surgical plane may be identified laterally rather than medially. In addition, retrograde filling of the bladder with 200–300 cc may help identify its margins. Of note, the

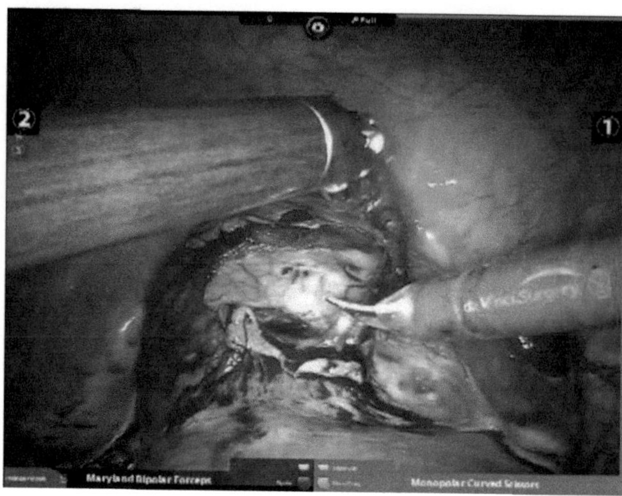

Fig. 62.6 Development of the bladder flap. The bladder flap is developed by holding the bladder upwards with a grasping instrument and applying sharp and blunt traction with the blunt end of the monopolar shears on the vesico-uterine fold

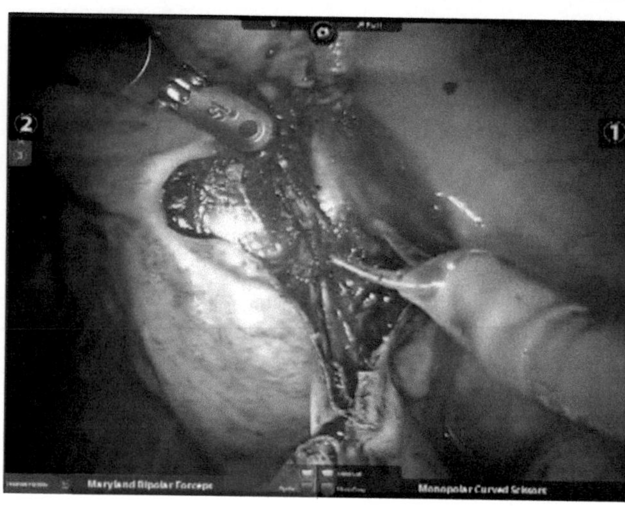

Fig. 62.7 Coagulation of the uterine arteries. After skeletonization of the uterine arteries, the vessel is grasped and coagulated with a bipolar instrument (in this figure, with robotic bipolar forceps)

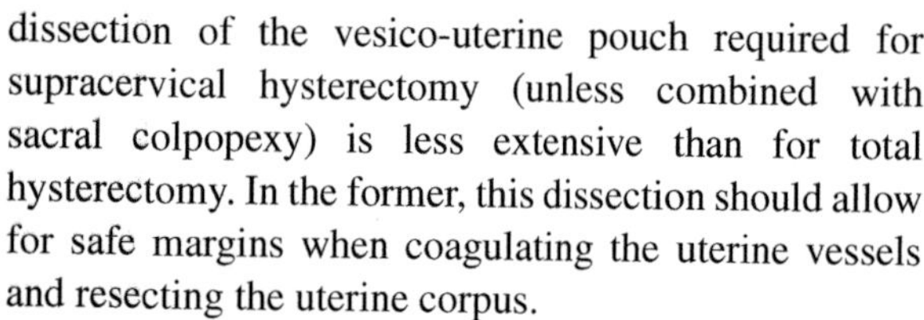

dissection of the vesico-uterine pouch required for supracervical hysterectomy (unless combined with sacral colpopexy) is less extensive than for total hysterectomy. In the former, this dissection should allow for safe margins when coagulating the uterine vessels and resecting the uterine corpus.

4. *Division of the posterior leaf of the broad ligament*: The incision of the round ligament is then carried posteriorly to the level of the colpotomy ring, just above the insertion of the sacro-uterine ligaments to the uterus. During this step, the serosa is separated from the underlying uterine vessels. This step may be performed using the bipolar Maryland forceps or PK forceps as a dissecting instrument.
5. *Skeletonization of the uterine vessels*: The areolar tissue surrounding the uterine vessels is taken down with sharp and blunt dissection in order to create a distinct vascular pedicle. This will allow to coagulate those vessels with less electro-surgery, resulting with decreased thermal spread (Fig. 62.7).
6. *Division of the uterine vessels*: During this step, the cephalad traction of manipulator increases the distance from the ureters. The uterine vessels are coagulated with bipolar or PK forceps, while ensuring that the coagulating instrument is placed at a 90° angle to the vessel. Before the vessels are divided, it is important to ensure that the distal portion of the pedicle is well coagulated. In addition, the proximal portion of the pedicle is also coagulated in order to decrease the "backflow" bleeding from the uterus.
7. *Division of the cardinal ligaments*: This step is minimal for supracervical hysterectomy. The cardinal ligaments are coagulated by placing the bipolar instrument at a 90 degree angle to the colpotomy ring. It is important to avoid excessive electro-surgery during this step due to the risk of thermal spread and thermal injury to the ureters. As before, cephalad traction on the manipulator will decrease this risk.
8. *Amputation of the uterine corpus*: The uterus is separated from the cervix by cutting it at its isthmus, above the insertion of the utero-ovarian ligaments to the uterus, using the monopolar shears (Fig. 62.8). The usual direction of the incision is from one side to the other. Due to extensive use of electro-surgery during this step, the

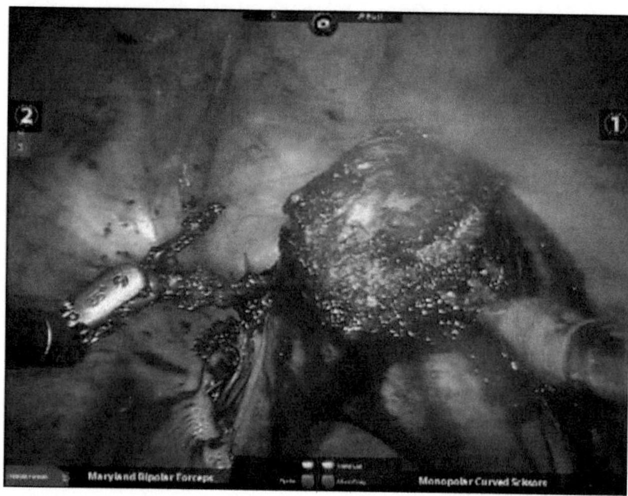

Fig. 62.8 Amputation of the uterine corpus. Once the uterine vessels are secured, the corpus is amputated at its isthmus with monopolar shears. The movement of the uterine manipulator as well as the use of grasping robotic and laparoscopic instruments for upwards traction of the uterus is helpful in maintaining the uterus in a safe distance from the bowel and the bladder, minimizing the risk of thermal injury through the extensive use of electro-surgery during this step of the surgery

adjacent organs (i.e., bowel, bladder, etc.) must be clearly visualized at all times. Movement of the manipulator in the appropriate direction may facilitate this step, which may be difficult when removing a large and bulky uterus. Monopolar loops are usually unnecessary for robotic supracervical hysterectomy. If the uterine manipulator is left in place during this step, its stem is encountered along the process, marking the midline of the isthmic incision. Most manipulators stems are manufactured from plastic or other non-conductive materials so that thermal injury through the monopolar shears is minimized. However, judicious use of monopolar energy and complete visualization of pelvic structure during this step is essential since inadvertent thermal injury to adjacent pelvic structure (i.e., bowel, bladder) may occur.

9. *Coagulation of the internal cervical os*: once the uterus is removed, the cervical canal may be coagulated with the bipolar forceps. This step may decrease the long term sequel of cyclic cervical bleeding originating from residual endometrial tissue within the cervical canal. Another option is to perform a "reverse cervical conization", where a cone-shaped cervical tissue is removed with monopolar shears. This technique may also decrease the rates of cyclic bleeding. The uterine manipulator may be removed vaginally once the uterine corpus has been amputated, and replaced by vaginal retractors such as a malleable retractor or rectal sizers (Fig. 62.2). Alternatively, some manipulators (such as the VCare) allow to retract the uterine stem, leaving in place the cervical ring which allows for some cervical manipulation vaginally.
10. *Adnexectomy or salpingectomy*: As explained above, prophylactic removal of the adnexa or the fallopian tubes should be discussed with the patient before surgery. Prior to coagulation of the ovarian vessels, the course of the ureters is again visualized. The ovarian vessels are coagulated with bipolar forceps, taking care to ensure adequate coagulated margins before the vessel are divided. The adnexa or the fallopian tubes may be removed through a 12 mm assistant laparoscopic port or with the use of a bag.
11. *Hemostasis*: the surgical pedicles are irrigated in a stepwise fashion and any bleeding is identified and coagulated. Further hemostasis control may be performed with a "low pressure check", whereby the intra-abdominal pressure is lowered to 4–5 mmHg.
12. *Specimen removal*: National guidelines should guide whether or not power morcellation is performed for specimen removal. Other options for specimen removal include cold knife morcellation through the largest abdominal port. For this technique, the uterus is placed in a specimen retrieval bag and brought with a grasper to the abdominal wall. For normal size uteri, a 12 mm incision may be sufficient. However, larger uteri containing fibroid may necessitate an enlargement of the abdominal incision to 2–3 cm.
13. *Routine cystoscopy*: Although routine cystoscopy has not been found to be cost-effective in all hysterectomy cases [22, 23], it may be performed with low surgical risks associated with the procedure and relatively quickly. Due to the higher rates of urethral injury in prolapse or incontinence surgery, routine cystoscopy may be justified in those cases.
14. *Port closure*: Fascial closure is often performed for laparoscopic ports larger than 10–12 mm. This may be performed with a laparoscopic needle. Smaller ports do not require fascial closure, and the skin may be closed with a continuous intradermal suture or with interrupted mattress sutures.

Surgical Steps for Concomitant Sacral Colpopexy

This procedure includes dissection of the anterior and posterior vaginal walls, followed by exposure of the longitudinal ligaments at the sacral promontory area, and placement of Y shaped mesh. Finally, the mesh may be covered by a peritoneal layer. The procedure begins with assessment of the pelvic anatomy, ease of visualizing the anterior and posterior vaginal walls, and the sacral promontory area.

1. Dissection of the anterior vaginal wall: similar to the technique described above for dissection of the bladder flap for hysterectomy, the bladder is taken down further using traction on the bladder with a grasping instrument (i.e., the robotic prograsp, or a laparoscopic grasper held by the bedside assistant) and combined sharp and blunt dissection with the monopolar shears (Fig. 62.9). In the correct surgical dissection plane, minimal bleeding is encountered. This dissection is aided by use of a wide curved vaginal obturator such as the end-to-end rectal anastomosis sizer (Fig. 62.2). The extent of the dissection is guided by the degree of prolapse of the anterior vaginal wall on pre-operative exam.
2. Dissection of the rectovaginal space: after the vaginal manipulator is placed in the posterior fornix, the loose peritoneal covering of the pouch of Douglas, in between the sacro-uterine ligaments, is grasped and a shallow incision is made in order to enter the rectovaginal space. This space usually contains loose areolar tissue which may be easily separated downward to the level of the rectum medially and the levator ani muscles laterally, while exposing the rectovaginal septum (also called Denonvilliers' fascia) (Fig. 62.10). As before, in the cor-

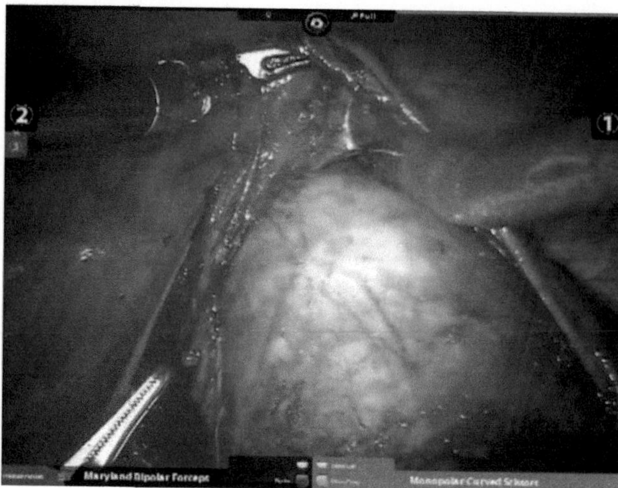

Fig. 62.9 Further exposure of the arterial vaginal wall. In this figure, the end-to-end anastomosis sizer is placed in the anterior fornix of the vagina, providing excellent demarcation of surgical plane between the vagina and the bladder

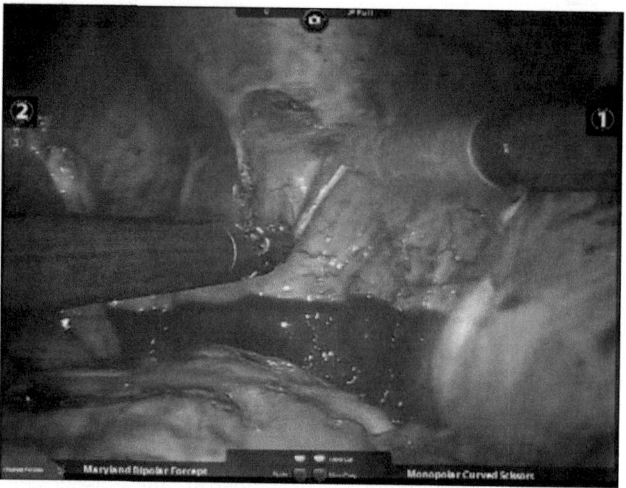

Fig. 62.10 Dissection of the rectovaginal space and exposure of the rectovaginal septum

rect surgical plane the bleeding is minimal during most of the dissection. However, in cases of extensive dissection (which may be required for advanced prolapse) some blood vessels are often encountered close to the rectum. We have found that use of the 30° optics pointed upwards aids in the visualization of the rectovaginal space. Likewise, a rectal probe may aid in recognizing the borders of the rectum. As for the dissection of the anterior vaginal wall, the extent of dissection of the rectovaginal space is guided by the degree of prolapse.

3. Dissection of the presacral area: this area is best visualized with a 30° optics pointed downwards, and after the sigmoid colon is retracted to the left with a grasping instrument (usually the prograsp) placed in the left robotic arm. In cases of a relatively mobile sigmoid colon the retraction of the sigmoid colon with grasping instruments may be insufficient for optimal visualization. In those cases, the sigmoid colon may be fixed to the left middle anterior abdominal wall by passing a suture on a straight long needle through the abdominal wall, to the sigmoid epiploica in 2–3 spots and back through the abdominal wall, close to the entry point. The suture is then tied and left in place for the duration of the surgery. Next, the bifurcation of the aorta, the course of the right common iliac artery and the course of the right ureter crossing over the pelvic brim are noted. The peritoneum above the dissection area in the sacral promontory is grasped and incised. The loose areolar tissue bellow is gently separated until the white anterior longitudinal ligament is seen. A dissection area of several centimeters is sufficient (Fig. 62.11). The major intraoperative complication during this step of the procedure is bleeding, which may originate from the middle sacral artery and vein or from smaller vessels. Thus, meticulous coagulation with bipolar forceps or the PK forceps combined with careful dissection is key. In addition, vascular clips or hemostatic agents should be available in the operating room in case they are required for hemostasis.
4. Dissection of the lateral peritoneum: the peritoneal incision on the presacral area is continued towards the Douglas pouch, medial to the right ureter and lateral to the rectum. This incision will be used to cover the mesh at the conclusion of the procedure. Alternatively, blunt dissection of this space while undermining the peritoneum with monopolar shears but without the peritoneal incision would allow to pass the mesh from the pelvic to the presacral area below the lateral peritoneum. This technique

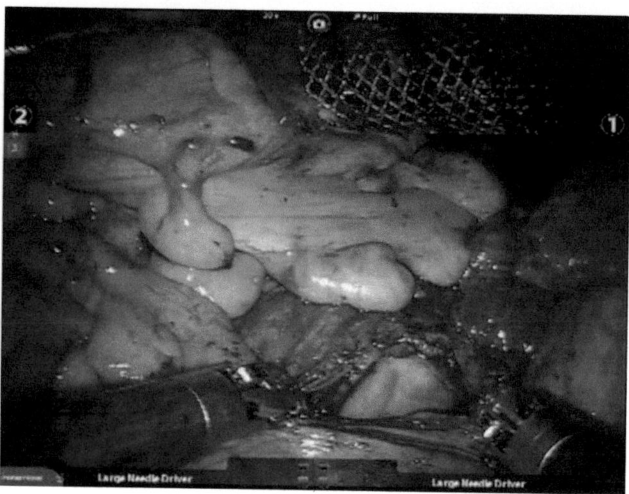

Fig. 62.11 Exposure of the anterior longitudinal ligament at the presacral area

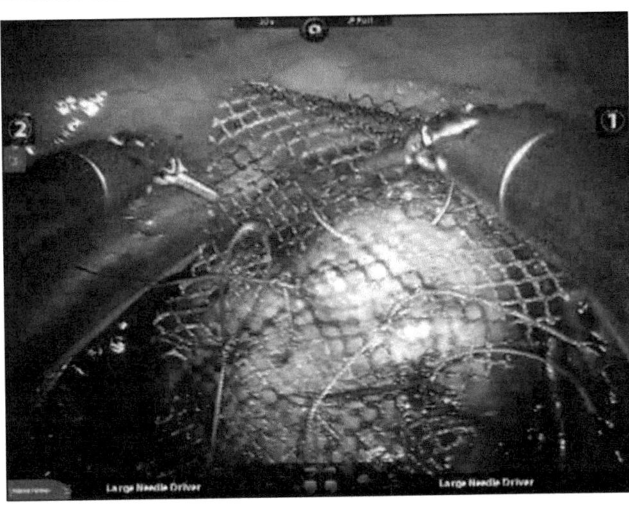

Fig. 62.12 Interrupted sutures anchoring the mesh to the cervical stump using a 2-0 non-absorbable suture and intracorporeal knots

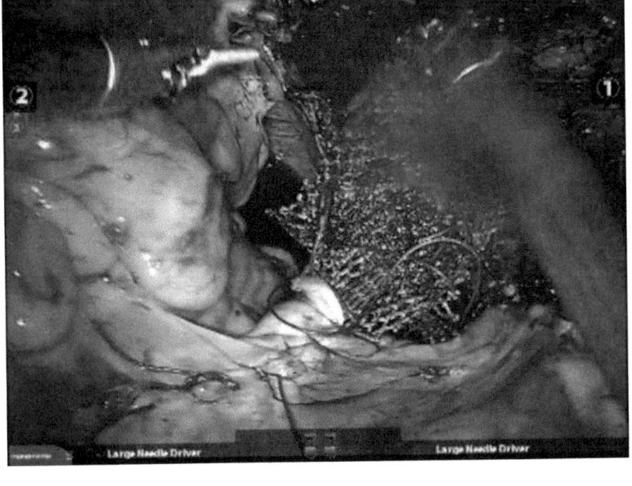

Fig. 62.13 The peritoneum is closed over the mesh using a running 2-0 or 1-0 absorbable suture

may shorten surgical time because peritoneal closure over the mesh with a continuous suture is unnecessary.

5. Tailoring of the mesh: the macroporous, polypropylene mesh, required for sacral colpopexy has a Y shape and include two rectangular pelvic arms (for the anterior and posterior vaginal walls) and one rectangular sacral arm. This mesh may be fashioned individually from a large 15*15 cm mesh square or purchased as a "ready to use" Y mesh. The commercially available Y meshes may also need some tailoring prior to their introduction into the abdominal cavity because their arms are too long for most patients.
6. Suturing of the Y mesh: the robotic monopolar shears and bipolar forceps are switched to needle drivers. The triangle of the Y mesh is placed on the cervical stump and 1–2 sutures are used to anchor it in place (Fig. 62.12). Subsequently, the mesh is anchored to the anterior vaginal wall, followed by the posterior vaginal wall, by a series of interrupted sutures using a small diameter suture (such as 2-0) and intracorporeal knotting. Use of the vaginal obturator to move the cervical stump according to the suturing area is very helpful. The choice of suture material is debatable: a non-absorbable polyester braided suture such as Ethibond (Ethicon, Somerville, New Jersey, USA) or a comparable absorbable suture (such a polyglactin suture). The former is easy to handle and knot, but should it protrude to the vaginal side of the vaginal wall, postoperative removal may be required. For the sake of efficiency, a relatively long suture (~35–40 cm) may be introduced into the abdominal cavity and used for several interrupted sutures.
7. Anchoring the mesh to the anterior longitudinal ligament: The sacral arm of the mesh is pulled cephalad, carrying the cervical stump upwards and correcting the prolapse. The position of the cervical stump is adjusted to ensure it is "tension free". At the chosen location, the sacral mesh arm is anchored to the anterior longitudinal ligament at the S1 region with a tacking instrument or with a couple of non-absorbable sutures. The tacking instrument is easy and quick to use, however, concerns have been raised regarding its possible role in the development of lumbosacral osteomyelitis and spondylodiscitis, a rare but severe complication of sacral colpopexy. Those concerns stem from the presumed deeper penetration of the bone tack compared to sutures. Nevertheless, since lumbosacral osteomyelitis has been reported with use of both tacking instruments and sutures, it is unclear whether one technique is safer than the other, and many surgeon continue to use tacking instruments until further evidence is available [24, 25]. If use of the tacking instrument is preferred, the best approach to operate it in terms of proximity to the presacral area and angle is offered by the right robotic port. This would require temporary undocking of the right robotic arm.
8. Peritoneal closure: any excess mesh is excised, and after hemostasis of the presacral area and the pelvic has been checked, the peritoneum is reapproximated over the entire length of the mesh with a running 2-0 absorbable suture (Fig. 62.13).

Surgical Outcomes and Complications of Robotic Sacral Colpopexy

Abdominal sacro colpopexy, whether by open, laparoscopic or robotic approach is considered superior in treatment of apical prolapse compared to the vaginal approach in terms of prolapse recurrence, residual prolapse [2]. However, the robotic approach is not necessarily superior to the conventional laparoscopic sacral colpopexy. In a randomized controlled trial by Paraiso et al. [26], 78 patients were randomized to the laparoscopic or robotic sacral colpopexy. There were no differences in vaginal support and functional outcomes at 1 year follow up, but the robotic surgery was significantly longer and more expensive than the laparoscopic one. Nevertheless, since laparoscopic sacral colpopexy is a technically demanding procedure requiring advanced suturing skills and a long learning curve, the robotic platform may allow additional surgeons to perform it.

A recent systematic review on the outcomes and complications of robotic sacral colpopexy included 1488 cases from 27 studies, published from 2006 to 2013 [27]. Intraoperative complication occurred in 3 % (including mostly vaginotomies, urinary tract injuries, and bowel injuries). Postoperative complications occurred in 11 % of cases overall, but only 2 % were graded as severe (such as bowel obstructions, port site hernia, port site nerve entrapment, and peritonitis due to bowel injury). Mesh erosion at the vaginal area was reported in 2 % of patients, and appeared to be related to the execution of total hysterectomy as opposed to supracervical hysterectomy, and to the use of a standard weight polypropylene mesh as opposed to a lightweight polypropylene mesh (the latter being a protective factor).

Finally, spondylodiscitis of the L5-S1 disc or vertebral osteomyelitis is rare complication of the procedure, with less than 30 cases reported in the literature for all sacral colpopexy surgical approaches [24]. This severe complication (which may or may not involve mesh erosion at the presacral area) is often preceded by a urinary tract or vaginal cuff infection. Patients present with back pain several weeks after the procedure and often require additional surgeries for drainage, debridement and mesh removal in addition to broad spectrum intravenous antibiotic treatment.

References

1. Lieng M, Qvigstad E, Istre O, Langebrekke A, Ballard K. Long-term outcomes following laparoscopic supracervical hysterectomy. BJOG. 2008;115:1605–10.
2. Maher C, Feiner B, Baessler K, Schmid C. Surgical management of pelvic organ prolapse in women. Cochrane Database Syst Rev. 2013;4:CD004014.
3. Osmundsen BC, Clark A, Goldsmith C, Adams K, Denman MA, Edwards R, Gregory WT. Mesh erosion in robotic sacrocolpopexy. Female Pelvic Med Reconstr Surg. 2012;18:86–8.
4. Thakar R, Ayers S, Clarkson P, Stanton S, Manyonda I. Outcomes after total versus subtotal abdominal hysterectomy. N Engl J Med. 2002;347:1318–25.
5. Andersen LL, Ottesen B, Alling Møller LM, Gluud C, Tabor A, Zobbe V, Hoffmann E, Gimbel HM, Danish Hysterectomy Trial Group. Subtotal versus total abdominal hysterectomy: randomized clinical trial with 14-year questionnaire follow-up. Am J Obstet Gynecol. 2015;212(6):758.e1–54.
6. Uccella S, Ghezzi F, Mariani A, Cromi A, Bogani G, Serati M, Bolis P. Vaginal cuff closure after minimally invasive hysterectomy: our experience and systematic review of the literature. Am J Obstet Gynecol. 2011;205:119.
7. Wallwiener M, Taran FA, Rothmund R, Kasperkowiak A, Auwärter G, Ganz A, Kraemer B, Abele H, Schönfisch B, Isaacson KB, Brucker SY. Laparoscopic supracervical hysterectomy (LSH) versus total laparoscopic hysterectomy (TLH): an implementation study in 1,952 patients with an analysis of risk factors for conversion to laparotomy and complications, and of procedure specific re-operations. Arch Gynecol Obstet. 2013;288:1329–39.
8. Gimbel H, Zobbe V, Andersen BM, Filtenborg T, Gluud C, Tabor A. Randomised controlled trial of total compared with subtotal hysterectomy with one-year follow up results. BJOG. 2003;110: 1088–98.
9. Donnez J, Nisolle M. Laparoscopic supracervical (subtotal) hysterectomy (LASH). J Gynecol Surg. 1993;9:91–4.
10. Liu FW, Galvan-Turner VB, Pfaendler KS, Longoria TC, Bristow RE. A critical assessment of morcellation and its impact on gynecologic surgery and the limitations of the existing literature. Am J Obstet Gynecol. 2015;212(6):717–24.
11. Food and Drug Administration. Quantitative assessment of the prevalence of unsuspected uterine sarcoma in women undergoing treatment of uterine fibroids. Available at: http://www.fda.gov/downloads/MedicalDevices/Safety/AlertsandNotices/UCM393589.pdf.
12. Lieng M, Berner E, Busund B. Risk of morcellation of uterine leiomyosacomas in laparoscopic supracervical hysterectomy and laparoscopic myomectomy, a retrospective trial including 4791 women. J Minim Invasive Gynecol. 2015;22:410–4.
13. Ton R, Kilic GS, Phelps JY. A medical-legal review of power morcellation in the face of the recent FDA warning and litigation. J Minim Invasive Gynecol. 2015;22(4):564–72.
14. Cohen SL, Greenberg JA, Wang KC, et al. Risk of leakage and tissue dissemination with various contained tissue extraction (CTE) techniques:an in vitro pilot study. J Minim Invasive Gynecol. 2014;21:935–9.
15. Morelli M, Venturella R, Mocciaro R, Di Cello A, Rania E, Lico D, D'Alessandro P, Zullo F. Prophylactic salpingectomy in premenopausal low-risk women for ovarian cancer: primum non nocere. Gynecol Oncol. 2013;129:448–51.
16. Vorwergk J, Radosa MP, Nicolaus K, Baus N, Jimenez Cruz J, Rengsberger M, Gajda M, Diebolder H, Runnebaum IB. Prophylactic bilateral salpingectomy (PBS) to reduce ovarian cancer risk incorporated in standard premenopausal hysterectomy: complications and re-operation rate. J Cancer Res Clin Oncol. 2014;140:859–65.
17. Parker WH, Broder MS, Chang E, Feskanich D, Farquhar C, Liu Z, Shoupe D, Berek JS, Hankinson S, Manson JE. Ovarian conservation at the time of hysterectomy and long-term health outcomes in the nurses' health study. Obstet Gynecol. 2009;113: 1027–37.
18. Rocca WA, Grossardt BR, de Andrade M, Malkasian GD, Melton 3rd LJ. Survival patterns after oophorectomy in premenopausal women: a population-based cohort study. Lancet Oncol. 2006;7:821–8.
19. Shuster LT, Gostout BS, Grossardt BR, Rocca WA. Prophylactic oophorectomy in premenopausal women and long-term health. Menopause Int. 2008;14:111–6.
20. Elective and risk-reducing salpingo-oophorectomy. ACOG Practice Bulletin No. 89. American College of Obstetricians and Gynecologists. Obstet Gynecol. 2008;111:231–41.
21. Berek JS, Chalas E, Edelson M, Moore DH, Burke WM, Cliby WA, Berchuck A, Society of Gynecologic Oncologists Clinical Practice Committee. Prophylactic and risk-reducing bilateral salpingo-oophorectomy: recommendations based on risk of ovarian cancer. Obstet Gynecol. 2010;116:733–43.

22. Visco AG, Taber KH, Weidner AC, Barber MD, Myers ER. Cost-effectiveness of universal cystoscopy to identify ureteral injury at hysterectomy. Obstet Gynecol. 2001;97:685–92.
23. Vakili B, Chesson RR, Kyle BL, Shobeiri SA, Echols KT, Gist R, Zheng YT, Nolan TE. The incidence of urinary tract injury during hysterectomy: a prospective analysis based on universal cystoscopy. Am J Obstet Gynecol. 2005;192:1599–604.
24. Propst K, Tunitsky-Bitton E, Schimpf MO, Ridgeway B. Pyogenic spondylodiscitis associated with sacral colpopexy and rectopexy: report of two cases and evaluation of the literature. Int Urogynecol J. 2014;25:21–31.
25. Nosseir SB, Kim YH, Lind LR, Winkler HA. Sacral osteomyelitis after robotically assisted laparoscopic sacral colpopexy. Obstet Gynecol. 2010;116:513–5.
26. Paraiso MF, Jelovsek JE, Frick A, Chen CC, Barber MD. Laparoscopic compared with robotic sacral colpopexy for vaginal prolapse. Obstet Gynecol. 2011;118:1005–13.
27. Serati M, Bogani G, Sorice P, Braga A, Torella M, Salvatore S, Uccella S, Cromi A, Ghezzi F. Robot-assisted sacrocolpopexy for pelvic organ prolapse: a systematic review and meta-analysis of comparative studies. Eur Urol. 2014;66:303–18.

Cervical Stump Extirpation with Regard to Robotic-Assisted Laparoscopic Hysterectomy

63

Hung-Cheng Lai and Yu-Chi Wang

Introduction

Over the past decades, minimally invasive surgery MIS) has become a trend in the field of surgery. The laparoscopic surgery boomed in the late 1980s and continued to gain popularity into the 1990s and this MIS have been successfully applied to the gynecological benign and malignant tumors. For many years, MIS appeared to represent an alternative approach in the gynecological surgery compared to the traditional exploratory laparotomy. Another novel MIS technology called "robotic surgery" which composed of patient-side cart, computer stand-interface and surgeon console is introduced in the 2000s and provide advantages for the surgeons. It is particular useful in obese patients, long-time surgeries and the operation required extensive suturing. This newly technology is similar to or better than previous laparoscopic surgery in shortened hospital stay, less blood loss, less surgical pain, a faster recovery and less scarring.

Since the approval by the US Food and Drug Administration (FDA) in 2005, robotic surgeries have been widely used in gynecologic field including benign and malignant disorders [1]. The first case of hysterectomy by robotic surgery was reported in 2002 [2]. By 2011, 37 % of hysterectomies in United State were performed by laparoscopy and 27 % were by robot. (Intuitive surgical Inc., Sunnyvale, CA, USA).

Although minimally invasive surgery provide many advantages, the extirpation of uterine cervix remains a challenge since the vicinity of cervix contains structures such as bladder, ureter and rectum which may subject to injuries (Fig. 63.1). The key of success include the identification of uterine artery, ureter and the plans of uterine-vesicle fold and recto-vaginal space. Here, we described the details of these procedures in this chapter.

H.-C. Lai (✉)
Obstetrics and Gynecology, Shuang Ho Hospital, Taipei Medical University, No. 291, Zhongzheng Rd., Zhonghe Dist., New Taipei City 235, Taiwan
e-mail: hclai@s.tmu.edu.tw; hclai30656@gmail.com

Y.-C. Wang
Obstetrics and Gynecology, Tri-Service General Hospital, 5F, 325, Sec 2, Cheng-Gong Rd., Neihu District, Taipei 114, Taiwan
e-mail: yuchitsgh@gmail.com

I. Alkatout, L. Mettler (eds.), *Hysterectomy*, DOI 10.1007/978-3-319-22497-8_63

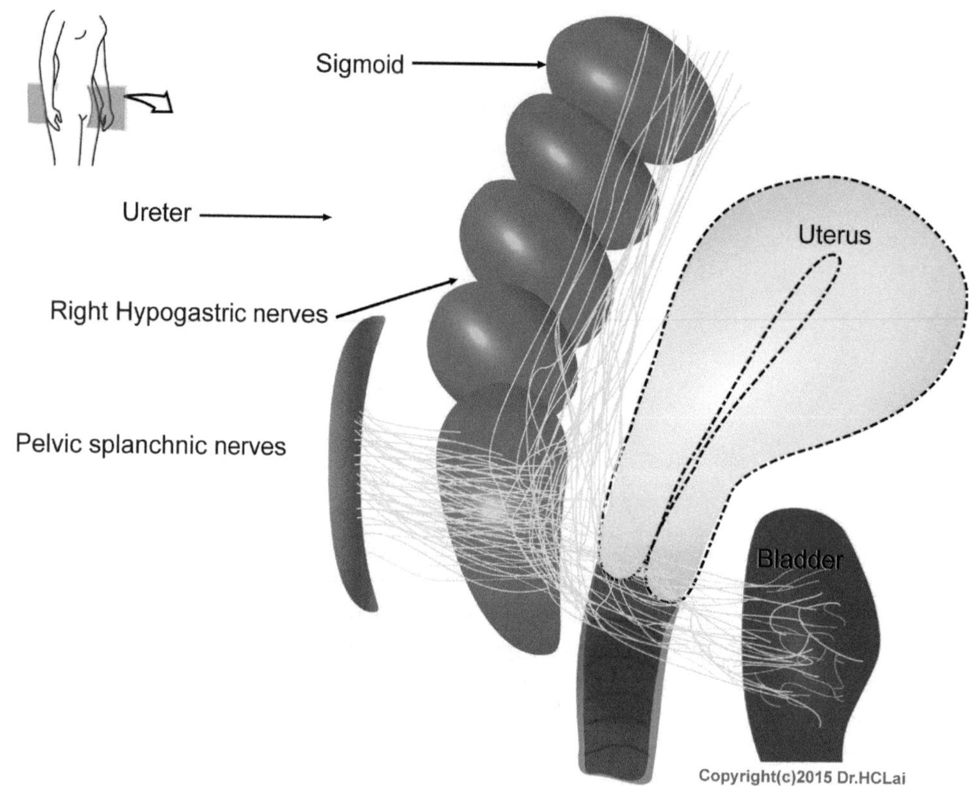

Fig. 63.1 The anatomy of the pelvic structures including bladder, uterus, cervix, bowel, ureter and pelvic nerve. The ureter comes across uterine cervix at about 2–3 cm lateral to the isthmus. Nerve innervation spread along and below ureter to the bladder

Hysterectomy

The uterus is elevated using manipulator (Fig. 63.2). Carefully checking the whole pelvis and avoid to trauma and tear the bowel, bladder and vessels. First, the round ligament and fallopian tubes are grasped and coagulated by a bipolar forceps and then cut using monopolar spatula or scissors at right side (Fig. 63.3). Then, the anterior leaf of broad ligament is subsequently separated down to the bladder peritoneum to the uterus. After opening the retroperitoneum, the ureter can be identified on the posterior leaf of the broad ligament The grasper can hold the peritoneum and the ureter can be dissected carefully using a blunt dissector or spatula. The uterine artery is then identified and clamped (Figs. 63.4 and 63.5). The ureter, then, can be bluntly pushed a little bit laterally to have more space when doing colpotomy. The bladder is pushed downward to expose the vaginal colpus. Then the anterior colpotomy can be made using the unipolar spetula or forceps, and, circumscribe the cervix (Fig. 63.6). The uterine manipulator can be pushed forward to get a little tension of tissues for better cutting. Then the cervix is clamped by a tenaculum forceps and retrieved it through vagina. If the specimen is large, the uterus can be removed piece by piece by vaginal or transumbilical morcellation. The sponge in a glove or a baby nose suction bulb is placed into the vagina to prevent the loss of pneumoperitoneum (Figs. 63.7 and 63.8). Finally, the edge of the vaginal cuff is sutured (Fig. 63.9).

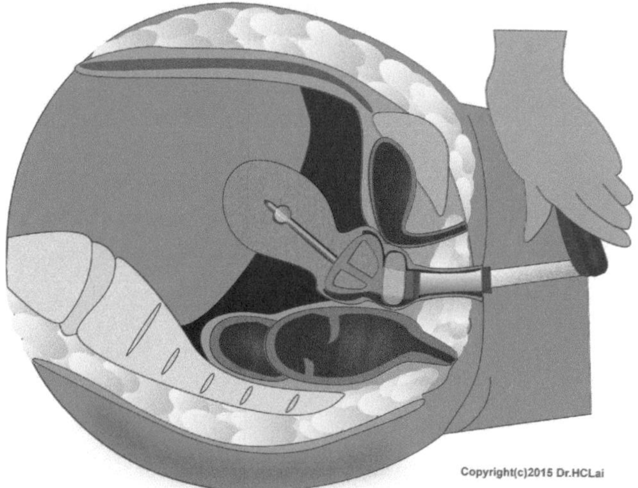

Fig. 63.2 The uterine manipulator is used to displace the uterus away from the bladder, ureter and rectum

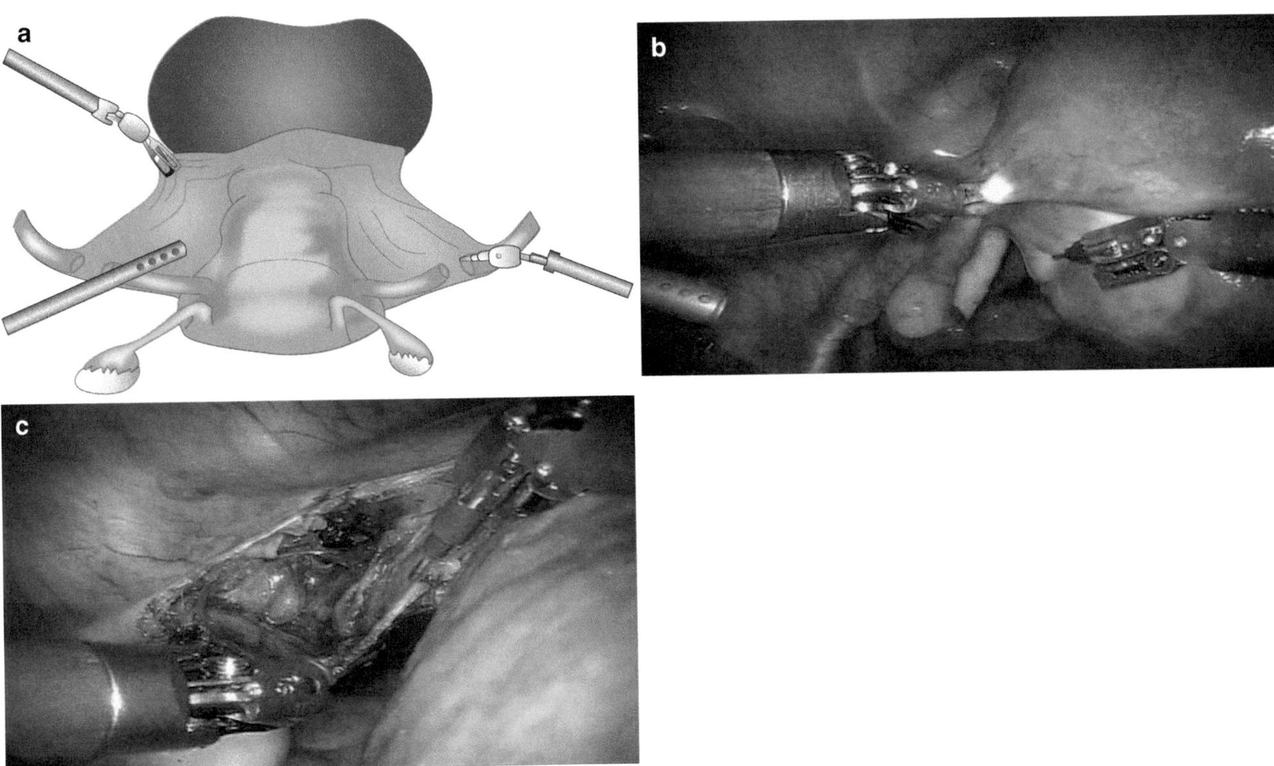

Fig. 63.3 (a) Illustration of round ligaments and the leaves of the broad ligament. (b) The round ligament and fallopian tubes are coagulated and then cut. (c) The anterior leaf of broad ligament is subsequently separated down to the bladder peritoneum to the uterus

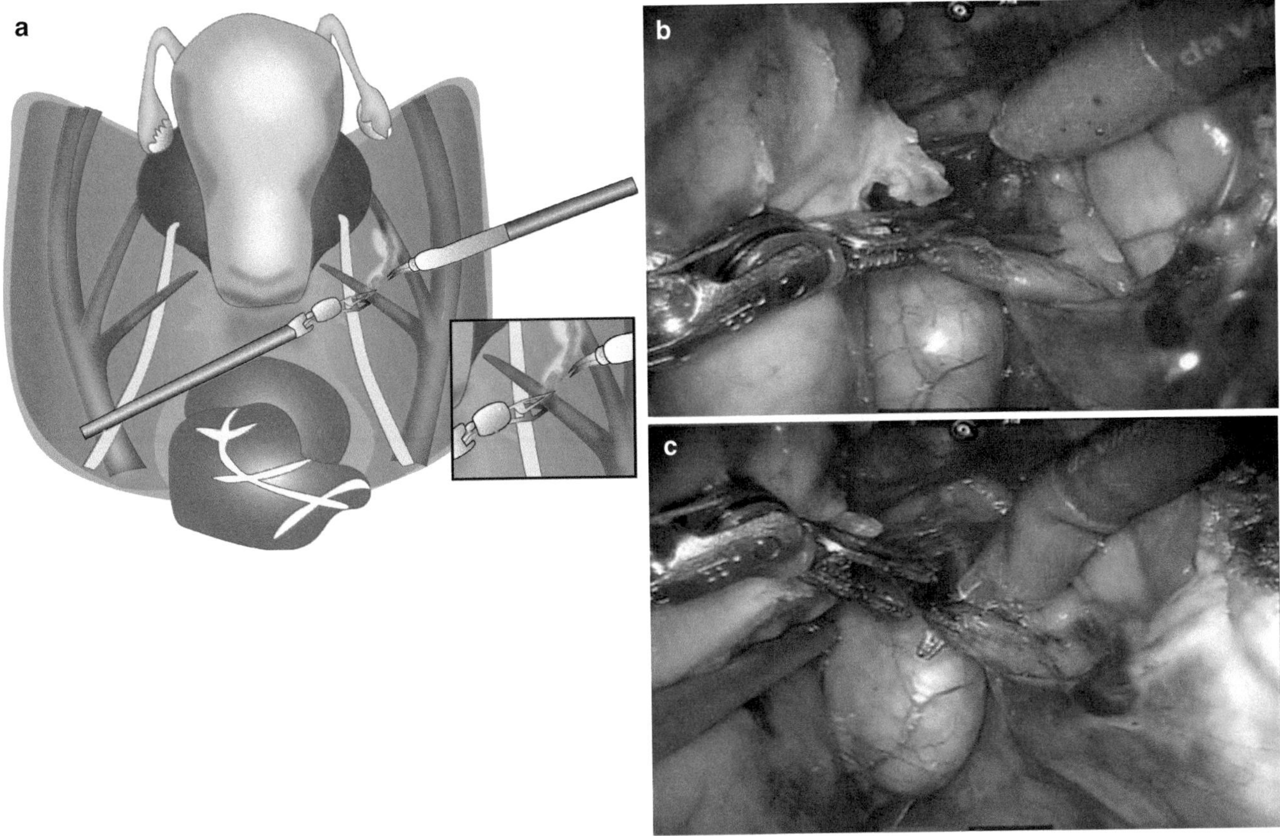

Fig. 63.4 (a) Illustration of uterine artery and ureter at the level of "bridge over trouble water". (b)The ureter can be identified at the level of pelvic brim and be bluntly dissected by scissor from its peritoneal attachment down to the parametrial level. (c) The uterine artery is then skeletonized as "the bridge over trouble water" and then coagulated using bipolar forceps

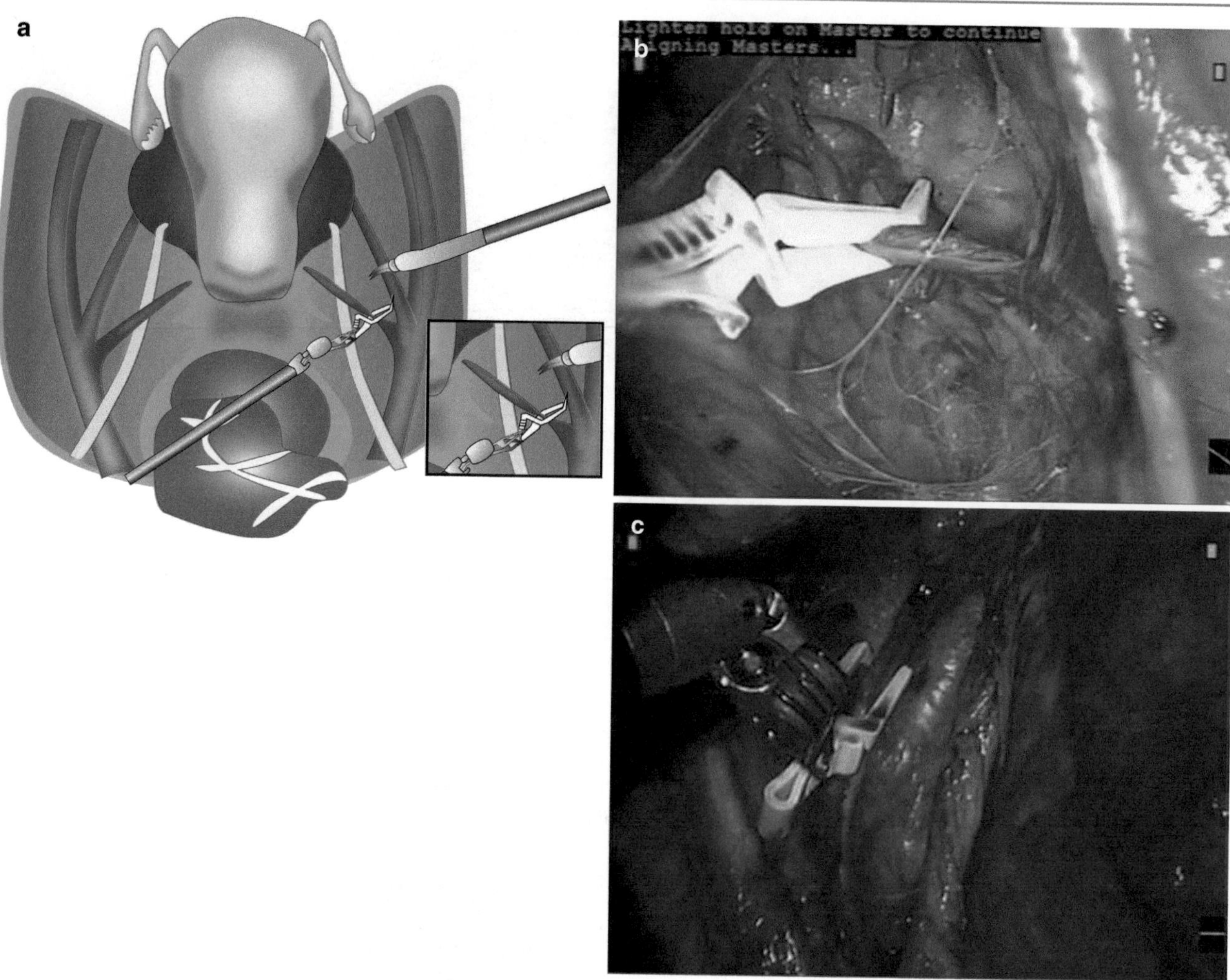

Fig. 63.5 (**a**) Illustration of clamping uterine artery at its origin from internal iliac artery. (**b**) The right ureter was bluntly dissected using a scissor dissector or spatula. The origin of uterine artery from internal iliac artery can be identified parallel to the ureter at this level. A bulldog clamp can be introduced using fenestrated forceps and temporarily clip the uterine artery until the uterine incision was sutured. The bulldog is removed after a complete homeostasis of the uterine body. (**c**) The clipped uterine artery and ureter, left

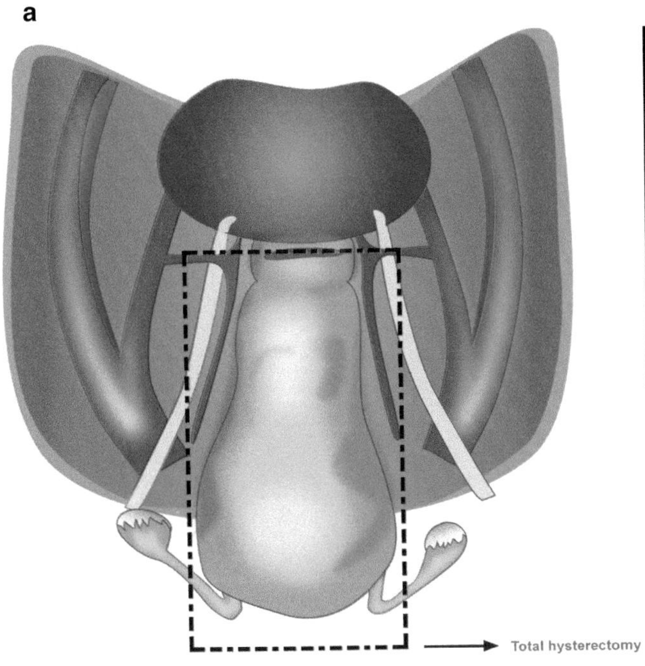

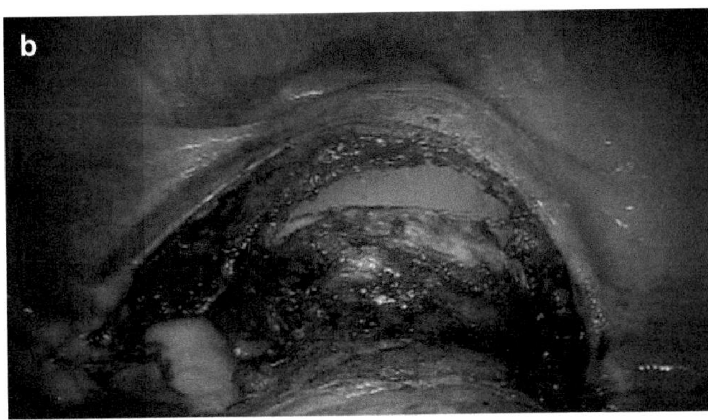

Fig. 63.6 (**a**) Illustration of the robotic view of total hysterectomy. (**b**) The placement of a baby nose sucker in vagina provides a good support for colpotomy. After the placement of a suction ball to the apex of the fornix, the bladder is released from the cervix by using scissors. Then the vagina is incised and opened by monopolar scissors

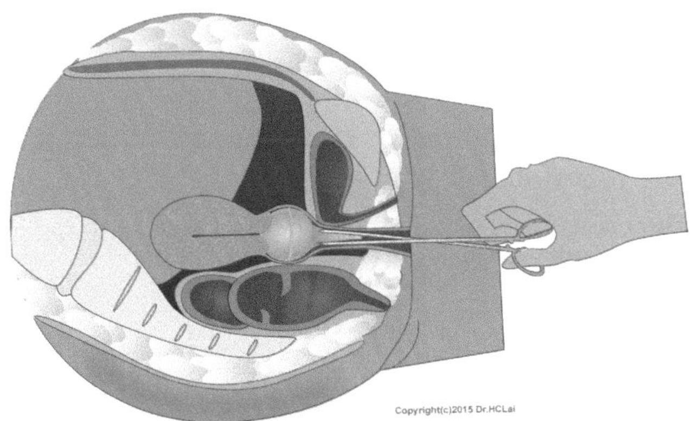

Fig. 63.7 The application of nose sucker as a pneumo-occluder

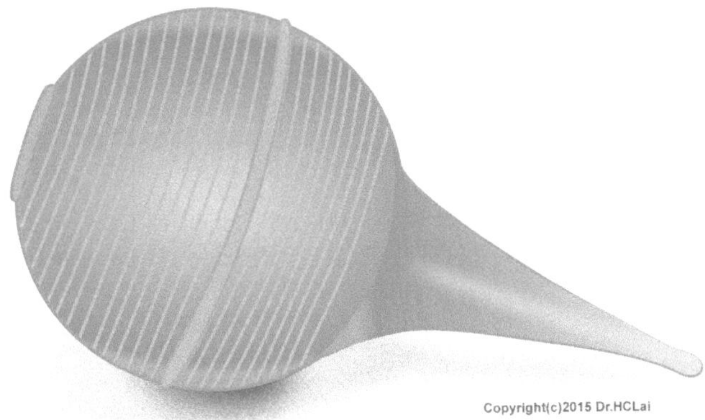

Fig. 63.8 The view of the suction bulb

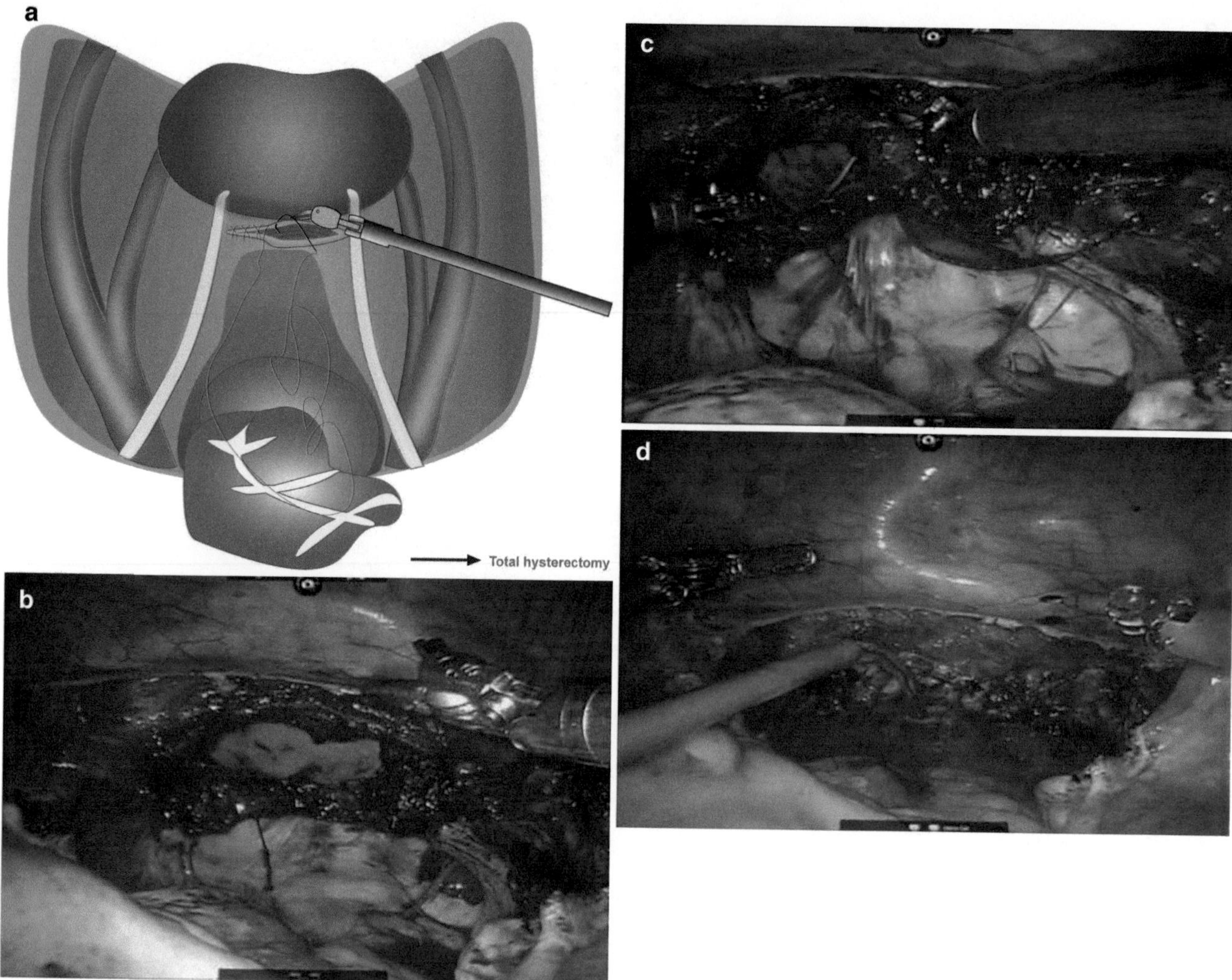

Fig. 63.9 (**a**) Illustration of the vaginal cuff closure. (**b**) The vaginal cuff after colpotomy and removal of uterus. (**c**) Closure of the first layer of vaginal cuff using V-lock suture. (**d**) Completion of double layered suture of vaginal cuff

Subtotal Hysterectomy

After the dissection of round ligament and ovarian ligament, the ureter can be identified at the posterior leaf of peritoneum. The peritoneum can be graped by bipolar grasper. Then, a gentle scratching using spatula or scissor on the medical aspect of peritoneum from the level around internal iliac artery may lead to the white peristalsing ureter covered by whirling vessels. Parallel to the ureter along the pelvic wall, the uterine artery can be identified by pulsation. The uterine artery can be skeletonized and dissected down to the cross above ureter (Figs. 63.4 and 63.5). Care should be taken to avoid tearing veins below. The uterine artery can be cauterized by bipolar forceps at any level of the course. For a large uterine mass, the origin of uterine artery can only be identified below the level around pelvic brim. Usually, using robot, the "bridge over trouble water" can be reached posteriorly. After uterine artery is cauterized, the ureter can be gently pushed laterally to release more space between cervix and ureter (Figs. 63.10 and 63.11). Then, the fundus is elevated by manipulator or tracted by tenaculum forceps or grasp. An incision is made anteriorly or posteriorly at the isthmus level above uterine artery. Ascending branches of uterine arteries and veins can be cauterized by bipolar forceps. After hemi-transection of the cervix, the manipulator can be removed.

The dragging of uterus due to deep Trendelenburg position exposes the cervical cannel. The cervix can be cut using unipolar spatula or scissor. The uterus can be removed by morcellator. Alternatively, a tenaculum forceps can be used to grasp the uterus to avoid wandering uterus in the abdominal cavity. Then, the robot can be detached. The uterus can be removed through a 2.5 cm umbilical incision with wound retractor.

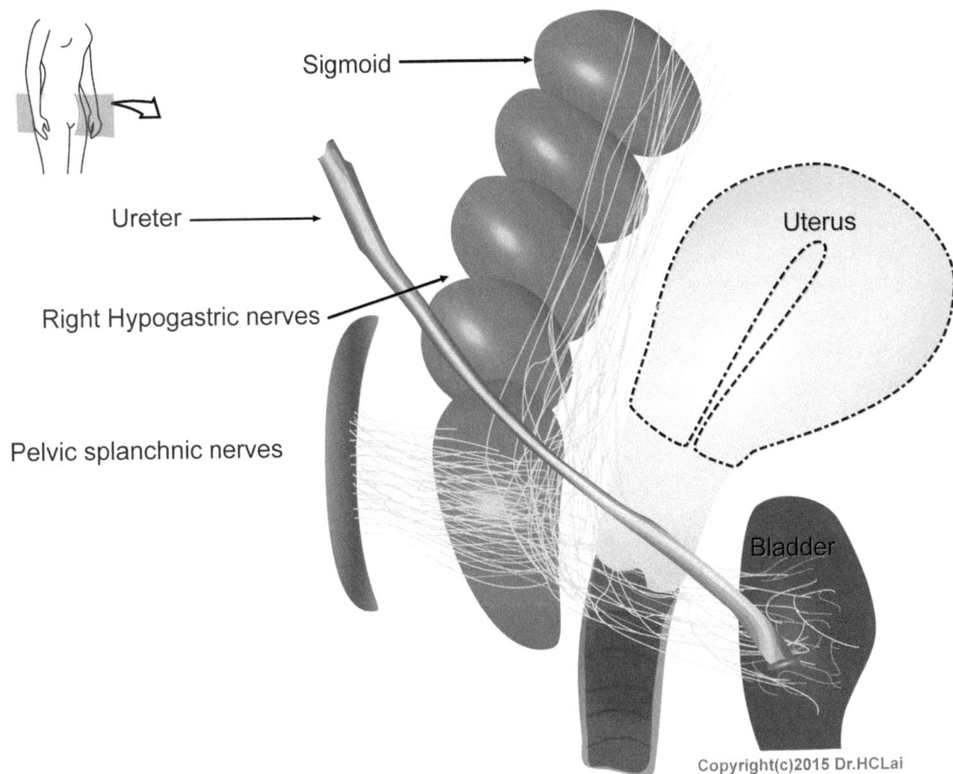

Fig. 63.10 Subtotal hysterectomy: After the uterine artery is clamped or ligated, the uterus is retracted by a grasper or a manipulator. The uterus and cervix is separated by the monopolar scissors at the isthmus where uterine artery enters uterus

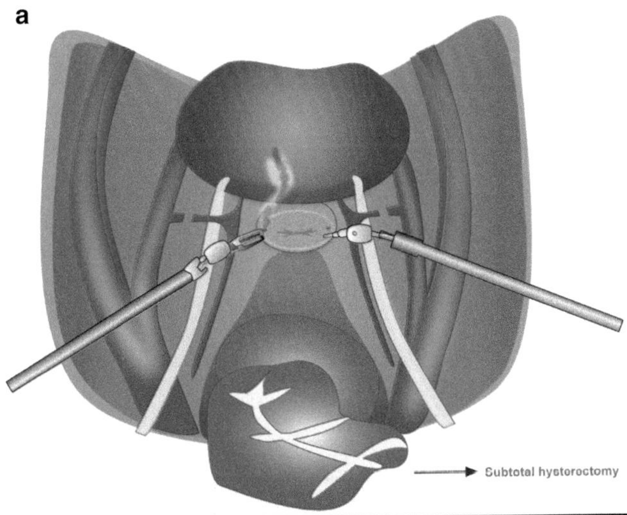

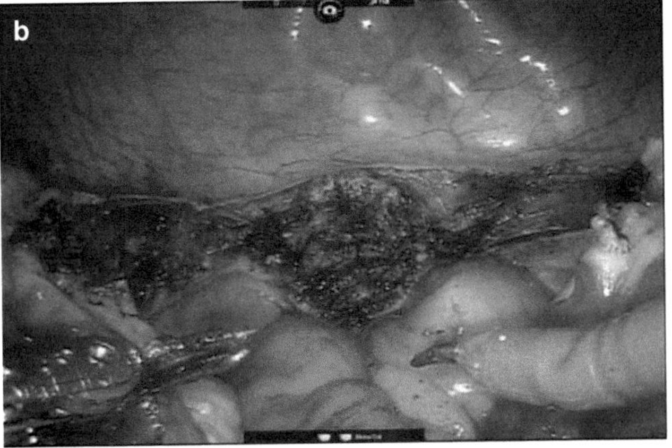

Fig. 63.11 (**a**) Illustration of cervical stump after supracervical hysterectomy. (**b**) Cervical stump after supracervical hysterectomy. Hemostasis is easier if the uterine arteries are ligated before the transection of uterine cervix

Radical Hysterectomy

The paravesical spaces are bounded by the external vessels laterally and the bladder medially (Fig. 63.12). The pararectal spaces are bounded by the rectum medially and the hypogastric artery laterally (Fig. 63.13). Then they are opened with gentle dissection using the monopolar spatula or scissors down to the pelvic wall. Furthermore, the uterine artery can be identified at the origin of hypogastric artery (Fig. 63.14). It is coagulated using bipolar forceps and cut. Then the uterine artery is elevated using grasper and the ureter can be identified below along the medial leaf of peritoneum. The ureter is pushed laterally along the tunnels and anterior leaf is exposed. The hypogastric nerve can be identified along the lateral aspect of rectal peritoneum (Fig. 63.15). The nerve fibers heading to the uterus is cut using monopolar scissor or spatula along the posterior leaf of tunnel. Then the recto-vaginal space is dissected and exposed at the middle, extended laterally to bilateral uterosacral ligament (Fig. 63.16). The uterosacral ligament are transected using the bipolar forceps ad scissors later. Finally, the bladder is pushed downward to expose the vaginal colpus. A circle colpotomy is made (Fig. 63.17). The uterus is dissected, extirpated through vagina (Fig. 63.18). The vaginal cuff is sutured (Fig. 63.19).

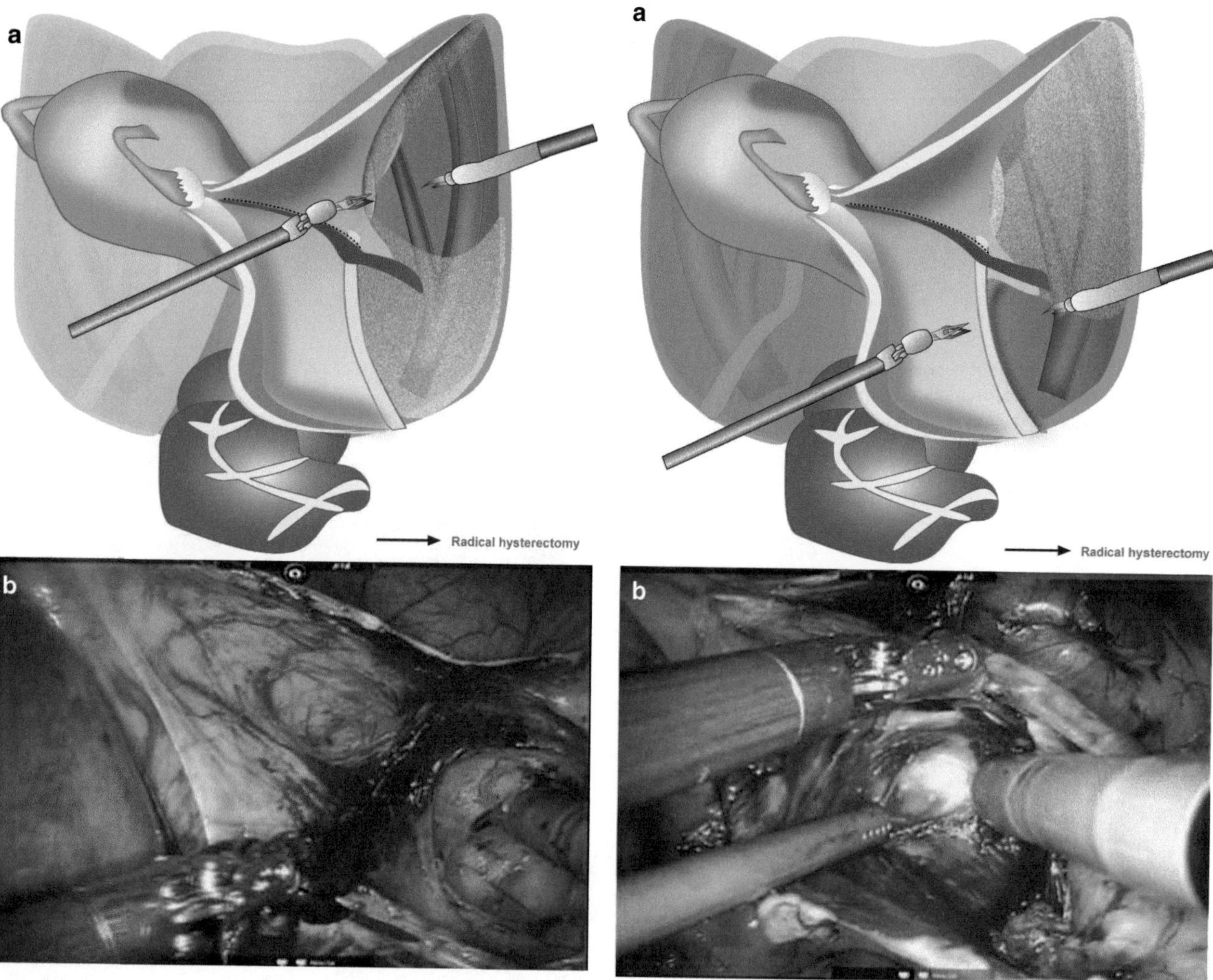

Fig. 63.12 (**a**) Illustration of paravesicle space. (**b**) The paravesical space is developed by a gentle dissection of bladder away from pelvic wall laterally. The umbilical artery can be identified and pushed laterally

Fig. 63.13 (**a**) Illustration of pararectal space. (**b**) The pararectal space is developed by dissection down along the medial aspect of peritoneum. The ureter can be identified at the peritoneum medially and the internal iliac artery is the boundary laterally. The space can be developed down to the pelvic floor

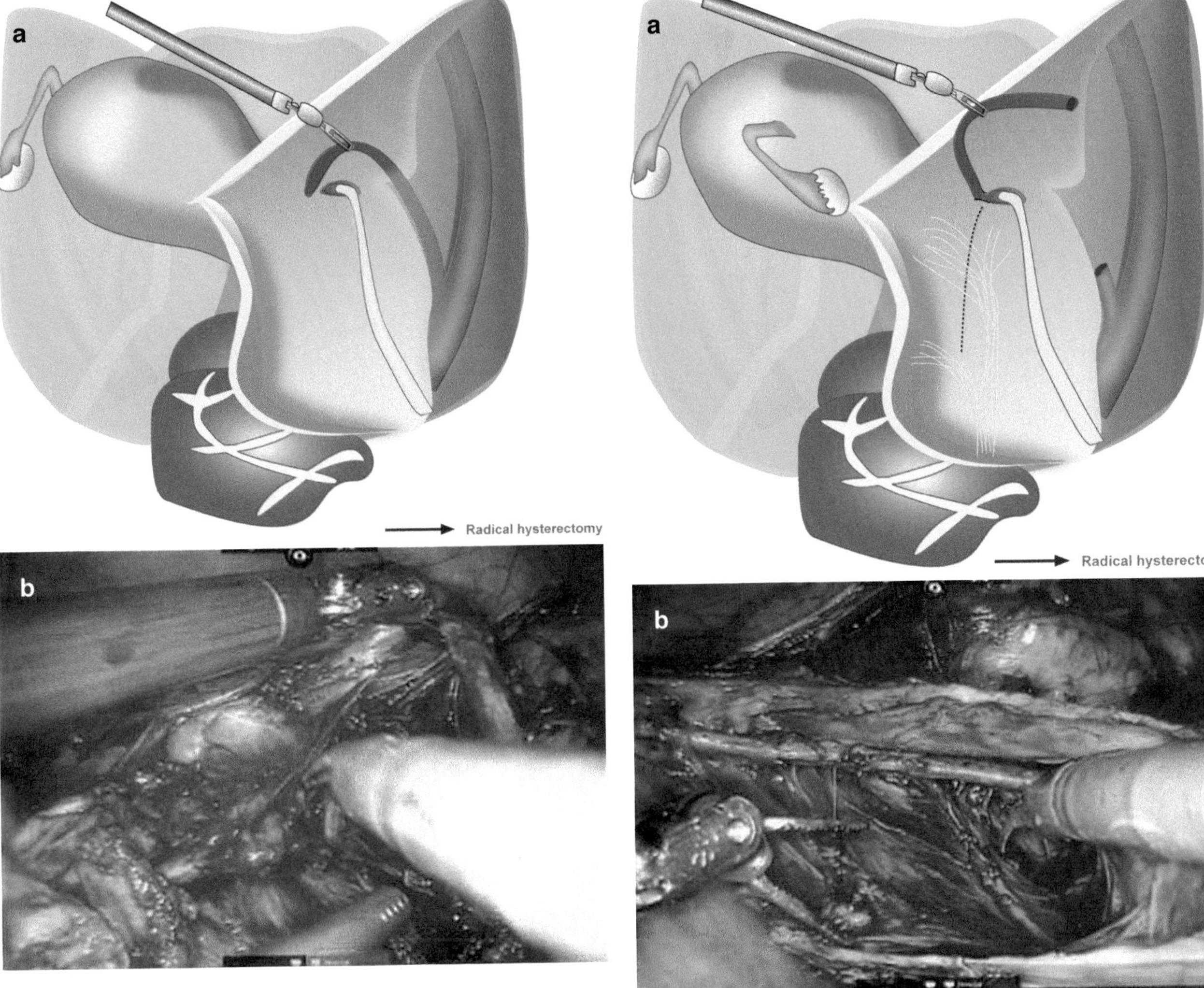

Fig. 63.14 (**a**) Development of anterior leaf of tunnel. (**b**) The ureter tunnel is identified by lifting the uterine artery and pushing downward the ureter until the complete separation of ureter and uterine artery. The anterior leaf is identified by the tissues covering ureter between bladder and uterus

Fig. 63.15 (**a**) Illustration of posterior leaf of tunnel and hyogastric nerve. (**b**) The ureter run from pelvic wall to the uterus along (along with a preserved uterine vein). The posterior leaf of tunnel can be identified at below the ureter. Nerve fibers spreading around the peritoneum, the hypogastric nerve, are identified along the medial aspect of peritoneum down to the posterior leaf. An incision perpendicular to ureter can be made from the pararectal peritoneum along the posterior leaf. Nerve fibers toward uterus are dissected whilst fibers toward bladder can be preserved

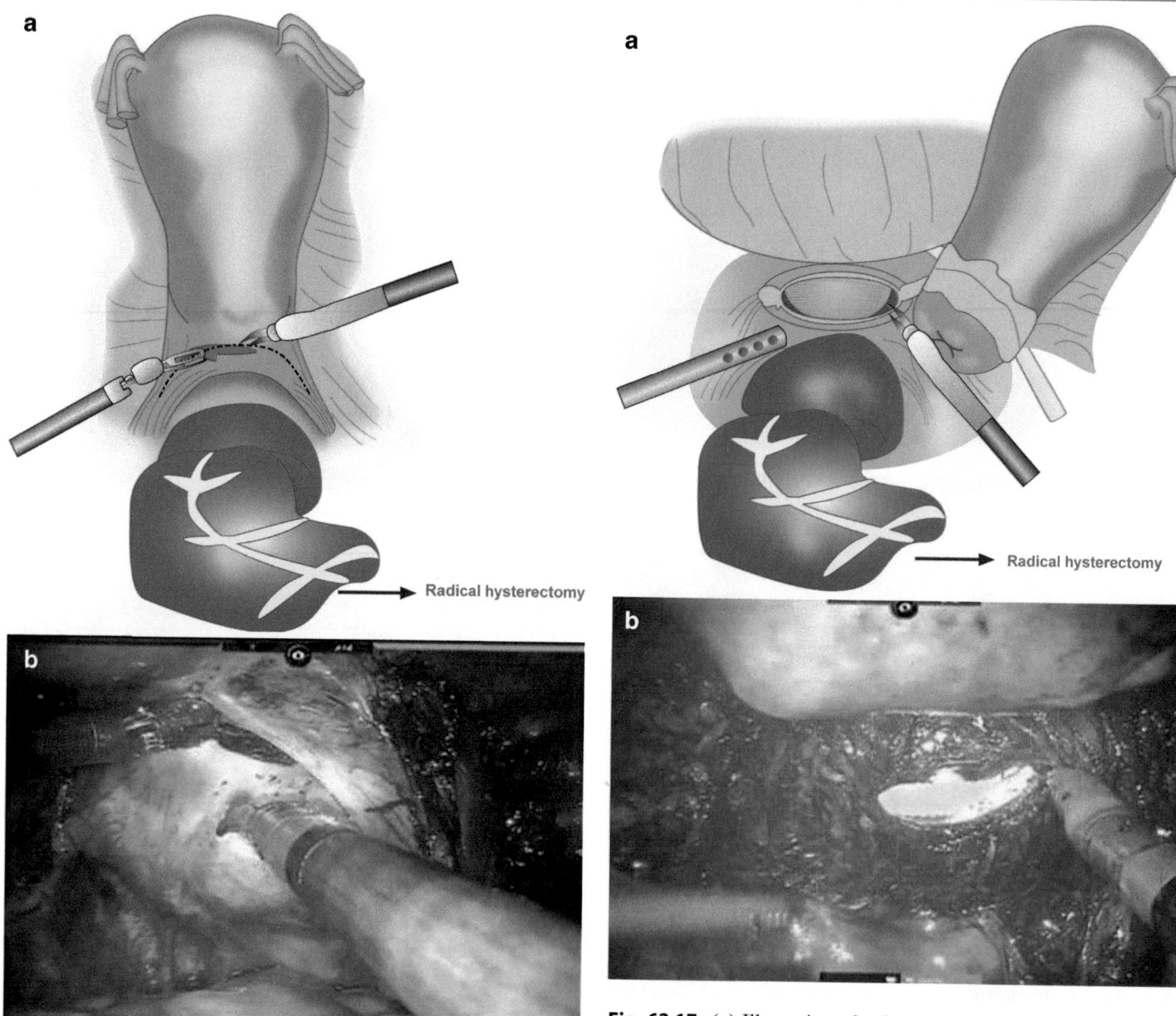

Fig. 63.16 (**a**) Illustration of posterior colpotomy. (**b**) The bulging of posterior fornex by pushing the nose sucker in vagina can be identified. An incision is made at the level of uterosacral ligaments and the recto-vaginal space can be developed downward. The space can be expanded laterally toward uterosacral ligaments. Then, uterosacral ligaments are transected, followed by the paracolpos below

Fig. 63.17 (**a**) Illustration of colpotomy. (**b**) The colpotomy is made using monopolar scissors at posteriorly and anteriorly. The dissection is completed by circumscribing the vagina on the sucker bulb

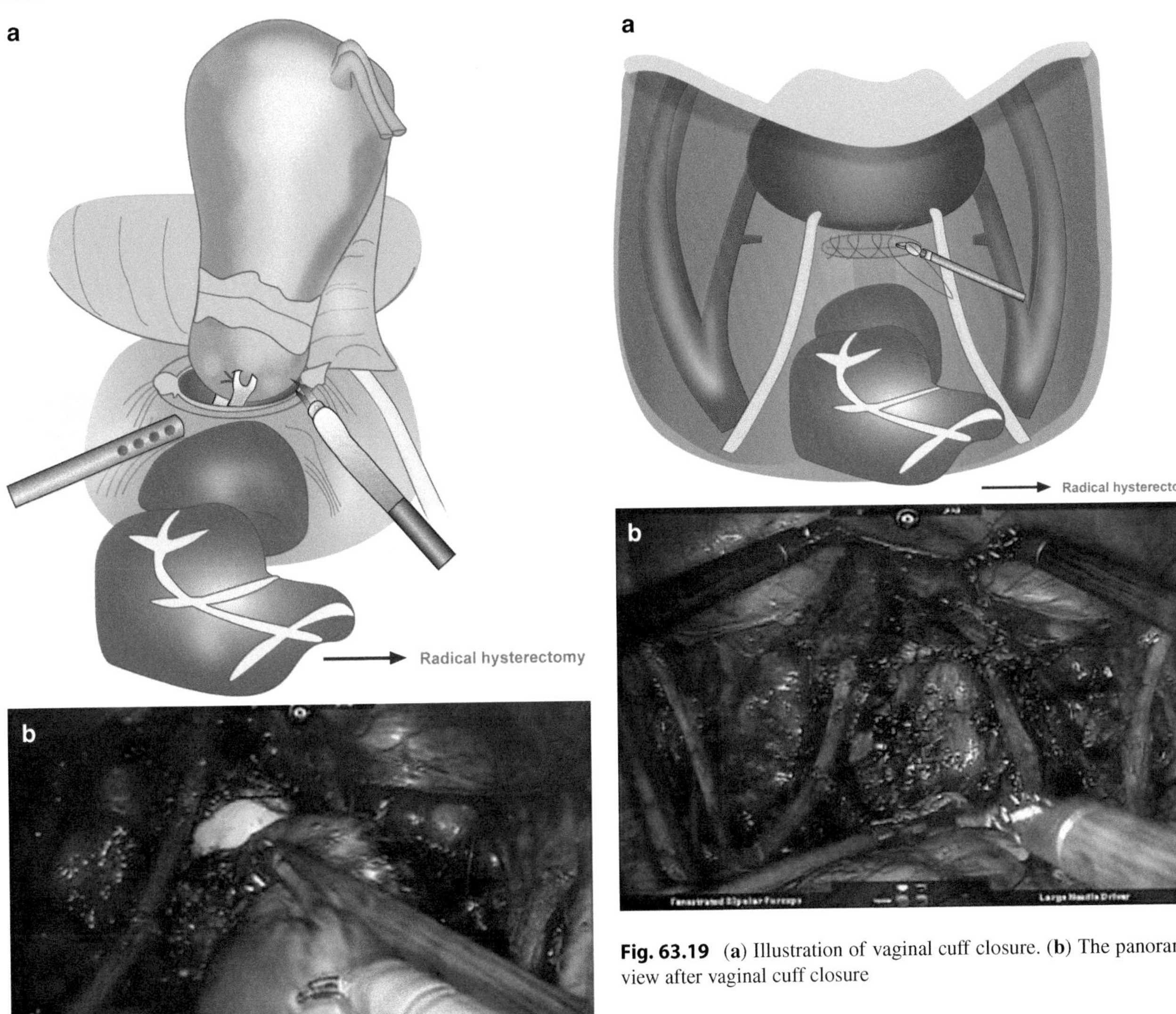

Fig. 63.18 (**a**) Illustration of removal of uterus. (**b**) The uterus is extirpated from the vagina using the Allis clamp or tenaculum forceps

Fig. 63.19 (**a**) Illustration of vaginal cuff closure. (**b**) The panoramic view after vaginal cuff closure

Acknowledgement The authors acknowledge Ms. Hui-Yin Su for the preparation of illustrations.

References

1. Tan SJ, Lin CK, Fu PT, Liu YL, Sun CC, Chang CC, Yu MH, Lai HC. Robotic surgery in complicated gynecologic diseases: experience of Tri-Service General Hospital in Taiwan. Taiwan J Obstet Gynecol. 2012;51:18–25.
2. Diaz-Arrastia C, Jurnalov C, Gomez G, Townsend Jr C. Laparoscopic hysterectomy using a computer-enhanced surgical robot. Surg Endosc. 2002;16:1271–3.

Robotic-Assisted Total Hysterectomy: Hysterectomy Techniques in the Normal-Sized and Small Uterus

64

Megan N. Wasson and Javier F. Magrina

Introduction

The introduction of robotic technology has dramatically altered the surgical approach to hysterectomy. Following introduction of the robotic surgical system, there has been a dramatic decrease in the proportion of hysterectomies being performed via laparotomy. Furthermore, a continually growing number of hysterectomies are being performed via laparoscopy both with and without the assistance of robotic technology [1].

Patient Positioning

The combination of Trendelenburg and dorsal lithotomy positioning and can result in neurologic injury if not performed correctly. Correct preparation of the operating room table prior to the patient entering the operating room is essential (Figs. 64.1, 64.2, 64.3 and 64.4). Following administration of anesthetic, methodical positioning of the patient in the dorsal lithotomy position is performed (Figs. 64.5, 64.6, 64.7, 64.8, 64.9, 64.10, 64.11 and 64.12).If the patient is obese, the arms may be supported on arm boards placed alongside the operating table.

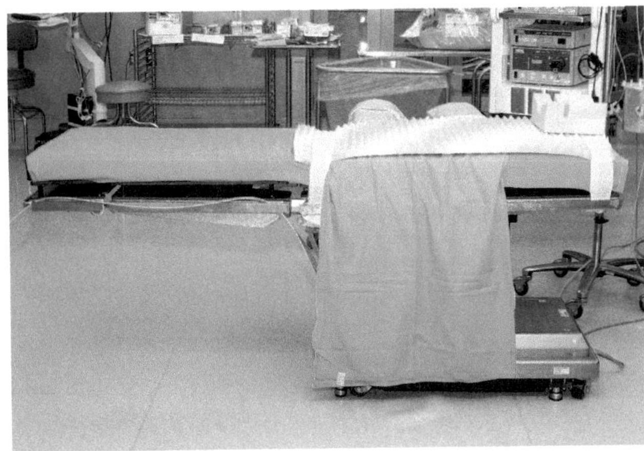

Fig. 64.1 The operating table is prepared for the patient by placing a draw sheet across the table. This will later be used to assist in securing the patient's arms at her side

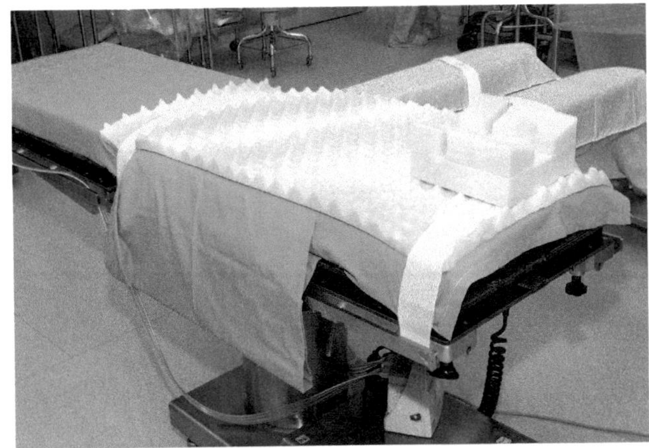

Fig. 64.2 A piece of egg crate foam is placed on top of the draw sheet and operating table padding

M.N. Wasson (✉) • J.F. Magrina
Department of Medical and Surgical Gynecology, Mayo Clinic Arizona, 5777 E, Mayo Blud, Phoenix, AZ 85054, USA
e-mail: Wasson.megan@mayo.edu; Magrina.javier@mayo.edu

I. Alkatout, L. Mettler (eds.), *Hysterectomy*, DOI 10.1007/978-3-319-22497-8_64

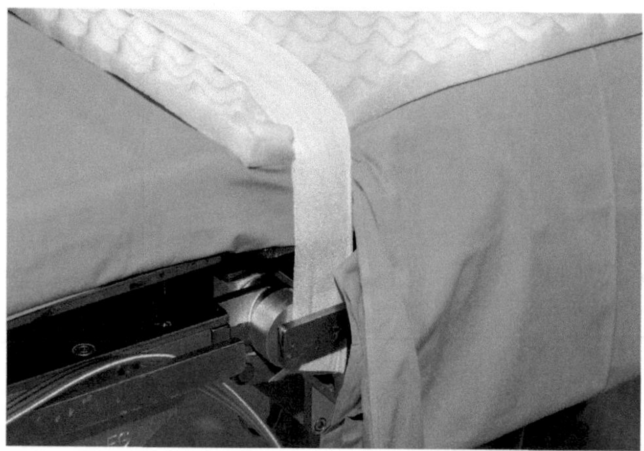

Fig. 64.3 The egg crate foam is then secured to the hand rails with tape

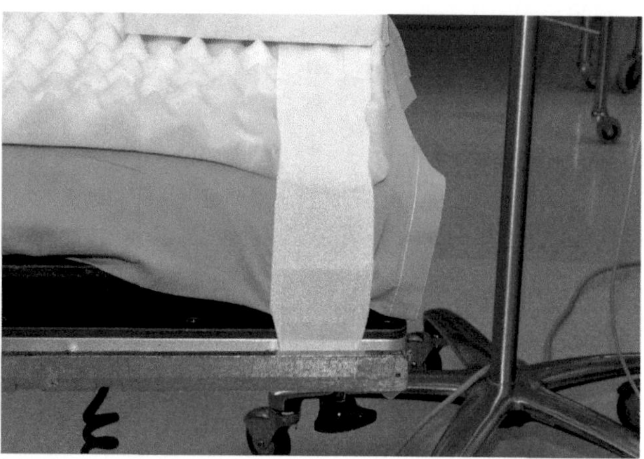

Fig. 64.4 Securing the egg crate foam to the hand rails will decrease the amount of sliding the patient will experience when placed in Trendelenburg

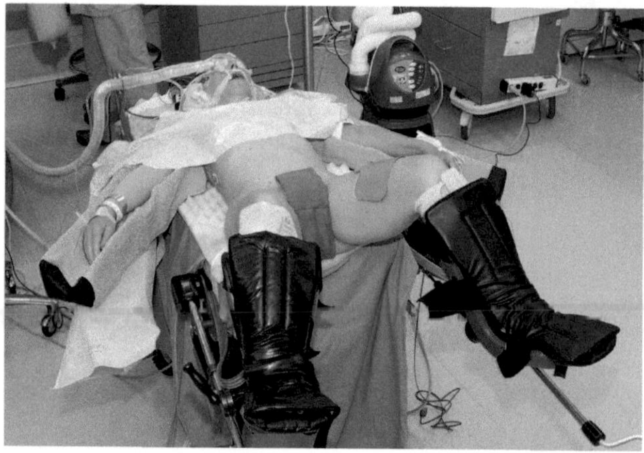

Fig. 64.5 After general anesthesia is achieved, the patient is placed in low dorsal lithotomy position using Allen stirrups

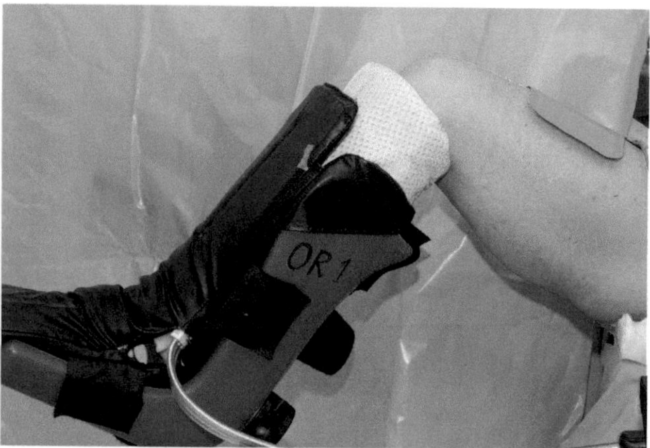

Fig. 64.6 It is ensured that the thighs and legs are gently flexed, the ankles and feet are evenly supported and hips are minimally abducted

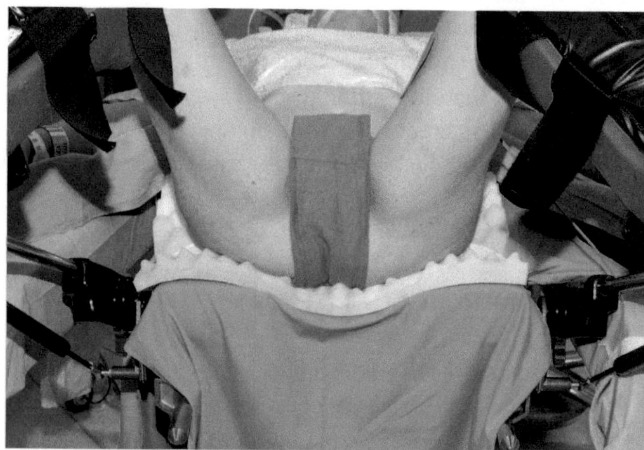

Fig. 64.7 Care is made to ensure the buttocks are firmly seated on the operating table. They must be at the edge of the table, but not overhanging

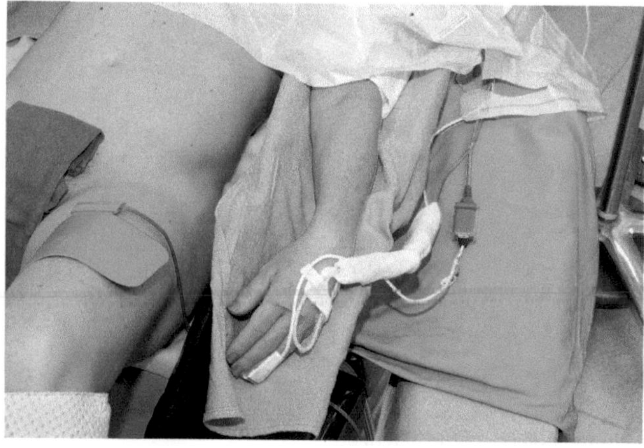

Fig. 64.8 The patient's arms are then padded with foam from the upper arm to her forearm

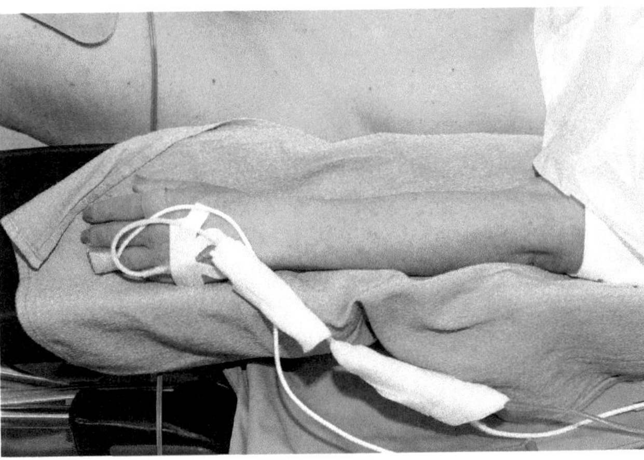

Fig. 64.9 The arm is the rested alongside the body, palm facing the thigh and fingers unclenched. Padding is provided to areas along the intravenous tubing which could result in pressure injury utilizing gauze wrapping

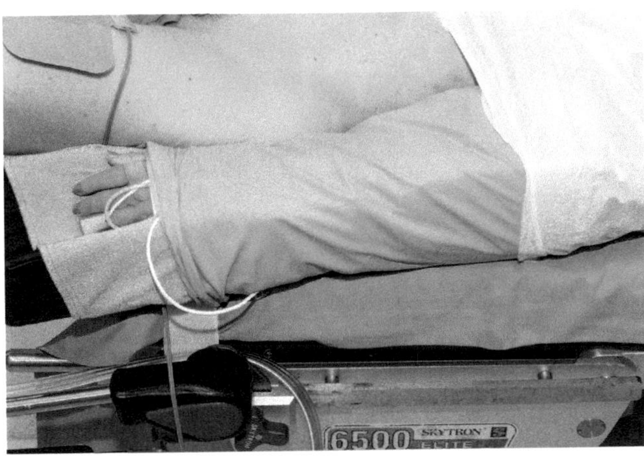

Fig. 64.10 The draw sheet is then wrapped over the arms and tucked underneath the patient's back. This securely fastens the arms to the side

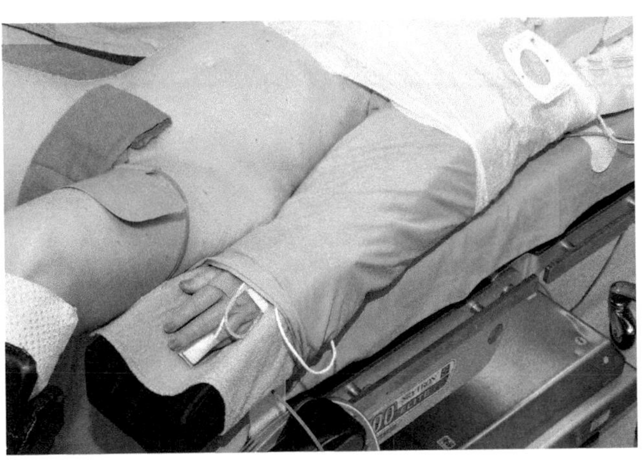

Fig. 64.11 Care is taken to ensure there are no areas of pressure or potential nerve compression

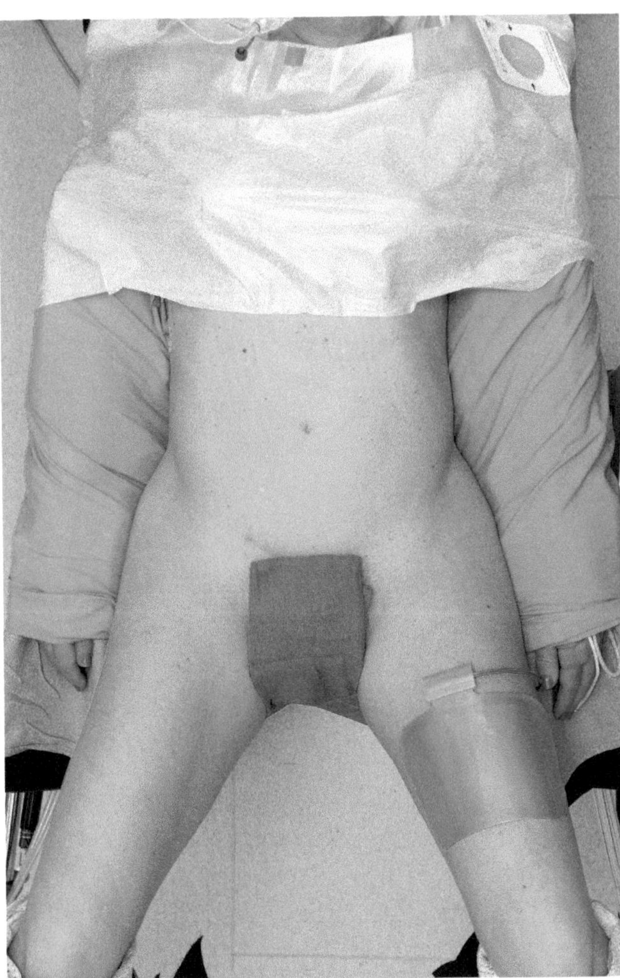

Fig. 64.12 Correct positioning ensures that there are no areas or pressure or potential nerve compression

Trocar Placement

When completing a hysterectomy for a normal-sized or small uterus, four trocars are typically required (Fig. 64.13). One serves as the optical trocar, one serves as the assistant port, and two are used for the robotic arms. Use of the third robotic arm is not routinely necessary in these cases.

Correct placement of the trocars is essential to prevent robotic arm collision during the procedure. A common configuration consists first of the optical trocar placed through the deepest aspect of the umbilicus. Two robotic trocars are placed at the level of the umbilicus, 12 cm to the right and left, respectively. A 5 or 10 mm assistant trocar is positioned equidistant and 3 cm cranial between the umbilicus and the left robotic trocar.

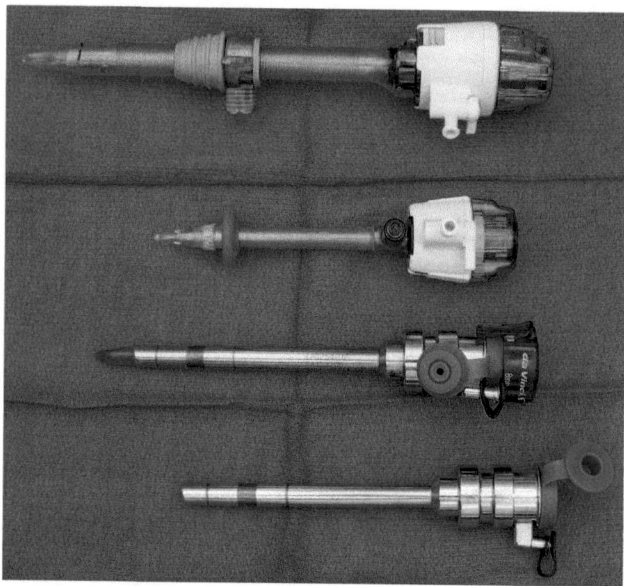

Fig. 64.13 Four trocars are typically required for completing a robotic hysterectomy

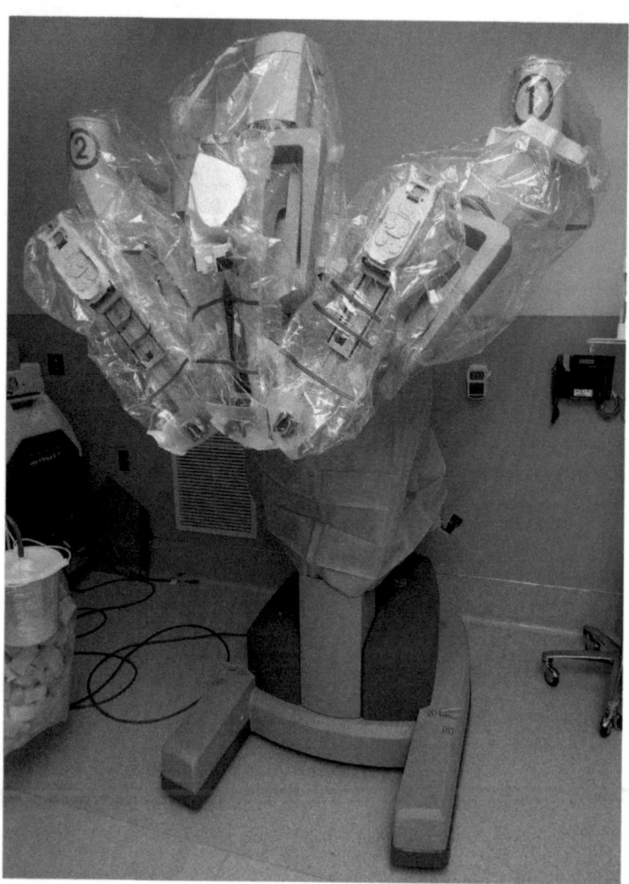

Fig. 64.14 The robotic column is maintained away from the operating table until the surgeon is ready for docking

Robotic Column Location

At the initiation of the hysterectomy, the robotic column is stored away from the surgical field (Fig. 64.14). When docking is performed, the robotic column can be placed in the midline or to the right or left of the patient. Midline placement is not ideal, as this impedes access to the vagina and thereby limits the ability for specimen removal or uterine manipulation (Fig. 64.15). Utilization of a template can assist in obtaining an optimal docking location (Figs. 64.16 and 64.17).

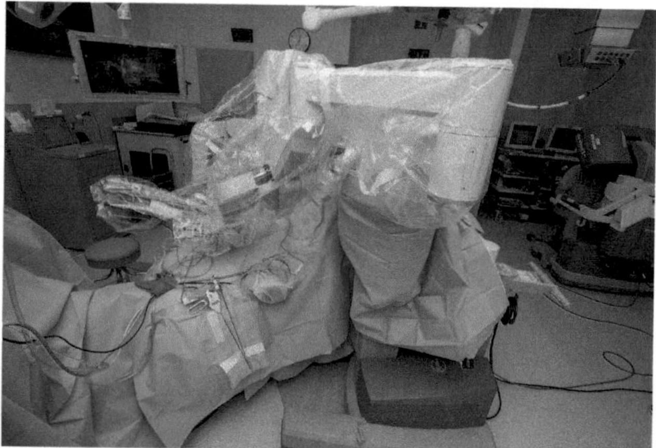

Fig. 64.15 Placing the robotic column to the left or right of the patient's legs eliminates the restriction faced with midline placement

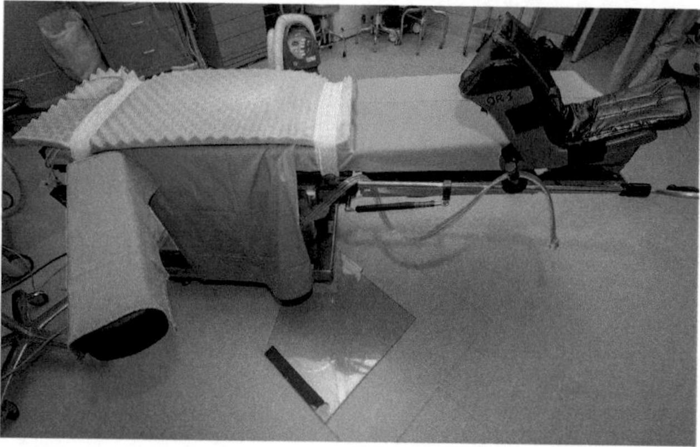

Fig. 64.16 The Mayo Clinic robotic template is placed in the area of desired robotic column location

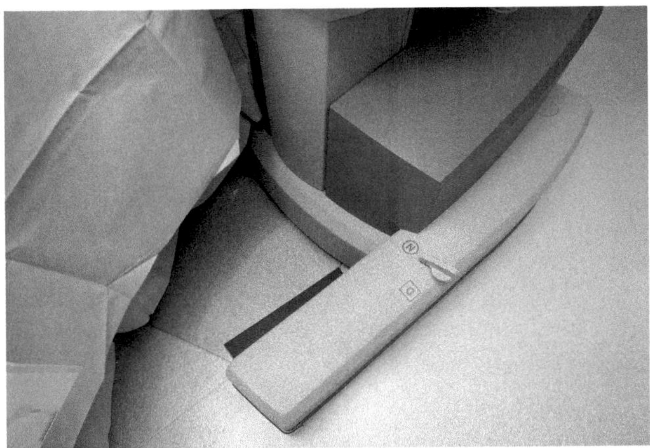

Fig. 64.17 Utilization of the Mayo Clinic robotic template facilitates accurate, efficient, and reproducible placement of the robotic column for all pelvic surgeries

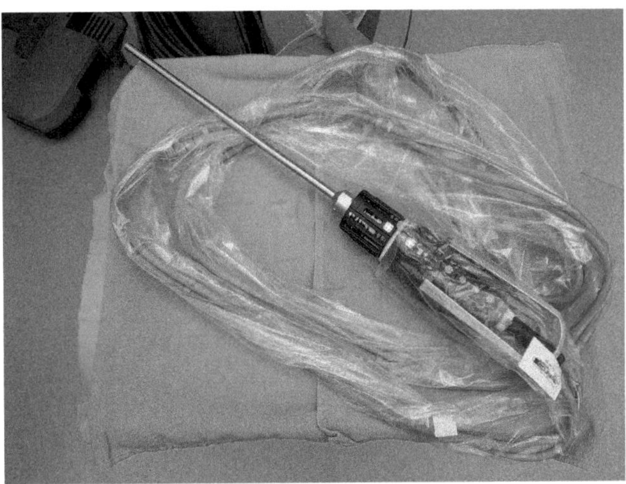

Fig. 64.18 The robotic laparoscope is 12 mm in diameter and is introduced through the optical trocar at the umbilicus

Robotic Instrumentation

Following docking of the robotic system, the robotic instruments are introduced through the robotic trocars. The first instrument introduced is the laparoscope as this allows for direct visualization of all subsequent manipulation of the robotic instruments (Fig. 64.18).

Utilization of a bipolar instrument, monopolar instrument, and needle driver are essential to completing a robotic hysterectomy (Fig. 64.19).Use of the monopolar scissors or spatula is dependent on the surgeon's preference.

Typical placement of the robotic instruments for a right-handed surgeon consists of the monopolar instrument in the right hand and the bipolar instrument in the left hand (Fig. 64.20).

Monopolar energy is ideal for opening thin tissue layers overlying larger structures, such as the vesicouterine peritoneum. Monopolar energy can also be utilized to achieve and maintain hemostasis when addressing small or superficial blood vessels.

Bipolar energy is ideal when larger vessels are encountered and able to be isolated from surrounding structures. Coagulation of the infundibulopelvic ligament or uterine arteries can be achieved with either bipolar energy or a vessel sealing device. If bipolar energy is utilized to coagulate large blood vessels, monopolar energy must be employed for vessel transection.

When the time comes for suturing, the monopolar instrument is exchanged for the meganeedle holder.

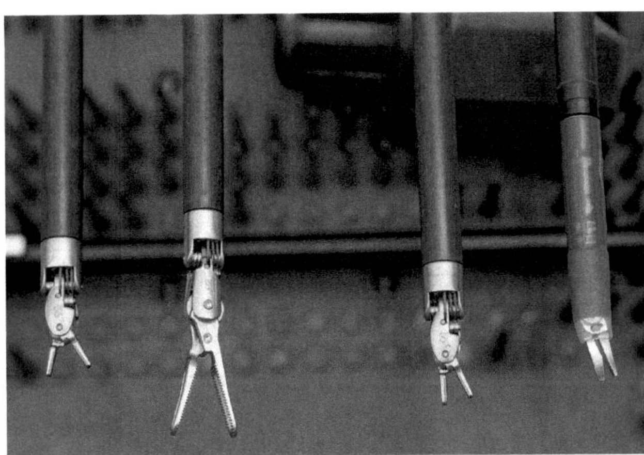

Fig. 64.19 For completion of a hysterectomy for a normal-sized or small uterus, the most commonly used instruments are the bipolar PK dissecting forceps, monopolar scissors or spatula, and meganeedle holder. When permitted, it is preferred that the meganeedle holder have the incorporated suture-cutting scissors

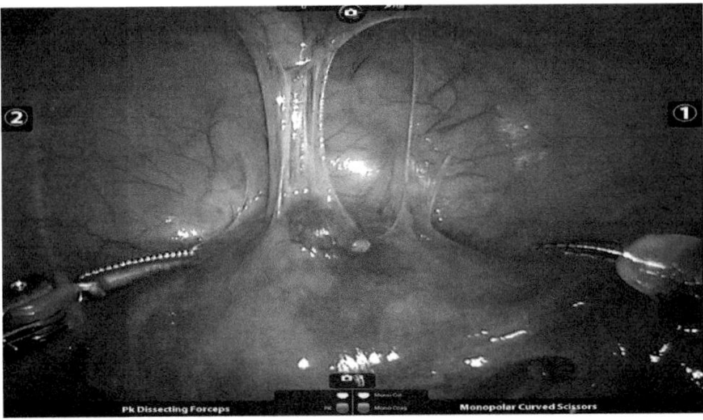

Fig. 64.20 The monopolar instrument is used with the right arm and a bipolar PK dissecting forceps is used with the left arm for right-handed surgeons

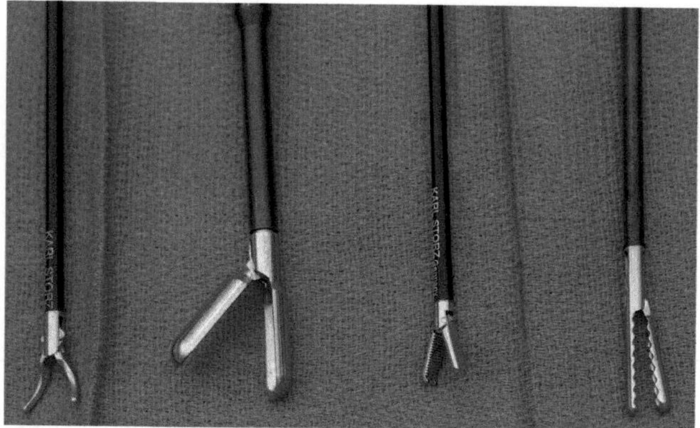

Fig. 64.21 Various laparoscopic instruments are utilized by the assistant

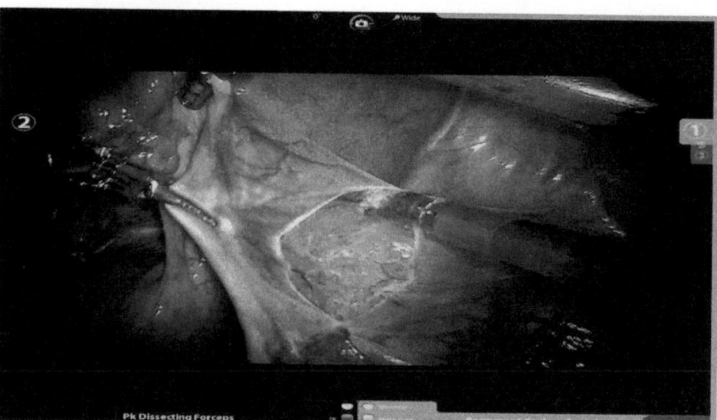

Fig. 64.22 Grasp the uterus by one of the round ligaments and pull it towards the patient's contralateral side. Make a peritoneal incision lateral and parallel to the infundibulopelvic ligament using monopolar energy

Use of Assistants

The efficiency and economy of the hysterectomy is improved by the use of a trained, knowledgeable assistant. The assistant provides assistance with vessel-sealing, suction and irrigation, tissue retraction, specimen retrieval, introduction and removal of suture and needles, and correcting malfunctions of the robotic instruments or arms (Fig. 64.21).

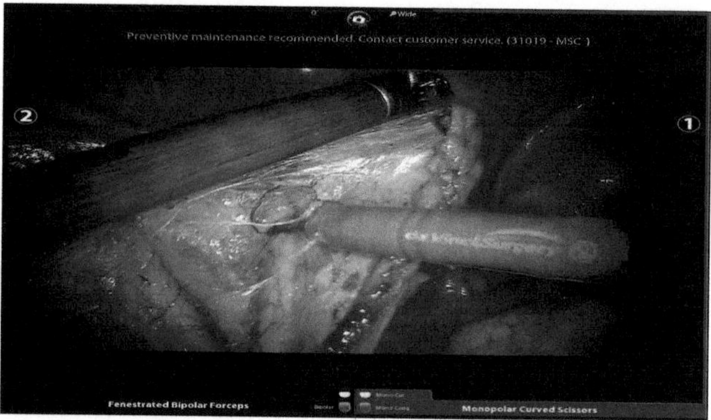

Fig. 64.23 Open the retroperitoneal space lateral to the infundibulopelvic ligament using monopolar energy and identify the ureter. Short bursts of monopolar energy followed by blunt dissection allows hemostasis to be maintained, while decreasing risk of injury to surrounding structures

Hysterectomy Procedure for a Normal or Small-Sized Uterus

To begin a robotic hysterectomy, first expose the pelvic side wall by placing traction on the round ligament. Enter the retroperitoneal space by incising the peritoneum adjacent to the infundibulopelvic ligament (Fig. 64.22). Further open the retroperitoneal space to identify the ureter (Fig. 64.23). Following identification of the ureter, the infundibulopelvic ligament can be easily isolated and divided if a salpingo-oophorectomy is desired (Figs. 64.24 and 64.25). The peritoneum is then opened further separating the uterus from the pelvic side wall (Fig. 64.26). The round ligament is then divided (Fig. 64.27). The vesicouterine peritoneum is then opened to develop the bladder flap (Fig. 64.28). Continue to open the broad ligament and skeletonize the uterine vessels (Fig. 64.29).Follow the ureter starting at the pelvic brim where it is most easily identified. The distance between the cervix, uterine vessels, and the ureter should be noted to estimate the risk of ureteral injury when dividing the cardinal ligament.

If the ureter appears coursing towards the cervix, divide the uterine artery over the ureter and displace the ureter laterally. Utilize the vessel sealing device to seal and divide the lower cardinal ligaments adjacent to the cervix bilaterally (Fig. 64.30).

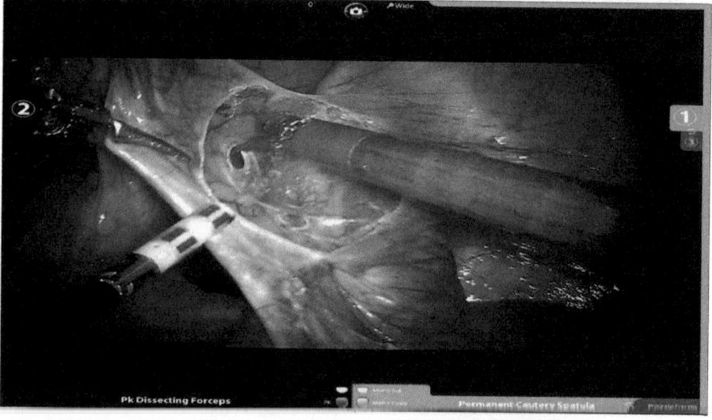

Fig. 64.24 Create a window in the medial leaf of the broad ligament above the ureter and below the infundibulopelvic ligament using monopolar energy

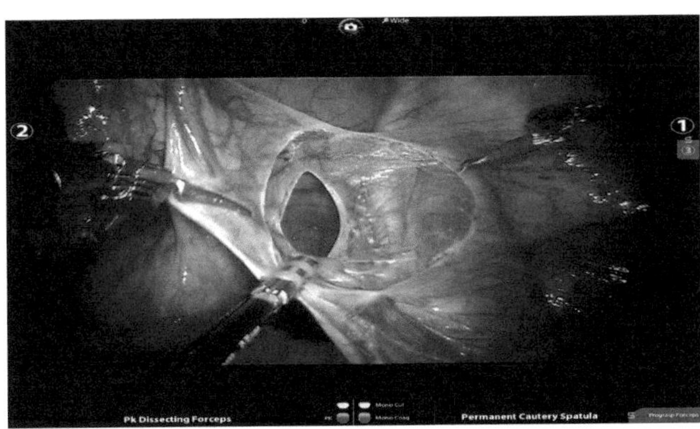

Fig. 64.25 Grasp and divide the infundibulopelvic ligament using a vessel sealing device

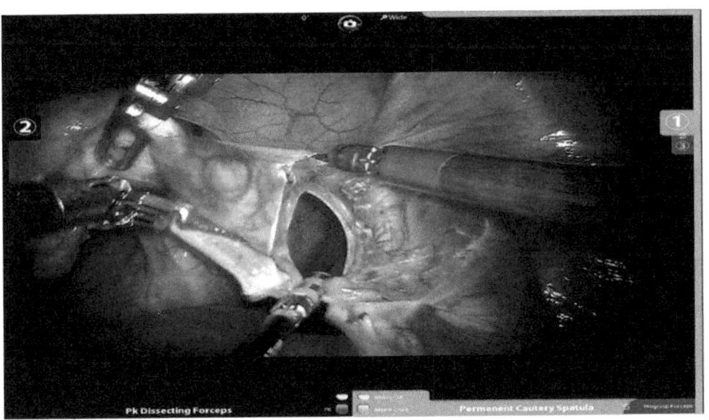

Fig. 64.26 Using monopolar energy, incise the peritoneum overlying the external iliac vessels towards the lateral aspect of the round ligament

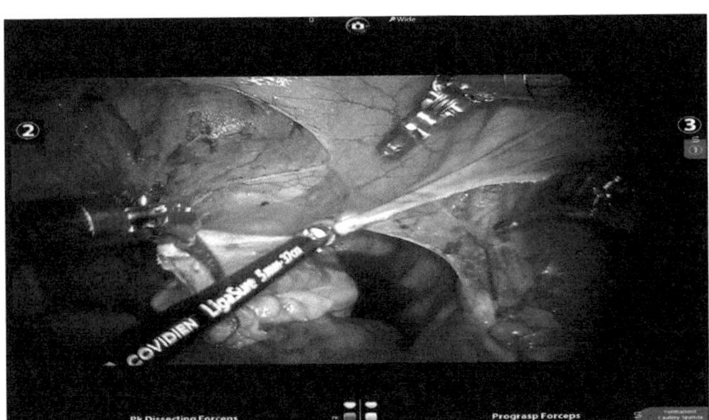

Fig. 64.27 Transect the round ligament at its lateral aspect using the bipolar PK dissecting forceps and monopolar energy or a vessel sealing device

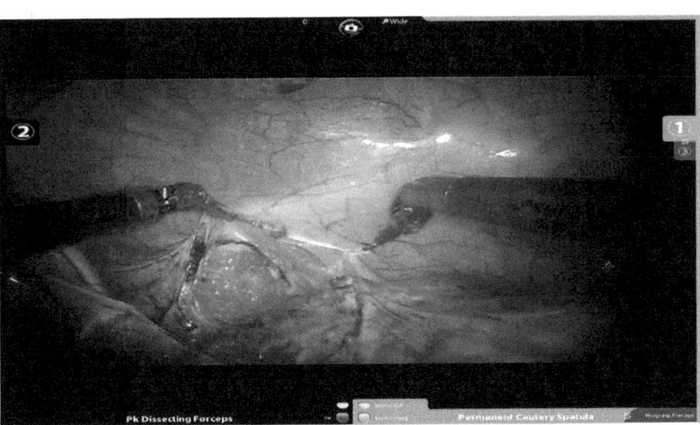

Fig. 64.28 Using monopolar energy from the scissors or the spatula incise the anterior leaf of the broad ligament towards the vesicouterine peritoneal reflection

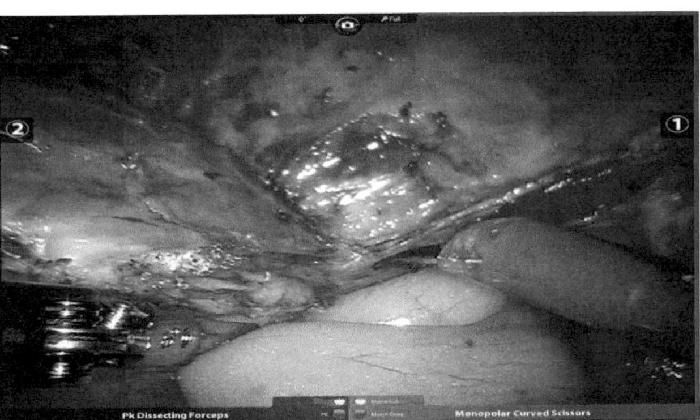

Fig. 64.29 Dissect the retroperitoneal areolar tissue in the broad ligament using monopolar energy until the uterine vessels are clearly visible along the lateral wall of the uterus

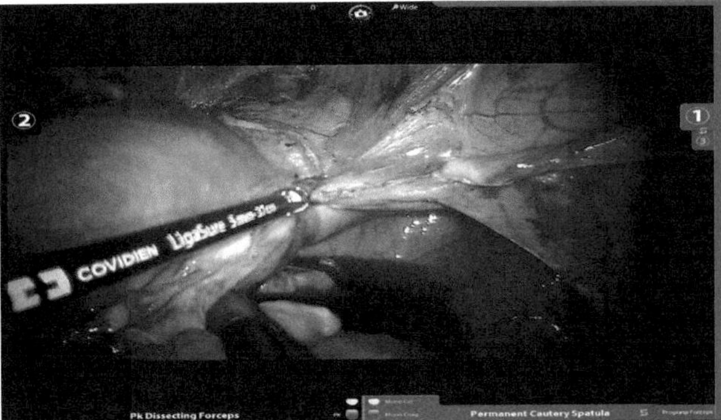

Fig. 64.30 Utilize a vessel sealing device to divide the upper cardinal ligament adjacent to the lateral cervical wall

All steps are then repeated on the opposite side.

Utilize a vaginal probe to assist with further development of the bladder flap (Figs. 64.31 and 64.32).

When performing a hysterectomy on a patient with history of cesarean delivery, adhesions between the bladder and uterus are likely to be encountered. Care must be employed to safely separate the bladder from the uterus (Figs. 64.33 and 64.34).

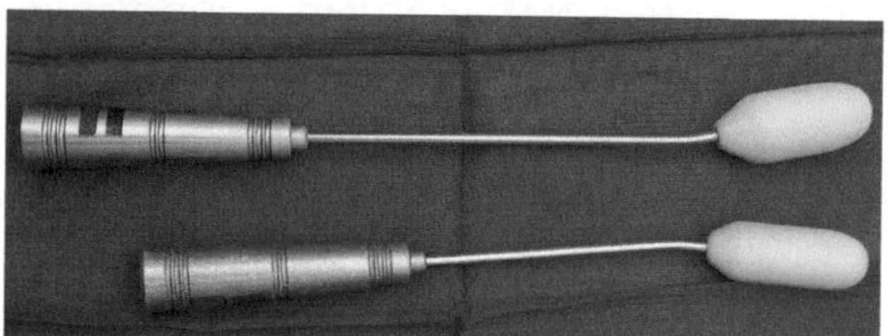

Fig. 64.31 To assist with bladder dissection, the surgical technician introduces a reusable vaginal probe or cervical cup. This helps to facilitate bladder dissection and identification of the cervicovaginal junction. A uterine manipulator is not required with this technique

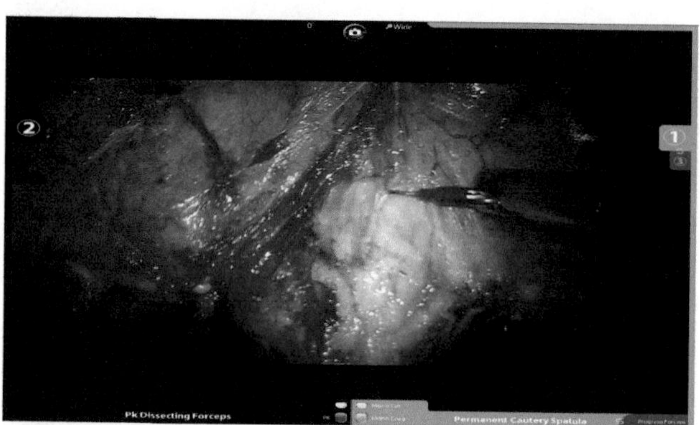

Fig. 64.32 The bladder is dissected from the anterior cervix and upper vagina at a distance of 1–2 cm from the cervicovaginal junction by separating the areolar tissue between the cervix and bladder using monopolar energy. The dissection is carried out first in the midline and then to the right and left

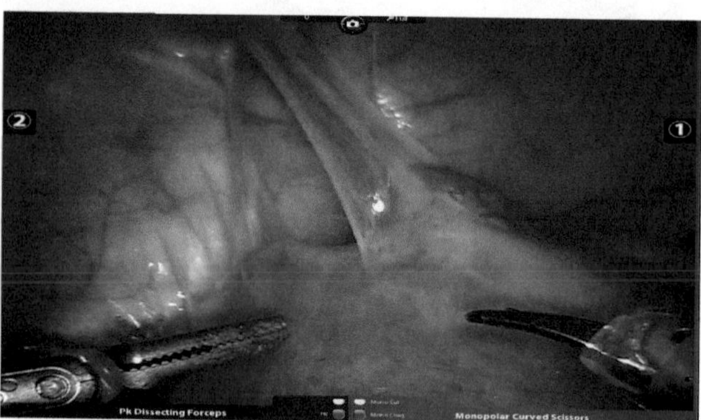

Fig. 64.33 Patients with a history of cesarean delivery can develop scar tissue between the bladder and uterus

The vaginal probe is also essential for identifying the cervicovaginal junction (Fig. 64.35). Monopolar energy is then utilized for perform a circumferential colpotomy (Figs. 64.36, 64.37, 64.38 and 64.39). When making the colpotomy, maintenance of pneumoperitoneum is achieved by

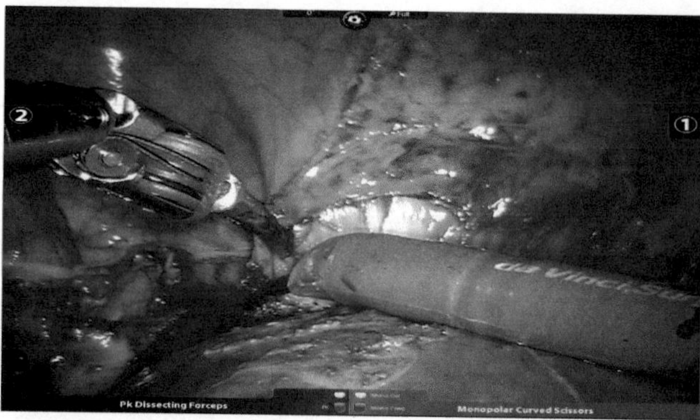

Fig. 64.34 In patients with a history of cesarean section, the dissection is carried out first on the right or left of the uterine scar and then in the midline

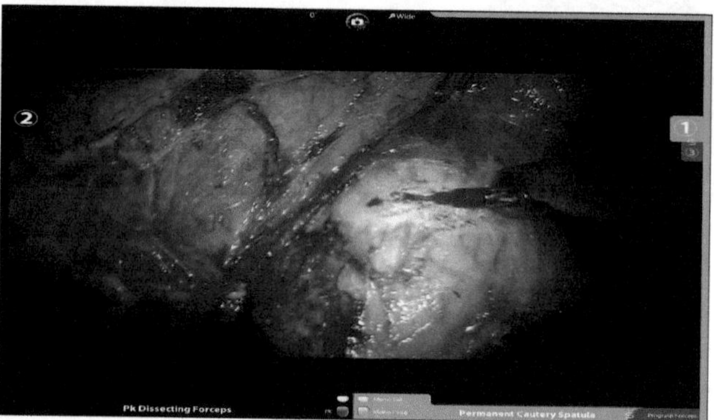

Fig. 64.35 The cervicovaginal junction is identified and marked with monopolar energy

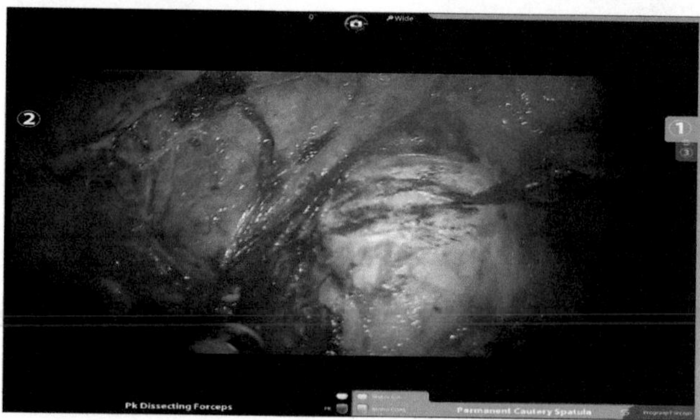

Fig. 64.36 Perform a colpotomy utilizing monopolar energy starting at the 12 o'clock position at the previously identified site on the cervicovaginal junction. It is preferred that this is completed on the "cut" monopolar energy setting

approximating the labia majora in the midline over a laparotomy sponge.

Following completion of the colpotomy, the uterus is delivered through the vagina (Fig. 64.40). Pneumoperitoneum is then maintained utilizing a vaginal occluder (Fig. 64.41).

The vaginal cuff is then closed with barbed suture in a continuous fashion, with a continuous suture using 2-0 PDS, or with interrupted figure-of-eight sutures (Figs. 64.41, 64.42, 64.43, 64.44, 64.45, 64.46, 64.47, 64.48, 64.49, 64.50, 64.51, 64.52, 64.53, 64.54, 64.55, 64.56, 64.57 and 64.58).

Assess for hemostasis including lowering the intraabdominal CO_2 pressure, allowing visualization of any venous bleeding. Any areas of bleeding should be identified. Small,

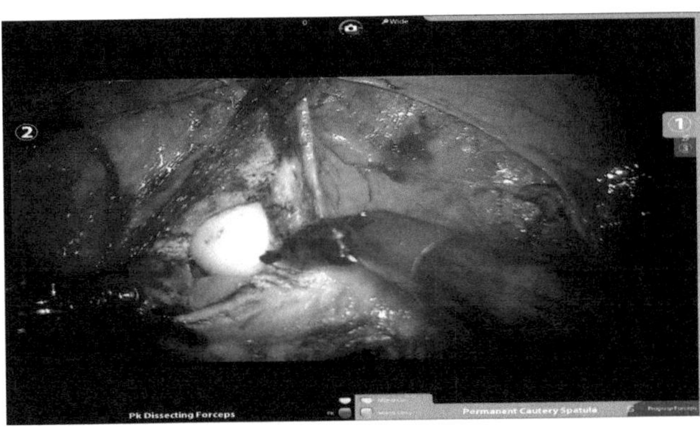

Fig. 64.37 Extend the colpotomy towards the right vaginal fornix

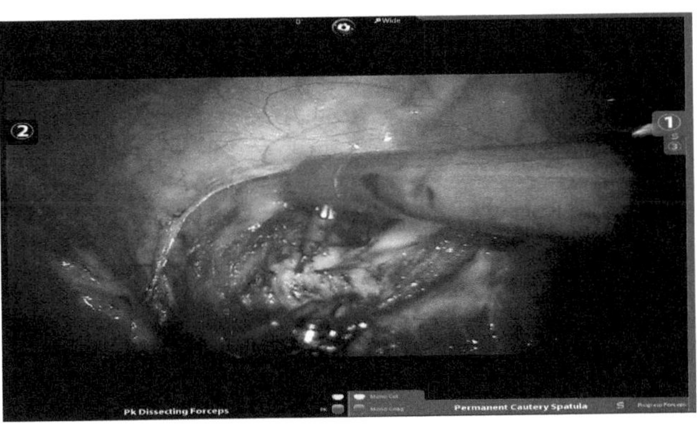

Fig. 64.38 Continue the colpotomy circumferentially along the cervico-vaginal junction

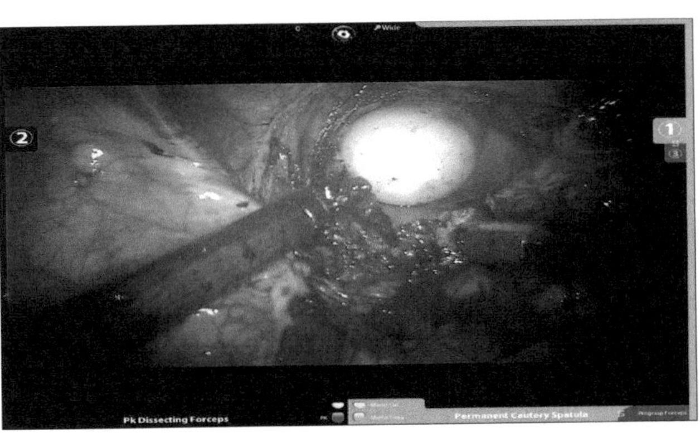

Fig. 64.39 Continue the colpotomy posteriorly until the previous site of transection is met on the opposite side

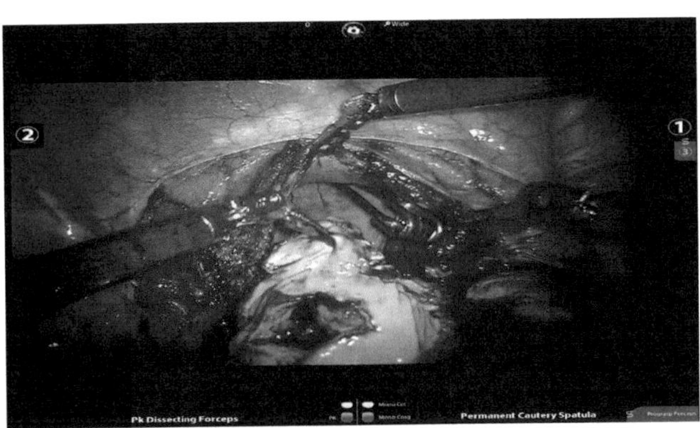

Fig. 64.40 Once the colpotomy is complete, a double-toothed tenaculum is introduced through the vagina, while maintaining approximation of the labia majora. The cervix is then grasped and the uterus is removed through the vagina

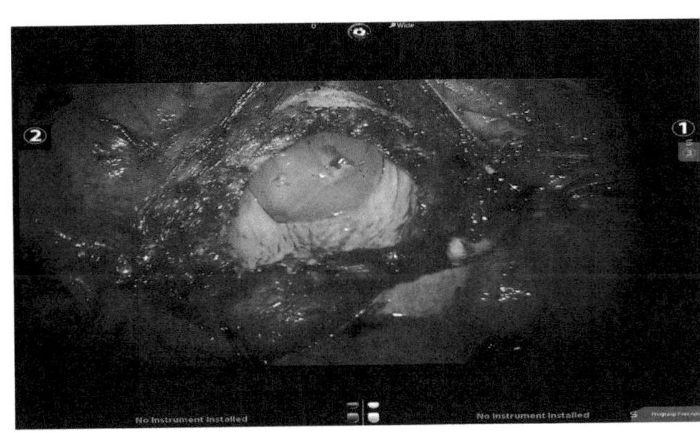

Fig. 64.41 Following specimen removal, a plastic balloon is placed in the vagina and filled with 60 mL of water. This allows pneumoperitoneum to be maintained throughout colpotomy closure

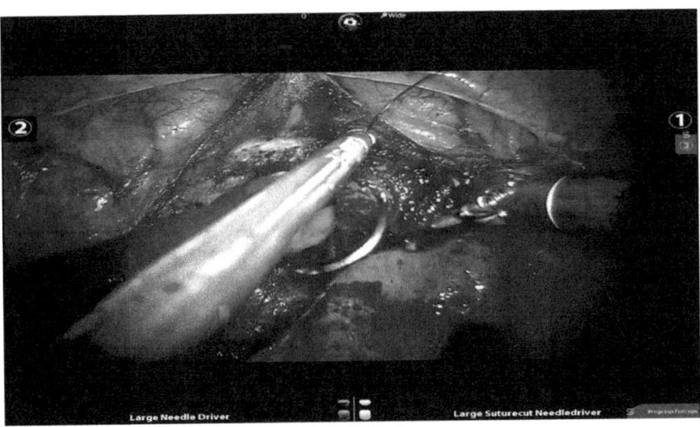

Fig. 64.42 The assistant then exchanges the monopolar device for the meganeedle holder and introduces the needle and suture for the vaginal cuff closure

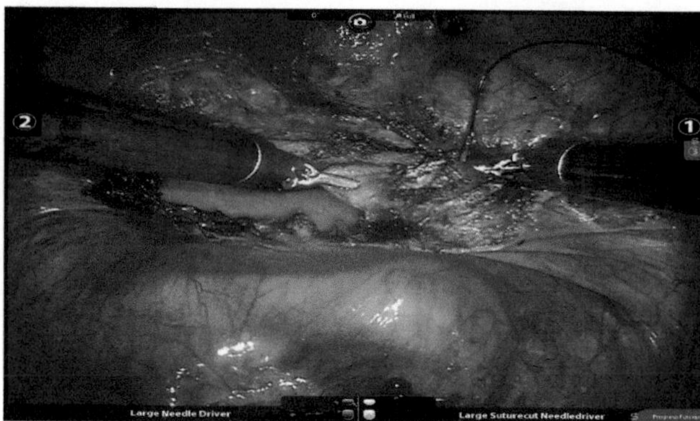

Fig. 64.43 To close the cuff with figure-of-eight sutures, the vaginal angle is first everted and the vaginal mucosa is exposed using the non-dominant hand. The needle is then placed laterally to the vaginal angle. Care is taken to avoid entrapment of the ureter

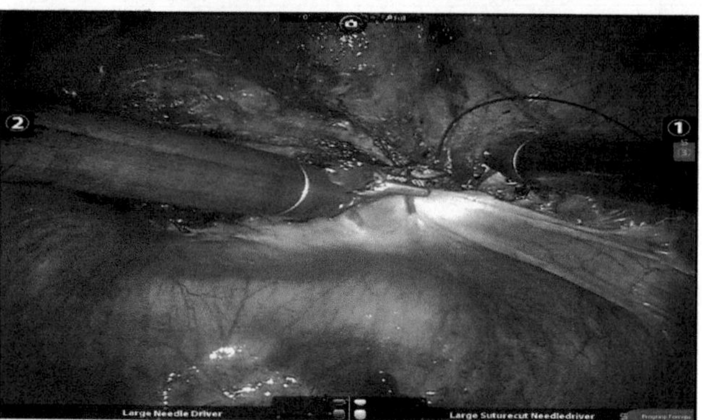

Fig. 64.44 The non-dominant hand then grasps the needle as it exits the uterosacral ligament and overlying peritoneum

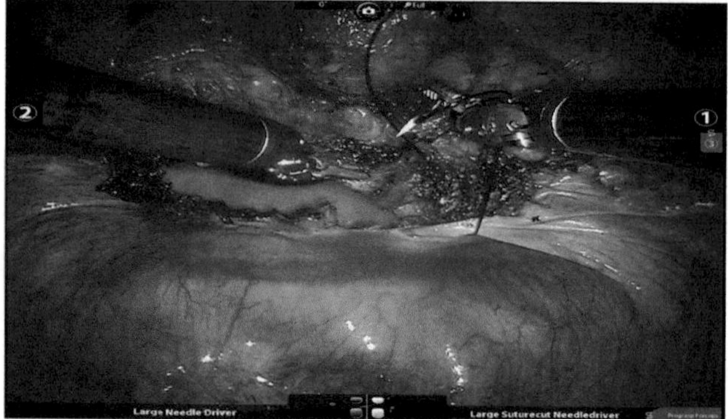

Fig. 64.45 The needle is transferred back to the dominant hand. The anterior portion of the vaginal cuff is then grasped and everted with the non-dominant hand. The needle is placed through the vaginal cuff using the dominant hand

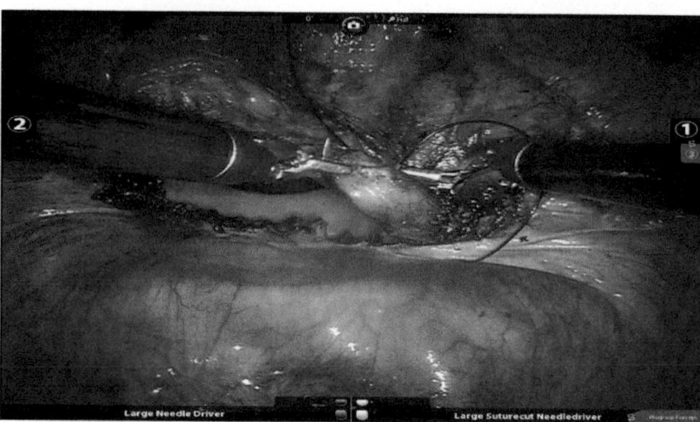

Fig. 64.46 The non-dominant hand then grasps the needle as it exits the vaginal mucosa

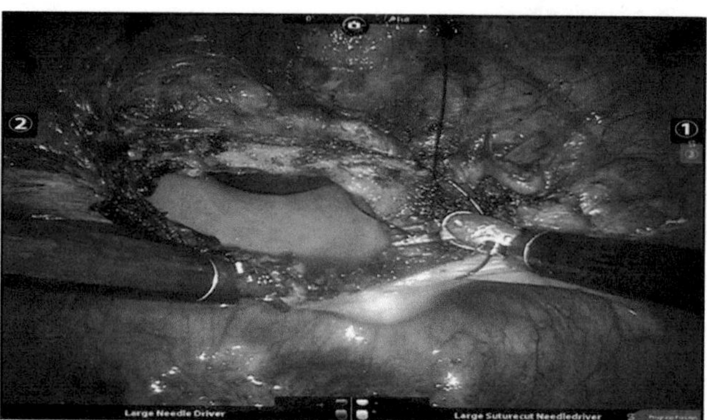

Fig. 64.47 The needle is transferred back to the dominant hand. The posterior portion of the vaginal cuff is then grasped and everted with the non-dominant hand. The needle is placed through the vaginal cuff using the dominant hand

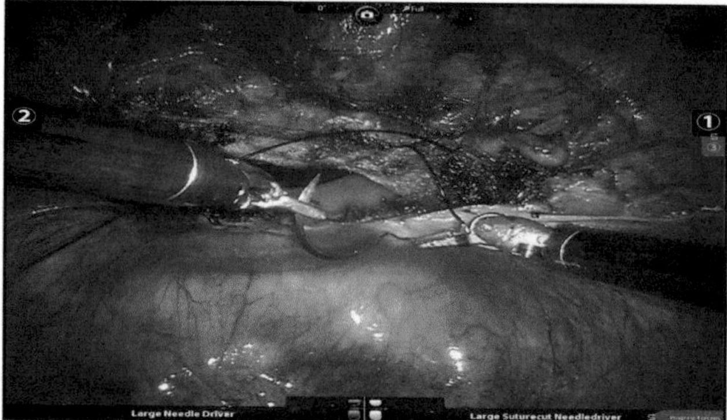

Fig. 64.48 This technique creates a figure-of-eight stitch

superficial vessels can be coagulated using monopolar energy. Larger vessels, such as the uterine artery, can be coagulated using bipolar energy or a vessel sealing device.

When assured of excellent hemostasis, undock the robotic arms from the trocars. The robotic column is then moved away from the patient to its initial parking location. The surgeon returns to the operating table to assist with closure.

During vaginal cuff closure, 5 mL of indigo carmine is injected intravascularly. Depending on the trained personnel available, cystoscopy is performed before, during, or after trocar closure to ensure bladder integrity and bilateral ureteral outflow.

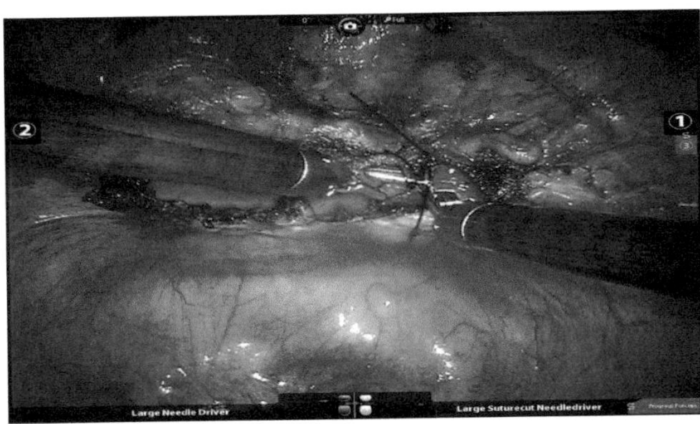

Fig. 64.49 The dominant hand is then placed along the suture line. The non-dominant hand is used to wrap the suture counter-clockwise around the dominant hand for two complete circles. This creates a surgeon's knot

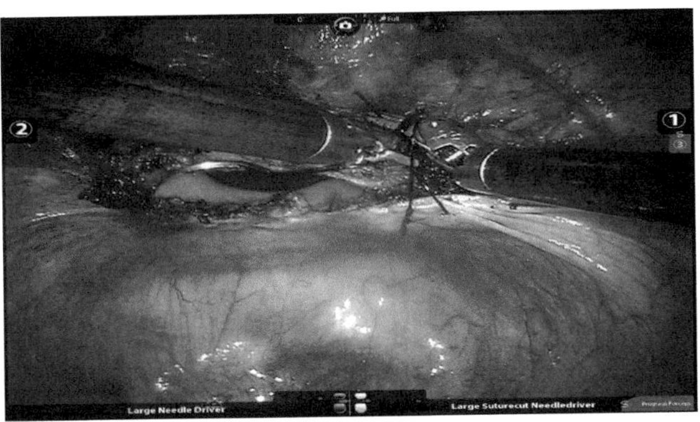

Fig. 64.50 The dominant hand then grasps the free end of the suture

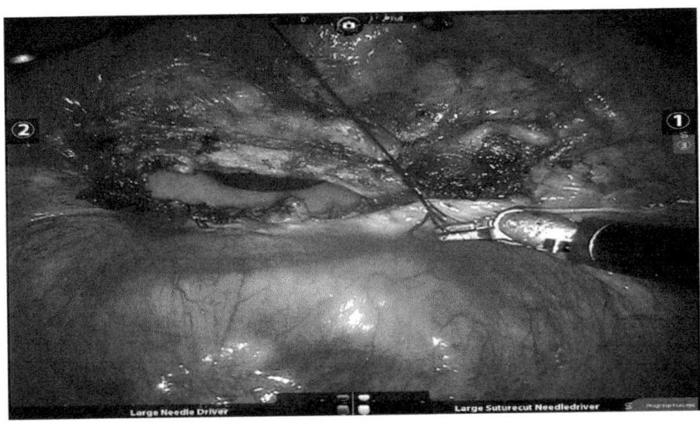

Fig. 64.51 The dominant and non-dominant hands are then pulled apart. The knot is laid flat

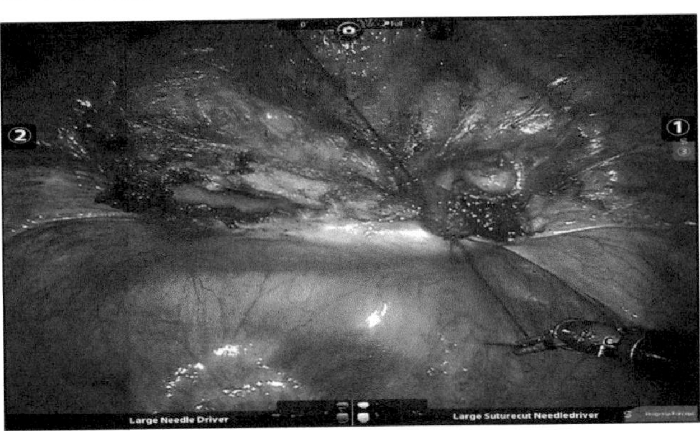

Fig. 64.52 Tension is applied to ensure tight approximation of the cuff edges

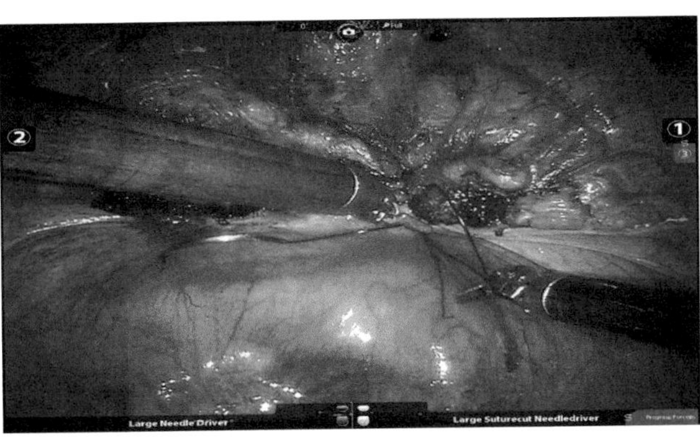

Fig. 64.53 The non-dominant hand is used to wrap the suture clockwise around the dominant hand. The dominant hand then grasps the free end of the suture

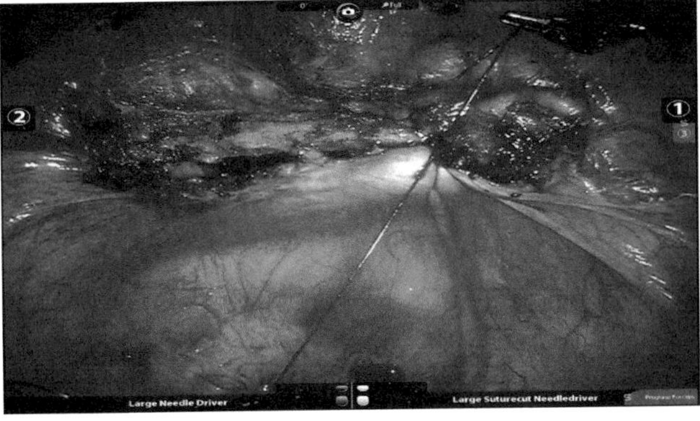

Fig. 64.54 The dominant and non-dominant hands are then pulled apart, creating a square knot. This is repeated for an additional two throws. The suture is then cut and the steps repeated along the entire length of the vaginal cuff

While performing cystoscopy, pneumoperitoneum is evacuated to decrease the intraabdominal pressure. Following cystoscopy reestablish pneumoperitoneum and evaluate for hemostasis.

Close the fascia on all laparoscopic ports greater than or equal to 10 mm using a delayed absorbable suture, such as 0-0 vicryl. A fascial closure device can be used to provide assistance.

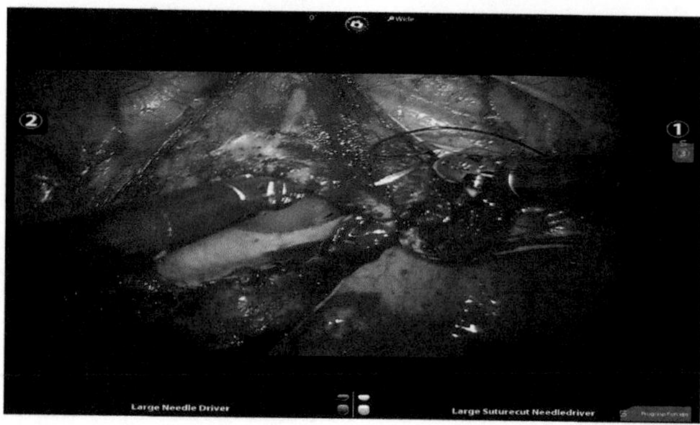

Fig. 64.55 Regardless of the technique, the needle is placed 5 mm from the outer (not mucosal) vaginal margin, which is easily identifiable by the cautery marking. The needle bites are placed at 5 mm intervals

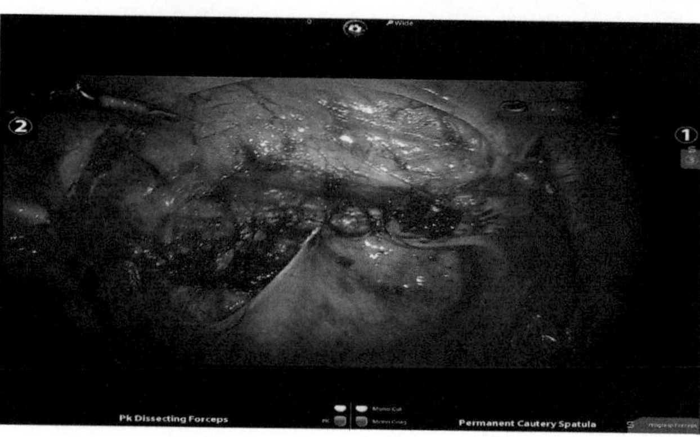

Fig. 64.57 Care is taken to incorporate the uterosacral ligaments at each vaginal angle

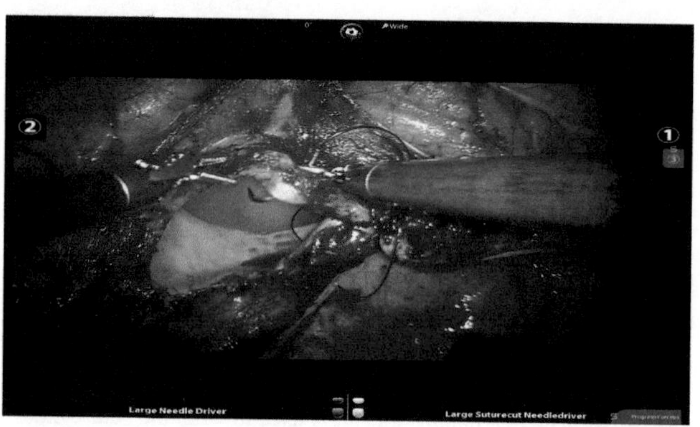

Fig. 64.56 Eversion of the vaginal mucosa confirms adequate distance from the vaginal margin

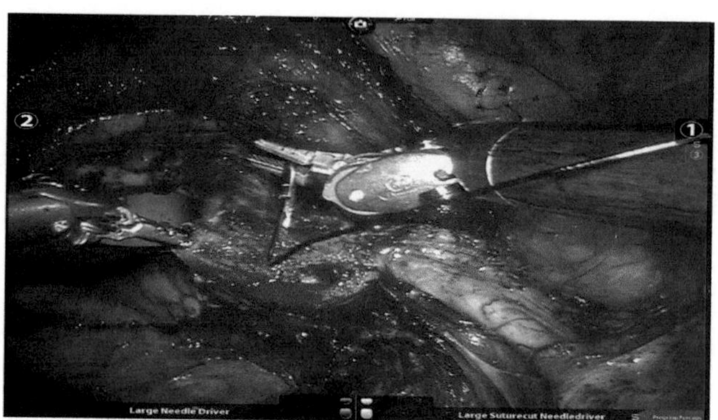

Fig. 64.58 Ensure adequate distance between the cuff closure and the ureters

Reference

1. Wright JD, Herzog TJ, Tsui J, Ananth CV, Lewin SN, YS L, Neugut AI, Hershman DL. Nationwide trends in the performance of inpatient hysterectomy in the United States. Obstet Gynecol. 2013;122:233–41.

Suggested Reading

Kho RM, Hilger WS, Hentz JG, Magtibay PM, Magrina JF. Robotic hysterectomy: technique and initial outcomes. Am J Obstet Gynecol. 2007;197(1):113.e1–4.

Magrina JF, Kho R, Magtibay PM. Robotic radical hysterectomy: technical aspects. Gynecol Oncologia. 2009;113(1):28–31. Epub 2009 Jan 26.

Robotic-Assisted Total Hysterectomy: Hysterectomy Techniques for the Large Uterus

65

Dan-Arin Silasi

Introduction

Uterine leiomyomata are common benign tumors in women of reproductive age. They can reach significant sizes and cause debilitating symptoms such as abnormal uterine bleeding, dysmenorrhea, pelvic pain, dyspareunia, or urinary and intestinal symptoms.

Hysterectomy is the definitive treatment for leiomyomata, and in the United States leiomyoma represents the leading indication for this operation [1, 2]. Published studies recognize laparoscopy as a surgical approach with better outcomes when compared with laparotomy [3].

However, the ability to perform a laparoscopic hysterectomy decreases as the uterine size increases [4–7]. Other deterrents for a laparoscopic approach are a history of abdominal or pelvic surgeries and morbid obesity [8].

In our practice, we believe that the robotic surgical system has significantly impacted patients who present with a surgical indication for very large uteri [9].

In our experience, a large uterine size does not constitute a contraindication for robotic surgery and none of our surgeries for uteri larger than 1000 grams have required laparotomy [10–13]. This chapter addresses the challenges in robotic surgery when treating patients with a very large myomatous uterus.

Preoperative Evaluation

Our routine preoperative evaluation includes taking a complete history and performing a physical examination. Aspects to consider are the size and mobility of the uterus and the vaginal caliber.

D.-A. Silasi, MD
Division of Gynecologic Oncology, Yale School of Medicine, New Haven, CT, USA
e-mail: Dan-arin.silasi@yale.edu

Uterine Mobility

Very large uteri are commonly wedged into the pelvis but in most cases, on examination, the uterus can be mobilized cephalad, sometimes by just a few millimeters. When uterine mobility is present, even when it is severely limited, access can be gained to the uterine vessels and to the ureters. A frozen pelvis should be addressed with caution. The most common cause of lack of mobility is the expansion of the leiomyomata deep into the retroperitoneum. In these cases, extensive retroperitoneal dissection will be necessary to free the uterus and gain access to the vascular pedicles and ureters (Fig. 65.1).

Vaginal Caliber

With the exception of a few patients who present with a very wide vaginal caliber or extensive uterine adenomyosis rendering the uterus soft and pliable, the uterus will be too large to be delivered transvaginally intact. In most cases, the uterus will be morcellated in the vagina. Morcellation via mini-laparotomy should be reserved for patients with unfavorable vaginal anatomy.

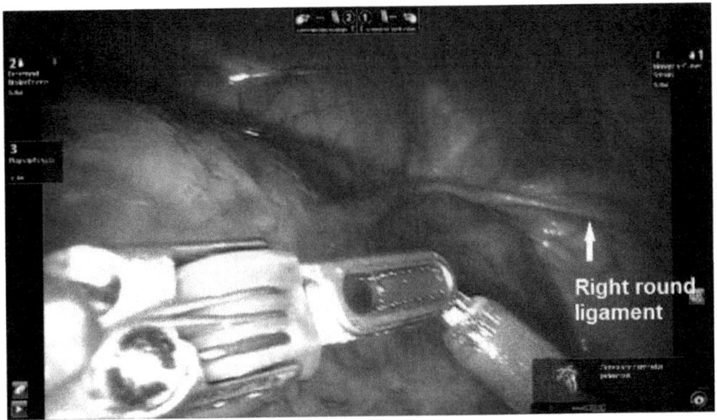

Fig. 65.1 The uterus is too large to fit into the operator's view. It is wedged into the pelvis. Extensive retroperitoneal dissection is necessary to free the uterus and gain access to the ureters and vessels

I. Alkatout, L. Mettler (eds.), *Hysterectomy*, DOI 10.1007/978-3-319-22497-8_65

Uterine Size

Imaging studies for evaluation of the pelvic anatomy and uterine size are not routinely ordered in our practice unless very large pelvic masses are identified preoperatively [14]. Large masses are not a contraindication to robotic surgery if they have a cystic component. This will allow the mass to be contained in a laparoscopic bag; the mouth of the bag will then be everted at the vaginal introitus and the mass will be partially drained without any spillage or contamination of the peritoneal cavity. The limiting factor is the diameter of the laparoscopic bags available to the surgeon from the supply room. The largest laparoscopic bag available at our institution is the 20 cm wide LapSac® Surgical Tissue Pouch by Cook Medical (Bloomington, IN) (Fig. 65.2).

GnRH Analogues

We do not routinely administer gonadotropin release hormone (GnRH) analogues. In most cases, they will decrease the uterine size and may improve the preoperative anemia. However, the uterine sizes addressed in this chapter are too large for GnRH analogues to make a meaningful impact at the time of surgery.

Preoperative Diagnosis of Cancer

Patients who present with abnormal uterine bleeding require endometrial sampling prior to hysterectomy. The tests available to diagnose uterine sarcomata preoperatively are unreliable.

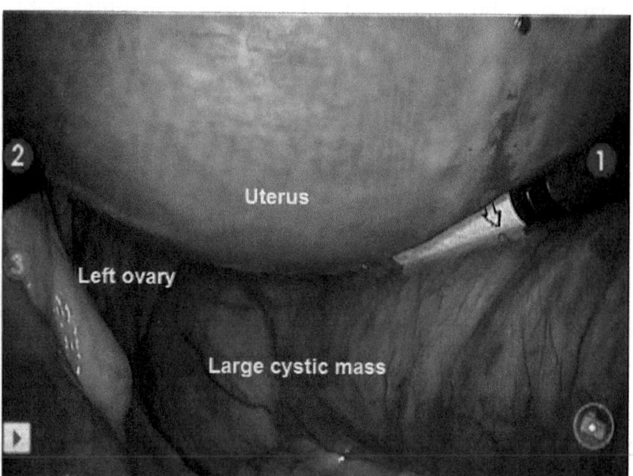

Fig. 65.2 Large myomatous uterus and large cystic mass. The cyst was densely adherent to the cul-de-sac peritoneum and rectum serosa

Bowel Preparation

Preoperative mechanical bowel preparation is common in the clinical practice of laparoscopic pelvic surgeons. Current clinical data, mostly obtained from colorectal surgery practice, offers no evidence to support the claim that preoperative colon cleansing reduces the risk of anastomotic leaks or infectious complications. On the contrary, doing so may increase the rate of anastomotic complications. For laparoscopic gynecologic procedures, randomized controlled trials have shown no improved exposure during the procedure [15]. Preoperatively, our patients are given instructions for a clear liquid diet the day before the procedure.

However, certain aspects related to the lack of exposure in these patients need to be mentioned. In obese patients, the mesentery and epiploica are heavily laden with fat and so the volume that the intestines occupy in the peritoneal cavity is much larger. This impairs the manipulation of the bowel and its storage in the upper abdomen during pelvic surgery. Also, the hypertrophic omentum also takes up more space in the upper abdomen, thus displacing the bowel towards the pelvis. In addition, the severely hypertrophic uterus takes up the entire pelvis and a good portion of the abdomen. For these reasons, in some cases, preoperative bowel preparation may be of value by decreasing the amount of intraluminal chime, hopefully allowing better exposure and visualization. In these cases, where the operator struggles to obtain visualization, considerations other than the preoperative patients' discomfort should be prioritized, such as intraoperative safety and reduced operative time.

Patient Positioning

We use two positioning methods:

- The patients are positioned on a gel pad over a bean bag (Vac-Pac® Olympic Medical, Seattle, WA) and then placed in a dorsal low lithotomy position using Yellofin® stirrups (Allen Medical Systems, Acton, MA). The disadvantage of using the bean bag is that a laparotomy retractor such as the Bookwalter retractor cannot be attached to the operating table's siderails in case of conversion to laparotomy (Fig. 65.3)
- Alternatively, a foam pad and padded shoulder braces can achieve the same stabilization of the patient (Figs. 65.4, 65.5 and 65.6)

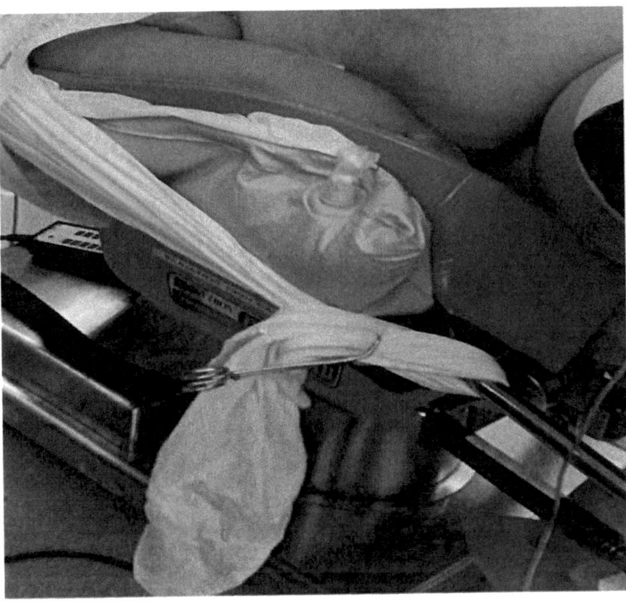

Fig. 65.3 The patient is stabilized on a bean bag with the help of a sling made from hospital sheets

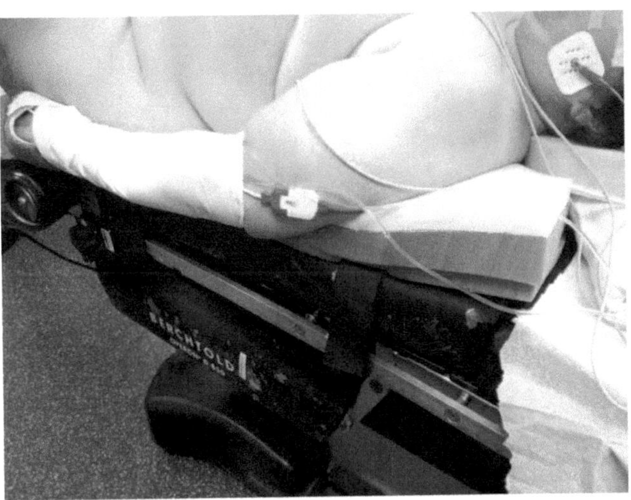

Fig. 65.4 The patient is placed on Devon™ Trendelenburg Positioning Kit (Medtronic, Minneapolis, MN)

Port Placement

Commonly we place the ports symmetrically, in an arch centered by the camera port ("sunrise or half-moon distribution"). The camera port is inserted at a level that is higher than the uterine fundus. If the uterine fundus extends to the xyphoid, the initial port can be placed in the left upper quadrant or left flank to achieve pneumoperitoneum and visualization.

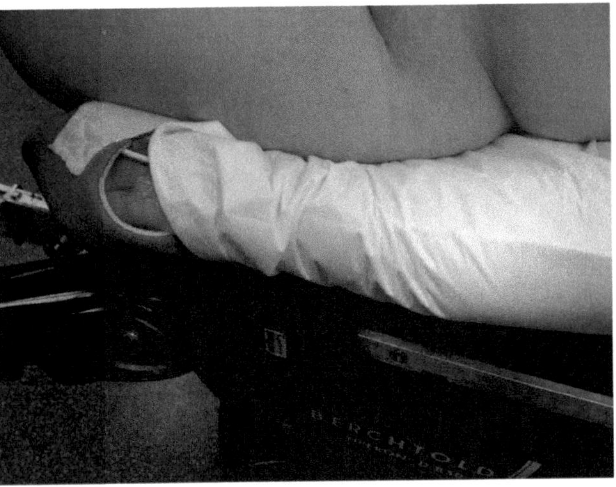

Fig. 65.5 The hands are protected and the arms are tucked

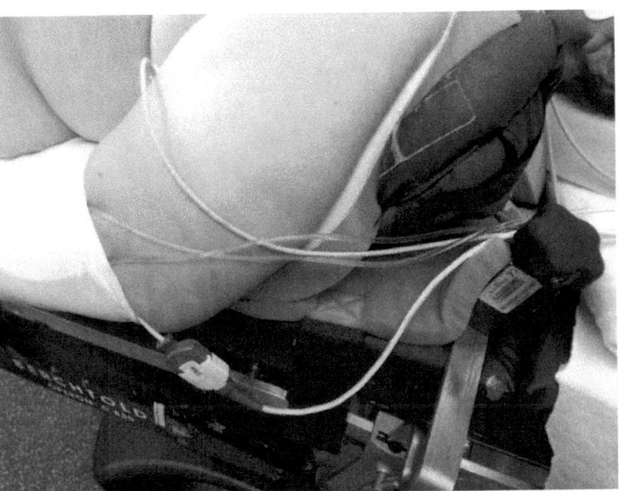

Fig. 65.6 Shoulder supports prevent the patient from sliding on the table. The pressure is on the infraspinous fossa, not on the acromion

These port configurations work well for all 3 robotic systems: S, Si, and Xi (Figs. 65.7, 65.8 and 65.9).

Sunrise placement of ports: Variations of the sunrise configuration can be used, depending on the particular anatomy of the patient (Figs. 65.10, 65.11, 65.12, 65.13, 65.14, 65.15 and 65.16).

The surgeon can oversee the entire operative field when performing hysterectomies for moderately sized uteri. This is not possible in most cases described in this chapter. The lack of access and visualization and particularities of each case dictate the strategy in each operation. The same operative routine will not be applicable in different patients. Instead, the surgeon must visualize in his/her mind the

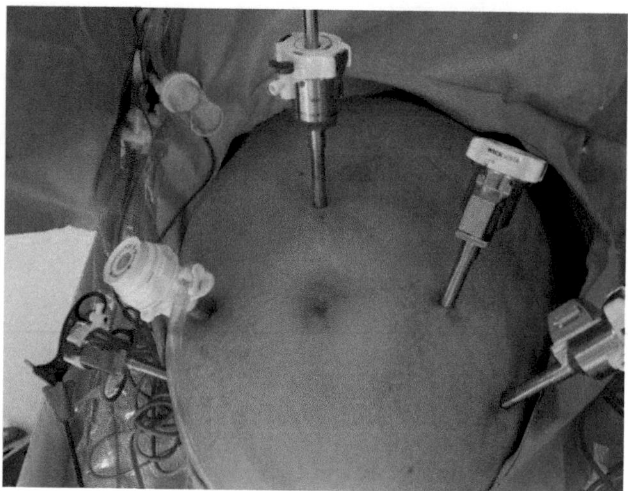

Fig. 65.7 The most common port placement (sunrise): the camera port located above the umbilicus, one robotic port and the assistant port on each side of the umbilicus and two robotic ports below the umbilicus. This is the Xi system; from right to left: arm 1 (Prograsp), arm 2 (fenestrated bipolar), arm 3 (camera port), 12 mm assistant port, arm 4 (monopolar scissors)

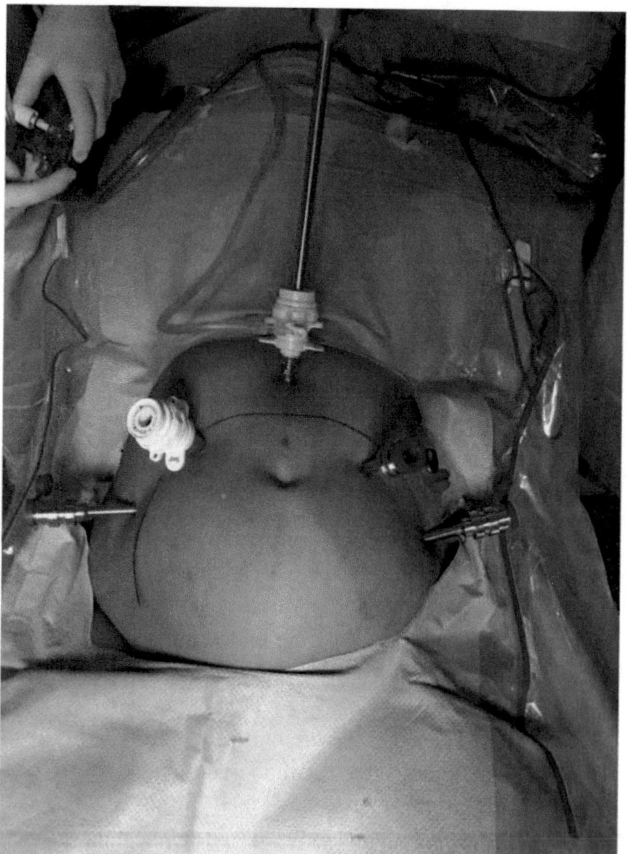

Fig. 65.8 The sunrise placement for the S and Si systems. From right to left: arm 3 (Prograsp), arm 2 (fenestrated bipolar), camera arm and port, 12 mm assistant port, arm 1 (monopolar scissors). The contour of the uterus is outlined on the abdominal wall for illustration purposes

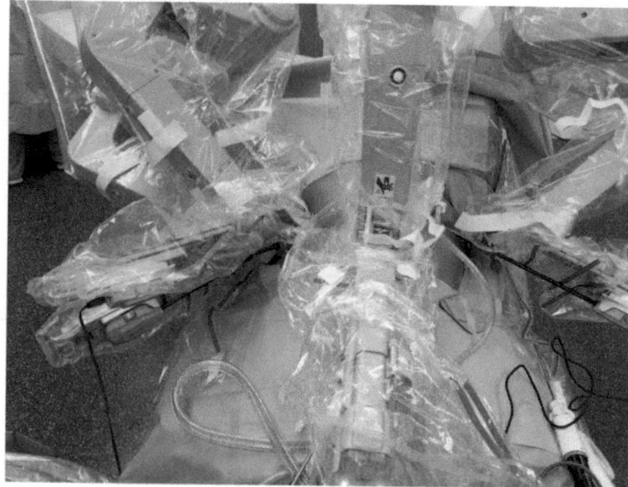

Fig. 65.9 The Si system after docking.

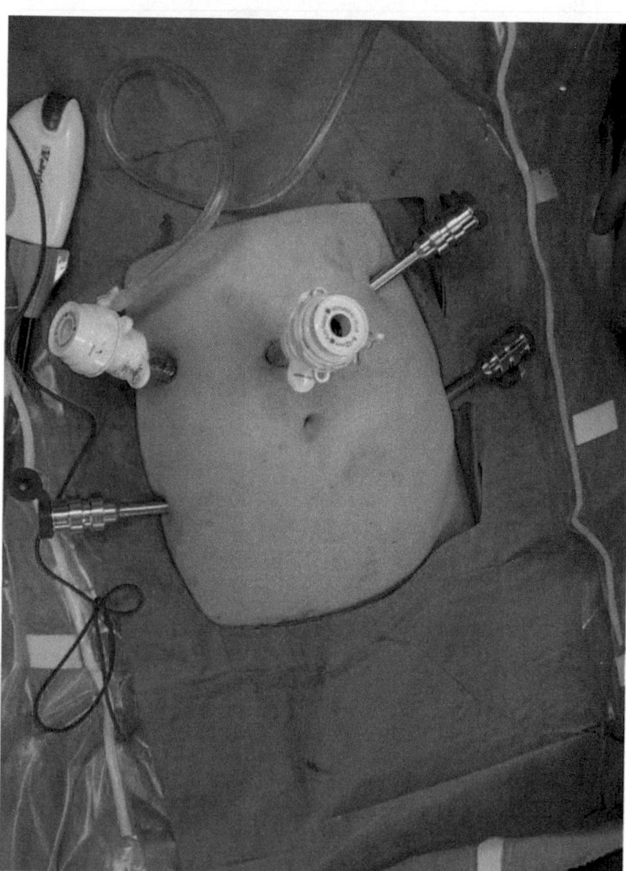

Fig. 65.10 The camera port is midline and above the umbilicus. The abdomen of this patient is long and narrow. For this patient, this port configuration is more favorable than the usual sunrise placement since the ports are closer to each other. This configuration prevents the arms clashing during the procedure

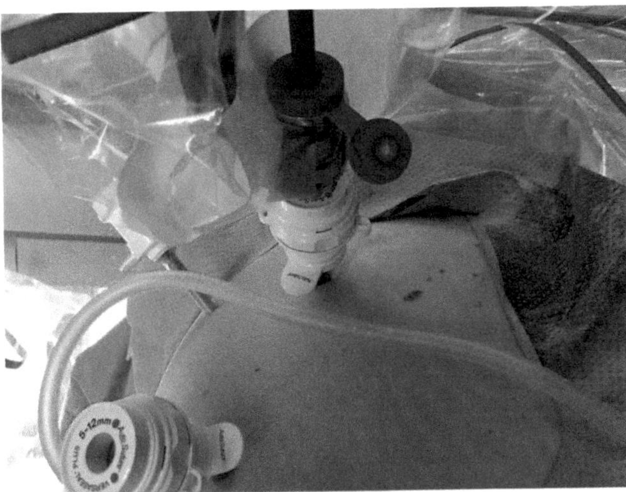

Fig. 65.11 Tips and tricks: Telescoping. Freehand laparoscopy and camera placement through several ports (for lysis of adhesions, etc.) may be needed prior to docking. The camera of the Xi system is 8 mm in diameter and fits through all ports. However, this is not the case for the S and Si systems. The figure shows the repurposing of a regular port into a robotic port. A port-in-a-port placement works well, without undue tension on the fascia

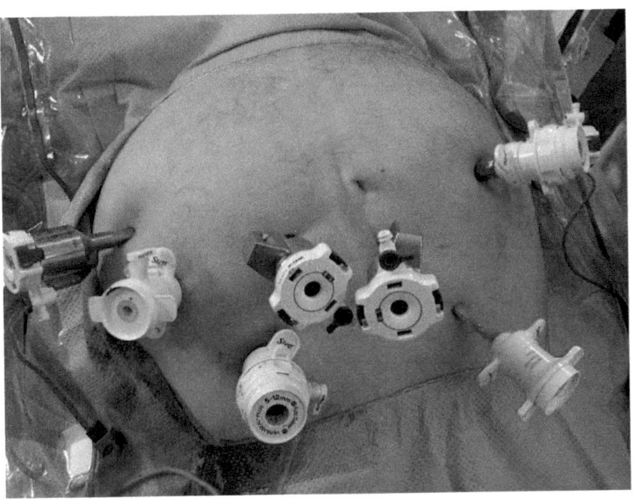

Fig. 65.12 Severe adhesions in the entire abdomen required placement of more ports. Additional laparoscopic incisions will have no detrimental impact on the patient's recovery

necessary to complete the procedure and the remaining surgical steps and bring everything together in the end.

Sometimes simple adjustments like switching a 0° degree to a 30° camera provide significant payback. The figures show how the visual field changes dramatically when switching cameras. One has to remember that the angle of the camera to the patient's body changes for different angles of the lens. The 30° camera is much closer to the patient's face and padding of the face and endotracheal tube is prudent (Fig. 65.17).

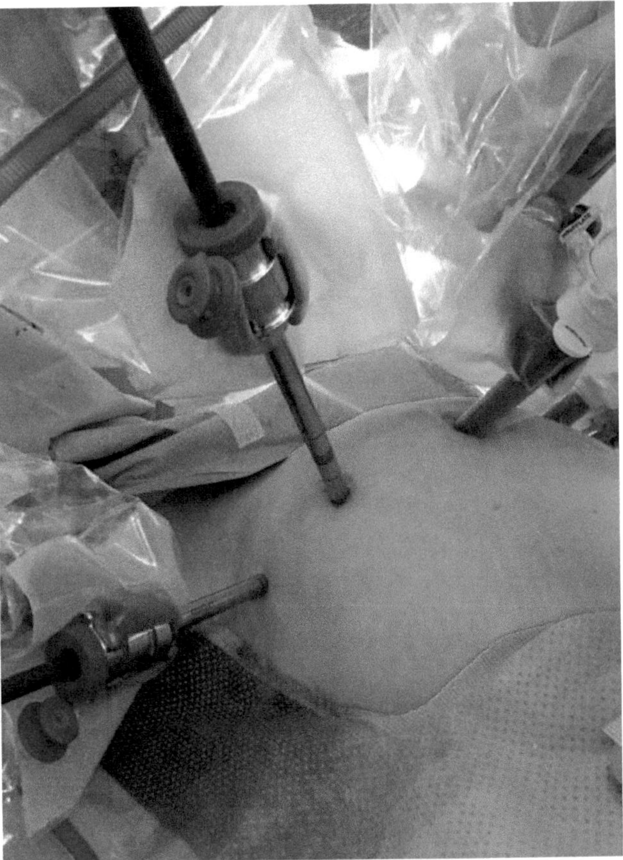

Fig. 65.13 Tips and tricks. S and Si systems: The best use of the obesity trocar is in very thin patients. In a patient with a narrow abdomen the ports will be very close to each other. The figure shows the camera port (right), the obesity trocar for arm 2 (middle) and a regular robotic port for arm 3 (left). This "stacking" will prevent clashing of the robotic arms during the procedure

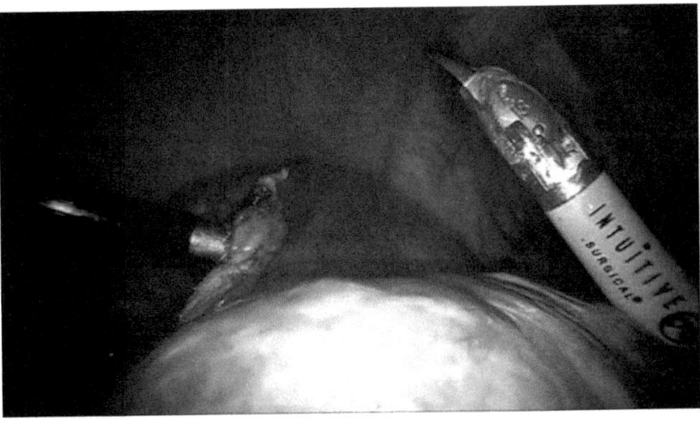

Fig.65.14 A large myoma causes ballooning of the lower uterine segment. In cases like this, changing the 0 ° to a 30 ° camera helps visualization when developing the bladder flap

Sometimes, additional ports may need to be inserted during difficult cases, mostly to assist with bowel retraction and exposure or when instruments cannot reach from one side of

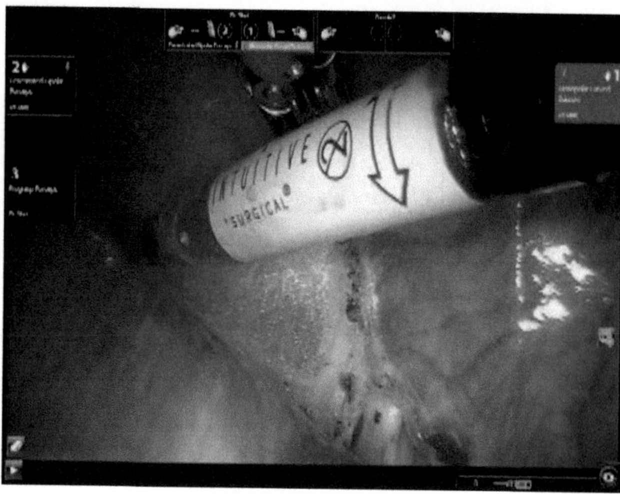

Fig. 65.15 This is an example of how visualization improves when changing the 0° degree to a 30 ° camera. Figure 65.15 shows the maximum achievable visualization with the 0 ° camera

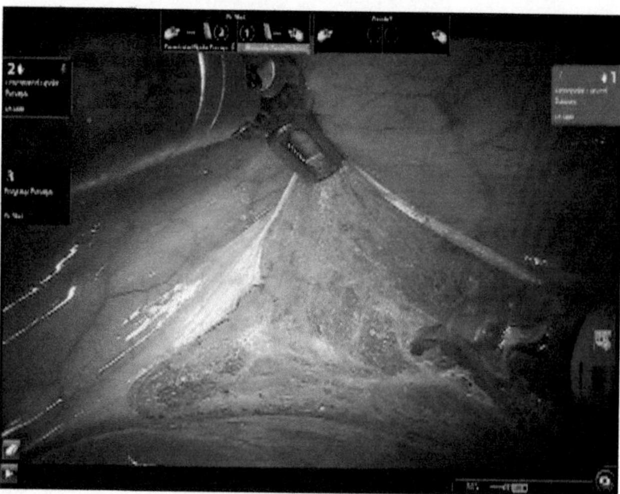

Fig. 65.16 It is easier to complete the bladder serosa incision by switching to the 30 ° down camera

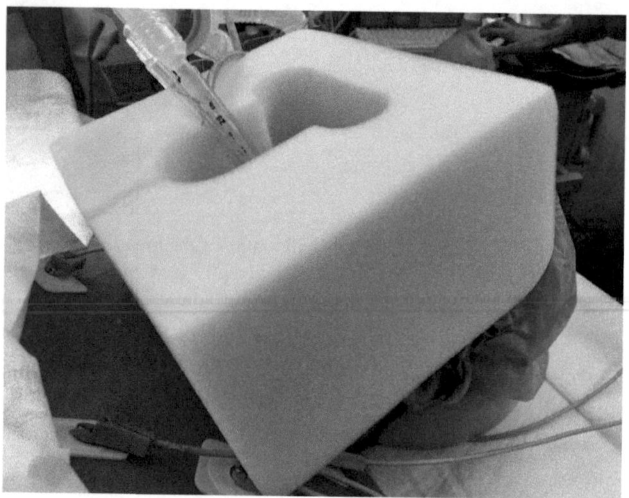

Fig. 65.17 Protection for the patient's face

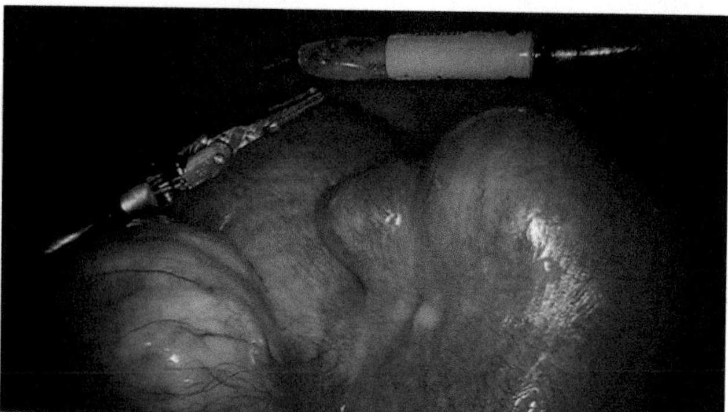

Fig. 65.18 The instruments' reach to the opposite side of the pelvis is severely impaired by the large uterine corpus

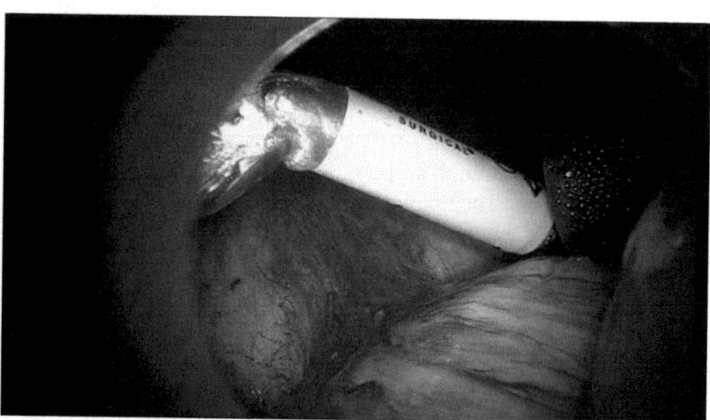

Fig. 65.19 Visualization and maneuvering can be severely impaired. The fat in the right lower corner is from high placement of the port into the falciform ligament

the abdomen over the massive uterus to the other side. In some cases, the uterine size precludes the access of the dissecting instrument used by the dominant hand all the way to the contralateral side across the uterine bulk. Switching the instruments and operating with the nondominant hand while grasping with the dominant hand can overcome this situation (Figs. 65.18 and 65.19).

In patients with previous scars from abdominoplasty, cholecystectomy, or other surgeries, we have inserted the ports through the existing scars, if feasible.

However, these are only guidelines and, depending on the torso length or overall width of the patient, as well as the goals to be achieved during the surgical procedure, the ports should be logically placed so as to maximize maneuverability and visualization.

The assistant port should measure 11 or 12 mm in diameter. This will facilitate insertion of sponges in the peritoneal cavity when needed. The 8 mm robotic ports or a 5 mm assistant port will make this task unfeasible.

The assistant trocar is used for insufflation, and one of the robotic ports is used to attach a smoke evacuator.

For patients with very large uteri, we recommend performing the operations using all four arms of the robotic surgical system. Also, we recommend positioning the robot between the patients' legs (S and Si models) since side-docking severely limits the reach of arm 3 into the upper abdomen. For this setting, the robotic system will be undocked for transvaginal delivery of the uterus. The boom of the Xi model allows side-docking with no impact on the arms' maneuverability.

Robotic Instruments

The main robotic instruments (Intuitive Surgical, Sunnyvale, CA, USA) used are Hot Shears (monopolar curved scissors) with a tip cover accessory and power setting of 50 W for arm 1, fenestrated bipolar forceps with a power setting of 50 W for arm 2, and Cadiere or ProGrasp (Intuitive Surgical, Sunnyvale, CA, USA) forceps for arm 3. The arm numbers are different for the Xi model. Vascular pedicles were coagulated and transected by the scrubbed assistant with a LigaSure sealer/divider (Valleylab, Boulder, CO, USA).

Grasping and traction and counter-traction should be generally avoided. The specimen is too heavy and the tissue will tear and bleed. Instead, manipulation by pushing the uterine corpus is effective in achieving exposure (Figs. 65.20, 65.21, 65.22 and 65.23).

Uterine Manipulator

The uterine manipulator is less useful for manipulation since the uterus is so large. However, when coupled with a cervical cup, it is an excellent tool for delineating the vaginal fornices prior to colpotomy. This is especially useful when the utero-cervical junction is extremely bulky or when abundant adiposity completely obscures the anatomical landmarks. I prefer the Koh Colpotomizer™ System (CooperSurgical, Trumbull, CT) in conjunction with a RUMI® Uterine Manipulator (CooperSurgical, Trumbull, CT) and a Colpo-pneumo Occluder™ balloon. These are inserted prior to port placement. When the manipulator is pushed by the assistant, the distance between the uterine vessels and ureters will increase by up to 1 cm. This additional maneuver helps to protect the ureters from thermal injury. Generally, in heavy patients, the distance between the cervix and ureters is slightly less than in thin patients, but this difference is clinically insignificant. Also, in many cases, as an added difficulty to the lack of visualization and exposure, the distances between the ureters and cervix are not the same on the right and left [18, 19].

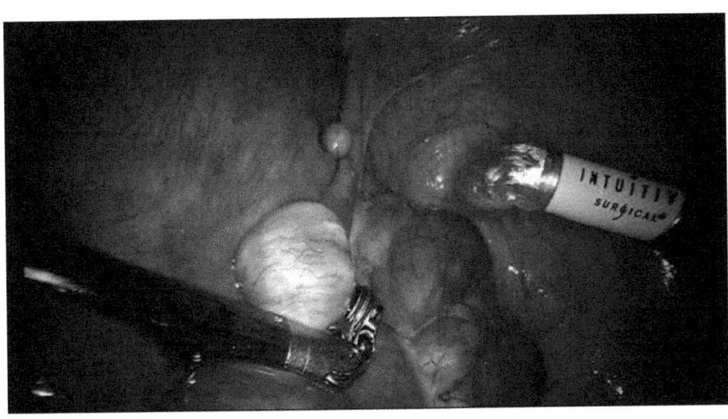

Fig. 65.20 Irregularities in the uterine contour are very helpful for providing grasp and manipulation

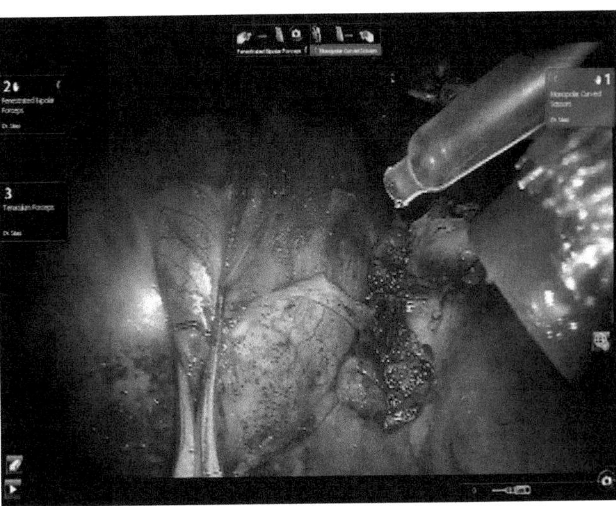

Fig. 65.21 The robotic tenaculum can be used when no other means of manipulation are available. This is frequently the case when lower uterine segments are ballooned out. The insertion site should be carefully chosen. A trial and error approach will result in profuse bleeding from every puncture site

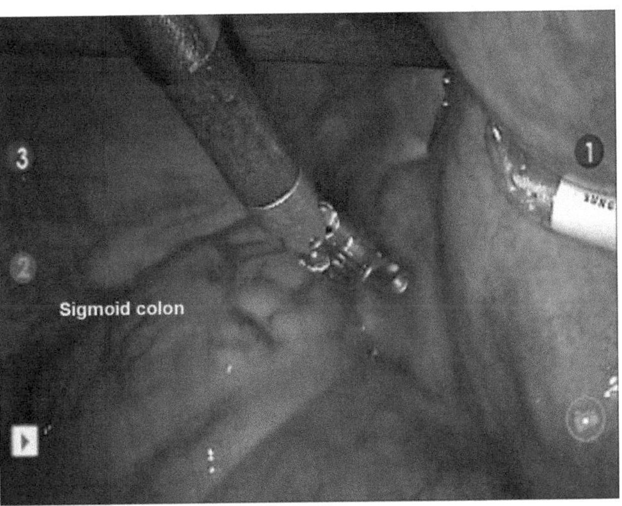

Fig. 65.22 The left ovary is engulfed by expanding leiomyomata. Pushing is a more effective strategy than grasping

Energy Instruments

The cost of the operating instruments is an important consideration for any surgical procedure. The use of the robotic bipolar cautery is effective and inexpensive. However, for the resection of very large uteri I recommend the use of an

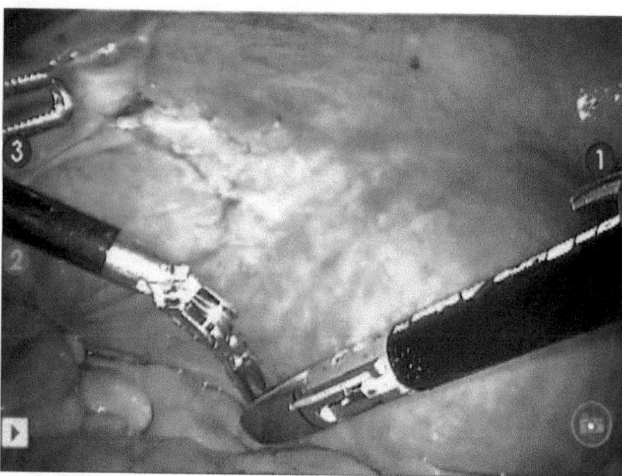

Fig. 65.23 The assistant can help with lifting and manipulation when the uterus is too heavy for the robotic instruments

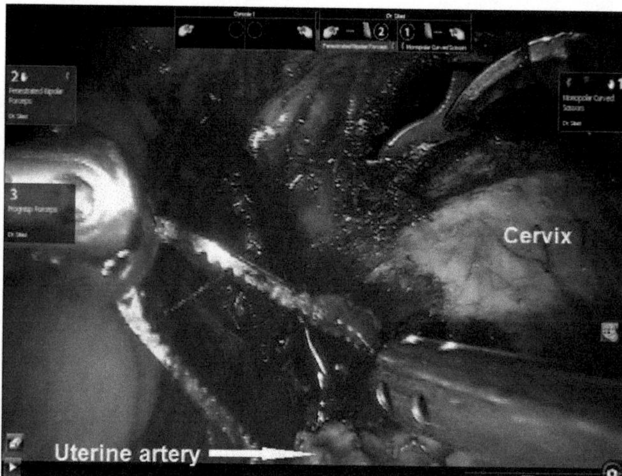

Fig. 65.24 The distal segment of the transected left uterine artery is actively bleeding after sealing was unsuccessful. The fenestrated bipolar cautery will grasp the bleeding vessel

advanced energy device in addition to the traditional bipolar cautery. A wristed vessel sealer is also available for the robotic system. The maneuverability of this device is outstanding but the tradeoff is poor grasping and dissection capabilities.

I prefer a free-hand 5 mm advanced vessel sealer, which will allow freehand laparoscopy when needed. Sometimes these complex procedures require a combination of freehand and robotic laparoscopy. The sealing capacity of the 5 mm instrument is close to that of the wider device with the advantage that this vessel sealer can be inserted through the 8 mm robotic port.

Frequently, one or several of the vessels' diameters will exceed the manufacturer's recommendations for the safe use of any sealing device. In addition, when pelvic edema is present, the vessel walls have a higher than normal water content as well. The efficacy of the sealing devices can be impaired in these circumstances. The vessel wall edema can be anticipated when the dissected retroperitoneal tissues are edematous and fluid is leaking from the open retroperitoneal spaces. Excessive amounts of steam will be released when sealing the vessels: because of the crowded space, the camera is very close to the operative site and the lens will fog. The edema and tissue weeping will resolve once the hysterectomy is completed, sometimes even before the vaginal apex is sutured.

For prevention of catastrophic hemorrhage of very large vessels, I grasp the pedicle with the bipolar cautery while the assistant applies the sealing device on the pedicle. Both ultrasonic and bipolar electrosurgical instruments employ tissue sensing technology and can seal blood vessels with supra-physiologic burst pressure equal to or higher than that of surgical clips or ligatures. The thermal impact to surrounding tissue is minimal [16, 17].

If the sealing is not complete and the vessel is still open after transection, the bipolar cautery will keep the vessels from retracting and can accomplish the following maneuvers:

- Coagulate the vessels held within the jaws of the instrument and achieve hemostasis. Desiccation of the tissues in bipolar diathermy is accomplished when the bubbling stops. The disadvantage of this approach is that when it fails the surgeon is left with the charred end of a (still) bleeding vessel (Fig. 65.24)
- Hold the vessels and apply Weck® Hem-o-lok® polymer clips on the pedicle. The titanium clips available for the robotic system are too small for this task. Alternatively, if the surgeon estimates that successful sealing of the vessels is improbable, the pedicle or individual vessels can be skeletonized and then transected after polymer clips have been applied, without any use of thermal energy (Fig. 65.25)
- One of the advantages of the wristed robotic instruments is the ease of suturing and knot-tying. However, for patients with very large uteri, this advantage is almost always lost because of the very limited space available to perform these maneuvers

Vessels

The most important aspect of hysterectomy for very large uteri is securing the vascular pedicles. Failure to achieve hemostasis in operations where the uterus is massive and extends into the abdominal cavity often leads to abandoning the laparoscopic approach and performing a laparotomy to control the bleeding. It is imperative that meticulous hemostasis is maintained throughout the entire case.

An important reminder is that the anatomy of the pelvic structures can be severely altered. The bladder location and

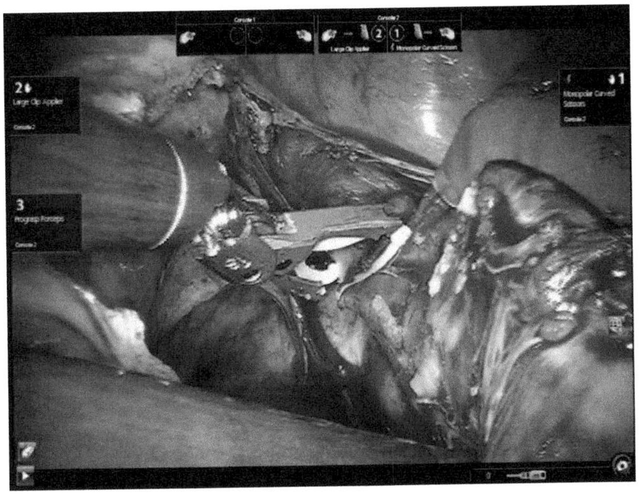

Fig. 65.25 Application of the Weck® Hem-o-lok® polymer clips using the specialized robotic instrument

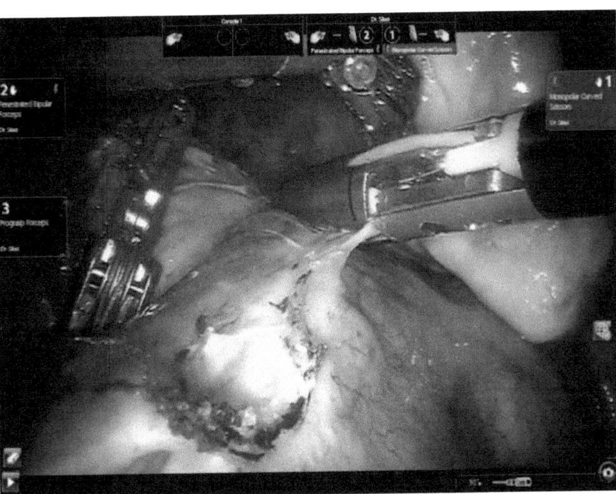

Fig. 65.26 The sealing instrument is applied on the hypertrophic utero-ovarian vascular arcade. The ProGrasp™ instrument is wrapped around the utero-cervical junction: it is very effective in moving the uterus out of the pelvis. I call it the 'choking maneuver'

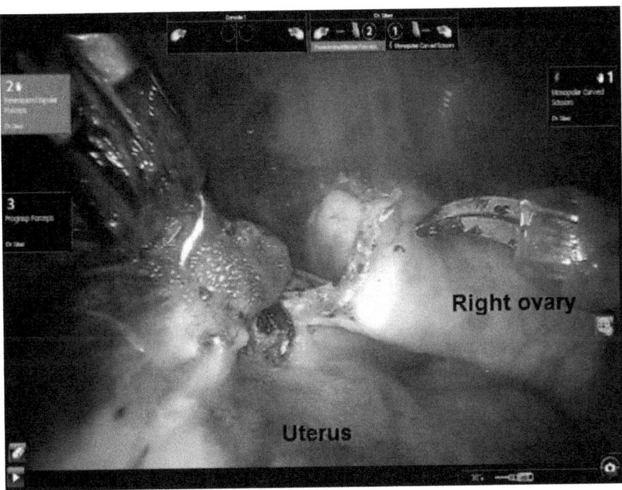

Fig. 65.27 Sealing was incomplete. The severed vessel retracts into the body of the uterus. A lengthy application of bipolar diathermy is necessary to control the bleeding. Ongoing bubbling means that complete desiccation has not occurred yet

contour, the trajectory of the ureters and sometimes even the course of the external iliac or hypogastric vessels can be different than expected. Meticulous dissection is the key to identify these structures and restore the normal anatomy. When the retroperitoneal tissues achieve the foamy appearance caused by pneumodissection, the vessels, ureters, and bladder are easier to identify. However, even a small hemorrhage will saturate the retroperitoneum with blood and obscure the surgical landmarks. Irrigation will also saturate the avascular planes, albeit with a clear and transparent fluid, and it should be avoided if possible. The best approach to improve visualization once the actively bleeding vessels have been secured and the blood is suctioned, is to insert a sponge through the assistant port and dab the bloody site.

Despite limited visualization from above because of the uterine bulk, the location of the four uterine pedicles is quite predictable.

Ovarian Vessels

Even if they are not visible initially, the ovarian vessels are easy to find by pushing the uterus forward.

The anatomy of these pedicles is the most consistent and the infundibulo-pelvic ligaments retain their usual location. They are the easiest to secure, whether the hysterectomy includes adnexectomy or it is performed with the intent of ovarian preservation. The diameter of these vessels is larger than normal. For ovarian preservation, the utero-ovarian arcade can be more difficult to secure if the ovaries are engulfed by the expanding uterus. In this case, care must be taken to seal the vessels thoroughly before transection. When transected without achieving complete hemostasis, the vessels will retract inside the uterine mass and will be out of reach for repeat thermal applications. This will cause profuse bleeding that is very difficult to contain. If there is enough room for maneuvering, it may be prudent to apply the energy device at adjacent spots on any pedicle and increase the probability of sealing. Redundant thermal sealing will increase the operative time but achieving complete hemostasis is very important since these complex procedures leave very little room for error (Figs. 65.26 and 65.27).

It is easier in these procedures, when compared to hysterectomy for normal-size uteri, to avoid thermal injury to the ureters at the pelvic brim while securing the infundibulo-pelvic ligaments. The ovarian vessels are elongated and stretched away from the ureters by the large uterus (Fig. 65.28).

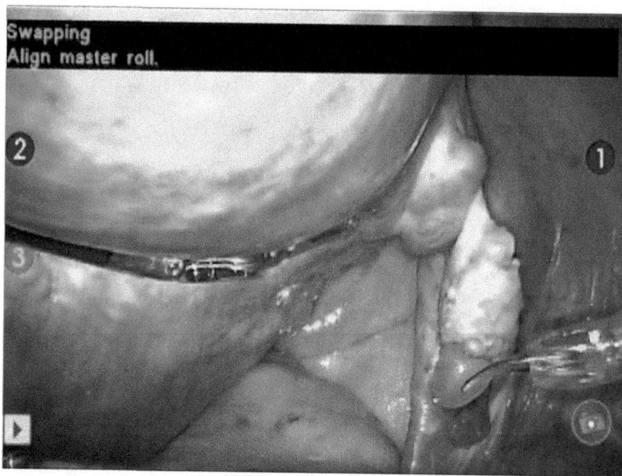

Fig. 65.28 The infundibulo-pelvic ligaments are exposed by lifting the uterus. Routinely they are elongated and stretched away from the ureters

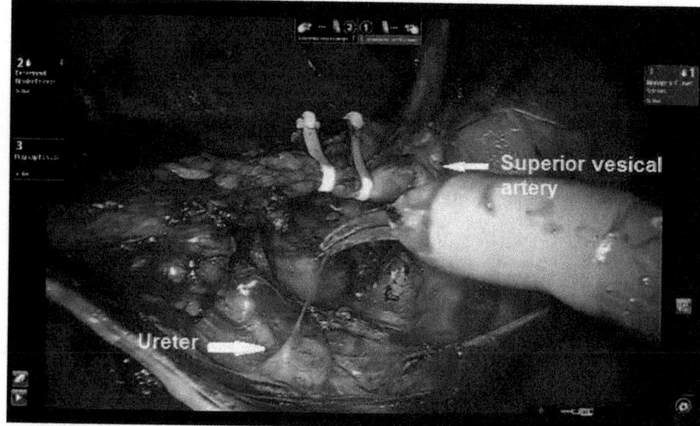

Fig. 65.29 The vessels can be secured at or close to their emergence

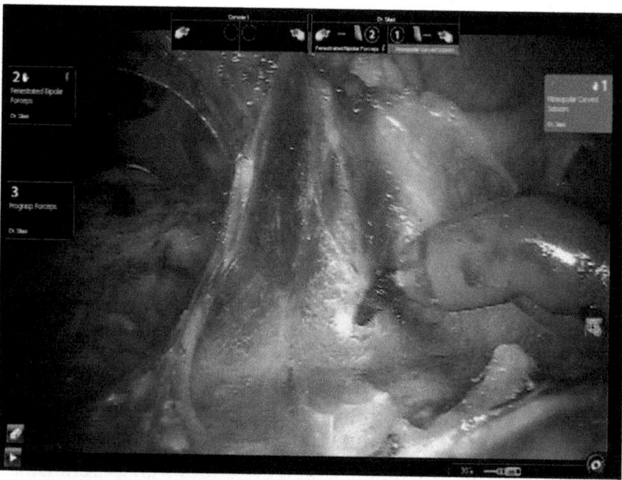

Fig. 65.30 The edema of the retroperitoneal tissues is pronounced as evidenced by the glistening and weeping areolar spaces

Uterine Vascular Supply Below the Pelvic Brim

Unless the anatomical presentation dictates otherwise, I recommend securing the left-sided uterine vessels first, followed by the right-sided ones. The reason is that once three out of four uterine pedicles have been sealed, the fourth will swell up, sometimes markedly so. The absence of the sigmoid colon on the right side of the pelvis allows for better exposure and increased room for maneuvering, which may be necessary to achieve hemostasis.

Arteries

The arteries are hypertrophic because of the increased blood supply and the surgeon will frequently encounter unusual branching. Even the ascending cervical artery, an insignificant vessel in normal circumstances, can flood the pelvis when transected without effective sealing.

Frequently, the uterine bulk completely obscures the utero-cervical junction. A simple strategy to find the uterine vessels is to follow the lateral uterine contour down into the pelvis after dissection of the avascular space of Graves. For better visualization of the vessels, the 0 ° camera may need to be changed to a 30 ° down camera. The camera will sneak in between the massively enlarged uterus and pelvic sidewall and may need to be rotated clockwise on the right and counterclockwise on the left to achieve visualization.

If the uterine vessels cannot be secured at the utero-cervical junction, the alternative is to coagulate them at the emergence from the superior vesical artery. At this proximal level, the arterial wall is less edematous and the success of thermal sealing with one application is higher. The ureter should be identified and mobilized if necessary. The para-vesical and para-rectal spaces should be developed in the same manner as in a radical hysterectomy and the skeletonized vessels can be sealed safely (Fig. 65.29).

Excessive blood loss can occur when the sealing device cannot achieve complete hemostasis of the uterine vessels, especially when the vessel diameter exceeds the recommended 7 mm size. In addition, the retroperitoneal tissues and the vessel walls can be quite edematous from impaired venous return, and although collagen denaturation will occur, tissue desiccation can be suboptimal after firing the sealing device (Fig. 65.30).

When the diameter of the vessels, especially of the veins, is too large, we recommend skeletonizing the components of the pedicle and sealing the vessels individually (Fig. 65.31).

For smaller vessels, if hemostasis is not complete, titanium clips can correct the problem when applied by the assistant or by the robotic arm while the operator holds and exposes the bleeding vessel. Despite the fact that placement of suture ligatures are facilitated by the articulated wrist, this is usually not possible because of the limited space.

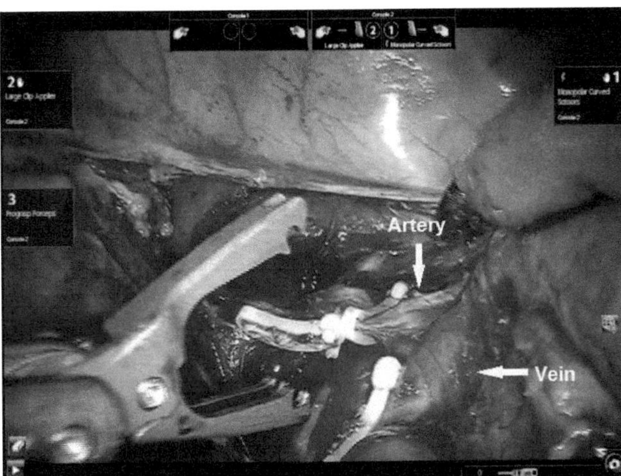

Fig. 65.31 The dilated uterine vein is secured first, followed by the artery

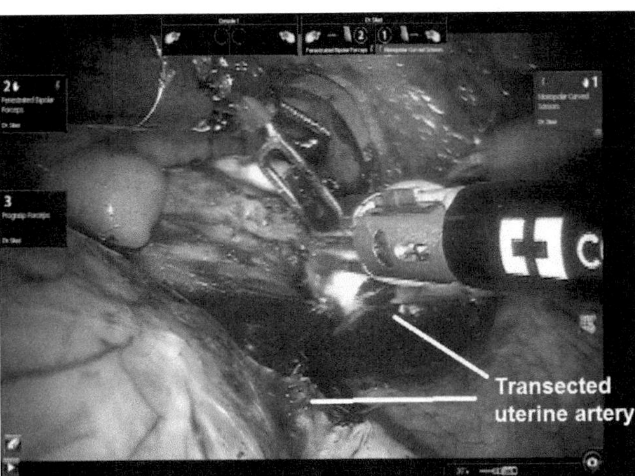

Fig. 65.33 The sealing was unsuccessful

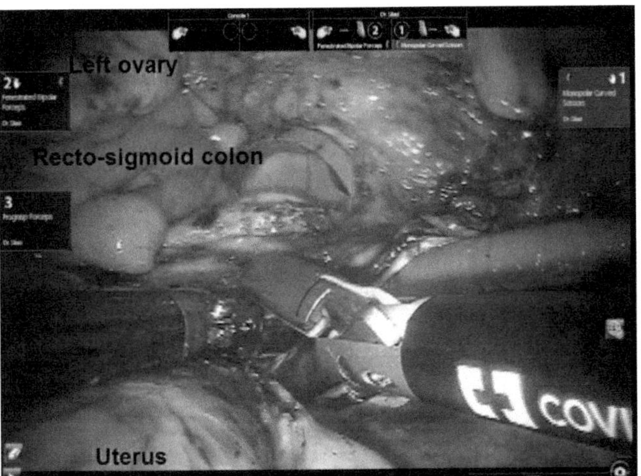

Fig. 65.32 The sealer divider is applied on the right uterine pedicle

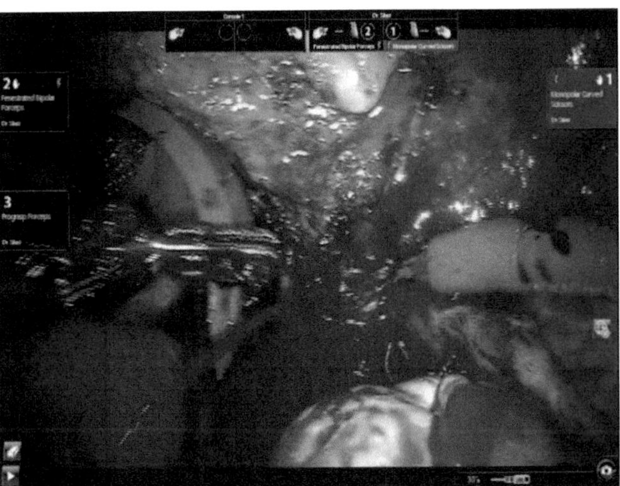

Fig. 65.34 Active bleeding from the uterine artery

In very difficult cases, when the surgeon is confronted with a lower uterine segment too large to allow access to both uterine arteries with the sealing device from the assistant port, the placement of a sixth port in a convenient location can provide the required access (Figs. 65.32, 65.33, 65.34 and 65.35). In morbidly obese patients this additional port can be used for a bowel retractor to improve exposure. Alternatively, the wristed vessel sealer of the robotic system can be used with any arm, for a multitude of angles.

Veins

The enlarged vein diameter is caused by the increased blood supply, but it is also compounded by the impaired venous return produced by the mechanical compression of the hypertrophic uterus resting on the great vessels in the pelvis. Special consideration needs to be given to the venous plexus

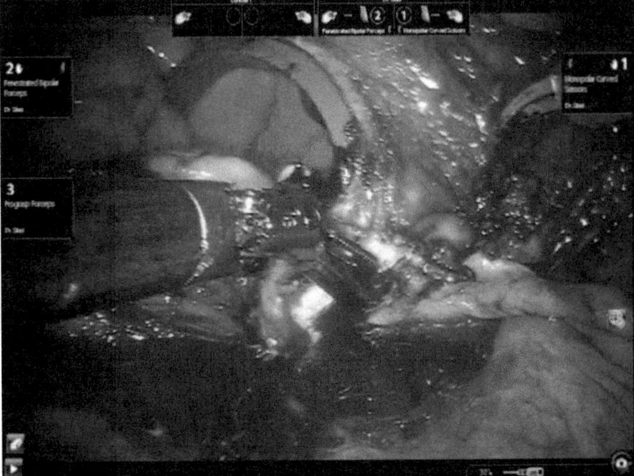

Fig. 65.35 The artery retracts, floods the pelvis and can be difficult to secure. Prior lateral mobilization of the ureter is essential to avoiding thermal injury when exposure is severely limited

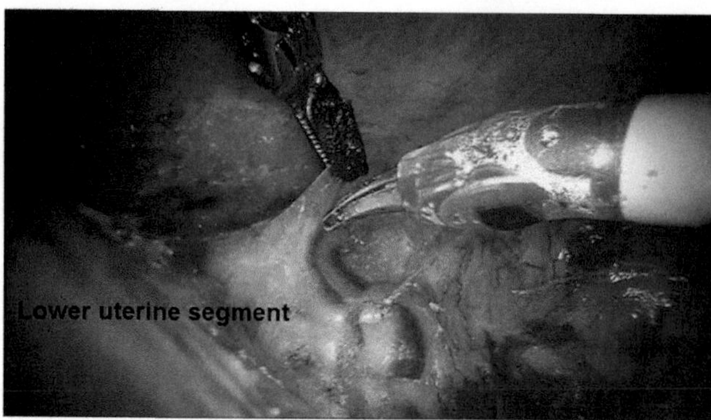

Fig. 65.36 The anatomy of the venous plexus of the bladder is unpredictable and meticulous dissection is required

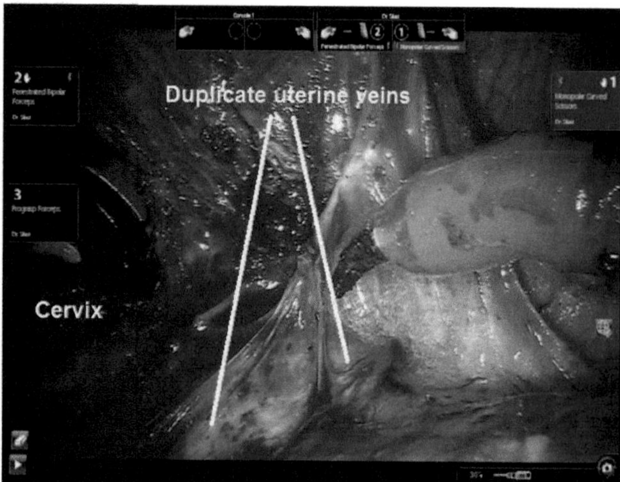

Fig. 65.37 The diameter of the very wide double veins can be estimated intraoperatively by comparing it to the known size of one of the instruments

of the bladder when leiomyomata are ballooning out the lower uterine segment. These vessels have highly irregular locations, are very tortuous, and tend to be severely engorged and prone to easy bleeding. Once injured, they will flood the pelvis and will be very difficult to secure (Fig. 65.36).

Indiscriminate suction to evacuate the blood will collapse the pneumoperitoneum and the intestines will slide from the upper abdomen over the sacral promontory and pile up on top of the pelvic organs. The trocars are fixed to the robotic arms and the collapse of the anterior abdominal wall may cause the loss of one or more ports at a time when complete access and visualization are critical (Fig. 65.37).

Special emphasis has to be placed on neovascularization when the uterine leiomyomata extend into the retroperitoneum, as is frequently the case. Vessels of various origins and calibers will feed and drain the leiomyomata that grow into the virtual spaces of the retroperitoneum. Most commonly, the location of these uterine extensions are deep within the broad ligaments and in the pararectal spaces. Involvement of the paravesical spaces or Waldeyer's space is less common. A thorough knowledge of the retroperitoneum is required if the uterine bulk extends into the retroperitoneal virtual spaces and distorts the normal anatomy.

Bleeding

Blood loss is inherent to surgery and while all surgeons strive for bloodless procedures and dry operative fields, heavy bleeding will happen occasionally, irrespective of the level of skill or experience. However, the level of skill and experience will determine how fast the hemorrhage will be stopped.

Prevention is key and one of the steps that should always be be accomplished is mobilization of the bladder and ureters laterally at enough distance to prevent thermal injury to these structures in case repeat application of heat is required. The classic teaching is to seal (or clamp) the uterine vessels intimately close to the cervix, and the residents are thought to bounce the instrument off the cervix while closing the jaws. This technique leaves no room for error if the vessels bleed after transection. They will inevitably retract and make re-grasping and sealing very difficult. Instead, the sealer/divider should be applied slightly more lateral to the cervix and this will compensate for vessel retraction in the event of non-sealing. However, this approach requires intraoperative knowledge of the ureter trajectory.

Other prevention methods that can be used:

- The surgeon develops the para vesical and para-rectal spaces similar to a radical hysterectomy and the uterine vessels are secured at this level. The linear segment of uterine artery as it crosses over the ureter is one of the most stable characteristics of this otherwise tortuous vessel (Figs. 65.38 and 65.39)
- An X-ray detectable sponge inserted into the peritoneal cavity prior to attempting to seal the vessels can be an useful adjunct in case the bleeding vessel is not easily discernible. It has a much greater surface than the robotic/laparoscopic instruments and can be used to tamponade the bleeding area. The robotic system provides the surgeon with the advantage of locking in place the arm with the sponge without getting tired. This time can be gainfully used to suction the pool of blood, dissect around the area with the other two arms, and have the circulator nurse bring needed supplies into the room (Fig. 65.40)

Arterial blood can squirt on the camera lens and completely obscure the view. This is unusual for venous hemorrhage.

If only one lens of the binocular camera is affected, there is no need to waste valuable time to clean the camera and the surgeon can continue to operate using only one eye until the hemorrhage is contained. If the loss of visualization is

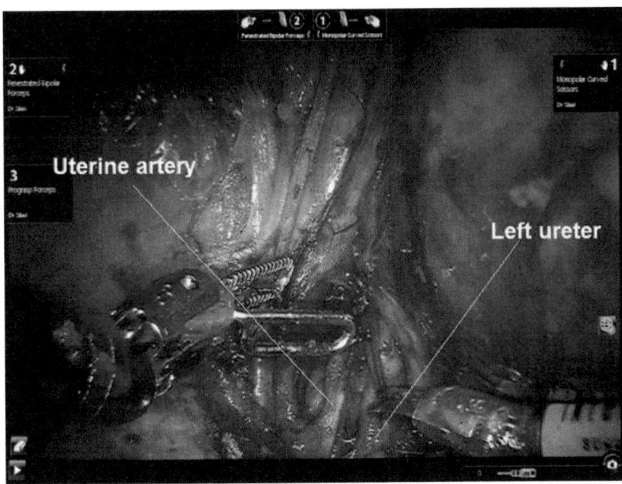

Fig. 65.38 Dissection of the retroperitoneum with emphasis on the ureter and uterine artery

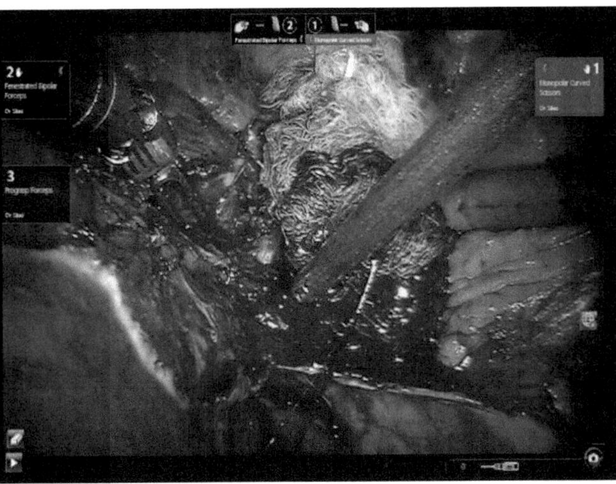

Fig. 65.40 The sponge is held in place with arm 1. Arm 2 with the bipolar cautery is holding one end of the bleeding vessel while the assistant uses the suction to clean the operative field

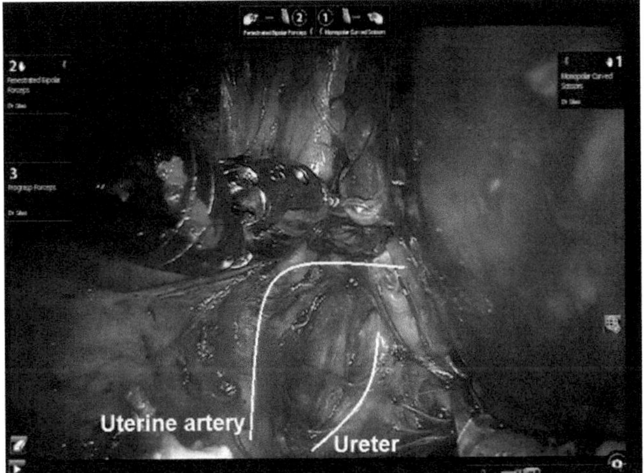

Fig. 65.39 Once dissection is completed, the uterine artery is easily elevated away from the ureter. The uterus is too large for the sealing device to reach from across the abdomen but the bipolar cautery in arm 2 will be used to desiccate the vessel

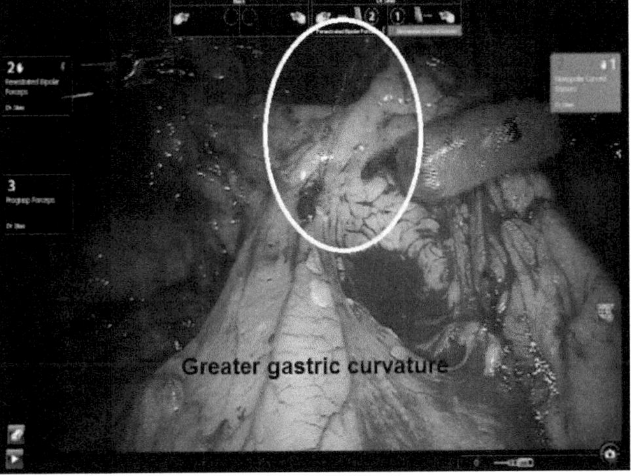

Fig. 65.41 No hysterectomy images were available for blood squirting onto the lens. However, the problem is the same regardless of the procedure. Blood from one of the short gastric vessels shoots towards the lens during omentectomy

complete, the surgeon will move the camera back and point it straight down. This simple move that changes the angle of the camera to the patient's axis will greatly facilitate the ability of the assistant to remove the camera and clean it at a time when seconds matter (Figs. 65.41 and 65.42).

In the rare event when the previously described intra-abdominal sponge was not damp or soaked, I have used it to clean the lens with the robotic arm, with inconsistent results.

If bleeding is uncontrollable, do not hesitate to undock the robot and perform a laparotomy. In most but the life-threatening cases, a Pfannenstiel or Maylard incision will be adequate to access the uterine vessels proper. The risk of bladder injury is minimal since the bladder was already mobilized caudad. There is no need to access the mid- and upper abdomen to reach the ovarian pedicles; they were already secured. Once the bleeding vessels are secured and the colpotomy completed, the specimen can be easily delivered through the new incision.

Lymphatics

Occasionally, the surgeon encounters massively distended lymphatic vessels with serpiginous channels of 1–2 cm diameter accompanying, wrapping around, and obscuring the blood vessels. Lymphatic drainage, even more so than venous drainage, can be severely impaired by the mechanical obstruction caused by the large and irregular uterus. There is

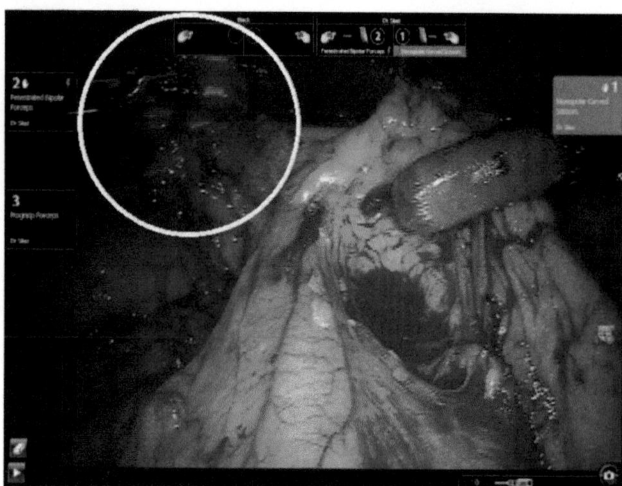

Fig. 65.42 The recording shows the blood drops immediately before they splash into the camera

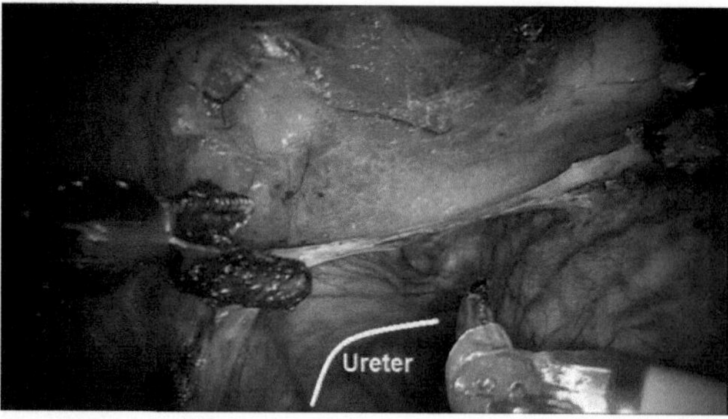

Fig. 65.43 Favorable situations like this one are rare: there is no edema or neovascularization, and the ureter can be easily identified

no corresponding lymphedema of the lower extremities, but cystic spaces of up to several centimeters in size surround the uterine vessels and are filled with clear straw-colored fluid. Their presence can surprise the operating physician. A sudden gush of this clear fluid can be misinterpreted as injury to urinary structures but is of no consequence.

Complications

The following retroperitoneal structures need to be identified and dissected with caution: the external iliac and hypogastric vessels and the ureters.

Injuries to the Ureter

The identification of the ureter trajectory is imperative before applying an energy source to seal any uterine vessels (Figs. 65.43 and 65.44).

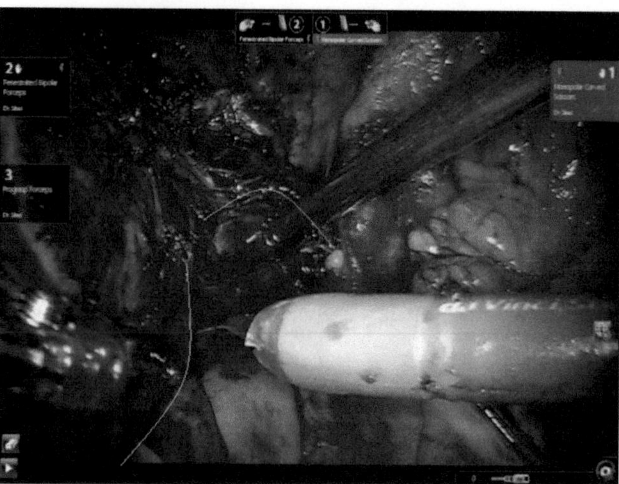

Fig. 65.44 This is an example of an unfavorable situation. There is bleeding, fibrosis, and poorly defined surgical planes. The trajectories of the ureter and uterine artery are more a guess than a certainty. In such cases, patience and meticulous dissection are required

The uterine vessels are pushed laterally by the expanding lower uterine segment and are in closer proximity than usual to the ureters. In addition, the anatomy can be significantly distorted and the ureters pushed cephalad by the uterus as it grows out of the pelvis. It is not unusual for the ureters to be at the same or higher level than the superior vesical artery. For this reason, sometimes it is easier to seal the uterine vessels at their origin from the anterior division of the hypogastric artery. The ureters are easiest to identify at the bifurcation of the common iliac arteries, as they dive into the pelvis. From there, their trajectory can be followed to the level of the uterine vessels and into the ureter tunnel. Another good landmark for ureter identification is where it crosses under the uterine artery.

Precise identification of the ureter course into the retroperitoneum has important practical implications. Incomplete sealing of the vessels requires re-application of thermal energy in a crowded pelvis, while the visualization is impaired from the accumulating blood. Knowledge of the ureters' trajectories will afford the opportunity to use energy more liberally.

Transperitoneal observation of ureteral peristalsis at the pelvic brim provides no assurance that thermal injury or transection below the pelvic brim has been avoided. While complete ureterolysis is not necessary in all cases, the surgeon should be proficient in this procedure and perform it when necessary (Figs. 65.45 and 65.46).

When extensive ureterolysis has been performed and the ureter is readily visible, injuries can easily be averted. However, comprehensive visualization of the ureter is not always possible. Ureter injury prevention relies heavily on mobilizing the ureter laterally, away from the vessels where thermal energy will be applied. Adequate mobilization of the

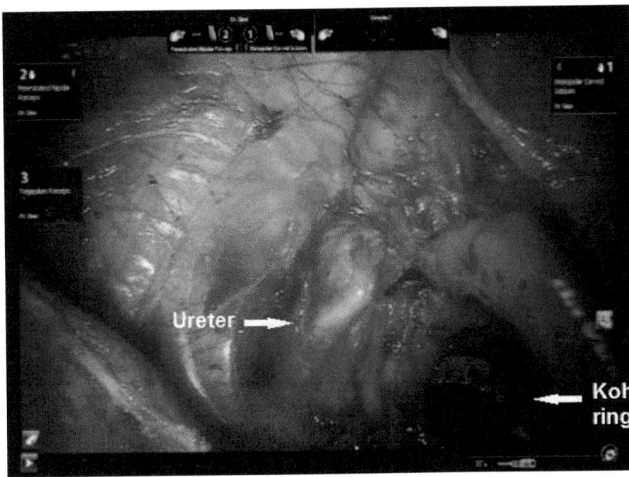

Fig. 65.45 The left ureter is very close to the colpotomy incision despite pushing the colpotomy ring from below

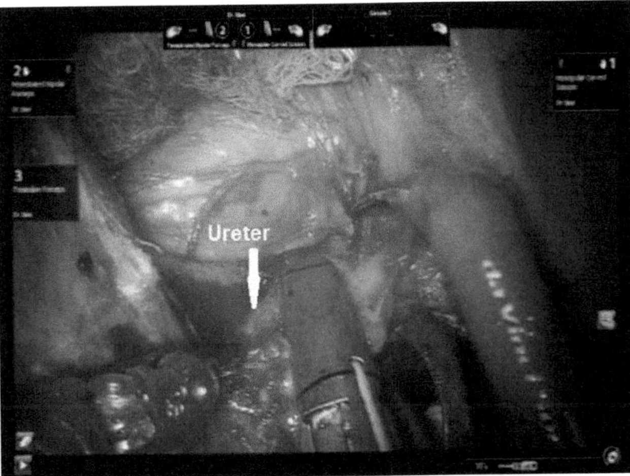

Fig. 65.46 The ureter is immediately adjacent to the vessels. An overzealous assistant attempts to apply the sealer divider on the vessels and ureter. Previous dissection of the left ureter allowed timely identification and prevention of thermal injury

bladder flap will move the ureters laterllay. Also, pushing the uterine manipulator cephalad will add up to 1 cm to the distance between the point of sealing the uterine vessels and the trajectory of the ureters, thus adding an additional maneuver of protecting the ureters from thermal injury [18].

A study performed at Ben-Gurion University in Israel evaluated this extremely important aspect in hysterectomy: the anatomical proximity between the cervix and the ureters. The distance between the ureters and the cervix was measured in 499 computerized tomography (CT) studies at the most dorsal reflection of the ureters. At least one ureter was within 0.5 cm of the cervix in 3.6 % of patients with normal CT scans and in 10.3 % of patients with cervical pathology. Overall, the right ureter was significantly closer to the cervix than the left (2.0 ± −0.8 cm vs. 2.2 ± 1.0 cm, $p < 0.05$). In cases were the pathology was limited to the cervix, the right ureter was more distant than the left (2.0 ± 0.6 cm vs. 1.7 ± 0.6 cm, $p < 0.05$). The distance between the ureters and the cervix was inversely correlated with the lateral diameter of the cervix ($r = 0.18$, $p < 0.001$) and its anterior-posterior diameter ($r = 0.11$, $p < 0.001$) [19].

A study from the University of Indianapolis in the United States was aimed at determining the distance of the ureter from the cervix and the influence of age and weight on this distance. In 52 patients, at the most dorsal reflection of the ureter, the average distance from ureter to cervical margin was 2.3 ± 0.8 cm (range, 0.1–5.3 cm). There was no relationship to age, but there was a linear relationship between this distance and body mass index (R2 = 0.075; P = .049); thus the ureter was slightly more proximal to the cervical margin in heavier women. They concluded that in women with apparently normal pelvic anatomy, the average distance between the ureter and cervix is >2 cm but this distance is <0.5 cm in 12 % of the patients studied [20].

We have not used the preoperative placement of regular or lighted ureteral stents to facilitate intraoperative ureter identification and we recommend against the practice of universal cystoscopy during major gynecologic cases.

Injuries to the Vessels

The prevention of injuries to the aorta or vena cava at the beginning of the procedure require full attention of the surgeon. Trivial aspects and sounds common to the start of any procedure such as the scrub technician setting up the instrumens, with the accompanying noise, the beeping of the monitors, and everybody talking at once, can distract the operator. However, no other surgical inadvertent situation can change the fate of the entire procedure within seconds and put the patient's life at risk.

My preference for insufflation is the Verres needle with the gas on high flow and as it penetrates the abdominal wall into the peritoneal cavity, the gas pressure readings provide the surgeon with useful information and decrease the 'blindness' of the blind insertion. Insertion injuries of the solid organs like liver, kidney, pancreas, are exceedingly rare and a clean needle stick does not need to be addressed. The only life-threatening injury that demands immediate attention is to the greater vessels. For obese patients, the point of entry into the abdomen in relationship to the retroperitoneal greater vessels is higher than for thin patients and for patients with very high BMI the needle is not long enough to reach the vessels. However, the surgeon should keep in mind the possibility of vessel injury and retroperitoneal hemorrhage. A retroperitoneal hematoma needs to be observed for expansion with the intra-abdominal pressure decreased to a minimum. If it appears stable, the surgeon can continue with the procedure. Re-insufflation of the peritoneal cavity for the duration of the procedure will add to the hemostatic effect. Retroperitoneal exploration is usually counterproductive in small injuries of the great vessels and should be reserved for large iatrogenic defects.

Other penetrating injuries of the great vessels are immediately evident. The uterine bulk severely limits exposure and maneuvering space and these injuries can be life-threatening. If feasible, one of the robotic graspers can hold and approximate the vessel defect tight while titanium clips are applied by the assistant or the robotic specialized instrument. Vessel suturing can be accomplished much easier with the robotic system than with conventional laparoscopic instruments.

In patients with very large uteri, the trajectory of the external iliac vessels is less affected than that of the ureters. The hypogastric vessels have the most stable presentation, with the exception of the anterior division.

When the uterus expands into the retroperitoneum, neovascularization is present and unpredictable. Meticulous and gentle dissection will avoid tears, especially of the veins. A previously inserted sponge is much more effective in applying pressure and containing the bleeding than the instrument alone.

The surgeon should notify the anesthesiology team immediately if a major injury occurs. Do not hesitate to perform an emergent laparotomy if the hemorrhage cannot be contained laparoscopically.

In patients with uteri up to 16–18 weeks' size, the organ can be visualized in its entirety at all times throughout the procedure. For very large uteri, 24–30 weeks' size and above, the organ is too large and extends beyond the visual field of the surgeon. For this reason, I strongly recommend periodic surveillance of the already sealed pedicles. While the operator is focused on the lower uterine segment, the pressure and traction applied on the corpus for manipulation and visualization purposes can force the previously sealed utero-ovarian vessels to re-open. The surgeon will not notice this extensive hemorrhage since the blood will be pooling into the upper abdomen because of the Trendelenburg position. This complication is unique to these procedures.

Injuries to the Bladder

The use of the 30° down laparoscope is helpful when developing the bladder flap.

If injured, the bladder can be easily repaired once the uterus is removed. The defect should be closed in several layers. The wristed instruments facilitate suturing greatly. Imbricating the tissues is aided by the redundancy of a bladder that was extensively stretched by the enlarged uterus (Figs. 65.47 and 65.48).

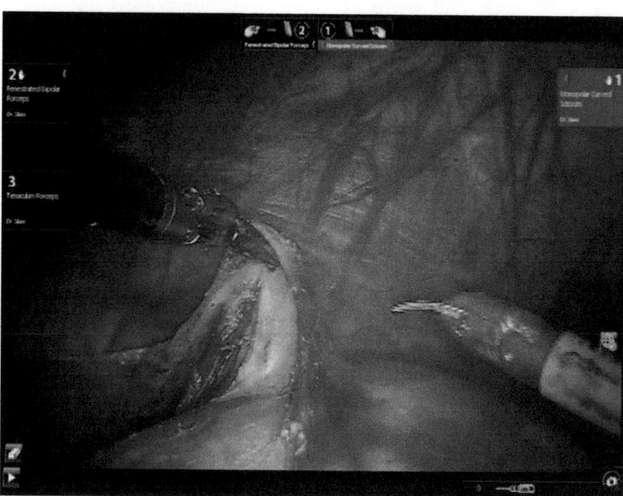

Fig. 65.47 A large anterior myoma has stretched the bladder and the bladder serosa reflection is almost at the level of the umbilicus

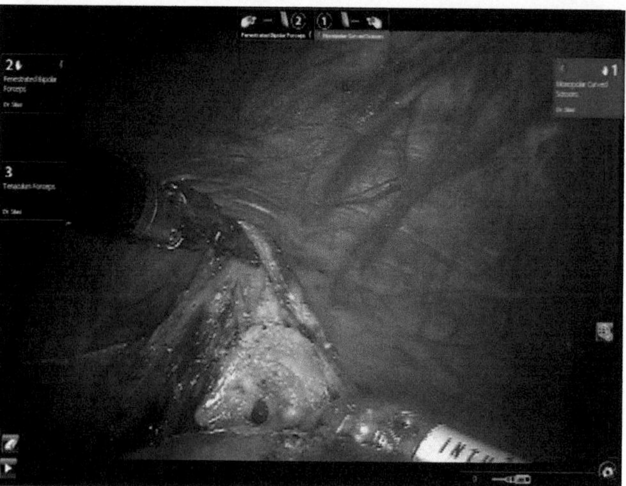

Fig. 65.48 The bladder wall is very thin at this level and a more careful dissection would have avoided the cystotomy

Delivery of the Specimen

The tests available to diagnose uterine sarcomas preoperatively are unreliable. The incidence of uterine sarcomas in patients with leiomyomata is the subject of significant controversy and the use of power morcellators has been the focus of the Federal Drug Administration [20].

The surgical presentations addressed in this chapter are not cases where the uterus can be delivered intact transvaginally. If cancer is diagnosed or suspected preoperatively, the hysterectomy should be accomplished by laparotomy. Techniques where the uterus with endometrial cancer is cored or spirally sliced to fit in the vagina and is delivered without intraperitoneal spillage have been described [21, 22].

However, these techniques are not applicable to uteri of this size when cancer is suspected or diagnosed.

The technique of power morcellation in a bag has been described but no commercially available bags exist for specimens this large.

After complete devascularization and separation of the uterus, the large specimens are removed by two methods: (1) piecemeal delivery of the uterus through the vagina or (2) piecemeal delivery of the uterus through mini-laparotomy.

Specimen removal, especially the transvaginal approach, accounts for a considerable part of the operative time. Delivery is facilitated when extensive adenomyosis is present, making the uterus soft. Also, multiple small leiomyomata can be individually shelled from their pseudocapsule and this will also aid delivery. The least desirable situation for delivery is the presence of a single very large and very firm leiomyoma.

Transvaginal Delivery

If the robotic system is docked between the patient's legs, undocking provides a much greater range of motion for the operator and assistant and allows the return of the patient to a horizontal or minimal Trendelenburg position for the duration of the specimen removal. The uterus is grasped and gradually brought into the vagina and cut piecemeal with scissors and/or a scalpel while Breisky-Navratil vaginal retractors provide exposure and protection of the vaginal walls. All cutting occurs in the vagina without contamination of the peritoneal cavity. Inevitably, blood and other fluids will run off from the uterus while it is being cut into pieces. Removing the patient from the Trendelenburg position will prevent contamination of the peritoneal cavity with these fluids. Any type of morcellation can be used: bisection, coring, "paper-roll" technique, or wedge morcellation [23–25].

Special consideration should be given to old and infarcted leiomyomata that are completely calcified and larger than the vaginal caliber. When sharp instruments are unable to cut through this tissue, monopolar cautery on high power can penetrate the tissue. Delivery of these specimens is very tedious.

Transabdominal Delivery

Some patients will present with a narrow and/or long vagina. In these cases, enlarging one of the port sites or performing a suprapubic mini-laparotomy allows piecemeal delivery of the uterus. However, this approach will contaminate the peritoneal cavity and abdominal wall with uterine debris.

Conclusion

Resection of very large uteri using the robotic system is a feasible alternative to laparotomy, regardless of the patients' body habitus. However, it requires sophisticated surgical skills and is a more time-consuming approach. Without doubt, the benefits of this approach to the patients surpass the longer operative times and the higher costs associated with the amortization of the robotic system.

References

1. Cohen SL, Vitonis AF, Einarsson JI. Updated hysterectomy surveillance and factors associated with minimally invasive hysterectomy. JSLS. 2014;18(3)
2. Vilos GA, Allaire C, Laberge PY, Leyland N; Special Contributors, Vilos AG, Murji A, Chen I. The management of uterine leiomyomas. J Obstet Gynaecol Can 2015; 37(2):157–181.
3. Smorgick N, Dalton VK, Patzkowsky KE, Hoffman MR, Advincula AP, As-Sanie S. Comparison of 2 minimally invasive routes for hysterectomy of large uteri. Int J Gynaecol Obstet. 2013;122(2):128–31.
4. Marana R, Busacca M, Zupi E, Garcea N, Paparella P, Catalano GF. Laparoscopically assisted vaginal hysterectomy versus total abdominal hysterectomy: a prospective, randomized multicenter study. Am J Obstet Gynecol. 1999;180:270–5.
5. Ferrari MM, Berlanda N, Mezzopane R, Ragusa G, Cavallo M, Pardi G. Identifying the indications for laparoscopically assisted vaginal hysterectomy: a prospective, randomized comparison with abdominal hysterectomy in patients with symptomatic uterine fibroids. BJOG. 2000;107:620–5.
6. Uccella S, Cromi A, Casarin J, Bogani G, Serati M, Gisone B, Pinelli C, Fasola M, Ghezzi F. Minilaparoscopic versus standard laparoscopic hysterectomy for uteri ≥ 16 weeks of gestation: surgical outcomes, postoperative quality of life, and cosmesis. J Laparoendosc Adv Surg Tech A. 2015;25(5):386–91.
7. Kovac SR. Route of hysterectomy: an evidence-based approach. Clin Obstet Gynecol. 2014;57(1):58–71.
8. Sinha R, Sundaram M, Lakhotia S, Hedge A, Kadam P. Total laparoscopic hysterectomy in women with previous cesarean sections. J Minim Invasive Gynecol. 2010;17(4):513–7.
9. Loring M, Morris SN, Isaacson KB. Minimally invasive specialists and rates of laparoscopic hysterectomy. JSLS. 2015;19(1):e2014.00221.
10. Silasi DA, Gallo T, Silasi M, Menderes G, Azodi M. Robotic versus abdominal hysterectomy for very large uteri. JSLS. 2013;17(3):400–6.
11. Uccella S, Cromi A, Serati M, Casarin J, Sturla D, Ghezzi F. Laparoscopic hysterectomy in case of uteri weighing ≥1 kilogram: a series of 71 cases and review of the literature. J Minim Invasive Gynecol. 2014;24(3):460–5.
12. Alperin M, Kivnick S, Poon KY. Outpatient laparoscopic hysterectomy for large uteri. J Minim Invasive Gynecol. 2012;19(6):689–94.
13. Uccella S, Cromi A, Bogani G, Casarin J, Formenti G, Ghezzi F. Systematic implementation of laparoscopic hysterectomy independent of uterus size: clinical effect. J Minim Invasive Gynecol. 2013;20(4):505–16.
14. Stoelinga B, Huirne J, Heymans MW, Reekers JA, Ankum WM, Hehenkamp WJ. The estimated volume of the fibroid uterus: a comparison of ultrasound and bimanual examination versus volume at MRI or hysterectomy. Eur J Obstet Gynecol Reprod Biol. 2015;184:89–96.
15. Ryan NA, Ng VS, Sangi-Haghpeykar H, Guan X. Evaluating mechanical bowel preparation prior to total laparoscopic hysterectomy. JSLS. 2015;19(3)

16. Paul PG, Prathap T, Kaur H, Shabnam K, Kandhari D, Chopade G. Secondary hemorrhage after total laparoscopic hysterectomy. JSLS 2014 Jul-Sep;18(3).
17. Camran Nezhat, MD, Michael Lewis, MD, Louise P. King, MD, JD. Laparoscopic vessel sealing devices. Prevention and management of laparoendoscopic surgical complications, 3rd edition.
18. DA Silasi. Robotic surgery in the morbidly obese patient: a surgeon's planning guide. Contemporary OB/GYN. http://contemporaryobgyn.modernmedicine.com/contemporary-obgyn/news/robotic-surgery-morbidly-obese-patient-surgeon-s-planning-guide
19. Hurd WW, Chee SS, Gallagher KL, Ohl DA, Hurteau JA. Location of the ureters in relation to the uterine cervix by computed tomography. Am J Obstet Gynecol. 2001;184(3):336–9.
20. Gemer O, Simonovsky A, Huerta M, Kapustian V, Anteby E, Linov L. A radiological study on the anatomical proximity of the ureters and the cervix. Int Urogynecol J Pelvic Floor Dysfunct. 2007;18(9):991–5.
21. Harris JA, Swenson CW, Uppal S, Kamdar N, Mahnert N, As-Sanie S, Morgan DM. Practice patterns and postoperative complications before and after food and drug administration safety communication on power morcellation. Am J Obstet Gynecol. 2015;214(1):98.e1–98.e13.
22. Favero G, Miglino G, Köhler C, Pfiffer T, Silva E, Silva A, Ribeiro A, Le X, Anton C, Baracat EC, Carvalho JP. Vaginal morcellation inside protective pouch: a safe strategy for uterine extration in cases of bulky endometrial cancers: operative and oncological safety of the method. J Minim Invasive Gynecol. 2015;22(6):938–43.
23. Montella F, Riboni F, Cosma S, Dealberti D, Prigione S, Pisani C, Rovetta E. A safe method of vaginal longitudinal morcellation of bulky uterus with endometrial cancer in a bag at laparoscopy. Surg Endosc. 2014;28(6):1949–53.
24. Montella F, Cosma S, Riboni F, Dealberti D, Benedetto C, Abate S. A safe and simple laparoscopic cold knife section technique for bulky uterus removal. J Laparoendosc Adv Surg Tech A. 2015;25(9):755–9.
25. Clark Donat L, Clark M, Tower AM, Menderes G, Parkash V, Silasi DA, Azodi M. Transvaginal morcellation. JSLS. 2015;19(2)

Robotic-Assisted Total Hysterectomy: Hysterectomy Techniques in Prolapse Situations

66

Emad Matanes, Roy Lauterbach, and Lior Lowenstein

Introduction

Pelvic organ prolapse (POP) is a protrusion of pelvic organs and their associating vaginal segments descend from their normal positions into the vagina [1]. This condition is common, being symptomatic in approximately 30 % of women 50–89 years of age and requiring a corrective procedure in 11 % of women by 80 years of age. In the next 30 years, the demand for treatment of POP will increase 45 % on the background of the increase of old women population [2]. Other associated risk factors for development of POP include: vaginal delivery, history of hysterectomy, obesity, race and history of previous operations [3].

Definitions

Cystocele: Herniation of the anterior vaginal wall. (Fig. 66.1)
Rectocele: Herniation of the posterior vaginal wall. (Fig. 66.1)
Enterocele: Protrusion of the small intestines and peritoneum into the vaginal canal. (Fig. 66.2)
Uterine prolapse: Downward protrusion of the cervix and uterus toward the introitus. (Fig. 66.3)

Pathophysiology

POP results from weakening of the supportive structures which is caused either by stretching and tearing of the supportive system or by neuromuscular dysfunction. The structures that support the vagina and the uterus are divided into three levels which correspond to differing areas of support [4]:

Level I: The upper part of the vagina and the cervix are suspended from above. The suspension referred to the **cardinal and uterosacral ligaments**.

E. Matanes • R. Lauterbach • L. Lowenstein (✉)
Obstetrics and Gynecology, Rambam Medical Center, Haifa, Israel
e-mail: lowensteinmd@gmail.com

Level II: The midline position of the vagina is maintained by the paravaginal attachments of the lateral vagina and the **endopelvic fascia** to **arcus tendineus**.

Level III: The distal vagina is supported by muscles and connective tissue which surround it. It is fused laterally to the levator muscle and posteriorly to the perineal body while anteriorly it blends with the urethra.

Anatomy

The pelvic organs are arranged in three compartments:

Anterior compartment: Contains the urinary bladder, the Urethra and the anterior wall of the vagina.
Posterior compartment: Includes the rectum and the vaginal posterior wall. It is supported by the pelvic floor musculature and connective tissue posteriorly and the pararectal fascia and its attachments to the lateral pelvic floor musculature and its fascia.
Apical compartment: Contains the uterus, cervix and the apical part of the vagina.

Treatment

The treatment for POP is based on both, surgical and nonsurgical approaches.

Nonsurgical Treatment

It is recommended in cases of:

- Mild to moderate POP.
- Patients who are still interested in having future pregnancies.
- Patients who are not interested in surgical approach.

I. Alkatout, L. Mettler (eds.), *Hysterectomy*, DOI 10.1007/978-3-319-22497-8_66

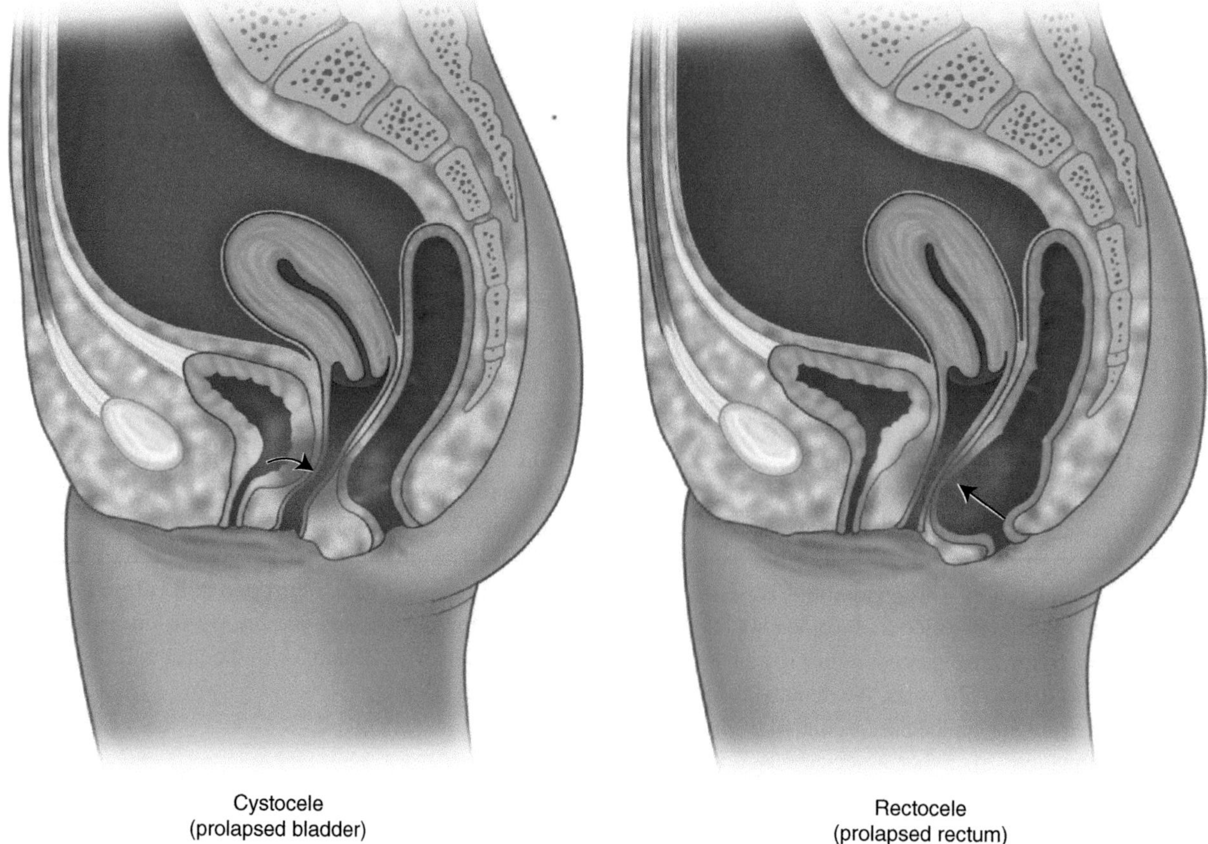

Fig. 66.1 Weak Vesico-vaginal and Recto-vaginal connective tissues result in a vaginal hernia that precedes the bladder (*left*) and rectum (*right*) herniation's that follow

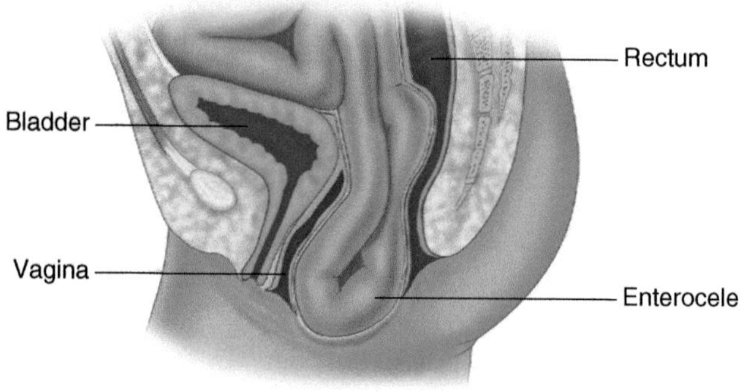

Fig. 66.2 Protrusion of the small intestines into the vagina

Options for treatment are:

1. Life style intervention:
   - Pelvic floor muscle training PFMT
   - Weight loss
2. Mechanical devices (Pessary)

Surgical management

The main purpose of surgical treatment is symptomatic relief by restoration of the vaginal anatomy. Three main surgical approaches for treatment of POP: vaginal, abdominal and laparoscopic (both conventional and robotic). The use of vaginal meshes was very common until October 2008, when the FDA published its` first warning regarding possible complications following the use of mesh in vaginal surgeries. Since then, many surgeons around the world converted their surgical approach from vaginal to abdominal and returned to use the traditional gold standard approach for POP repair thus sacrocolpopexy [5].

Sacrocolpopexy can be performed by abdominal approach, conventional laparoscopy or robotic laparoscopy.

The principle of the procedure is to lay a Y shaped mesh over the prolapsed organ, whether it is the vaginal wall, the cervix (in cases in which Supra cervical hysterectomy is performed) or the uterus (in cases in which the uterus is not excised). The upper arms of the Y shaped mesh embrace the prolapsed organ and the remaining part of the mesh is fixated to the anterior longitudinal ligament of the sacrum.

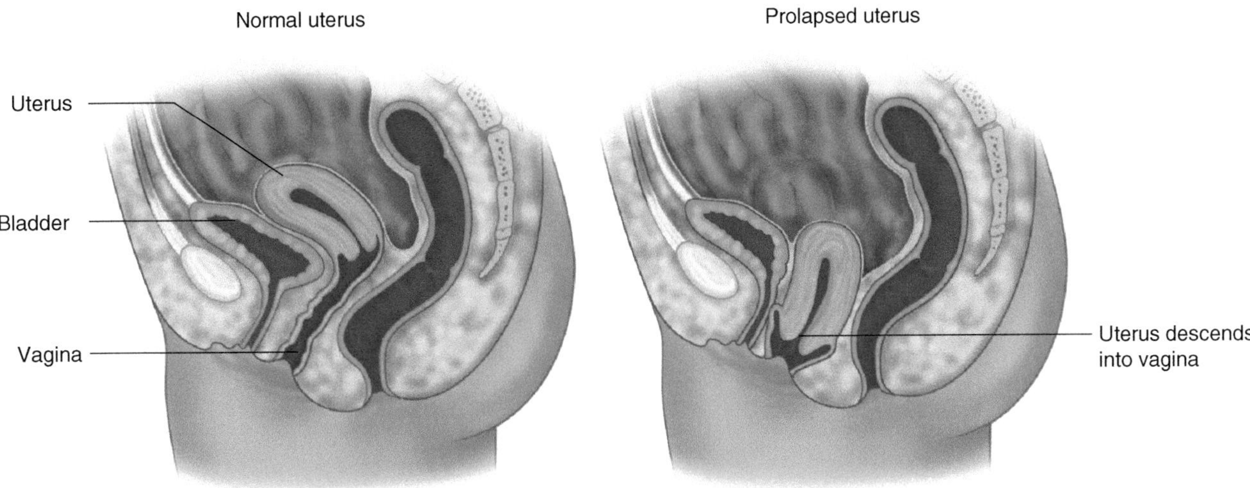

Fig. 66.3 Weakened cardinal and utero-sacral ligaments may lead to uterine prolapse

In the past two decades, the open approach has been replaced by the laparoscopic one due to its` proven advantages, and recently, there has been another shift from conventional laparoscopy to robotic laparoscopy [6] .

The Robot Evolution

- 1985: The first robotic surgical operation was presented, Kwoh and his associates reported performing a brain biopsy with a robotic arm PUMA560 successfully [1]
- 1993: Robodec was the first robot to be granted FDA approval for a hip replacement surgery.
- 2001: The first Telerobotic cholecystectomy was performed successfully with the ZEUS robot.
- 2005: The FDA approved robotic technology for gynecologic surgery.
- 12/2011: The FDA accepted the specific Single-Site equipment for use with the Da Vinci Surgical System (Fig. 66.4).

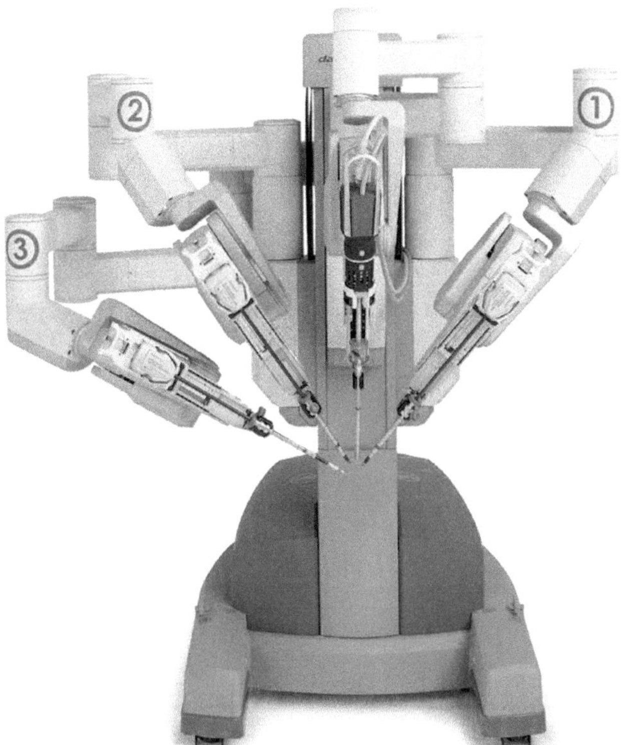

Fig. 66.4 The Da Vinci Robot is the most utilized robot today in the surgical world. The arms marked "1", "2", "3" are the operating arms, and the 4th arm is the camera holder. During single port surgery the arm marked "3" is not in use during surgery. ©2016 Intuitive Surgical, Inc.

Robotic Sacrocolpopexy and Supracervical Hysterectomy–Multiport

Insertion of the veress needle and creation of pneumoperitoneum. Before inserting the veress needle in, it is necessary to identify the possible insertion points based on the patient's medical and surgical history. The common approach is by making a small medial incision approximately 2 centimeters above the umbilicus. In patients with a history of previous abdominal surgery, it may be wise to consider approaching the abdomen with an incision at palmer's point, located at the left mid-clavicular line, approximately 2–3 centimeters under the rib cage.

During the insertion of trocars at the site of the first incision, RUQ, RLQ and LLQ (Fig. 66.5), it is imperative to

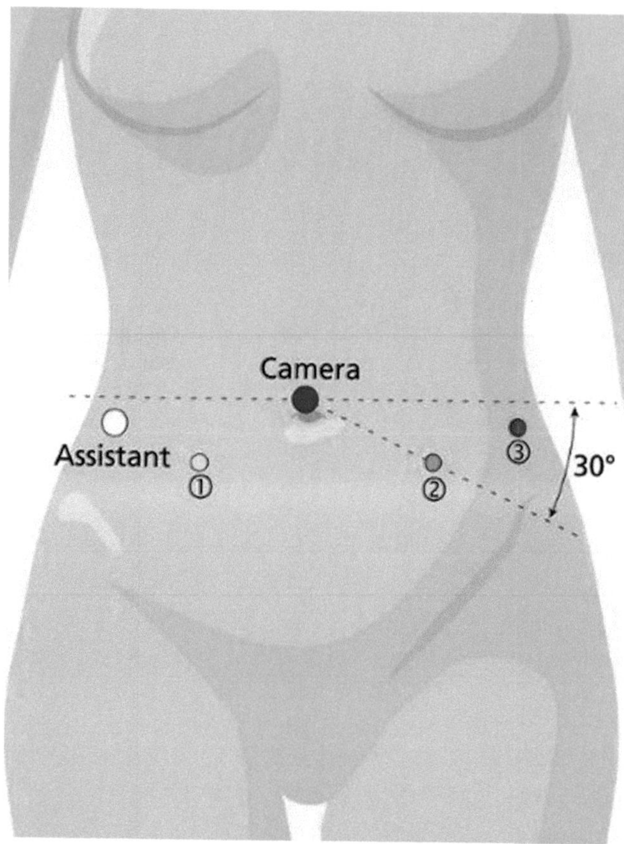

Fig. 66.5 During multi-port surgery 5 incisions are made in the abdomen, in the shape of a "W", 4 incisions are designated for the insertion of the robot arms, and the 5th incision is designated as the assistant port, allowing the insertion and extraction of surgical tools (needles/mesh/instruments) that otherwise assist the surgeon during surgery. Single port surgery utilizes a single supra-umbilical incision, thus making the other incisions redundant. ©2016 Intuitive Surgical, Inc.

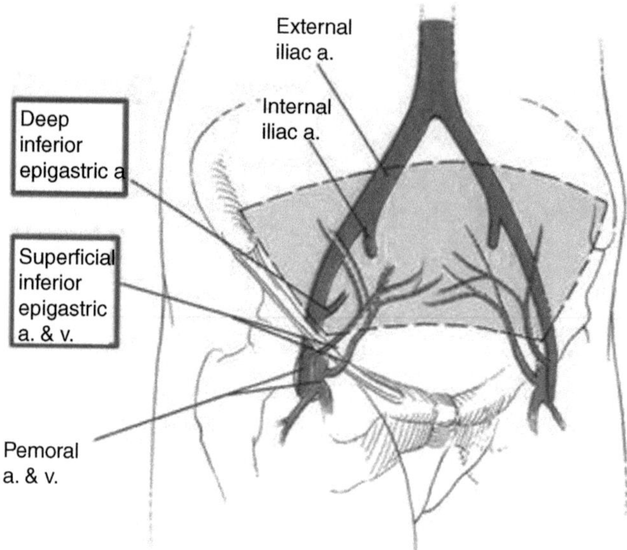

Fig. 66.6 Make an effort to avoid making incisions on the course of the DEEP INFERIOR EPIGASTRIC ARTERY AND SUPERFICIAL INFERIOR EPIGASTRIC VESSELS- that run down the abdominal wall

avoid perforating 2 significant arteries that pass through the abdominal wall:

(a) Inferior Epigastric vessels that originate from the External Iliac arteries run superiorly and enter the rectus sheath deep to the rectus abdominis, while supplying the rectus abdominis muscle, and the deep abdominal wall of the pubic and inferior umbilical regions.
(b) Superficial Epigastric arteries that originate from the Femoral artery run in the subcutaneous tissue toward the umbilicus, while supplying the superficial abdominal wall of the pubic and inferior umbilical regions (Fig. 66.6).

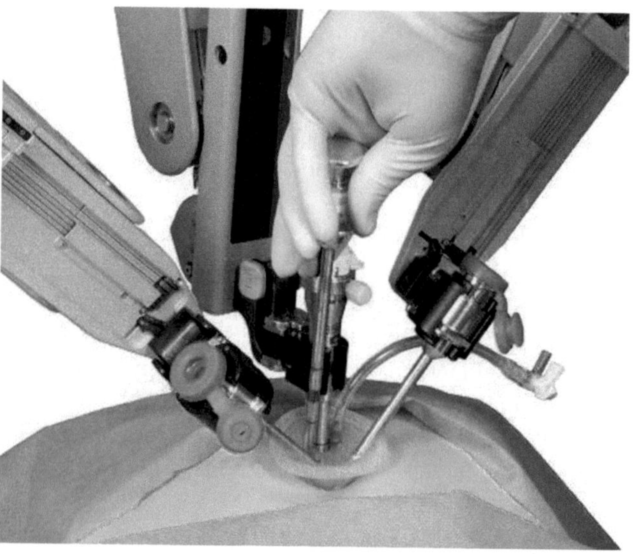

Fig. 66.7 Two robot instruments are inserted through the single port on top of a camera, an assistant trocar and the gas tube attached to the port, thus making the extra 4 incisions made in multi-port surgery redundant. ©2016 Intuitive Surgical, Inc.

Single-Port Surgery

The next generation of robotic assisted laparoscopy is the single port access, in which the surgeon operates almost exclusively through a single entry point, typically the patient's navel, leaving only a single small scar (Figs. 66.7, 66.8 and 66.9). Benefits of single-port robotic assisted sacrocolpopexy surgery may include:

- Faster recovery.
- Shorter hospitalization.
- Minimal post op pain.

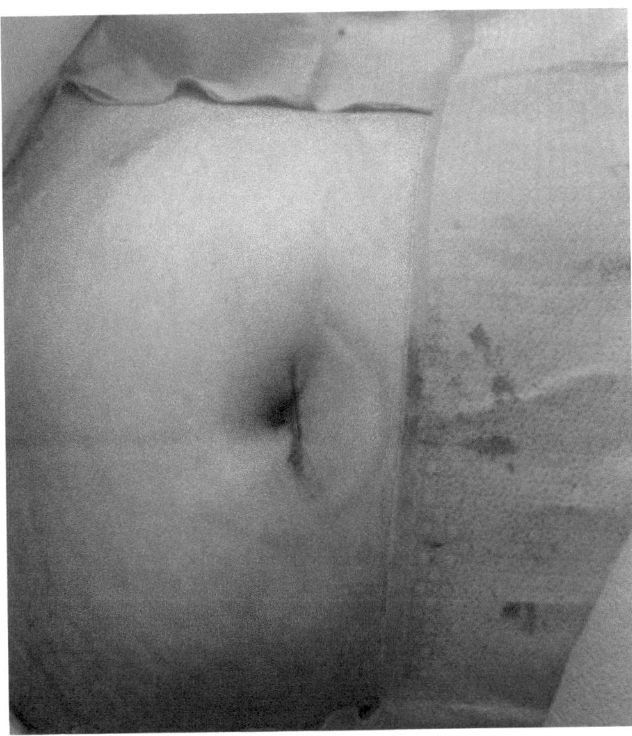

Fig. 66.8 The post-surgical minimal scar after single port surgery

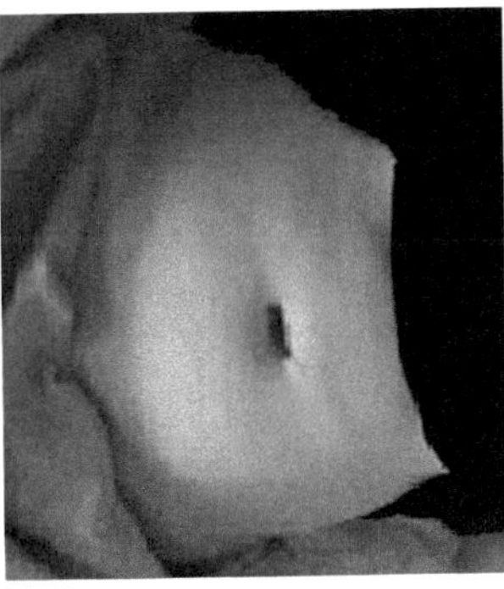

Fig. 66.9 Three weeks post-surgery, the scar is embedded into the umbilicus and is barely recognizable

- Virtually Scar free results.
- Minimal blood loss.

Four instruments are inserted via the single port in addition to the CO2 tube creating the pneumoperitoneum.

During Surgery

On visualization of the pelvic cavity it is crucial to keep in mind the course of the ureters. The ureters descend subperitoneally into the pelvis, passing inferior of the uterine artery. They then penetrate the bladder wall obliquely from its` posterio-inferior angle. The pelvic portion of each ureter is served by the vaginal artery and the internal iliac veins.

Upon entering the peritoneal cavity, it is very important to orientate anatomically (Fig. 66.10):

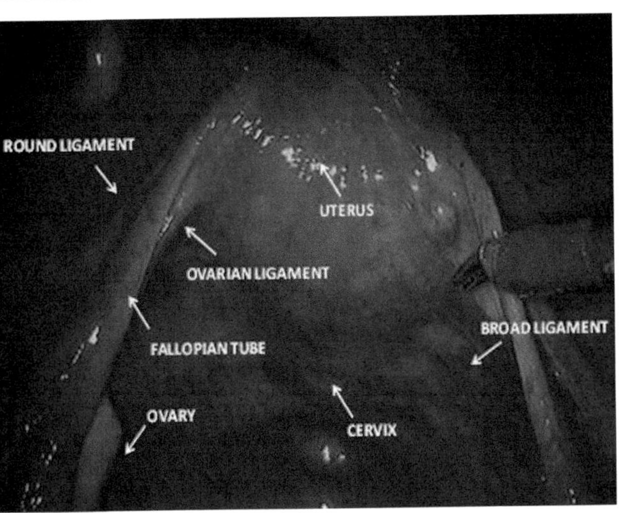

Fig. 66.10 Anatomical orientation: The posterior plane of the uterus, attached on both sides to the ovarian ligaments (connecting the uterus and the ovaries); the round ligament lies anterior to the fallopian tubes that are connect at the superior-lateral aspects of the uterus on their medial part and run laterally to the ovaries, which can be recognized on the left side as an oval, white structure. The broad ligament is the peritoneal sheet that covers the uterus anteriorly and posteriorly and contains several important structures including uterine blood vessels, ovarian blood vessels, ligaments and fallopian tubes

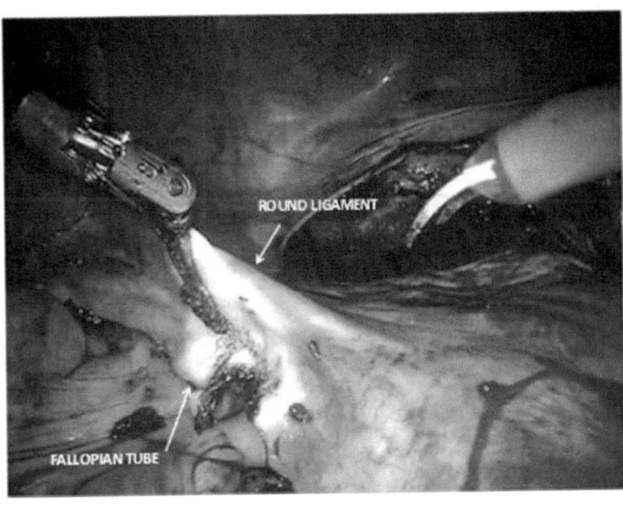

Fig. 66.11 Bipolar (searing) in the right arm, and scissors (cutting) in the left arm utilized to detach the round ligament, a preliminary step during Hysterectomy

Surgery Steps

1. Sealing and cutting of the round ligament and the fallopian tube (Fig. 66.11).

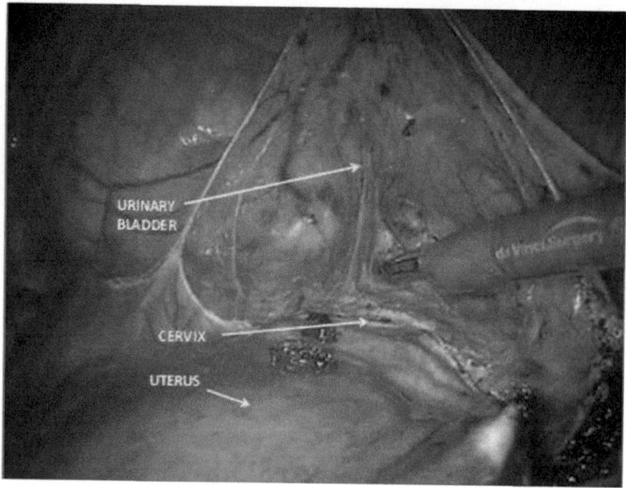

Fig. 66.12 Peeling of the bladder off the cervix

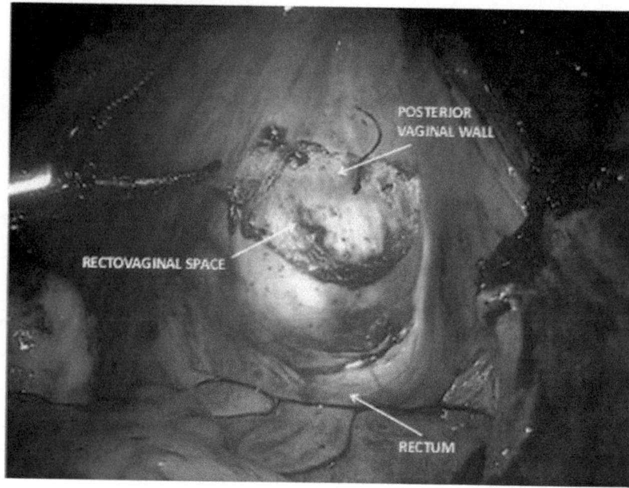

Fig. 66.14 Preparation of the posterior vaginal wall for the fixation of the posterior portion of the mesh

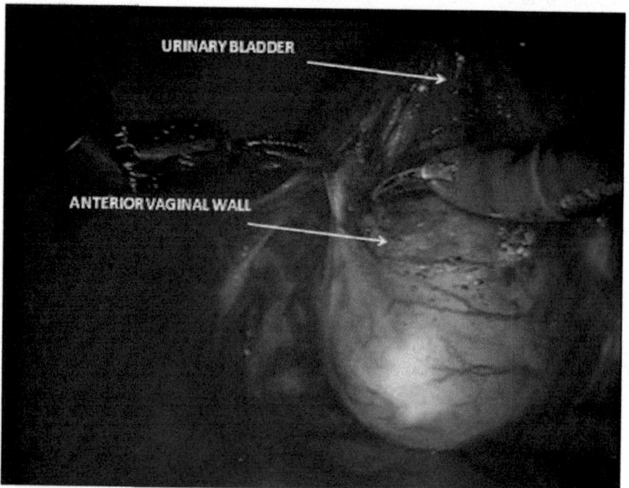

Fig. 66.13 Preparation for the fixation of the anterior portion of the mesh, an important step during surgery that serves a double purpose: avoiding damage to the bladder, and optimal fixation of the mesh, thus allowing better prolapse fixation results

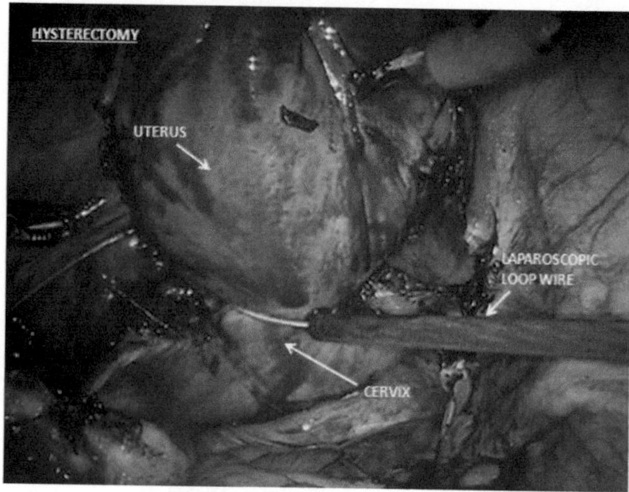

Fig. 66.15 Hysterectomy: usually performed supra-cervically. After detaching the uterus from its` supplying blood vessels, a loop wire is manipulated around the uterus, until reaching the upper part of the cervix, where uterine detachment is facilitated

2. Opening of the broad ligament and the posterior sheet.
3. The same actions need to be repeated on the other side of the uterus.
4. Opening of the bladder fold and pushing it over the anterior vaginal wall and the bladder's neck (Figs. 66.12 and 66.13).
5. Sealing and cutting the uterine arteries.
6. Developing the posterior rectovaginal space- opening the peritoneum on the posterior vaginal wall. (Fig. 66.14)
7. Total removal of the uterus using a loop wire while leaving the cervix intact (Figs. 66.15 and 66.16).
8. The anterior longitudinal ligament is exposed. The middle sacral vessels should be visualized to avoid inadvertent injury (Figs. 66.17 and 66.18).
9. Open the peritoneum from the sacral promontory downward toward the cul-de-sac and the posterior vaginal wall in order to cover the mesh with peritoneum.
10. Sewing the surgical mash to the posterior vaginal wall, the cervical stump and the anterior vaginal wall.

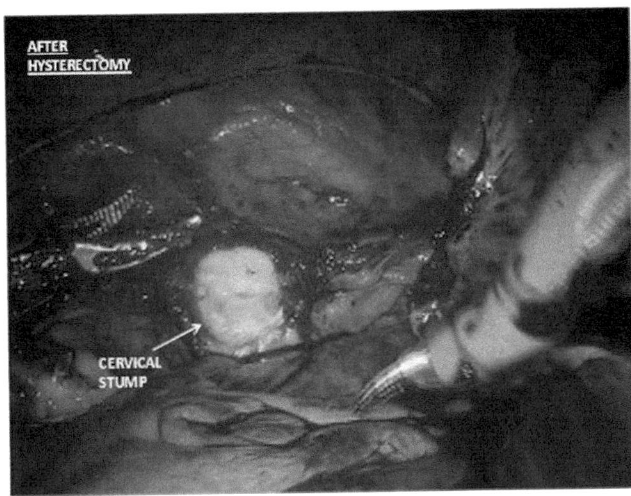

Fig. 66.16 The cervical stump is utilized later in surgery as an anchor for mesh fixation

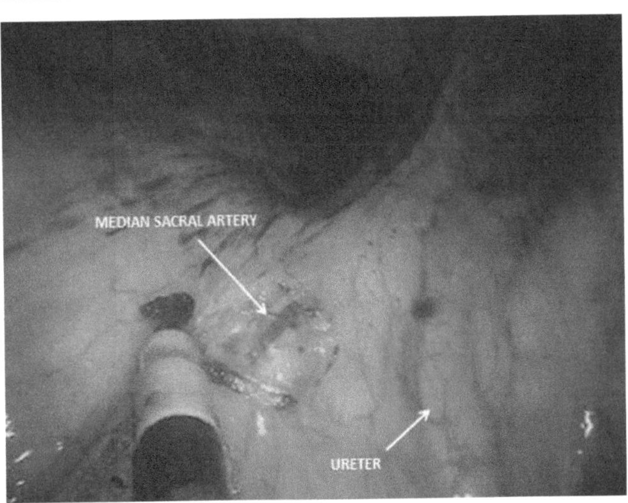

Fig. 66.18 Avoid damage to the median sacral vessels

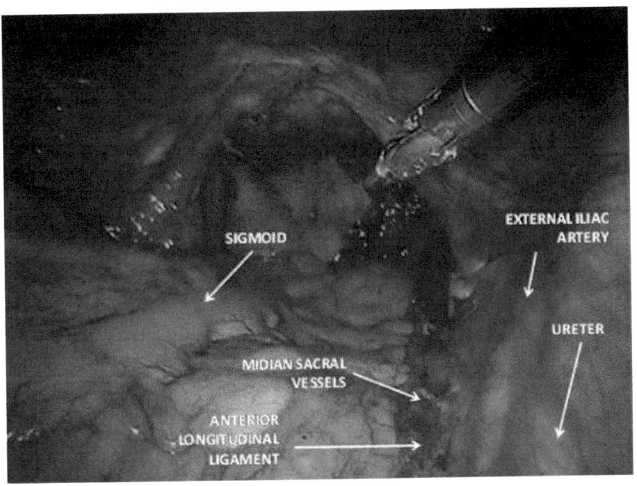

Fig. 66.17 Preparation of the promontorium for mesh fixation-anatomical landmarks that the surgeon must identify in order to avoid complications-ureter on the right side of the picture (usually identified by it's peristalsis; the common iliac artery in its` bifurcation to internal and external iliac arteries. Peeling the peritoneum off the promontorium to identify the longitudinal ligament

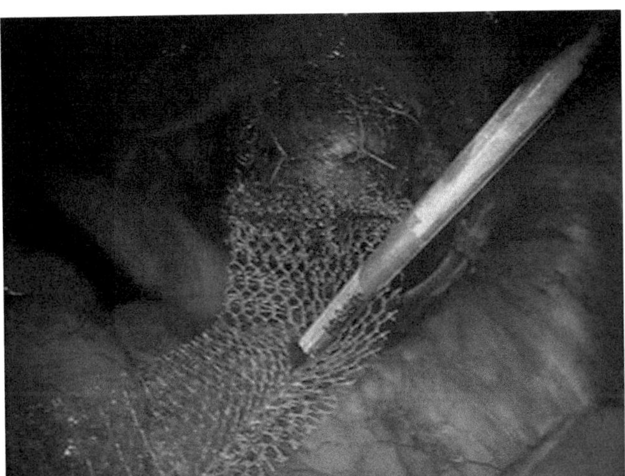

Fig. 66.19 Fixation of the inferior portion of the "Y" shaped mesh to the longitudinal ligament with tacks

11. Fixation of the surgical mesh to the promontory of the sacrum with tacks (Fig. 66.19).
12. Peritoneal closure: Fixation of the mesh to the sacral promontory, followed by re approximation of the peritoneal edges, and concealment of the mesh retroperitoneally.

Covering the mesh with peritoneum is in debate, while some consider this as a preventive measure for bowel adhesions to the mesh, this was not proven to be evidence based.

Opening the peritoneum along the promentriom toward posterior vaginal wall can result in bleeding and rarely to damage the sigmoid colon or the ureter. Closure the peritoneum over the mesh needs to be learned. Injury to adjacent vessels or the ureter can also occur during the procedure (Figs. 66.20 and 66.21).

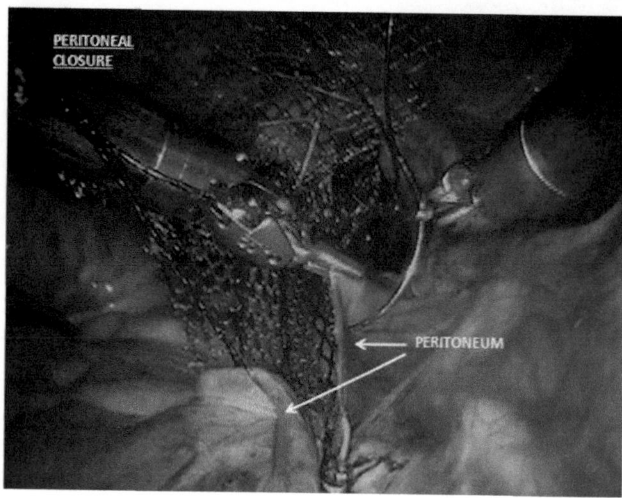

Fig. 66.20 After peeling the peritoneum and fixating the mesh to the promontorium, the mesh is "buried" under the peritoneum by suturing both ends of the peritoneum with a v-lock suture

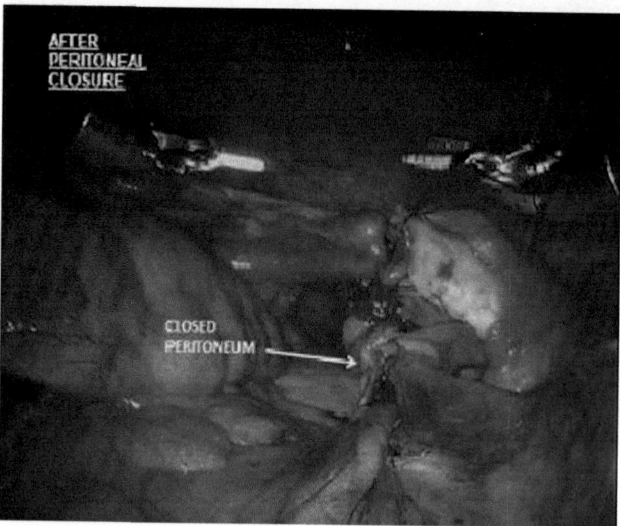

Fig. 66.21 The sutured peritoneum after peritonization (the mesh is buried under the peritoneum)

References

1. Jelovsek JE, Maher C, Barber MD. Pelvic organ prolapse. Lancet. 2007;369(9566):1027–38.
2. Luber KM, Boero S, Choe JY. The demographics of pelvic floor disorders: current observations and future projections. Am J Obstet Gynecol. 2001;184(7):1496–501. discussion 1501–3
3. Swift SE, Pound T, Dias JK. Case–control study of etiologic factors in the development of severe pelvic organ prolapse. Int Urogynecol J Pelvic Floor Dysfunct. 2001;12:187–92.
4. Young SB, Daman JJ, Bony LG. Vaginal paravaginal reapair: one-year outcomes. Am J Obstet Gynecol. 2001;185:1360–6.
5. Wang LC, Awamlh BA, et al. Trends in Mesh Use for Pelvic Organ Prolapse Repair from the Medicare Database. Urology. 2015;86(5):885–91. doi:10.1016/j.urology.2015.08.022. pii: S0090-4295(15)00834-1. [Epub ahead of print]
6. Nezhat CH, Nezhat F, Nezhat C. Laparoscopic sacral colpopexy for vaginal vault prolapse. Obstet Gynecol. 1994;84:885–8.

Robotic-Assisted Radical Hysterectomy

67

Emma L. Barber and John F. Boggess

Indications for Robotic Radical Hysterectomy

Piver, Rutledge and Smith originally described five types of hysterectomy for treatment of cervical cancer in 1974 [1]. A type I hysterectomy is an extrafascial or simple hysterectomy and is appropriate for the treatment of stage IA1 carcinoma of the cervix without lymph-vascular space invasion. In a type II hysterectomy, the uterine artery is ligated at its junction with the ureter and the para-cervical tissue medial to this is removed. This allows for preservation of the blood supply to the ureter and a decreased risk for ureteral vaginal fistula formation. A type II radical hysterectomy along with pelvic lymphadenectomy is appropriate treatment for IA2 carcinoma of the cervix, with or without lymph-vascular space invasion. A type III radical hysterectomy mandates removal of the parametria medial to the origin of the uterine artery as it branches off the internal iliac artery, removal of the uterosacral ligaments at their origin and an upper vaginectomy. A type III radical hysterectomy along with pelvic lymphadenectomy is the standard treatment for IB1 cervical cancer and may also be used for select IB2 as well as IIA lesions. Radical hysterectomy, either type II or type III can also be used to treat cases of uterine cancer with gross cervical involvement (Table 67.1).

Soon after the introduction of the robotic platform in 2005, Sert and Abeler published the first case report of robotic assisted type III radical hysterectomy [2]. The technique was later described in a series of 51 patients where robotic hysterectomy was found to decrease complications, specifically blood loss, and to shorten hospital stay when compared to open radical hysterectomy [3]. In addition, retrospective studies have shown that robotic assisted radical hysterectomy has equivalent survival to open radical hysterectomy [4–6]. The oncologic indications for robotic type III radical hysterectomy are the same as those for the open procedure. Laparoscopy and the robotic platform also require appropriate patient selection. Insufflation and steep Trendelenberg positioning promote physiologic cardiopulmonary changes that can result in increased hypercarbia, decreased cardiac output, and decreased pulmonary compliance. Thus, patients with significant pulmonary or cardiac conditions may not be able to tolerate the required positioning for the duration of the operation. This patient positioning also increases both the intraocular pressure and intracranial pressure. Thus, any intracranial pathology associated with intracranial hypertension or disruption of the blood-brain barrier are contraindications (Table 67.2). Additionally, among patients with glaucoma, preoperative tonometry should ensure that intraocular pressure is not increased, as robotic surgery in addition to an already elevated intraocular pressure can result in permanent ocular damage (Fig. 67.1).

Uterine size is another contraindication to a minimally invasive approach. A large bulky uterus can limit visualization and given that morcellation should be avoided in the case of cervical carcinoma, the uterine specimen must be able to be delivered through the vagina at the conclusion of the surgery. Previously described contraindications include increased patient BMI and extensive prior surgical history. While it is true that patients with a high BMI can provide a challenge in terms of increased weight on the diaphragm and the resulting decreased pulmonary compliance, we have found that many morbidly obese patients without significant cardiopulmonary co-morbidities are able to tolerate required positioning and do not experience an increased risk of perioperative pulmonary complications based on the degree of obesity [7]. Additionally, the surgical benefits of wristed instruments within the abdomen and pelvis as well as a camera that is able to descend into the pelvis actually offers increased visualization and dexterity in the obese patient over open surgery. Extensive prior surgical history has also been noted as a contraindication to minimally invasive surgery, however, we do not consider this a contraindication.

E.L. Barber (✉) • J.F. Boggess
Obstetrics and Gynecology, Division of Gynecologic Oncology, University of North Carolina, Chapel Hill, NC, USA
e-mail: embarber@med.unc.edu; jboggess@med.unc.edu

I. Alkatout, L. Mettler (eds.), *Hysterectomy*, DOI 10.1007/978-3-319-22497-8_67

Table 67.1 Types of radical hysterectomy

	Indications	Location of uterine artery ligation	Uterosacral ligaments	Vaginal margin
Type I (extrafascial)	IA1 cervical carcinoma without LVSI	Insertion into the cervix	Insertion into cervix	At cervico-vaginal junction
Type II (modified radical)	IA2 cervical carcinoma, uterine cancer with cervical involvement	Junction with the ureter	Midpoint between cervix and sacral attachments	1–2 cm of vaginal margin
Type III (radical)	IB1 cervical carcinoma and select IB2 and IIA lesions, uterine cancer with cervical involvement	Origin at the internal iliac artery	At sacral attachment	2–3 cm of vaginal margin

Table 67.2 Contraindications to a robotic approach

	Degree of contraindication	Rationale
Uterine size	Absolute	Morcellation should not be performed. Therefore, the specimen must be able to be delivered vaginally at the conclusion of the procedure
Conditions with increased ICP	Absolute	Required positioning will exacerbate intracranial hypertension ad can result in disruption of blood-brain barrier
Glaucoma with increased IOP	Absolute	Required positioning increases the intraocular pressure and can result in permanent vision loss and even blindness
Morbid obesity without cardiopulmonary compromise	None	These patients are generally able to be ventilated and the benefits of minimally invasive surgery and the wristed instruments of the robotic platform are even more pronounced in the morbidly obese
Cardiopulmonary compromise	Relative	Depending on the degree of compromise, patients may not be able to tolerate the required positioning, however, this is difficult to predict preoperatively and thus patients should have a trial of positioning before deeming this a contraindication
Extensive surgical history	None	Robotic platform allows for increased dexterity and visualization allowing the surgeon to perform lysis of adhesions

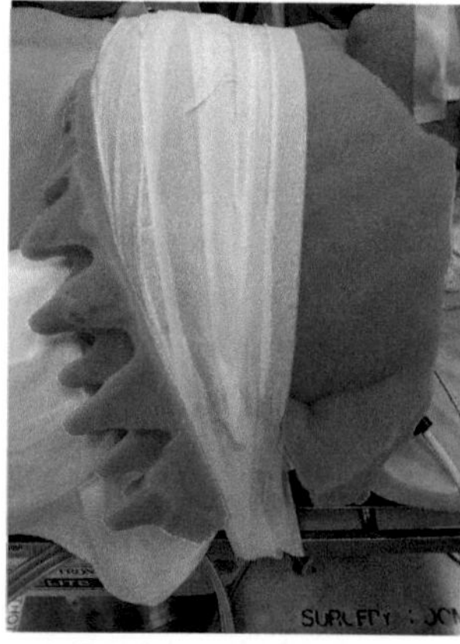

Fig. 67.1 Securing patient for steep Trendelenberg positioning. The patient's chest is padded and she is secured to the bed using thick cloth tape. The tape is passed around the patient and the bed 3–5 times depending on the patient's weight

Robotic Versus Laparoscopic Versus Abdominal Radical Hysterectomy

Minimally invasive radical hysterectomy, including both robotic and laparoscopic radical hysterectomy, offers advantages over abdominal radical hysterectomy. Minimally invasive radical hysterectomy has been associated with decreased blood loss, lower rates of transfusion, decreased length of hospital stay, equal or lower rates of postoperative complication, and an equal or increased number of lymph nodes sampled when compared with an open procedure [8–11].

Studies examining robotics versus traditional laparoscopy have found that traditional laparoscopy is associated with similar postoperative outcomes, but longer operative times. In addition, most laparoscopic radical hysterectomy series are limited to patients with a BMI under 30 whereas robotic papers include obese and morbid obese patients in their cohorts. Traditional laparoscopy is also associated with a longer learning curve and does not offer the same ergonomic benefits as robotic surgery. In contrast with other surgical procedures such as benign hysterectomy, robotic radical hysterectomy is not associated with increased cost compared with traditional laparoscopy [11]. In the only study to examine the cost of robotic, abdominal and laparoscopic radical hysterectomy for the treatment of cervical cancer using a large national database, the authors found that laparoscopic radical hysterectomy was associated with median costs of $11,774 whereas robotic radical hysterectomy actually had a statistically significant lower median cost of $10,176 [11].

Data on oncologic outcomes are similarly reassuring. One study showed no difference in 3-year overall and recurrence free survival for patients undergoing robotic versus abdominal radical hysterectomy [4]. A multicenter retrospective study examined 517 patients and demonstrated no difference in recurrence or survival between patients undergoing open or robotic radical hysterectomy with a median follow up of 34 months [12]. The same is true for laparoscopic versus open radical hysterectomy with both having similar risk of recurrence and mortality [6].

Surgical Procedure

Clinic Evaluation and Patient Counseling

History and physical examination are essential to identify patients who are good candidates for robotic radical hysterectomy. Evidence of parametrial spread on examination or imaging that reveals metastatic disease necessitates primary treatment with pelvic chemoradiation or systemic chemotherapy. Preoperative assessment should also screen for the previously mentioned contraindications to robotic surgery. Standard preoperative assessment with indicated laboratory work including a type and screen should be performed. Bowel preparation is not necessary.

As with any surgical procedure, patients should have an informed consent discussion regarding the risks and benefits of robotic radical hysterectomy. Standard risks such as bleeding, infection and injury to blood vessels, nerves, bladder, ureter, and bowels should be discussed. Additionally, for robotic radical hysterectomy, the risk of conversion to a laparotomy, risk of fistula formation and risk of both short-term and long-term bladder dysfunction should all be discussed. Patients should also be informed of the possibility of post-operative radiation depending on the final surgical pathology.

Preoperative Positioning

The patient is brought to the operating room and placed under general anesthesia. Prior to induction, sequential compression devices are placed on the lower extremities. She is then positioned in the low dorsolithotomy position using Allen stirrups to allow for adequate space to bring the robot to the bedside. Examination under anesthesia is performed prior to beginning the surgery to reorient the surgeon to the patient's anatomy and to confirm the absence of parametrial or pelvic sidewall disease, which would preclude a surgical approach. After the patient is positioned in the dorsolithotomy position, she is secured to the table to allow for steep Trendelenberg positioning. This can be done using shoulder blocks, chest padding with taping or a beanbag device which molds to the patient. Given the risk of brachial plexus injuries relying only on shoulder blocks and the cost of bean bag devices, we prefer to use chest padding and taping to secure the patient to the bed. Although uterine manipulation is standard in robotic hysterectomy, for a robotic radical hysterectomy, we prefer to avoid disruption of the tumor and instead place a large rectal dilator (EEA sizer) in the vagina prior to draping for use at the time of colpotomy. A pneumo-occluder balloon is also placed in the vagina to prevent loss of pneumoperitoneum during the colopotomy. A foley catheter is also placed to decompress with bladder and decrease the risk of bladder injury. Prophylactic antibiotics are administered prior to skin incision (Fig. 67.2).

Abdominal Entry

We routinely enter the abdomen in the left upper quadrant at Palmer's point (left upper quadrant 2 cm below the costal margin in the mid-clavicular line) after an orogastric tube has been placed to suction. This allows us to avoid adhesions from prior surgery and will be the site for our assistant port [13]. We inject the skin with local anesthetic prior to incision and enter the abdomen with a 2 mm miniport. Once the abdomen is insufflated, a 2 mm camera is inserted into the abdomen and an abdominal survey is performed focusing on the anterior abdominal wall and presence of any adhesive disease. An alternative technique is to insufflate at this site with a veress needle and place a 5 mm visiport under direct visualization.

Port Placement

Five total trocars are used. Two traditional laparoscopic trocars are used for the camera and assistant port and three robotic trocars are used for the robotic arms. A 12 mm trocar is placed in the umbilicus and functions as the camera port. The robotic camera is introduced through this port and a complete abdominopelvic survey is completed to identify any evidence of metastatic disease or adhesive disease that

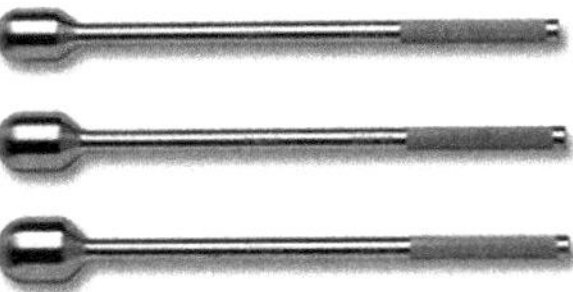

Fig. 67.2 EEA sizer and vaginal balloon. A rectal end-to-end anastomosis (EEA) sizer is placed into the vagina to allow for uterine manipulation and to assist in identification of the cervico-vaginal junction. A pneumo-occluder balloon is placed around the handle and inflated to prevent the loss of pneumoperitoneum during colpotomy

will prevent port placement. Any abnormalities encountered in the abdomen or pelvis that are suspicious for metastatic disease should be biopsied and sent for frozen section. Confirmation of metastatic disease should prompt the surgeon to consider aborting the surgery in favor of radiation therapy depending on the clinical scenario. Any encountered adhesive disease, which prevents port placement or will not be accessible with the robot is taken down laparoscopically. Additional robotic trocars are placed as follows: arm 1 is placed 8–10 cm lateral to the camera port in the right upper abdomen, arm 2 is placed in the left upper abdomen again, 8-10 cm lateral to the camera port, mirroring arm 1, and arm 3 is placed in the left lower quadrant just superior to the anterior iliac spine and at least 8 cm in distance from arm 2. A 10/12 mm assistant port is placed in the left upper quadrant at the site of laparoscopic entry. All trocars are placed under direct visualization and all ports are advanced to the thick black line on the trocar cannula to allow for optimal range of motion for the robotic arms. The patient is then placed in steep Trendelenberg. If tolerated, we use 30 ° of Trendelenberg. The robot is moved into position either between the patient's legs or over the left leg in a side docking position. The camera arm is docked first. The robotic arm clutch button is pressed and the angle of the camera arm is aligned with the angle of the trocar. The trocar is stabilized with one hand and the other hand is used to press the robotic arm clutch button and deliver the arm to the trocar, clipping both wings to secure the robotic arm to the trocar. The remaining three robot arms are docked to their respective trocars in the same fashion (Fig. 67.3).

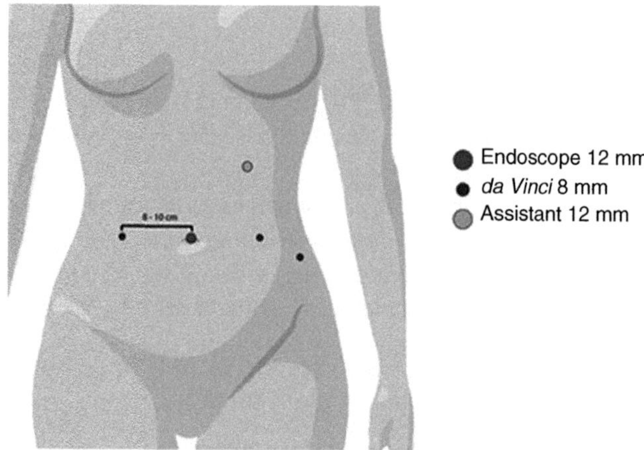

Fig. 67.3 Port placement. A 12 mm trocar is placed in the umbilicus and functions as the camera port. Arm 1 is placed 8–10 cm lateral to the camera port in the right upper abdomen and arm 2 is placed in the left upper abdomen mirroring arm 1. Arm 3 is placed in the left lower quadrant just superior to the anterior iliac spine and at least 8 cm in distance from arm 2. A 10/12 mm assistant port is placed in the left upper quadrant at the site of laparoscopic entry (With kind permission from John F. Boggess, MD 2007)

Robotic Instruments

Once the robot arms have been docked, the robotic camera is introduced through the camera port. We use a 0-degree camera throughout the surgery. The robotic instruments are then introduced. The monopolar scissors are used in the right hand and the fenestrated bipolar in the left hand. A blunt grasper, such as a prograsp or a cadiere, is used in arm 3. All instruments are introduced into the abdomen under direct visualization.

Opening the Retroperitoneum and Avascular Spaces of the Pelvis

The uterus is manipulated with the fourth robotic arm. The right uterine cornua is grasped and moved to the patient's left. The right round ligament is transected using monopolar cautery as far laterally as possible and this peritoneal incision is extended cephalad parallel to the infundibulopelvic ligament. The medial umbilical ligament is placed on tension medially and caudad to allow for identification of the superior vesical artery. The peritoneum just lateral to the artery is incised cephalad to its origin. The monopolar scissors and fenestrated bipolar graspers are then used to spread perpendicular to the pelvic sidewall to bluntly open the paravesicle space down to the level of the levator muscles. The pararectal space is opened in a similar fashion by spreading in a perpendicular manner in between the ureter and internal iliac artery and vein. After the paravesical and pararectal spaces have been opened, the parametria to be resected can be easily identified as the remaining tissue between the two spaces. At this time, any extension of tumor into the parametrial tissues is evaluated and as evidence of extension indicates the need for postoperative radiation and the surgeon evaluates whether or not to proceed depending on the clinical scenario (Fig. 67.4).

Pelvic Lymphadenectomy

A bilateral pelvic lymphadenectomy is then performed. The fourth robotic arm is used to reflect the superior vesical artery medially and open the paravesical space. The operative assistant using a laparoscopic grasper retracts the proximal peritoneum at the pelvic brim to expose the entire area of nodal dissection. The nodal tissue just inferior to the bifurcation of the common iliac artery is grasped and elevated with the fenestrated bipolar forceps. The monopolar scissors are used to make an incision overlying the psoas muscle just lateral to the artery and the genitofemoral nerve is mobilized laterally. Once the sur-

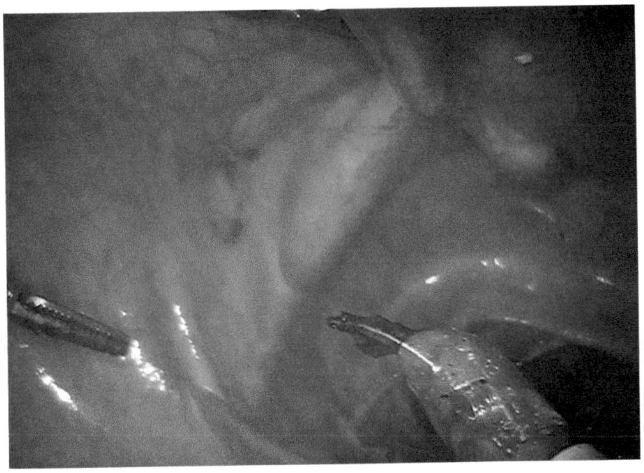

Fig. 67.4 Identification of the superior vesical artery. The median umbilical ligament is identified on the anterior abdominal wall. It is placed on tension medially and caudad which in turn pulls the superior vesical artery medially and away from the pelvic sidewall to allow for easy identification

face of the external iliac artery is identified, the nodal tissue is dissected free from the artery caudally using a combination of blunt dissection and cautery, as appropriate, until the deep circumflex iliac vein is encountered. The nodal bundle is reflected medially and gentle dissection is used to identify the surface of the external iliac vein and the nodal tissue is freed from its attachments to the vein cephalad to the bifurcation. The nodal bundle is grasped at the midpoint between the bifurcation of the common iliac artery and the crossing of the deep circumflex iliac vein. The vein is pushed laterally in order to enter the space between the nodal bundle and the pelvic sidewall. The obturator nerve is identified and the caudad portion of the nodal bundle in the obturator space is grasped with the fenestrated bipolar forceps and reflected medially and cephalad. The surface of the vein is pushed laterally and the obturator nerve is pushed inferiorly to free the nodal bundle from the obturator space. This process is continued cephalad until the bifurcation is reached and the specimen is freed. It is placed in a specimen bag in the upper abdomen for subsequent removal. The same is done on the left side (Figs. 67.5 and 67.6).

Ureteral Dissection

The ureter is identified along the medial leaf of the broad ligament. It is dissected free from its medial attachments and mobilized laterally to the level of the uterine artery and cardinal ligament in order to allow adequate visualization for the origin of the uterine artery. Care is taken to preserve the blood supply, adventitia and muscularis of the ureter to decrease the risk of fistula (Fig. 67.7).

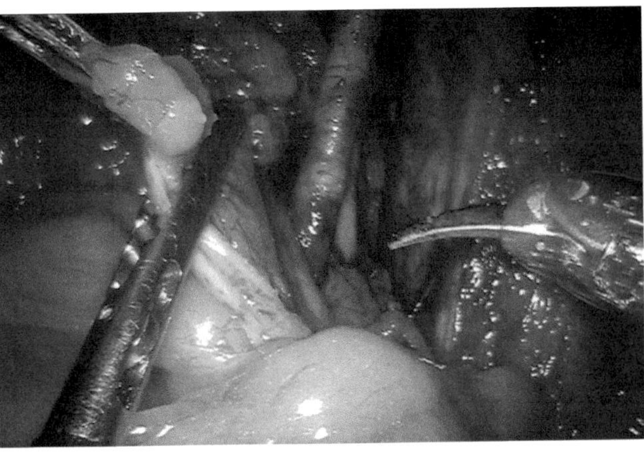

Fig. 67.5 Peritoneal retraction. The assistant retracts the peritoneum at the pelvic brim medially to allow for exposure to perform the nodal dissection

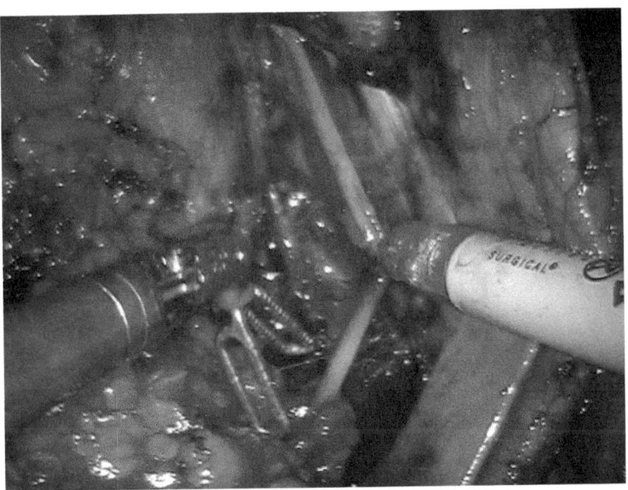

Fig. 67.6 Obturator nerve. The obturator nerve is identified and the nodal bundle is dissected free by grasping the nodal bundle, moving it cephalad and medially, and pushing the nerve laterally and inferiorly

Bladder Flap, Uterine Artery Transection and Parametrial Dissection

The vesico-uterine fold is incised with monopolar cautery and extended laterally to create the bladder flap. The vesico-uterine peritoneum is elevated and the vesico-uterine space is entered using a combination of blunt and sharp dissection with use of cautery as appropriate. This space is further dissected caudally until the bladder has been taken down sufficiently off the anterior vaginal wall to achieve an adequate margin. The uterine artery is identified at its origin from the internal iliac artery. The origin is isolated by dissecting away the surrounding tissue with blunt dissection with the fenestrated bipolar forceps. The artery and vein are then cauterized with bipolar cautery and transected. The artery is then freed from its attachments to the ureter and the ureter is

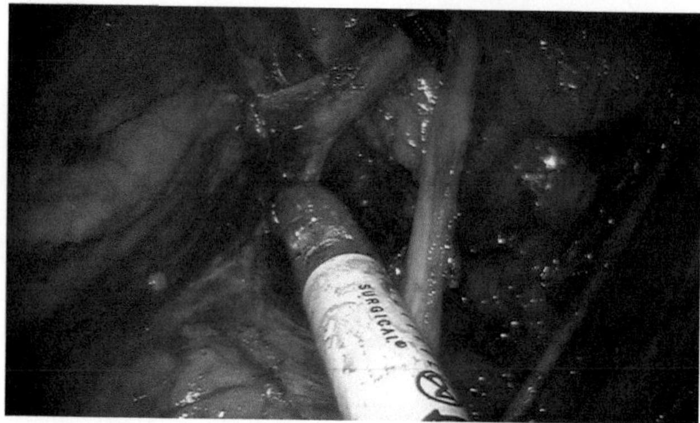

Fig. 67.7 Ureteral dissection. The ureter is reflected laterally and dissected free from its medial attachments

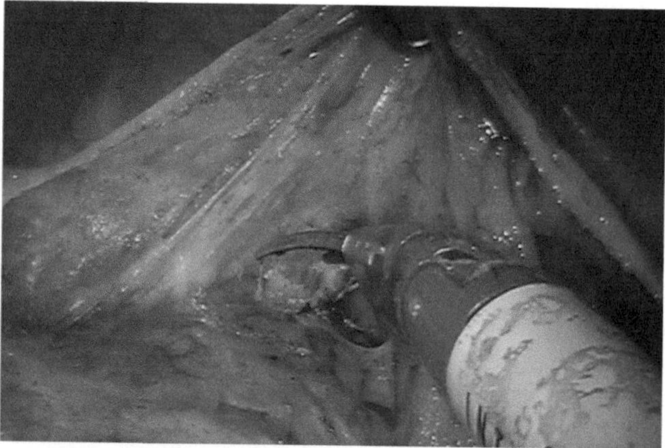

Fig. 67.8 Bladder flap. The vesico-uterine peritoneum is elevated and the bladder is dissected off the cervix and vagina

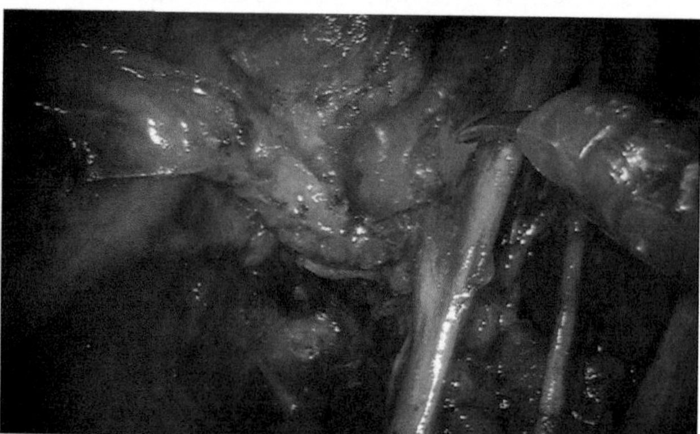

Fig. 67.9 Uterine artery isolation. The uterine artery is isolated at its origin

further mobilized laterally. The parametrial tissue is dissected off the ureter and mobilized medially. This allows for exposure of the ureteral tunnel of Wertheim and the ureter is unroofed to its insertion into the bladder by bipolar coagulating the anterior vesico-uterine ligament (Figs. 67.8, 67.9 and 67.10).

Transect the Utero-Ovarian Ligament or Infundibulopelvic Ligament

At this time, either the infudibulopelvic ligament or the utero-ovarian ligament is transected depending on the patient's age and the clinical circumstance. If the ovary is preserved, salpingectomy should be considered in order to reduce the future risk of ovarian cancer [14]. The paravesical space has been previously opened and the ureter is again identified. A window is made in the broad ligament below the infundibulopelvic ligament and above the ureter using the monopolar scissors. Blunt traction is used to extend this incision along the length of the infundibulopelvic ligament. Bipolar cautery followed by transection with the monopolar scissors is used to transect either the infundibulopelvic ligament at its origin or the utero-ovarian ligament (Fig. 67.11).

Transect Uterosacral Ligaments While Preserving the Sacral Nerve Plexus

The uterus is retracted anteriorly using the third robotic arm. The incision along the posterior broad ligament is continued medially towards the uterosacral ligament. As this is performed, the endopelvic fascia containing the hypogastric nerve plexus is dissected laterally. The peritoneum overlying the rectovaginal space between the two uterosacral ligaments is incised and the rectovaginal space is developed with blunt dissection. The uterosacral ligaments are cauterized with bipolar cautery at their insertion into the posterior vaginal wall and the remainder of the cardinal ligament is resected to the pelvic sidewall (Figs. 67.12, 67.13 and 67.14).

Colpotomy with Upper Vaginectomy

The EEA sizer which was previously placed in the vagina is advanced to identify the cervicovaginal margin. An incision is made along the anterior vaginal wall 2–3 cm inferior to the cervicovaginal junction to allow for an adequate margin. This incision is made with the monopolar cautery and continued around circumferentially, freeing the specimen. The specimen is removed through the vagina as are the specimen bags with the previously dissected pelvic lymph node specimens (Fig. 67.15).

Vaginal Cuff Closure

A mega suture cut needle driver is introduced into the right hand and a 0-vicryl suture on a CT-1 needle cut to 25 cm is passed through the assistant port. The vaginal cuff is closed in a running unlocked fashion from right to left. It is important

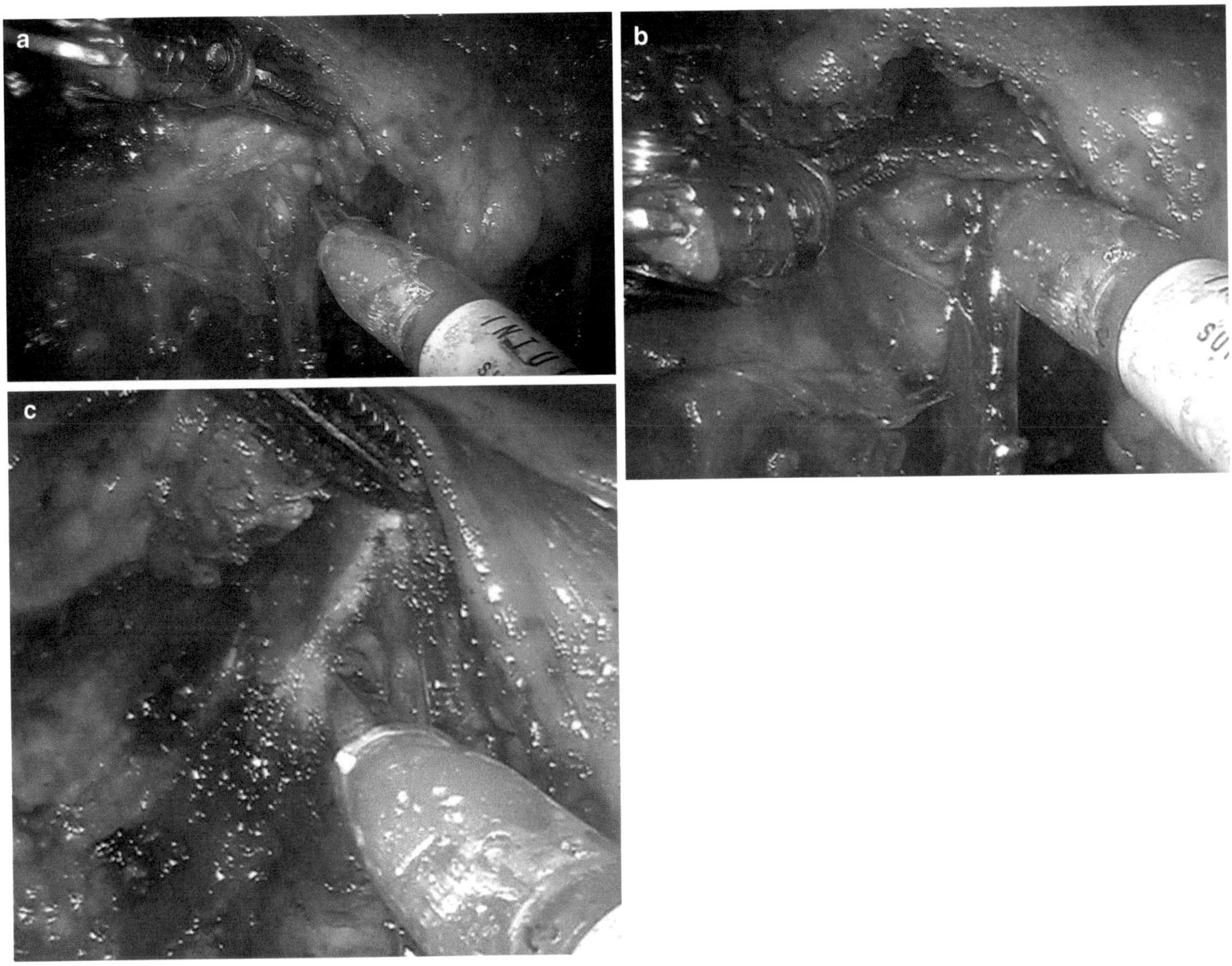

Fig. 67.10 Anterior vesicouterine ligament and tunnel of Wertheim. The ureter is unroofed through the tunnel of Wertheim (**a**). The anterior vesicouterine ligament is coagulated (**b**) and transected (**c**) exposing the insertion of the ureter into the bladder

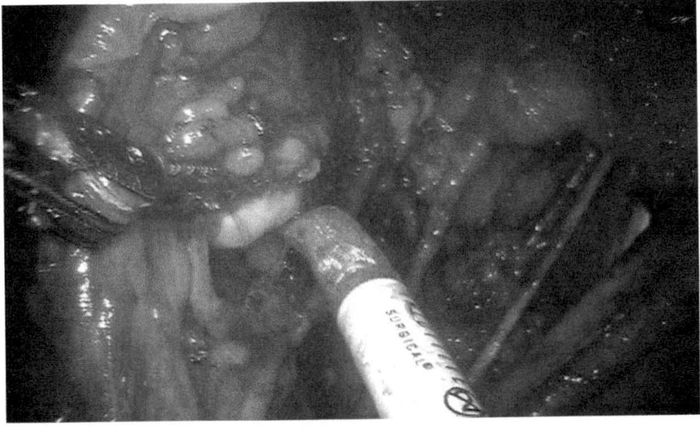

Fig. 67.11 Infundibulopelvic ligament. A window is made in the broad ligament and the infundibulopelvic ligament is cauterized and transected

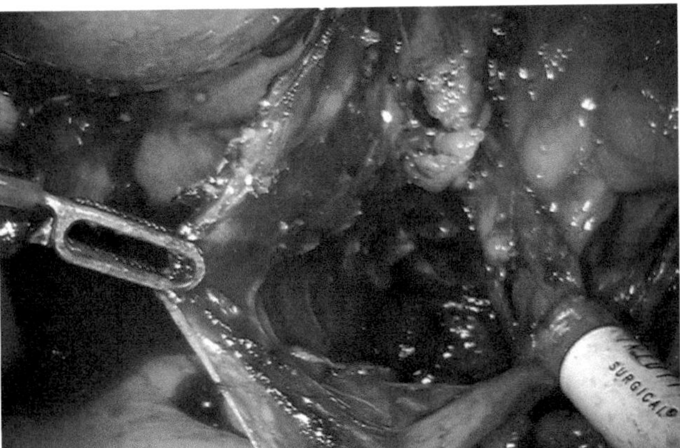

Fig. 67.12 Preserve the hypogastric plexus. The peritoneum is grasped and the endopelvic fascia containing the hypogastric nerve plexus is dissected off the peritoneum by sweeping laterally

to incorporate approximately 1 cm of vagina in each suture bite, to include the fascia and to keep the running closure on tension throughout by having the surgical assist "follow" with a laparoscopic needle driver holding the suture. The suture cut needle driver is used to cut the suture and the needle is

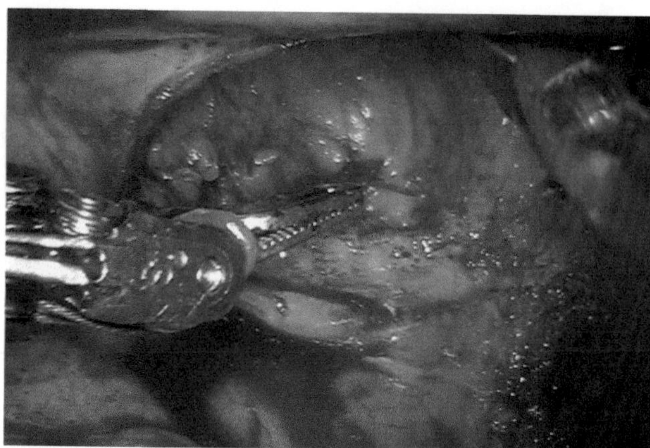

Fig. 67.13 Open rectovaginal space. The rectovaginal space is developed using blunt dissection

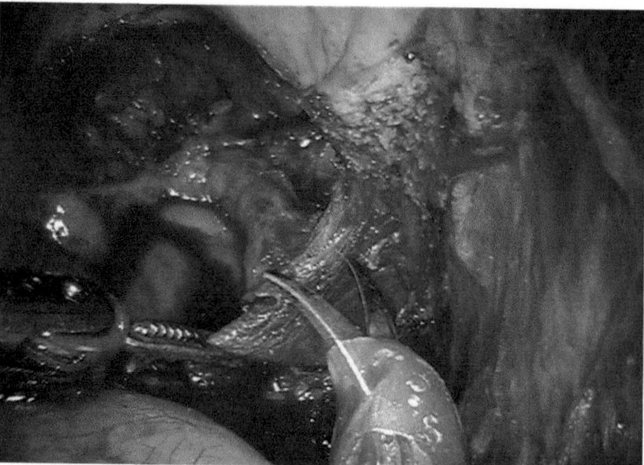

Fig. 67.14 Uterosacral transection. The uterosacral ligaments are transected at their sacral insertion after the hypogastric nerve plexus has been dissected laterally

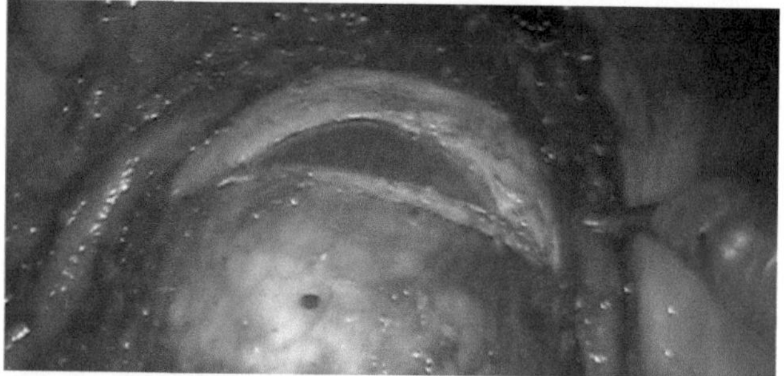

Fig. 67.15 Colpotomy. An incision is made along the vaginal wall 2–3 cm inferior to the cervico-vaginal junction. The EEA sizer is used to provide anatomic orientation

passed out of the assistant port. The abdomen and pelvis are irrigated and all operative sites are assessed for hemostasis (Fig. 67.16).

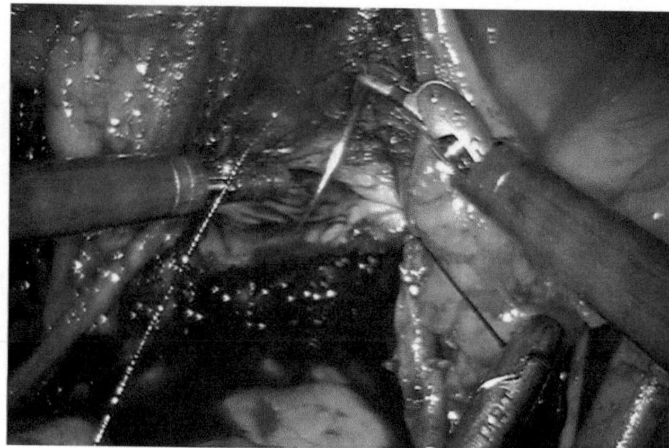

Fig. 67.16 Vaginal cuff closure. The assistant follows the surgeon using a laparoscopic needle driver to ensure continuous tension is maintained

Oophoropexy

If the ovaries are left in situ, oophoropexy may be performed to protect ovarian function in the event that adjuvant radiation is required. The peritoneum surrounding the infundibulopelvic ligament is further skeletonized using the monopolar scissors to allow increased mobility. The adnexa is mobilized above the pelvic brim. A 0-vicryl suture is passed through the assistant port and the ovary is sutured and tied to the pelvic peritoneum above the pelvic brim using a figure of eight stich. If desired, the ovaries can be marked with surgical clips for identification in radiation planning. The needle is removed via the assistant port.

Closing

After the abdomen and pelvis are irrigated and hemostasis is achieved, all robotic instruments are removed from the patient's abdomen. The robotic arms are undocked from the trocars and the robot is moved from the bedside. The abdomen is desufflated and manual breaths are given by the anesthesiologist to decrease residual intra-abdominal gas. The fascia at the 12 mm ports is closed with 0-vicryl to prevent hernia formation. The skin is closed in a subcuticular fashion with 4–0 vicryl or using dermabond (Fig. 67.17).

Postoperative Care

The postoperative management and recovery after a robotic radical hysterectomy mirrors that of other minimally invasive surgery. Patients are given a general diet on postoperative day zero and in our experience, all patients are able to tolerate oral pain medications and do not require any intravenous narcotics.

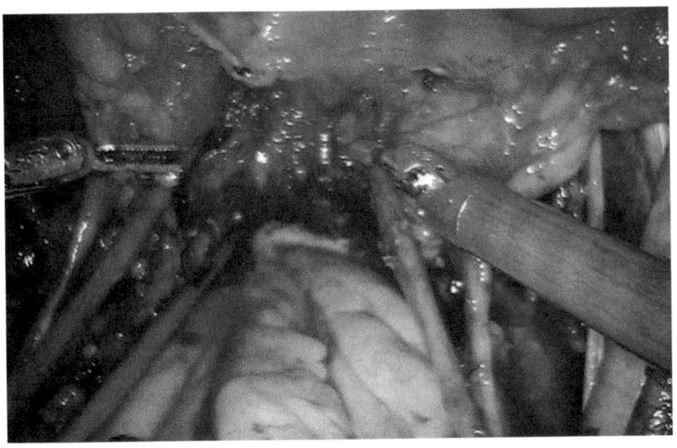

Fig. 67.17 Irrigation and hemostasis. At the conclusion of the procedure, irrigation is performed and hemostasis is assured

Patients do not require intravenous fluids by early postoperative day one. The vast majority of patients are able to go home on postoperative day one. Given the extensive bladder dissection and resulting parasympathetic and sympathetic denervation required for type III radical hysterectomy, all patients are sent home with a foley catheter and present to clinic four to seven days postoperatively for a voiding trial to ensure adequate bladder function prior to catheter removal.

References

1. Piver MS, Rutledge F, Smith JP. Five classes of extended hysterectomy for women with cervical cancer. Obstet Gynecol 1974;44:265–72.
2. Sert BM, Abeler VM. Robotic-assisted laparoscopic radical hysterectomy (Piver type III) with pelvic node dissection–case report. Eur J Gynaecol Oncol. 2006;27:531–3.
3. Boggess JF, Gehrig PA, Cantrell L, et al. A case-control study of robot-assisted type III radical hysterectomy with pelvic lymph node dissection compared with open radical hysterectomy. Am J Obstet Gynecol. 2008;199:357 e1–7.
4. Cantrell LA, Mendivil A, Gehrig PA, Boggess JF. Survival outcomes for women undergoing type III robotic radical hysterectomy for cervical cancer: a 3-year experience. Gynecol Oncol. 2010;117:260–5.
5. Hoogendam JP, Verheijen RH, Wegner I, Zweemer RP. Oncological outcome and long-term complications in robot-assisted radical surgery for early stage cervical cancer: an observational cohort study. BJOG. 2014;121:1538–45.
6. Li G, Yan X, Shang H, Wang G, Chen L, Han Y. A comparison of laparoscopic radical hysterectomy and pelvic lymphadenectomy and laparotomy in the treatment of Ib-IIa cervical cancer. Gynecol Oncol. 2007;105:176–80.
7. Wysham WZ, Kim KH, Roberts JM, et al. Obesity and perioperative pulmonary complications in robotic gynecologic surgery. Am J Obstet Gynecol. 2015;213(1):33.e1–7.
8. Estape R, Lambrou N, Diaz R, Estape E, Dunkin N, Rivera A. A case matched analysis of robotic radical hysterectomy with lymphadenectomy compared with laparoscopy and laparotomy. Gynecol Oncol. 2009;113:357–61.
9. Ko EM, Muto MG, Berkowitz RS, Feltmate CM. Robotic versus open radical hysterectomy: a comparative study at a single institution. Gynecol Oncol. 2008;111:425–30.
10. Lowe MP, Chamberlain DH, Kamelle SA, Johnson PR, Tillmanns TD. A multi-institutional experience with robotic-assisted radical hysterectomy for early stage cervical cancer. Gynecol Oncol. 2009;113:191–4.
11. Wright JD, Herzog TJ, Neugut AI, et al. Comparative effectiveness of minimally invasive and abdominal radical hysterectomy for cervical cancer. Gynecol Oncol. 2012;127:11–7.
12. Sert BM, Boggess JF, Ahmad S, Jackson AL, Stavitzski NM, Dahl AA, Holloway RW. Robotic versus open yype III radical hysterectomy: a multi-institutional experience for early stage cervical cancer. Soc Gyencol Oncol. Chicago, IL2015
13. Vilos GA, Ternamian A, Dempster J, Laberge PY, The Society of O, Gynaecologists of C. Laparoscopic entry: a review of techniques, technologies, and complications. J Obstet Gynaecol Can(JOGC = Journal d'obstetrique et gynecologie du Canada : JOGC). 2007;29:433–65.
14. Committee on Gynecologic Practice. Committee opinion no. 620: Salpingectomy for ovarian cancer prevention. Obstet Gynecol. 2015;125:279–81.

Robotic-Assisted Radical Hysterectomy (RRH) as Nerve-Sparing Procedure

68

Gun Oh Chong and Yoon S. Lee

Radical hysterectomy is a well-accepted treatment modality of early-stage cervical cancer. Radical hysterectomy is defined as the en bloc removal of the uterus and cervix with the surrounding parametrial tissue, upper vagina. The term radical hysterectomy has been used to refer to a wide range of procedures that act with different degrees of radicality. In 1974, Piver and Rutledge describe five different types of extended abdominal radical hysterectomy [1].

A new classification has recently been proposed by Querleu and Morrow in 2008 (Table 68.1) [2].

Because conventional radical hysterectomy (CRH) involves dividing and disrupting the cardinal and utersacral ligament, which contain the autonomic nerves, urinary, anorectal, and sexaul dysfunction can be developed. One thrid of patients report bladder dysfunction after radical hysterectomy such as difficulty emptying the bladder, incomplete emptying and urgency [3]. Furthermore, anorectal dysfuction, including constipation, have been reported in 5–10 % of patients after CRH [4]. Considerable sexual dysfunction, including decrease in sexual interest and organism, and vaginal dryness, are also noticed after CRH, which compromise sexual activity and result in subtantial distress [5].

Japanese surgeons first introduced the nerve-sparing radical hysterectomy (NSRH) procedure to preserve pelvic autonomic nerves, with desire to prevent disabling long-term adverse effect [6]. Subsequently, most international investigators who described their experiences using NSRH reported favorable outcomes, including earlier return of bladder function [7, 8], better vaginal blood flow [9], and fewer symptoms related to anorectal function [10]. A recent meta-analysis also showed that NSRH may decrease intraoperative complications, and urinary and anorectal dysfunction [11, 12]. However, NSRH has been suggested to decrease the resection scope of radical hysterectomy, so that the narrowed resection scope may compromise therapeutic effect [13]. Possover et al. and Höckel et al. provided type III NSRH including meticulous cleansing of the neural part of the cardinal ligament from all fatty and lymphoid tissue [7, 14]. Whether leaving neural part of the cardinal ligament poses an increased risk for recurrence or lowers chances of survival remains a matter debate in the literature [15–17]. A recent meta-analysis demonstrated that NSRH may have similar clinical safety and extent of resection compared with CRH and not affect prognosis [11, 12]. However, Basaran et al. provided that the evidence adressing the oncological safety of NSRH over that of CRH is neither adequate nor statistically relevant in their systemic review [18]. A properly disigned, prospective randomized noninferiority trial is needed to assess the oncological outcomes of NSRH.

Since the introduction of the conventional laparoscopy, improvements in gynecologic surgery have been notable. However, laparoscopic radical hysterectomy is not a popular choice among gynecologic oncologist because of the increased operative time and the steep learning curve required for competency [18]. Moreover, laparoscopic NSRH has a higher urological complication rate, longer operating times, and much blood loss than does CRH, especilly during the initial learning perioid [8]. Robotic technology has recently come into wide-spread use to overcome the limitations of laparoscopic surgery. Robotic surgery gives more surgical options, such as nerve-sparing technique, due to its superior visualization (3-dimensional imaging of the operative field), mechanical improvement (seven degree of instrument mobility inside the body) and stabilization/tremor filtration of the instrument within the surgical field which lead to easier identification and preservation of anatomical structures. Marchal et al. [19] performed the robotic radical hysterectomy (RRH) in 2005, and more recently Magrina et al. [20] described techniques of robotic NSRH. It has been reported that RRH is a feasible and safe surgical modality compared with the existing radical abdominal hysterectomy and laparoscopic radical hysterectomy for the treatment of early-stage cer-

G.O. Chong • Y.S. Lee (✉)
Gynecologic Cancer Center, Kyungpook National University Medical Center, Daegu, Korea
e-mail: gochong@knu.ac.kr; yslee@knu.ac.kr

I. Alkatout, L. Mettler (eds.), *Hysterectomy*, DOI 10.1007/978-3-319-22497-8_68

Table 68.1 Classification of radical hysterectomy by Querleu and Morrow

Q-M classification	Ureter mobilization	Transection of paracervix	Transection of uterosacral and vesicouterine ligament	Vaginal resection	Piver-Smith classification
A	Not done	Medial to ureter and lateral to cervix	At the level of cervix	<10 mm	Extrafascial hysterectomy
B	Unroofed and rolled laterally	At the level of the ureteral tunnel	Partial resection	At least 10 mm	Modified radical hysterectomy
C	Mobilised completely	Transected completely	At the level of rectum and bladder	15–20 mm	Classical radical hysretecomy
C1	With autonomic nerve preservation				
C2	Without autonomic nerve preservation				

Table 68.2 Comparison of surgical outcomes between nerve-sparing robotic radial hysterectomy and total laparoscopic radical hysterectomy

	RRH (n=50)	TLRH (n=50)	*P* value
Operating time (min)	230.1±35.8	211.2±46.7	0.025[a]
Blood loss (ml)	54.9±31.5	201.9±148.4	<0.001[a]
Pelvic node (n)	25.0±9.9	23.1 ±10.4	0.361[a]
Length of hospital stay (days)	9.6±5.6	8.7±3.1	0.325[a]
Time to normal residual urine (days)	9.6±6.4	11.0±6.2	0.291[a]
Transfusion (n, %)	1 (2 %)	4 (8 %)	0.169[b]

Data are presented as the mean ± SD or as a percentage of the total number
RRH robotic radical hysterectomy, *TLRH* total laparoscopic radical hysterectomy
[a]Student t-test
[b]Chi-square test

Table 68.3 Comparison of intraoperative and postoperative complications between nerve-sparing robotic radial hysterectomy and total laparoscopic radical hysterectomy

	RRH (n=50)	TLRH (n=50)	*P* value
Intraoperative complications (n)	0	4	0.041[a]
Bladder injury	0	3	
Major vessels injury	0	1	
Postoperative complications (n)	7	9	0.585[a]
Febrile morbidity	1	2	
Ileus	2	1	
Ureterovaginal fistula	1	2	
Hydronephrosis	2	0	
Lymphedema	0	2	
Vaginal cuff dehiscence	0	1	
Postoperative bleeding	1	0	
Trocar site herniation	0	1	
Total complications (n)	7	13	0.134[a]

Data are presented as a percentage of the total number
RRH robotic radical hysterectomy, *TLRH* total laparoscopic radical hysterectomy
[a]Chi-square test

vical cancer. [21–24]. Chong et al. reported that mean blood loss and intraoperative complication rate in the robotic group were significantly lower than those of laparoscopic group during initial phase of NSRH (Tables 68.2 and 68.3) [25]. Furthermore, no differences in cervical cancer recurrences occured in patients who undergone robotic, conventional laparoscopic, or abdominal radical hysterectomy in long-term follow-up data [22, 26].

If we focus on the advantages of robotic NSRH, esay differentiation between the fine sacral afferent fibers and the deep uterine veins due to articulating movement of the robotic arms ; stable traction and conter-traction of robotic arms, which enable us to expose the surgical plane consistently and precisely ; and an excellent 3-dimensional viwe of the robotic system within the narrow space. Furthermore, these technical advantages have given us improved dissection of the posterior vesicouterine ligament. The vesical branch of the inferiror hypogastric plexus can be preserved after dissecting several fragile veins step-by-step.

Anatomy of Pelvic Autonomic Nerves

1. Superior hypogatric plexus

Superior hypogatric plexus (SHP) is an unpaired structure situated anterior to the fifth lumbar vertebra and the sacral promontory, between the two common iliac arteries, and is formed by the union of numerous filaments, which descend on either side from the aortic plexus, and from the lumbar ganglia [27]. The SHP divides into right and left branch at or below the sacral promontory.

2. Pelvic splanchnic nerves

Pelvic splanchnic nerves (PSN) are parasympathetic nerve fibers arising near the sacral foramina from the ventral rami of the sacral nerve S2-S4. They are variable number and not always found arising from S2-S4 [28]. The S3 and S4 branches are the main contributors to the inferior hypogastric plexus (IHP) [29], the S3 branch being the largest one [28].

3. Sacral splanchnic nerves

The sacral splanchnic nerves are orginated from S2 sympathetic ganglion and contributes to the IHP [29]. Their primary function is to provide sympathetic component to the sacral plexus nerves for vasomotor, pilomotor, and sudomotor innervation of the lower extremity.

4. Inferior hypogastric plexus

IHP is composed of three different component : SHP via the hypogastric nerve, the sympathetic trunk via sacral splanchnic nerves, and the parasympathetic nerves via pelvic splanchnic nerves. IHP contains sympathetic and parasympathetic innervation. Symphathetic innervation from the SHP projects to the two IHPs via the bilateral fiber bundles of the hypogastric nerves. The sacral splanchinc nerve is originated from S2 symphathetic ganglion and contributes to the IHP. The hypogastric nerve fuses with parasympathetic splanchnic nerves originating from S2-S4 to the inferior hypogastric plexus (IHP). In the horizontal plane the IHP is located at about the level of S4 and S5. In the sagittal plane, the IHP is observed more commonly in the uterosacral ligament (57 %) and less commonly at the level of the parametrium (30 %), or between the lateral vaginal wall and the bladder (11 %) or at the rectal wall (2 %) [29]. The IHP continues inferior the vagina and bladder along with posterior vesicouterine ligament and the lateral wall of the vagina [30, 31].

Functions of Pelvic Autonomic Nerves

The pelvic autonomic nerves are essential for a normal physiologic function of the pelvic organs. For urinary function, parasymphathetic nerve disruption causes a hypocontractile of acontractile bladder with decreased sensation. Symphathetic nerve disruption results in a bladder with decreased compliance and high storage pressures. Moreover, sympathetic denervation may cause bladder neck incompetence and incontinenec. Disruption of the autonomic nerve supply to the rectum results in colorectal motility disorder [32, 33]. Autonomic nerve disruption results in altered vascular function during sexual arousal, and possibly disordered orgasm [34]. The exact role of SHP still remains unclear. However, Virtanen et al. reported an increase in the frequency of constipation and defecation problems after sacrocoloplexy [35]. Moreover, damage to the SHP could lead to urinary incontinence, especially due to incompetence and leakage at the internal urethral sphincter [36]. Hence, we should make an effort to preserve SHP during para-aortic lymphadenectomy.

Procedures of Robtoic NSRH: Step-by-Step

Patient Preparation, Docking and Instrumentation

The patients were placed in the a 20–30° Trendelenburg position. Proper initial positioning is essential because the robot must be disengaged before any change in position of the oprating table can be made. A 5-puncture technique was used with 4 robotic arms. A 12-mm primary trocar for 30 degree telescope was directly placed though the umbilicus. For lower para-aortic lymphadenectomy, a 12-mm primary trocar was placed 1–3 cm above the umbilicus. Two 8-mm lateral trocars were placed 7–8 cm lateral to the primary trocar for the 2 robotic arms. A fourth robotic tracar was placed 7–8 cm lateral and caudal to the right robotic trocar. An accessory 12-mm trocar was placed in the left upper quardrant for assistance, such as suctioning, irrigation, retraction, or grasping (Fig. 68.1). An EndoWrist monopolar scissors (Intuituve Inc., Sunnyvale, CA) was used in the right hand, and EndoWrist fenestrated bipolar forceps (Intuituve Inc., Sunnyvale, CA) in the left hand. An EndoWrist Prograsper (Intuituve Inc., Sunnyvale, CA) was placed in the fourth robotic arm. For vaginal cuff closure, the monopolar scissor was replaced by an EndoWrist needle holder (Intuituve Inc., Sunnyvale, CA).

The assistant, sitting to the left of the patient, at shoulder level, performed important tasks using an accessory torcar, such as sealing and division vascular structure using a Ligasure system (Covidien, Valleylab, Boulder, CO) or an Enseal device (SurgRx Inc., Redwood City, CA), suction and irrigation, removal of biopsy specimens, tissue retraction and grasping, and introduction and retrieval of sutures for vagianl cuff closure. The second assistant was situated between the patients' legs and moved the uterine manipulator. The robotic column was positioned between the legs of the patient, behind the second assistant.

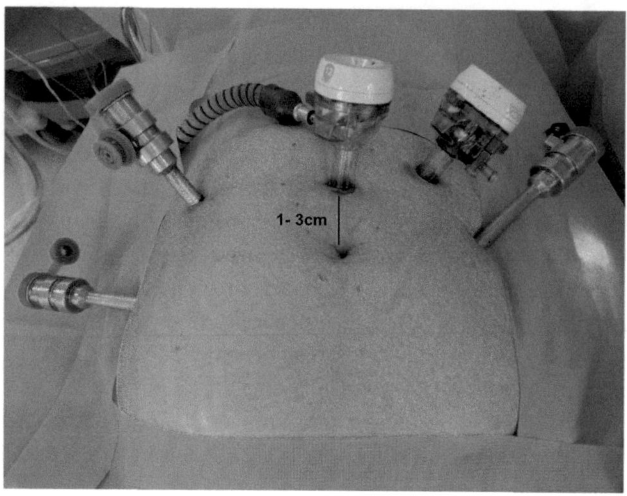

Fig. 68.1 Positioning of trocars for robotic nerve-sparing radical hysterectomy.

Identification of Superior Hypogsatric Plexus (SHP)

After left upward traction of rectosigmoid mesentery using EndoWrist Prograsper, a peritoneal incision is made at below inferior mesenteric artery. The SHP is found overlying the aorta and sacral promontory, medial to both ureters (Fig. 68.2). Rectosigmoid is mobilized, and then the avascular space of the lateral rectal portion is found by using the upward traction of rectosigmoid mesentery. The SHP is isolated by vessel loop. The SHP divides into right and left branches at or below the sacral promontory. A continuous downward dissection is then made uint the hypogastric nerve is identified. Using this approach, communication between the SHP and hypogatric nerve could be found.

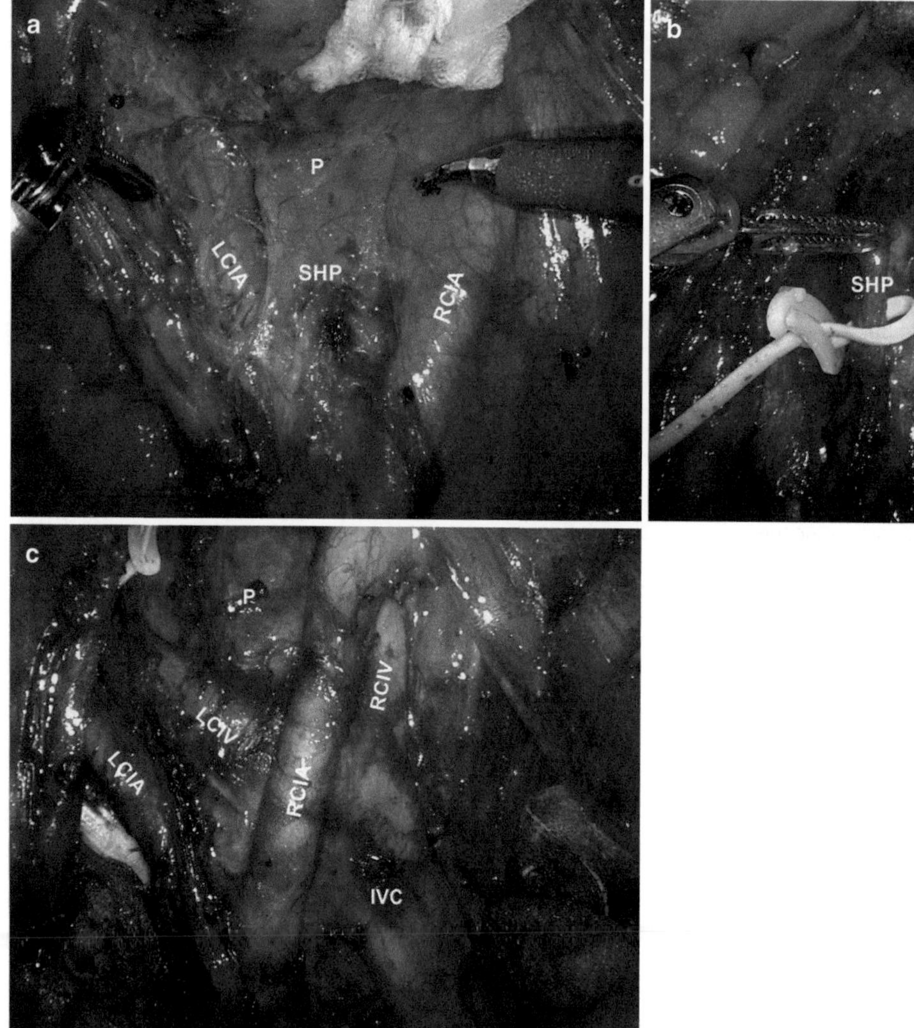

Fig. 68.2 Identification of Superior hypogastric plexus. (**a**) After traction of rectosigmoid, peritoneal incision is made and we can identify the common iliac artery, superior hypogastric plexus, and promontory. (**b**) Superior hypogastric plexus is isolated by vessel loop. (**c**) Final view of lower para-aortic lymphadenectomy and the superior hypogastric plexus (isolated by vessel loop). *IVC* inferior vena cava, *LCIA* left common iliac artery, *LCIV* left common iliac vein, *P* promontory, *RCIA* right common iliac artery, *RCIV* right common iliac vein, *SHP* superior hypogastric plexus

Identification of Pelvic Splanchnic Nerve (PSN), Inferior Hypogastric Plexus (IHP) and Hypogastric Nerve

Between the paravesical and pararectal spaces, the cardinal ligament was sperated by a scissor dissector. The uterine artery is dissected at the level of the hypogatric artery and several deep uterine veins are coagulated with bipolar graspers and transected. After careful seperation of deep uterine vessels to the base of the cardinal ligament, PSNs that communicated with the IHP and hypogastric nerve are observed. PSNs are variable in number 3–4. Sometimes PSN are indistinguishable to fibrotic connective structure. Then, the hypogastic nerve appears as a thickened band and is identified approximately 2–5 cm below the ureter (Fig. 68.3).

Identification of the Hypogastric Nerve and IHP During the Dissection of the Uterosacal and Rectovaginal Ligaments

After well dissection of the rectovaginal space, both uterosacral ligaments clearly identified. The hypogastric nerve is located in the lateral portion of the uterosacral ligament. The hypogastric nerve is mobilized laterally from the the lateral aspect of the uterosacral ligament. A space between medial part of uterosacral ligament and hypogastric nerve is developed. Only the medial fibrous component of the uterosacral ligament is divided, and the lateral nervous compartment is perserved (Fig. 68.4).

Identification of Vesical Branch of the IHP from Posterior Vesicouterine Ligament

This step is the most critical step in the nerve-sparing procedure. After unroofing the ureter with dissection of the anterior vesicouterine ligament, the ureter is mobilized laterally to identify and isolate the posterior vesicouterine ligament. Posterior vesicouterine ligament is exposed by anterior and lateral retraction of the ureter. And then, several vesical veins (lateral, middle, medial, inferior) in the posterior vesicouterine ligament are identified and these veins are carefully separated and skeletonized step-by-step. The vesical branches of the IHP may be easily damaged during extensive removal of paravaginal tissue. To spare the vesical branches of the IHP completely, only the uterovaginal branches of the IHP should be resected. After the cut edge of the inferior vesical vein is pulled medially with upward traction, the vesical branches of the IHP are exposed, which divided into medial and lateral branches [37]. In advanced cases, the medial branches of the IHP could be sacrificed to obtain an adequate cancer-free margin [37]. After these procedures, the vesical branches of the IHP are preserved (Fig. 68.5). After nerve-sparing RRH, the entire course of pelvic autonomic nerves could be examined cleary incluing SHP, hypogatric nerve communicating with parasympathetic nerves, and vesical branch of the IHP (Fig. 68.5e).

Extended Lymphadenectomy

The areas of extended lymphadenectomy are the superior and inferior gluteal, presacral (subaortic), common iliac, and lower paraaortic nodes. Extended lymphadenectomy is started without injury to the SHP and hypogastric nerve. Right paraaortic lymph nodes are dissected at the level of the inferior mesenteric artery. The inferior mesenteric artery and SHP are then identified, and a space is created between the inferior mesenteric artery and SHP that enable the ureter to be displaced laterally and the left paraaortic node to be displaced medially. Inframesenteric nodes are removed without injury to the ureter and the left common iliac nodes are easily removed due to the upward traction of the rectosigmoid. Through the left upward traction of the SHP, the right side of presacral nodes on the promontory is removed without injury to the presacral vein. By using the right upward traction of the SHP, the left side of the presacral nodes and left common iliac nodes are removed. After further dissection of the hypogastric vessels, we can identify the posterior branches of the hypogastric artery, the superior gluteal artery which locates between lumboscaral plexus and S1, and inferior gluteal artery which locates between S2 and S3. After extended lymphadenectomy, the pelvic anatomy could be examined more clearly including the SHP, promontory, lower part of aorta, common iliac vessels, hypogastric vessels, hypogastric nerve communicating with parasympathetic nerves, and vesical branches of the IHP (Fig. 68.6).

Extended lymphadenectomy may contribute to the prevention of locoregional relapse [38]. Recent study showed the the prevalence of internal iliac vein anomalies was 26.7 % in the presacral area [39]. To prevent life-threatening the internal iliac vein injury, the anatomical variations of the internal iliac vein should be known exactly during lymphadenectomy at presacral area.

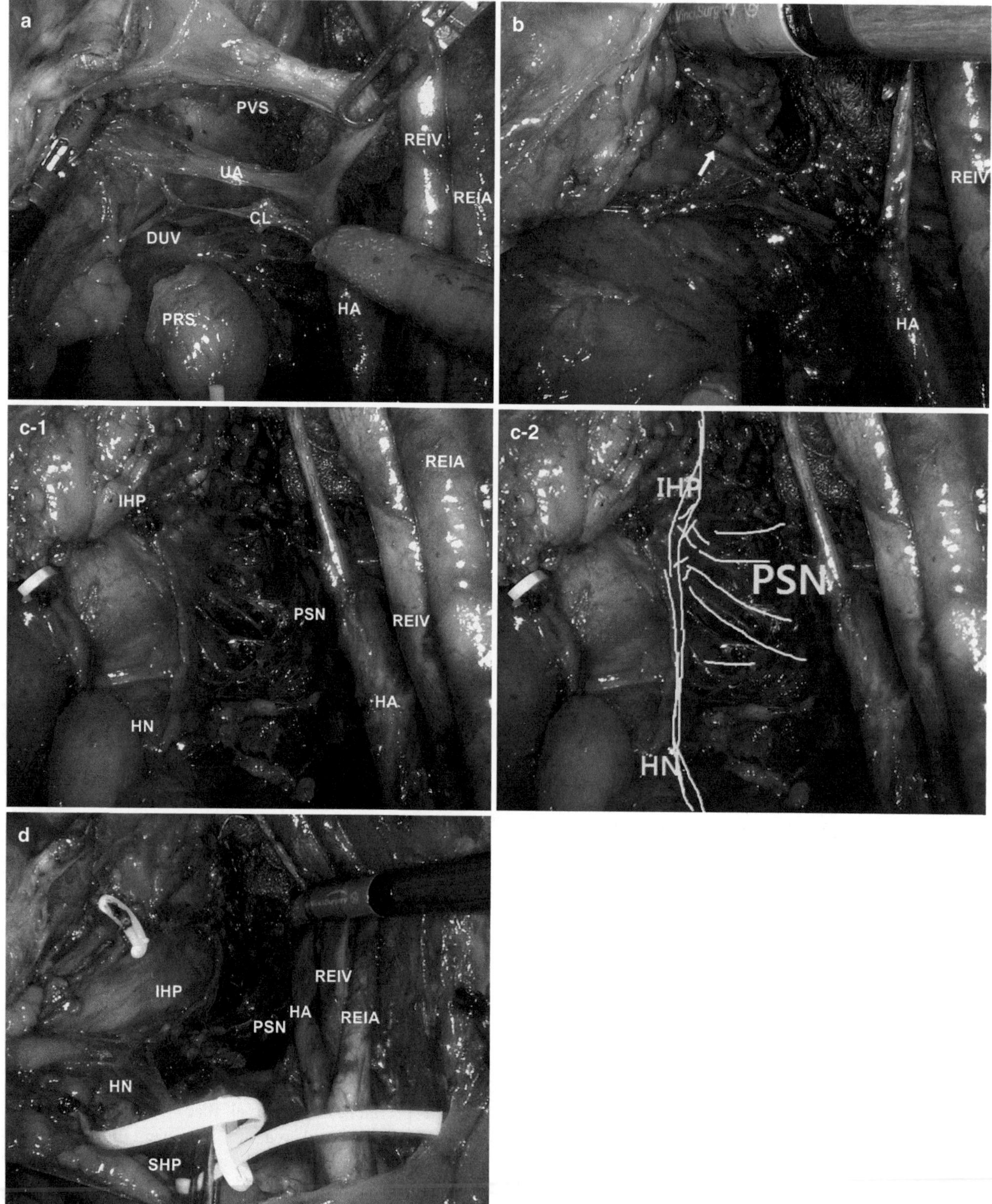

Fig. 68.3 Identification of pelvic splanchnic nerve, hypogastric nerve and inferior hypogastric plexus. (**a**) Between paravesical and pararectal space, the uterine artery and deep uterine veins which are located in the cardinal ligament are divided by step by step. (**b**) Uterine veins (white arrow) are isolated by robotic scissor, then divided by bipolar or Ligasure system. (**c1**) Pelvic splanchnic nerves are communicated with the inferior hypogastric plexus and hypogastric nerve. (**c2**) Schematic view of **c1**. (**d**) Hypogastric nerve is communicated with superior hypogastric plexus (isolated by vessel loop). *CL* cardinal ligament, *DUV* deep uterine vein, *HA* hypogastric artery, *IHP* inferior hypogastric plexus, *PSN* pelvic splanchnic nerve, *PRS* pararectal space, *PVS* paravesical space, *SHP* superior hypogastric plexus, *UA* uterine artery

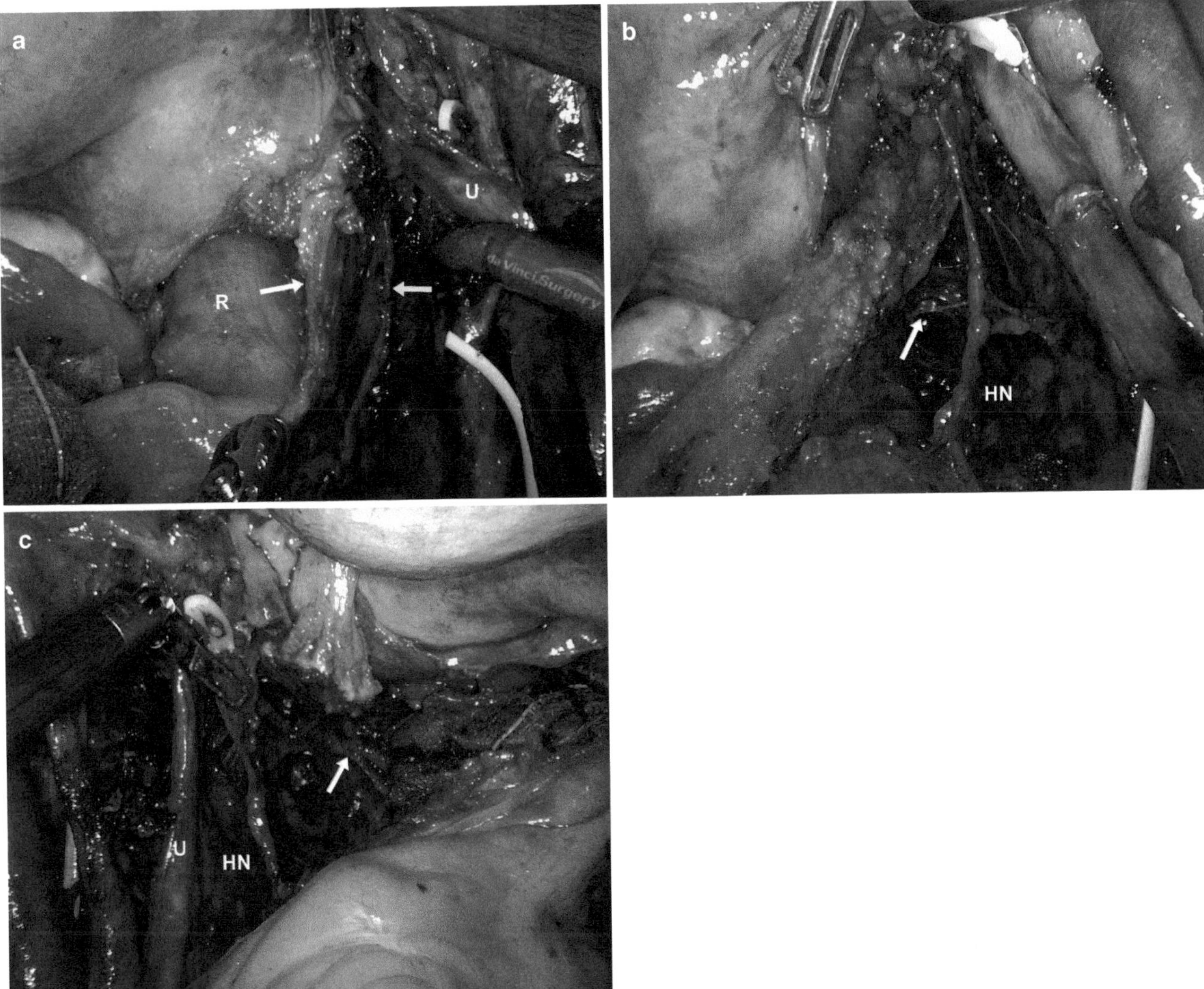

Fig. 68.4 Identification of hypogastric nerve during dissection of uterosacral and rectovaginal ligament. (**a**) After dissection of rectovaginal space, rectovaginal and uterosacral ligaments (*white arrow*) and hypogastric nerve (*yellow arrow*) are identified (*right side*). (**b**) After dissection of rectovaginal and uterosacral ligaments, rectal branches of hypogastric nerve (*white arrow*) are clearly preserved (*right side*). (**c**) Rectal branches of hypogastric nerve (*white arrow, left side*). *HN* hypogastric nerve, *R* rectum, *U* ureter

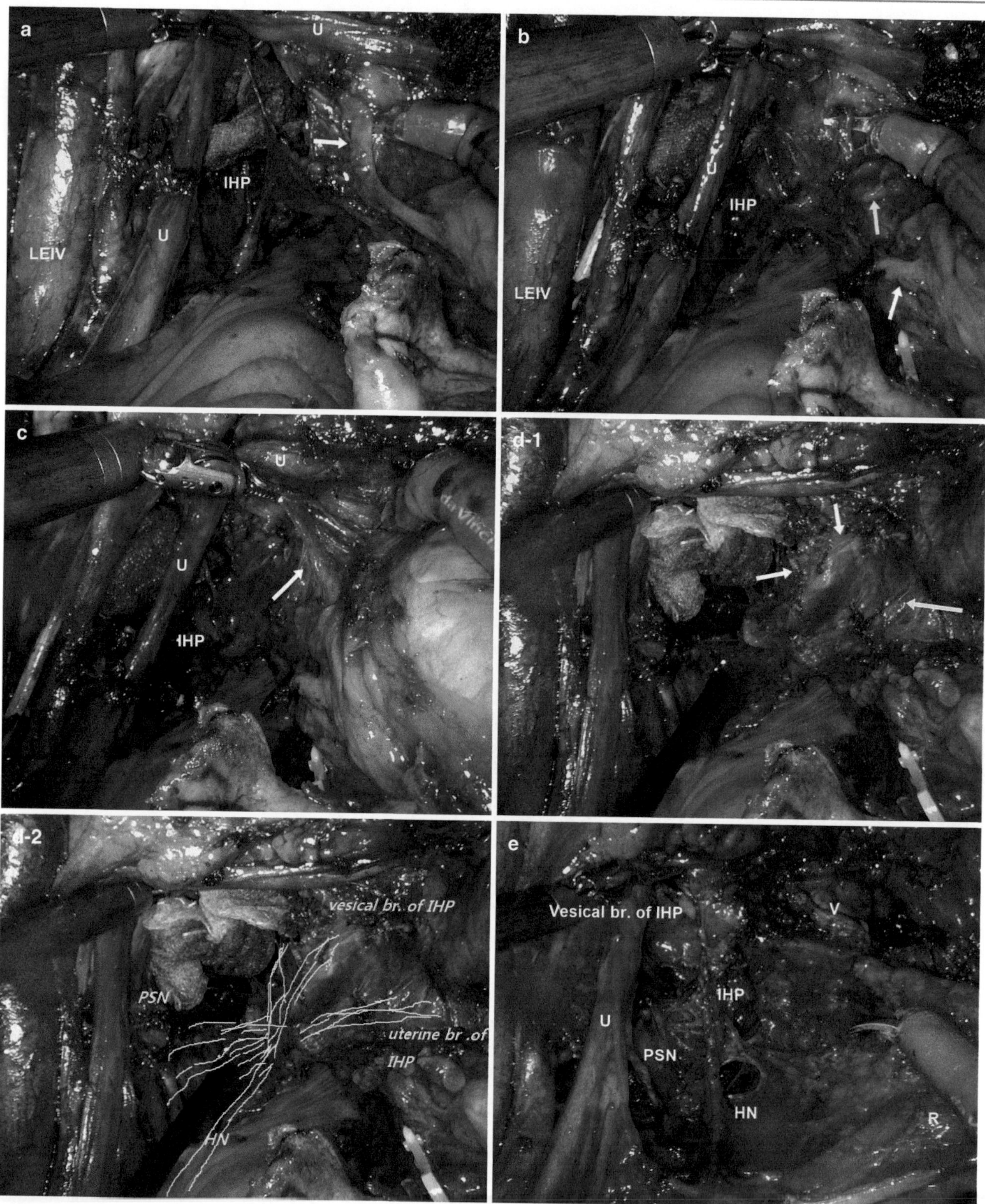

Fig. 68.5 Identification of vesical branches of inferior hypogastric plexus from posterior vesicouterine ligament. (**a**) Several veins in posterior vesicouterine ligament are identified by fine movement of robotic scissor and skeletonized by step by step. First, lateral vein (*white arrow*) is isolated (*left side*). (**b**) Lateral (*white arrow*) and middle (*yellow arrow*) veins are isolated (*left side*). (**c**) Medial vein (*white arrow*) is isolated (*left side*). (**d1**) After all veins are divided and isolated, veins are retracted upward. Vesical (*white arrow*) and uterine branches (*yellow arrow*) of inferior hypogastric plexus are identified (*left side*). (**d2**) Schematic view of **d1**. (**e**) After removal of the uterus, preserved pelvic autonomic nervous parts are clearly identified (*left side*). *HN* hypogastric nerve, *IHP* inferior hypogastric plexus, *LEIV* left external iliac vein, *PSN* pelvic splanchnic nerve, *R* rectum, *U* ureter.

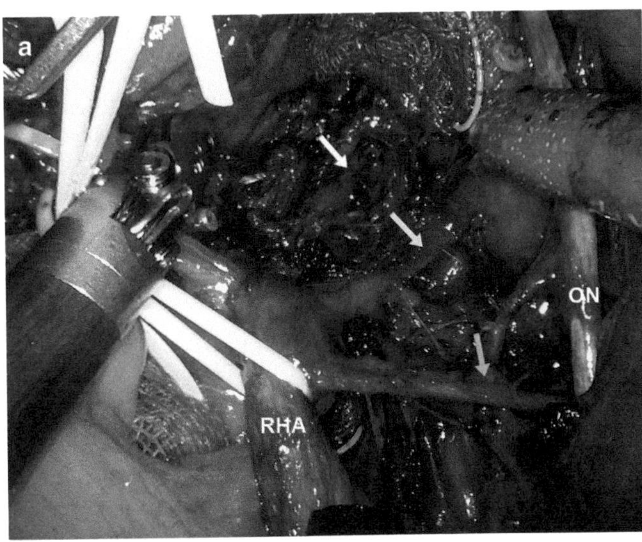

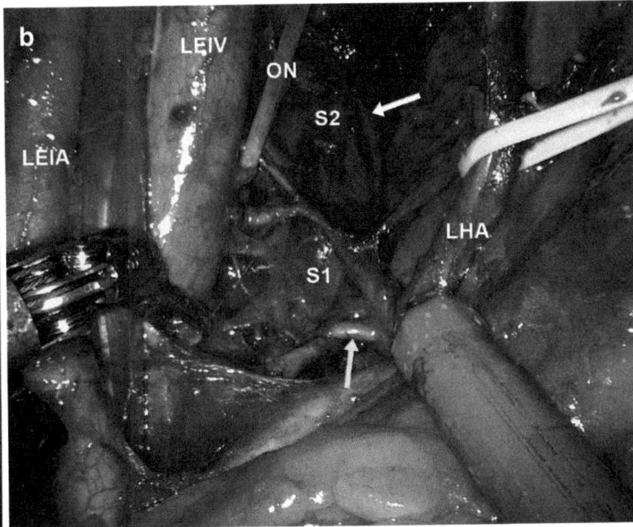

Fig. 68.6 After traction of hypogastric artery, branches of hypogastric artery are clearly identified. (**a**) Common trunk of inferior gluteal artery and internal pudendal artery (*white arrow*), superior gluteal artery (*yellow arrow*), and iliolumbar artery with veins (*green arrow, right side*). (**b**) Common trunk of inferior gluteal and internal pudendal artery (*white arrow*), and superior gluteal artery with veins (*yellow arrow, left side*). *LEIA* left external iliac artery, *LEIV* left external iliac vein, *LHA* left hypogastric artery, *ON* obturator nerve, *RHA* right hypogastric artery

Table 68.4 Systemic review of robotic radical hysterectomy versus abdominal radical hysterectomy and robotic radical hysterectomy versus laparoscopic radical hysterectomy

Variables	RRH vs. ARH	RRH vs. LRH
Estimated blood loss	RRH – Pro ARH – Con	RRH – Pro LRH - Con
Operative time	Equivalent	Equivalent
Lymph nodes count	Equivalent	Equivalent
Intraoperative complications	Equivalent	Equivalent
Hospital stay	RRH – Pro ARH – Con	Equivalent

RRH robotic radical hysterectomy, *ARH* abdominal radical hysterectomy, *LRH* laparoscopic radical hysterectomy

Robotic NSRH

Recent systemic review and meta-analysis shows that RRH may be superior to abdominal radical hysterectomy (ARH) with lower estimatated blood loss, shorter hospital stay, less febrile morbidity and wound-related complications [38]. Although RRH was associated with less estimated blood loss than laparosocpic radical hysterectomy (LRH), mean differnenc was of borderline significance. There was no significant differece in operative time or intraoperative complications. RRH and LRH appear equivalent in intraoperative and short-term postoperative outcomes (Table 68.4) [40].

Robotic NSRH is a feasible and safe modality for the treatment of early cervical cancer without compromising radicality. Excellent 3-dimensional image amplification facilitates visualization and the teaching of the pelvic autonomic nerves. Moreover, articulating movement of the robotic arms, lack of tremor, stable traction and counter-traction of robotic arms provide us to expose the surgical plane consistently and precisely.

References

1. Piver MS, Rutledge F, Smith JP. Five classes of extended hysterectomy for women with cervical cancer. Obstet Gynecol. 1974;44:265–72.
2. Querleu D, Morrow CP. Classification of radical hysterectomy. Lancet Oncol. 2008;9:297–303.
3. Pieterse QD, Maas CP, ter Kuile MM, Lowik M, van Eijkeren MA, Trimbos JB, Kenter GG. An observational longitudinal study to evaluate miction, defecation, and sexual function after radical hysterectomy with pelvic lymphadenectomy for early-stage cervical cancer. Int J Gynecol Cancer. 2006;16:1119–29.
4. Barnes W, Waggoner S, Delgado G, Maher K, Potkul R, Barter J, Benjamin S. Manometric characterization of rectal dysfunction following radical hysterectomy. Gynecol Oncol. 1991;42:116–9.
5. Bergmark K, Avall-Lundqvist E, Dickman PW, Henningsohn L, Steineck G. Vaginal changes and sexuality in women with a history of cervical cancer. N Engl J Med. 1999;340:1383–9.

6. Fujii S, Takakura K, Matsumura N, Higuchi T, Yura S, Mandai M, Baba T, Yoshioka S. Anatomic identification and functional outcomes of the nerve sparing Okabayashi radical hysterectomy. Gynecol Oncol. 2007;107:4–13.
7. Possover M, Stöber S, Plaul K, Schneider A. Identification and preservation of the motoric innervation of the bladder in radical hysterectomy type III. Gynecol Oncol. 2000;79:154–7.
8. Chong GO, Park NY, Hong DG, Cho YL, Park IS, Lee YS. Learning curve of laparoscopic radical hysterectomy with pelvic and/or para-aortic lymphadenectomy in the early and locally advanced cervical cancer: comparison of the first 50 and second 50 cases. Int J Gynecol Cancer. 2009;19:1459–64.
9. Pieterse QD, Ter Kuile MM, Deruiter MC, Trimbos JB, Kenter GG, Maas CP. Vaginal blood flow after radical hysterectomy with and without nerve sparing. A preliminary report. Int J Gynecol Cancer. 2008;18:576–83.
10. Cibula D, Velechovska P, Sláma J, Fischerova D, Pinkavova I, Pavlista D, Dundr P, Hill M, Freitag P, Zikan M. Late morbidity following nerve-sparing radical hysterectomy. Gynecol Oncol. 2010;116:506–11.
11. Long Y, Yao DS, Pan XW, Ou TY. Clinical efficacy and safety of nerve-sparing radical hysterectomy for cervical cancer: a systematic review and meta-analysis. PLoS One. 2014;9:–e94116.
12. Kim HS, Kim K, Ryoo SB, Seo JH, Kim SY, Park JW, Kim MA, Hong KS, Jeong CW, Song YS, Study Group FUSION. Conventional versus nerve-sparing radical surgery for cervical cancer: a meta-analysis. J Gynecol Oncol. 2015;26:100–10.
13. Landoni F, Maneo A, Cormio G, Perego P, Milani R, Caruso O, Mangioni C, Class II. versus class III radical hysterectomy in stage IB-IIA cervical cancer: a prospective randomized study. Gynecol Oncol. 2001;80:3–12.
14. Höckel M, Konerding MA, Heussel CP. Liposuction-assisted nerve-sparing extended radical hysterectomy: oncologic rationale, surgical anatomy, and feasibility study. Am J Obstet Gynecol. 1998;178:971–6.
15. Girardi F, Lichtenegger W, Tamussino K, Haas J. The importance of parametrial lymph nodes in the treatment of cervical cancer. Gynecol Oncol. 1989;34:206–11.
16. Landoni F, Bocciolone L, Perego P, Maneo A, Bratina G, Mangioni C. Cancer of the cervix, FIGO stages IB and IIA: patterns of local growth and paracervical extension. Int J Gynecol Cancer. 1995;5:329–34.
17. Hagen B, Shepherd JH, Jacobs IJ. Parametrial resection for invasive cervical cancer. Int J Gynecol Cancer. 2000;10:1–6.
18. Frumovitz M, Ramirez PT, Greer M, Gregurich MA, Wolf J, Bodurka DC, Levenback C. Laparoscopic training and practice in gynecologic oncology among Society of Gynecologic Oncologists members and fellows-in-training. Gynecol Oncol. 2004;94:746–53.
19. Marchal F, Rauch P, Vandromme J, Laurent I, Lobontiu A, Ahcel B, Verhaeghe JL, Meistelman C, Degueldre M, Villemot JP, Guillemin F. Telerobotic-assisted laparoscopic hysterectomy for benign and oncologic pathologies: initial clinical experience with 30 patients. Surg Endosc. 2005;19:826–31.
20. Magrina JF, Pawlina W, Kho RM, Magtibay PM. Robotic nerve-sparing radical hysterectomy: feasibility and technique. Gynecol Oncol. 2011;121:605–9.
21. Boggess JF, Gehrig PA, Cantrell L, Shafer A, Ridgway M, Skinner EN, Fowler WCA. case-control study of robot-assisted type III radical hysterectomy with pelvic lymph node dissection compared with open radical hysterectomy. Am J Obstet Gynecol. 2008;199:357.e1–7.
22. Magrina JF, Kho RM, Weaver AL, Montero RP, Magtibay PM. Robotic radical hysterectomy: comparison with laparoscopy and laparotomy. Gynecol Oncologia. 2008;109:86–91.
23. Ko EM, Muto MG, Berkowitz RS, Feltmate CM. Robotic versus open radical hysterectomy: a comparative study at a single institution. Gynecol Oncol. 2008;111:425–30.
24. Estape R, Lambrou N, Diaz R, Estape E, Dunkin N, Rivera A. A case matched analysis of robotic radical hysterectomy with lymphadenectomy compared with laparoscopy and laparotomy. Gynecol Oncol. 2009;113:357–61.
25. Chong GO, Lee YH, Hong DG, Cho YL, Park IS, Lee YS. Robot versus laparoscopic nerve-sparing radical hysterectomy for cervical cancer: a comparison of the intraoperative and perioperative results of a single surgeon's initial experience. Int J Gynecol Cancer. 2013;23:1145–9.
26. van den Tillaart SA, Kenter GG, Peters AA, Dekker FW, Gaarenstroom KN, Fleuren GJ, Trimbos JB. Nerve-sparing radical hysterectomy: local recurrence rate, feasibility, and safety in cervical cancer patients stage IA to IIA. Int J Gynecol Cancer. 2009;19:39–45.
27. Correia JA, De-Ary-Pires B, Pires-Neto MA, De Ary-Pires R. The developmental anatomy of the human superior hypogastric plexus: a morphometrical investigation with clinical and surgical correlations. Clin Anat. 2010;23:962–70.
28. Havenga K, DeRuiter MC, Enker WE, Welvaart K. Anatomical basis of autonomic nerve-preserving total mesorectal excision for rectal cancer. Br J Surg. 1996;83:384–8.
29. Baader B, Herrmann M. Topography of the pelvic autonomic nervous system and its potential impact on surgical intervention in the pelvis. Clin Anat. 2003;16:119–30.
30. Maas CP, Trimbos JB, DeRuiter MC, van de Velde CJ, Kenter GG. Nerve sparing radical hysterectomy: latest developments and historical perspective. Crit Rev Oncol Hematol. 2003;48:271–9.
31. Fujii S. Anatomic identification of nerve-sparing radical hysterectomy: a step-by-step procedure. Gynecol Oncologia. 2008;111:S33–41.
32. Yalla SV, Andriole GL. Vesicourethral dysfunction following pelvic visceral ablative surgery. J Urol. 1984;132:503–9.
33. Smith AN, Varma JS, Binnie NR, Papachrysostomou M. Disordered colorectal motility in intractable constipation following hysterectomy. Br J Surg. 1990;77:1361–5.
34. Levin RJ. The physiology of sexual function in women. Clin Obstet Gynaecol. 1980;7:213–52.
35. Virtanen H, Hirvonen T, Mäkinen J, Kiilholma P. Outcome of thirty patients who underwent repair of posthysterectomy prolapse of the vaginal vault with abdominal sacral colpopexy. J Am Coll Surg. 1994;178:283–7.
36. Johnson RM, McGuire EJ. Urogenital complications of anterior approaches to the lumbar spine. Clin Orthop Relat Res. 1981;154:114–8.
37. Park NY, Cho YL, Park IS, Lee YS. Laparoscopic pelvic anatomy of nerve-sparing radical hysterectomy. Clin Anat. 2010;23:186–91.
38. Lee YS, Chong GO, Lee YH, Hong DG, Cho YL, Park IS. Robot-assisted total preservation of the pelvic autonomic nerve with extended systematic lymphadenectomy as part of nerve-sparing radical hysterectomy for cervical cancer. Int J Gynecol Cancer. 2013;23:1133–8.
39. Chong GO, Lee YH, Hong DG, Cho YL, Lee YS. Anatomical variations of the internal iliac veins in the presacral area: clinical implications during sacral colpopepxy or extended pelvic lymphadenectomy. Clin Anat. 2015;28:661–4.
40. Shazly SA, Murad MH, Dowdy SC, Gostout BS, Famuyide AO. Robotic radical hysterectomy in early stage cervical cancer: a systematic review and meta-analysis. Gynecol Oncol. 2015;138:457–71.

Robotic-Assisted Radical Hysterectomy as Compartmental Resection According to rTMMR and rPMMR

69

Rainer Kimmig

Introduction

On the basis of ontogenetic compartmental development the findings about compartmental border control in malignant tumour progression led to the concept of "compartmental resection" in solid malignant tumors [1–4]. Since loco-regional recurrence usually occurs in compartment remnants or in the associated lymph compartments total "compartments of risk" have to be removed completely, whereas neighbouring compartments may left entirely untouched. The first tumour resected following this concept was rectal cancer by total mesorectal excision (TME) resulting in dramatically reduced loco-regional recurrence [5]. At present this procedure has become standard in rectal cancer surgery [6]. For cervical cancer M. Höckel has convincingly shown by his monocentric data that the corresponding method named total mesometrial resection (TMMR) also reduces efficiently locoregional recurrences compared to standard treatment – without any additional radiation therapy even in risk situations [7, 8]. The Method is described for open surgery in a separate chapter. Together with M. Höckel total mesometrial resection (rTMMR) has been translated to robotic surgery [9]. On parallel, the modification of compartmental resection for endometrial cancer as peritoneal mesometrial resection (PMMR) according to the different lymph drainage has also been adopted to robotic surgery as rPMMR [10]. Although, the two methods have to be applied together with therapeutic pelvic or pelvic and paraaortic lymphadenectomy to control not only for local but also for regional disease, in this chapter the technique of radical hysterectomy only is described; however technique of therapeutic lymphonodectomy has already been published elsewhere, and will be described step by step in the following chapter 70.

R. Kimmig
Gynecology and Obstetrics, West German Cancer Center, University Hospital Essen, University Duisburg-Essen, Hufelandstr. 55, Essen, NRW D-45122, Germany
e-mail: Rainer.kimmig@uk-essen.de

Anatomical Basis of Müllerian Compartment and Local Lymph Drainage

For uterine cancer removal of the Müllerian compartment and its draining lymphatic compartments has to be performed completely. Embryological development, compartment borders and type of resection in uterine cancer is perfectly described by M. Höckel [4, 7]. As shown in Fig. 69.1, the uterus has to be removed together with the vascular mesometrium (corresponding to the uterine vessel system including vesicouterine anastomoses) and the ligamentous mesometrium (corresponding to the rectovaginal and sacrouterine ligament). However, there is no longer any modification with respect to the tumor size, as the concept requires always complete resection. There is only one part of the Müllerian compartment left in situ for functional reasons – the vagina. The vaginal resection margin is the only intracompartmental resection has directly to be controlled for clear margins (>10 mm recommended) in compartment confined tumors [4]. According to the different lymph drainage of the upper and lower Müllerian compartment in cervical cancer vascular and ligamentous mesometria have to be resected. In endometrial cancer without cervical involvement there is no drainage along the ligamentous mesometria; on the other hand there is drainage along the mesonephric pathway on parallel to the ovarian vessel system. Thus, ligamentous mesometria may be preserved, but infundibulopelvic ligaments have to be resected completely in corporal uterine disease as can be seen from Fig. 69.1 a–d.

Due to the lymphatic network which develops embryologically by sprouting from embryonal veins [11], compartment visualization can be achieved by fluorescent agents. Isocyanine-green (ICG) may be injected into the uterine cervix or corpus according to the tumour site and fluorescence will be detectable in the lymphatic system from minutes to many hours from application during surgery [12]. In short, 0.3 ml of a solution of 1.25 mg/ml ICG had injected ´0.5–1 cm deep either into cervical stroma at 3, 6, 9 and 12 o'clock in cervical cancer or at 3 and 9 o'clock twice at the fundal and midcorporal part in endometrial cancer. Lymphatic drainage is

I. Alkatout, L. Mettler (eds.), *Hysterectomy*, DOI 10.1007/978-3-319-22497-8_69

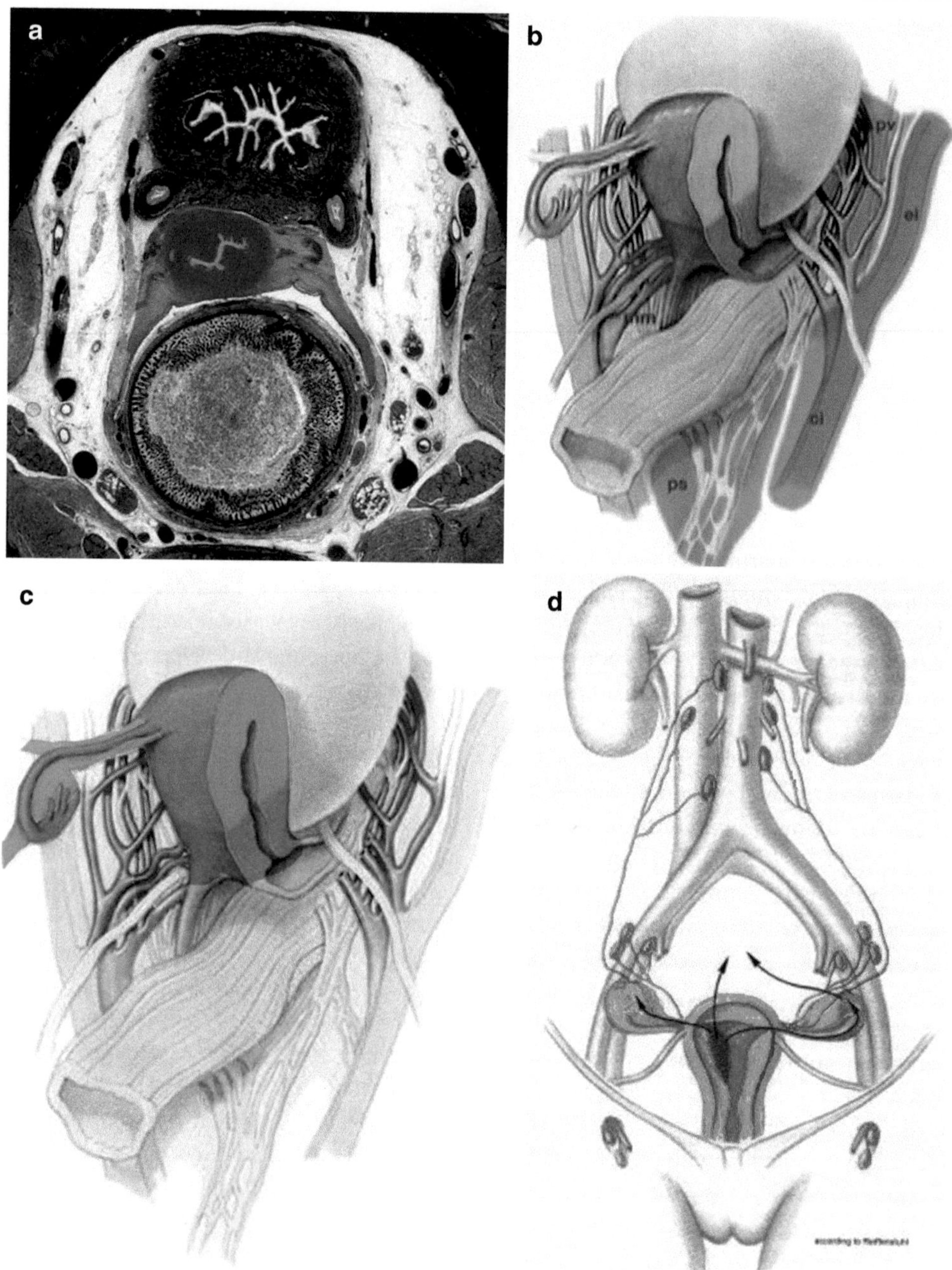

Fig. 69.1 (**a**) Embryologic development of Müllerian compartment (*red*). (**b**) Müllerian compartment in the adult (*green*). Draining pelvic lymphatic compartments: mesometrial (*mm*), paravisceral (*pv*), external iliac (*ei*), common iliac (*ci*) and presacral (*ps*). (**c**) Involvement of Müllerian compartment in endometrial cancer (*green*). (**d**) Lymphatic drainage in endometrial cancer (*green*). (**a**) Reprinted from The Lancet, 6(10), Höckel M, Horn LC, Fritsch H, Association between the mesenchymal compartment of uterovaginal organogenesis and local tumour spread in stage IB-IIB cervical carcinoma: a prospective study, 751–6, Copyright 2005, with permission from Elsevier; (**b**) Reprinted from Lancet Oncol, 10, Michael Höckel, Lars-Christian Horn, Norma Manthey, Ulf-Dietrich Braumann, Ulrich Wolf, Gero Teichmann, Katrin Frauenschläger, Nadja Dornhöfer, Jens Einenkel, Resection of the embryologically defined uterovaginal (Müllerian) compartment and pelvic control in patients with cervical cancer: a prospective analysis, 683–92, Copyright 2009, with permission from Elsevier. (**c**) Reprinted from Gynecologic Oncology, vol. 107, supplement 1, Höckel M, Do we need a new classification for radical hysterectomy? Insights in surgical anatomy and local tumor spread from human embryology, S106–S112, Copyright 2007, with permission from Elsevier. (**d**) (Modified from Hepp et al. [14], with permission)

directed from midline to lateral and drains primarily either to the iliac nodes along the vascular and ligamentous mesometria or to the paraaortic nodes along the mesonephric ovarian vessel system, or both. Up to now we never observed a drainage into the vesical or rectal compartment, neither via the vesicouterine nor the rectovaginal ligament. For better understanding of compartmental resection visualization by fluorescence will be added to the anatomical illustrations of the technique.

Technique of Total Mesometrial Resection and Peritoneal Mesometrial Resection [9, 10]

Principles of TMMR are described already in detail by Michael Höckel. The compartmental resection of the Müllerian compartment with respect to cervical and endometrial cancer does not differ in principle but only with respect to sub-compartments and their route of lymph drainage. Therefore, the technique of TMMR and PMMR adapted to robotic surgery will be described "Step by Step" for both procedures together. Steps only valid for cervical cancer or endometrial cancer will be indicated, common steps will be highlighted. As already mentioned, intention of compartmental surgery in uterine cancer is invariably to remove the local and regional compartment of risk entirely. Thus, the therapeutic lymphadenectomy is intrinsically tied to the radical hysterectomy, although not described in this chapter. The radical hysterectomy will usually be preceded by the therapeutic pelvic and – if indicated – paraaortic lymphadenectomy (technique [13]). Dependent on the sub-compartmental origin of the tumor either TMMR or PMMR or a combination of the two is performed. Differences and common steps are summarized in Table 69.1.

Surgical steps for TMMR are described in Steps 6 and 8–20, for PMMR in Steps 1–7 and 12–20, whereas all common steps are high-lighted in the text.

General Remarks and Trocar Placement

Robotic surgery usually starts cranially and proceeds caudally for technical reasons due to the steep Trendelenburg positioning to guarantee a clear visual field throughout the surgery. Four robotic arms (camera and three instruments) are used and one 10 mm trocar for assistance. The incision for the camera has to be made about 8–10 cm cranially to the upper limit of surgery, if possible. A typical setting of Incisions is shown in Fig. 69.2 for TMMR and pelvic lymphadenectomy for the da Vinci SI system. In the da Vinci Xi System this is no longer necessary since surgery can be performed in the entire abdomen without any change in docking.

Steps one to seven are dedicated to the therapeutic resection of the mesonephric sub-compartment of infundibulopelvic ligaments, therapeutic pelvic and paraaortic lymphadenectomy and peritoneal incision strategy. Except for lymphadenectomy these steps refer exclusively on PMMR for endometrial cancer.

Lymphatic drainage of uterine corpus may be visualized by intracorporal injection of Indocyanine green (ICG) solution made visible by near infrared excitation during surgery. As demonstrated in Fig. 69.3 lymphatic drainage from uterine corpus via infundibulopelvic ligaments runs along the mesosalpinx and mesovarian lymphatic network (A/B) and consists of two main lymphatic truncs accompanying the ovarian artery and vein (C/D) with variable intercalated nodes. They drain to the preaortic nodes inferior to the right ovarian artery and the precaval nodes medially of the ovarian vein on the right and to the left "renal angle" on the left (not shown).

Step 1

Incision of the peritoneum lateral to the right infundibulopelvic ligament superior to the crossing of right common iliac artery and division of peritoneum along the border to the right mesocolic fat tissue (Fig. 69.4) to expose the anterior aspect of the caval vein, the right ureter, the right infundibulopelvic ligament and the right colon mesentery (Fig. 69.5).

Step 2

The border between the mesonephric compartment of the ovarian vessel system and the compartment of right colon is identified; anastomosing vessels of the ovarian and right colonic vessels – which always are present - have to be identified and dissected (Fig. 69.6).

Step 3

The infundibulopelvic ligament is elevated and mobilized from laterally to medially keeping the connections to the paraaortic lymphatic system intact and separating it dorsolaterally from the right ureter and mesureter. Ureteral supplying vessels should kept intact (Fig. 69.7).

Table 69.1 Common and different steps in TMMR and PMMR

	Uterus	Vascular mesometrium	Ligamentous mesometrium	Fallopian tubes	Ovaries	IP ligaments
TMMR and therapeutic LNE	Yes	Yes	Yes	Yes	No[a]	No
PMMR and therapeutic LNE	Yes	Yes	No[a]	Yes	Yes	Yes

[a]This is usually not part of the procedure, but may be indicated based on the individual situation

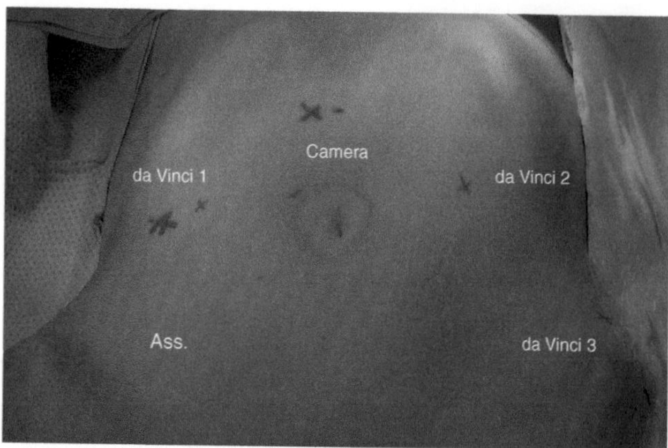

Fig. 69.2 Trocar postitioning for robotic TMMR

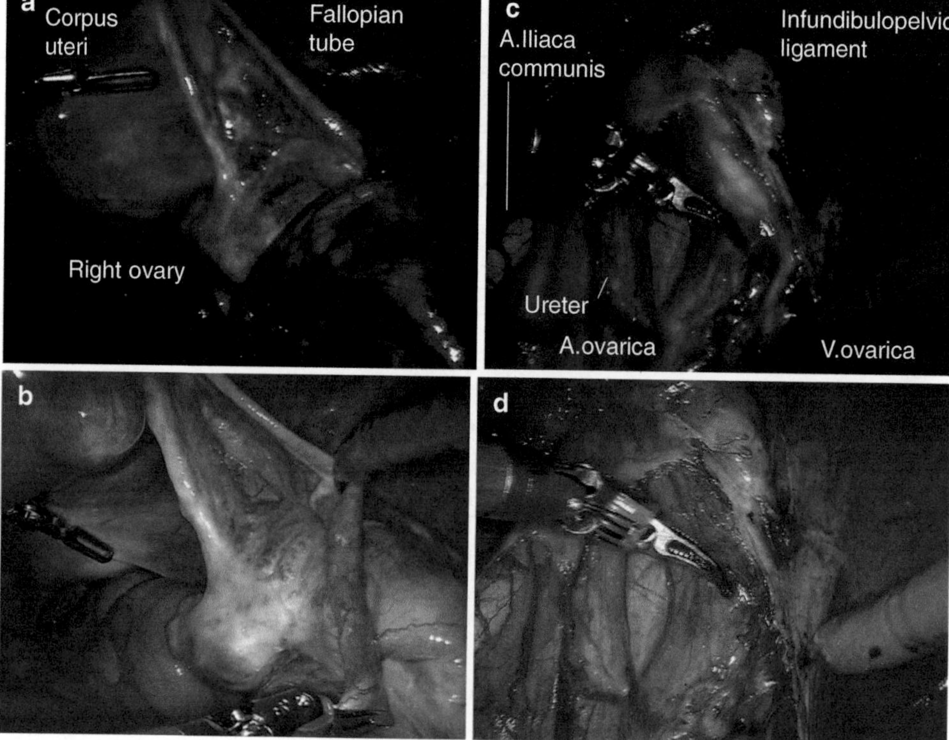

Fig. 69.3 Lymph drainage right infundibulopelvic ligament: mesovary and mesosalpinx (**a**, **b**) and infundibulopelvic ligament (**c**, **d**) each in normal light and infrared induced ICG fluorescence

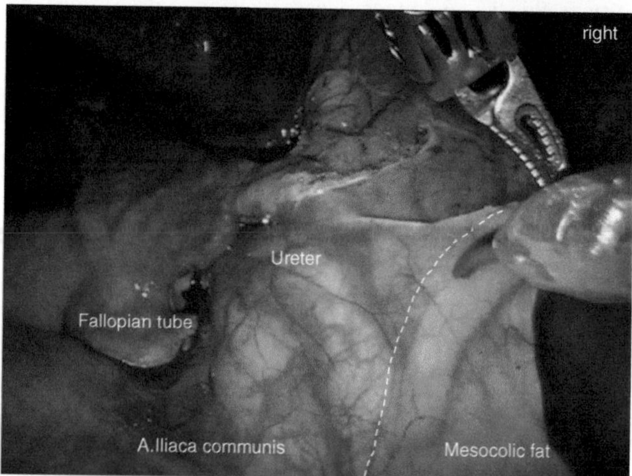

Fig. 69.4 Peritoneal incision between right infundibulopelvic ligament and mesocolon

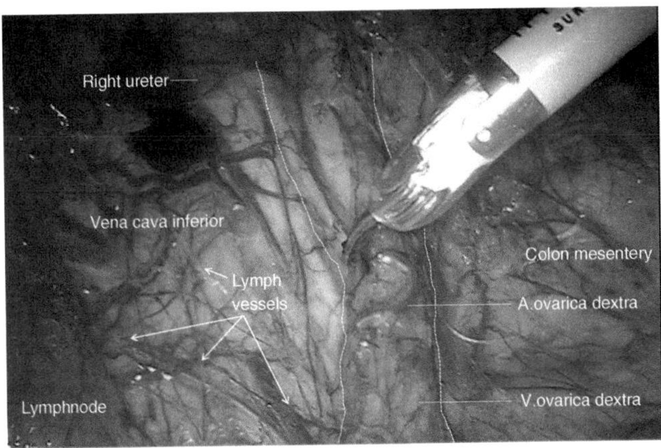

Fig. 69.5 Identification of right infundibulopelvic ligament, ureter and right colon mesentery

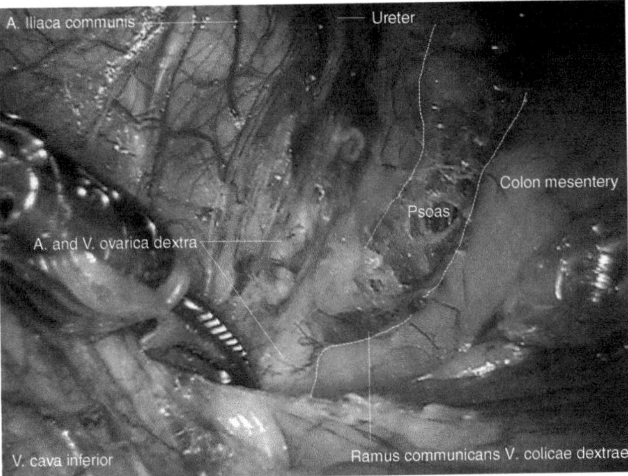

Fig. 69.6 Separation of right infundibulopelvic ligament from right colon mesentery

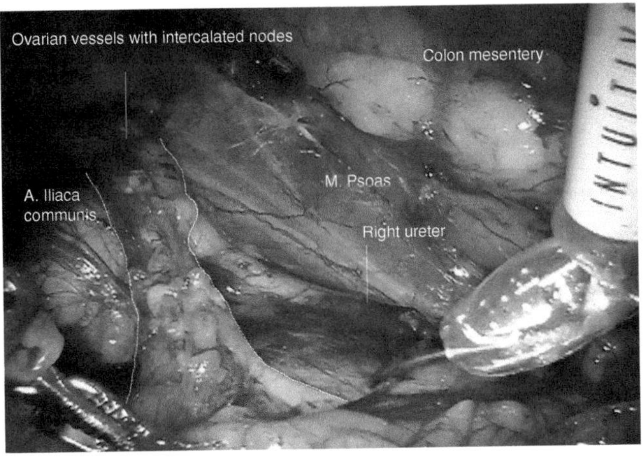

Fig. 69.7 Separation of ovarian vessel system from mesocolon, psoas muscle, ureter and caval vein

Step 4

Resection of the right infundibulopelvic ligament following the dissection of ovarian vessels at their origin together (Fig. 69.8) with periaortic lymphadenectomy which has to be performed completely up to the renal vessels. The right infundibulopelvic mesonephric compartment is completely mobilized together with adherent compartment of right periaortic nodes (Fig. 69.9).

Step 5

On the left side preparation of the infudibulopelvic ligament will start cranially. Following mobilization and dissection of the left paraaortic lymph compartment the left ovarian vein and artery (Fig. 69.8 c, d) are resected at their origin and mobilized from laterally to medially; again vessel anastomoses to the left colon mesentery have to be resected and the left ureter has to be prepared identically to the right (Fig. 69.10). The ligament is developed to the left pelvis dorsally of the mesosigma and pulled though the so-called "sigmoid tunnel". Since there are no lymphatic connections to the infundibulopelvic ligament below the left common iliac vessels the further moblization to the uterus now may be done as usual.

Step 6

Completion of therapeutic pelvic and paraaortic lymphadenectomy as previously described for endometrial cancer and/or cervical cancer [13].

Step 7

Incision of the peritoneum covering the round ligament, the ovarian vessels, the utero-ovarian junctions and the vascular mesometrium. This maneuver assures a complete resection of Müllerian compartment together with the connecting structures to the mesonephric compartment containing the lymphatic network together with the ovaries and the infundibulopelvic ligaments (Fig. 69.11).

Step 8

Radical hysterectomy with complete resection of the vascular mesometrium will now be performed as described

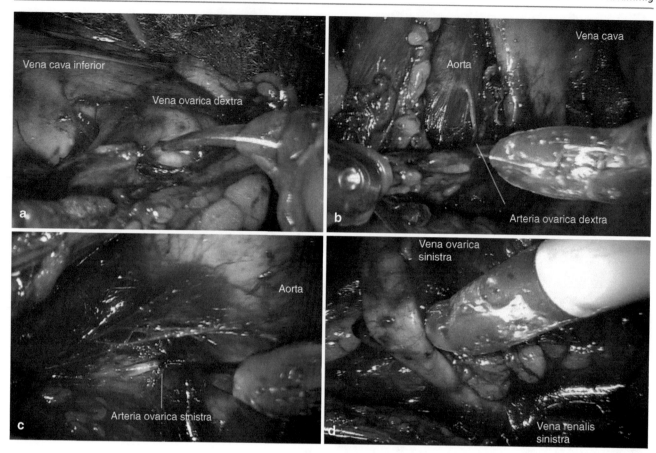

Fig. 69.8 (a–d) Dissection of ovarian veins and arteries from caval and renal veins and aorta

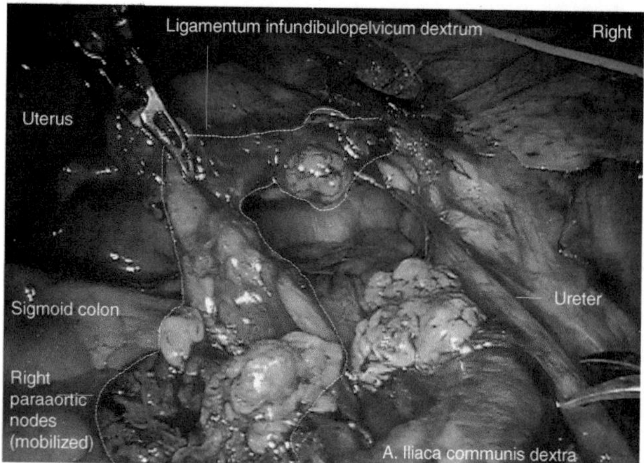

Fig. 69.9 Completely mobilized right ovarian vessel system with right paraaortic nodes

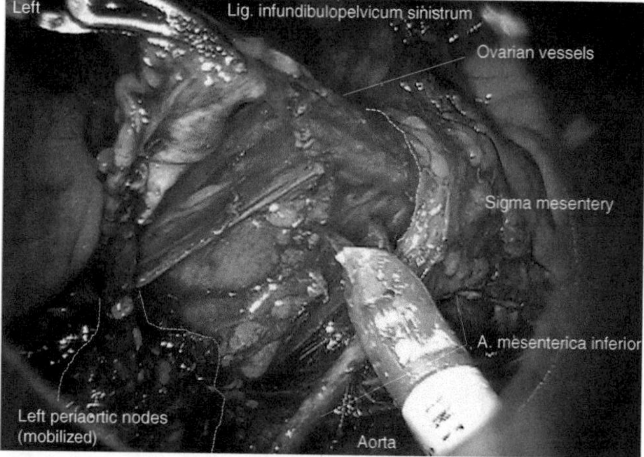

Fig. 69.10 Mobilized left ovarian vessel system entering the "sigmoid tunnel"

in detail for rTMMR [9]. If ovaries should be preserved in cervical cancer, fallopian tubes will be dissected along the mesosalpinx and ligg. Ovarii propria will be dissected.

Step 9

Preferably preparation starts posteriorly. Peritoneum will be incised in the pouch of Douglas and the rectum is mobilized medially from the vaginal wall. Preparation should free the

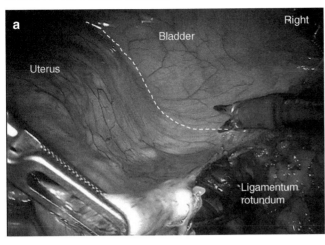

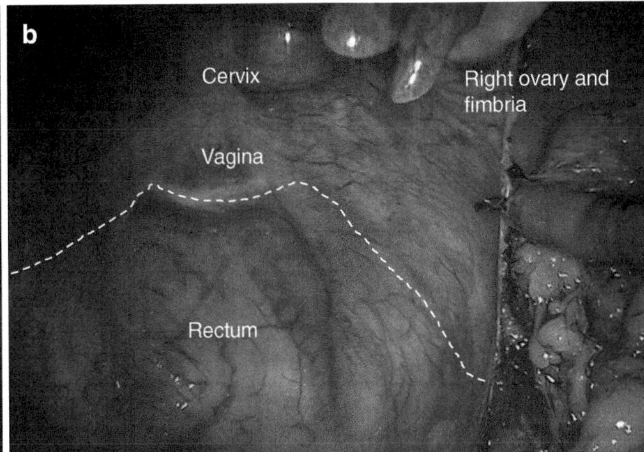

Fig. 69.11 Ventral (a) and dorsal (b) peritoneal incision in PMMR covering the utero-ovarian vessels

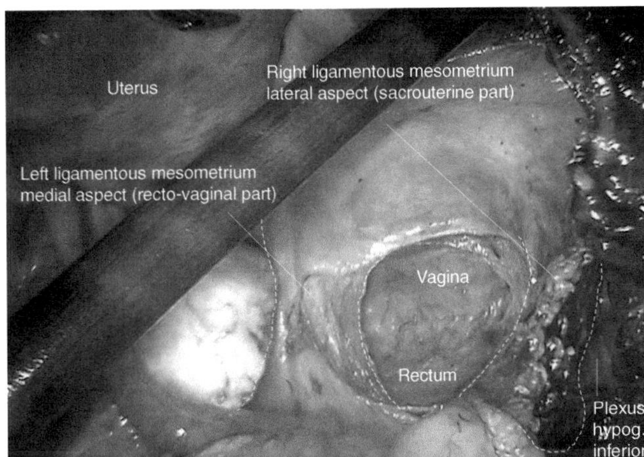

Fig. 69.12 Incision of peritoneum of Douglas pouch and separation of vagina and rectum and preparation of ligamentous mesometria

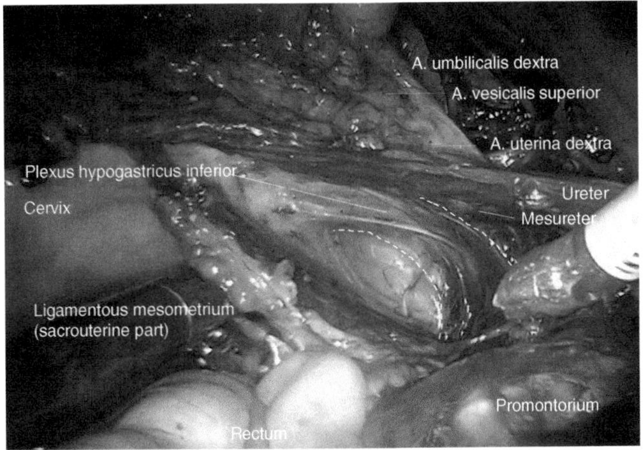

Fig. 69.13 Detaching of right ureter, mesureter and plexus hypogastricus inferior from right ligamentous mesometrium

vaginal wall at least 1 cm more caudally as intended resection line. The ligamentous mesometria (Fig. 69.12) which correspond medially to rectovaginal and rectouterine ligament are lateralized until their insertion to the perirectal tissue is reached usually ventrally to the descendent branch of the rectal artery.

Step 10

Starting on the right side the ureter is identified at its attachment to the pararectal peritoneum and detached together with the mesureter and the adherent inferior hypogastric plexus and nerve without separating these structures from each other. Thus, the avascular plain between the lateral part of the ligamentous mesometrium (anatomically corresponding to the sacrouterine ligament) may easily be opened and the nerve plain can be dissociated laterally from the ligamentous mesometrium (Fig. 69.13). The lymphatic drainage from uterine cervix is demonstrated by ICG fluorescence and is limited to the ligamentous mesometrium and postponed lymph compartment not draining to the rectal compartment, the ureteral or nerve plains (Fig. 69.14).

Step 11

The medial and lateral part of the ligamentous mesometrium may now be completely exposed (left, Fig. 69.15) and resected first laterally, pararectally along the pelvic side wall (sacrouterine part, along the mm. coccygeus and iliococcygeus and the endopelvic fascia); second, prerectally along the descending branch of the rectal artery (rectouterine/vaginal part).

Step 12

To detach the vesico-uterine attachment, the anterior surface of the uterus has to be exposed and put under tension to facilitate incision of the peritoneum at the vesico-uterine fold. The

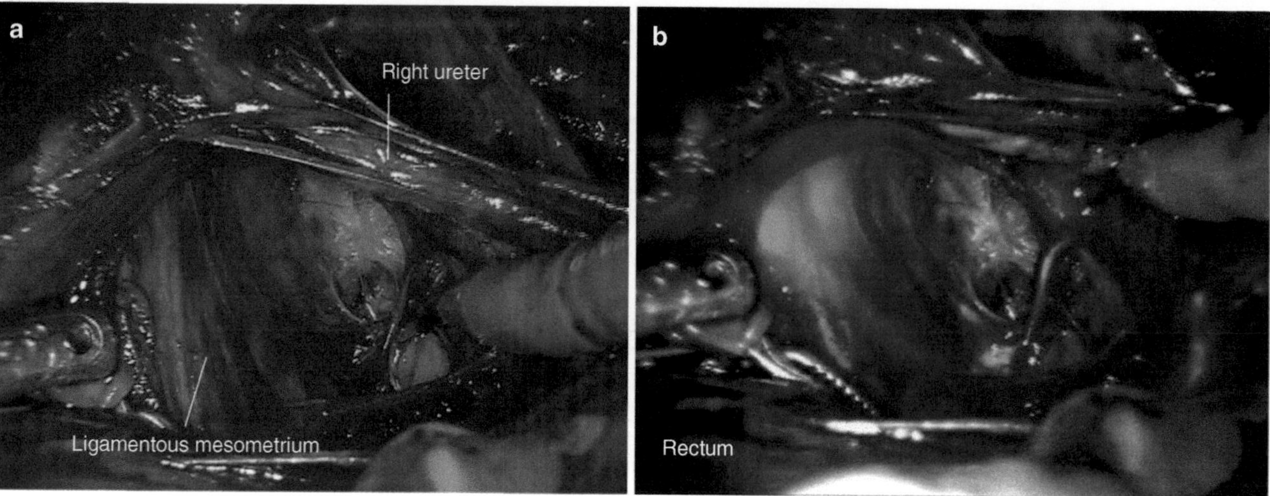

Fig. 69.14 Lateral (sacrouterine) part of right ligamentous mesometrium in cervical cancer and its connections to deep paravisceral lymph node compartments ((**a**) normal light, (**b**) ICG Fluorescence in near infrared light)

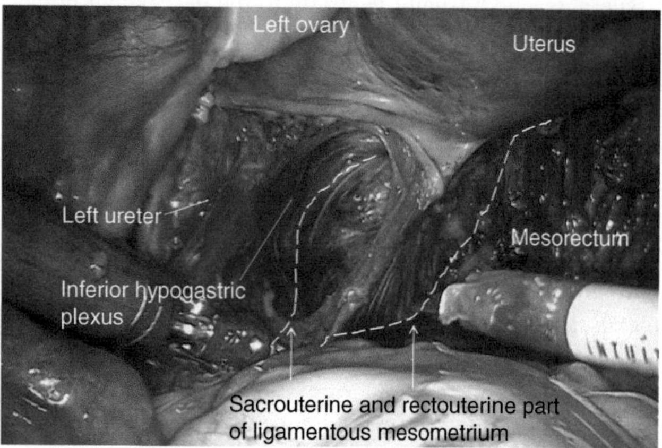

Fig. 69.15 Ligamentous mesometrium on the left side. Overview and resection lines of ligamentous mesometrium in cervical cancer

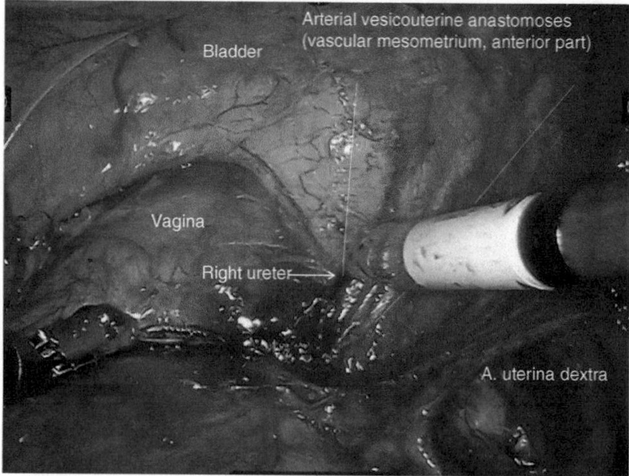

Fig. 69.16 Dissection of the vesicouterine and vesicovaginal tissue plain and preparation of vesicoureteral junctions

peritoneum has to be incised in direction to the lateral part of the round ligaments to divide these at the entrance to the inguinal channel. The loose connective tissue of the vesicouterine and vesicovaginal tissue plain is dissected caudally until the ureters are identified entering the vesical wall (Fig. 69.16). The preparation is extended then laterally and the border of the vesical and Müllerian compartments is identified.

Step 13

The right umbilical artery is identified and completely exposed to its origin from the internal iliac artery. Thus, branching of uterine artery and one or more superior vesical arteries can easily be identified (Fig. 69.17). Now, the ventral border of the vascular mesometrium may be prepared between the uterine and superior vesical vessels, the dorsal border between the uterine artery and the hypogastric plexus, laterally to the ureter.

As it has been shown already for the ligamentous mesometrium in Fig. 69.17, the vascular mesometrium will also be identified by ICG transporting lymph vessels from uterine cervix (Fig. 69.18). There is sharp delineation and no lymphatic drainage to the bladder compartment or along the superior vesical artery.

Step 14

The vascular mesometrium can now be exposed, first by developing the avascular space between its anterior surface and the bladder mesentery containing the superior vesical artery (Fig. 69.17); secondly, by developing the avascular space between the posterior surface and the plain of the ureter, mesureter and inferior hypogastric plexus (Fig. 69.19). The caudal border of the vascular mesometrium is marked by

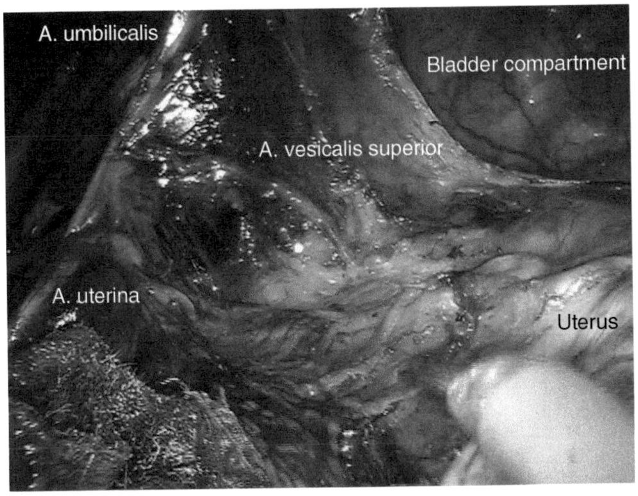

Fig. 69.17 Ventral aspect of vascular mesometrium separated from the bladder compartment

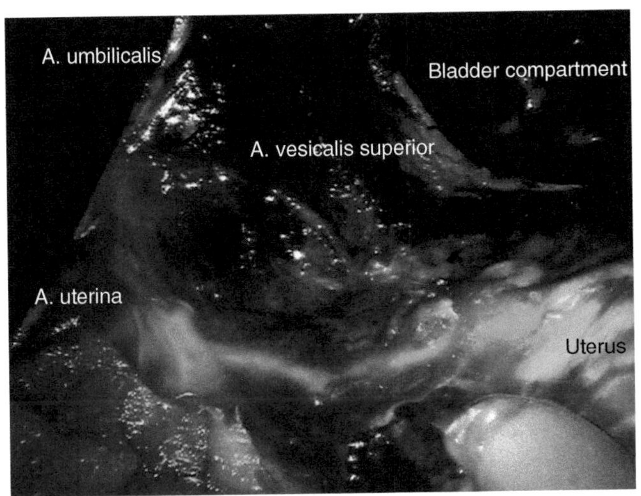

Fig. 69.18 Corresponding ICG lymphography of left vascular mesometrium (Fig. 69.17)

the deep uterine vein, which should also be resected in cervical cancer, but may be left in endometrial cancer (Fig. 69.20). The deep uterine vein often is branching from a common trunc with superior vesical vein. It should be prepared and coagulated before dissection to avoid bleeding. Splanchnic nerves always cross below the vein, thus never will be damaged, if the level of deep uterine vein is taken as the caudal border of resection – with or without resection of the vein.

Step 15

The complete resection of the vascular mesometrium including all paracervical/mesometrial intercalated nodes starts with the coagulation and division of the uterine artery and superficial uterine veins at their origin from the iliacal vessels. This step should be carried out without separating

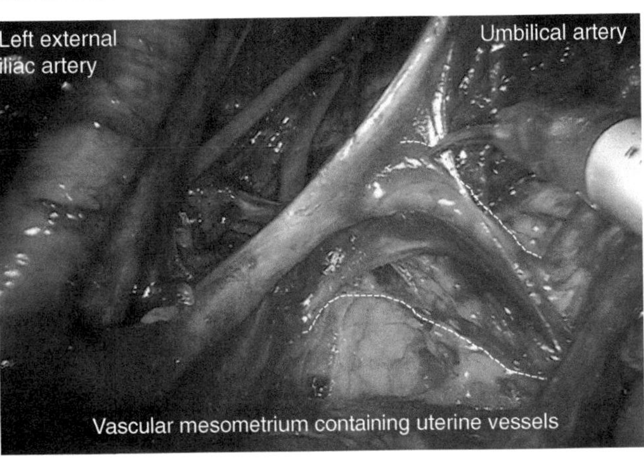

Fig. 69.19 Left vascular mesometrium (lateral part, dorsal aspect)

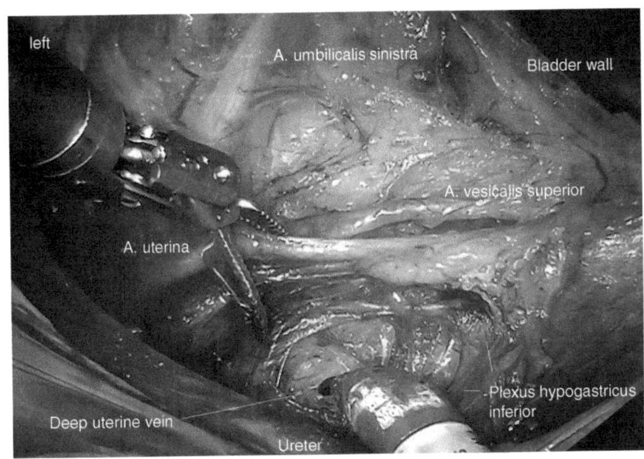

Fig. 69.20 Resection of left vascular mesometrium

the vessels in order to remove all perivascular lymphatic tissue “en bloc” (Fig. 69.20). The deep uterine vein is identified and coagulated separately.

Step 16

Dissection of the ureteral branch of the uterine artery (and vein) following elevation of the uterine bundle is necessary to mobilize the ureter in its “tunnel” (Fig. 69.21). Coagulation and dissection of vesicouterine/vaginal arterial anastomoses in the anterior part of vesicouterine ligament will separate the Müllerian from the vesical compartment ventrally, carefully preserving the ureteral branches of the bladder mesentery (Fig. 69.22).

Step 17

Dissection of the uterine nerve fibers of the hypogastric nerve at the lateral posterior aspect of the cervix will enable to preserve the bladder branches of the hypogastric nerve.

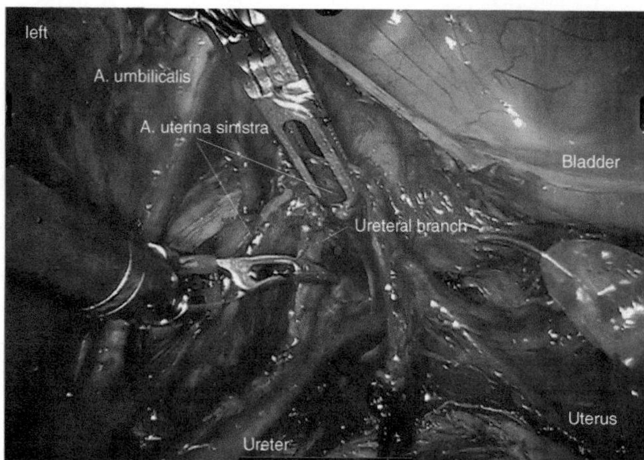

Fig. 69.21 Disection of ureteral branch of uterine artery, left vascular mesometrium

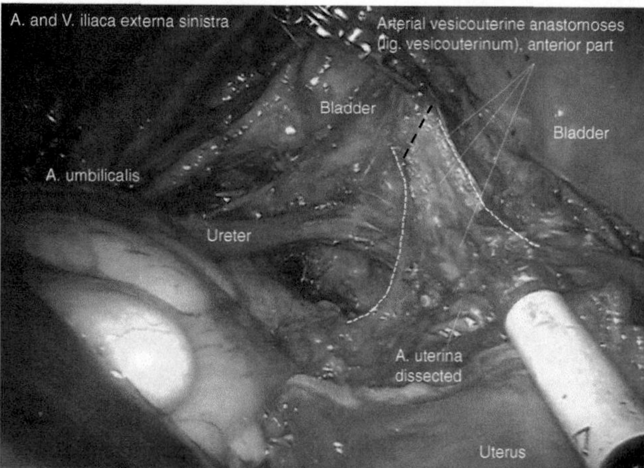

Fig. 69.22 Preparation of anterior part of left vascular mesometrium corresponding to vesico-uterine ligament

They will be lateralized and pushed caudally together with the ureter (Fig. 69.23).

Step 18

Dissection of the "ladder-like" arranged vesicovaginal venous anastomoses (Fig. 69.24), if not already done during separation of the ventral aspect of vascular mesometrium from the bladder mesentery (so called "posterior leaf of vesicouterine ligament").

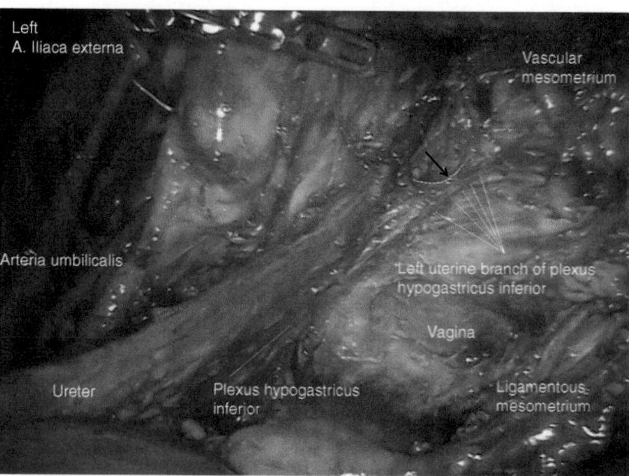

Fig. 69.23 Dissection of left uterine branching nerves to lateralize inferior hypogastric nerve

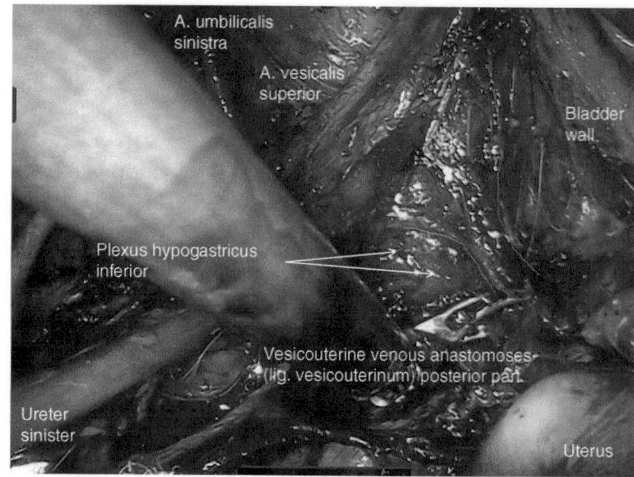

Fig. 69.24 Dissection of venous vesico-uterine anastomoses of vascular mesometrium on the left

Step 19

Definition of the vaginal resection plane and dissection of the mesocolpium if necessary. Opening the vagina from dorsally and resection of vaginal cuff with sufficiently clear margins confirmed by frozen section (Fig. 69.25).

Step 20

Removal of resected tissue, bags and sponges vaginally, and confirmation of clear margins. The vagina is closed by running suture.

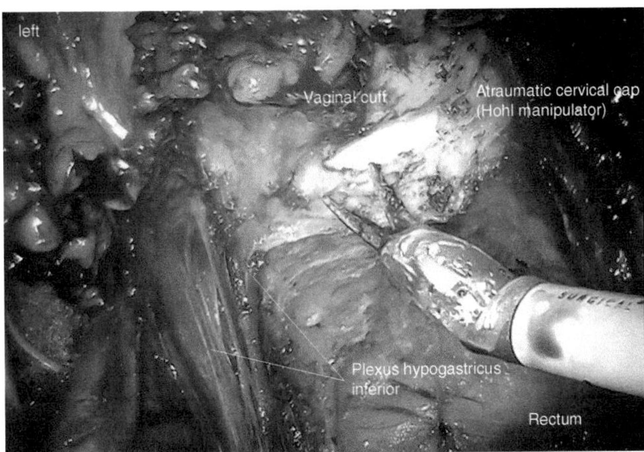

Fig. 69.25 Definition of length of vaginal cuff and colpotomy

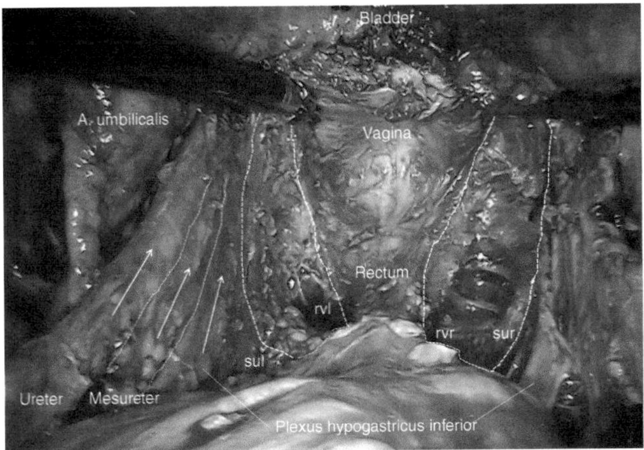

Fig. 69.26 Final situation following TMMR: resection lines ligamentous mesometria su (sacrouterine), rv (recto-vaginal), l/r

Finally, all tissue of Müllerian compartment has been removed completely - except for the vaginal part for functional reasons - but adjacent structures of neighbouring compartments such as ureter, mesureter, hypogastric plexus, rectal and vesical mesentery are entirely preserved whereas the vascular and ligamentous mesometria are entirely removed (Fig. 69.26). Thus, this procedure may be performed identically for all compartment defined cervical and endometrial cancers ensuring maximum radicalness with respect to tumor resection without increasing morbidity by extending surgery to neighboring structures. Adaption of surgery to compartments instead of tumor size and extent may enhance loco-regional tumor control, whereas unnecessary morbidity is prevented.

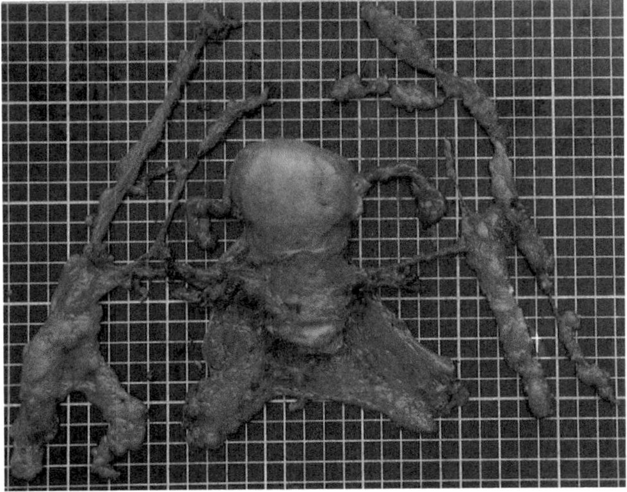

Fig. 69.27 Typical specimen following TMMR in cervical cancer with vascular and ligamentous mesometria and pelvic lymph node compartments

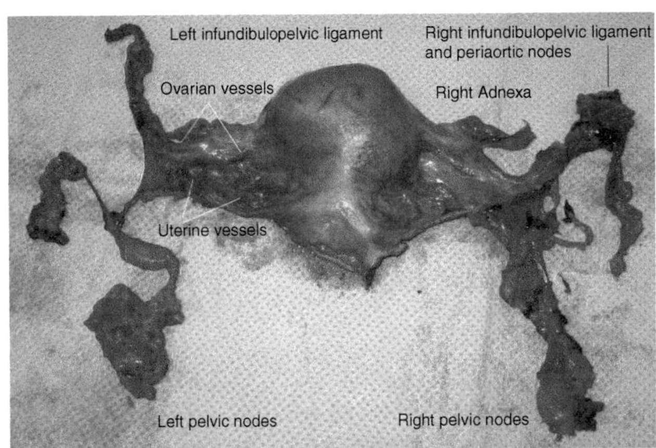

Fig. 69.28 Typical specimen following PMMR in endometrial cancer with vascular mesometria, uteroovarian vessel network and mesonephric compartment of infundibulopelvic ligaments

Finally, typical specimens following TMMR (Fig. 69.27) and PMMR (Fig. 69.28) are shown. Figure 69.29 demonstrates that ICG labeling of the Müllerian compartment reliably persists over hours during cancer surgery for intraoperative orientation and postoperative control.

To compare clinical results of surgical techniques in practice and even more in studies the procedure has to be named and exactly standardized. Thus, in this chapter the technique of TMMR and PMMR performed by robotically assisted laparoscopic surgery has been defined and described step by step.

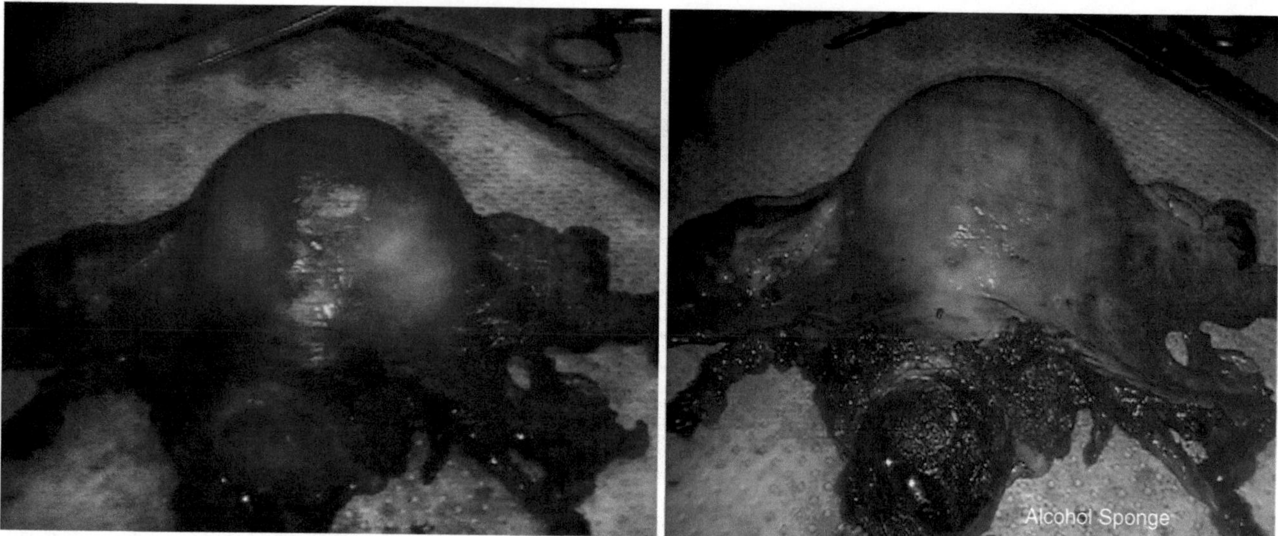

Fig. 69.29 Green ICG fluorescence of Müllerian compartment after corporal injection in endometrial cancer, PMMR specimen

References

1. Wolpert L. Positional information and spatial pattern of cellular differentiation. J Theor Biol. 1969;25:1–47.
2. Garcia-Bellido A, Ripoll P, Morata G. Developmental compartmentalization of the wing disk of Drosophila. Nature. 1973;245:251–3.
3. Dahmann C, Oates AC, Brand M. Boundary formation and maintenance in tissue development. Nat Rev Genet. 2011;12:43–55.
4. Höckel M. Morphogenetic fields of embryonic development in locoregional cancer spread. Lancet Oncol. 2015;16(3):e148–51. doi:10.1016/S1470-2045(14)71028-9.
5. Heald RJ, Rayan DRH. Recurrence and survival after total mesorectal excision for rectal cancer. Lancet. 1986;327:1479–82.
6. Weaver KL, Grimm Jr LM, Fleshman JW. Changing the way we manage rectal cancer-standardizing TME from open to robotic (including laparoscopic). Clin Colon Rectal Surg. 2015;28(1):28–37. doi:10.1055/s-0035-1545067.
7. Höckel M, Horn L-C, Manthey N, Braumann U-D, Wolf U, Teichmann G, Frauenschläger K, Dornhöfer N, Einenkel J. Resection of the embryologically defined uterovaginal (Müllerian) compartment and pelvic control in patients with cervical cancer: a prospective analysis. Lancet Oncol. 2009;10:683–92.
8. Höckel M, Horn LC, Tetsch E, Einenkel J. Pattern anlaysis of regional spread and therapeutic lymph node dissection in cervical cancer based on ontogenetic anatomy. Gynecol Oncol. 2012;125:168–74.
9. Kimmig R, Wimberger P, Buderath P, Aktas B, Iannaccone A, Heubner M. Definition of compartment-based radical surgery in uterine cancer: radical hysterectomy in cervical cancer as 'total mesometrial resection (TMMR)' by Michael Höckel translated to robotic surgery (rTMMR). World J Surg Oncol. 2013;11(1):211.
10. Kimmig R, Aktas B, Buderath P, Wimberger P, Iannaccone A, Heubner M. Definition of compartment-based radical surgery in uterine cancer: modified radical hysterectomy in intermediate/high-risk endometrial cancer using peritoneal mesometrial resection (PMMR) by M Höckel translated to robotic surgery. World J Surg Oncol. 2013;11(1):198.
11. Kimmig R, Aktas B, Buderath P, Rusch P, Heubner M. Lymphatic network visualized by Indocyanine-green (ICG) as in vivo marker for embryologically derived organ compartments and their drainage in uterine cancer surgery. J Surg Oncol. 2016;113(5):554–9. doi: 10.1002/jso.24174.
12. Yang Y, Oliver G. Development of the mammalian lymphatic vasculature. J Clin Invest. 2015;124:888–97.
13. Kimmig R, Iannaccone A, Buderath P, Aktas B, Wimberger P, Heubner M. Definition of compartment based radical surgery in uterine cancer-part I: therapeutic Pelvic and periaortic lymphadenectomy by Michael Höckel translated to robotic surgery. ISRN Obstet Gynecol. 2013;2013:297921. doi:10.1155/2013/297921.
14. B. U. Sevin. Kap 2. H. Hepp, P. Scheidel, J. M. Monaghan, editors. Lymphonodektomie in der gynäkologischen Onkologie. Indikation, Technik und Konsequenzen für die Therapieplanung. Urban&Schwarzenberg; 1988. p. 24, ISBN 3-541-12351-6.

Robotically Assisted Therapeutic Pelvic and Paraaortic Lymphadenectomy in Uterine Cancer

70

Rainer Kimmig

Introduction

There are several strategies in lymphadenectomy and even more techniques all named "pelvic lymphadenectomy" or "paraaortic lymphadenectomy."

Thus, first it has to be defined what will be the intention of lymphadenectomy – diagnostic or therapeutic? In case of diagnostic intent sentinel node biopsy may be an adequate approach for reduction of morbidity, other forms of staging lymphadenectomy may be too but are more or less undefined. To confirm a "sufficient" lymphadenectomy indication of numbers of nodes retrieved has been proposed. However, on the contrary, in case of therapeutic intention it makes no sense to define any number of nodes to be taken out, but to define not to leave any node in with respect to the compartment of risk.

In conjunction with compartmental resection of "organ compartments at risk" which have to be resected entirely, only resection of the entire "node compartments at risk" may considered adequate for maximum potential therapeutic effect.

Just to remember the basis of compartmental resection from Chapter 69: On the basis of ontogenetic compartmental development the findings about compartmental border control in malignant tumour progression led to the concept of "compartmental resection" in solid malignant tumors [1–4]. Since loco-regional recurrence usually occurs in compartment remnants or in the associated lymph compartments total "compartments of risk" have to be removed completely, whereas neighbouring compartments may left entirely untouched. The first tumour resected following this concept was rectal cancer by total mesorectal excision (TME) resulting in dramatically reduced loco-regional recurrence [5]. At present this procedure has become standard in rectal cancer surgery [6]. For cervical cancer M. Höckel has convincingly shown by his monocentric data that the corresponding method named total mesometrial resection (TMMR) also reduces efficiently locoregional recurrences compared to standard treatment – without any additional radiation therapy even in risk situations [7, 8]. The Method is described for open surgery in a separate chapter. Together with M. Höckel total mesometrial resection (rTMMR) has been translated to robotic surgery [9]. On parallel, the modification of compartmental resection for endometrial cancer as peritoneal mesometrial resection (PMMR) according to the different lymph drainage has also been adopted to robotic surgery as rPMMR [10]. Although, the two methods have to be applied together with therapeutic pelvic or pelvic and paraaortic lymphadenectomy to control not only for local but also for regional disease, in this chapter the technique of therapeutic lymphonodectomy (tLNE) only is described; however technique of TMMR and PMMR has already been described step by step in Chapter 69.

Anatomical Basis of Müllerian Compartment and Local Lymph Drainage

For uterine cancer removal of the Müllerian compartment and its draining lymphatic compartments has to be performed completely. Embryological development, compartment borders and type of resection in uterine cancer is perfectly described by M. Höckel [4, 7]. As shown in Fig. 70.1 the uterus has to be removed together with the vascular mesometrium (corresponding to the uterine vessel system including vesicouterine anastomoses) and the ligamentous mesometrium (c+orresponding to the rectovaginal and sacrouterine ligament). However, there is not any longer any modification with respect to the tumor size, as the concept requires always complete resection. There is only one part of the Müllerian

R. Kimmig
Gynecology and Obstetrics, West German Cancer Center, University Hospital Essen, University Duisburg-Essen, Hufelandstr. 55, Essen, NRW D-45122, Germany
e-mail: Rainer.kimmig@uk-essen.de

I. Alkatout, L. Mettler (eds.), *Hysterectomy*, DOI 10.1007/978-3-319-22497-8_70

compartment left in situ for functional reasons – the vagina. The vaginal resection margin is the only intracompartmental resection has directly to be controlled for clear margins (>10 mm recommended) in compartment confined tumors [4]. According to the different lymph drainage of the upper and lower Müllerian compartment in cervical cancer vascular and ligamentous mesometria have to be resected. In endometrial cancer without cervical involvement there is no drainage along the ligamentous mesometria; on the other hand there is drainage along the mesonephric pathway on parallel to the ovarian vessel system. Thus, ligamentous mesometria may be preserved, but infundibulopelvic ligaments have to be resected completely in corporal uterine disease as can be seen from Fig. 70.1 a–d.

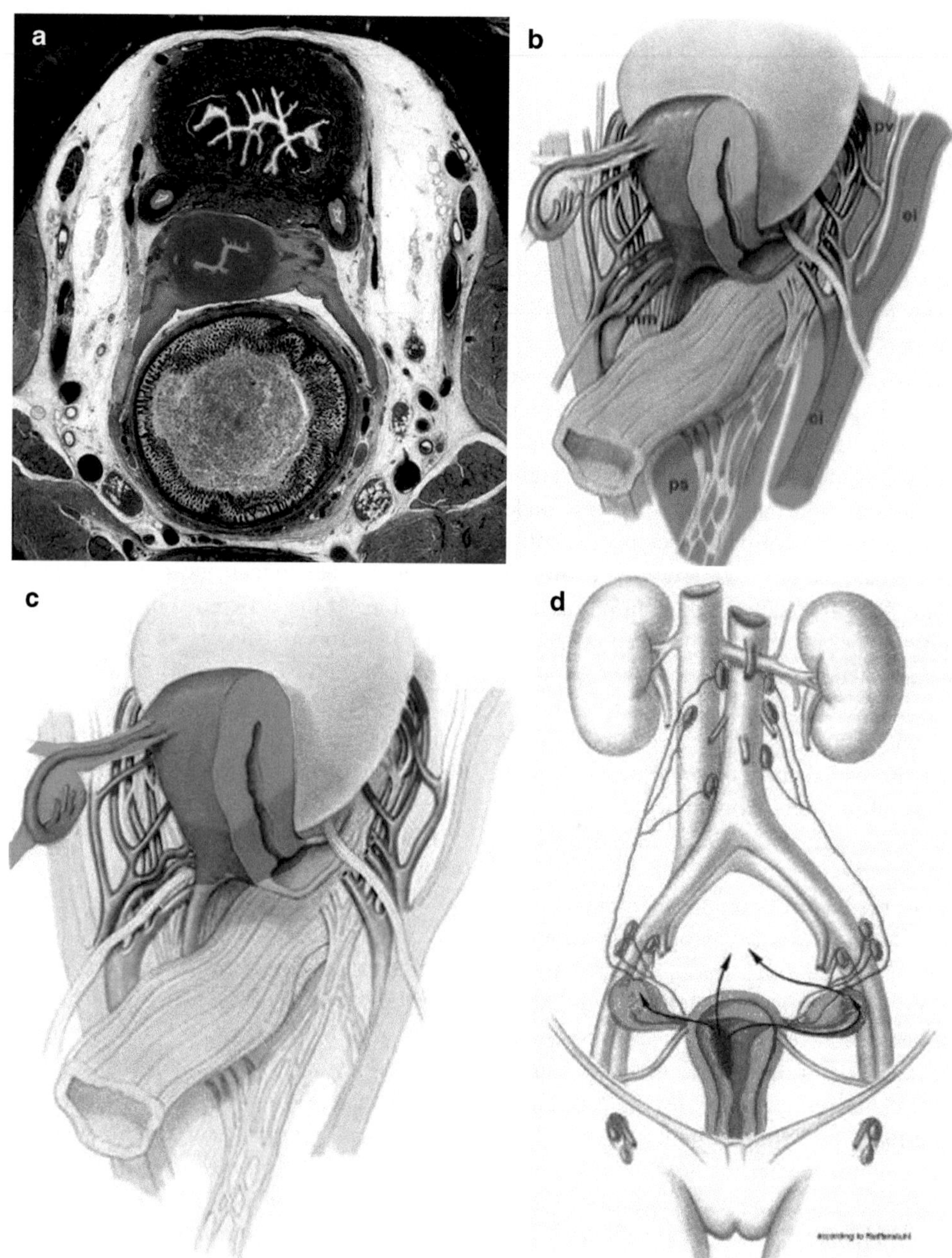

Fig. 70.1 (**a**) Embryologic development of Müllerian compartment (*red*); (**b**) Müllerian compartment in the adult (*green*); (**c**) Involvement of Müllerian compartment in endometrial cancer (*green*); (**d**) Additional lymphatic drainage in endometrial cancer (*green*)

Therapeutic Lymphadenectomy

In this chapter this type of "therapeutic lymphadenectomy" as described by M. Höckel will be demonstrated using robotically-assisted laparoscopy exclusively for the different pelvic and paraaortic lymph compartments. This has already been published in [9–17].

As outlined in Chapter 69 the lymphatic network of the Müllerian system derives from embryonal veins [18] and thus covers the whole compartment and may visualized by fluorescence lymphography intraoperatively. In mammals, embryologic development is suggested as a stepwise process starting from the embryonic veins, where lymphatic endothelial cells (LEC) are initially specified [19]. The lymphatic system develops by budding from "cardinal veins" and thus, necessarily parallels the venous system, although no open connection remains between the two systems except for the iugular lymph sacs to the subclavian veins which enable lymph drainage back to the blood circulation. There is some evidence that the origin of the very first draining lymphatic capillaries may arise not only by sprouting but also by scattered local mesenchymal cells expressing lymphoendothelial markers [19]. Very important is the fact, that collecting lymph vessels and also main transporting lymph vessels develop lymphatic valves which guarantee a directed "downstream" lymph flow [19]. This is also true for the connecting lymph vessels from the organ compartment to the lymph compartments (basins of first or subsequent order). Thus, visualization of the lymphatic vessel network of a distinct organ should be able to mark the organ compartment and the compartments of specific lymphatic drainage "downstream" from a defined localization resembling functional aspects. This should have dramatic clinical impact on surgical oncology with respect on individual radical compartmental surgery in cancer due to the compartmental order of tumor progression [20] and the tremendous impact of the lymphatic system on local, regional and distant tumor progression.

Uterine Cervix and upper vagina is drained via two different pathways: first, along the uterine and vaginal arteries and veins to the pelvic side wall, using mainly the lymph vessels running along of the uterine artery. They drain primarily into the paravisceral and external iliac lymph basin which are the lymph compartments of first order for these organ (sub) compartments and contain the respective site information. The second pathway runs along the posterior ligamentous mesometrium and mesocolpium (corresponding to the sacrouterine and rectovaginal ligaments) and drains primarily to the deep paravisceral nodes ventrally to the ischiadic spine and the nerve roots of the ischiadic nerve. There are collecting lymph channels transporting the lymph fluid to the common iliac lymph basin, ventrally and dorsally of the common iliac vessels and again connecting this compartment of second order to the inferior paracaval and paraaortic lymph node compartment (third order) connected again to the infrarenal lymph paraaortic and paracaval nodes (forth order) which may also serve as first order lymph compartment for the mesonephric and colonic system, for example.

We have to keep in mind, that the draining lymph channels of the lower Müllerian compartment (Cervix, Vagina) run caudally and dorsally, thus involving rather the posterior nodes along the vessels; Anatomically the paraaortic and paracaval nodes are separated in two subcompartments on each side: the anterior (mesenteric) and the posterior (lumbar) part. Although, lymphatic spread is found in cervical and vaginal cancer predominantly in the lumbar subcompartment there are a lot of anastomoses between the lymphatic systems, which can be shown anatomically and by ICG fluorescence, that ther may be also metastatic spread to the mesenteric subcompartment.

In endometrial cancer lymphatic spread is different. From the upper part of Müllerian compartment lymphatic drainage runs cranially of the uterine artery and predominantly ventrally to the main vessels. In addition, there is a mesonephric pathway along the ovarian vessels directly to the paraaortic lymph compartment. Consequently, tumor spread is predominantly found in the ventral, mesenteric subcompartments; same is true for ovarian cancer where more or less the same lymphatic pathways are used.

If we respect that in a functional intact lymphatic system the lymphatic flow is unidirectional due to valves consequent and complete removal of the lymph compartments at risk should be able to control for locoregional disease. This may no longer be true in macroscopically bulky disease since in that situation due to tumor barriers in the downstream system may lead to upstream dissemination by valve insufficiency.

For systematic reasons it makes sense to define pelvic and paraaortic lymphadenectomy as different entities. However, with respect to the compartmental order of lymph basins in ontogenetic development it seems to be more appropriate to define pelvic and paraaortic lymph compartments draining the respective organ (sub) compartments of the tumor origin.

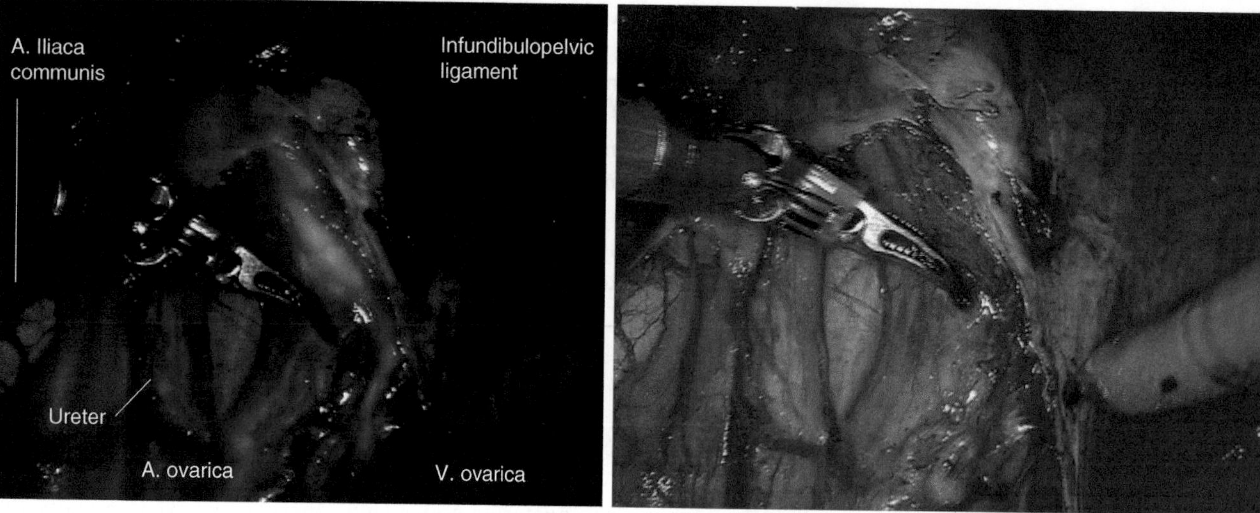

Fig. 70.2 Lymph drainage right infundibulopelvic ligament (ICG and real light comparison)

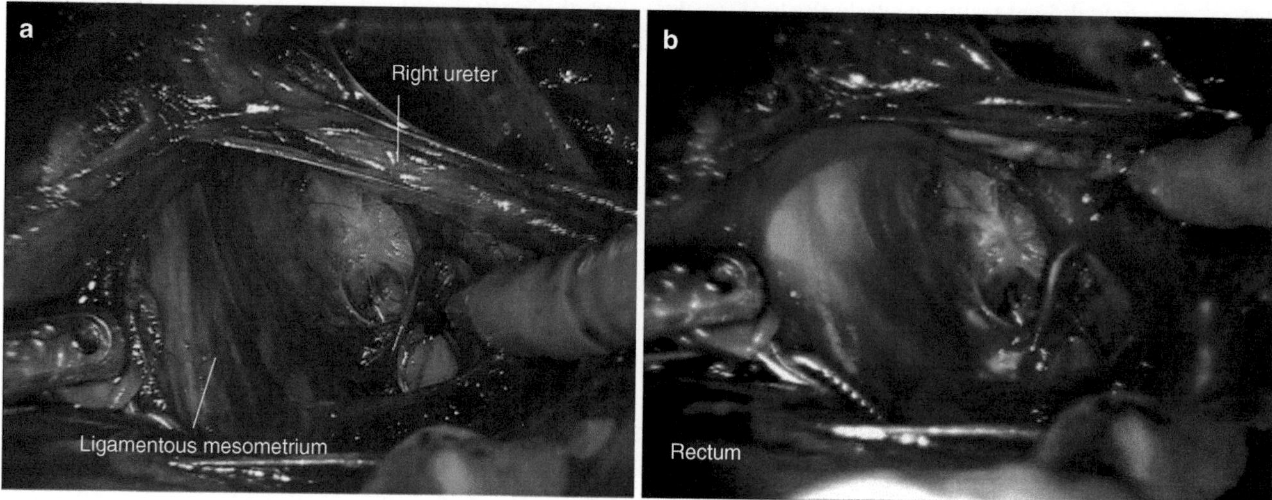

Fig. 70.3 Lateral (sacrouterine) part of right ligamentous mesometrium in cervical cancer and its connections to deep paravisceral lymph node compartments (*A* normal light, *B* ICG Fluorescence in near infrared light)

Lymph Compartments at Risk for Endometrial and Cervical Cancer

Due to the embryological development of lymphatic drainage of the Müllerian compartment there are three main pathways to reach the pelvic and paraaortic basins. First, Müllerian pathway along the vascular mesometrium to the paravisceral and external iliac basin, second along the ligamentous mesometrium to the paravisceral basin, predominantly along obturator and gluteal vessels to posterior part of internal iliac vessels. Third, the mesonephric pathway along the infudibulopelvic ligaments. Wheras cervical subcompartment drains to the lower vascular and ligamentous mesometrium, the corporal subcompartment drains to the upper vascular mesometrium and the infundibulopelvic ligament. Typical situations of intraoperative visualization using ICG in cervical and endometrial cancer are shown in Figs. 70.2, 70.3, 70.4, and 70.5.

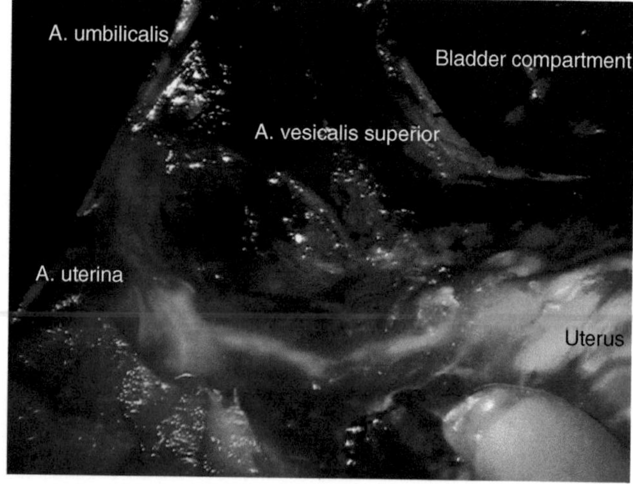

Fig. 70.4 Ventral aspect of vascular mesometrium separated from the bladder compartment

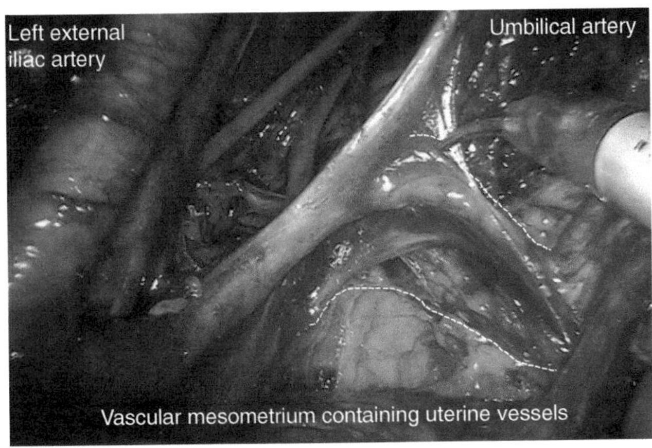

Fig. 70.5 Corresponding ICG lymphography of left vascular mesometrium (Fig. 70.4)

Therapeutic Pelvic Lymphadenectomy: Step by Step

The pelvic lymph basins draining the uterine compartment are: External iliac basin, paravisceral basin including preischiadic and prespinal region, common iliac basin including subaortic nodes (Fig. 70.1).

Thus, the lymph compartment of first order is represented by the paravisceral and external iliac lymph basin and of highest risk, postponed (second order) are the common iliac basins including subaortic nodes getting at risk following involvement of first order lymph basins.

Surgical Strategy and Technique

Step 1

Usually, pelvic lymphadenectomy starts at the level of the right common iliac artery. Following opening of the peritoneum laterally to the artery but medial to the ureter the complete retroperitoneal lymph basins are exposed from the aortic bifurcation to the bifurcation of the common iliac vessels down to S2 (Fig. 70.6, before dissection). Following peritoneal incision the superior hypogastric plexus will be elevated ventrally together with the mesosigma, forming the so-called sigmoid tunnel and the intact retroperitoneal lymphatic compartments are exposed (Fig. 70.7).

Step 2

Lateral borders of the dissection dorsally are defined by the psoas muscle, the ureter, the genitofemoral nerve and if preserved, ventrally the infundibulopelvic ligament (Fig. 70.8). All structures have to be separated from the lymphatic compartment.

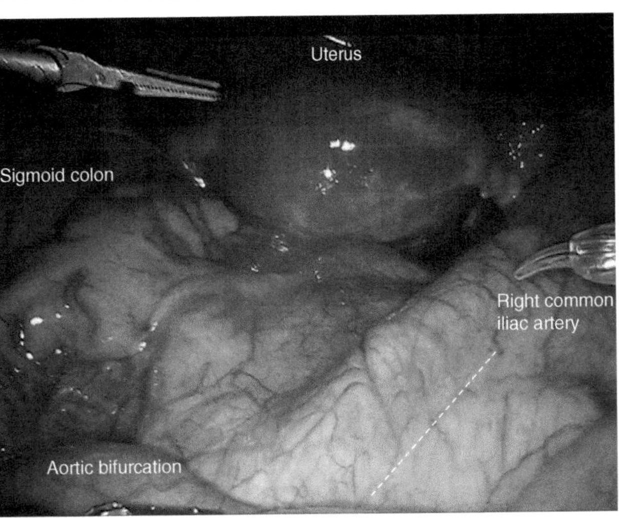

Fig. 70.6 Exposition prior to peritoneal incision at the level of right common ilac artery

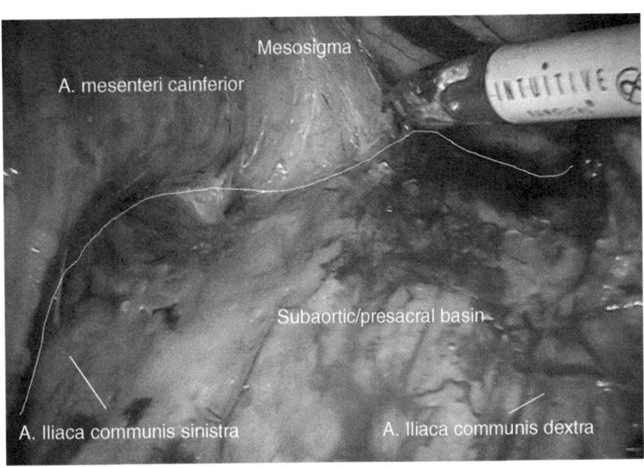

Fig. 70.7 Subaortic and caudal mesenteric paraaortic lymph compartment exposed

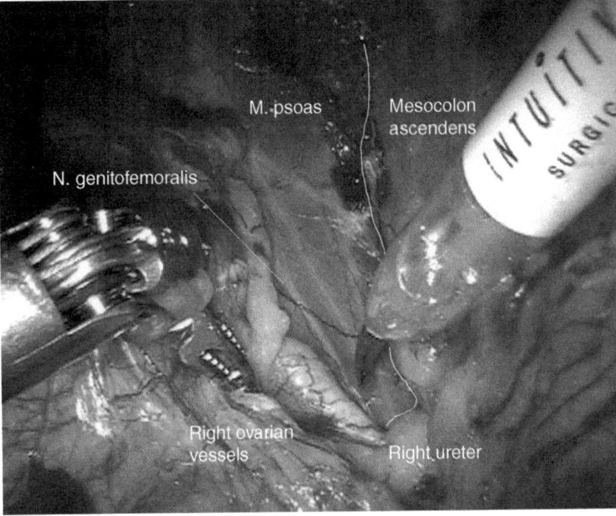

Fig. 70.8 Right lateral border of common iliac lymph basin

Step 3

Common iliac lymph basins will be resected "en bloc" from right to left, starting at the level of aortic bifurcation. Following structures should be exposed and detached from right to left: ureter, left sympathetic chain, n. genitofemoralis, n. obturatorius, truncus lumbosacralis, a. and v. iliaca communis, promontorium, A. sacralis media and same to the left (Figs. 70.8, 70.9, 70.10, 70.11, and 70.12). The connection to the inferior lumbar and mesenteric aortic basins can be taken as upper border for the dissection (Fig. 70.13). The lower border of dissection will be the ureter crossing at the common iliac bifurcation; medially, however, internal iliac nodes should be resected already down to the level of S2 (Fig. 70.14); lower crossing splanchnic nerves will thus be preserved.

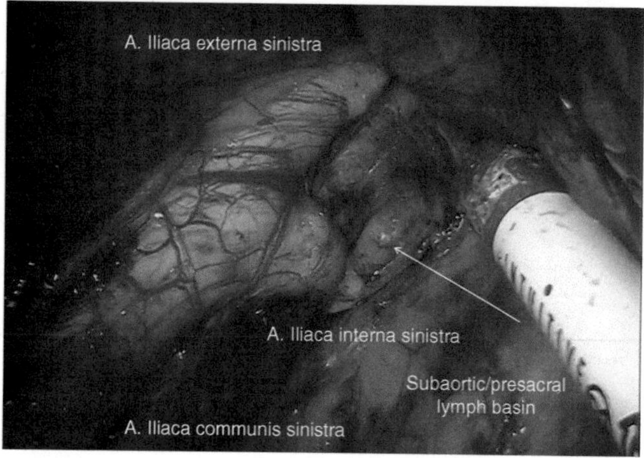

Fig. 70.11 Subaortic (left medial common iliac) and upper paravisceral lymph compartment to S2

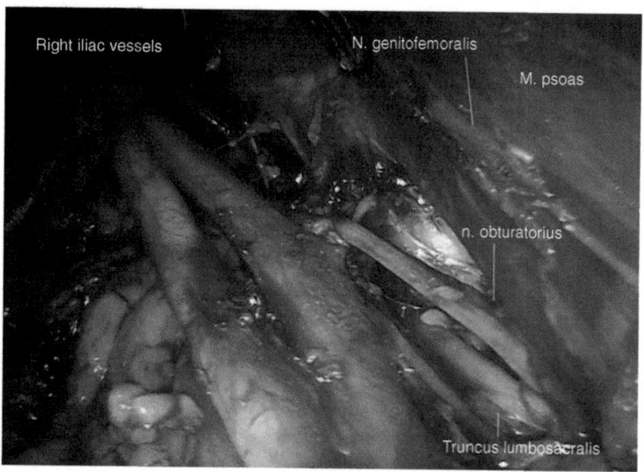

Fig. 70.9 Lateral common iliac lymph basin partially dissected on the right

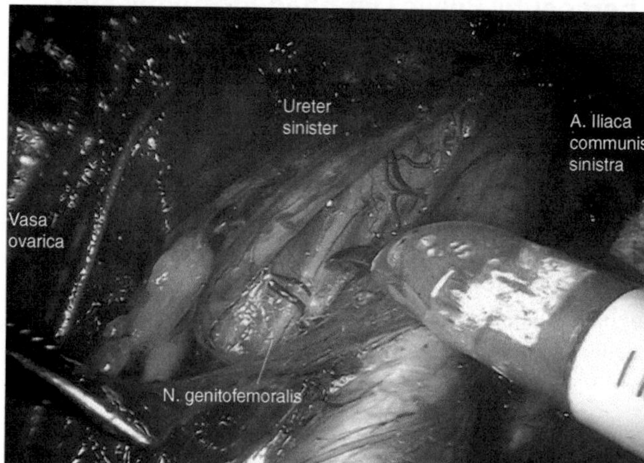

Fig. 70.12 Left lateral border of common iliac lymph basin

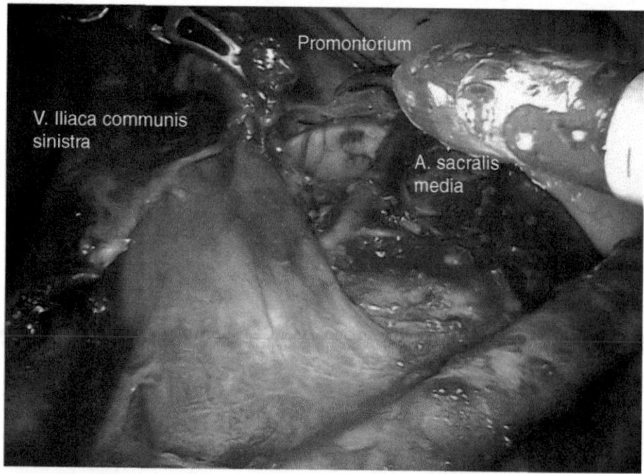

Fig. 70.10 Subaortic (medial common iliac) lymph basin partially dissected

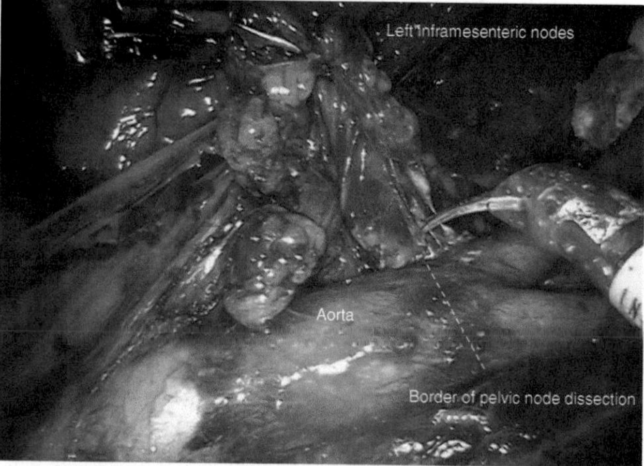

Fig. 70.13 Cranial border of common iliac lymph basin

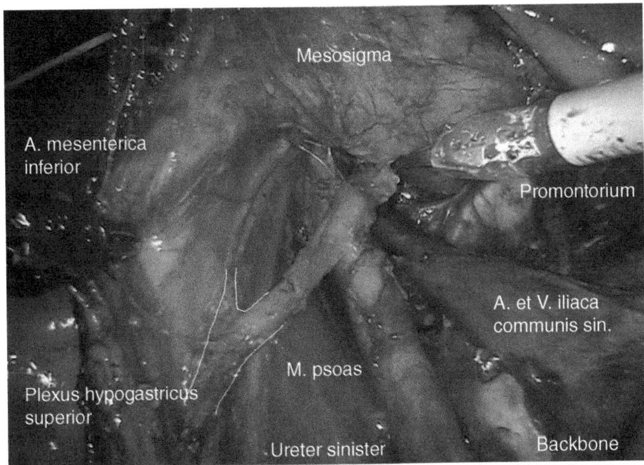

Fig. 70.14 Left caudal border of common iliac lymph basin

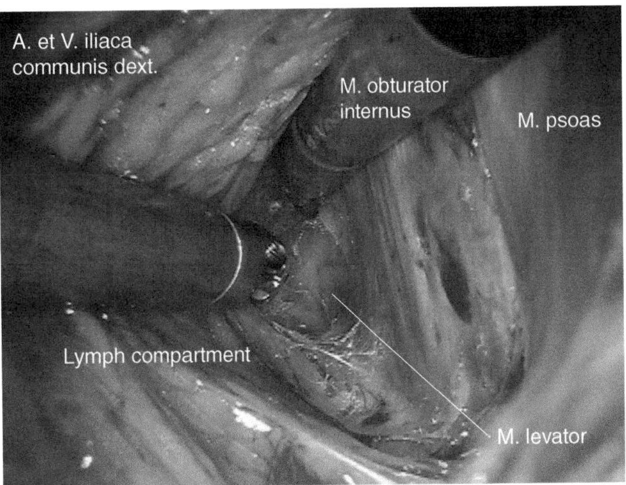

Fig. 70.15 Lateral border of right pelvic paravisceral lymph compartment

Step 4

Lateral exposition of external and paravisceral lymph basin on the right. Lateral border again is represented by the genitofemoral nerve and the psoas fascia. These structures will be separated from the lymph compartment. Next, the lymph compartment will be detached from the pelvic side wall by following the psoas muscle to the internal obturator muscle, passing the arcus tendineus to the levator muscle and the endopelvic fascia. This can easily be achieved lateral to the external iliac vessels, inferior to the gluteal vessels and the ischiadic nerve since this region is more or less avascular (Fig. 70.15).

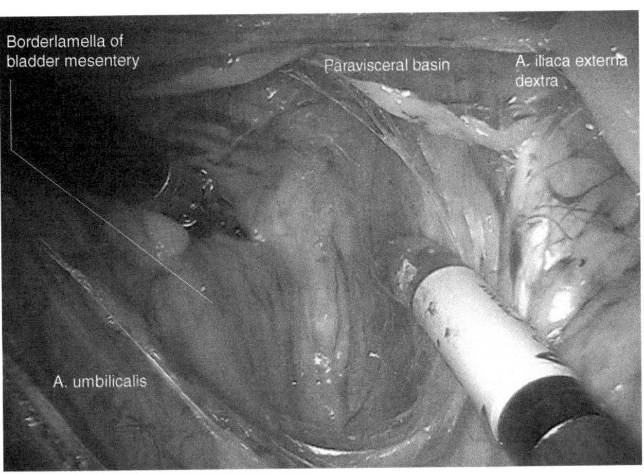

Fig. 70.16 Medial border of right pelvic paravisceral lymph compartment

Step 5

Medial exposition of external and paravisceral lymph basin on the right. Medial border is represented by the bladder mesentery containing the umbilical artery. The avascular space beween the border lamella and the lymphatic compartment will be opened again down to the endopelvic fascia (Fig. 70.16). Now the caudal resection of external iliac nodes is defined and the compartment border is detached in the avascular space separating it from the parainguinal fat tissue ventrally to the iliac vessels. At this level the inferior epigastric and the circumflex iliac vessels can be visualized (Fig. 70.17). The connecting lymph vessels of the medial femoral channel will be dissected and the connecting vein from external iliac to obturator vein can easily be followed to the obturator nerve and vessels.

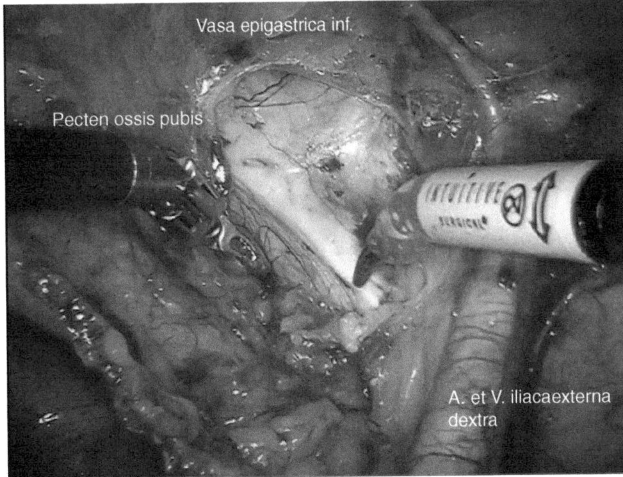

Fig. 70.17 Caudal border of right pelvic external iliac lymph compartment

Step 6

Resection of external and paravisceral lymph basin "en bloc".

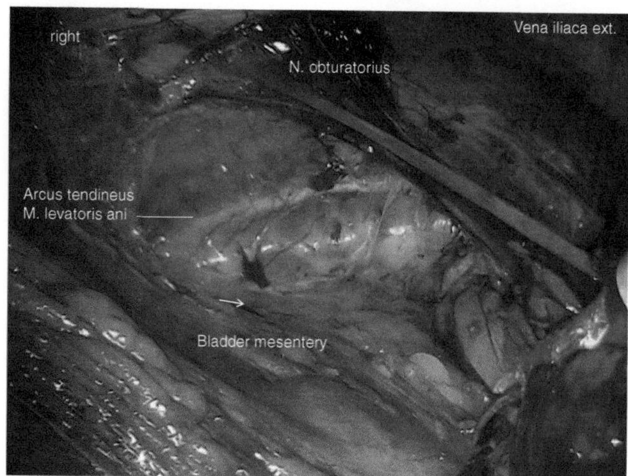

Fig. 70.18 Caudal part of right paravisceral lymph compartment removed

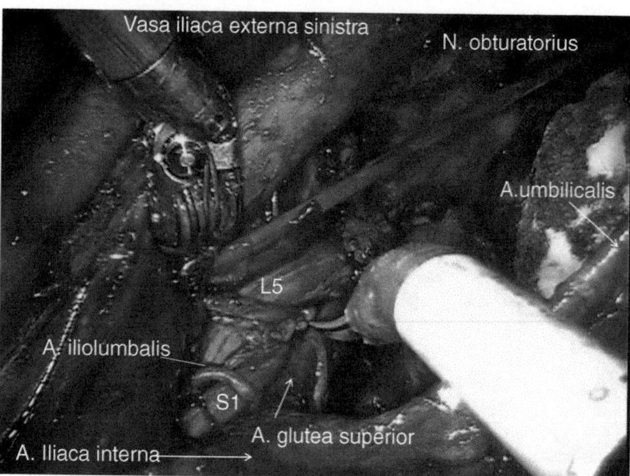

Fig. 70.19 Cranial part of left paravisceral lymph compartment removed (**a**)

To unwrap the external iliac vessels lymphatic tissue of the medial and lateral part is divided best along external iliac artery. Pulling the nodal tissue medially it may be detached from the iliac vein and the obturator bundle is exposed. Due to the prior lateral detachment, the whole tissue can now be detached completely from the obturator bundle and the obturator fossa from caudally to cranially reaching the posterior internal iliac region laterally and the anterior branches ventrally. At this level, all the lymphatic tissue up to the dissection border of common iliac nodes can now be retrieved from medially (Fig. 70.18).

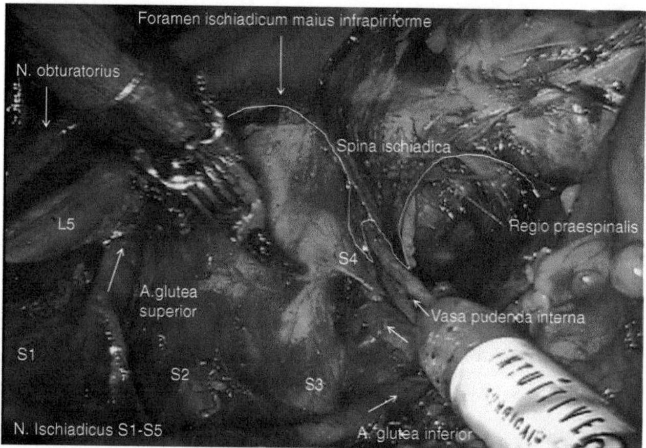

Fig. 70.20 Cranial part of left paravisceral lymph compartment removed (**b**)

Step 7

Resection of upper posterior paravisceral lymph basin preischiadically.

Whereas the prespinal nodes are already resected with the obturator nodes it is more challenging to remove all the preischiadic nodes between the gluteal and pudendal vessels. If necessary veins can be dissected but arteries normally can be preserved. The tissue has to be removed and the sacral roots and main stem of ischiadic nerve are cleaned (Figs. 70.19 and 70.20, shown on the left).

Steps 8–11 on the Left Side Are as Described for Step 4–7 on the Right

The surgical steps on the left side will be identically performed as desrcibed for the right.

Therapeutic Paraaortic Lymphadenectomy: Step by Step

There are two different types of paraaortic lymphadenectomy; with or without mesonephric lymph system along the ovarian vessels; this has to be removed additionally in endometrial and ovarian cancer, whereas in cervical cancer it will be not necessary.

Trocar Placement

With respect to trocar placement it is important to define preoperatively to define at which level nodes have to be removed, predominantly using a “da Vinci Si” system. The camera trocar has to be placed about 8–10 cm more cranially as the most cranial point of planned dissection and the instrument trocars have to be placed more cranially but in the same configuration as in demonstrated in Fig. 70.21. If this is not possible, trocars have to be placed around the umbilicus (mostly a little bit lower) and the patient cart has to be re-docked to reach the higher abdominal regions. Using the "da Vinci Xi" system this is no longer mandatory; placing the trocars at the level of the umbilicus in one straight line the whole abdomen is accessible without re-docking, facilitating the procedure in the cranial part and allowing easily to extent the surgery to the upper abdomen, if necessary.

Differences of Paraaortic Lymphatic Drainage in Cervical and Endometrial Cancer

Again to keep in mind: In endometrial cancer lymph drainage primary lymph basins are pelvic and paraaortic and have to be removed entirely since lymphatic drainage follows the vascular mesometrium and the infundibulopelvic ligament. Thus, whereas in cervical cancer, paraaortic lymph basins are of third or higher order postponed to pelvic basins and may be spared in case of negative pelvic nodes, in endometrial cancer paraaortic nodes are of first order. That means the compartment at high risk for nodal metastases comparable to the pelvic lymph compartments.

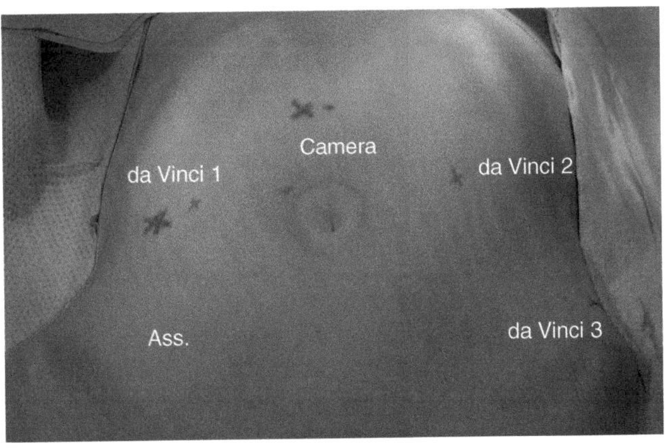

Fig. 70.21 Trocar postitioning for robotic TMMR and therapeutic pelvic LNE

Consequently, in the therapeutic approach – analogous to cervical cancer – in endometrial cancer together with the vascular mesometrium also the network for vascular and lymphatic anastomoses between uterus and adnexa has to be removed, at best covered by the peritoneal leaves of the broad ligament (PMMR). The vascular and lymphatic drainage system along the ovarian vessels has also to be removed in analogy to the vascular mesometrium up to its connection to the periaortic and pericaval lymph basins. Whereas the vascular anastomoses to the mesenteric vessel system (right and left colon) are dissected the connections to the periaortic lymph basins are preserved and removed together "en bloc." Since there is no drainage from uterine corpus to the ligamentous mesometrium the deep gluteal, pudendal, and rectal nodes may be preserved. As already outlined lymphatic tumor spread in endometrial cancer will take place predominantly in the ventral part of lymph compartment such as the mesenteric paraaortic and paracaval nodes, due to embryologically derived anatomy.

Table 70.1 illustrates lymph compartments to be removed in cervical and endometrial cancer.

Step 12

In case of cervical cancer inframesenteric periaortic lymphadenectomy may be performed following elevation of the superior hypogastric plexus (Fig. 70.22), the inferior mesenteric artery, and the sigmoid colon ventrally, thus continuing lymphadenectomy from common iliac vessels (Figs. 70.13 and 70.23). It has to be ascertained to remove the interaortocaval nodes (Fig. 70.24) and the lumbar chains dorsolaterally of vena cava (Fig. 70.25) and aorta; the connecting branches from right sympathetic chain to the superior hypogastric plexus may be maintained (Fig. 70.26).

Step 13

For infrarenal lymphadenectomy dissection has to be extended cranially to the renal vessels. In principle, retroperitoneal compartments will be exposed by defining right lateral border (ureter and psoas muscle), cranial border (renal veins, detaching duodenum). The ventral border by elevating

Table 70.1 Common and different steps in therapeutic lymphadenectomy in cervical and endometrial cancer

	External iliac and paravisceral nodes	preischiadic and prespinal nodes	Common iliac nodes	Subaortic/ presacral nodes	Inframesenteric paraaortic nodes	infrarenal paraaortic nodes
TMMR and therapeutic LNE	Yes	Yes	Yes	Yes	No, only if common iliac nodes are positive	No, only if im paraarotic nodes are positive
PMMR and therapeutic LNE	Yes	No	Yes	Yes	Yes	Yes

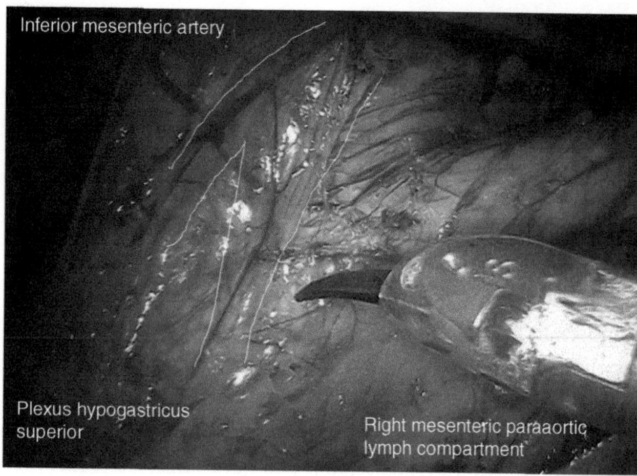

Fig. 70.22 Plexus hypogastricus superior crossing Aorta inframesenterically

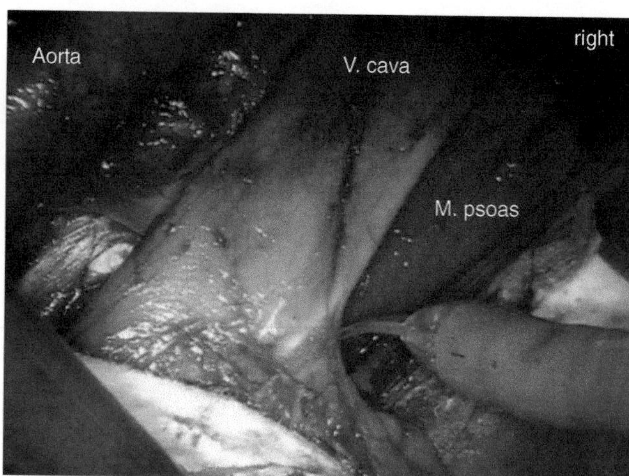

Fig. 70.25 Removal of infrarenal paracaval lumbar lymph compartment on the right

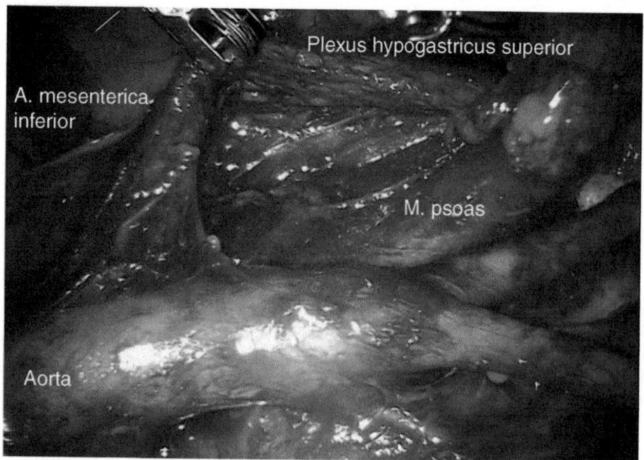

Fig. 70.23 Inframesenteric paraaortic lymph mesenteric and lumbar lymph compartment removed

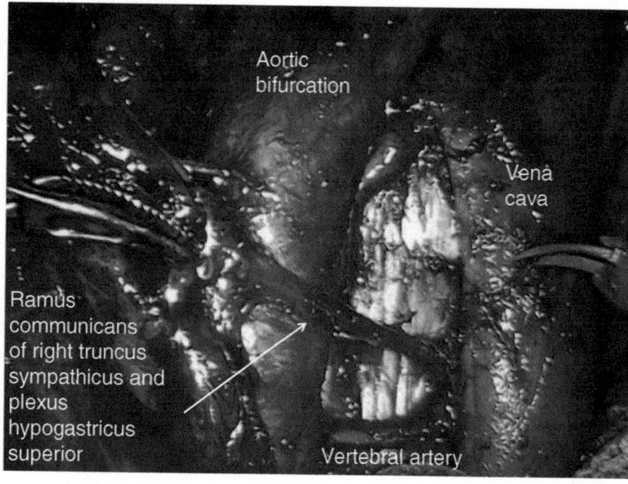

Fig. 70.26 Removal of mesenteric interaortocaval lumbar lymph compartment

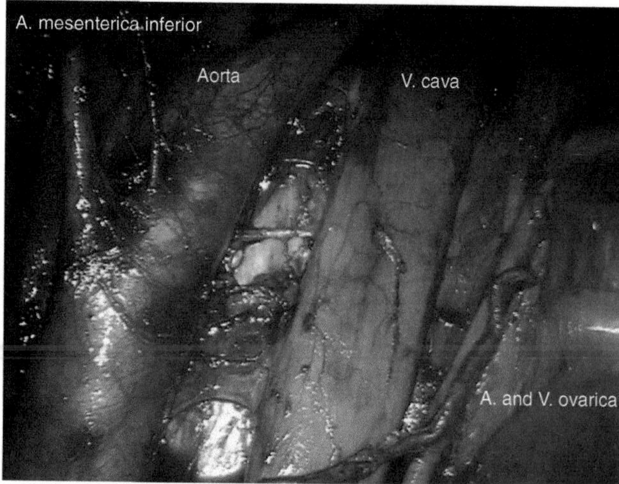

Fig. 70.24 Infrarenal interaortocaval mesenteric and lumbar lymph compartment removed

the plexus mesentericus inferior and hypogastricus superior together with inferior mesenteric artery and vein. Usually, connecting nerve branches to the right sympathetic chain (Fig. 70.26) have now to be dissected to allow ventral elevation of the plexus. Finally, left lateral border will be defined by the ovarian vein, ureter and psoas muscle; now interaortocaval infrarenal nodes and left infrarenal nodes can be removed; connecting nerve fibres to the left sympathetic chain may be preserved (Fig. 70.27).

Step 14

Complete resection of paraaortic infrarenal lumbar and mesenteric lymph compartments from right to left is now completed (Fig. 70.28) in cervical cancer without the need of resecting the mesonephric ovarian vessel system.

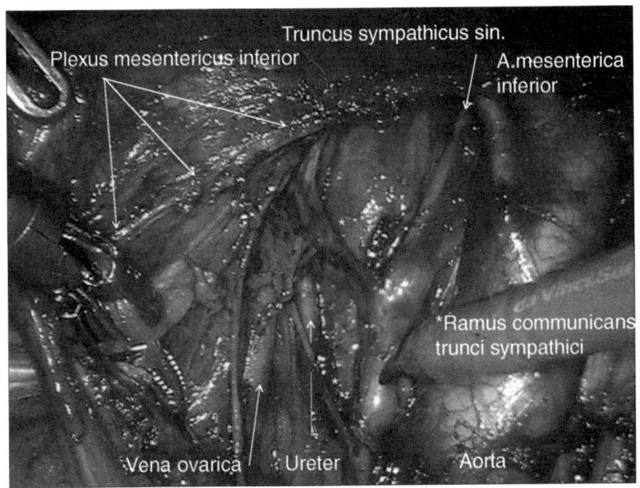

Fig. 70.27 Removal of left infrarenal paraaortic lumbar lymph compartment

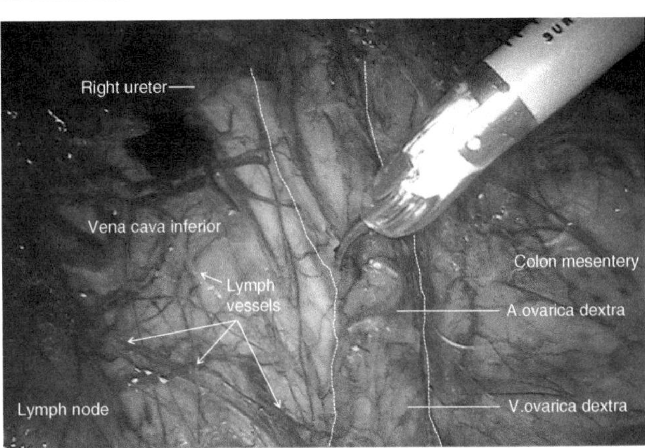

Fig. 70.29 Identification of right infundibulopelvic ligament, ureter and right colon mesentery

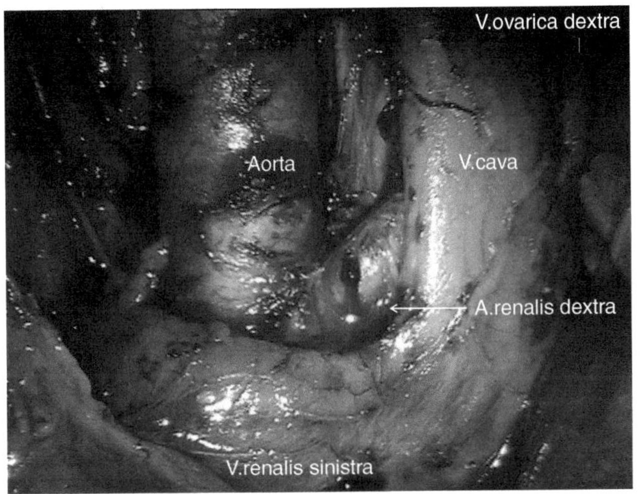

Fig. 70.28 Removal of left infrarenal mesenteric and lumbar lymph compartment (renal angle)

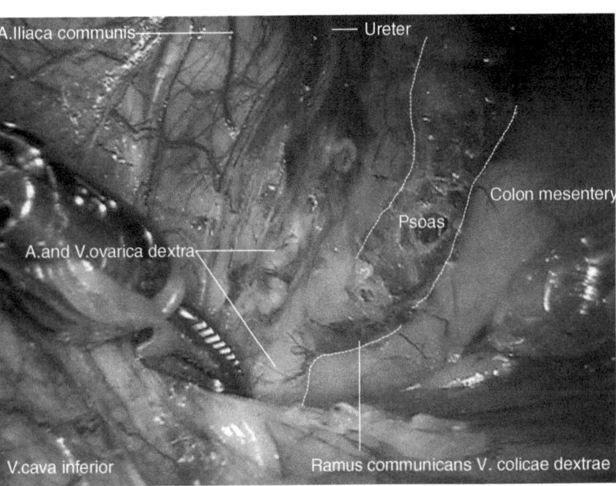

Fig. 70.30 Separation of right infundibulopelvic ligament from right colon mesentery

Step 15 in Endometrial and Ovarian Cancer (Instead of Steps 12–14)

In case of endometrial or ovarian cancer the infundibulopelvic ligaments have to be resected first; aorta, vena cava, the right ureter, and the right infundibulopelvic ligament are identified (Fig. 70.29). Mobilization of the right colic mesentery allows to identify vessel anastomoses to the ovarian vessel system and can be divided (Fig. 70.30). Following the ovarian vein the lateral border of the ovarian lymphovascular drainage bundle can be mobilized until the caval vein is reached (Fig. 70.31). Thus all anastomoses to the periaortic lymph basin will be kept intact. The duodenum usually is loosely attached to the preaortic region and has to be mobilized.

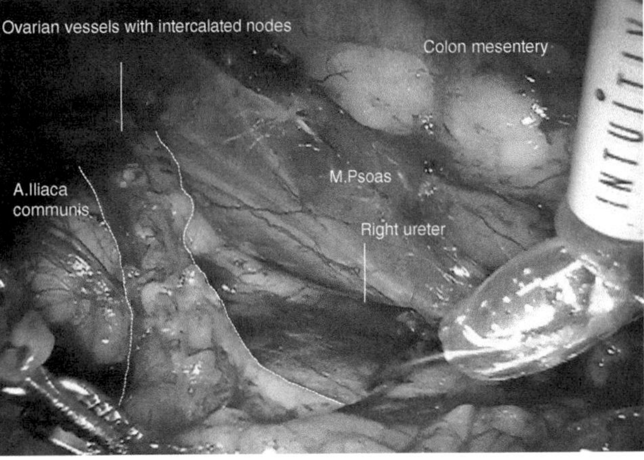

Fig. 70.31 Separation of ovarian vessel system from mesocolon, psoas muscle, ureter and caval vein

Step 16

The right ovarian vein is dissected at the level of caval vein and dissected (Fig. 70.32a). The lymphatic downstream channels may be dissected cranially along the right renal vein and dorsally to the right paracaval region to expose the back bone. The mobilized right lymphatic paraaortic compartment may now be pulled to the left, and the interaortocaval region will be exposed. The vertebral vessels will identified and and detached from lymphatic tissue as it is the case with the caval vein. Care has to be taken to remove the lumbar lymph node chain running dorsolaterally draining from deep right pelvis, which is not directly connected to the ventral chain of the mesenteric compartment. The right ovarian artery will be exposed, coagulated and divided (Fig. 70.32b). The left renal vein will be followed from its caval angle to lateral, and again the lymph channels will be dissected along the left renal vein until the left ovarian vein can be identified. The nerve fibres of the inferior mesenteric plexus are crossing ventrally, should be elevated and preserved (Fig. 70.33). The left ovarian vein is coagulated, and cut ((Fig. 70.32c). Now moving downward using the ovarian vein as lateral border and the aorta as medial border for mobilization and resection of left periaortic lymphatic basin left ovarian artery will be identified approximately at the level of right ovarian artery, coagulated, and cut (Fig. 70.32d). As described in the Chapter PMMR, the mesonephric vessel system will be removed together with the adjacent paraaortic lymph nodes.

Most important, in therapeutic lymphadenectomy, is to keep the surgical field dry to be able to safely remove the entire compartment. Although, there are plenty of vessels, which may be injured, normally it is no problem to perform surgery in a way that the vessels are kept intact or coagulated before dissected. To prevent problems prophylactically, sponges should be used instead of suction/irrigation since those are not at risk to cause additional injury and keep the field try; in addition, in venous bleeding compression with a sponge for some minutes may be very effective in controlling bleeding from smaller vessels; in larger venous lesions the application of a hemostatic patch such as Tachosil® instead of a suture is most efficient in our hands. In arterial lesions, however, a suture using 4-0 to 5-0 monofilamental unresorbable material is usually the best way to control the bleeding following clamping the proximal and distal part of the vessel transiently for endoscopic suture. Most bleedings may be managed endoscopically; prevention of any bleeding, however, is the safest way, to avoid further complications. Specifically for robotic surgery: don't risk bleeding

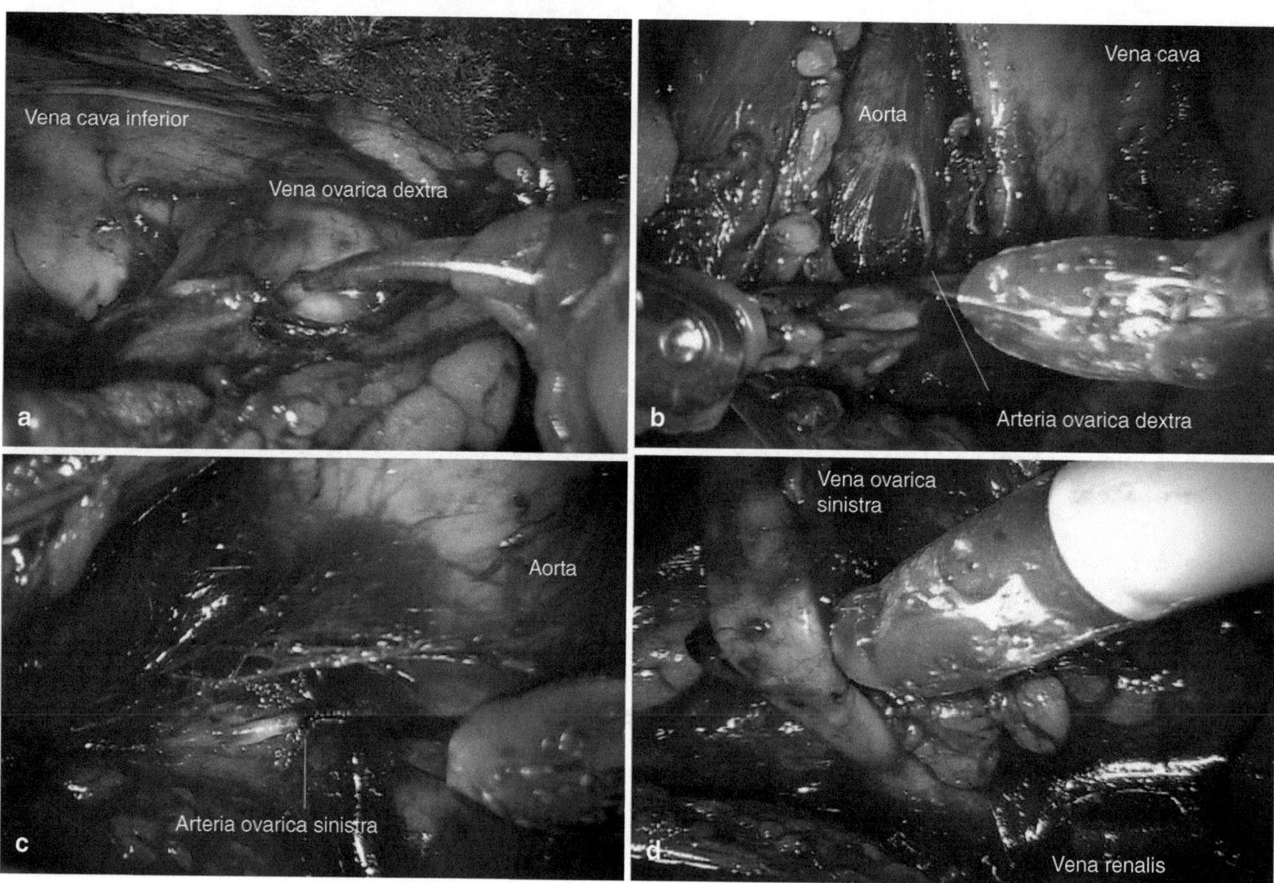

Fig. 70.32 Dissection of ovarian veins and arteries from caval and renal veins and aorta

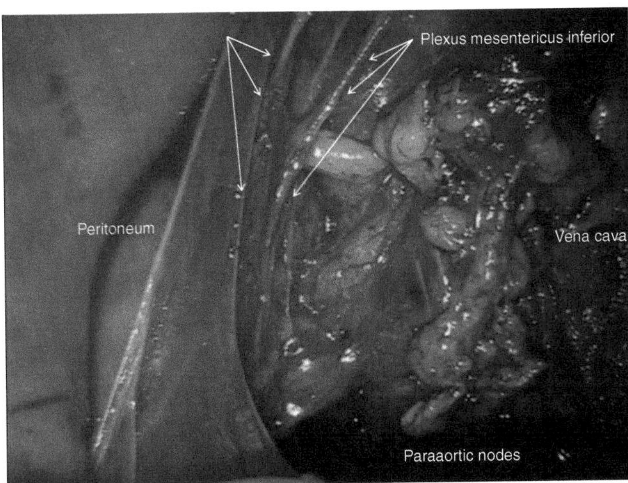

Fig. 70.33 Inferior mesenteric plexus in preparation at the infrarenal level

when you are close to the border of range of motion with your instruments! This will primarily be true using the "da Vinci SI" instead of the "da Vinci Xi".

In summary, therapeutic lymphadenectomy in cervical cancer consists of: external iliac, paravisceral, common iliac and subaortic lymph compartments. In case of positive nodes additionally the inframesenteric lumbar and mesenteric lymph compartments and if also involved the infrarenal lumbar and mesenteric lymph compartments. In endometrial and ovarian cancer all the compartments correspond to primary sites but the preischiadic and prespinal nodes of the paravisceral compartment may be spared since they will not be involved in the drainage of these subcompartments as long as lymphatic valves are intact. However, additionally, the mesonephric ovarian vascular and lymph vessel system has to be removed.

References

1. Wolpert L. Positional information and spatial pattern of cellular differentiation. J Theor Biol. 1969;25:1–47.
2. Garcia-Bellido A, Ripoll P, Morata G. Developmental compartmentalization of the wing disk of Drosophila. Nature. 1973;245:251–3.
3. Dahmann C, Oates AC, Brand M. Boundary formation and maintenance in tissue development. Nat Rev Genet. 2011;12:43–55.
4. Höckel M. Morphogenetic fields of embryonic development in locoregional cancer spread. Lancet Oncol. 2015;16(3):e148–51. doi:10.1016/S1470-2045(14)71028-9.
5. Heald RJ, Rayan DRH. Recurrence and survival after total mesorectal excision for rectal cancer. Lancet. 1986;327:1479–82.
6. Weaver KL, Grimm Jr LM, Fleshman JW. Changing the way we manage rectal cancer-standardizing TME from open to robotic (including laparoscopic). Clin Colon Rectal Surg. 2015;28(1):28–37. doi:10.1055/s-0035-1545067.
7. Höckel M, Horn L-C, Manthey N, Braumann U-D, Wolf U, Teichmann G, Frauenschläger K, Dornhöfer N, Einenkel J. Resection of the embryologically defined uterovaginal (Müllerian) compartment and pelvic control in patients with cervical cancer: a prospective analysis. Lancet Oncol. 2009;10:683–92.
8. Höckel M, Horn LC, Tetsch E, Einenkel J. Pattern anlaysis of regional spread and therapeutic lymph node dissection in cervical cancer based on ontogenetic anatomy. Gynecol Oncol. 2012;125:168–74.
9. Kimmig R, Wimberger P, Buderath P, Aktas B, Iannaccone A, Heubner M. Definition of compartment-based radical surgery in uterine cancer: radical hysterectomy in cervical cancer as 'total mesometrial resection (TMMR)' by Michael Höckel translated to robotic surgery (rTMMR). World J Surg Oncol. 2013;11(1):211.
10. Kimmig R, Aktas B, Buderath P, Wimberger P, Iannaccone A, Heubner M. Definition of compartment-based radical surgery in uterine cancer: modified radical hysterectomy in intermediate/high-risk endometrial cancer using peritoneal mesometrial resection (PMMR) by M Höckel translated to robotic surgery. World J Surg Oncol. 2013;11(1):–198.
11. Kimmig R, Iannaccone A, Buderath P, Aktas B, Wimberger P, Heubner M. Definition of compartment based radical surgery in uterine cancer-part I: therapeutic pelvic and periaortic lymphadenectomy by Michael Höckel translated to robotic surgery. ISRN Obstet Gynecol. 2013;2013:297921. doi:10.1155/2013/297921.
12. Kimmig R, Aktas B, Buderath P, Rusch P, Heubner M. Lymphatic network visualized by Indocyanine-green (ICG) as *in vivo* marker for embryologically derived organ compartments and their drainage in uterine cancer surgery. J Surg Oncol. 2016;113(5):554-9. doi: 10.1002/jso.24174.
13. Kimmig R. Diagnostische und therapeutische Lymphonodektomie, Kap. 8, S. 97–108; Totale mesometriale Resektion nach Höckel, Kap. 12, S. 119–128 und Fertilitätserhaltende mesometriale Resektion", Kap. 13, S. 129–136. In: Wagner U, Hofmann R, Bartsch DK, Boekhoff J, Hrsg. Operationsatlas Gynäkologische Onkologie. Springer verlag; 2013, Berlin, Heidelberg. ISBN 978-3-642-35127-3.
14. Kimmig R. Compartment based surgery: the TMMR, FMMR and PMMR family in uterine cancer. In: Kilic SG, Ertan K, Kose FM, editors. Robotic surgery: practical examples in gynecology, Chapter 23. Berlin/Boston: de Gruyter Verlag; 2013. p. 287–318. ISBN 3110306557.
15. Kimmig R. Innovationen in der operativen Therapie von Genitalkarzinomen. Gynakologe. 2014;12:932–41.
16. Kimmig R, Aktas B, Heubner M. Endometriumkarzinom – operative Strategie und Adjuvanz. Gynakologe. 2013;46:339–44.
17. Kimmig R.. Robotic surgery for cervical cancer. Endoscopic total mesometrial resection and therapeutic lymphonodectomy [Robotic Surgery beim Zervixkarzinom. Endoskopische totale mesometriale Resektion und therapeutische Lymphonodektomie]. Gynakologe. 2012;45:707–711, (German).
18. Ribatti D, Crivellato E. The embryonic origins of lymphatic vessels: an historical review. Br J Haematol. 2010;149:669–74.
19. Yang Y, Oliver G. Development of the mammalian lymphatic vasculature. J Clin Invest. 2015;124:888–97.
20. Höckel M. Cancer permeates locally within ontogenetic compartments: clinical evidence and implications for cancer surgery. Future Oncol. 2012;8(1):29–36. doi:10.2217/fon.11.128.

Robot Assisted Laparoscopic Fertility Sparing Radical Trachelectomy

71

Jan Persson

Introduction

In 1994 Daniel Dargent described vaginal radical trachelectomy in conjunction with laparoscopic pelvic lymphadenectomy to preserve fertility in women with early stage cervical cancer [1]. A trachelectomy can also be performed abdominally either as an open procedure or by laparoscopy. The latter approach has not gained any popularity, probably due to its complexity [2–5]. Robot assisted laparoscopic trachelectomy was first described in 2008 and may help overcome some of the surgical difficulties associated with traditional laparoscopy [6]. More than 900 cases of fertility sparing trachelectomy have been published, of those 760 with the laparoscopic/vaginal approach [7]. The procedure is considered as safe as a radical hysterectomy, with a recurrence rate of less than 5 % and a mortality of less than 3 % given strict selection criteria [7–13].

As a rule, only well informed women with a wish for preserved fertility and no previous history of infertility are candidates for fertility sparing trachelectomy. Selection criteria include cervical squamous or adenosquamous epithelial cancers from stage IAI (with lymphovascular space invasion) to stage 1B1 ≤2 cm. A more restrictive policy is advocated in case of adenocarcinomas and in particular in case of rare high risk histologies such as clear cell or neuroendocrine cancers. The tumor should be possible to resect with sufficient margins still leaving an adequate length of the remaining cervix which may disqualify women with previous large cone biopsies from being candidates for trachelectomy. If applying the aforementioned criteria, around 45 % of women younger than 40 years and with operable cervical cancer are estimated as potential candidates for fertility sparing surgery [8]. As age at first childbirth is increasing in many countries the proportion of women being candidates for trachelectomy will most likely increase further over time.

J. Persson
Geneccological and Robotic Surgery, Department of Genecology and Obstetrics, Skåne University Hospital, Lund, Sweden
e-mail: Jan.persson@med.lu.se

Surprisingly, and despite the use of recommended fecundity criteria as above, Ramirez et al. report that only 43 % of women attempt to get pregnant following a trachelectomy. A 70 % pregnancy rate is reported among those with an active wish to conceive [7, 8, 14–17].

There are no studies evaluating the risk of premature birth related to the remaining cervical length but it is generally believed that the remaining cervix should be at least 10 mm to avoid a too high prematurity rate. The use of a permanent cervical cerclage may compensate for a short cervical length but may cause problems in case of a late spontaneous abortion. A cerclage placed to distally may erode to the vaginal and cause a foreign body reaction usually necessitating removal in particular if multifilament materials are used for the cerclage. The association between cervical stenosis and cervical cerclage is however unclear.

Due to the importance of radical resection and still an adequate remaining cervix, it is cruzial that the surgical approach is reproducible, allows an exact resection level and an optimal placement of the cervical cerclage.

So far, the da manufacturer of the da Vinci robot (da Vinci ® Surgical System, Intuitive Surgical Inc, CA, USA) has so far launched four different robot systems (DaVinci standard, S, Si and Xi systems) all four providing instruments with a wrist function at the tip, movement downgrading, tremor elimination, a stable 3-dimension view of the operative field and an ergonomic working position. These features may help the surgeon overcome some of the limitations associated with traditional laparoscopic surgery. As most women candidates for radical trachelectomy are nulliparous vaginal access may be restricted. Therefore a radical vaginal trachelectomy may be difficult to perform in a standardized manner and times between procedures may be long making surgical training for this particular approach insufficient. In a setting where robot assisted surgery is frequently used for other advanced gyneoncological procedures a robot assisted laparoscopic abdominal approach for the trachelectomy seems reproducible and accurate and experience from other advanced procedures helpful [18–21].

I. Alkatout, L. Mettler (eds.), *Hysterectomy*, DOI 10.1007/978 3 319-22497-8_71

Patient Selection and Preoperative Assessment

A careful selection is mandatory to achieve the desired oncological and fertility outcome and includes women with a desire to preserve fertility and with beneficial tumor characteristics. It is important that the woman and her partner are well informed about preoperative examinations, situations in which a planned trachelectomy concept may have to be abandoned (i.e. metastatic lymph nodes or inadequate surgical margins) as well as alternative treatment in such situations. It is also important to discuss the risk of premature delivery. The cervical cancer should have diameter less than two cm (FIGO stage IAI with LVSI, IA2, IBI), preferably squamous cell cancers. IBI cancers requires a beneficial localization in the distal part of the cervix and with tumor invasion less than half the cervical stroma. A more restrictive attitude should be advocated in case of adenocarcinomas. Patients with clear cell and neuroendocrine cancers should not primarily be candidates for fertility sparing surgery. Therefore a review by an expert gynecological pathologist with focus on the histological subtype, lymphovascular space invasion, depth of invasion and in case of a cone biopsy the proximal and distal tumor margins is important. To evaluate the tumor diameter, the degree of stromal invasion against outer cervical margins and to evaluate the possibility to achieve adequate negative surgical margins a MRI is recommended. A CT scan of the thorax and abdomen should be performed to rule out disseminated disease. It is also strongly recommended that the surgeon him/herself estimates the length of the whole cervix with the use of high resolution vaginal ultrasonography to ensure both the possibility of adequate surgical margins and ideally 10 mm remaining cervix after a completed trachelectomy. A preoperative evaluation of the cervix is particularly important after a previous cone biopsy. A colposcopy is recommended to rule out cancer spread or severe dysplasia in the vagina.

Intraoperative Assessment

A radical trachelectomy may be performed in two separate sessions, an initial lymphadenectomy, and if lymph nodes are free from metastases at final histology, the trachelectomy in a second session. From a logistic and patients' perspective this approach is not ideal. Given appropriate selection, women planned for fertility sparing trachelectomy have a low risk for lymph node metastases. The sentinel lymph node concept allows an intraoperative detection of the nodes with the highest risk for metastases and a reversal of the fertility sparing approach if nodes are found metastatic at frozen section. It is still under debate whether it is safe to remove the sentinel nodes only but if used in tumors less than two cm the sentinel node technique has shown a high sensitivity and low false negative detection rate [22].

The transsection level of the cervix is cruzial. On one hand, the remaining cervix should be at least 10 mm to minimize premature childbirth and on the other hand, the tumor should be removed with adequate proximal (and distal) surgical margins to ensure safe oncological outcome without need for adjuvant treatment. The importance of the preoperative workout and surgeons' experience cannot be overestimated. It is recommended that the trachelectomy specimen and in some cases also a separate proximal disc of the remaining cervix are evaluated as frozen section as well as a being subject for an elaborate final histological workout. Finally, during surgery it is important also to investigate for and describe the presence and extent of possible factors that may impair fertility, i.e endometriosis, tubal pathology and pelvic adhesions, for proper postoperative fertility guidance and to avoid a delayed instigation of necessary assisted reproduction measures.

Surgical Technique

All models of the da Vinci robots can be used but we recommend a da Vinci Si or Xi system adapted for the near infrared fluorescent technique with the use of Indocyanine green as detecting dye. Ports should be placed for standard pelvic surgery as recommended for the respective systems. The Si robot may be docked centrally or side docked at surgeons' discretion whereas the Xi robot usually is docked 90° from the side. Suitable robot instruments are; a monopolar scissors, a bipolar forceps, a grasper and a needle holder. For the assistant one 10–12 mm trocar is needed for suction/ irrigation, insertion of sponges and loops and for retrieval of lymph nodes. We recommend to always use a nodal retrieval bag. For identification of the vaginal fornices a vaginal tube or another type of fornix presenter without an intracervical part is placed at onset of surgery.

The operation may be divided into three steps; the pelvic lymphadenectomy with detection of sentinel lymph nodes, the radical trachelectomy including dissection and lateralization of the ureters pelvic hypogastric nerve fibres and the reconstructive part including readaptation of the vagina to the remaining cervix and placement of a permanent cerclage. To avoid time loss during waiting for frozen section, it is important to perform the different steps in a correct order depending on local logistics for frozen section.

For detection of sentinel lymph nodes we inject a total of one mL Indocyanine green (diluted to 2.5 mg/mL in sterile water) slowly submucosally at 2-4-8-10 o'clock in the cervix immediately before docking the robot.

The identification of nodes starts with a careful development of the pararectal and paravesical spaces during which

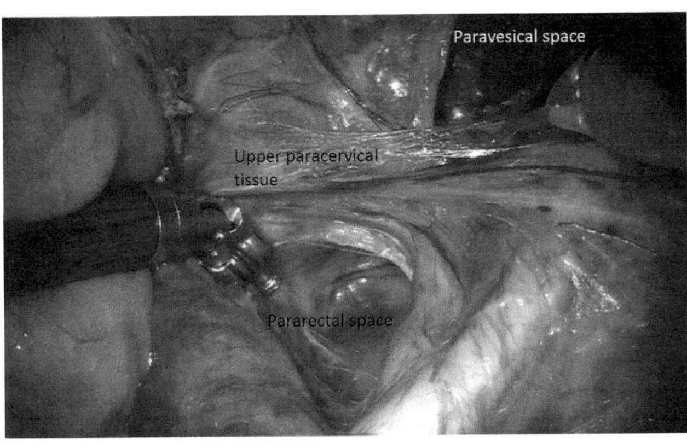

Fig. 71.1 The upper paracervical tissue is kept intact by opening the avascular paravesical and pararectal spaces

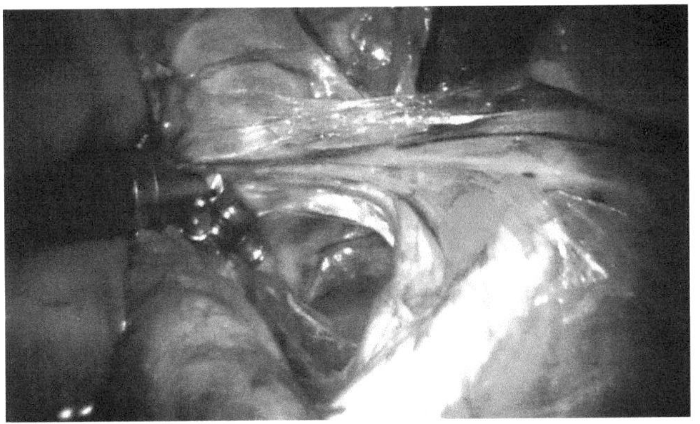

Fig. 71.2 Lymphatic vessels and a sentinel lymph node appears green with the use of the near infrared fluorescent technique and indocyanine green injected into the cervix

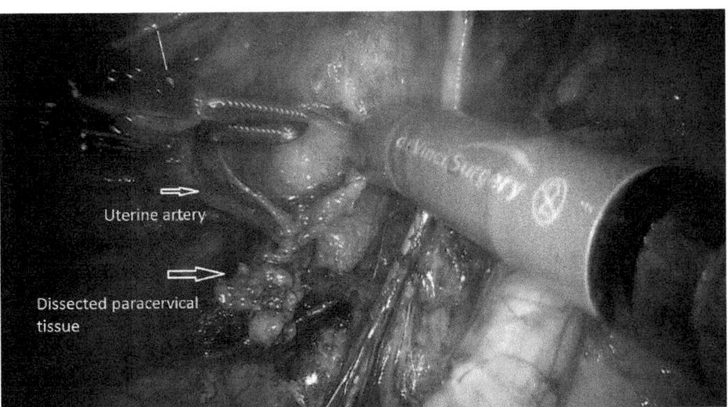

Fig. 71.3 The upper paracervical tissue is removed separately sparing the uterine artery

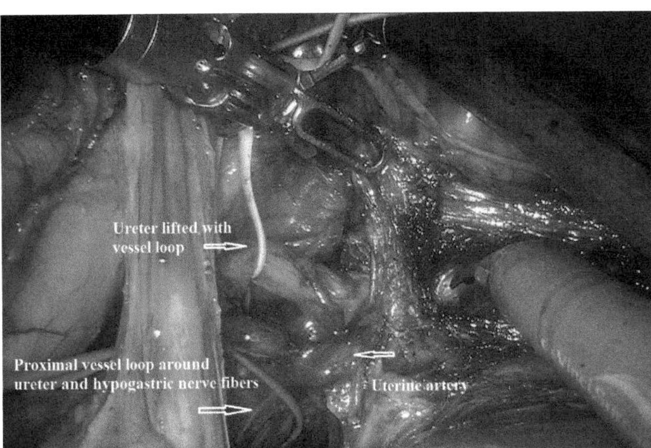

Fig. 71.4 Vessel loop placed around the ureter distal of the uterine artery

it is important to leave the upper paracervical tissue and lymph vessels intact to avoid spillage of dye and to enable a detection of individual lymph vessels (Fig. 71.1). The sentinel nodes are removed separately and sent for frozen section along with any clinically suspect nodes (Fig. 71.2). In case of a no uptake of Indocyanine green a full pelvic lymphadenectoomy has to be performed at the respective pelvic side wall and in this situation it is particularly important to look for macroscopically suspicious nodes for analyse during surgery. Awaiting frozen section results, the common iliac nodes are removed bilaterally. This is most easily done by opening the peritoneum along the medial part of the right common iliac artery to the level of the aortic bifurcation and on the left side by lifting the sigmoid colon together with the ureter and infundibulopelvic ligament with the fourth robot arm to get full access to the nodes. Local treatment protocol and the histology and size of the cervical cancer decide whether removal of the sentinel nodes only should be considered safe or if the frozen section results should be used only for tailoring of the further lymphadenccomy and abortion of the trachelectomy concept if sentinel lymph nodes are metastatic. After the remaining pelvic lymphadenectomy (if so required) the uterine arteries are identified together with the upper paracervical tissue. The ureters are then dissected and visualized also at the ventral and distal side of the uterine arteries to enable a careful removal of the upper paracervical tissue sparing the uterine arteries and visualizing the descending uterine artery (Fig. 71.3). Vessel loops are placed around the ureter distal of the uterine artery to facilitate later dissection of the lower paracervical tissue and bladder pillar (Fig. 71.4).

The posterior dissection starts with a further dissection of the pararectal space to identify the hypogastric nerves. The medial broad ligament is then opened and by developing the Okabayashi space the lateral nervous part of the sacrouterine ligament is separated from the medial fibrous part (Fig. 71.5). Vessel loops are then placed around the ureter and the nervous part of the ligament for retraction and to help identification of the hypogastric nerve fibers during further dissection (Fig. 71.6). The rectovaginal space is then opened to facilitate division of the fibrous parts of the sacrouterine ligaments at the desired level. Then the anterior peritoneum is opened (leaving the round ligaments intact) and a strict

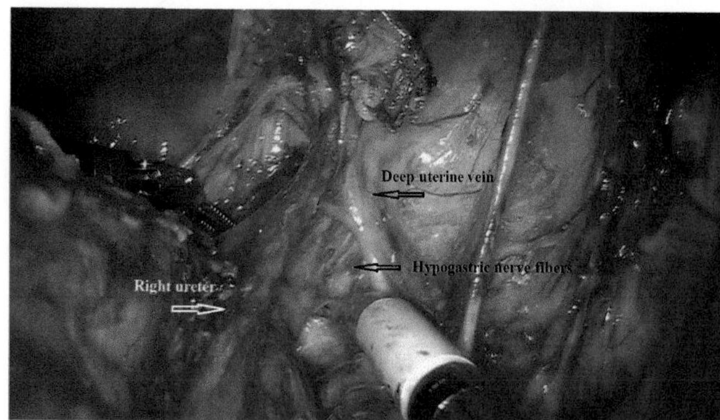

Fig. 71.5 The Okabayashi space is opened to separate the medial fibrous and lateral nervous parts of the sacrouterine ligament followed by lateralization of the ureter and nerves with a vessel loop (Jan Persson 2012)

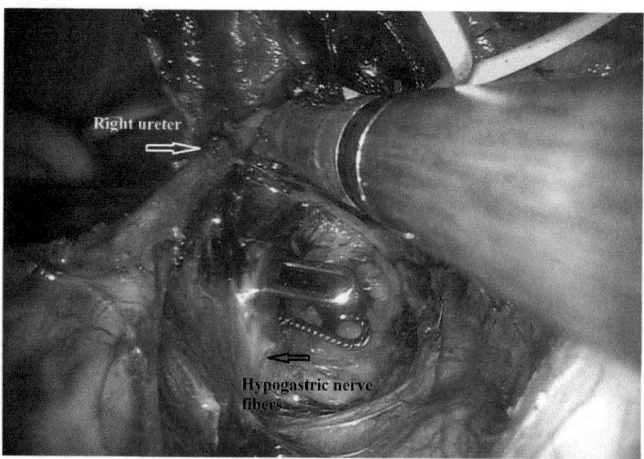

Fig. 71.6 Identification and dissection of the lower paracervical tissue and bladder pillar (left side)

midline dissection of the bladder is performed to separate the bladder pillars for later division. Before the final lateral dissection the descending uterine arteries are identified and ligated twice on each side allowing to allow cutting in between them without blood loss. The further lateral dissection (lower paracervical tissue) and dissection of the bladder pillar is facilitated by the aid of the previously placed second vessel loop around the ureter distal of the intact uterine artery (Fig. 71.7). By the use of separate vessel loops around the hypogastric nerves and the distal ureters the bladder branches of the nerves may be identified and saved along their course in the lower paracervical tissue. Finally, the vagina is dissected distally approximately 1.5 cm further than the desired vaginal cuff specimen length to mobilize enough vaginal tissue for a sufficient reattachment to the cervix (Fig. 71.8). With the preoperative vaginal ultrasonography and tumor localization in mind a careful planning of the cervical transsection level is important. The outer contour of the uterus as well as the level of the approaching main uterine branches is

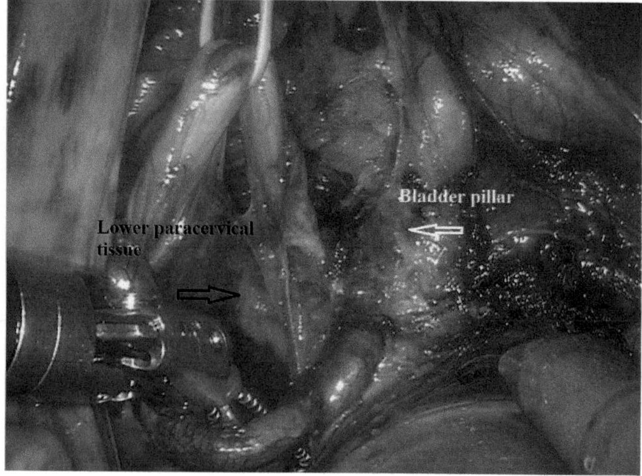

Fig. 71.7 The vaginal tube helps identification of the vaginal fornices and estimation of an appropriate length of the vagina

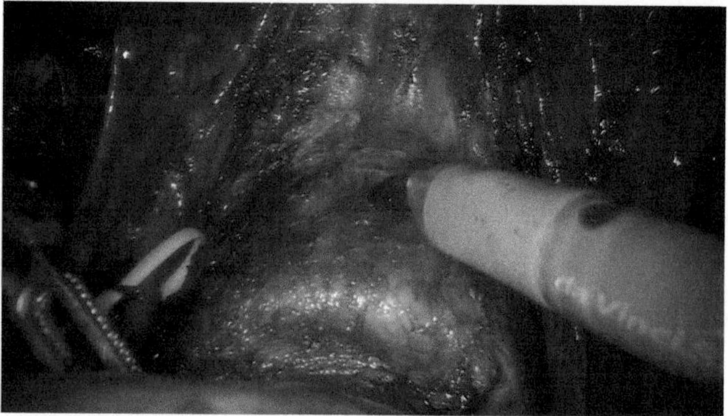

Fig. 71.8 The level of cervical transsection is dediced with help of the uterine contour after the vagina is opened

a good help for defining the level of the proximal uterine isthmus (Fig. 71.9). The vagina is opened at the desired level to facilitate the transsection of the cervix by visualization from the vaginal and abdominal side. The whole trachelectomy specimen is sent for frozen section to ensure negative margins. It is recommended to dye the proximal and distal edges of the specimen to simplify its orientation for the pathologist. Awaiting the final frozen section results the vagina is reattached to the remaining cervix with resorbable mattress sutures in order to cover most of the cut cervix but still leaving the new external orifice free. The suturing should start at the lateral corners of the vagina to ensure an even distribution of the opened larger vaginal circumference around the smaller cervix (Fig. 71.10). Finally, a permanent monofilament non resorbable cerclage (i.e 0 Prolene) is placed at the level of the inner os. The cerclage is placed medial of the uterine arteries. The tension of the cerclage suture is decided visually with the aid of a posterior sliding locking knot gradually tightened to achieve a slight induration of the tissue (Fig. 71.11). No intracervical device is

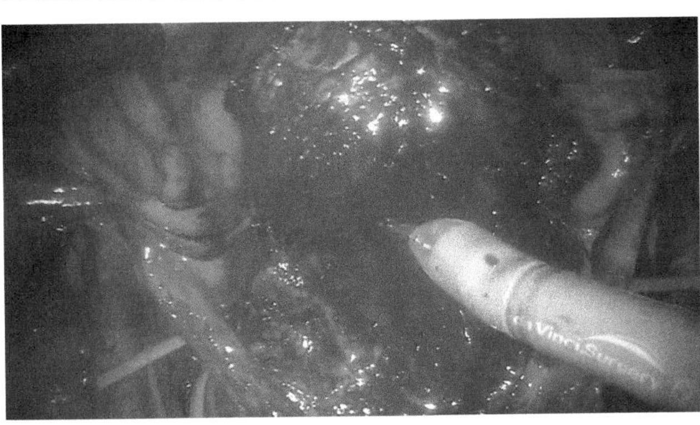

Fig. 71.9 The vagina is sutured to the remaning cervix starting at the lateral corners to ensure an even distribution of vagina anteriorly and posteriorly

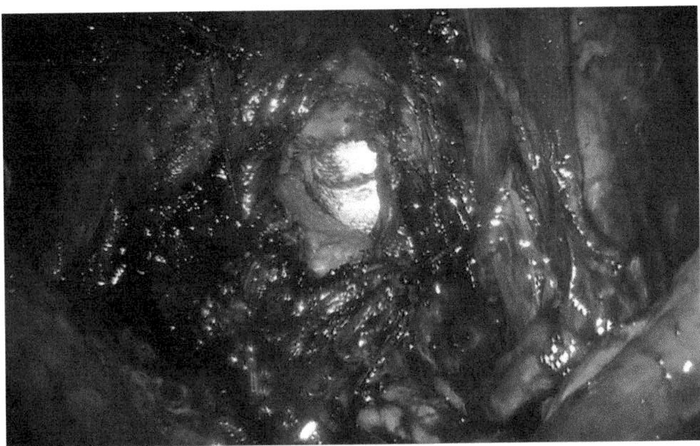

Fig. 71.10 A permanent monofilament suture is placed medial of the vessels at the level of the upper uterine isthmus

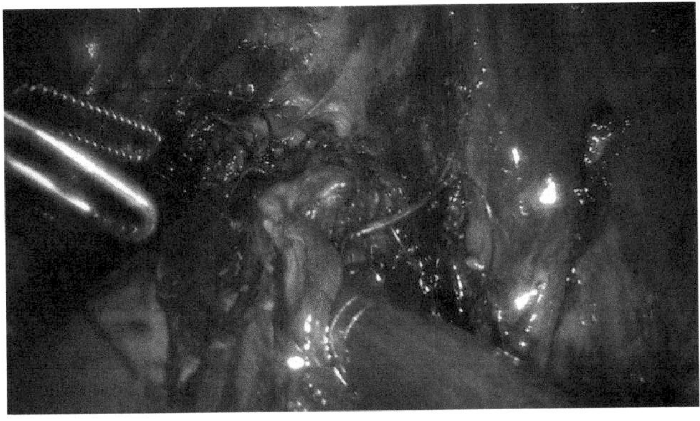

Fig. 71.11 Laparoscopic view three weeks after a robotic radical trachelectomy

necessary to secure patency of the cervical canal. A final check of the readapted uterus should be done.

If proximal margins are insufficient it may in selected cases be place for removal of an extra part of the cervix. If the margins are tumor involved a conversion to a radical hysterectomy is recommended, simply by releasing the vaginal/cervical sutures and cutting the round ligaments and by releasing the ovaries. The ovaries can then be tunnelled retroperitoneally and transpositioned in the paracolic gutters at desired level. Figure 71.11 shows a laparoscopic view of the pelvis three weeks after a robotic trachelectomy.

Postoperative Care and Follow Up

Postoperative surgical morbidity is low frequent after a vaginal or laparoscopic trachelectomy. Most side effects are due to the lymphadenectomy. An early onset moderate abdominal swelling or a proximal lymphedema of the vulvar area, labiae and inner thighs may be scaring for the patient but are usually self limiting. Postoperative urinary retention is rarely a problem but should be controlled. Bleeding from the cut cervix may occur similar to after a large cone biopsy. Fertility sparing trachelectomy is associated with cervical stenosis and rejection/exteriorization of the cervical cerclage. A cervical stenosis is associated with subsequent infertility and may hinder retrieval of intracervical cells for Pap-smear during follow up. Rejection of parts of the suture used for cervical cerclage is likely associated with a too distal placement of the suture. One study indicates that robotic trachelectomy, compared with vaginal trachelectomy, results in a cerclage placement closer to the inner cervical os, theoretically beneficial for reducing both the rate of cerclage erosion and the rate of preterm delivery [19].

No commonly used criteria for timing of pregnancy after surgery exist. It may be advisable to await a negative Pap-smear at first follow up 3 months after surgery. It is unclear whether antibiotic prophylaxis and general advise during pregnancy reduces the risk for prematurity. Some centers advocate the use of oral Metronidazol from gestational week 16 to 22, no sexual intercourse and in case of a strenuous work sick leave from week 22 + 0 and throughout the pregnancy.

All patients should be planned for a Cesarean delivery and informed to seek immediate help in case of premature uterine contractions. A particular problem with the permanent cervical cerclage is late first trimester or second trimester miscarriages necessitating a removal/ division of the cerclage to enable a complete transvaginal evacuation of the fetus and placenta without the need for a Sectio Parva. Cutting of the cerclage can be performed via a posterior culdotomy or laparoscopy and the cerclage may later be replaced laparoscopically. In general we discourage from the use of IUD as contraceptive due to a potentially increased risk for ascending infections.

Protocols for follow up usually advocate controls every 3–4 months the first 2 years, then every 6 months until 5 years after which the patient may be subject to routine controls or on an individual basis. It is important to harvest intracervical cells for Pap-smear. It should be indicated that the patient has been subject to a trachelectomy as the cytological evaluation may be more difficult to interpret. A HPV test may add further information. A colposcopy and guided biopsies or cervical curettage should be performed in case of aberrant bleeding and a pathological Pap-smear. It is however common with aberrant vaginal bleedings in particular the first 6–12 months due to exteriorization of intracervical mucosa. As quality control, a vaginal ultrasonography can be performed to evaluate the length of the remaining cervix, the placement of the cerclage and to rule out retention of menstrual blood in the uterus as a sign of a cervical stenosis. MRI or PET-CT investigations should be performed if clinically indicated.

Some patients ask for a post trachelectomy hysterectomy after finalizing childbirth. This may be performed after proper counselling as a second operation will further shorten the vagina. As a post-trachelectomy hysterectomy, preferably by a second robot assisted laparoscopic approach, may be complex the operation should be performed by an experienced gynecological oncologist and include a thorough inspection of the whole pelvis.

References

1. Dargent D, Burn JL, Roy M, Remi I. Pregnancies following radical trachelectomy for invasive cervical cancer. Gynecol Oncol. 1994;52:105. (Abstract)
2. Abu-Rustum NR, Sonoda Y, Black D, Levine DA, Chi DS, Barakat RR. Fertility-sparing radical abdominal trachelectomy for cervical carcinoma: technique and review of the literature. Gynecol Oncol. 2006;103:807–13.
3. Ungár L, Smith JR, Pálfalvi L, Del Priore G. Abdominal radical trachelectomy during pregnancy to preserve pregnancy and fertility. Obstet Gynecol. 2006;108:811–4.
4. Martin A, Torrent A. Laparoscopic nerve-sparing radical trachelectomy: surgical technique and outcome. J Minim Invasive Gynecol. 2010;17:37–41.
5. Kim JH, Park JY, Kim DY, Kim YM, Kim YT, Nam JH. Fertility-sparing laparoscopic radical trachelectomy for young women with early stage cervical cancer. BJOG. 2010;117:340–7.
6. Persson J, Kannisto P, Bossmar T. Robot-assisted abdominal laparoscopic radical trachelectomy. Gynecol Oncol. 2008;111:564–7.
7. Shepherd JH, Milliken DA. Conservative surgery for carcinoma of the cervix. Clin Oncol (R Coll Radiol). 2008;20:395–400.
8. Ramirez PT, Schmeler KM, Soliman PT, Frumovitz M. Fertility preservation in patients with early cervical cancer: radical trachelectomy. Gynecol Oncol. 2008;110:25–8.
9. Rob L, Skapa P, Robova H. Fertility-sparing surgery in patients with cervical cancer. Lancet Oncol. 2011;12:192–200.
10. Martinez A, Poilblanc M, Ferron G, De Cuypere M, Jouve E, Querleu D. Fertility-preserving surgical procedures, techniques. Best Pract Res Clin Obstet Gynecol. 2012;26:407–24.
11. Dursun P, LeBlanc E, Nogueira MC. Radical vaginal trachelectomy (Dargent's operation): a critical review of the literature. Eur J Surg Oncol. 2007;33:933–41.
12. Diaz JP, Sonoda Y, Leitao MM, Zivanovic O, Brown CL, Chi DS, Barakat RR, Abu-Rustum NR. Oncologic outcome of fertility-sparing radical trachelectomy versus radical hysterectomy for stage IB1 cervical carcinoma. Gynecol Oncol. 2008;111:255–60.
13. Plante M, Gregoire J, Renaud MC, Roy M. The vaginal radical trachelectomy: an update of a series of 125 cases and 106 pregnancies. Gynecol Oncol. 2011;121:290–7.
14. Dargent D, Martin X, Sacchetoni A, Mathevet P. Laparoscopic vaginal radical trachelectomy: a treatment to preserve the fertility of cervical carcinoma patients. Cancer. 2000;88:1877–82.
15. Jolley JA, Battista L, Wing DA. Management of pregnancy after radical trachelectomy: case reports and systematic review of the literature. Am J Perinatol. 2007;24:531–9.
16. Kim CH, Abu-Rustum NR, Chi DS, Gardner GJ, Leitao MM Jr, Carter J, Barakat RR, Sonoda Y. Reproductive outcomes of patients undergoing radical trachelectomy for early-stage cervical cancer. Gynecol Oncol 2012;125(3):585-588
17. Boss EA, van Golde RJ, Beerendonk CC, Massuger LF. Pregnancy after radical trachelectomy: a real option? Gynecol Oncol. 2005;99:152–6.
18. Persson J, Imboden S, Reynisson P, Andersson B, Borgfeldt C, Bossmar T. Reproducibility and accuracy of robot-assisted laparoscopic fertility sparing radical trachelectomy. Gynecol Oncol. 2012;127(3):484–8. Epub 2012 Aug 28
19. Nick AM, Frumovitz MM, Soliman PT, Schmeler KM, Ramirez PT. Fertility sparing surgery for treatment of early-stage cervical cancer: open vs. robotic radical trachelectomy. Gynecol Oncol. 2012;124:276–80.
20. Al-Niaimi AN, Einstein MH, Perry L, Hartenbach EM, Kushner DM. Uterine artery sparing robotic radical trachelectomy (AS-RRT) for early cancer of the cervix. Int J Gynaecol Obstet. 2011;112:76–80.
21. Ramirez PT, Schmeler KM, Malpica A, Soliman PT. Safety and feasibility of robotic radical trachelectomy in patients with early-stage cervical cancer. Gynecol Oncol. 2010;116:512–5.
22. Darlin L, Persson J, Bossmar T, Lindahl B, Kannisto P, Måsbäck A, Borgfeldt C. The sentinel node concept in early cervical cancer performs well in tumors smaller than 2 cm. Gynecol Oncol. 2010;117:266–9.

Robotic-Assisted Radical Hysterectomy with Anterior and Posterior Exenteration-Urological Perspectives

72

Saad Hatahet, Ahmad Shabsigh, Dimitrios Moschonas, and Petros Sountoulides

Introduction

Pelvic exenteration (PE) describes a radical surgery involving the en bloc resection of the pelvic organs, including the internal reproductive organs, the urinary bladder and the rectosigmoid. Indications include advanced primary or recurrent pelvic malignancies, most commonly local or locally advanced cervical and bladder carcinomas.

From an urological point of view, PE has been utilized for the treatment of localized or locally advanced bladder cancer. Bladder cancer is one of the most common urologic malignancies in the world. In the USA, about 74,000 new cases are expected to be diagnosed in 2015, with an estimated 16,000 deaths related to them [1]. At initial diagnosis, more than 70 % of patients have Non-Muscle-Invasive Bladder Cancer (NMIBC). These less aggressive neoplasms are generally treated with transurethral resection of bladder (TURB) with or without intravesical immuno or chemotherapy [2]. Radical cystectomy (RC) with bilateral pelvic lymphadenectomy is still the gold standard treatment for the local control of non-metastatic muscle invasive bladder cancer (pT2-T4aN0M0) [3]. Radical cystectomy is one of the most morbid surgeries in urologic oncology. It is associated with high post-operative complication rates (27–64 %) [4], high risk of readmission, and re-operation. Over the last few decades, numerous modifications of the surgery were developed to reduce the post-operative morbidity and the long-term impact of this major operation. Minimally invasive techniques, continent urinary diversions, and better perioperative management all aim to achieve these goals. In the following few pages we review the history, surgical steps and outcomes of robotic assisted radical cystectomy in the setting of total pelvic exenteration.

Saad Hatahet • Ahmad Shabsigh (✉)
Department of Urology, The Ohio State University, Wexner Medical Center, Columbus, OH, USA
e-mail: saadhatahet@yahoo.com; Ahmad.shabsigh@osumc.edu

D. Moschonas • P. Sountoulides
Department of Urology, Royal Surrey County Hospital, Guildford, Surrey, UK
e-mail: dmoschonas1@yahoo.gr; sountp@hotmail.com

History of Laparoscopy and Robotic Surgery in Bladder Cancer Management

The first laparoscopic simple cystectomy was reported by Para in 1992 [5]. A year later, de Badajoz performed the first laparoscopic radical cystectomy for bladder cancer with an ileal conduit urinary diversion [6]. By the year 2000, experienced minimally invasive surgeons took advantage of better laparoscopic instruments, and performed the first two cases of laparoscopic radical cystoprostatectomy with intracorporeal ileal conduit [7].

Shortly after the Da Vinci surgical system was approved by the Food and Drug Administration (FDA) in 2000, the Vattikuti Urology Institute in Henry Ford Hospital reported the nerve-sparing robot-assisted radical cystectomy (RRC) for in 17 bladder cancer patients (14 men and 3 women) [8]. In 2003, Beecken and his colleagues performed the first robotic radical cystectomy and completely intra-abdominal formation of an orthotopic neobladder [9].

Over the last decade, the use of the Da Vinci system became more prevalent. By 2012, more than 400,000 robotic surgeries were done in the USA, triple the number just four years earlier. In 2013 almost 1,400 U.S. hospitals (nearly 1 out of 4) had at least one Da Vinci system. By June 30, 2015, there were 3,398 units worldwide, 2,295 of them in the United States (Intuitive LLC).

The early reports of RRC were promising. Not surprisingly, the operation took more time than open radical cystectomy. More importantly, RRC was associated with lower post-operative morbidity. As expected, there was a rapid adaptation of technology. Data from 279 hospitals across the United States revealed an increase in RRC rates from 0.6 % in 2004 to 12.8 % in 2010 [10]. Currently, most, if not all, large oncology centers in the USA utilize robotic assisted radical cystectomy.

I. Alkatout, L. Mettler (eds.), *Hysterectomy*, DOI 10.1007/978-3-319-22497-8_72

Laparoscopic Radical Cystectomy (LAR): Benefits and Difficulties

Since its inception, laparoscopic radical cystectomy remained a technically challenging procedure. The inherent constraints of laparoscopic instruments and the challenging nature of minimally invasive pelvic surgery prevented the wide adaptation of this technique. Even with these difficulties, most published studies have shown LAR to be feasible with less morbidity and mortality, and comparable oncologic outcomes compared to open surgery.

Recently, a meta-analysis of sixteen eligible case series reports comparing LRC vs ORC was performed. The study confirmed the safety and feasibility of LRC. It was clear that while the average operative time for LRC was longer, laparoscopic radical cystectomy was associated with significantly fewer overall complications, less blood loss, shorter length of hospital stay, less need of blood transfusion, shorter time to ambulation, shorter time to regular diet, and less narcotic requirement [20]. Surprisingly, there were fewer positive surgical margins, positive lymph node, lower distant metastasis rate, and lower mortality with LRC. These findings are more likely to be related to patients' selection than true better oncologic outcome with laparoscopic surgery [11].

Robotic Radical Cystectomy Benefits

The robotic systems provided reliable solutions for most of the difficulties encountered during laparoscopic surgery. Surgeons can benefit from the magnified 3D high-definition vision system and special wristed instruments that bend and rotate far greater than the human wrist, allowing the surgeon to perform difficult dissections and suturing. A surgeon's hands tremors or sudden strong moves are not transmitted to the robotic arms, protecting patients from accidental errors and enhancing their safety. Despite the surgeon's loss of real tactile sensation of the tissue with the Da Vinci system, surgeons were able to use the visual clues to perform safe and efficient surgeries. More importantly, there was a significantly shorter learning curve compared to laparoscopy, increasing the benefit of minimally invasive surgery for patients with bladder cancer.

Pelvic Lymph Node Dissection (PLND) in Radical Cystectomy

General Aspects

Bilateral pelvic lymph node dissection is an essential part of surgical therapy for bladder, prostate and gynecologic malignancies [3, 12, 13]. To develop the needed skills to perform adequate lymph node dissection, surgeons need to commit significant time and effort to learn the subtleties of systematic and efficient dissection. In most cases, skilled surgeons spend more time performing pelvic lymph node dissection than the time required to complete the exenteration. Unless cystectomy alone is considered, it is recommended that PLND is done first. This sets the surgical fossa for a fast and easy radical cystectomy, helps define the vascular pedicels of the bladder and the prostate, and gets the pelvis ready for urinary diversion.

Technically, there is no reason that the same lymph node dissection done in open surgery is not duplicated robotically. With appropriate port placement and exposure, robotic pelvic lymph node dissection achieves comparable results to open surgery [14].

How Many Lymph Nodes Should Be Dissected?

The number of lymph nodes identified after surgery depends on multiple factors, including the limits of the dissection and its thoroughness, the pathologic processing, and how meticulous the pathological examination is. In practice, wider and more systematic resection leads to an increase in the likelihood of identifying positive LNs. Furthermore, extended LNs dissection not only provides the most accurate staging but may also offer the patient the best chance of survival [15–17].

With increased experience, the number of lymph nodes dissected during RC increased substantially between 1988 and 2010 (≥10 nodes removed as an adequate number). However, a minority of patients still do not receive LND, and removing >14 lymph nodes has been shown to improve progression-free survival [18].

Limited (Standard) Pelvic Lymph Node Dissection

Standard PLND was described by "Stewart's Operative Urology" and includes the pelvic sidewall between the genitofemoral and obturator nerves, and bifurcation of the iliac vessels to the circumflex iliac vein [19], including all lymphatic tissues around the common iliac, intercommon iliac, and internal iliac groups, and the obturator group bilaterally [20, 21] (Fig. 72.1).

Up to one-third of all positive lymph nodes are located around the common iliac artery. About 80 % of all positive nodes could be cleared completely by standard PLND, including all lymphatic tissues along the common, external, and internal iliac regions [14, 16, 22]. Some experts recommend doing frozen section on the true pelvis LNs; if the frozen section examination revealed no positive LNs, LN dissection does not need to be carried out further. If, however, the frozen section examination is not performed, or if it identifies positive nodes, an extended PLND is done [21].

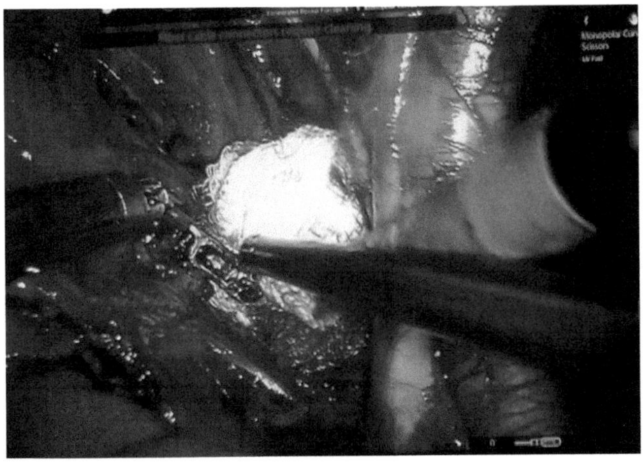

Fig. 72.1 Taking care of minor bleeding during robot-assisted lymph node dissection at the time of radical cystectomy

Extended PLND Limits and Benefits

Extending the dissection up to the aortic bifurcation or the inferior mesenteric artery increased the detection of positive nodes by 13–16 % [16, 20].

A recent lymphatic bladder mapping study suggests that the template for an appropriate PLND at cystectomy should include the external iliac (including the fossa of Marcille), obturator and internal iliac region (lateral and medial to the internal iliac vessels), as well as the common iliac vessels up to at least the uretero-iliac junction bilaterally [17].

Standard PLND is associated with suboptimal staging, and a higher rate of local progression. In contrast, extended PLND provides better 5-year recurrence-free survival for patients with lymph node positive disease. Even patients with pT2N0 or pT3N0 bladder cancer have better prognosis after RC and extended pelvic lymph node dissection [16, 17, 23].

The possible benefits of higher resection must be weighed against the potential increased demands in both time and extent of surgical field, the increased risk of complications, and injury to the autonomic sympathetic nerves, threatening both sexual function and continence in patients who are candidates for orthotopic bladder substitution [17].

Robotic Radical Cystectomy: Surgical Technique

Patient Preparation

Bowel preparation before radical cystectomy and urinary diversion does not provide any advantage. It does not seem to impact the rates of perioperative infectious, wound, and bowel complications [24, 25]. Omitting bowel preparation before ileal urinary diversion is safe, and not associated with bacterial overgrowth or added complications [24]. To the contrary, avoidance of preoperative bowel preparation led to early restoration of intestinal function and shorter hospital stay [25, 26].

Improving performance status prior to surgery is essential. Proper nutrition, ambulation, and relieving ureteral obstruction with ureteral stent or nephrostomy tube are all good measures that should be considered if possible. Post radical cystectomy venous thrombus events are common [4, 27]. Thus, wearing compression socks, using sequential compression devices, and perioperative anticoagulation are indicated for these patients [28].

Positioning

Lithotomy position with legs in Allen Yellowfins stirrups (Allen Medical Systems, Acton, Massachusetts) is the standard position during RRC. This allows the Robot cart to be moved between the patient's legs. All pressure points should be padded for safety and the patient should be secured to the table. The patient should then be put in a steep Trendelenburg position, which helps in mobilization of the small bowel for better access to the pelvis. The assistant can stand on either side of the patient. After prepping and draping the patient, a 20–22 Fr Foley catheter should be inserted in the bladder. In female patients a sponge on stick can be placed in the vagina to help in identification of vaginal cuff. We personally like to use EEA reusable stainless steel sizer and vaginal pneumo-occluder.

Port Placement in Four-Arm Robotic Approach

To facilitate proximal lymph node and ureteral dissection, the port placement is considerably more cephalad in comparison with robotic assisted radical prostatectomy. The camera 12-mm port is placed 3–8 cm above the umbilicus while the three working 8 mm robotic ports are placed 2–5 cm above the level of the umbilicus in an arch line. If the patient had prior surgeries, the first port is usually placed under direct vision away from the scars. The abdomen is then inspected, and any adhesions are taken down.

A 12 or 15-mm assistant port is placed slightly more caudal and lateral; this positioning allows for improved angulation during stapling of the bowel reconstruction. The 15-mm port is used to pass the 15-mm Endocatch bag as well. In females, if possible, the specimen is extracted via the vagina. Additional 12 mm assistant port could be used and placed laterally in the level of robotic ports on the side of the assistant [29].

Bladder Removal and Extended PLND

Right Ureter Dissection

The posterior peritoneum is incised around the cecum. The incision is extended laterally at the white line of Told and medially anterior to the right common iliac artery. The right ureter is identified over the common iliac artery. The ureter is dissected off the common iliac artery. A vessel loop is used to to mobilize the ureter by the assistant. The ureter is dissected distally all the way to the superior vesical artery. It is very important to preserve as much of the peri-ureteral tissue as possible to avoid ureteral ischemic injury. The ureter can be clipped distally with two clips and cut between them at this time, or just prior to taking the bladder pedicels. Distal ureteral margin can be sent for frozen section. It is recommended to use Hem-o-lock to clip the ureter and take a suture at the corner of the distal ureter end; this will help in handling the ureter and reduce traumatic injury to the ureter [30].

Extended PLND

The first important role of a thorough and efficient pelvic lymph node dissection is exposure and setting up the field. After isolation of the right ureter, the hypogastric artery is dissected to the obliterated medial umbilical ligament. This is usually retracted medially, to expose the medial side of the external iliac and obturator lymph nodes. The dissection is carried on both sides of hypogastric vessels to the perirectal fat. This will isolate the obturator fossa from the hypogastric lymph node packet. Attention is then paid to the lateral limits of the dissection. The femoro-genital nerve is identified and isolated. The external iliac lymph nodes are pushed medially. We recommend that the lateral limit of the dissection is developed at this point by dissecting the right external iliac and obturator lymph nodes medially of the pelvic side wall. Small vessels and lymphatics should be cauterized. Splitting the lymphatic tissue over the entire extent of the right common iliac artery and right external iliac artery is recommended. The tissue is dissected on both sides of the right external iliac artery and vein. The distal side of the external iliac packets should be clipped to reduce the formation of symptomatic lymphocele. Next the right obturator nerve and vessels are identified. The obturator lymph node packet is then dissected off the posterior edge of the external iliac vein all the way from the bifurcation of the iliac arteries to the lymph node of cloquet. The lymph nodes are then dissected off the anterior side of the obturator nerve. It is strongly recommended that the proximal end of the packet is dissected first. This will prevent the obturator lymph nodes from dropping and making the dissection of the proximal end more difficult. The distal side of the packet is then clipped. The lateral hypogastric lymph nodes are then dissected. The right common iliac lymph nodes are dissected all the way to the lateral edge of the right common iliac vein and IVC. Followed by the dissection of the right fossa of Marcille, this is done by retracting the right common iliac vein medially. Attention to the proximal end of the obturator nerve is important. The tissue is then dissected in a medial direction exposing the left common iliac vein and anterior surface of the sacrum. The lymph nodes of the left common iliac vein are then removed. Use of bipolar is recommended to control the small vessels at the inferior side of the left common iliac vein toward the sacrum. The lymph nodes anterior to the sacrum and at the medial side of the hypogastric lymph nodes are removed. The right and left common iliac node packets are clipped and divided at the anterior side of the bifurcation of the aorta and also starts the left pelvic lymph node dissection by exposing the medial aspect of the left common iliac artery which will serve as a landmark after the leftcolon is reflected. This will help in developing the mesenteric window that is used to pass the left ureter to the right side of the pelvis. After completion of the medial dissection, the lymphatic packet is mobilized laterally.

Additionally, this approach allows improved exposure of the internal iliac vein. The lymph nodes should be placed in a 10 mm specimen retrieval bag and can be removed in appropriate packets through the 12 or 15 mm port. In order to limit cost, a reusable 10 mm bag can be used for all lymph node packets [30].

Left Ureter Dissection

The sigmoid colon is mobilized at the white line of Told, then it is mobilized medially with the forth arm (Prograsp forceps). This usually exposes the left ureter anterior to the left common iliac artery. The ureter is dissected all the way to the superior vesical artery. At this point we usually develop the mesenteric window caudal to the inferior mesenteric artery. Caution should be taken to avoid injury to the colon blood supply. The left pelvic lymph node dissection is then performed.

The Posterior Dissection in Women

Unless fertility preservation is a consideration, the surgeon should remove the uterus, ovaries, and Fallopian tubes with or without anterior vaginectomy. This depends on the location of the bladder cancer and the stage of the disease. Examination under anesthesia and pre-operative imaging are essential in this decision. If the female genital organs are spared, the peritoneum is incised at the posterior bladder wall between the bladder and the uterus. The plane is developed inferiorly and laterally to reach the lower ureters which should be dissected. The rest of the surgery is similar to the full pelvic exenteration.

Since cystectomy is much more common in elderly patients, sparing the female genitalia is rare and full pelvic exenteration is usually done. In this case the gonadal vessels are clipped at the time of ureteral dissection. Attention should be to the infindibulopelvic (IP) ligaments, which should be clipped and cut. By continuing dissection inferiorly, the uterine artery should be identified and clipped. The sponge stick or the vaginal sizer is pushed anteriorly in the posterior fornix. If the anterior vaginal wall is removed with hysterectomy, the vaginal sizer is pushed and the vaginal cuff is incised posterior to the cervix. The vascular pedicles of the bladder are defined, dissected, clipped and cut bilaterally. Then the vesico-vaginal space is dissected inferiorly, all the way to the urethra, and if vagina is persevered then performing a supra-cervical hysterectomy. After the anterior dissection (discussed in a following section), the vagina is closed with figure of eight absorbable sutures.

Bladder Pedicles and Neurovascular Bundles Dissection Nerve-Sparing Technique

The anterior peritoneum is incised lateral to the medial umblilical ligaments and the urachus. The bladder should not be dropped at this point, as it would increase the difficulty of bladder pedicle dissection and control.

The right and left ureters are double clipped with Hem-o-loc clips and incised as close as possible to the bladder. The endopelvic fascia is incised and opened to the prostato-urethral junction. At this point the vascular pedicles of the bladder are defined, clipped or stapled with an Endo-GIA or bipolar device like the Ligasure.

Unless nerve sparing is contraindicated, the neurovascular bundles should be identified close to the tips of the seminal vesicles. The dissection starts immediately next to the walls of the seminal vesicle, between the vesicle and the posterior layer of Denonvillier's fascia; high anterior dissection is preferred. A combination of antegrade and retrograde dissection of the neurovascular bundle is done similar to robotic radical prostatectomy. Use of electrocautery during dissection of the pedicles is controversial. Some surgeons recommend avoiding any thermal injury, while others advocate the safety of bipolar devices [8, 31–33]. Finally, nerve sparing should be carried down to the genitourinary diaphragm to prevent injury during the apical and urethral dissection.

Anterior Bladder Wall Dissection

The urachus is incised; attention to the small vessels at the proximal end is important. The bladder is dropped from the anterior abdominal wall all the way to the space of Retzius towards the bladder neck.

If neobladder urinary diversion is planned, the pubourethral suspensory ligaments should be spared to avoid extensive dissection of the urethra for better preservation of the urethral sphincter complex and its nerve supply.

Urethral Dissection and Removal of the Bladder Specimen

When reaching the anterior wall of the bladder neck, the Dorsal Vein complex should be identified and ligated with 0 polysorb suture or stapled with EndoGIA. In females, flexible cystoscopy helps to identify the proximal limit of the urethra and the relationship to the tumor. This facilitates excellent preservation of the urethra and improves the recovery of continence after neobladder diversion. Preservation of the neurovascular bundles lateral to the urethral is achieved by blunt and gentle dissection. Similarly, for male patients, the apex of the prostate is dissected superiorly to obtain adequate urethral stump. Avoidance of spillage is achieved by leaving a catheter balloon inflated, grabbing the catheter with Prograsp forceps and cutting distally. The catheter can then be used to lift the specimen until it is placed in an Endobag. Alternatively, the catheter can be removed and the bladder neck can be closed with a figure of eight suture. If neobladder urinary diversion is planned, urethral margin sample should be sent for frozen section. This can be taken from the bladder neck.

Urinary Diversion

One of the main questions when performing a urinary diversion after a robot-assisted cystectomy, is whether to create the urinary diversion intra- or extracorporeally? The standard types of urinary diversion that are used in a classical open radical cystectomy could be performed in RRC. The first extracorporeal ileal conduit was described by Menon et al. [8]. In this approach, a periumbilical extraction incision is usually sufficient. We would recommend that the ureters are tagged with full length 2-0 suture robotically prior to opening the abdomen. This will help in bringing the ureters to the extraction incision for anastomosis. An Alexis retractor can be used to facilitate the extracorporeal construction of the ileal conduit. It is recommended that a continent cutaneous urinary diversion should be done in an extracorporeal fashion as well.

Intracorporeal Ileal Conduit Formation

Isolate the Bowel Segment

To isolate the bowel segment, the ileocecal valve is identified first. Using a marked umbilical tape, the distal end of the bowel segment is defined approximately 15–20 cm from the ileocecal valve. Some surgeons prefer Intraoperative fluorescence imaging to evaluate the segment's blood supply [34]. Double 3-0 silk sutures are placed on both the proximal and distal end of the ileal conduit for retraction. The bowel segment is then isolated and stapled using a 60 mm Endo-GIA stapler with bowel staples.

The bowel continuity is restored by a standard side-to-side anastomosis using a 60 mm Endo-GIA stapler through the assistant 12 mm assistant port. Three 3–0 silk sutures are placed spaced 2 cm apart on the anti-mesenteric sides to re-approximate the segments of bowel and to aid in completing the side-to-side anastomosis. The stapler should be applied at the anti-mesenteric ileum border. Finally the mesenteric window is closed with interrupted 3-0 silk sutures.

Uretero-Intestinal Anastomosis

The anastomosis between the ureters and the bowel segment could be performed by either Wallace technique or Bricker techniques [7, 30].

Wallace Technique

A stay suture is placed to hold the two ureters ends together. The ureters are spatulated 2 cm long. The posterior walls of the ureters are sutured side-to-side using a 4-0 polyglactin suture. Two single-J, 90-cm ureteric stents or 8 Fr pediatric feeding tubes are introduced over a guide wire. Double J stents can also be used. Using the Prograsp forceps, the stents are pulled through the afferent limb and pushed up into the ureters on each side. The uretero-ileal anastomosis between the Wallace plate and the pouch is performed according to a modified van Velthoven et al. technique. A suture is placed close to the distal end of the conduit to help with maturation of the stoma. Finally, the stoma is performed in the standard method after de-inflating the abdomen [30]

Bricker Anastomosis

Two small incisions are made in the ileal conduit near its proximal edge. The ureters are spatulated as mentioned before. We prefer to place a 5-0 silk suture as a sty suture between the peri-ureteral tissue and the ileal conduit. This can facilitate the anastomosis. The uretero-enteric anastomosis is done by placing one 4–0 polyglactin sutures at each sides of the anastomosis, and then continue the anastomosis with some interrupted sutures. Stents are placed and the anastomosis is completed (Fig. 72.2).

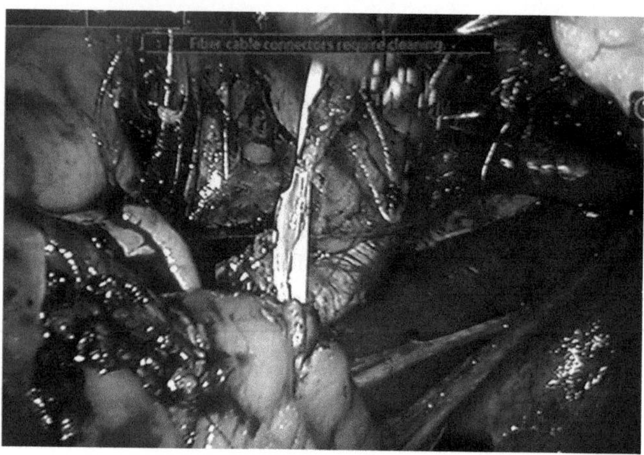

Fig. 72.2 Uretero-iliac anastomosis during a Bricker urinary diversion. The stented ureter is ready to be anastomosed to the isolated ileal segment

Intracorporeal Neobladder Formation

Robotic intracorporeal neobladder reconstruction is more challenging. Initial perioperative results seem to be comparable to open series [35]. Some researcher reported that it can be performed in a safeand reproducible fashion, even during the early learning curve [36].

There are general concepts that are used in all types of intracorporeal neobladders. The first general step is returning the patient's position from the Trendelenburg position to the supine position. This allows the bowels to move back to the lower abdomen cavity, reducing the tension off the urethro-enteric anastomosis. Second, isolating the bowel segment is done in the same fashion as described earlier. The length of the bowel segment depends on the type of the neobladder that is planned. Third, we recommend that a 3-0 silk suture is placed at the most depended part of the segment to advance the pouch into the pelvis for the anastomosis. Finally, the uretero-enteric anastomoses are performed in a similar fashion as the anastomoses performed during a robot-assisted ileal conduit.

U-shaped Pouch

A 60 cm segment is isolated. The distal 45 cm of the bowel segment is detubularized in the standard fashion for a Studer neobladder [34]. The proximal limb of 15 cm of ileum is left intact for the chimney and the eventual site for the ureteral anastomoses. The posterior plate of the bowel is then sutured together with a barbed suture in a running fashion to achieve a watertight closure [37]. The inferior side of the anterior plate should also be closed prior to the urethro-enteric anastomosis. A 2 cm incision at the most depended part of the pouch is made. Using the midpoint silk suture, the pouch is advanced into the pelvis using the Prograsp forceps.

A figure of eight 2-0 polysorb or barbed suture is then tied down from the posterior side of the most dependent portion of the pouch to posterior plate to Denonvillier's fascia just adjacent to the rectrourethralis muscle. This releases the tension from the urethro-eneteric anastomosis [38]. The urethro-enteric anastomosis is performed by placing a double armed 3-0 barbed sutures (or double armed 3-0 Monocryl) on a small tapered needle. The closure is usually started at a 4–5 o'clock position of the right side of the pouch's neck. In a running counterclockwise fashion, the posterior closure is completed. The assistant should facilitate the closure with the tip of a Foley catheter. The right arm of the suture is then used to close the anterior part of the anastomosis.

Modified Ileum Studer Neobladder

In a modified Studer neobladder the anastomosis between the urethra and bowel is performed at the beginning, before detubularisation of the bowel segment. This will stabilize the bowel loop and enhance forming the neobladder. First, the most dependent part of the bowel segment is identified, this is usually more than 35 cm proximal to the ileocecal valve. This part is brought down to the urethra and a small incision at the contra-mesenteric side is made to perform the urethral anastomosis according to the Van Velthoven technique with a two-times 2-0 suture. First, the suture is placed at the 5:30-o'clock position by passing the needle from the outside to the inside of the bowel's opening, and from inside to outside in urethral lumen. Then, the other suture is put at the 6:30- o'clock position by the other needle. The rest of the anastomosis is done in standard fashion. A 22 Fr Foley catheter is passed through the anastomosis and the balloon is inflated to 5 ml. Then an ileal segment of 20–25 cm from the ileocecal valve and 15 cm from the urethral–enteric anastomosis is selected and isolated as before. For the afferent reservoir loop, a distance of about 40 cm from the urethral–enteric anastomosis is selected and cut with a stapler in the same way. The rest of the procedure is similar to the standard Studer pouch [35, 36, 39].

Robotic Radical Cystectomy Versus Open Radical Cystectomy Outcomes

Retrospective Cohort Studies

Over the last few years, multiple reports of case cohorts were published, as is common for a new surgical technique. These focused on defining the perioperative benefits, morbidity, and mortality of RRC compared to gold standard ORC. Most of these studies were small in numbers and represented single center experiences. Recently, a good systematic literature review was conducted. The study focused on reports published within the last 5 years [40]. In summary, the review showed that robotic radical cystectomy consistently had less estimated blood loss, faster time to bowel activity, and reduced hospital stay; however, these improvements come with increased operative time and cost [40].

Retrospective comparative studies showed statistically significant reduction in operative **Estimated Blood Loss** (EBL) in RRC (<300 ml) [41, 42]. As a consequence, the rate of perioperative blood transfusion was lower [42–45]. Most studies indicated a longer **Operation Time** in RRC [40, 46, 47]. The average operation time was between 349–393 min in ORC compared to 415–455 min in RRC [47, 48].

Regarding post-operative morbidity and mortality, results were mixed. Some researchers reported favorable rates of low grade complications after RRC. However, these favorable trends did not translate to a decrease in major complications [46, 49, 50]. Others reported lower risk of mortality and minor and major complications after RRC [43, 44].

Patients who underwent RRC have quicker **bowel function recovery**, and shorter time to passing flatus [46, 51]. They used less **analgesics** [40, 52]. Finally, most studies reported a shorter **hospital stay** after RRC [43, 49].

Short term oncological outcomes of RRC were similar to ORC [41, 50]. Due to the short follow up in these studies, their focus was on pathologic stage, number of nodes harvested, and positive surgical margin rates [22, 52, 53]. Short term survival rates were also similar in both approaches. The Kaplan-Meier estimate for 2-year recurrence-free, disease-specific, and overall survival were 67 %, 75 %, and 68 % for robotic radical cystectomy, and 58 %, 63 % , and 63 % for open radical cystectomy [49]. In one small study, the long-term oncologic outcome of 14 RRC patients who were followed for more than 5 years was comparable to these for ORC (overall survival of 64 %, disease-specific survival of 75 %, and disease-free survival of 50 %) [48].

Health-related quality-of-life measures were not significantly different between ORC and RRC. Aboumohamed et al. used validated instruments (cancer body image scale (BIS) and the bladder cancer index (BCI)) to evaluate urinary, bowel, sexual function, and body image after RRC and ORC. Prospectively collected data from 182 patients from multiple institutions showed no difference between the two groups [51].

Prospective Randomized Control Trials

Up till now, only three randomized trials were performed to compare RRC and ORC. All of these trials agree on the benefits of RRC in lowering the EBL and in cost of longer operating time. None of the randomized trials showed statically significant benefits for RRC over ORC in reducing complications rate or improving the oncological outcomes.

The first trial was published in **2009 by Nix J** in University of North Carolina [45]. 41 patients were randomly assigned to one of the two techniques. The study showed that RRC was associated with lower EBL (258cc vc 575cc), significantly longer operation time (4.20 h vs 3.51 h), and less need for inpatient narcotic requirements. Other variables including complication rates were almost similar between the two procedural groups [45].

The second randomized surgical trial was published in 2012 by Parekh DJ et al, at The University of Texas Health Sciences Center at San Antonio. Again, this was a small trial of 40 patients. There was decreased estimated blood loss with RRC (400cc vs. 800) and decreased hospital stay with no significant differences in surrogates of oncologic efficacy [54].

The last and largest randomized trial was published in 2014 by Bochner et al. from Memorial Sloan Kettering

Cancer Center, New York. The study was a superiority trial of 118 patients. Although there was a trend for lower low grade complications after RRC, the authors concluded that the RRC is associated with lower mean intraoperative blood loss and significantly longer operative time. But it is similar in 90-d complication rates, hospital stay, pathologic outcomes, and 3- and 6-mo health-related quality-of-life outcomes between the two surgical techniques. Of note, the trial was designed to prove a 20 % improvement of post-operative morbidity after RRC. Thus the trial failed to identify a large advantage for RRC over ORC [54].

Finally a multi-institutional, randomized, non-inferiority NCI sponsored Trial (RAZOR) finished accrual of 350 patients in 2014. Fifteen institutions used standardized measures to evaluate cancer outcomes, surgical complications and HRQL of ORC vs. RRC with a primary endpoint of 2-year progression free survival. Full data from the RAZOR trial is not expected until 2016–2017 [55].

Costs

Few studies evaluated the financial burden of robotic surgeries. A recent systematic study compared the cost effectiveness of robotic surgeries (not only RRC) to open surgeries. The authors found that robotic surgeries' costs were consistently higher than open and laparoscopic surgery [56].

Smith and his colleagues looked specifically at the economics of RRC as part of the first randomized surgical trial in 2010. RRC was associated with an overall higher financial cost (+$1,640) than the ORC in the perioperative setting. (Robotic $16,248 vs open $14,608) [57]. A larger study that compared the cost of 1444 ORCs to 224 RRCs have also shown that the robotic approach is significantly more costly [58]. This increase of expenses in the robotic surgery itself were related to the high purchase and maintenance cost of the robotic platform[58], longer operating time, and the higher costs of robotic supplies [49, 59]. In a well done analysis, Martin et al. found that RRC was 16 % more expensive than ORC when only comparing direct operative costs[60].

The two main drivers of higher cost after radical cystectomy cited in the published data were hospital length of stay and operative durations [59, 60]. Although RRC was consistently associated with shorter length of stay, the cost deference was insufficient to offset the increased cost of robotic surgery [59]. Interestingly, there was a 38 % cost advantage found favoring RRC in the actual total patient costs in the Martin AD study [60].

It is possible that cost of robotic surgery will drop with the increased competition between manufacturers and wider dissemination of the technology [61]. When that happens, it is expected that the impact of indirect costs of post-operative complications and the longer hospital stay of ORC may deem RRC to be a more cost efficient treatment for invasive bladder cancer [43, 58].

The Future of RRC

The use of the robot in urologic surgery continues to increase. With the facilities that this technology provide for surgeons and the comparable outcomes between RRC and ORC that have shown by the available studies, RRC continues to be more popular and favorable. The improvement of surgeons' experience was quick and obvious with the decrease in operative time [61] and the performance of more complicated procedures, such as intra corporeal urinary diversion, robotically and successfully. The short learning curve of RRC compared with laparoscopic radical cystectomy as minimally invasive approaches helps new physicians and residents to perform radical cystectomy more efficiently [62]. All these factors and many others make the RRC a promising surgery either in regards to the quality of health care, or in surgeon's preference. And who knows – if RRC shows more significant clinical and statistical outcomes, it could become the gold standard approach in management of muscle invasive bladder cancer!

Comments

Because it includes many different surgical steps and techniques, radical cystectomy is a comparatively unique surgery in urology. The high morbidity and mortality rates make this procedure more challenging. Now, 12 years after the initial RRC was performed, urologists have formed a more inclusive understanding of the advantages and disadvantages of RRC. It is clear that the technical advantages, lower EBL, and faster recovery after RRC comes at the price of increased operative time and financial burden. However, it is promising that the perioperative and oncological outcomes of RRC were similar or better but not worse when compared with the gold standard ORC.

The results of a valuable multi-institutional, non-inferiority, randomized surgical trial (**RAZOR**) designed to compare RRC with ORC is expected in the near future. This trial is promising because of its statistical design and large cohort. It remains to be seen if it will support the RRC as an acceptable minimally invasive alternative to the classical ORC.

Urological Complications of Radical Hysterectomy and P.E

Injuries to the Bladder and Ureters

Ureteral injuries as well as bladder injuries may happen during any type of hysterectomy, particularly during the learning curve, and are estimated to occur with a frequency of 1.2% (range 0–6%) for ureteral injuries and 2 % (range 0.6–4%) for bladder injuries [63, 64]. Ureter injuries are in 70% of cases detected after surgery, often resulting in an unintended emergency laparotomy or second laparoscopy [65].

The ureters are always at risk during any type of radical pelvic surgery as they lie close to the rectum and the female reproductive organs. During laparoscopic hysterectomy, in particular, the distal ureters may be injured during ligation of the uterine arteries, or at the time of dissection and division of the cardinal ligaments below the uterine vessels [66]. However it is the cases with abnormal anatomy that pose the highest risk for ureteral injury. Special caution should be exercised in patients with severe prolapse where the pelvic anatomy is distorted and the ureter may lie just 0.5 cm lateral to the cervix. Cystoscopic evaluation with administration of i.v Indigo carmine dye may be helpful in these cases in order to confirm bilateral ureteral integrity.

Steps to be taken in order to avoid ureteral injury include (a) staying in the midline when incorporating the perivesical fascia as sutures placed too lateral may cause ureteral injury, (b) placing the clamps close to the uterus, (c) removing the uterus intact with surgical margins in close proximity to the uterus, thereby avoiding ureteral injury.

Ureteral injuries are much less likely to be recognized intraoperatively, and in some cases can be missed despite the use of intraoperative cystoscopy. The surgical treatment for ureteral injuries follows established operative principles, which include resecting devitalized injured ureteral tissue, establishing tensionless mucosal apposition over a stented ureter, isolating the anastomotic repair with omentum or fat, and placing of a drain in close proximity to the repair. The operative technique is dependent upon the location of the ureteral injury. Distal ureteral injuries, which are usually the case in R.E, can be managed with direct uretero-utereral anastomosis, ureteroneocystostomy with psoas hitch or Boari flap.

Lately, minimally invasive surgery using the robot is leading to a paradigm shift in the management of urinary tract injuries, which has been traditionally approached with open surgery. There are reported cases of robotic total hysterectomy and concomitant repair of incidental ureteral injury via ureteroureterostomy using standard end-to-end anastomosis technique and intracorporeal retrograde double J stent placement [67–69].

Bladder injuries may occur during attempt to enter the vesicouterine peritoneal space and are more frequent in women with history of cesarean section and scarring in this area. In transvaginal procedures, injuries to the bladder most commonly occur when perforating into the retropubic space. In general the risk of cystotomy can be reduced when one makes sure that the bladder is empty prior to perforation. Usually these cystotomies are at the base of the bladder and generally above the trigone. When repairing bladder injuries, care must be taken to close the cystotomy in two layers using absorbable sutures and test for watertightness using methylene blue dye instilled through the catheter. A bladder catheter is such cases should be kept for 7–10 days postoperatively [70].

In patients with a history of pelvic irradiation, an omental flap of labial fat pad interposition should be considered in order to prevent fistula formation [71]. If a bladder injury however is not detected intraoperatively, a trial of conservative management with an indwelling Foley catheter can be attempted. It is important to remember that early identification of bladder, or ureteral injury is crucial, considering that the best time for repair is at the time of injury when the tissues are in their best condition and all options for repair are still available.

Delayed Complications-Ureteral Stricture

Ureteral strictures are the usual long-term complications of iatrogenic injuries to the ureters. Upper urinary tract obstruction from a stricture may encounter months to years after hysterectomy. The treatment options include either an immediate percutaneous nephrostomy in case of a severely obstructed urinary tract or efforts to dilate the ureter and pass a retrograde stent over a guidewire in cases of mild dilatation and short stricture length [72, 73].

According to some, delayed recognition of a ureteral injury should be best managed by percutaneous drainage and definitive surgical repair should be postponed until after several months, depending again on the location and length of the strictured area. Percutaneous ureteral dilatation followed by antegrade stent placement has been reported with good success rates especially in strictures that are short in length [74].

Finally in challenging cases when other options are not available, a short segment of the ileum can be used for the creation of an ileal ureter. Ileal-ureter substitution is a valuable option in selected patient with complex ureteral defects that are not amenable to or have failed endourological approaches. Avoiding the complexity of tailored and tunnelled anastomoses may reduce the potential morbidity and re-intervention rate in patients with challenging surgical fields [75, 76].

References

1. Siegel RL, Miller KD, Jemal A. Cancer statistics, 2015. CA Cancer J Clin. 2015;65(1):5–29.
2. Babjuk M, Oosterlinck W, Sylvester R, Kaasinen E, Böhle A, Palou-Redorta J, et al. EAU guidelines on non-muscle-invasive urothelial carcinoma of the bladder, the 2011 update. Eur Urol. 2011;59(6):997–1008.
3. Witjes JA, Compérat E, Cowan NC, Santis M, Gakisi G, Lebret T, et al. EAU guidelines on muscle-invasive and metastatic bladder cancer: summary of the 2013 guidelines. Eur Urol. 2014;65(4):778–92.

4. Shabsigh A, Korets R, Vora KC, Brooks CM, Cronin AM, Savage C, et al. Defining early morbidity of radical cystectomy for patients with bladder cancer using a standardized reporting methodology. Eur Urol. 2009;55(1):164–74.
5. Parra RO, Andrus CH, Jones JP, Boullier JA. Laparoscopic cystectomy: initial report on a new treatment for the retained bladder. J Urol. 1992;148(4):1140–4.
6. Sánchez de Badajoz E, Reche Rosado A, Gutiérrez de la Cruz JM, Jiménez Garrido A. Radical cystectomy and laparoscopic ileal conduit. Arch Esp Urol. 1993;4(7):4.
7. Gill IS, Fergany A, Klein EA, Kaouk JH, Sung GT, Meraney AM, et al. Laparoscopic radical cystoprostatectomy with ileal conduit performed completely intracorporeally: the initial 2 cases. Urology. 2000;56(1):26–9.
8. Menon M, Hemal AK, Tewari A, Shrivastava A, Shoma AM, El-Tabey NA, et al. Nerve-sparing robot-assisted radical cystoprostatectomy and urinary diversion. BJU Int. 2003;92(3):232–6.
9. Beecken WD, Wolfram M, Engl T, Bentas W, Probst M, Blaheta R, et al. Robotic-assisted laparoscopic radical cystectomy and intra-abdominal formation of an orthotopic ileal neobladder. Eur Urol. 2003;44(3):337–9.
10. Leow JJ, Reese SW, Jiang W, Lipsitz SR, Bellmunt J, Trinh QD, et al. Propensity-matched comparison of morbidity and costs of open and robot-assisted radical cystectomies: a contemporary population-based analysis in the United States. Eur Urol. 2014;66(3):569–76.
11. Tang K, Li H, Xia D, Hu Z, Zhuang Q, Liu J, et al. Laparoscopic versus open radical cystectomy in bladder cancer: a systematic review and meta-analysis of comparative studies. PLoS One. 2014;9(5):e95667.
12. Kim HS, Suh DH, Kim MK, Chung HH, Park NH, Song YS. Systematic lymphadenectomy for survival in patients with endometrial cancer: a meta-analysis. Jpn J Clin Oncol. 2012;42(5):405–12.
13. Briganti A, Blute ML, Eastham JH, et al. Pelvic lymph node dissection in prostate cancer. Eur Urol. 2009;55(6):1251–65.
14. Abaza R, Dangle PP, Gong MC, Bahnson RR, Pohar KS. Quality of lymphadenectomy is equivalent with robotic and open cystectomy using an extended template. J Urol. 2012;187(4):1200–4.
15. Herr HW, Bochner BH, Dalbagni G, Donat SM, Reuter VE, Bajorin DF. Impact of the number of lymph nodes retrieved on outcome in patients with muscle invasive bladder cancer. J Urol. 2002;167(3):1295–8.
16. Leissner J, Ghoneim MA, Abol-Enein H, Thüroff JW, Franzaring L, Fisch M, et al. Extended radical lymphadenectomy in patients with urothelial bladder cancer: results of a prospective multicenter study. J Urol. 2004;171(1):139–44.
17. Stein JP. The role of lymphadenectomy in patients undergoing radical cystectomy for bladder cancer. Curr Oncol Rep. 2007;9(3):213–21.
18. Cole AP, Dalela D, Hanske J, Mullane SA, Choueiri TK, Meyer CP, et al. Temporal trends in receipt of adequate lymphadenectomy in bladder cancer 1988 to 2010. Urol Oncol. 2015;33(12):504 e9–504 e17.
19. Pontes JE. Lymphadenectomy technique. In: Novick AC, Streem SB, Pontes JE, editors. Operative urology, vol. 2. Baltimore: Williams & Wilkins; 1989. p. 451.
20. Abol-Enein H, El-Baz M, Abd El-Hameed MA, Abdel-Latif M, Ghoneim MA. Lymph node involvement in patients with bladder cancer treated with radical cystectomy: a patho-anatomical study-a single center experience. J Urol. 2004;172(5 Pt 1):1818–21.
21. Axel Heidenreich DP. Anatomic extent of pelvic lymphadenectomy in bladder cancer. Eur Urol Suppl. 2010;9(3):419–23.
22. Wang L, Mudaliar K, Mehta V, Barkan GA, Quek ML, Flanigan RC, et al. Seeking a standard for adequate pathologic lymph node staging in primary bladder carcinoma. Virchows Arch. 2014;464(5):595–602.
23. Dhar NB, Klein EA, Reuther AM, Thalmann GN, Madersbacher S, Studer UE. Outcome after radical cystectomy with limited or extended pelvic lymph node dissection. J Urol. 2008;179(3):873–8.
24. Hashad MM, Atta M, Elabbady A, Elfiky S, Khattab A, Kotb A. Safety of no bowel preparation before ileal urinary diversion. BJU Int. 2012;110(11 Pt C):E1109–13.
25. Shafii M, Murphy DM, Donovan MG, Hickey DPI. Mechanical bowel preparation necessary in patients undergoing cystectomy and urinary diversion? BJU Int. 2002;89(9):879–81.
26. Maffezzini M, Campodonico F, Canepa G, Gerbi G, Parodi D. Current perioperative management of radical cystectomy with intestinal urinary reconstruction for muscle-invasive bladder cancer and reduction of the incidence of postoperative ileus. Surg Oncol. 2008;17(1):41–8.
27. Alberts BD, Woldu SL, Weinberg AC, Danzig MR, Korets R, Badani KK. Venous thromboembolism after major urologic oncology surgery: a focus on the incidence and timing of thromboembolic events after 27,455 operations. Urology. 2014;84(4):799–806.
28. Pridgeon S, Allchorne P, Turner B, Peters J, Green J. Venous thromboembolism (VTE) prophylaxis and urological pelvic cancer surgery: a UK national audit. BJU Int. 2015;115(2):223–9.
29. Chopra S, Metcalfe C, Castro Abreu AL, Azhar RA, Satkunasivam R, Desai M, et al. Port placement and docking for robotic surgery: the University of Southern California approach. J Endourol. 2015;29(8):868–72.
30. Collins JW, Hosseini A, Sooriakumaran P, Nyberg T, Sanchez-Salas R, Adding C, et al. Tips and tricks for intracorporeal robot-assisted urinary diversion. Curr Urol Rep. 2014;15(11):457.
31. Savera AT, Kaul S, Badani K, Stark AT, Shah NL, Menon M. Robotic radical prostatectomy with the "Veil of Aphrodite" technique: histologic evidence of enhanced nerve sparing. Eur Urol. 2006;49(6):1065–73. discussion 1073–4
32. Tewari A, Peabody JO, Fischer M, Sarle R, Vallancien G, Delmas V, et al. An operative and anatomic study to help in nerve sparing during laparoscopic and robotic radical prostatectomy. Eur Urol. 2003;43(5):444–54.
33. Ahlering TE, Eichel L, Skarecky D. Evaluation of long-term thermal injury using cautery during nerve sparing robotic prostatectomy. Urology. 2008;72(6):1371–4.
34. Goh AC, Gill IS, Lee DJ, Castro Abreu AL, Fairey AS, Leslie S, et al. Robotic intracorporeal orthotopic ileal neobladder: replicating open surgical principles. Eur Urol. 2012;62(5):891–901.
35. Fahmy O, Asri K, Schwentner C, Stenzl A, Gakis G. Current status of robotic assisted radical cystectomy with intracorporeal ileal neobladder for bladder cancer. J Surg Oncol. 2015;112(4):427–9.
36. Desai MM, Abreu AL, Goh AC, Fairey A, Berger A, Leslie S, et al. Robotic intracorporeal urinary diversion: technical details to improve time efficiency. J Endourol. 2014;28(11):1320–7.
37. Shah HN, Nayyar R, Rajamahanty S, Hemal AK. Prospective evaluation of unidirectional barbed suture for various indications in surgeon-controlled robotic reconstructive urologic surgery: Wake Forest University experience. Int Urol Nephrol. 2012;44(3):775–85.
38. Pham KN, Sack BS, O'Connor RC, Guralnick ML, Langenstroer P, See WA, Jacobsohn K. V-Loc urethro-intestinal anastomosis during robotic cystectomy with orthotopic urinary diversion. Can Urol Assoc J. 2013;7(11-12):E663–6.
39. Abreu AL, Chopra S, Azhar RA, Berger AK, Miranda G, Cai J, et al. Robotic radical cystectomy and intracorporeal urinary diversion: The USC technique. Indian J Urol. 2014;30(3):300–6.
40. Luchey AM, Agarwal G, Poch MA. Robotic-assisted radical cystectomy. Cancer Control. 2015;22(3):301–6.
41. Smith AB, Raynor M, Amling CL, Busby JE, Castle E, Davis R, et al. Multi-institutional analysis of robotic radical cystectomy for

bladder cancer: perioperative outcomes and complications in 227 patients. J Laparoendosc Adv Surg Tech A. 2012;22(1):17–21.
42. Pruthi RS, Nielsen ME, Nix J, Smith A, Schultz H, Wallen EM. Robotic radical cystectomy for bladder cancer: surgical and pathological outcomes in 100 consecutive cases. J Urol. 2010;183(2):510–4.
43. Ng CK, Kauffman EC, Lee MM, Otto BJ, Portnoff A, Ehrlich JR, et al. A comparison of postoperative complications in open versus robotic cystectomy. Eur Urol. 2010;57(2):274–81.
44. Yu HY, Hevelone ND, Lipsitz SR, Kowalczyk KJ, Nguyen PL, Choueiri TK, et al. Comparative analysis of outcomes and costs following open radical cystectomy versus robot-assisted laparoscopic radical cystectomy: results from the US Nationwide Inpatient Sample. Eur Urol. 2012;61(6):1239–44.
45. Nix J, Smith A, Kurpad R, Nielsen ME, Wallen EM, Pruthi RS. Prospective randomized controlled trial of robotic versus open radical cystectomy for bladder cancer: perioperative and pathologic results. Eur Urol. 2010;57(2):196–201.
46. Guru KA, Wilding GE, Piacente P, Thompson J, Deng W, Kim HL, et al. Robot-assisted radical cystectomy versus open radical cystectomy: assessment of postoperative pain. Can J Urol. 2007;14(6):3753–6.
47. Styn NR, Montgomery JS, Wood DP, Hafez KS, Lee CT, Tallman C, et al. Matched comparison of robotic-assisted and open radical cystectomy. Urology. 2012;79(6):1303–8.
48. Khan MS, Elhage O, Challacombe B, Murphy D, Coker B, Rimington P, et al. Long-term outcomes of robot-assisted radical cystectomy for bladder cancer. Eur Urol. 2013;64(2):219–24.
49. Wang GJ, Barocas DA, Raman JD, Scherr DS. Robotic vs open radical cystectomy: prospective comparison of perioperative outcomes and pathological measures of early oncological efficacy. BJU Int. 2008;101(1):89–93.
50. Niegisch G, Albers P, Rabenalt R. Perioperative complications and oncological safety of robot-assisted (RARC) vs. open radical cystectomy (ORC). Urol Oncol. 2014;32(7):966–74.
51. Aboumohamed AA, Raza SJ, Al-Daghmin A, Tallman C, Creighton T, Crossley H, et al. Health-related quality of life outcomes after robot-assisted and open radical cystectomy using a validated bladder-specific instrument: a multi-institutional study. Urology. 2014;83(6):1300–8.
52. Xia L, Wang X, Xu T, Zhang X, Zhu Z, Qin L, et al. Robotic versus open radical cystectomy: an updated systematic review and meta-analysis. PLoS One. 2015;10(3):e0121032.
53. Kader AK, Richards KA, Krane LS, Pettus JA, Smith JJ, Hemal AK. Robot-assisted laparoscopic vs open radical cystectomy: comparison of complications and perioperative oncological outcomes in 200 patients. BJU Int. 2013;112(4):E290–4.
54. Messer JC, Punnen S, Fitzgerald J, Svatek R, Parekh DJ. Health-related quality of life from a prospective randomised clinical trial of robot-assisted laparoscopic vs open radical cystectomy. BJU Int. 2014;114(6):896–902.
55. Smith ND, Castle EP, Gonzalgo ML, Svatek RS, Weizer AZ, Montgomery JS, et al. The RAZOR (randomized open vs robotic cystectomy) trial: study design and trial update. BJU Int. 2015;115(2):198–205.
56. Tandogdu Z, Vale L, Fraser C, Ramsay CA. Systematic review of economic evaluations of the use of robotic assisted laparoscopy in surgery compared with open or laparoscopic surgery. Appl Health Econ Health Policy. 2015;13(5):457–67.
57. Smith A, Kurpad R, Lal A, Nielsen M, Wallen EM, Pruthi RS. Cost analysis of robotic versus open radical cystectomy for bladder cancer. J Urol. 2010;183(2):505–9.
58. Mmeje CO, Martin AD, Nunez-Nateras R, Parker AS, Thiel DD, Castle EP. Cost analysis of open radical cystectomy versus robot-assisted radical cystectomy. Curr Urol Rep. 2013;14(1):26–31.
59. Lee R, Ng CK, Shariat SF, Borkina A, Guimento R, Brumit KF, et al. The economics of robotic cystectomy: cost comparison of open versus robotic cystectomy. BJU Int. 2011;108(11):1886–92.
60. Martin AD, Nunez RN, Castle EP. Robot-assisted radical cystectomy versus open radical cystectomy: a complete cost analysis. Urology. 2011;77(3):621–5.
61. Hayn MH, Hellenthal NJ, Seixas-Mikelus SA, Mansour AM, Stegemann A, Hussain A, et al. Is patient outcome compromised during the initial experience with robot-assisted radical cystectomy? Results of 164 consecutive cases. BJU Int. 2011;108(6):882–7.
62. Ahmed K, Ibrahim A, Wang TT, Khan N, Challacombe B, Khan MS, et al. Assessing the cost effectiveness of robotics in urological surgery – a systematic review. BJU Int. 2012;110(10):1544–56.
63. Johnson N, Barlow D, Lethaby A, Tavender E, Curr L, Garry R. Methods of hysterectomy: systematic review and meta-analysis of randomised controlled trials. BMJ. 2005;330(7506):1478.
64. Harkki-Siren P, Sjoberg J, Kurki T. Major complications of laparoscopy: a follow-up Finnish study. Obstet Gynecol. 1999;94:94–8.
65. Janssen PF, Brölmann HA, Huirne JA. Recommendations to prevent urinary tract injuries during laparoscopic hysterectomy: a systematic Delphi procedure among experts. J Minim Invasive Gynecol. 2011;18(3):314–21.
66. Tamussino K, Lang P, Breinl E. Ureteral complications with operative gynecologic laparoscopy. Am J Obstet Gynecol. 1998;178:967–71.
67. Menderes G, Clark LE, Azodi M. Incidental ureteral injury and repair during robotic-assisted total laparoscopic hysterectomy. J Minim Invasive Gynecol. 2015;22(3):320.
68. Magrina JF, Kho R, Magtibay PM. Robotic radical hysterectomy: technical aspects. Gynecol Oncol. 2009;113(1):28–31.
69. Lim PCW. Robotic assisted total pelvic exenteration: a case report. Gynecol Oncol. 2009;115(2):310–1.
70. Gomez RG, Ceballos L, Coburn M, et al. Consensus statement on bladder injuries. BJU Int. 2004;94:27–32.
71. Kniery KR, Johnson EK, Steele SR. Operative considerations for rectovaginal fistulas. World J Gastrointest Surg. 2015;7(8):133–7.
72. Koukouras D, Petsas T, Liatsikos E, Kallidonis P, Sdralis EK, Adonakis G, et al. Percutaneous minimally invasive management of iatrogenic ureteral injuries. J Endourol. 2010;24(12):1921–7.
73. Zhang Z, Zhang C, Wu C, Yang B, Wang H, Hou J, et al. Progressive ureteral dilations and retrograde placement of single-j stent guided by flexible cystoscope for management of ureteroenteral anastomotic stricture in patients after radical cystectomy and bricker urinary diversion. J Endourol. 2015;29(1):90–4.
74. Uflacker A, Sheeran D, Khaja M, Patrie J, Elias G, Saad W. Outcomes of percutaneous management of anastomotic ureteral strictures in renal transplantation: chronic nephroureteral stent placement with and without Balloon dilatation. Cardiovasc Intervent Radiol. 2015;38(3):693–701.
75. Xu YM, Feng C, Kato H, Xie H, Zhang XR. Long-term outcome of ileal ureteric replacement with an iliopsoas muscle tunnel antirefluxing technique for the treatment of long-segment ureteric strictures. Urology. 2016;88:201–6. pii: S0090-4295(15)01052-3
76. Gomez-Gomez E, Malde S, Spilotros M, Shah PJ, J Greenwell T, Ockrim JL. A tertiary experience of ileal-ureter substitution: contemporary indications and outcomes. Scand J Urol. 2016;50(3):192–9.

Robotic-Assisted Radical Hysterectomy with Anterior and Posterior Exenteration: Surgical Perspective

73

Sanghoon Lee, Seok Ho Kang, Seon Hahn Kim, and Jae Yun Song

Introduction

Cervical cancer is the fourth most common cancer in women, with an estimated 528,000 new cases/yr. worldwide. In 2012, it was also the fourth most common cause of cancer deaths in women worldwide. More than 70 % of all cervical cancers occur in underdeveloped areas [1]. Human papillomavirus (HPV) infection is regarded as the major cause of cervical intraepithelial neoplasia (CIN) and cervical cancer. Genital HPV infection is common in sexually active young women and persistent infection with carcinogenic HPV causes almost all cervical cancers. A minority of women with precancerous lesions develop invasive cancer [2–4]. The establishment of causal links between HPV and cervical cancer has helped to guide age-appropriate interventions for preventing cervical cancer [5].

The rates of incidence and death of cervical cancer have decreased gradually over the last decade due to early detection and treatment in most developed countries [6]. In the past, open radical hysterectomy (RH) through a midline incision, was the standard operative management for early stage cervical cancer. However, minimally invasive surgery for RH has recently become widespread as the result of advances in laparoscopic instrumentation and surgical techniques [7–10]. Many studies have demonstrated the safety, feasibility, and benefits of laparoscopic RH. The advantages of laparoscopic surgery include decreased blood loss, shorter recovery time, shorter hospital stay, earlier return of bowel and bladder function, and higher quality of life [9, 11, 12]. An increasing number of studies comparing the feasibility and advantages of robot-assisted surgery for early stage cervical cancer with conventional laparoscopy or laparotomy have appeared during recent years [13–16].

Here, we reviewed published articles to assess the current role of robotic surgery including RH and pelvic exenteration in women with cervical cancer.

Robotic Radical Hysterectomy

RH is one of the most complex surgeries in gynecologic oncology and is the standard surgical treatment for early stage cervical cancer. More than a century ago, the first abdominal RH was reported by Wertheim. The technique was then modified by Meigs in the 1950s [44]. Later, vaginal RH was described by Schauta in 1901. Laparoscopic RH with pelvic and paraaortic lymphadenectomy was introduced by Canis et al. in 1989. In the early 1990s, and over the last two decades, numerous studies have indicated that total laparoscopic RH is feasible.

Traditionally, RH has been associated with higher complication rates due to the numerous dissections required for the bladder, ureter, parametrium, and rectum. In the past two decades, gynecologic oncologic surgeons have utilized minimally invasive techniques to decrease morbidity while maintaining surgical and oncological outcomes. Many studies have demonstrated the safety and feasibility of laparoscopic RH as the treatment for early-stage cervical cancer. Although the laparoscopic approach provides long-term outcomes comparable to those of open radical hysterectomy, this approach was not widely adopted in surgical practice, due to disadvantages such as: long learning curve, two dimensional view, poor ergonomic position for surgeons, and limited movements of instruments. These conditions negatively influenced the surgical performance, resulting in tremor, fatigue, and less accuracy [37]. Laparoscopic RH also poses difficulties in ureteral and parametrial dissection similar to conventional laparoscopy [17]. Dissection is technically easier with robotic approaches [18]. The concept of robotic assisted surgery started in 1994 [45]. Initially developed for

S. Lee, MD, PhD (✉) • S.H. Kang, MD, PhD
S.H. Kim, MD, PhD • J.Y. Song, MD, PhD
Department of Obstetrics and Gynecology, Korea University College of Medicine, 73 Inchon-ro, Seongbuk-gu Seoul 02841, South Korea
e-mail: mdleesh@gmail.com; drkimsh@korea.ac.kr; sjyuni105@gmail.com

I. Alkatout, L. Mettler (eds.), *Hysterectomy*, DOI 10.1007/978-3-319-22497-8_73

battlefield medicine, robot-assisted surgery was approved by the U.S. Food and Drug Administration in 1999 for urologic and cardiac procedures [43]. Robotic surgery has several advantages over laparoscopy: three dimensional vision, wristed instrumentation, less tremor, and ergonomic positioning for the surgeon while performing the surgical procedures [19]. Such benefits enhance dexterity and decrease skill-based error. Since 2005, the role of robots in gynecological surgery has increased, with robot assistance being used in many traditional procedures, including hysterectomy, prolapse surgery, myomectomy, tubal surgery, endometriotic and adnexal surgery, pelvic and paraaortic lymph node dissection, and sacrocolpopexy [26]. In procedures such as RH, that are technically challenging by laparoscopy [37, 38], the enhanced visualization provided by the robotic technique gives surgeons improved ability to identify tissue planes, blood vessels, and nerves during surgery [20]. Therefore, robotic surgery is reported to be associated with decreased blood loss in comparative studies.

The female pelvis is a confined space for surgeons to perform procedures. Standard laparoscopic instruments have more limited degrees of freedom than human hands, and they may hamper surgeons' procedures. Standard laparoscopic instruments have limited degree of positioning for the surgeon during intracorporeal knot tying. On the other hand, wristed robotic instrumentation, like human hands, provides greater dexterity with seven degrees of movement. Three degrees are provided by the robotic arms attached to the abdominal wall trocars (insertion, pitch, yaw) and 4 ° result from the "wristed" instruments (pitch, yaw, roll and grip). The degrees provided by the robotic arms attached to the abdominal wall trocars around the robotic instruments coordinate system origin and the center of mass. Pitch is the rotation around the lateral or transverse axis; yaw is the rotation around the vertical axis; and roll is the rotation around the longitudinal axis. The resultant improved dexterity allows finer, more delicate and tremor-free manipulation, dissection, removal, or resection of tissue. In addition, fatigue and physical discomfort can limit any surgical procedure. During laparoscopy, surgeons have to pose uncomfortably to successfully complete the surgical procedure because they need to reach over the patient. With robotic surgery, surgeons may sit comfortably at the surgical console from the vantage point of standing at the patient's head, and manipulate the hand controls and foot pedals in an ergonomic position. This may reduce fatigue and discomfort during complex surgical procedures.

The major disadvantages of robotic surgery include the cost, large volume of robots and consoles, limited availability within some health systems, and the need to train the residents, attending surgeons, and operating room personnel in the use of such technology. Another limitation of robotic surgery is the lack of haptic or tactile feedback. This has been noted to be a limitation for novice robotic surgeons, but they most quickly adapt and obtain heightened visual feedback from the magnified, three-dimensional vision system. If there are particular structures that surgeons desire to palpate, such as the cervicovaginal colpotomy ring during hysterectomy or sacral promontory during sacrocolpopexy, they can do so by laparoscopy before docking robots, or by asking the bedside assistant to palpate and confirm the location.

The first robotic assisted RH for cervical cancer was reported by Sert and Abeler in 2006 [21]. Since then, there have been several case series focusing on cervical cancer management. Kim et al. examined 10 patients with cervical cancer, and Fanning et al. included 20 patients in their analysis. These patients underwent robotic laparoscopic RH with only a few intraoperative complications; one patient had a cystectomy, which was repaired. They also had only a few postoperative issues; one patient had an uterovaginal fistula and one patient developed pneumonia, with operating time 355–390 min, and mean blood loss 207 and 300 ml, respectively. Recent systematic reviews and meta-analyses suggest that robotic RH may be superior to abdominal RH with less estimated blood loss, shorter hospital stays, less febrile morbidities, and wound-related complications. The percentage of robotic-assisted hysterectomies is increasing; while 0.5 % of total hysterectomies were performed robotically in 2007, 9.5 % utilized robotic techniques in 2010 [42].

Robotic RH and laparoscopic RH appear to have equivalent intraoperative and short-term postoperative outcomes [22]. Longer operative time and learning curve are among the reasons why the robotic technique has not yet been adopted worldwide in gynecologic oncology practice. In robotic surgery, total operation time consists of docking and console time. Docking time is the time needed to assemble instruments, attach patient to the robot, advance column to the operating table, fasten the robotic arms to the inserted trocars, and introduce the laparoscope. Console time is defined as the surgical time needed to perform the entire operation at the console. Operative time is defined by the anesthesiologists as the time between the insertion of the Foley catheter and the closing of the last trocar site. Sert and Eraker described 25 patients with early stage cervical cancer who had undergone robot-assisted RH and pelvic lymph node dissection, showing a total mean time of 219 min, with a mean console time of 170 min. Estape et al. compared 32 RH by robotic approach with 17 by laparoscopy and 14 by open surgery; the mean console time in the robotic, laparoscopic, and laparotomy groups was 2.4 h, 2.2 h, and 1.9 h, respectively [16]. Magrina et al. compared 27 patients who underwent robotic or modified RH with patients who underwent RH via laparoscopic and laparotomic approach. They found similar operative time from skin incision to skin closure between robotic (189.6 min) and laparotomic RH, but it was significantly shorter than the time required for the laparoscopic approach [20]. From a multi-institutional experience, Lowe and Chamberlain et al. found the median operative time of robotic-assisted RH to be 215 min. From a prospective study of seven patients who underwent robot-assisted RH, Lowe and Hoekstra et al. found no statistically significant difference in operative times; 260 min in robot-assisted RH and 264 min in traditional RH [45]. Overall, surgical experience and personal learning curve may influence the operative time. Several studies demonstrated that the robotic docking time decreases significantly as surgeons and assistants gain experience, with the reported mean docking time being 10 min at the beginning and 2–3 min at the end of the learning curve [20, 38].

There is a general agreement on the significant decrease in intraoperative bleeding in minimally invasive surgery. An article reported similar levels of blood loss between robotic with laparoscopic RH; which were, importantly, different from those of open surgery. In patients who underwent robotic or laparoscopic RH, the overall rate of blood transfusion was very low. Sert and Abeler compared 35 patients who underwent hysterectomy via robotic radical (RRH), laparoscopic (TLRH) and laparotomic (ORH) approaches. The mean estimated blood loss was significantly reduced in the group of patients who received robot-assisted surgeries compared with those who received laparoscopic and laparotomy surgeries [41]. Blood transfusion rates for symptomatic postoperative anemia after robotic RH vary from 5 to 35 % [16, 39]. Magrina et al. reported that in the robotic group, one patient with an operative blood loss of 180 ml had an unexplained drop of Hb to 6.6 g on her first postoperative day. The patient was transfused and discharged the following day. In the laparotomy group, all three patients were transfused postoperatively, while one of them had preoperative anemia (Hgb 9.0 g/ml) secondary to postmenopausal bleeding [20]. Gortchev et al. compared 294 T1b1 cervical cancer patients; robot assisted RH was performed in 73 patients, laparoscopic-assisted vaginal RH in 46 patients, and abdominal RH in 175 patients. No significant differences between the three operative methods were found in the values of the postoperative hematocrit ($p = 0.153$), and between the pre- and postoperative hematocrit ($p = 0.253$). In a systematic literature review and meta-analysis by Geetha et al., 21 studies (1339 patients) of laparoscopic RH, 14 open RH (1552 patients) and 12 robotic RH (327 patients) were compared. Mean blood loss was significantly higher in open RH than in both laparoscopic and robotic RH (ANOVA $F(2.44) = 21.6$; $P<0.001$). The difference in blood loss between laparoscopic and robotic RH was not statically significant. Both laparoscopic and robotic RH had a significantly lower proportion of patients with blood transfusion compared with the open method (ANOVA $F(2.24) = 20.5$; $P<0.001$). Although the robotic RH appears to require less blood transfusion, the difference in transfusion percentage between laparoscopic and robotic RH was not statistically significant [46]. Moreover, Estape at al. compared 32 cases of RH by robotic approach with 17 by laparoscopy and 14 by open surgery. The results showed that the incidence of blood transfusion was highest (35.7 %) in the cases of laparotomy, with one patient given a blood transfusion pre-operatively due to anemia [16].

Lower rates of intraoperative complications occur in minimally invasive surgery compared with the open approach, due to more accurate tissue manipulation and better anatomic visualization [37]. The complication rates in radical robotic surgery vary in a wide range-from 7.8 to 59 %. Different criteria for defining minor complications and different periods of follow-up are the main reasons for the variations observed. Definitions of early and late postoperative complications also vary. Magrina et al. define early complications as those that occur in the first 6 weeks after the operation, while Maggioni et al. define them as those that occur in the first month after the operation [38]. Urinary injury, which may happen during ureterolysis and bladder isolation steps, is frequently reported in RH. Sert and Eraker described three cases of bladder perforation among 25 cases of robotic RH, which were successfully repaired robotically. A recent review comparing robotic versus total laparoscopic RH for early stage cervical cancer found similar overall rates (~6 %) of major intraoperative complications, with lower rates of vascular and bladder injury during robotic RH [37]. Estape et al. reported one cystotomy in the robotic group in a patient with three cesarean sections, and two cystotomies in the laparoscopic group. Another recent review article described a significant difference in the number of major postoperative complications between RRH (9.6 %) and TLRH (5.5 %). The RRH group included 11 cases of vaginal dehiscence, 10 cases of vaginal cuff abscess, and 5 cases of port site hernia [39]. On the contrary, no significant differences in the frequency of the complications were established in publications that compared the robotic with the open and/or laparoscopic surgery [16, 41].

An increased relative risk of vaginal cuff complication has been observed for minimally invasive hysterectomy techniques when compared with vaginal or abdominal ones. The study that observed this risk is controversial, due to the lack of a standardized method of classification and registration of postoperative injuries. A recent review showed a higher rate of vaginal dehiscence in the RRH group than in the laparoscopic group, which may be associated with the extensive use of monopolar and bipolar electrosurgery, which may increase thermal damage and devascularization of the cuff site. Other studies disagree with the above review and describe a similar incidence of vaginal cuff separation in laparoscopic and robotic hysterectomies [39]. Other organs are also under the risk of thermal injury. Thermal injury to bowel may be more difficult to diagnose intraoperatively [47]. Person et al. reported the leaking of lymphatic fluid through the vagina and/or vaginal cuff dehiscence in 10 out of 80 women (12 %) who underwent robotic RH with pelvic lymphadenectomy. The frequency of this complication was significantly different between three surgeons who performed robotic RH [37].

Magrina et al. reported that intraoperative injuries were noted in the laparoscopy group and laparotomy group only. One patient from the laparoscopy group had rectotomy during the resection of an invasive endometriotic lesion of the anterior rectal wall, and was included as complication, but was the only readmission. Another patient had an umbilical trocar site infection. In the laparotomy group, one patient developed pneumonia, one had sterile wound seroma, and one had ileus. Minor early complications (<6 weeks) in the robotic group consisted of one case of urinary retention and two of urinary tract infection. In the laparoscopic group, one patient had a corneal abrasion, one experienced urinary retention and one had passage of lymphatic fluid through the vagina on the fifth postoperative day through an intact vaginal cuff. In the laparotomy group, one patient had urinary retention, and two had vomiting [20]. Sert and Abeler et al. reported that three robot-assisted RH patients and one laparoscopic patient had accidental cystotomy, which was repaired peri-operatively. No readmission was required, and no bowel or ureter injuries happened [41].

Geetha et al. reported the mean percentage of patients with infectious morbidity for the three types of RH studies. Post-operative infectious morbidity was significantly higher among patients who underwent open RH compared with those who underwent RH via other methods (ANOVA F (2.36) = 6.24; P = 0.005). The difference in infectious morbidity between laparoscopy and robotic RH was well within the range for chance fluctuations. The mean percentage of patients with non-infectious morbidity for the three types of RH was similar (ANOVA F (2.37) = 1.80; P = 0.179). No cases of bowel injury were reported among patients who underwent robotic RH. The mean number of patients with ureteric injury after all three types of RH was similar (ANOFA F (2.39) = 1.21; P = 0.309). Ureteric injury was reported in 7/13 (53.9 %), 6/19 (31.6 %) and 2/10 (20 %) of ARH, LRH, and RRH studies, respectively [46].

Shorter hospital stay is one of the most important advantages of minimally invasive surgery. The length of hospital stay reflects the difference in the postoperative outcomes of the patients with different operative procedures. Factors that determine the hospital stay are: the ability of the patient to ambulate independently, recovery of the functions of the gastrointestinal tract and the ability to use oral drugs. Recovery of urinary bladder function (residual urine <50 ml) is not a determinant. All comparative studies of robotic RH reported a mean length of hospital stay of 1–2 days, which was similar in the laparoscopic RH group, but significantly shorter than in the open RH group [16, 37–40, 42]. Table 73.1 summarizes reports on robot assisted laparoscopic radical hysterectomy for early stage cervical cancer.

Increased maneuverability of the instruments with a robotic platform is most likely the reason for increased lymph node yield in the robotic group when compared with both laparoscopic and laparotomy groups [41]. Oncological outcomes after RH for early stage cervical cancer are determined by the number of lymph nodes retrieved and the recurrence rate. Results concerning the number of lymph nodes retrieved by the different surgical approaches are controversial. Several comparative studies found no significant differences in the number of lymph nodes retrieved between robotic, laparoscopic, and open techniques. A case control study which compared robotic to open type III RH found a better node retrieval outcome in the robotic approach. On the contrary, Maggioni et al. showed a reduced number of lymph nodes in the RRH group compared with the ORH group [37]. More recently, Estape et al. reported a case-matched comparative analysis between laparoscopic, robotic, and abdominal RH with lymphadenectomy, and reported a significantly higher number of nodes retrieved in the robotic approach and equivalent rates of positive surgical margins [37]. The increased lymph node yield may be explained by the agility of the robotic instruments that allows more comprehensive and accurate node dissection. The number of lymph nodes obtained may increase further following a learning curve [42].

Data about the follow-up period and recurrence rates in patients with cervical cancer who underwent robotic RH have been reported in a few articles [48, 51, 47, 49] Estape et al. reported that mean patient follow up was shortest for the robotic group (242.2 days) followed by the laparoscopic (941.6 days) and laparotomy groups (1382 days) [16]. Gortchev et al. reported that the mean follow-up period was significantly shorter in the robotic group (316 days), followed by the laparotomy (808 days) and laparoscopy groups (1531 days) [38]. All patients were followed according to the routine study protocol, including clinical examination, vaginal ultrasound, smear from the vaginal cuff, routine blood tests, and chest x-ray. The follow up examination was performed every 3 months during the first 3 years, every 6 months until 5 years and once a year thereafter. In some cases, MR scans of the pelvis, additional PET-CTs or CT scans were required [41].

Although robotic assisted-technology is theoretically an enhancement of conventional laparoscopy, several studies have reported the conversion of the robotic approach to laparotomy, not laparoscopy. There were six cases of conversion from robot-assisted laparoscopy to laparotomy in two studies due to: dense adhesions (n = 1), tumor erosion into the rectosigmoid colon (n = 2), non-life threatening bleeding from the vena cava (n = 2), and uterine myomas and obliterated cul-de-sac to avoid morcellation (n = 1). Some physicians are comfortable using the robot, while those who are not, continue the procedure using the traditional laparoscopic technique. This is of concern because the advantages of laparoscopy and robotic technology are comparable, whereas laparotomy leads to greater complications, such as more blood loss and longer hospital stay. Robotic assisted laparoscopy and traditional laparoscopy have differences.

Table 73.1 Summary of reports on RALPH for early stage cervical cancer

Study	Parameters	Patients (n)	OP time (min)	EBL (ml)	Transfusion rate (%)	LOS (days)	Complications (%)
Sert and Abeler [21]	Robot	7	241	71	0	4	57.1
	Lap	7	300	160	0	8	85.7
Magrina et al. [20]	Robot	27	190	131	3.7	1.7	7.4
	Lap	31	220	208	0	2.4	9.7
	Open	35	267	444	8.6	3.6	14.3
Ricardo et al. [16]	Robot	32	200	130	1	2.6	6
	Lap	17	180	209	0	2.3	4
	Open	14	120	621	5	4	4
Grigor et al. [38]	Robot	73	152	NM	NM	4	3
	Lap	46	232	NM	NM	4	1
	Open	175	168	NM	NM	9	9
Lambaudie et al. [52]	Robot	20	190	100	0	3	4
	Lap	12	210	400	0	7	2
Sert and Abeler [41]	Robot	35	263	82	2.8	3.8	20
	Lap	7	364	160	0	8.4	85.7
	Open	26	163	595	7	9.2	46.1
Estape et al. [39]	Robot	32	144	130	3.1	2.6	18.8
	Lap	17	132	209	0	2.3	23.5
	Open	14	114	621	35.7	4.0	28.6

Abbreviations: *RALRH* robot-assisted laparoscopic radical hysterectomy, *Lap* laparoscopy, *Op time* operation time, *EBL* estimated blood loss, *LOS* length of hospital stay, *NM* not mentioned

Because of the bulkiness and limitations unique to the robot, certain procedures, such as achieving hemostasis of uncontrolled bleeding and performing dissection and resection of bulky tissue (e.g., bowel resection and large tumors), are easier with traditional laparoscopy than with the robot. The robotic surgical approach may have negative effects on the training of surgical fellows, because some institutions rarely choose the traditional laparoscopic approach and, instead, choose the robotic approach when considering minimally invasive surgery. Future surgeons should be trained in both laparoscopy and robotic technology to take advantage of both techniques [42].

Surgical Procedure for Radical Hysterectomy

The round ligaments are clamped and divided, and a bladder flap is developed on either side. The top of the broad ligament is incised in a cranial direction. The infundibulopelvic ligament is clamped, transected, and doubly suture-ligated. At this point, the peritoneum on the lateral aspect of the broad ligament is dissected further laterally to expose the psoas major muscle. During the course of the dissection, the ureter is identified and dissected free at the point where it crosses the common iliac artery, which is then identified and cleared of fat, as is the external iliac vein. During the course of the dissection, the ureter is located posterior to the ovarian vascular complex. As the external iliac node dissection proceeds towards the iliac bifurcation, the internal iliac artery is identified and cleared of fat. Elevation of the external iliac vein exposes the obturator fossa, which is filled with fat and lymph nodes. The fat is dissected out of the fossa, and the obturator nerve and artery are cleaned of fat and lymph tissue. The dissection is carried laterally until the fascia of the obturator internus muscle is reached. Great care must be taken not to tear or otherwise injure the tributaries of the internal iliac veins because they bleed profusely and are very difficult to secure. When the obturator dissection is completed, the operator turns their attention to the common iliac node dissection. Again, great care must be taken not to injure the left common iliac vein. Next, the ureter is dissected inferiorly, removing the encompassing fibrofatty tissue, and reflecting it medially to be removed with the uterus. The uterine arteries and veins are clamped far laterally, just distal to their origin from the anterior division of the hypogastric artery. If the hypogastric artery is to be clamped, this should be performed distal to the origin of the superior and inferior gluteal arteries. At this point, the ureter is entering its tunnel through the cardinal ligament just cephalad to where it enters the wall of the bladder. The ureter is now free of the parametria. Next, the bladder pillars are identified, cut, and secured. The vesicouterine space is dissected downward well below the uterine cervix. The peritoneum between the uterosacral ligaments is divided, and the rectouterine space is developed and dissected downward below the cervix. The uterosacral ligaments are cut and suture-ligated. The lower cardinal ligament, deep parametrial fat, and fascia are clamped and cut medial to the

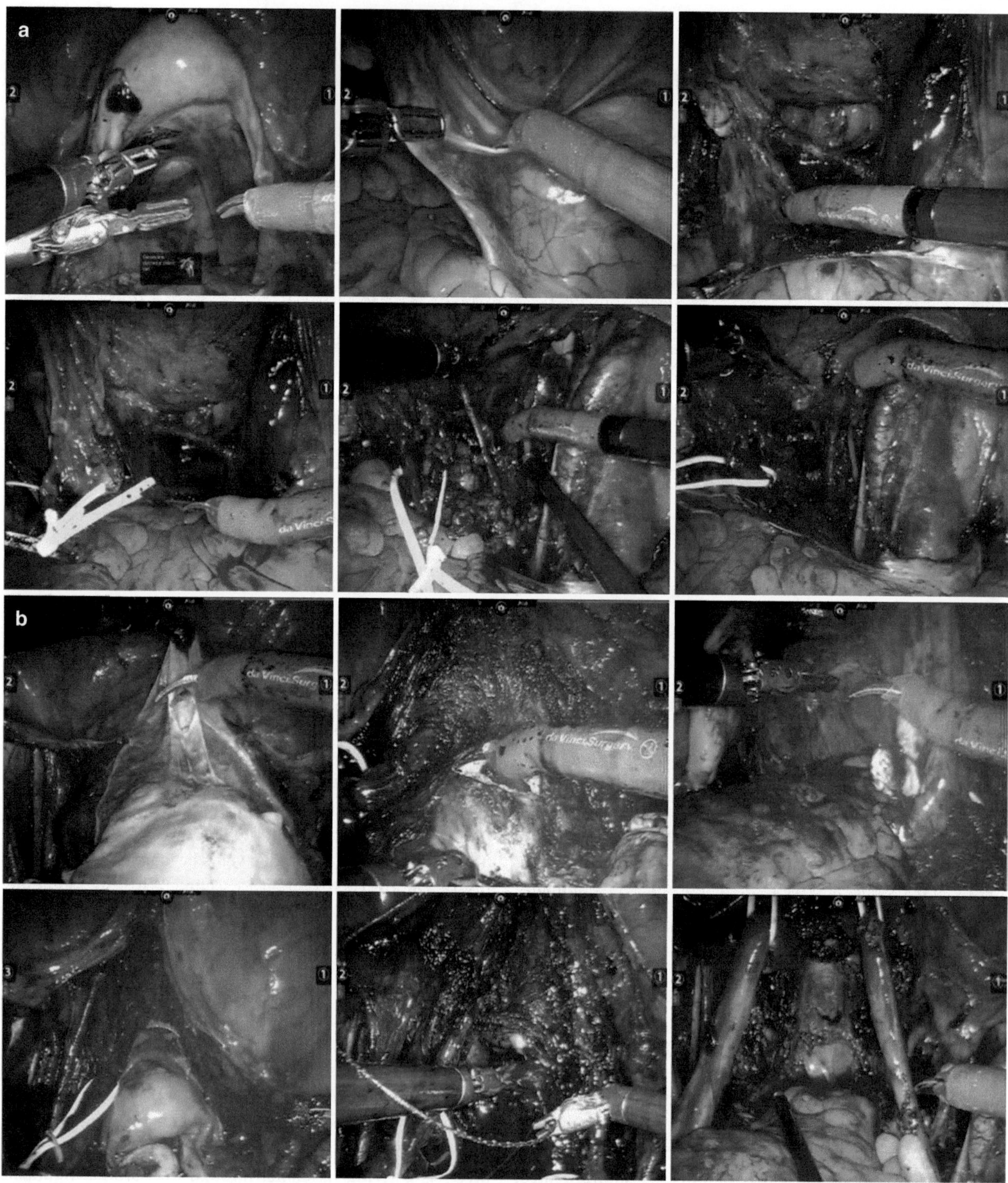

Fig. 73.1 Robotic radical hysterectomy. (**a**) Opening of the paravesical and pararectal spaces and dissection of the ureter (yellow rubber band ligation) and vessels. Resection of pelvic lymph nodes and the right lateral parametrium. (**b**) Dissection of the urinary bladder and vaginal wall. Removal of the specimen and closure of the vaginal cuff

ureter. The vagina is clamped approximately 4 cm below the cervix, and the specimen is removed. The peritoneum is drained with catheter and the abdominal incision closed [48] (Fig. 73.1).

Robotic Pelvic Exenteration

Pelvic exenteration (PE) has been used for 60 years to treat cancers of the lower and middle female genital tract in radiated pelvis [27]. PE is a radical surgery involving the en bloc resection of the pelvic organs, including the internal reproductive organs, bladder, and rectosigmoid. The indications for PE include advanced primary or recurrent pelvic malignancies, among which centrally recurrent cervical carcinomas are most common; while other gynecologic, urologic, and rectal cancers are also included [28]. The following are contra-indications for PE: patients with major medical, psychiatric, or emotional co-morbidity, and incapacity; lower extremity lymphedema indicating unresectable disease; extrapelvic disease associated with poor prognosis; immobile tumors fixed to the pelvic sidewall (relative if bone can be resected); invasion of the proximal (S1 or higher) lumbosacral spine or lumbosacral plexus/sciatic nerves; and encasement of the external or common iliac vessels by the tumor [31]. Distant metastasis has also traditionally been a contraindication for PE with curative intent [28].

In 1948, Brunshwing introduced PE as the treatment for persistent or recurrent gynecological cancer [27]. The first study of this technique reported that among 22 patients studied, 5 died from the operation itself [30]. In the following 50 years, the criteria for selecting patients that would benefit the most from this extensive surgery were defined. Improvements in surgical techniques and peri-operative care, and implementation of reconstructive procedures reduced the operative mortality to 0–5.3 % [29]. PE is now considered a safe and feasible procedure that can help selected patients with no other options for cure, although the reported morbidity rates remain high (38–65 %) [32]. PE is associated with a significant complication rate, with ~40–50 % major complications and ~80 % minor complications [28]. The most common morbidity is infection (19–86 %), which includes wound infection, urinary tract infection, sepsis, and abscess. The most common late morbidities are intestinal obstruction and fistula (5–10 %) [30]. Mortality rate is 1–16 %, with disparate causes including sepsis, thromboembolic disease, and cardiopulmonary failure. Death in the perioperative period occurs in less than 5 % of patients, while women over the age of 65 have the highest risk [28]. Relative contra-indications are: ureteral obstruction, poor candidate for surgery because of medical comorbidities, or poor candidate for surgery because of inability to care for stomas or senility. Advanced age has previously been considered a relative contraindication to exenterative surgery, probably because older patients are more likely to have pre-existing medical conditions, such as heart disease, obstructive pulmonary disease, decreased renal function, and altered immunologic response [49].

The 5 year survival rate of patients who underwent PE for recurrent or persistent cervical cancer following surgery and radiotherapy or radiation therapy alone was 52 % [28, 29]. This result confirms that cervical cancer patients are appropriate candidates for PE. Even though vaginal, vulvar, and endometrial cancer patients can benefit from the operation, it is still debatable whether they are good candidates for such an aggressive surgery, given that their usual bad prognosis maybe due to the different biology and pathways of diffusion of their cancers.

The recent development of laparoscopic pelvic surgery and robotically assisted laparoscopic pelvic surgery, particularly in uro-oncology and colorectal cancer, has created new possibilities. Minimally invasive therapy can offer operative and early postoperative advantages, although the long-term oncological and palliative outcomes still have to be evaluated. Blood loss and transfusion rate are significantly reduced, and the time needed to recover oral intake and bowel function are reduced. The patients generally return to normal activity more quickly, although complication rates are more or less equivalent [31]. Careful selection of patients is vital for robotic-assisted PE to be successful. The tumor should be removed according to strict oncologic criteria (en-bloc removal of cancer, obtaining free margins, avoiding dissemination of tumor by manipulation of cancer mass) and correct surgical technique should be used in order to achieve urinary and fecal diversion [32]. Table 73.2 summarizes reports on robot assisted pelvic exenteration for cervical cancer.

Surgical Procedures for Pelvic Exenteration

PE is classified as anterior (APE), posterior (PPE), and total (PE). APE is the removal of the reproductive tract and bladder; PPE is the removal of the reproductive tract along with the rectosigmoid colon; and TPE is the removal of the reproductive tract, bladder, and rectosigmoid colon [29]. Here, we describe the surgical techniques for all three procedures.

Pelvic exenteration consists of three important and distinct components: determination of resectability, resection, and reconstruction. The procedure begins with the patient in a low lithotomy position to allow for abdominal and perineal portions of the surgery. Combined epidural and general anesthesia may be considered for additional postoperative pain control. PE is traditionally performed as an open abdominal procedure, but recent developments in laparoscopy and robotics have allowed for the minimally-invasive adaptation of the technique. First, the abdomen and pelvis are thoroughly examined for evidence of metastatic disease. Washings may be sent for cytology. Any suspicious lesion is biopsied and sent for frozen section to exclude the possibility of distant metastatic disease that would preclude complete resection or alter the surgical plan. For recurrent cervical cancer, low para-aortic and pelvic lymph node dissection may be performed again to preclude metastatic spread beyond the pelvis. Lateral involvement of disease to the pelvic sidewall should be assessed at this time [27, 28, 50]. The round ligaments are divided, and the paravesicular and pararectal spaces are

Table 73.2 Summary of reports on robotic pelvic exenteration for cervical cancer

Study	Publication type	Histologic type	Type of operation	Procedure duration, (min)	Blood loss, (ml)	Complications	Postoperative stay (days)
Lambaudie et al. [25]	Case report	Squamous cell carcinoma	Anterior pelvic exenteration	480	200	Perineal abscess, Miami pouch fistula, ureteral stenosis	53
Akhil et al. [30]	Case report	Squamous cell carcinoma	Total pelvic exenteration	240	300	NM	11
Davis et al. [36]	Case report	Squamous cell carcinoma	Anterior pelvic exenteration	540	550	NM	8
Lim et al. [24]	Case report	Squamous cel carcinoma	Total pelvic exenteration	375	375	None	10
Lavazzo et al. [33]	Cases	Squamous cervical cancer	Anterior pelvic exenteration	375–600	200–550	Postoperative complications-perineal abscess, ureteral stenosis	3–53

NM not mentioned

developed. At this time, the pelvic sidewalls may again be examined. At this point, the extent of PE must be determined. Total PE includes removal of the bladder and distal uterus, portions of rectum and sigmoid colon, internal reproductive organs, and vagina.

En bloc resection Removal of the specimen begins with the ligation and division of the fibrovascular pedicle containing the uterine vessels, cardinal ligament, and ureter bilaterally. The uterine artery is ligated at its origin from the hypogastric artery, lateral to the ureter. The infundibulopelvic ligaments are ligated above the level of the common iliac vessels. The sigmoid is then mobilized and transected with a gastrointestinal anastomotic stapler, and the sigmoid vessels are identified and ligated. Care must be taken to preserve blood flow to the remaining colon-usually the sigmoid and the sacrum are developed to the level of the levator ani muscles. The avascular plane between the sigmoid and the sacrum is developed to the level of the levator ani muscles. The prevesicular space is extended bluntly. At this point, the specimen should be freely mobile in the pelvis. The perineal portion of the procedure is then performed. An incision is marked to include the urethra, vaginal opening, anus, and possibly the vulva. The muscles of the pelvic floor are transected circumferentially. The pubococcygeal and anococcygeal ligaments are identified and divided. Upon completion of the dissection, the entire specimen is free to be removed.

Anterior pelvic exenteration Anterior PE involves the removal of the bladder and internal reproductive organs but spares the gastrointestinal tract. The rectosigmoid, anus, and lower portion of the posterior vagina are left intact. Bimanual palpation, in which the pelvic hand inserts one finger into the vagina and another into the rectum, while the abdominal hand palpates the posterior cul-de-sac and retracts the rectum posteriorly, will confirm the initial impression that an anterior resection is advisable. If the space posterior to the cervix feels free, then an incision can be made in the cul-de-sac to allow the rectum to drop away from the upper vagina, leaving at least 4 cm margin on the vagina. The potential space between the rectum and posterior vagina is developed abdominally, and adequacy of the margin is confirmed by direct vision vaginally. The posterior vaginal incision is made from below, with the cancer in view, to ensure adequate margin. Biopsies of the vagina, which will be left intact over the rectum, are sent for frozen section. The perineal incision is made, removing the urethra and surrounding soft tissue, but preserving the clitoris and labia (Fig. 73.2).

Posterior pelvic exenteration Posterior exenterations are rarely performed, except for primary stage IVA cancers of the cervix invading the rectum. Posterior PE removes the internal reproductive organs and rectosigmoid, but spares the anterior vagina, urinary bladder, and uterus. After dividing the round ligaments and developing the perivesicular and perirectal spaces, the peritoneum between the bladder and uterus is incised, and the bladder is reflected as inferiorly as possible with sharp dissection. The uterus is then mobilized and dissected free of soft tissue attachments, similar to the technique for RH. The uterine arteries are divided at their origin and reflected medially, trying to preserve other branches of the internal iliac arteries. The cardinal ligaments are then divided laterally, the ureteral dissection is completed to the bladder, and the anterior vagina is entered. The rectosigmoid is freed posteriorly, the parametrium is mobilized medially, and the dissection is carried down to the levator muscles, identical to the posterior dissection in a total exenteration. The perineal incision will involve only the posterior aspect of the vulva and anus. An omental flap and small pack

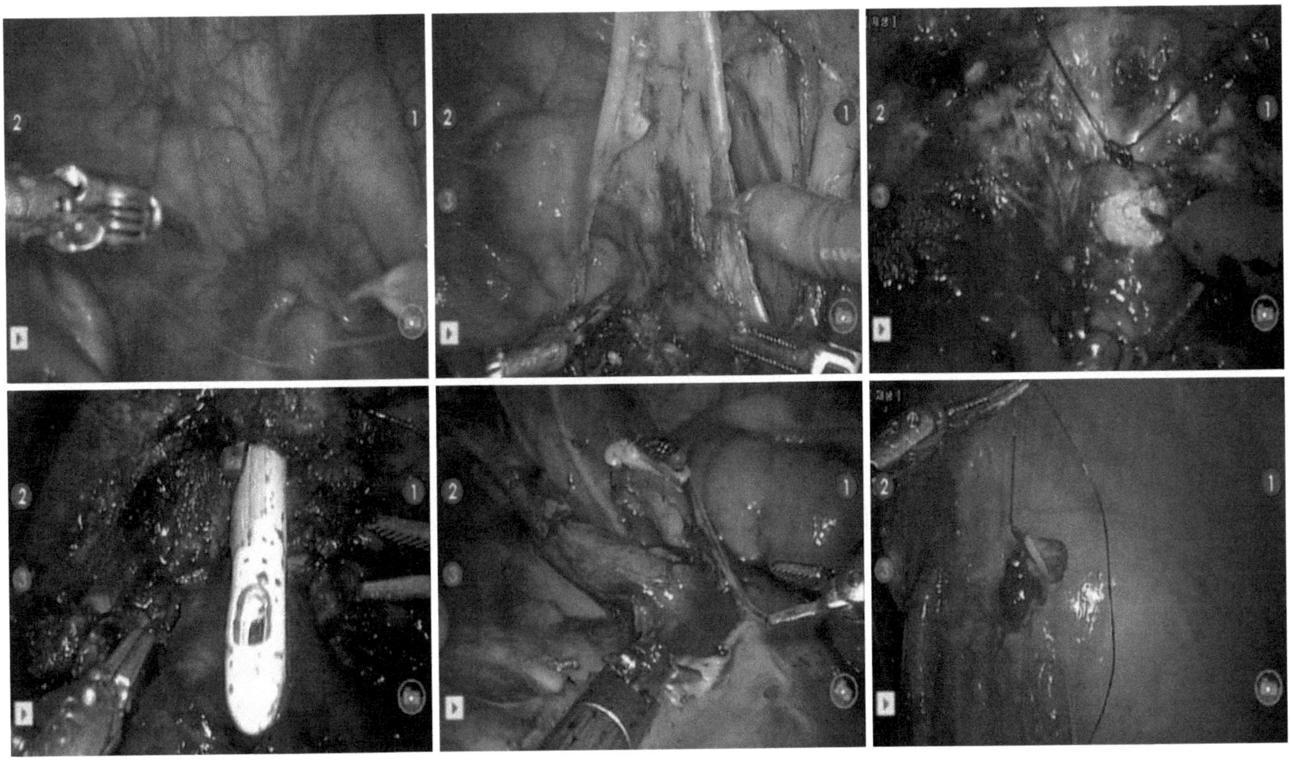

Fig. 73.2 Robot-assisted pelvic exenteration-Anterior PE. Dissection of the lateral pelvic wall and urinary bladder. Resection of the urinary bladder and mobilization of the ureter. Preparing of the urinary diversion to the lower abdominal wall

can be used to complete the management of the defect, and colostomy is performed (Fig. 73.3).

Supralevator pelvic exenteration Women with disease extending posteriorly from the cervix onto the vaginal epithelium or into the rectal wall are candidates for this procedure, provided the cancer does not extend to the lower third of the vagina posteriorly. After the bladder, urethra, and anterior vagina are mobilized, as previously described, the posterior vaginal wall incision is made 4 cm below the tumor. The vaginal epithelium is mobilized for 1–2 cm away from the rectal muscularis. The hand then encircles the mobilized rectum and pulls it cephalad. The specimen side is clamped to reduce spillage of feces and divided, leaving an anal and rectal stump. The length of the anal rectal stump from the anal sphincter is ideally 6 cm or greater. If less than 6 cm in length, the risk of fistula and incontinence is greater. After mobilization of this lower specimen, the sigmoid colon is divided along with the sigmoidal arteries and the superior rectal artery. Ample mobilization for reanastomosis is accomplished by incising the lateral attachments of the sigmoid and descending colon, mobilizing it and, if necessary, sacrificing some of the sigmoidal vessels. The major blood supply is from the inferior mesenteric artery, which has significant anastomoses between it and the middle colic artery. After the sigmoid and left colon are mobilized, the colon should be observed for adequacy of blood supply and viability while the urinary diversion is done, and the flaps for neovaginal construction are harvested. The anastomosis is accomplished using 28–31 mm-diameter circular staplers. Following anastomosis, the omentum is mobilized and brought into the pelvis as an omental graft. It is used to wrap the low rectal anastomosis and to fill the presacral space.

Reconstruction

Urinary Diversion The standard urinary diversion for several decades was the urinary conduit using a segment of the ileum to which the ureters would be anastomosed, and a stoma created in the right lower abdomen. Currently, the preferred method of urinary diversion is a continent pouch, created from the distal ileum, ascending colon, and a portion of the transverse colon. The ileum is divided 10–12 cm proximal to the ileocecal valve, and the transverse colon is divided just distal to the middle colic artery (Miami pouch). An ileotransverse colon enterostomy is performed to restore continuity to the gastrointestinal tract. The isolated segment of bowel is opened with cautery along the tenia. The bowel is then folded on itself in a U-shape conduit and the edges closed with a stapling device. This formation of the colon creates a reservoir and interrupts the ability of the bowel to peristalsis and increase the pouch pressure.

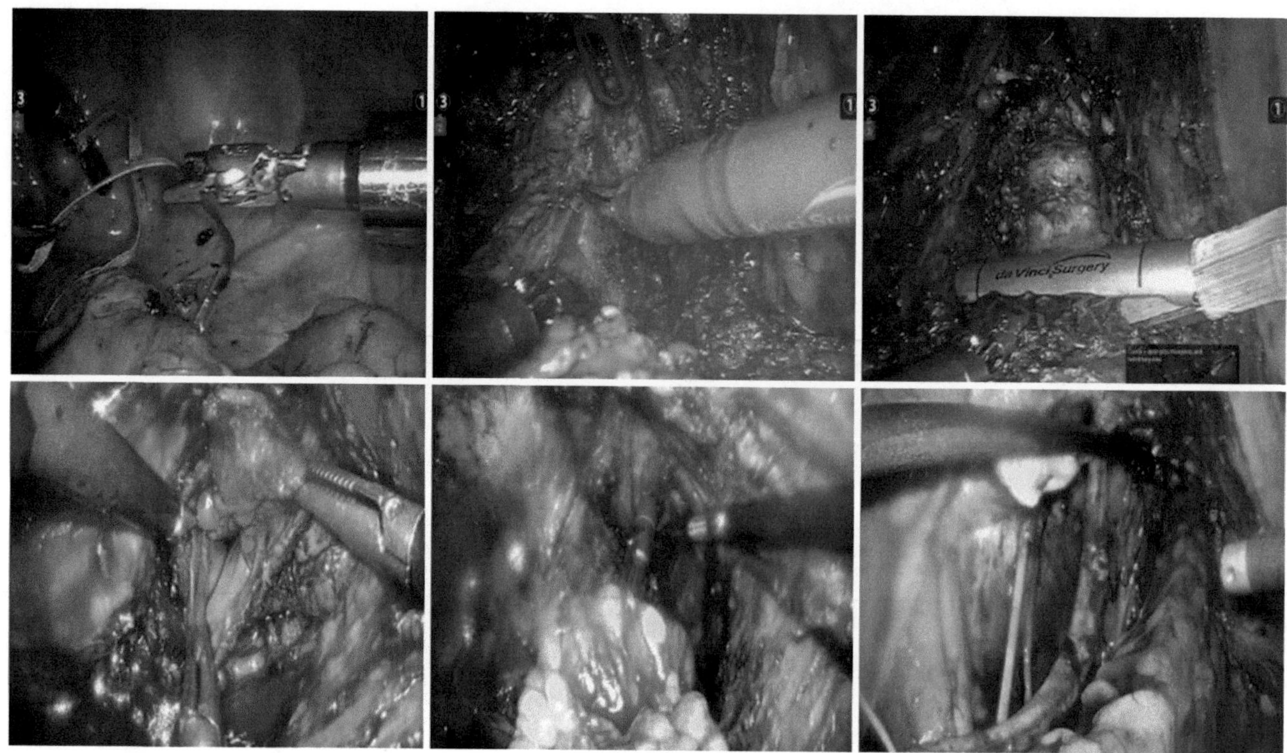

Fig. 73.3 Robot-assisted pelvic exenteration-Posterior PE. Developing of the perirectal spaces and dissection of the rectosigmoid colon. Resection of the rectosigmoid colon above the levator muscles. Reconstruction of the proximal sigmoid colon to the rectal stump

The ureters brought through stab wounds into the bowel reservoir, and the spatulated ends are anastomosed mucosa to mucosa. The left ureter is brought through the sigmoid mesentery to reach the reservoir. A 14 French catheter is placed into the ileum and passed through into the reservoir. Excess ileum is excised from the antimesenteric edge with a stapling device, and three purse string sutures are placed at the ileocecal valve to tighten the ileum. The tapered end of the ilium is brought out as a stoma. The ureters are stented and, with a Malecot catheter, are brought out through the anterior wall of the reservoir and through a separate opening in the abdominal wall. Stents and catheter are removed 2 weeks postoperatively.

Fecal diversion For patients whose disease requires infralevator dissection posteriorly, permanent end colostomy will be required because the anal sphincter is compromised or excised. If the sphincter and enough rectum may be spared without compromising the chance at complete disease resection, low rectal anastomosis with circular staplers is a reasonable option, if enough healthy tissue remains. To improve the frequency of stooling by improving the reservoir of the rectum, a colonic J-pouch may be used, particularly in patients with very little rectum remaining (less than 5 cm) [27, 28, 50, 51].

Robotic systems maintain the advantages of conventional laparoscopy while enabling the surgeon to dissect down and into the narrow pelvic floor. 3D stereoscopic vision (facilitated by the use of binocular optical systems), tremor filtration, and reduced operators' fatigue are the obvious advantages of robotic technology. The articulated instruments permit a wide range of motions while increasing the ability of the operator to work efficiently within the confines of the pelvic floor. All of these advantages can help procedures to preserve anatomic structures of the pelvis and make both destruction and reconstruction phases of PE easier [31, 32]. Moreover, the harmonic scalpel enables control of the pelvic sidewall vessels and transaction of the ligamentous attachments around the extirpated pelvic structures. Intestinal anastomosis after colorectal cancer resection can be performed by an experienced surgeon, in accordance with current oncologic guidelines. In addition, the 360° motion of a robotic wrist permits fine suturing that is necessary for performing ureteral iliostomy and ideal loop urinary diversion [34]. Robotic assisted laparoscopic surgery is associated with significantly less blood loss, less pain, shorter recovery time, shorter hospital stay, and better aesthetic results. Furthermore, shorter hospital stays and quicker return to normal activity may mean that postoperative chemotherapy or radiation can begin earlier, and complications related to bowel adhesions caused by radiation can be reduced [28, 32].

The cases of robotic-assisted laparoscopic PE with urinary diversion performed extracorporeally (ileal conduit diversion + orthotopic neobladder) were first described by Pruthi et al. [23] in 12 women with localized bladder cancer. Lim [24] reported the first case of robotic assisted total PE with ileal loop urinary diversion and end colostomy for the treatment of recurrent cervical cancer. Lavazzo et al. reported eight patients between 43 and 67 years of age treated with robotic-assisted PE for IB2 to IVA squamous cell carcinoma of the cervix. In 7 out of the 8 patients, anterior PE was performed; the other woman underwent total PE, with the duration ranging from 375 to 600 min, and blood loss from 200 to 550 ml. Postoperative complications occurred in two patients and included perineal abscess, Miami pouch fistula, and ureteral stenosis. Postoperative hospital stay ranged from 3 to 53 days, while postoperative follow-up ranged from 2 to 31 months [32].

Lawande et al. reported a 35 year old female with advanced cervical cancer who presented with vesicovaginal and rectovaginal fistula. They performed total robotic PE with colo-anal anastomosis and uretero-sigmoidostomy. The total operation time was 240 min and the console time was 120 min. The estimated blood loss was 300 ml and the intensive care unit stay was 2 days. Post-operatively, the patient had good fecal and urinary continence and high quality of life [26].

Davis et al. reported two women, 50 and 58 years old respectively, who required anterior PE for recurrent cervical cancer (squamous cervical cancer-IVB). Mean operation time was 9 h, mean blood loss was 550 ml, and postoperative hospital stay was 8 days. Postoperative complications were not mentioned. The authors reported that the robotic system is promising in patients needing surgery for recurrent cervical cancer. It provides improved visualization of the deep pelvis, enhanced manipulation of radiated fibrotic tissue, and reduced blood loss [36]. Subsequently, Lambaudie et al. reported a case series of three patients who underwent robot-assisted total PE [25]. Interestingly, the urinary diversion was made extracorporeal by transrectal laparotomy. The authors reported that with regard to hospital stay, there was no benefit compared with laparotomy, essentially due to urinary diversion management (catheterization) and self-catheterization to preserve the nerve.

Given the radical and prolonged nature of this procedure, patients and providers must be prepared for a long and potentially complicated hospital course. Many patients, after operation, need to stay in the intensive care unit immediately for close monitoring, particularly for dramatic fluid shifts. Blood loss may be high with transfusion required in most patients. Special attention to prophylaxis for thromboembolism, respiratory care, and nutrition is required. Some patients will require total parenteral nutrition due to prolonged inability to eat postoperatively to prevent relatively common ileus [43].

All series show that about 25–40 % of well selected patients with no metastatic disease survive for a minimum of 5 years. Patients who had palliative exenteration may still benefit from surgery in terms of quality of life and life expectancy of 18–24 months. The organ and histological subtypes often have significant influence on long-term prognosis. As a rule, exenteration for colonic and rectal adenocarcinomas results in better survival. This may be partly due to better responsiveness to chemotherapy and new small molecule-targeting agents. Cervical cancer also shows reasonably good survival due to its response to radiation therapy [31].

Considering the novelty of this minimally invasive procedure, several principles and standards must be rigorously evaluated and maintained. First, it remains paramount to observe and maintain the oncologic principles of such procedure without surgical modifications. That is, pathologic endpoints and consequent oncologic outcomes must never be compromised with such new techniques. Second, such procedures should have appropriate perioperative outcomes including operation time, blood loss, and length of hospital stay. Such measures may reflect and influence morbidity, recovery, and operative difficulty (i.e., the learning curve) of surgeons. For example, in robotic prostatectomy procedures, operation time has been used as an indirect measure of surgical difficulty and progress in overcoming the learning curve [35].

Conclusions

In summary, laparoscopy and robotics are preferable to laparotomy for patients requiring RH, with some advantages noted for robotics over laparoscopy. Current evidence demonstrates the safety and feasibility of robotic-assisted RH for early stage cervical cancer. Robotic approach provides clear benefits of minimally invasive surgery, such as lower morbidity, reduced blood loss, and faster recovery than open surgery. Further studies are necessary to evaluate long term survival and to analyze morbidity after surgery and adjuvant therapies.

Despite the apparent encouraging early results suggesting the advantage of minimally invasive surgery for PE, questions remain about the surgical effectiveness of this approach. Further studies on minimally invasive techniques for PE are needed prior to widespread clinical application of these techniques. Furthermore, research should also focus on the postoperative quality of life and other benefits for the patient.

References

1. GLOBOCAN Cancer Fact Sheet- globocan 2012. Available at: http://www.iarc.fr/en/media-centre/pr/2013/pdfs/pr223_E.pdf.
2. Schiffman M, Castle PE, Jeronimo J, Rodriguez AC, Wacholder S. Human papillomavirus and cervical cancer. Lancet. 2007;370:890–970.

3. Winer RL, Hughes JP, Feng Q, et al. Condom use and the risk of genital human papillomavirus infection in young women. N Engl J Med. 2006;354:2645–54.
4. Min KJ, Lee JK, Lee S, Kim MK. Alcohol consumption and viral load are synergistically associated with CIN1. J Open Access. 2013; doi:10.1371/journal. pone.0072142.
5. Lee S, Kim JW, Hong JH, et al. Clinical significance of HPV DNA contesting in Korean women with ASCUS or ASC-H. Diagn Cytopathol. 2014;23:1058–62.
6. Vizcaino AP, Moreno V, Bosch FX, et al. International trends in incidence of cervical cancer: II. Squamous-cell carcinoma. Int J Cancer. 2000;86:429–35.
7. Canis M, Mage G, Pouly JL, et al. Laparoscopic radical hysterectomy for cervical cancer. Baillieres Clin Obstet Gynaecol. 1995;9:675–89.
8. Nezhat CR, Burrell MO, Nezhat FR, et al. Laparoscopic radical hysterectomy with paraaortic and pelvic node dissection. Am J Obstet Gynecol. 1992;166:864–5.
9. Frumovitz M, dos Reis R, CC S, et al. Comparison of total laparoscopic and abdominal radical hysterectomy for patients with early-stage cervical cancer. Obstet Gynecol. 2007;110:96–102.
10. Nezhat F, Mahdavi A, Nagarsheth NP. Total laparoscopic radical hysterectomy and pelvic lymphadenectomy using harmonic shears. J Minim Invasive Gynecol. 2006;13:20–5.
11. Obermair A, Ginbey P, McCartney AJ. Feasibility and safety of total laparoscopic radical hysterectomy. J Am Assoc Gynecol Laparosc. 2003;10:345–9.
12. Ramirez PT, Slomovitz BM, Soliman PT, et al. Total laparoscopic radical hysterectomy and lymphadenectomy: the M. D. Anderson Cancer Center experience. Gynecol Oncol. 2006;102:252–5.
13. Sert MB. Comparison between robot-assisted laparoscopic radical hysterectomy (RRH) and abdominal radical hysterectomy (ARH): a case control study from EIO/Milan. Gynecol Oncol. 2010;117:389–90.
14. Geisler JP, Orr CJ, Khurshid N, et al. Robotically assisted laparoscopic radical hysterectomy compared with open radical hysterectomy. Int J Gynecol Cancer. 2010;20:438–42.
15. Maggioni A, Minig L, Zanagnolo V, et al. Robotic approach for cervical cancer: comparison with laparotomy: a case control study. Gynecol Oncol. 2009;115:60–4.
16. Estape R, Lambrou N, Diaz R, et al. A case matched analysis of robotic radical hysterectomy with lymphadenectomy compared with laparoscopy and laparotomy. Gynecol Oncol. 2009;113:357–61.
17. Swan K, Advincula AP. Role of robotic surgery in urogynecologic surgery and radical hysterectomy: how far can we go? Curr Opin Urol. 2011;21:78–83.
18. Sert BM, Abeler VM. Robotic-assisted laparoscopic radical hysterectomy (Piver type III) with pelvic node dissection: case report. Eur J Gynaecol Oncol. 2006;27:531–3.
19. Corcione F, Esposito C, Cuccurullo D, et al. Advantages and limits of robot-assisted laparoscopic surgery: preliminary experience. Surg Endosc. 2005;19:117–9.
20. Magrina JF, Kho RM, Weaver AL, Montero RP, Magtibay PM. Robotic radical hysterectomy: comparison with laparoscopy and laparotomy. Gynecol Oncol. 2008;109:86–91.
21. Sert B, Abeler V. Robotic radical hysterectomy in early-stage cervical carcinoma patients, comparing results with total laparoscopic radical hysterectomy cases. The future is now? Int J Med Robot. 2007;3:224–8.
22. Shzly SA, Murad MH, Dowdy SC, Gostout BS, Famuyide AO. Robotic radical hysterectomy in early stage cervical cancer: a systemic review and meta-analysis. Gynecol Oncol. 2015;138:457–71.
23. Pruthi RS, Stefaniak H, Hubbard JS, Wallen EM. Robot-assisted laparoscopic anterior pelvic exenteration for bladder cancer in the female patient. J Endourol. 2008;22:2397–402.
24. Lim PC. Robotic assisted total pelvic exenteration: a case report. Gynecol Oncol. 2009;115:310–1.
25. Lambaude E, Narducci F, Leblanc E, Bannier M, Houvenaeghel G. Robotically-assisted laparoscopic anterior pelvic exenteration for recurrent cervical cancer: report of three first cases. Gynecol Oncol. 2010;116:582–3.
26. Lawande A, Kenawadekar R, Desai R, et al. Case report. Robotic total pelvic exentration. J Robot Surg. 2014;8:93–6. doi:10.1007/s11701-013-0404-5.
27. Hockel M, Dornhofer N. Pelvic exentration for gynecological tumors; achievements and unanswered guestions. Lancet Oncol. 2006;7:837–47.
28. Diver EJ, . Alejanro Rauh-Hain J, Del Carmen MG. Total pelvic exentration for gynecologic malignancies. Int J Surg Oncol. 2012; doi:10.1155/2012/693535.
29. Maggioni A, Roviglione G, Landoni F, et al. Pelvic exenteration; ten-year experience at the Europan Institute of Oncology in Milan. Gynecol Oncol. 2009;114:64–8.
30. Jonathan S. Berek, Candace Howe, Leo D. Lagasse, Neville F. Hacker Gyncol Oncol. 2005;99:153–9.
31. Boustead GB, Feneley MR. Pelvic exentrative surgery for palliation of malignant disease in Robotic Era. Clin Ongol. 2010;22:740–6.
32. Lavazzo C, Gkegks ID. Review article Robotic technology for pelvic exentration in cases of cervical cancer. Int J Obstet Gynecol. 2014;125:15–7.
33. Kaufmann OG, Young JL, Sountoulides P, Kaplan AG, Dash A, Ornstein DK. Roboic radical anterior pelvic exentration: the UCI experience. Mini Invasive Therapy. 2011;20:240–6.
34. Guru KA, Nogueira M, Piacente P, Nyquist J, Mohler JL, Kim HL. Rapid communication: Robot-assisted anterior exentration: technique and initial series. J Endourol. 2007;21:633–9.
35. Herrell SD, Smith Jr JA. Robotic assisted laparoscopic prostatectomy: what is the learning curve? Urology. 2005;66:105–7.
36. Davis MA, Adams S, Eun D, Lee D, Randall TC. Robotic-assisted laparoscopic exenteration in recurrent cervical cancer Robotics improved the surgical experience for 2 women with recurrent cervical cancer. Am J Obstet Gynecol. 2010;202:582–3.
37. Renato S, Mohamed M, Serena S, et al. Robot assisted radical hysterectomy for cervical cancer: review of surgical and ongological outcomes. ISRN Obstet Gynecol. 2011; doi:10.5402/2011/872434.
38. Gortchev G, Tomov S, Tantchev L, Velkova A, Radionova Z. Robot-assisted radical hysterectomy-perioperative and survival outcomes in patients with cervical cancer compared to laparoscopic and open radical surgery. Gynecol Surg. 2012;9:81–8. doi:10.1007/s10397-011-0683-7.
39. Estape R, Lambrou N, Diaz R, et al. A case matched analysis of robotic radical hysterectomy and pelvic lymphadenectomy compared with laparoscopy and laparotomy. Gynecol Oncol. 2009;113:357–61.
40. Pasic RP, Rizzo JA, Fang H, Ross S, Moore M, Gunnarsson C. Comparing robot-assisted with convntional laparoscopic hyserectomy: impact on cost and clinical outcomes. J Minim Invasive Gynecol. 2010; doi:10.1016/j.jmig.2010.06.009.
41. Bilal Sert M, Abeler V. Robot-assisted laparoscopic radical hysterectomy: comprison with total laparoscopic hysterectomy and abdominal radical hysterectomy; one surgeone's experience at the Norwegian Radium Hospital. Gynecol Oncol. 2011;121:600–4.
42. Cho JE, Nezhat FR. Robotic and gynecologic oncology: review of the literature. J Minim Invasive Gynecol. 2009; doi:10.1016/j.jmig.2009.06.024.
43. Committee opinion. The American College of Obstetricians and Gynecologists, Committee Opinion, Number 628, March 2015.
44. E. Ancuta, Codrina Ancuta, L. Gutu. Robotic surgery versus abdominal and laparoscopic radical hysterectomy in cervical cancer. 2012. http://www.intechopen.com/books/.

45. Lowe MP, Chamberlain DH, Kamelle SA, Johnson PR, Tillmans TD. A multiinstitutional experience with robotic-assisted radical hysterectomy for early stage cervical cancer. Gynecol Oncol. 2009;113:191–4.
46. Geetha P, M. KN. Laparoscopic, robotic and open method of radical hysterectomy for cervical cancer: a systematic review. J Mini Access Surg. 2012;8:67–73.
47. Busmar B. Comparison between Robotic radical Hysterectomy with laparoscopic and open abdominal radical hysterectomy in the treatment of early stage cervical cancer. World J Lap Surg. 2015;8:26–31.
48. Michael S. Baggish, Mickey M. Karram. Atlas of pelvic anatomy and gynecologic surgery. 2nd edn. Saunders. 2006. p. 184–98.
49. Gressel GM, Partride EE, Makhiji S. Pelvic exenteration. Glob Lib Women's Med. 2015; doi:10.103843/GLOWM.10233.
50. Rock J, Jones H. Te Line's operative gynecology. 10th ed. Philadelphia: Lippincott, Williams, and Milkins; 2011.
51. Exentreation for gynecologic cancer: guidance for healthcare workers.c2014 [updated 2014 Jul 21]. Available from: http://www.uptodate.com/.
52. Lambaudie E, Houvenaeghel G, Walz J, et al. Robot-assisted laparoscopy in gynecologic ongology. Surg Endosc. 2008;22:2743–7.

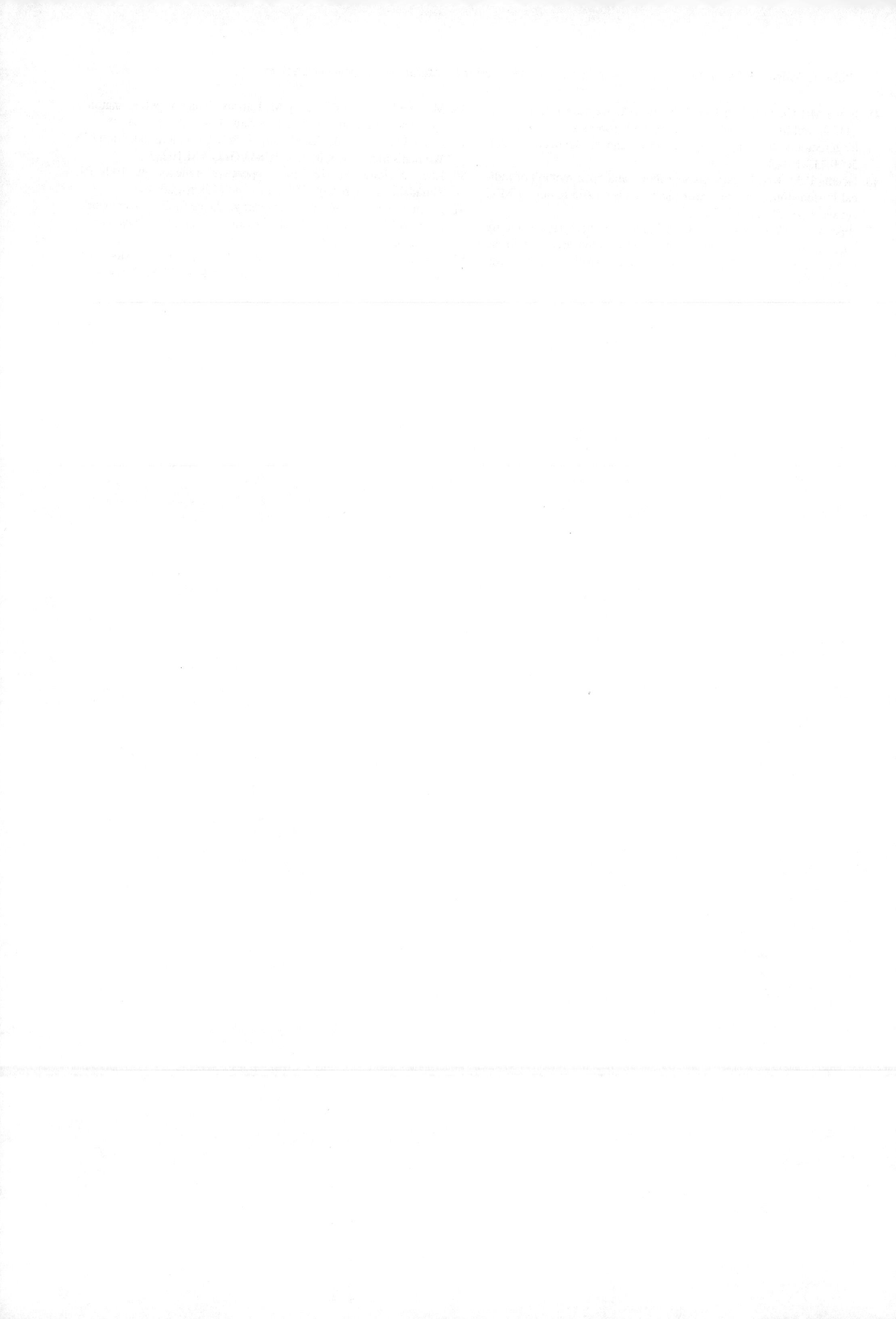

Robotic-Assisted Laparoscopic Hysterectomy and Endometriosis

74

Camran Nezhat, Erika Balassiano, Ceana H. Nezhat, and Azadeh Nezhat

Introduction of Robotic Surgery in the Field of Gynecology

Leonardo da Vinci sketched the first prototype of a robot in 1464 when he was 12 years old (Fig. 74.1). His life-sized armored robot knight was not realized until 1495 when it was built for the entertainment of his patron, the Duke of Sforza, at a celebration in the Court of Milan [1]. Five hundred years later, the field of robotics is not limited to entertainment, but has improved many aspects of everyday life. In medicine, for example, robotics has brought advancements to minimally invasive surgery.

The da Vinci robot was developed by the Medical Technology Laboratory (MTL) team, at the Stanford Research Institute (SRI), under the direction of Dr. Ajit Shah in early 1990s [2]. In collaboration with the Department of Defense and the National Aeronautics and Space Administration, the initial objective was to allow military surgeons to perform surgery from a remote location on wounded soldiers in mobile medical facilities close to the battlefield [3]. As the technology further developed with improved visual systems, articulating instrument manipulators, and better ergonomics, new uses for the robotic telepresence technology evolved and the robotic system was adapted to civilian surgical use as a new minimally invasive surgical technology.

The da Vinci® Robotic Surgical System (Intuitive Surgical® Inc., Sunnyvale, CA) pioneered as the first integrated three-dimensional viewing systems for minimally invasive surgery. The first successful telesurgery with the da Vinci® was a cholecystectomy performed in 1997 by Jacques Himpens and Guy Cardier in Brussels, Belgium [4]. A few years later in 2000, the U.S. Food and Drug Administration approved the da Vinci® Surgical Robotic device for laparoscopy, and in 2005, it was specifically approved for laparoscopic hysterectomy. Its current breadth of medical applications includes minimally invasive cardiothoracic surgery, urology, colorectal, general surgery, otolaryngology, and gynecology.

In the field of gynecology, the da Vinci® surgical system assists with a number of procedures including hysterectomy, myomectomy, complex resections of endometriotic lesions, tubal reversal, sacral colpopexy, and oncology surgery [5]. Since its introduction in 2000 to the U.S. market, the number

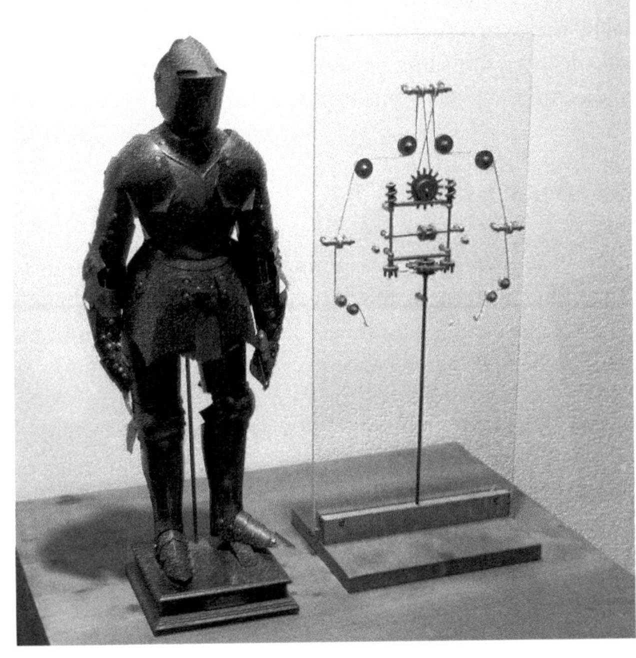

Fig. 74.1 A recreation of da Vinci's robot, fashioned in German-Italian medieval armor, was able to make several human-like movements. This model is on display in Berlin

C. Nezhat (✉) • A. Nezhat
Center for Special Minimally Invasive and Robotic Surgery, Palo Alto, CA, USA
e-mail: drnezhat@gmail.com; Azadeh.Nezhatmd@gmail.com

E. Balassiano
Deptartment of Gynecology, Center for Special Minimally Invasive and Robotic Surgery, Palo Alto, CA, USA
e-mail: erikabalassiano@gmail.com

C.H. Nezhat
Nezhat Medical Center, Atlanta, GA, USA
e-mail: ceana@nezhat.com

I. Alkatout, L. Mettler (eds.), *Hysterectomy*, DOI 10.1007/978-3-319-22497-8_74

of surgeon users has exponentially increased. Its widespread acceptance and application to gynecologic surgery can be attributed to its ease of use over conventional laparoscopy which subjects surgeons to counterintuitive hand movements, 2-dimensional video images, limited degrees of instrument motion, in addition to ergonomic challenges and tremor amplification [5]. Currently, there are over 3000 da Vinci® Systems installed worldwide and more than 2000 in the U.S. alone. The number of da Vinci® procedures performed in 2009 was 180,000 and within 1 year the number of procedures increased by 35 % to 278,000 in 2010 [6].

Advantages

The most obvious advantages of minimally invasive surgery are smaller incisions, less pain, shorter hospital stays, faster postoperative recovery, and improved patient satisfaction. Specific features of the da Vinci® Robotic System that enhance laparoscopic surgery are the immersive, high definition, 3-dimensional visual imaging which allows the surgeon to have better depth of perception and ability to magnify (x2 to x10). The computer can translate the surgeon's hand movements into the same movements of the robotic instruments. The robotic wrist can roll (twisting motion), pitch (up/down), yaw (side-to-side), and grip, allowing the surgeon 7° of freedom for each hand. Dexterity is further enhanced through computer motion scaling which allows the surgeon to make large macroscopic movements that the computer translates into microscopic movements of the instrument tips in the surgical field. In addition, the computer filters out high frequency hand motion and decreases operator tremor. The surgeon console decreases operator fatigue by allowing the surgeon to sit and comfortably perform the procedure.

Disadvantages

Certainly, there are some drawbacks to robotic surgery. The initial cost for the hospital system is high. A da Vinci® Robotic Surgical System costs slightly under $two million with an annual maintenance average cost of $140,000 per year. The cost-per-case for drapes and instruments is approximately $1000 [6]. The three component robotic system is bulky and requires large operating room space to comfortably accommodate and maneuver the system components. The unwieldy robotic arms have large excursion arcs that lead to frequent collisions and limitations on the placement of ports on the patient's torso. Furthermore, the bedside surgical assistant has to maneuver around the large robot and manage the uterine manipulation. Technical disadvantages are lack of tactile feedback to the surgeon operating from the console, and the inability to regulate the force applied to the tissue. Another drawback is that neither the patient nor the surgical table can be moved or repositioned once the robot is docked.

Preoperative Preparation, Patient Selection, and Anesthesia Considerations

Preoperative preparation can help assess the patient's ability to successfully undergo a robotic-assisted laparoscopic surgical procedure. Cardiovascular and pulmonary comorbidities should be thoroughly evaluated with appropriate preoperative testing. Although there is no data to support the use of preoperative mechanical bowel preparation, we believe that it helps to decompress the bowel for better visualization, decreases the risk of contamination due an unintended bowel injury, and allows for primary repair of the bowel, if needed. Specifically in cases of severe and deep infiltrating endometriosis involving the posterior cul-de-sac and the recto-sigmoid colon, adhesion formation and anatomy distortion can be very prominent, making bowel preparation extremely helpful.

In order to provide safe patient care, surgeons and anesthesiologists must understand the physiologic derangements that robotic-assisted laparoscopic surgery can have on anesthetic management. Several important issues specifically related to robotic surgeries include patient medical comorbidities, especially cardiovascular and pulmonary diseases, patient positioning, duration of the procedure, development of hypothermia, hemodynamic and respiratory effects of the pneumoperitoneum, and blood loss.

Intraoperative anesthesia considerations during robotic surgery are similar to traditional laparoscopy. Gynecologic procedures such as hysterectomy are performed in lithotomy with steep Trendelenburg position to take advantage of gravity that allows the bowel to drop down and out of the surgical field. It also helps to run the bowel in order to search for endometriotic lesions. Several hemodynamic changes occur with insufflation of the abdomen and the steep Trendelenburg position. The compressive effects of CO_2 insufflation on arterial vasculature result in a dramatic increase in systemic vascular resistance (SVR), particularly during the initial phase of insufflation. Using impedance cardiography, Westerband et al. reported a 30 % reduction in cardiac index (CI) and a 79 % increase in SVR immediately after peritoneal insufflation to 15 mm Hg [7]. In addition, patient position can markedly affect the cardiovascular system; a 10–30 % reduction in cardiac output occurs when a patient is placed in Trendelenburg [8].

The respiratory system is also impacted by CO_2 insufflation and pulmonary compliance is reduced by 30–50 % in both healthy and obese patients [8]. Peak airway pressure, plateau pressure, and intrathoracic pressure are increased [9]. Maintenance of normocarbia and acid-base status may be challenging in patients with poor pre-operative respiratory statuses. The main factors contributing to an increase in $PaCO_2$ and respiratory acidosis are the peritoneal absorption of CO_2, increased dead space in patients with coexisting lung disease, increased metabolism during surgery, inadequate ventilation, subcutaneous emphysema, and CO_2 embolism.

Obese patients undoubtedly benefit from minimally invasive surgery; however, there are challenges to anesthesia in this population. Arterial oxygenation is significantly impaired in overweight patients under general anesthesia in Trendelenburg position. Fluid replacement is also challenging, as crystalloids cause edema to form quickly around the face, eyes, and upper airway. Post extubation respiratory distress has been described, requiring emergent reintubation. Thus, fluid replacement should be restricted to 1–2 l over the course of the surgery using sufficient colloids. At the end of the surgery, it is crucial to ensure that significant laryngeal edema has not occurred while in steep Trendelenburg, and that the patient can breathe around the endotracheal tube with a deflated cuff prior to extubation [10].

Basic Set up for the Da Vinci® Robotic System

The da Vinci® Robotic System is composed of three components: the surgeon console, the patient-side robotic cart, and the InSite vision console (Fig. 74.2). The surgeon sits at the console away from the patient and uses a stereoscopic 3-dimensional viewer with hand manipulators and foot pedals, which control the robotic-assisted instruments within the patient. Ergonomic hand controls translate the 3-dimensional motion of the surgeon's hands into signals that directly control the robotic arms. The ratio of the surgeon hand motions to robotic arm motion can be modified through motion scaling. For example, a 5:1 ratio translates 5 inches of movement by surgeon into 1 inch of movement by the robotic arm. These ratios are preset. Foot pedals within the console are used for activation of electrosurgery, "clutching" or readjusting the hand controls, and switching between functioning robotic arms [11].

The patient-side robotic cart has telerobotic arms to which the EndoWrist® instruments attach. The robotic cart has four arms; one of the arms holds the laparoscope while the other two to three arms hold various laparoscopic surgical instruments. The InSite® vision console processes the images from the endoscope containing the stereoscopic cameras and dual optical lenses to the surgeon console where the operator has a 3-dimensional image of the surgical field.

Three people are directly involved in the robotic surgery: the surgeon, the bedside surgical assistant, and the scrub nurse. However, an anesthesiologist and circulating nurse familiar with the robotic laparoscopy can assist in making the procedure run efficiently (Fig. 74.3).

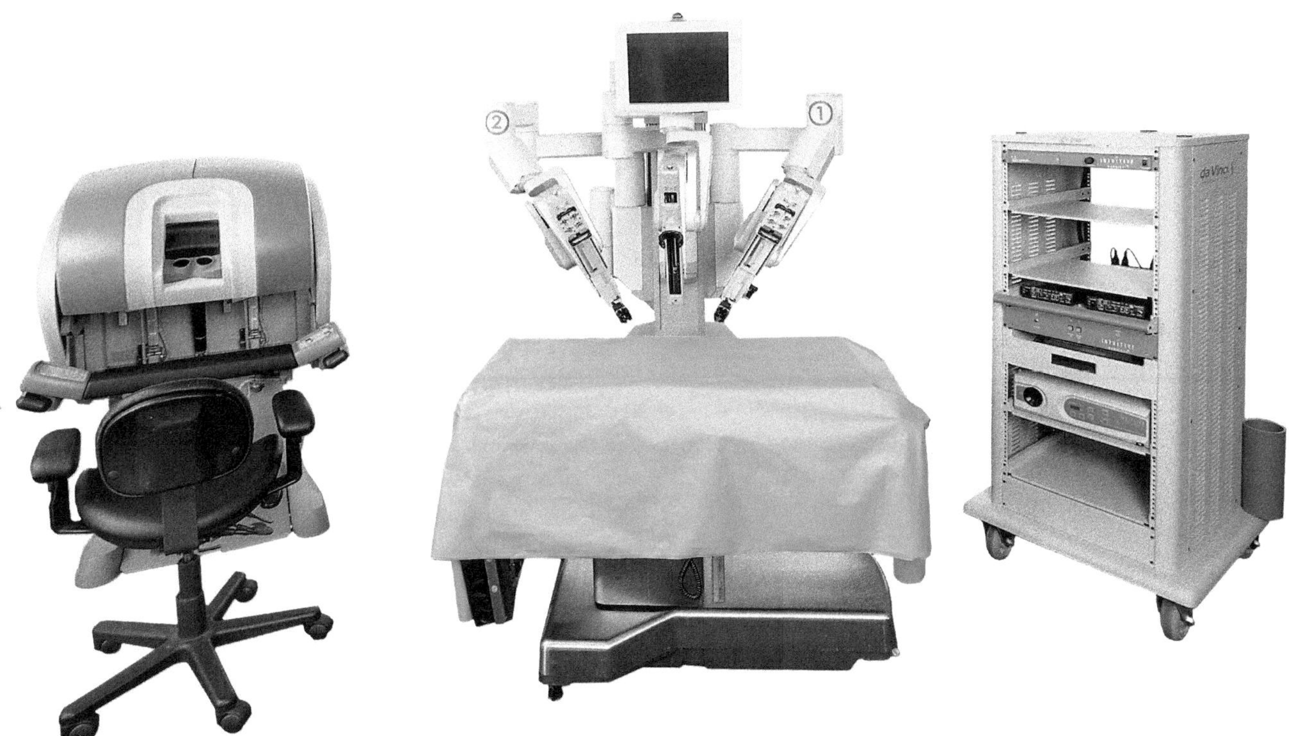

Fig. 74.2 The da Vinci Surgical System by Intuitive Surgical® Inc. (Sunnyvale, CA). The three main components are: surgeon console (*left*), the patient-side robotic cart (*middle*), and the InSite® vision console (*right*)

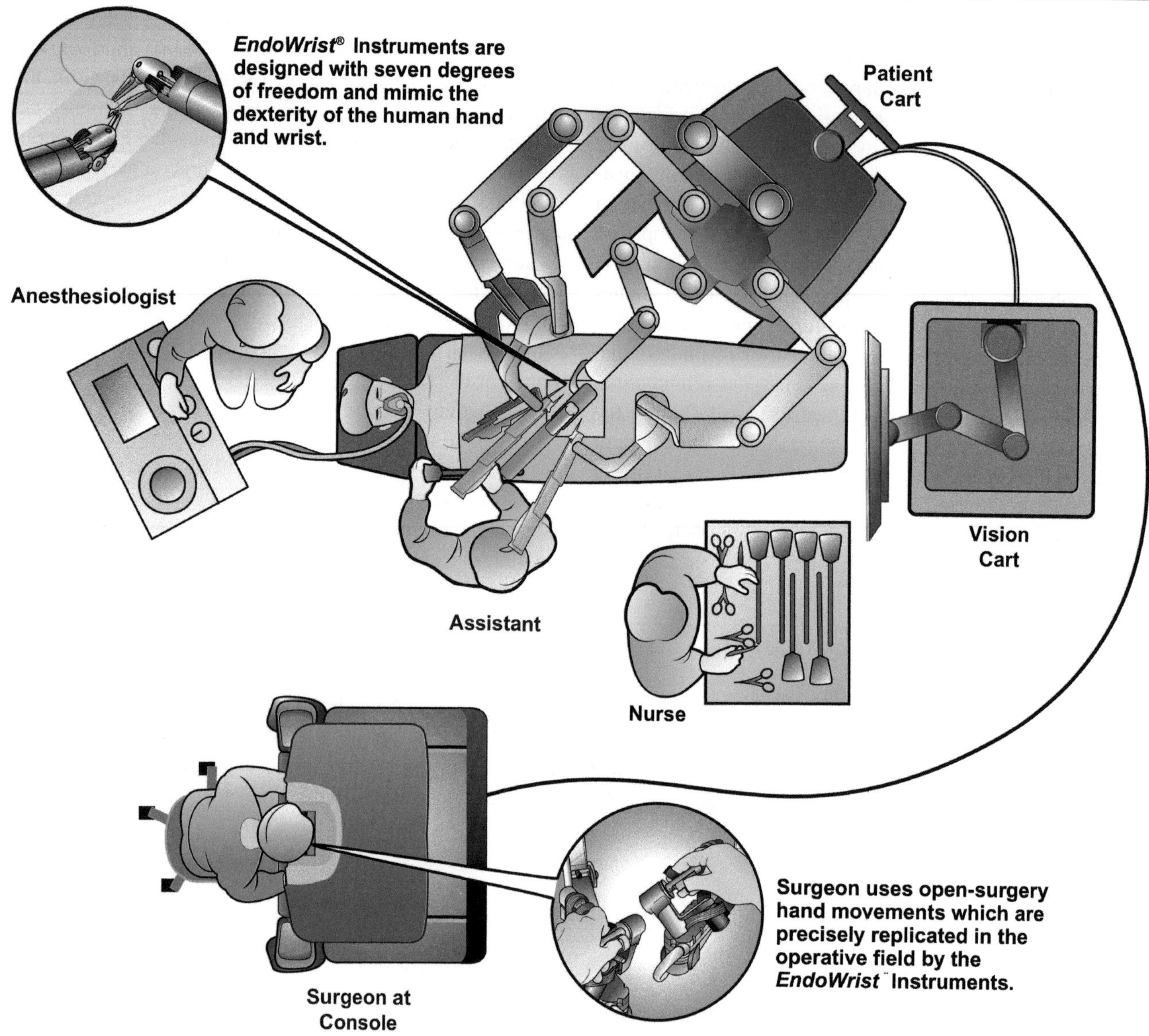

Fig. 74.3 General operating room set-up for the da Vinci® surgical system

The Robotic-Assisted Laparoscopic Hysterectomy (RALH)

Hysterectomy continues to be the most common gynecologic surgery in the United States. An estimated 600,000 women each year undergo hysterectomies for benign indications, most commonly uterine myomas, endometriosis, and uterine prolapse [12]. The goal of laparoscopic hysterectomy and laparoscopic-assisted vaginal hysterectomy is to convert abdominal hysterectomies to endoscopic ones [13]. A cross-sectional analysis of national discharge data in 2005 found that the most common route of hysterectomy was total abdominal hysterectomy (64 %), followed by vaginal hysterectomy (22 %), and laparoscopic hysterectomy (14 %) [14].

Though vaginal hysterectomy is the optimal and most minimally invasive approach, the inability to visualize the abdominal-pelvic anatomy is a disadvantage. The benefit of laparoscopic hysterectomy is the ability to visualize *in situ* the abdominal and pelvic pathology prior to removing the uterus and adnexa, if needed.

Different studies have compared laparoscopic hysterectomy with and without robotic assistance [15, 16]. It has been shown that the use of the robot is more time consuming and it could also be more expensive, however surgical outcomes are the same, except for a higher rate of vaginal cuff dehiscence associated with robotic assistance. In our experience, the robotic platform can be regarded as an "another instrument for laparoscopic surgery". It potentially allows to master suturing in lesser time and is less tiring when operating on obese patients instead of adhering to the old fashioned exploratory laparotomy. It is simply another tool available to the gynecologic surgeon.

Patient Positioning

Similar to laparoscopic-assisted hysterectomy, preparing for a robotic-assisted hysterectomy begins with safe and appropriate patient positioning. The operating room table should be configured for gynecological procedures, with the ability to lower the bottom of the bed. A gel pad or another non-slip device should be placed between the operating room table and the patient in order to prevent the patient from sliding down after steep Trendelenburg has been established. Obese patients are especially prone to shift down the operating room table during surgery. This movement is problematic for both uterine manipulation and surgical field displacement. Shoulder braces should be avoided because of the risk of brachial plexus nerve injuries.

For the RALH, the patient is placed in low dorsal lithotomy position with arms padded and tucked to the side of the table (Fig. 74.4). Proper padding of pressure points prior to draping is extremely important to prevent tissue and nerve injury especially during longer procedures. A Foley catheter is placed to drain the bladder. A nasogastric tube (NGT) or orogastric tube (OGT) is placed to decompress the stomach and reduce the risk of visceral injury upon entry. Antibiotic prophylaxis should be given prior to the start of the case, cefazolin 1–2 g IV or clindamycin 600 mg IV plus gentamycin 1.5 mg/kg IV for patients with penicillin allergies [17]. Though it is a laparoscopic procedure, the RALH is still considered a surgical wound Class 2, a clean-contaminated wound.

Uterine Manipulation

An exam under anesthesia is performed to reassess the size and position of the uterus, to sound the uterus, and to measure the size of the cervix. The cervix size is assessed visually or with a hand held cervical sizer. There are several commonly used uterine manipulators which have a colpotomy ring that is essential for a successful colpotomy at the end of the laparoscopic hysterectomy procedure. The VCare® Uterine Manipulator (ConMed Corporation, Utica, NY) and the RUMI (Cooper Surgical, Trumbull, CT) are two examples. The VCare® is a disposable unit with its own colpotomy ring attached to a handle and vaginal occludes (Fig. 74.5). The KOH colpotomizer system® incorporates the RUMI handle, a choice of different sized colpotomy rings, and a selection of different sized tips. A vaginal balloon pneumo-occluder should also be assembled on the RUMI® uterine manipulator and inflated in the vagina to maintain pneumoperitoneum as the colpotomy is made (Fig. 74.6).

Laparoscopic Entry and Port Placement

After the uterine manipulator is placed and the colpotomy ring sits securely in the cervicovaginal junction, the surgeon can return to the patient's abdomen and establish pneumoperitoneum by various methods. A 12 mm port (Fig. 74.7. location A) is usually placed at the umbilicus, or higher depending on the size of the uterus, after pneumoperitoneum is obtained to 15 mmHg. A survey of the abdomen and pelvis is performed, noting the liver edge, gallbladder, fundus of the stomach, and appendix, in order to thoroughly search for extragenital endometriosis. Two 8 mm robotic trocars are placed bilaterally 10 cm lateral to the umbilicus and 2 cm

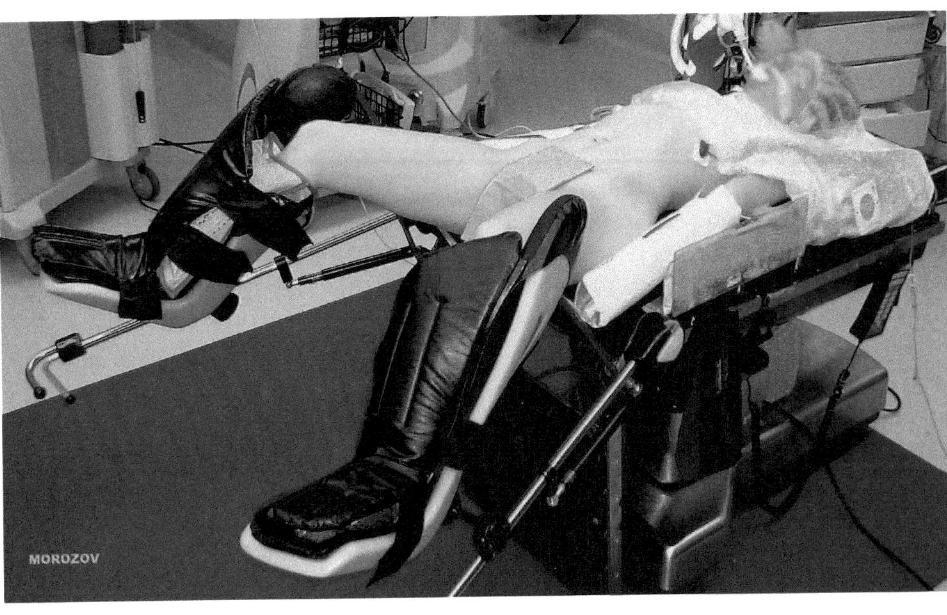

Fig. 74.4 Patient positioning for gynecologic robotic procedures. The patient is positioned in dorsal lithotomy using Allen stirrups with arms tucked to the side. Later on, steep Trendelenburg will be used

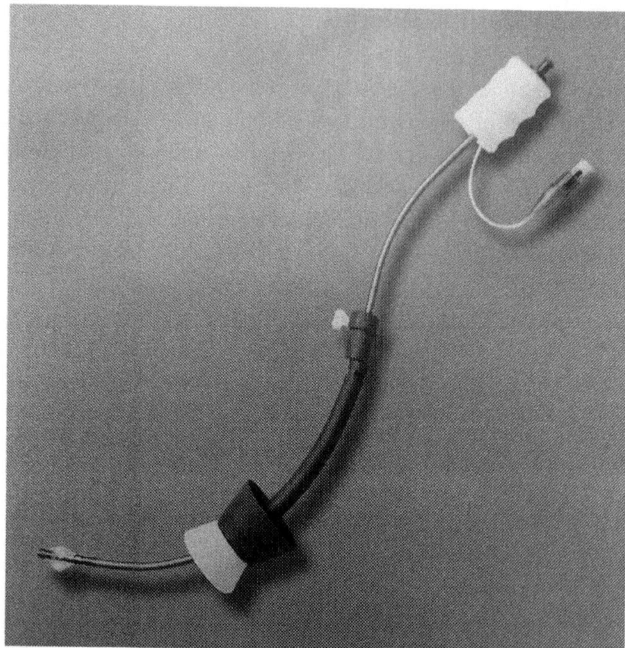

Fig. 74.5 VCare®, a commonly used uterine manipulator with a colpotomy ring

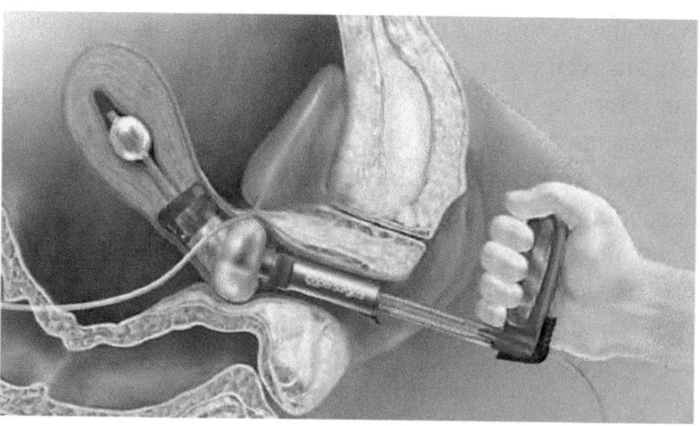

Fig. 74.6 RUMI®, a commonly used uterine manipulator with a colpotomy ring

above the level of the uterine fundus (Fig. 74.7. location B) under direct laparoscopic visualization. An accessory 5 mm trocar is placed between the umbilical port and the lateral port 3 cm caudal to the umbilicus (Fig. 74.7. location C). When the fourth robotic arm is used, that trocar is placed at least 8 cm lateral to the umbilicus and 8 cm cephalad to the right robotic trocar.

The operating room table is lowered, and the patient is placed in the maximum amount of Trendelenburg to allow optimal visualization with the bowel falling away from the pelvis into the upper abdomen. After the final degree of Trendelenburg is established and the patient-side robotic cart has been docked, no further table movements can be made.

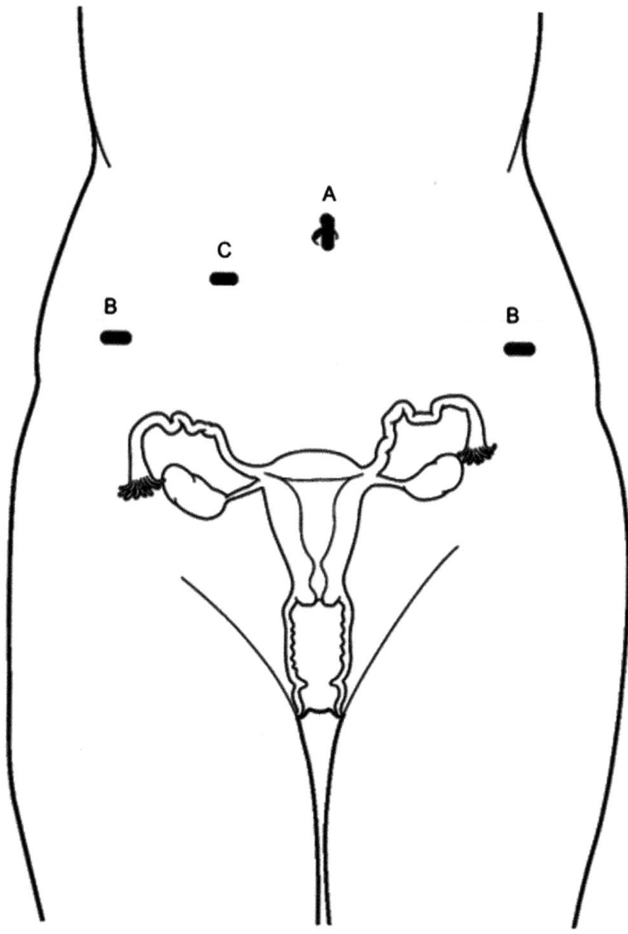

Fig. 74.7 Robotic port site placement for gynecologic surgery

The average set up time, defined as the time between switching from laparoscopy to the robot, is 16–18 min for an experienced OR team. This process includes docking the sterile draped robot, switching trocars, changing the camera, and attaching the surgical instruments. Disassembly time is 2.5–3 min on average [18, 19].

Docking the Bedside Robot

The traditional docking of the robotic cart for gynecological procedures is between the patient's legs. The advantage of this docking position is that the camera and working arms are placed in the same axis as the patient's torso. However, this position poses challenges for gynecologic procedures, as the bedside assistant is unable to access to the vagina and provide good uterine manipulation and exposure.

An alternative for gynecologic surgery is side docking at a 45° angle from the midline, with the central column of the robotic cart and the camera arm in line with the patient's contra lateral shoulder. This configuration allows the bedside assistant easier access to the uterine manipulator and the vagina, should the uterine manipulator need to be adjusted during the surgery or if there is difficulty removing the uterus after the hysterectomy is completed. It also provides room for an intraoperative rectovaginal exam if needed to localize and palpate endometriotic nodules, in an attempt to overcome one of the drawbacks of the current robotic platform: the lack of haptics. This is an important disadvantage when considering treatment and resection of endometriotic nodules in the rectovaginal space using robotic assistance. The fibrotic tissue, consequence of severe disease, cannot be felt in the rectovaginal septum.

Once the patient-side robotic cart is docked, the robotic arms can be attached to the 8 mm trocars and the robotic endoscope and instruments can be inserted. Careful attention should be given to the robotic arms to prevent them from contacting the patient directly. Crush injuries to the patient may occur unintentionally if the robot is improperly positioned.

Switching the Laparoscopic Camera to the Robotic Scope

The endoscope typically used for gynecologic procedures, including hysterectomy, is the 12 mm 0-degree laparoscope that is introduced through the 12 mm umbilical port. There is a 30° laparoscope that is helpful for urogynecology cases in the lower pelvis. As in traditional laparoscopy, the camera and light source should be carefully monitored and never left directly on drapes in order to avoid fires and thermal injury to the patient. If the tip of the robotic endoscope becomes dirty or fogged during surgery, it should be removed from its robotic arm and cleaned with a proper solution and lens cloth in order to prevent scratching of the optics. Wiping the tip of the robotic endoscope on internal organs should not be done because the robotic endoscope is significantly hotter than standard endoscopes and will cause thermal damage to the viscera.

EndoWrist Instruments

The da Vinci® Robotic System has a selection of 8 mm EndoWrist® instruments for gynecologic surgery. Most of the robotic instruments (Fig. 74.8) have been adapted from traditional laparoscopic equipment. Among the most common and useful for RALH procedures are the monopolar curved scissors, fenestrated bipolar forceps, tenaculum forceps, mega needle driver, Gyrus PK® grasper (Olympus Company, Southborough, MA) (not pictured), and Harmonic scalpel® (Ethicon Endo-Surgery, Cincinnati, OH) (not pictured). These instruments can be snapped into the robotic 8 mm ports.

Robotic-Assisted Laparoscopic Hysterectomy Technique

The RALH technique is similar to the open hysterectomy. Initially, the round ligament is identified, desiccated with bipolar forceps at 25-35 W current and cut with the monopolar scissors (Fig. 74.9). The anterior leaf of the broad ligament is then incised towards the bladder and the vesicouterine reflection (bladder flap) is created. If the ovaries are to be removed, the infundibulopelvic (IP) ligament is identified along with the ipsilateral ureter, isolated and desiccated with bipolar electrosurgery or ultrasonic energy and cut with shears. The laparoscopic surgeon should skeletonize the ureter and uterine vessels, so their courses are properly identified and injures avoided (Fig. 74.10a, b). Ureterolysis is performed after proper identification of the ureter as it enters the pelvis at the pelvic brim. The retroperitoneum is then opened in the ovarian fossa superiorly to the ureter with aid of the CO2 laser. Hydrodissection is then accomplished with the Nezhat-Dorsey probe which is also used for blunt dissection if needed in case of dense scar tissue in this area. The ureter is then pushed inferiorly from the dissection area to a safe location after hydrodissection is completed. Small bleeders are cauterized at the same time dissection is performed with the CO_2 laser.

If the ovaries are to be conserved, then the utero-ovarian ligament is desiccated and cut. The anterior leaf of the broad ligament is then fully incised, completing the vesicouterine reflection anteriorly. The vesicouterine reflection is tented up using fenestrated bipolar and the bladder is gently dissected off the lower uterine segment and cervix using sharp dissection with the Endoshears or bluntly. The tendinous attachments between the bladder, cervix, and upper vagina may be dissected or desiccated (Fig. 74.11).

The uterine arteries are identified and skeletonized, allowing the ureters to fall further laterally for safe vessel sealing and division of the vessels. The cardinal ligaments are subsequently desiccated and divided. The uterine manipulator is helpful in retracting the uterus in the opposite direction, facilitating exposure of the uterine vessels. After the uterine arteries are divided, the bedside assistant performing the uterine manipulation should push the uterine manipulator cephalad to accentuate the edges of the colpotomy cup (Fig. 74.12). Deep infiltrating endometriosis can be dissected off the retrocervical areas with the CO2 laser and the Nezhat-Dorsey probe. Very careful dissection is performed specially if bowel adhesions are encountered.

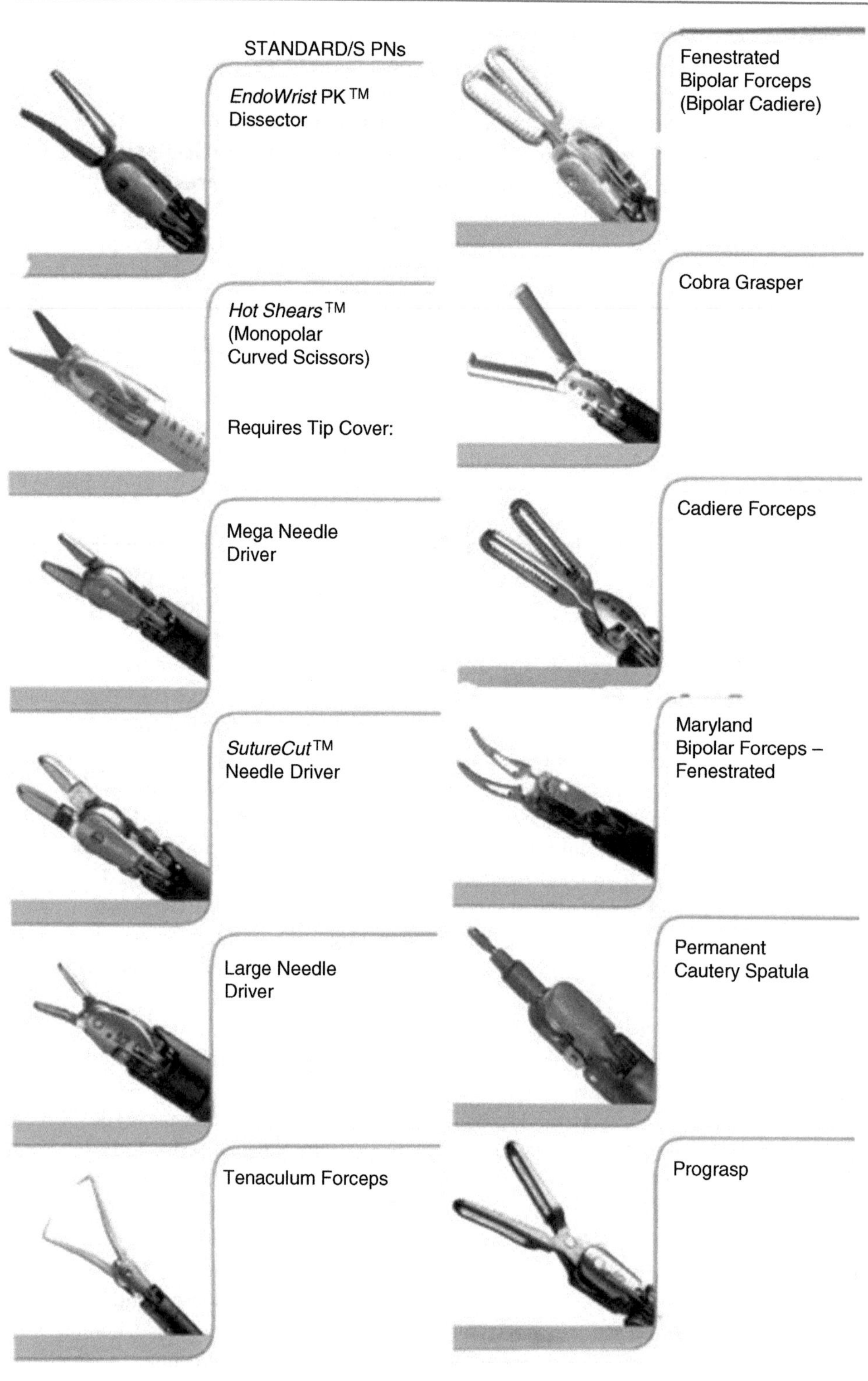

Fig. 74.8 Selection of EndoWrist® instruments

At this point, the experience of the surgeon plays a major role in order to avoid bowel injuries.

The colpotomy is performed with the monopolar hot shears at 30 W cutting current. The uterus (and ovaries) can then be pulled through the vaginal cuff or if too large, it may be removed through extracorporeal morcellation in the vagina. Vaginal morcellation is performed with a long knife handle and a #10 blade, making circumferential incisions into the uterus while pulling outwards on the cervix. It is important to always keep the blade inside the myometrium and away from the surrounding vagina. A self retained retractor (Alexis® retractor, Applied Medical, CA) can also be used to protect the vaginal walls during morcellation.

If supracervical hysterectomy is requested or vaginal access is limited, morcellation can be done through the anterior abdominal wall in a similar fashion.

A mini-laparotomy is performed (no more than 3–4 cm long) and a self retained retractor also used for exposure plus or minus a specimen bag for contained morcellation. Lahey clamps are used to exteriorize the uterus and extracorporeal morcellation is then performed in the same manner previously described. In light of the current controversy regarding uterine morcellation and the possibility of diagnosing a leiomyosarcoma, we recommend against the use of electromechanical devices for intracorporeal morcellation [20, 21].

If the uterus is small enough to be left in the vagina just below the vaginal cuff, then it can serve as a pneumo-occluder

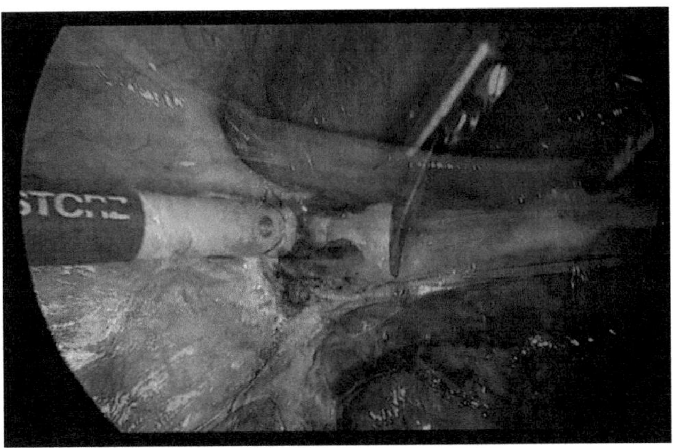

Fig. 74.9 The round ligament is identified, desiccated and cut with the monopolar scissors

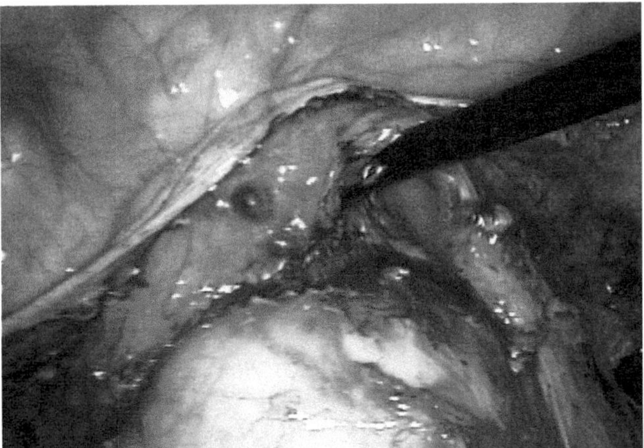

Fig. 74.11 Vesicouterine space after complete dissection

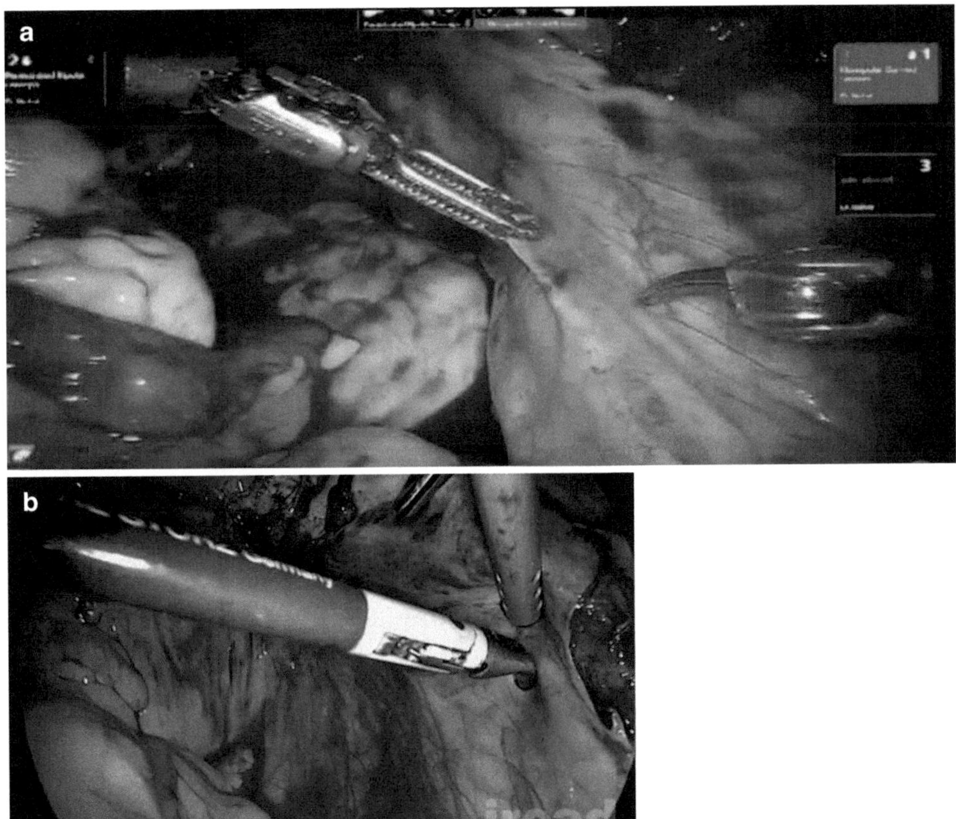

Fig. 74.10 (**a**, **b**) Ureterolysis. It is important to skeletonize the ureter in order to properly identify its course

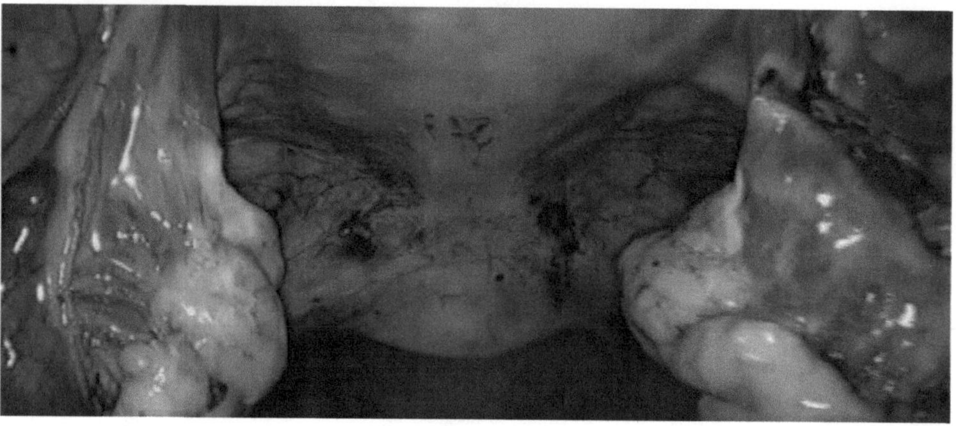

Fig. 74.12 The colpotomy cup edges were accentuated with the correct placement and use of the uterine manipulator, allowing good exposure for colpotomy

or the balloon occluder can be replaced into the vagina after removing the specimen. Irrigation of the abdomen and pelvis and control of bleeding are performed prior to closing the vaginal cuff. Minor bleeding at the cuff can be controlled with cuff closure.

Excessive desiccation at the cuff should be avoided in order to prevent thermal damage to tissue and poor tissue healing which may lead to cuff breakdown and vaginal cuff dehiscence. The vaginal cuff can be securely closed with 2–0 Vicryl on at CT-1 needle via interrupted figure of eight stitches or with a running stitch and use of Lapra-ty® suture clips (Ethicon Endo-surgery, Cincinnati, OH).

Once the vaginal cuff is closed, the pelvis is irrigated a final time and examined for hemostasis. Desufflation of the abdomen and reinsufflation is another method of examining hemostasis under a physiologic lower intraabdominal pressure. For vaginal cuff support and prolapse prevention, the Moskowitz procedure is performed. The uterosacral ligaments are identified and a string suture is placed. Firstly, it transverses the right uterosacral ligament, then goes to the cardinal ligament under the uterine artery, followed by a very small bite posteriorly into the rectovaginal fascia, then over the left cardinal fascia and finally concludes its course at the left uterosacral ligament. An extracorporeal tie brings the cardinal ligaments, uterosacral ligaments and posterior vaginal fascia together in the midline. It provides excellent support for the vaginal cuff apex.

Cystoscopy at the conclusion of the hysterectomy is routinely performed to confirm the patency of the ureters and integrity of the bladder. Rates of bladder and ureteral injury during laparoscopic hysterectomy have been reported to be as high as 2.9 and 1.75 %, respectively [22]. One ampule of indigo carmine (1 ampule, 40 mg in 5 ml) is injected by IV approximately 5–10 min prior to the cystoscopy to aid in visualizing the patency of the ureters. If indigo carmine is not available, 200 mg of over the counter phenazopyridine (Pyridium®) given 30 min prior to procedure exerts the same effect. The dye should be visualized through both ureteral orifices. The bladder should also be inspected for sutures and thermal injuries.

Port sites larger than 10 mm should be closed to prevent trocar site herniation. These sites can be laparoscopically closed with a fascial closure device such as a Carter-Thomason CloseSure® System (Cooper Surgical, Trumbull, CT). A 0-Vicryl suture in a UR-6 needle can also be used for closure of the umbilicus fascia if the subcutaneous fat layer is not too thick, allowing proper identification of the fascia layer. The skin can be closed with Dermabond® (Ethicon Inc., Menlo Park, CA) or a subcutaneous stitch using 4–0 Monocryl suture.

Postoperative Care

The average length of stay for a robotic hysterectomy is less than 24 h. After the surgery and patient's recovery in PACU are completed, the patient can be restarted on a clear or regular diet if she is not experiencing nausea. Patients may ambulate on postoperative day 0. The Foley catheter can be removed immediately postoperatively, but more often it is left in the bladder overnight and removed the next morning. The patient can be discharged to home on postoperative day 1 with precautions for vaginal bleeding, vaginal discharge, abdominal pain, and fever. Six to eight weeks is recommended before the patient can resume vaginal intercourse to allow the vaginal apex to heal properly.

Complications of Robotic Surgery

According to Jonsdottir et al., the rates of intraoperative and minor postoperative complications have significantly decreased with the RALH procedure versus abdominal hysterectomy, while there was no difference in overall mean costs [23]. Comparing RALH to laparoscopic hysterectomy in a meta-analysis, the estimated blood loss, length of postoperative

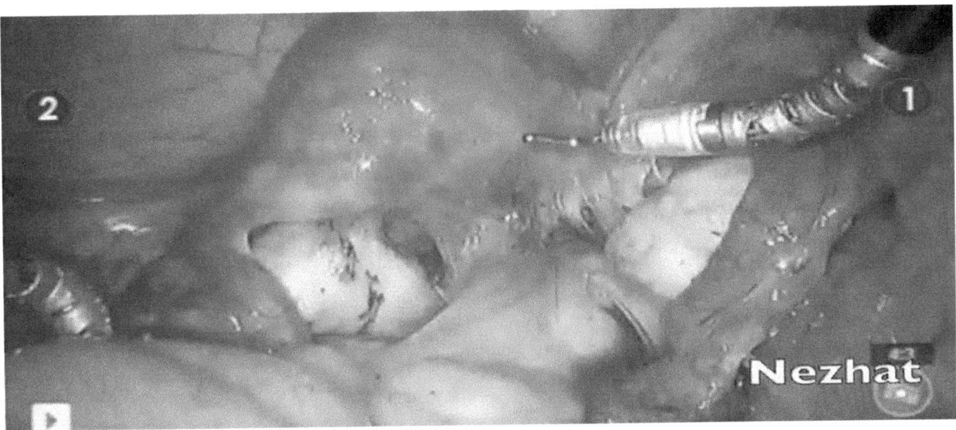

Fig. 74.13 Example of pelvic adhesions distorting the normal pelvic anatomy and increasing the risk of complications

hospital stay, and complications were comparable [24]. One perioperative complication found more frequently with both RALH and laparoscopic hysterectomy is vaginal cuff dehiscence with small bowel evisceration.

Though vaginal cuff dehiscence is rare, it is a serious and potentially life-threatening condition. Incidences of vaginal cuff dehiscence after robotic hysterectomy have been reported as high as 4.1 % (95 % CI 2.3–5.8 %) [25]. However, more recent literature suggests a lower incidence in laparoscopic hysterectomies 0.75 % (95 % CI 0.09–1.4), but the incidence is higher than that of abdominal 0.38 % (95 % CI 0.16–0.61) and vaginal 0.11 % (95 % CI 0.0–0.32) hysterectomies [26]. This difference suggests that vaginal cuff dehiscence may be occurring due to the use of electro-surgery to perform the colpotomy. The electro-surgery creates thermal cuff tissue damage and the devascularized tissue delays or even halts wound healing.

Ureter complications are another potential problem with laparoscopic and robotic-assisted hysterectomy. The ureters are commonly injured at the level of the IP ligament when this is transected prior to performing an oophorectomy. Another potential location for injury is where the ureters travel under the uterine arteries during uterine artery ligation, at the level of the uterosacral ligaments and during ureter insertion at the bladder dome when creating the vesicouterine space. If the anatomy is distorted due to the presence of leiomyomas or endometriosis, or adhesions from previous surgeries or history of pelvic inflammatory disease (Fig. 74.13), the risk for ureteral injury is even higher.

Most ureteral injuries are not identified or even suspected without cystoscopy [27–29]. Prompt recognition and management is essential in order to prevent further sequelae and patient morbitity, including multiple surgeries and organ loss. From our experience, we strongly recommended routine cystoscopy after every laparoscopic or robotic-assisted laparoscopic hysterectomy.

When dealing with endometriosis, prevention and recognition are the most important steps in order to avoid serious postoperative complications. Due to the severe adhesion formation that can be encountered, knowing the pelvic anatomy is crucial. Identification of the pelvic organs needs to be accomplished prior to attempting lysis of adhesions, ligation of vessels or treatment of the disease. Then, after the procedure is completed, we inspect the pelvic once again and perform cystoscopy and proctoscopy as indicated.

Conclusion

There is a clear trend in surgery, driven by patient demand, to perform less invasive approaches to common gynecologic procedures such as hysterectomy. The da Vinci® Robotic Surgical System enables gynecologic surgeons to convert complex cases such as hysterectomy, myomectomy, incontinence, microsurgical tubal anastomosis, and endometriosis cases, to endoscopic ones. Performing endoscopic surgery on the da Vinci® Robotic Surgical System has several advantages over traditional laparoscopy, such as high definition 3-dimensional visual imaging, greater dexterity with more degrees of freedom, and intuitive hand movements, which provide less-experienced laparoscopists with the confidence and technological support to master difficult endoscopic suturing and knot tying.

The advent of robotic surgery has enabled conversion of even more complex gynecologic procedures, including radical hysterectomy and fistula repair, especially in obese patients, to minimally invasive techniques [30–34]. This new technology may allow lower volume gynecologic surgeons to offer their patients procedures with clear health advantages – less pain, shorter hospital stay, fewer complications, and earlier return to activity and work [34].

References

1. Rosheim ME. Leonardo's lost robots. Berlin: Springer; 2006.
2. Shah A and Schipper E. A History of Telepresence Surgery. In: Nezhat's video-assisted and robotic-assisted laparoscopy and hysteroscopy, Chapter 23.1, 4th ed. 2013. p. 629–31.
3. Satava RM. Robotic surgery: from past to future – a personal journey. Surg Clin North Am. 2003;83:1491–500. xii
4. Cadiere GB, Himpens J, Germay O, et al. Feasibility of robotic laparoscopic surgery: 146 cases. World J Surg. 2001;25:1467–77.
5. Nezhat C, Hajhosseini B, King LP. Robotic-assisted laparoscopic treatment of bowel, bladder, and ureteral endometriosis. JSLS J Soc Laparoendosc Surg/Soc Laparoendosc Surg. 2011;15:387–92.
6. Intuitive Surgical Inc. Frequently asked questions. 2015. Accessed 20 Jan 2015, at http://www.intuitivesurgical.com/company/faqs.html.
7. Westerband A, Van De Water J, Amzallag M, et al. Cardiovascular changes during laparoscopic cholecystectomy. Surg Gynecol Obstet. 1992;175:535–8.
8. Hirvonen EA, Nuutinen LS, Kauko M. Hemodynamic changes due to Trendelenburg positioning and pneumoperitoneum during laparoscopic hysterectomy. Acta anaesthesiol Scandinavica. 1995;39:949–55.
9. Irgau I, Koyfman Y, Tikellis JI. Elective intraoperative intracranial pressure monitoring during laparoscopic cholecystectomy. Arch Surg. 1995;130:1011–3.
10. Sullivan MJ, Frost EA, Lew MW. Anesthetic care of the patient for robotic surgery. Middle East J Anesthesiol. 2008;19:967–82.
11. Sroga J, Patel SD, Falcone T. Robotics in reproductive medicine. Front Biosci J Virtual Library. 2008;13:1308–17.
12. Whiteman MK, SD H, Jamieson DJ, et al. Inpatient hysterectomy surveillance in the United States, 2000-2004. Am J Obstet Gynecol. 2008;198:34 e1–7.
13. Reich H and Katz A. Total Laparoscopic Hysterectomy–indications, techniques, and outcomes. In: Nezhat's video-assisted and robotic-assisted laparoscopy and hysteroscopy, Chapter 14, 4th ed. 2013. p. 370–85.
14. Jacoby VL, Autry A, Jacobson G, Domush R, Nakagawa S, Jacoby A. Nationwide use of laparoscopic hysterectomy compared with abdominal and vaginal approaches. Obstet Gynecol. 2009;114:1041–8.
15. Reynolds RK, Advincula AP. Robot-assisted laparoscopic hysterectomy: technique and initial experience. Am J Surg. 2006;191:555–60.
16. Pasic RP, Rizzo JA, Fang H, Ross S, Moore M, Gunnarsson C. Comparing robot-assisted with conventional laparoscopic hysterectomy: impact on cost and clinical outcomes. J Minim Invasive Gynecol. 2010;17(6):730–8.
17. ACOG Committee on Practice Bulletins--Gynecology. ACOG practice bulletin No. 104: antibiotic prophylaxis for gynecologic procedures. Obstet Gynecol. 2009;113:1180–9.
18. Nezhat C, Saberi NS, Shahmohamady B, Nezhat F. Robotic-assisted laparoscopy in gynecological surgery. JSLS J Soc Laparoendosc Surg/Soc Laparoendosc Surg. 2006;10:317–20.
19. Nezhat C, Lavie O, Hsu S, Watson J, Barnett O, Lemyre M. Robotic-assisted laparoscopic myomectomy compared with standard laparoscopic myomectomy – a retrospective matched control study. Fertil Steril. 2009;91:556–9.
20. Kho KA, Nezhat CH. Evaluating the risks of electric uterine morcellation. JAMA. 2014;311(9):905–6.
21. Kho KA, Shin JH, Nezhat C. Vaginal extraction of large uteri with the Alexis retractor. J Minim Invasive Gynecol. 2009;16(5):616–7.
22. Gilmour DT, Das S, Flowerdew G. Rates of urinary tract injury from gynecologic surgery and the role of intraoperative cystoscopy. Obstet Gynecol. 2006;107:1366–72.
23. Jonsdottir GM, Jorgensen S, Cohen SL, et al. Increasing minimally invasive hysterectomy: effect on cost and complications. Obstet Gynecol. 2011;117:1142–9.
24. Sarlos D, Kots LA. Robotic versus laparoscopic hysterectomy: a review of recent comparative studies. Curr Opin Obstet Gynecol. 2011;23:283–8.
25. Kho RM, Akl MN, Cornella JL, Magtibay PM, Wechter ME, Magrina JF. Incidence and characteristics of patients with vaginal cuff dehiscence after robotic procedures. Obstet Gynecol. 2009;114:231–5.
26. Hur HC, Donnellan N, Mansuria S, Barber RE, Guido R, Lee T. Vaginal cuff dehiscence after different modes of hysterectomy. Obstet Gynecol. 2011;118:794–801.
27. McMaster-Fay RA, Jones RA. Laparoscopic hysterectomy and ureteric injury: a comparison of the initial 275 cases and the last 1000 cases using staples. Gynecol Surg. 2006;3:118–21.
28. Sharon A, Auslander R, Brandes-Klein O, et al. Cystoscopy after total and subtotal laparoscopic hysterectomy: the value of a routine cystoscopy. Gynecol Surg. 2006;3:122–7.
29. Wu HH, Yang PY, Yeh GP, et al. The detection of ureteral injuries after hysterectomy. J Minim Invasive Gynecol. 2006;13:403–8.
30. Falcone T, Goldberg JM. Robotics in gynecology. Surg Clin North Am. 2003;83:1483–9. xii
31. Chang-Jackson SC, Acholonu Jr UC, Nezhat FR. Robotic-assisted laparoscopic repair of a vesicouterine fistula. JSLS J Soc Laparoendosc Surg/Soc Laparoendosc Surg. 2011;15:339–42.
32. Nezhat C, Xie J, Aldape D, Balassiano E, Soliemannjad R, Nezhat F. Use of Laparoscopic modified nerve-sparing radical hysterectomy for the treatment of extensive endometriosis. Cureus. 6(1):e159. doi:10.7759/cureus.159.
33. Nezhat FR, Sirota I. Perioperative outcomes of robotic assisted laparoscopic surgery versus conventional laparoscopy surgery for advanced-stage endometriosis. JSLS. 2014;18(4):e2014.00094.
34. Nezhat C, Lavie O, Lemyre M, et al. Laparoscopic hysterectomy with and without a robot: stanford experience. JSJS. 2009; 13:125–8.

Hysterectomy Techniques for Obese Patients

75

Amanda M. Hill, Lindsay Clark Donat, and Masoud Azodi

Introduction

Obesity poses certain challenges and risks to patients and surgeons in the perioperative period. Patients with obesity often have other comorbidities, which increase the risks of surgery and anesthesia. The increased adipose tissue makes positioning and surgical exposure more difficult. Patients are also at higher risk of cardiopulmonary events in the postoperative period.

The use of a robotic system such as the Da Vinci Surgical System (Intuitive Surgical, Sunnyvale, CA, USA) affords possible advantages when used for hysterectomy in obese patients [1–4]. While traditional laparoscopy can be ergonomically challenging, the robotic system allows the surgeon to sit comfortably at the console, providing improved ergonomics [5]. Robotic surgery also conveys the advantage of a third arm, controlled by the primary surgeon, which aids in visualization despite the increased adipose tissue obscuring the surgical field. Patients experience faster recovery when compared to open surgery, which is especially important in the obese population [6]. Women are able to ambulate and tolerate a regular diet more rapidly, decreasing the risk of venous thromboembolism (VTE) and ileus.

This chapter will outline the challenges, advantages, and additional considerations in the preoperative, intraoperative, and postoperative periods in patients with obesity undergoing robotically-assisted hysterectomy.

A.M. Hill
Department of Obstetrics and Gynecology, Yale University, Bridgeport Hospital, Bridgeport, CT, USA
e-mail: AmandaHillMD@gmail.com

L.C. Donat
Deptarment of Obstetrics and Gynecology, Rhode Island Hospital, Warwick, RI, USA
e-mail: Lclarkdonat@gmail.com

Masoud Azodi (✉)
Department of Obstetrics and Gynecology, Yale University, Yale New Haven Hospital, New Haven, CT, USA
e-mail: Masoud.Azodi@yale.edu

Preoperative Considerations

Like all surgical procedures, proper patient selection is an important consideration when planning to perform a robotic--assisted laparoscopic hysterectomy. Patients with obesity often have other comorbidities that must be considered when deciding on treatment options and optimally managed before proceeding with surgery. Typical indications for benign hysterectomy such as abnormal uterine bleeding, pelvic pain from adenomyosis or endometriosis, and even endometrial hyperplasia may be more appropriately managed medically (Table 75.1). It is important to weigh the risks and benefits of surgery in these patients to avoid potential complications of anesthesia and recovery. That being said, studies have shown no increased risk of surgical complications in obese patients compared with those of normal BMI [4, 7].

Obesity is associated with cardiovascular, pulmonary, and metabolic conditions. Patients with obesity are more likely to suffer from hypertension, coronary and peripheral vascular disease, ventricular hypertrophy, obstructive sleep apnea (OSA), hypoventilation due to restrictive or obstructive respiratory syndromes, dyslipidemias, diabetes mellitus, and decreased exercise tolerance [7–9]. It is essential that patients are evaluated by their medical doctor for a medical risk assessment prior to proceeding with elective surgery. They should also see a cardiologist and/or pulmonologist if they suffer from more severe cardiopulmonary disease or if specific conditions are uncovered during the preoperative evaluations. These specialists can offer recommendations to optimize the patient's clinical condition and thus reduce the risk of adverse perioperative cardiopulmonary outcomes.

Patients may also be unaware of existing medical problems due to lack of screening or if they have not seen a primary care physician. All patients with obesity planning elective surgery should be seen by a primary care physician to have appropriate screening tests prior to surgery. It is also beneficial for the patient to have a preoperative assessment with the anesthesiologist that will be caring for

I. Alkatout, L. Mettler (eds.), *Hysterectomy*, DOI 10.1007/978-3-319-22497-8_75

Table 75.1 Alternatives to hysterectomy

Diagnosis	Alternative to hysterectomy
Abnormal uterine bleeding	
Endometrial polyps	Hysteroscopic polypectomy
	Global endometrial ablation
Submucosal leiomyoma	Hysteroscopic myomectomy
	Global endometrial ablation
Ovulatory dysfunction	Oral contraceptive pills
	Depo medroxyprogesteroneacetate
	Levonorgestrel intrauterine system
	Leuprolide
Endometrial dysfunction (heavy, regular bleeding with no structural pathology)	Oral contraceptive pills
	Depo medroxyprogesteroneacetate
	Levonorgestrel intrauterine system
	Leuprolide
	Tranexamic acid
	Global endometrial ablation
Dysmenorrhea / Adenomyosis	NSAIDs
	Oral contraceptive pills
	Depo medroxyprogesteroneacetate
	Levonorgestrel intrauterine system
	Leuprolide
Endometriosis	NSAIDs
	Oral contraceptive pills
	Depo medroxyprogesterone acetate
	Levonorgestrel intrauterine system
	Leuprolide
Leiomyoma	Myomectomy
	Radiofrequency ablation
	Uterine artery embolization
	Magnetic resonance guided focused ultrasound
Endometrial hyperplasia	Progestin therapy
	Medroxyprogesterone acetate
	Megestrol acetate
	Levonorgestrel intrauterine system
	Aromatase inhibitors
	Hysteroscopy resection

them. The anesthesiologist may request additional tests or evaluation by specialists in order to prepare a safe plan to manage the patient's cardiopulmonary needs in the perioperative period.

Routine preoperative assessment should include a clinical evaluation, indicated routine blood work (complete blood count, blood type and antibody screen, basic metabolic panel), electrocardiogram, and chest x-ray [7–10]. Some authors suggest that routine chest x-ray is not necessary as it does not alter perioperative management [7, 8]. However, most recommendations call for chest x-ray in those over the age of 50, those with known heart or lung disease, or those with abnormal physical exam findings. Electrocardiogram is recommended for all patients with obesity given that obesity is a risk factor for heart disease [7, 8].

Patients with known cardiac disease or those with abnormal findings on routine preoperative assessment should be referred to a cardiologist for further testing such as echocardiography or a stress test. Routine echocardiogram and stress test are not recommended due to the low rate of abnormalities and lack of consequence on perioperative management [8].

Impaired pulmonary mechanisms due to obesity increase the risk of complications such as pneumonia, respiratory failure, pulmonary hypertension, and pulmonary embolism after surgery [9]. It also makes mechanical ventilation more difficult due to decreased compliance and increased intra--abdominal pressure leading to reduced lung volumes [9]. Patients with known pulmonary disease should be evaluated by their pulmonologist preoperatively. Polysomnography (or sleep study) should be strongly considered due to the high prevalence (up to 40 %) of OSA in patients with obesity [8]. CPAP should ideally be initiated 6 weeks prior to surgery [8]. Routine spirometry is not recommended, unless COPD is suspected [8, 9]. Abnormal pulmonary function tests, when severe, can prompt planned intensive care unit admission [7].

As with any patient, patients with obesity undergoing robotic-assisted laparoscopic hysterectomy should have complete preoperative counseling including the indication for surgery, alternatives, and risks. The risk of complications related to the patient's underlying medical conditions should be clearly addressed, and special attention should be paid to risks of VTE and infectious complications, since obesity increases these risks [4, 9]. There is also an increased risk of conversion to an open procedure in obese patients [4]. Bowel preparation may be advisable to decompress the bowel, improving visualization of the surgical field [3]. Patients should have a good understanding and realistic expectations of the preparation for and recovery from surgery.

When operating on morbidly obese patients, the surgeon should be aware of the resources and limitations of the facility in which they operate. With the increasing prevalence of obesity, many hospitals and surgery centers are equipped with bariatric wheelchairs, lifts, and beds. The surgeon should be aware of the weight limits of the operating room tables and other special equipment required. Specially designed OR tables do exist in the case that a patient's weight exceeds the standard limit. However, some of these models have mobility limitations which could interfere with the degree of trendelenburg required for robotic-assisted laparoscopic hysterectomy. OR table accessories such as table extenders are often required for the obese patient. Most robotic-assisted laparoscopic hysterectomies will be done in lithotomy position using stirrups. The weight limit of the Basic Stirrups and Yellofins® Stirrups (Allen Medical Systems, Acton, MA) is 350 pounds (159 kilograms), while the Yellofins® Elite Stirrups (Allen Medical Systems, Acton, MA) can accommodate a patient up to 500 pounds (227 kilograms). Specially designed for larger patients, Ultrafins® (Allen Medical Systems, Acton, MA) can be used for patients up to 800 pounds (363 kilograms). The OR staff should be alerted to the special needs of the obese or morbidly obese patient to adequately prepare for transporting, positioning, and transferring the patient to prevent delays or embarrassment for the patient.

Intraoperative Considerations

Obesity adds complexity to all aspects of robotic-assisted laparoscopic hysterectomy, including patient positioning, anesthesia, and exposure and visualization. Robotic-assisted laparoscopic hysterectomy has many measurable benefits over laparotomy, including shorter hospital stay, less pain, faster return to normal activity, decreased incidence of post--operative ileus, fever, and wound infection, and improved quality of life [1–3]. This is particularly true for the obese patient. In this section we will address how obesity affects various aspects of robotic-assisted laparoscopic hysterectomy and strategies for combating obesity in the operating room.

Anesthetic Considerations

Obesity significantly increases the risk of preexisting medical conditions in women undergoing robotic-assisted laparoscopic hysterectomy. Adults with a BMI > 40 are at increased risk of diabetes mellitus, hypercholesterolemia, hypertension, and asthma [7]. Women with obesity have an increased oxygen demand, increased cardiac output, larger stroke volumes, increased vascular resistance, increased cardiovascular work and ultimately increased risk of heart disease [11]. These women are also at increased risk for congestive heart failure, pulmonary edema, and arrhythmias. The pulmonary system is also affected by obesity. The respiratory function in obese patients is characterized by reduced functional vital capacity, functional residual capacity, total lung volume, total lung capacity, and expiratory reserve volume [4]. Compromises to lung function are compounded in women with OSA or obesity hyperventilation syndrome [4]. Additionally, obese patients are at higher risk for aspiration, due to increase gastric volumes and delayed emptying [12].

Due to these physiologic changes, induction of general anesthesia is a critical step in the care of the obese patient undergoing robotic-assisted laparoscopic hysterectomy. Women with obesity experience a more rapid desaturation during the apneic episodes that take place during induction of anesthesia [13]. This can be counteracted by optimal pre--oxygenation of obese patients [4]. With induction of anesthesia, ventilation with a facemask is considerably more difficult as a result of the decreased lung compliance and increased airway resistance associated with obesity. It is notable that most patients who tolerate induction of anesthesia and supine positioning are able to tolerate pneumoperitoneum and trendelenburg positioning [4].

During the procedure, the anesthesiologist may employ specific ventilation techniques. Pressure control ventilation may be used to improve the lung ventilation-perfusion ratio, generate higher flow peaks, and improve alveolar recruitment [14]. Additionally, higher inspiratory pressures may need to be used if ventilatory compliance is reduced secondary to the weight of abdominal viscera when the patient is in steep trendelenburg position [15]. Breaks from trendelenburg positioning may be necessary to prevent unsafe elevations of arterial carbon dioxide levels [4]. If the partial pressure of arterial carbon dioxide level increases, the robot should be undocked, the patient should be taken out of Trendelenburg position, and the abdomen should be desufflated. Once the partial pressure of arterial carbon dioxide level returns to normal, the patient can be placed back into Trendelenburg position, the abdomen can be insufflated, and the robot re-docked, allowing surgery to continue [4]. Obese women are also at increased risk of laryngeal edema, which may require prolonged intubation postoperatively [4].

In addition to considerations regarding airway management, intravenous access must also be considered. Multiple IV lines may be placed once the patient is in the operating room. Many anesthesiologists prefer to use invasive patient monitoring [4]. This may be particularly true for robotic--assisted laparoscopy, where the patient is more difficulty to access during surgery.

Positioning

Positioning obese and morbidly obese women for robotic--assisted laparoscopic hysterectomy can be challenging and may take additional time [3, 16]. In preparation for robotic--assisted laparoscopic hysterectomy, women are traditionally positioned in the dorsal lithotomy position with arms tucked at military position at the patient's sides. When positioning the patient, the use of a bariatric bed should be considered. Bariatric beds are wider, allowing for easier tucking of the arms, and have a lower profile to the floor. Bed extenders or sleds should be utilized if needed in order to ensure that the arms are secured [4]. Furthermore, moving the asleep obese patient into the dorsal lithotomy position can be challenging. It may take a team approach to safely position the patient. If airway management is not an issue, patient "self--positioning" into stirrups prior to anesthesia induction may be considered [3].

The patient should be securely positioned in order to prevent movement while in steep trendelenburg position. Downward movement may make the surgery more difficult and lead to nerve stretch injuries to the brachial plexus [17]. Anti-skid materials such as egg crate foam, gel pad, or surgical beanbag should be used to prevent slippage. Some surgeons prefer the use of shoulder braces. These should only be used when the patient's arms are tucked at the side [17, 18]. They should be placed over the acromioclavicular joint, as inappropriate placement can lead to brachial plexus injury [17, 18].

It is important to ensure correct positioning with ample padding, as obese patients are at greater risk for pressure sores and nerve injuries as compared to non-obese patients [4]. To reduce the risk of ulnar nerve injury, the arm should be pronated and liberally padded [18]. Care should be taken to pad the lateral aspect of the knee to avoid peroneal nerve injuries. Excess flexion (> 90°) of the hip and external rotation of the thigh should be avoided, as this can lead to sciatic, femoral, and lateral femoral cutaneous nerve injuries. Due to the complexities associated with positioning, surgeons should be aware of the increased time this may add to the surgical case [16, 19]. Figure 75.1 demonstrates some aspects of patient positioning.

Surgical Prophylaxis

Most surgical procedures for benign gynecologic indications are considered intermediate risk for VTE [20, 21]. Sequential compression devices are the standard prophylactic treatment for moderate risk procedures, defined as major abdominal

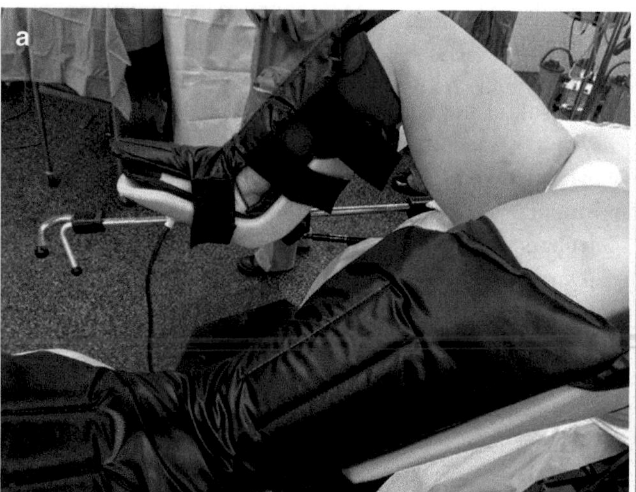

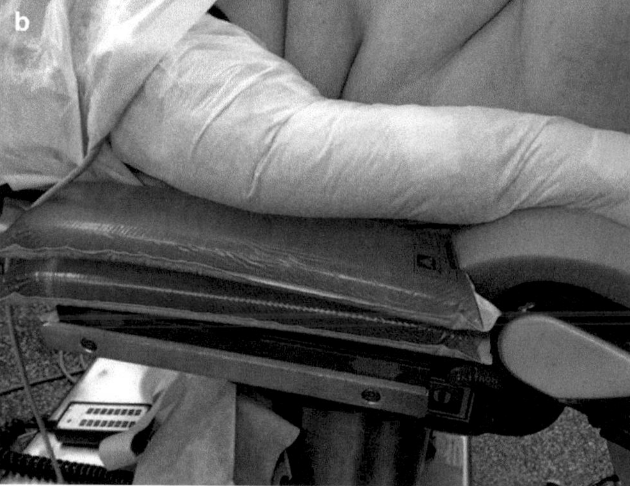

Fig. 75.1 Patient positioning utilizing Yellofins® Stirrups (**a**) and additional padding and a bed extender (**b**)

procedures lasting longer than 30 minutes [21]. It is important to ensure that there are appropriately sized devices available to adequately protect against VTE. If appropriately fitting devices are not available, pharmacologic prophylaxis with 5000 units of subcutaneous unfractionated heparin or 30–40 mg subcutaneous enoxaparin should be given prior to incision.

All women undergoing hysterectomy should receive appropriate preoperative antibiotics, adjusted for weight, for the prevention of postoperative infection. Antibiotics should be re-dosed after 3 hours or with an estimated blood loss over 1500 mL [22]. While there is no data in the gynecology literature, 2 g cefazolin has been shown to provide adequate coverage for clean-contaminated procedures in morbidly obese patients [23].

Abdominal Access and Trocar Placement

Abdominal access may be more challenging in obese patients. This is secondary to an increased distance from the skin to fascia and from the fascia to the peritoneum. Understanding the changes in anatomy is an important for ensuring a safe entry. The shortest distance between the skin and the peritoneal cavity is always through the umbilicus. As BMI increases it has been demonstrated that the umbilicus drifts caudad in relation to the aortic bifurcation [24, 25]. If choosing to enter at the umbilicus, a 90-degree entry should be utilized in order to maximize triangulation [4, 25]. In women with a large pannus, a supra-umbilical or left upper quadrant entry may be preferable, in order to maximize triangulation and access to the anatomy. Obesity is a risk factor for failed entry and pre-peritoneal insufflation [26]. Utilization of the open Hassan technique or left upper quadrant entry may minimize this risk [26]. If a left upper quadrant entry technique is chosen, the entry point should be in the mid-clavicular line, 2–3 cm below the subcostal margin [27]. An orogastric or nasogastric tube should be placed, and the stomach should be drained prior to entry.

When placing accessory trocars for robotic-assisted hysterectomy, it is important to consider the mechanics of the robotic movements as well as the anterior abdominal wall anatomy in the obese patient. When operating on the Da Vinci Surgical System, it is recommended that trocars be placed approximately 8–10 cm apart when moving laterally across the abdomen. The increased diameter of the abdomen may aid in appropriate trocar placement, and decrease the risk of arm collision. Additionally, as morbidly obese patients may have increased subcutaneous fat in the lower part of the abdomen or a pannus, trocar placement will be higher on the abdomen, closer to the level of the umbilicus [4] (Fig. 75.2). The use of long or bariatric trocars should be considered to overcome the increased thickness of the anterior abdominal wall [4]. Additionally, while placement of accessory trocars under direct visualization minimizes risk of injury, visualization of the inferior epigastric vessels and bladder may be limited [28] (Fig. 75.3).

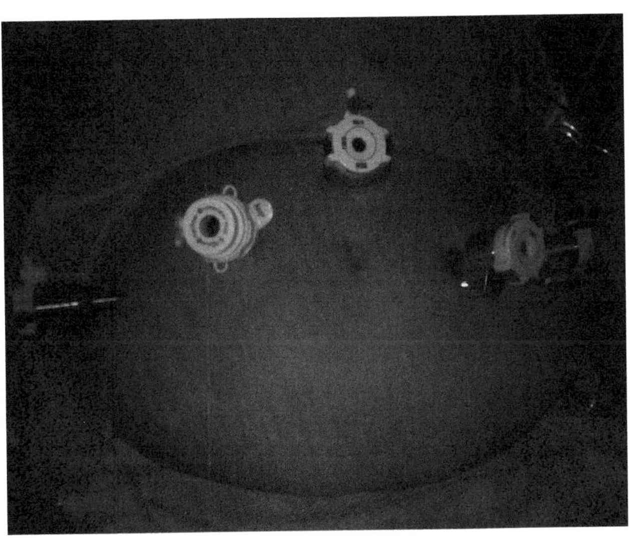

Fig. 75.2 Example of proper trocar placement for robotic assisted laparoscopic hysterectomy

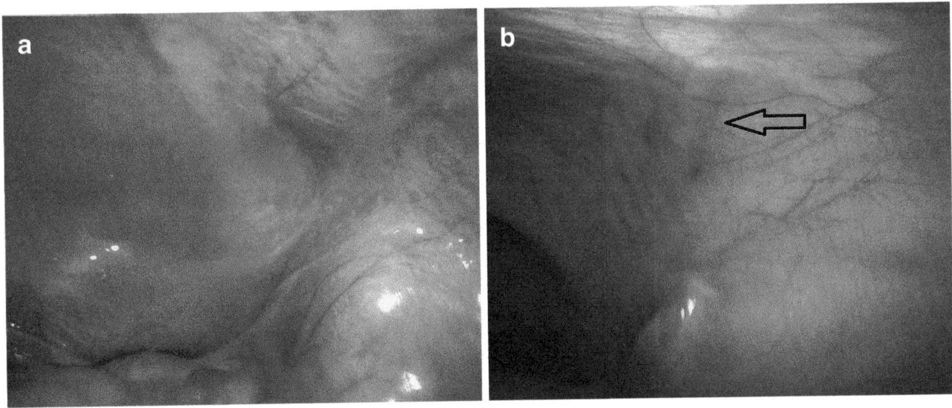

Fig. 75.3 The inferior epigastric vessels are unable to be visualized in an obese patient (**a**) compared to a patient with normal BMI (**b**)

Exposure and Visualization

Excess adiposity effects visualization and exposure of the surgical field (Fig. 75.4). During placement of the accessory trocars, the inferior epigastric vessels are not reliably visualized due to larger amounts of preperitoneal adipose tissue [28]. A comprehensive understanding of anterior abdominal wall anatomy is necessary to minimize risks of injury to these vessels.

Robotic-assisted laparoscopic hysterectomy traditionally requires the patient to be placed in steep trendelenburg position in order to displace the bowel cephalad and gain access to the pelvis [29]. Prior to beginning the surgery, a 2–5 minute trial of steep trendelenburg may be useful to assure the patient can tolerate the trendelenburg position. This should also be done after insufflation, but prior to beginning the operation. Generally if a patient is able to tolerate this trial, the patient is able to tolerate robotic-assisted laparoscopic surgery [30]. Often, despite steep trendelenburg positioning, exposure may be inadequate due to extra fat on the sigmoid colon (Fig. 75.5). This may be managed by utilizing additional assistant ports to introduce a laparoscopic fan to hold the bowel, or a stitch placed through the epiploic appendices and attached to the anterior abdominal wall drawing the bowel away from the surgical field [4, 19] (Fig. 75.6). Additionally, robotic-assisted surgery allows the surgeon to use the third arm as a retractor, which may be useful in the setting of a redundant colon or extra epipolic appendices.

Increased adiposity may also affect the urinary system. Studies have shown that identification of the bladder margins may be more difficult in obese patients [28]. This may lead to injury at the time of trocar placement or bladder dissection. Understanding anatomic landmarks, careful dissection of the bladder away from the uterine vessels, and skeletonization of the vessels may reduce the likelihood of injury. Backfilling the bladder may also allow the surgeon to better delineate bladder margins. While no studies have shown an increase in ureteral injury, transperitoneal visualization of the ureters is reduced in obese patients. Retroperitoneal identification may be required to appropriately identify the ureter (Fig. 75.7).

In general, increasing obesity is associated with prolonged operative time, prolonged time under anesthesia, and increased blood loss for patients undergoing laparoscopic and robotic-assisted laparoscopic hysterectomy [16, 29]. Interestingly one study by Siedhoff et al. demonstrated an increasing severity of complications in women undergoing laparoscopic hysterectomy with increasing BMI [16]. This may also be true in robotic surgery. In studies comparing robotic and laparoscopic surgery for the treatment of endometrial cancer, robotic-assisted surgery has been shown to have advantages, including decreased operative time and decreased estimated blood loss [29]. This may be related to improved visualization, improved dexterity to maneuver around fatty tissue, less surgeon fatigue, and improved exposure through retracting excess tissue with the 3rd robotic arm [19].

In summary, the surgeon should perform the same steps when performing a robotic-assisted laparoscopic hysterectomy on an obese patient, as compared to a non-obese patient. What differs is that anatomy may be obscured by increased adiposity. A complete understanding of pelvic anatomy and meticulous surgical technique can improve the surgeon's ability to identify the essential structure and safely complete a robotic-assisted laparoscopic hysterectomy in the obese patient.

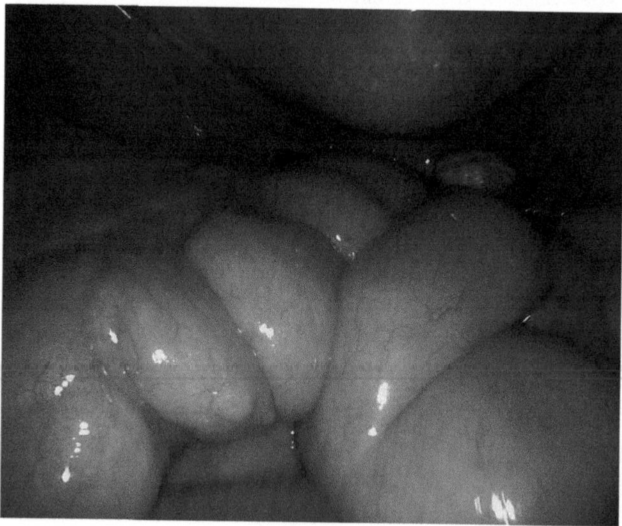

Fig. 75.4 Excess adipose tissue obscuring surgical field

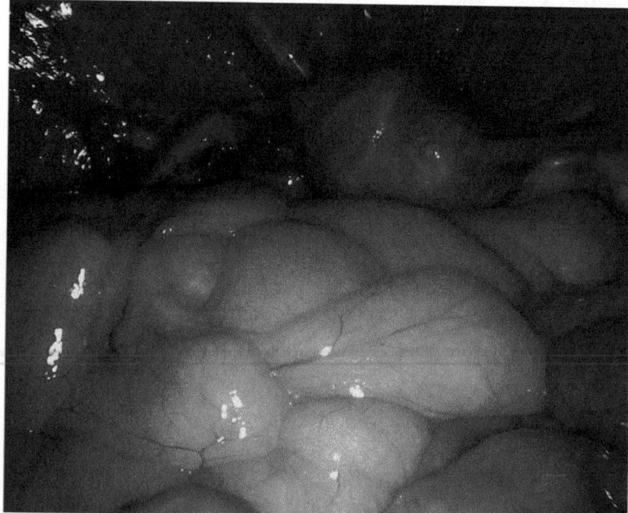

Fig. 75.5 Excess adipose tissue on the colon

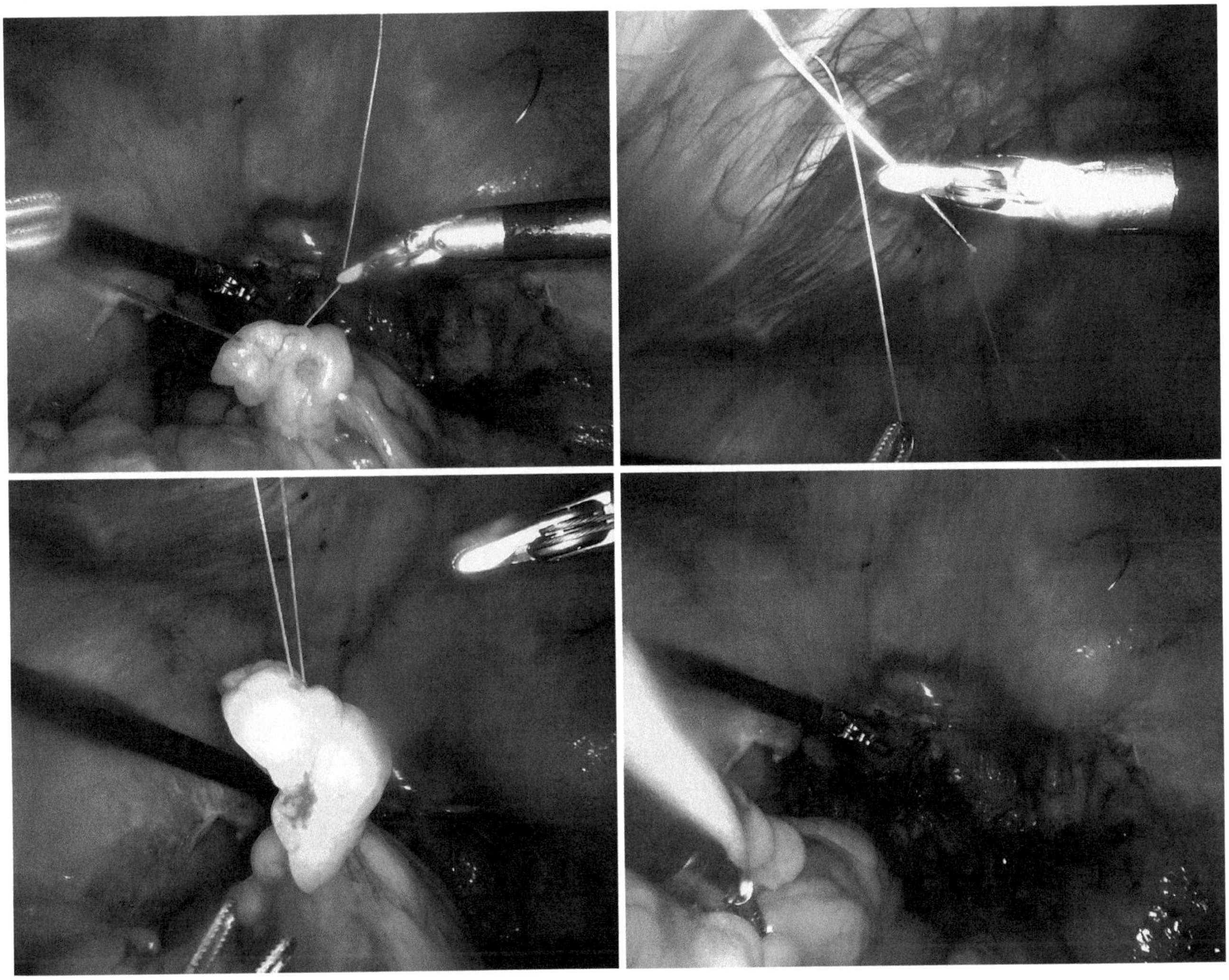

Fig. 75.6 Temporary suture through sigmoid colon epiploica to tack it to the anterior abdominal wall to aid in visualization of the pelvis

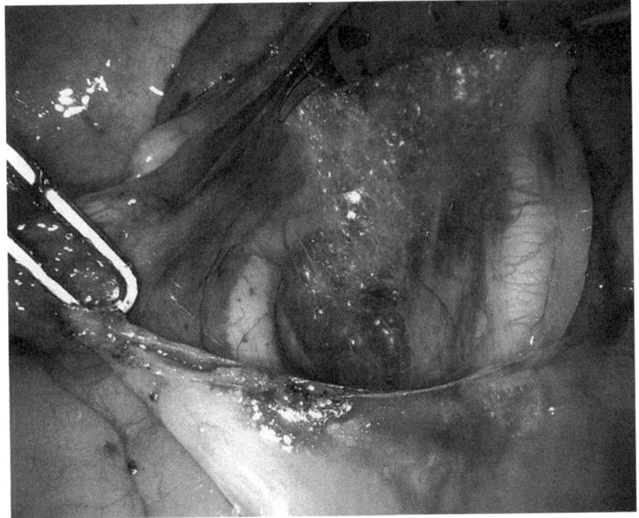

Fig. 75.7 Identification of the ureter by retroperitoneal dissection. Technical skill and knowledge of anatomy is required to complete this procedure

Postoperative Considerations

Patients with obesity are at higher risk for postoperative complications. They have a higher rate of venous thromboembolism and resumption of ambulation may be more difficult particularly for the morbidly obese patient [9, 31]. They are also at higher risk of cardiopulmonary and metabolic problems related to underlying comorbidities. Routine postoperative recommendations should be encouraged in this population, in addition to some special considerations outlined below.

Postoperatively, patients are at risk of pneumonia and postoperative fever attributed to atelectasis [8, 9]. Incentive spirometer use is important to prevent atelectasis. Pain control is also essential to prevent splinting, which leads to poor lung expansion and atelectasis. One of the advantages of robotic surgery is the lower pain level that patients experience compared to open surgery [1–3]. This decreases the amount of narcotic use, and minimizes the risk of decreased respiratory drive [9]. Many patients with obesity also suffer from OSA, and use of CPAP should be continued or initiated in the postoperative period [8, 9]. Even for patients without a diagnosis of OSA, positive pressure noninvasive ventilation may be required in the immediate postoperative period. Additionally, OSA increases the risk of coronary heart disease and heart failure, and these patients should be closely monitored for at least 23 hours after surgery [4, 8].

Obesity increased the risk of VTE, especially in women [31, 32]. Proposed mechanisms include enhanced platelet activity, increased clotting factors, and impaired fibrinolysis [32]. Early ambulation will decrease the rate of VTE by removing stasis of blood flow from Virchow's triad. Additionally, VTE prophylaxis is recommended in all patients hospitalized after surgery [4]. According to the 2012 CHEST Evidence-Based Clinical Practice Guideline, patients undergoing gynecologic surgery who are at moderate risk for VTE (Caprini score 3–4) should receive low--molecular-weight heparin (LMWH) or mechanical prophylaxis; those at high risk (Caprini score ≥5) should receive both; those undergoing surgery for cancer require 4 weeks of LMWH [33]. The Caprini score includes points for BMI greater than 25 and additional point for BMI over 40. Of note, the CHEST guidelines are not specific for laparoscopic surgery, and use of LMWH is controversial after laparoscopic or robotic surgery for benign disease [4, 34].

Starting a regular diet as soon as tolerated after surgery will decrease the rate of postoperative ileus, as well as expedite the resumption of the patient's home medications for diabetes, hypertension, and dyslipidemia. Most patients undergoing a robotic-assisted laparoscopic hysterectomy will be able to resume their usual diet the same day. Patients with diabetes mellitus should have a carbohydrate-consistent diet and tight blood glucose control, as elevated blood glucose levels can impair healing and increase the risk of infection [35].

In conclusion, robotic-assisted laparoscopic hysterectomy is an attractive option for the obese population, with many advantages such as decreased pain, shorter hospital stay, and faster return to daily activities. While these factors decrease the rate of complications, proper patient selection and attention to the unique challenges and comorbidities of this patient population are essential.

References

1. Nawfal K, Orady M, Eisenstei D, Wegienka G. Effect of body mass index on robotic assisted total laparoscopic hysterectomy. J Minim Invasive Gynecol. 2011;18:328–32.
2. Gallo T, Kashani S, Patel D, Elsahwi K, Silasi D, Azodi M. Robotic--assisted laparoscopic hysterectomy: outcomes in obese and morbidly obese patients. JSLS. 2012;16:421–7.
3. Almeida O. Robotic hysterectomy strategies in the morbidly obese patient. JSLS. 2013;17:418–22.
4. Scheib S, Tanner E, Green I, Fader A. Laparoscopy in the morbidly obese: physiologic considerations and surgical techniques to optimize success. J Minim Invasive Gynecol. 2014;21:182–95.
5. Lee GI, Lee MR, Clanton T, Sutton E, Park AE, Marohn MR. Comparative assessment of physical and cognitive ergonomics associated with robotic and traditional laparoscopic surgeries. Surg Endosc. 2014;28(2):456–65.
6. Wright KN, Jonsdottier GM, Jorgensen S, Shah N, Einarsson JI. Costs and outcomes of abdominal, vaginal, laparoscopic and robotic hysterectomies. JSLS. 2012;16:519–24.
7. Ramaswamy A, Gonzalez R, Smith D. Extensive preoperative testing is not necessary in morbidly obese patients undergoing gastric bypass. J Gastrointest Surg. 2004;8:159–65.
8. Catheline J, Bihan H, Quang T, Sadoun D, Charniot J, Onnen I, Fournier J, Bénichou J, Cohen R. Preoperative cardiac and pulmonary assessment in bariatric surgery. Obes Surg. 2008;18:271–7.
9. Kaw R, Aboussouan L, Auckley D, Bae C, Gugliotti D, Grant P, Jaber W, Schauer P, Sessler D. Challenges in pulmonary risk assessment and perioperative management in bariatric surgery patients. Obes Surg. 2008;18:134–8.
10. Maddox T. Preoperative cardiovascular evaluation for noncardiac surgery. Mt Sinai J Med. 2005;72(3):185–92.
11. Kral JG. Morbidity of severe obesity. Surg Clin North Am. 2001;81(5):1039–61.
12. Sugerman HJ. Effects of increased intra-abdominal pressure in severe obesity. Surg Clin North Am. 2001;81:1063–75.
13. Juvin P, Lavaut E, Dupont H, Lefevre P, Demetriou M, Dumoulin JL, et al. Difficult tracheal intubation is more common in obese than in lean patients. Anesth Analg. 2003;97(2):595–600.
14. Cadi P, Guenoun T, Journois D, Chevallier JM, Diehl JL, Safran D. Pressure-controlled ventilation improves oxygenation during laparoscopic obesity surgery compared with volume-controlled ventilation. Br J Anaesth. 2008;100:709–16.
15. Talib HF, Zabani IA, Abdelrahman HS, et al. Intraoperative ventilatory strategies for prevention of pulmonary atelectasis in obese patients undergoing laparoscopic bariatric surgery. Anesth Analg. 2009;109:1511–6.
16. Siedhoff MT, Carey ET, Findley AD, Riggins LE, Garrett JM, Steege JF. Effect of extreme obesity on outcomes in laparoscopic hysterectomy. J Minim Invasive Gynecol. 2012;19(6):701–7.
17. Coppieters MW. Shoulder restraints as a potential cause for stretch neuropathies: biomechanical support for the impact of shoulder girdle depression and arm abduction on nerve strain. Anesthesiology. 2006;104:1351–2.
18. Bradshaw AD, Advincula AP. Postoperative neuropathy in gynecologic surgery. Obstet Gynecol Clin N Am. 2010;27:451–9.
19. Stone P, Burnett A, Burton B, Roman J. Overcoming extreme obesity with robotic surgery. Int J Med Robot. 2010;6(4):382–5.
20. Rahn DD, Mamik MM, Sanses TV et al. Society of Gynecologic Surgeons Systematic Review Group. Venous thromboembolism prophylaxis in gynecologic surgery: a systemic review. Obstet Gynecol 2011: 118:1111–25
21. Geerts WH, Bergqvist D, Pineo GF, et al. American College of Chest Physicians Evidence-Based Clinical Practice Guidelines (8th edition). Chest. 2008;133(6 Suppl):381S–453S.
22. ACOG Committee on Practice Bulletins: Gynecology. ACOG practice bulletin No. 104. Antibiotic prophylaxis for gynecologic procedures. Obstet Gynecol. 2009;113:1180–9.
23. Forse RA, Karam B, MacLean LD, Christou NV. Antibiotic prophylaxis for surgery in morbidly obese patients. Surgery. 1989;106:750–6.
24. Hurd W, Burde R, DeLancey J, Gauvin J, Aisen A. Abdominal wall characterization with magnetic resonance imaging and computer

tomography: the effect of obesity on the laparoscopic approach. J Reprod Med. 1991;36:473–6.
25. Hurd W, Bude R, DeLancey J, Pearl M. The relationship of the umbilicus to the aortic bifurcation: implications for laparoscopic technique. Obstet Gynecol. 1992;80:48–51.
26. Ahmad G.O'Flynn H, Duffy JM, Phillips K, Watson A. Laparoscopic entry techniques. Cochrane Database Syst Rev. 2012: 2:CD006583.
27. Tulikangas PK, Nicklas A, Falcone T, Price LL. Anatomy of the left upper quadrant for cannula insertion. J Am Assoc Gynecol Laparosc. 2000;7:211–4.
28. Hurd WW, Amesse LS, Gruber JS, Horowitz GM, Cha GM, Hurteau JA. Visualization of the epigastric vessels and bladder before laparoscopic trocar placement. Fertil Steril. 2003;80(1):209–12.
29. Boggess JF, Gehrig PA, Cantrell L, Shafer A, Ridgway M, Skinner EN, Fowler WC. A comparative study of 3 surgical methods for hysterectomy with staging for endometrial cancer: robotic assistance, laparoscopy, laparotomy. Am J Obstet Gynecol. 2008;199(4):360.
30. Lamvu G, Zolnoun D, Boggess J, JF S. Obesity: physiologic changes and challenges during laparoscopy. Am J Obstet Gynecol. 2004;191:669–74.
31. Stein P, Beemath A, Olson R. Obesity as a risk factor in venous thromboembolism. Am J Med. 2005;118:978–80.
32. Freeman A, Pendleton R, Rondina M. Prevention of venous thromboembolism in obesity. Expert Rev Cardiovasc Ther. 2010;8(12):1711–21.
33. Guyatt G, Akl E, Crowther M, Gutterman D, Schuunemann H, American College of Chest Physicians. Antithrombotic therapy and prevention of thrombosis, 9th ed: American College of check physicians evidence-based clinical practice guidelines. Chest. 2012;141:7s.
34. Ramirez P, Nick A, Frumovitz M, Schmeler K. Venous thromboembolic events in minimally invasive gynecologic surgery. J Minim Invasive Gynecol. 2013;20:766–9.
35. Pomposelli JJ, Baxter JK, Babineau TJ, Pomfret EA, Driscoll DF, Forse RA, et al. Early postoperative glucose control predicts nosocomial infection rate in diabetic patients. JPEN. 1998;22(2):77–81.

Robotic-Assisted Single-Port Laparoscopic Hysterectomy

76

Vito Cela, Nicola Pluchino, and Letizia Freschi

Introduction

The recent phenomenon of laparo-endoscopic single-site surgery (LESS) opened a new way to perform minimally invasive gynaecological surgery presenting a number of advantages over traditional laparoscopic surgery. However, LESS is challenging due to the lack of port triangulation, two dimensional view, poor ergonomic position for the surgeon and a steep learning curve overall for suturing. To potentially overcome these challenges, single-site robotic surgical platforms have been developed recently. Robotic surgical platforms may shorten the minimally invasive learning curve for select surgeons compared with traditional laparoscopy. A single-site robotic platform may also help to overcome some of the technical limitations of LESS (learning curve, instrument crowding, lack of triangulation, and loss of depth of perception/instability with current 2-dimensional flexible optics). Furthermore, the introduction of the da Vinci robotic system to single-site surgery, will further diminish the impediments that limit this minimally invasive technique.

Robotic-Assisted Single-Port Laparoscopic Hysterectomy

During the past years, the field of laparoscopy has undergone several changes and continuous efforts have been made to improve the morbidity and cosmesis of laparoscopic surgery with a special focus on miniaturization of equipment, evolution of robotic surgical units, and reduction of port size and number. Laparoendoscopic single-site surgery (LESS) is a term that covers a spectrum of surgical techniques that perform laparoscopic surgery by consolidating all ports into only one surgical incision. Although early results are encouraging, this should not disguise the technical difficulties associated with performing LESS procedure. LESS is challenging due to the lack of port triangulation (which lead to the clashing of laparoscopic instruments), two dimensional view, poor ergonomic position for the surgeon and a steep learning curve overall for suturing. New technologies such as flexible scopes, angle instruments and novel robotic platforms have improved the success and consistency of the single-port approach, leading to the inevitable hybridization of robotic technology with LESS surgery. As result, employment of the da Vinci surgical system (Intuitive Surgical, Inc., Sunnyvale, CA) allows greater surgical maneuverability and improves ergonomics during LESS. Preliminary advances in R-LESS (robotic laparoendoscopic single-site surgery) have been already documented in urologic and general, but just in last years have been analyzed the possible application of the robotic laparoendoscopic single-site technology to the gynecological surgery.

In 2011 Nam et al. described a series of seven women with a diagnosis of benign or malignant gynaecological disease concluding that RSSH is feasible and offers some potential advantages over standard robotic or laparoscopic surgery, i.e. minimally invasive access with a smaller scar, less pain and results comparable to those obtained using classical procedures [1]. In the same year, Escobar et al. published a pilot study aiming to evaluate the possible application of robotic laparoendoscopic single-site technology to gynecological surgery, analyzing feasibility and reproducibility of a dedicated da Vinci single-port robotic platform in cadavers for the performance of various gynecologic oncology procedures [2]. All surgical procedures were performed through a single 3–4 cm umbilical incision with a multichannel system that consisted of a wound retractor, surgical gloves, and two 10/12 mm and two 8-mm trocars. A 3–4 cm vertical umbilical skin incision via an open Hasson approach was made and then, the Alexis Wound Retractor (Applied

V. Cela, MD, PhD (✉) • L. Freschi
Obstetrics and Gynecology Unit, Department of Maternal Fetal, University of Pisa, Via Roma 35, Pisa 56123, Italy
e-mail: celav2001@gmail.com

N. Pluchino, MD, PhD
Obstetrics and Gynecology, University Hospital of Geneva, Bd de la Cluse, 30, Geneva 1211, Switzerland
e-mail: nicola.pluchino@gmail.com

I. Alkatout, L. Mettler (eds.), *Hysterectomy*, DOI 10.1007/978-3-319-22497-8_76

Medical, Rancho Santa Margarita, CA, USA) was inserted into the peritoneal cavity. The wrist portion of a size 7.5 surgical glove was fixed to the outer ring of the wound retractor. After making a small hole in the fingertips of the glove, two 10/12-mm and two 8-mm trocars were inserted, and the abdomen was insufflated with CO2 gas. After placing the robotic single-port access system, the overall procedure was similar to that of single-port transumbilical laparoscopic surgery.

However, in October 2011, has been performed the first worldwide case of robot-assisted laparoscopic single-site hysterectomy (RSSH) with the newly designed multichannel port (Intuitive Surgical) for the da Vinci surgical system [3].

Single-site instruments and accessories are designed for the Si version of the da Vinci Surgical System. The single-site port is a multichannel disposable access port with a target anatomy arrow indicator and room for four cannulae and an insufflation valve. Two curved cannulae are for robotically controlled instruments whereas the other two cannulae are straight: one is 8.5 mm and accommodates the high-definition three-dimensional endoscope, and the other is a 5-mm bedside-assistant surgeon port (Fig. 76.1). The docking clamps of the robot automatically recognize the shape of the single-site curved cannulas and reassign each master control to the slave instrument on the opposite side, compensating for the crossing of the curved cannulas. The system includes a range of 5-mm nonwristed, semirigid, and reposable instruments, including a monopolar hook, two bipolar instrument options (a fenestrated bipolar and a Maryland dissector), different types of graspers, curved scissors, a medium-large Hem-o-lok clip applier (Teleflex Medical), needle drivers, and a suction irrigator. Patients are placed in a modified dorsal lithotomy position, and extremities are separated and flexed using adjustable boot stirrups. Anti-skid methods (e.g., vacuum bean bag and gel pad) can be used, and maximum Trendelenburg position (>30°) has to be attained before the Da Vinci Si robot is docked between the legs. After the placament of bladder catheter, an uterine manipulator device ha sto be placed, when possible, in order to improve uterine mobilization. Port placement is performed by using Hasson's technique modified with a 2.0-cm omega-shaped intraumbilical incision (Fig. 76.2) down to the level of the fascia; this is entered and a finger sweep to check for adhesions is performed. Prelubrication of the single-site port with a sterile saline solution prior to introduction is recommended, then, port insertion can be reached utilizing two techniques, the "unfolded" and the "folded" port-clamping technique using an atraumatic clamp and grasping just above the lower rim before proceeding with insertion (Fig. 76.3); at last the arrow marking on the port is aligned with the target anatomy (uterus/pelvis). After an initial pneumoperitoneum at 20 mmHg, it can be reduced to 8 mmHg taking advantage of the strength of the its mobility before curved cannulae's insertion (Fig. 76.4). This step is important to ensure that there is adequate working space for the curved cannulae during the entire surgical procedure and that the instruments are fully supported. Adhesions have to be removed as necessary and loops of small bowel have to be folded, not pushed, back into the upper abdomen to expose the root of the mesentery.

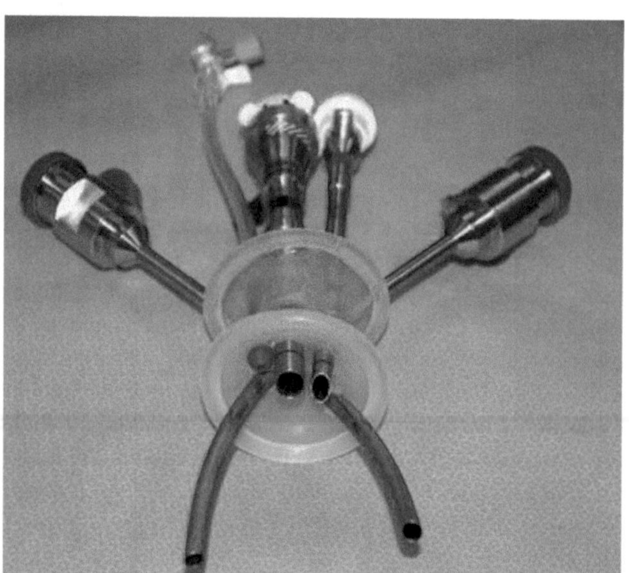

Fig. 76.1 A Single-port cluster

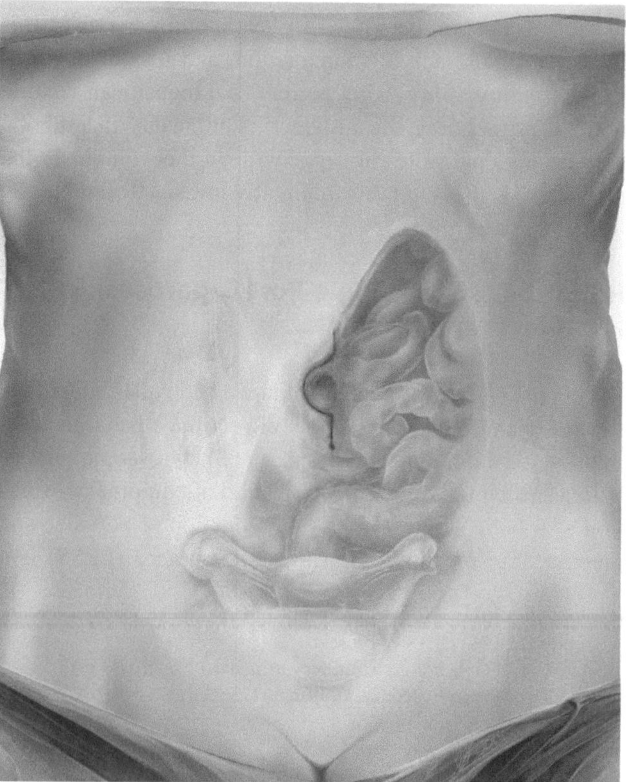

Fig. 76.2 Omega-shape umbelical incision

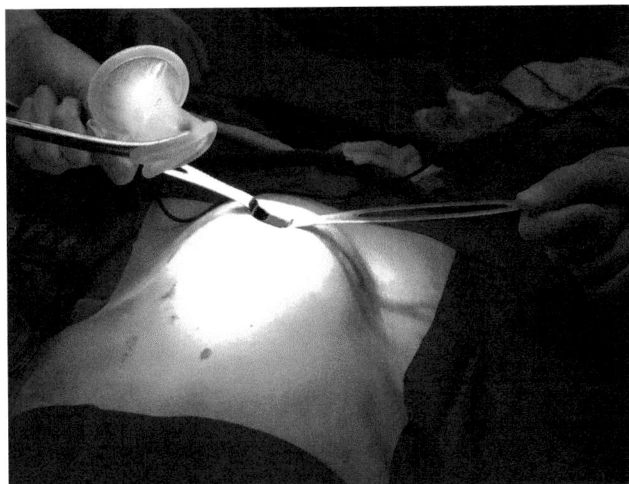

Fig. 76.3 Single-site port introduction with the "folded" port-clamping technique using an atraumatic clamp

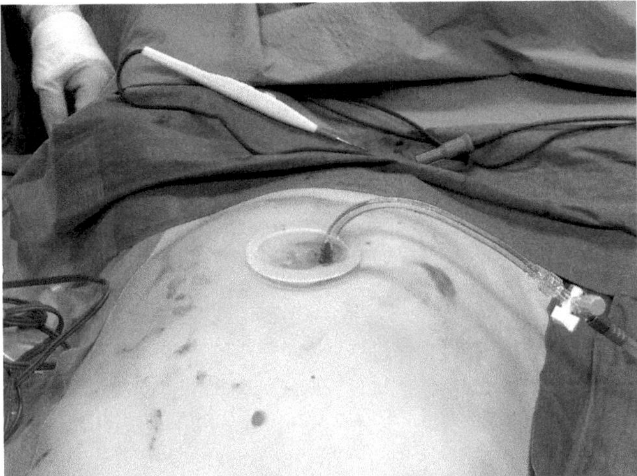

Fig. 76.4 Pneumoperitoneum induction after the umbelical placement of the single-site port

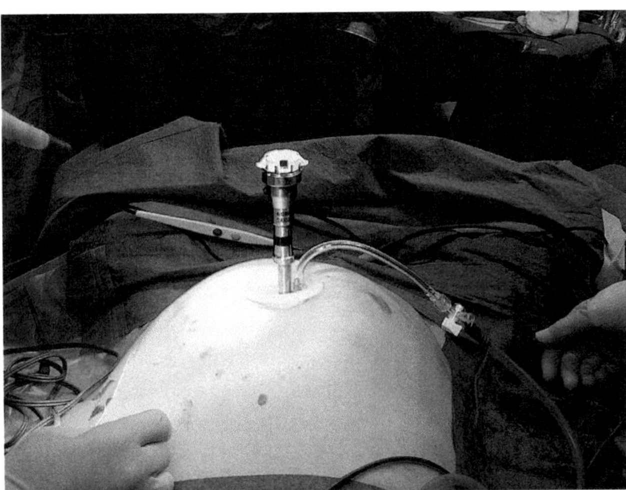

Fig. 76.5 Positioning of the 12-mm lubricated trocar for the robotic 30-degree scope

Once sufficient initial exposure is achieved, the cart can be docked and the 12-mm lubricated trocar for the robotic 30-degree scope and two 8-mm trocars for the robotic instruments are placed in a triangular way under direct visualization (Figs. 76.5 and 76.6). Through the 5-mm bedside-assistant port endoscopic suction, coagulation and cutting with electrothermal bipolar vessel sealer can performed. Placing the robotic single-port access system, As far as the surgical technique, the procedure is similar to that of multiport robot-assisted surgery: The ovaries are examined. The right round ligament is coagulated and transected (Fig. 76.7) and the retroperitoneal space is opened to identify the ureter (Fig. 76.8). Then, the infundibulopelvic ligament is securely skeletonized, coagulated and transected. The uterine arteries are skeletonized, coagulated and transected. The bladder and the attached peritoneal flap are developed using a monopolar hook and dissected below the colpotomy cup (Fig. 76.9). Both uterosacral ligaments are excised with the monopolar hook and the peritoneum on the posterior cervix is excised and divided from the cervix. Similar steps are performed

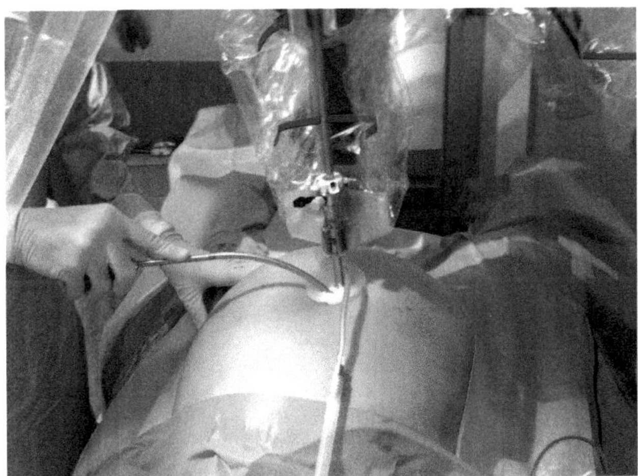

Fig. 76.6 One of the two 8-mm trocars for the robotic instruments placed under direct visualization

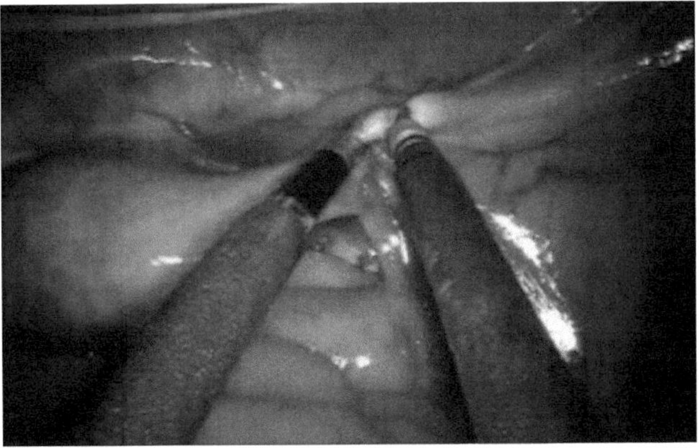

Fig. 76.7 Coagulation and section right broad ligament

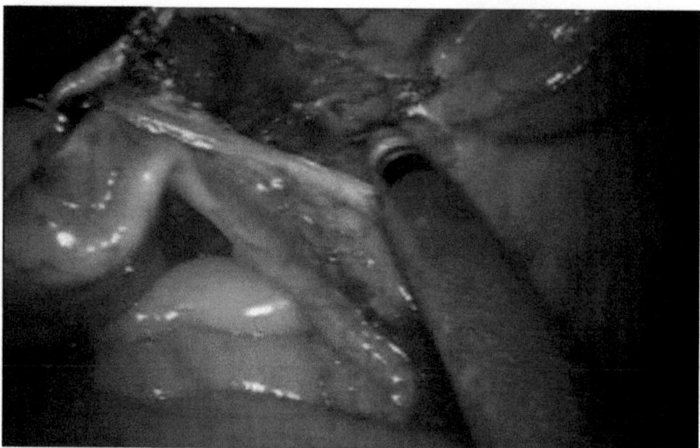

Fig. 76.8 Retroperitoneal space opening and identification of the ureter

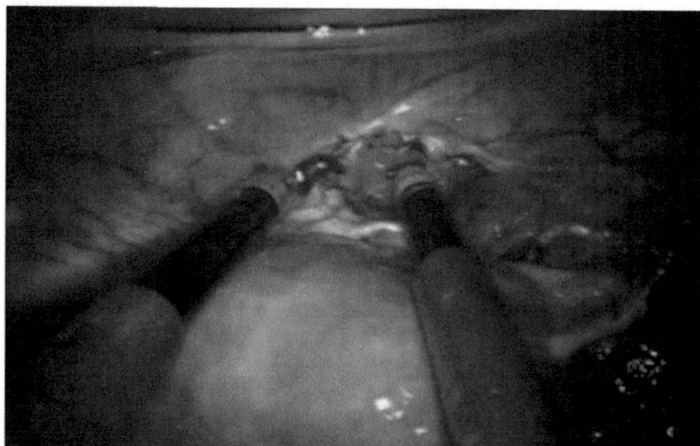

Fig. 76.9 Opening of the vescico-uterine space

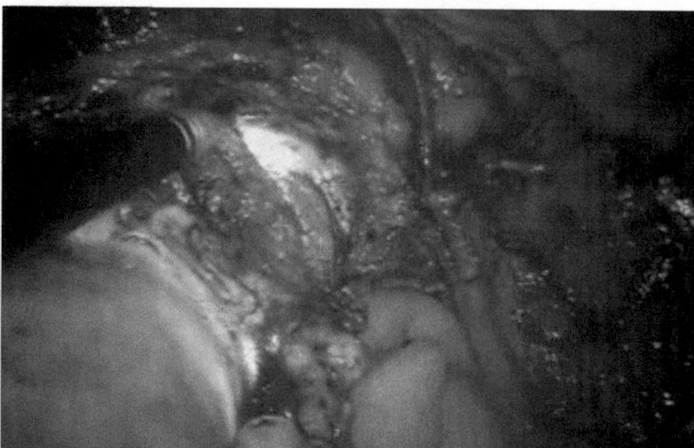

Fig. 76.10 Anterior colpotomy

contralaterally. The anterior colpotomy (Fig. 76.10) and posterior colpotomy are performed with the monopolar hook and the vagina delineated with colpotomizer. The uterus and adnexae are then removed through the vagina. In cases of younger patients the ovaries could be preserved to avoid menopausal symptoms. (Fig. 76.11). As far as the vaginal cuff closure, it can be obtained in different ways according to

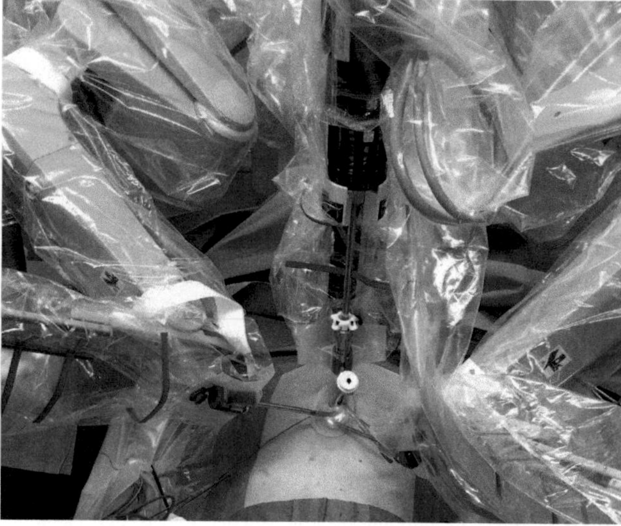

Fig. 76.11 Final single-site robotic port dock

the anatomical features of the vagina itself: with an intracorporeal barbed suture or intracorporeal interrupted figure-of-eight sutures (0 Vicryl™, Ethicon) or transvaginally with interrupted delayed absorbable suture of Vicryl 2/0 (Ethicon Inc., Somerville, NJ).

Discussion

Bogliolo et al. proposed also in some circumstances, such as a narrow vagina or the need of vaginal vault suspension, requiring a robotic approach to colporraphy, an intracorporeal suture with extracorporeal knots a particolar way to close the vaginal vuff. The procedure was performed introducing the 0 caliber polyglycolic acid suture (Vicryl ™; Ethicon) by the 10 mms trocar through the single site port. The number of suture in vaginal cuff closure was four and was performed with interrupted figure-of-eight sutures. The knots were pushed in to the pelvis by the use of Knot Pusher Storz device [4]. Undoubtedly, one of the greatest limitations of the single-site platform is that the semiflexible robotic instruments are not currently capable of articulation (as in multiport robotic surgery), ad the cannulas are rather long. This means that there are fewer degrees of freedom than with multiport robotic surgery and a very small distance between the instrument and the uterus. This makes the suture really demanding, not only in the tying of the incorporeal knots but also in the pulling of the vaginal tissue in the right direction (i.e., parallel to the needle) during the needle's passage.

Another important aspect, is that, according to current evidence, transvaginal suturing of the vaginal stump is associated with a lower incidence of vaginal dehiscence or general cuff complications compared with both laparoscopic and robotic suturing. Anyhow, the method of vaginal cuff closure during robotic total hysterectomy should be simple and time efficient, with the risks of infection and vaginal cuff dehiscence minimized.

After hemostasis, the fascia was repaired with a 2/0 Vicryl interrupted stitches (Ethicon Inc.) and skin closed with 3/0 Ethilon interrupted stitches.

Cela et al. analyzed, in vivo, using a CUSUM method, the learning curve of robot-assisted single-site hysterectomy identifing two different phases of the learning curve of the procedure: phase 1, found to require six cases, can represent the initial learning curve phase, and phase 2 can represent the mastery phase, with a reduction in OT (operative time). When comparing the six initial cases with the last six cases any statistical difference in terms of morbidity was revealed, but a trend has been reported in terms of OT and CT (console time). These data suggest that after a learning curve phase, the surgeon may achieve a higher level of competence and consider offering this approach to patients presenting with more complicated cases. Furthermore, data demonstrated that large BMI or high uterine weight would have a negative impact on the surgical performance of RSSH by increasing the operative times, console times, or docking times. Based on these results, an increased BMI as well as high uterine weight is not associated with prolonged operative times.

These data are confirmed also by Bogliolo et al. in a recent retrospective analysis in which large BMI and short stature seemed not to have a negative impact on the surgical performance, suggesting that this innovative surgical technique should also be used for obese patients to achieve the goal of very minimally invasive surgery. Indeed, regarding overweight and obese patients, although they reported BMI ≥ 25 in 20 cases and BMI ≥ 30 in seven patients, laparoscopic conversion was required in only one case.

High uterine weight was significantly correlated with longer operative time, but it seemed not to prejudice good surgical outcome. Sixteen weeks were chosen as the size limitation because, according to our standard laparoscopic experience, large uteri could require supra-umbilical access, which is technically not recommended in single-site surgery.

Regarding hospital stays in their series, Bogliolo et al. reported a long hospitalization time on average because the two patients who experienced a complication were discharged on days 8 and 14 [5].

Two recent studies analyzed the role of robotic single-site approach to endometrial cancer.

Abdulrahman et al. [6] proposed the sentinel lymph node (SLN) biopsy as a safe and less morbid approach to full lymphadenectomy in endometrial cancer (EC) and demonstrated SLN biopsy and extrafascial hysterectomy utilizing the single-site robotic system, to be feasible and able to offer some benefits over traditional robotic surgery.

Mereu et al., instead, treated four patients with histological diagnosis of endometrial adenocarcinoma G1 and instrumental FIGO stage IA or IB with total single access robotic laparoscopic extra-fascial hysterectomy and bilateral salpingo-oophorectomy. The procedure was performed through a single trans-umbilical incision of 35 mm using a Da Vinci Robotic S System and a Gelport device with one 12 mm trocar for robotic 3D optic, two 8-mm trocars and one 5-mm trocar. Data confirmed the procedure to be technically feasible and reproducible in patients with low-stage endometrial cancer with optimal surgical outcome and postoperative course [7].

In 2014 Bogliolo et al. published an interesting retrospective series of perioperative data from ten consecutive patients who underwent robotic-assisted single-site laparoscopic hysterectomy (RSSH) for female-to-male transsexualim (FMT). Single-site robotic surgery was confirmed to be a valid choice in FMT reassignment surgery, with a low rate of complications, good pain control, and excellent aesthetic results with only a minor perioperative complication occurred and not directly related to single-site technique [8].

Recently, has been published a case of combined cholecystectomy and hysterectomy using the da Vinci surgical system with the single site platform providing a critical analysis of the technique, including limitations of current single-site technology. Data demonstrated the feasibility of performing general surgery and gynecologic procedures concomitantly using a robotic single site (RSS) surgical approach. Cholecystectomy and total hysterec-tomy were conducted uneventfully and they were performed in a relatively short time by surgeons with previous experience of RSS, working in a multidisciplinary robotic center [9].

In conclusion, over the past 10 years, many efforts have been made to reduce the surgical invasiveness of minimally invasive surgery. The evolution of the single-port technique in laparoscopy achieved the goal of reducing the number of ports, improving the cosmetic benefits, avoiding the potential morbidity associated with multiple incisions and minimizing postoperative pain and recovery time. However, LESS surgery is characterized by a longer operative time that is partially justified by the lack of the third operative instrument. Single-site robotic surgery has the same advantages as LESS, but the automatic reversion of the crossed instruments allows for far greater manoeuvrability and ergonomics compared with other single-site methods. However, actually we are still far from having a perfect system and are rather in the infancy of robotic single site. The robotic single-site platform has several limitations, including reduced extracorporeal triangulation and a limited repertoire of non-articulating instruments and electrosurgical options compared with conventional multiport robotic surgery [10, 11] (Table 76.1). Taken together, these limitations may require significant modifications in technique for the traditional robotic surgeon. Each aspect of the set-up, including the exact umbilical incision length and positioning of the port

Table 76.1 Pros and Cons of robot-assisted single site hysterectomy

PROS	CONS
Minimally invasive approach	Limited repertoire of non-articulating instruments and electrosurgical options
3D visualization	Costs
Improved surgeon dexterity	Reduced extracorporeal triangulation
Enhanced ergonomics	
Short learning curve	

and platform, had to be precise for the RSS instrumentation to operate efficiently.

The possible future use of flexible endoscopes will improve the practicality of robotic LESS and will may increase the range of its applications.

Advances in the field of robotics will hopefully overcome these limitations and provide improved triangulation, degrees of freedom, dexterity, visualization, and new instruments with different kind of energies. However, the introduction of the da Vinci robotic system to single-site surgery, will further diminish the impediments that limit this minimally invasive technique. Prospective comparison studies are needed, but preliminary results are encouraging and the development of robotic systems specific to RSS may define the new horizon of single-site surgery.

References

1. Nam EJ, Kim SW, Lee M, et al. Robotic single-port transumbilical total hysterectomy: a pilot study. J Gynecol Oncol. 2011;22:120–6.
2. Escobar PF, Kebria M, Falcone T. Evaluation of a novel single port robotic platform in the cadaver model for the performance of various procedures in gynecologic oncology. Gynecol Oncol. 2011;120:380–4.
3. Cela V, Freschi L, Simi G, et al. Robotic single-site hysterectomy: feasibility, learning curve and surgical outcome. Surg Endosc. 2013;27:2638–43.
4. Bogliolo S, Cassani C, Babilonti L, Spinillo A. Vaginal cuff closure during robotic single-port hysterectomy: is the vaginal route always the best one? Surg Endosc. 2013;27(12):4754–5. doi:10.1007/s00464-013-3106-1. Epub 2013 Aug 13.
5. Bogliolo S, Mereu L, Cassani C, Gardella B, Zanellini F, Dominoni M, Babilonti L, Delpezzo C, Tateo S, Spinillo A. Robotic single-site hysterectomy: two institutions' preliminary experience. Int J Med Robot. 2015;11(2):159–65.
6. Sinno AK et al. Single site robotic sentinel lymph node biopsy and hysterectomy in endometrial cancer. Gynecol Oncol. 2015;137(1):190.
7. Mereu L, Carri G, Khalifa H. Robotic single port total laparoscopic hysterectomy for endometrial cancer patients. Gynecol Oncol. 2012;127(3):644. doi:10.1016/j.ygyno.2012.07.129. Epub 2012 Aug 4.
8. Bogliolo S, Cassani C, Babilonti L, Gardella B, Zanellini F, Dominoni M, Santamaria V, Nappi RE, Spinillo A. Robotic single-site surgery for female-to-male transsexuals: preliminary experience. ScientificWorldJournal. 2014;2014:674579. doi:10.1155/2014/674579. Epub 2014 Apr.
9. Pluchino N, Buchs NC, Drakopoulos P, Wenger JM, Morel P, Dällenbach P. Robotic single-site combined cholecystectomy and hysterectomy: advantages and limits. Int J Surg Case Rep. 2014;5(12):1025–7. doi:10.1016/j.ijscr.2014.10.001. Epub 2014 Oct 29.
10. Verit A, Rizkala E, Autorino R, Stein RJ. Robotic laparoendoscopic single-site surgery: from present to future. Indian J Urol. 2012;28:76–81.
11. White MA, Haber GP, Autorino R, Khanna R, Altunrende F, Yang B, Stein RJ, Kaouk JH. Robotic laparoendoscopic single-site surgery. BJU Int. 2010;106(6 Pt B):923–7.

Robot-assisted Laparoscopic Pelvic and Paraaortic Lymphadenectomy

77

Jan Persson

Introduction

Pelvic and paraaortic lymphadenectomy is mainly used for staging of genital and other pelvic cancers. Both pelvic and paraaortic lymphadenectomy are well suited for laparoscopy with a low complication rate reported in large series from centers of excellence [1, 2]. Still, despite being described more than 20 years ago, traditional laparoscopic lymphadenectomy, in particular, the paraaortic type, has not been performed at most centers. This is probably due to the complexity of traditional laparoscopy and/or a lack of large enough volumes to introduce and maintain a new surgical approach. The da Vinci surgical robot (da Vinci ® Surgical System, Intuitive Surgical Inc., CA, USA) was approved for gynecological procedures in 2005. So far, four robot systems have been launched (da Vinci standard, S, Si and Xi systems) of which the first (standard) model is no longer kept active by the manufacturer. All models provide instruments with a wrist function at the tip, movement downgrading, tremor elimination, a stable 3-dimensional view of the operative field and an ergonomic working position. These features may help the surgeon overcome some of the limitations associated with traditional laparoscopic surgery.

As no prospective randomized studies compare robotic and laparoscopic pelvic and paraaortic lymphadenectomy alone, available data is restricted to case series with or without retrospective control groups, not seldom data from early robot adopters even using the first robot model with its limitations. Still, the overall conclusion is that robot assistance results in the same or better nodal yield, less bleeding and less conversions to open surgery, in particular in obese patients. [3–8].

J. Persson
Department of Obstetrics and Gynecology, Skåne University Hospital, Lund, Sweden
e-mail: jan.persson@med.lu.se

Robot Assisted Laparoscopic Pelvic Lymhadenectomy

All models of the da Vinci robots can be used, although preferably a da Vinci Si or Xi system adapted for the near infrared fluorescent technique (Firefly) which allows for the use of Indocynaine green for detection of sentinel lymph nodes [9]. Ports should be placed for standard pelvic surgery as recommended for the respective systems. The S-Si robot may be docked centrally or side docked at surgeons' discretion whereas the Xi robot can be docked at various positions, usually from the side of the patient. In case of a simultaneous paraaortic lymphadenectomy port placement is adjusted accordingly as described below. Suitable robot instruments are; a monopolar scissors, a bipolar forceps and a grasper. For the assistant one or two trocars are needed for suction/irrigation, grasping, insertion of sponges and for retrieval of lymph nodes, the latter usually requiring a 12–15 mm trocar diameter. The procedure starts with inspection of the whole abdomen and pelvis to rule out disseminated disease. This is best performed before the robot arms and instruments are docked as this allows a complete abdominal overview including the liver and diaphragm and avoids unnecessary cost for robot instruments in case an immediate conversion to open surgery should be indicated.

The pelvic lymphadenectomy starts with developing the avascular planes and identifying landmarks from the aortic bifurcation and distally before any lymphadenectomy is performed. Sentinel lymph nodes (if such technique is applied) or otherwise cancer suspect nodes should be looked for and removed separately for frozen section. Lymph nodes should always be retrieved in a protective bag. It is important to avoid grasping directly on the lymph nodes with robot instruments as this otherwise may crush a potentially metastatic node with risk of tumor spread. In general, the dissection is most easily performed if tension of the tissue is applied and with dissection close to the adjacent vessels.

The presacral and common iliac node dissection starts with opening the peritoneum medial of the right common iliac artery to the level of the aortic bifurcation (Fig. 77.1).

I. Alkatout, L. Mettler (eds.), *Hysterectomy*, DOI 10.1007/978-3-319-22497-8_77

This way, the right ureter and infundibulopelvic ligament are visualized and lateralized. The third robot instrument (usually the grasper) can be used to lift the sigmoid colon, the infundibulopelvic ligament and the ureter to expose the left common lymph node chain (Fig. 77.2). It is usually helpful to retract the sigmoid colon towards the left abdominal side wall with a sponge reinforced stitch. The hypogastric nerve should be identified at the level of the aortic bifurcation and saved (Fig. 77.3). With the whole presacral and common iliac nodal areas exposed the lymphadenectomy is performed starting with the area medial of the common iliac arteries and the presacral area (Fig. 77.4) followed by the lateral common iliac lymph node chains saving the genitofemoral nerves visualized as they run along the psoas muscles (Fig. 77.2).

The paravesical and pararectal spaces are then opened. This is most easily performed by lifting the round ligament cranially and medially creating a fold of the lateral broad ligament as a starting point (Fig. 77.5). The broad ligament is then incized laterally along the infundibulopelvic ligament and if needed the incision is prolonged lateral of the caecum/sigmoid colon for slight mobilization of the colon. The paravesical space, limited by the pubic bone, the obliterated umbilical artery, the upper paracervical tissue and the exter-

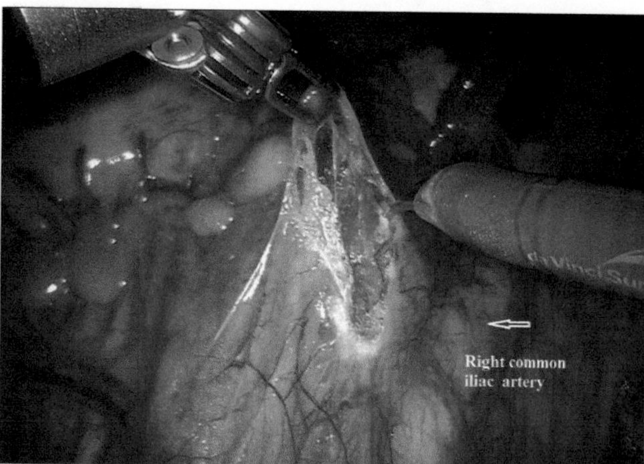

Fig. 77.1 The presacral and common iliac node dissection starts with opening of the peritoneum medial of the right common iliac artery

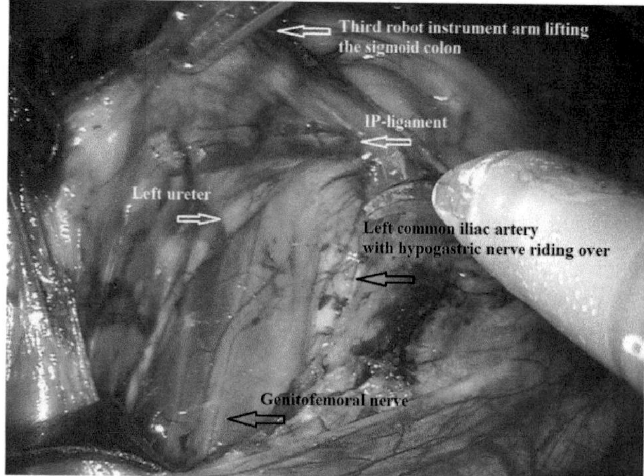

Fig. 77.2 The third robot arm is used for lifting the sigmoid colon to expose the left side common iliac area

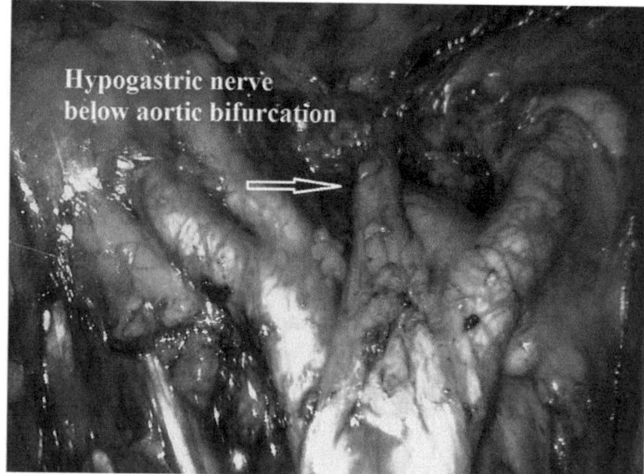

Fig. 77.3 The hypogastric nerve shall be isolated and saved

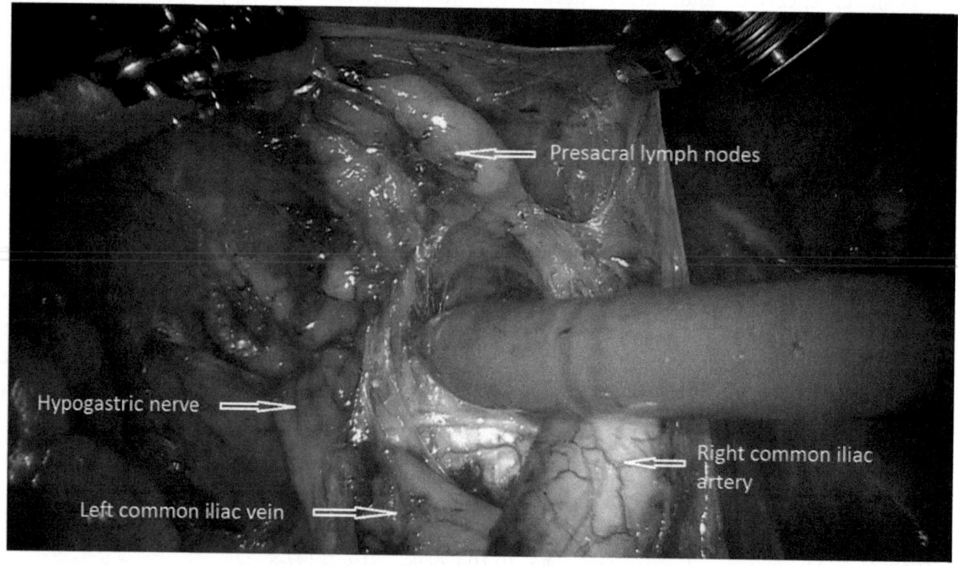

Fig. 77.4 Presacral nodal dissection

nal iliac vessels, is developed bluntly visualizing the course of the obturator nerve and associated deep blood vessels and lymph nodes (Fig. 77.6). Then the pararectal space is opened starting by identifying the ureter running along the medial broad ligament (ideally kept intact until later) and the hypogastric artery as medial and lateral borders (Fig. 77.7). Opened deeper, the pararectal space will display the deep uterine vein, the hypogastric nerve fibers and the origin of the obliterated umbilical artery where the uterine artery is usually found (Fig. 77.8). It is important to keep the upper parametrium (paracervical tissue) intact between the paravesical and pararectal spaces for a later radical hysterectomy or a separate upper paracervical parametrectomy and for not disrupting the lymphatics in case a sentinel node technique is applied (Figs. 77.7 and 77.9). The external iliac node dissection starts with the identification of genitofemoral nerve, usually serving as a lateral border. The superficial lateral lymph chain is then released from lateral to medial and folded over the external iliac artery and completed with the medial nodes and ideally removed en bloc (Fig. 77.10). The deep external nodes and the proximal obturator nodes are removed after the iliac vessels are mobilized medially to expose the obturator fossa and the proximal course of the obturator nerve (Fig. 77.11). Vessels from the ileopsoas muscle to the obturator nodal tissues can be coagulated at this stage as they are a common cause of bleeding during later lymphadenectomy in the obturator fossa (Fig. 77.11). Then, the remaining obturator nodes are removed en bloc following the obturator nerve sparing the obturator vein and exposing the pelvic floor (Fig. 77.12). A check of the whole pelvic retrieval area should be performed at the end.

Finally, it is worth mentioning some risks: It is important to avoid grasping the obturator nerve with the robot instruments as the constant grip force will risk damaging

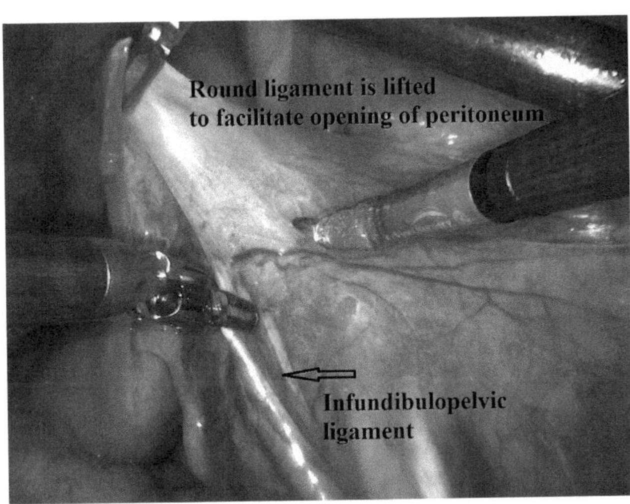

Fig. 77.6 The paravesical space

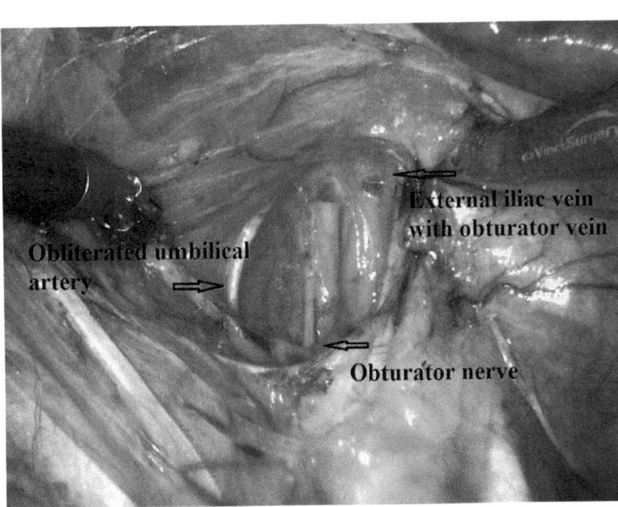

Fig. 77.7 The pararectal space

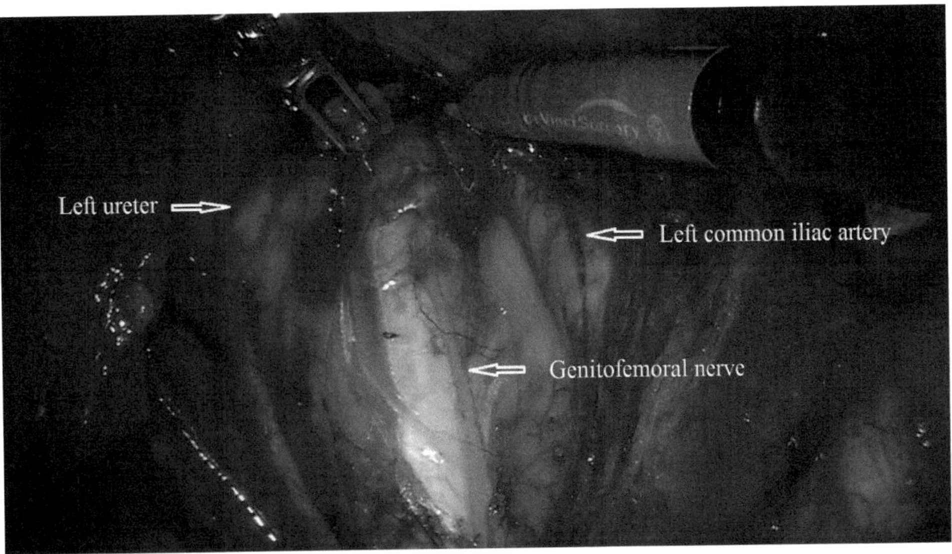

Fig. 77.5 Opening of the pelvic side wall avascular planes is facilitated by lifting the round ligament to create a fold of the lateral broad ligament

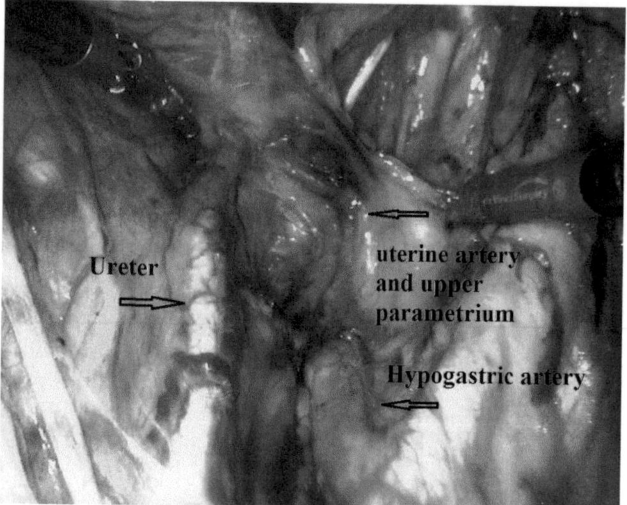

Fig. 77.8 Deeper dissection of the pararectal space

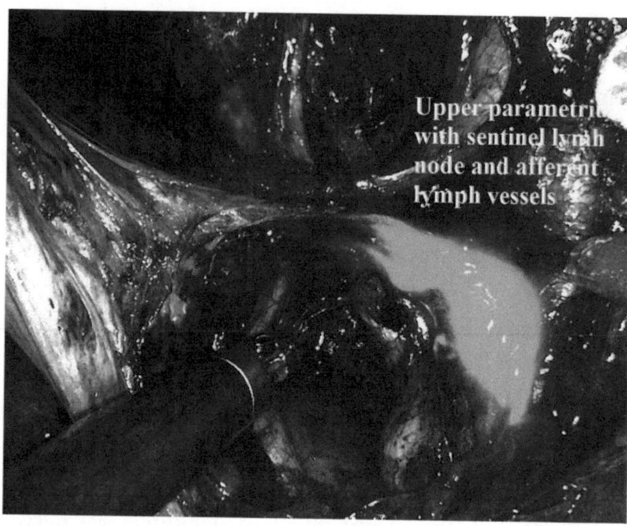

Fig. 77.10 Right side superficial external iliac nodes

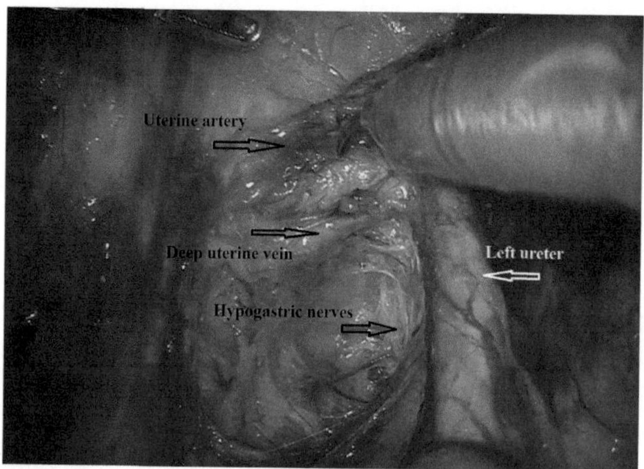

Fig. 77.9 Upper parametrial lymphatics and a sentinel lymph node displayed with the firefly technique

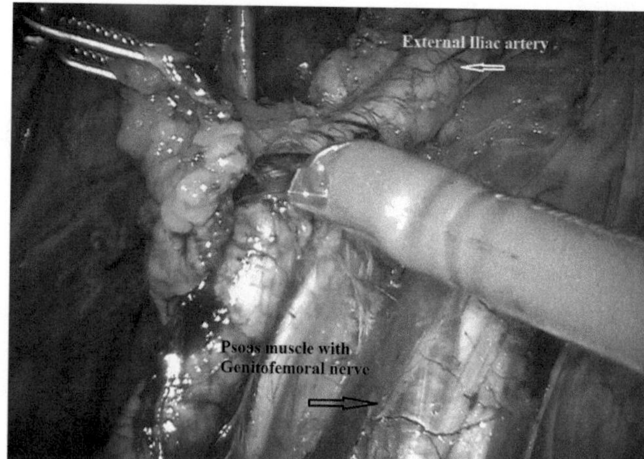

Fig. 77.11 Right side deep external and proximal obturator lymph nodes. *Black arrow* shows blood vessels from the ileopsoas muscle often causing bleeding during obturator node dissection

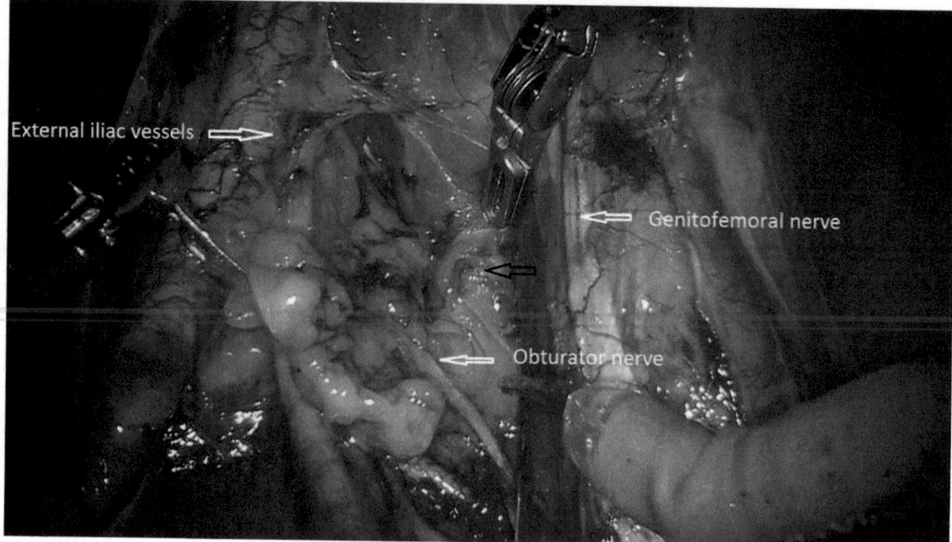

Fig. 77.12 Right side obturator lymph nodes

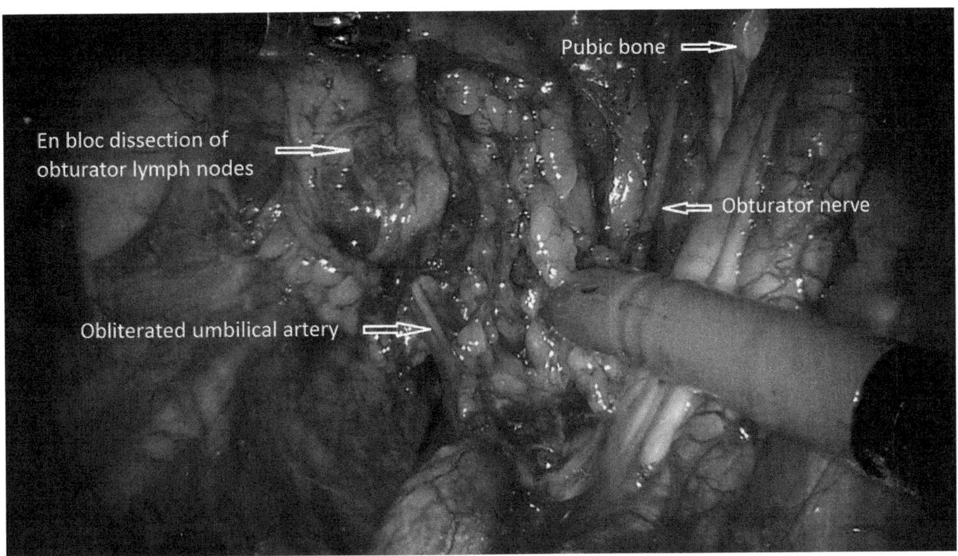

Fig. 77.13 Close proximity between obturator nerve and proximal obturator lymph nodes (left side)

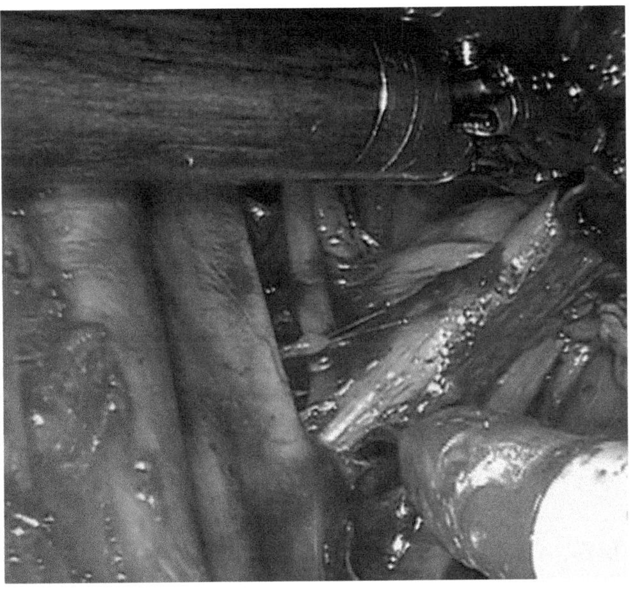

Fig. 77.14 Genitofemoral nerve and Lateralcutaneous femoral nerve (left side).

the nerve. During the final proximal part of the obturator node dissection, if performed from the medial side, extra attention should be given to the nerve to avoid damage of the obturator nerve and hypogastric vein due to their close proximity (Fig. 77.13). A too deep and lateral dissection during the external node removal risks harming the lateral cutaneous femoral nerve (Fig. 77.14).

Robot Assisted Laparoscopic Paraaortic Lymphadenectomy

Paraaortic lymphadenectomy can be performed as a single procedure or in conjunction with pelvic lymphadenectomy and removal of pelvic organs. A retroperitoneal approach may be clinically beneficial in case the paraaortic lymphadenectomy is a single procedure, in particular in case of intraabdominal adhesions and in obese patients. However, with the retroperitoneal approach the space for robot arms is limited and there are no obvious overall advantages with the use of robots compared with traditional laparoscopy [9]. It is likely that the more slender robot arms of the new da Vinci Xi model will be advantageous but this remains to be seen. Therefore, and due to the fact that other procedures are often planned in the same session, a transperitoneal approach will most often be the choice for the robotic paraaortic lymphadenecomy. Principally, this can be performed in two ways: as a proximal prolongation of the pelvic lymphadenectomy along the aorta with the robot docked centrally between the patients legs or side docked for pelvic surgery. This requires ports placed higher than for pelvic surgery only and a steep Trendelenburg position of the patient (Fig. 77.15 and 77.16). This approach may be technically difficult, mainly due to obscuring bowel, and restricted access to the inframesenteric area particularly in obese and short patients [10, 11].

The alternative transperitoneal approach is to place the S or Si robot at the patients head or shoulder and dissect from caudal to cranial through a smaller opening of the

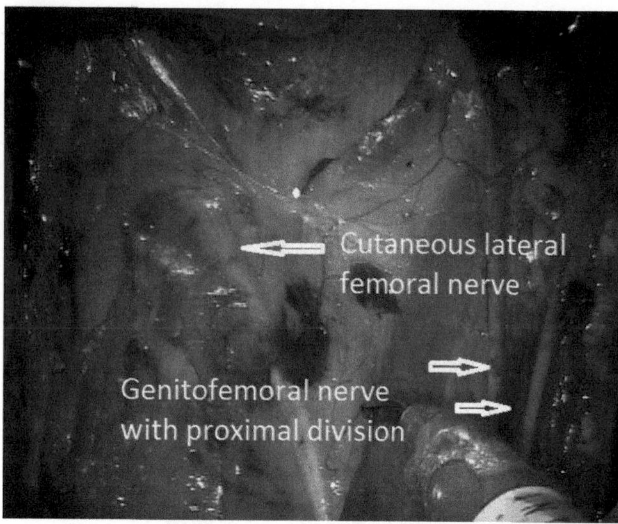

Fig. 77.15 Port placement for paraaortic and pelvic lymph node dissection with pelvic docking of a S-Si robot

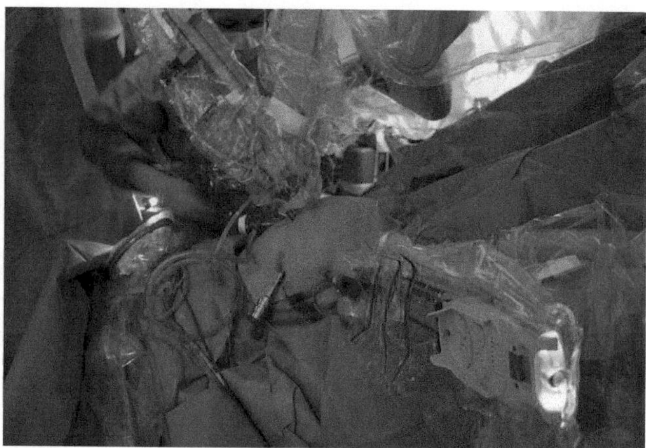

Fig. 77.17 A paraaortic lymphadenectomy with the Xi robot or S-Si robots with double docking starts with creating a tunnel under the bowel along the aorta starting opening the peritoneum below the aortic bifurcation.

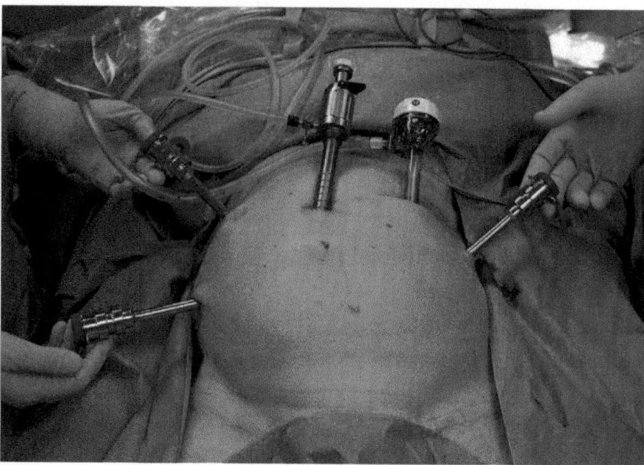

Fig. 77.16 The robot arms should be adjusted to reach the upper abdomen during paraaortic and pelvic lymph node dissection with pelvic docking of the S-Si robot

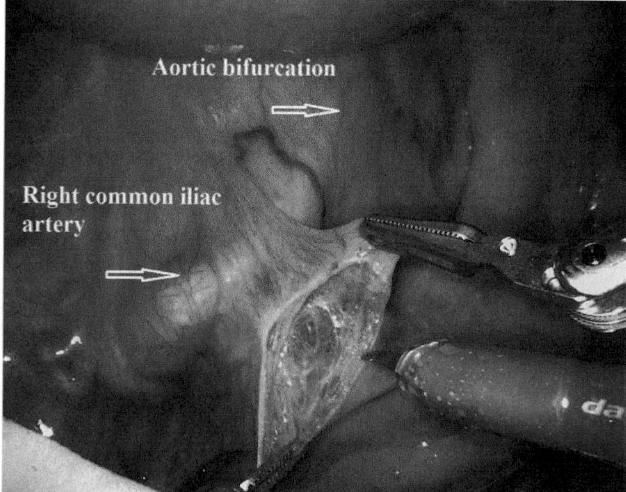

Fig. 77.18 The paraarotic lymph node dissection with the Xi robot starts with a small opening of the peritoneum just below the aortic bifurcation

peritoneum at the level of the bifurcation (Fig. 77.17). This may be beneficial to prevent the bowel from interfering with the surgical field but sometimes requires an additional higher port for optics and a separate upper abdominal assistant's port in case pelvic surgery will be performed during the same session. With the S-Si robots a de-redocking for later pelvic position after the patient has been rotated 180 degrees will be necessary ("double docking"). Alternatively, with the robot initially placed at patients shoulder it can be redocked in a pelvic side position with a smaller adjustment of patients position sideways ("double side docking") and a full 180 degree rotation, often time consuming and cumbersome for the anesthetist, can be avoided.

Using the da Vinci Xi model both these double docking alternatives can be omitted due to the " roof hanged" robot arm boom and the increased range of motion of the robot arms. Instead of a cumbersome rotation of the patient or double docking the robot arm boom can be rotated 180 degrees, either via a swift de-redocking and rotating the whole robot arm boom or by using the increased range of motion of the arms, with the robot fundament unchanged. A rotation of the whole robot arm set provides more space for the assistant using at least one suprapubic port which is necessary for assisting parallel to the robot instruments and for lifting the roof of the peritoneal tunnel created over the aorta (Figs. 77.18, 77.19 and 77.20).

The basic surgical principle for all approaches is similar. All surgery requires a good anatomical knowledge and awareness that approximately one third of patients have some vascular anomaly in the paraaortic area [12–14]. A preoperative

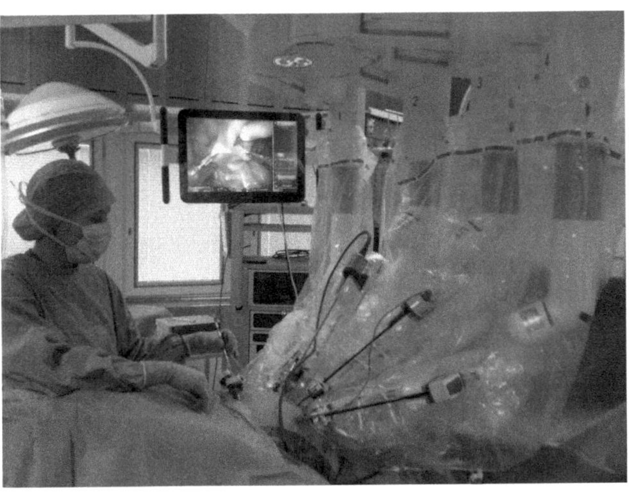

Fig. 77.19 Paraaortic lymphadenectomy with the Xi robot. Note position of the robot arm boom

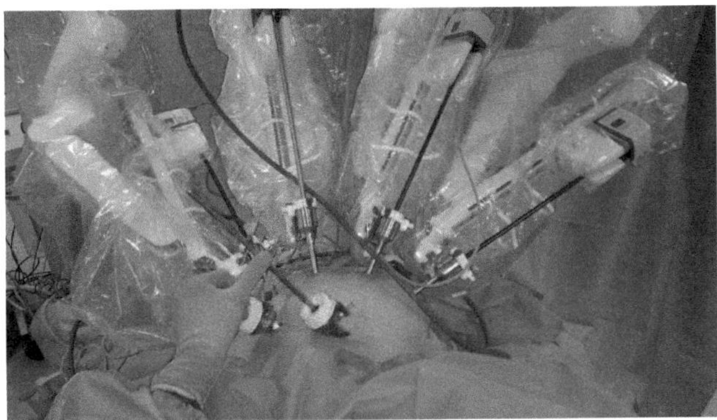

Fig. 77.20 Position of assistant and assistants trocars for a paraarotic lymph nodes dissection with the Xi robot

CT scan of the abdomen should include information on any major blood vessel anomalies and in case of enlarged lymph nodes an exact position of those related to easily identified vascular landmarks. It is particularly important that the whole staff is familiar with all used assistants instruments, hemostatic agents and that an emergency de-docking plan is implemented. Although conversion to open surgery due to bleeding rarely occurs, a laparotomy set including vessel repairing instruments should be readily available. The anesthetist should be asked to keep fluid balance on the negative side to avoid too distended veins. In all, everyone should be prepared and experienced with their respective tasks.

Usually, it is beneficial to use the Palmers' point entry and a similar position of the 12 mm assistants' trocar as this allows an intraabdominal overview of the position of the optics trocar and a partial removal of the lower falciform ligament that sometimes hinders an optimal position of the optics trocar. This entry point also allows for the release of midline oriented adhesions as well as diagnosing a previously unknown umbilical hernia. The incision for the optics

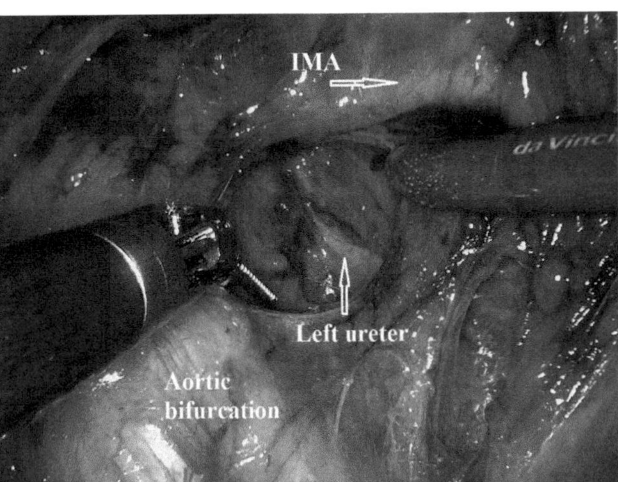

Fig. 77.21 Visualization of the left ureter and the IMA

trocar should be kept minimal to avoid leaking of gas and minimize the risk for the optics trocar to slide out if some retraction is necessary. For the same reason, it is often beneficial to use an optics trocar with outer ridges or a balloon trocar. The remaining trocars are then placed (Fig. 77.15). An overview of the abdomen to rule out disseminated disease should be performed before docking the robot instruments. The necessary degree of Trendelenburg is controlled from inside with the optics. After docking the robot the range of motion of the robot arms should be optimized to reach the paraaortic area (Fig. 77.16).

With the Xi robot or in case of double docking/patient rotation it is recommended to initiate the procedure as described above but also place at least one suprapubic assistant's port for the paraaortic dissection (Figs. 77.19 and 77.20). The paraaortic dissection starts with making a 5–6 centimeter peritoneal incision just below the aortic bifurcation as a tunnel opening (Fig. 77.18). With the aid of the fourth arm and instruments inserted via the supraumbilical assistant's port the roof of the tunnel is elevated simply by using the shafts of closed instruments inserted to the apex of the created tunnel. Then, before any attempts of lymphadenectomy, a gradual further cranial dissection to fully visualize the anatomical landmarks and potential vessel anomalies to the level of the left renal vein is performed (Figs. 77.21, 77.22 and 77.23). For finding the left supramesenteric part of the ureter, which is often runs deep, it is usually helpful to dissect the left ureter as far cranially as possible when exploring the left side inframesenteric part. The main left and right side hypogastric nerve branches is usually possible to preserve without compromising the lymphadenectomy (Fig. 77.24). The lymphadenectomy is performed from cranial to distal. The upper limit of the dissection can be marked with a titanium clip.

With this approach, the access is usually good, and with less obscuring bowel compared with the technique described

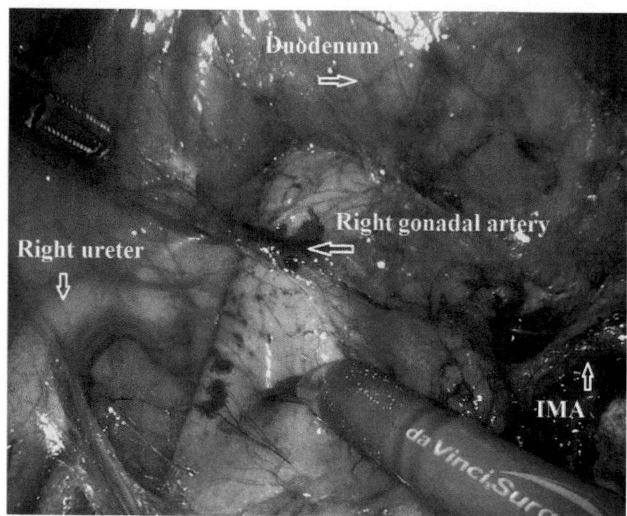

Fig. 77.22 Dissection of the paracaval right side visualizing the right ureter and gonadal vessels

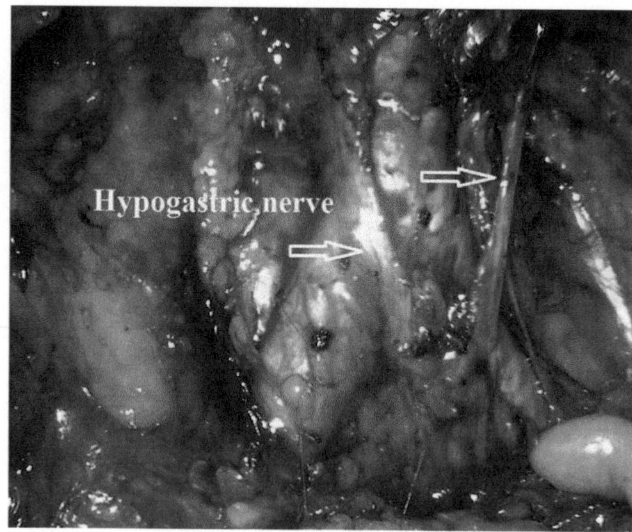

Fig. 77.24 The right and left branches of the hypogastric nerves can usually be preserved

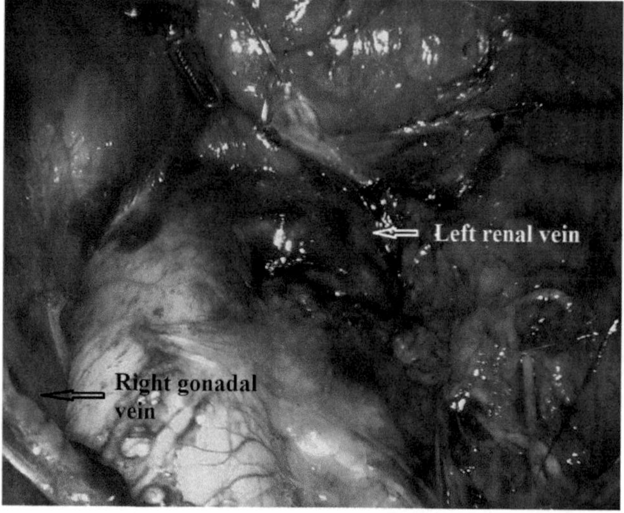

Fig. 77.23 Reaching the left renal vein with requires a gentle lift of the duodenum

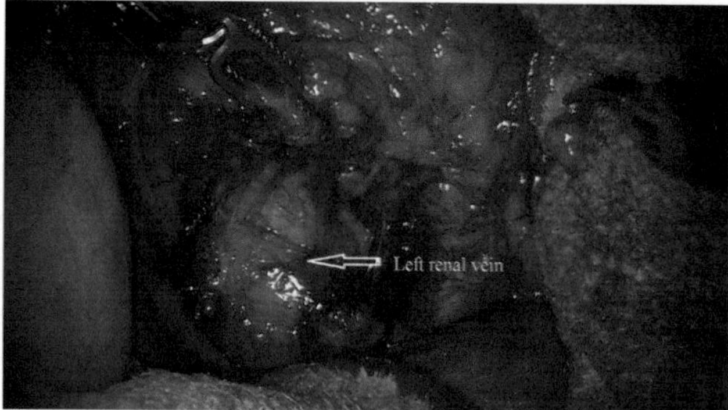

Fig. 77.25 Reaching the left renal vein with pelvic position of the S-Si robots usually requires help of two assistants retractors and sponges

below. The disadvantages are the need for one or two suprapubic assistant's ports, the need for rotation of the patient, and the lower robot port placement needed for an adequate angle related to the aorta. This results in a more perpendicular instrument angle for the lower paraaortic and upper pelvic lymphadenectomy and a shorter distance from the pelvic operative area to the optics with a decreased overview and more need for cleaning of the lens.

With the pelvic position of the robot, the operation starts with retracting the sigmoid colon against the left abdominal wall with one or two sponge reinforced sutures through appendices epiploicae. Then the caecum and ascending colon are mobilized by incizing the lateral peritoneum as far up as possible. The small bowel mesentery is often adherent to the IP-ligament and has to be released to allow the small bowel to retract cranially. The peritoneum is then opened medial of the right common iliac artery to the level of the aortic bifurcation and further to the inferior mesenteric artery (IMA) and the ureters, the IP-ligaments and the hypogastric nerve are visualized similar to the onset of a pelvic lymphadenectomy (Figs. 77.1, 77.2 and 77.3). The third robot arm grasper is useful for further lifting the sigmoid or retracting the right ureter and IP-ligament. The lower paraaortic and paracaval lateral areas are then opened carefully to clearly explore the vessel anatomy. Then the IMA is skeletonized and the dissection continued to reach the level of the left renal vein (Fig. 77.25). The role of the assistant at this stage is to lift the proximal peritoneal fold to prevent the small bowel from interfering with the surgical field, sometimes

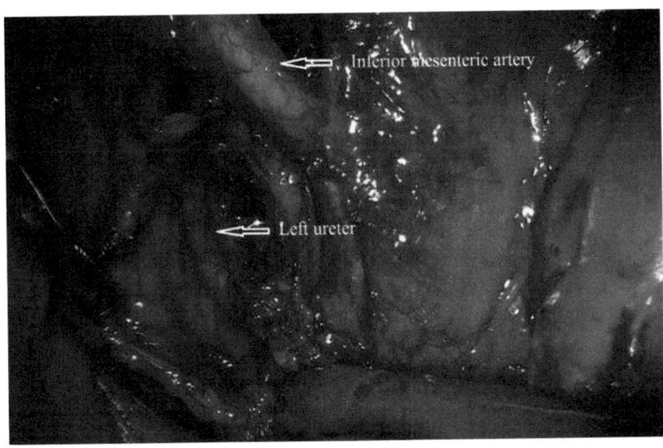

Fig. 77.26 The left supramesenteric part of the ureter must be visualized and lateralized before removing lymph nodes

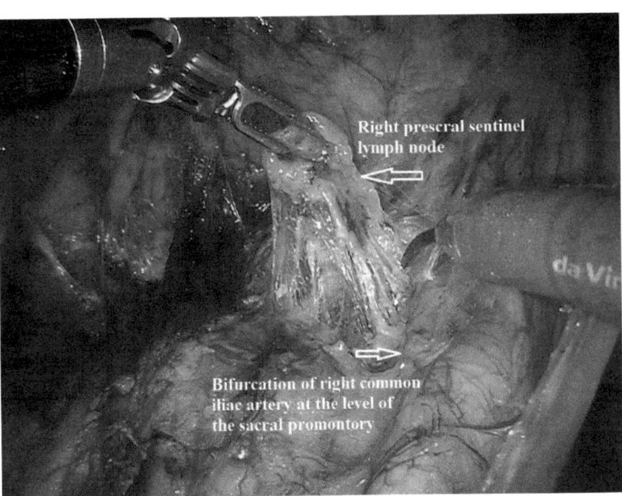

Fig. 77.27 Right side presacral dissection

requiring a second assistants' port and a several sponges. The third arm is used for retracting the left side of the peritoneal opening at desired level. The origin of the IP-ligaments and the gonadal arteries are identified as well as the ureters in the supramesenteric area, in particular on the left side where the course of the ureter is deeper (Fig. 77.26). The ureter must be lateralized before removal of the lymph nodes.

After exploring the whole operative field a final view of the vessel anatomy is obtained before the lymphadenectomy begins. The order of dissection is optional but it usually a good idea to start cranially and with the left supramesenteric paraaortic area as this tends to be the most difficult part, followed by the intraaortacaval and finally the precaval parts. Any bleeding from previous distal dissection may also be cumbersome when the supramesenteric dissection is performed. In case leaking of large amount of lymphatic fluid occurs, in particular if opaque/chylous, it is important to find the leak and close it with clips as it may be associated with later development of chylous ascites. A metal clip marking the proximal limit for the dissection is often appreciated by the radiooncologists. Finally the inframesenteric nodal dissection is performed compartmentwize. Attention should be given to free nodal tissue under the IMA which is easily overseen. It is usually possible to free and save the main branches of the hypogastric nerve running from right to left over the inframesenteric aorta via the aortic bifurcation and then further on presacrally (Fig. 77.24).

Effort should be made to achieve good hemostasis throughout the procedure, not only to reduce the risk for a major bleeding and conversion but to avoid time consuming hemostatic actions. Before nodal dissection it is recommended to have a laparoscopic sponge in the abdomen practical for simultaneous suction and compression of smaller bleeds i.e. from Fellows veins that usually stops with compression with or without help of surgical hemostatic agents. Smaller arterial bleeds are best controlled with clips or bipolar diathermia whereas vessel damage considered inappropriate for compression or diathermia may be sutured. Any attempt to repair a larger bleed should include a temporary control, i.e. by grasping with the robot instruments and only after optimizing the surgical and anesthesiological situation the actual repair should be attempted. It is for safety reasons important to strongly discourage from repeated unsuccessful attempts to control a bleed.

The near infrared fluorescent technique for detection of sentinel lymph nodes is available with the Xi and Si systems. By the use of an adapted light source, optics and software the used tracer (Indocyanine green) will appear green against a grey background. So far, no standardized technique of injection sites, dosing and timing for the use within gynecology are agreed on but several centers perform studies. A standardization must include knowledge of the lymphatic anatomy, a clear definition of sentinel lymph nodes and a defined stepwise surgical algorithm. The tracer has a rapid spread leading to many coloured lymph nodes which cannot all be defined as sentinel lymph nodes. Therefore, the afferent lymph vessel in each major lymphatic chain must be identified to define the node closest to the tumour (the sentinel lymph node). Hence the retroperitoneal dissection must be performed meticulously to avoid cutting lymph vessels. To avoid disturbance from tracer leakage during sentinel node remove, dissection of nodes preferably starts cranially, i.e. with the presacral nodes (Figs. 77.27 and 77.28) followed by the pelvic side walls (Figs. 77.29 and 77.30). In case of no uptake of tracer a full lymphadenectomy shall be performed. In this situation it is particularly important to look for macroscopically cancer suspect nodes.

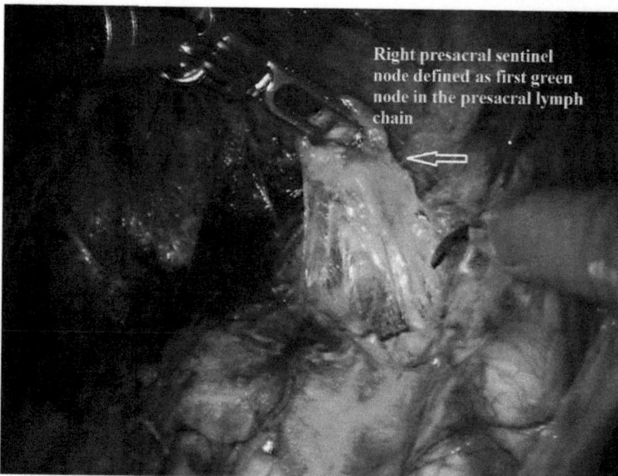

Fig. 77.28 Right side presacral dissection with the firefly technique

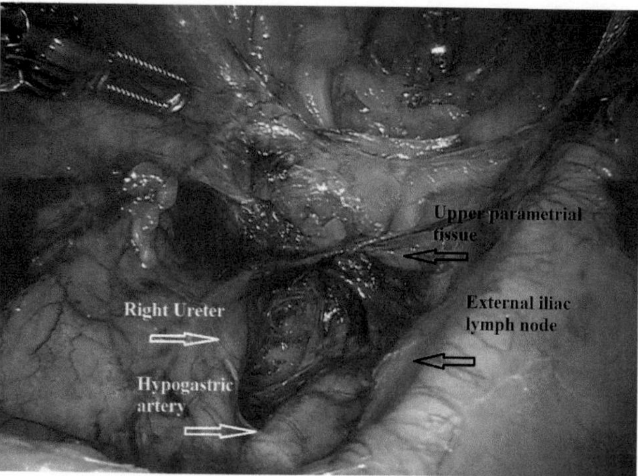

Fig. 77.29 Right upper paracervical/parametrial tissue

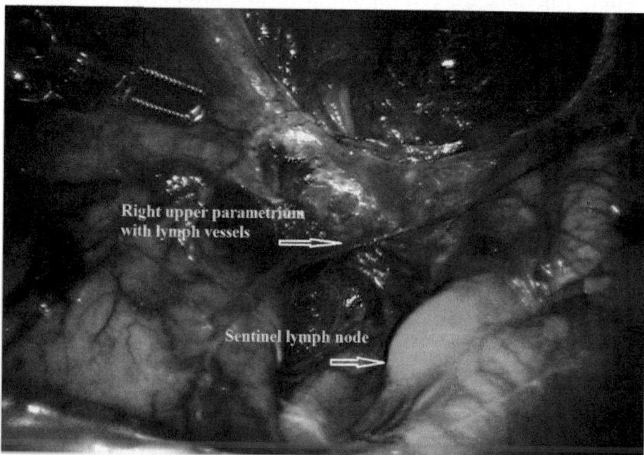

Fig. 77.30 Right upper parametrium seen with the firefly technique

References

1. Köhler C, Klemm P, Schau A, Possover M, Krause N, Tozzi R, Schneider A. Introduction of transperitoneal lymphadenectomy in a gynecologic oncology center: analysis of 650 laparoscopic pelvic and/or paraaortic transperitoneal lymphadenectomies. Gynecol Oncol. 2004;95(1):52–61.
2. Querleu D, Leblanc E, Cartron G, Narducci F, Ferron G, Martel P. Audit of preoperative and early complications of laparoscopic lymph node dissection in 1000 gynecologic cancer patients. Am J Obstet Gynecol. 2006;195(5):1287–92. Epub 2006 May 3
3. Boggess JF, Gehrig PA, Cantrell L, Shafer A, Ridgway M, Skinner EN, Fowler WC. A comparative study of 3 surgical methods for hysterectomy with staging for endometrial cancer: robotic assistance, laparoscopy, laparotomy. Am J Obstet Gynecol. 2008;199(4):360.e1–9. doi:10.1016/j.ajog.2008.08.012.
4. Somashekhar SP, Jaka RC, Zaveri SS. Prospective randomized study comparing robotic-assisted hysterectomy and regional lymphadenectomy with traditional laparotomy for staging of endometrial carcinoma -initial Indian experience. Indian J Surg Oncol. 2014;5(3):217–23. doi:10.1007/s13193-014-0321-8. Epub 2014 Jun 21
5. Chiou H, Chiu L, Chen C, Yen Y, Chang C, Liu W. Comparing robotic surgery with laparoscopy and laparotomy for endometrial cancer management: a cohort study. Int J Surg. 2014;13C:17–22. doi:10.1016/j.ijsu.2014.11.015. [Epub ahead of print].
6. Abaza R, Dangle PP, Gong MC, Bahnson RR, Pohar KS. Quality of lymphadenectomy is equivalent with robotic and open cystectomy using an extended template. Urol. 2012;187(4):1200–4. doi:10.1016/j.juro.2011.11.092. Epub 2012 Feb 15.
7. Lim PC, Kang E, Park DH. A comparative detail analysis of the learning curve and surgical outcome for robotic hysterectomy with-lymphadenectomy versus laparoscopic hysterectomy with lymphadenectomy in treatment of endometrial cancer: a case-matched controlled study of the first one hundred twenty two patients. Gynecol Oncol. 2011;120(3):413–8. doi:10.1016/j.ygyno.2010.11.034. Epub 2010 Dec 30.
8. Seamon LG, Bryant SA, Rheaume PS, Kimball KJ, Huh WK, Fowler JM, Phillips GS, Cohn DE. Comprehensive surgical staging for endometrial cancer in obese patients: comparing robotics and laparotomy. Obstet Gynecol. 2009;114(1):16–21. doi:10.1097/AOG.0b013e3181aa96c7.
9. Gehrig PA, Cantrell LA, Shafer A, Abaid LN, Mendivil A, Boggess JF. What is the optimal minimally invasive surgical procedure for endometrial cancer staging in the obese and morbidly obese woman? Gynecol Oncol. 2008;111(1):41–5. doi:10.1016/j.ygyno.2008.06.030. Epub 2008 Aug 9.
10. Rossi EC, Ivanova A, Boggess JF. Robotically assisted fluorescence-guided lymph node mapping with ICG for gynecologic malignancies: a feasibility study. Gynecol Oncol. 2012;124(1):78–82. doi:10.1016/j.ygyno.2011.09.025. Epub 2011 Oct 11.
11. Bats AS, Mimouni M, Bensaïd C, Seror J, Douay-Hauser N, Nos C, Lécuru F. Robotic extraperitoneal paraaortic lymphadenectomy in gynecological cancers: feasibility, safety, and short-term outcomes of isolated and combined procedures. Int J Gynecol Cancer. 2014;24(8):1486–92. doi:10.1097/IGC.0000000000000240.
12. Franké O, Narducci F, Chereau-Ewald E, Orsoni M, Jauffret C, Leblanc E, Houvenaeghel G, Lambaudie E. Role of a double docking to improve lymph node dissection: when robotically assisted laparoscopy for para-aortic lymphadenectomy is associated to a

pelvic procedure. Int J Gynecol Cancer. 2014. [Epub ahead of print].

13. James JA, Rakowski JA, Jeppson CN, Stavitzski NM, Ahmad S, Holloway RW. Robotic transperitoneal infra-renal aortic lymphadenectomy in early-stage endometrial cancer. Gynecol Oncol. 2014; pii: S0090–8258(14)01625–4. doi: 10.1016/j.ygyno.2014.12.028. [Epub ahead of print].

14. Klemm P, Fröber R, Köhler C, Schneider A. Vascular anomalies in the paraaortic region diagnosed by laparoscopy in patients with gynaecologic malignancies. Gynecol Oncol. 2005;96(2):278–82.

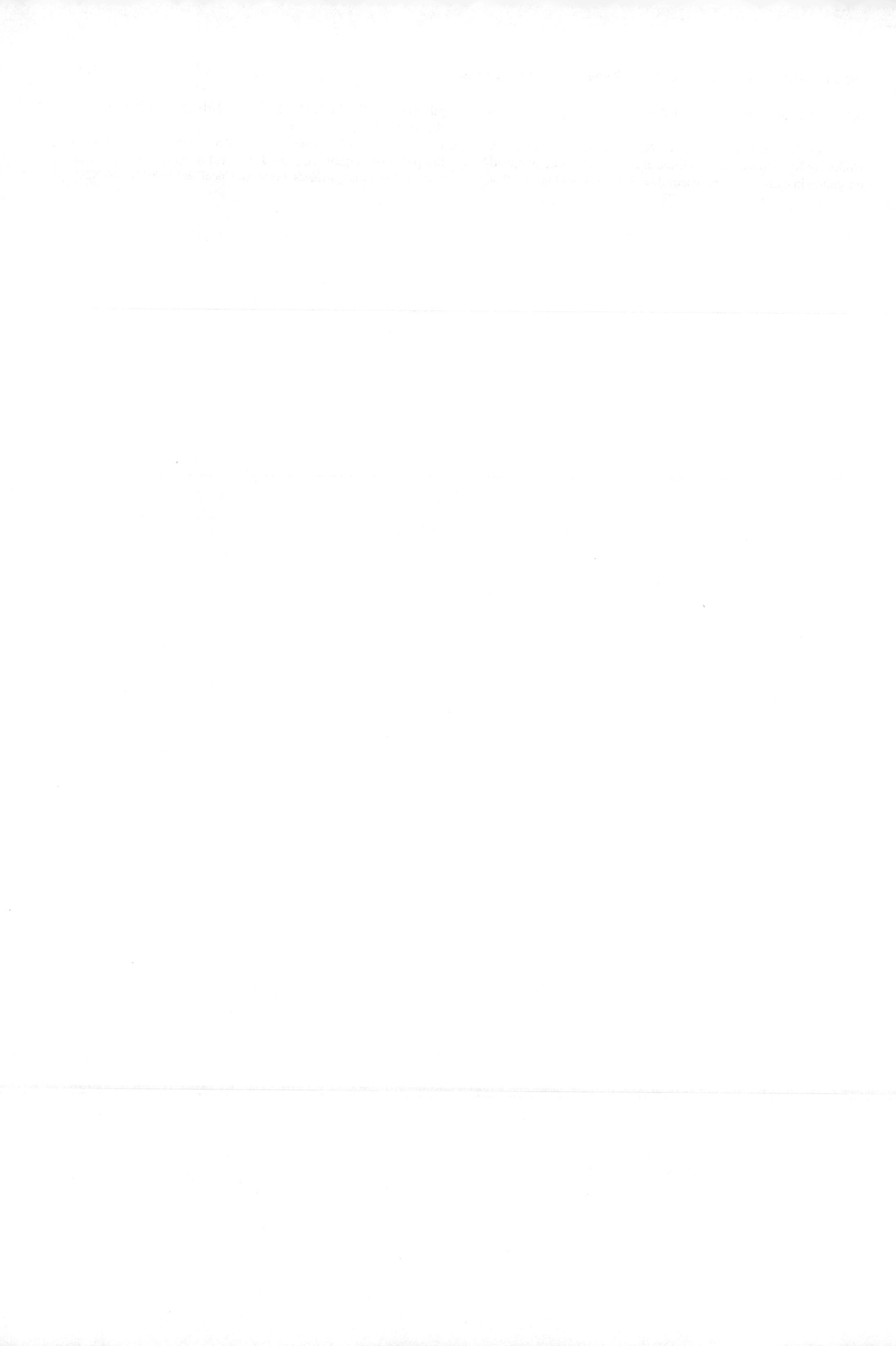

Techniques for Gastrocolic and Infracolic Robotic Omentectomy

78

Gerald Feuer and Nisha Lakhi

Anatomy

The greater omentum is composed of a double layer of peritoneum and mainly fatty tissue. It extends from the greater curvature of the stomach, passes in front of the small intestines, and reflects on itself to ascend to the transverse colon (Fig. 78.1). The gastrocolic omentum extends from the greater curvature of the stomach to the superior aspect of the transverse colon [1]. When performing an omentectomy, the right border of the omentum can normally be identified at the ceacum and the left border at the splenic flexure. Identifying these landmarks may be useful for acquiring orientation during dissection.

Blood Supply

The right and left gastroepiploic vessels traverse the greater curvature of the stomach and provide the sole blood supply to the greater omentum. Three dominant omental vessels, along with smaller branches, arise from the gastroepiploic system and provide vascular supply to the omentum (Fig. 78.2) [1].

Function of the Omentum

The omentum has three main functions:

1. Fat deposition.
2. Functions as a secondary lymphoid organ.

The omentum contains secondary lymphoid tissue called “milky spots”. It has been demonstrated that this tissue is a rich source of lymphocytes, macrophages and monocytes, which may aid in the removal of foreign material and bacteria. In addition, this tissue possesses antimicrobial and angiogenic properties through release of fibroblast growth factors and hence has a role in healing inflamed or ischemic tissue [2, 3].

3. Infection and Wound Isolation

The omentum is a mobile organ in the peritoneum. It serves to fix the viscera and isolate abnormal tissue or infection to limit its spread [2, 3].

Indications for Omentectomy

An omentectomy is indicated as part of the standard surgical staging for malignant ovarian neoplasms, borderline tumors, and primary peritoneal cancers (Table 78.1). It should be performed in cases even if there is not macroscopically visible disease [4]. The safety and feasibility of an omentectomy as part of a robotic staging operation for ovarian cancer has been documented in the literature [5]. Omentectomy should also be performed as part of the staging operation for serous papillary endometrial cancer, as this histological subtype of uterine cancer tends to spread transperitoneally and behaves in a manner similar to epithelial ovarian cancer [6].

In cases where there is no macroscopically visible disease on the omentum, the extent of omentectomy has not been elucidated, as there has been no study comparing total omentectomy, subtotal omentectomy, or omental biopsies alone for the purposes of staging and treatment of epithelial ovarian cancer [4]. In our practice, we perform an infracolic omentectomy as part of the general staging procedure, and include resection of the gastrocolic omentum in cases where

G. Feuer (✉)
Department of Gynaecologic Oncology, Northside Hospital, 980 Johnson Ferry Road NE, Suite 900, Atlanta, GA 30342, USA
e-mail: gfeuer@aol.com

N. Lakhi
Department of Obstetrics and Gynaecology, Richmond University Medical Center, 355 Bard Avenue, Staten Island, NY 10310, USA
e-mail: nlakhi@yahoo.com

I. Alkatout, L. Mettler (eds.), *Hysterectomy*, DOI 10.1007/978-3-319-22497-8_78

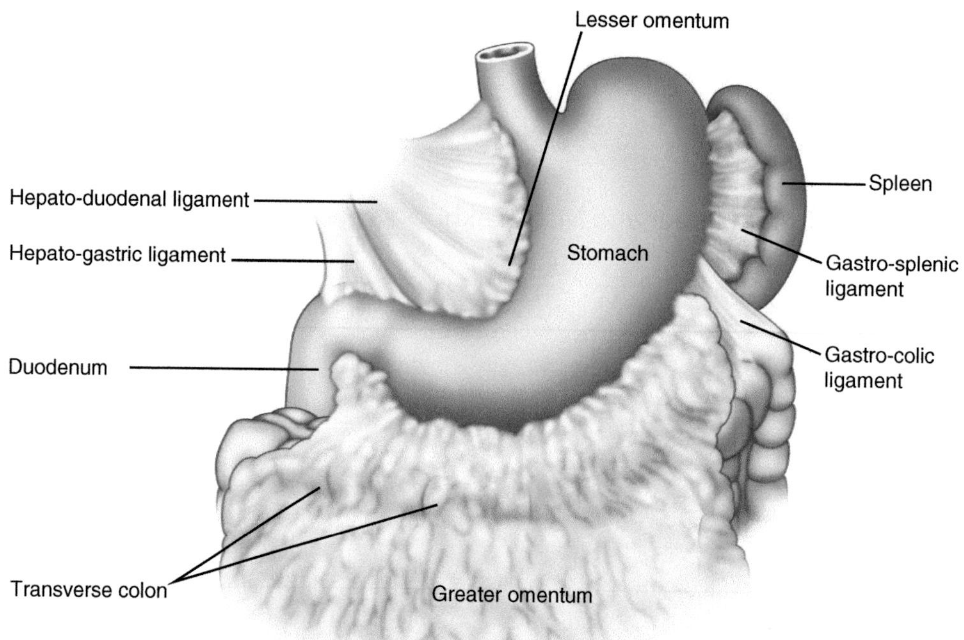

Fig. 78.1 Relationship of omentum to surrounding structures

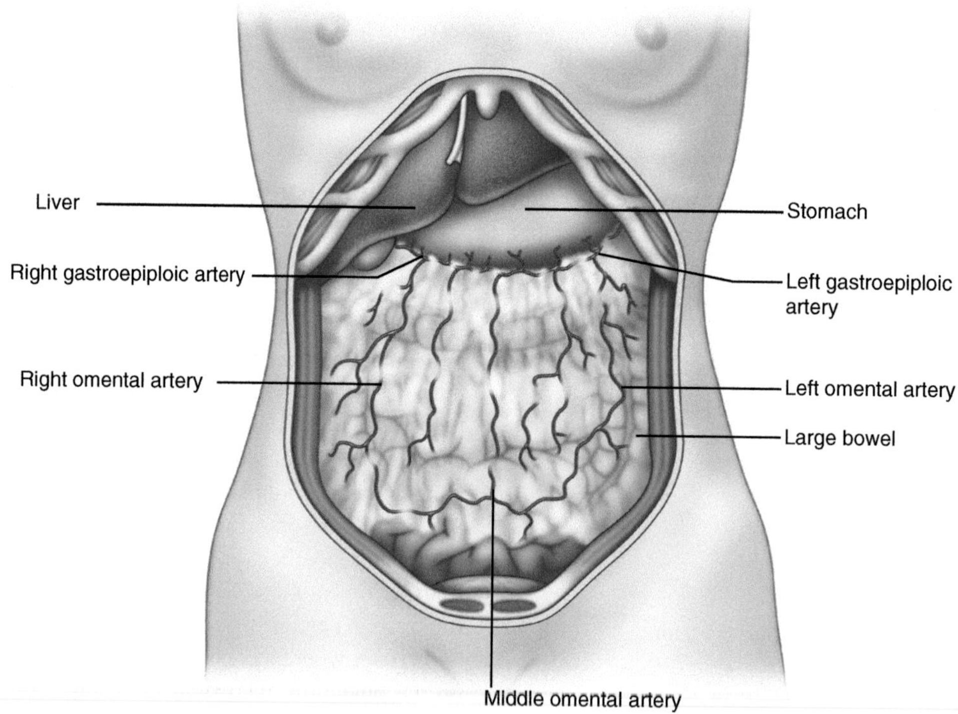

Fig. 78.2 Blood supply to the omentum

Table 78.1 Indications for omentectomy

Indications for Omentectomy
Epithelial ovarian cancer
Borderline ovarian tumors
Sex cord stromal ovarian tumors
Germ cell ovarian tumors
Primary peritoneal cancer
Uterine serous papillary/clear cell tumors
Uterine sarcoma

there is extensive upper abdominal disease or macroscopically visible disease on the gastrocolic omentum.

Note: The technique described is for performing an omentectomy utilizing the da Vinci® Si System (Si). Modifications of technique and port placement that are necessary when utilizing the da Vinci® Xi System (Xi) are mentioned where appropriate.

Robotic Infracolic Omentectomy

Port Placement and Docking

The optical port is positioned midline, approximately 22–24 cm (9 inches) above the symphysis pubis. Two lateral 8 mm robotic ports are introduced. The right 8 mm robotic port is positioned 10 cm lateral and 2 cm inferior to the optical port. The left 8 mm robotic port is placed 11–12 cm lateral and 2 cm inferior to the optical port. The left port is further lateralized in order to optimize dissection at the splenic flexure. If an assistant utilizes two ports, one 12 mm port is placed at the right lateral side of the patient 10 cm from the robotic port, and one 5 mm port in the right upper quadrant below the costal margin and midway between the left lateral port and the midline port. (Fig. 78.3).

The robot is centrally docked between the patient's legs, as this placement provides more range on the right side as compared to side docking (Fig. 78.4).

If utilizing the *da Vinci® Xi System* (Xi), the two lateral 8 mm robot ports are placed at the same plane as the optical port, each 9–10 cm lateralized from the midline (Fig. 78.5). It is not necessary to further lateralize the left robotic port to adequately reach the splenic flexure as in the Si model. For the Xi model, the robot can be docked centrally, but preferably from the patient's left side (Fig. 78.6).

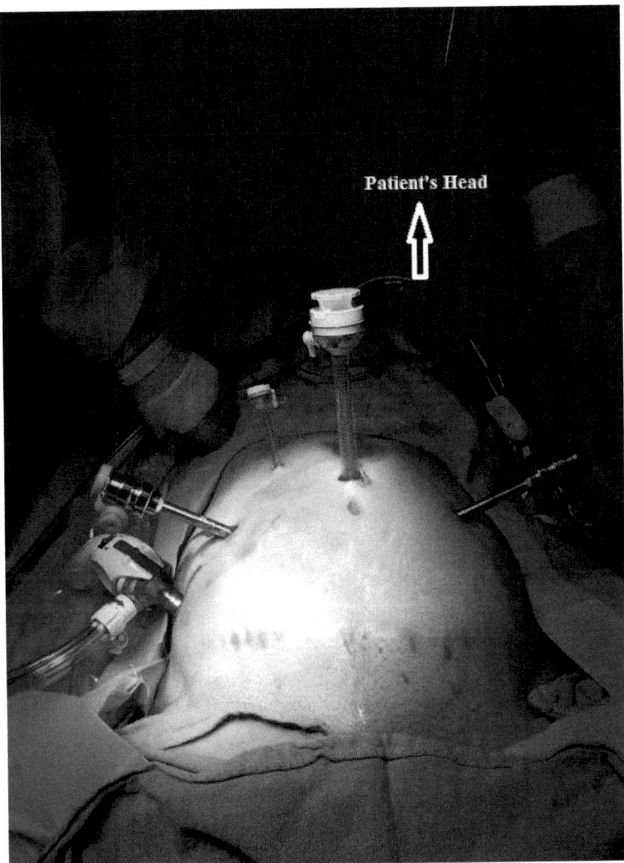

Fig. 78.3 Port position of infracolic omentectomy using the *da Vinci® SI System*

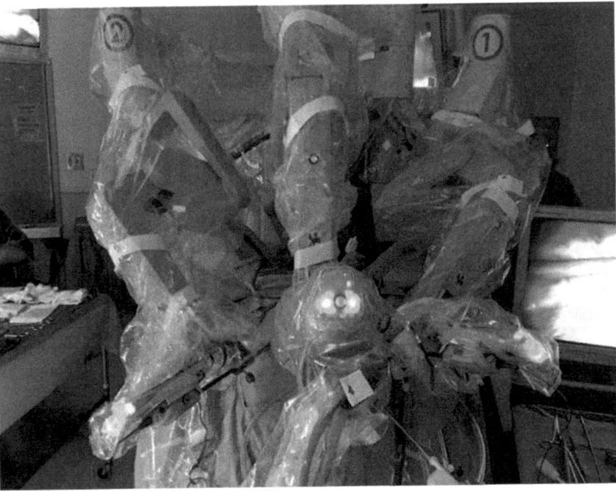

Fig. 78.4 *da Vinci® SI System* docked between the patient's legs in preparation for infracolic omentectomy.

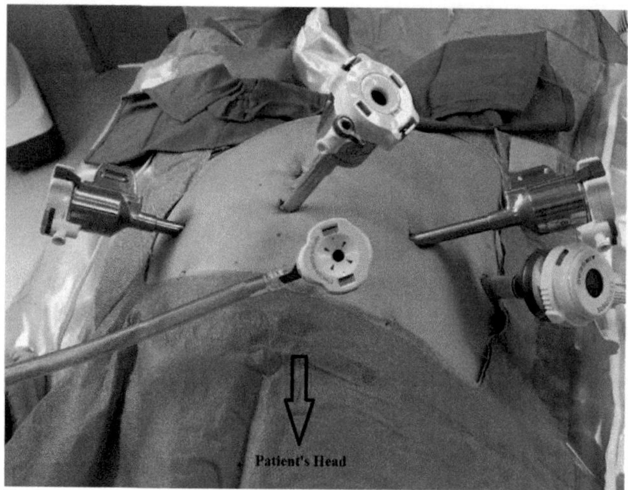

Fig. 78.5 Port position of infracolic omentectomy using the *da Vinci® XI System*

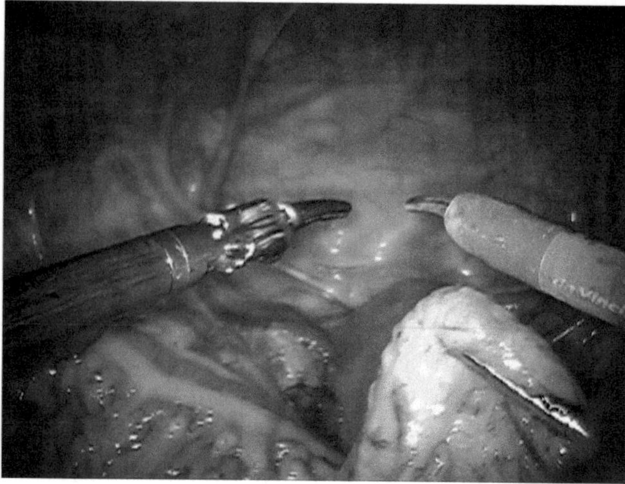

Fig. 78.7 Assistant laparoscopically grasping the omentum

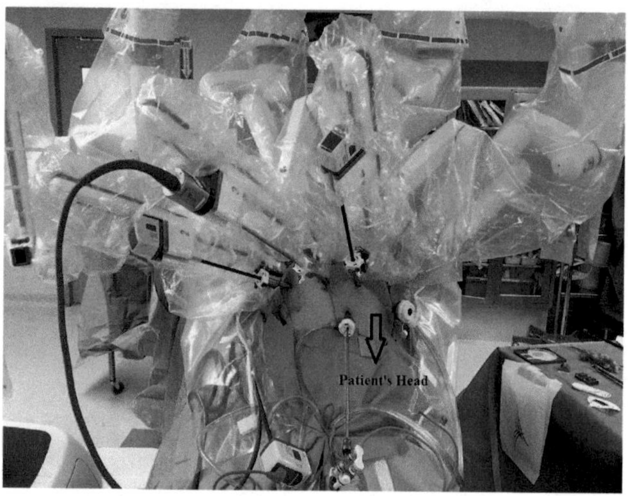

Fig. 78.6 *da Vinci® XI System* docked between the patient's legs in preparation for infracolic omentectomy.

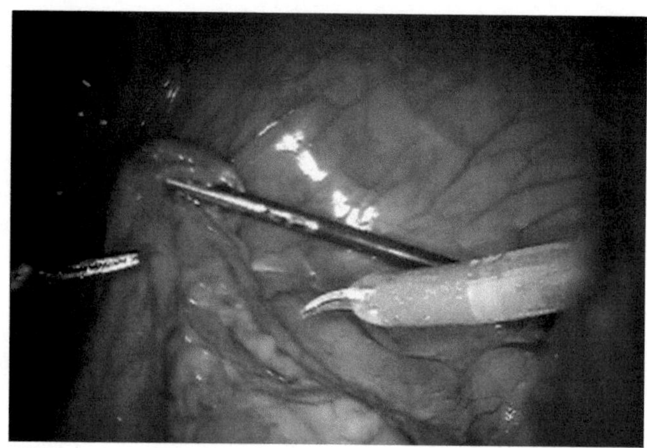

Fig. 78.8 Assistant pulling the omentum towards the pelvis

Role of the Assistant in Robotic Omentectomy

We describe a three arm technique for a robotic infracolic omentectomy. In this technique, the assistant has a critical role: The assistant laparoscopically maintains the omentum midline, pulls it deep into the pelvis, and provides countertraction. This allows for easier dissection and visualization throughout the procedure. It is important that the surgeon and the assistant work in tandem, maintaining equal traction and countertraction. If a skilled assistant is not available, a fourth arm can be employed to provide countertraction in the direction of the pelvis. The port would be placed in the same plane as the other robotic port on the left side, approximately 9–10 cm lateral for the Xi system and 10–12 cm lateral for the Si system. However the use of a fourth arm is less effective, as the fine, real-time adjustments a skilled assistant can make are difficult to duplicate with an additional robotic arm.

Procedure

At the start of the procedure, the assistant grasps the omentum at an area to the right of the mid-transverse colon and places it within the pelvis (Fig. 78.7).

The assistant or fourth arm maintains the position of the omentum toward the pelvis (Fig. 78.8), while the surgeon utilizes the left robotic arm to provide gentle traction immediately adjacent to area to be incised (Fig. 78.9). This aids in exposure of the anterior and posterior peritoneal reflections of the omentum, where the point of entry is made (Fig. 78.10).

The surgeon commences dissection at the mid-transverse colon (Fig. 78.11). Monopolar scissors are used to cut

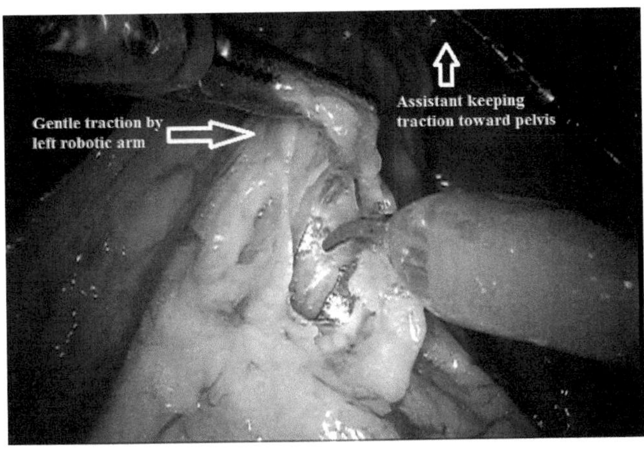

Fig. 78.9 Assistant maintaining the position of omentum in pelvis as the surgeon exerts gentle traction with the left robotic arm to reveal the peritoneal folds.

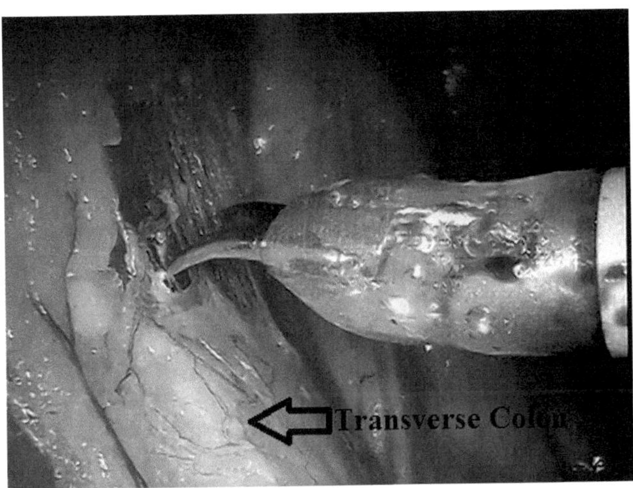

Fig. 78.10 The point of entry is made at the mid-transverse colon where the thin anterior posterior peritoneal fold can be visualized

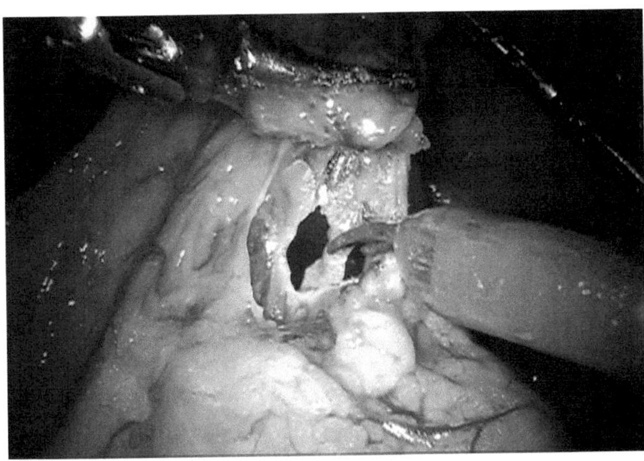

Fig. 78.11 Surgeon begins dissection by incising the peritoneal folds with the robotic scissors

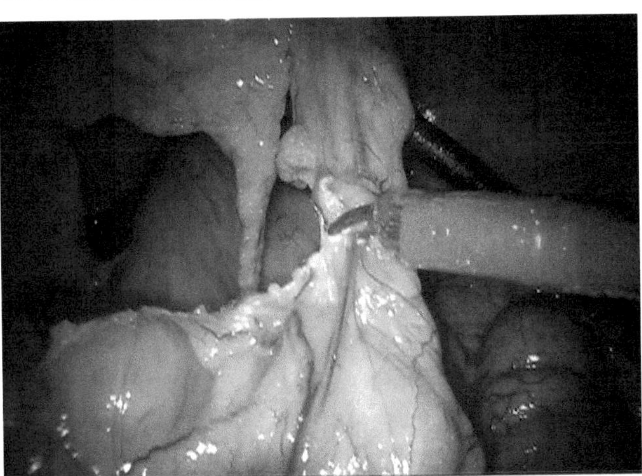

Fig. 78.12 Cutting current is used along the mid-transverse colon to incise the peritoneal folds. The assistant maintains traction of the omentum towards the pelvis.

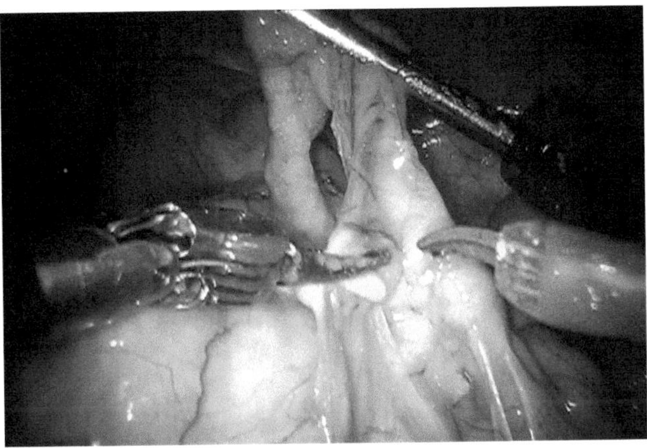

Fig. 78.13 Bipolar current being used to coagulate larger pedicles

the thin anterior and posterior peritoneal reflections (Fig. 78.12). Thicker vascular pedicles are first desiccated with bipolar cautery (Fig. 78.13). It is important to keep the bowel in direct visualization to avoid thermal injury (Fig. 78.14). In order to avoid thermal injury to the bowel, a distance of 3–5 mm from the bowel should be kept when using cutting current. A distance of 1 cm should be maintained when using coagulation current due to its increased thermal spread.

The surgeon continues dissection from the mid-transverse colon towards the ceacum (Fig. 78.15). This step can be more difficult in cases where the bowel is inadequately prepared or in obese patients that have abundant abdominal fat. In the obese patient, a useful trick to identify the peritoneal reflection along the transverse colon is to flip to omentum so that its posterior surface is visualized. The posterior surface can be followed to identify the transverse colon and find the peritoneal reflections.

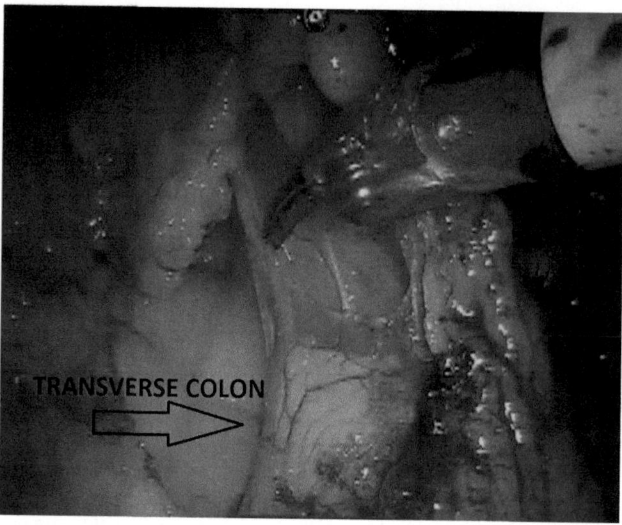

Fig. 78.14 A distance of 3–5 mm from the bowel should be maintained when using cutting current.

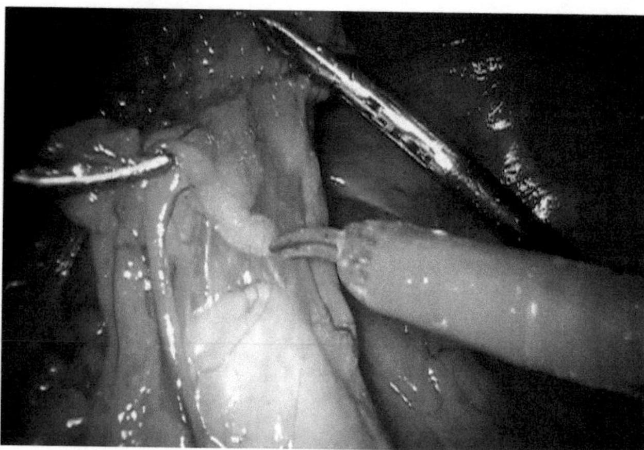

Fig. 78.16 Near the splenic flexure, the assistant is pulling the omentum towards the right lower quadrant as the surgeon uses the left robotic arm to pull up on the omentum, thereby revealing the peritoneal reflection.

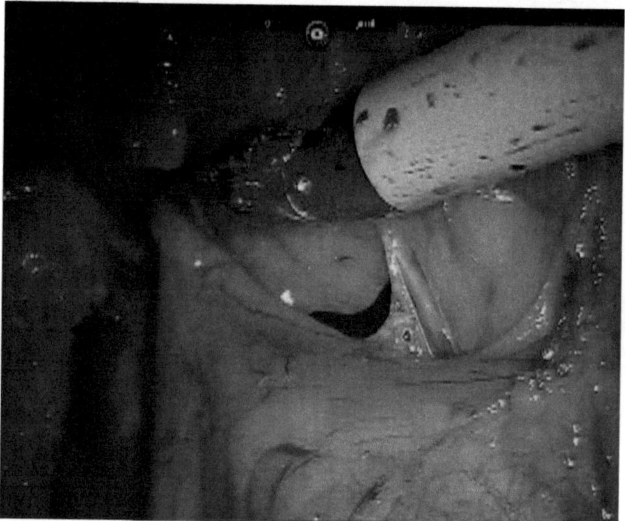

Fig. 78.15 Dissection along the mid-transverse colon towards the ceacum

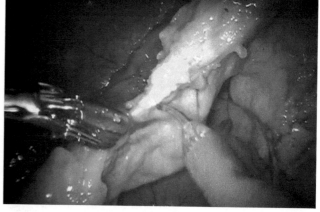

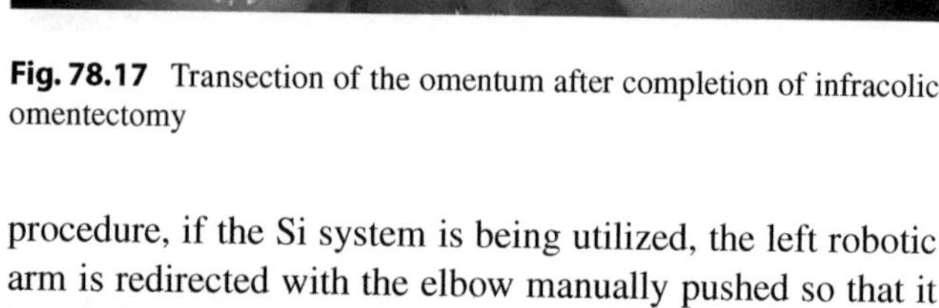

Fig. 78.17 Transection of the omentum after completion of infracolic omentectomy

In order for the procedure to be successful, the surgeon and the assistant have to make periodic adjustments in the amount and direction of traction and countertraction, so that the peritoneal reflections and transverse colon can be easily visualized.

After completion of dissection at the ceacum, the surgeon returns to the mid-transverse colon and dissects towards the splenic flexure. The ability to reach the splenic flexure is dependent on optimal placement of the left robotic arm. The first consideration is during the initial port placement, where the arm is placed 11–12 cm lateral left from the midline for the Si system. Placement of this port 9–10 cm from the midline is sufficient for Xi system. Second, at this point in the procedure, if the Si system is being utilized, the left robotic arm is redirected with the elbow manually pushed so that it is pointing toward the robot.

As dissection continues toward the splenic flexure, the assistant or fourth arm provides countertraction towards the right lower quadrant as the surgeon maintains upward traction (Fig. 78.16). The anterior and posterior peritoneal reflections are identified and cut with monopolar cautery. Vascular pedicles are identified and initially desiccated with bipolar cautery and cut with the robotic scissors with or without the utilization of cautery. Once one satisfactorily accomplishes the extent of dissection towards the splenic flexure similar to an open procedure, the specimen is transected using bipolar current or monopolar in combination with the robotic scissors (Fig. 78.17).

At the completion of the infracolic omentectomy, the omentum is tacked to the left pelvic sidewall using a surgical clip or a stitch. It is extracted vaginally at the completion of the hysterectomy and staging procedure. The omentum is grasped with a sponge stick and rotated clockwise during extraction. The key steps for infracolic omentectomy are summarized below (Table 78.2).

Robotic omentectomy, once mastered, can be performed with operative times similar to open and faster than laparoscipic omentectomies. However, some differences between robotic and other approaches should be noted. Compared to the laparoscopic approach, port positioning for robotic omentectomy is usually higher, as described. This is important, especially for the placement of the optical port, since its position is not easily interchangeable as it is in conventional laparoscopy. The higher position of the optical port in robotic surgery allows for visualization of both the upper abdomen as well as the pelvis. Laparoscopiclly, the camera can be moved to a suprapubic port and the surgeon can dissect in the upper abdomen via accessory ports. With the robotic approach, the optical port is fixed; therefore, the surgeon is more dependent on the assistant maintaining the position of the omentum in the pelvis. Additionally, access to the left upper quadrant toward the splenic flexure can be more difficult with the robotic approach. If there is no macroscopically visible disease, we generally terminate the infracolic omentectomy 10–15 cm (4–6 inches) from the splenic flexure, which is similar to an open procedure. Access to the left upper quadrant when using the Si model is optimized by further lateralizing the left robotic port and when approaching the splenic flexure, manually re-directing the left robotic arm, so that its elbow points towards the robot. Coordination between the surgeon and assistant, the robotic omentectomy can accomplished with efficiency similar to open and faster than laparoscopic approaches.

Robotic Gastrocolic Omentectomy

A gastrocolic omentectomy is performed when there is upper abdominal disease or macroscopic disease on the gastrocolic omentum. We initially make a laparoscopic assessment prior to docking the robot and decide if this procedure needs to be undertaken. If necessary, it is performed prior to the infracolic omentectomy that is described above. For the Si system, a double docking technique is necessary: first docking the robot over the patient's right shoulder for the gastrocolic dissection (Fig. 78.18), and then centrally docking the robot

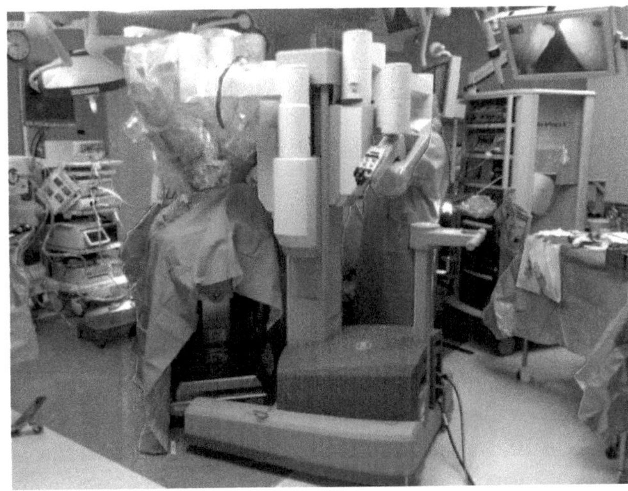

Fig. 78.18 Docking of the *da Vinci® SI System* over the patient's right shoulder in preparation for a gastrocolic omentectomy

Table 78.2 Key steps for infracolic omentectomy procedure

Beginning of procedure 1. The omentum is laparoscopically placed in the pelvis. The assistant maintains traction throughout the procedure to keep the omentum in the pelvis rather than the upper abdomen. 2. Dissection begins at the mid-transverse colon, where the anterior and posterior peritoneal folds are identified and entered. 3. In order to identify the peritoneal folds, the left robotic arm pulls up on the omentum, exerting upward traction to assist in revealing the peritoneal reflections.
Middle of procedure 1. Dissection begins from the point of entry along mid-transverse colon and continues toward the caecum. 2. Cutting current with the monopolar scissors is used to dissect along the anterior and posterior peritoneal folds. 3. Once dissection to the caecum is complete, we return to the point of entry along the mid-transverse colon in order to dissect in the opposite direction, towards the splenic flexure. 4. At this point, if the Si system is being used, manually re-directing the left robotic arm, so that its elbow points towards the robot, can optimize dissection towards the splenic flexure. 5. Dissection continues along the anterior and posterior peritoneal folds as previously.
End of procedure 1. The extent of dissection is variable; however, if there is no grossly visible disease, we normally terminate dissection 10–15 cm (4–6 inches) from the splenic flexure. 2. In order to terminate the procedure, a point of transection is determined. Bipolar current is used to desiccate the thick fatty area of the omentum being transected, and robotic scissors are used to cut and free the specimen.

between the patient's legs to accomplish the infracolic portion. This is not necessary with the Xi system as the boom of the robot can be turned to approach multiple quadrants.

Procedure

To begin the gastrocolic omentectomy, the stomach is tented up (Fig. 78.19) and the peritoneal folds of the omentum are incised to the right of the midline with cutting current in order to enter the lesser sac (Fig. 78.20). It is useful to identify a thin area of peritoneum along the greater curvature of the stomach and enter the lesser sac from this point.

A robotic vessel sealer is helpful for dissection and maintaining hemostasis. The sealer is used in the left robotic arm and an atraumatic fenestrated grasper is placed in the right incised to the right of the midline robotic arm. The role of the assistant is to exert upwards traction on the stomach with an atraumatic grasper while the right robotic arm places downward traction on the omentum. This dynamic should be maintained throughout the dissection (Fig. 78.21).

The omentectomy is commenced from the point where the lesser sac was entered. The sealer is placed approximately 1–1.5 cm away from the short gastric arteries (Fig. 78.22). A double seal technique is used, in which the sealer is fired twice before cutting; this allows for a more hemostatic dissection. Dissection is continued along the greater curvature of the stomach toward the splenic flexure (Fig. 78.23).

Upon reaching the splenic flexure, the dissection is directed towards the transverse colon (Fig. 78.24). This facilitates the infra-colic omentectomy that can be continued from the pelvis. In order to define the limit of the omentetomy, it is important to make a detailed visual inspection of any residual disease so that it can be included with the specimen.

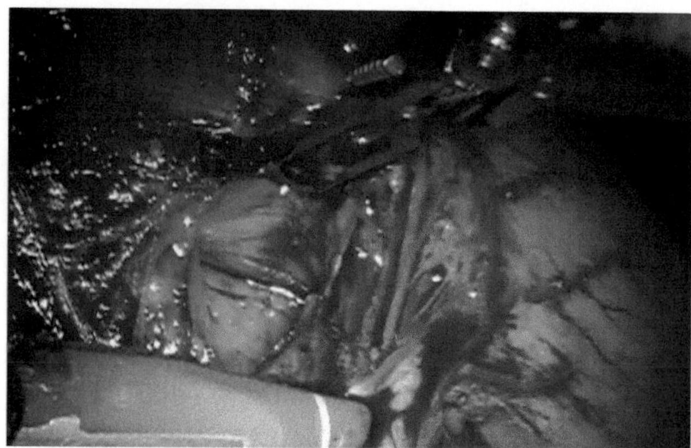

Fig. 78.20 Cutting current used to enter lesser sac

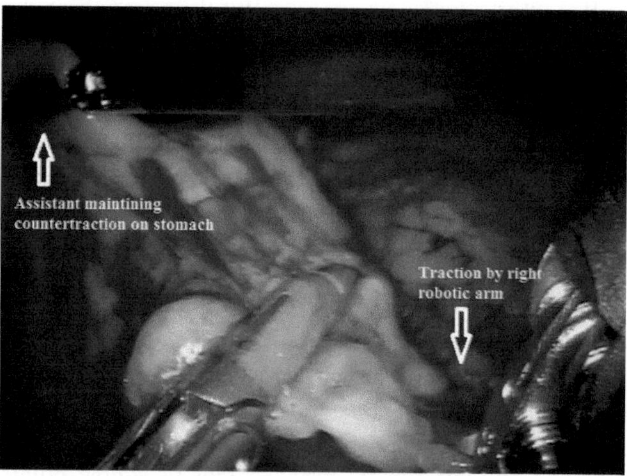

Fig. 78.21 The sealer is used in the left robotic arm. The assistant maintains upward traction on the stomach as the surgeon uses an atraumatic grasper in the right robotic arm to pull the omentum downwards

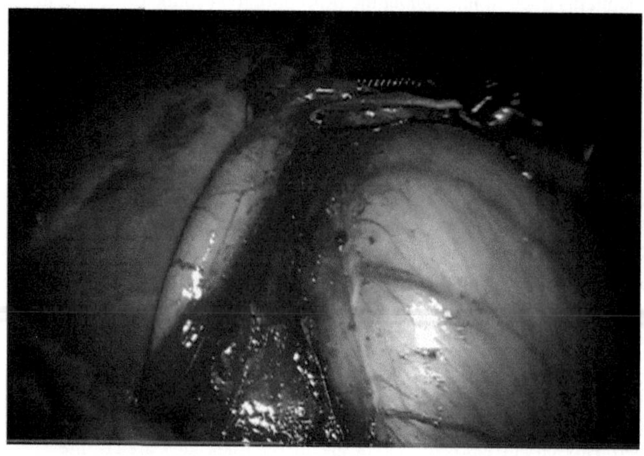

Fig. 78.19 The surgeon uses the robotic arm to grasp and tent up the stomach in order to identify point of entry to lesser sac

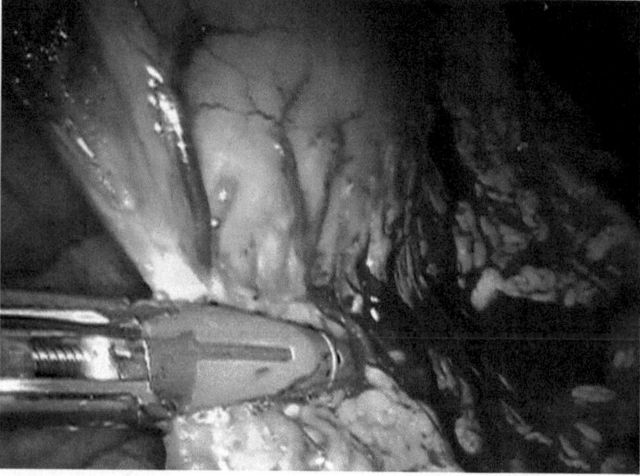

Fig. 78.22 The sealer is placed approximately 1–1.5 cm away from the short gastric arteries

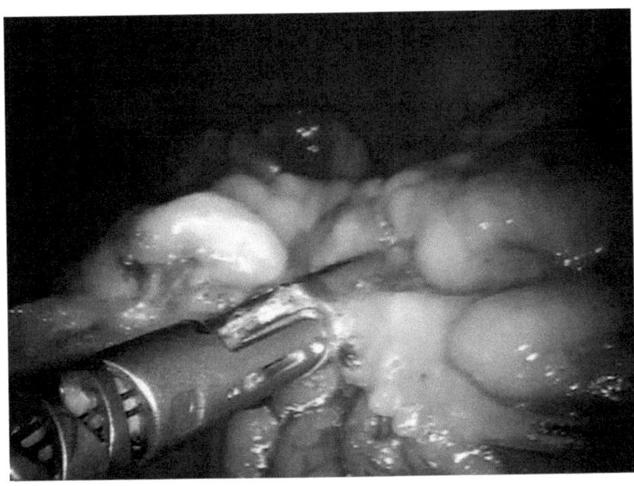

Fig. 78.23 Dissection with the sealer along the greater curvature of the stomach towards the splenic flexure

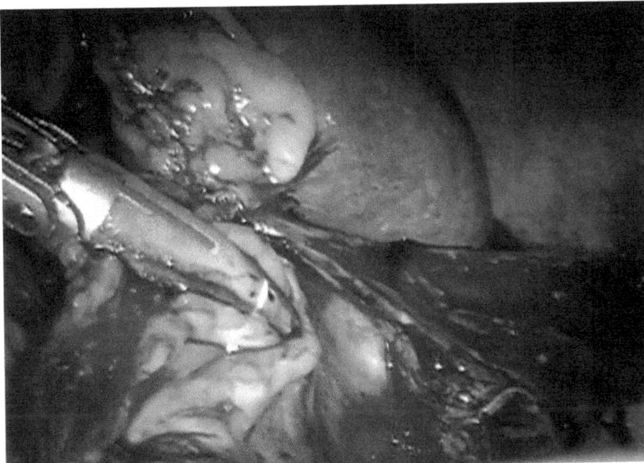

Fig. 78.24 Direction of dissection directed towards the transverse colon after reaching the splenic flexure

At this point the sealer is placed in the right arm and the atraumatic grasper in the left arm and dissection is continued for a short while to the right and then towards the transverse colon. This sets up dissection for the infracolic omentectomy as described above, and allows the entire omentum to be removed en bloc. If using the Si system, the robot is undocked from over the patient's right shoulder and re-docked centrally. This can be accomplished by either turning the patient's bed (with cooperation from the anesthesiologist) or mobilizing of the robot. For the Xi system one undocks, simply rotates the boom, re-docks, and then redirects the orientation for the new anatomy targeted.

References

1. Liebermann-Meffert D. The greater omentum. anatomy, embryology, and surgical applications. Surg Clin North Am. 2000;80(1):275–93 xii.
2. Shah S, Lowery E, Braun RK, Martin A, Huang N, Medina M, Sethupathi P, Seki Y, Takami M, Byrne K, Wigfield C, Love RB, Iwashima M. Cellular basis of tissue regeneration by omentum. PLoS One. 2012;7(6):e38368.
3. Arie AB, McNally L, Kapp DS, Teng NN. The omentum and omentectomy in epithelial ovarian cancer: a reappraisal. Part I--Omental function and history of omentectomy. Gynecol Oncol. 2013; 131(3):780–3.
4. Arie AB, McNally L, Kapp DS, Teng NN. The omentum and omentectomy in epithelial ovarian cancer: a reappraisal: part II--the role of omentectomy in the staging and treatment of apparent early stage epithelial ovarian cancer. Gynecol Oncol. 2013;131(3):784–90.
5. Feuer GA, Lakhi N, Barker J, Salmieri S, Burrell M. Perioperative and clinical outcomes in the management of epithelial ovarian cancer using a robotic or abdominal approach. Gynecol Oncol. 2013; 131(3):520–4.
6. Feuer GA, Lakhi N, Woo A, Salmieri SS, Beryl MO, Serur E. Robotic surgery for staging of serous papillary and clear cell carcinoma of the endometrium. Int J Med Robot. 2014;10(3):306–13.

Robotic-Assisted Laparoscopic Hysterectomy: Final Steps and Postoperative Considerations

79

Bahriye Aktas

Robotic surgery provides all the benefits of the laparoscopic technique with greater precision and effectiveness with no major difference regarding postoperative considerations and complications.

When the surgery is completed, an exploration of the upper abdomen and pelvis is required to control that there is no damage. Immediate intraoperative management of any damage is recommended for the best postoperative outcome.

Performing cystoscopy should not be done routinely, but in select cases cystoscopy is helpful after vaginal closure to check ureteral patency and for any signs of bladder injury. Please note that a normal cystoscopy does not exclude a delayed thermal injury to either the ureters or the bladder [1].

Vaginal cuff dehiscence after hysterectomy is a rare but severe postoperative complication. The rate of vaginal cuff dehiscence seems to have been shown to increase after both robotic and laparoscopic surgeries compared with that after the open approach [2]. However the incidence is significantly higher in total laparoscopic hysterectomy than laparoscopy assisted vaginal hysterectomy. Thus the vaginal closure technique is essential to avoid any cuff dehiscence. The intra – corporeal cuff suture seems to be superior to the vaginal suture to prevent the vaginal cuff complications [3]. Additionally abstaining from vaginal intercourse should be recommended to decrease the rate for postcoital vaginal cuff dehiscence.

Whereas adhesions are common after hysterectomies and could be the reason for delayed abdominal pain. To avoid accumulation of seroma a soft plastic drain sometimes is placed through one of the incisions, which usually will be removed before the patient goes home. There are a lot of ambiguous data with on the efficacy of agents against adhesions, but only a few of the various available pharmacological and non – pharmacological agents have been studied in randomized controlled trials [4].

Once the robotic assisted procedure is finished, all instruments and endoscopes and cannulas are removed. The cannulas will be removed after disconnecting the roboter arms. Subcutaneous emphysema could result from placement of the Veress needle into the extraperitoneal space or during prolonged procedures after using robotic assisted or laparoscopic techniques when cannulas are dislocated. Patient's companions should be told that during laparoscopic hysterectomy may secondarily occur subcutaneous emphysema as gas gains access through enlargement of the trocar incision in the parietal peritoneum and usually dissolves in 12–24 hours [5–8].

The port site skin incisions are closed with dissolving sutures or skin glue. Any 12 mm incisions and extended incisions for delivering specimen retrieval bag require fascial closure using 0 vicryl sutures to prevent incisional hernias. The skin is closed with 4–0 monocryl sutures in a continuous subcutaneous or intracutaneous fashion. The 5 mm incisions generally do not require fascial closure and are closed with single sutures with 4–0 monocryl or glue for better cosmetic results.

For reducing immediate postoperative pain, injection of local analgesia at all post incision sites is possible [9] but not necessary.

Subsequently, the sterile accessories and drapes can be removed and the patient will be transferred to the recovery room. The nurses and doctors will monitor patients' recovery as she wakes up and will continue monitoring until she is discharged from the hospital.

A post – operative assessment should be done at the same day of the surgery, including palpation of the abdomen, checking the drainage, if any was placed and looking for any vaginal bleeding. Checking the blood values is not necessary; accept there are clinical signs for postoperative hemorrhage.

In cases of postoperative vaginal cuff hematoma usage of antibiotics could be necessary to prevent any infections.

B. Aktas
Department of Gynecology and Obstetrics, University Hospital Essen, Hufelandstrasse 55, Essen 45147, Germany
e-mail: bahriye.aktas@uk-essen.de

I. Alkatout, L. Mettler (eds.), *Hysterectomy*, DOI 10.1007/978-3-319-22497-8_79

Single prophylactic doses and additional intraoperative doses in prolonged surgeries are useful and recommended.

The main indications to extend the application of antibiotics postoperatively are intraoperative interventions on the intestines or urinary tract.

In patients who underwent general anesthesia, the Foley catheter should be removed postoperatively when the patient is awake and no longer immobile. Mobilization of the patients should also be performed as soon as possible to prevent thrombosis, if indicated heparin should be given in patients at risk, especially patients with cancer diagnosis. During hospitalization patients should receive thrombosis prophylaxis, because thromboembolism is relatively common in gyneco – oncological surgery.

Against the past there are no special steps for rebuilding the diet after hysterectomy but flatulent foods should be avoided.

A discharge assessment will be performed including abdominal sonography to check the kidneys and a vaginal sonography to exclude any hematoma.

In most cases patients return to their routine activities 2 weeks after the operation. Final pelvic examination is usually indicated after 6–12 weeks, mainly are indicated for pain or pyrexia. Sexual activity may be allowed after a recovery time to avoid postcoital vaginal cuff dehiscence and infections as previously described. In general, patients can resume sexual relations after 8 weeks, may be later for patients at risk for impaired healing like obese patients and patients with diabetes.

A review of the literature published 2011 described a significant difference in number of major postoperative complications between robotic radical hysterectomy (9.6 %) and total laparoscopic radical hysterectomy (5.5 %). In the robotic procedure group were included 11 cases of vaginal cuff dehiscence, 10 cases of vaginal cuff abscess, and 5 cases of port site hernia [10]. Despite to these data, Estape et al. demonstrated that the incidence of postoperative complications was less in the robotic group (18.8 %) than either the laparoscopic group (23.5 %) or the laparotomy group (28.6 %). In the first group, one patient developed a pelvic abscess and another one a vaginal evisceration [11]. Two other studies did not observe any significant differences in postoperative outcomes [12, 13]. Similar early, less than 6 weeks, major postoperative complications in robotic radical hysterectomy (7 %), laparoscopic radical hysterectomy (6 %), and open radical hysterectomy (9 %) groups was described by Magrina et al. [13]. Overall postoperative complications rate of 12 %, including deep venous thrombosis (2.4 %), pyelonephritis (2.4 %), prolonged bladder catheterization of 21 days (2.4 %), and infection (4.8 %) was demonstrated by Lowe et al. [14]. Early mobilization and administering heparin in patients at risk for developing deep venous thrombosis, removing of the Foley catheter and treating prophylactically with an antibiotic intraoperatively could help to prevent these complications.

Robotic approach provides clear benefits of minimally invasive surgery, such as a reduced blood loss, a lower morbidity, and a faster recovery than open surgery. Although surgical outcomes are similar or slightly improved when compared to laparoscopy [15]. Complication rates and hospital stay are also similar for robotic and conventional laparoscopic surgery [16], indeed, current studies shows faster recovery time for patients underwent robotic surgery [17].

Overall there is no major difference between robotic – assisted hysterectomy and the laparoscopic hysterectomy regarding postoperative considerations and complications [18, 19].

References

1. Einarsson JI, Suzuki Y. Total laparoscopic hysterectomy: 10 steps toward a successful procedure. Rev Obstet Gynecol. 2009;2(1):57–64.
2. Zapardiel I, Zanagnolo V, Peiretti M, Maggioni A, Bocciolone L. Avoiding vaginal cuff dehiscence after robotic oncological surgery: reliable suturing technique. Int J Gynecol Cancer. 2010;20:1264–7.
3. Kim MJ, Kim S, Bae HS, Lee JK, Lee NW, Song JY. Evaluation of risk factors of vaginal cuff dehiscence after hysterectomy. Obstet Gynecol Sci. 2014;57(2):136–43.
4. Hirschelmann A, Tchartchian G, Wallwiener M, Hackethal A, De Wilde RL. A review of the problematic adhesion prophylaxis in gynaecological surgery. Arch Gynecol Obstet. 2012;285(4):1089–97.
5. Jhingran A, Levenback C. Malignant disease of the cervix. Microinvasive and invasive cancers. In: Katz VL, Lentz GM, Lobo RA, Gershenson DM, editors. 5th comprehensive gynecology. Philadelphia: Mosby/Elsevier ; 2007. p. 759–81.ISBN: 978-0-323-02951-3
6. Kim,Y.T. (2007).Robotic radical hysterectomy with pelvic lymphadenectomy for cervical carcinoma: a pilot study, Gynecol Oncol, Vol. 105, pp. 176-180, ISSN: 0090-8258.
7. Li G, Yan X, Shang H. A comparison of laparoscopic radical hysterectomy and pelvic lymphadenectomy and laparotomy in the treatment of Ib-IIa cervical cancer. Gynecol Oncol. 2007;105:176–80. ISSN: 0090-8258.
8. Tang A, Obermair A. Technique of laparoscopic radical hysterectomy and comparison of three techniques: laparotomy, laparoscopy and robotics. In: Textbook of Gynaecological Oncology; 2009.
9. Einarsson JI, Sun J, Orav J, Young AE. Local analgesia in laparoscopy: a randomized trial. Obstet Gynecol. 2004;104:1335–9.
10. Kruijdenberg CBM, Van Den Einden LCG, Hendriks JCM, Zusterzeel PL, Bekkers RL. Robot-assisted versus total laparoscopic radical hysterectomy in early cervical cancer, a review. Gynecol Oncol. 2011;120(3):334–9.
11. Estape R, Lambrou N, Diaz R, Estape E, Dunkin N, Rivera A. A case matched analysis of robotic radical hysterectomy with lymphadenectomy compared with laparoscopy and laparotomy. Gynecol Oncol. 2009;113(3):357–61.

12. Nezhat FR, Datta MS, Liu C, Chuang L, Zakashansky K. Robotic radical hysterectomy versus total laparoscopic radical hysterectomy with pelvic lymphadenectomy for treatment of early cervical cancer. JSLS. 2008;12(3):227–37.
13. Magrina JF, Kho RM, Weaver AL, Montero RP, Magtibay PM. Robotic radical hysterectomy: comparison with laparoscopy and laparotomy. Gynecol Oncol. 2008;109(1):86–91.
14. Lowe MP, Chamberlain DH, Kamelle SA, Johnson PR, Tillmanns TD. A multi-institutional experience with robotic-assisted radical hysterectomy for early stage cervical cancer. Gynecol Oncol. 2009;113(2):191–4.
15. Renato S, Mohamed M, Serena S, et al. Robot-assisted radical hysterectomy for cervical cancer: review of surgical and oncological outcomes. ISRN Obstet Gynecol. 2011;2011:872434.
16. Sarlos D, Kots LV, Stevanovic N, Schaer G. Robotic hysterectomy versus conventional laparoscopic hysterectomy: outcome and cost analyses of a matched case–control study. Eur J Obstet Gynecol Reprod Biol. 2010;150:92–6.
17. Buderath P, Aktas B, Heubner M, Kimmig R. Robot-assisted hysterectomy: a critical evaluation. Robot Surg:Res Rev. 2015;2:59–63. Dove Press
18. Basil J, Pavelka J. Robotic gynecologic surgery. In: Baggish MS, Karram MM, editors. Atlas of pelvic anatomy and gynecologic surgery. 3 ed. Saunders: Elsevier; 2011. p. 1327–34 .ISBN: 978-1-4160-5909-7.
19. Orady M, Hrynewych A, Nawfal AK, Wegienka G. Comparison of robotic-assisted hysterectomy to other minimally invasive approaches. JSLS. 2012;16(4):542–8.

PGSTL 10/12/2017